CASTLE CONNOLLY

TOP DOCTORS

New York Metro Area

17th Edition

Top Doctors Make A Difference

America's Trusted Source For Identifying Top Doctors

The selection of medical providers for inclusion in this book was based in part on opinions solicited from physicians, nurses, and other healthcare professionals. The author and publishers cannot assure the accuracy of information provided to them by third parties, since such opinions are necessarily subjective and may be incomplete. The omission from this book of particular healthcare providers does not mean that such providers are not competent or reputable.

The purpose of this book is educational and informational. It is not intended to replace the advice of your physician or to assist the layman in diagnosing or treating illness, disease, or injury. Following the advice or recommendations set forth in this book is entirely at the reader's own risk. The author and publishers cannot ensure accuracy of, or assume responsibility for, the information in the book as such information is affected by constant change. Liability to any person or organization for any loss or damage caused by errors or omissions in this book is hereby disclaimed. Whenever possible, readers should consult their own primary care physician when selecting healthcare providers, including any selection based upon information contained in this book. In order to protect patient privacy, the names of patients cited in anecdotes throughout the book have been omitted.

The confidence of our readers in our editorial integrity is crucial to the success of the Castle Connolly Guides. Any use of the Castle Connolly name, or of any list or listing (or portion of either) from any Castle Connolly Guide, for advertising or for any commercial purpose, without prior written consent, is strictly prohibited and may result in legal action.

For more information, please contact:

Castle Connolly Medical Ltd., 42 West 24th St, New York, New York 10010
212-367-8400x110
E-mail: info@castleconnolly.com
Web site: http://www.castleconnolly.com.

Library of Congress Control Number: 2013919421
ISBN 1-883769-34-5 978-1-883769-34-5 (paperback)
Printed in the United States of America

Table of Contents

Table of Contents

Table of Contents

Table of Contents

Hippocratic Oath

I swear by Apollo the physician, and Asklepios, and health, and All-Heal and all the gods and goddesses, that, according to my ability and judgement, I will keep this Oath and this stipulation — to reckon him who taught me this Art equally dear to me as my parents, to share my substance with him, and relieve his necessities if required; to look upon his offspring in the same footing as my own brothers, and to teach them this Art, if they should wish to learn it, without fee or stipulation; and that by precept, lecture and every other mode of instruction, I will impart a knowledge of the Art to my own sons, and those of my teachers, and to disciples bound by a stipulation and oath according to the law of medicine, but to none others.

I will follow that system of regimen which, according to my ability and judgement, I consider for the benefit of my patients, and abstain from whatever is deleterious and mischievous. I will give no deadly medicine to anyone if asked nor suggest any such counsel; and in like manner I will not give to a woman a pessary to produce abortion. With purity and wholeness I will pass my life and practice my Art.

I will not cut persons labouring under the stone, but will leave this to be done by men who are practitioners of this work. Into whatever houses I enter, I will go into them for the benefit of the sick, and will abstain from every voluntary act of mischief and corruption; and, further, from the seduction of females or males, of freemen and slaves. Whatever, in connection with my professional practice, or not in connection with it, I see or hear, in the life of men, which ought not to be spoken of abroad, I will not divulge, as reckoning that all such should be kept secret. While I continue to keep this Oath unviolated, may it be granted to me to enjoy life and the practice of the art, respected by all men, in all times! But should I trespass and violate this Oath, may the reverse be my lot!

From Dorland's Illustrated Medical Dictionary. 27th ed. (Philadelphia) W.B. Saunders Co., 1988. Hippocratic Oath. [Hippocrates. Greek physician, 460-377 B.C.]

About the Publishers

John K. Castle, the Chairman of Castle Connolly Medical Ltd., has spent much of the last three decades involved with healthcare institutions and issues. Mr. Castle served as Chairman of the Board of New York Medical College for eleven years, an institution where he served on the Board of Trustees for twenty-two years.

Mr. Castle has been extensively involved in other healthcare and voluntary activities as well. He served for five years as a commissioner and officer of the Joint Commission formerly known as (JCAHO), the body which accredits most public and private hospitals throughout the United States. Mr. Castle has also served as a trustee of five different hospitals in the metropolitan New York region, including NewYork Presbyterian Hospital, where he continues to serve.

Mr. Castle has also served as the Chairman of the Columbia Presbyterian Science Advisory Council and as a Director of the Whitehead Institute for Biomedical Research. He is a Fellow of New York Academy of Medicine and has served as a Trustee of the Academy. He was Chairman of the United Hospital Fund of New York's Capital Campaign and continues as Director Emeritus of the United Hospital Fund. He is a Life Member of the MIT Corporation, the governing body of the Massachusetts Institute of Technology.

Mr. Castle received his bachelor's degree from the Massachusetts Institute of Technology, his MBA as a Baker Scholar with High Distinction from Harvard, and two Honorary Doctorate degrees.

Mr. Castle's goal, as is the goal of Dr. John Connolly and all the Castle Connolly team, is to publish ***America's Top Doctors®, America's Top Doctors® for Cancer, Top Doctors: New York Metro Area***, and other materials as well as build websites to help the public identify the very best in healthcare resources.

John J. Connolly, Ed.D., - the nation's foremost expert on identifying top physicians, is the President & CEO of Castle Connolly Medical Ltd. publisher of *America's Top Doctors*® and other consumer guides to help people find the best healthcare. He is also Vice-Chairman of Castle Connolly Graduate Medical Ltd., which publishes review manuals to assist resident physicians and fellows in preparing for their board exams.

Dr. Connolly served as President of New York Medical College, the nation's second largest private medical college, for more than ten years. He is a Fellow of the New York Academy of Medicine, a Fellow of the New York Academy of Sciences, a Director of the Northeast Business Group on Health, a member of the President's Council of the United Hospital Fund, and a member of the Board of the American Swiss Foundation.

Dr. Connolly has served as trustee of two hospitals and as Chairman of the Board of one. He is extensively involved in healthcare and community activities and has served on a number of voluntary and corporate boards including the Board of the American Lyme Disease Foundation, of which he is a founder and past chairman, and the Culinary Institute of America for over 20 years where he is now Chairman Emeritus. He also served as a director and Chairman of the Professional Examination Service and is presently on the board of the American Swiss Foundation. His current corporate board service includes: Baker and Taylor; Air Methods Corporation; Dearborn Risk Management and the Advisory Board of the Hudson Group. He holds a Bachelor of Science degree from Worcester State College, a Master's degree from the University of Connecticut, and a Doctor of Education degree in College and University Administration from Teacher's College, Columbia University, honorary doctorates (LHD) from Mercy College and Worcester State University.

Over the years, Dr. Connolly has served on the boards of, and as an officer of, numerous not for profit organizations including: President, Sullivan County Association for Retarded Children; Director and Chairman United Way of Dutchess County; Director and Founding Chairman Dutchess County Industrial Development Agency; Director and Founder Dutchess County Economic Development Association, President, Westchester County Historical Society.

Medical Advisory Board

Castle Connolly Medical Ltd. is pleased to be associated with a distinguished group of medical leaders who offer invaluable advice and wisdom in its efforts to assist consumers in making good healthcare choices. We thank each member of the Medical Advisory Board for their valuable contributions.

Jeremiah A. Barondess, M.D.
President Emeritus
New York Academy of Medicine,
Professor of Clinical Medicine
Emeritus, Weill-Cornell Medical
College

Menard M. Gertler, M.D., D.Sc.
Clinical Professor of Medicine
Cornell University Medical School

Yutaka Kikkawa, M.D.
Professor and Chairman (Emeritus)
Department of Pathology
University of California
Irvine College of Medicine

Edward D. Miller, M.D.
Dean/CEO Emeritus
Johns Hopkins Medicine
Professor of Anesthesiology &
Critical Care Medicine

Ronald Pion, M.D.
Chairman and CEO
Medical Telecommunications
Associates

Leon G. Smith, M.D.
Chairman of Medicine
St. Michael's Medical Center, NJ

Ralph Snyderman, M.D.
Former President and CEO
Duke University Health System

Roger Bulger, M.D.
National Institutes of Health (Ret.)

Leo Hennikoff, M.D.
President and CEO (Ret.)
Rush Presbyterian-St. Luke's
Medical Center

David Paige, M.D.
Professor
Bloomberg School of Public Health
John Hopkins University

Richard L. Reece, M.D.
Editor
Physician Practice Options

Helen Smits, M.D.
Former Deputy Director
Health Care Financing
Administration (HCFA)

Foreword

Dear Reader:

Choosing a doctor is one of the most important choices in your life. However, most of us put little effort into this selection. We simply pick a name from a list or get a recommendation from a friend.

Most of us have very little information about our doctors, and/or don't know where to get it. With the publication of this Castle Connolly Guide—Top Doctors: New York Metro Area, you can learn about doctors' medical school education, residency, training, fellowships, board certifications, hospital appointments and much more. The Guide also describes in simple terms what information you should ascertain about each doctor and how to evaluate it. This information gathering is essential for anyone who wants to find a good doctor to truly meet his or her healthcare needs.

As an administrator and nurse who deals with the problems of health on a daily basis, I know well the importance of getting the best healthcare. Our center assists medical malpractice victims. The human tragedy we often encounter is heartbreaking.

In many cases, had the patient taken a few minutes to make a modest effort to learn more about his or her doctor's background, a serious incident may have been avoided.

That is why *Top Doctors: New York Metro Area* is so important to consumers. In this new and rapidly changing healthcare environment, patients must be well informed. Many do not trust the healthcare system. They are not confident that their health plan, their hospital, or even their doctor, is motivated to protect them and to ensure that they get excellent care.

The Castle Connolly Guide is a comprehensive guide chock full of valuable information. It is completely consumer-friendly, giving readers all that they need to know to make intelligent, informed choices.

Use it well and in good health!

Sincerely,

Sandra Gainer, R.N.
Associate Director
National Center for Patient Rights

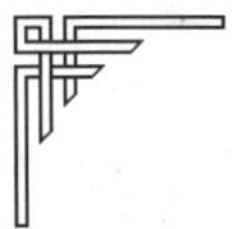

The Best in American Medicine
www.CastleConnolly.com

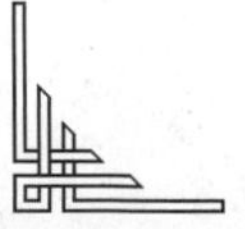
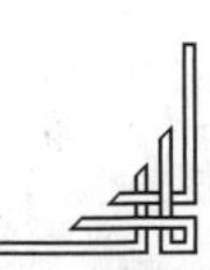

Why Top Doctors Make A Difference:

A Message for Employers and Families

Most people would agree that gambling with their health is a dangerous idea. When it comes to medical care, excellence and expertise are crucially important. Yet Americans receive top-quality care from their doctors and hospitals only about half of the time. From inadequate screening during routine checkups to subpar treatment of critical illnesses, inferior care can have costly and tragic results. Too often, patients simply don't know how to find the best doctor to deliver the best care.

Castle Connolly takes this challenge seriously. Since the company's founding in 1991, our "Top Doctors" guides have been identifying the nation's best doctors and hospitals in every part of the country and in every medical specialty. Our lists are based on peer nominations and professional assessments by our physician-led research team – not on hype, advertising, or third parties that have something to gain by recommending a particular provider. Castle Connolly's Top Doctors are rigorously selected from among hundreds of thousands of physicians. Our intensive research methodology is designed to identify doctors that will speed patients' healing, minimize pain and discomfort, shorten recovery periods and enhance and lengthen lives – in other words, achieve the best possible health outcomes.

Today, such independent assessment of medical care is more important than ever. Anyone can draw up a "best of" list – and many organizations do. Pharmaceutical companies favor those physicians who are high prescribers of their drugs. To many health insurers a physician's fees are often a more important factor than quality. Many publications and websites recommend health care providers who pay to get their names mentioned. But Castle Connolly has no such conflicts of interest. Our sole purpose is to help patients, their families and their employers find health care providers who deliver superior results.

Some people believe that patient ratings are the best source of information on doctors. Unfortunately, that is a misguided assumption. Patients may be able to rate a doctor's "bedside manner," but they know little about the complexity of medical care. In fact, an article in Forbes magazine pointed out - "The current system might just kill you. Many doctors, in order to get high ratings (and a higher salary), over-prescribe and over-test, just to "satisfy" patients, who probably aren't qualified to judge their care. And there's a financial cost, as flawed survey methods and the decisions they induce, produce billions more in waste."

After a physician's name is submitted by colleagues as part of our nomination process for consideration as a Top Doctor, our physician-led research team delves into the professional records of top nominated physicians in order to ascertain those that have exceptional training, experience and are highly regarded by their peers. In addition, disciplinary histories and malpractice actions, when available, are also carefully scrutinized.

Why Top Doctors Make A Difference

Top Doctors can have an enormous impact. For patients and their families, the value of receiving first-class medical care is great but unquantifiable – it's measured in quality and even length of life. Employers, however, can see the results in their bottom line. Faulty diagnoses and improper treatment take a toll in productivity and ripple out into higher workplace costs. No company should have to make do for weeks or months without a key employee or executive, when a Top Doctor may have solved the patient's problem efficiently and simply.

Castle Connolly has dozens of examples, some dramatic and lifesaving, that demonstrate the point that finding the best doctor or hospital can make a significant difference in patients' lives. The few that follow clearly demonstrate this point.

- Kay was examined by her local physician, who advised her that lumps in her breast were very likely malignant and recommended an immediate mastectomy. Closer investigation by a Castle Connolly specialist showed that the lumps were in fact benign and Kay avoided the cost, trauma and pain of a radical mastectomy.
- After Bill was diagnosed with kidney stones, his family doctor recommended surgery. Bill got a second opinion from a Castle Connolly Top Doctor who treated the condition with medication instead – and five years later, he is still doing fine without surgery.
- Jim was scheduled for surgery to amputate his foot. A relative contacted Castle Connolly to check out his doctor. The research team quickly identified the surgeon as one who had lost his license in one state and was disciplined in another. The surgery was rescheduled with a different surgeon.
- Rose and Liz, both in their 60's and carrying a few extra pounds, needed knee surgery. Rose chose a physician who practiced near her home, while Liz picked a Castle Connolly Top Doctor. Two years after her operation, Rose still uses a cane much of the time. Six months following surgery, Liz was back to her old self and feeling terrific. No doubt, a Top Doctor had a major impact on Liz's favorable outcome.
- Karl, the manager of a horse farm, suddenly had a problem with one of his eyes. A local ophthalmologist diagnosed glaucoma and told Karl he needed immediate surgery. Castle Connolly referred him to a Top Doctor, who has been successfully treating Karl with eye drops ever since.

Expertise and leading-edge technology are especially important in diagnosing and treating cancer, stroke and cardiovascular patients. Administered by a Top Doctor, sophisticated techniques may keep pancreatic and brain cancer sufferers alive for years, compared with the few months that conventional chemotherapy normally achieves. Top Doctors often have higher cure rates for prostate and breast cancer, thanks in part to early detection, but also due to more advanced treatment options.

Patients with cardiac disease can frequently avoid open-heart or multiple-bypass surgery with stents and other less-invasive technologies. And although many physicians will counsel elderly patients to avoid surgery under any circumstances, a Top Doctor may be able to operate on people 90 years of age or older and still achieve excellent outcomes. Stroke victims, in the hands of a Top Doctor, can recover to a degree unheard of just a few years ago. World-class neurosurgeons can deal with bleeding strokes that were formerly inoperable. Early detection through imaging and swift treatment with drugs can dissolve clots blocking critical blood flow to the brain before permanent damage is done – and without invasive procedures. Men operated on at hospitals and by surgeons with high volumes of particular procedures, specifically radical prostatectomy, had a 7.7 percent risk of recurrence of prostate cancer as compared to 10.9 percent for surgeries done by physicians with lower surgical volumes.

As further evidence of this principle, consider the following statistics, all reported in a recent Newsweek article and based on professional journal reports.

At one leading specialty hospital, the five year survival rate for Stage IV prostate cancer is 71 percent vs. 38 percent nationally.

At a major academic health center for Stage IV cervical cancer the survival rate is 33 percent vs. 16 percent nationally. For breast cancer, after a mastectomy, 81 percent of women treated at top centers are still alive after five years compared to 77 percent nationally.

In addition, a recent study in the *Journal of the National Cancer Institute* found that treatment variation from surgeon to surgeon is significant and may account for up to 30% of recurrences of the cancer. Also, in late 2011, "The Annals of Surgery" published a study that demonstrated that patients with an uneventful course of surgery and recovery had a mean cost per case of $27,946.00 versus $159,345.00 for those patients with complications.

A significant study was recently published in the *New England Journal of Medicine.* It reviewed the actual surgery results of gastric bypass surgery on 10,343 patients by the same 20 surgeons, between 2006 and 2012.

The differences between the most skilled and least skilled surgeons were remarkable. Comparing the top 25% to the bottom 25%, the researchers found:

- The least-skilled surgeons had nearly triple the rate of complications, 14.5% versus 5.2%.
- The least-skilled surgeons required longer operations, 137 minutes versus 98 minutes.
- Although death is a very rare outcome for gastric bypass surgery, patients had a higher risk of dying if their operations were done by the least-skilled doctors, 0.26% versus 0.05%.

Across the board, the most skilled surgeons had better results.

The bottom line: Top Doctors can help patients in ways not generally available in the medical community. But while people intuitively know this to be true, most lack the resources to make the best choices when they fall ill. Many people rely on referrals from the family physician, yet even a trusted and competent physician may not be the best source of information. Doctors are busy with their practices, and their referral contacts are usually limited to their plan network or hospital. Few have time to research who, wherever in the nation, is really the best for a particular procedure or problem. That often leaves patients who need a top specialist at the mercy of advertising and hearsay. They may even pick a name at random from their insurer's directory or website, or even respond to advertising.

Knowledgeable employers realize that providing employees and their families with access to the best medical care, as well as avoiding the worst, impacts a company's bottom line in a positive way. Money saved on the wrong treatment, unnecessary surgery, days lost from work, or the focus on the illness of a loved one or oneself instead of work, are worth the effort to identify the best doctors.

Castle Connolly is committed to helping such patients get the care they need and deserve. Our professional staff, with years of experience, has earned us the trust and respect of the medical and lay communities alike. We are in a unique position to assist individuals and companies in accessing the best and most efficient healthcare available today. Castle Connolly Guides and our website are comprehensive, user-friendly resources that let consumers find a doctor by name, specialty, and geographic location – or even by special expertise in a particular disease or procedure. Hospital affiliations and contact information are presented clearly and concisely. The guides and website also include helpful tools for choosing a Top Doctor, with tips on how to evaluate a physician's education, experience, and personal suitability.

When it comes to healthcare, cutting corners rarely pays off. Unlike its imitators, Castle Connolly provides thorough and unbiased research by trained professionals. We believe that choosing a Top Doctor is the most important decision a patient can make and we work tirelessly to facilitate that decision.

Introduction

A savvy consumer, searching for a car, restaurant, house or even a spouse, can easily find a guidebook to help. Yet, when it comes to choosing healthcare providers, the bookshelves are nearly bare.

Top Doctors: New York Metro Area has been written to fill that void. It will guide you in making critical —even lifesaving—choices.

This Guide Has Two Goals:

- To provide you with a base of information and a framework of understanding so that you can participate in the important healthcare choices that will maximize your own health, your family's health and the quality of your life.
- To provide detailed information on more than 6,400 well-trained, highly competent physicians from which you may confidently choose your personal best doctors for your own healthcare needs and those of your family.

Medicine is often described as a combination of art and science. This description holds true for the process of selecting the best medical care. This book describes the "science" of making that selection. It is not magical or even difficult. It is simply a matter of knowing what information you should have and where to find it.

The "art" is what you will bring to the selection process. It is based upon your feelings, your needs and the chemistry that develops between you and those who provide your healthcare. Castle Connolly's *Top Doctors: New York Metro Area* will help you prepare for that interaction and will guide you in getting the most from it.

Most importantly, Castle Connolly's *Top Doctors: New York Metro Area* will tell you how to combine the art and science so that you can make the best choices.

How to Use This Guide

This book has been written as a basic, "how to" guide for selecting the best healthcare. Section One provides important information on how to choose the best doctors. Doctors are the most important providers of healthcare and regardless of the type of medical insurance you have, you want the very best doctors to attend to your healthcare needs. Section Three contains listings of doctors as well as information on hospitals invited to participate in the Guide's Partnership for Excellence program. Section Four includes information on "Centers of Excellence"—special programs and services—offered by a number of the hospitals participating in the Partnership for Excellence program. Section Five contains seven appendices with important and interesting information.

There Are Two Effective Ways to Use This Guide:

- Start at the beginning. This method will give you a broad understanding of the healthcare field and a clearer perspective of where you, the patient, fit in it. This method will arm you with necessary information for making informed choices and will help you find the best doctors.
- Study the doctor listings. While at least a brief reading of some or all of the introductory chapters is recommended so that, in the end, you will make well-informed choices, it is understandable that you may wish to go straight to the physician listings. The organization of these listings is outlined on pages 71 to 79. You will find guidelines for effectively using the listings on these pages.

Each chapter begins with explanations of terms that may be new to you. Reviewing these terms will help you read the section more easily.

In preparing this book, we've left little to chance or question. We hope to inspire you to assume a curious and insistent attitude as you make the healthcare choices that will take you and your family through life.

SECTION ONE

The Doctor of Choice

Primary Care Physicians

Chapter 1

Quick Tips

The time to establish a relationship with a doctor is while you are healthy. The top doctor to establish your relationship with is the one who is most likely to keep you healthy: A primary care doctor.

Primary means first, so a primary care doctor is the first one you see for most health problems.

It is difficult for any doctor, however skilled, to make judgements based on only one visit or a single test.

Your primary care doctor can educate you about the "hows" and "whys" of health maintenance and disease prevention and follow up to help you stay faithful to the course the two of you have agreed upon.

Any doctor with a license can practice in any specialty he/she chooses. Board certification is your assurance that the doctor has appropriate training in the specialty.

When considering recommendations, use the old navigational technique of triangulation: focus on doctors whose names are mentioned by three or more people.

Hospital telephone referral lines are not designed to distinguish among hundreds of doctors who may be more or less well regarded by other doctors, or who may be better suited to a particular caller when factors other than location, insurance coverage and office hours are taken into consideration.

Many local medical societies publish directories, some of which are intended primarily for doctor-to-doctor referrals, while others are distributed to the public. They provide information but do not address quality.

The internet provides many websites that provide lists of doctors: some are of questionable quality. Be careful that the information is from a trusted source.

Quick Take

... Primary care physician. That's a hot term in healthcare today. Who is this physician? How do you find one?...

Key Terms

Lupus Erythematosus - An autoimmune disorder, also referred to as SLE, or simply "lupus". It can cause inflammation and possible damage to a number of vital organs and is commonly marked by joint pain, facial and other rashes, abnormally high antibody levels, and diminished red blood cell levels.

Lyme Disease - An infectious disease, transmitted through the bite of a deer tick, which may or may not produce a distinctive bull's-eye rash at the site of the tick bite. First identified in Lyme, Connecticut, the infection may also produce other symptoms, including flu-like aches, arthritic joint pain, and, in complicated cases, cardiac abnormalities.

Managed Care - The process of integrating the finance and delivery of healthcare to control costs and improve quality. A managed care plan typically involves a group of practitioners who "manage" care for a specified population.

Osteopath - A healthcare professional who has earned a degree in osteopathic medicine, a D.O. Osteopathic medicine emphasizes massage and bone manipulation while traditional western allopathic medicine emphasizes treatment with drugs and surgery.

Preventive Medicine/Care - Health services that are aimed at maintaining good health and preventing illness. These services include routine physical examinations, immunizations, certain screening tests such as mammograms or Pap tests, as well as the practice of good health habits.

Primary Care Physician - The first doctor consulted for any health problem, a Primary Care Physician is a specialist who offers basic, including preventive, medical care. It is important to maintain an ongoing relationship with your primary care physician.

Specialist - A physician who practices in one or more of the 25 specialties defined by the American Board of Medical Specialties (ABMS). The term is also used to denote a physician's area of practice, such as pediatrics, geriatrics, surgery, etc.

Subspecialist - A specialist who obtains further training and certification in one or more of the 70 subspecialties approved by the American Board of Medical Specialties. The physician must first be certified in a specialty. For example, a board certified internist may become certified in cardiology or gastroenterology.

Primary Care Physicians

When it comes to choosing a doctor, too many people let the decision slide until they are sick or hurt and need immediate medical attention. That's unfortunate if an illness that could have been managed successfully develops to a stage where it becomes difficult to control or cure. It's even more unfortunate if the illness could have been prevented in the first place.

The time to establish a relationship with a doctor is while you are healthy, and the best one to establish your relationship with is the one who is most likely to keep you healthy: a primary care doctor.

Primary means first, so a primary care doctor is the first one you see for any health problem. Primary also means basic, so a primary care doctor offers the kind of fundamental care that can keep you healthy.

Yes, You Do Need a Doctor When You're Healthy.

Here are four good reasons why you should start your search for a primary care doctor now:

Reason One

A primary care doctor can put your current medical condition into a context that consists of your medical history, current condition as compared with past medical status, and changes in your body and environment over time. It is difficult for any doctor, however skilled, to make informed medical judgments based on only one visit or a single test. Conditions well out of normal range are easy to pick up, but extreme variations do not always occur and a serious illness may develop slowly with only a gradual increase in symptoms. The operative word is continuity: ideally, your medical care should not be interrupted by changes in providers.

Reason Two

A primary care doctor is better able to treat you as a whole person. Medicine has become very specialized and procedure-oriented, but the human body is not a loose collection of unrelated parts. It is a "whole" with strong interrelationships among all biological systems. Some of the poorest medical care results from people jumping from subspecialist to subspecialist. Despite talent, skill and training, no specialist knows the patient well enough, or for long enough, to be able to take the whole person into consideration and track the normal patterns of evolution and change. We end up with a specialist for every organ and system instead of a doctor who will care for the whole person.

Reason Three

A primary care doctor can establish preventive programs. Our healthcare system does not place enough emphasis on preventing illness; most healthcare dollars are spent on curative, rather than preventive, medicine. However, the status quo is slowly changing, and it is within primary care that the change is most evident. Your primary care doctor can educate you about the hows and whys of health maintenance and disease prevention and can follow up to help you stay faithful to the course the two of you have agreed upon. Only an ongoing relationship makes this possible.

Reason Four

A primary care doctor can save you money. Managed care advocates, among others, have long deplored the waste inherent in a system in which patients can simply call any specialist any time they have an ache or pain or are not feeling well. Primary care doctors can monitor referrals to specialists, following the patient closely to put together a variety of observations, opinions, and test results in order to treat each person on an individual basis. This improves the quality of care and also controls costs.

Patients who visit specialists without some guidance from a primary care doctor may choose the wrong specialist based on a general observation and self-diagnosis about the problem or illness they're experiencing. While in some cases the problem may be obvious (for example, an eye injury), in others it may be more subtle. Diseases such as lupus erythematosus and Lyme disease, for example, often have a myriad of symptoms that are easily misinterpreted by laypersons; in fact, they are often difficult even for doctors to diagnose accurately. While certain problems may require the collaboration of several specialists, it is important to have a primary care doctor navigating the course.

Finally, it is estimated that almost half of all emergency room visits in some areas are for non-emergencies; it's the most expensive place to receive primary care. When people have primary care doctors, they tend to turn to them rather than to hospital emergency departments.

If you are enrolled in any kind of managed care program, health maintenance organization (HMO) or other program, you will almost always be required to select a primary care doctor from its roster. Managed care executives recognize the necessity of a primary care doctor, not only for delivering quality healthcare, but also for controlling costs.

How to Find a Doctor

Unless you already have a primary care doctor you are satisfied with, you will have to find one. How? Here are five possible avenues to begin the process of finding the doctor that best suits your needs; each has limits, however.

Doctor Referrals

If you are moving and are leaving a trusted doctor behind, get a recommendation or two before you go. Furthermore, ask in what context and how well your doctor knows the new doctor—they may not have met since medical school.

Friends and Relatives

Always keep in mind that such recommendations are based largely on what may be "simpatico," or a personal affinity. Ask why your friend likes the doctor. It might be because the fees are low or the doctor makes house calls or is warm and sociable—all valid considerations, but certainly not principal determinants. So be wary of the generalized recommendation that "Dr. Jones is just wonderful." When considering recommendations, use the old navigational technique of triangulation: focus on doctors whose names are mentioned by three or more people.

Hospital Referral Services

Hospital telephone referral lines are not designed to distinguish among hundreds of doctors who may be more or less well regarded by other doctors, or who may be better suited to a particular caller when factors other than location, insurance coverage and office hours are taken into consideration. It would be impolitic for hospital referral services to rate their doctors. Their recommendations are based on specialty and geographic proximity, usually by way of a computer that rotates through the lists to "recommend" the next three names in line, and all members of the medical staff are eligible to participate.

Medical Society Directories

Many local medical societies publish directories, some of which are intended primarily for doctor-to-doctor referrals, while others are distributed to the public. These directories usually provide names, addresses, phone numbers and specialties and can be useful sources. However, they do not distinguish among doctors in any way. All members of the medical society, usually a countywide organization, are eligible for inclusion. This also applies to the referral lines offered by many medical societies.

The Internet

There are many websites that provide information on doctors. Some are directories or internet phone books. These can be helpful. Some claim to be based on quality measures. Many of these require physicians to pay, others are of questionable quality. Be sure the site sponsor or source is a trusted one.

Many Ways to Say Doctor

In this guide, the term "doctor" is used to describe only medical doctors who have received a Doctor of Medicine degree (MD) and osteopaths who have received a Doctor of Osteopathic Medicine degree (DO). Doctors who have been trained in the British system may hold a degree of Bachelor of Medicine (MB), Bachelor of Surgery (BS), or Bachelor of Chirurgia (BCh), which is based on the ancient Greek term that refers to surgery.

The more formal term for any of these practitioners is "physician." However, most people use the more popular term "doctor," which is the one generally used in this book. Our discussions do not include other kinds of doctors such as dentists, podiatrists, psychologists or chiropractors, who also deliver healthcare.

Primary Care: The Fundamental Four

There is not complete agreement in medicine on which specialties are practiced by the group of doctors known as primary care specialists. For the purposes of this book, we have included the following specialties: Internal Medicine, Pediatrics, Family Practice and Obstetrics and Gynecology. Most adults choose general internists as their primary care doctors and select pediatricians for their children. There is also another type of specialist, the family practitioner, who cares for both children and adults. In addition to such generalists, many women also select an obstetrician/gynecologist as their primary care providers.

- A **general internist**, specializing in internal medicine, is trained to treat all internal organs and systems of the body. Many internists also are board certified in a subspecialty such as cardiology, gastroenterology or geriatric medicine. Therefore, if you have a history of heart disease, you may wish to select an internist who has additional training in cardiology, but who primarily practices general internal medicine. On the other hand, your primary care doctor may refer you to a cardiologist when necessary, and both may treat you over a period of years. In fact, it is not unusual for a patient with a serious or complex illness to be followed by two or three doctors, with the primary care doctor "quarterbacking" the team.

- A **family practitioner** is very broadly trained. Such doctors come closest to the general practitioner of the past. They are qualified to treat all family members, including children.

- A **pediatrician** is the doctor you would choose for the care of your children. As with doctors in internal medicine, pediatricians often have a subspecialty such as cardiology, rheumatology or endocrinology.

- **Obstetricians and Gynecologists** are the subject of significant debate in terms of their appropriateness as primary care doctors. The American Board of Obstetrics and Gynecology states that these doctors are specialists and are not generally trained for primary care. However, the reality is that many, particularly those who solely practice gynecology, often serve as a woman's primary care doctor. Gynecologists are divided on the issue. One recent study showed that 95 percent of visits to ob-gyns are self-referred and that about 60 percent of visits to these specialists are for diagnostic services and preventive services. Another study, by the American College of Obstetricians and Gynecologists, showed that 54 percent of women who see a gynecologist use these doctors for primary care. Reflecting the reality of current medical practice, we have included these specialists in the primary care category.

A businessman in his late fifties, a long-time competitive runner, had surgery in one of New York's top hospitals to repair a badly torn Achilles tendon. At his first follow-up visit to the orthopaedic surgeon, he was assured that "everything was healing perfectly," that he had nothing to be concerned about, and that he would soon be up and running again. Shortly thereafter, just before a summer camping trip, he decided to have his yearly physical examination. The primary care doctor examined the site of the surgery, probing up and down the whole length of the leg. Explaining that he was concerned about certain swelling and discoloration, the doctor arranged for a further examination with ultrasound imaging. This sophisticated test showed that a blood clot had formed in the upper part of the leg, which could have caused severe disability and even death had it gotten into the bloodstream and traveled to the heart or brain. It was the primary care doctor, who knew the patient well, who discovered the potentially fatal condition while carefully conducting a full physical exam.

What Makes A "Top" Doctor

Chapter 2

Quick Tips

- If in doubt about a doctor's training, ask the doctor if the residency completed was in the specialty of his/her practice. If not, ask why not.

- Board certification and recertification are the best ways to measure competence and training.

- The easiest way you can assess the quality of a doctor's residency program is to see if it took place in a large medical center with a name you recognize.

- If a doctor does not have admitting privileges or is not on the attending staff of a hospital, you might consider choosing another doctor.

- There are many excellent, well-trained doctors at community hospitals and they should be as carefully evaluated and considered in your search as a doctor at a teaching hospital.

- Doctors who are full-time academicians may be in the forefront of new techniques and research, but they are not necessarily better doctors.

- The best care is provided by a combination of primary care doctors and other specialists and subspecialists.

- Do not hesitate to ask how frequently your doctor has performed a procedure and with what degree of success. Practice may not lead to perfection, but it improves skills and enhances the probability of success.

- Check the date of graduation from medical school or completion of residency if you want to know precisely how long a doctor has been in practice.

Quick Take

... If a doctor does not have admitting privileges or is not on the attending staff of a hospital, you might consider choosing another doctor. ...

Key Terms

Academic Medical Center - A large medical complex that centers around a teaching hospital in which residency and fellowship programs are offered, where the medical school faculty practices full time and where major clinical research activities occur.

Board Certified - Term signifying that a doctor is qualified for specialization by one of the American Board of Medical Specialties (ABMS) boards. Qualification includes completing an approved residency and passing a rigid exam.

Board Eligible - Term signifying that a doctor has completed an approved residency but has not yet taken the exam given by one of the ABMS recognized boards. The term conveys no official status in the eyes of the ABMS.

Clinical - Medical care that involves direct contact with patients.

Credentialing - A process of screening conducted by hospitals wherein they review the training and licenses of doctors applying to practice on their medical staffs.

Indemnity - A form of health insurance coverage that pays for healthcare but permits the patients to select their provider. Until 1990, indemnity insurance covered most insured people in the United States.

Licensure - Official credentials by individual states that permit a doctor to practice medicine in that state. In some states, doctors may be licensed with no more than one year of post-graduate training.

Residency - A training period spent in a hospital by a graduate of a medical school before going into practice. Residents have earned a medical degree and, therefore, are doctors, but must complete an approved residency and pass an exam to become board certified.

Tertiary Care - Medical services provided by a hospital or medical center that include complex treatments and procedures such as open heart surgery, organ transplants and burn care.

What Makes A "Top" Doctor

Castle Connolly's Top Doctors™ selection process begins with surveys of physicians and healthcare professionals. Each year, Castle Connolly surveys thousands of physicians and other healthcare professionals and asks them to identify excellent doctors in every specialty in their region and throughout the nation. When we began the research for the first edition of America's Top Doctors®, we surveyed over 230,000 of the nation's leading medical specialists, department chairs, residency program directors, vice presidents of medical affairs and presidents of the nation's leading medical centers and specialty hospitals.

In addition to mail and online surveys, the Castle Connolly physician-led research team makes thousands of phone calls each year, talking with leading specialists, chairs of clinical departments and vice presidents of medical affairs, seeking to identify top specialists for most diseases and procedures.

The Castle Connolly physician-led research team carefully reviews the credentials of every physician being considered for inclusion in Castle Connolly Guides, magazine articles and website. The review includes, among other factors, scrutiny of medical education, training, hospital appointments, administrative posts, professional achievements, and malpractice and disciplinary history.

Information on outcomes, procedure volume and malpractice is becoming increasingly available, but the public disclosure varies from state to state. Castle Connolly uses its best efforts to gather the information that is available and use it effectively. Ultimately, however, it is the professional judgment of the Castle Connolly editors, the Chief Medical and Research Officer and the research staff, which determines Castle Connolly Top Doctor™ selection.

Physicians may also be removed from the Castle Connolly lists if, in the judgment of the selection team, that is warranted. Some of the reasons physicians are removed include retirement, change in practice (taking a full time administrative post, for example), unavailability to patients, malpractice or disciplinary issues, negative physician or patient feedback, professional demeanor or a change in the "mix" of specialists Castle Connolly will present for a given community. Being removed from a Castle Connolly list does not necessarily indicate something negative about the physician. At the same time, Castle Connolly does not claim to identify every excellent physician in the nation or a region. The physicians identified through the Castle Connolly research process are clearly among the very best, but there are always other very good physicians not identified by Castle Connolly and that is why our guides, websites and other distribution channels for this critical information describe a process whereby consumers can identify excellent physicians using their own efforts.

There are four basic criteria for selecting your own best doctor: professional preparation, professional reputation, office and practice arrangements and personal or bedside manner. The first three of these assessments can be made prior to your first visit, which is when you can make your fourth evaluation.

Chapter 2

Professional Preparation

Education

Your review of your prospective doctor's education and training should begin with medical school. While you may feel that the institution where someone earned a bachelor's degree could be an indication of the quality of the doctor, most people in the medical field do not believe it plays a major role. A degree from a highly selective undergraduate college or university will help an aspiring doctor gain admission to a medical school, but once there, all students are peers. However, the information on undergraduate colleges, if important to you, is available in the American Board of Medical Specialties (ABMS) Compendium of Certified Medical Specialists and other medical directories.

American medical schools are highly standardized, at least in terms of minimum quality. All U.S. medical schools that grant medical degrees (MDs) and osteopathic degrees (DOs) are accredited by a group known as the LCME (Liaison Committee for Medical Education). Most are also accredited by the appropriate state agency, if one exists, and by regional accrediting agencies that accredit colleges and universities of all kinds.

Furthermore, U.S. medical schools have universally high standards for admission, including success on the undergraduate level and on the Medical College Admissions Tests (MCATs). Although frequently criticized for being slow to change and for training too many specialists, the system of medical education in the United States has insured high quality in medical practice. One recent positive change is a strong effort in most medical schools to diversify the composition of the student body. While these schools have been less successful in enrolling racial minorities, the number of women in U.S. medical schools has increased to the point where they now make up about 50 percent of most classes. In certain specialties preferred by female medical graduates (pediatrics, for example), it is possible that, in coming years, the majority of specialists will be female.

Most doctors practicing in the United States are graduates of U.S. medical schools. There are two other groups of doctors in practice who make up a substantial proportion of the total doctor population. They are: (1) foreign nationals who graduated from foreign schools; and (2) U.S. nationals who graduated from foreign schools (Canadian medical schools are not considered foreign). About one out of three physicians currently practicing in the U.S. represent these groups.

Foreign Medical Graduates

Foreign medical schools vary greatly in quality. Even some of the oldest and finest European schools have become virtually "open door institutions," with huge numbers of unscreened students who make teaching and learning difficult. Others are excellent and provided the model for our own system of medical education.

The fact that someone graduated from a foreign school does not mean that he or she is a poor doctor. Foreign schools, like U.S. schools, produce good doctors and poor doctors. Foreign medical graduates must pass the same exam taken by U.S. graduates for licensure, but the failure rate for foreign graduates is significantly higher. In the first year of using the new United States Medical Licensing Exam (USMLE), 93 percent of U.S. medical school graduates passed Step II, the clinical exam, as compared with 39 percent of foreign graduates. It is clear that the quality of foreign schools, if not individual doctors, is not the same as U.S. medical schools, at least as measured by our standards. Nonetheless, many communities and patients have been well served by foreign medical graduates practicing in this country—often in areas where it has been difficult to attract graduates of American schools.

Residency

Most doctors practicing today have at least three years of postgraduate training (following the MD or DO) in an approved residency program. This is not only an important step in the process of becoming a competent doctor, but it is also a requirement for board (specialty) certification. Most people assume that a prospective doctor needs to complete a three-year residency program to obtain a medical license. This is not true in some states. New York State, for example, requires only one postgraduate year. However, since all approved residencies last at least three years, and some, such as neurosurgery, general surgery, orthopaedic surgery and urology, may extend for five or more years, it is important to know the details of a doctor's training. Licensure alone is not enough of a basis on which to make a good choice.

Without undertaking extensive and detailed research on every residency program, the best assessment you can make of a doctor's residency program is to see if it took place in a large medical center whose name you recognize. The more prestigious institutions tend to attract the best medical students, sometimes regardless of the quality of the individual residency program. If in doubt about a doctor's training, ask the doctor if the residency completed was in the specialty of his/her practice. If not, ask why.

It is also important to be certain that a doctor completed a residency that has been approved by the appropriate governing board of the specialty such as the American Board of Surgery, the American Board of Radiology or the American Osteopathic Board of Pediatrics. These board groups are listed in Appendix A. If you are really concerned about a doctor's training, you should first call the hospital that offered the residency and ask if the residency was approved by the appropriate specialty group. If still in doubt, review the publication Directory of Graduate Medical Education Programs, often called the "green book," found in medical school or hospital libraries, which lists all approved residencies.

Board Certification

With an MD or DO degree and a license, an individual may practice any kind of medicine—with or without additional special training. For example, doctors with a license but no special training may call themselves cardiologists or pediatricians. This is why board certification is such an important factor. Twenty-five specialties are recognized by the American Board of Medical Specialties (ABMS). (Visit www.abms.org or call (312) 436-2600 for more information.) Eighteen boards certify in 106 specialties under the aegis of the American Osteopathic Association (AOA). (Visit www.osteopathic.org or call 800-621-1773 for more information.) Doctors who have qualified for such specialization are called board certified; they have completed an approved residency and passed the board's exam. (See Appendix A for an approved ABMS and AOA list; see pages 81-87 for a description of each specialty and subspecialty.) While many doctors who are not board certified do call themselves specialists, board certification is the best standard by which to measure competence and training.

You can be confident that doctors who are board certified have at a minimum the proper training in their specialty and have demonstrated their proficiency through supervision and testing. While there are many non-board certified doctors who are highly competent, it is more difficult to assess the level of their training. Board certification alone does not guarantee competence, but it is a standard that reflects successful completion of an appropriate training program.

Recertification

A relatively new focus of the specialty boards is the area of recertification. Until recently, board certification lasted for an unlimited time period. Now, almost all of the boards have put time limits on the certification period. For example, in internal medicine, it is ten years; in family practice seven years. In osteopathic medicine, some of the boards need to set a recertification period within 10 years. Many have done so already. These more stringent standards reflect an increasing emphasis, by both the medical boards and state agencies responsible for licensing doctors, on recertification.

Since the policies of the boards vary widely, it is good procedure to ask a doctor if certification was awarded and when. If the date was seven to ten years ago, ask if he/she has been recertified. Note: The most recent date of board certification or recertification is indicated in each physician's listing in this guide.

Unfortunately, many boards permit "grandfathering," whereby already certified doctors do not have to be recertified, and recertification demands apply only to newly certified doctors. Appendix A contains a list of the names and addresses of the boards and the certification period for each board specialty. Even if recertification is not required, it is good professional practice for doctors to undertake the process. It assures you, the patient, that they are attempting to stay current.

Many states have a continuing medical education (CME) requirement for doctors. These states typically require a minimum number of CME credits for a doctor to maintain a medical license. Seven states require 150 CME credits over a three-year period. Osteopathic doctors are required to take 120 hours of CME credits within three years to maintain certification.

Board Eligibility

Many doctors who have been recently trained are waiting to take the boards. They are sometimes described as "board eligible," a common term that the ABMS advocates abandoning because of its ambiguity. Board eligible means that the doctor has completed an approved residency and is qualified to sit for the related board's exam.

Each member board of the ABMS has its own policy regarding the use and recognition of the board eligible term. Therefore, the description "board eligible" should not be viewed as a genuine qualification, especially if a doctor has been out of medical school long enough to have taken the certification exam. To the boards, a doctor is either board certified or not. Furthermore, most of the specialty boards permit unlimited attempts to pass the exam and, in some cases, doctors who have failed the exam twice or even ten times continue to call themselves board eligible. In osteopathic medicine, the board eligible status is recognized only for the first six years after completion of a residency.

Self-Designated Medical Specialties

In addition to the ABMS and AOA-approved list of specialties and subspecialties, there is a wide variety of other doctors, and groups of doctors, who may call themselves "specialists". There are, at present, at least 100 such groups called self-designated medical specialties. They range from doctors who are working to create a recognized body of knowledge and subspecialty training to less formal groups interested in a particular approach to the practice of medicine. These groups may or may not have standards for membership. There is no way of determining the true extent of their members' training, and they are not recognized by the ABMS* or the AOA. While you should be cautious of doctors who claim they are specialists in these areas, many do have advanced training and the groups at least offer a listing of people interested in a particular approach to medical care. Rely on board certification to assure yourself of basic competence and use membership in one of these groups to indicate strong interest and possible additional training in a particular aspect of medicine. A list of these self-designated medical specialties may be found in Appendix B.

Fellowships

The purpose of a fellowship is to provide advanced training in the clinical techniques and research of a particular subspecialty. In the U.S. there are a variety of fellowship programs available to doctors, and they fall into two broad categories: approved and unapproved. Approved fellowships are those approved by the appropriate medical specialty board (e.g., the American Board of Radiology) and that lead to a subspecialty certificate. Fellowship programs that are not approved are often in the same areas of training as those that are, but they do not lead to a subspecialty

* One subspecialty, not yet recognized by the ABMS - Pediatric Neurosurgery - has been included because the retaining and certification process is rigorous and meaningful.

certificate. Unfortunately, all too often, unapproved fellowships exist only to provide relatively inexpensive labor for the research and/or patient care activities of a clinical department in a medical school or hospital. In such cases, the learning that takes place is secondary and may be a good deal less than in an approved fellowship. On the other hand, any fellowship is better than none at all and some unapproved fellowships have that status for a valid reason, which should not reflect negatively on the program. For example, the fellowship may have been recently created with approval being sought. To check that a fellowship is an approved one, call the hospital where the training took place or the medical board for that specialty.

Professional Reputation

There are doctors who meet every professional standard on paper, but who are simply not good doctors. In all probability, the medical community has ascertained that while the individual may still practice medicine, his or her reputation will reflect that collective assessment. There are also doctors who are outstanding leaders in their fields because of research or professional activities, but who are not particularly strong or perhaps even active in patient care. It is important to distinguish that kind of professional reputation from a reputation as a competent, caring doctor in delivering patient care. In a consumer survey conducted by the management consulting firm Towers Perrin, the chief criterion by which the respondents selected doctors was reputation. This was the most important factor for those enrolled in either managed care or indemnity plans.

Hospital Appointment

Most doctors are on the medical staff of one or more hospitals and are known as attendings. If a doctor does not have admitting privileges or is not on the attending staff of a hospital, you may wish to consider choosing another doctor. It can be very difficult to ascertain whether the lack of hospital appointment is for a good reason or not. For example, it is understandable that some doctors who are raising families or heading toward retirement choose not to meet the demands (meetings, committees, etc.) of being an attending. However, if you need care in a hospital, the lack of such an appointment means that another doctor will have to oversee that care. In some specialties such as dermatology and psychiatry, doctors may conduct their entire practices in the office, and a hospital appointment is not as essential, or as good a criterion for assessment, as in other specialties.

While mistakes are made, most hospitals are quite careful about admissions to their medical staffs. The best hospitals are highly selective, so a degree of screening (or "credentialing") has been done for you. In other words, the best doctors practice at the best hospitals. Since caring for a patient in the hospital is often a team effort involving a number of specialists, the reputation of the hospital where the doctor admits patients carries special weight. Hospital medical staffs also review their colleagues credentials before authorizing them to perform specific procedures. In addition, they typically reappoint their medical staffs—and review them—every two or three years. In effect, this is an additional screening to protect patients. It is especially true of hospitals that have what are known as closed staffs, where it is impossible to obtain admitting privileges unless there is a vacancy that the administration and medical staff deem necessary to fill. If you are having some type of surgical procedure and are concerned about the doctor's skill or experience with it, it may be worthwhile to call the Medical Affairs office at the doctor's hospital to see if he or she is authorized to perform that procedure in the hospital.

The reasons for a hospital's selectivity are easy to understand: every hospital wants to have the best reputation possible in order to attract patients, and no hospital, excellent or not, wishes to expose itself to liability. Obviously, the quality of the medical staff is immensely important in creating that reputation. Unfortunately, some hospitals are less diligent when a major group practice of doctors, all of whom have previously been affiliated with the institution, adds new members. In such cases, the hospital may almost automatically grant privileges without conducting the same intensive review given to individual doctors who are not members of a group practice. Also, some hospitals are less selective in granting privileges when beds are empty than when beds are full, since additional attendings provide additional patients.

A last and very important reason why a hospital appointment is an essential requirement in your choice of a doctor is that many states permit doctors to practice without malpractice insurance. If you are injured as a result of the doctor's poor care, you could be without recourse. However, few hospitals permit doctors to practice in them unless they carry malpractice insurance. This not only protects the hospital, but the patient as well.

Many people believe that they should choose a doctor with an appointment at a major medical center as opposed to a community hospital. This assumption is incorrect on two counts. For one thing, there are many excellent, well-trained doctors at community hospitals and they should be as carefully evaluated and considered in your search as a doctor at a large institution. What's more, the term "medical center" has less significance today than it did years ago when the term was used to describe only the major university hospitals of medical schools. A true medical center is a teaching hospital that offers multiple residency programs and at which the medical school faculty practices full-time, with fellowship programs and major clinical research activities an integral part of the teaching of medical students. These large centers also are involved in tertiary care, offering services such as organ transplants, burn care and cardiovascular surgery.

Today many community hospitals have added the term medical center to their name. They do this for two purposes: to indicate that they, too, offer advanced and sophisticated medical programs, and to compete for patients with the academic medical centers. With academic medical centers turning out many well-trained specialists and subspecialists who establish practices in nearby communities and then want to continue the highly specialized techniques they have learned, many community hospitals have initiated tertiary care programs of their own, further blurring the distinction between medical centers and hospitals.

In any case, most of our healthcare today is delivered outside of the hospital in ambulatory outpatient settings. Those who are hospitalized for acute illness (e.g., surgery, serious infection) will find that community hospitals and their staffs are well-suited to the task.

When extremely difficult and complex problems develop, or when tertiary care is needed, many communities have excellent academic medical centers. Of course, they offer primary care as well, especially to those who live nearby. This illustrates the point, once again, that medical care is a local issue.

Medical School Faculty Appointment

Many doctors have appointments on the faculties of medical schools. There is a range of categories from "straight" appointments—meaning full-time appointment as professor, associate professor, assistant professor or instructor—to clinical ranks that may reflect lesser degrees of involvement in teaching or research. If someone carries what is known as a straight academic rank (i.e., professor of surgery, without "clinical" in the title), this usually means that the individual is engaged full-time in medical school research and/or teaching activities. The title "professor of clinical surgery" usually describes a doctor who has a full-time appointment in a medical school, but who puts a greater emphasis on clinical practice (patient care) than on research or teaching. The title "clinical professor of surgery" usually specifies a part-time or adjunct appointment and less direct involvement in medical school activities.

Doctors who are full-time academicians may be in the forefront of new techniques and research, but they are not necessarily better doctors. Nonetheless, you can be assured that they have the support of other faculty, residents and medical students.

When you are seeking a subspecialist, a doctor's relationship to a medical school becomes more meaningful since medical school faculties tend to be made up of subspecialists. You are less likely to find large numbers of general or primary care practitioners engaged full-time on a medical school faculty. The newest approaches and techniques in medicine, for the most part, are explored and developed by medical school faculties in their laboratories and clinical practice settings. This is where they practice their subspecialties, as well as teach and perform research. Such leading specialists are not necessarily better doctors than community doctors—they are trained to provide a different kind of medical care. The best care is provided by a combination of primary care doctors and other specialists and subspecialists.

Medical Society Membership

Most medical society memberships sound very prestigious and some are; however, there are many societies that are not selective and which virtually any doctor can join. In addition, membership in many of the more prestigious societies is based on research and publication, or on leadership in the field, and may have little to do with direct patient care. While it is clearly an honor to be invited to join these groups, membership may be less than helpful in discerning whether a doctor can meet your needs.

Board certified doctors are referred to as Diplomates of the Board. Some of the colleges of medical specialties (e.g., the American College of Radiology and the American College of Surgeons) have multiple levels of recognition. The first is basic membership and the second, more prestigious and difficult to obtain, is status as a Fellow. Fellowship status in the colleges is meaningful and is based on experience, professional achievement and recognition by one's peers, including extensive experience in patient care. It should be viewed as a significant professional qualification.

Experience

Experience is difficult to assess. Obviously, in most cases, an older doctor has more experience; on the other hand, a younger doctor has been more recently immersed in residency, the challenge of medical school, or even a fellowship, and may be the most up-to-date. If a doctor is board certified, you may assume that assures at least a minimal amount of experience, but it could be as little as a year. In this guide the board certification date may reflect a doctor's most recent recertification, so check the date of graduation from medical school or completion of residency if you want to know precisely how long a doctor has been in practice.

There is a good deal of evidence that there is a positive relationship between quantity of experience and quality of care. That is, the more often a doctor performs a procedure, the better he/she becomes at it. That is why it is important to ask a doctor about his or her experience with the procedure that you need. Does the doctor see and treat similar cases every day, every week or only rarely? Of course, with some rare conditions, rarely is the only possible answer, but it is relative frequency that is critical. Major metropolitan areas, especially New York and San Francisco, became leaders in the treatment of AIDS because of the large number of patients seen in those metropolitan areas. Doctors in the suburbs of New York City (especially in New York's Westchester, Nassau and Suffolk counties) and in Fairfield County, Connecticut became leaders in the research and treatment of Lyme disease because that region is the epicenter of the disease.

In some states, data is available on volume or numbers of certain procedures performed at hospitals. Likewise, The Leapfrog Group (www.leapfroggroup.org) compares hospitals' performance on the national standards of safety, quality and efficiency - areas of healthcare that are most relevant to consumers and this information is later used to improve hospital quality, save healthcare spending and assist hospital employees with purchasing strategies. The federal government has posted outcome data for hospitals, but for a limited number of procedures, on a website www.hospitalcompare.hhs.gov/hospital-search.aspx. There is a good deal of controversy, however, on the validity and usefulness of such data. Opponents cite the fact that some of the data is produced from Medicare patient records only and, thus, is based solely on an elderly population that does not represent the total activity of a hospital or doctor. Proponents of the use of such volume data agree that it is not perfect, but suggest that it can be one useful criterion in selecting the best places to receive care for these specific problems. Recognizing the limitations of such data, the healthcare consumer may, nonetheless, find it of interest and use.

Office and Practice Arrangements

Although clearly not as important as training or reputation, office and practice arrangements are usually of great significance to patients. Practice arrangements include office hours, office location, billing procedures and office testing among the many factors that result in how well the office is run.

Many years ago most doctors practiced independently in private offices. They were called solo practitioners and usually had agreements with other doctors to respond to their patients' calls when they were unavailable. In recent decades, most doctors have entered group practices; indeed, this is becoming the most common way for young doctors to begin to practice. Two or more doctors in the same specialty, or in different specialties (a multi-specialty group), share offices and staff to lower their costs of operations. They also cover for each other on rotation for weekends, evenings and vacations. As a patient you may prefer one of the following: a solo practitioner who is covered occasionally; a group where you usually, but not always, see the same doctor; or a multi-specialty group where, if a consultation or referral is necessary, the specialist is at the same location. The choice is really one of personal preference.

There are other factors relating to practice arrangements that may or may not be important to an individual when choosing a doctor. One is the location of the office. A consumer poll conducted for the Robert Wood Johnson Foundation identified office location as one of the two most important factors in the selection of a doctor (the other was a recommendation by a relative or friend). Actually, the site of the office can be very important in choosing a doctor you may visit on a regular basis. If the location is inconvenient, you may be discouraged from making needed visits.

Another important factor concerns the use of nurse practitioners and physician's assistants in the office. Licensed nurse practitioners are advanced practice nurses in primary care. They have additional training beyond the basic requirements for nursing licensure, usually a master's degree or special certificate. They perform a broad range of nursing functions as well as functions that, historically, have been performed by doctors, including assessing and diagnosing, conducting physical examinations, ordering diagnostic tests, implementing treatment plans and monitoring patient status. Physician's assistants are licensed to provide medical care in many states. However, unlike nurses, they may practice only under a doctor's direction and supervision. According to an article in the professional journal Family Practice Management, these "midlevel providers," as they are called, "can handle 80 to 90 percent of the problems that occasion office visits." These providers have become more of a presence in healthcare in recent years, especially in medical groups and HMOs. If you don't think you will be satisfied having your office visit and examination conducted by anyone but the doctor, you should determine up front how many midlevel providers are on staff and how extensive their responsibilities are.

Narrowing the Choice

Here are 10 additional questions that will guide you in assessing if the practice patterns or arrangements of a doctor meet your needs. If there are other items not listed that are important to you, add them to the list before you make your initial appointment. You should try to obtain as much of the information as possible from the staff.

- Are you currently accepting new patients and, if so, is a referral required?
- On average, how long does a patient have to wait for an appointment?
- Are you open on weekends? In the evening?
- If lab work and X-rays are performed in the office what are the qualifications of the people doing the tests?
- Are full payment, deductibles or co-payments required at the time of the appointment?
- Do you accept my insurance plan? Medicare? Medicaid? Workers' compensation? No-fault insurance?
- Do you accept credit cards and, if so, which do you accept?
- Do you accept patient phone calls?
- Do you use electronic medical records?
- Is your office handicapped-accessible?

If you have a chronic illness or disease, there may be certain additional aspects of a doctor's practice that could be particularly important to you. You should discuss any chronic problems when first establishing a relationship with a doctor. In fact, you may want to find a doctor with special interest or training in that problem.

House calls also continue to be important to some people. Yes, some doctors still do make house calls! In fact, a recent American Medical News article suggested that 43 percent of internal medicine specialists and 65 percent of family practice specialists made one or more house calls a year. However, it is important to point out that the number of doctors making house calls has declined because of technology, liability risks and time pressures. Important diagnostic equipment often cannot be carried around in a doctor's little black bag and is only available in the office or hospital. Also, the time required to visit one patient at home markedly reduces the time available to see other patients.

Personal or Bedside Manner

To many patients, once they have determined that a doctor is competent, the doctor's professional manner—also known as bedside manner—is the most important part of their choice. The Towers Perrin report cited earlier indicated that after reputation, skill in communicating was the most important factor sought in doctors. Patients prefer sensitive and caring doctors who listen carefully and demonstrate their concern. Studies show that such doctors are sued less often than others!

What characteristics make up a doctor's personal manner? The four described below may, when considered together, give you a clear idea of whether a particular doctor will be your personal "top" doctor.

- **Listening**. Professional manner includes the doctor's willingness to listen to patients, be supportive and understanding, explain procedures and exhibit concern and respect. These skills are expressed at the bedside, in the office, or in any setting where there is doctor/patient contact. Listening is also a valuable diagnostic tool. Unfortunately, these skills often have not been taught well in medical schools and the lack of them forms the primary basis for complaints from patients. However, there is growing emphasis on these vital interpersonal and communications skills in medical schools today and with good reason. They are critically important to most patients.
- **Cultural Sensitivity.** Some patients may prefer doctors who speak their language or are familiar with their cultural background. The term "culturally competent physician" is a relatively new one describing doctors who have the needed skills and attitudes to effectively treat patients from minority cultures.
- **Ethical, Religious and Philosophical Views.** Religion, or at least views on issues such as abortion, utilization of life-sustaining measures, natural childbirth, breast-feeding and other such matters can also be important. It is perfectly appropriate to ask doctors their views on sensitive issues.
- **Decision-making Procedures.** Years ago patients took the words of the doctor as law, not to be questioned or perhaps even discussed. That is not the case today. Consumers are better informed about health issues and may want to be actively involved in the decision making that affects their health. Some patients do not feel this way and are comfortable accepting a doctor's diagnosis or course of treatment without question. Some doctors—in diminishing numbers, thankfully—feel uncomfortable with patients who want everything explained to them or want to be involved in decision-making. Consider how you feel about this issue and discuss it with your doctor to be certain you are on compatible wavelengths.

Of course, what ultimately makes a "top" doctor are the results, the "outcomes," of care. Unfortunately, there is relatively little information available to consumers on the outcomes of physicians and hospitals. Some states, New York for example, have produced studies on outcomes for cardiac surgery. Also, some HMOs are talking about producing report cards for doctors. Generally, however, consumers will have difficulty finding outcome studies for individual doctors.

On the other hand, there is a growing movement to track and publish outcomes data on hospitals. The federal government has taken the lead by releasing outcomes data by hospitals for selected procedures. Visit www.hospitalcompare.hhs.gov.

One woman—a long-time City resident who moved to the suburbs to be near her children—found out the hard way about advice when she selected a doctor on the basis of her neighbor's glowing praise. During the initial visit, the patient's numerous questions about her chronic arthritis condition went unanswered while the doctor merely patted her on the shoulder and assured her that he would "take care of everything." While the paternalistic attitude might have suited the neighbor's needs, it fell far short for this senior patient, who was used to a good give-and-take with her former internist. She resumed her search for a doctor—this time with the assistance of the Castle Connolly guide, a more reliable source than a friend's recommendation.

The Best in American Medicine
www.CastleConnolly.com

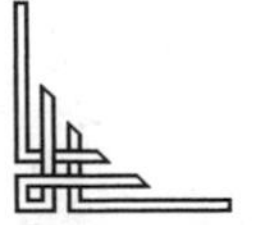
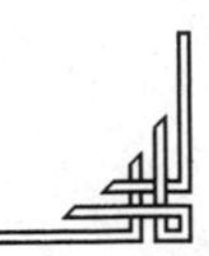

You And Your Doctor: A Team

Chapter 3

Quick Tips

- Always obtain copies of all medical records and tests for your files.
- When selecting a doctor, especially a primary care doctor, it is appropriate to request an interview to get acquainted.
- Good doctors listen, good patients talk.
- Always bring a pad and pencil with you to medical appointments. When the doctor gives you instructions, take notes.
- The Physician's Desk Reference, commonly known as the PDR, is available in most libraries and is an excellent resource for learning more about medications. (The PDR web page is at http://www.pdr.net)
- Do not hesitate to ask your pharmacist about side effects, generic substitutions and other questions related to your medications.

Quick Take

... The best doctor-patient relationship is based on a two-way dialogue. Be open and honest and seek a doctor who is the same. ...

Key Terms

American Medical Association - A membership organization of physicians and their professional associations dedicated to promoting the art and science of medicine and the betterment of public health through establishing and promoting ethical, educational, and clinical standards for the medical profession. It represents the interests of physicians on the national level.

Baseline Tests - A series of basic, routine medical tests—such as electrocardiogram, complete blood count, blood pressure measurement, weight measurement, and chest X-ray—that are usually completed by a physician upon a patient's initial visit in order to provide a standard for comparison during subsequent health examinations.

Generic Drugs - Prescription medications that have been marketed by one company under a proprietary or brand name and which may be sold, after the original exclusive patent expires, under a generic name or the name assigned to it during an early stage of development. Most generic drugs are less expensive than proprietary versions and are just as effective except in cases when, because of different manufacturing processes, they are not bioequivalent or handled by the body in an identical manner.

Third Party Payer - An organization such as indemnity insurance company or managed care organization that provides individual and group health insurance, or a governmental department which assumes responsibility for the payment of an individual's healthcare, either directly to the healthcare provider or by means of reimbursement to the individual (Medicare and Medicaid are such government programs).

You And Your Doctor: A Team

Trust and respect between doctors and patients have reached a low point in modern American society. A recent poll of consumers sponsored by the American Medical Association (AMA) concluded that approximately 70 percent of those who responded agreed with the statement that "people are beginning to lose faith in their doctors." (Despite concerns about doctors in general, much research has shown that patients tend to rate their own doctors well.)

Trust between doctors and patients has declined for many reasons, including unrealistic expectations on the part of some patients and the patronizing attitudes of some doctors, which clash with the higher education level and medical sophistication of many patients. This has been further complicated by changing financial arrangements, particularly those involving the government and third-party payers, and the perception that some doctors seem to be motivated not by the values of the Hippocratic Oath (See page xv), but by those of the marketplace. The AMA poll cited earlier found that 69 percent of respondents agreed that doctors "are too interested in making money." Perhaps a significant factor in creating this atmosphere is that in many cases the relationship between doctor and patient now has another dimension, the managed care organization. Another significant contributor is the huge amount of paperwork required from doctors. Generated by quality-assurance efforts, regulation, complex billing and managed care procedures, this burden reduces the time doctors are able to spend with patients.

Given the formidable obstacles, it might seem impossible to find a primary care doctor who is well suited to your needs. If you have carefully read the preceding chapters, your work is half done. What remains is to find that special individual who fits the criteria.

The Initial Interview

When selecting a doctor, especially a primary care doctor, it is appropriate to request an exploratory interview. Frequently, doctors will engage in such brief interviews at no charge, at a reduced fee or by telephone. It is preferable to find out about a doctor's credentials, office hours and billing procedures from the staff beforehand so you don't waste time asking about basic facts. This leaves time to ask the doctor questions that will allow you to determine what kind of relationship could develop. It is interesting that many parents will insist on interviewing a pediatrician for their child but wouldn't think of interviewing a physician for themselves.

Ask the Right Questions

The most important aspect of this session is to see if you can develop a positive doctor/patient relationship. Are you comfortable with the doctor's manner, style and general personality? Do you feel a strong sense of trust in the doctor? Here are five questions to ask the doctor plus two questions to ask yourself that may lead you closer to a selection.

- What is your experience in treating __________ (if you are seeking care for a particular illness or condition)?
- Are you open to treatments and therapies that do not rely heavily on medication?
- What preventive programs do you suggest for someone of my age, sex and health status?
- How do you feel about involving patients in decision-making?
- What are your views on__________(ethical and moral issues of importance to you as a patient)?

Even when the doctor is responding to your questions, you should ask yourself:

- Is the doctor paying attention to me and really considering my questions or do the impersonal "stock" answers indicate that the doctor's thoughts are elsewhere?
- Does this doctor speak about good health and prevention with the personal knowledge of someone who seems to practice it?

If your prospective doctor seems to measure up to your standards, get the relationship off to a good start by making an appointment for a complete check-up. During this appointment, you will have an opportunity to share your medical and family history and baseline tests will be performed to serve as a standard in the years ahead.

Talking with Your Doctor

After you have selected your doctor, your first appointment should include an extensive review of your medical history. Your doctor should spend time with you, ask questions and listen to your responses carefully.

Medical students are often told, "Listen to your patients. They'll tell you what's wrong with them." This conveys an important lesson not only for doctors, but for patients: Good doctors listen; good patients talk.

Analysis of doctor/patient conversations has revealed that many patients wait until the end of a conversation, even until they are saying goodbye, to tell their doctors what is really bothering them. This is just a small example of the dynamics of doctor/patient relationships. It is also a good example of a waste of valuable time—the doctor's and the patient's. One reason doctors need to be trained to be good listeners is that they frequently must ascertain what is troubling the patient not by what is said directly, but by what is said indirectly, not at all or through body language and other signs. However, it is always easier, less time-consuming and certainly more effective if a patient can describe problems completely and accurately.

Before you even see a doctor, you should prepare thoroughly. You should have a complete record of your medical history, including a record of X-rays and any other diagnostic tests, as well as blood workups. You need information about childhood diseases, chronic conditions, hospitalizations, past and present medications, doses and drug reactions, if any, and, if possible, something about the health history of your parents and even their siblings. Except for the last item, these are available to patients from their previous doctors or hospitals. That is why it is useful to obtain copies of all medical records and tests for your own files. Not only will this save you time and effort, but may avoid additional testing and expense. Your doctor will also ask many seemingly personal questions about your work, education, sex life and even drug and alcohol use. These are all part of a complete medical history and will help your doctor better understand you and your state of health.

If you have a particular problem or concern, describe all your symptoms. Try not to minimize or exaggerate and, most of all, don't deny.

If you have questions to ask your doctor, make a list. Always bring a pad and pencil with you to medical appointments. When the doctor gives you instructions, take notes or ask the doctor to write them down for you. If a prescription is written, ask about doses, side effects, efficacy and alternative medications as well as generic substitutes. The Physician's Desk Reference, commonly known as the PDR, is available in most libraries and is an excellent resource for learning more about medications. There is also a PDR web page on the Internet at http://www.pdr.net. You can also get a great deal of information on medications from another health professional, your pharmacist. Do not hesitate to ask your pharmacist about side effects, generic substitutions and other questions related to your medications. However, if the information you receive conflicts with that given by your doctor, consult with the doctor and follow his or her directions.

A Matter of Time

Patients want and expect doctors who listen, express concern, explain conditions and procedures in a clear and understandable manner, discuss medications and their effects and side effects thoroughly, return calls, are available when needed and, perhaps most importantly, spend sufficient time with them. With increasing demands on their time, many doctors are left with an uneasy feeling of "running to stay in place." The end result may be a tendency, unintended for the most part, to rush through a patient visit. This situation contributes to the erosion of the doctor/patient relationship.

Also contributing to this problem is pervasive lateness on the part of doctors. Patients frequently complain that they spend hours in a doctor's waiting room, long past the appointed hour (research has shown the average wait is 20 minutes).

Unfortunately, the duration of a patient visit is not always predictable and unexpected delays may occur if the diagnosis is complicated or if a patient needs to discuss what is on his or her mind. The doctor who spends extra time with another patient is probably the doctor you want for yourself. If the lateness is excessive, persistent and without apparent good reason, discuss it with your doctor and, if it is interfering with your relationship, consider changing doctors.

Today many primary care physicians are changing their practices to a new model known as concierge or "private medicine." In this model, physicians reduce their practice patient load from, say, 2,200 patients to 600. Each patient who remains in, or enters, a concierge practice is required to pay an annual fee typically ranging from $1,500 to $5,000, or even more. As a function of the reduced patient load, the physicians have far greater time to spend with each patient and can offer faster appointments or better access sometimes even around the clock. The physician can also focus more on preventive medicine and other aspects of sound patient care, a luxury and benefit to the patient that many physicians in a primary care practice cannot enjoy.

After a delay of two hours in his doctor's office, one patient, a self-employed marketing consultant, made sure that it would never happen again. Did he have a showdown with the doctor? Did he decide never to return? Not at all. He simply made it a point to call the doctor's office two hours before his scheduled appointment to see how the schedule was running. He then adjusted his own schedule to coincide with the doctor's.

Strengthening Your Team

Chapter 4

Quick Tips

- The more complex and difficult the problem, the more important reputation is. In fact, you might well narrow your focus to doctors on the staffs of certain medical centers noted for excellence with specific problems.
- Doctors typically refer patients to doctors on the staffs of the same hospitals where they practice.
- If the lateness of your doctor is excessive, persistent and without apparent good reason, discuss it with him or her.
- If you are not comfortable with your primary care doctor's referral, ask for a number of options. If necessary, you may consider going "out of network" even if you have to pay some or all of the fee.
- In many cases, insurance companies will pay for second opinions, but check ahead of time to make sure your insurance plan does cover them.
- One way HMOs control costs is by limiting second opinions.
- Doctors may have different solutions to the same problem — and any one or more could work.

Quick Take

... The old adage, two heads are better than one, often applies in healthcare, too. Expanded options include referrals, second opinions, alternative therapies and clinical trials. ...

Key Terms

Alternative Therapy - Non-traditional forms of healthcare — including acupuncture, homeopathy, naturopathy, massage, reflexology, biofeedback, hypnotherapy, herbology, therapeutic touc, and prayer — that are often based on ancient healing methods and have not been tested in a conventional scientific manner.

Clinical Trial - An experimental trial of a new drug or therapy in a selected group of human volunteers who suffer from the condition for which the experimental drug or treatment is to be used.

Double Blind Study - One form of a clinical trial in which two groups of volunteers — one group receiving the real drug or treatment and the other receiving a placebo or dummy — are followed for a specific period of time by researchers who do not know themselves who is receiving which therapy.

Protocol - A rigid set of rules set up for a clinical trial by the Food and Drug Administration (FDA) which must be followed strictly by all researchers and volunteers participating in the trial.

Strengthening Your Team

When You Need a Specialist

For the most part, selecting a specialist is similar to choosing a primary care doctor. There is one major difference, however; typically you will be referred to a specialist by your primary care doctor. Suggesting a consultation does not show a weakness on the part of the doctor. On the contrary, the real weakness lies in a doctor's reluctance to suggest consultations when advisable. Your primary care doctor will receive a written report from any consultation or referral. You should request a copy as well.

Ask your doctor why this particular specialist is being recommended. Find out about the specialist's training and experience. If your doctor has sent many patients to the same doctor for the same treatment, you should find out how successful the treatment was and if the patients were satisfied. You might also ask if the specialist would be the one selected for your doctor's own personal care. You should feel comfortable about seeing the specialist and, if you are not, ask for another recommendation or find a different one on your own.

Frequently, patients do seek out specialists on their own. If you are attempting to find a specialist or subspecialist without the guidance of your primary care doctor, use the various selection procedures described in Chapters One, Two and Three. When selecting a physician on your own, even greater emphasis should be placed on board certification in the relevant specialty. If you are trying to find someone to treat a very specific problem, make certain that the individual is well trained in that area. You may check to see if a doctor is board certified by calling the American Board of Medical Specialties at (312) 436-2600 or visiting their web site at www.abms.org.

You will also want to know if the specialist you select is well respected. The more complex and difficult the problem, the more important reputation is. In fact, you might narrow your focus to doctors on the staffs of certain medical centers noted for excellence in treating your specific problem. There are a number of books and magazine articles such as the annual U.S. News & World Report issue on America's best hospitals that offer views on the best medical centers for specific problems.

Finally, make certain your doctor and the specialist communicate easily about your case. If you should have a problem with a specialist, or if you are not pleased with the care given, let your primary care doctor know about it right away.

Doctors typically refer patients to doctors on the staffs of the same hospitals at which they practice. There are good and poor reasons for this, as explained below.

Why Doctors Usually Refer to Doctors in the Same Hospitals

Good Reasons:

- They know the doctors better.
- They continue to be involved in the case.
- Coordination of multiple specialists may be easier.

Poor Reasons:

- It is easier.
- They will get referrals back.
- It reduces the chance of losing the patient to another doctor.
- It may help build social or professional relationships.
- The hospital may pressure doctors to refer within the institution.

In today's managed care environment doctor referrals usually are restricted to other doctors in the managed care organization's network. Sometimes the referring doctor may not even be familiar with the other doctor's qualifications. If you are not comfortable with your primary care doctor's referral, ask for a number of options. If necessary, you may consider going "out of network" even if you have to pay some or all of the fee.

Second Opinions

Second opinions are a valuable medical tool, infrequently used in many instances, overused in others. Clearly, you do not want to get another doctor's opinion on every ailment or problem, but there are definitely times you should seek out a second opinion:

- Before major surgery.
- When the diagnosis is serious or life-threatening.
- If a rare disease is diagnosed.
- If the diagnosis is uncertain.
- If you think the number of tests or procedures recommended is excessive.
- If a test result has serious implications—a positive Pap smear for example—have the test re-done immediately before taking further action.
- If the treatment suggested is risky or expensive.

- If you are uncomfortable with the diagnosis and treatment recommended.
- If a course of treatment is not working.
- If you question your doctor's competence.
- If your insurance company requires it.

Most doctors will be supportive if you request a second opinion and many will even recommend it. In many cases, insurance companies will pay for second opinions, but check ahead of time to make sure your insurance plan does indeed cover them. In an HMO, you may have to be more assertive because one way that HMOs control costs is by limiting second opinions. This is especially true if you want an opinion outside the plan's network.

Often, the opinion of a second doctor will affirm the opinion of the first, but the reassurance may be worth the time and extra cost. On the other hand, if the second opinion differs from the first, you have two remaining alternatives: seek the opinion of a third doctor, or educate yourself as much as possible by talking with both doctors and reading up on the problem (trusting your instincts about which diagnosis is correct). If the diagnosis is the same but the recommended treatments differ, remember that doctors may have different solutions to the same problem—and any one or more could be efficient. For example, an orthopaedic surgeon may recommend surgery to correct a knee injury while a physiatrist (a doctor certified in physical medicine and rehabilitation) may recommend rehabilitation. One might work better than the other or they could both work equally well. The choice may be based on your preference. Remember, however, that surgical solutions can rarely be reversed. It usually is best to try a non-surgical solution first, if possible.

Complementary Medicine: Exploring Your Options

A recent study conducted by the University of Florida estimated that 86 percent of households in the U.S. use some type of complementary therapies (a term that implies that these therapies are used along with conventional medical treatment rather than in place of them). Total out-of-pocket expenditures for complementary/alternative medicine approach $30 billion annually, estimates David Eisenberg, MD and colleagues at the Harvard/Beth Israel Center for the Study of Alternative Medicine Research. They further point out that total visits to complementary/alternative providers numbered 629 million in 1997 as compared to 386 million visits to primary care physicians.

One of the reasons conventional medical therapies are conventional is that most have been proven to be effective in a rigorous scientific manner, while many complementary/alternative therapies have not been tested under accepted scientific conditions. You should always consider the possibility that some alternative therapies, since they are unproven, may do more harm than good. The alternative approaches in use today range from legitimate searches for new therapies to outright quackery and fraud. Without the guidance of the scientific and medical community, it is sometimes impossible for doctors, let alone consumers, to tell the difference.

Nonetheless, doctors are becoming more open to the use of complementary/alternative approaches. One study reported that about 30 percent of doctors questioned in the Los Angeles area said that they were open to complementary/alternative practices in one form or another and that acceptance is growing. Medical scientists are also indicating a new interest in studying approaches to health that may complement the strengths of Western medicine. Some of the therapies being explored include mind-body medicine, hypnotherapy, biofeedback, chiropractic, vital energy, metabolic therapy, naturopathy, homeopathy, therapeutic touch, acupuncture, prayer and the use of herbs.

Alternative healthcare often complements rather than replaces Western medicine. As such, the terms complementary or integrative, which accurately describe the relationship between Western and alternative healthcare, are used with increased frequency as this type of approach towards medicine becomes more commonplace.

In a New England Journal of Medicine study, 72 percent of the respondents who used unconventional therapies did not inform their medical doctor that they had done so. That is unfortunate, because such treatments could be greatly enhanced with the support and advice of a primary care doctor. More worrisome is the great danger that some people may use alternative treatments in lieu of, rather than as a supplement to, more conventional and proven medical therapies. A classic and tragic example of this was the surge of patients who traveled to Mexico to seek a "magic bullet" cure for cancer promised by the drug Laetrile (made from apricot pits). There was no magic; indeed, patients lost money, hope and, in some cases, the opportunity for timely use of proven treatment. If you do explore alternative therapies, be certain to let your doctor know about it. Some may be harmful, especially if you are undergoing another treatment under your doctor's direction.

To learn more about complementary/alternative medicine, contact the National Center for Complementary and Alternative Medicine Clearinghouse to locate a source of reliable information on the practice you are considering (see Appendix E).

How to Use Complementary/Alternative Medicine Wisely and Well

- Try to learn everything you can about the particular therapy that interests you. Your local library and the Internet both have substantial materials on complementary/alternative medicine.
- Discuss your plans with your doctor. You might gain some insight into the therapy in terms of its possible risks. Furthermore, if you are currently under medical treatment, you should make certain that the two approaches will not conflict in some way.
- If you start an alternative therapy and it does not appear to be providing relief, or seems to be worsening the condition, contact your doctor immediately.

Clinical Trials: Should You Participate?

Each year, more than half a million Americans, some of them sick, but even more of them healthy, volunteer to take part in experimental trials of new drugs and therapies. Before drugs, vaccines, biological agents and medical devices are made available for general use by doctors and their patients, they must go through extensive testing on animals and humans called "clinical trials." There is probably at least one clinical trial in process at some medical center for almost every serious disease.

On the plus side, a clinical trial offers the opportunity for prompt use of a drug or other treatment that seems promising, and comes with the bonus of regular and thorough medical examinations at no cost to you (some trials even make allowances for participants' travel and other expenses). Moreover, patients are encouraged to discuss all of their experiences regarding the trial. You will probably learn more about your condition and feel more in control, which can have a very positive effect. On the downside, you may be giving up standard treatment for something that may or may not be better. There is even the possibility that you will not get a drug at all, because most trials are conducted by the double-blind method, in which half of the participants get the drug and half get a placebo, or "dummy" medicine. Even the doctors conducting the trials do not know who is getting which drug.

What to Know Before You Get Involved

If you are considering participating in a clinical trial, you will want to know:

- Who is the sponsor? Look for a federal government, major health organization, drug company or university-sponsored trial.
- Do any impartial authorities monitor the trial? Every hospital conducting research has an institutional review board (IRB) consisting of medical professionals and community leaders who approve that hospital's participation. There are also data and safety monitoring boards that oversee trials.
- What is the financial relationship, if any, between the doctor, hospital and the company or agency sponsoring the trial?

- Will there be pain or discomfort? Will diagnostic tests be involved? Get detailed answers to these concerns before you sign any form.
- How often will I be examined? This depends on the guidelines of the trial (called the protocol). You should make every effort to keep your appointments.
- Does my own doctor get a record of my participation in the trial? Routine health information is sent to your doctor, but details relevant to a "blinded" trial are not disclosed until the trial is over.
- Is the drug in this trial approved for treatment of any other disorder? If the answer is yes, you then know that the drug has a prior safety record.
- After the study has ended, if I have responded well to the drug, will I be able to continue using it, even before it is approved?
- Can I drop out?

If you are interested in participating in a clinical trial, make your desire known to your doctor, who can track down openings in trials being conducted by medical centers, private foundations, drug companies, physician groups and the federal government. You can also access information on clinical trials by visiting the CenterWatch Clinical Trials Listing Service at www.centerwatch.com or the web site of the National Cancer Institute at www.cancer.gov/clinicaltrials.

Easy Access to specialists and subspecialists, especially in large metropolitan areas, presents certain problems in coordination of care that a patient should be aware of. This difficulty is probably epitomized by one woman who was treated by a dermatologist, an ophthalmologist, a rheumatologist, a psychiatrist and an allergist, all of whom had office space in her very large apartment complex on Manhattan's upper west side-thus eliminating her need to even put on her coat. Fortunately, all were quite competent and had all the necessary qualifications. Unfortunately, each was affiliated with a different medical center, which made coordinating her care with her primary care doctor very complex.

Changing Your Doctor

Chapter 5

Quick Tips

Surgical solutions can rarely be reversed. It usually is best to try a non-surgical solution first, if possible.

You should always consider the possibility that alternative therapies - simply because they are unproven - may do more harm than good.

If you do explore alternative therapies, be certain to let your doctor know about it. Some may be harmful, especially if you are undergoing another treatment under your doctor's direction.

Before you decide to part company with your doctor, ask yourself if you've been a responsible patient.

A doctor-patient relationship is like a marriage — both sides have to work to make it successful.

Expressing your dissatisfaction may open the communication lines between you and your doctor; you might even end up in a better relationship with your present doctor

Unless the situation is intolerable or the doctor is impaired, stay with your current doctor until you have found another one that you like

When changing doctors, you may have to sign a release with your new doctor approving the transfer of all your medical records to the new office. These records cannot be withheld for any reason, even if you have not yet paid your last bill.

Quick Take

... There's a big difference between doctor-hopping and changing doctors for a good reason. Most failed doctor-patient relationships can be attributed to some common complaints but sometimes are a matter of self-defense...

Key Terms

National Practitioner Data Bank - A computerized listing, created by an Act of Congress, to track health professionals who are disciplined for unprofessional behavior and to deter them from simply moving their practicies from one state to another.

Public Citizen Health Research Group - A Washington, D.C. based consumer advocacy group that has been publicly critical of many medical practices that the group considers detrimental to public healthcare.

Changing Your Doctor

Obviously, at times there are good reasons for changing doctors. Some are very simple and straightforward, such as a doctor's retirement, illness or death, your own relocation or a change in your health plan. About 40 percent of people enrolling in managed care plans have to change their doctor to one who is affiliated with their plan.

The onset of a chronic condition may also prompt a change to a different medical specialist, such as a rheumatologist or cardiologist, if a condition needs to be managed by a specialist other than a primary care doctor.

If you have continuing symptoms that your doctor has been unable to diagnose or if, after a diagnosis, your problems continue to linger without improvement, you should at least consider getting a second opinion and, depending on that opinion, possibly change doctors. Doctors often have different approaches to the same problem. A different doctor may offer a different perspective and, perhaps, a solution.

You might also change doctors in order to find one who includes complementary/alternative medicine in the treatment or to find one who can help you enroll in a clinical trial.

People who have hostile feelings toward organized medicine tend to change doctors frequently; their complaints then become a self-fulfilling prophecy. They don't get continuous, quality care because it's impossible for anyone to deliver it. On the other hand, negative feelings may be prompted by unfortunate encounters with incompetent doctors or by the patronizing or otherwise inappropriate attitudes expressed by some doctors toward patients. Patients on the receiving end of such a relationship should continue their search for a doctor who better meets their needs.

Eight Reasons to Say Goodbye

Here are the eight most common complaints about "doctors I don't go to anymore."

Poor Bedside Manner

Good medical care is more than diagnosis and treatment; it's also an attitude on the part of the doctor that sparks a sense of trust in the patient. Being under the care of a doctor who is impersonal, abrupt, bored, arrogant, condescending or sarcastic may, in the end, be counterproductive.

The doctor's aloofness could have a more serious explanation: substance abuse or psychological impairment, which, according to a recent American Medical Association report, affect 30,000 to 40,000 physicians. Mood swings and detachment are signs to watch for.

Too Vague and Evasive

A doctor who dismisses problems with "it's nothing to worry about" or "let me take care of it" or who uses medical jargon isn't interested in having you as a partner in your healthcare. The effect of this evasiveness can be anger, fear and confusion, leading to failure to follow directions and failure of treatment.

Never on Schedule

Medical emergencies can make appointment scheduling an inexact science, but when snafus become chronic, it's a sign of trouble. An explanation can ease the frustration, but make-up time should not be at your expense.

Couldn't Diagnose the Problem

Some conditions can't be diagnosed on-the-spot. Others aren't attributable to one specific cause. That doesn't excuse an incomplete workup, however, which may leave you with a condition that could have been treated earlier.

Ordered too Many Tests

Sophisticated technology is available and doctors tend to use it, although some testing may not be necessary. The number of tests performed for diagnosis seems to be reduced in patient-doctor relationships where communication is strong.

Discouraged Second Opinions

A doctor who dissuades you from talking to another doctor may perceive it as questioning his or her professional abilities.

Didn't Protect My Medical Privacy

No patient should have to discuss the reason for a visit, payment or payment problems within earshot of other patients or staff.

Under certain conditions, medical records can be requested by and turned over to insurance companies, lawyers, employers and certain others without your consent, but you can certainly see them, too, to make sure they contain the proper information. In all 50 states and the District of Columbia, federal law grants patients access to their medical records.

Unpleasant Office Staff

Repeated incidents such as rudeness over the telephone, a brusque physician's assistant or being kept waiting in an examining room for a long time before the doctor shows up are all annoying indications that a staff could do better.

The staff takes its cues from the chief. A doctor who doesn't demand the highest level of performance from a staff may be sending a message about his or her own laxity in diagnosis and treatment.

Should You Switch?

If these conditions exist in your doctor-patient relationship, it may be time to consider finding a new doctor. But before you decide to part company with your doctor, ask yourself if you've been a responsible patient. Often problems arise when patients don't reveal their full medical history or if they forget to alert their doctor about other drugs they are taking. A doctor-patient relationship is like a marriage—both sides have to work to make it successful.

If you're sure the problem isn't on your side, however, confront your doctor with your grievances. Or, if it's easier for you, you may want to write them in a letter. Expressing your dissatisfaction may open the communication lines between you and your doctor. You might even end up in a better relationship with your present doctor. Sometimes doctors aren't aware that they are in the midst of a deteriorating relationship until a patient wants to leave.

But if you are still unhappy with your doctor and you've decided a change is necessary, you can make a clean break by simply going to another doctor. Keep in mind, however, that your most important concern should be continuity of care. So, unless the situation is intolerable or the doctor is impaired, stay with your current doctor until you have found another one that you like.

Generally, medical records are kept by your doctor until you have found a new one. You will then have to sign a release with your new doctor approving the transfer of all your medical records to the new office. These records cannot be withheld for any reason, even if you have not yet paid your last bill.

Finally, don't feel embarrassed or guilty if you decide to change doctors. Remember, good quality medical care is your right!

Self Defense: Avoiding Questionable Doctors

In addition to finding good doctors, you also want to be able to identify and avoid doctors who have a history of professional problems. One way to do this is to make certain a doctor has not been disciplined by your state or, in fact, any state. You can call the appropriate state agency (listed in Appendix E) or check the web sites of those state agencies that make this information available. These sites list the names of doctors who have been disciplined by their state or by the federal government. The disciplinary actions were taken for a variety of reasons, including overprescribing or misprescribing medications, criminal convictions, alcohol or drug abuse and patient sexual abuse.

You also may visit the 'Vital Healthcare Info' section of the Castle Connolly Medical Ltd. web site (www.CastleConnolly.com) for links to those states with discipline information on their sites. You may also visit the American Medical Association (AMA) at www.ama-assn.org and American Board of Medical Specialities (ABMS) at www.abms.org. For the websites for biographical information about doctors, including board certification see Appendix D.

The Public Citizen Health Research Group, which publishes a report on the number of physicians disciplined in each state, believes that many states are not aggressive enough in monitoring doctors. They have been leading the call for public access to the National Practitioner Data Bank. The Data Bank was created in 1986 by an Act of Congress to track professionals who are disciplined for unprofessional behavior and to deter them from simply moving their practices from one state to another. The Data Bank became operational in 1990 and contains a record of adverse actions such as license removal, loss of clinical privileges and professional society membership actions taken against doctors and other licensed health professionals such as dentists. It contains the names of more than 170,000 health practitioners who have either a licensing action or malpractice judgment or settlement against them. There is strong pressure from some medical groups either to do away with the Data Bank or to place even stricter controls on access to it. They support their position with examples of errors in the handling of sensitive information. It is unlikely that Congress would permit the elimination of the Data Bank. In fact, it is possible that at some time in the future, access may be made more available to the public. However, at the present time there is no public general access to this information. After intense pressure a restricted data bank can now be accessed by research and journalism groups, provided they agree to newly imposed restrictions, which may be found unworkable.

A data service used by lawyers to check on a doctor's or hospital's malpractice history is LEXIS/NEXIS, the computerized legal information service. Some libraries will do a LEXIS/NEXIS search for a fee. Public access to the listing of malpractice payments is one issue on which doctors are very sensitive, and rightfully so. Many malpractice payments are made by insurance companies over the objections of doctors because the insurers feel it's cheaper to settle than to fight. Yet, doctors who feel they are blameless contend that these settlements reflect negatively on them. Also, since so many specialists, such as those in obstetrics and gynecology, are subject to more frequent lawsuits because of the nature of their practices, doctors are concerned about how patients will interpret a malpractice settlement. A few states, for example Massachussetts, make this information available on the State Health Department website. Check to see if it is available in your state. (See Vital Healthcare Information on the Castle Connolly Medical Ltd website (www.CastleConnolly.com.)

People who believe they have a problem with a doctor, whether in regard to fees, treatment or ethics, may contact the appropriate local medical society in the county in which the doctor practices or the state medical society. State health departments are also places consumers may turn to for assistance or information on disciplinary actions taken against doctors. The health department, typically, will only divulge that an action has been taken but will not give you any specific information about it (See Appendix E for phone numbers and addresses).

Changing your doctor should not be considered a setback in your search for the best doctor to meet your needs. As you may have come to understand throughout preceding chapters in this book, the personal and treatment styles doctors bring to their practices vary greatly. What is important for you, as a patient, to realize is that these subtle and immeasurable characteristics can be as important as clinical skills. There is, in fact, substantial empirical and anecdotal evidence demonstrating that confidence in the healer and the healing process plays a major role in many cures. Your main objective is to find the therapy—in combination with the professional who is providing the therapy—that works best for you.

In one case involving a woman in her mid-thirties, the doctor-patient relationship was severed over what was basically a conflict in personalities: the woman wished to have more control over her healthcare, and the doctor was reluctant to give it. The impasse was reached before the two could attempt any kind of a compromise, and the woman went off in search of a doctor who would better suit her personal needs. A year later, after a fruitless search for a doctor whose medical expertise she respected, she returned to her original doctor.

The Best in American Medicine
www.CastleConnolly.com

Choosing a Doctor in a Health Plan

Quick Tips

A data service used by lawyers to check on a doctor's or hospital's malpractice history is Lexis/Nexis, the computerized legal information service. Lexis will do a search and issue a report on any malpractice awards or settlements ordered by a court.

State health departments are also places consumers may turn to for assistance or information on disciplinary actions taken against doctors.

There is substantial empirical and anecdotal evidence demonstrating that confidence in the healer and the healing process plays a major role in many cures.

People who belive they have a problem with a doctor in regard to fees, treatment, or ethics, may contact the appropriate local medical society in the county in which the doctor practices, or the state medical society.

When choosing a doctor in a health plan, use the same criteria you would apply to selecting a doctor in a fee-for-service practice.

Typically, you will be sent a list with little information other than the doctor's name, specialty and address. Find out more about those doctors you may be considering.

In some cases, a health plan will agree to pay at least a consultation fee if you feel strongly that you need to discuss your problem with another doctor outside of the health plan network

If method of health plan payment to physicians is an issue of concern to you, it may be wise to ask your doctor about the method of compensation in the health plan in which you are enrolled.

Quick Take

... The rules are different but they are not difficult to play by. The first step is to sort out the alphabet soup of models. The model of health plan usually determines how your care will be delivered and often your satisfaction with it ...

Key Terms

Capitation - A method of payment to physicians and other healthcare providers whereby a fixed amount of money is allotted for each patient served.

EPO - An Exclusive Provider Organization is similar to a PPO except the patients must use only providers in the EPO.

Group Model HMO - A model of an HMO in which the HMO contracts with large multi-specialty groups of doctors to provide care, usually from a number of central locations.

Health Maintenance Organization (HMO) - One type of managed care organization that provides for a wide range of comprehensive healthcare services for its members in return for a fixed, predetermined fee. The care is provided by a network or group of physicians affiliated with the organization and possibly other healthcare professionals. The term "health plan" is a more common name in use today, which applies to all of the various health insurance organizations described in this list.

IPA - An Independent Practice Association is one model of health maintenance organization (HMO) in which the organization contracts with individual doctors, or groups of doctors, to provide care for the enrolled patients in the doctors' own offices.

PHO - A Physician Hospital Organization is an organization of a hospital and its physicians that may contract with managed care organizations (MCO) or may become licensed as an MCO itself.

PPO - A Preferred Provider Organization is a managed care model that offers healthcare provided by a group of doctors and/or hospitals that have negotiated discounted rates, either capitated or fee-for-service, for enrollees while continuing to provide care for other patients. Patients typically pay less if they use the PPO provider.

PSO - A Provider Service Organization, sometimes called a provider service network (PSN), is a group of doctors that are organized to provide care to a large number of patients, typically under contract to managed care organizations.

Staff Model HMO - A managed care model where the HMO employs the doctors, usally on salary. Care is provided out of a number of centralized locations.

Choosing a Doctor in a Health Plan

At one time only doctors looking for new patients joined HMOs. Today, there is a new reality. Although HMO's still exist, a more common name is health plan. Almost all doctors—more than 80 percent—participate in some kind of managed care arrangement. So it is likely that you will find the best for your own care if you know how to work the system.

When managed care achieves a significant market penetration and begins to control the flow of large numbers of patients, more doctors sign on. Also, many hospitals encourage their doctors to sign on with as many different plans as possible in order to ensure that the hospital does not lose any potential patients. Managed care now enrolls more than one out of every three people in the country, and more than 80 percent of workers who get health insurance through their employer are in some form of managed care. Today, more people are enrolled in PPOs (Preferred Provider Organization), which tend to be more flexible in choices of physicians, than are enrolled in HMOs. However, we will use health plan as "shorthand" for both.

The main factors to focus on in assessing a health plan or a PPO are its resources, primarily doctors and hospitals. First, is there an ample selection of primary care doctors near where you live and work? Second, are the doctors well qualified? This can be answered by following the approach outlined in this book for finding the best doctors. When choosing doctors, it is usually a good idea to call their offices to confirm they are still affiliated with the particular plan. Doctors frequently change affiliations with managed care plans. Also, it is a good idea to check on the procedure for using the doctor listed.

Health plans may list hundreds of doctors but not all of them are necessarily accessible to all members. A large health plan, for example, may restrict the number of specialists that primary care doctors can refer to for various reasons, including location, hospital capacity and general resource allocation. So although you may see the name of an ophthalmologist, gynecologist or other specialist you want to use, and indeed that doctor may be affiliated with the health plan, it does not necessarily follow that your primary care doctor is free to refer you to them. Those specialists may see health plan patients only on a certain basis—for specific procedures, for example, or in a certain geographic region—and then possibly only after a rigorous screening process. These possibilities illustrate the varying styles of operation you will find in managed care plans.

Doctors in health plans are bound by the same professional ethics that guide all doctors. However, there is a major difference; in a health plan, the plan is responsible for providing you with care as well as with a doctor. If your doctor leaves the plan, you don't follow him or her. The plan provides a new doctor for you.

Selecting Doctors in a Health Plan

Selecting a doctor in a health plan can be a greater challenge than selecting one when you have indemnity insurance that leaves you free to select a doctor without the restrictions of the plan. Obviously, in a health plan arrangement you need to select a doctor who belongs to that plan. Studies have shown that about 40 percent of enrollees in managed care plans have to choose a new doctor when they join. However, even in a plan of small size, you will usually have the option of choosing among a number of primary care doctors as well as other specialists and subspecialists. In doing so, utilize the same criteria you would apply to selecting a doctor in a fee-for-service practice.

The first doctor you select in a health plan is your primary care doctor. Typically, you will be sent a list with little information other than the doctor's name, specialty and address. Find out more about those doctors you may be considering. Use the process described earlier in this book. If you make a selection and are not satisfied, request a change. Ask about the procedure for changing doctors before you join the plan.

When you need a specialist, it is your primary care doctor who will refer you, as in traditional indemnity plans. But, unlike indemnity plans in which you can find a specialist on your own if you choose, in managed care plans you must be referred to see a specialist. Again, your choices will be limited in selecting specialists, but be assertive. Ask for a choice of doctors and ask why your primary care doctor recommends a particular specialist. One disadvantage to the IPA model and the network referral process is that primary care doctors can end up making referrals to specialists and/or subspecialists that they do not know. This may result in poor communication between the primary care doctor and the specialist, which is not in the patient's best interest. If you are not satisfied with the choices offered, ask to go outside the plan. Choice of providers outside a plan is built into certain managed care plans (PPOs or POS, Point of Service) and is permitted in many others under certain conditions.

However, if you do not have a choice, or if the choices are not ones with which you agree, consider going outside the health plan. Although you are likely to have to pay more, it may be worth it if you get a correct diagnosis and appropriate treatment for your problem. In some cases, the health plan will agree to pay at least a consultation fee if you feel strongly that you need to discuss your problem with another doctor outside the health plan network. After the consultation, if you still feel the need for a different doctor, at least your choice will be based on more complete information.

One of the most popular options offered by health plans permits going outside of the network of doctors and hospitals—but at an added cost. The point of service, or POS plan, one of the fastest growing offerings of many health plans, permits the health plan member to use doctors, hospitals, and other services that are not part of the health plan network. Typically, the member will pay an additional fee for this choice—for example, 20 percent or 30 percent of the cost—whereas if the member stays "in-network" the health plan will pay all or close to all of the cost.

When leaving the network of a POS, however, patients should find out exactly how much it will cost to do so. Some health plans will pay a percentage of "usual and customary fees" while others will pay a percentage of their own fee schedule, which is usually lower.

HMO Models

Although a large alphabet soup of health plan models has appeared since the big move toward managed care began in the late 1980s, and we now have PPOs, PSOs, and EPOs, two models are most important to the healthcare consumer. One is the staff or group model where patients visit their doctors in a single, or perhaps in a few, locations and where all the doctors and most, if not all, diagnostic and treatment facilities are located. The second is the independent practice association or IPA model where doctors see patients in their private offices. Organizations such as PPOs, EPOs and PSOs tend to be organized on the IPA model.

Whether a group/staff model or an IPA, all health plans require a primary care physician and all have certain protocols, usually involving referral by the primary care physician, to access a specialist.

Doctor Compensation

There is virtually no difference in the types of doctors who practice in the two plan models and each should be evaluated in terms of benefits to the individual patient. There is, however, a separate matter of how doctors in HMOs are compensated, and this issue has become a major concern to both patients and doctors.

Health plans compensate doctors in a number of ways. Doctors who are employed by staff model health plans are usually on salary, perhaps with a quality bonus based on patient satisfaction. In group model health plans, the physician group has a contract with the health plan and the doctors are employed by the group, usually on salary and, again, often with a quality bonus.

In the IPA model, or in PPOs, EPOs, PSOs and other types of managed care organizations the doctors are usually paid in one of two ways. In the past, the predominant payment method was a negotiated fee schedule, typically designed at some discount to the doctor's normal fee. Doctors simply traded the promise of higher volume for a reduced fee. Today, a major method of payment in an IPA is capitation. While this is fast becoming the most common method of payment in IPAs it is also the one generating the most controversy.

Under a capitated or capitation system doctors are paid a set amount per month or per year to provide care to a patient during that time period. So, for example, a primary care physician may be paid $25 per member per month.

Health plans have moved toward capitation as a method of payment because they found that discounted fee-for-service payment methods did not reduce costs as much as had been hoped, if at all. To make up for discounted fees of 20 percent, for instance, some doctors simply scheduled 20 percent more patient visits so that their incomes would not decrease. Doctors openly comment that discounted fees translate to discounted time with patients!

Capitation has helped to control costs. However, it also has introduced a number of important ethical issues for doctors, other healthcare providers, and for patients. Many are troubled by the notion that a doctor could be placed in a situation that appears to promise rewards for not providing care. It is generally recognized that under a fee-for-service system doctors have an incentive to provide more care, even if it is not necessary, because they are paid by the amount of care they deliver. But the reverse is not accepted in such a benign fashion: the concept of a doctor being rewarded to provide less care is of major concern to many people, including many doctors.

Another technique involved in payment systems utilized by managed care companies is called "withholds" or "set-asides." This method is also used to motivate doctors to control costs and, as in capitation, raises similar ethical concerns. Under this method, for example, a group of pediatricians is contracted to care for 1,000 children. That contract is based on a budget of $15,000 a month. A certain amount of that budget, say 20 percent, is reserved for referrals to subspecialists and another 20 percent is set aside or withheld. If the group of doctors uses fewer subspecialist referrals than budgeted they receive the 20 percent that was set aside. If they use more subspecialist referrals than were budgeted the extra amount comes out of the set-aside. The more set-aside that is used for referrals, the less doctors will be able to receive from it.

A great deal of controversy has ensued over these payment mechanisms. Some states, in fact, are legislating to prohibit or restrict these practices. Individual "horror stories" of patients who have been denied appropriate care, such as not being referred to a subspecialist in a timely manner, have been used to demonstrate the issue in human terms.

Some studies demonstrate that when physician-run health plans are paid by capitation and are in control they reduce costs more substantially than other plans. Some doctors strongly support capitation. They believe it makes them, rather than managers, responsible for allocating resources and making medical decisions.

And, despite the outcry, most of the studies of health plan patients versus non-plan patients demonstrate no differences in their health status.

In fact, there is a substantial body of research suggesting that health plan members receive more in the way of preventive services than do non-health plan populations.

If method of payment is an issue of concern to you, it may be wise to ask your doctor about the method of compensation in the health plan in which you are enrolled. If you believe the method would work against you as a patient you should discuss it with your doctor and ask if and how it influences the manner of care for patients. If you are not satisfied by the answer you may want to change doctors or, better yet, change health plans, if possible.

While the wisest course of action is to ask about this issue before joining a health plan, rather than after you have become a member, most plan members have not done this. If you believe you are not receiving appropriate care because of a health plan policy, you can contact your state health insurance department (see Appendix E).

In response to patient and physician concerns about payment policies, groups of doctors in various parts of the country have formed organizations to receive and investigate complaints against HMOs. You can contact them with any grievances you have about your plan (see Physicians Who Care, Appendix D).

How Doctors and Patients Feel about Managed Care

People enrolled in health plans tend to be satisfied by their plans. However, most doctors do not like managed care—and understandably so! Managed care organizations negotiate deep discounts in fees for doctors. There is no reason doctors should prefer this process, but when managed care controls so many patients there is little choice but to join managed care and negotiate.

Managed care organizations also require doctors to do a substantial amount of paperwork and to follow policies and procedures that control costs and monitor quality. All of this creates a level of business management most doctors resent.

At least a portion of these negative attitudes toward managed care can be ascribed to differences in the organization of medical practices in different parts of the country.

The northeast, south, and southwest regions have been the slowest to accept managed care because doctors generally resisted it more strongly than those in other parts of the country. Doctors in large group practices, which are more common in the far west and midwest than in the east, adapted to managed care more readily. In the northeast, where doctors practice solo or in small groups, the change has been greater and the adjustment more difficult.

Most doctors have adapted and learned to practice successfully in this new medical environment. According to a survey conducted by the American Medical Association, just over a third (210,811) of physicians in this country are now members of group practices. In 1995 group practices numbered 19,788, an increase of 361 percent since 1965. From 1991 to 1995, the number of groups increased by 16.4 percent and the number of group physicians by 14.3 percent.

The survey shows that, in an environment that is organizationally complex, medical groups have changed how they are organized legally, with partnerships declining to 13.8 percent and professional corporations increasing to 77.9 percent. In the latter group, control of decision making remains largely in the physician's hands. This ability to retain decision making power has dramatically altered physicians' attitudes towards managed care.

The view of patients and the public, however, is decidedly more positive about managed care.

A study sponsored by the Medstat Group, J.D. Power and Associates and the New England Medical Center reported that in 20 markets across the United States, health plans received more top scores than PPOs and fee-for-service plans.

The study asked plan members to assess their health plans on choice of providers, physician care, premiums and deductibles and access to care. Health plans topped fee-for-service and point-of-service plans in more than half of the markets.

One of the findings uncovered in a Louis Harris Associates poll of consumers was that of the majority surveyed, 59 percent, believed the trend toward managed care was a good thing as compared to 28 percent who viewed it as a bad thing. Also, 48 percent as compared to 39 percent believed managed care would improve quality, and 59 percent versus 30 percent believed it would help contain the costs of care. Of note was that the response of those people in communities with a high penetration by managed care tended to be the most positive!

There are many studies that have examined the quality of care and the satisfaction of patients in managed care settings. Most show that members of health plans and other managed care organizations are at least as satisfied or more satisfied with their care than people covered by indemnity insurance. Some studies have shown indemnity-covered people are more satisfied, particularly when it relates to choice of doctors. In fact, the issue of greatest concern to health plan enrollees is usually access, particularly to specialists. Advocates of either view can point to studies to support managed care or to criticize it. The key may lay in the studies that have demonstrated that when individuals have a choice, and select a managed care plan, they tend to be more satisfied than those who have no choice.

In terms of quality, the conclusion is similar. While critics may contend that the care delivered by managed care organizations is not adequate, and a study of Medicaid patients is frequently cited to support this view, the overwhelming majority of studies demonstrate no difference in the health status and quality of care of those people covered by managed care plans or by indemnity insurance.

The variability in the results of all of the studies on quality and satisfaction in managed care reinforces the important premise that, as there are good doctors and poor doctors, there are good health plans and poor health plans. It is important for consumers to know how to discern the difference and to put some effort, however modest, into finding the best.

Points to Remember

- To summarize, there is basically no difference in quality between doctors who participate in health plans and those who do not accept insurance. You can find excellent doctors if you're a member of a health plan and you can find poor ones, just as you can find excellent and poor doctors if you carry indemnity insurance. The key is making sure that you find the best available for your own needs and the needs of your family.

Some simple guidelines to remember:

- Review the credentials and training of any doctor who cares for you.
- Make certain that a doctor you select is taking new patients and the waiting period for an appointment is not unreasonable.
- Be sure the health plan has a sufficient number of specialists and subspecialists you may need to see and that they are of high quality. For example, if you have diabetes, you will want to make sure that the plan has endocrinologists on staff or as part of its network. If you have coronary heart disease, you will want to make sure that the plan has first rate cardiologists and an arrangement with an outstanding center where the doctors perform invasive and non-invasive diagnostic techniques and which has a good record for open heart surgery.
- Determine beforehand the health plan's policy for patient referral to subspecialists, especially whether or not you will have a choice and how it may be exercised.
- Inquire about the rules for changing doctors in the plan if you are not satisfied with your initial choice. You will want to know not only the procedure but how often such change is allowed.
- Ask about your options to go out of network and what your additional percentage of payment will be if you exercise this option. In determining what percentage the health plan pays, try to find out whether their payment is based on the health plan fee scale or "usual and customary" fees.
- Ask your doctor about the health plan's compensation system. You want to be sure that the system for paying your doctor will not have a negative influence on your care.

The Best in American Medicine
www.CastleConnolly.com

SECTION TWO

Directory of Doctors

Includes
Partnership for Excellence
Program

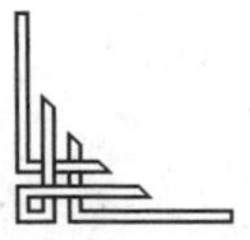
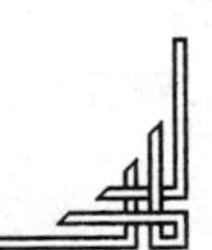

The Best in American Medicine
www.CastleConnolly.com

How to use the Directory of Doctors

Castle Connolly Medical Ltd. provides healthcare consumers with an invaluable source of information to identify leading physicians in their own community. This thirteenth edition of the Castle Connolly Guide, *Top Doctors: New York Metro Area*, contains vital information on more than 6,000 of the finest doctors in the region. Our guides are the result of a methodical process requiring a complete credential, licensing and disciplinary review of all doctors nominated for inclusion in the guide.

Why This Book Is Your Best Guide

Top Doctors: New York Metro Area is unique in a number of ways. The first edition of the Guide, published in 1994, was the first selective directory of doctors who practice in the New York metropolitan region. Castle Connolly recognizes that most healthcare is provided locally and people generally obtain their healthcare where they live or work. Therefore, by identifying excellent, caring physicians in every community and in every hospital, we apprise consumers of the best healthcare available to them within their own communities. Healthcare consumers in the New York metropolitan region are very fortunate with the abundance of doctors—approximately 55,000—who practice in the area. On the other hand, making a selection of one out of such a multitude can be a daunting task; it's hard even to know where to start. With *Top Doctors: New York Metro Area* in hand, you are already well on your way to finding the very best doctor for your individual needs and the needs of your family members.

With the profusion of outstanding academic medical centers, tertiary care teaching hospitals and fine regional hospitals in the New York metropolitan area, virtually any medical procedure or treatment can be found close to home. By virtue of this fact, it would be a simple matter to compile a book identifying the outstanding leaders in medical research and academic medicine in the region. Although many of these doctors are included in the listings, their names are to be found among the many excellent and caring doctors who deliver outstanding patient care in every community in the area. The goal—first and foremost—is to help you find the best doctors to meet your healthcare needs where you live and work. Again, a good reason why the Castle Connolly Guide is exceptional.

Further, the Castle Connolly Guide is different from most other listings of doctors in its selection process. Our selection is predicated on an extensive nomination procedure and a set of exacting standards which each nominated doctor was required to meet. To you, this means that the basis for inclusion of every one of the doctors in the listings was twofold: respect of their peers and medical excellence. Doctors do not pay to be listed. Our goal is to serve consumers, not doctors, hospitals or health plans.

How Castle Connolly Selects the Top Doctors

The basis of the Castle Connolly selection process is peer nomination. In some ways, this resembles an enhancement of the process in which a personal physician provides a patient with a referral to another physician for a particular problem. However, if the recommendation of one doctor is good, the recommendation of many doctors is even better. So, we ask thousands of randomly-selected physicians in the New York metropolitan area for their nominations.

How do we accomplish this enormous task? Over the years, the Castle Connolly physician-directed research team developed its extensive database of physicians through periodic mail, telephone and email surveys in the following counties:

New York State: New York, Bronx, Kings, Queens, Richmond, Nassau, Suffolk, Rockland, Westchester

New Jersey: Bergen, Essex, Hudson, Mercer, Middlesex, Monmouth, Morris, Passaic, Somerset, Union

Connecticut: Fairfield, New Haven

This cumulative database is systematically maintained and continuously updated. Surveyed physicians nominate top doctors in both their own and related specialties—especially those to whom they would refer their patients and their own family members. The database is also updated through further mail and telephone surveys. Each year we build on our prior research and supplement our database by inviting leading physicians at major medical centers in the metropolitan area, the thousands of top doctors included in earlier editions of our guide, and local leaders in the various medical specialties to offer their nominations for *Top Doctors: New York Metro Area*.

In addition to nominations obtained directly from practicing physicians, Castle Connolly solicits nominations from each area hospital's:

- President or Chief Executive Officer
- Vice President of Medical Affairs or the equivalent position
- Chief of Service in:
  - Anesthesiology
  - Medicine
  - Neurology
  - Obstetrics/Gynecology
  - Pathology
  - Pediatrics
  - Radiology
  - Surgery

Considerations for Inclusion Among the Top Doctors

Castle Connolly considers the following among the varied criteria used to determine physician eligibility for inclusion in our guides.

Professional Qualifications

- Education
- Residency
- Board certification
- Fellowships
- Professional reputation
- Hospital appointment
- Medical school faculty appointment
- Experience
- Disciplinary history

Personal Characteristics/Qualities

Not only do we seek nominations of physicians who excel in academic medicine and research, but most importantly, those who exhibit excellence in patient care. We ask physicians in our survey to consider not only the training and clinical skills of the physicians they nominate, but also interpersonal skills such as the following:

- Listening and communicating effectively
- Demonstrating empathy
- Educating and informing
- Instilling trust and confidence

Verification/Credential Review

The Castle Connolly research staff reviews and refines the pool of nominated physicians in a region, validates nominations and verifies credentials. This results in the development of a preliminary list of physicians. Each provisionally selected physician is then required to complete a comprehensive professional biographical form including their special practice interests (see the "SPECIALTY & SPECIAL EXPERTISE INDEX"). The information contained in the biographical form becomes an integral part of each selected physician's listing in the guide.

The last phase of the process refines the list of provisionally selected doctors by cross-referencing their names against a variety of databases providing confirmation of:

- Board certification and recertification
- Licensing
- Disciplinary history

In some regions, a small number of peer-nominated physicians who are not board-certified may be included in a guide. These are doctors recognized by their colleagues as having exceptional demonstrated clinical practice experience.

Physicians ultimately selected for inclusion in *Top Doctors: New York Metro Area* receive formal notification of their nomination for listing upon completion of the final confirmation of their professional credentials.

How You Can Select the Top Doctors

How can you begin to make a choice from such a compilation of names? There is, in fact, a basic step-by-step process which varies somewhat depending on your individual needs as you approach the list. Here are the possibilities:

ONE: If You are Looking for a Doctor in a Particular County

The key: Physicians listed in the following pages are organized under the county in which their office is located so that you can go directly to the section listing doctors in your county of residence.

Key fact: Like most healthcare consumers, you probably receive your healthcare locally. If you think about it, you usually have been treated by doctors close to where you live and in community hospitals. If necessary, you may be referred to regional specialists and nearby medical centers.

TWO: If You are Looking for a Primary Care Physician — a Generalist

The key: The doctors who practice predominantly primary care, in the specialties of internal medicine, family practice, pediatrics, and obstetrics/gynecology, are designated by the notation a in the listing.

Key fact: Every board certified physician is a specialist. The term "having boards" signifies that a physician has completed an approved residency in a given specialty and has passed a rigorous examination given by that particular board. Therefore, doctors who practice primary care—internists, family practitioners, pediatricians, and Ob/Gyns—are specialists in their respective fields, as are urologists, otolaryngologists and radiologists. These specialists are considered primary care physicians.

THREE: If You are Looking for a Physician in a Particular Specialty

The key: Each entry contains the specialty practiced by the doctor and, in most cases, the most recent year of board certification.

Key fact: Many physicians specialize in fields of medicine that are not primary care. These specialists have completed an approved residency in a given specialty and have passed a rigorous exam given by that specialty board. For example, some physicians are board certified in psychiatry, surgery, allergy and immunology or dermatology.

Many doctors choose to specialize further. They choose an additional training program called a fellowship and upon completion of the program, they are required to take another exam in order to be certified as a subspecialist. An example of such subspecialization is an internist (initially board certified in internal medicine) who subspecialize in nephrology or cardiology. This doctor would be termed "double boarded" and would very likely practice nephrology or cardiology rather than internal medicine as a primary care physician.

FOUR: If You are Looking for a Doctor with Expertise in a Particular Disease or Technique

The key: Particular skills and interests of the doctors are found under the heading "SPECIALTY & SPECIAL EXPERTISE INDEX."

Key fact: A physician may have a special expertise interest in a particular field of medicine without actually being board certified in that area. Special expertise interests should not be confused with a board certified medical specialty. For example, cosmetic surgery is not an American Board of Medical Specialties recognized specialty, but it may constitute a major practice activity for many plastic surgeons. Certain doctors may develop a reputation as "specialists" in AIDS, diabetes or arthroscopic surgery. None of these are recognized medical specialties, yet they are indications of a doctor's expertise in a disease or medical or surgical procedure which may be helpful if you have the disease or need the procedure.

Many doctors who have a strong interest in, or consider themselves "specializing in," a particular health problem or medical technique form special interest groups referred to as "self-designated medical specialties." These groups are often confused with recognized medical specialties, which they are not. Some of the groups would like to be recognized by the ABMS and may even work toward that goal. For example, adolescent medicine was a special interest and self-designated specialty that is now an ABMS recognized subspecialty.

Choosing a doctor with a special practice interest is an additional step to be considered after you have already narrowed your choices to particular specialists and/or subspecialists. The "SPECIALTY & SPECIAL EXPERTISE INDEX" lists the doctors' special area or areas of expertise and can be particularly useful in identifying physicians who embrace alternative or complementary practices. Self-designated medical specialties are listed in Appendix B.

FIVE: If You are Looking for a Doctor by Name

The key: The "ALPHABETICAL LISTING OF DOCTORS" indicates the page on which information on the doctor's credentials can be found. The listing is arranged in last name, first name order.

Key fact: Most people start their search for a doctor through recommendation by family and friends. As a savvy healthcare consumer you realize that such recommendations are often based on personal "chemistry" and may be made by someone who actually knows very little about doctors or healthcare. Therefore, you will want to check the credentials of any recommended doctor and follow the additional recommendations that we have outlined in Sections one and two.

SIX: If You want Detailed Information on a Particular Doctor

The key: Each doctor's listing includes a substantial amount of information about the doctor.

Key fact: Wise choices in healthcare are made by consumers who have gathered as much information as possible about a particular doctor. If a professional information form was not returned by a doctor in time for inclusion in the book, our research staff verified certain major points of information (name, address, telephone, hospital affiliation, and specialty) from public sources and we have included this limited information. Even if a doctor's full credentials are included in this book, it is possible that, since the time of publication, the doctor has moved his or her office(s), changed telephone number(s), joined new medical groups, resigned from or joined hospital staffs, and, especially, changed relationships with HMOs and PPOs. Nonetheless, you can, in most cases, track down the doctor by using the following sources:

- Doctor's office—call the office number listed in the directory and ask for a new number.
- Hospitals—call the hospital listed in the directory and ask for help in locating a particular doctor.
- State Health Department—all state health department numbers are listed in Appendix E.
- American Board of Medical Specialties—a complete listing of ABMS Specialty Boards is found in Appendix A.
- American Osteopathic Association—a complete listing of AOA Specialty Boards is found in Appendix A.

Conclusion

You are now ready to work with our directory of more than 6,000 of the finest doctors in the New York metropolitan area. Although you may be well-informed as a result of reading Sections one and two of this book, it is possible that choosing the doctor will seem to be a complex endeavor. The tendency might be to try to get the job done as quickly as possible by choosing a doctor based solely on the convenience of the office's location. To do so would be a big mistake. You want the best healthcare. You deserve it. A little effort will help you to get the best.

There are many excellent doctors in the region not listed in this book. You can identify them by using the process we have described in Sections one and two or, if a doctor in this book is unable to meet your needs, ask about other physicians highly regarded by that doctor.

We believe that this book will educate and enlighten you throughout its pages and that it will prove its value in the end—when you decide on the doctor with whom you plan to have a lasting relationship.

Obtaining Additional Doctor Information

You may wish to call a doctor's office to make an appointment or to help determine if the doctor is the one you want to care for you. Here are some questions you may want to ask:

1. Is a referral required?
2. Are you accepting new patients?
3. Which health plans/insurance do you accept?
4. Do you accept Medicare? Medicaid? Workers' compensation? No-fault insurance?
5. Are payments of deductible and co-payments required at the time of appointment?
6. Do you accept credit cards?
7. Do you see patients in the evening? On weekends?
8. Is the office handicapped-accessible?
9. Do you accept phone calls from patients?
10 Do you communicate with patients via the internet?
11. If you are not comfortable addressing the doctor in English, ask if your native language is spoken by the doctor or by someone else in the office.

Sample Listing

Smith, John MD [IM] *PCP - Spec Exp: Ulcers; Crohn's Disease;*

Name [specialty] & Primary Care Physician indication — Special Expertise(s)

Hospital: NYU Med Ctr (page 130); **Address:** 100 Tenth St, FL 5 - Ste 3A, MC-1234, New York, NY 10010;

admitting hospital(s) & Hospital Information page(s) — Office address — Mail code — City, state zip

Phone: (904) 296-0000; **Board Cert:** IM 70, GE 74; **Med School:** U Fla Coll Med 66;

Office phone — *Board certification(s) & date(s) — Medical school & year of degree

Resid: IM, NYU Med Ctr, 69; **Fellow:** GE, Lenox Hill Hosp, 72;

Residency(ies) & location(s) — Fellowship(s) & location(s)

Fac Appt: Assoc Clin Prof Med, NYU Sch Med

Faculty appointment & location

* Indicates the most recent date of board certification or recertification.

In our listings of the professional information on doctors, we have abbreviated hospitals and medical schools. The abbreviations are designed to be self-explanatory, but if you need assistance, refer to Appendix D: Hospitals Listings.

Note on Special Expertise(s):

These are not medical specialties as described on pages 81-87, but the areas of expertise or practice interests indicated by the doctor.

The information reported in each doctor's listing is, for the most part, provided by the doctor or his/her office staff. Castle Connolly attempts to verify the data through other sources but cannot guarantee that in all cases all data have been so verified or are accurate. All such information is subject to change from time to time due to changes in physician practices. Many doctors participate in several health plans and/or switch plans frequently. Therefore, you should verify with the doctor's office whether your health plan is currently accepted.

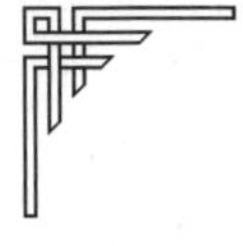

The Best in American Medicine
www.CastleConnolly.com

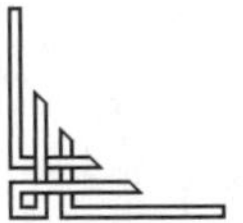
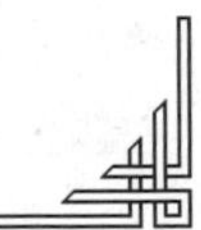

Medical Specialties and Subspecialties

In the pages that follow, each list of doctors in a medical specialty or subspecialty is preceded by a brief description of that specialty (or subspecialty) and the training required for board certification.

Critical Care Medicine has been excluded because in emergency situations there is neither time nor opportunity for choice. A number of other specialities not relevant to most patients (e.g., Forensic Psychiatry) have not been included as well.

The following descriptions of medical specialties and subspecialties were provided by the American Board of Medical Specialties (ABMS), an organization comprised of the 24 medical specialty boards that provide certification in 25 medical specialties. A complete listing of all specialists certified by the ABMS can be found in The Official ABMS Directory of Board Certified Medical Specialists, is published by Marquis Who's Who. It is available (either in a multi-volume directory or on CD-ROM) in most public libraries, hospital libraries, university libraries and medical libraries. The ABMS also operates a toll-free phone line at 1-866-275-2267 and a website at www.abms.org to verify the certification status of individual doctors.

The following important policy statement, approved by the ABMS Assembly on March 19, 1987, remains valid.

The Purpose Of Certification

The intent of the certification process, as defined by the member boards of the American Board of Medical Specialties, is to provide assurance to the public that a certified medical specialist has successfully completed an approved educational program and an evaluation, including an examination process designed to assess the knowledge, experience and skills requisite to the provision of high quality patient care in that specialty.

Medical Specialty and Subspecialty Descriptions and Abbreviations

The following medical specialties and subspecialties are indicated in the doctors' listings by their abbreviations. Specialties are indicated in bold, subspecialties in italics, and the four primary care specialties in bold capitals. To review the official American Board of Medical Specialties (ABMS) organization of specialties, refer to Appendix A.

Addiction Psychiatry *AdP*

Deals with habitual psychological and physiological dependence on a substance or practice which is beyond voluntary control.

Adolescent Medicine *AM*

Involves the primary care treatment of adolescents and young adults.

Allergy & Immunology **A&I**

Diagnosis and treatment of allergies, asthma and skin problems such as hives and contact dermatitis.

Cardiac Electrophysiology (Clinical) *CE*

Involves complicated technical procedures to evaluate heart rhythms and determine appropriate treatment for them.

Cardiovascular Disease *Cv*

Involves the diagnosis and treatment of disorders of the heart, lungs and blood vessels.

Child & Adolescent Psychiatry *ChAP*

Deals with the diagnosis and treatment of mental diseases in children and adolescents.

Child Neurology *ChiN*

Diagnosis and medical treatment of disorders of the brain, spinal cord and nervous system in children.

Clinical Genetics **CG**

Deals with identifying the genetic causes of inherited diseases and ailments and preventing, when possible, their occurrence.

Colon and Rectal Surgery **CRS**

Surgical treatment of diseases of the intestinal tract, colon and rectum, anal canal and perianal area.

Critical Care Medicine *CCM*

Involves diagnosing and taking immediate action to prevent death or further injury of a patient. Examples of critical injuries include shock, heart attack, drug overdose and massive bleeding.

Dermatology **D**
Diagnosis and treatment of benign and malignant disorders of the skin, mouth, external genitalia, hair and nails, as well as a number of sexually transmitted diseases.

Diagnostic Radiology *DR*
Involves the study of all modalities of radiant energy in medical diagnoses and therapeutic procedures utilizing radiologic guidance.

Endocrinology, Diabetes & Metabolism *EDM*
Involves the study and treatment of patients suffering from hormonal and chemical disorders.

FAMILY MEDICINE **FMed**
Deals with and oversees the total healthcare of individual patients and their family members. Family practitioners are more common in rural areas and may perform procedures more commonly performed by specialists (e.g., minor surgery).

Gastroenterology *Ge*
The study, diagnosis and treatment of diseases of the digestive organs including the stomach, bowels, liver and gallbladder.

Geriatric Medicine *Ger*
Deals with diseases of the elderly and the problems associated with aging.

Geriatric Psychiatry *GerPsy*
Involves the diagnosis, prevention and treatment of mental illness in the elderly.

Gynecologic Oncology *GO*
Deals with cancers of the female genital tract and reproductive systems.

Hematology *Hem*
Involves the diagnosis and treatment of diseases and disorders of the blood, bone marrow, spleen and lymph glands.

Hospice and Palliative Medicine *H&PM*
Palliative care relieves the suffering and provides the best quality of life to people suffering from serious and severe chronic illness. Hospice care focuses on the palliation of a terminally ill patient's symptoms and also provides passionate support to both the patient and their surrounding loved ones.

Infectious Disease *Inf*
The study and treatment of diseases caused by a bacterium, virus, fungus or animal parasite.

INTERNAL MEDICINE **IM**

Diagnosis and nonsurgical treatment of diseases, especially those of adults. Internists may act as primary care specialists, highly trained family doctors or they may subspecialize in specialties such as cardiology or nephrology.

Interventional Cardiology *IC*

A cardiologist with special training who uses minimally invasive and non-surgical procedures to treat cardiovascular diseases.

Maternal & Fetal Medicine *MF*

Involves the care of women with high-risk pregnancies and their unborn fetuses.

Medical Oncology *Onc*

Refers to the study and treatment of tumors and other cancers.

Neonatal-Perinatal Medicine *NP*

Involves the diagnosis and treatments of infants prior to, during and one month beyond birth.

Nephrology *Nep*

Concerned with disorders of the kidneys, high blood pressure, fluid and mineral balance, dialysis of body wastes when the kidneys do not function and consultation with surgeons about kidney transplantation.

Neurological Surgery **NS**

Involves surgery of the brain, spinal cord and nervous system.

Neurology **N**

Diagnosis and medical treatment of disorders of the brain, spinal cord and nervous system.

Neuroradiology *NRad*

Involves the utilization of imaging procedures during diagnosis as they relate to the brain, spine and spinal cord, head, neck and organs of special sense in adults and children.

Nuclear Medicine **NuM**

Evaluation of the functions of all the organs in the body and treatment of thyroid disease, benign and malignant tumors and radiation exposure through the use of radioactive substances.

OBSTETRICS & GYNECOLOGY **ObG**

Deals with the medical aspects of and intervention in pregnancy and labor and the overall health of the female reproductive system.

Occupational Medicine *OM*
Concentrates on the effect of the work environment on the health of employees.

Ophthalmology **Oph**
Diagnosis and treatment of diseases of and injuries to the eye.

Orthopaedic Surgery **OrS**
Involves operations to correct injuries which interfere with the form and function of the extremities, spine and associated structures.

Otolaryngology **Oto**
Explores and treats diseases in the interrelated areas of the ears, nose and throat.

Pain Medicine *PM*
Involves providing a high level of care for patients experiencing problems with acute or chronic pain in both hospital and ambulatory settings.

Pathology **Path**
A doctor trained to examine tissue specimens microscopically and in clinical laboratory tests, to diagnose and monitor diseases.

Pediatric Cardiology *PCd*
Involves the diagnosis and treatment of heart disease in children.

Pediatric Critical Care Medicine *PCCM*
Involves the care of children who are victims of life threatening disorders such as severe accidents, shock and diabetes acidosis.

Pediatric Endocrinology *PEn*
Involves the study and treatment of children with hormonal and chemical disorders.

Pediatric Gastroenterology *PGe*
The study, diagnosis and treatment of diseases of the digestive tract in children.

Pediatric Hematology-Oncology *PHO*
The study and treatment of cancers of the blood and blood-forming parts of the body in children.

Pediatric Infectious Disease *PInf*
The study and treatment of diseases caused by a virus, bacterium, fungus or animal parasite in children.

Pediatric Nephrology *PNep*
Deals with the diagnosis and treatment of disorders of the kidneys in children.

Pediatric Otolaryngology *PO*
Involves the diagnosis and treatment of disorders of the ear, nose and throat which affect children.

Pediatric Pulmonology *PPul*
Involves the diagnosis and treatment of diseases of the chest, lungs, and chest tissue in children.

Pediatric Rheumatology *PRhu*
Involves the treatment of diseases of the joints and connective tissues in children.

Pediatric Surgery *PS*
Treatment of disease, injury or deformity in children through surgical techniques.

Pediatric Urology *Ped Uro*
Treatment of urologic congenital anomilies, and childhood and adolescent acquired urologic problems such as disease and trauma.

PEDIATRICS **Ped**
Diagnosis and treatment of diseases of childhood and monitoring of the growth, development and well-being of preadolescent.

Physical Medicine & Rehabilitation **PMR**
The use of physical therapy and physical agents such as water, heat, light electricity and mechanical manipulations in the diagnosis, treatment and prevention of disease and body disorders.

Plastic Surgery **PlS**
Involves reconstructive and cosmetic surgery of the face and other body parts.

Preventive Medicine **PrM**
A specialty focusing on the prevention of illness and on the health of groups rather than individuals.

Psychiatry **Psyc**
Examination, treatment and prevention of mental illness through the use of psychoanalysis and/or drugs.

Pulmonary Disease *Pul*
Involves the diagnosis and treatment of diseases of the chest, lungs and airways.

Radiation Oncology *RadRO*
Involves the use of radiant energy and isotopes in the study and treatment of disease, especially malignant cancer.

Reproductive Endocrinology *RE*

Deals with the endocrine system (including the pituitary, thyroid, parathyroid, adrenal glands, placenta, ovaries and testes) and how its failure relates to infertility.

Rheumatology *Rhu*

Involves the treatment of diseases of the joints, muscles, bones and associated structures.

Sports Medicine *SM*

Refers to the practice of an orthopedist or other physician who specializes in injuries to the bone or other soft tissues (muscles, tendons, ligaments) caused by participation in athletic active.

Surgery **S**

Treatment of disease, injury and deformity by surgical procedures.

Surgery of the Hand *HS*

Involves providing appropriate care for all structures in the upper extremity directly affecting the hand and wrist function.

Thoracic & Cardiac Surgery **T&CS**

Involves surgery on the heart, lungs and chest area.

Urology **U**

Diagnosis and treatment of diseases of the genitals in men and disorders of the urinary tract and bladder in both men and women.

Vascular & Interventional Radiology *VIR*

Involves diagnosing and treating diseases by percutaneous methods guided by various radiologic imaging modalities.

Vascular Surgery *VascS*

Involves the operative treatment of disorders of the blood vessels excluding those to the heart, lungs or brain.

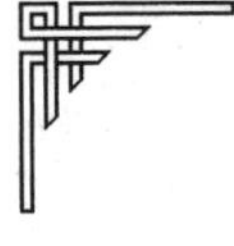

The Best in American Medicine
www.CastleConnolly.com

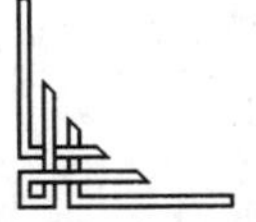

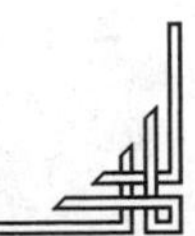

Partnership for Excellence

The Hospital Information Program

There are more than 200 acute care and specialty hospitals in the New York metropolitan area, many of which have extraordinary capabilities for superior patient care. Castle Connolly Medical Ltd. has received many requests from book buyers to provide information about hospitals. In response, we have invited a select group of outstanding hospitals to profile their services in this guide through the medium of paid advertorials. This program, called the Hospital Information Program is totally separate from the physician selection process, which is based upon a completely independent review system. Hospitals that sponsored pages in the Hospital Information Program are organized into three groups: Major Medical Centers, Specialty Hospitals and Regional Medical Centers.

Major Medical Centers begin on the next page and are followed by the Specialty Hospital pages. This section is followed by the listings of doctors. Regional Medical Centers and Hospitals are found at the beginning of each county section - within the doctor listings. The information gives you an overview of programs and services offered by these hospitals, as well as vital information related to their accreditation and sponsorship. Each hospital profile also contains a physician referral number, should you wish to ask the hospitals for recommendations of physicians not listed in the Castle Connolly Guide.

The "Centers of Excellence" section was also developed in response to requests from our readers who want to know which hospitals have special programs or services focusing on a particular illness or health need. The "Centers of Excellence" described here are also offered by hospitals participating in the Partnership for Excellence section of this guide. They reflect the depth of commitment of these hospitals, which provides the staff, resources and financial support necessary to develop these special programs. We believe you will find this information helpful in your search for the best healthcare — from both physicians and hospitals— for you and your family.

We are pleased to have these distinguished institutions as partners in our effort to help you meet your healthcare needs.

The following pages contain vital information on ten of the region's Major Medical Centers. A Major Medical Center is an acute care hospital with tertiary care services, residency programs, a major affiliation with a medical school and clinical research programs. A major medical center draws its patients from a broad geographic region, even nationally and internationally and, in many instances, is the center of a network or consortium of hospitals.

The New York metropolitan region is nationally and internationally known for its major medical centers and their excellent programs and services. Some of the nation's leading academic centers are in this region and, in addition to superior patient care and cutting edge patient research, they produce thousands of talented, well trained physicians and other health professionals each year. Castle Connolly Medical Ltd. has invited a number of major medical centers in the region to sponsor the profiles and information that follows.

Major Medical Centers

Atlantic Health System

Continuum Health Partners

Hackensack University Medical Center

Maimonides Medical Center

Montefiore Medical Center

Mount Sinai Medical Center

NewYork-Presbyterian Hospital

North Shore-LIJ Health System

NYU Langone Medical Center

The Best in American Medicine
www.CastleConnolly.com

ATLANTIC HEALTH SYSTEM

Morristown Medical Center • Overlook Medical Center • Newton Medical Center • Goryeb Children's Hospital

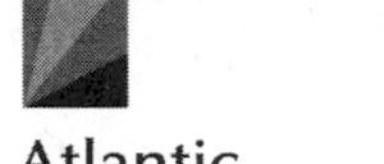

Atlantic
Health System

Atlantic Neuroscience Institute • Carol G. Simon Cancer Center • Gagnon Cardiovascular Institute • Atlantic Rehabilitation • Atlantic Sports Health

Atlantic Health System, 475 South Street, P.O. Box 1905, Morristown, NJ 07962
www.atlantichealth.org

To find a doctor, call 1-800-247-9580 or visit us online

Sponsorship: Voluntary Not–for-Profit • Beds: 1,315 • Accreditation: The Joint Commission

Atlantic Health System is at the forefront of medicine, setting standards for quality health care in New Jersey and beyond. The nationally recognized physicians, experienced nurses and skilled staff provide outstanding and compassionate care. Through our vision, we empower our communities to be the healthiest in the nation. Atlantic Health System includes Morristown Medical Center in Morristown, NJ; Overlook Medical Center in Summit, NJ; Newton Medical Center in Newton, NJ; and Goryeb Children's Hospital in Morristown, NJ. Official health care partner of the New York Jets, an official health care provider of the New Jersey Devils and official sports medicine and rehabilitation partner of the New Jersey Interscholastic Athletic Associations, the Atlantic Sports Health program has established itself as a leader in the field of sports medicine. Atlantic Integrative Medicine combines mind/body therapies with medical knowledge to enhance your health and everyday life. Atlantic Health System is a clinical and academic affiliate of The Mount Sinai Hospital and the Icahn School of Medicine at Mount Sinai; a Major Clinical Affiliate of Rutgers Cancer Institute of New Jersey; and is a member of AllSpire Health Partners.

Morristown Medical Center – 100 Madison Avenue, Morristown, NJ 07960
Morristown Medical Center provides high-level patient care in first-rate facilities with a full range of medical specialties and services.

Morristown Medical Center is named a Level 1 Regional Trauma Center by the American College of Surgeons and a Level II Trauma Center by the state. Home to Gagnon Cardiovascular Institute, it performs more cardiac surgeries than any other hospital in NJ, placing its cardiac program in the top two percent in the country.

Designated a Regional Perinatal Center, Morristown Medical Center treats the most complicated obstetrical cases and providing specialized care to sick or premature infants.

In 2013, U.S. News & World Report ranked Morristown Medical Center as a top hospital nationwide for cardiology, heart surgery, gynecology and geriatrics. Morristown Medical Center also ranked as a "Best Regional Hospital" for cancer, diabetes & endocrinology, neurology and neurosurgery, orthopedics as well as gastroenterology & GI surgery, nephrology, pulmonology and urology. In 2013, NJBIZ recognized Morristown Medical Center as "Hospital of the Year."

Carol G. Simon Cancer Center offers advanced methods to diagnose, treat and manage all types of cancers. Our dedicated breast center is equipped with all-digital mammograms and breast tomosynthesis 3D mammography to provide the most precise images available and dedicated fellowship-trained breast radiologists. We also offer a wide array of clinical trials, genetic counseling, psychosocial support, dietary assistance, and integrative medicine therapies, as well as nurse navigators to help guide patients and families through the treatment plan and to survivorship.

Morristown Medical Center performs more than 1,600 joint replacements a year. Surgical success rates are among the highest in the country, earning the Gold Seal from The Joint Commission. Morristown Medical Center was re-designated a Magnet Hospital for Excellence in Nursing Service, the highest level of recognition by American Nurses Credentialing Center for facilities that provide acute care services, a distinction awarded to less than five percent of U.S. hospitals.

Part of Morristown Medical Center, Urgent Care at Hackettstown equipped with on-site lab and X-ray services, provides immediate medical services.

Overlook Medical Center - 99 Beauvoir Avenue, Summit, NJ 07901
Overlook Medical Center is a nationally recognized regional medical center in Summit, New Jersey. The Atlantic Neuroscience Institute serves as the hub for the New Jersey Stroke Network, treating 40 percent of the state's stroke patients, is home to a comprehensive Level IV Epilepsy Center, as well as research and

treatment programs in Movement and Memory Disorders. Overlook treats more aneurysm cases than any other institution in New Jersey, is the only NY/NJ hospital with specialists trained in MEG for functional brain mapping. The largest neuro-interventional radiology service in New Jersey also is housed at Overlook.

Gagnon Cardiovascular Institute offers diagnostic services such as cardiac catheterization and advanced imaging to cardiac and peripheral angioplasty and vascular surgery.

The Minimally Invasive Surgery Program utilizes a wide range of robotics in the operating room, including the first robot, ViKY, in New Jersey to use voice recognition technology for surgeries in the gastrointestinal, urologic, thoracic and gynecologic regions.

Carol G. Simon Cancer Center offers the most advanced methods to diagnose, treat, and manage all types of cancers. Board-certified physicians and oncology-trained professionals provide multidisciplinary care in surgical, medical, and radiation oncology using state-of-the-art technology, including CyberKnife® radiosurgery technology, which offers noninvasive, highly accurate and painless treatment for many kinds of tumors. Overlook is one of a select group of hospitals throughout the country to be certified for wound healing.

In 2013, U.S. News & World Report ranked Overlook Medical Center among the best hospitals in central New Jersey and as a "Best Regional Hospital" for neurology and neurosurgery as well as gastroenterology & GI surgery, gynecology, geriatrics, nephrology, pulmonology and urology.

Newton Medical Center – 175 High Street, Newton, NJ 07860

Newton Medical Center is a fully accredited, acute care hospital serving Sussex and Warren counties in New Jersey, Pike County in Pennsylvania, and southern Orange County in New York. Specialty service areas include cardiology, general and vascular surgery, orthopedics, gastroenterology, nephrology, oncology, neurology, mental health and sleep medicine.

As the premier medical facility in the region, Newton Medical Center has earned multiple accolades, including three-year accreditations by the American College of Surgeons' Commission on Cancer for cancer treatment and by the American College of Radiology for digital mammography services. The hospital also received the 2012 Outstanding Achievement Award by the Commission on Cancer. The echocardiography services at the Charles L. Tice Heart Center for Diagnostic Services have been accredited three consecutive times by the Intersocietal Accreditation Commission (IAC).

Newton Medical Center in 2013 was named Top Hospital overall in New Jersey and No. 1 for treatment of prostate and breast cancers, congestive heart failure treatment, hip and knee repair, high-risk pregnancy and treatment of neurological disorders, among hospitals with 350 beds or fewer by Inside Jersey magazine partnered with Castle Connolly Medical Ltd.

The new Physical/Occupational Therapy Center and Wound Care Center, including a suite with two hyperbaric oxygen chambers, offer state-of-the-art technology and treatments for healing. The hospital also offers state-of-the-art imaging services, including a wide-bore magnetic resonance imaging (MRI) scanner.

Newton Medical Center's renowned Emergency Department provides state-of-the-art care to the region. Newton Medical Center's new Telemedicine Electronic Stroke System, a remote presence robot, offers immediate access to stroke specialists in the emergency department.

Newton Medical Center also operates Sparta Health & Wellness and Vernon Health & Wellness/Urgent Care in New Jersey, and Milford Health & Wellness/Urgent Care in Pennsylvania, offering a variety of quality care services close to home, including Urgent Care at Vernon and Milford.

Goryeb Children's Hospital – 100 Madison Avenue, Morristown, NJ 07960

Upon opening its doors in 2002, Goryeb Children's Hospital quickly became the hospital of choice for families throughout the area, and today treats more than 50,000 pediatric patients annually across 20 different areas of medical and surgical care, including 750 patients annually in the Foley Pediatric Intensive Care Unit and more than 2,500 inpatients. Goryeb Children's Hospital is a state-designated children's hospital. More than 100 board certified pediatric specialists at Goryeb provide care to patients at multiple locations throughout the state. In addition, Goryeb has more than 250 community pediatricians on staff.
The physicians and staff at Goryeb subscribe to a patient- and family-centered philosophy of care, partnering together with families to generate the best possible outcomes. Families and caregivers are educated, supported and empowered to make informed decisions about their child's care and to cope confidently with their child's condition or illness.

PHYSICIAN REFERRAL **For a physician referral or for more information please contact Atlantic Health System at: 1-800-247-9580 or atlantichealth.org**

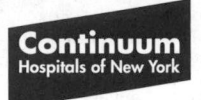

Beth Israel Medical Center
Beth Israel Brooklyn
Roosevelt Hospital
St. Luke's Hospital
NY Eye and Ear Infirmary

800.420.4004 www.chpnyc.org

Sponsorship: Voluntary Not-for-profit **Beds:** 2,180 certified beds
Accreditation: Joint Commission of Accreditation of Healthcare Organizations (JCAHO), Accreditation Council for Graduate Medical Education, Medical Society of New York, in conjunction with the Accreditation Council for Continuing Medical Education

A STRONG PARTNERSHIP WITH A PROUD HERITAGE

Continuum Health Partners is a partnership of five venerable health care providers: Beth Israel Medical Center-Milton and Carroll Petrie Division, Beth Israel Brooklyn, St. Luke's Hospital, Roosevelt Hospital, and The New York Eye and Ear Infirmary. Each of the five partner institutions was established more than a century ago by individuals committed to improving health and health care in their communities. Today, the system represents over 4,000 physicians and dentists and is superbly equipped to respond to the health care needs of the populations we serve. Continuum providers also see patients in group and private practice settings and in ambulatory centers in New York City and Westchester County.

LOCATIONS

Continuum Health Partners has campuses in Manhattan and Brooklyn. Beth Israel Medical Center has two divisions: the Milton and Caroll Petrie Division on the East Side, and Beth Israel Brooklyn. The Phillips Ambulatory Care Center, a state-of-the-art outpatient center, is located at Union Square. St. Luke's Hospital is in Morningside Heights and Roosevelt Hospital is in the Columbus Circle and Lincoln Center neighborhoods on the West Side. The New York Eye and Ear Infirmary is located on Second Avenue and 14th Street.

ACADEMIC AFFILIATIONS

Beth Israel Medical Center is the University Hospital and Manhattan Campus for the Albert Einstein College of Medicine. St. Luke's-Roosevelt Hospital Center is an Academic Affiliate of Columbia University College of Physicians and Surgeons. The New York Eye and Ear Infirmary is the primary teaching center of the New York Medical College and affiliated teaching hospitals in the areas of ophthalmology and otolaryngology.

For a referral to a great doctor in your neighborhood, call 800.420.4004.
Our Physician Referral Service can help you find a primary care
physician or specialist affiliated with
Beth Israel, St. Luke's, Roosevelt, or The New York Eye and Ear Infirmary.
Visit our Website at www.chpnyc.org

Centers of Excellence at Continuum Hospitals of New York

Cancer	The Continuum Cancer Centers of New York offer early detection, diagnosis, and treatment of a wide range of cancers. Our nationally recognized physicians offer innovative and highly successful programs coupled with superb support services. Our cancer services are state of the art, supported by sophisticated programs in medical oncology, surgical oncology, and radiation oncology.
Cardiac Services	The cardiology, cardiac surgery, and cardiac rehabilitation experts at Continuum offer a full range of diagnostic and treatment services. Some highlights of our cardiac programs are minimally invasive robotic cardiac surgery, arrhythmia services, 24-hour cardiac catheterization labs, and expertise in congestive heart failure.
Neurological Services	Continuum is home to many world leaders in neurology, neurosurgery and interventional neuroradiology. Our physicians are recognized authorities who establish innovative care protocols, chart new venues in therapy and develop the technologies that set the standards in the neuroscience fields.
Orthopedic Services	Continuum's orthopedic physicians are leading providers of general orthopedic, sports medicine, spine and rheumatologic care. Our specialists offer state-of-the-art care to patients throughout the New York metropolitan region. Many of our orthopedic surgeons are leaders in their field and are fellowship trained in their areas of sub-specialty.
Ear, Nose and Throat	Continuum offers eye, ear, nose and throat services throughout our system. The New York Center for Head and Neck combines the formidable medical and surgical capabilities of the five hospitals of Continuum. The center comprises 45 physicians across 14 specialties and subspecialties, including world-renowned surgeons and educators.
HIV/AIDS	We are one of the largest providers of HIV/AIDS care in New York City, with comprehensive-care clinics and facilities in multiple locations. Our facilities offer a complete range of health care services for individuals with HIV: diagnostic procedures, the latest treatments, and support services.
Pain Management	Our Department of Pain Medicine and Palliative Care offers a broad array of therapies for chronic pain of all types. The highly trained medical team includes pain specialists with backgrounds in neurology, rehabilitation medicine, anesthesiology and psychology.
Substance Abuse	Continuum offers extensive chemical dependency treatment services through The Addiction Institute of New York, the Stuyvesant Square Chemical Dependency Treatment Program, and the Department of Psychiatry and Behavioral Health. Our services include inpatient detoxification and outpatient programs, services for the mentally ill, family services, and after-care programs.

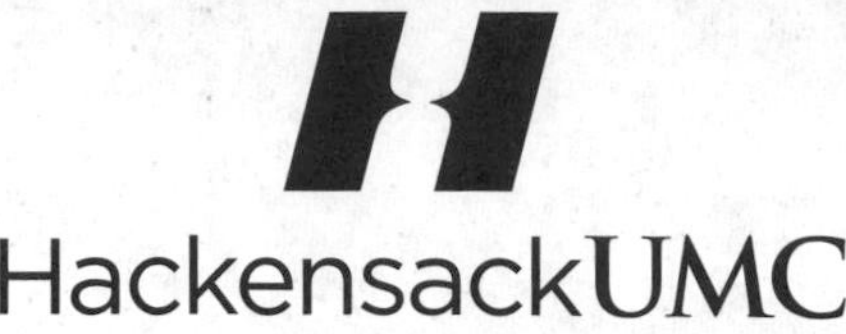

30 Prospect Avenue, Hackensack, NJ 07601 • 551-996-2000
www.HackensackUMC.org

Number of beds: 775
Number of employees: 7,619
2012 Admissions: 45,322
Sponsorship: A not-for-profit, teaching and research hospital affiliated with Georgetown University School of Medicine, Rutgers Medical School, St. George's University School of Medicine, and Stevens Institute of Technology.
Beds: A 775-bed, Level II Trauma Center, providing tertiary and regional services for the New York/New Jersey metropolitan area.
Accreditation: Joint Commission

HackensackUMC is the recipient of 19 Gold Seals of Approval™ for healthcare quality from the Joint Commission, the only medical facility in the United States to achieve this record-number of the Joint Commission Disease-Specific Care Certifications.

The medical center holds the Joint Commission Disease-Specific Care Certifications in: Acute Myocardial Infarction, Asthma, Asthma (Pediatrics), Bone Marrow Transplant, Breast Cancer, Chronic Obstructive Pulmonary Disease, Colorectal Cancer, Coronary Artery Bypass Graft, Depression, End Stage Renal Disease, Heart Failure, Inpatient Diabetes, Joint Replacement - Hip, Joint Replacement - Knee, Multi-System Trauma, Palliative Care, Pneumonia, Stroke (Primary Stroke Center), and Uterine-Ovarian Cancer.

BACKGROUND

Hackensack University Medical Center (HackensackUMC) is a 775-bed teaching and research hospital that provides the largest number of admissions in New Jersey. Founded 125 years ago with 12 beds and as Bergen County's first hospital, HackensackUMC has demonstrated more than a century of growth and progress. At HackensackUMC, quality means pushing medicine further to lead the pursuit of excellence in healthcare. HackensackUMC is a nationally recognized healthcare organization offering patients the most comprehensive services, state-of-the-art technologies, and facilities. Honors include being named one of America's 50 Best Hospitals™ by Healthgrades® for seven years in a row. HackensackUMC is the only hospital in New Jersey, New York and New England to receive this honor for seven consecutive years. *U.S. News & World Report* ranked HackensackUMC the number one hospital in New Jersey and one of the top three New York metro hospitals. The medical center also received ten national rankings and three New York metro area rankings. The American College of Surgeons National Surgical Quality Improvement Program (ACS NSQIP®) has recognized HackensackUMC as one of 37 ACS NSQIP participating hospitals that have achieved meritorious outcomes for surgical patient care. It was also named one of the 100 Great Hospitals in America by *Becker's Hospital Review,* and is the only hospital in New Jersey to be listed among The Leapfrog Group's Top Hospitals for three consecutive years. HackensackUMC is a Magnet® recognized hospital for nursing excellence - the first in New Jersey and second in the nation - receiving its fourth designation in April 2009. It is the Hometown Hospital of the New York Football Giants as well as the New York Red Bulls soccer team.

MEDICAL AND DENTAL STAFF

Since HackensackUMC is one of the region's most comprehensive and progressive medical centers, it easily attracts many of the area's leading physicians - nearly 1,600 of them. These doctors, many of whom are on the cutting-edge in their fields and have received their training at our nation's most prominent institutions, have selected HackensackUMC as their place to practice their best medicine.

NURSING EXCELLENCE

Our medical staff is joined by a team of extraordinary nurses. As a Magnet® Hospital, HackensackUMC attracts and retains nurses who are tops in their fields. Making history in 1995 as the first official Magnet® Hospital in New Jersey, HackensackUMC is the only hospital in New Jersey with four designations from the American Nurses Credentialing Center.

WORLD-CLASS CARDIAC CARE

HackensackUMC is home to one of America's most comprehensive cardiac and vascular hospitals: its Heart & Vascular Hospital, a "hospital within a hospital," integrates preventive, diagnostic and treatment services, with a special focus on cardiovascular disease management and breakthrough research. Inpatients and outpatients are treated for all types of cardiac and vascular diseases, including heart problems, such as: blocked arteries and irregular heartbeats; peripheral vascular disease; and neurovascular diseases, such as stroke and aneurysm. Housing all of these services within one specialized location allows for more efficient, effective patient care.

U.S. News & World Report ranked HackensackUMC #33 out of more than 700 hospitals in the nation for Cardiology & Heart Surgery in their 2013-14 Best Hospitals rankings. HackensackUMC is also one of Healthgrades® America's 100 Best Hospitals for Cardiac Care™ and Coronary Intervention in 2013, and was ranked #1 in NJ by Healthgrades for Cardiology Services in 2013. HackensackUMC was also named among one of *Becker's Hospital Review's* 100 Hospitals With Great Heart Programs.

ONE OF THE NATION'S LARGEST AND MOST COMPREHENSIVE CANCER CENTERS

At John Theurer Cancer Center, we believe cancer is hard enough for patients and their loved ones. It is this belief that drives our passion to deliver extraordinary care every day, helping us to become one of the nation's top 50 cancer centers, ranked #31 out of more than 900 hospitals by *U.S. News & World Report* - the highest-ranked cancer center in New Jersey with this recognition. It was also listed among the 100 Hospitals and Health Systems With Great Oncology Programs by *Becker's Hospital Review*.

In January 2011, we opened a new building that houses 14 specialty divisions, research and support services. This state-of-the-art facility offers a wide range of free resources to help patients become active participants in their treatment and support their fight against cancer. These resources include yoga, fitness, interactive nutrition classes in the Cooking Studio, art workshops, a patient resource librarian to help patients find credible health information online, and more.

During the past 25 years, we have become one of the largest cancer centers in the United States, but we have kept our focus on the unique needs of our patients. Prevention, treatment, and research advances have grown exponentially during this time. We are not only keeping up with the change of pace, we are at the forefront of providing tomorrow's treatment today by:

- Taking multidisciplinary care to a new level with teams of disease-specific experts under one roof;
- Delivering personalized medicine focused on novel therapies, participatory treatment, predictive measures, and preventive care;
- Advancing research through biomarker-driven clinical trials and translational research;
- Providing holistic care that includes a wide range of complementary services important to the well-being of our patients that can be easily integrated into their care; and
- Creating a comforting environment in a new high-tech, high-touch building.

We believe our model is the next step towards the future of patient care, changing the cancer care experience one patient at a time. To receive information on John Theurer Cancer Center's services, call 551-996-5900 or visit jtcancercenter.org.

ONE OF THE NATION'S RENOWNED PEDIATRIC PROGRAMS

The Joseph M. Sanzari Children's Hospital at HackensackUMC is a state-designated children's hospital and an award-winning facility that has been recognized as one of the top-ranked children's hospitals in New Jersey and in the country. It ranked 29th among the Best Children's Hospitals for Neurology and Neurosurgery in the 2013-14 Best Children's Hospitals rankings by *U.S. News & World Report* — the first hospital in New Jersey to be ranked in any Best Children's Hospitals specialty, and the only hospital in the state to be ranked in Neurology and Neurosurgery.

The Joseph M. Sanzari Children's Hospital was one of the first hospitals in New Jersey to have a separate, dedicated pediatric emergency room (PER) and is an American College of Surgeons designated Level II Trauma Center that cares for pediatric patients. The PER is staffed 24 hours a day, seven days a week with physicians and nurses who are specialized in the care of children requiring emergency medical services. It houses more than 30 specialties in a patient- and family-centered environment that includes children's play and family kitchen areas, and private inpatient rooms with computers, Internet access, and flat-screen plasma televisions.

The cutting-edge technologies facilities, expert staff, dedicated PER and specialty units that distinguish the Joseph M. Sanzari Children's Hospital are second to none.

For more information on any of the services offered at HackensackUMC, please call 551-996-2000, or visit www.HackensackUMC.org.

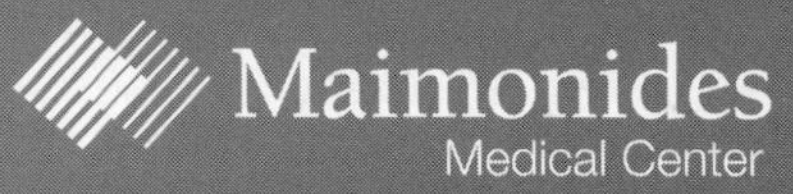

4802 Tenth Avenue
Brooklyn, New York 11219
Phone: 718.283.6000
Physician Referral:
888.MMC.DOCS (662.3627)
www.maimonidesmed.org

Sponsorship: Voluntary, Not-for-Profit
Beds: 711 acute, 70 psychiatric
Accreditation: The Joint Commission
American College of Surgeons
American Council
for Graduate Medical Education (ACGME)

Maimonides Medical Center is the Brooklyn clinical campus of the Albert Einstein College of Medicine and is among the largest independent teaching hospitals in the U.S., training more than 400 medical and surgical residents each year. Widely recognized for major achievements in medical technology and patient safety, Maimonides conducts clinical trials for new treatments and therapies, and cited for overall clinical excellence by numerous health care evaluation services. Cardiovascular, Stroke, Cancer and Critical Care services at Maimonides are rated among the best in the nation.

SIGNIFICANT ACCOMPLISHMENTS

Our excellence in cardiac care is historic. The first successful human heart transplant in the U.S. was performed at Maimonides in 1967, and Maimonides is ranked by the Centers for Medicare & Medicaid Services as one of only 25 hospitals in the U.S. that consistently achieve excellent ratings in heart attack, heart failure and pnuemonia patient outcomes.

Physicians at Maimonides were among the first in the U.S. to use computers to enter patient orders, thereby reducing the risk of errors, increasing efficiency, and speeding the healing process.

Maimonides has appeared on the American Hospital Association's "Most Wired" list for advanced information technology more often than any other health care institution in the metropolitan area.

More babies are born at Maimonides than at any other single-campus hospital in New York State. We are designated as a Regional Perinatal Center and the quality of our Obstetric and Pediatric services are unrivaled in the region.

CENTERS OF EXCELLENCE

Cancer Center
The Maimonides Cancer Center offers a fully integrated approach to cancer care that includes prevention, screening, diagnostics, treatment, palliative care and clinical research. Staffed by leading oncologists, radiologists, surgeons, nurses and social workers, the Center provides compassionate, patient-centered, state-of-the-art care. The newly built Breast Cancer Center is located just around the corner and features a spa-like decor in which our dedicated team of breast cancer specialists treat patients.

Heart & Vascular Center
Renowned for its Catheterization Lab and pioneering new surgical procedures, the Maimonides Heart & Vascular Center includes an Electrophysiology (EP) Lab, Hybrid OR, two ICUs, Vascular Laboratory, Advanced Cardiac Care Unit, Congestive Heart Failure program and Atrial Fibrillation Center. The first successful heart transplant in America was performed at Maimonides in 1967. Today, its Cardiology and Cardiothoracic Surgery divisions continue to innovate. Maimonides has been ranked by the Centers for Medicare & Medicaid Services among those hospitals achieving excellent ratings in both heart attack and heart failure patient outcomes. Its Left Ventricular Assist Device (LVAD) Program, the first and only one in Brooklyn, recently received advanced certification from the Joint Commission.

The Center also offers comprehensive diagnostic, clinical and surgical services for patients with vascular disease and associated conditions. An Aortic Program was opened in 2013. In addition to traditional open surgery, the Center utilizes minimally invasive, endovascular and catheter-directed techniques whenever possible. Our physicians are board-certified, highly-experienced and make use of innovative technologies, such as our accredited Vascular Diagnostics Laboratory and our new Hybrid OR.

Stroke Center
The Jaffe Stroke Center at Maimonides is ranked among the best in the nation. It is currently the site of clinical trials for new stroke medications, medical devices and stroke protocols. Listed among the top 100 stroke centers in the nation by the American Stroke Association, it is *Five-Star* rated by HealthGrades.

Infants & Children's Hospital
The Maimonides Infants & Children's Hospital, one of only five accredited children's hospitals in NYC, includes comprehensive inpatient services and over 30 pediatric subspecialties. Our Child Life & Creative Arts therapies are fully integrated with a family-centered approach to care. The Maimonides Infants & Children's Hospital also includes a Pediatric ICU, Neonatal ICU, Outpatient Services and a Pediatric ER.

Stella & Joseph Payson Birthing Center
More babies are delivered at Maimonides than at any other single-campus hospital in New York State. The Payson Birthing Center offers a home-like setting with physicians, nurses, midwives and doulas, combined with advanced technology including a perinatal testing center with 3-D ultrasound and 24/7 neonatology.

Geriatrics Program
Maimonides serves one of the oldest inpatient populations in New York State, with one quarter of inpatients over the age of 75. The Geriatrics Program is fully equipped to meet the special needs of these seniors, including the assessment of memory loss and expertise in geriatric syndromes that result in incontinence, falls and frailty. The Program encompasses inpatient and outpatient services, features the Acute Care for Elderly (ACE) Unit, the Safe at Home program and home-visiting.

Montefiore
Inspired Medicine

111 East 210th Street
Bronx, New York 10467
1-800-MD-MONTE
www.montefiore.org

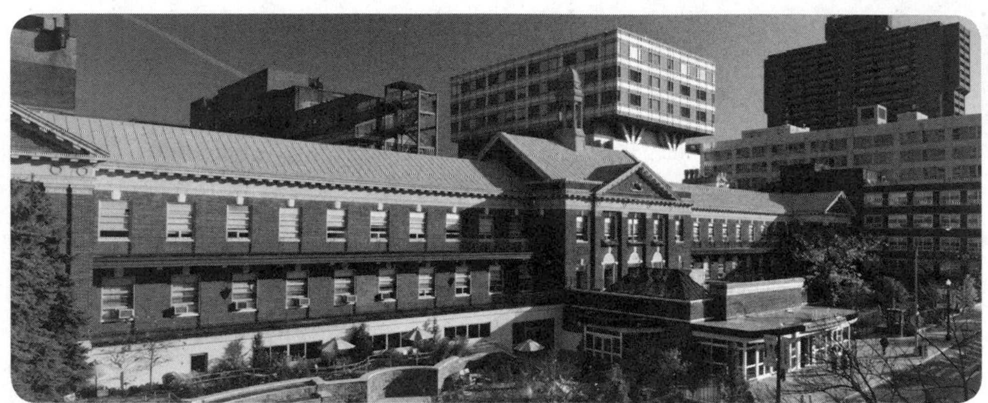

Montefiore Medical Center serves as a tertiary care referral center for patients from across the New York metropolitan area and beyond, and offers a full range of healthcare services to two million residents throughout the neighboring counties of Westchester and the Bronx, one of the most culturally and economically diverse urban communities in the United States. As the University Hospital and academic medical center for Albert Einstein College of Medicine, Montefiore is recognized by *U.S. News & World Report* as a national and regional leader in specialty and chronic care for both adults and children. The Children's Hospital at Montefiore was ranked among the best in the country by *U.S. News & World Report* for the fifth consecutive year.

Comprising four hospitals with 1,491 beds, Montefiore has more than 90,000 annual hospital admissions and provides more than 2.6 million ambulatory visits through a network of over 130 locations. Montefiore's emergency department is one of the busiest in the nation, with approximately 300,000 visits annually, and its nationally renowned home healthcare program provides more than 500,000 visits annually. In addition to having one of the largest school health programs in the country, Montefiore Medical Center includes a 23-site medical group practice integrated throughout the Bronx and Westchester and a care management organization providing services to nearly 200,000 health plan members.

Montefiore is a national leader in the research and treatment of acute and chronic diseases and is known and respected for its model of care emphasizing accountability and interdisciplinary programs. With notable centers of excellence in heart and vascular care, cancer care, transplantation, children's health, surgery, neurosciences, orthopaedics, ophthalmology and women's health, Montefiore defines clinical excellence and delivers premier care in a compassionate environment.

Montefiore Medical Center Hospitals

Montefiore Hospital
111 East 210th Street
Bronx, New York 10467

Wakefield Hospital
600 East 233rd Street
Bronx, New York 10466

Weiler Hospital
1825 Eastchester Road
Bronx, New York 10461

The Children's Hospital at Montefiore
3415 Bainbridge Avenue
Bronx, New York 10467

The Children's Hospital at Montefiore

Since opening its doors to the Bronx, Westchester and surrounding communities in 2001, The Children's Hospital at Montefiore has garnered significant attention for its clinical innovation, state-of-the-art care and exceptional outcomes. CHAM's specialty services are consistently recognized by *U.S. News & World Report* and organizations such as the American Diabetes Association and the Muscular Dystrophy Association, to name a few. Backed by more than $20 million in active National Institutes of Health (NIH) research grants, CHAM investigators are working to advance treatments for childhood diseases and disabilities.

Montefiore Einstein Center for Cancer Care

The Montefiore Einstein Center for Cancer Care skillfully blends advanced cancer treatment with a patient-centered environment to achieve exceptional outcomes for adults and children. At Montefiore, specialists from medical, surgical and radiation oncology draw upon the latest treatments and research to develop personalized care plans for patients with both common and rare forms of cancer. Their efforts are supported by a multidisciplinary team that includes a dedicated psychiatrist and psychological social worker. The Center is a national leader in the use of targeted immunotherapies and is involved in NIH-funded research studying the use of inhaled chemotherapy for lung cancer, the benefits of high-intensity focused ultrasound guided by magnetic resonance imaging in the treatment of bone cancer, and nanomedicines.

Montefiore Einstein Center for Heart & Vascular Care

Offering novel treatments and intricate, life-saving procedures, the Center for Heart & Vascular Care is a nationally respected leader in its field. The Center's specialists in adult and pediatric cardiology and cardiovascular surgery provide care for patients with the full spectrum of cardiovascular conditions, including complex valve conditions and advanced heart failure. It is a four-time recipient of the Society of Thoracic Surgeons' prestigious "three-star" ranking for its commitment to surgical excellence, and it has been funded through the NIH/National Heart, Lung, and Blood Institute's Cardiothoracic Surgical Trials Network for 10 consecutive years.

Montefiore Einstein Center for Transplantation

The Center for Transplantation is one of the most established transplant programs in the United States. It provides comprehensive organ failure management and performs heart, liver, kidney and pancreas transplants for adults and children. In all areas of transplant, the Center achieves one-year survival rates that are equal to or better than national benchmarks. To ensure the well-being of its patients, the Center consistently works to overcome social, economic and linguistic barriers to transplant. In partnership with the Marion Bessin Liver Research Center at Albert Einstein College of Medicine, the Center is conducting pioneering work in the area of liver disease.

Neurosciences at Montefiore

The Neurosciences Program at Montefiore brings together state-of-the-art technology and nationally respected specialists to improve outcomes and quality of life for children and adults with neurological disorders. Its services range from endovascular coiling, stereotactic-guided radiosurgery and complex craniofacial reconstructions to specialized programs in neuro-oncology, epilepsy, neuroimmunology, and sleep-wake disorders. The program is bolstered by a robust research enterprise that includes NIH- and foundation-sponsored studies.

Surgery at Montefiore

High volumes and exceptional surgical outcomes have made the Department of Surgery a magnet for referral. It is recognized by the American College of Surgeons' National Surgical Quality Improvement Program for exemplary outcomes in several categories and is a leader in the use of novel minimally invasive surgical approaches. Each of its five Divisions—breast, general, pediatric, transplant and plastic and reconstructive surgery—is led by renowned surgeons who possess unparalleled experience and expertise.

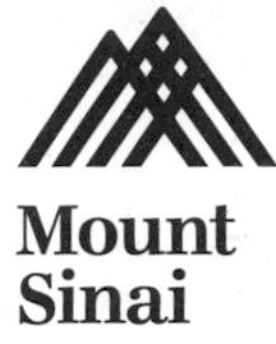

The Mount Sinai Medical Center

One Gustave L. Levy Place
Fifth Avenue and 100th Street
New York, NY 10029-6574

Physician Referral:
1-800-MD-SINAI (637-4624)
www.mountsinai.org

Sponsorship: Voluntary Not-for-Profit
Beds: 1,171
Accreditation:
The Joint Commission; Commission for Accreditation of Rehabilitation Facilities;
Magnet Award for Nursing Excellence

For over 160 years, **THE MOUNT SINAI MEDICAL CENTER** in New York City has been committed to delivering outstanding health care to patients locally and globally. Encompassing both The Mount Sinai Hospital and Icahn School of Medicine at Mount Sinai, the institution is a leader in medical breakthroughs, innovations in care, and translational research. The Icahn School of Medicine has consistently been ranked by *U.S. News & World Report* as one of the nation's top 20 medical schools, and it is among the top five in the nation in National Institutes of Health funding per investigator. The Mount Sinai Hospital is nationally ranked as one of the top 25 hospitals in 7 specialties in the 2013-2014 "Best Hospitals" issue of *U.S. News & World Report*. Mount Sinai's Kravis Children's Hospital also ranks in seven out of ten pediatric specialties by *U.S. News & World Report*. Located between the Upper East Side and East and Central Harlem—New York City's most and least affluent communities—Mount Sinai provides services to meet the needs of every patient.

Under the direction of Valentin Fuster, MD, PhD, **Mount Sinai Heart** incorporates world-class resources, interdisciplinary programs, and innovative approaches to prevent and treat cardiovascular diseases. In New York State, our Cardiac Catheterization Laboratory was deemed both the busiest and the safest, with the lowest 30-day risk-adjusted mortality rate for percutaneous coronary interventions (PCI). Building on the expertise of our internationally renowned cardiologists, interventionalists, and cardiac surgeons, we provide patients with the most advanced evidence-based medicine, treatments, and personalized care.

The Tisch Cancer Institute coordinates a full-service diagnostic and treatment program for cancer patients. Our programs include those in cancer of the liver, breast, prostate, and head and neck, as well as hematological malignancies, such as myeloproliferative disorders. In 2011, we opened the **Dubin Breast Center**, which provides advanced detection and treatment - and addresses every aspect of breast health – all in one centralized location. In October 2012, the **Derald H. Ruttenberg Treatment Center**, the Institute's outpatient cancer facility, will double in size upon its move one block north to the new **Leon and Norma Hess Center for Science and Medicine**. In addition, the Hess Center will house two full floors dedicated to cancer research.

Recognized as a national leader in organ transplantation, **The Recanati/Miller Transplantation Institute** is one of the few places in the country that provides multi-organ transplantation. Our surgeons were the first in New York State to perform many combined transplant procedures, including liver and kidney transplantation, pediatric liver transplantation, and living adult- and pediatric-donor liver transplantation.

The Department of Genetics and Genomic Sciences conducts basic research, trains fellows who specialize in research or counseling, and educates the next generation of doctors and genetic counselors in cutting-edge precision medicine techniques. **The Mount Sinai Genetic Testing Laboratory** is the leading referral center for clinical genetics and metabolic disorders in the New York tri-state area and one of the largest newborn screening referral centers in the United States. Our Department's genetic testing lab and medical genetics clinic provide expert diagnostic, therapeutic, and counseling services for patients and families with genetic disorders, birth defects, and pregnancy loss.

Geriatrics and Palliative Medicine specialists at Mount Sinai promote healthy aging and provide a balanced and integrated approach to improving the quality of life for New York's elderly. Ranked fourth in the country for geriatrics by *U.S. News & World Report* in 2012, we remain a national pioneer in geriatric medicine.

Our internationally recognized **Neurosurgery and Neurology** services rank as premier destinations for care. Our neurosurgeons have expertise in skull-base surgery, cerebrovascular disease, pituitary disorders, acoustic

Continued on next page

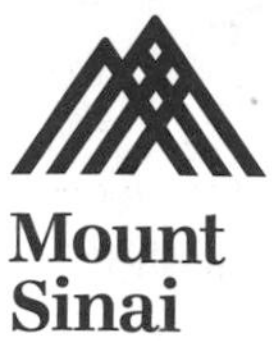

Mount Sinai

(continued)

tumors, spinal reconstruction, epilepsy, radiosurgery, stereotactic and primary brain tumor surgery, and neuroendoscopy. Our neurologists lead internationally recognized centers for patient care, research and physician training that provide interdisciplinary expertise on brain and nervous system disorders including Parkinson's disease, dystonia, multiple sclerosis, epilepsy, headache, stroke, dementia, and neuromuscular disease.

Mount Sinai's **Gastrointestinal and Surgical** specialists have developed and advanced numerous techniques to help patients with Crohn's disease, ulcerative colitis, Barrett's esophagus and other digestive disorders lead healthier lives. They have led the way in caring for patients in need of advanced gastrointestinal endoscopy procedures and in developing innovative medical and surgical approaches for inflammatory bowel disease.

Rehabilitation Medicine offers comprehensive care for people with spinal cord injuries, brain injuries, major limb amputations and a variety of other neuromuscular, musculoskeletal, and chronic conditions. We are accredited by the Commission on Accreditation of Rehabilitation Facilities for the treatment of inpatient spinal cord and brain injury and amputations. We also offer comprehensive outpatient rehabilitation services, including physical, occupational, speech and neuropsychological therapies.

Dedicated to the preservation and restoration of the musculoskeletal system, members of our **Department of Orthopaedics** provide personalized treatments using the latest technology. They excel in total joint replacement, microvascular, cancer, and minimally invasive procedures, and surgeries of the foot and ankle, knee, hip, hand, elbow, shoulder, and spine. Our Joint Replacement Center offers easy access to care at all levels: pre-operative assessment, recovery, and therapy.

Mount Sinai's **Department of Urology** provides diagnosis and treatment for many conditions including prostate, bladder and kidney cancers. Our urologists are leaders in advancing emerging diagnostic techniques and treatments, and rank as experts in open, laparoscopic and robotic surgery. This combination of skills makes them uniquely qualified to determine the best approach for each patient. Consistently voted among the country's top doctors, our team has been recognized for the depth of its knowledge, experience and compassion.

A leader in diabetes treatment, management, and research, our **Division of Endocrinology, Diabetes, and Bone Disease** provides a full range of services to treat this epidemic. Patients with type 1 or type 2 diabetes are cared for by accomplished endocrinologists, nurse practitioners, and registered dietitians, who provide specialized, state-of-the-art treatment to help patients manage their condition safely.

Our **Department of Surgery** boasts highly skilled and talented clinicians and educators, who are pioneers in their respective fields. We are one of the oldest surgical departments in the country, and celebrate a rich history of offering unsurpassed patient care. We also train the next generation of surgeons, and have the highest caliber of surgical residents who graduate and go on to become leaders at institutions across the globe.

The Kravis Children's Hospital was named among the best children's hospitals in the country by *U.S. News & World Report*, and ranked in seven specialties: cardiology & heart surgery, gastroenterology, diabetes and endocrinology, urology, nephrology, cancer, and pulmonology. We offer advanced treatment, supported by research, community outreach, and advocacy programs. We treat heart, brain, and spine disorders; epilepsy; cancers and blood diseases; diabetes; gastrointestinal tract conditions; renal diseases; hypertension; asthma and other respiratory system illnesses; sleep problems; allergies; fetal and newborn conditions, and perform life-saving organ transplantations.

NewYork-Presbyterian Heart—The optimal care of patients with heart disease is achieved by combining an experienced team of clinicians with the latest advances in technology. Basic science and clinical research efforts are aimed at developing more effective, less invasive ways to prevent, diagnose, and treat the full spectrum of cardiac disorders.

NewYork-Presbyterian Neuroscience Centers—Our team provides the most sophisticated diagnostic and treatment services for Alzheimer's disease, multiple sclerosis, Parkinson's disease, aneurysms, epilepsy, brain tumors, strokes, and other neurological disorders. Our scientific investigators are conducting research aimed at better understanding these diseases and further improving patient care.

NewYork-Presbyterian Psychiatry—NewYork-Presbyterian Hospital's behavioral health and psychiatric services for adults, children, and adolescents offer a full continuum of programs at all levels of care—including inpatient, outpatient, partial hospital, day treatment, and residential services. Specialized services are available in neuropsychiatry, chemical dependency, and eating disorders.

NewYork-Presbyterian Transplant Institute—NewYork-Presbyterian Hospital features the largest transplant program in the country. Our experts are internationally known for performing adult and pediatric heart, liver, kidney, pancreas, lung, bone marrow/stem cell, and intestinal and ex vivo transplantation.

NewYork-Presbyterian Vascular Care Center—We provide comprehensive, multidisciplinary preventive, diagnostic, and treatment services for aortic aneurysm, carotid artery disease, blood clots, peripheral vascular diseases, venous insufficiency, and venous ulcers. We take a minimally invasive approach to these diseases whenever possible.

William Randolph Hearst Burn Center—NewYork-Presbyterian Hospital is home to the largest and busiest burn center in the nation, caring for more than 5,000 outpatients annually. Our investigators also conduct research to improve survival and enhance the quality of life of burn victims.

In addition, the Hospital offers extraordinary expertise, comprehensive programs, and specialized resources in the fields of:

AIDS—The Center for Special Studies at NewYork-Presbyterian/Weill Cornell and the AIDS Care Program at NewYork-Presbyterian/Columbia provide comprehensive care for men, women, and children with HIV/AIDS. Both sites are designated as AIDS centers by New York State and by the National Institutes of Health.

Reproductive Medicine and Infertility—Our leading physicians and scientists in reproductive medicine use innovative technology for the comprehensive treatment of infertility in women and men. Our prestigious program is renowned for achieving success rates that are among the best in the world.

Trauma Center—Level 1 designations as an Adult Trauma Unit and a Pediatric Trauma Unit ensure the Hospital upholds the highest standards of 24-hour preparedness and treatment.

Women's Health Care—One of the first hospitals dedicated to women's health, NewYork-Presbyterian has established comprehensive programs which provide health care to women through all stages of their lives. The Hospital offers outstanding services in maternal-fetal health, gynecologic oncology, and a full range of preventive, primary, and specialty care.

NewYork-Presbyterian Healthcare System

NewYork-Presbyterian provides a comprehensive network of healthcare providers throughout the New York metropolitan area, including northern New Jersey, Westchester County, and Fairfield, Connecticut. The full-service system includes 15 acute-care, community hospitals, specialty institutions, 4 long-term facilities, and over 100 outpatient care centers.

Physician Referral: To find a NewYork-Presbyterian Hospital affiliated physician to meet your needs, call toll free **1-877-NYP-WELL** (1-877-697-9355) or visit our website at **www.nyp.org**

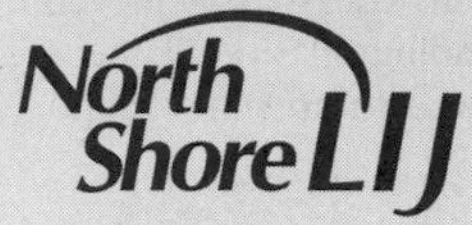

North Shore-LIJ Health System
Administration Offices
145 Community Drive
Great Neck, NY 11021
northshorelij.com
(516) 465-8000

A Network of Award-Winning Hospitals and Programs.
Your Partner in Quality Care.

One of the nation's largest healthcare systems, North Shore-LIJ Health System delivers world-class clinical care throughout the New York metropolitan area, pioneering research at The Feinstein Institute for Medical Research and a visionary approach to medical education highlighted by Hofstra North Shore-LIJ School of Medicine. With nearly $7 billion in revenue and a workforce of more than 46,000, North Shore-LIJ is the largest employer on Long Island and the third-largest private employer in New York City.

North Shore-LIJ cares for people at every stage of life at 16 hospitals including a dedicated children's hospital, long-term care facilities and nearly 400 ambulatory and physician practices throughout the region. North Shore-LIJ's hospitals and long-term care facilities house more than 6,000 beds, employ more than 10,000 nurses and have affiliations with more than 9,440 physicians. **In the most recent rankings by *U.S. News & World Report*, North Shore-LIJ hospitals were recognized with national and regional designations in a wide range of specialties.**

In addition to our network of hospitals, our health system delivers clinical care through the North Shore-LIJ Medical Group, the nation's sixth-largest physician group practice with more than 2,400 full-time physicians.

North Shore-LIJ Network of Hospitals

- **Five tertiary hospitals**
  - **Lenox Hill Hospital,** Manhattan
    — Manhattan Eye, Ear and Throat Hospital
  - **Long Island Jewish Medical Center,** New Hyde Park
  - **North Shore University Hospital,** Manhasset
  - **Southside Hospital,** Bay Shore
  - **Staten Island University Hospital** (North)
- **Three specialty care hospitals**
  - **South Oaks Hospital,** Amityville
  - **Steven & Alexandra Cohen Children's Medical Center of New York,** New Hyde Park
  - **The Zucker Hillside Hospital,** Glen Oaks
- **Seven community hospitals**
  - **Forest Hills Hospital**
  - **Franklin Hospital,** Valley Stream
  - **Glen Cove Hospital**
  - **Huntington Hospital**
  - **Plainview Hospital**
  - **Staten Island University Hospital** (South)
  - **Syosset Hospital**
- **One affiliate hospital**
  - **Nassau University Medical Center,** East Meadow

To find a doctor: **1-888-321-DOCS** or **northshorelij.com**

A Home to Learning and Discovery

Beyond care delivery, North Shore-LIJ is home to The Feinstein Institute for Medical Research, which ranks among the nation's top 5 percent of all institutions that receive funding from the National Institutes of Health. At The Feinstein, scientists and investigators are conducting breakthrough research in oncology, immunology, psychiatry, neurology and many other specialties, and are leading 2,100 research studies with 15,000 participants.

As an academic medical center, North Shore-LIJ is also committed to educating the next generation of physicians. Hofstra North Shore-LIJ School of Medicine is the nation's 133rd medical school and New York State's first new allopathic medical school in nearly 40 years.

Find the North Shore-LIJ Healthcare Provider That's Right for You

We make it easy to find the North Shore-LIJ specialist you need. Our knowledgeable staff will provide information on specialists, primary care physicians and special services. We're available to take your call 24 hours a day, 7 days a week.

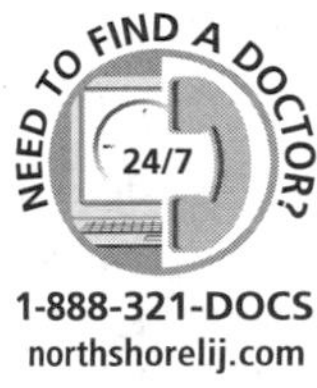

1-888-321-DOCS
northshorelij.com

North Shore-LIJ's Award-Winning Programs and Services Include:

- The Arthur Smith Institute for Urology
- Bariatric Surgery
- Behavioral Health
- Cohen Children's Medical Center of NY (Pediatrics)
- Cushing Neuroscience Institute
- The Feinstein Institute for Medical Research
- North Shore-LIJ Katz Institute for Women's Health
- North Shore-LIJ Cancer Institute
- North Shore-LIJ Cardiovascular Services
- North Shore-LIJ Center for Emergency Medical Services
- North Shore-LIJ Home Care Network
- North Shore-LIJ Imaging
- North Shore-LIJ Laboratories
- North Shore-LIJ Medical Group Urgent Care Centers
- North Shore-LIJ Orthopaedic Institute
- North Shore-LIJ Rehabilitation Network
- Obstetrics & Gynecology
- Radiation Medicine
- Robotic Surgery

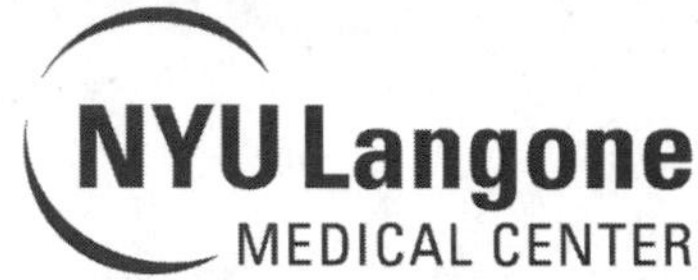

NYU LANGONE MEDICAL CENTER

NYU Langone Medical Center—a world-class, patient-centered, integrated, academic medical center—is one of the nation's premier destinations for excellence in patient care, biomedical research, and medical education. Located in the heart of Manhattan, NYU Langone is composed of Tisch Hospital, its flagship acute care facility; the Hospital for Joint Diseases, a dedicated inpatient orthopaedic hospital; Hassenfeld Children's Hospital, a comprehensive pediatric hospital supporting a full array of children's health services; Rusk Rehabilitation, the #1 rehab program in New York since *U.S. News & World Report* began its hospital rankings in 1989; and a growing ambulatory care network with locations throughout Manhattan, the outer boroughs, and the tri-state area, bringing services directly to where its patients live and work.

In a culture where treating the whole person and not simply the disease is the norm, NYU Langone Medical Center is renowned for clinical excellence across a wide array of specialties, including cancer, cardiology, cardiac and vascular surgery, musculoskeletal (including orthopaedics and rehabilitation), neurosurgery and children's services.

An integral part of NYU Langone, NYU School of Medicine has trained thousands of physicians and scientists who have helped to shape the course of medical history and enrich the lives of countless people since 1841. NYU Langone's tri-fold mission to serve, teach, and discover is achieved 365 days a year. For more information, go to www.NYULMC.org, Facebook, Twitter, and YouTube.

550 First Avenue *(at 31st Street)*
New York, NY 10016

www.NYULMC.org

Physician Referral: **888-7-NYU-MED** *(888-769-8633)*

Additional Areas of Expertise:

Alzheimer's, Brain Aging and Dementia

Cancer

Cardiovascular Services

Children's Health Services

Dermatology

Diabetes

Endocrinology

Fertility/IVF

Gastroenterology

Geriatrics

Internal Medicine

Hematology and Medical Oncology

Men's Health

Nephrology

Neurology

Neurosurgery

Obstetrics and Gynecology

Orthopaedics and Orthopaedic Surgery

Otolaryngology

Pain Medicine

Palliative Care

Psychiatry

Radiation Oncology

Radiology

Reconstructive Plastic Surgery

Rheumatology

Rehabilitation Medicine

Sleep Disorders

Stroke

Surgery

Transplant

Women's Health

Urology

Looking for information on our expert physicians? 1-888-769-8633

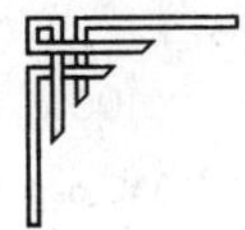

The Best in American Medicine
www.CastleConnolly.com

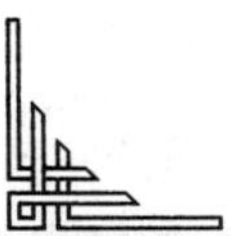
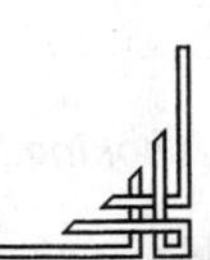

Specialty Hospitals

The New York metropolitan region is unique in its concentration of excellent Specialty Hospitals. Specialty Hospitals include those with a specific patient and disease focus such as cardiac care, psychiatric care and care of diseases and problems of eyes and ears. Many of these hospitals are nationally and internationally known for their outstanding care in these specialty areas and draw patients from the region and beyond who seek their excellent specialized care.

Castle Connolly Medical Ltd. has invited the following outstanding Specialty Hospitals to present important facts and information on their hospitals by sponsoring the profiles that follow.

Specialty Hospitals

Calvary Hospital

Hospital for Special Surgery

Memorial Sloan-Kettering Cancer Center

New York Eye & Ear Infirmary

St Francis Hospital - The Heart Center

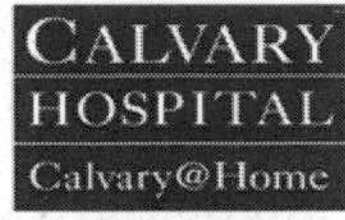

1740 Eastchester Road
Bronx, NY 10461
Tel: (718) 518-2000
Fax: (718) 518-2674

150 55th Street
Brooklyn, NY 11220
Tel: (718) 518-2000
Fax: (718) 518-2670

www.calvaryhospital.org

Beds:	225 (200 in Bronx, 25 at Brooklyn Satellite located at Lutheran Medical Center)
Accreditation:	The Joint Commission, College of American Pathologists (CAP)

SETTING THE STANDARD FOR PALLIATIVE CARE

Founded in 1899, Calvary Hospital is the nation's only fully accredited acute care specialty hospital dedicated to providing palliative care to adult advanced cancer patients. We care for patients at a 200-bed Bronx facility and a 25-bed satellite at Lutheran Medical Center in Brooklyn. Calvary's family-centric approach helps more than 6,000 patients and families each year with inpatient care, outpatient care, Calvary Home Care and Hospice, and the Center for Curative and Palliative Wound Care. The Joint Commission gave Calvary Hospital and our Home Care/Hospice program the Gold Seal of Approval™ in 2013. Press Ganey consistently ranks Calvary in the top one percent of its peers in patient satisfaction. Calvary received a 2012 Circle of Life Award® for innovative palliative and end-of-life care. To learn more or sign up for the e-newsletter, *Calvary Life*, please go to www.calvaryhospital.org.

Acute Inpatient Care

One-page form expedites admissions process. Adults with advanced cancer are assigned a primary physician and a care team: nurse, social worker, dietitian, and case manager. Goal is to maximize physical, spiritual, and emotional comfort. Pastoral care and bereavement support are integral to care.

Calvary@Home: Home Care, Hospice, Nursing Home Hospice

Certified Home Health Agency

We provide a full range of home care services, not limited to patients with advanced cancer, in all five boroughs as well as Westchester, Rockland, Putnam, and Nassau counties. Care is coordinated by patient's community physician or Calvary doctor. Nurse is available 24/7 for telephone consults.

Hospice & Nursing Home Hospice (NHH)

For people with all terminal diagnoses who are primarily cared for at home. Emphasis on quality of life, control of pain and symptoms, and support for family. Serves patients in Bronx, Brooklyn, Manhattan, Queens, Westchester, Nassau, and Rockland. Care may be coordinated by community physician or Calvary doctor. Nurse is available 24/7 by telephone. Bereavement support. Short-term hospitalization is available for acute symptom management. NHH is for nursing home residents suffering from all end-stage illnesses. Goal is to promote quality of life. Through a partnership with Mary Manning Walsh Home in Manhattan, Calvary provides an inpatient level of care for a select number of patients.

Family Care

Focuses on the impact of cancer on the family. Extensive bereavement support for adults, teens, and children, including bereavement camp for children and teens who participate in our support groups.

Pastoral Care

Calvary's Clinical Pastoral Education (CPE) program achieved certification by the Association for Clinical Pastoral Education – less than 2 years after the program was re-established. The 20-week, 400-hour program is the country's only CPE program exclusively focused on giving students hands-on experience solely with terminally ill patients in a hospital and home hospice setting.

Palliative Care Institute

Calvary's research and education arm, offers a curriculum for medical students, residents, postdoctoral fellows, and senior health practitioners, as well as health lectures for the community.

Outpatient and Wound Care

Outpatient clinic for cancer patients undergoing active treatment or who do not require acute inpatient care. The Center for Curative and Palliative Wound Care treats complex wounds related to cancer, diabetes, vascular disease, and other illnesses.

HOSPITAL
FOR
SPECIAL
SURGERY

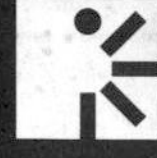

HOSPITAL FOR SPECIAL SURGERY

535 East 70th Street • New York, NY 10021
Physician Referral: 800.854.0071 • www.HSS.edu
Facebook, Twitter and YouTube @ HSpecialSurgery

Sponsorship: Private, Non-Profit
Beds: 205
Accreditation: The Joint Commission
Web Site: HSS.edu

HSS.edu

Every Musculoskeletal Specialty.

One Comprehensive Web Site.

FIRST IN ITS FIELD

Founded in 1863, Hospital for Special Surgery is a leading tertiary care academic medical center for orthopedics, rheumatology, and rehabilitation.

PIONEERS IN ORTHOPEDIC SURGERY

HSS performs more joint replacements than any other hospital in the world, and more hip and knee procedures than any other hospital in the nation. Surgeries that are rare at other hospitals are routine procedures here. HSS pioneered designs and surgical techniques for the modern artificial knee replacement in the 1970's and has been leading total knee replacement ever since. HSS also pioneered minimally invasive spine surgery techniques that reduce the need for spinal fusion. Our surgeons are also innovators in hand, elbow, shoulder, and spine surgery techniques and are leading experts in arthroscopy and hip preservation.

GLOBAL LEADERS IN RHEUMATOLOGY

HSS rheumatologists are international authorities, academic leaders, and pioneering researchers in rheumatological and autoimmune conditions. They are recognized for their depth of experience in diagnosing and treating the full spectrum of rheumatological diseases, including osteoarthritis, lupus, antiphospholipid syndrome, rheumatoid arthritis, scleroderma, vasculitis, gout, and pediatric inflammatory arthritis, and are valued resources for evaluation of patients who are diagnostic dilemmas. Cutting edge research and treatment centers include the Mary Kirkland Center for Lupus Research, the Barbara Volcker Center for Women and Rheumatic Diseases, the Inflammatory Arthritis Center, the Scleroderma, Vasculitis, & Myositis Center, and the Osteoporosis and Metabolic Bone Health Center.

WORLD'S MOST EXPERIENCED MUSCULOSKELETAL RADIOLOGISTS

HSS is the world's largest academic center dedicated to musculoskeletal imaging. Our experts developed novel MRI techniques that detect early failure of joint arthroplasty and implants. HSS innovations in ultrasound and MRI also allow earlier diagnosis of autoimmune conditions and arthritis.

RECOGNIZED FOR QUALITY

HSS has one of the lowest surgical complication rates in the country as well as top scores for patient safety. For the fourth consecutive year, HSS was recognized by the state for having an infection rate that is significantly lower than the New York State average for hip replacement. 95% of our hip and knee replacement patients receive regional anesthesia, shown to provide superior outcomes with less pain and complications, compared to 11% elsewhere. 92% of patients say they would recommend HSS to their friends and family, compared to 71% for other U.S. hospitals.

Ranked #1 in the Nation for Orthopedics in *U.S.News & World Report* "Best Hospitals" 2013-14 issue. Among the top ranked in Orthopedics & Rheumatology for 23 consecutive years

First hospital in NY State to receive Magnet Recognition for Nursing Excellence by the American Nurses Credentialing Center three consecutive times

Official Hospital of the NY Mets, NY Giants, NY Knicks, NY Liberty, NY Red Bulls, The PGA of America, New York Road Runners for the ING New York City Marathon, St. John's Athletics, CUNY Athletic Conference, and other professional and college teams

Designated as the first National Medical Center of the United States Olympic Committee's National Medical Network

Memorial Sloan-Kettering Cancer Center

The Best Cancer Care. Anywhere.

1275 York Avenue
New York, NY 10065
Make an Appointment: (800) 525-2225
www.mskcc.org

Beds: 469
Sponsorship/Network Affiliation: Private, Non-Profit
Make an Appointment: (800) 525-2225

THE MEMORIAL SLOAN-KETTERING ADVANTAGE: CANCER IS OUR ONLY FOCUS

At Memorial Sloan-Kettering Cancer Center, our only focus is cancer. Internationally recognized as one of the world's premier facilities for cancer care, we are consistently ranked as one of the nation's top cancer centers by *U.S. News & World Report.* We are proud to be a National Cancer Institute Comprehensive Cancer Center and a member of the National Comprehensive Cancer Network.

A TEAM APPROACH TO CANCER CARE

Our patients benefit from individualized treatment plans developed by a team of specialists with unsurpassed depth and breadth of experience. Teams include surgeons, medical and radiation oncologists, radiologists, pathologists, nurses, and others who are specialists in a specific type of cancer. They develop treatment plans that reflect their combined expertise, so patients who need several different types of therapy will receive the best combination for them.

GREATER PRECISION IN DIAGNOSIS

Getting the correct diagnosis right from the start is crucial. We use the most advanced imaging technologies, such as combined PET/CT and nuclear medicine scans, to accurately detect and precisely locate cancer. Our highly specialized pathologists analyze some 60,000 tumor samples annually to determine an exact diagnosis and the extent of disease. Increasingly, they use new technology to identify molecular differences among tumors, allowing even greater precision in diagnosis.

UNPARALLELED SURGICAL EXPERTISE

Recent studies have shown that, for many cancers, patients have fewer complications and better outcomes if they have surgery at a hospital where high volumes of these operations are performed by surgeons experienced in the procedure. Our surgeons are among the most experienced cancer surgeons in the world. They use the latest surgical technology, including robotic and minimally invasive techniques, as well as interventional radiology for embolization, thermal ablation, and chemical ablation of tumors. In their quest to spare or reconstruct organs and preserve function, they are renowned for not only saving lives, but preserving the quality of life.

ADVANCES IN CHEMOTHERAPY

Our medical oncologists are leaders in developing new chemotherapy drugs that are safer and more effective than standard therapies. They also help manage any side effects of chemotherapy, such as nausea and fatigue, so patients can continue their usual activities wherever possible. Increasingly, our medical oncologists use advanced technologies, such as immunotherapies or vaccines, often in combination with chemotherapy.

LEADERS IN RADIATION THERAPY

Our radiation oncologists are skilled in complex treatment planning and delivery techniques. Through their efforts, intensity-modulated radiation therapy was enhanced with image guidance (IGRT). IGRT enables our radiation oncologists to precisely sculpt multiple radiation beams to the contours of a tumor, sparing nearby normal tissue. The higher doses of radiation possible in IGRT also have a greater chance of killing tumors. Our doctors may use radiation combined with chemotherapy to make tumors more sensitive to the radiation, enhancing the chances of success.

RESEARCH EXPANDS TREATMENT OPTIONS

Through close collaboration between clinicians and research scientists, new therapies developed in the laboratory can be quickly translated into improved treatment options for patients.

INSURANCE

Memorial Sloan-Kettering Cancer Center is in-network with most New York–area insurance plans.

MAKE AN APPOINTMENT: (800) 525-2225

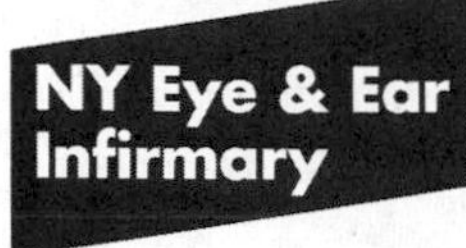

THE NEW YORK EYE AND EAR INFIRMARY

310 East 14th Street
New York, New York 10003
Tel. 212.979.4000 Fax. 212.228.0664
www.nyee.edu

BEDS:	**69; Operating Rooms: 19; Surgical Cases: 31,000+ a year**
Sponsorship:	**Voluntary Not-for-Profit**
Accreditation:	**The Joint Commission**
	College of American Pathologists

GENERAL OVERVIEW

The New York Eye and Ear Infirmary is one of the world's leading facilities for the diagnosis and treatment of diseases of the eyes, ears, nose, throat and related conditions. Founded in 1820, it is the first and most historic specialty hospital in the nation, as well as one of the busiest.

ACADEMIC AFFILIATIONS

The New York Eye and Ear Infirmary has some of the nation's most competitive and highly regarded residency programs in Ophthalmology and Otolaryngology/ Head & Neck Surgery, plus more than two dozen post-graduate fellowships in subspecialties of Ophthalmology, Otolaryngology and Plastic & Reconstructive Surgery. NYEE is an affiliated teaching hospital of New York Medical College. The Accreditation Council for Continuing Medical Education has awarded NYEE's Institute for Continuing Medical Education its highest accreditation status – "Accreditation with Commendation" as a provider of continuing medical education for physicians.

THE MEDICAL STAFF

The Medical Staff includes more than 600 board-certified attending physicians and surgeons throughout the metropolitan area. Many are renowned for their breakthrough research introducing widely practiced techniques.

SPECIALTIES

Ophthalmology: Within this area are comprehensive eye care, cataract, cornea & external disease, refractive surgery, eye trauma, glaucoma, pediatric glaucoma, low vision, neuro-ophthalmlogy, ophthalmic oncology, ophthalmic pathology, oculoplastic & orbital surgery, pediatric ophthalmology & strabismus, retinal vitreous, and uveitis/ocular immunology. Laser treatments, photographic and imaging services, and electrophysiological testing are among the most advanced anywhere.

Otolaryngology: The department is in the forefront of treatment modalities using highly sophisticated endoscopic and laser equipment. Subspecialties include rhinology, laryngology, head & neck surgery, otology/neurotology, facial plastic surgery, pediatric otolaryngology, audiology, speech therapy and hearing aid dispensing.

Plastic & Reconstructive Surgery: Microsurgical capabilities and premium patient accommodations provide an optimum environment for facial plasty, liposuction, breast surgery and repair of defects from disease or trauma.

RELATED SERVICES

New York Eye Trauma Center: An advanced program for emergency treatment of eye injuries, it also is the Eye Injury Registry of New York State and leading collector of data which will help develop preventative strategies.

Ambulatory Surgery: A comprehensive Ambulatory Surgery Center is designed to expedite admission testing, pre-op preparation and post-op recovery in an efficient and comfortable setting.

Pediatric Specialty Care: Services of eye and ear, nose and throat specialists are coordinated with other professional and support staff especially sensitive to the youngest patients.

RESEARCH AND EDUCATION

The New York Eye and Ear Infirmary is a national and international leader in research in its specialties, achieving many "firsts" in successful surgical procedures and medical treatments. Laboratories include Cell Culture, Ocular Imaging, and Microsurgical Education. Over a hundred studies and clinical trials are currently being conducted.

Physician Referral: Call 1.800.449.HOPE (4673)

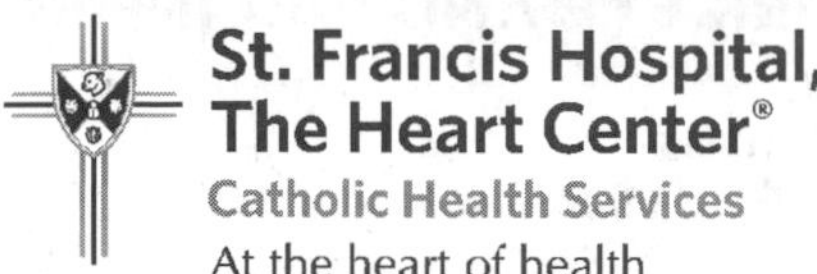

100 Port Washington Blvd.
Roslyn, New York 11576
www.stfrancisheartcenter.com
(516) 562-6000
1-888-HEARTNY

St. Francis Hospital, The Heart Center® is New York State's only specialty designated cardiac center and a nationally recognized leader in cardiac care. Founded in 1922 by the Franciscan Missionaries of Mary, the Hospital is an innovator in the delivery of specialized cardiovascular services in an environment where excellence and compassion are emphasized. St. Francis also offers a nationally recognized program in non-cardiac surgery, including some of the most advanced technology and minimally invasive techniques available for vascular, prostate, ear-nose-throat (ENT), abdominal, oncologic, gastrointestinal, and orthopedic surgery and procedures.

Cardiac Diagnostics and Treatment

St. Francis Hospital performs one of the highest volumes of cardiac surgical, interventional and arrhythmia procedures in the nation and has been consistently recognized for its outstanding quality of care. In 2013-14, St. Francis Hospital was ranked one of America's top 10 hospitals in cardiology and heart surgery by *U.S. News & World Report*.

Cardiac surgery: In 2012, 1,337 open-heart surgeries were performed at St. Francis Hospital. The Hospital's cardiothoracic surgical staff has the combined experience of over 16,000 open-heart procedures in the last 10 years alone and are experts in all types of heart surgery, from conventional, open-heart bypass to off-pump coronary artery bypass (OPCAB) to the newest, minimally invasive valve procedures, including surgical techniques designed to treat certain cardiac arrhythmias or irregular heart rhythms.

Cardiac catheterization: In 2012, St. Francis interventional cardiologists performed 10,025 cardiac catheterizations and 2,719 percutaneous coronary interventions (angioplasty with stents) and other cardiac and peripheral vascular interventions. The Hospital is also recognized as one of the East Coast's highest volume centers for catheter-based techniques to repair congenital heart defects.

Arrhythmia and Pacemaker Center: St. Francis has a leading national program for pacemaker implantation and the diagnosis and treatment of cardiac rhythm abnormalities. The Center has unparalleled expertise in radiofrequency cardiac ablation, including treatment of atrial fibrillation.

Research and Technology: At the St. Francis Cardiac Research Institute, a team of world-renowned researchers is working with the latest noninvasive imaging technology, including advanced techniques and world-class expertise in cardiac CT angiography, cardiac magnetic resonance imaging (MRI), cardiac PET/CT and three-dimensional echocardiography. This multimodality approach to investigating the heart's function and disease processes is aimed at improving methods of diagnosing heart disease.

Broad-Based Excellence

St. Francis Hospital is also ranked one of America's best hospitals in ear, nose and throat; gastroenterology and GI surgery; geriatrics; neurology and neurosurgery; orthopedics; pulmonology; and urology by *U.S. News & World Report*. In 2012, the Hospital opened a new Cancer Institute, which brings together all of the essential elements for an integrated approach to treating cancer with the Hospital's signature commitment to quality and compassionate care.

Physician referral:	**1-888-HEARTNY**
Sponsorship:	Voluntary not-for-profit
Beds:	306
Accreditation:	Awarded accreditation from the Joint Commission.

New York Metropolitan Regional Medical Centers and Hospitals

The New York metropolitan region is fortunate to have a large number of truly excellent Regional Medical Centers and Hospitals. Many of these institutions offer sophisticated services that in years past were offered only at academic medical centers. However, with advancements in medical technology, Regional Medical Centers and Hospitals have access to the equipment, and by virtue of the medical schools and teaching hospitals in the region, the well-trained physicians and staff, to offer these programs.

Regional Medical Centers and Hospitals range in size from the small (100 beds) to the very large (800 beds) but they share a common theme: a primary focus on patient care.

We have invited a select number of excellent Regional Medical Centers and Hospitals to provide readers of the Castle Connolly Guide with information on their institutions and services by sponsoring profiles, which are included at the end of individual county sections in the physician listings that follow.

Regional Medical Centers and Hospitals

Children's & Women's Physicians of Westchester, LLP

Greenwich Hospital

Hackensack University Health Network

Hackensack UMC at Pascack Valley

Hackensack UMC Mountainside

Holy Name Medical Center

New York Hospital Queens

New York Methodist Hospital

Northern Westchester Hospital

Stamford Hospital

SUNY Downstate Medical Center (Univ Hosp of Brooklyn)

Trinitas Regional Medical Center

Valley Hospital

White Plains Hospital Center

Winthrop-University Hospital

SECTION THREE

Physician Listings

The State of New York

New York (Manhattan)

New York (Manhattan)

Addiction Psychiatry

Collins, Eric D MD (AdP) - **Spec Exp:** Addiction/Substance Abuse; Opiate Addiction; Dual Diagnosis; Alcohol Abuse; **Hospital:** NY-Presby/Columbia Univ Med Ctr, NY (page 104), Silver Hill Hosp; **Address:** 180 Ft Washington Ave, Box HP-260, New York, NY 10032; **Phone:** 212-305-8732; **Board Cert:** Psychiatry 2005; Addiction Psychiatry 2007; Psychosomatic Medicine 2008; **Med School:** Columbia P&S 1990; **Resid:** Psychiatry, NY State Psyc Inst 1995; **Fellow:** Psychosomatic Medicine, NY-Presby/Columbia Univ Med Ctr 1996; Addiction Psychiatry, NY State Psyc Inst 1997; **Fac Appt:** Assoc Clin Prof Psyc, Columbia P&S

Frances, Richard J MD (AdP) - **Spec Exp:** Addiction/Substance Abuse; Anxiety & Mood Disorders; Forensic Psychiatry; **Hospital:** Silver Hill Hosp, NYU Langone Med Ctr (page 108); **Address:** 510 E 86th St, Ste 1D, New York, NY 10028; **Phone:** 212-861-0570; **Board Cert:** Psychiatry 1976; Addiction Psychiatry 2012; **Med School:** NYU Sch Med 1971; **Resid:** Psychiatry, Jacobi Med Ctr 1974; **Fellow:** Psychoanalysis, NY Psychoanalytic Inst 1983; **Fac Appt:** Clin Prof Psyc, NYU Sch Med

Galanter, I Marc MD (AdP) - **Spec Exp:** Alcohol Abuse; Drug Abuse; Anxiety & Depression; **Hospital:** NYU Langone Med Ctr (page 108); **Address:** 285 Central Park West, New York, NY 10024-3006; **Phone:** 212-877-4093; **Board Cert:** Psychiatry 1974; Addiction Psychiatry 2011; **Med School:** Albert Einstein Coll Med 1967; **Resid:** Pediatrics, UCLA Med Ctr 1978; Psychiatry, Bronx Muni Hosp-Einstein 1971; **Fac Appt:** Prof Psyc, NYU Sch Med

Kleber, Herbert D MD (AdP) - **Spec Exp:** Opiate Addiction; Cocaine Addiction; Drug Abuse; **Hospital:** NY-Presby/Columbia Univ Med Ctr, NY (page 104), NY State Psychiatric Inst; **Address:** NY State Psychiatric Inst, 1051 Riverside Drive, Rm 3713, Unit 66, New York, NY 10032-1007; **Phone:** 732-235-7729; **Med School:** Jefferson Med Coll 1960; **Resid:** Psychiatry, Yale-New Haven Hosp 1964; **Fac Appt:** Prof Psyc, Columbia P&S

Levin, Frances R MD (AdP) - **Spec Exp:** Addiction/Substance Abuse; Dual Diagnosis; Substance Abuse in ADHD Patients; Alcohol Abuse; **Hospital:** NY State Psychiatric Inst, NY-Presby/Columbia Univ Med Ctr, NY (page 104); **Address:** NYS Psychiatric Inst, 1051 Riverside Drive, rm 3625, Box 66, New York, NY 10032; **Phone:** 212-543-5896; **Board Cert:** Psychiatry 1990; Addiction Psychiatry 2013; **Med School:** Cornell Univ-Weill Med Coll 1985; **Resid:** Psychiatry, Payne Whitney Clin 1989; **Fellow:** Substance Abuse, Univ MD Med Ctr/NIDA 1990; **Fac Appt:** Prof Psyc, Columbia P&S

Paul, Edward MD (AdP) - **Spec Exp:** Opiate Addiction; Alcohol Abuse; Smoking Cessation; Cocaine Addiction; **Hospital:** NYU Langone Med Ctr (page 108); **Address:** 155 E 31st St, Ste 25J, New York, NY 10016; **Phone:** 212-447-5712; **Board Cert:** Psychiatry 1987; Addiction Psychiatry 2013; **Med School:** Columbia P&S 1982; **Resid:** Psychiatry, Payne Whitney Clin 1987; Psychoanalysis, NYU Med Ctr 1993; **Fellow:** Substance Abuse, NY-Presby/Weill Cornell Med Ctr 1987; **Fac Appt:** Asst Clin Prof Psyc, NYU Sch Med

Rosenberg, Kenneth P MD (AdP) - **Spec Exp:** Addiction/Substance Abuse; Sexual Dysfunction; **Hospital:** NY-Presby/Weill Cornell Med Ctr, NY (page 104); **Address:** 49 E 78th St, Ste 2A, New York, NY 10075; **Phone:** 212-861-8807; **Board Cert:** Psychiatry 1992; Addiction Psychiatry 2009; **Med School:** Albert Einstein Coll Med 1983; **Resid:** Psychiatry, NY-Presby/Weill Cornell Med Ctr 1988; **Fellow:** Substance Abuse, NY-Presby/Weill Cornell Med Ctr 1991; Public Health, NY-Presby/Weill Cornell Med Ctr 1992; **Fac Appt:** Assoc Clin Prof Psyc, Cornell Univ-Weill Med Coll

Scimeca, Michael M MD (AdP) - **Spec Exp:** Addiction/Substance Abuse; Alcohol Abuse; **Hospital:** Mt Sinai Med Ctr (page 102), James J. Peters VA Med Ctr-Bronx; **Address:** 200 W 90th St, New York, NY 10024; **Phone:** 212-580-9605; **Board Cert:** Psychiatry 2007; Addiction Psychiatry 2007; **Med School:** Univ Tex, San Antonio 1978; **Resid:** Psychiatry, Montefiore Med Ctr 1981; **Fac Appt:** Assoc Clin Prof Psyc, Mount Sinai Sch Med

Weiss, Carol J MD (AdP) - **Spec Exp:** Drug Abuse; Alcohol Abuse; **Hospital:** NY-Presby/Weill Cornell Med Ctr, NY (page 104); **Address:** 1044 Madison Ave, Ste PH1, New York, NY 10075; **Phone:** 212-988-1209; **Board Cert:** Psychiatry 1989; Addiction Psychiatry 2013; Addiction Medicine 2009; **Med School:** Johns Hopkins Univ 1983; **Resid:** Psychiatry, NY-Presby/Weill Cornell Med Ctr 1987; **Fellow:** Addiction Psychiatry, NY-Presby/Weill Cornell Med Ctr 1989; **Fac Appt:** Asst Clin Prof Psyc, Cornell Univ-Weill Med Coll

Adolescent Medicine

Bell, David L MD (AM) - **Spec Exp:** Men's Health; **Hospital:** Morgan Stanley Children's Hosp of NY-Presby, NY (page 104); **Address:** Audobon Primary Care, 21 Audobon Ave, New York, NY 10032; **Phone:** 212-304-7737; **Board Cert:** Pediatrics 2010; **Med School:** Univ Tex SW, Dallas 1989; **Resid:** Pediatrics, Bellevue Hosp 1993; **Fellow:** Adolescent Medicine, UCSF Med Ctr 1996; **Fac Appt:** Asst Prof Ped, Columbia P&S

Catallozzi, Marina MD (AM) - **Spec Exp:** AIDS/HIV in Adolescents; Adolescent Gynecology; Sexually Transmitted Diseases; **Hospital:** Morgan Stanley Children's Hosp of NY-Presby, NY (page 104); **Address:** Audubon Primary Care Practice, 21 Audubon Ave, New York, NY 10032; **Phone:** 212-342-3200; **Board Cert:** Pediatrics 2007; Adolescent Medicine 2013; **Med School:** Brown Univ 1996; **Resid:** Pediatrics, CHOP 2000; **Fellow:** Adolescent Medicine, CHOP 2004; **Fac Appt:** Asst Prof Ped, Columbia P&S

Cohall, Alwyn T MD (AM) - **Spec Exp:** AIDS/HIV in Adolsecents; Adolescent Behavior-High Risk; **Hospital:** Morgan Stanley Children's Hosp of NY-Presby, NY (page 104), NY-Presby/Columbia Univ Med Ctr, NY (page 104); **Address:** 3959 Broadway, Ste 106, New York, NY 10032; **Phone:** 646-284-9725; **Board Cert:** Pediatrics ; Adolescent Medicine 2010; **Med School:** UMDNJ-NJ Med Sch, Newark 1980; **Resid:** Pediatrics, Montefiore Med Ctr 1983; **Fellow:** Adolescent Medicine, Mount Sinai Med Ctr 1984; **Fac Appt:** Clin Prof Ped, Columbia P&S

Ipp, Lisa S MD (AM) - **Spec Exp:** Adolescent Gynecology; **Hospital:** NY-Presby/Weill Cornell Med Ctr, NY (page 104), Hosp For Special Surgery (page 113); **Address:** NY Presby Hosp-Pediatrics, 505 E 70th St, Helmsley Tower Fl 5, New York, NY 10021; **Phone:** 212-746-3303; **Board Cert:** Pediatrics 2007; Adolescent Medicine 2011; **Med School:** Cornell Univ-Weill Med Coll 1996; **Resid:** Pediatrics, Hasbro Children's Hosp 1999; **Fellow:** Adolescent Medicine, Mt Sinai Med Ctr 2002; **Fac Appt:** Assoc Clin Prof Ped, Cornell Univ-Weill Med Coll

Lopez, Ralph I MD (AM) - **Spec Exp:** Growth/Development Disorders; Eating Disorders; Learning Disorders; Parenting Issues; **Hospital:** NY-Presby/Weill Cornell Med Ctr, NY (page 104); **Address:** 418 E 71st St, New York, NY 10021-4894; **Phone:** 212-772-8989; **Board Cert:** Pediatrics 1972; **Med School:** NYU Sch Med 1967; **Resid:** Pediatrics, Bellevue Hosp 1969; Pediatrics, Chldns Hosp 1970; **Fellow:** Adolescent Medicine, Chldns Hosp 1971; **Fac Appt:** Clin Prof Ped, Cornell Univ-Weill Med Coll

Marks, Andrea M MD (AM) - **Spec Exp:** Eating Disorders; Adolescent Gynecology; Psychosomatic Disorders; Parenting Issues; **Hospital:** Mt Sinai Med Ctr (page 102); **Address:** Adolescent-Young Adult Medicine, 14 E 90th St, Ste 1B, New York, NY 10128; **Phone:** 212-987-1414; **Board Cert:** Pediatrics 1977; **Med School:** Univ Pennsylvania 1972; **Resid:** Pediatrics, Chldns Hosp 1974; **Fellow:** Adolescent Medicine, Chldns Hosp 1975; **Fac Appt:** Assoc Clin Prof Ped, Mount Sinai Sch Med

Nucci-Sack, Anne T MD (AM) - **Spec Exp:** Adolescent Gynecology; Vaccines; **Hospital:** Mt Sinai Med Ctr (page 102); **Address:** Mt Sinai, Adolescent Hlth Ctr, 312 E 94th St, New York, NY 10128; **Phone:** 212-423-3000; **Board Cert:** Pediatrics 1986; Adolescent Medicine 2009; **Med School:** NY Med Coll 1981; **Resid:** Pediatrics, Montefiore Med Ctr 1984; **Fellow:** Adolescent Medicine, Montefiore Med Ctr 1990; **Fac Appt:** Asst Prof Ped, Mount Sinai Sch Med

Pastore, Doris R MD (AM) - **Spec Exp:** Nutrition; Eating Disorders; **Hospital:** Mt Sinai Med Ctr (page 102); **Address:** Adolescent-Young Adult Medicine, 14 E 90 St, Ste 1B, New York, NY 10128; **Phone:** 212-987-1414; **Board Cert:** Pediatrics 2012; Adolescent Medicine 2009; **Med School:** NY Med Coll 1985; **Resid:** Pediatrics, Montefiore Med Ctr 1988; **Fellow:** Adolescent Medicine, N Shore Univ Hosp/Cornell 1990

Pegler, Cynthia R MD (AM) - **Spec Exp:** Adolescent Gynecology; Eating Disorders; **Hospital:** NY-Presby/Weill Cornell Med Ctr, NY (page 104); **Address:** 992 5th Ave, New York, NY 10028; **Phone:** 212-517-5313; **Board Cert:** Pediatrics 2010; Adolescent Medicine 2009; **Med School:** Albany Med Coll 1984; **Resid:** Pediatrics, N Shore Univ Hosp 1987; **Fellow:** Adolescent Medicine, N Shore Univ Hosp 1990

Rosewater, Karen M MD (AM) - **Spec Exp:** Eating Disorders; **Hospital:** Mt Sinai Med Ctr (page 102); **Address:** Adolescent-Young Adult Medicine, 14 E 90th St, Ste 1B, New York, NY 10128; **Phone:** 212-987-1414; **Board Cert:** Adolescent Medicine 2009; **Med School:** Yale Univ 1994; **Resid:** Pediatrics, Chldns Hosp 1997; **Fellow:** Adolescent Medicine, Chldns Natl Med Ctr 2000

Rudy, Bret J MD (AM) - **Spec Exp:** HIV in Adolescents; AIDS/HIV; **Hospital:** NYU Langone Med Ctr (page 108), Bellevue Hosp Ctr; **Address:** 145 E 32nd St, rm 1408, 14th Fl Penthouse, New York, NY 10016; **Phone:** 212-263-6425; **Board Cert:** Adolescent Medicine 2009; **Med School:** Univ Pittsburgh 1985; **Resid:** Pediatrics, Chldns Hosp 1988; **Fellow:** Hematology & Oncology, Chldns Hosp 1989; Internal Medicine, Chldns Hosp 1994

Soren, Karen MD (AM) - **Spec Exp:** Adolescent Gynecology; Behavioral Disorders; **Hospital:** Morgan Stanley Children's Hosp of NY-Presby, NY (page 104), NY-Presby/Columbia Univ Med Ctr, NY (page 104); **Address:** Audobon Primary Care, 21 Audobon Ave, New York, NY 10032; **Phone:** 212-342-3200; **Board Cert:** Pediatrics ; Adolescent Medicine 2009; **Med School:** NYU Sch Med 1982; **Resid:** Pediatrics, Chldn's Hosp Natl Med Ctr 1985; **Fellow:** Adolescent Medicine, Univ Chicago Med Ctr 1987; **Fac Appt:** Assoc Prof Ped, Columbia P&S

Steever, John B MD (AM) - **Spec Exp:** Adolescent Gynecology; Adolescent Behavior-High Risk; Abuse/Neglect; **Hospital:** Mt Sinai Med Ctr (page 102); **Address:** Mt Sinai Adolescent Hlth Ctr, 312 E 94 St Fl 2, New York, NY 10128; **Phone:** 212-423-2900; **Board Cert:** Pediatrics 2013; Adolescent Medicine ; **Med School:** Geo Wash Univ 1993; **Resid:** Pediatrics, Chldn's Hosp 1996; **Fellow:** Adolescent Medicine, Chldn's Hosp 1999; **Fac Appt:** Asst Prof Ped, Mount Sinai Sch Med

Allergy & Immunology

Bassett, Clifford MD (A&I) - **Spec Exp:** Asthma & Sinusitis; Food Allergy; Pet Allergy; Skin Allergies; **Hospital:** NYU Langone Med Ctr (page 108); **Address:** Allergy & Asthma Care NY, 381 Park Ave S, Ste 1020, New York, NY 10016; **Phone:** 212-260-6078; **Board Cert:** Allergy & Immunology 2006; **Med School:** NY Med Coll 1985; **Resid:** Internal Medicine, Hackensack Univ Med Ctr 1989; **Fellow:** Allergy & Immunology, LI Coll Hosp 1993; **Fac Appt:** Asst Clin Prof Med, NYU Sch Med

Buchbinder, Ellen M MD (A&I) - **Spec Exp:** Asthma & Allergy; Rhinitis; Hives; Food & Drug Allergy; **Hospital:** Mt Sinai Med Ctr (page 102); **Address:** 111 E 88th St, Ste 1-B, New York, NY 10128; **Phone:** 212-410-3246; **Board Cert:** Internal Medicine 1981; Allergy & Immunology 1983; **Med School:** Tulane Univ 1978; **Resid:** Internal Medicine, New England Deaconess Hosp 1981; **Fellow:** Allergy & Immunology, Mass Genl Hosp 1983; **Fac Appt:** Asst Clin Prof Med, Mount Sinai Sch Med

Burton, Daniel A MD (A&I) - **Spec Exp:** Rhinitis; Asthma; Food & Drug Allergy; Urticaria; **Hospital:** NY-Presby/Weill Cornell Med Ctr, NY (page 104), Hosp For Special Surgery (page 113); **Address:** 235 E 67th St, Ste 203, New York, NY 10065; **Phone:** 212-288-9300; **Board Cert:** Internal Medicine 1989; Allergy & Immunology 2003; **Med School:** Wright State Univ 1984; **Resid:** Internal Medicine, St Lukes-Roosevelt Hosp Ctr 1987; **Fellow:** Allergy & Immunology, NY Hosp 1989; **Fac Appt:** Asst Prof Med, Cornell Univ-Weill Med Coll

Chandler, Michael J MD (A&I) - **Spec Exp:** Asthma; Sinus Disorders; Airway Disorders; **Hospital:** Mt Sinai Med Ctr (page 102); **Address:** City Allergy, 115 E 61st St Fl 12, New York, NY 10065; **Phone:** 212-486-6715; **Board Cert:** Internal Medicine 1984; Allergy & Immunology 1987; **Med School:** Wayne State Univ 1981; **Resid:** Internal Medicine, Northwestern Meml Hosp 1984; **Fellow:** Allergy & Immunology, Northwestern Meml Hosp 1986; **Fac Appt:** Asst Clin Prof Med, Mount Sinai Sch Med

Corn, Beth E MD (A&I) - **Spec Exp:** Asthma; Rhinitis; Food Allergy; **Hospital:** Mt Sinai Med Ctr (page 102); **Address:** Mt Sinai, Allergy & Immunology Dept, 5 E 98th St Fl 11, New York, NY 10029; **Phone:** 212-241-0764; **Board Cert:** Allergy & Immunology 2005; **Med School:** Albert Einstein Coll Med 1989; **Resid:** Internal Medicine, St Lukes-Roosevelt Hosp 1992; **Fellow:** Clinical Immunology, Mount Sinai Med Ctr 1994; **Fac Appt:** Asst Prof Med, Mount Sinai Sch Med

Cunningham-Rundles, Charlotte MD/PhD (A&I) - **Spec Exp:** Immunotherapy; Immunodeficiency Disorders; **Hospital:** Mt Sinai Med Ctr (page 102); **Address:** Mt Sinai Hosp, Dept of Med-Allergy & Immunology, 5 E 98th St Fl 11, New York, NY 10029; **Phone:** 212-659-9268; **Board Cert:** Internal Medicine 1972; **Med School:** Columbia P&S 1969; **Resid:** Internal Medicine, Bellevue Hosp Ctr 1972; **Fellow:** Allergy & Immunology, NYU Med Ctr 1974; **Fac Appt:** Prof Med, Mount Sinai Sch Med

Frenkel, Renata MD (A&I) - **Spec Exp:** Asthma; Allergy; Sinus Disorders; Urticaria; **Hospital:** St. Luke's - Roosevelt Hosp Ctr - Roosevelt Div (page 94), Lenox Hill Hosp (page 106); **Address:** 30 W 60th St, Ste 1U, New York, NY 10023; **Phone:** 212-265-1990; **Board Cert:** Allergy & Immunology 1979; **Med School:** Austria 1968; **Resid:** Allergy & Immunology, St Lukes-Roosevelt Hosp 1975; **Fac Appt:** Assoc Clin Prof Ped, Columbia P&S

Grubman, Samuel MD (A&I) - **Spec Exp:** Asthma & Allergy; Food Allergy; Immunodeficiency Disorders; Pediatric Allergy & Immunology; **Hospital:** NYU Langone Med Ctr (page 108); **Address:** NY Downtown Allergy, 154 W 14th St Fl 4, New York, NY 10011; **Phone:** 212-616-4122; **Board Cert:** Pediatrics 1987; Allergy & Immunology 2009; **Med School:** Mount Sinai Sch Med 1983; **Resid:** Pediatrics, NYU Med Ctr 1986; **Fellow:** Allergy & Immunology, Montefiore Med Ctr 1988; **Fac Appt:** Assoc Clin Prof Ped, NYU Sch Med

Lubitz, Arthur M MD (A&I) - **Spec Exp:** Allergy; Asthma; Immunotherapy; **Hospital:** Lenox Hill Hosp (page 106), NYU Langone Med Ctr (page 108); **Address:** 315 W 57th St, Ste 309, New York, NY 10019; **Phone:** 212-247-7447; **Board Cert:** Internal Medicine 1984; Allergy & Immunology 2013; **Med School:** SUNY Downstate 1980; **Resid:** Internal Medicine, Coney Island Hosp 1983; **Fellow:** Allergy & Immunology, LI Coll Hosp 1985

Mazza, David S MD (A&I) - **Spec Exp:** Asthma; Sinus Disorders; Eczema; **Hospital:** St. Luke's - Roosevelt Hosp Ctr - Roosevelt Div (page 94); **Address:** 7 Lexington Ave, Ste P3, New York, NY 10010-5517; **Phone:** 212-677-7170; **Board Cert:** Pediatrics 1983; Allergy & Immunology 2008; **Med School:** Univ VT Coll Med 1977; **Resid:** Pediatrics, NYU-Bellevue Hosp 1980; **Fellow:** Pediatric Allergy & Immunology, Bellevue Hosp 1982; **Fac Appt:** Asst Prof Ped, Columbia P&S

Shepherd, Gillian M MD (A&I) - **Spec Exp:** Food & Drug Allergy; Rhinosinusitis & Asthma; Urticaria; Insect Allergies; **Hospital:** NY-Presby/Weill Cornell Med Ctr, NY (page 104); **Address:** 235 E 67th St, Ste 203, New York, NY 10065; **Phone:** 212-288-9300; **Board Cert:** Internal Medicine 1979; Allergy & Immunology 1981; **Med School:** NY Med Coll 1976; **Resid:** Internal Medicine, Lenox Hill Hosp 1979; **Fellow:** Allergy & Immunology, New York Hosp-Cornell 1981; **Fac Appt:** Assoc Clin Prof Med, Cornell Univ-Weill Med Coll

Slankard, Marjorie L MD (A&I) - **Spec Exp:** Sinus Disorders; Asthma; Food Allergy; **Hospital:** NY-Presby/Columbia Univ Med Ctr, NY (page 104), Valley Hosp (page 721); **Address:** 51 W 51st St, Ste 360, New York, NY 10019; **Phone:** 212-326-8410; **Board Cert:** Internal Medicine 1974; Allergy & Immunology 1977; **Med School:** Univ MO-Columbia Sch Med 1971; **Resid:** Internal Medicine, New York Hosp 1974; **Fellow:** Allergy & Immunology, New York Hosp-Cornell 1976; Neoplastic Diseases, Mount Sinai Med Ctr 1980; **Fac Appt:** Clin Prof Med, Columbia P&S

Tolston, Evelyn MD (A&I) - **Spec Exp:** Rhinitis; Asthma; Allergy; Sinusitis; **Hospital:** NYU Langone Med Ctr (page 108), Beth Israel Med Ctr - Petrie Div (page 94); **Address:** 161 Madison Ave, Ste 3A, New York, NY 10016; **Phone:** 646-424-0400, **Board Cert:** Allergy & Immunology 2005; **Med School:** Ukraine 1982; **Resid:** Internal Medicine, Cabrini Med Ctr 1993; Allergy & Immunology, Albert Einstein Coll Med 1995

Young, Stuart H MD (A&I) - **Spec Exp:** Asthma; Nasal & Sinus Disorders; Urticaria; Eczema; **Hospital:** Mt Sinai Med Ctr (page 102); **Address:** 121 E 60th St, New York, NY 10022-1102; **Phone:** 212-826-0815; **Board Cert:** Pediatrics 1968; Allergy & Immunology 1972; **Med School:** SUNY Downstate 1963; **Resid:** Pediatrics, Kings Co Hosp 1966; **Fellow:** Allergy & Immunology, Natl Jewish Hosp 1970; **Fac Appt:** Assoc Clin Prof Med, Mount Sinai Sch Med

Cardiac Electrophysiology

Bernstein, Neil E MD (CE) - **Spec Exp:** Arrhythmias; Atrial Fibrillation; Pacemakers; **Hospital:** NYU Langone Med Ctr (page 108); **Address:** NYU Heart Rhythm Ctr, 403 E 34 St Fl 4, New York, NY 10016; **Phone:** 212-263-3600; **Board Cert:** Internal Medicine 1989; Cardiovascular Disease 2004; Cardiac Electrophysiology 2005; **Med School:** NYU Sch Med 1986; **Resid:** Internal Medicine, NYU/Bellevue Med Ctr 1990; **Fellow:** Cardiovascular Disease, NYU/Bellevue Med Ctr 1994; **Fac Appt:** Asst Prof Med, NYU Sch Med

Biviano, Angelo MD (CE) - **Spec Exp:** Catheter Ablation; Defibrillators; Pacemakers; Atrial Fibrillation; **Hospital:** NY-Presby/Columbia Univ Med Ctr, NY (page 104); **Address:** 161 Fort Washington Ave, Ste 648, New York, NY 10032; **Phone:** 212-305-8559; **Board Cert:** Cardiovascular Disease 2004; Cardiac Electrophysiology 2006; **Med School:** Harvard Med Sch 1997; **Resid:** Internal Medicine, NewYork-Presby Hosp/Columbia Univ Med Ctr 2001; Cardiovascular Disease, NewYork-Presby Hosp/Columbia Univ Med Ctr 2004; **Fellow:** Cardiac Electrophysiology, NewYork-Presby Hosp/Columbia Univ Med Ctr 2005; **Fac Appt:** Asst Prof Med, Columbia P&S

Chinitz, Larry A MD (CE) - **Spec Exp:** Arrhythmias; Pacemakers; Defibrillators; Atrial Fibrillation; **Hospital:** NYU Langone Med Ctr (page 108); **Address:** Heart Rhythm Ctr, 403 E 34th St Fl 4, New York, NY 10016-6402; **Phone:** 212-263-7149; **Board Cert:** Internal Medicine 1982; Cardiovascular Disease 1985; **Med School:** NYU Sch Med 1979; **Resid:** Internal Medicine, Bellevue Hosp Ctr 1983; **Fellow:** Cardiovascular Disease, NYU Med Ctr/Bellevue Hosp Ctr 1985; Cardiac Electrophysiology, Montefiore Hosp 1986; **Fac Appt:** Assoc Prof Med, NYU Sch Med

Garan, Hasan MD (CE) - **Spec Exp:** Arrhythmias; Cardiac Catheterization; Pacemakers/Defibrillators; **Hospital:** NY-Presby/Columbia Univ Med Ctr, NY (page 104); **Address:** NY-Presby, Arrhythmia Svc, 161 Fort Washington Ave, Ste 648, New York, NY 10032; **Phone:** 212-305-7646; **Board Cert:** Internal Medicine 1977; Cardiovascular Disease 1979; **Med School:** Harvard Med Sch 1974; **Resid:** Internal Medicine, Hosp Univ Penn 1976; **Fellow:** Cardiovascular Disease, Mass Genl Hosp 1978; Cardiac Electrophysiology, Mass Genl Hosp 1979; **Fac Appt:** Prof Med, Columbia P&S

Gomes, Joseph Anthony MD (CE) - **Spec Exp:** Arrhythmias; Heart Attack; Atrial Fibrillation; Pacemakers; **Hospital:** Mt Sinai Med Ctr (page 102); **Address:** Cardiovascular Medicine Assocs, 1190 Fifth Ave, 1-South, Guggenheim Pavilion, New York, NY 10029-6500; **Phone:** 212-241-7272; **Board Cert:** Internal Medicine 1974; Cardiovascular Disease 1975; **Med School:** India 1969; **Resid:** Internal Medicine, Mt Sinai Med Ctr 1973; **Fellow:** Cardiovascular Disease, Mt Sinai Med Ctr 1975; Cardiac Electrophysiology, USPHS Cardio-Pulmonary Lab 1976; **Fac Appt:** Prof Med, Mount Sinai Sch Med

Hanon, Samuel MD (CE) - **Spec Exp:** Arrhythmias; Defibrillators; Heart Failure; Atrial Fibrillation; **Hospital:** Beth Israel Med Ctr - Petrie Div (page 94), St. Luke's - Roosevelt Hosp Ctr - Roosevelt Div (page 94); **Address:** Beth Israel Med Ctr, 16th at 1st Ave, 5 Baird Hall, New York, NY 10003; **Phone:** 212-844-1266; **Board Cert:** Cardiovascular Disease 2005; Cardiac Electrophysiology 2006; **Med School:** Albert Einstein Coll Med 1998; **Resid:** Internal Medicine, Beth Israel Med Ctr 2001; **Fellow:** Cardiovascular Disease, Beth Israel Med Ctr 2005; Cardiac Electrophysiology, NY Presby-Columbia Med Ctr 2006

Harnick, David J MD (CE) - **Spec Exp:** Arrhythmias; **Hospital:** Mt Sinai Med Ctr (page 102); **Address:** 148 E 38 St, New York, NY 10003; **Phone:** 212-679-4488; **Board Cert:** Cardiovascular Disease 2012; Cardiac Electrophysiology 2003; **Med School:** Mount Sinai Sch Med 1996; **Resid:** Internal Medicine, NY Presby-Columbia Med Ctr 1999; **Fellow:** Cardiovascular Disease, Mount Sinai Med Ctr 2002; Cardiac Electrophysiology, Mount Sinai Med Ctr 2003

Lerman, Bruce MD (CE) - **Spec Exp:** Catheter Ablation; Atrial Fibrillation; Defibrillators; Arrhythmias; **Hospital:** NY-Presby/Weill Cornell Med Ctr, NY (page 104); **Address:** NY Presby/Weill Cornell Med Ctr, 520 E 70th St, Starr 4, New York, NY 10021-9800; **Phone:** 212-746-2169; **Board Cert:** Internal Medicine 1980; Cardiovascular Disease 1985; Cardiac Electrophysiology 2012; **Med School:** Loyola Univ-Stritch Sch Med 1977; **Resid:** Internal Medicine, Northwestern Univ Hosp 1980; Internal Medicine, Univ Michigan Med Ctr 1981; **Fellow:** Cardiovascular Disease, Hosp Univ Penn 1982; Cardiovascular Disease, Johns Hopkins Hosp 1983; **Fac Appt:** Prof Med, Cornell Univ-Weill Med Coll

Markowitz, Steven M MD (CE) - **Spec Exp:** Arrhythmias; Syncope; **Hospital:** NY-Presby/Weill Cornell Med Ctr, NY (page 104); **Address:** NY-Presby, Cardiac Electrophysiology, 520 E 70th St Starr Bldg Fl 4, New York, NY 10021; **Phone:** 212-746-2655; **Board Cert:** Cardiovascular Disease 2005; Cardiac Electrophysiology 2006; **Med School:** Harvard Med Sch 1988; **Resid:** Internal Medicine, NY-Presby/Weill Cornell Med Ctr 1991; **Fellow:** Cardiovascular Disease, NY-Presby/Weill Cornell Med Ctr 1995; Cardiac Electrophysiology, NY-Presby/Weill Cornell Med Ctr 1996; **Fac Appt:** Prof Med, Cornell Univ-Weill Med Coll

Matos, Jeffrey A MD (CE) - **Spec Exp:** Arrhythmias; Pacemakers; Defibrillators; **Hospital:** Lenox Hill Hosp (page 106); **Address:** Arrhythmia Assocs NY, 1421 3rd Ave Fl 5, New York, NY 10028; **Phone:** 212-772-6384; **Board Cert:** Internal Medicine 1980; Cardiovascular Disease 1983; **Med School:** Harvard Med Sch 1975; **Resid:** Internal Medicine, Beth Israel Med Ctr 1978; **Fellow:** Cardiovascular Disease, Brigham & Womens Hosp 1980; **Fac Appt:** Assoc Clin Prof Med, NYU Sch Med

Mehta, Davendra MD/PhD (CE) - **Spec Exp:** Arrhythmias; Congenital Heart Disease-Adult; Atrial Fibrillation; Heart Failure; **Hospital:** Mt Sinai Med Ctr (page 102); **Address:** Cardiovascular Medicine Assocs, 1190 Fifth Ave, 1-South, Guggenheim Pavilion, New York, NY 10029-6501; **Phone:** 212-241-3559; **Board Cert:** Cardiovascular Disease 2009; Cardiac Electrophysiology 2009; **Med School:** India 1976; **Resid:** Internal Medicine, Leicester Royal Infirmary 1983; **Fellow:** Cardiovascular Disease, Groby Road Hosp 1986; Electrocardiography, St George's Hosp 1989; **Fac Appt:** Prof Med, Mount Sinai Sch Med

Reddy, Vivek Yerrapu MD (CE) - **Spec Exp:** Arrhythmias; Atril Fibrillation; Cardiac Catheterization; **Hospital:** Mt Sinai Med Ctr (page 102); **Address:** 1190 Fifth Ave, Guggenheim Pavilion, New York, NY 10029; **Phone:** 212-241-7114; **Med School:** Univ Mich Med Sch 1995; **Resid:** Internal Medicine, Yale-New Haven Hosp 1997; **Fellow:** Cardiovascular Disease, Univ Chicago Med Ctr 1999; Cardiac Electrophysiology, Mass Genl Hosp 2001; **Fac Appt:** Prof Med, Mount Sinai Sch Med

Suri, Ranjit MD (CE) - **Spec Exp:** Arrhythmias; Atrial Fibrillation; Pacemakers; Sudden Death Prevention; **Hospital:** Lenox Hill Hosp (page 106), NY Hosp Queens (page 488); **Address:** Heart Rhythm Center, Lenox Hill Hosp, 100 E 77th St, New York, NY 10075; **Phone:** 212-434-6500; **Board Cert:** Internal Medicine 2007; Cardiovascular Disease 2006; Cardiac Electrophysiology 2011; **Med School:** India 1982; **Resid:** Internal Medicine, Univ Conn Sch Med 1994; **Fellow:** Cardiovascular Disease, Univ Conn Sch Med 1993; Cardiac Electrophysiology, Mass Genl Hosp 2000; **Fac Appt:** Asst Clin Prof Med, Cornell Univ-Weill Med Coll

Whang, William MD (CE) - **Spec Exp:** Catheter Ablation; Arrhythmias; Atrial Fibrillation; Pacemakers/Defibrillators; **Hospital:** NY-Presby/Columbia Univ Med Ctr, NY (page 104); **Address:** 161 Fort Washingon Ave, Fl 6, rm 648, New York, NY 10032; **Phone:** 212-305-8559; **Board Cert:** Cardiovascular Disease 2004; Cardiac Electrophysiology 2005; **Med School:** Columbia P&S 1998; **Resid:** Internal Medicine, NY-Presby Hosp/Columbia Univ Med Ctr 2001; **Fellow:** Cardiovascular Disease, Mass Genl Hosp 2004; Cardiac Electrophysiology, Mass Genl Hosp 2006; **Fac Appt:** Asst Clin Prof Med, Columbia P&S

Cardiovascular Disease

Andersen, Holly S MD (Cv) - **Spec Exp:** Preventive Cardiology; Women's Health; Mitral Valve Prolapse; **Hospital:** NY-Presby/Weill Cornell Med Ctr, NY (page 104); **Address:** 425 E 61st St Fl 6, New York, NY 10065; **Phone:** 212-752-2000; **Board Cert:** Internal Medicine 2012; Cardiovascular Disease 2005; **Med School:** Univ Rochester 1989; **Resid:** Internal Medicine, NY Presby-Cornell Med Ctr 1992; **Fellow:** Cardiovascular Disease, NY Presby-Cornell Med Ctr 1995; **Fac Appt:** Assoc Clin Prof Med, Cornell Univ-Weill Med Coll

Berdoff, Russell L MD (Cv) - **Spec Exp:** Coronary Artery Disease; Heart Valve Disease; Preventive Cardiology; **Hospital:** Beth Israel Med Ctr - Petrie Div (page 94); **Address:** 67 Irving Pl, Fl 7, New York, NY 10003; **Phone:** 212-979-9224; **Board Cert:** Internal Medicine 1978; Cardiovascular Disease 1981; **Med School:** NY Med Coll 1975; **Resid:** Internal Medicine, DC Genl Hosp 1978; **Fellow:** Cardiovascular Disease, Johns Hopkins Hosp 1980; **Fac Appt:** Assoc Clin Prof Med, Albert Einstein Coll Med

Berger, Marvin MD (Cv) - **Spec Exp:** Echocardiography; **Hospital:** Beth Israel Med Ctr - Petrie Div (page 94); **Address:** BIMC, Heart Inst, 10 Union Square, Ste 2A, New York, NY 10003; **Phone:** 212-420-2068; **Board Cert:** Internal Medicine 1969; Cardiovascular Disease 1977; **Med School:** Ros Franklin Univ/Chicago Med Sch 1961; **Resid:** Internal Medicine, Beth Israel Med Ctr 1964; **Fellow:** Cardiovascular Disease, Mount Sinai Med Ctr 1965; **Fac Appt:** Prof Med, Albert Einstein Coll Med

Bergmann, Steven R MD/PhD (Cv) - **Spec Exp:** Nuclear Cardiology; Cardiac Imaging; Cardiac Stress Testing; **Hospital:** Beth Israel Med Ctr - Petrie Div (page 94); **Address:** BIMC, Heart Inst, 10 Union Square E, Ste 2A, New York, NY 10003; **Phone:** 212-420-4681; **Board Cert:** Internal Medicine 2013; **Med School:** Washington Univ, St Louis 1985; **Resid:** Internal Medicine, Barnes-Jewish Hosp 1988; **Fellow:** Cardiovascular Disease, Barnes-Jewish Hosp 1990; **Fac Appt:** Prof Med, Albert Einstein Coll Med

Blake, James A MD (Cv) - **Spec Exp:** Congestive Heart Failure; Nuclear Cardiology; Echocardiography; Hypertension; **Hospital:** NY-Presby/Weill Cornell Med Ctr, NY (page 104), Hosp For Special Surgery (page 113); **Address:** 133 E 58th St, Ste 301, New York, NY 10022; **Phone:** 212-755-8700; **Board Cert:** Internal Medicine 1984; Cardiovascular Disease 1987; Echocardiography 2009; Nuclear Cardiology 2009; **Med School:** Albert Einstein Coll Med 1981; **Resid:** Internal Medicine, NY-Presby/Weill Cornell Med Ctr 1984; **Fellow:** Cardiovascular Disease, NY-Presby/Weill Cornell Med Ctr 1987; **Fac Appt:** Assoc Clin Prof Med, Cornell Univ-Weill Med Coll

Blumenthal, David S MD (Cv) - **Spec Exp:** Heart Valve Disease; Preventive Cardiology; Coronary Artery Disease; **Hospital:** NY-Presby/Weill Cornell Med Ctr, NY (page 104); **Address:** 407 E 70th St, Fl 1, New York, NY 10021-5302; **Phone:** 212-861-3222; **Board Cert:** Internal Medicine 1978; Cardiovascular Disease 1981; **Med School:** Cornell Univ-Weill Med Coll 1975; **Resid:** Internal Medicine, NY Hosp 1978; Internal Medicine, NY Hosp 1981; **Fellow:** Cardiovascular Disease, Johns Hopkins Hosp 1980; **Fac Appt:** Clin Prof Med, Cornell Univ-Weill Med Coll

Campagna, Robert MD (Cv) - **Spec Exp:** Coronary Artery Disease; **Hospital:** NY-Presby/Weill Cornell Med Ctr, NY (page 104); **Address:** New York Cardio Assocs, 425 E 61st St Fl 6, New York, NY 10021; **Phone:** 212-752-2000; **Board Cert:** Internal Medicine 2003; Cardiovascular Disease 2005; **Med School:** Cornell Univ-Weill Med Coll 1989; **Resid:** Internal Medicine, NY Presby-Cornell Med Ctr 1992; **Fellow:** Cardiovascular Disease, NY Presby-Cornell Med Ctr 1995; **Fac Appt:** Assoc Clin Prof Med, Cornell Univ-Weill Med Coll

Cemaletin, Nevber S MD (Cv) - **Hospital:** Lenox Hill Hosp (page 106); **Address:** 110 E 59th St, Ste 9B, New York, NY 10022; **Phone:** 212-583-2899; **Board Cert:** Internal Medicine 1988; Cardiovascular Disease 1989; **Med School:** NY Med Coll 1984; **Resid:** Internal Medicine, Lenox Hill Hosp 1987; **Fellow:** Cardiovascular Disease, Lenox Hill Hosp 1989

Cohen, Michael H MD (Cv) - **Spec Exp:** Congestive Heart Failure; Coronary Artery Disease; Hypertension; Cholesterol/Lipid Disorders; **Hospital:** NY-Presby/Columbia Univ Med Ctr, NY (page 104); **Address:** 161 Fort Washington Ave, rm 328, New York, NY 10032-3713; **Phone:** 212-305-5440; **Board Cert:** Internal Medicine 1971; **Med School:** Johns Hopkins Univ 1965; **Resid:** Internal Medicine, NY-Presby Hosp/Columbia Univ 1971; **Fellow:** Cardiovascular Disease, NY-Presby Hosp/Columbia Univ 1970; **Fac Appt:** Clin Prof Med, Johns Hopkins Univ

Cole, William J MD (Cv) - **Spec Exp:** Coronary Artery Disease; Hypertension; Cholesterol/Lipid Disorders; **Hospital:** NYU Langone Med Ctr (page 108); **Address:** 530 First Ave, Ste 3-D, New York, NY 10016; **Phone:** 212-263-7071; **Board Cert:** Internal Medicine 1983; Cardiovascular Disease 1987; **Med School:** NYU Sch Med 1980; **Resid:** Internal Medicine, Bellevue Hosp-NYU Med Ctr 1984; **Fellow:** Cardiovascular Disease, Bellevue Hosp-NYU Med Ctr 1986; **Fac Appt:** Asst Clin Prof Med, NYU Sch Med

Coppola, John T MD (Cv) - **Spec Exp:** Cardiac Catheterization; Angioplasty; **Hospital:** NYU Langone Med Ctr (page 108), Bellevue Hosp Ctr; **Address:** 275 7th Ave Fl 3, New York, NY 10001; **Phone:** 646-660-9999; **Board Cert:** Internal Medicine 1981; Cardiovascular Disease 1983; Interventional Cardiology 2009; **Med School:** NY Med Coll 1978; **Resid:** Internal Medicine, St Vincent Catholic Med Ctr 1981; **Fellow:** Cardiovascular Disease, St Vincent Catholic Med Ctr 1983

Dangas, George MD/PhD (Cv) - **Spec Exp:** Acute Coronary Syndromes; Angioplasty & Stent Placement; Endovascular Therapy; Percutaneous Vascular Interventions; **Hospital:** Mt Sinai Med Ctr (page 102), Mount Sinai Hosp of Queens (page 102); **Address:** Cardiovascular Med Assocs, 1190 5th Ave, rm GP1 South, New York, NY 10029; **Phone:** 212-241-7014; **Board Cert:** Interventional Cardiology 2009; Cardiovascular Disease 2007; Vascular Medicine 2006; Endovascular Medicine 2005; **Med School:** Greece 1989; **Resid:** Internal Medicine, Miriam Hosp 1994; **Fellow:** Cardiovascular Disease, Mount Sinai Med Ctr 1997; Interventional Cardiology, Mount Sinai Med Ctr 1998; **Fac Appt:** Prof Med, Mount Sinai Sch Med

Deutsch, Adam MD (Cv) - **Spec Exp:** Hypertension; Cholesterol/Lipid Disorders; Echocardiography; Congestive Heart Failure; **Hospital:** NY-Presby/Weill Cornell Med Ctr, NY (page 104), Lenox Hill Hosp (page 106); **Address:** Park Avenue Cardiology, 1036 Park Ave, Ste 1A, New York, NY 10028; **Phone:** 212-879-9000; **Board Cert:** Internal Medicine 2006; Cardiovascular Disease 2009; **Med School:** Albert Einstein Coll Med 1992; **Resid:** Internal Medicine, NY-Presby/Columbia Univ Med Ctr 1995; **Fellow:** Cardiovascular Disease, NY-Presby/Columbia Univ Med Ctr 1998

Devereux, Richard B MD (Cv) - **Spec Exp:** Marfan's Syndrome; **Hospital:** NY-Presby/Weill Cornell Med Ctr, NY (page 104); **Address:** 525 E 68th St, rm K-415, New York, NY 10065; **Phone:** 212-746-4655; **Board Cert:** Internal Medicine 1974; Cardiovascular Disease 1977; **Med School:** Univ Pennsylvania 1971; **Resid:** Internal Medicine, New York Hosp 1974; **Fellow:** Cardiovascular Disease, Hosp Univ Penn - UPHS 1976; **Fac Appt:** Prof Med, Cornell Univ Weill Med Coll

Drusin, Ronald MD (Cv) - **Spec Exp:** Cholesterol/Lipid Disorders; Coronary Artery Disease; Heart Valve Disease; Transplant Medicine-Heart; **Hospital:** NY-Presby/Columbia Univ Med Ctr, NY (page 104); **Address:** NY-Presby, Cardiology Dept, 161 Fort Washington Ave, Ste 647, New York, NY 10032; **Phone:** 212-305-5371; **Board Cert:** Internal Medicine 1973; Cardiovascular Disease 1975; **Med School:** Columbia P&S 1966; **Resid:** Internal Medicine, NY-Presby/Columbia Univ Med Ctr 1969; **Fellow:** Cardiovascular Disease, NY-Presby/Columbia Univ Med Ctr 1973; **Fac Appt:** Clin Prof Med, Columbia P&S

Dubois, Nicholas B MD (Cv) - **Spec Exp:** Hypertension; Coronary Artery Disease; Nuclear Cardiology; **Hospital:** Mt Sinai Med Ctr (page 102), Lenox Hill Hosp (page 106); **Address:** Mt Sinai Manhattan Heart, 177 E 87th St, Ste 507, New York, NY 10128; **Phone:** 212-828-3200; **Board Cert:** Cardiovascular Disease 2005; **Med School:** Cornell Univ 1999; **Resid:** Internal Medicine, Montefiore Med Ctr 2002; **Fellow:** Cardiovascular Disease, Cleveland Clinic 2005; **Fac Appt:** Assoc Prof Med, Mount Sinai Sch Med

Friedman, Howard S MD (Cv) - **Spec Exp:** Atrial Fibrillation; Coronary Artery Disease; Hypertension; **Hospital:** NYU Langone Med Ctr (page 108); **Address:** 650 First Ave, Fl 3, New York, NY 10016-3240; **Phone:** 212-889-9393; **Board Cert:** Internal Medicine 1971; Cardiovascular Disease 1974; Geriatric Medicine 2004; **Med School:** SUNY Buffalo 1966; **Resid:** Internal Medicine, Barnes-Jewish Hosp 1968; **Fellow:** Cardiovascular Disease, Mt Sinai Med Ctr 1970; Cardiovascular Disease, Mt Sinai Med Ctr 1973; **Fac Appt:** Clin Prof Med, NYU Sch Med

Friedman, Sanford J MD (Cv) - **Spec Exp:** Preventive Cardiology; **Hospital:** Mt Sinai Med Ctr (page 102); **Address:** 941 Park Ave, New York, NY 10028; **Phone:** 212-988-3772; **Board Cert:** Internal Medicine 1980; Cardiovascular Disease 1977; **Med School:** Tufts Univ 1971; **Resid:** Internal Medicine, Mt Sinai Hosp 1974; **Fellow:** Cardiovascular Disease, Mt Sinai Hosp 1976; **Fac Appt:** Assoc Clin Prof Med, Mount Sinai Sch Med

Fuchs, Richard MD (Cv) - **Spec Exp:** Coronary Artery Disease; Heart Valve Disease; Preventive Cardiology; **Hospital:** NY-Presby/Weill Cornell Med Ctr, NY (page 104); **Address:** 310 E 72nd St, New York, NY 10021; **Phone:** 212-717-2254; **Board Cert:** Internal Medicine 1979; Cardiovascular Disease 1981; **Med School:** Harvard Med Sch 1976; **Resid:** Internal Medicine, New York Hosp 1979; **Fellow:** Cardiovascular Disease, Johns Hopkins Hosp 1982; **Fac Appt:** Clin Prof Med, Cornell Univ-Weill Med Coll

Fuster, Valentin MD/PhD (Cv) - **Spec Exp:** Coronary Artery Disease; Heart Valve Disease; Congenital Heart Disease; Preventive Cardiology; **Hospital:** Mt Sinai Med Ctr (page 102); **Address:** Cardiovascular Med Assocs, 1190 Fifth Ave Fl 1, New York, NY 10029-6500; **Phone:** 212-241-7911; **Board Cert:** Internal Medicine 1976; Cardiovascular Disease 1977; **Med School:** Spain 1967; **Resid:** Internal Medicine, Mayo Clin 1972; Cardiovascular Disease, Mayo Clin 1974; **Fellow:** Cardiovascular Disease, Univ Edinburgh 1971; **Fac Appt:** Prof Med, Mount Sinai Sch Med

Gliklich, Jerry MD (Cv) - **Spec Exp:** Heart Valve Disease; Arrhythmias; **Hospital:** NY-Presby/Columbia Univ Med Ctr, NY (page 104); **Address:** NY-Presby, Heart Ctr, 173 Fort Washington Ave, Ste 606, New York, NY 10032; **Phone:** 212-305-5588; **Board Cert:** Internal Medicine 1978; Cardiovascular Disease 1981; **Med School:** Columbia P&S 1975; **Resid:** Internal Medicine, NY-Presby/Weill Cornell Med Ctr 1978; **Fellow:** Cardiovascular Disease, NY-Presby/Columbia Univ Med Ctr 1981; **Fac Appt:** Clin Prof Med, Columbia P&S

Goldberg, Harvey L MD (Cv) - **Spec Exp:** Coronary Artery Disease; **Hospital:** NY-Presby/Weill Cornell Med Ctr, NY (page 104), Lenox Hill Hosp (page 106); **Address:** New York Cardio Assocs, 425 E 61st St Fl 6, New York, NY 10021-8795; **Phone:** 212-752-2000; **Board Cert:** Internal Medicine 1979; Cardiovascular Disease 1981; **Med School:** Cornell Univ 1976; **Resid:** Internal Medicine, New York Hosp 1979; **Fellow:** Cardiovascular Disease, New York Hosp-Cornell 1981; **Fac Appt:** Assoc Clin Prof Med, Cornell Univ-Weill Med Coll

Goldberg, Nieca MD (Cv) - **Spec Exp:** Women's Health; Preventive Cardiology; Heart Disease in Women; **Hospital:** NYU Langone Med Ctr (page 108), Lenox Hill Hosp (page 106); **Address:** Joan H. Tisch Ctr for Women's Hlth, 207 E 84th St, New York, NY 10028; **Phone:** 212-289-2045; **Board Cert:** Internal Medicine 1987; Cardiovascular Disease 2005; **Med School:** SUNY Downstate 1984; **Resid:** Internal Medicine, St. Luke's - Roosevelt Hosp Ctr - Roosevelt Div 1987; **Fellow:** Cardiovascular Disease, SUNY Downstate Affil Hosp 1990; **Fac Appt:** Assoc Clin Prof Med, NYU Sch Med

Goldman, Martin E MD (Cv) - **Spec Exp:** Heart Valve Disease; Echocardiography; Diagnostic Problems; **Hospital:** Mt Sinai Med Ctr (page 102); **Address:** Mt Sinai, Cardiology Dept, 1190 5th Ave, New York, NY 10029; **Phone:** 212-241-3078; **Board Cert:** Internal Medicine 1979; Cardiovascular Disease 1981; **Med School:** Albert Einstein Coll Med 1976; **Resid:** Internal Medicine, Brigham & Womens Hosp 1978; **Fellow:** Cardiovascular Disease, Mount Sinai Med Ctr 1980; **Fac Appt:** Prof Med, Mount Sinai Sch Med

Goodman, Dennis A MD (Cv) - **Spec Exp:** Preventive Cardiology; Cholesterol/Lipid Disorders; Complementary Medicine; **Hospital:** NYU Langone Med Ctr (page 108), Lenox Hill Hosp (page 106); **Address:** 635 Madison Ave, Fl 3, New York, NY 10022; **Phone:** 212-784-5998; **Board Cert:** Internal Medicine 1984; Cardiovascular Disease 1989; Integrative Medicine 2006; **Med School:** South Africa 1979; **Resid:** Internal Medicine, Montefiore Med Ctr 1984; **Fellow:** Cardiovascular Disease, Baylor Coll Med 1987; **Fac Appt:** Assoc Clin Prof Med, NYU Sch Med

Halperin, Jonathan L MD (Cv) - **Spec Exp:** Vascular Disease; Atrial Fibrillation; **Hospital:** Mt Sinai Med Ctr (page 102); **Address:** Cardiology Associates, 1190 Fifth Ave, New York, NY 10029; **Phone:** 212-241-7243; **Board Cert:** Internal Medicine 1980; Cardiovascular Disease 1981; **Med School:** Boston Univ 1975; **Resid:** Internal Medicine, Boston Univ Med Ctr 1977; **Fellow:** Vascular Medicine, Boston Univ Med Ctr 1978; Cardiovascular Disease, Boston Univ Med Ctr 1980; **Fac Appt:** Prof Med, Mount Sinai Sch Med

Hecht, Alan MD (Cv) - **Spec Exp:** Heart Valve Disease; Coronary Artery Disease; Arrhythmias; **Hospital:** Mt Sinai Med Ctr (page 102); **Address:** 1075 Park Ave, New York, NY 10128; **Phone:** 212-876-0845; **Board Cert:** Internal Medicine 1984; Cardiovascular Disease 1987; **Med School:** Northwestern Univ 1981; **Resid:** Internal Medicine, Mt Sinai Hosp 1984; **Fellow:** Cardiovascular Disease, Mt Sinai Hosp 1986; **Fac Appt:** Assoc Clin Prof Med, Mount Sinai Sch Med

Horn, Evelyn M MD (Cv) - **Spec Exp:** Pulmonary Hypertension; Heart Failure; Ventricular Assist Device (LVAD); **Hospital:** NY-Presby/Weill Cornell Med Ctr, NY (page 104); **Address:** 520 E 70th St Starr Bldg Fl 4 - Ste 443, New York, NY 10021; **Phone:** 212-746-2381; **Board Cert:** Internal Medicine 1983; Cardiovascular Disease 1985; Advanced Heart Failure & Transplant Cardiology 2010; **Med School:** Mount Sinai Sch Med 1980; **Resid:** Internal Medicine, Mt Sinai Hosp 1983; **Fellow:** Cardiovascular Disease, Cedars-Sinai Med Ctr 1985; **Fac Appt:** Clin Prof Med, Cornell Univ-Weill Med Coll

Inra, Lawrence A MD (Cv) - **Spec Exp:** Coronary Artery Disease; Preventive Cardiology; Cholesterol/Lipid Disorders; Hypertension; **Hospital:** NY-Presby/Weill Cornell Med Ctr, NY (page 104), Hosp For Special Surgery (page 113); **Address:** 407 E 70th St, New York, NY 10021; **Phone:** 212-249-1011; **Board Cert:** Internal Medicine 1979; Cardiovascular Disease 1981; **Med School:** Johns Hopkins Univ 1976; **Resid:** Internal Medicine, Presby/Weill Cornell Med Ctr 1979; **Fellow:** Cardiovascular Disease, Mt Sinai Med Ctr 1981; **Fac Appt:** Assoc Clin Prof Med, Cornell Univ-Weill Med Coll

Jorde, Ulrich MD (Cv) - **Hospital:** NY-Presby/Columbia Univ Med Ctr, NY (page 104); **Address:** NY Presby/Columbia, Cardiology Dept, 622 W 168 St, PH12 rm 134, New York, NY 10032; **Phone:** 212-305-9264; **Board Cert:** Cardiovascular Disease 2011; **Med School:** Germany 1991; **Resid:** Internal Medicine, Mount Sinai Med Ctr 1995; **Fellow:** Cardiovascular Disease, Albert Einstein Coll Med 1999; **Fac Appt:** Assoc Prof Med, Columbia P&S

Kalman, Jill MD (Cv) - **Spec Exp:** Heart Failure; Cardiomyopathy; Heart Disease in Women; **Hospital:** Mt Sinai Med Ctr (page 102); **Address:** Mt Sinai, Cardiology Dept, 1190 5th Ave, rm 6-178B, New York, NY 10029; **Phone:** 212-241-0511; **Board Cert:** Cardiovascular Disease 2005; **Med School:** Mount Sinai Sch Med 1987; **Resid:** Internal Medicine, Mount Sinai Med Ctr 1991; **Fellow:** Cardiovascular Disease, Mount Sinai Med Ctr 1995; **Fac Appt:** Assoc Prof Med, Mount Sinai Sch Med

Kamen, Mazen O MD (Cv) - **Spec Exp:** Heart Valve Disease; Cholesterol/Lipid Disorders; Hypertension; Coronary Artery Disease; **Hospital:** NY-Presby/Weill Cornell Med Ctr, NY (page 104); **Address:** 1021 Park Ave, Ste 101, New York, NY 10028; **Phone:** 212-427-5800; **Board Cert:** Cardiovascular Disease 2006; **Med School:** NYU Sch Med 1983; **Resid:** Surgery, NYU Med Ctr 1984; Internal Medicine, NYU Med Ctr 1986; **Fellow:** Cardiovascular Disease, NY-Presby/Weill Cornell Med Ctr 1990; **Fac Appt:** Asst Clin Prof Med, Cornell Univ-Weill Med Coll

Katz, Edward S MD (Cv) - **Spec Exp:** Echocardiography; Cholesterol/Lipid Disorders; Coronary Artery Disease; **Hospital:** NYU Langone Med Ctr (page 108), NYU Hosp For Joint Dis (page 108); **Address:** NYU Cardiology Associates, 530 1st Ave, Ste 9U, New York, NY 10016; **Phone:** 212-263-7751; **Board Cert:** Cardiovascular Disease 2011; Internal Medicine 1988; Echocardiography 2005; **Med School:** NYU Sch Med 1985; **Resid:** Internal Medicine, NYU Med Ctr 1988; **Fellow:** Cardiovascular Disease, NYU Med Ctr 1991; **Fac Appt:** Assoc Prof Med, NYU Sch Med

Katz, Stuart D MD (Cv) - **Spec Exp:** Heart Failure; Transplant Medicine-Heart; **Hospital:** NYU Langone Med Ctr (page 108); **Address:** NYU Cardiology Assocs, 530 First Ave Skirball Bldg - Ste 9U, New York, NY 10016; **Phone:** 212-263-7751; **Board Cert:** Internal Medicine 1986; Cardiovascular Disease 1989; Advanced Heart Failure & Transplant Cardiology 2010; **Med School:** SUNY Downstate 1983; **Resid:** Internal Medicine, Johns Hopkins Bayview Med Ctr 1986; **Fellow:** Cardiovascular Disease, Montefiore Med Ctr-Moses Campus 1989; **Fac Appt:** Prof Med, NYU Sch Med

Kligfield, Paul MD (Cv) - **Hospital:** NY-Presby/Weill Cornell Med Ctr, NY (page 104); **Address:** NY-Presby, Cardiology Dept, 525 E 68th St, Ste L195, New York, NY 10021; **Phone:** 212-746-4686; **Board Cert:** Internal Medicine 1973; Cardiovascular Disease 1975; **Med School:** Harvard Med Sch 1970; **Resid:** Internal Medicine, Beth Israel Deaconess Med Ctr 1972; **Fellow:** Cardiovascular Research, St Georges Hosp 1973; Cardiovascular Disease, NY-Presby/Weill Cornell Med Ctr 1975; **Fac Appt:** Prof Med, Cornell Univ-Weill Med Coll

Kronzon, Itzhak MD (Cv) - **Spec Exp:** Heart Valve Disease; Echocardiography; Cardiac Imaging; Pericardial Disease; **Hospital:** Lenox Hill Hosp (page 106); **Address:** Lenox Hill Hosp, Cardiology Dept, 100 E 77th St Fl 2, New York, NY 10075; **Phone:** 212-434-6119; **Board Cert:** Internal Medicine 1979; Cardiovascular Disease 1981; Echocardiography 2013; **Med School:** Israel 1964; **Resid:** Internal Medicine, Hadassah Hosp 1969; **Fellow:** Cardiovascular Disease, Montefiore Med Ctr 1973; Cardiovascular Disease, NYU Med Ctr 1974; **Fac Appt:** Prof Med, NYU Sch Med

Kutnick, Richard T MD (Cv) - **Spec Exp:** Echocardiography; **Hospital:** Lenox Hill Hosp (page 106); **Address:** 1421 3rd Ave, Fl 6, New York, NY 10028; **Phone:** 212-879-2628; **Board Cert:** Internal Medicine 1979; Cardiovascular Disease 1981; **Med School:** Tufts Univ 1976; **Resid:** Internal Medicine, Lenox Hill Hosp 1979; **Fellow:** Cardiovascular Disease, Lenox Hill Hosp 1981; **Fac Appt:** Asst Prof Med, NYU Sch Med

Lewis, Benjamin H MD (Cv) - **Spec Exp:** Cardiac Stress Testing; Heart Disease & Gender; Echocardiography; Preventive Cardiology; **Hospital:** NY-Presby/Columbia Univ Med Ctr, NY (page 104), Lenox Hill Hosp (page 106); **Address:** 51 W 51st St, Fl 3, Ste 365, New York, NY 10019; **Phone:** 212-326-8425; **Board Cert:** Internal Medicine 1980; Cardiovascular Disease 1983; **Med School:** UCSF 1977; **Resid:** Internal Medicine, Columbia-Presby Hosp 1980; **Fellow:** Cardiovascular Disease, Brigham Womens Hosp 1982; **Fac Appt:** Assoc Prof Med, Columbia P&S

Mancini, Donna M MD (Cv) - **Spec Exp:** Congestive Heart Failure; Transplant Medicine-Heart; **Hospital:** NY-Presby/Columbia Univ Med Ctr, NY (page 104); **Address:** NY-Presby, Ctr Advanced Cardiac Care, 622 W 168th St Fl 12 - rm 134, New York, NY 10032; **Phone:** 212-305-4600; **Board Cert:** Internal Medicine 1983; Cardiovascular Disease 1987; Advanced Heart Failure & Transplant Cardiology 2010; **Med School:** Albert Einstein Coll Med 1980; **Resid:** Internal Medicine, Jacobi Med Ctr 1983; **Fellow:** Cardiovascular Disease, Jacobi Med Ctr 1986; **Fac Appt:** Prof Med, Columbia P&S

Masri, Bassem M MD (Cv) - **Spec Exp:** Cholesterol/Lipid Disorders; Coronary Artery Disease; Preventive Cardiology; Hypertension; **Hospital:** NY-Presby/Weill Cornell Med Ctr, NY (page 104); **Address:** NY-Presby, Cardiac Prevention Ctr, 1305 York Ave Fl 8, New York, NY 10021; **Phone:** 646-962-6004; **Med School:** Lebanon 1988; **Resid:** Internal Medicine, Ameri Univ Beirut 1991; **Fellow:** Cardiovascular Disease, Baylor Med Ctr 1991; **Fac Appt:** Asst Prof Med, Cornell Univ-Weill Med Coll

Matta, Raymond J MD (Cv) - **Hospital:** Mt Sinai Med Ctr (page 102); **Address:** 1120 Park Ave, Ste 1C, New York, NY 10128; **Phone:** 212-410-5800; **Board Cert:** Internal Medicine 1973; Cardiovascular Disease 1975; **Med School:** Univ Pittsburgh 1969; **Resid:** Internal Medicine, Mass Genl Hosp 1971; **Fellow:** Cardiovascular Disease, Brigham & Womens Hosp 1975; **Fac Appt:** Assoc Clin Prof Med, Mount Sinai Sch Med

Mattes, Leonard MD (Cv) - **Hospital:** Mt Sinai Med Ctr (page 102); **Address:** 1199 Park Ave, Ste 1F, New York, NY 10128; **Phone:** 212-876-7045; **Board Cert:** Internal Medicine 1972; Cardiovascular Disease 1975; **Med School:** Tulane Univ 1962; **Resid:** Internal Medicine, Mount Sinai Med Ctr 1967; Cardiovascular Disease, Mount Sinai Med Ctr 1969; **Fellow:** Cardiovascular Disease, Mount Sinai Med Ctr 1968; **Fac Appt:** Asst Clin Prof Med, Mount Sinai Sch Med

Meller, Jose MD (Cv) - **Spec Exp:** Preventive Cardiology; Coronary Artery Disease; Heart Disease in Pregnancy; Heart Valve Disease; **Hospital:** Mt Sinai Med Ctr (page 102); **Address:** 941 Park Ave, New York, NY 10028; **Phone:** 212-988-3772; **Board Cert:** Internal Medicine 1973; Cardiovascular Disease 1975; **Med School:** Chile 1969; **Resid:** Internal Medicine, Elmhurst Hosp 1971; Internal Medicine, Mt Sinai Med Ctr 1972; **Fellow:** Cardiovascular Disease, Mt Sinai Med Ctr 1974; **Fac Appt:** Clin Prof Med, Mount Sinai Sch Med

Messerli, Franz Hannes MD (Cv) - **Spec Exp:** Hypertension; Heart Failure; Coronary Artery Disease; **Hospital:** St. Luke's - Roosevelt Hosp Ctr - Roosevelt Div (page 94); **Address:** University Medical Practice Assocs, Div Cardiology, 425 W 59th St, Ste 9C, New York, NY 10019; **Phone:** 212-492-5550; **Board Cert:** Internal Medicine 1978; **Med School:** Switzerland 1970; **Resid:** Internal Medicine, Univ of Bern Inselspital 1973; **Fellow:** Cardiovascular Disease, Hotel Dieu Hospital 1975

Miller, David H MD (Cv) - **Spec Exp:** Hypertension; Coronary Artery Disease; **Hospital:** NY-Presby/Weill Cornell Med Ctr, NY (page 104); **Address:** NY-Presby, Cardiology Dept, 520 E 70th St, Ste 443, New York, NY 10021; **Phone:** 212-746-2144; **Board Cert:** Internal Medicine 1980; Cardiovascular Disease 1981; **Med School:** Univ VA Sch Med 1976; **Resid:** Internal Medicine, NY-Presby/Weill Cornell Med Ctr 1979; **Fellow:** Cardiovascular Disease, NY-Presby/Weill Cornell Med Ctr 1981; **Fac Appt:** Assoc Prof Med, Cornell Univ-Weill Med Coll

Mueller, Richard L MD (Cv) - **Spec Exp:** Vein Disorders; Stress Echocardiography; Hypertension; Echocardiography; **Hospital:** NY-Presby/Weill Cornell Med Ctr, NY (page 104), St. Luke's - Roosevelt Hosp Ctr - St Luke's Hosp (page 94); **Address:** Cardiovascular Diagnostics, PC, Cosmetic Vein Solutions - Sutton Place Laser Vein Removal, 401 E 55th St, New York, NY 10022-6158; **Phone:** 212-593-9800; **Board Cert:** Internal Medicine 2010; Cardiovascular Disease 2000; Echocardiography 1999; Vascular Medicine 2006; **Med School:** UCSF 1987; **Resid:** Internal Medicine, North Shore Univ Hosp 1991; Internal Medicine, Meml Sloan Kettering Cancer Ctr 1990; **Fellow:** Cardiovascular Disease, New York Hosp 1994; **Fac Appt:** Asst Clin Prof Med, Cornell Univ-Weill Med Coll

Myerson, Merle MD (Cv) - **Spec Exp:** Preventive Cardiology; Cholesterol/Lipid Disorders; **Hospital:** St. Luke's - Roosevelt Hosp Ctr - Roosevelt Div (page 94), St. Luke's - Roosevelt Hosp Ctr - St Luke's Hosp (page 94); **Address:** 425 W 59th St, Ste 9C, Ctr for CV Disease Prevention, New York, NY 10019; **Phone:** 212-492-5550; **Board Cert:** Cardiovascular Disease 2003; **Med School:** SUNY Downstate 1993; **Resid:** Internal Medicine, Duke Univ Med Ctr 1996; **Fellow:** Cardiovascular Epidemiology, Mary Imogene Basset Hosp 1997; Cardiovascular Disease, Columbia Univ Med Ctr 2001

Nash, Ira S MD (Cv) - **Spec Exp:** Preventive Cardiology; Coronary Artery Disease; **Hospital:** Lenox Hill Hosp (page 106), NS-LIJ Hlth Sys (page 106); **Address:** Park East Cardiovascular, 158 E 84th St, New York, NY 10028; **Phone:** 212-535-6340 x204; **Board Cert:** Internal Medicine 1987; Cardiovascular Disease 1989; **Med School:** Harvard Med Sch 1984; **Resid:** Internal Medicine, Beth Israel Hosp 1987; **Fellow:** Cardiovascular Disease, Beth Israel Hosp 1990

O'Brien, Francis J MD (Cv) - **Spec Exp:** Preventive Cardiology; **Hospital:** NYU Langone Med Ctr (page 108), Bellevue Hosp Ctr; **Address:** 347 E 37th St Fl 2, New York, NY 10016; **Phone:** 212-726-7457; **Board Cert:** Internal Medicine 1985; Cardiovascular Disease 1989; **Med School:** Harvard Med Sch 1982; **Resid:** Internal Medicine, NYU Med Ctr 1986; **Fellow:** Cardiovascular Disease, Bellevue-NYU Hosp 1988; **Fac Appt:** Assoc Clin Prof Med, NYU Sch Med

Pinney, Sean MD (Cv) - **Spec Exp:** Transplant Medicine-Heart; Heart Failure; Pulmonary Hypertension; Congenital Heart Disease; **Hospital:** Mt Sinai Med Ctr (page 102); **Address:** Mt Sinai, Cardiovascular Med Assocs, 5 E 98th St Fl 3, New York, NY 10029; **Phone:** 212-241-7300; **Board Cert:** Cardiovascular Disease 2011; Advanced Heart Failure & Transplant Cardiology 2012; **Med School:** Georgetown Univ 1994; **Resid:** Internal Medicine, Bet Israel Deaconess Med Ctr 1999; **Fellow:** Cardiovascular Disease, NY-Presby/Columbia Univ Med Ctr 2001; Transplant Medicine, NY-Presby/Columbia Univ Med Ctr 2002; **Fac Appt:** Assoc Prof Med, Mount Sinai Sch Med

Poon, Michael MD (Cv) - **Spec Exp:** Coronary Artery Disease; Pulmonary Hypertension; Cardiac CT Angiography; Cardiac Imaging; **Hospital:** Stony Brook Univ Med Ctr, Mt Sinai Med Ctr (page 102); **Address:** 70 Bowery, Ste 303, New York, NY 10013; **Phone:** 212-925-4088; **Board Cert:** Cardiovascular Disease 2007; Cardiovascular Computed Tomography 2008; **Med School:** Mount Sinai Sch Med 1987; **Resid:** Internal Medicine, Mount Sinai Med Ctr 1991; **Fellow:** Cardiovascular Disease, Mount Sinai Med Ctr 1993; **Fac Appt:** Prof Med, SUNY Stony Brook

Post, Martin R MD (Cv) - **Spec Exp:** Coronary Artery Disease; Cholesterol/Lipid Disorders; **Hospital:** NY-Presby/Weill Cornell Med Ctr, NY (page 104); **Address:** 425 E 61st St Fl 6, New York, NY 10021-8722; **Phone:** 212-752-2000; **Board Cert:** Internal Medicine 1974; Cardiovascular Disease 1974; **Med School:** SUNY Upstate Med Univ 1967; **Resid:** Internal Medicine, Ohio State Univ Hosp 1970; **Fellow:** Cardiovascular Disease, New York Hosp 1972

Radwaner, Bradley A MD (Cv) - **Spec Exp:** Preventive Cardiology; Cholesterol/Lipid Disorders; Interventional Cardiology; **Hospital:** Lenox Hill Hosp (page 106); **Address:** 136 E 57th St, Suite 1001, New York, NY 10022; **Phone:** 212-717-0666; **Board Cert:** Internal Medicine 1983; Cardiovascular Disease 1985; **Med School:** Cornell Univ-Weill Med Coll 1980; **Resid:** Internal Medicine, Lenox Hill Hosp 1983; **Fellow:** Cardiovascular Disease, St Lukes Hosp 1985; Interventional Cardiology, NYU Med Ctr 1986; **Fac Appt:** Asst Clin Prof Med, Cornell Univ-Weill Med Coll

Reichstein, Robert P MD (Cv) - **Spec Exp:** Preventive Cardiology; Atrial Fibrillation; Hypertension; **Hospital:** Mt Sinai Med Ctr (page 102); **Address:** 1185 Park Ave, Ste 1L, New York, NY 10128; **Phone:** 212-996-2900; **Board Cert:** Internal Medicine 1980; Cardiovascular Disease 1983; **Med School:** Ros Franklin Univ/Chicago Med Sch 1977; **Resid:** Internal Medicine, Mt Sinai Hosp 1981; **Fellow:** Cardiovascular Disease, Mt Sinai Hosp 1984; **Fac Appt:** Asst Clin Prof Med, Finch/Chicago Med Sch

Rentrop, K. Peter MD (Cv) - **Spec Exp:** Nuclear Cardiology; **Hospital:** NYU Langone Med Ctr (page 108); **Address:** 920 Broadway, Ste 600, New York, NY 10010; **Phone:** 212-475-8066; **Board Cert:** Internal Medicine 1973; Nuclear Cardiology 2013; **Med School:** Germany 1966; **Resid:** Internal Medicine, Detroit Med Ctr 1970; Internal Medicine, Cleveland Clin 1971; **Fellow:** Cardiovascular Disease, Cleveland Clin 1973; **Fac Appt:** Prof Med, NY Med Coll

Romanello, Paul P MD (Cv) - **Spec Exp:** Cholesterol/Lipid Disorders; Coronary Artery Disease; Hypertension; Nuclear Cardiology; **Hospital:** Lenox Hill Hosp (page 106); **Address:** Park East Cardiovascular, 158 E 84th St, New York, NY 10028; **Phone:** 212-535-6340; **Board Cert:** Internal Medicine 1987; Cardiovascular Disease 1989; Nuclear Cardiology 2008; **Med School:** SUNY Upstate Med Univ 1983; **Resid:** Internal Medicine, Lenox Hill Hosp 1987; **Fellow:** Cardiovascular Disease, Lenox Hill Hosp 1989

Rosenbaum, Marlon S MD (Cv) - **Spec Exp:** Congenital Heart Disease-Adult; Heart Valve Disease; **Hospital:** NY-Presby/Columbia Univ Med Ctr, NY (page 104); **Address:** NY-Presby, Adult Congential Heart Ctr, 161 Fort Washington Ave, rm 627, New York, NY 10032; **Phone:** 212-305-6936; **Board Cert:** Internal Medicine 1983; Cardiovascular Disease 1985; **Med School:** NYU Sch Med 1980; **Resid:** Internal Medicine, NY-Presby/Columbia Univ Med Ctr 1983; **Fellow:** Cardiovascular Disease, Westchester Med Ctr 1985; Cardiovascular Disease, Mass Genl Hosp 1986; **Fac Appt:** Assoc Clin Prof Med, Columbia P&S

Rozanski, Alan MD (Cv) - **Spec Exp:** Nuclear Cardiology; Stress Management; **Hospital:** St. Luke's - Roosevelt Hosp Ctr - Roosevelt Div (page 94); **Address:** 1111 Amsterdam Ave, New York, NY 10025; **Phone:** 212-523-4011; **Board Cert:** Internal Medicine 1978; Cardiovascular Disease 1983; Nuclear Medicine 1983; **Med School:** Tufts Univ 1975; **Resid:** Internal Medicine, Mt Sinai Hosp 1978; **Fellow:** Cardiovascular Disease, Mt Sinai Hosp 1980; Nuclear Medicine, Cedars-Sinai Med Ctr 1982; **Fac Appt:** Prof Med, Columbia P&S

Ruiz, Carlos E MD/PhD (Cv) - **Spec Exp:** Interventional Cardiology; Transplant Medicine-Heart; Cardiac Catheterization; **Hospital:** Lenox Hill Hosp (page 106); **Address:** Lenox Hill Hosp, Cardiac & Vascular, 130 E 77th St Fl 4, New York, NY 10075; **Phone:** 212-434-2606; **Board Cert:** Internal Medicine ; **Med School:** Spain 1972; **Resid:** Pediatrics, Univ Barcelona 1973; Internal Medicine, LAC & USC Med Ctr 1978; **Fellow:** Cardiovascular Disease, Univ Barcelona 1975; Critical Care Medicine, LAC & USC Med Ctr 1977

Schiffer, Mark B MD (Cv) - **Spec Exp:** Preventive Cardiology; Cholesterol/Lipid Disorders; Coronary Artery Disease; **Hospital:** Lenox Hill Hosp (page 106); **Address:** Park East Cardiovascular, 158 E 84th St, New York, NY 10028; **Phone:** 212-535-6340; **Board Cert:** Internal Medicine 1980; Cardiovascular Disease 1983; **Med School:** Northwestern Univ 1977; **Resid:** Internal Medicine, Lenox Hill Hosp 1981; **Fellow:** Cardiovascular Disease, Lenox Hill Hosp 1983

Schulman, Ira C MD (Cv) - **Spec Exp:** Angina; Heart Failure; Cholesterol/Lipid Disorders; **Hospital:** NYU Langone Med Ctr (page 108), NY-Presby/Lower Manhattan Hosp (page 104); **Address:** 111 Broadway, Fl 2, New York, NY 10006; **Phone:** 212-263-9700; **Board Cert:** Internal Medicine 1977; Cardiovascular Disease 1979; **Med School:** NYU Sch Med 1974; **Resid:** Internal Medicine, Bellevue Hosp 1977; **Fellow:** Cardiovascular Disease, Montefiore Med Ctr 1979; **Fac Appt:** Assoc Prof Med, NYU Sch Med

Schwartz, Allan MD (Cv) - **Hospital:** NY-Presby/Columbia Univ Med Ctr, NY (page 104); **Address:** 173 Fort Washington Ave, Ste 4-600C, New York, NY 10032; **Phone:** 212-305-5367; **Board Cert:** Internal Medicine 1977; Cardiovascular Disease 1979; **Med School:** Columbia P&S 1974; **Resid:** Internal Medicine, Columbia-Presby Med Ctr 1976; **Fellow:** Cardiovascular Disease, Mass Genl Hosp 1978; **Fac Appt:** Clin Prof Med, Columbia P&S

Schwartz, William J MD (Cv) - **Spec Exp:** Coronary Artery Disease; Cardiac Catheterization; Congestive Heart Failure; **Hospital:** Mt Sinai Med Ctr (page 102); **Address:** Mt Sinai Multispecialty Physicians, 150 E 77th St, Ste 1E, New York, NY 10075; **Phone:** 212-439-6000; **Board Cert:** Internal Medicine 1978; Cardiovascular Disease 1981; **Med School:** Albert Einstein Coll Med 1975; **Resid:** Internal Medicine, Bronx Municipal Hosp 1978; **Fellow:** Cardiovascular Disease, Bronx Municipal Hosp 1981; **Fac Appt:** Asst Prof Med, Mount Sinai Sch Med

Seinfeld, David MD (Cv) - **Spec Exp:** Preventive Cardiology; **Hospital:** Lenox Hill Hosp (page 106); **Address:** 20 E 68th St, Ste 214, New York, NY 10065; **Phone:** 212-288-1538; **Board Cert:** Internal Medicine 1976; Cardiovascular Disease 1979; **Med School:** Albert Einstein Coll Med 1973; **Resid:** Internal Medicine, Montefiore Med Ctr 1976; **Fellow:** Cardiovascular Disease, Montefiore Med Ctr 1978; **Fac Appt:** Assoc Clin Prof Med, Albert Einstein Coll Med

Sherman, Warren MD (Cv) - **Spec Exp:** Angioplasty; Interventional Cardiology; **Hospital:** NY-Presby/Columbia Univ Med Ctr, NY (page 104); **Address:** NY-Presby, Cardiology Dept, 161 Fort Washington Ave Fl 6, New York, NY 10032; **Phone:** 212-304-5697; **Board Cert:** Internal Medicine 1980; Cardiovascular Disease 1983; **Med School:** SUNY Upstate Med Univ 1977; **Resid:** Internal Medicine, Rochester Genl Hosp 1980; **Fellow:** Cardiovascular Disease, OR Hlth Sci Univ 1982; **Fac Appt:** Assoc Prof Med, Columbia P&S

Shimony, Rony MD (Cv) - **Spec Exp:** Coronary Artery Disease; Arrhythmias; Heart Failure; Non-Invasive Cardiology; **Hospital:** Mt Sinai Med Ctr (page 102); **Address:** 485 Madison Ave Fl 17, New York, NY 10022; **Phone:** 212-752-2700; **Board Cert:** Internal Medicine 1987; Cardiovascular Disease 1989; **Med School:** SUNY Buffalo 1984; **Resid:** Internal Medicine, Lenox Hill Hosp 1987; **Fellow:** Cardiovascular Disease, Lenox Hill Hosp 1989; Cardiac Electrophysiology, Lenox Hill Hosp 1992; **Fac Appt:** Asst Prof Med, Mount Sinai Sch Med

Siegal, Michael S MD (Cv) - **Spec Exp:** Coronary Artery Disease; **Hospital:** St. Luke's - Roosevelt Hosp Ctr - Roosevelt Div (page 94); **Address:** 30 Central Park S, Ste 13A, New York, NY 10019; **Phone:** 212-319-1700; **Board Cert:** Internal Medicine 1980; Cardiovascular Disease 1983; **Med School:** Columbia P&S 1977; **Resid:** Internal Medicine, Bellevue/NYU Med Ctr 1980; **Fellow:** Cardiovascular Disease, Mt Sinai Hosp 1982

Siegel, Stephen A MD (Cv) - **Spec Exp:** Sports Medicine-Cardiology; Preventive Cardiology; Cholesterol/Lipid Disorders; Hypertension; **Hospital:** NYU Langone Med Ctr (page 108); **Address:** 245 E 35th St, New York, NY 10016; **Phone:** 212-684-1108; **Board Cert:** Internal Medicine 1981; Cardiovascular Disease 1983; **Med School:** Med Coll VA 1978; **Resid:** Internal Medicine, NYU Med Ctr/Bellevue Hosp Ctr 1981; **Fellow:** Cardiovascular Disease, NYU Med Ctr/Bellevue Hosp Ctr 1983; **Fac Appt:** Asst Clin Prof Med, NYU Sch Med

Sklaroff, Herschel J MD (Cv) - **Spec Exp:** Angina; Syncope; Hypertension; Diagnostic Problems; **Hospital:** Mt Sinai Med Ctr (page 102); **Address:** 1175 Park Ave, New York, NY 10128; **Phone:** 212-289-6500; **Board Cert:** Internal Medicine 1969; Cardiovascular Disease 1977; **Med School:** Univ Pennsylvania 1961; **Resid:** Internal Medicine, Mount Sinai Med Ctr 1965; Cardiovascular Disease, Mount Sinai Med Ctr 1966; **Fac Appt:** Clin Prof Med, Mount Sinai Sch Med

Slater, William R MD (Cv) - **Spec Exp:** Arrhythmias; Heart Valve Disease; Cardiac Electrophysiology; **Hospital:** NYU Langone Med Ctr (page 108); **Address:** NYU Medical Ctr, Div Cardiology, 530 First Ave Skirball Bldg - Ste 9U, New York, NY 10016; **Phone:** 212-263-7463; **Board Cert:** Internal Medicine 1981; Cardiovascular Disease 1985; **Med School:** Harvard Med Sch 1978; **Resid:** Internal Medicine, Bellevue Hosp Ctr 1981; **Fellow:** Cardiovascular Disease, Mt Sinai Hosp 1984; Cardiovascular Disease, Mass Genl Hosp/Brigham & Womens Hosp 1986; **Fac Appt:** Assoc Prof Med, NYU Sch Med

Spiegel, Alan MD (Cv) - **Spec Exp:** Arrhythmias; Heart Valve Disease; Cholesterol/Lipid Disorders; Preventive Cardiology; **Hospital:** NYU Langone Med Ctr (page 108); **Address:** Concorde Medical Grp-Cardiology Division, 38 E 32nd St, Ste 801, New York, NY 10016; **Phone:** 212-684-7172; **Board Cert:** Internal Medicine 1981; Cardiovascular Disease 1987; **Med School:** Albert Einstein Coll Med 1978; **Resid:** Internal Medicine, Bellevue Hosp Ctr 1982; **Fellow:** Cardiovascular Disease, Univ of Penn 1984; **Fac Appt:** Asst Clin Prof Med, NYU Sch Med

Stein, Richard A MD (Cv) - **Spec Exp:** Preventive Cardiology; Coronary Artery Disease; Cardiac Rehabilitation; **Hospital:** NYU Langone Med Ctr (page 108); **Address:** NYU Cardiology Associates, 530 First Ave, Ste 9U, New York, NY 10016; **Phone:** 212-263-7751; **Board Cert:** Internal Medicine 1973; Cardiovascular Disease 1975; Sports Medicine 2007; **Med School:** NYU Sch Med 1967; **Resid:** Internal Medicine, Univ Hosp 1969; **Fellow:** Cardiovascular Disease, Univ Hosp 1974; **Fac Appt:** Prof Med, NYU Sch Med

Steinbaum, Suzanne R DO (Cv) - **Spec Exp:** Heart Disease in Women; Cholesterol/Lipid Disorders; Preventive Cardiology; Nutrition; **Hospital:** Lenox Hill Hosp (page 106); **Address:** Heart & Vascular Institute, Lenox Hill Hosp, 110 E 59th St, Ste 8A, New York, NY 10022; **Phone:** 212-434-6902; **Board Cert:** Cardiovascular Disease 2005; **Med School:** Kirksville Coll Osteo Med 1994; **Resid:** Internal Medicine, Beth Israel Med Ctr 1998; **Fellow:** Preventive Medicine, Beth Israel Med Ctr 1999; Cardiovascular Disease, Beth Israel Med Ctr 2002

Steingart, Richard M MD (Cv) - **Spec Exp:** Heart Failure; Heart Disease in Cancer Patients; Cardiac Effects of Cancer/Cancer Therapy; Amyloid Heart Disease; **Hospital:** Meml Sloan-Kettering Canc Ctr (page 114); **Address:** 1275 York Ave, New York, NY 10065; **Phone:** 212-639-8488; **Board Cert:** Internal Medicine 1977; Cardiovascular Disease 1979; **Med School:** Mount Sinai Sch Med 1974; **Resid:** Internal Medicine, Yale-New Haven Hosp 1977; **Fellow:** Cardiovascular Disease, Mt Sinai Med Ctr 1979; **Fac Appt:** Prof Med, Cornell Univ-Weill Med Coll

Tenenbaum, Joseph MD (Cv) - **Spec Exp:** Heart Valve Disease; Coronary Artery Disease; Atrial Fibrillation; Critical Care; **Hospital:** NY-Presby/Columbia Univ Med Ctr, NY (page 104); **Address:** 173 Ft Washington Ave, MHC Bldg - Fl 4 - Ste 606, Irving Pavilion, New York, NY 10032; **Phone:** 212-305-5288; **Board Cert:** Internal Medicine 1977; Cardiovascular Disease 1979; **Med School:** Harvard Med Sch 1974; **Resid:** Internal Medicine, Columbia-Presby Med Ctr 1977; **Fellow:** Cardiovascular Disease, Mt Sinai Hosp 1979; **Fac Appt:** Prof Med, Columbia P&S

Tyberg, Theodore MD (Cv) - **Spec Exp:** Coronary Artery Disease; Cholesterol/Lipid Disorders; **Hospital:** NY-Presby/Weill Cornell Med Ctr, NY (page 104); **Address:** 425 E 61st St, Fl 6, New York, NY 10065; **Phone:** 212-752-2000; **Board Cert:** Internal Medicine 1978; Cardiovascular Disease 1981; **Med School:** Rush Med Coll 1975; **Resid:** Internal Medicine, New York Hosp 1978; **Fellow:** Cardiovascular Disease, Yale-New Haven Hosp 1980; **Fac Appt:** Assoc Clin Prof Med, Cornell Univ-Weill Med Coll

Unger, Allen MD (Cv) - **Spec Exp:** Cholesterol/Lipid Disorders; Hypertension; Preventive Cardiology; Coronary Artery Disease; **Hospital:** Mt Sinai Med Ctr (page 102); **Address:** 12 E 86th St, New York, NY 10028; **Phone:** 212-734-6000; **Board Cert:** Internal Medicine 1968; Cardiovascular Disease 1977; **Med School:** SUNY Upstate Med Univ 1960; **Resid:** Internal Medicine, Mount Sinai Med Ctr 1967; **Fellow:** Cardiovascular Disease, Mount Sinai Med Ctr 1966; **Fac Appt:** Asst Clin Prof Med, Mount Sinai Sch Med

Varriale, Philip MD (Cv) - **Spec Exp:** Coronary Artery Disease; Arrhythmias; Congestive Heart Failure; Pacemakers; **Hospital:** Beth Israel Med Ctr - Petrie Div (page 94); **Address:** 222 E 19th St, Ste 2D, New York, NY 10003; **Phone:** 212-777-3219; **Board Cert:** Internal Medicine 1966; Cardiovascular Disease 1970; **Med School:** SUNY Hlth Sci Ctr 1959; **Resid:** Internal Medicine, Brooklyn VA Hosp 1962; Internal Medicine, St Vincents Hosp 1963; **Fellow:** Cardiovascular Disease, St Vincents Hosp 1964; **Fac Appt:** Assoc Clin Prof Med, Mount Sinai Sch Med

Weintraub, Howard S MD (Cv) - **Spec Exp:** Cholesterol/Lipid Disorders; Hypertension; Preventive Cardiology; Metabolic Syndrome; **Hospital:** NYU Langone Med Ctr (page 108); **Address:** 345 E 37th St, Ste 308, New York, NY 10016-3217; **Phone:** 212-599-5030; **Board Cert:** Internal Medicine 1979; Cardiovascular Disease 1985; **Med School:** NYU Sch Med 1976; **Resid:** Internal Medicine, NYU Med Ctr 1979; **Fellow:** Pulmonary Disease, NYU Med Ctr 1980; Cardiovascular Disease, NYU Med Ctr 1982; **Fac Appt:** Clin Prof Med, NYU Sch Med

Weisenseel Jr, Arthur C MD (Cv) - **Spec Exp:** Coronary Artery Disease; Cholesterol/Lipid Disorders; Congestive Heart Failure; Preventive Cardiology; **Hospital:** Mt Sinai Med Ctr (page 102); **Address:** 12 E 86th St, New York, NY 10028; **Phone:** 212-734-6000; **Board Cert:** Internal Medicine 1969; Cardiovascular Disease 1973; **Med School:** Georgetown Univ 1963; **Resid:** Internal Medicine, Mount Sinai Med Ctr 1966; **Fellow:** Cardiovascular Disease, Mount Sinai Med Ctr 1967; **Fac Appt:** Assoc Clin Prof Med, Mount Sinai Sch Med

Wolk, Michael Jay MD (Cv) - **Spec Exp:** Coronary Artery Disease; Heart Failure; Hypertension; **Hospital:** NY-Presby/Weill Cornell Med Ctr, NY (page 104); **Address:** 425 E 61st St, Fl 6, New York, NY 10021; **Phone:** 212-752-2000; **Board Cert:** Internal Medicine 1971; Cardiovascular Disease 1973; **Med School:** Columbia P&S 1964; **Resid:** Internal Medicine, Univ Hosp 1967; **Fellow:** Cardiovascular Disease, New England Med Ctr 1969; Cardiovascular Disease, New York Hosp-Cornell 1970; **Fac Appt:** Clin Prof Med, Cornell Univ-Weill Med Coll

Child & Adolescent Psychiatry

Abright, A. Reese MD (ChAP) - **Spec Exp:** Mood Disorders; ADD/ADHD; Anxiety Disorders; **Hospital:** Elmhurst Hosp Ctr; **Address:** 140 E 40th St, Ste 1B, New York, NY 10016; **Phone:** 212-867-3131; **Board Cert:** Psychiatry 1978; Child & Adolescent Psychiatry 1981; **Med School:** Univ Tex SW, Dallas 1973; **Resid:** Psychiatry, St Vincent's Hosp 1974; Psychiatry, Presby/Weill Cornell Med Ctr 1977; **Fellow:** Child & Adolescent Psychiatry, Presby/Weill Cornell Med Ctr 1979; **Fac Appt:** Clin Prof Psyc, NY Med Coll

Bartell, Abraham MD (ChAP) - **Spec Exp:** Psychiatry in Cancer; Psychiatry in Physical Illness; **Hospital:** Meml Sloan-Kettering Canc Ctr (page 114); **Address:** 1275 York Ave Fl 9, New York, NY 10065; **Phone:** 646-888-0060; **Board Cert:** Psychiatry 2010; Child & Adolescent Psychiatry 2012; **Med School:** SUNY Downstate 1993; **Resid:** Psychiatry, Emma P Bradley Hosp 1996; **Fellow:** Child & Adolescent Psychiatry, Emma P Bradley Hosp 1998

Becker, Ina MD (ChAP) - **Spec Exp:** Anxiety Disorders; Mood Disorders; ADD/ADHD; **Hospital:** NY-Presby/Columbia Univ Med Ctr, NY (page 104); **Address:** 49 W 24th St, Ste 1010, New York, NY 10010; **Phone:** 917-441-0880; **Board Cert:** Psychiatry 2005; Psychosomatic Medicine 2008; **Med School:** Germany 1987; **Resid:** Psychiatry, Montefiore Med Ctr 1993; **Fac Appt:** Asst Clin Prof Psyc, Columbia P&S

Boorady, Roy J MD (ChAP) - **Spec Exp:** Psychopharmacology; Anxiety & Mood Disorders; ADD/ADHD; **Address:** Child Mind Institute, 445 Park Ave at 56th St, New York, NY 10022; **Phone:** 212-308-3118; **Board Cert:** Psychiatry 1993; Child & Adolescent Psychiatry 1994; **Med School:** SUNY Buffalo 1987; **Resid:** Psychiatry, Mass Mental Hlth Ctr 1991; **Fellow:** Child & Adolescent Psychiatry, Mass Genl Hosp 1993

Burkes, Lynn MD (ChAP) - **Spec Exp:** Diagnostic Problems; ADD/ADHD; Divorce/Family Issues; Developmental Disorders; **Hospital:** NYU Langone Med Ctr (page 108); **Address:** 185 West End Ave, Ste 1E, New York, NY 10023-5539; **Phone:** 212-362-5920; **Board Cert:** Psychiatry 1977; Child & Adolescent Psychiatry 1978; **Med School:** Med Coll PA 1970; **Resid:** Psychiatry, Albert Einstein Affil Hosp 1973; **Fellow:** Psychiatry, Bellevue Hosp 1975; **Fac Appt:** Assoc Clin Prof Psyc, NYU Sch Med

Coffey, Barbara J MD (ChAP) - **Spec Exp:** Tourette's Syndrome; ADD/ADHD; Obsessive-Compulsive Disorder; Psychopharmacology; **Hospital:** Mt Sinai Med Ctr (page 102); **Address:** Tics & Tourette's Clin & Rsch Program, 1240 Park Ave, New York, NY 10029; **Phone:** 212-659-1663; **Board Cert:** Psychiatry 1981; Child & Adolescent Psychiatry 1986; **Med School:** Tufts Univ 1975; **Resid:** Psychiatry, Boston Med Ctr 1978; **Fellow:** Child & Adolescent Psychiatry, Tufts Med Ctr 1980; **Fac Appt:** Prof Psyc, Mount Sinai Sch Med

Fox, Sarah J MD (ChAP) - **Spec Exp:** Anxiety & Mood Disorders; Eating Disorders; Psychoanalysis; **Hospital:** NY-Presby/Columbia Univ Med Ctr, NY (page 104); **Address:** 210 W 89th St, New York, NY 10024; **Phone:** 212-874-4558; **Board Cert:** Psychiatry 1991; Child & Adolescent Psychiatry 1994; **Med School:** Tufts Univ 1982; **Resid:** Psychiatry, Bronx Psych Ctr 1984; Psychiatry, Montefiore Med Ctr 1985; **Fellow:** Child & Adolescent Psychiatry, Columbia-Presby Med Ctr 1987

Gabbay, Vilma MD (ChAP) - **Spec Exp:** Depression; Mood Disorders; Tourette's Syndrome; **Hospital:** Mt Sinai Med Ctr (page 102); **Address:** Pediatric Mood & Anxiety Disorders Prog, 1240 Park Ave, New York, NY 10029; **Phone:** 212-659-1660; **Board Cert:** Psychiatry 2005; Child & Adolescent Psychiatry 2007; **Med School:** Israel 1994; **Resid:** Psychiatry, Montefiore Med Ctr 2001; **Fellow:** Child & Adolescent Psychiatry, NYU Med Ctr 2003; **Fac Appt:** Assoc Prof Psyc, Mount Sinai Sch Med

Grice, Dorothy MD (ChAP) - **Spec Exp:** Obsessive-Compulsive Disorder; Tourette's Syndrome; Autism; **Hospital:** Mt Sinai Med Ctr (page 102); **Address:** 1240 Park Ave Fl 1 - rm 1, New York, NY 10029; **Phone:** 212-659-1660; **Board Cert:** Psychiatry ; Child & Adolescent Psychiatry 2007; **Med School:** Med Univ SC 1988; **Resid:** Psychiatry, Med Univ SC Med Ctr 1992; **Fellow:** Child & Adolescent Psychiatry, Yale Child Study Ctr 1996

Havens, Jennifer MD (ChAP) - **Spec Exp:** Bereavement/Traumatic Grief; **Hospital:** Bellevue Hosp Ctr, NYU Langone Med Ctr (page 108); **Address:** NYU Child Study Ctr, One Park Ave, Fl 7th, New York, NY 10016; **Phone:** 212-263-6622; **Board Cert:** Psychiatry 1991; Child & Adolescent Psychiatry 1993; **Med School:** Tufts Univ 1986; **Resid:** Psychiatry, NY Presby Hosp 1988; **Fellow:** Child & Adolescent Psychiatry, NY Presby Hosp 1991; **Fac Appt:** Assoc Prof ChAP, NYU Sch Med

Hirsch, Glenn S MD (ChAP) - **Spec Exp:** Anxiety & Mood Disorders; Tourette's Syndrome; Bipolar/Mood Disorders; ADD/ADHD; **Hospital:** NYU Langone Med Ctr (page 108), Bellevue Hosp Ctr; **Address:** NYU Child Study Center, 1 Park Ave, Fl 7, New York, NY 10016; **Phone:** 212-263-8704; **Board Cert:** Psychiatry 1984; Child & Adolescent Psychiatry 1985; **Med School:** Albert Einstein Coll Med 1979; **Resid:** Psychiatry, New York Hosp-Cornell 1982; **Fellow:** Child & Adolescent Psychiatry, Columbia-Presby Med Ctr 1984; **Fac Appt:** Asst Prof ChAP, NYU Sch Med

Koplewicz, Harold S MD (ChAP) - **Spec Exp:** Anxiety & Mood Disorders; Psychopharmacology; ADD/ADHD; **Address:** Child Mind Inst, 445 Park Ave at 56th St, New York, NY 10022; **Phone:** 212-308-3118; **Board Cert:** Psychiatry 1983; Child & Adolescent Psychiatry 1984; **Med School:** Albert Einstein Coll Med 1978; **Resid:** Psychiatry, Presby/Westchester Div 1981; Psychiatry, NY State Psych Inst 1983; **Fellow:** Psychiatric Research, NY State Psych Inst 1985

Kron, Leo L MD (ChAP) - **Spec Exp:** Psychopharmacology; Psychotherapy; **Hospital:** St. Luke's - Roosevelt Hosp Ctr - Roosevelt Div (page 94); **Address:** 30 E 76th St, Ste 3A, New York, NY 10021; **Phone:** 212-861-7001; **Board Cert:** Psychiatry 1977; Child & Adolescent Psychiatry 1986; **Med School:** Univ British Columbia Fac Med 1971; **Resid:** Psychiatry, Montefiore Med Ctr 1976; **Fellow:** Child & Adolescent Psychiatry, St Lukes Hosp 1978; **Fac Appt:** Asst Clin Prof Psyc, Columbia P&S

Lewis, Owen MD (ChAP) - **Spec Exp:** Psychotherapy; Psychopharmacology; **Hospital:** NY-Presby/Columbia Univ Med Ctr, NY (page 104); **Address:** 11 E 87th St, New York, NY 10128; **Phone:** 212-996-8196; **Board Cert:** Psychiatry 1982; Child & Adolescent Psychiatry 1986; **Med School:** Mount Sinai Sch Med 1976; **Resid:** Psychiatry, NY-Presby/Weill Cornell Med Ctr 1980; **Fellow:** Child & Adolescent Psychiatry, NY-Presby/Weill Cornell Med Ctr 1982; **Fac Appt:** Clin Prof Psyc, Columbia P&S

Moreau, Donna L MD (ChAP) - **Spec Exp:** Psychotherapy & Psychopharmacology; Anxiety & Mood Disorders; **Hospital:** Morgan Stanley Children's Hosp of NY-Presby, NY (page 104); **Address:** 110 East End Ave, New York, NY 10028-7412; **Phone:** 212-772-9205; **Board Cert:** Psychiatry 1985; Child & Adolescent Psychiatry 1991; **Med School:** SUNY Hlth Sci Ctr 1980; **Resid:** Psychiatry, NY Hosp/Payne Whitney Clin 1983; **Fellow:** Child & Adolescent Psychiatry, NY Hosp/Payne Whitney Clin 1985; **Fac Appt:** Assoc Clin Prof Psyc, Columbia P&S

Perry, Richard MD (ChAP) - **Spec Exp:** Pervasive Development Disorders; Behavioral Disorders; Psychopharmacology; **Hospital:** Bellevue Hosp Ctr, NYU Langone Med Ctr (page 108); **Address:** 55 W 74th St, New York, NY 10023-2429; **Phone:** 212-595-0116; **Board Cert:** Psychiatry 1976; Child & Adolescent Psychiatry 1985; **Med School:** Belgium 1970; **Resid:** Psychiatry, Bellevue Hosp 1972; **Fellow:** Child & Adolescent Psychiatry, Bellevue Hosp 1974; **Fac Appt:** Clin Prof Psyc, NYU Sch Med

Ravitz, Alan J MD (ChAP) - **Spec Exp:** Psychopharmacology; Anxiety Disorders; **Address:** Child Mind Inst, 445 Park Ave at 56th St, New York, NY 10022; **Phone:** 212-308-3118; **Board Cert:** Psychiatry 1984; Child & Adolescent Psychiatry 1986; Forensic Psychiatry 2007; **Med School:** Mich State Univ 1978; **Resid:** Psychiatry, Univ Chicago Med Ctr 1982; **Fellow:** Child & Adolescent Psychiatry, Univ Chicago Med Ctr 1984; **Fac Appt:** Assoc Prof Psyc, NYU Sch Med

Shatkin, Jess P MD (ChAP) - **Spec Exp:** Behavioral Disorders; Anxiety & Mood Disorders; ADD/ADHD; Autism; **Hospital:** NYU Langone Med Ctr (page 108), Bellevue Hosp Ctr; **Address:** One Park Ave, 7th Fl, New York, NY 10016; **Phone:** 646-754-4900; **Board Cert:** Psychiatry 2011; Child & Adolescent Psychiatry 2003; **Med School:** SUNY Hlth Sci Ctr 1996; **Resid:** Psychiatry, UCLA NPI 1999; **Fellow:** Child & Adolescent Psychiatry, UCLA NPI 2001; **Fac Appt:** Assoc Clin Prof ChAP, NYU Sch Med

Spencer, Elizabeth Kay MD (ChAP) - **Hospital:** NYU Langone Med Ctr (page 108); **Address:** 121 E 31st St, Ste 1B, New York, NY 10016-6835; **Phone:** 212-684-3810; **Board Cert:** Psychiatry 1990; Child & Adolescent Psychiatry 1992; **Med School:** Geo Wash Univ 1979; **Resid:** Pediatrics, Univ Maryland Hosp 1982; Psychiatry, NYU Med Ctr 1986; **Fellow:** Behavioral Pediatrics, Univ Maryland Hosp 1984; Child & Adolescent Psychiatry, NYU Med Ctr 1988

Turecki, Stanley K MD (ChAP) - **Spec Exp:** Temperamentally Difficult Child; ADD/ADHD; Parenting Issues; **Hospital:** Lenox Hill Hosp (page 106); **Address:** 136 E 64th St, Ste 1B, New York, NY 10065; **Phone:** 212-355-2535; **Board Cert:** Psychiatry 1978; Child & Adolescent Psychiatry 1981; **Med School:** South Africa 1961; **Resid:** Psychiatry, Tara Hospital 1969; Psychiatry, Mt Sinai Hosp 1971

Walkup, John T MD (ChAP) - **Spec Exp:** Anxiety Disorders; **Hospital:** NY-Presby/Weill Cornell Med Ctr, NY (page 104); **Address:** NY Presby/Weill Cornell Med Ctr, Div Child and Adolescent Psychiatry, 525 E 68th St, rm F-1109, New York, NY 10065; **Phone:** 212-746-1891; **Board Cert:** Psychiatry 1987; Child & Adolescent Psychiatry 1992; **Med School:** Univ Minn 1982; **Resid:** Psychiatry, Yale Univ Med Sch 1985; **Fellow:** Child Psychiatry, Yale Chld Study Ctr 1988; **Fac Appt:** Prof Psyc, Cornell Univ-Weill Med Coll

Walsh, Peter MD (ChAP) - **Hospital:** NY-Presby/Columbia Univ Med Ctr, NY (page 104); **Address:** 115 Central Park W, Ste 5, New York, NY 10023; **Phone:** 212-579-5552; **Med School:** Georgetown Univ 1991; **Resid:** Psychiatry, NY Presby-Columbia Med Ctr 1994; **Fellow:** Child & Adolescent Psychiatry, NY Presby-Columbia Med Ctr 1996

Child Neurology

Akman, Cigdem I MD (ChiN) - **Spec Exp:** Epilepsy; **Hospital:** NY-Presby/Columbia Univ Med Ctr, NY (page 104); **Address:** Harkness Pavilion, 180 Fort Washington Ave Fl 5, New York, NY 10032; **Phone:** 212-305-8549; **Board Cert:** Child Neurology ; Clinical Neurophysiology ; **Med School:** Turkey 1988; **Resid:** Pediatrics, Maimonides Med Ctr 1996; Neurology, SUNY Hlth Sci Ctr 1999; **Fellow:** Child Neurology, Columbia-Presy Med Ctr 2000; Epilepsy, Chlidren's Hosp 2002; **Fac Appt:** Assoc Clin Prof N, Columbia P&S

Allen, Jeffrey MD (ChiN) - **Spec Exp:** Neuro-Oncology; Brain Tumors; Neurofibromatosis; **Hospital:** NYU Langone Med Ctr (page 108); **Address:** Hassenfeld Childrens Ctr, 160 E 32nd St Fl 2 - Ste L3, New York, NY 10016; **Phone:** 212-263-9907; **Board Cert:** Child Neurology 1977; **Med School:** Harvard Med Sch 1969; **Resid:** Pediatrics, Montreal Chldns Hosp 1973; Pediatric Neurology, Montreal Neur Inst/McGill 1976; **Fac Appt:** Prof Ped, NYU Sch Med

Aron, Alan MD (ChiN) - **Spec Exp:** Neurofibromatosis; Movement Disorders; Developmental Delay; **Hospital:** Mt Sinai Med Ctr (page 102); **Address:** Mt Sinai Hosp, Child Neurology, 5 E 98th St Fl 10, Box 1206, New York, NY 10029; **Phone:** 212-831-4393; **Board Cert:** Pediatrics ; Neurology ; Child Neurology ; **Med School:** Columbia P&S 1958; **Resid:** Pediatrics, Babies Hosp-Columbia-Presby Hosp 1961; **Fellow:** Pediatric Neurology, Babies Hosp-Columbia Presby Hosp 1964; **Fac Appt:** Prof N, Mount Sinai Sch Med

Chiriboga-Klein, Claudia MD (ChiN) - **Spec Exp:** Developmental Disorders; Movement Disorders; Spasticity Management; **Hospital:** NY-Presby/Columbia Univ Med Ctr, NY (page 104); **Address:** 180 Fort Washington Ave Fl 5, Harkness Pavilion, New York, NY 10032; **Phone:** 212-305-8549; **Board Cert:** Child Neurology ; **Med School:** Argentina 1982; **Resid:** Pediatrics, St Lukes-Roosevelt Med Ctr 1985; Neurology, Columbia-Presby Med Ctr 1988; **Fac Appt:** Assoc Clin Prof N, Columbia P&S

DeVivo, Darryl C MD (ChiN) - **Spec Exp:** Metabolic Disorders; Neuromuscular Disorders; Spinal Muscular Atrophy (SMA); **Hospital:** NY-Presby/Columbia Univ Med Ctr, NY (page 104); **Address:** Neurological Inst, 710 W 168th St, Ste NI 201, New York, NY 10032; **Phone:** 212-305-5244; **Board Cert:** Child Neurology 1972; **Med School:** Univ VA Sch Med 1964; **Resid:** Pediatrics, Mass Genl Hosp 1966; Neurology, Mass Genl Hosp 1967; **Fellow:** Neurology, Natl Inst Hlth 1969; Child Neurology, Chldns Hosp 1970; **Fac Appt:** Prof N, Columbia P&S

Engel, Murray MD (ChiN) - **Spec Exp:** Neurophysiology; Neurodevelopmental Disabilities; Epilepsy; **Hospital:** NY-Presby/Weill Cornell Med Ctr, NY (page 104), Stamford Hosp (page 939); **Address:** 525 E 68th St, Box 91, New York, NY 10021; **Phone:** 212-746-3278; **Board Cert:** Pediatrics 1979; Neurology 1980; Clinical Neurophysiology 2005; **Med School:** Univ Chicago-Pritzker Sch Med 1972; **Resid:** Pediatrics, Yale-New Haven Hosp 1974; Child Neurology, NY-Presby/Columbia Univ Med Ctr 1977; **Fac Appt:** Prof Ped, Cornell Univ-Weill Med Coll

Kairam, Ram MD (ChiN) - **Spec Exp:** Autism; Behavioral Disorders; **Hospital:** NY-Presby/Columbia Univ Med Ctr, NY (page 104); **Address:** NY-Presby, Child Neurology, 180 Ft Washington Ave Fl 5, New York, NY 10032; **Phone:** 212-342-6867; **Board Cert:** Pediatrics 1981; Child Neurology 1989; Neonatal-Perinatal Medicine 1981; **Med School:** India 1970; **Resid:** Pediatrics, Harlem Hosp Ctr 1977; Neonatal-Perinatal Medicine, NY-Presby/Columbia Univ Med Ctr 1979; **Fellow:** Pediatric Neurology, NY-Presby/Columbia Univ Med Ctr 1982; **Fac Appt:** Asst Prof Ped, Columbia P&S

Kaufman, David M MD (ChiN) - **Spec Exp:** Epilepsy/Seizure Disorders; Headache; Learning Disorders; Autism; **Hospital:** Mt Sinai Med Ctr (page 102), Lenox Hill Hosp (page 106); **Address:** 3 E 83rd St, New York, NY 10028-0459; **Phone:** 212-737-4911; **Board Cert:** Pediatrics 1980; **Med School:** Boston Univ 1975; **Resid:** Pediatrics, New York Hosp 1977; Neurology, Mount Sinai Hosp 1978; **Fellow:** Child Neurology, Mount Sinai Hosp 1980; **Fac Appt:** Assoc Clin Prof N, Mount Sinai Sch Med

Khakoo, Yasmin MD (ChiN) - **Spec Exp:** Neuro-Oncology; Brain Tumors-Pediatric; **Hospital:** Meml Sloan-Kettering Canc Ctr (page 114); **Address:** Meml Sloan-Kettering, Ped Neuro-Onc, 1275 York Ave, New York, NY 10065; **Phone:** 212-639-8292; **Board Cert:** Pediatrics 2008; Child Neurology 2007; **Med School:** Columbia P&S 1990; **Resid:** Pediatrics, UCSF Med Ctr 1993; **Fellow:** Child Neurology, UCSF Med Ctr 1996; Neuro-Oncology, Meml Sloan-Kettering Cancer Ctr 1999

Kosofsky, Barry E MD/PhD (ChiN) - **Spec Exp:** Developmental Disorders; Autism; Stroke; **Hospital:** NY-Presby/Weill Cornell Med Ctr, NY (page 104); **Address:** Cornell Med Ctr, Dept Pediatrics, 505 E 70th St, Helmsley Tower Fl 3, New York, NY 10021; **Phone:** 212-746-3321; **Board Cert:** Child Neurology 1993; **Med School:** Johns Hopkins Univ 1985; **Resid:** Pediatrics, Chldns Hosp 1987; Child Neurology, Mass Genl Hosp 1990; **Fellow:** Neurological Biology, Mass Genl Hosp 1992; **Fac Appt:** Prof Ped, Cornell Univ-Weill Med Coll

Miles, Daniel K MD (ChiN) - **Spec Exp:** Tuberous Sclerosis; Epilepsy; **Hospital:** NYU Langone Med Ctr (page 108); **Address:** New York Epilepsy & Neurology, 223 E 34th St Fl 1, New York, NY 10016; **Phone:** 646-558-0808; **Board Cert:** Child Neurology 1994; **Med School:** UMDNJ-NJ Med Sch, Newark 1983; **Resid:** Pediatrics, St Christopher's Hosp 1986; **Fellow:** Pediatric Neurology, Chlds Meml Hosp 1989; Epilepsy, Boston Chlds Hosp 1990

Molofsky, Walter J MD (ChiN) - **Spec Exp:** Seizure Disorders; Headache; ADD/ADHD; Stroke; **Hospital:** Beth Israel Med Ctr - Petrie Div (page 94), St. Luke's - Roosevelt Hosp Ctr - Roosevelt Div (page 94); **Address:** Beth Israel Medical Center, 10 Union Square East, Ste 5G, New York, NY 10003; **Phone:** 212-844-6944; **Board Cert:** Pediatrics 1982; Child Neurology 1986; **Med School:** NYU Sch Med 1976; **Resid:** Pediatrics, Columbia-Presby Med Ctr 1978; **Fellow:** Child Neurology, Columbia-Presby Med Ctr 1981; **Fac Appt:** Assoc Prof N, Albert Einstein Coll Med

Nass, Ruth D MD (ChiN) - **Spec Exp:** Autism; ADD/ADHD; Learning Disorders; Migraine; **Hospital:** NYU Langone Med Ctr (page 108); **Address:** 1 Park Ave Fl 7, New York, NY 10016; **Phone:** 212-263-6622; **Board Cert:** Pediatrics 1980; Child Neurology 1981; **Med School:** Albert Einstein Coll Med 1975; **Resid:** Pediatrics, NY-Presby/Weill Cornell Med Ctr 1977; Child Neurology, NY-Presby/Weill Cornell Med Ctr 1980; **Fellow:** Neurology, NY-Presby/Weill Cornell Med Ctr 1982; **Fac Appt:** Prof N, NYU Sch Med

Riviello Jr, James J MD (ChiN) - **Spec Exp:** Epilepsy/Seizure Disorders; Epilepsy in Tuberous Sclerosis; Electrical Status Epilepticus Of Sleep; **Hospital:** Morgan Stanley Children's Hosp of NY-Presby, NY (page 104); **Address:** NY-Presby, Child Neurology, 180 Fort Washington Ave, rm 542, New York, NY 10032; **Phone:** 646-426-3876; **Board Cert:** Pediatrics 1984; Child Neurology 1985; Clinical Neurophysiology 2006; **Med School:** Tufts Univ 1978; **Resid:** Pediatrics, St Christopher Hosp Chldn 1980; Neurology, Temple Univ Hosp 1983; **Fellow:** Pediatric Neurology, St Christopher Hosp Chldn 1983; **Fac Appt:** Prof N, Columbia P&S

Wolf, Steven M MD (ChiN) - **Spec Exp:** Epilepsy; Headache; Migraine; **Hospital:** Beth Israel Med Ctr - Petrie Div (page 94), St. Luke's - Roosevelt Hosp Ctr - Roosevelt Div (page 94); **Address:** Beth Israel Med Ctr, Dept Ped Neurology, 10 Union Square East, Ste 5J, New York, NY 10003; **Phone:** 212-844-6944; **Board Cert:** Child Neurology 2006; Pediatrics 2011; Clinical Neurophysiology 2008; **Med School:** Albany Med Coll 1989; **Resid:** Pediatrics, Montefiore Med Ctr 1991; **Fellow:** Child Neurology, Montefiore Med Ctr 1994; Epilepsy, Montefiore Med Ctr 1995; **Fac Appt:** Assoc Prof N, Albert Einstein Coll Med

Clinical Genetics

Anyane-Yeboa, Kwame MD (CG) - **Spec Exp:** Dysmorphology; Prenatal Diagnosis; **Hospital:** Morgan Stanley Children's Hosp of NY-Presby, NY (page 104); **Address:** Morgan Stanley Chldn's Hosp NY, 3959 Broadway, rm 718N, New York, NY 10032; **Phone:** 212-305-6731; **Board Cert:** Pediatrics 1979; Clinical Genetics 1982; **Med School:** Ghana 1972; **Resid:** Pediatrics, Harlem Hosp Ctr 1977; **Fellow:** Clinical Genetics, Columbia P&S 1980; **Fac Appt:** Assoc Prof Ped, Columbia P&S

Chung, Wendy Kay MD (CG) - **Spec Exp:** Cancer Genetics; Metabolic Genetic Disorders; **Hospital:** NY-Presby/Columbia Univ Med Ctr, NY (page 104); **Address:** 3959 Broadway Ave, New York, NY 10032; **Phone:** 212-305-6731; **Board Cert:** Clinical Genetics 2002; Clinical Molecular Genetics 2005; **Med School:** Cornell Univ 1998; **Resid:** Clinical Genetics, NY-Presby/Columbia Univ Med Ctr 2002; **Fellow:** Genetics, NY-Presby/Columbia Univ Med Ctr 2003; **Fac Appt:** Asst Prof Ped, Columbia P&S

Davis, Jessica G MD (CG) - **Spec Exp:** Marfan's Syndrome; Mental Retardation; Neurofibromatosis; Ehlers-Danlos Syndrome; **Hospital:** NY-Presby/Weill Cornell Med Ctr, NY (page 104), Hosp For Special Surgery (page 113); **Address:** 505 E 70th St, Box 128, New York, NY 10065; **Phone:** 646-962-2205; **Board Cert:** Clinical Genetics 1984; **Med School:** Columbia P&S 1959; **Resid:** Pediatrics, St Luke's Hosp 1962; Clinical Genetics, Albert Einstein Coll Med Affil Hosp 1965; **Fellow:** Cytogenetics, Albert Einstein Coll Med Affil Hosp 1966; Pediatrics, Albert Einstein Col Med Affil Hosp 1968; **Fac Appt:** Assoc Clin Prof Ped, Cornell Univ-Weill Med Coll

Desnick, Robert J MD/PhD (CG) - **Spec Exp:** Inherited Metabolic Disorders; Lysosomal Diseases; Gaucher Disease; Porphyria; **Hospital:** Mt Sinai Med Ctr (page 102); **Address:** Mount Sinai Med Ctr, Icahn Med Inst, 1425 Madison Ave, Fl 14, rm 14-34, Box 1498, New York, NY 10029; **Phone:** 212-659-6700; **Board Cert:** Clinical Genetics 1982; Clinical Biochemical Genetics 1982; Clinical Molecular Genetics 2009; **Med School:** Univ Minn 1971; **Resid:** Pediatrics, Univ Minn Affil Hosp 1973; **Fac Appt:** Prof Emeritus CG, Mount Sinai Sch Med

Pappas, John Georgios MD (CG) - **Spec Exp:** Genetic Disorders; Growth Disorders; **Hospital:** NYU Langone Med Ctr (page 108), NYU Hosp For Joint Dis (page 108); **Address:** 301 E 17th St Fl 3, New York, NY 10009; **Phone:** 212-598-6040; **Board Cert:** Pediatrics 2007; Clinical Genetics 2010; **Med School:** Greece 1985; **Resid:** Pediatrics, Beth Israel Med Ctr 1991; **Fellow:** Clinical Genetics, Mt Sinai Med Ctr 1995; **Fac Appt:** Asst Prof Ped, NYU Sch Med

Wasserstein, Melissa MD (CG) - **Spec Exp:** Phenylketonuria (PKU); Fabry's Disease; Metabolic Genetic Disorders; **Hospital:** Mt Sinai Med Ctr (page 102); **Address:** Mt Sinai Med Ctr, Clin Genetics, 1428 Madison Ave, rm AB1-12, New York, NY 10029; **Phone:** 212-241-6947; **Board Cert:** Pediatrics 2010; Clinical Biochemical Genetics 2010; **Med School:** NYU Sch Med 1992; **Resid:** Pediatrics, Mt Sinai Med Ctr 1995; **Fellow:** Clinical Genetics, Mt Sinai Med Ctr 1997; **Fac Appt:** Assoc Prof CG, Mount Sinai Sch Med

Colon & Rectal Surgery

Arnell, Tracey D MD (CRS) - **Spec Exp:** Laparoscopic Surgery; Diverticulitis; Inflammatory Bowel Disease; Anorectal Disorders; **Hospital:** NY-Presby/Columbia Univ Med Ctr, NY (page 104); **Address:** 161 Fort Washington Ave, New York, NY 10032; **Phone:** 212-342-1734; **Board Cert:** Surgery 2009; Colon & Rectal Surgery 2010; **Med School:** Univ Wash 1992; **Resid:** Surgery, Harbor-UCLA Med Ctr 1998; **Fellow:** Colon & Rectal Surgery, Lahey Clinic 1999; **Fac Appt:** Asst Prof S, Columbia P&S

Brandeis, Steven Z MD (CRS) - **Spec Exp:** Hemorrhoids; Anal Disorders & Reconstruction; Colon & Rectal Cancer; Anorectal Disorders; **Hospital:** NYU Langone Med Ctr (page 108); **Address:** 251 E 33rd St Fl 2 - Ste 2N, New York, NY 10016; **Phone:** 212-696-5411; **Board Cert:** Colon & Rectal Surgery 1982; **Med School:** NYU Sch Med 1975; **Resid:** Surgery, NYU Med Ctr-Bellevue Hosp 1980; **Fellow:** Colon & Rectal Surgery, RWJ Univ Hosp 1981; **Fac Appt:** Asst Prof S, NYU Sch Med

Feingold, Daniel L MD (CRS) - **Spec Exp:** Colon & Rectal Cancer; Minimally Invasive Surgery; Inflammatory Bowel Disease/Crohn's; Diverticulitis; **Hospital:** NY-Presby/Columbia Univ Med Ctr, NY (page 104); **Address:** NY Presby Hosp-Columbia, 161 Fort Washington Ave, New York, NY 10032; **Phone:** 212-342-1155; **Board Cert:** Surgery 2012; Colon & Rectal Surgery ; **Med School:** Ros Franklin Univ/Chicago Med Sch 1996; **Resid:** Surgery, Barnes-Jewish Hosp 1998; Surgery, NY-Presby/Columbia Univ Med Ctr 2003; **Fellow:** Surgical Oncology, NIH Natl Cancer Inst 2000; Colon & Rectal Surgery, Robert Wood Johnson Affil Hosp 2004; **Fac Appt:** Assoc Clin Prof S, Columbia P&S

Gorfine, Stephen R MD (CRS) - **Spec Exp:** Anal Disorders & Reconstruction; Hemorrhoids; Rectal Cancer; Anal Cancer; **Hospital:** Mt Sinai Med Ctr (page 102); **Address:** 25 E 69th St, New York, NY 10021-4925; **Phone:** 212-517-8600; **Board Cert:** Internal Medicine 1981; Surgery 2007; Colon & Rectal Surgery 1988; **Med School:** Univ Mass Sch Med 1978; **Resid:** Internal Medicine, Mt Sinai Hosp 1981; Surgery, Mt Sinai Hosp 1985; **Fellow:** Colon & Rectal Surgery, Ferguson Hosp 1987; **Fac Appt:** Clin Prof S, Mount Sinai Sch Med

Guillem, Jose G MD (CRS) - **Spec Exp:** Colon & Rectal Cancer; Rectal Cancer/Sphincter Preservation; Colon & Rectal Cancer-Hereditary; Peritoneal Mucinous Carcinomatosis; **Hospital:** Meml Sloan-Kettering Canc Ctr (page 114); **Address:** 1275 York Ave, New York, NY 10065; **Phone:** 212-639-8278; **Board Cert:** Surgery 2004; Colon & Rectal Surgery 2005; **Med School:** Yale Univ 1983; **Resid:** Surgery, Columbia-Presby Med Ctr 1990; **Fellow:** Colon & Rectal Surgery, Lahey Clinic 1991; **Fac Appt:** Prof CRS, Cornell Univ-Weill Med Coll

Lee, Sang Won MD (CRS) - **Spec Exp:** Inflammatory Bowel Disease; Diverticulitis; Anorectal Disorders; Colon & Rectal Cancer & Surgery; **Hospital:** NY-Presby/Weill Cornell Med Ctr, NY (page 104); **Address:** NY-Presby/Weill Cornell Med Ctr, 1315 York Ave, New York, NY 10021; **Phone:** 212-746-6030; **Board Cert:** Surgery 2012; Colon & Rectal Surgery 2013; **Med School:** NYU Sch Med 1993; **Resid:** Surgery, Beth Israel Deaconess Med Ctr 2001; **Fellow:** Laparoscopic Surgery, NY-Presby/Weill Cornell Med Ctr 2002; Colon & Rectal Surgery, NY-Presby/Weill Cornell Med Ctr 2003; **Fac Appt:** Asst Prof S, Cornell Univ-Weill Med Coll

Martz, Joseph E MD (CRS) - **Spec Exp:** Laparoscopic Surgery; Gastrointestinal Surgery; Colon & Rectal Cancer; Minimally Invasive Surgery; **Hospital:** Beth Israel Med Ctr - Petrie Div (page 94); **Address:** 10 Union Square E, New York, NY 10003; **Phone:** 212-420-3960; **Board Cert:** Surgery 2010; Colon & Rectal Surgery 2011; **Med School:** NYU Sch Med 1995; **Resid:** Surgery, Beth Israel Med Ctr 2000; **Fellow:** Colon & Rectal Surgery, Lahey Clinic 2001

Milsom, Jeffrey W MD (CRS) - **Spec Exp:** Laparoscopic Surgery; Inflammatory Bowel Disease/Crohn's; Colon & Rectal Cancer & Surgery; **Hospital:** NY-Presby/Weill Cornell Med Ctr, NY (page 104); **Address:** NY Cornell Med Ctr, Div Colorectal Surg, 1315 York Ave Fl 2, New York, NY 10065-5304; **Phone:** 646-962-2993; **Board Cert:** Colon & Rectal Surgery 1986; **Med School:** Univ Pittsburgh 1979; **Resid:** Surgery, St Luke's-Roosevelt Hosp 1981; Surgery, Univ Virginia Med Ctr 1984; **Fellow:** Colon & Rectal Surgery, Ferguson Hosp 1985; **Fac Appt:** Prof S, Cornell Univ-Weill Med Coll

Penzer, Jason MD (CRS) - **Spec Exp:** Hemorrhoids; Colon & Rectal Cancer; Diverticulitis; Inflammatory Bowel Disease; **Hospital:** Lenox Hill Hosp (page 106), Beth Israel Med Ctr - Petrie Div (page 94); **Address:** 515 Madison Ave, Ste 705, New York, NY 10022; **Phone:** 212-675-2997; **Board Cert:** Surgery 2010; Colon & Rectal Surgery 2011; **Med School:** Yale Univ 1996; **Resid:** Surgery, St Vincent's Hosp 2001; **Fellow:** Colon & Rectal Surgery, UMDNJ Med Ctr 2002; **Fac Appt:** Asst Clin Prof S, NY Med Coll

Sonoda, Toyooki MD (CRS) - **Spec Exp:** Inflammatory Bowel Disease; Laparoscopic Surgery; Colon & Rectal Cancer & Surgery; Crohn's Disease; **Hospital:** NY-Presby/Weill Cornell Med Ctr, NY (page 104); **Address:** Weill Cornell-Colon & Rectal Surgery, 1315 York Ave, New York, NY 10021; **Phone:** 212-746-6030; **Board Cert:** Surgery 2010; Colon & Rectal Surgery 2011; **Med School:** Yale Univ 1993; **Resid:** Surgery, UCSF Med Ctr 1995; Surgery, Cleveland Clinic 1998; **Fellow:** Laparoscopic Surgery, Mt Sinai Med Ctr 1999; Colon & Rectal Surgery, Cleveland Clinic 2000; **Fac Appt:** Assoc Clin Prof S, Cornell Univ-Weill Med Coll

Steinhagen, Randolph M MD (CRS) - **Spec Exp:** Colon & Rectal Cancer & Surgery; Crohn's Disease; Hemorrhoids; Ulcerative Colitis; **Hospital:** Mt Sinai Med Ctr (page 102), St. John's Riverside Hosp-Andrus Pavil; **Address:** Div Colon & Rectal Surgery, 5 E 98th St Fl 14 - Ste D, Box 1259, New York, NY 10029-6501; **Phone:** 212-241-3547; **Board Cert:** Surgery 2012; Colon & Rectal Surgery 1985; **Med School:** Wayne State Univ 1977; **Resid:** Surgery, Mount Sinai Hosp 1982; **Fellow:** Colon & Rectal Surgery, Cleveland Clinic 1983; **Fac Appt:** Prof S, Mount Sinai Sch Med

Temple, Larissa MD (CRS) - **Spec Exp:** Colon & Rectal Cancer; Anal Cancer; Laparoscopic Surgery; **Hospital:** Meml Sloan-Kettering Canc Ctr (page 114); **Address:** 1275 York Ave Fl 10, New York, NY 10065; **Phone:** 212-639-6081; **Board Cert:** Surgery 2011; Colon & Rectal Surgery 2005; **Med School:** Univ Calgary 1994; **Resid:** Surgery, Univ Toronto 2000; **Fellow:** Surgical Oncology, Meml Sloan Kettering Cancer Ctr 2002

Weiser, Martin R MD (CRS) - **Spec Exp:** Colon & Rectal Cancer; Laparoscopic Surgery; Cancer Surgery; **Hospital:** Meml Sloan-Kettering Canc Ctr (page 114); **Address:** Meml Sloan-Kettering Cancer Ctr, 1275 York Ave, Ste C1075, New York, NY 10065; **Phone:** 646-639-6698; **Board Cert:** Surgery 2009; Colon & Rectal Surgery 2012; **Med School:** Univ Chicago-Pritzker Sch Med 1991; **Resid:** Surgery, Brigham & Women's Hosp 1998; Colon & Rectal Surgery, Mount Sinai Med Ctr 2002; **Fellow:** Research, Harvard Med Sch 1995; Surgical Oncology, Meml Sloan Kettering Cancer Ctr 2000; **Fac Appt:** Assoc Prof S, Cornell Univ-Weill Med Coll

Whelan, Richard L MD (CRS) - **Spec Exp:** Laparoscopic Surgery; Colon & Rectal Cancer; Colonoscopy; Diverticulitis; **Hospital:** St. Luke's - Roosevelt Hosp Ctr - Roosevelt Div (page 94), NY-Presby/Columbia Univ Med Ctr, NY (page 104); **Address:** St Luke-Roosevelt Hosp, 425 W 59th St, Ste 7B, Brodsky Bldg, New York, NY 10019; **Phone:** 212-523-8172; **Board Cert:** Colon & Rectal Surgery 1989; **Med School:** Columbia P&S 1982; **Resid:** Surgery, NY-Presby/Columbia Univ Med Ctr 1987; **Fellow:** Colon & Rectal Surgery, Univ Minn Med Ctr 1988; **Fac Appt:** Prof S, Columbia P&S

Critical Care Medicine

Halpern, Neil A MD (CCM) - **Hospital:** Meml Sloan-Kettering Canc Ctr (page 114), Mt Sinai Med Ctr (page 102); **Address:** 1275 York Ave, Ste C-1179H, New York, NY 10065; **Phone:** 212-639-6731; **Board Cert:** Internal Medicine 1984; Critical Care Medicine 2009; **Med School:** Mount Sinai Sch Med 1981; **Resid:** Internal Medicine, Mount Sinai Hosp 1984; **Fellow:** Critical Care Medicine, Univ Pittsburgh Med Ctr 1985; **Fac Appt:** Prof Med, Cornell Univ-Weill Med Coll

Wagner, Ira J MD (CCM) - **Hospital:** Lenox Hill Hosp (page 106); **Address:** Lenox Hill Hospital, East Bldg, 100 E 77th St Fl 4, New York, NY 10021; **Phone:** 212-434-4130; **Board Cert:** Internal Medicine 1980; Critical Care Medicine 2009; **Med School:** SUNY Downstate 1976; **Resid:** Internal Medicine, St Vincent's Hosp 1979; **Fellow:** Critical Care Medicine, Univ Pittsburgh 1980

Dermatology

Albom, Michael J MD (D) - **Spec Exp:** Mohs' Surgery; Cosmetic Dermatology; Botox Therapy; Reconstructive Surgery; **Hospital:** NYU Langone Med Ctr (page 108), Lenox Hill Hosp (Manh Eye, Ear & Throat Hosp) (page 106); **Address:** 33 E 70th St, New York, NY 10021; **Phone:** 212-517-2121; **Board Cert:** Dermatology 1976; **Med School:** Boston Univ 1970; **Resid:** Dermatology, Boston Univ Med Ctr 1974; **Fellow:** Mohs Surgery, NYU Med Ctr 1975; **Fac Appt:** Clin Prof D, NYU Sch Med

Amin, Snehal P MD (D) - **Spec Exp:** Skin Laser Surgery; Mohs' Surgery; Skin Cancer; **Hospital:** NY-Presby/Weill Cornell Med Ctr, NY (page 104); **Address:** 800 Second Ave, Ste 200A, New York, NY 10017; **Phone:** 212-661-3376; **Board Cert:** Dermatology 2013; **Med School:** Albert Einstein Coll Med 2000; **Resid:** Dermatology, NY Presby-Weill Cornell Med Ctr 2004; **Fellow:** Mohs Surgery, Skin Laser Surgery Spec-NY/NJ 2005; **Fac Appt:** Asst Prof D, Cornell Univ-Weill Med Coll

Aranoff, Shera M MD (D) - **Spec Exp:** Skin Cancer; Cosmetic Dermatology; Acne; Dermatologic Surgery; **Hospital:** Lenox Hill Hosp (page 106); **Address:** 975 Park Ave, Ste 1-A, New York, NY 10028; **Phone:** 212-772-9305; **Board Cert:** Dermatology 1980; **Med School:** NY Med Coll 1973; **Resid:** Dermatology, Westchester Co Med Ctr 1980

Avram, Marc R MD (D) - **Spec Exp:** Hair Restoration/Transplant; Skin Laser Surgery; Cosmetic Dermatology; Botox Therapy; **Hospital:** NY-Presby/Weill Cornell Med Ctr, NY (page 104); **Address:** 905 5th Ave, MS 10021, New York, NY 10021-2650; **Phone:** 212-734-4007; **Board Cert:** Dermatology 2012; Hair Restoration Surgery 2007; **Med School:** SUNY Downstate 1989; **Resid:** Dermatology, Mass Genl Hosp 1994; **Fac Appt:** Clin Prof D, Cornell Univ-Weill Med Coll

Becker, David S MD (D) - **Spec Exp:** Mohs' Surgery; Dermatologic Surgery; Skin Cancer; Laser Surgery; **Hospital:** NY-Presby/Weill Cornell Med Ctr, NY (page 104); **Address:** The Dermatologic Society of Greater NY, 205 E 69th St, Ste 1C, New York, NY 10021; **Phone:** 212-772-3600; **Board Cert:** Dermatology 2001; **Med School:** UCSF 1989; **Resid:** Dermatology, UCSF Med Ctr 1993; **Fellow:** Dermatologic Surgery, Mass Genl Hosp 1994

Belsito, Donald V MD (D) - **Spec Exp:** Contact Dermatitis; Cutaneous Lymphoma; Psoriasis; Atopic Dermatitis; **Hospital:** NY-Presby/Columbia Univ Med Ctr, NY (page 104); **Address:** Columbia Dermatology Associates, 51 W 51st St, Fl 3, Ste 390, New York, NY 10019; **Phone:** 212-305-5293; **Board Cert:** Internal Medicine 1979; Dermatology 1983; Clinical & Laboratory Dematologic Immunology 1985; **Med School:** Cornell Univ-Weill Med Coll 1976; **Resid:** Internal Medicine, Case West Res Univ Hosps 1979; Dermatology, NYU Med Ctr 1982; **Fellow:** Dermatologic Research, NYU Med Ctr 1983; **Fac Appt:** Prof D, Columbia P&S

Berkowitz, Eric Z MD (D) - **Spec Exp:** Skin Cancer; Mohs' Surgery; Cosmetic Dermatology; **Hospital:** Mt Sinai Med Ctr (page 102); **Address:** 390 West End Ave, Ste 1G, New York, NY 10024; **Phone:** 212-877-0171; **Board Cert:** Dermatology ; **Med School:** Albert Einstein Coll Med 2001; **Resid:** Dermatology, Mount Sinai Med Ctr 2005; **Fellow:** Dermatologic Surgery, Mount Sinai Med Ctr 2006

Bernstein, Robert M MD (D) - **Spec Exp:** Hair Restoration/Transplant; Hair Loss in Women; Hair Transplant-Robotic Surgery; **Hospital:** NY-Presby/Columbia Univ Med Ctr, NY (page 104); **Address:** 110 E 55th St, Fl 11, New York, NY 10022; **Phone:** 212-826-2400; **Board Cert:** Dermatology 1982; Hair Restoration Surgery 1998; **Med School:** UMDNJ-NJ Med Sch, Newark 1978; **Resid:** Dermatology, Einstein Affil Hosp 1982; **Fac Appt:** Clin Prof D, Columbia P&S

Berson, Diane S MD (D) - **Spec Exp:** Aging Skin; Acne; Skin Cancer; **Hospital:** NY-Presby/Weill Cornell Med Ctr, NY (page 104); **Address:** 211 E 53rd St, Ste 3, New York, NY 10022-4803; **Phone:** 212-355-3511; **Board Cert:** Dermatology 2009; **Med School:** NYU Sch Med 1984; **Resid:** Dermatology, SUNY Hlth Sci Ctr 1988; **Fac Appt:** Assoc Prof D, Cornell Univ-Weill Med Coll

Bickers, David R MD (D) - **Spec Exp:** Skin Cancer-Consult by Referral Only; **Hospital:** NY-Presby/Columbia Univ Med Ctr, NY (page 104); **Address:** 51 W 51st St, Ste 390, New York, NY 10104; **Phone:** 212-326-8465; **Board Cert:** Dermatology 2006; **Med School:** Univ VA Sch Med 1967; **Resid:** Dermatology, NYU Med Ctr 1974; **Fac Appt:** Prof D, Columbia P&S

Brademas, Mary Ellen MD (D) - **Spec Exp:** Cosmetic Dermatology; Nail Diseases; **Hospital:** NYU Langone Med Ctr (page 108), Bellevue Hosp Ctr; **Address:** 11 5th Ave, Ste F, New York, NY 10003; **Phone:** 212-477-1515; **Board Cert:** Dermatology 1983; **Med School:** Georgetown Univ 1979; **Resid:** Dermatology, Johns Hopkins Hosp 1981; Dermatology, NYU Med Ctr 1983; **Fac Appt:** Assoc Clin Prof D, NYU Sch Med

Brandt, Fredric S MD (D) - **Spec Exp:** Botox Therapy; Cosmetic Dermatology; **Address:** Laser & Skin Surgery Ctr, 323 E 34th St Fl 2, New York, NY 10016; **Phone:** 212-889-7096; **Board Cert:** Internal Medicine 1978; Dermatology 1981; **Med School:** Hahnemann Univ 1975; **Resid:** Internal Medicine, NYU Sch Med Affil Hosp 1978; Dermatology, Jackson Meml Hosp 1981

Buchness, Mary Ruth MD (D) - **Spec Exp:** Skin Infections; Skin Cancer; Cosmetic Dermatology; Psoriasis; **Hospital:** NY-Presby Hosp/The Allen Hosp (page 104); **Address:** 560 Broadway, Ste 406, New York, NY 10012; **Phone:** 212-822-3515; **Board Cert:** Dermatology 1986; **Med School:** Columbia P&S 1982; **Resid:** Dermatology, Columbia Univ Med Ctr 1986; **Fac Appt:** Assoc Prof Med, NY Med Coll

Burke, Karen E MD/PhD (D) - **Spec Exp:** Skin Cancer; Cosmetic Dermatology; Aging Skin; **Hospital:** Mt Sinai Med Ctr (page 102); **Address:** 429 E 52nd St, New York, NY 10022; **Phone:** 212-754-1100; **Board Cert:** Dermatology 1985; **Med School:** NYU Sch Med 1978; **Resid:** Dermatology, NYU Med Ctr 1983; **Fac Appt:** Asst Clin Prof D, Mount Sinai Sch Med

Carucci, John A MD/PhD (D) - **Spec Exp:** Mohs' Surgery; **Hospital:** NYU Langone Med Ctr (page 108); **Address:** 240 E 38th St Fl 12, New York, NY 10016; **Phone:** 212-263-7019; **Board Cert:** Dermatology 2007; **Med School:** SUNY Downstate 1994; **Resid:** Dermatology, NYU Med Ctr 1998; **Fellow:** Mohs Surgery, Yule-New Haven Hosp 2000; **Fac Appt:** Asst Prof D, Cornell Univ-Weill Med Coll

Clark, Sheryl MD (D) - **Spec Exp:** Melanoma; Skin Cancer; Skin Laser Surgery; Cosmetic Dermatology; **Hospital:** NY-Presby/Weill Cornell Med Ctr, NY (page 104); **Address:** 109 E 61st St, New York, NY 10065; **Phone:** 212-750-2905; **Board Cert:** Dermatology 1988; **Med School:** Case West Res Univ 1982; **Resid:** Dermatology, Barnes Hosp-Wash Univ 1988; **Fac Appt:** Asst Clin Prof D, Cornell Univ-Weill Med Coll

Cohen, David E MD (D) - **Spec Exp:** Occupational Dermatology; Contact Dermatitis; **Hospital:** NYU Langone Med Ctr (page 108); **Address:** NYU Dermatologic Assocs, 530 1st Ave, Ste 7R, New York, NY 10016; **Phone:** 212-263-5889; **Board Cert:** Dermatology 2003; Occupational Medicine 1996; **Med School:** SUNY Stony Brook 1989; **Resid:** Dermatology, NYU Med Ctr 1993; **Fellow:** Occupational Medicine, Columbia Univ Sch of Public Hlth 1994; **Fac Appt:** Assoc Prof D, NYU Sch Med

Cook-Bolden, Fran Elesha MD (D) - **Spec Exp:** Black/Asian Skin Care; **Hospital:** St. Luke's - Roosevelt Hosp Ctr - Roosevelt Div (page 94); **Address:** 150 E 58th St Fl 3rd Annex, New York, NY 10155; **Phone:** 212-223-6599; **Board Cert:** Dermatology 2008; **Med School:** Howard Univ 1987; **Resid:** Internal Medicine, Univ Hosp-SUNY Hlth Ctr 1990; **Fellow:** Dermatology, NYU Med Ctr 1996; **Fac Appt:** Asst Clin Prof D, Columbia P&S

Davis, Joyce MD (D) - **Spec Exp:** Acne; Hair loss; Cosmetic Dermatology; **Hospital:** Beth Israel Med Ctr - Petrie Div (page 94), Mt Sinai Med Ctr (page 102); **Address:** 69 Fifth Ave, New York, NY 10003; **Phone:** 212-242-3066; **Board Cert:** Dermatology 1983; **Med School:** Albert Einstein Coll Med 1979; **Resid:** Dermatology, Mount Sinai Med Ctr 1983

DeLeo, Vincent A MD (D) - **Spec Exp:** Contact Dermatitis; **Hospital:** St. Luke's - Roosevelt Hosp Ctr - Roosevelt Div (page 94), Beth Israel Med Ctr - Petrie Div (page 94); **Address:** 1090 Amsterdam Ave, Fl 11, New York, NY 10025; **Phone:** 212-523-5898; **Board Cert:** Dermatology 2009; **Med School:** Louisiana State U, New Orleans 1969; **Resid:** Dermatology, NY-Presby/Columbia Univ Med Ctr 1976; **Fac Appt:** Clin Prof D, Columbia P&S

Demar, Leon K MD (D) - **Spec Exp:** Skin Cancer; Acne; Cosmetic Dermatology; Pediatric Dermatology; **Hospital:** Lenox Hill Hosp (page 106), NY-Presby/Columbia Univ Med Ctr, NY (page 104); **Address:** 985 5th Ave, New York, NY 10075; **Phone:** 212-988-9010; **Board Cert:** Dermatology 1977; **Med School:** NYU Sch Med 1973; **Resid:** Dermatology, Stanford Med Ctr 1975; Dermatology, Columbia-Presby Med Ctr 1977; **Fac Appt:** Asst Clin Prof D, Columbia P&S

Felderman, Lenora MD (D) - **Spec Exp:** Cosmetic Dermatology; Facial Rejuvenation; Acne & Rosacea; Skin Cancer; **Hospital:** NY-Presby/Weill Cornell Med Ctr, NY (page 104); **Address:** 1317 3rd Ave, Fl 8, New York, NY 10021-2995; **Phone:** 212-734-0091; **Board Cert:** Dermatology 2009; **Med School:** NY Med Coll 1981; **Resid:** Dermatology, Montefiore Med Ctr 1985; **Fac Appt:** Asst Clin Prof D, Cornell Univ-Weill Med Coll

Franks Jr, Andrew G MD (D) - **Spec Exp:** Lupus/SLE; Raynaud's Disease; Scleroderma; Dermatomyositis; **Hospital:** NYU Langone Med Ctr (page 108); **Address:** NYU Dermatologic Assocs, 240 E 38th St, New York, NY 10016; **Phone:** 212-263-5015; **Board Cert:** Internal Medicine 1975; Dermatology 1977; Rheumatology 1978; **Med School:** NY Med Coll 1971; **Resid:** Internal Medicine, Beth Israel Med Ctr 1974; Dermatology, Columbia-Presby Med Ctr 1975; **Fellow:** Rheumatology, Columbia-Presby Med Ctr 1977; **Fac Appt:** Prof D, NYU Sch Med

Garzon, Maria C MD (D) - **Spec Exp:** Pediatric Dermatology; Vascular Malformations/Birthmarks; Mycosis Fungoides; **Hospital:** NY-Presby/Columbia Univ Med Ctr, NY (page 104); **Address:** Columbia Univ, Dept Dermatology, 161 Ft Washington Ave Fl 12, New York, NY 10032; **Phone:** 212-305-5293; **Board Cert:** Dermatology 2013; Pediatric Dermatology 2004; Pediatrics 2009; **Med School:** Columbia P&S 1988; **Resid:** Pediatrics, Columbia Presby-Babies Hosp 1991; **Fellow:** Dermatology, Columbia Presby Med Ctr 1995; **Fac Appt:** Assoc Clin Prof D, Columbia P&S

Gendler, Ellen C MD (D) - **Spec Exp:** Cosmetic Dermatology; Contact Dermatitis; Botox Therapy; Facial Rejuvenation; **Hospital:** NYU Langone Med Ctr (page 108); **Address:** 1035 Fifth Ave, New York, NY 10028; **Phone:** 212-288-8222; **Board Cert:** Dermatology 1985; **Med School:** Columbia P&S 1981; **Resid:** Dermatology, NYU Med Ctr 1985; **Fac Appt:** Assoc Clin Prof D, NYU Sch Med

Geronemus, Roy G MD (D) - **Spec Exp:** Skin Cancer; Mohs' Surgery; Cosmetic Dermatology; **Hospital:** New York Eye & Ear Infirm (page 115), NYU Langone Med Ctr (page 108); **Address:** Laser Skin Surgical Ctr of NY, 317 E 34th St, Ste 11N, New York, NY 10016-4974; **Phone:** 212-686-7306; **Board Cert:** Dermatology 1983; **Med School:** Univ Miami Sch Med 1979; **Resid:** Dermatology, NYU-Skin Cancer Unit 1983; **Fellow:** Mohs Surgery, NYU-Skin Cancer Unit 1984; **Fac Appt:** Clin Prof D, NYU Sch Med

Gmyrek, Robyn S MD (D) - **Spec Exp:** Cosmetic Dermatology; Photodynamic Therapy; Skin Laser Surgery-Resurfacing; Varicose Veins; **Hospital:** NY-Presby/Columbia Univ Med Ctr, NY (page 104); **Address:** Columbia Univ Skin & Laser Ctr, 51 W 51st St, Ste 390, New York, NY 10020; **Phone:** 212-326-8889; **Board Cert:** Dermatology 2009; **Med School:** Columbia P&S 1996; **Resid:** Dermatology, NY-Presby/Columbia Univ Med Ctr 2000; **Fac Appt:** Asst Clin Prof D, Columbia P&S

Goldberg, David J MD (D) - **Spec Exp:** Mohs' Surgery; Skin Cancer; Cosmetic Dermatology; Laser Surgery; **Hospital:** Mt Sinai Med Ctr (page 102), Hackensack Univ Med Ctr (page 718); **Address:** 115 E 57th St, Ste 400, New York, NY 10022; **Phone:** 212-750-8900; **Board Cert:** Dermatology 1984; Clinical & Laboratory Dematologic Immunology 1987; **Med School:** Yale Univ 1980; **Resid:** Dermatology, NYU Med Ctr 1984; **Fellow:** Mohs Surgery, NYU Med Ctr 1985; **Fac Appt:** Clin Prof D, Mount Sinai Sch Med

Gordon, Marsha L MD (D) - **Spec Exp:** Cosmetic Dermatology; Botox Therapy; Facial Rejuvenation; **Hospital:** Mt Sinai Med Ctr (page 102); **Address:** 5 E 98th St Fl 5, New York, NY 10029-6574; **Phone:** 212-241-9728; **Board Cert:** Dermatology 1988; **Med School:** Univ Pennsylvania 1984; **Resid:** Dermatology, Mt Sinai Med Ctr 1988; **Fac Appt:** Clin Prof D, Mount Sinai Sch Med

Green, Michele S MD (D) - **Spec Exp:** Cosmetic Dermatology; Skin Laser Surgery; Facial Rejuvenation; Botox Therapy; **Hospital:** Lenox Hill Hosp (page 106); **Address:** 156 E 79th St, Ste 1B, New York, NY 10075; **Phone:** 212-535-3088; **Board Cert:** Dermatology 2013; **Med School:** Mount Sinai Sch Med 1991; **Resid:** Dermatology, Mt Sinai Hosp 1995

Greenspan, Alan H MD (D) - **Spec Exp:** Skin Cancer; Dermatologic Surgery; Phototherapy; **Hospital:** NYU Langone Med Ctr (page 108); **Address:** 39 Broadway, Ste 3005, New York, NY 10006; **Phone:** 212-509-5200; **Board Cert:** Dermatology 2009; **Med School:** Northwestern Univ 1979; **Resid:** Internal Medicine, Northwestern Univ 1981; Dermatology, NYU Med Ctr 1984; **Fac Appt:** Asst Clin Prof D, NYU Sch Med

Gross, Dennis F MD (D) - **Hospital:** NYU Langone Med Ctr (page 108); **Address:** 900 Fifth Ave, New York, NY 10021; **Phone:** 212-725-4555; **Board Cert:** Dermatology 1990; **Med School:** SUNY Stony Brook 1986; **Resid:** Dermatology, NYU Med Ctr 1990; **Fac Appt:** Asst Clin Prof D, NYU Sch Med

Grossman, Melanie MD (D) - **Spec Exp:** Skin Laser Surgery; Facial Rejuvenation; Body Contouring; Cosmetic Dermatology; **Hospital:** NY-Presby/Columbia Univ Med Ctr, NY (page 104); **Address:** 161 Madison Ave, Ste 4NW, New York, NY 10016-5405; **Phone:** 212-725-8600; **Board Cert:** Dermatology 2010; **Med School:** NYU Sch Med 1988; **Resid:** Internal Medicine, Yale-New Haven Hosp 1989; Dermatology, Columbia-Presby Med Ctr 1992; **Fellow:** Laser Surgery, Mass Genl Hosp 1995; **Fac Appt:** Asst Clin Prof D, Columbia P&S

Hale, Elizabeth K MD (D) - **Spec Exp:** Skin Cancer; Mohs' Surgery; Cosmetic Dermatology; **Hospital:** NYU Langone Med Ctr (page 108); **Address:** 317 E 34th St, Fl 11, New York, NY 10016; **Phone:** 212-686-7306; **Board Cert:** Dermatology 2012; **Med School:** NYU Sch Med 1998; **Resid:** Dermatology, NYU Med Ctr 2002; **Fellow:** Mohs Surgery, NYU Med Ctr 2003; **Fac Appt:** Assoc Clin Prof D, NYU Sch Med

Halpern, Allan C MD (D) - **Spec Exp:** Skin Cancer; Melanoma; Melanoma Early Detection/Prevention; **Hospital:** Meml Sloan-Kettering Canc Ctr (page 114); **Address:** Memorial Sloan-Kettering Cancer Ctr, 160 E 53rd St, Fl 2, New York, NY 10022; **Phone:** 212-610-0766; **Board Cert:** Internal Medicine 1984; Dermatology 1988; **Med School:** Albert Einstein Coll Med 1981; **Resid:** Internal Medicine, Montefiore Hosp 1985; Dermatology, Hosp Univ Penn 1989; **Fellow:** Epidemiology, Hosp Univ Penn 1989; **Fac Appt:** Assoc Prof Med, Cornell Univ-Weill Med Coll

Hatcher, Virgil MD (D) - **Spec Exp:** Cosmetic Dermatology; Psoriasis; Viral Infections; **Hospital:** NYU Langone Med Ctr (page 108); **Address:** 420 W 23rd St, Ste A-GF, New York, NY 10011-2172; **Phone:** 212-675-4244; **Board Cert:** Dermatology 2009; **Med School:** UCSF 1978; **Resid:** Dermatology, NYU Med Ctr 1982; **Fellow:** Virology, NYU Med Ctr 1983; **Fac Appt:** Asst Clin Prof D, NYU Sch Med

Hochman, Herbert A MD (D) - **Spec Exp:** Cosmetic Dermatology; Skin Laser Surgery; Skin Cancer; **Hospital:** Lenox Hill Hosp (page 106); **Address:** 1020 Park Ave, New York, NY 10028-0913; **Phone:** 212-861-1656; **Board Cert:** Dermatology 1977; **Med School:** Tulane Univ 1970; **Resid:** Dermatology, Montefiore Med Ctr 1976

Jacobs, Michael Ira MD (D) - **Spec Exp:** Skin Cancer; Melanoma; Cosmetic Dermatology; **Hospital:** NY-Presby/Weill Cornell Med Ctr, NY (page 104); **Address:** 407 E 70th St Fl 2, New York, NY 10021-5302; **Phone:** 212-772-7190; **Board Cert:** Dermatology 1981; **Med School:** Cornell Univ-Weill Med Coll 1977; **Resid:** Dermatology, New York Hosp 1981; **Fac Appt:** Assoc Clin Prof D, Cornell Univ-Weill Med Coll

Katz, Bruce MD (D) - **Spec Exp:** Laser Surgery; Cosmetic Surgery; Liposuction & Body Contouring; Cosmetic Dermatology; **Hospital:** Mt Sinai Med Ctr (page 102); **Address:** Juva Skin, Laser & Body Contouring Center, 60 E 56th St, Fl 2, New York, NY 10022-3350; **Phone:** 212-688-5882; **Board Cert:** Dermatology 1983; **Med School:** McGill Univ 1977; **Resid:** Internal Medicine, Columbia Presby Med Ctr 1979; Dermatology, Columbia Presby Med Ctr 1982; **Fac Appt:** Clin Prof D, Mount Sinai Sch Med

Katz, Susan MD (D) - **Spec Exp:** Psoriasis; Skin Cancer & Moles; Cutaneous Lymphoma; Cosmetic Dermatology; **Hospital:** NYU Langone Med Ctr (page 108); **Address:** 111 Broadway Fl 2, New York, NY 10006; **Phone:** 212-263-9700; **Board Cert:** Dermatology 2009; **Med School:** NYU Sch Med 1977; **Resid:** Internal Medicine, Roosevelt Hosp 1979; Dermatology, Montefiore Med Ctr 1983; **Fac Appt:** Asst Clin Prof D, NYU Sch Med

Kauvar, Arielle B MD (D) - **Spec Exp:** Laser Surgery; Cosmetic Dermatology; Mohs' Surgery; Botox Therapy; **Hospital:** NYU Langone Med Ctr (page 108), New York Eye & Ear Infirm (page 115); **Address:** 1044 Fifth Ave, New York, NY 10028; **Phone:** 212-249-9440; **Board Cert:** Dermatology 2011; **Med School:** Harvard Med Sch 1989; **Resid:** Dermatology, NYU Med Ctr 1993; **Fellow:** Mohs Surgery, Laser & Skin Surgery Ctr 1994; **Fac Appt:** Assoc Clin Prof D, NYU Sch Med

Kenet, Barney J MD (D) - **Spec Exp:** Dermatologic Surgery; Cosmetic Dermatology; Liposuction; **Hospital:** NY-Presby/Weill Cornell Med Ctr, NY (page 104); **Address:** 25 E 86th St, Lobby A, New York, NY 10028; **Phone:** 212-535-9753; **Board Cert:** Dermatology 2012; **Med School:** Brown Univ 1988; **Resid:** Dermatology, New York Hosp 1992

Kline, Mitchell A MD (D) - **Spec Exp:** Melanoma; Skin Cancer; Mohs' Surgery; Cosmetic Dermatology; **Hospital:** NY-Presby/Weill Cornell Med Ctr, NY (page 104); **Address:** 700 Park Ave, New York, NY 10021; **Phone:** 212-517-6555; **Board Cert:** Dermatology 2009; **Med School:** Univ Pennsylvania 1985; **Resid:** Internal Medicine, Graduate Hosp 1987; Dermatology, New York Hosp 1990

Kriegel, David A MD (D) - **Spec Exp:** Mohs' Surgery; Skin Cancer; **Hospital:** Mt Sinai Med Ctr (page 102); **Address:** Manhattan Ctr for Dermatology, 250 W 57th St, Ste 825, New York, NY 10107-0809; **Phone:** 212-489-6669; **Board Cert:** Dermatology 2003; **Med School:** Boston Univ 1987; **Resid:** Dermatology, New England Med Ctr 1991; **Fellow:** Mohs Surgery, Stony Brook Univ Hosp 1993; **Fac Appt:** Assoc Prof D, Mount Sinai Sch Med

Lebwohl, Mark G MD (D) - **Spec Exp:** Skin Cancer; Psoriasis; Pseudoxanthoma Elasticum; **Hospital:** Mt Sinai Med Ctr (page 102); **Address:** Dermatology Assocs, 5 E 98th St Fl 5, New York, NY 10029-6501; **Phone:** 212-241-9728; **Board Cert:** Internal Medicine 1981; Dermatology 1983; **Med School:** Harvard Med Sch 1978; **Resid:** Internal Medicine, Mt Sinai Hosp 1981; Dermatology, Mt Sinai Hosp 1983; **Fellow:** Dermatology, Mt Sinai Hosp 1983; **Fac Appt:** Prof D, Mount Sinai Sch Med

Lombardo, Peter C MD (D) - **Spec Exp:** Skin Cancer; Cosmetic Dermatology; **Hospital:** St. Luke's - Roosevelt Hosp Ctr - Roosevelt Div (page 94), NY-Presby/Columbia Univ Med Ctr, NY (page 104); **Address:** Sutton Place Dermatology, 445 E 58th St, New York, NY 10022-2302; **Phone:** 212-838-0270; **Board Cert:** Dermatology 2009; **Med School:** Albany Med Coll 1959; **Resid:** Dermatology, Columbia-Presby 1965; Internal Medicine, St Luke's-Roosevelt Hosp Ctr 1966; **Fac Appt:** Assoc Clin Prof D, Columbia P&S

Marmur, Ellen S MD (D) - **Spec Exp:** Cosmetic Dermatology; Mohs' Surgery; Laser Surgery; Skin Cancer; **Hospital:** Mt Sinai Med Ctr (page 102); **Address:** 12 E 87th St, Ste 1-A, New York, NY 10028; **Phone:** 212-996-6900; **Board Cert:** Dermatology 2013; **Med School:** Albert Einstein Coll Med 1999; **Resid:** Dermatology, New York Hosp 2003; **Fellow:** Mohs Surgery, Hackensack Hosp 2004; Cosmetic Dermatology, Hackensack Hosp 2004; **Fac Appt:** Assoc Prof D, Mount Sinai Sch Med

Morel, Kimberly D MD (D) - **Spec Exp:** Pediatric Dermatology; Vascular Birthmarks; Atopic Dermatitis; Psoriasis; **Hospital:** NY-Presby/Columbia Univ Med Ctr, NY (page 104), Morgan Stanley Children's Hosp of NY-Presby, NY (page 104); **Address:** Columbia Univ, Dept Dermatology, 161 Fort Washington Ave Fl 12, New York, NY 10032; **Phone:** 212-305-5293; **Board Cert:** Pediatrics 2007; Dermatology 2003; Pediatric Dermatology 2008; **Med School:** SUNY Downstate 1996; **Resid:** Pediatrics, NY Presby Hosp/Columbia 1999; Dermatology, NY Presby Hosp/Columbia 2003; **Fellow:** Pediatric & Adolescent Dermatology, Chldn's Hosp 2003; **Fac Appt:** Assoc Clin Prof D, Columbia P&S

Myskowski, Patricia L MD (D) - **Spec Exp:** Cutaneous Lymphoma; AIDS-Kaposi's Sarcoma; Skin Cancer; **Hospital:** Meml Sloan-Kettering Canc Ctr (page 114); **Address:** 160 E 53 St, New York, NY 10022; **Phone:** 212-610-0768; **Board Cert:** Dermatology 1980; Clinical & Laboratory Dematologic Immunology 1985; **Med School:** Brown Univ 1975; **Resid:** Internal Medicine, Bronx VA Hosp 1977; Dermatology, NY Hosp-Cornell Med Ctr 1980; **Fellow:** Dermatology, Meml Sloan Kettering Cancer Ctr 1981; **Fac Appt:** Assoc Prof D, Cornell Univ-Weill Med Coll

Orbuch, Philip MD (D) - **Spec Exp:** Pediatric Dermatology; Skin Cancer; **Hospital:** NYU Langone Med Ctr (page 108), Bellevue Hosp Ctr; **Address:** 345 E 37th St, Ste 307, New York, NY 10016; **Phone:** 212-532-5355; **Board Cert:** Dermatology 2009; **Med School:** Israel 1981; **Resid:** Dermatology, NYU Med Ctr 1985; **Fellow:** Dermatology, NYU Med Ctr 1986; **Fac Appt:** Assoc Clin Prof D, NYU Sch Med

Orentreich, David S MD (D) - **Spec Exp:** Dermatologic Surgery; Liposuction; Hair Restoration/Transplant; Laser Surgery; **Hospital:** Mt Sinai Med Ctr (page 102); **Address:** 909 5th Ave, New York, NY 10021; **Phone:** 212-794-0800; **Board Cert:** Dermatology 1984; **Med School:** Columbia P&S 1980; **Resid:** Dermatology, Mt Sinai Med Ctr 1984; **Fac Appt:** Asst Clin Prof D, Mount Sinai Sch Med

Orlow, Seth J MD/PhD (D) - **Spec Exp:** Pediatric Dermatology; Birthmarks/Hemangiomas; Psoriasis/Eczema; **Hospital:** NYU Langone Med Ctr (page 108); **Address:** NYU Dermatologic Assocs, Faculty Practice Twr, 530 First Ave Fl 7 - Ste 7R, New York, NY 10016-6402; **Phone:** 212-263-5889; **Board Cert:** Dermatology 2009; Pediatric Dermatology 2004; **Med School:** Albert Einstein Coll Med 1986; **Resid:** Pediatrics, Mt Sinai Med Ctr 1987; Dermatology, Yale-New Haven Hosp 1989; **Fellow:** Pediatric Dermatology, Yale-New Haven Hosp 1990; **Fac Appt:** Prof D, NYU Sch Med

Ostad, Ariel MD (D) - **Spec Exp:** Skin Cancer; Mohs' Surgery; Skin Laser Surgery; Cosmetic Dermatology; **Hospital:** NYU Langone Med Ctr (page 108), Lenox Hill Hosp (page 106); **Address:** 897 Lexington Ave, New York, NY 10065; **Phone:** 212-517-7900; **Board Cert:** Dermatology 2004; **Med School:** NYU Sch Med 1991; **Resid:** Dermatology, NYU Med Ctr 1995; **Fellow:** Dermatologic Surgery, UCLA Med Ctr 1996; **Fac Appt:** Asst Prof D, NYU Sch Med

Podwal, Mark H MD (D) - **Spec Exp:** Skin Cancer; **Hospital:** NYU Langone Med Ctr (page 108); **Address:** 55 E 73rd St, New York, NY 10021; **Phone:** 212-288-7488; **Board Cert:** Dermatology 1975; **Med School:** NYU Sch Med 1970; **Resid:** Dermatology, Kings Co Hosp Ctr 1972; Dermatology, Bellevue Hosp 1974; **Fac Appt:** Assoc Clin Prof D, NYU Sch Med

Polis, Laurie MD (D) - **Spec Exp:** Cosmetic Dermatology; Skin Laser Surgery; Facial Rejuvenation; **Hospital:** Mt Sinai Med Ctr (page 102); **Address:** 62 Crosby St, New York, NY 10012; **Phone:** 212-431-1600 x227; **Board Cert:** Dermatology 1989; **Med School:** Mount Sinai Sch Med 1983; **Resid:** Dermatology, Montefiore Med Ctr 1989; **Fac Appt:** Asst Prof D, Mount Sinai Sch Med

Prioleau, Philip G MD (D) - **Spec Exp:** Melanoma; Skin Cancer; Mohs' Surgery; **Hospital:** NY-Presby/Weill Cornell Med Ctr, NY (page 104); **Address:** 1035 Fifth Ave, Ste C, New York, NY 10028; **Phone:** 212-794-3548; **Board Cert:** Surgery 1973; Anatomic Pathology 1979; Dermatopathology 1980; Dermatology 1983; **Med School:** Med Univ SC 1967; **Resid:** Surgery, Univ VA Med Ctr 1972; Plastic Surgery, Duke Univ Hosp 1975; **Fellow:** Dermatopathology, Barnes Jewish Hosp 1980; Dermatology, NYU Med Ctr 1981; **Fac Appt:** Assoc Clin Prof D, Cornell Univ-Weill Med Coll

Prystowsky, Janet MD (D) - **Spec Exp:** Mohs' Surgery; Cosmetic Dermatology; Skin Cancer; Laser Surgery; **Hospital:** St. Luke's - Roosevelt Hosp Ctr - Roosevelt Div (page 94); **Address:** 110 E 55th St Fl 7, New York, NY 10022; **Phone:** 212-230-1212; **Board Cert:** Dermatology 1987; **Med School:** Univ Chicago-Pritzker Sch Med 1983; **Resid:** Dermatology, Hosp Univ Penn 1987; **Fellow:** Mohs Surgery, SUNY Stony Brook Med Ctr 1998

Ramsay, David L MD (D) - **Spec Exp:** Cutaneous Lymphoma; Skin Cancer; Mycosis Fungoides; **Hospital:** NYU Langone Med Ctr (page 108); **Address:** 530 1st Ave, Ste 7G, New York, NY 10016-6402; **Phone:** 212-683-6283; **Board Cert:** Dermatology 1974; **Med School:** Indiana Univ 1969; **Resid:** Dermatology, NYU Med Ctr 1973; **Fellow:** Dermatology, Univ Illinois Hosp 1974; **Fac Appt:** Clin Prof D, NYU Sch Med

Ratner, Desiree MD (D) - **Spec Exp:** Mohs' Surgery; Skin Cancer; **Hospital:** Beth Israel Med Ctr - Petrie Div (page 94); **Address:** 325 W 15th St, New York, NY 10011; **Phone:** 212-367-0145; **Board Cert:** Dermatology 2003; **Med School:** Johns Hopkins Univ 1989; **Resid:** Internal Medicine, Beth Israel Deaconess Med Ctr 1990; Dermatology, Univ Michigan Med Ctr 1993; **Fellow:** Mohs Surgery, New England Med Ctr 1994; Mohs Surgery, Lahey Clinic 1995; **Fac Appt:** Prof D, Columbia P&S

Rigel, Darrell S MD (D) - **Spec Exp:** Melanoma; Skin Cancer; Cosmetic Dermatology; **Hospital:** NYU Langone Med Ctr (page 108); **Address:** 35 E 35th Street, Ste 208, New York, NY 10016-3823; **Phone:** 212-684-5964; **Board Cert:** Dermatology 1983; **Med School:** Geo Wash Univ 1978; **Resid:** Dermatology, NYU Med Ctr 1982; **Fellow:** Dermatologic Surgery, NYU Med Ctr 1983; **Fac Appt:** Clin Prof D, NYU Sch Med

Rokhsar, Cameron K MD (D) - **Spec Exp:** Skin Laser Surgery; Skin Cancer; Liposuction; Mohs' Surgery; **Hospital:** Winthrop Univ Hosp (page 524), Montefiore Med Ctr-Einstein Campus (page 100); **Address:** NY Cosmetic, Skin & Laser Surgery Ctr, 328 E 75th St, Ste A, New York, NY 10021; **Phone:** 212-285-1110; **Board Cert:** Dermatology 2012; **Med School:** NYU Sch Med 1998; **Resid:** Dermatology, Albert Einstein Affil Hosp 2002; **Fellow:** Dermatologic Surgery, Laser & Skin Surgery Ctr of La Jolla 2004; **Fac Appt:** Asst Prof D, Albert Einstein Coll Med

Romano, John MD (D) - **Spec Exp:** Cosmetic Dermatology; **Hospital:** NY-Presby/Weill Cornell Med Ctr, NY (page 104); **Address:** 58 W 15th St, Grnd Fl, New York, NY 10011; **Phone:** 212-242-5815; **Board Cert:** Dermatology 1980; **Med School:** Cornell Univ-Weill Med Coll 1973; **Resid:** Internal Medicine, St Vincents Hosp 1976; Dermatology, New York Hosp 1978; **Fac Appt:** Asst Clin Prof D, Cornell Univ-Weill Med Coll

Roth, Jeffrey S MD/PhD (D) - **Spec Exp:** Melanoma; Skin Cancer; HIV-Related Skin Disorders; Cosmetic Dermatology; **Hospital:** Mt Sinai Med Ctr (page 102); **Address:** Park Avenue Dermatology Assocs, 580 Park Ave, New York, NY 10065-7313; **Phone:** 212-752-3692; **Board Cert:** Dermatology 2013; **Med School:** Columbia P&S 1989; **Resid:** Dermatology, Columbia-Presby Hosp 1993; **Fac Appt:** Asst Clin Prof D, Mount Sinai Sch Med

Safai, Bijan MD (D) - **Spec Exp:** Dermatologic Surgery; Skin Cancer; Skin Laser Surgery; Cosmetic Dermatology; **Hospital:** Metropolitan Hosp Ctr - NY; **Address:** 625 Park Ave, New York, NY 10065; **Phone:** 212-988-8918; **Board Cert:** Dermatology 1974; **Med School:** Iran 1965; **Resid:** Internal Medicine, VA Med Ctr 1970; Dermatology, NYU Med Ctr 1973; **Fellow:** Immunology, Meml Sloan-Kettering Cancer Ctr 1974; **Fac Appt:** Prof D, NY Med Coll

Schultz, Neal B MD (D) - **Spec Exp:** Cosmetic Dermatology; Melanoma Early Detection/Prevention; Skin Laser Surgery; Tattoo Removal; **Hospital:** Mt Sinai Med Ctr (page 102); **Address:** Park Avenue Skin Care, 1130 Park Ave, New York, NY 10128; **Phone:** 212-369-9600; **Board Cert:** Dermatology 1978; **Med School:** Columbia P&S 1973; **Resid:** Internal Medicine, Mt Sinai Hosp 1975; Dermatology, Mt Sinai Hosp 1978; **Fac Appt:** Clin Prof D, Mount Sinai Sch Med

Schweiger, Eric S MD (D) - **Spec Exp:** Cosmetic Dermatology; Acne; Facial Rejuvenation; Skin Laser Surgery-Resurfacing; **Hospital:** Mt Sinai Med Ctr (page 102); **Address:** Schweiger Dermatology, 110 E 55th St Fl 14, New York, NY 10022; **Phone:** 212-283-3000; **Board Cert:** Dermatology 2008; **Med School:** Albert Einstein Coll Med 2003; **Resid:** Dermatology, Univ Kansas Med Ctr 2008; **Fac Appt:** Asst Clin Prof D, Mount Sinai Sch Med

Seidenberg, Roy Stern MD (D) - **Spec Exp:** Cosmetic Dermatology; Acne; **Hospital:** NYU Langone Med Ctr (page 108); **Address:** 317 E 34th St Fl 6, New York, NY 10016; **Phone:** 212-421-7546; **Board Cert:** Dermatology 2008; **Med School:** NY Med Coll 1991; **Resid:** Internal Medicine, Montefiore Med Ctr 1994; Dermatology, Cooper Hosp 1998; **Fellow:** Dermatologic Surgery, Boston Univ Med Ctr 1995; **Fac Appt:** Asst Clin Prof D, NYU Sch Med

Shelton, Ronald M MD (D) - **Spec Exp:** Cosmetic Dermatology; Mohs' Surgery; Skin Laser Surgery; Skin Cancer; **Hospital:** Mt Sinai Med Ctr (page 102); **Address:** 260 E 66 St, New York, NY 10065; **Phone:** 212-593-1818; **Board Cert:** Dermatology 1990; **Med School:** SUNY Upstate Med Univ 1984; **Resid:** Dermatology, Brooke Army Med Ctr 1990; **Fellow:** Mohs Surgery, UCSF Med Ctr 1993; **Fac Appt:** Assoc Clin Prof D, Mount Sinai Sch Med

Shim-Chang, Helen MD (D) - **Spec Exp:** Dermatopathology; **Hospital:** Mt Sinai Med Ctr (page 102); **Address:** Dermatology Assocs, 5 E 98th St Fl 5, New York, NY 10029; **Phone:** 212-241-9728; **Board Cert:** Anatomic Pathology 1997; Dermatopathology 1998; Dermatology 2008; **Med School:** Hahnemann Univ 1991; **Resid:** Internal Medicine, Mt Sinai Sch Med 1993; Dermatology, Mt Sinai Sch Med 1997; **Fellow:** Dermatopathology, Mt Sinai Hosp 1998

Shupack, Jerome L MD (D) - **Spec Exp:** Rare Skin Disorders; Psoriasis; Eczema; Blistering Diseases; **Hospital:** NYU Langone Med Ctr (page 108); **Address:** 530 1st Ave, HCC 7F, New York, NY 10016-6402; **Phone:** 212-263-7344; **Board Cert:** Dermatology 1970; **Med School:** Columbia P&S 1963; **Resid:** Internal Medicine, Mt Sinai Hosp 1965; Dermatology, NYU Med Ctr 1970; **Fac Appt:** Prof D, NYU Sch Med

Silverberg, Nanette B MD (D) - **Spec Exp:** Pediatric Dermatology; Vitiligo; Atopic Dermatitis; Viral Infections; **Hospital:** Beth Israel Med Ctr - Petrie Div (page 94), St. Luke's - Roosevelt Hosp Ctr - St Luke's Hosp (page 94); **Address:** 10 Union Square E, Ste 3C, New York, NY 10003; **Phone:** 212-844-8800; **Board Cert:** Dermatology 2006; Pediatric Dermatology 2004; **Med School:** SUNY Downstate 1994; **Resid:** Dermatology, SUNY Downstate Med Ctr 1998; **Fellow:** Pediatric Dermatology, Chldn's Meml Hosp 1999; **Fac Appt:** Clin Prof D, Columbia P&S

Sobel, Howard MD (D) - **Spec Exp:** Cosmetic Dermatology; Botox Therapy; Liposuction; Skin Laser Surgery; **Hospital:** Lenox Hill Hosp (page 106), Beth Israel Med Ctr - Petrie Div (page 94); **Address:** 960A Park Ave, New York, NY 10028-0325; **Phone:** 212-288-0060; **Med School:** Albert Einstein Coll Med 1975; **Resid:** Dermatology, Emory Univ Hosp 1979

Soter, Nicholas A MD (D) - **Spec Exp:** Urticaria; Psoriasis; Vasculitis; Phototherapy; **Hospital:** NYU Langone Med Ctr (page 108); **Address:** 240 E 38th St, Fl 12, New York, NY 10016-6402; **Phone:** 212-263-5015; **Board Cert:** Dermatology 1970; Diagnostic Lab Immunology 1985; **Med School:** Univ Tex SW, Dallas 1965; **Resid:** Dermatology, Baylor Med Ctr 1968; Dermatology, Mass Genl Hosp 1969; **Fellow:** Immunology, Harvard Med Sch 1973; **Fac Appt:** Prof D, NYU Sch Med

Tanenbaum, Diane G MD (D) - **Spec Exp:** Skin Cancer; **Hospital:** Lenox Hill Hosp (page 106), NYU Langone Med Ctr (page 108); **Address:** 16 E 79th St, Ste 22, New York, NY 10075-0150; **Phone:** 212-249-6122; **Board Cert:** Dermatology 1971; **Med School:** SUNY Downstate 1964; **Resid:** Dermatology, NYU Med Ctr 1970; **Fac Appt:** Assoc Clin Prof D, NYU Sch Med

Unger, Walter P MD (D) - **Spec Exp:** Hair Restoration/Transplant; **Hospital:** Mt Sinai Med Ctr (page 102); **Address:** 710 Park Ave, New York, NY 10021-6591; **Phone:** 212-249-9393; **Board Cert:** Dermatology 1968; Hair Restoration Surgery 2008; **Med School:** Univ Toronto 1963; **Resid:** Dermatology, Philadelphia Skin-Cancer Hosp 1967; Internal Medicine, Sunny Brook Hosp 1968; **Fac Appt:** Clin Prof D, Mount Sinai Sch Med

Vogel, Louis N MD (D) - **Spec Exp:** Cosmetic Dermatology; Botox Therapy; Hair Removal-Laser; **Hospital:** NYU Langone Med Ctr (page 108); **Address:** 16 Park Ave, Ste 1D, New York, NY 10016-4329; **Phone:** 212-447-5443; **Board Cert:** Internal Medicine 1980; Dermatology 1983; **Med School:** Boston Univ 1977; **Resid:** Internal Medicine, NYU Med Ctr 1980; Dermatology, NYU Med Ctr 1983; **Fac Appt:** Asst Clin Prof D, NYU Sch Med

Walther, Robert MD (D) - **Spec Exp:** Acne; Skin Cancer; Psoriasis; **Hospital:** NY-Presby/Columbia Univ Med Ctr, NY (page 104); **Address:** 161 Ft Wahington Ave Fl 12, New York, NY 10032; **Phone:** 212-326-8465; **Board Cert:** Dermatology 2009; Internal Medicine 1977; **Med School:** Univ NC Sch Med 1973; **Resid:** Internal Medicine, Univ Miami Hosps 1975; Dermatology, Columbia-Presby Hosp 1978; **Fellow:** Dermatology, Rockefeller Univ Hosp 1980; **Fac Appt:** Clin Prof D, Columbia P&S

Warner, Robert MD (D) - **Spec Exp:** Laser Surgery; Laser Hair Removal; Cosmetic Dermatology; Botox Therapy; **Hospital:** Mt Sinai Med Ctr (page 102); **Address:** 580 Park Ave, New York, NY 10065; **Phone:** 212-752-3692; **Board Cert:** Dermatology 1981; **Med School:** SUNY Hlth Sci Ctr 1977; **Resid:** Dermatology, Mount Sinai Hosp 1981; **Fac Appt:** Asst Clin Prof D, Mount Sinai Sch Med

Wattenberg, Debra J MD (D) - **Spec Exp:** Cosmetic Dermatology; Botox Therapy; Skin Laser Surgery; Acne; **Hospital:** Mt Sinai Med Ctr (page 102); **Address:** 875 Fifth Ave, New York, NY 10065; **Phone:** 212-288-3200; **Board Cert:** Dermatology 2011; **Med School:** Mount Sinai Sch Med 1988; **Resid:** Dermatology, Mount Sinai Hosp 1992; **Fac Appt:** Assoc Clin Prof D, Mount Sinai Sch Med

Wechsler, Amy B MD (D) - **Spec Exp:** Cosmetic Dermatology; Acne; Skin Laser Surgery; **Address:** 3 E 69th St, New York, NY 10021; **Phone:** 212-396-2500; **Board Cert:** Psychiatry 2010; Dermatology 2005; **Med School:** Cornell Univ 1995; **Resid:** Psychiatry, Payne Whitney Clinic 1999; Dermatology, SUNY Downstate Med Ctr 2005; **Fellow:** Child & Adolescent Psychiatry, Payne Whitney Clinic 2001

Wexler, Patricia MD (D) - **Spec Exp:** Facial Rejuvenation; Liposuction; Botox Therapy; Acne; **Hospital:** Mt Sinai Med Ctr (page 102); **Address:** 145 E 32nd St Fl 7, New York, NY 10016; **Phone:** 212-684-2626; **Board Cert:** Internal Medicine 1983; Dermatology 1986; **Med School:** Belgium 1979; **Resid:** Internal Medicine, Beth Israel Med Ctr 1982; Dermatology, Mt Sinai Hosp 1986; **Fellow:** Infectious Disease, Beth Israel Med Ctr 1983; **Fac Appt:** Assoc Clin Prof D, Mount Sinai Sch Med

Diagnostic Radiology

Abramson, Sara J MD (DR) - **Spec Exp:** Pediatric Radiology; **Hospital:** Meml Sloan-Kettering Canc Ctr (page 114); **Address:** 444 E 68th St, New York, NY 10065; **Phone:** 212-639-2184; **Board Cert:** Diagnostic Radiology 1976; **Med School:** Mount Sinai Sch Med 1971; **Resid:** Pediatrics, Mt Sinai Hosp 1973; Diagnostic Radiology, Chldns Mercy Hosp 1976; **Fellow:** Pediatric Radiology, Chldns Hosp 1981

Adler, Ronald S MD/PhD (DR) - **Spec Exp:** Musculoskeletal Imaging; Ultrasound; Power Doppler Imaging; **Hospital:** NYU Langone Med Ctr (page 108), NYU Hosp For Joint Dis (page 108); **Address:** Ctr for Musculoskeletal Care-Radiology Dept, 333 E 38th St Fl 6, New York, NY 10016; **Phone:** 646-501-7440; **Board Cert:** Diagnostic Radiology 1988; **Med School:** Wayne State Univ 1984; **Resid:** Diagnostic Radiology, Univ Mich Med Ctr 1988; **Fellow:** Ultrasound/CT/MRI, Univ Mich Med Ctr 1989; **Fac Appt:** Prof Rad, Cornell Univ-Weill Med Coll

Akin, Oguz MD (DR) - **Spec Exp:** Prostate Cancer; Kidney Cancer; Genitourinary Cancer; MRI; **Hospital:** Meml Sloan-Kettering Canc Ctr (page 114); **Address:** Meml Sloan-Kettering Cancer Ctr, 1275 York Ave, rm C276H, New York, NY 10065; **Phone:** 212-639-3458; **Board Cert:** Diagnostic Radiology 2007; **Med School:** Turkey 1996; **Resid:** Diagnostic Radiology, Baskent Univ Sch Med 2001; **Fellow:** Body Imaging, Meml Sloan Kettering Cancer Ctr 2004

Austin, John H. M. MD (DR) - **Spec Exp:** Lung Cancer; Thoracic Radiology; **Hospital:** NY-Presby/Columbia Univ Med Ctr, NY (page 104); **Address:** 177 Fort Washington Ave, Milstein Hosp Bldg 3-202C, New York, NY 10032-3784; **Phone:** 212-305-2639; **Board Cert:** Diagnostic Radiology 1970; **Med School:** Yale Univ 1965; **Resid:** Diagnostic Radiology, UCSF Med Ctr 1968; **Fellow:** Diagnostic Radiology, UCSF Med Ctr 1970; **Fac Appt:** Prof Emeritus Rad, Columbia P&S

Barone, Clement M MD (DR) - **Spec Exp:** Women's Imaging; Mammography; Bone Densitometry; **Hospital:** Mt Sinai Med Ctr (page 102); **Address:** 1440 York Ave, Ste P-1, New York, NY 10075; **Phone:** 212-988-1303; **Board Cert:** Diagnostic Radiology 1974; **Med School:** NY Med Coll 1968; **Resid:** Diagnostic Radiology, Mt Sinai Hosp 1970; Diagnostic Radiology, Mt Sinai Hosp 1974; **Fac Appt:** Asst Clin Prof, Mount Sinai Sch Med

Berson, Barry MD (DR) - **Spec Exp:** Mammography; Breast Imaging; Bone Densitometry; **Hospital:** Mt Sinai Med Ctr (page 102); **Address:** 165 E 84th St, New York, NY 10028-0302; **Phone:** 212-535-9770; **Board Cert:** Diagnostic Radiology 1990; **Med School:** Mount Sinai Sch Med 1984; **Resid:** Diagnostic Radiology, Mount Sinai Hosp 1990; **Fellow:** Neuroradiology, NYU Med Ctr 1992

Brill, Paula W MD (DR) - **Spec Exp:** Pediatric Radiology; Ultrasound; **Hospital:** NY-Presby/Weill Cornell Med Ctr, NY (page 104); **Address:** 525 E 68th St, New York, NY 10065; **Phone:** 212-746-2554; **Board Cert:** Pediatrics 1970; Diagnostic Radiology 1971; Pediatric Radiology 2005; **Med School:** Cornell Univ-Weill Med Coll 1962; **Resid:** Pediatrics, New York Hosp 1968; Diagnostic Radiology, New York Hosp 1971; **Fellow:** Diagnostic Radiology, Cornell Univ 1971; **Fac Appt:** Prof Rad, Cornell Univ-Weill Med Coll

Brown, Marc G MD (DR) - **Spec Exp:** Breast Imaging; **Hospital:** NY-Presby/Columbia Univ Med Ctr, NY (page 104); **Address:** Columbia Doctors Midtown-Radiology, 51 W 51st St, Ste 300, New York, NY 10019; **Phone:** 212-326-8517; **Board Cert:** Diagnostic Radiology ; **Med School:** Columbia P&S 1992; **Resid:** Diagnostic Radiology, NY Presby Hosp/Columbia 1996; **Fellow:** Breast Imaging, NY Presby Hosp/Columbia 1997; **Fac Appt:** Assoc Clin Prof Rad, Columbia P&S

Chaim, Joshua L DO (DR) - **Spec Exp:** CT Scan; Ultrasound; MRI; **Hospital:** Meml Sloan-Kettering Canc Ctr (page 114); **Address:** Meml Sloan Kettering Cancer Ctr, Dept of Radiology, 1275 York Ave Fl 2nd, New York, NY 10065; **Phone:** 646-888-4530; **Board Cert:** Diagnostic Radiology 2007; **Med School:** NY Coll Osteo Med 2002; **Resid:** Diagnostic Radiology, St Barnabas Hosp 2007

Cohen, Burton A MD (DR) - **Spec Exp:** CT Scan; MRI; PET Imaging; **Hospital:** Mt Sinai Med Ctr (page 102); **Address:** New York Medical Imaging Associates, 165 E 84th St, New York, NY 10028; **Phone:** 212-535-9770; **Board Cert:** Diagnostic Radiology 1979; **Med School:** NY Med Coll 1975; **Resid:** Diagnostic Radiology, Mt Sinai Hosp 1979; **Fac Appt:** Assoc Clin Prof Rad, Mount Sinai Sch Med

Dershaw, D David MD (DR) - **Spec Exp:** Breast Imaging; Breast Cancer; Mammography; **Hospital:** Meml Sloan-Kettering Canc Ctr (page 114); **Address:** 300 E 66th St, rm 727, New York, NY 10065; **Phone:** 646-888-4505; **Board Cert:** Diagnostic Radiology 1978; Radiology 1974; **Med School:** Jefferson Med Coll 1974; **Resid:** Diagnostic Radiology, New York Hosp 1978; **Fellow:** Ultrasound, Thos Jefferson Univ Hosp 1979; **Fac Appt:** Prof Rad, Cornell Univ-Weill Med Coll

Edelstein, Barbara A MD (DR) - **Spec Exp:** Breast Cancer; Women's Imaging; **Address:** 1045 Park Ave, New York, NY 10028; **Phone:** 212-860-7700; **Board Cert:** Diagnostic Radiology 1983; **Med School:** NY Med Coll 1977; **Resid:** Diagnostic Radiology, Montefiore Hosp 1982

Fefferman, Nancy R MD (DR) - **Spec Exp:** Pediatric Radiology; **Hospital:** NYU Langone Med Ctr (page 108); **Address:** 660 1st Ave Fl 3, New York, NY 10016; **Phone:** 212-263-5362; **Board Cert:** Radiology 1996; Pediatric Radiology 2009; **Med School:** NYU Sch Med 1991; **Resid:** Radiology, NYU Langone Med Ctr 1996; **Fellow:** Pediatric Radiology, NYU Langone Med Ctr 1997; **Fac Appt:** Asst Prof Rad, NYU Sch Med

Fried, Karen O MD (DR) - **Spec Exp:** Ultrasound; Thyroid Ultrasound; Vascular Ultrasound; **Address:** Lenox Hill Radiology, 61 E 77th St, New York, NY 10075; **Phone:** 212-772-3111; **Board Cert:** Diagnostic Radiology 1990; **Med School:** Albany Med Coll 1985; **Resid:** Diagnostic Radiology, LIJ Med Ctr 1990; **Fellow:** Cross Sectional Imaging, LIJ Med Ctr 1991

Fuqua III, James L MD (DR) - **Spec Exp:** CT Body Scan; Gastrointestinal Imaging; **Hospital:** Meml Sloan-Kettering Canc Ctr (page 114); **Address:** Meml Sloan Kettering Cancer Ctr, Dept of Radiology, 1275 York Ave Fl 2nd, New York, NY 10065; **Phone:** 646-888-4529; **Board Cert:** Diagnostic Radiology 2007; **Med School:** Univ Tenn Coll Med 2002; **Resid:** Diagnostic Radiology, Methodist Hosp 2007; **Fellow:** Body Imaging, Meml Sloan Kettering Cancer Ctr 2008

Ginsberg, Michelle S MD (DR) - **Spec Exp:** Lung Cancer; Thoracic Radiology; Pulmonary Embolism; Gastrointestinal Imaging; **Hospital:** Meml Sloan-Kettering Canc Ctr (page 114); **Address:** Meml Sloan Kettering Cancer Ctr, 1275 York Ave, Dept Radiology, New York, NY 10021; **Phone:** 212-639-7292; **Board Cert:** Diagnostic Radiology 1995; **Med School:** Brown Univ 1990; **Resid:** Radiology, Montefiore Med Ctr- Weiler Div 1995; **Fellow:** Diagnostic Radiology, Meml Sloan Kettering Cancer Ctr 1996; **Fac Appt:** Assoc Prof Rad, Cornell Univ-Weill Med Coll

Henschke, Claudia L MD/PhD (DR) - **Spec Exp:** Lung Cancer; Lung Disease; Thoracic Radiology; **Hospital:** Mt Sinai Med Ctr (page 102); **Address:** Mt Sinai Med Ctr, Radiology Dept, 1 Gustave Levy Pl, Box 1234, New York, NY 10029; **Phone:** 212-241-2420; **Board Cert:** Diagnostic Radiology 1981; **Med School:** Howard Univ 1977; **Resid:** Diagnostic Radiology, Brigham & Womens Hosp 1982; **Fac Appt:** Prof Rad, Mount Sinai Sch Med

Herman, Zeva W MD (DR) - **Spec Exp:** Breast Imaging; Ultrasound; MRI; **Hospital:** Mt Sinai Med Ctr (page 102); **Address:** 525 Park Ave, New York, NY 10065; **Phone:** 212-888-1000 x1574; **Board Cert:** Diagnostic Radiology 1993; **Med School:** Mount Sinai Sch Med 1988; **Resid:** Diagnostic Radiology, Lenox Hill Hosp 1992; **Fellow:** Body Imaging, Meml Sloan Kettering Cancer Ctr 1993

Holliday, Roy A MD (DR) - **Spec Exp:** Head & Neck Imaging; **Hospital:** New York Eye & Ear Infirm (page 115), Beth Israel Med Ctr - Petrie Div (page 94); **Address:** New York Eye & Ear Infirmary, Dept Radiology, 310 E 14th St, North Bldg - Ground Fl, New York, NY 10003; **Phone:** 212-979-4397; **Board Cert:** Diagnostic Radiology 1986; **Med School:** NYU Sch Med 1982; **Resid:** Diagnostic Radiology, NYU Med Ctr 1986; **Fellow:** Neuroradiology, NYU Med Ctr 1987; **Fac Appt:** Prof Rad, Albert Einstein Coll Med

Hricak, Hedvig MD/PhD (DR) - **Spec Exp:** Prostate Cancer-MR Spectroscopy (MRSI); Breast Imaging; Breast Cancer; Gynecologic Cancer; **Hospital:** Meml Sloan-Kettering Canc Ctr (page 114); **Address:** 1275 York Ave, Ste C278, New York, NY 10065; **Phone:** 800-525-2225; **Board Cert:** Diagnostic Radiology 1978; **Med School:** Yugoslavia 1970; **Resid:** Diagnostic Radiology, St Joseph Mercy Hosp 1977; **Fellow:** Ultrasound/CT, Henry Ford Hosp 1978; **Fac Appt:** Prof Rad, Cornell Univ-Weill Med Coll

Jacobs, Morton MD (DR) - **Spec Exp:** Neuroradiology; Head & Neck Imaging; Musculoskeletal Imaging; **Address:** Manhattan Diagnostic Radiology, 400 E 66th St, New York, NY 10065; **Phone:** 212-838-4243; **Board Cert:** Diagnostic Radiology 1976; Neuroradiology 2006; **Med School:** Ros Franklin Univ/Chicago Med Sch 1972; **Resid:** Diagnostic Radiology, New York Hosp 1976; **Fellow:** Neuroradiology, New York Hosp 1979

Levy, Miriam MD (DR) - **Spec Exp:** Breast Imaging; Mammography; Women's Imaging; **Address:** Medical Imaging of Manhattan, 635 Madison Ave, Fl 16, New York, NY 10022; **Phone:** 212-794-2500; **Board Cert:** Diagnostic Radiology 1983; **Med School:** Albert Einstein Coll Med 1979; **Resid:** Diagnostic Radiology, Geo Wash Univ Hosp 1982; Diagnostic Radiology, St Vincents Hosp 1983; **Fellow:** Ultrasound/CT/MRI, New York Hosp 1984; **Fac Appt:** Asst Clin Prof Path, Mount Sinai Sch Med

Math, Kevin R MD (DR) - **Spec Exp:** Musculoskeletal Imaging; MRI; **Hospital:** Beth Israel Med Ctr - Petrie Div (page 94); **Address:** East Manhattan Diagnostic Imaging, 424 E 89th St, New York, NY 10128; **Phone:** 212-410-5100; **Board Cert:** Diagnostic Radiology 1993; **Med School:** SUNY Upstate Med Univ 1988; **Resid:** Diagnostic Radiology, SUNY Hlth Sci Ctr 1993; **Fellow:** Musculoskeletal Imaging, Hosp Special Surgery/Weill Cornell Med Ctr 1994; **Fac Appt:** Assoc Clin Prof Rad, Albert Einstein Coll Med

Megibow, Alec J MD (DR) - **Spec Exp:** Abdominal Imaging; Gastrointestinal Imaging; CT Body Scan; **Hospital:** NYU Langone Med Ctr (page 108), Bellevue Hosp Ctr; **Address:** 550 1st Ave, HHC 232, New York, NY 10016; **Phone:** 212-263-5222; **Board Cert:** Diagnostic Radiology 1978; **Med School:** SUNY Upstate Med Univ 1974; **Resid:** Diagnostic Radiology, Bellevue/NYU Langone Med Ctr 1978; **Fellow:** Abdominal Imaging, NYU Langone Med Ctr 1978; **Fac Appt:** Prof Rad, NYU Sch Med

Miller, Theodore T MD (DR) - **Spec Exp:** Interventional Radiology; Ultrasound; CT Scan; **Hospital:** Hosp For Special Surgery (page 113); **Address:** Dept Radiology, 535 E 70th St, New York, NY 10021; **Phone:** 212-606-1127; **Board Cert:** Diagnostic Radiology 1993; **Med School:** Vanderbilt Univ 1987; **Resid:** Radiology, Mt Sinai Hosp 1992; **Fellow:** Radiology, Hosp for Spec Surg 1993; **Fac Appt:** Prof Rad, Cornell Univ-Weill Med Coll

Mintz, Douglas N MD (DR) - **Spec Exp:** Musculoskeletal Imaging; Bone Tumors; Trauma Radiology; **Hospital:** Hosp For Special Surgery (page 113); **Address:** Hospital for Special Surgery, Rediology & Imaging Dept, 535 E 70th St Fl 3, New York, NY 10021; **Phone:** 212-606-1828; **Board Cert:** Diagnostic Radiology 1997; **Med School:** Columbia P&S 1988; **Resid:** Radiology, Lenox Hill Hosp 1997; **Fellow:** Musculoskeletal Imaging, Hosp for Special Surgery 1998

Mitnick, Julie S MD (DR) - **Spec Exp:** Mammography; Breast Cancer; **Address:** Murray Hill Radiology & Mammography, 650 First Ave Fl 2, New York, NY 10016; **Phone:** 212-686-4440; **Board Cert:** Diagnostic Radiology 1977; **Med School:** NYU Sch Med 1972; **Resid:** Diagnostic Radiology, NYU Med Ctr 1977; **Fellow:** Pediatric Radiology, NYU Med Ctr 1978; **Fac Appt:** Assoc Clin Prof Rad, NYU Sch Med

Morris, Elizabeth A MD (DR) - **Spec Exp:** Breast Imaging; Breast MRI; Breast Cancer; **Hospital:** Meml Sloan-Kettering Canc Ctr (page 114); **Address:** 300 E 66th St, Fl 7, Department of Radiology, New York, NY 10065; **Phone:** 646-888-4510; **Board Cert:** Diagnostic Radiology 1994; **Med School:** UCSF 1989; **Resid:** Diagnostic Radiology, NY-Cornell Med Ctr 1994; **Fellow:** Breast Imaging, Meml Sloan-Kettering Cancer Ctr 1995; **Fac Appt:** Prof Rad, Cornell Univ-Weill Med Coll

Naidich, David P MD (DR) - **Spec Exp:** Chest Radiology; Chronic Lung Disease; Lung Cancer; Pulmonary Embolism; **Hospital:** NYU Langone Med Ctr (page 108), Bellevue Hosp Ctr; **Address:** NYU Medical Center, Dept Radiology, 560 1st Ave, rm 236, New York, NY 10016; **Phone:** 212-263-5229; **Board Cert:** Diagnostic Radiology 1980; **Med School:** NYU Sch Med 1975; **Resid:** Diagnostic Radiology, Johns Hopkins Hosp 1979; **Fellow:** Cross Sectional Imaging, Johns Hopkins Hosp 1980; **Fac Appt:** Prof Rad, NYU Sch Med

Neistadt, L Daniel MD (DR) - **Spec Exp:** CT Body Scan; Gastrointestinal Imaging; Ultrasound; PET Imaging; **Address:** Manhattan Diagnostic Radiology, 400 E 66th St, New York, NY 10065; **Phone:** 212-838-4243; **Board Cert:** Internal Medicine 1975; Nuclear Medicine 1977; Diagnostic Radiology 1980; **Med School:** Stanford Univ 1972; **Resid:** Nuclear Medicine, New York Hosp 1977; Diagnostic Radiology, New York Hosp 1980; **Fellow:** Ultrasound/CT, New York Hosp 1981

Newhouse, Jeffrey H MD (DR) - **Spec Exp:** Abdominal Imaging; **Hospital:** NY-Presby/Columbia Univ Med Ctr, NY (page 104); **Address:** 622 W 168th St, New York, NY 10032; **Phone:** 212-305-7898; **Board Cert:** Diagnostic Radiology 1972; **Med School:** Harvard Med Sch 1967; **Resid:** Diagnostic Radiology, Mass Genl Hosp 1972; **Fac Appt:** Prof, Columbia P&S

Novick, Mark D MD (DR) - **Spec Exp:** Mammography; Breast Imaging; MRI; **Address:** Lenox Hill Radiology, 61 E 77th St, New York, NY 10075; **Phone:** 212-772-3111; **Board Cert:** Diagnostic Radiology 1983; **Med School:** Univ Tenn Coll Med 1978; **Resid:** Diagnostic Radiology, Univ Tenn Med Ctr 1982

Panicek, David M MD (DR) - **Spec Exp:** Bone Cancer; Soft Tissue Tumors; Musculoskeletal Tumors; **Hospital:** Meml Sloan-Kettering Canc Ctr (page 114); **Address:** Meml Sloan Kettering Cancer Ctr, Dept of Radiology, 1276 York Ave, Ste C276G, New York, NY 10065; **Phone:** 800-525-2225; **Board Cert:** Diagnostic Radiology 1984; **Med School:** Cornell Univ-Weill Med Coll 1980; **Resid:** Diagnostic Radiology, NY Hosp-Cornell Med Ctr 1984; **Fac Appt:** Prof Rad, Cornell Univ-Weill Med Coll

Pavlov, Helene MD (DR) - **Spec Exp:** Sports Medicine Radiology; Musculoskeletal Imaging; Orthopaedic Imaging; **Hospital:** Hosp For Special Surgery (page 113), NY-Presby/Weill Cornell Med Ctr, NY (page 104); **Address:** Hosp for Special Surgery, 535 E 70th St Fl 3, New York, NY 10021-4892; **Phone:** 212-606-1132; **Board Cert:** Diagnostic Radiology 1976; **Med School:** Temple Univ 1972; **Resid:** Diagnostic Radiology, Germantown Hosp 1976; **Fellow:** Musculoskeletal Imaging, Hosp For Special Surg 1977; **Fac Appt:** Prof Rad, Cornell Univ-Weill Med Coll

Pfaff, H Charles MD (DR) - **Spec Exp:** Musculoskeletal Imaging; Neuroradiology; **Hospital:** Beth Israel Med Ctr - Petrie Div (page 94), New York Eye & Ear Infirm (page 115); **Address:** New York Radiology Partners, 147 W 15th St, New York, NY 10011; **Phone:** 212-473-5323; **Board Cert:** Diagnostic Radiology 1992; **Med School:** Univ NC Sch Med 1987; **Resid:** Diagnostic Radiology, NY Presby/Columbia Med Ctr 1992; **Fellow:** Neuroradiology, NY Presby/Columbia Med Ctr 1993; **Fac Appt:** Asst Prof Rad, Albert Einstein Coll Med

Potter, Hollis G MD (DR) - **Spec Exp:** Musculoskeletal Imaging; Cartilage Damage; Arthroplasty Imaging; **Hospital:** Hosp For Special Surgery (page 113); **Address:** Hosp for Special Surgery, MRI-basement, 535 E 70th St, Ste MRI, New York, NY 10021-4892; **Phone:** 212-606-1023; **Board Cert:** Diagnostic Radiology 1990; **Med School:** NY Med Coll 1985; **Resid:** Diagnostic Radiology, N Shore Univ Hosp 1990; **Fellow:** Diagnostic Radiology, Hosp for Special Surgery 1991; **Fac Appt:** Prof Rad, Cornell Univ-Weill Med Coll

Prince, Martin R MD/PhD (DR) - **Spec Exp:** MRI Angiography; Abdominal Imaging; **Hospital:** NY-Presby/Weill Cornell Med Ctr, NY (page 104), NY-Presby/Columbia Univ Med Ctr, NY (page 104); **Address:** 416 E 55th St, New York, NY 10022; **Phone:** 212-746-6880; **Board Cert:** Diagnostic Radiology 1993; **Med School:** Harvard Med Sch 1985; **Resid:** Radiology, Mass Genl Hosp 1988; **Fellow:** Magnetic Resonance Imaging, Mass Genl Hosp 1989; Angiography, Mass Genl Hosp 1993; **Fac Appt:** Prof Rad, Cornell Univ-Weill Med Coll

Recht, Michael MD (DR) - **Spec Exp:** Musculoskeletal Imaging; **Hospital:** NYU Langone Med Ctr (page 108); **Address:** NYU Sch Med, Dept Radiology, 660 First Ave Fl 3, New York, NY 10016; **Phone:** 212-263-9530; **Board Cert:** Diagnostic Radiology 1987; **Med School:** Univ Pennsylvania 1983; **Resid:** Radiology, Hosp Univ Penn 1987; **Fellow:** Interventional Radiology, Hosp Univ Penn 1988; Musculoskeletal Imaging, UCSD Med Ctr 1992; **Fac Appt:** Prof Rad, NYU Sch Med

Rosenberg, Zehava S MD (DR) - **Spec Exp:** Musculoskeletal Imaging; **Hospital:** NYU Langone Med Ctr (page 108), NYU Hosp For Joint Dis (page 108); **Address:** NYU Hosp for Joint Diseases, 301 E 17th St, rm 600, New York, NY 10003; **Phone:** 212-598-6112; **Board Cert:** Diagnostic Radiology 1985; **Med School:** Univ Conn 1980; **Resid:** Diagnostic Radiology, Einstein Affil Hosp 1984; **Fellow:** Musculoskeletal Imaging, NY Columbia-Presby Hosp 1986; **Fac Appt:** Prof Rad, NYU Sch Med

Rosenblatt, Ruth MD (DR) - **Spec Exp:** Breast Cancer; **Hospital:** NY-Presby/Weill Cornell Med Ctr, NY (page 104); **Address:** 425 E 61st St Fl 9, New York, NY 10065; **Phone:** 212-821-0661; **Board Cert:** Diagnostic Radiology 1969; **Med School:** Med Coll PA Hahnemann 1964; **Resid:** Diagnostic Radiology, Montefiore Med Ctr 1968; **Fac Appt:** Clin Prof Rad, Cornell Univ-Weill Med Coll

Rosenfeld, Stanley MD (DR) - **Spec Exp:** Mammography; Ultrasound; Breast MRI; **Hospital:** Mt Sinai Med Ctr (page 102); **Address:** Rosetta Radiology, 1421 3rd Ave, New York, NY 10028; **Phone:** 212-744-5538; **Board Cert:** Diagnostic Radiology 1978; **Med School:** Albert Einstein Coll Med 1974; **Resid:** Diagnostic Radiology, Montefiore Hosp Med Ctr 1978; **Fac Appt:** Asst Prof Rad, Mount Sinai Sch Med

Ruzal-Shapiro, Carrie MD (DR) - **Spec Exp:** Pediatric Radiology; **Hospital:** NY-Presby/Columbia Univ Med Ctr, NY (page 104); **Address:** NY Presby/Columbia-Dept Radiology, 3959 Broadway, Chony 3 North, New York, NY 10032; **Phone:** 212-305-9665; **Board Cert:** Diagnostic Radiology 1988; Pediatric Radiology 2004; **Med School:** Columbia P&S 1982; **Resid:** Radiology, NY-Presby/Columbia Univ Med Ctr 1988; **Fellow:** Pediatric Radiology, NY-Presby/Columbia Univ Med Ctr 1989; **Fac Appt:** Clin Prof Rad, Columbia P&S

Schwartz, Lawrence H MD (DR) - **Spec Exp:** Prostate Cancer; MRI; **Hospital:** NY-Presby/Columbia Univ Med Ctr, NY (page 104); **Address:** 180 Ft Washington Ave, Harkness Pav, rm 320, New York, NY 10032; **Phone:** 212-305-8994; **Board Cert:** Diagnostic Radiology 1991; **Med School:** Boston Univ 1986; **Resid:** Diagnostic Radiology, NY-Presby/Weill Cornell Med Ctr 1991; **Fellow:** Ultrasound/CT/MRI, Brigham & Women's Hosp 1991; **Fac Appt:** Prof Rad, Columbia P&S

Som, Peter MD (DR) - **Spec Exp:** CT Scan; PET Imaging; MRI; Cancer Imaging; **Hospital:** Mt Sinai Med Ctr (page 102); **Address:** Radiology Associates, 1176 Fifth Ave, New York, NY 10029; **Phone:** 212-241-8333; **Board Cert:** Diagnostic Radiology 1972; **Med School:** NYU Sch Med 1967; **Resid:** Diagnostic Radiology, Mt Sinai Hosp 1971; **Fac Appt:** Prof Rad, Mount Sinai Sch Med

Sonnenblick, Emily B MD (DR) - **Spec Exp:** Breast Imaging; Breast MRI; **Hospital:** Mt Sinai Med Ctr (page 102); **Address:** Mount Sinai Medical Center, 1176 Fifth Ave, New York, NY 10029; **Phone:** 212-744-5538; **Board Cert:** Diagnostic Radiology 1987; **Med School:** Cornell Univ-Weill Med Coll 1982; **Resid:** Diagnostic Radiology, Hosp U Penn 1984; Diagnostic Radiology, Columbia-Presby Med Ctr 1986; **Fellow:** Ultrasound, Mt Sinai Med Ctr 1987

Wolff, Steven D MD/PhD (DR) - **Spec Exp:** Cardiovascular Imaging; Cardiac MRI; **Hospital:** Lenox Hill Hosp (page 106), NY-Presby/Columbia Univ Med Ctr, NY (page 104); **Address:** 170 E 77th St, New York, NY 10075; **Phone:** 212-369-9200; **Board Cert:** Diagnostic Radiology 1994; **Med School:** Duke Univ 1989; **Resid:** Diagnostic Radiology, Johns Hopkins Hosp 1994

Yankelevitz, David F MD (DR) - **Spec Exp:** Lung Cancer; Thoracic Radiology; **Hospital:** Mt Sinai Med Ctr (page 102); **Address:** Mt Sinai Med Ctr, Radiology Dept, 1 Gustave Levy Pl, Box 1234, New York, NY 10029; **Phone:** 212-241-2420; **Board Cert:** Diagnostic Radiology 1987; Nuclear Medicine 1987; **Med School:** SUNY Hlth Sci Ctr 1981; **Resid:** Diagnostic Radiology, Long Island Coll Hosp 1984; Nuclear Medicine, NY-Cornell Med Ctr 1986; **Fellow:** Diagnostic Radiology, NY-Cornell Med Ctr 1987; **Fac Appt:** Prof Rad, Cornell Univ-Weill Med Coll

Endocrinology, Diabetes & Metabolism

Bergman, Donald MD (EDM) - **Spec Exp:** Osteoporosis; Thyroid Disorders; Calcium Disorders; Paget's Disease of Bone; **Hospital:** Mt Sinai Med Ctr (page 102); **Address:** 1199 Park Ave, Ste 1F, New York, NY 10128; **Phone:** 212-876-7333; **Board Cert:** Internal Medicine 1975; Endocrinology, Diabetes & Metabolism 1977; **Med School:** Jefferson Med Coll 1971; **Resid:** Obstetrics & Gynecology, Mt Sinai Hosp 1972; Internal Medicine, Mt Sinai Hosp 1975; **Fellow:** Endocrinology, Diabetes & Metabolism, Mt Sinai Hosp 1977; **Fac Appt:** Clin Prof Med, Mount Sinai Sch Med

Bilezikian, John P MD (EDM) - **Spec Exp:** Osteoporosis; Bone Disorders-Metabolic; **Hospital:** NY-Presby/Columbia Univ Med Ctr, NY (page 104); **Address:** Columbia Metabolic Bone Disease Program, Harkness Pavilion, 180 Ft Washington Ave Fl 9 - Ste 904, New York, NY 10032; **Phone:** 212-305-2663; **Board Cert:** Internal Medicine 1975; Endocrinology, Diabetes & Metabolism 1977; **Med School:** Columbia P&S 1969; **Resid:** Internal Medicine, NY-Presby/Columbia Univ Med Ctr 1975; **Fellow:** Endocrinology, Diabetes & Metabolism, Natl Inst Health 1977; **Fac Appt:** Prof Med, Columbia P&S

Bloomgarden, Zachary T MD (EDM) - **Spec Exp:** Diabetes; Diabetic Kidney Disease; Cholesterol/Lipid Disorders; **Hospital:** Mt Sinai Med Ctr (page 102); **Address:** 35 E 85th St, New York, NY 10028-0954; **Phone:** 212-879-5933; **Board Cert:** Internal Medicine 1977; Endocrinology, Diabetes & Metabolism 1979; **Med School:** Albert Einstein Coll Med 1974; **Resid:** Internal Medicine, Montefiore Med Ctr 1977; **Fellow:** Endocrinology, Diabetes & Metabolism, Vanderbilt Univ Med Ctr 1979; **Fac Appt:** Clin Prof Med, Mount Sinai Sch Med

Blum, Conrad B MD (EDM) - **Spec Exp:** Cholesterol/Lipid Disorders; Thyroid Disorders; Diabetes; **Hospital:** NY-Presby/Columbia Univ Med Ctr, NY (page 104); **Address:** 51 W 51 St, rm 360, New York, NY 10022-1002; **Phone:** 212-326-8421; **Board Cert:** Internal Medicine 1976; Endocrinology, Diabetes & Metabolism 1977; **Med School:** Northwestern Univ 1971; **Resid:** Internal Medicine, Brigham & Women's Hosp 1976; **Fellow:** Endocrinology, Diabetes & Metabolism, Northwestern Meml Hosp 1977; **Fac Appt:** Clin Prof Med, Columbia P&S

Bockman, Richard S MD/PhD (EDM) - **Spec Exp:** Bone Disorders-Metabolic; Osteoporosis; Parathyroid Disorders; Paget's Disease of Bone; **Hospital:** Hosp For Special Surgery (page 113), NY-Presby/Weill Cornell Med Ctr, NY (page 104); **Address:** 519 E 72nd St, Ste 206, New York, NY 10021; **Phone:** 212-606-1458; **Board Cert:** Internal Medicine 1975; **Med School:** Yale Univ 1968; **Resid:** Internal Medicine, NYU Langone Med Ctr 1973; **Fellow:** Endocrinology, Diabetes & Metabolism, NY-Presby/Weill Cornell Med Ctr 1975; **Fac Appt:** Prof Med, Cornell Univ-Weill Med Coll

Brett, Elise M MD (EDM) - **Spec Exp:** Diabetes; Osteoporosis; **Hospital:** Mt Sinai Med Ctr (page 102); **Address:** 1192 Park Ave, New York, NY 10128; **Phone:** 212-831-2100; **Board Cert:** Internal Medicine 2007; Endocrinology, Diabetes & Metabolism 2009; **Med School:** Mount Sinai Sch Med 1994; **Resid:** Internal Medicine, Mt Sinai Hosp 1997; **Fellow:** Endocrinology, Diabetes & Metabolism, Mt Sinai Hosp 1999; **Fac Appt:** Assoc Clin Prof Med, Mount Sinai Sch Med

Brillon, David J MD (EDM) - **Spec Exp:** Diabetes; Thyroid Disorders; Clinical Trials; **Hospital:** NY-Presby/Weill Cornell Med Ctr, NY (page 104); **Address:** Cornell-Weill Physicians-Endocrinology, 525 E 68th St Fl 20, Baker Pavilion, New York, NY 10065; **Phone:** 212-746-6290; **Board Cert:** Internal Medicine 1983; Endocrinology, Diabetes & Metabolism 1987; **Med School:** Brown Univ 1980; **Resid:** Internal Medicine, Rochester Genl Hosp 1983; **Fellow:** Endocrinology, Rochester Genl Hosp 1986; Endocrinology, Diabetes & Metabolism, UCSD Med Ctr 1988; **Fac Appt:** Clin Prof Med, Cornell Univ-Weill Med Coll

Bukberg, Phillip MD (EDM) - **Spec Exp:** Diabetes; Cholesterol/Lipid Disorders; **Hospital:** Beth Israel Med Ctr - Petrie Div (page 94); **Address:** 317 E 17th St Fl 7, Fierman Hall, New York, NY 10003; **Phone:** 212-420-2777; **Board Cert:** Internal Medicine 1977; Endocrinology, Diabetes & Metabolism 1979; **Med School:** SUNY Downstate 1973; **Resid:** Internal Medicine, St Vincent's Hosp & Med Ctr 1977; **Fellow:** Endocrinology, Meml Sloan Kettering Cancer Ctr 1979; Endocrinology, Mt Sinai Hosp 1982

Davies, Terry F MD (EDM) - **Spec Exp:** Thyroid Disorders in Pregnancy; Graves' Disease; Hashimoto's Disease; Thyroid Cancer; **Hospital:** Mt Sinai Med Ctr (page 102), VA Hudson Valley-FDR/Montrose; **Address:** 5 E 98th St, Box 1055, New York, NY 10029-6500; **Phone:** 212-241-7975; **Med School:** England, UK 1971; **Resid:** Internal Medicine, Univ Newcastle Affil Hosp 1975; **Fellow:** Endocrinology, Diabetes & Metabolism, Univ Newcastle Affil Hosp 1977; Endocrinology, Diabetes & Metabolism, Natl Inst Hlth 1979; **Fac Appt:** Prof Med, Mount Sinai Sch Med

Fagin, James A MD (EDM) - **Spec Exp:** Thyroid Cancer; **Hospital:** Meml Sloan-Kettering Canc Ctr (page 114); **Address:** Meml Sloan-Kettering Cancer Ctr, 1275 York Ave, New York, NY 10065; **Phone:** 646-888-2718; **Board Cert:** Internal Medicine ; Endocrinology, Diabetes & Metabolism 2010; **Med School:** Argentina 1973; **Resid:** Internal Medicine, Hammersmith/W Middlesex Hosp 1981; Endocrinology, Diabetes & Metabolism, Hosp Italiano 1983; **Fellow:** Endocrinology, Diabetes & Metabolism, VA Wadsworth Hosp/Cedars-Sinai Med Ctr 1985

Goland, Robin S MD (EDM) - **Spec Exp:** Diabetes; **Hospital:** NY-Presby/Columbia Univ Med Ctr, NY (page 104); **Address:** 1150 St Nicholas Ave Fl 2, Naomi Berrie Diabetic Ctr, New York, NY 10032; **Phone:** 212-851-5494; **Board Cert:** Internal Medicine 1983; Endocrinology 1989; **Med School:** Columbia P&S 1980; **Resid:** Internal Medicine, Columbia-Presby Med Ctr 1984; **Fellow:** Endocrinology, Diabetes & Metabolism, Columbia-Presby Med Ctr 1987; **Fac Appt:** Prof Med, Columbia P&S

Greene, Loren Wissner MD (EDM) - **Spec Exp:** Thyroid Disorders; Osteoporosis; Pituitary Disorders; Diabetes; **Hospital:** NYU Langone Med Ctr (page 108), NY-Presby/Lower Manhattan Hosp (page 104); **Address:** 650 First Ave, Fl 7th, New York, NY 10016-6402; **Phone:** 212-263-7449; **Board Cert:** Internal Medicine 1978; Endocrinology, Diabetes & Metabolism 1981; **Med School:** NYU Sch Med 1975; **Resid:** Internal Medicine, Bellevue Hosp Ctr-NYU 1978; **Fellow:** Endocrinology, Bellevue Hosp Ctr-NYU 1980; **Fac Appt:** Assoc Clin Prof Med, NYU Sch Med

Haber, Richard S MD (EDM) - **Spec Exp:** Thyroid Disorders; Thyroid Cancer; Parathyroid Disorders; Parathyroid Cancer; **Hospital:** Mt Sinai Med Ctr (page 102); **Address:** Mt Sinai Med Ctr, Dept Medicine, Div of Endocrinology, 5 E 98th St Fl 11, New York, NY 10029; **Phone:** 212-241-7975; **Board Cert:** Endocrinology, Diabetes & Metabolism 1983; Internal Medicine 1980; **Med School:** NYU Sch Med 1977; **Resid:** Internal Medicine, SUNY Health Sci Ctr 1980; **Fellow:** Endocrinology, Diabetes & Metabolism, NY Presby-Columbia Med Ctr 1983; **Fac Appt:** Prof Med, Mount Sinai Sch Med

Jacobs Jr, Thomas P MD (EDM) - **Spec Exp:** Adrenal Disorders; Pituitary Disorders; Calcium Disorders; Thyroid Disorders; **Hospital:** NY-Presby/Columbia Univ Med Ctr, NY (page 104); **Address:** 161 Fort Washington Ave, rm 210, MS 10032, New York, NY 10032-3713; **Phone:** 212-305-5578; **Board Cert:** Internal Medicine 1973; Endocrinology, Diabetes & Metabolism 1975; **Med School:** Johns Hopkins Univ 1968; **Resid:** Internal Medicine, Columbia Presby Hosp 1973; **Fellow:** Endocrinology, Diabetes & Metabolism, Univ Wash Med Ctr 1975; **Fac Appt:** Clin Prof Med, Columbia P&S

Kleinberg, David L MD (EDM) - **Spec Exp:** Pituitary Disorders; Neuroendocrinology; **Hospital:** NYU Langone Med Ctr (page 108); **Address:** 650 1st Ave Fl 4, New York, NY 10016; **Phone:** 212-263-6772; **Board Cert:** Internal Medicine 1972; Endocrinology 1975; **Med School:** Univ Miami Sch Med 1966; **Resid:** Internal Medicine, Maimonides Med Ctr 1968; Internal Medicine, NY-Presby/Columbia Univ Med Ctr 1971; **Fellow:** Endocrinology, Diabetes & Metabolism, NY-Presby/Columbia Univ Med Ctr 1970; **Fac Appt:** Prof Med, NYU Sch Med

Klyde, Barry J MD (EDM) - **Spec Exp:** Thyroid Disorders; Adrenal Disorders; Reproductive Endocrinology; Bone Disorders-Metabolic; **Hospital:** NY-Presby/Weill Cornell Med Ctr, NY (page 104); **Address:** 520 E 72nd St, Ste LO, New York, NY 10021-4840; **Phone:** 212-772-3333; **Board Cert:** Internal Medicine 1977; Endocrinology, Diabetes & Metabolism 1981; **Med School:** Stanford Univ 1974; **Resid:** Internal Medicine, New York Hosp 1977; **Fellow:** Endocrinology, Diabetes & Metabolism, New York Hosp & Rockefeller Univ 1979; **Fac Appt:** Asst Clin Prof Med, Cornell Univ-Weill Med Coll

Levine, Alice C MD (EDM) - **Spec Exp:** Adrenal Disorders; Pituitary Disorders; Reproductive Endocrinology; **Hospital:** Mt Sinai Med Ctr (page 102); **Address:** Mt Sinai School of Med, Dept of Medicine - Endocrinology, 5 E 98th St Fl 11, New York, NY 10029; **Phone:** 212-241-7975; **Board Cert:** Internal Medicine 1984; Endocrinology, Diabetes & Metabolism 1987; **Med School:** Columbia P&S 1981; **Resid:** Internal Medicine, NYU/Manhattan VA Hosp 1984; **Fellow:** Endocrinology, Diabetes & Metabolism, Mt Sinai Med Ctr 1986; **Fac Appt:** Prof Med, Mount Sinai Sch Med

Maclaren, Noel Keith MD (EDM) - **Spec Exp:** Diabetes; Obesity; Thyroid Disorders; Addison's Disease; **Hospital:** Lenox Hill Hosp (page 106), NY-Presby/Weill Cornell Med Ctr, NY (page 104); **Address:** Bioseek Endocrine Clinic, 200 W 57th St, Ste 605, New York, NY 10019; **Phone:** 212-371-0658; **Board Cert:** Pediatrics 1977; Pediatric Endocrinology 1978; **Med School:** New Zealand 1963; **Resid:** Internal Medicine, Wellington Public Hosp 1967; **Fellow:** Pediatric Endocrinology, Johns Hopkins Hosp 1973; Pediatric Endocrinology, Univ MD Hosp 1974; **Fac Appt:** Prof Ped, Cornell Univ-Weill Med Coll

McConnell, Robert J MD (EDM) - **Spec Exp:** Thyroid Disorders; Thyroid Ultrasound; **Hospital:** NY-Presby/Columbia Univ Med Ctr, NY (page 104); **Address:** 161 Fort Washington Ave, Ste 210, New York, NY 10032-3713; **Phone:** 212-305-5579; **Board Cert:** Internal Medicine 1978; Endocrinology, Diabetes & Metabolism 1981; **Med School:** Columbia P&S 1973; **Resid:** Internal Medicine, Barnes Hosp 1975; **Fellow:** Endocrinology, Diabetes & Metabolism, Columbia-Presby Hosp 1978; **Fac Appt:** Clin Prof Med, Columbia P&S

Mechanick, Jeffrey I MD (EDM) - **Spec Exp:** Nutrition; Thyroid Disorders; Thyroid Cancer; Bone Disorders-Metabolic; **Hospital:** Mt Sinai Med Ctr (page 102); **Address:** 1192 Park Ave, New York, NY 10128; **Phone:** 212-831-2100; **Board Cert:** Internal Medicine 1988; Endocrinology, Diabetes & Metabolism 2003; **Med School:** Mount Sinai Sch Med 1985; **Resid:** Internal Medicine, Baylor Affil Hosp 1988; **Fellow:** Endocrinology, Diabetes & Metabolism, Mt Sinai Hosp 1990; **Fac Appt:** Clin Prof Med, Mount Sinai Sch Med

Peck, Valerie H MD (EDM) - **Spec Exp:** Osteoporosis; Thyroid Disorders; Obesity; Weight Management; **Hospital:** NYU Langone Med Ctr (page 108); **Address:** 135 E 37th St, New York, NY 10016; **Phone:** 212-213-3233; **Board Cert:** Internal Medicine 1977; Endocrinology, Diabetes & Metabolism 1979; **Med School:** NYU Sch Med 1974; **Resid:** Internal Medicine, Bellevue Hosp Ctr 1977; **Fellow:** Endocrinology, Bellevue Hosp Ctr 1978; **Fac Appt:** Assoc Clin Prof Med, NYU Sch Med

Poretsky, Leonid MD (EDM) - **Spec Exp:** Diabetes; Thyroid Disorders; **Hospital:** Beth Israel Med Ctr - Petrie Div (page 94); **Address:** 317 E 17th St Fl 7, New York, NY 10003; **Phone:** 212-420-2226; **Board Cert:** Internal Medicine 1983; Endocrinology, Diabetes & Metabolism 1985; **Med School:** Russia 1977; **Resid:** Internal Medicine, Coney Island Hosp 1983; **Fellow:** Endocrinology, Beth Israel Hosp 1985; **Fac Appt:** Prof Med, Albert Einstein Coll Med

Rayfield, Elliot J MD (EDM) - **Spec Exp:** Diabetes; Hypoglycemia; **Hospital:** Mt Sinai Med Ctr (page 102); **Address:** Park Avenue Diabetes Care, 1150 Park Ave Fl 1, New York, NY 10128; **Phone:** 212-427-9191; **Board Cert:** Internal Medicine 1971; Endocrinology, Diabetes & Metabolism 1973; **Med School:** Jefferson Med Coll 1967; **Resid:** Internal Medicine, Univ Mich Hosp 1970; **Fellow:** Endocrinology, Diabetes & Metabolism, Peter Bent Brigham Hosp 1971; **Fac Appt:** Clin Prof Med, Mount Sinai Sch Med

Seltzer, Terry F MD (EDM) - **Spec Exp:** Diabetes; Thyroid Disorders; Calcium Disorders; Adrenal Disorders; **Hospital:** NYU Langone Med Ctr (page 108); **Address:** 530 1st Ave, Ste 4D, New York, NY 10016-6402; **Phone:** 212-263-8717; **Board Cert:** Internal Medicine 1980; Endocrinology 1983; **Med School:** Harvard Med Sch 1977; **Resid:** Internal Medicine, NYU-Bellevue Hosp 1980; **Fellow:** Endocrinology, Diabetes & Metabolism, NYU-Bellevue Hosp 1982; **Fac Appt:** Asst Prof Med, NYU Sch Med

Seplowitz, Alan H MD (EDM) - **Spec Exp:** Thyroid Disorders; Cholesterol/Lipid Disorders; Diabetes; **Hospital:** NY-Presby/Columbia Univ Med Ctr, NY (page 104); **Address:** 161 Fort Washington Ave, Ste 4-422, New York, NY 10032-3729; **Phone:** 212-305-5503; **Board Cert:** Internal Medicine 1975; Endocrinology 1977; **Med School:** Columbia P&S 1972; **Resid:** Internal Medicine, Columbia-Presby Med Ctr 1974; **Fellow:** Lipid Metabolism, Natl Inst Hlth 1976; Endocrinology, Diabetes & Metabolism, Columbia-Presby Med Ctr 1978; **Fac Appt:** Assoc Prof Med, Columbia P&S

Shane, Elizabeth J MD (EDM) - **Spec Exp:** Bone Disorders-Metabolic; Osteoporosis; Parathyroid Disorders; **Hospital:** NY-Presby/Columbia Univ Med Ctr, NY (page 104); **Address:** 180 Ft Washington Ave, rm 904, New York, NY 10032; **Phone:** 212-305-2663; **Board Cert:** Internal Medicine 1978; Endocrinology 1981; **Med School:** Univ Toronto 1975; **Resid:** Internal Medicine, Columbia-Presby Hosp 1978; **Fellow:** Endocrinology, Columbia-Presby Hosp 1981; **Fac Appt:** Clin Prof Med, Columbia P&S

Silverberg, Shonni J MD (EDM) - **Spec Exp:** Parathyroid Disorders; Osteoporosis; Calcium Disorders; **Hospital:** NY-Presby/Columbia Univ Med Ctr, NY (page 104); **Address:** 180 Fort Washington Ave, Ste 920, New York, NY 10032; **Phone:** 212-305-2663 x8; **Board Cert:** Internal Medicine 1983; Endocrinology, Diabetes & Metabolism 1985; **Med School:** Cornell Univ-Weill Med Coll 1980; **Resid:** Internal Medicine, NY Hosp 1983; **Fellow:** Endocrinology, Diabetes & Metabolism, Columbia-Presby Med Ctr 1986; **Fac Appt:** Prof Med, Columbia P&S

Siris, Ethel S MD (EDM) - **Spec Exp:** Osteoporosis; Paget's Disease of Bone; Bone Disorders-Metabolic; **Hospital:** NY-Presby/Columbia Univ Med Ctr, NY (page 104); **Address:** 180 Ft Washington Ave, HP Bldg Fl 9 - Ste 903, New York, NY 10032-3710; **Phone:** 212-305-9531; **Board Cert:** Internal Medicine 1974; Endocrinology, Diabetes & Metabolism 1977; **Med School:** Columbia P&S 1971; **Resid:** Internal Medicine, NY-Presby/Columbia Univ Med Ctr 1974; **Fellow:** Research, Natl Inst of Hlth - Clin Ctr 1976; Endocrinology, Diabetes & Metabolism, NY-Presby/Columbia Univ Med Ctr 1977; **Fac Appt:** Prof Med, Columbia P&S

Tuttle, R Michael MD (EDM) - **Spec Exp:** Thyroid Cancer; **Hospital:** Meml Sloan-Kettering Canc Ctr (page 114); **Address:** Meml Sloan Kettering Cancer Ctr, 1275 York Ave, New York, NY 10065; **Phone:** 646-888-2716; **Board Cert:** Endocrinology, Diabetes & Metabolism 2004; **Med School:** Univ Louisville Sch Med 1987; **Resid:** Internal Medicine, DD Eisenhower Army Med Ctr 1990; **Fellow:** Endocrinology, Diabetes & Metabolism, Madigan Army Med Ctr 1993; **Fac Appt:** Prof Med, Cornell Univ-Weill Med Coll

Wardlaw, Sharon L MD (EDM) - **Spec Exp:** Neuroendocrinology; Pituitary Disorders; **Hospital:** NY-Presby/Columbia Univ Med Ctr, NY (page 104); **Address:** 180 Fort Washington Ave, rm 970, New York, NY 10032; **Phone:** 212-305-2254; **Board Cert:** Internal Medicine 1978; Endocrinology, Diabetes & Metabolism 1979; **Med School:** Cornell Univ-Weill Med Coll 1975; **Resid:** Internal Medicine, Case Western Univ Hosp 1977; **Fellow:** Endocrinology, Diabetes & Metabolism, Columbia-Presby 1980; **Fac Appt:** Prof Med, Columbia P&S

Zweig, Susan B MD (EDM) - **Spec Exp:** Thyroid Disorders; Diabetes; Polycystic Ovarian Syndrome; Osteoporosis; **Hospital:** NYU Langone Med Ctr (page 108), Bellevue Hosp Ctr; **Address:** 135 E 37th St, New York, NY 10016; **Phone:** 212-725-7841; **Board Cert:** Internal Medicine 2010; Endocrinology, Diabetes & Metabolism 2002; **Med School:** Israel 1997; **Resid:** Internal Medicine, St Lukes Roosevelt Hosp Ctr 2000; **Fellow:** Endocrinology, Beth Israel Med Ctr 2002; **Fac Appt:** Asst Clin Prof Med, NYU Sch Med

Family Medicine

Calman, Neil S MD (FMed) *PCP* - **Hospital:** Beth Israel Med Ctr - Petrie Div (page 94); **Address:** Sidney Hillman & Phillips Fam Practice, 16 E 16th St, New York, NY 10003-3105; **Phone:** 212-924-7744; **Board Cert:** Family Medicine 2003; **Med School:** Rush Med Coll 1975; **Resid:** Family Medicine, Montefiore Hosp Med Ctr 1978; **Fac Appt:** Prof FMed, Mount Sinai Sch Med

Kligler, Benjamin E MD (FMed) *PCP* - **Spec Exp:** Complementary Medicine; Acupuncture; **Hospital:** Beth Israel Med Ctr - Petrie Div (page 94); **Address:** Continuum Ctr for Health & Healing, 245 Fifth Ave, Fl 2, New York, NY 10016; **Phone:** 646-935-2257; **Board Cert:** Family Medicine 2008; **Med School:** Boston Univ 1990; **Resid:** Family Medicine, Albert Einstein Affil Hosps 1994; **Fac Appt:** Asst Prof FMed, Albert Einstein Coll Med

Levy, Albert MD (FMed) *PCP* - **Spec Exp:** Hypertension; Diabetes; Sexual Dysfunction; **Hospital:** Mt Sinai Med Ctr (page 102), Lenox Hill Hosp (page 106); **Address:** 911 Park Ave, New York, NY 10075; **Phone:** 212-288-7193; **Board Cert:** Family Medicine 2006; **Med School:** Brazil 1973; **Resid:** Surgery, Maimonides Hosp 1978; Family Medicine, Kings County Hosp 1980; **Fac Appt:** Asst Prof Med, Mount Sinai Sch Med

Lyon, Valerie K MD (FMed) *PCP* - **Spec Exp:** Preventive Medicine; **Hospital:** NYU Langone Med Ctr (page 108), Lenox Hill Hosp (page 106); **Address:** 59 E 54th St Fl 2, New York, NY 10022; **Phone:** 212-750-8330; **Board Cert:** Family Medicine 2006; **Med School:** Temple Univ 1986; **Resid:** Family Medicine, South Nassau Comm Hosp 1989

Prine, Linda W MD (FMed) *PCP* - **Hospital:** Beth Israel Med Ctr - Petrie Div (page 94); **Address:** The Institute for Family Health, 16 E 16th St, New York, NY 10003-3105; **Phone:** 212-924-7744; **Board Cert:** Family Medicine 2004; **Med School:** Cornell Univ-Weill Med Coll 1987; **Resid:** Family Medicine, Montefiore Med Ctr 1990; **Fac Appt:** Assoc Clin Prof FMed, Albert Einstein Coll Med

Schiller, Robert M MD (FMed) *PCP* - **Spec Exp:** Complementary Medicine; **Hospital:** Beth Israel Med Ctr - Petrie Div (page 94); **Address:** 16 E 16th St Fl 3, New York, NY 10003-3105; **Phone:** 212-924-7744; **Board Cert:** Family Medicine 2006; **Med School:** NYU Sch Med 1982; **Resid:** Family Medicine, Montefiore Med Ctr 1985; **Fac Appt:** Asst Prof FMed, Albert Einstein Coll Med

Shepard, Richard DO (FMed) *PCP* - **Hospital:** St. Luke's - Roosevelt Hosp Ctr - Roosevelt Div (page 94); **Address:** Manhattan Medical Care, 140 W 69th St, New York, NY 10023; **Phone:** 212-496-9620; **Board Cert:** Family Medicine 2008; Pediatrics 1980; **Med School:** Univ Osteo Med & Hlth Sci, Des Moines 1974; **Resid:** Pediatrics, St Vincent Hosp Med Ctr 1977; Family Medicine, Stony Brook Univ Med Ctr 1985

Gastroenterology

Ackert, John MD (Ge) - **Spec Exp:** Endoscopy; Colonoscopy; Gastroesophageal Reflux Disease (GERD); **Hospital:** NYU Langone Med Ctr (page 108); **Address:** 232 E 30th St, Grnd Fl, New York, NY 10016; **Phone:** 212-889-5544; **Board Cert:** Internal Medicine 1975; Gastroenterology 1977; **Med School:** NYU Sch Med 1972; **Resid:** Internal Medicine, Bellevue Hosp Ctr 1975; **Fellow:** Gastroenterology, Bellevue Hosp Ctr 1977

Adler, Howard MD (Ge) - **Spec Exp:** Colon Cancer; Colonoscopy; Endoscopy; **Hospital:** Montefiore Med Ctr-Einstein Campus (page 100); **Address:** 1020 Park Ave, New York, NY 10028; **Phone:** 646-373-5428; **Board Cert:** Internal Medicine 1967; Gastroenterology 1977; **Med School:** Albert Einstein Coll Med 1960; **Resid:** Internal Medicine, Herbert C Moffitt Hosp 1962; Internal Medicine, Bronx Municipal Hosp 1965; **Fellow:** Gastroenterology, Cornell U-Bellevue Hosp 1967

Agus, Saul G MD (Ge) - **Spec Exp:** Endoscopy; Inflammatory Bowel Disease; Celiac Disease; **Hospital:** Mt Sinai Med Ctr (page 102); **Address:** 1080 5th Ave, New York, NY 10128; **Phone:** 212-860-0841; **Board Cert:** Internal Medicine ; Gastroenterology ; **Med School:** NYU Sch Med 1968; **Resid:** Internal Medicine, Mass Genl Hosp 1972; **Fellow:** Gastroenterology, Mt Sinai Med Ctr 1974; **Fac Appt:** Asst Clin Prof Med, Mount Sinai Sch Med

Aisenberg, James MD (Ge) - **Spec Exp:** Colon Cancer Screening; Inflammatory Bowel Disease; Gastroesophageal Reflux Disease (GERD); Crohn's Disease; **Hospital:** Mt Sinai Med Ctr (page 102); **Address:** 311 E 79th St, Ste 2-A, New York, NY 10075; **Phone:** 212-996-6633; **Board Cert:** Gastroenterology 2000; **Med School:** Harvard Med Sch 1987; **Resid:** Internal Medicine, Columbia-Presby Med Ctr 1990; **Fellow:** Gastroenterology, Mt Sinai Hosp 1993; **Fac Appt:** Clin Prof Med, Mount Sinai Sch Med

Anandasabapathy, Sharmila MD (Ge) - **Spec Exp:** Endoscopy; Barrett's Esophagus; Gastroesophageal Reflux Disease (GERD); **Hospital:** Mt Sinai Med Ctr (page 102); **Address:** Mount Sinai Gastroenterology, 5 E 98th St Fl 11, New York, NY 10029; **Phone:** 212-241-4299; **Board Cert:** Gastroenterology 2004; **Med School:** Albert Einstein Coll Med 1998; **Resid:** Internal Medicine, NY Weill-Cornell Med Ctr 2001; **Fellow:** Gastroenterology, Mt Sinai Med Ctr 2004; **Fac Appt:** Assoc Prof Med, Mount Sinai Sch Med

Baiocco, Peter J MD (Ge) - **Spec Exp:** Inflammatory Bowel Disease; Colon Cancer Screening; Gastroesophageal Reflux Disease (GERD); Endoscopy; **Hospital:** Lenox Hill Hosp (page 106); **Address:** 1317 3rd Ave Fl 5, New York, NY 10021-2995; **Phone:** 212-734-8811; **Board Cert:** Internal Medicine 1981; Gastroenterology 1983; **Med School:** Mount Sinai Sch Med 1978; **Resid:** Internal Medicine, Lenox Hill Hosp 1981; **Fellow:** Gastroenterology, Lenox Hill Hosp 1983; **Fac Appt:** Asst Clin Prof Med, NYU Sch Med

Basuk, Paul M MD (Ge) - **Spec Exp:** Gallbladder Disease; Pancreatic Disease; Esophageal Disorders; **Hospital:** NY-Presby/Weill Cornell Med Ctr, NY (page 104); **Address:** 210 E 86th St, Ste 201, New York, NY 10028; **Phone:** 212-861-9715; **Board Cert:** Internal Medicine 1983; Gastroenterology 1987; **Med School:** Northwestern Univ 1980; **Resid:** Internal Medicine, UCSF Med Ctr 1983; **Fellow:** Gastroenterology, UCSF Med Ctr 1987; **Fac Appt:** Asst Clin Prof Med, Cornell Univ-Weill Med Coll

Bednarek, Karl T MD (Ge) - **Spec Exp:** Colon & Rectal Cancer Detection; **Hospital:** Beth Israel Med Ctr - Petrie Div (page 94); **Address:** 10 Union Square E, Ste 2G, New York, NY 10003; **Phone:** 212-844-6335; **Board Cert:** Internal Medicine 1985; **Med School:** Mount Sinai Sch Med 1982; **Resid:** Internal Medicine, Beth Israel Med Ctr 1986; **Fellow:** Gastroenterology, Beth Israel Med Ctr 1988; **Fac Appt:** Asst Prof Med, Albert Einstein Coll Med

Bernstein, Brett B MD (Ge) - **Spec Exp:** Gastroesophageal Reflux Disease (GERD); Capsule Endoscopy; Colon Cancer Screening; **Hospital:** Beth Israel Med Ctr - Petrie Div (page 94); **Address:** 10 Union Square East, Ste 2G, New York, NY 10003; **Phone:** 212-844-6330; **Board Cert:** Gastroenterology 2005; **Med School:** Mount Sinai Sch Med 1988; **Resid:** Internal Medicine, Beth Israel Med Ctr 1992; **Fellow:** Gastroenterology, Beth Israel Med Ctr 1994; **Fac Appt:** Asst Prof Med, Albert Einstein Coll Med

Borcich, Anthony S MD (Ge) - **Spec Exp:** Liver Disease; Hepatitis C; HIV & Hepatitis co-infection; **Hospital:** Mt Sinai Med Ctr (page 102), Lenox Hill Hosp (page 106); **Address:** 800A 5th Ave, New York, NY 10065; **Phone:** 212-722-8400; **Board Cert:** Internal Medicine 1987; Gastroenterology 1989; **Med School:** Northwestern Univ-Feinberg Sch Med 1984; **Resid:** Internal Medicine, St Lukes-Roosevelt Hosp 1987; **Fellow:** Gastroenterology, St Lukes-Roosevelt Hosp 1989; **Fac Appt:** Asst Clin Prof Med, Mount Sinai Sch Med

Brown Jr, Robert S MD (Ge) - **Spec Exp:** Hepatitis; Liver Disease; Transplant Medicine-Liver; Autoimmune Liver Disease; **Hospital:** NY-Presby/Columbia Univ Med Ctr, NY (page 104), NY-Presby/Weill Cornell Med Ctr, NY (page 104); **Address:** Ctr for Liver Disease & Transplantation, 622 W 168th St PH Bldg Fl 14 - rm 105, New York, NY 10032; **Phone:** 212-305-1305; **Board Cert:** Internal Medicine 2012; Gastroenterology 2005; Transplant Hepatology 2010; **Med School:** NYU Sch Med 1989; **Resid:** Internal Medicine, Beth Israel Deaconess Med Ctr 1992; **Fellow:** Gastroenterology, UCSF Med Ctr 1994; Hepatology, UCSF Med Ctr 1995; **Fac Appt:** Prof Med, Columbia P&S

Cantor, Michael C MD (Ge) - **Spec Exp:** Colon Cancer; Hepatitis; Liver Disease; **Hospital:** NY-Presby/Weill Cornell Med Ctr, NY (page 104); **Address:** 310 E 72nd St Fl Level C, New York, NY 10021-4703; **Phone:** 212-472-3333; **Board Cert:** Internal Medicine 1985; Gastroenterology 1989; **Med School:** Columbia P&S 1982; **Resid:** Internal Medicine, New York Hosp 1985; **Fellow:** Gastroenterology, New York Hosp 1988; **Fac Appt:** Asst Clin Prof Med, Cornell Univ-Weill Med Coll

Carr-Locke, David L MD (Ge) - **Spec Exp:** Pancreatic/Biliary Endoscopy (ERCP); Pancreatic & Biliary Disease; Endoscopy; **Hospital:** Beth Israel Med Ctr - Petrie Div (page 94); **Address:** 10 Union Square E, Ste 2G, New York, NY 10003; **Phone:** 212-420-4015; **Board Cert:** Internal Medicine 1974; **Med School:** England, UK 1972; **Resid:** Obstetrics & Gynecology, Orsett Hosp 1974; Internal Medicine, Leicester Hosp 1976; **Fellow:** Gastroenterology, Leicester Hosp 1978; Research, New Eng Baptist Hosp 1979; **Fac Appt:** Prof Med, Albert Einstein Coll Med

Chang, Peter K MD (Ge) - **Spec Exp:** Endoscopy; **Hospital:** Mt Sinai Med Ctr (page 102); **Address:** 1049 Park Ave, Ste 1C, New York, NY 10028-1061; **Phone:** 212-427-9888; **Board Cert:** Gastroenterology ; **Med School:** Mount Sinai Sch Med 1996; **Resid:** Internal Medicine, Mt Sinai Med Ctr 2000; **Fellow:** Gastroenterology, Mt Sinai Med Ctr 2003

Chapman, Mark L MD (Ge) - **Spec Exp:** Inflammatory Bowel Disease/Crohn's; Peptic Ulcer Disease; Gastrointestinal Motility Disorders; **Hospital:** Mt Sinai Med Ctr (page 102); **Address:** 12 E 86th St, New York, NY 10028-0506; **Phone:** 212-861-2000; **Board Cert:** Internal Medicine 1968; Gastroenterology 1970; **Med School:** SUNY Downstate 1961; **Resid:** Internal Medicine, Montefiore Med Ctr 1963; Internal Medicine, Mt Sinai Hosp 1964; **Fellow:** Gastroenterology, Mt Sinai Hosp 1966; **Fac Appt:** Assoc Clin Prof Med, Mount Sinai Sch Med

Cohen, Jonathan MD (Ge) - **Spec Exp:** Pancreatic/Biliary Endoscopy (ERCP); Colonoscopy; Barrett's Esophagus; Gastrointestinal Cancer; **Hospital:** NYU Langone Med Ctr (page 108); **Address:** Concorde Medical Group, 232 E 30th St, New York, NY 10016-8202; **Phone:** 212-889-5544; **Board Cert:** Gastroenterology 2005; **Med School:** Harvard Med Sch 1990; **Resid:** Internal Medicine, Beth Israel Hosp 1993; **Fellow:** Gastroenterology, UCLA Med Ctr 1995; Endoscopy, Wellesley Hosp 1995; **Fac Appt:** Clin Prof Med, NYU Sch Med

Cohen, Lawrence B MD (Ge) - **Spec Exp:** Gastroesophageal Reflux Disease (GERD); Esophageal Disorders; Colon & Rectal Cancer; Endoscopy; **Hospital:** Mt Sinai Med Ctr (page 102); **Address:** 311 E 79th St, Ste 2A, New York, NY 10075; **Phone:** 212-996-6633; **Board Cert:** Internal Medicine 1981; Gastroenterology 1983; **Med School:** Hahnemann Univ 1978; **Resid:** Internal Medicine, Mt Sinai Med Ctr 1981; **Fellow:** Gastroenterology, Mt Sinai Med Ctr 1983; **Fac Appt:** Clin Prof Med, Mount Sinai Sch Med

Cohen, Seth A MD (Ge) - **Spec Exp:** Pancreatic/Biliary Endoscopy (ERCP); Colonoscopy; Endoscopy; **Hospital:** Beth Israel Med Ctr - Petrie Div (page 94), Lenox Hill Hosp (page 106); **Address:** 305 Second Ave, Lower Level Suite #3, New York, NY 10003; **Phone:** 212-734-8874; **Board Cert:** Internal Medicine 1989; Gastroenterology 2004; **Med School:** Columbia P&S 1986; **Resid:** Internal Medicine, Mount Sinai Med Ctr 1989; **Fellow:** Gastroenterology, St Luke's-Roosevelt Hosp Ctr 1991; Gastroenterology, Beth Israel Hosp 1992

Connor, Bradley A MD (Ge) - **Spec Exp:** Travel Medicine; Parasitic Infections; Diarrheal Diseases; Tropical Diseases; **Hospital:** NY-Presby/Weill Cornell Med Ctr, NY (page 104); **Address:** 50 E 69th St, New York, NY 10021; **Phone:** 212-988-2800; **Board Cert:** Internal Medicine 1982; Gastroenterology 1985; **Med School:** Univ Tex SW, Dallas 1978; **Resid:** Internal Medicine, UT Hlth Sci Ctr-Bexar Co/A Murphy VA Hosps 1981; **Fellow:** Gastroenterology, NY Hosp 1984; **Fac Appt:** Assoc Clin Prof Med, Cornell Univ-Weill Med Coll

Cooper, Robert B MD (Ge) - **Spec Exp:** Colon Cancer Screening; Gastroesophageal Reflux Disease (GERD); Celiac Disease; Gallbladder Disease; **Hospital:** NY-Presby/Weill Cornell Med Ctr, NY (page 104); **Address:** 635 Madison Ave Fl 17, New York, NY 10022; **Phone:** 212-717-4967; **Board Cert:** Internal Medicine 1984; Gastroenterology 1989; **Med School:** Cornell Univ-Weill Med Coll 1981; **Resid:** Internal Medicine, NY Hosp/Weill Cornell Med Ctr 1984; **Fellow:** Gastroenterology, NY Hosp/Weill Cornell Med Ctr 1987; **Fac Appt:** Asst Clin Prof Med, Cornell Univ-Weill Med Coll

Dieterich, Douglas T MD (Ge) - **Spec Exp:** Hepatitis; AIDS/HIV-Gastrointestinal Complications; Liver Disease; Endoscopy; **Hospital:** Mt Sinai Med Ctr (page 102); **Address:** 5 E 98th St Fl 11, New York, NY 10029; **Phone:** 212-241-7270; **Board Cert:** Internal Medicine 1981; Gastroenterology 1987; **Med School:** NYU Sch Med 1978; **Resid:** Internal Medicine, Bellevue Hosp Ctr 1981; **Fellow:** Gastroenterology, Bellevue Hosp Ctr 1983; **Fac Appt:** Prof Med, Mount Sinai Sch Med

Faust, Michael J MD (Ge) - **Spec Exp:** Gastrointestinal Disorders; **Hospital:** NYU Langone Med Ctr (page 108); **Address:** 345 E 37th St, Ste 207, New York, NY 10016-3256; **Phone:** 212-986-3330; **Board Cert:** Internal Medicine 1981; Gastroenterology 1983; **Med School:** NYU Sch Med 1978; **Resid:** Internal Medicine, Bellevue Hosp/NYU Med Ctr 1981; **Fellow:** Gastroenterology, Bellevue Hosp 1983; **Fac Appt:** Asst Clin Prof Med, NYU Sch Med

Ferran, Elena Nascimbeni MD (Ge) - **Spec Exp:** Colonoscopy; Endoscopy; Irritable Bowel Syndrome; Liver Disease; **Hospital:** NYU Langone Med Ctr (page 108); **Address:** NYU-Tisch Ctr for Womens Hlth, 207 E 84 St, New York, NY 10028; **Phone:** 646-754-3300; **Board Cert:** Gastroenterology 2008; **Med School:** Italy 1988; **Resid:** Internal Medicine, St Vincent's Hosp 1994; **Fellow:** Gastroenterology, St Vincent's Hosp 1997; Hepatology, Mt Sinai Hosp 1998

Fochios, Steven E MD (Ge) - **Spec Exp:** Endoscopy; **Hospital:** Lenox Hill Hosp (page 106); **Address:** 117 E 65th St, New York, NY 10065; **Phone:** 212-861-4278; **Board Cert:** Internal Medicine 1980; Gastroenterology 1985; **Med School:** Geo Wash Univ 1976; **Resid:** Internal Medicine, Lenox Hill Hosp 1979; **Fellow:** Gastroenterology, Lenox Hill Hosp 1981

Foong, Anthony MD (Ge) - **Spec Exp:** Endoscopy; Colonoscopy; Gastrointestinal Disorders; Hemorrhoids; **Hospital:** Beth Israel Med Ctr - Petrie Div (page 94); **Address:** 210 Canal St, Ste 601, New York, NY 10013; **Phone:** 212-693-2100; **Board Cert:** Internal Medicine 1984; Gastroenterology 1987; **Med School:** Tufts Univ 1981; **Resid:** Internal Medicine, Univ Md Hosp 1984; **Fellow:** Gastroenterology, St Luke's-Roosevelt Hosp Ctr 1986

Frank, Michael S MD (Ge) - **Spec Exp:** Inflammatory Bowel Disease/Crohn's; Colonoscopy; Endoscopy; **Hospital:** Lenox Hill Hosp (page 106); **Address:** 9 E 63rd St, New York, NY 10065; **Phone:** 212-593-7170; **Board Cert:** Internal Medicine 1977; Gastroenterology 1979; **Med School:** Albert Einstein Coll Med 1974; **Resid:** Internal Medicine, Bronx Municipal Hosps 1977; **Fellow:** Gastroenterology, Montefiore Med Ctr 1979; **Fac Appt:** Assoc Clin Prof Med, NYU Sch Med

Freiman, Hal MD (Ge) - **Spec Exp:** Gastroesophageal Reflux Disease (GERD); Colon Cancer Screening; Irritable Bowel Syndrome; Hepatitis; **Hospital:** Beth Israel Med Ctr - Petrie Div (page 94), NYU Langone Med Ctr (page 108); **Address:** 59 W 12th St, Ste 1D, New York, NY 10011-8520; **Phone:** 212-206-0074; **Board Cert:** Internal Medicine 1981; Gastroenterology 1983; **Med School:** Albany Med Coll 1978; **Resid:** Internal Medicine, St Vincent's Hosp 1981; **Fellow:** Gastroenterology, Westchester Co Med Ctr 1983

Friedlander, Charles N MD (Ge) - **Spec Exp:** Colonoscopy; Irritable Bowel Syndrome; **Hospital:** NYU Langone Med Ctr (page 108); **Address:** 232 E 30th St, New York, NY 10016-8202; **Phone:** 212-889-5544; **Board Cert:** Internal Medicine 1974; Gastroenterology 1977; **Med School:** SUNY Downstate 1968; **Resid:** Internal Medicine, Bellevue Hosp 1974; **Fellow:** Gastroenterology, NYU Med Ctr 1976; **Fac Appt:** Assoc Clin Prof Med, NYU Sch Med

Gerdes, Hans MD (Ge) - **Spec Exp:** Endoscopy; Endoscopic Ultrasound; Barrett's Esophagus; Gastrointestinal Cancer; **Hospital:** Meml Sloan-Kettering Canc Ctr (page 114); **Address:** 1275 York Avenue, New York, NY 10065; **Phone:** 212-639-7108; **Board Cert:** Internal Medicine 1987; Gastroenterology 1989; **Med School:** Cornell Univ-Weill Med Coll 1983; **Resid:** Internal Medicine, New York Hosp 1986; **Fellow:** Gastroenterology, Meml Sloan Kettering Cancer Ctr 1989; **Fac Appt:** Prof Med, Cornell Univ-Weill Med Coll

Gerson, Charles MD (Ge) - **Spec Exp:** Irritable Bowel Syndrome; Diarrheal Diseases; **Hospital:** Mt Sinai Med Ctr (page 102); **Address:** 80 Central Park West, Ste B, New York, NY 10023-5204; **Phone:** 212-496-6161; **Board Cert:** Internal Medicine 1970; Gastroenterology 1972; **Med School:** SUNY Downstate 1962; **Resid:** Internal Medicine, Bellevue Hosp 1964; Internal Medicine, Mount Sinai Hosp 1965; **Fellow:** Gastroenterology, Bellevue Hosp 1968; Gastroenterology, Mount Sinai Hosp 1969; **Fac Appt:** Clin Prof Med, Mount Sinai Sch Med

Goldberg, Myron D MD (Ge) - **Spec Exp:** Colon Cancer Screening; Colonoscopy; Endoscopy; Hepatitis B & C; **Hospital:** Lenox Hill Hosp (page 106), NYU Langone Med Ctr (page 108); **Address:** 110 E 59th St, Ste 10C, New York, NY 10022-1304; **Phone:** 212-583-2900; **Board Cert:** Internal Medicine 1977; Gastroenterology 1979; **Med School:** Albert Einstein Coll Med 1971; **Resid:** Internal Medicine, Montefiore Med Ctr 1973; Internal Medicine, Lenox Hill Hosp 1974; **Fellow:** Gastroenterology, Columbia-Presby Hosp 1977; Gastroenterology, Lenox Hill Hosp 1978; **Fac Appt:** Asst Clin Prof Med, NYU Sch Med

Goldin, Howard MD (Ge) - **Spec Exp:** Inflammatory Bowel Disease/Crohn's; Endoscopy; Liver Disease; **Hospital:** NY-Presby/Weill Cornell Med Ctr, NY (page 104), Rockefeller Univ; **Address:** 646 Park Ave, New York, NY 10065; **Phone:** 212-249-0404; **Board Cert:** Internal Medicine 1968; Gastroenterology 1973; **Med School:** Cornell Univ-Weill Med Coll 1961; **Resid:** Internal Medicine, New York Hosp 1964; **Fellow:** Gastroenterology, New York Hosp 1966; **Fac Appt:** Clin Prof Med, Cornell Univ-Weill Med Coll

Green, Peter H R MD (Ge) - **Spec Exp:** Celiac Disease; Endoscopy; Colonoscopy; Malabsorption Syndrome; **Hospital:** NY-Presby/Columbia Univ Med Ctr, NY (page 104); **Address:** Celiac Dis Ctr, Harkness Bldg, 180 Fort Washington Ave, Ste 936, New York, NY 10032-3713; **Phone:** 212-305-5590; **Med School:** Australia 1970; **Resid:** Internal Medicine, North Shore Med Ctr 1974; **Fellow:** Gastroenterology, North Shore Med Ctr 1976; Gastroenterology, Beth Israel Deaconess Med Ctr 1977; **Fac Appt:** Prof Med, Columbia P&S

Gress, Francis G MD (Ge) - **Spec Exp:** Endoscopy; Pancreatic/Biliary Endoscopy (ERCP); Pancreatic Disease; Barrett's Esophagus; **Hospital:** NY-Presby/Columbia Univ Med Ctr, NY (page 104); **Address:** The Pancreas Center, 161 Fort Washington Ave, rm 852A, Herbert Irving Pavilion, New York, NY 10032; **Phone:** 212-305-1909; **Board Cert:** Gastroenterology 2012; **Med School:** Mount Sinai Sch Med 1988; **Resid:** Internal Medicine, Montefiore Med Ctr 1991; **Fellow:** Gastroenterology, Brooklyn Hosp Ctr 1993; Advanced Endoscopy, Indiana Univ Med Ctr 1994; **Fac Appt:** Prof Med, SUNY Downstate

Haber, Gregory B MD (Ge) - **Spec Exp:** Endoscopy; Pancreatic/Biliary Endoscopy (ERCP); Endoscopic Ultrasound; Barrett's Esophagus; **Hospital:** Lenox Hill Hosp (page 106); **Address:** 100 E 77th St Fl 2, New York, NY 10075; **Phone:** 212-434-6279; **Med School:** Univ Toronto 1970; **Resid:** Internal Medicine, Univ Toronto Med Ctr 1975; **Fellow:** Gastroenterology, Univ Toronto Med Ctr 1978

Hammerman, Hillel S MD (Ge) - **Spec Exp:** Swallowing Disorders; Liver Disease; Colonoscopy; **Hospital:** Lenox Hill Hosp (page 106); **Address:** 210 E 73rd St, Ste 1C, New York, NY 10021; **Phone:** 212-288-1030; **Board Cert:** Internal Medicine 1981; Gastroenterology 1983; **Med School:** Cornell Univ-Weill Med Coll 1978; **Resid:** Internal Medicine, Baltimore City Hosps 1981; **Fellow:** Gastroenterology, Lahey Clin 1983

Harary, Albert M MD (Ge) - **Spec Exp:** Endoscopy & Colonoscopy; Gastroesophageal Reflux Disease (GERD); Swallowing Disorders; **Hospital:** Lenox Hill Hosp (page 106), NYU Langone Med Ctr (page 108); **Address:** 110 E 55th St Fl 17, New York, NY 10022; **Phone:** 212-702-0123; **Board Cert:** Internal Medicine 1982; Gastroenterology 1985; **Med School:** Columbia P&S 1979; **Resid:** Internal Medicine, Univ Miami Affil Hosp 1982; **Fellow:** Gastroenterology, Univ Miami Affil Hosp 1984; **Fac Appt:** Asst Clin Prof Med, NYU Sch Med

Itzkowitz, Steven H MD (Ge) - **Spec Exp:** Colon & Rectal Cancer; Colon & Rectal Cancer Detection; Inflammatory Bowel Disease; Hereditary Cancer; **Hospital:** Mt Sinai Med Ctr (page 102); **Address:** 5 E 98th St, Box 1625, New York, NY 10029-6501; **Phone:** 212-241-4299; **Board Cert:** Internal Medicine 1982; Gastroenterology 1985; **Med School:** Mount Sinai Sch Med 1979; **Resid:** Internal Medicine, Bellevue Hosp/NYU Med Ctr 1982; **Fellow:** Gastroenterology, UCSF Med Ctr 1984; **Fac Appt:** Prof Med, Mount Sinai Sch Med

Jacobson, Ira M MD (Ge) - **Spec Exp:** Liver & Biliary Disease; Hepatitis; Hepatitis C; **Hospital:** NY-Presby/Weill Cornell Med Ctr, NY (page 104); **Address:** 1305 York Ave Fl 4, New York, NY 10021-5016; **Phone:** 646-962-4040; **Board Cert:** Internal Medicine 1982; Gastroenterology 2009; Transplant Hepatology 2006; **Med School:** Columbia P&S 1979; **Resid:** Internal Medicine, UCSF Med Ctr 1982; **Fellow:** Gastroenterology, Mass Genl Hosp 1984; **Fac Appt:** Prof Med, Cornell Univ-Weill Med Coll

Jaffin, Barry W MD (Ge) - **Spec Exp:** Gastrointestinal Motility Disorders; Inflammatory Bowel Disease; **Hospital:** Mt Sinai Med Ctr (page 102); **Address:** 620 Columbus Ave, New York, NY 10024; **Phone:** 212-721-2600; **Board Cert:** Internal Medicine 1984; Gastroenterology 1987; **Med School:** Mount Sinai Sch Med 1981; **Resid:** Internal Medicine, Med Ctr Hosp 1984; **Fellow:** Gastroenterology, Boston Univ Med Ctr 1986; **Fac Appt:** Asst Clin Prof Med, Mount Sinai Sch Med

Kahaleh, Michel MD (Ge) - **Spec Exp:** Pancreatic Disease; Pancreatic Cancer; **Hospital:** NY-Presby/Weill Cornell Med Ctr, NY (page 104); **Address:** 1305 York Ave Fl 4, New York, NY 10065; **Phone:** 646-962-4000; **Board Cert:** Internal Medicine 2009; Gastroenterology 2009; **Med School:** Belgium 1994; **Resid:** Internal Medicine, Univ Chicago Med Ctr 1999; **Fellow:** Gastroenterology, Esrasme Hosp/Univ Brussels; **Fac Appt:** Clin Prof Med, Cornell Univ-Weill Med Coll

Kairam, Indira R MD (Ge) - **Spec Exp:** Colon Cancer; Peptic Ulcer Disease; Hepatitis C; **Hospital:** St. Luke's - Roosevelt Hosp Ctr - St Luke's Hosp (page 94), St. Luke's - Roosevelt Hosp Ctr - Roosevelt Div (page 94); **Address:** 945 West End Ave, Ste 1D, New York, NY 10025-3573; **Phone:** 212-865-7355; **Board Cert:** Internal Medicine 1978; **Med School:** India 1973; **Resid:** Internal Medicine, St Clare's Hosp 1978; **Fellow:** Gastroenterology, Lahey Clinic 1980

Kim, Michelle K MD (Ge) - **Spec Exp:** Endscopic Ultrasound; Endoscopy; Gastrointestinal Cancer; **Hospital:** Mt Sinai Med Ctr (page 102); **Address:** Mt Sinai Faculty Practice, 5 E 98th St Fl 11, Box 1069, New York, NY 10029; **Phone:** 212-241-4299; **Board Cert:** Internal Medicine 2002; Gastroenterology 2005; **Med School:** Stanford Univ 1999; **Resid:** Internal Medicine, Weill Cornell Med Ctr 2002; **Fellow:** Gastroenterology, Weill Cornell Med Ctr 2005; **Fac Appt:** Asst Prof Med, Mount Sinai Sch Med

Kim-Schluger, Hyung Leona MD (Ge) - **Spec Exp:** Transplant Medicine-Liver; Liver Disease; Hepatitis C; **Hospital:** Montefiore Med Ctr-Moses Campus (page 100); **Address:** 5 E 98 St, Fl 12, New York, NY 10029; **Phone:** 212-659-8031; **Board Cert:** Gastroenterology 2003; Transplant Hepatology 2008; **Med School:** Columbia P&S 1988; **Resid:** Internal Medicine, NY-Presby/Columbia Univ Med Ctr 1991; **Fellow:** Gastroenterology, NY-Presby/Columbia Univ Med Ctr 1993; Transplant Hepatology, Mount Sinai Med Ctr 2008

Kimball, Annetta J MD (Ge) - **Spec Exp:** Hepatitis; Inflammatory Bowel Disease/Crohn's; Irritable Bowel Syndrome; **Hospital:** St. Luke's - Roosevelt Hosp Ctr - Roosevelt Div (page 94); **Address:** 315 W 57th St, Ste 301, New York, NY 10019; **Phone:** 212-371-8900; **Board Cert:** Internal Medicine 1972; Gastroenterology 1973; **Med School:** Boston Univ 1968; **Resid:** Internal Medicine, Roosevelt Hosp 1970; Internal Medicine, Mount Sinai Hosp 1971; **Fellow:** Gastroenterology, Mount Sinai Hosp 1973; **Fac Appt:** Assoc Clin Prof Med, Columbia P&S

Knapp, Albert B MD (Ge) - **Spec Exp:** Colonoscopy/Polypectomy; Endoscopy; Liver Disease; Transplant Medicine-Liver; **Hospital:** NYU Langone Med Ctr (page 108), Lenox Hill Hosp (page 106); **Address:** 760 Park Ave, New York, NY 10021-4152; **Phone:** 212-737-3446; **Board Cert:** Internal Medicine 1982; Gastroenterology 1987; **Med School:** Columbia P&S 1979; **Resid:** Internal Medicine, Albert Einstein Med Ctr 1982; **Fellow:** Gastroenterology, Brigham & Women's Hosp 1985; Virology, Pasteur Inst 1975; **Fac Appt:** Clin Prof Med, NYU Sch Med

Kornbluth, Arthur Asher MD (Ge) - **Spec Exp:** Ulcerative Colitis; Crohn's Disease; Colonoscopy; Inflammatory Bowel Disease; **Hospital:** Mt Sinai Med Ctr (page 102), Beth Israel Med Ctr - Petrie Div (page 94); **Address:** 1751 York Ave, New York, NY 10128-6812; **Phone:** 212-369-2490; **Board Cert:** Internal Medicine ; Gastroenterology 2012; **Med School:** SUNY Hlth Sci Ctr 1984; **Resid:** Internal Medicine, Montefiore-Einstein Div Med Ctr 1988; **Fellow:** Gastroenterology, Mt Sinai Hosp 1990; **Fac Appt:** Clin Prof Med, Mount Sinai Sch Med

Kotler, Donald P MD (Ge) - **Spec Exp:** Esophageal Disorders; Nutrition & AIDS; Hepatitis; **Hospital:** St. Luke's - Roosevelt Hosp Ctr - St Luke's Hosp (page 94); **Address:** 1111 Amsterdam Ave, SR 12, New York, NY 10025; **Phone:** 212-523-3670; **Board Cert:** Internal Medicine 1976; Gastroenterology 1979; **Med School:** Albert Einstein Coll Med 1973; **Resid:** Internal Medicine, Jacobi Med Ctr 1976; **Fellow:** Gastroenterology, Hosp Univ Penn - UPHS 1978; **Fac Appt:** Prof Med, Columbia P&S

Krumholz, Michael MD (Ge) - **Spec Exp:** Colonoscopy; Colon Cancer Screening; **Hospital:** Lenox Hill Hosp (page 106), Mt Sinai Med Ctr (page 102); **Address:** 111 E 80th St, Ste 1C, New York, NY 10021-0350; **Phone:** 212-734-5533; **Board Cert:** Internal Medicine 1983; Gastroenterology 1987; **Med School:** Mount Sinai Sch Med 1980; **Resid:** Internal Medicine, Beth Israel Hosp 1984; **Fellow:** Gastroenterology, Lenox Hill Hosp 1986

Kummer, Bart A MD (Ge) - **Spec Exp:** Colonoscopy; Endoscopy; **Hospital:** NYU Langone Med Ctr (page 108), NY-Presby/Lower Manhattan Hosp (page 104); **Address:** NYU Langone Trinity Ctr, 111 Broadway, Fl 2, New York, NY 10006; **Phone:** 212-263-9700; **Board Cert:** Internal Medicine 1982; Gastroenterology 1985; **Med School:** Cornell Univ-Weill Med Coll 1979; **Resid:** Internal Medicine, Harlem Hosp 1982; **Fellow:** Gastroenterology, St Luke's-Roosevelt Hosp Ctr 1985; **Fac Appt:** Asst Prof Med, NYU Sch Med

Kurtz, Robert C MD (Ge) - **Spec Exp:** Pancreatic Cancer (Familial); Gastrointestinal Cancer; Endoscopy; Cancer Prevention; **Hospital:** Meml Sloan-Kettering Canc Ctr (page 114); **Address:** 1275 York Ave, New York, NY 10065; **Phone:** 212-639-7620; **Board Cert:** Internal Medicine 1971; Gastroenterology 1977; **Med School:** Jefferson Med Coll 1968; **Resid:** Internal Medicine, NY Hosp/Meml Sloan Kettering Cancer Ctr 1971; **Fellow:** Gastroenterology, Meml Sloan Kettering Cancer Ctr 1973; **Fac Appt:** Prof Med, Cornell Univ-Weill Med Coll

Lambroza, Arnon MD (Ge) - **Spec Exp:** Achalasia; Gastroesophageal Reflux Disease (GERD); Barrett's Esophagus; Swallowing Disorders; **Hospital:** NY-Presby/Weill Cornell Med Ctr, NY (page 104), Lenox Hill Hosp (page 106); **Address:** 1085 Park Ave, New York, NY 10128-0320; **Phone:** 212-517-7570; **Board Cert:** Internal Medicine 1987; Gastroenterology 2011; **Med School:** Albert Einstein Coll Med 1984; **Resid:** Internal Medicine, Hosp Univ Penn 1987; **Fellow:** Gastroenterology, New York Hosp 1990; **Fac Appt:** Assoc Clin Prof Med, Cornell Univ-Weill Med Coll

Lax, James D MD (Ge) - **Spec Exp:** Liver Disease; Gastroesophageal Reflux Disease (GERD); Barrett's Esophagus; Eosinophilic Esophagitis; **Hospital:** St. Luke's - Roosevelt Hosp Ctr - Roosevelt Div (page 94); **Address:** 160 E 72nd St Fl Ground, New York, NY 10021-4364; **Phone:** 212-988-5740; **Board Cert:** Internal Medicine 1984; Gastroenterology 1987; **Med School:** NYU Sch Med 1981; **Resid:** Internal Medicine, St Luke's-Roosevelt Hosp Ctr 1984; **Fellow:** Gastroenterology, St Luke's-Roosevelt Hosp Ctr 1986; **Fac Appt:** Asst Clin Prof Med, Columbia P&S

Lebwohl, Oscar MD (Ge) - **Spec Exp:** Endoscopy; Inflammatory Bowel Disease/Crohn's; Ulcerative Colitis; Gastrointestinal Cancer; **Hospital:** NY-Presby/Columbia Univ Med Ctr, NY (page 104); **Address:** 161 Fort Washington Ave, rm 420, New York, NY 10032-3713; **Phone:** 212-305-5363; **Board Cert:** Internal Medicine 1975; Gastroenterology 1977; **Med School:** Harvard Med Sch 1972; **Resid:** Internal Medicine, Mt Sinai Med Ctr 1975; **Fellow:** Gastroenterology, Columbia-Presby Med Ctr 1976; Hepatology, Mt Sinai Med Ctr 1977; **Fac Appt:** Prof Med, Columbia P&S

Lewis, Blair MD (Ge) - **Spec Exp:** Endoscopy; Capsule Endoscopy; **Hospital:** Mt Sinai Med Ctr (page 102); **Address:** 1067 5th Ave, New York, NY 10128-0101; **Phone:** 212-369-6600; **Board Cert:** Internal Medicine 1985; Gastroenterology 1987; **Med School:** Albert Einstein Coll Med 1982; **Resid:** Internal Medicine, Montefiore Med Ctr 1985; **Fellow:** Gastroenterology, Mt Sinai Med Ctr 1987; **Fac Appt:** Clin Prof Med, Mount Sinai Sch Med

Lightdale, Charles J MD (Ge) - **Spec Exp:** Barrett's Esophagus; Gastrointestinal Cancer; Endoscopic Ultrasound; **Hospital:** NY-Presby/Columbia Univ Med Ctr, NY (page 104); **Address:** Columbia-Presby Med Ctr, Irving Pavilion, 161 Fort Washington Ave, rm 812, New York, NY 10032-3713; **Phone:** 212-305-3423; **Board Cert:** Internal Medicine 1972; Gastroenterology 1973; **Med School:** Columbia P&S 1966; **Resid:** Internal Medicine, Yale-New Haven Hosp 1968; Internal Medicine, NY Hosp-Cornell 1969; **Fellow:** Gastroenterology, NY Hosp-Cornell 1973; Gastroenterology & Nutrition, Meml Sloan-Kettering Cancer Ctr 1973; **Fac Appt:** Prof Med, Columbia P&S

Loria, Jeffrey Michael MD (Ge) - **Hospital:** Lenox Hill Hosp (page 106); **Address:** 178 E 85th St, Fl 4, New York, NY 10028; **Phone:** 212-288-2278; **Board Cert:** Internal Medicine 2012; Gastroenterology 2005; **Med School:** NY Med Coll 1987; **Resid:** Internal Medicine, Lenox Hill Hosp 1991; **Fellow:** Gastroenterology, Elmhurst Hosp Ctr 1994

Lucak, Susan L MD (Ge) - **Spec Exp:** Irritable Bowel Syndrome; Liver Disease; **Hospital:** Lenox Hill Hosp (page 106); **Address:** 903 Park Ave, New York, NY 10075; **Phone:** 212-861-0481; **Board Cert:** Internal Medicine 1984; Gastroenterology 2011; **Med School:** Albert Einstein Coll Med 1981; **Resid:** Internal Medicine, Montefiore Med Ctr 1985; **Fellow:** Gastroenterology, Montefiore Med Ctr 1987; Research, Columbia Presby Med Ctr 1991

Lustbader, Ian J MD (Ge) - **Spec Exp:** Hepatitis C; Colonoscopy; Crohn's Disease; **Hospital:** NYU Langone Med Ctr (page 108); **Address:** 245 E 35th St Fl 1, New York, NY 10016-4283; **Phone:** 212-685-5252; **Board Cert:** Internal Medicine 1985; Gastroenterology 1987; **Med School:** Columbia P&S 1982; **Resid:** Internal Medicine, St Luke's-Roosevelt Hosp Ctr 1985; **Fellow:** Gastroenterology, Bellevue Hosp 1987; **Fac Appt:** Asst Clin Prof Med, NYU Sch Med

Magun, Arthur M MD (Ge) - **Spec Exp:** Hepatitis; Ulcerative Colitis; Endoscopy; Crohn's Disease; **Hospital:** NY-Presby/Columbia Univ Med Ctr, NY (page 104); **Address:** 161 Fort Washington Ave, Herbert Irving Pavillion Fl 3 - rm 338, New York, NY 10032-3713; **Phone:** 212-305-5287; **Board Cert:** Internal Medicine 1980; Gastroenterology 1983; **Med School:** Mount Sinai Sch Med 1977; **Resid:** Internal Medicine, Presby/Columbia Univ Med Ctr 1980; **Fellow:** Gastroenterology, Presby/Columbia Univ Med Ctr 1983; **Fac Appt:** Clin Prof Med, Columbia P&S

Marion, James F MD (Ge) - **Spec Exp:** Colonoscopy; Colitis; Crohn's Disease; **Hospital:** Mt Sinai Med Ctr (page 102); **Address:** 12 E 86th St, New York, NY 10028; **Phone:** 212-861-2000; **Board Cert:** Internal Medicine 2003; Gastroenterology 2005; **Med School:** Columbia P&S 1989; **Resid:** Internal Medicine, Columbia Presby Hosp 1992; **Fellow:** Gastroenterology, Mt Sinai Hosp 1995; **Fac Appt:** Assoc Clin Prof Med, Mount Sinai Sch Med

Markowitz, Arnold J MD (Ge) - **Spec Exp:** Hereditary Cancer; Colon Cancer Screening; Gastrointestinal Cancer; **Hospital:** Meml Sloan-Kettering Canc Ctr (page 114); **Address:** 1275 York Avenue, New York, NY 10065; **Phone:** 212-639-2901; **Board Cert:** Gastroenterology 2003; **Med School:** NYU Sch Med 1987; **Resid:** Internal Medicine, NYU Med Ctr 1990; **Fellow:** Gastroenterology, Univ Mich Med Ctr 1992; Gastroenterology, Univ Penn Med Ctr 1994; **Fac Appt:** Clin Prof Med, Cornell Univ-Weill Med Coll

Markowitz, David D MD (Ge) - **Spec Exp:** Gastroesophageal Reflux Disease (GERD); Esophageal Disorders; **Hospital:** NY-Presby/Columbia Univ Med Ctr, NY (page 104); **Address:** 161 Ft Washington Ave, Ste 853, New York, NY 10032; **Phone:** 212-305-1024; **Board Cert:** Internal Medicine 1988; Gastroenterology 2011; **Med School:** Columbia P&S 1985; **Resid:** Internal Medicine, Presby/Columbia Univ Med Ctr 1988; **Fellow:** Gastroenterology, Presby/Columbia Univ Med Ctr 1991; **Fac Appt:** Assoc Prof Med, Columbia P&S

Marsh Jr, Franklin MD (Ge) - **Spec Exp:** Liver Disease; Endoscopy; Colon Cancer; Gastrointestinal Motility Disorders; **Hospital:** NY-Presby/Weill Cornell Med Ctr, NY (page 104); **Address:** 342 E 67th St, Ste 1D, New York, NY 10065-6238; **Phone:** 212-288-8820; **Board Cert:** Internal Medicine 1981; Gastroenterology 1985; **Med School:** SUNY Buffalo 1978; **Resid:** Internal Medicine, Harlem Hosp 1982; **Fellow:** Gastroenterology, New York Hosp 1984

Milano, Andrew MD (Ge) - **Spec Exp:** Endoscopy; Inflammatory Bowel Disease/Crohn's; Esophageal Disorders; **Hospital:** NYU Langone Med Ctr (page 108); **Address:** NYU, Gastroenterology Dept, 530 1st Ave, Ste 4K, New York, NY 10016; **Phone:** 212-263-7483; **Board Cert:** Internal Medicine 1977; Gastroenterology 1972; **Med School:** NYU Sch Med 1964; **Resid:** Internal Medicine, Bellevue Hosp 1967; **Fellow:** Gastroenterology, Bellevue Hosp 1968; **Fac Appt:** Clin Prof Med, NYU Sch Med

Min, Albert D MD (Ge) - **Spec Exp:** Hepatitis B & C; Liver Disease; **Hospital:** Beth Israel Med Ctr - Petrie Div (page 94); **Address:** Beth Israel Medical Ctr, 1st Ave at 16th St, New York, NY 10003; **Phone:** 212-420-4751; **Board Cert:** Internal Medicine 1988; Gastroenterology 2002; **Med School:** Univ Rochester 1985; **Resid:** Gastroenterology, SUNY Stony Brook 1988; **Fellow:** Hepatology, Montefiore Med Ctr 1991; **Fac Appt:** Assoc Clin Prof Med, Albert Einstein Coll Med

Miskovitz, Paul F MD (Ge) - **Spec Exp:** Endoscopy; Liver Disease; Biliary Disease; **Hospital:** NY-Presby/Weill Cornell Med Ctr, NY (page 104); **Address:** 635 Madison Ave, Fl 17, New York, NY 10022; **Phone:** 212-717-4966; **Board Cert:** Internal Medicine 1978; Gastroenterology 1981; **Med School:** Cornell Univ-Weill Med Coll 1975; **Resid:** Internal Medicine, Presby/Columbia Univ Med Ctr 1978; **Fellow:** Gastroenterology, Presby/Columbia Univ Med Ctr 1980; **Fac Appt:** Clin Prof Med, Cornell Univ-Weill Med Coll

Nagler, Jerry MD (Ge) - **Spec Exp:** Inflammatory Bowel Disease; Irritable Bowel Syndrome; **Hospital:** NY-Presby/Weill Cornell Med Ctr, NY (page 104); **Address:** 407 E 70th St, Fl 5 Bldg, New York, NY 10021-5302; **Phone:** 212-628-7777; **Board Cert:** Internal Medicine 1976; Gastroenterology 1983; **Med School:** Yale Univ 1973; **Resid:** Internal Medicine, Columbia-Presby Hosp 1976; **Fellow:** Gastroenterology, NY Hosp/Cornell Med Ctr 1978; **Fac Appt:** Assoc Clin Prof Med, Cornell Univ-Weill Med Coll

Ottaviano, Lawrence MD (Ge) - **Spec Exp:** Peptic Ulcer Disease; Colitis; **Address:** 60 Gramercy Park N, Ste 1B, New York, NY 10010; **Phone:** 212-254-1220; **Board Cert:** Internal Medicine 1988; Gastroenterology 2006; **Med School:** Grenada 1984; **Resid:** Internal Medicine, Cabrini Med Ctr 1987; **Fellow:** Gastroenterology, Cabrini Med Ctr 1989; **Fac Appt:** Asst Clin Prof Med, NY Med Coll

Pochapin, Mark B MD (Ge) - **Spec Exp:** Pancreatic Cancer; Endoscopic Ultrasound; Colon & Rectal Cancer Detection; **Hospital:** NYU Langone Med Ctr (page 108); **Address:** NYU Women's Ctr, 207 E 84th St Fl 2, New York, NY 10028; **Phone:** 646-501-6760; **Board Cert:** Gastroenterology 2004; **Med School:** Cornell Univ-Weill Med Coll 1988; **Resid:** Internal Medicine, NY Hosp-Cornell Med Ctr 1991; **Fellow:** Gastroenterology, Montefiore Med Ctr 1993; **Fac Appt:** Prof Med, Cornell Univ-Weill Med Coll

Poneros, John M MD (Ge) - **Spec Exp:** Malabsorption Syndrome; Barrett's Esophagus; Pancreatic & Biliary Disease; **Hospital:** NY-Presby/Columbia Univ Med Ctr, NY (page 104); **Address:** NY Presby, Gastroenterology Dept, 161 Fort Washington Ave, Ste 862, New York, NY 10032; **Phone:** 212-305-1021; **Board Cert:** Gastroenterology 2011; **Med School:** Columbia P&S 1995; **Resid:** Internal Medicine, NY-Presby/Columbia Univ Med Ctr 1998; **Fellow:** Gastroenterology, Mass Genl Hosp 2001; Advanced Endoscopy, Brigham & Womens Hosp 2002; **Fac Appt:** Asst Prof Med, Columbia P&S

Rieber, Jonathan M MD (Ge) - **Spec Exp:** Gastroesophageal Reflux Disease (GERD); Inflammatory Bowel Disease; Colonoscopy; **Hospital:** NY-Presby Hosp/The Allen Hosp (page 104), Lawrence Hosp Ctr; **Address:** 5030 Broadway, Ste 707, New York, NY 10034; **Phone:** 718-412-3445; **Board Cert:** Internal Medicine 2008; Gastroenterology 2010; **Med School:** NY Med Coll 1994; **Resid:** Internal Medicine, NY Presby-Columbia Med Ctr 1997; **Fellow:** Gastroenterology, NYU Med Ctr 2000; **Fac Appt:** Asst Clin Prof Med, Columbia P&S

Robilotti Jr, James G MD (Ge) - **Spec Exp:** Irritable Bowel Syndrome; Peptic Ulcer Disease; Gastroesophageal Reflux Disease (GERD); Colon Cancer Screening; **Hospital:** Beth Israel Med Ctr - Petrie Div (page 94); **Address:** 29 Washington Sq West, New York, NY 10011-9180; **Phone:** 212-475-4030; **Board Cert:** Internal Medicine 1972; Gastroenterology 1981; **Med School:** UMDNJ-NJ Med Sch, Newark 1965; **Resid:** Internal Medicine, St Vincent's Hosp 1968; **Fellow:** Gastroenterology, St Vincent's Hosp 1970; **Fac Appt:** Assoc Clin Prof Med, NY Med Coll

Romeu, Jose N MD (Ge) - **Spec Exp:** Colonoscopy/Polypectomy; Colonoscopy; Gastrointestinal Cancer; Gastroesophageal Reflux Disease (GERD); **Hospital:** Mt Sinai Med Ctr (page 102), Lenox Hill Hosp (page 106); **Address:** 1107 5th Ave, Ste 1N, New York, NY 10128-0145; **Phone:** 212-534-6747; **Board Cert:** Internal Medicine 1973; Gastroenterology 1975; **Med School:** NYU Sch Med 1970; **Resid:** Internal Medicine, Mt Sinai Hosp 1973; **Fellow:** Gastroenterology, Mt Sinai Hosp 1976; **Fac Appt:** Asst Clin Prof Med, Mount Sinai Sch Med

Rubin, Moshe MD (Ge) - **Spec Exp:** Enteroscopy-Small Bowel; Colonoscopy; Celiac Disease; Inflammatory Bowel Disease/Crohn's; **Hospital:** NY Hosp Queens (page 488), NY-Presby/Weill Cornell Med Ctr, NY (page 104); **Address:** 1020 Park Ave, Fl 1, New York, NY 10028; **Phone:** 212-772-1012; **Board Cert:** Internal Medicine 1986; Gastroenterology 1989; **Med School:** Yale Univ 1983; **Resid:** Internal Medicine, NY Hosp 1986; **Fellow:** Gastroenterology, Columbia-Presby Hosp 1988; **Fac Appt:** Assoc Prof Med, Cornell Univ-Weill Med Coll

Ruoff, Michael MD (Ge) - **Spec Exp:** Esophageal Disorders; Malabsorption; **Hospital:** NYU Langone Med Ctr (page 108); **Address:** 232 E 30 St Fl 1, New York, NY 10016-8202; **Phone:** 212-889-5544 x145; **Board Cert:** Internal Medicine 1980; Gastroenterology 1972; **Med School:** NYU Sch Med 1963; **Resid:** Internal Medicine, Bellevue Hosp 1966; **Fellow:** Gastroenterology, NYU Med Ctr 1967; **Fac Appt:** Clin Prof Med, NYU Sch Med

Sachar, David B MD (Ge) - **Spec Exp:** Inflammatory Bowel Disease-Consult; **Hospital:** Mt Sinai Med Ctr (page 102); **Address:** One Gustave L Levy Pl, MS 1069, New York, NY 10029; **Phone:** 212-241-4514; **Board Cert:** Internal Medicine 1969; Gastroenterology 1972; **Med School:** Harvard Med Sch 1963; **Resid:** Internal Medicine, Beth Israel Hosp 1965; Internal Medicine, Beth Israel Hosp 1968; **Fellow:** Gastroenterology, Mount Sinai Hosp 1970; **Fac Appt:** Clin Prof Med, Mount Sinai Sch Med

Salik, James MD (Ge) - **Spec Exp:** Colonoscopy; Liver Disease; Inflammatory Bowel Disease; **Hospital:** NYU Langone Med Ctr (page 108); **Address:** 232 E 30th St, New York, NY 10016-8202; **Phone:** 212-889-5544 x145; **Board Cert:** Internal Medicine 1983; Gastroenterology 1985; **Med School:** NYU Sch Med 1980; **Resid:** Internal Medicine, Bellevue Hosp 1983; **Fellow:** Gastroenterology, Bellevue Hosp 1985; **Fac Appt:** Asst Clin Prof Med, NYU Sch Med

Scherl, Ellen MD (Ge) - **Spec Exp:** Inflammatory Bowel Disease; Crohn's Disease; Ulcerative Colitis; **Hospital:** NY-Presby/Weill Cornell Med Ctr, NY (page 104); **Address:** 1315 York Ave, Mezzanine Level, New York, NY 10021; **Phone:** 212-746-5077; **Board Cert:** Internal Medicine 1983; **Med School:** NY Med Coll 1977; **Resid:** Internal Medicine, Beth Israel Med Ctr 1981; **Fellow:** Gastroenterology, Mt Sinai Med Ctr 1983; **Fac Appt:** Prof Med, Cornell Univ-Weill Med Coll

Schiano, Thomas D MD (Ge) - **Spec Exp:** Liver Disease; Transplant Medicine-Liver; Transplant Medicine-Bowel; Hepatitis; **Hospital:** Mt Sinai Med Ctr (page 102); **Address:** 5 E 98th St Fl 12, Box 1104, MS 10029, New York, NY 10029; **Phone:** 212-241-8035; **Board Cert:** Transplant Hepatology 2006; Gastroenterology 2005; **Med School:** Mexico 1987; **Resid:** Internal Medicine, Maimonides Med Ctr 1992; Gastroenterology, Temple Univ 1995; **Fellow:** Nutrition, Meml Sloan-Kettering Cancer Ctr 1993; Hepatology, Mt Sinai Med Ctr 1996; **Fac Appt:** Prof Med, Mount Sinai Sch Med

Schmerin, Michael J MD (Ge) - **Spec Exp:** Colonoscopy; Gastroscopy; Gastroesophageal Reflux Disease (GERD); **Hospital:** NY-Presby/Weill Cornell Med Ctr, NY (page 104), Lenox Hill Hosp (page 106); **Address:** 1060 Park Ave, Ste 1G, New York, NY 10128-1095; **Phone:** 212-348-3166; **Board Cert:** Internal Medicine 1976; Gastroenterology 1977; **Med School:** Jefferson Med Coll 1973; **Resid:** Internal Medicine, New York Presby Hosp 1976; **Fellow:** Gastroenterology, New York Presby Hosp 1977; **Fac Appt:** Asst Clin Prof Med, Cornell Univ-Weill Med Coll

Schneebaum, Cary MD (Ge) - **Spec Exp:** Colon Cancer Screening; **Hospital:** Beth Israel Med Ctr - Petrie Div (page 94); **Address:** 155 5th Ave, Fl 2, New York, NY 10010; **Phone:** 212-741-6100; **Board Cert:** Internal Medicine 1984; **Med School:** SUNY Hlth Sci Ctr 1981; **Resid:** Internal Medicine, Beth Israel Med Ctr 1984; **Fellow:** Gastroenterology, Beth Israel Med Ctr 1986

Schneider, Lewis P MD (Ge) - **Spec Exp:** Colon Cancer; Gastroesophageal Reflux Disease (GERD); Colon & Rectal Cancer; Capsule Endoscopy; **Hospital:** NY-Presby/Columbia Univ Med Ctr, NY (page 104); **Address:** 51 W 51 St, Ste 360, New York, NY 10022; **Phone:** 212-326-8426; **Board Cert:** Internal Medicine 1981; **Med School:** SUNY Downstate 1978; **Resid:** Internal Medicine, Columbia-Presby Hosp 1981; **Fellow:** Gastroenterology, Columbia-Presby Hosp 1983

Sherman, Alex MD (Ge) - **Spec Exp:** Liver Disease; Hepatitis; Endoscopy; Pancreatic/Biliary Endoscopy (ERCP); **Hospital:** NYU Langone Med Ctr (page 108); **Address:** Concorde Medical Group, 232 E 30th St, New York, NY 10016-8202; **Phone:** 212-889-5544; **Board Cert:** Internal Medicine ; Gastroenterology ; **Med School:** NYU Sch Med 1983; **Resid:** Internal Medicine, Bronx Municipal Hosp 1986; **Fellow:** Gastroenterology, NYU Med Ctr 1988; **Fac Appt:** Assoc Clin Prof Med, NYU Sch Med

Solny, Meyer MD (Ge) - **Spec Exp:** Endoscopy; **Hospital:** NY-Presby/Weill Cornell Med Ctr, NY (page 104), Lenox Hill Hosp (page 106); **Address:** 1 E 68th St, Ste 1E, New York, NY 10065; **Phone:** 212-570-6945; **Board Cert:** Internal Medicine ; Gastroenterology ; **Med School:** Columbia P&S 1974; **Resid:** Internal Medicine, NY Presby Hosp/Cornell 1977; **Fellow:** Gastroenterology, NY Presby Hosp/Cornell 1979

Starpoli, Anthony A MD (Ge) - **Spec Exp:** Gastroesophageal Reflux Disease (GERD); **Hospital:** Lenox Hill Hosp (page 106), NYU Langone Med Ctr (page 108); **Address:** 80 5th Ave, Ste 1605, New York, NY 10011; **Phone:** 212-673-2721; **Board Cert:** Internal Medicine 1989; Gastroenterology 2003; **Med School:** Univ IL Coll Med 1986; **Resid:** Internal Medicine, Sound Shore Med Ctr 1989; **Fellow:** Gastroenterology, St Vincents Hosp 1991; **Fac Appt:** Asst Clin Prof Med, NY Med Coll

Stein, Jeffrey A MD (Ge) - **Spec Exp:** Gallbladder Disease; Pancreatic Disease; **Hospital:** NY-Presby/Columbia Univ Med Ctr, NY (page 104); **Address:** 161 Ft Washington Ave, New York, NY 10032; **Phone:** 212-305-5444; **Board Cert:** Internal Medicine 1971; Gastroenterology 1973; **Med School:** Harvard Med Sch 1965; **Resid:** Internal Medicine, Presbyterian Hosp 1970; **Fellow:** Gastroenterology, Presbyterian Hosp 1971; **Fac Appt:** Clin Prof Med, Columbia P&S

Tobias, Hillel MD (Ge) - **Spec Exp:** Liver Disease; Hepatitis B & C; Liver & Biliary Disease; **Hospital:** NYU Langone Med Ctr (page 108); **Address:** 232 E 30th St, New York, NY 10016-8202; **Phone:** 212-889-5544; **Board Cert:** Internal Medicine 1967; Gastroenterology 1979; Transplant Hepatology 2006; **Med School:** Washington Univ, St Louis 1960; **Resid:** Internal Medicine, Bellevue Hosp Ctr 1963; Hepatology, Royal Free Hosp 1965; **Fellow:** Hepatology, Mt Sinai Hosp 1967; **Fac Appt:** Prof Med, NYU Sch Med

Traube, Morris MD (Ge) - **Spec Exp:** Esophageal Disorders; Swallowing Disorders; Gastroesophageal Reflux Disease (GERD); **Hospital:** NYU Langone Med Ctr (page 108); **Address:** NYU Gastroenterology Associates, 530 First Ave, Ste 9N, New York, NY 10016; **Phone:** 212-263-3095; **Board Cert:** Internal Medicine 1981; Gastroenterology 1983; **Med School:** SUNY Downstate 1978; **Resid:** Internal Medicine, Maimonides Med Ctr 1981; **Fellow:** Gastroenterology, Yale-New Haven Hosp 1984; **Fac Appt:** Prof Med, NYU Sch Med

Ullman, Thomas A MD (Ge) - **Spec Exp:** Irritable Bowel Syndrome; Ulcerative Colitis; Inflammatory Bowel Disease/Crohn's; Colon & Rectal Cancer; **Hospital:** Mt Sinai Med Ctr (page 102); **Address:** 5 E 98th St Fl 11, New York, NY 10028; **Phone:** 212-241-4299; **Board Cert:** Gastroenterology 2009; **Med School:** Cornell Univ-Weill Med Coll 1992; **Resid:** Internal Medicine, New York Hosp 1995; **Fellow:** Gastroenterology, Yale-New Haven Hosp 1999; **Fac Appt:** Assoc Prof Med, Mount Sinai Sch Med

Wang, Timothy C MD (Ge) - **Spec Exp:** Gastrointestinal Cancer; **Hospital:** NY-Presby/Columbia Univ Med Ctr, NY (page 104); **Address:** 161 Fort Washington Ave, Ste 862, New York, NY 10032; **Phone:** 212-305-1021; **Board Cert:** Internal Medicine 1986; Gastroenterology 1989; **Med School:** Columbia P&S 1983; **Resid:** Internal Medicine, Barnes Jewish Hosp 1986; **Fellow:** Gastroenterology, Mass General Hosp 1989; Research, Harvard Medical School 1989; **Fac Appt:** Prof Med, Columbia P&S

Waye, Jerome D MD (Ge) - **Spec Exp:** Endoscopy; Colon Cancer; Colonoscopy; **Hospital:** Mt Sinai Med Ctr (page 102), Lenox Hill Hosp (page 106); **Address:** 650 Park Ave, New York, NY 10065; **Phone:** 212-439-7779; **Board Cert:** Internal Medicine 1965; Gastroenterology 1970; **Med School:** Boston Univ 1958; **Resid:** Internal Medicine, Mt Sinai Hosp 1961; **Fellow:** Gastroenterology, Mt Sinai Hosp 1962; **Fac Appt:** Clin Prof Med, Mount Sinai Sch Med

Weiss, Robert A MD (Ge) - **Spec Exp:** Colon Cancer; Gastroesophageal Reflux Disease (GERD); Endoscopy; **Hospital:** Beth Israel Med Ctr - Petrie Div (page 94); **Address:** 380 2nd Ave, Ste 1004, New York, NY 10010; **Phone:** 212-473-4100; **Board Cert:** Internal Medicine 1987; Gastroenterology 1989; **Med School:** Mount Sinai Sch Med 1983; **Resid:** Internal Medicine, Beth Israel Med Ctr 1986; **Fellow:** Gastroenterology, Elmhurst Hosp Ctr-Mt Sinai 1988; **Fac Appt:** Asst Clin Prof Med, Albert Einstein Coll Med

Geriatric Medicine

Adelman, Ronald D MD (Ger) - **Spec Exp:** Geriatric Care; Palliative Care; Preventive Medicine; **Hospital:** NY-Presby/Weill Cornell Med Ctr, NY (page 104); **Address:** Irving Sherwood Wright Ctr on Aging, 1484-1486 1st Ave, New York, NY 10075; **Phone:** 212-746-7000; **Board Cert:** Internal Medicine 1982; Geriatric Medicine 2009; Hospice & Palliative Medicine 2012; **Med School:** Albert Einstein Coll Med 1978; **Resid:** Internal Medicine, Montefiore Med Ctr 1982; **Fac Appt:** Prof Med, Cornell Univ

Babitz, Lisa E MD (Ger) *PCP* - **Spec Exp:** Geriatric Medicine; **Hospital:** St. Luke's - Roosevelt Hosp Ctr - Roosevelt Div (page 94); **Address:** 457 W 57th St, New York, NY 10019; **Phone:** 212-265-1471; **Board Cert:** Internal Medicine 1984; **Med School:** Yale Univ 1981; **Resid:** Internal Medicine, Yale-New Haven Hosp 1984; **Fellow:** Geriatric Medicine, NYU Med Ctr 1986; **Fac Appt:** Assoc Clin Prof Med, Columbia P&S

Bloom, Patricia A MD (Ger) - **Spec Exp:** Complementary Medicine; Dementia; **Hospital:** Mt Sinai Med Ctr (page 102); **Address:** Martha Stewart Ctr for Living, 1440 Madison Ave, New York, NY 10029-6542; **Phone:** 212-659-8552; **Board Cert:** Internal Medicine 1978; Geriatric Medicine 2011; **Med School:** Univ Minn 1975; **Resid:** Internal Medicine, Montefiore Med Ctr 1978; **Fac Appt:** Assoc Prof Med, Mount Sinai Sch Med

Callahan, Eileen H MD (Ger) - **Spec Exp:** Frail Elderly; Preventive Medicine; Dementia; **Hospital:** Mt Sinai Med Ctr (page 102); **Address:** Martha Stewart Ctr for Living, 1440 Madison Ave, New York, NY 10029; **Phone:** 212-659-8552; **Board Cert:** Internal Medicine 2004; Geriatric Medicine 2008; **Med School:** UMDNJ-NJ Med Sch, Newark 1991; **Resid:** Internal Medicine, St Vincents Cath Med Ctr 1994; **Fellow:** Geriatric Medicine, Mt Sinai Med Ctr 1996; **Fac Appt:** Assoc Prof Med, Mount Sinai Sch Med

Chang, Christine MD (Ger) *PCP* - **Spec Exp:** Alzheimer's Disease; Dementia; **Hospital:** Mt Sinai Med Ctr (page 102); **Address:** 1440 Madison Ave, New York, NY 10029; **Phone:** 212-659-8552; **Board Cert:** Internal Medicine 2008; Geriatric Medicine 2010; **Med School:** Duke Univ 1995; **Resid:** Internal Medicine, Univ Pitt Hlth Sys 1998; **Fellow:** Geriatric Medicine, Johns Hopkins Hosp 2000; **Fac Appt:** Asst Prof Med, Mount Sinai Sch Med

Chun, Audrey K MD (Ger) - **Spec Exp:** Dementia; Depression; **Hospital:** Mt Sinai Med Ctr (page 102); **Address:** Martha Stewart Center for Living, 1440 Madison Ave, New York, NY 10029; **Phone:** 212-659-8552; **Board Cert:** Geriatric Medicine 2012; Internal Medicine 2013; **Med School:** Baylor Coll Med 1998; **Resid:** Internal Medicine, Baylor Affil Hosp 2001; **Fellow:** Geriatric Medicine, Mt Sinai Hosp 2003; **Fac Appt:** Asst Prof Med, Mount Sinai Sch Med

Feher, Laszlo A DO (Ger) *PCP* - **Spec Exp:** Preventive Medicine; Geriatric Care; **Hospital:** NYU Langone Med Ctr (page 108); **Address:** 251 E 33rd St, Ste 2F, New York, NY 10016; **Phone:** 212-686-4212; **Board Cert:** Internal Medicine 2007; Geriatric Medicine 2008; **Med School:** NY Coll Osteo Med 1993; **Resid:** Internal Medicine, St Lukes Roosevelt Hosp 1996; **Fellow:** Geriatric Medicine, NYU Med Ctr 1998

Finkelstein, Martin S MD (Ger) - **Spec Exp:** Geriatric Care; Preventive Medicine; **Hospital:** NYU Langone Med Ctr (page 108); **Address:** 314 E 30th St, New York, NY 10016-6402; **Phone:** 646-370-2000; **Board Cert:** Internal Medicine 1970; **Med School:** NYU Sch Med 1964; **Resid:** Internal Medicine, Bellevue Hosp 1966; Internal Medicine, Stanford Univ Med Ctr 1967; **Fellow:** Infectious Disease, Stanford Univ Med Ctr 1968; **Fac Appt:** Assoc Clin Prof Med, NYU Sch Med

Fogel, Joyce F MD (Ger) *PCP* - **Spec Exp:** Memory Disorders; Geriatric Functional Assessment; Preventive Medicine; **Hospital:** Beth Israel Med Ctr- Kings Hwy Div (page 94); **Address:** 275 8th Ave, New York, NY 10011-8305; **Phone:** 212-463-0101; **Board Cert:** Internal Medicine 1985; Geriatric Medicine 2011; **Med School:** SUNY Downstate 1982; **Resid:** Internal Medicine, Kings Co Hosp 1985; **Fellow:** Geriatric Medicine, Bellevue/NYU Med Ctr 1989; **Fac Appt:** Assoc Clin Prof Med, NY Med Coll

Karp, Adam H MD (Ger) *PCP* - **Spec Exp:** Falls in the Elderly; Geriatric Care; Preventive Medicine; **Hospital:** NYU Hosp For Joint Dis (page 108), NYU Langone Med Ctr (page 108); **Address:** 301 E 17th St, rm 208A, New York, NY 10003; **Phone:** 212-598-6738; **Board Cert:** Internal Medicine 2010; Geriatric Medicine 2012; **Med School:** Albert Einstein Coll Med 1987; **Resid:** Internal Medicine, Maimonides Med Ctr 1990; **Fellow:** Geriatric Medicine, Bellevue Hosp/NYU Med Ctr 1992; **Fac Appt:** Asst Clin Prof Med, NYU Sch Med

Korc-Grodzicki, Beatriz MD/PhD (Ger) - **Spec Exp:** Alzheimer's Disease; Preventive Medicine; Cancer in the Elderly; **Hospital:** Meml Sloan-Kettering Canc Ctr (page 114); **Address:** Meml Sloan Kettering Cancer Ctr, 1275 York Ave, New York, NY 10065; **Phone:** 646-888-3154; **Board Cert:** Internal Medicine 2007; Geriatric Medicine 2012; **Med School:** Uruguay 1983; **Resid:** Internal Medicine, Univ Rochester Med Ctr 1997; **Fellow:** Geriatric Medicine, Univ Rochester Med Ctr 2002; **Fac Appt:** Assoc Prof Med, Mount Sinai Sch Med

Lachs, Mark S MD (Ger) - **Spec Exp:** Abuse/Neglect; **Hospital:** NY-Presby/Weill Cornell Med Ctr, NY (page 104); **Address:** Irving Sherwood Wright Med Ctr on Aging, 1484 First Ave, New York, NY 10075; **Phone:** 212-746-7000; **Board Cert:** Internal Medicine 1988; Geriatric Medicine 2002; **Med School:** NYU Sch Med 1985; **Resid:** Internal Medicine, Hosp Univ Penn - UPHS 1988; **Fellow:** Geriatric Medicine, Yale-New Haven Hosp 1990; **Fac Appt:** Prof Med, Cornell Univ-Weill Med Coll

Leipzig, Rosanne M MD (Ger) *PCP* - **Spec Exp:** Medications in the Elderly; Alzheimer's Disease; Dementia; **Hospital:** Mt Sinai Med Ctr (page 102); **Address:** Martha Stewart Center for Living, 1440 Madison Ave, New York, NY 10029; **Phone:** 212-689-8552; **Board Cert:** Internal Medicine 1982; Geriatric Medicine 2008; Hospice & Palliative Medicine 2012; **Med School:** Univ Mich Med Sch 1978; **Resid:** Internal Medicine, Strong Meml Hosp 1982; **Fellow:** Clinical Pharmacology, New York Hosp 1985; **Fac Appt:** Prof Med, Mount Sinai Sch Med

Morrison, R Sean MD (Ger) - **Spec Exp:** Palliative Care; Alzheimer's Disease; Dementia; Frail Elderly; **Hospital:** Mt Sinai Med Ctr (page 102); **Address:** Martha Stewart Center for Living, 1440 Madison Ave, New York, NY 10029; **Phone:** 212-659-8552; **Board Cert:** Internal Medicine 2003; Geriatric Medicine 2006; Hospice & Palliative Medicine ; **Med School:** Univ Chicago-Pritzker Sch Med 1990; **Resid:** Internal Medicine, NY Hosp/Cornell Med Ctr 1993; **Fellow:** Geriatric Medicine, Mt Sinai Med Ctr 1996; **Fac Appt:** Prof Med, Mount Sinai Sch Med

Peterson, Monte H MD (Ger) *PCP* - **Hospital:** Beth Israel Med Ctr - Petrie Div (page 94); **Address:** Beth Israel Senior Health Ctr, 275 8th Ave, New York, NY 10011; **Phone:** 212-463-0101; **Board Cert:** Internal Medicine 1982; Geriatric Medicine 2009; **Med School:** Univ Iowa Coll Med 1979; **Resid:** Internal Medicine, UCSF/San Joaquin Vly Hosp 1982; **Fellow:** Geriatric Medicine, NY Presby-Cornell Med Ctr 1983; Geriatric Medicine, Mt Sinai Med Ctr 1984; **Fac Appt:** Asst Prof Med, Albert Einstein Coll Med

Raman, Bharathi MD (Ger) - **Spec Exp:** Long Term Care; Palliative Care; **Hospital:** NY-Presby/Weill Cornell Med Ctr, NY (page 104); **Address:** Irving Sherwood Wright Ctr on Aging, 1484-1486 1st Ave, New York, NY 10075; **Phone:** 212-746-7000; **Board Cert:** Internal Medicine 1988; Geriatric Medicine 2011; Hospice & Palliative Medicine 2012; **Med School:** India 1973; **Resid:** Internal Medicine, Woodhill Med Ctr 1988; **Fellow:** Geriatric Medicine, Mt Sinai Med Ctr 1990; **Fac Appt:** Asst Prof Med, Cornell Univ-Weill Med Coll

Sherman, Fredrick T MD (Ger) *PCP* - **Spec Exp:** Frail Elderly; Falls in the Elderly; Polypharmacology (Excess Medications); Memory Disorders; **Hospital:** Mt Sinai Med Ctr (page 102); **Address:** Coffey Geriatrics Assocs, 1440 Madison Ave, New York, NY 10029; **Phone:** 212-659-8552; **Board Cert:** Internal Medicine 1975; **Med School:** Temple Univ 1972; **Resid:** Internal Medicine, Med Coll Penn Hosp 1975; **Fac Appt:** Clin Prof Med, Mount Sinai Sch Med

Siegler, Eugenia L MD (Ger) *PCP* - **Spec Exp:** Dementia; Geriatric Care; **Hospital:** NY-Presby/Weill Cornell Med Ctr, NY (page 104); **Address:** Irving Sherwood Wright Ctr on Aging, 1484-1486 First Ave, New York, NY 10075; **Phone:** 212-746-7000; **Board Cert:** Internal Medicine 1986; Geriatric Medicine 2010; **Med School:** Johns Hopkins Univ 1983; **Resid:** Internal Medicine, Bellevue Hosp 1986; **Fellow:** Geriatric Medicine, Hosp Univ Penn 1989; **Fac Appt:** Assoc Prof Med, Cornell Univ-Weill Med Coll

Geriatric Psychiatry

Devanand, Davangere MD (GerPsy) - **Spec Exp:** Memory Disorders; Alzheimer's Disease; Depression; Cognitive Loss in Aging; **Hospital:** NY State Psychiatric Inst; **Address:** NY State Psychiatric Inst, 1051 Riverside Dr, Unit 126, New York, NY 10032; **Phone:** 212-543-5612; **Board Cert:** Psychiatry 1985; Geriatric Psychiatry 2010; **Med School:** India 1979; **Resid:** Psychiatry, SUNY Upstate Med Ctr 1982; Psychiatry, Yale-New Haven Hosp 1984; **Fellow:** Biological Psychiatry, NY Presby-Columbia Med Ctr 1985; **Fac Appt:** Clin Prof Psyc, Columbia P&S

Reisberg, Barry MD (GerPsy) - **Spec Exp:** Alzheimer's Disease; Dementia; Cognitive Loss in Aging; Depression; **Hospital:** NYU Langone Med Ctr (page 108); **Address:** NYU Med Ctr, Dept Psychiatry, 145 E 32nd St, Ste 508, New York, NY 10016; **Phone:** 212-263-8550; **Board Cert:** Psychiatry 1976; Geriatric Psychiatry 2012; **Med School:** NY Med Coll 1972; **Resid:** Psychiatry, Metropolitan Hosp 1975; **Fellow:** Psychiatric Research, Univ London 1975; **Fac Appt:** Prof Psyc, NYU Sch Med

Serby, Michael J MD (GerPsy) - **Spec Exp:** Alzheimer's Disease; Depression; Parkinson's Disease; **Hospital:** Beth Israel Med Ctr - Petrie Div (page 94); **Address:** 317 E 17th St, Fl 9, New York, NY 10003; **Phone:** 212-420-2421; **Board Cert:** Psychiatry 1979; Geriatric Psychiatry 2010; **Med School:** Emory Univ 1969; **Resid:** Psychiatry, Bellevue Hosp-NYU 1976; **Fac Appt:** Clin Prof Psyc, Albert Einstein Coll Med

Gynecologic Oncology

Abu-Rustum, Nadeem R MD (GO) - **Spec Exp:** Ovarian Cancer; Uterine Cancer; Cervical Cancer; Vulvar Disease/Cancer; **Hospital:** Meml Sloan-Kettering Canc Ctr (page 114); **Address:** 1275 York Ave, Ste H-1308, New York, NY 10065; **Phone:** 212-639-7051; **Board Cert:** Obstetrics & Gynecology 2012; Gynecologic Oncology 2012; **Med School:** Lebanon 1990; **Resid:** Obstetrics & Gynecology, Greater Baltimore Med Ctr 1994; **Fellow:** Gynecologic Oncology, Meml Sloan-Kettering Cancer Ctr 1997; **Fac Appt:** Prof ObG, Cornell Univ-Weill Med Coll

Barakat, Richard R MD (GO) - **Spec Exp:** Robotic Surgery; Ovarian Cancer; Uterine Cancer; Cervical Cancer; **Hospital:** Meml Sloan-Kettering Canc Ctr (page 114); **Address:** 1275 York Ave, rm H1305, New York, NY 10065; **Phone:** 646-497-9055; **Board Cert:** Obstetrics & Gynecology 2012; Gynecologic Oncology 2012; **Med School:** SUNY Hlth Sci Ctr 1985; **Resid:** Obstetrics & Gynecology, Bellevue Hosp 1989; **Fellow:** Gynecologic Oncology, Meml Sloan Kettering Cancer Ctr 1991; **Fac Appt:** Prof ObG, Cornell Univ-Weill Med Coll

Blank, Stephanie V MD (GO) - **Spec Exp:** Gynecologic Cancer; **Hospital:** NYU Langone Med Ctr (page 108); **Address:** NYU Clinical Cancer Center, 240 E 38th St, New York, NY 10016; **Phone:** 212-731-5705; **Board Cert:** Obstetrics & Gynecology 2012; Gynecologic Oncology 2012; **Med School:** UCSD 1994; **Resid:** Obstetrics & Gynecology, NY-Presby/Weill Cornell Med Ctr 1998; **Fellow:** Gynecologic Oncology, Hosp Univ Penn 2001; **Fac Appt:** Assoc Clin Prof NuM, NYU Sch Med

Brown, Carol MD (GO) - **Spec Exp:** Ovarian Cancer; Cervical Cancer; Uterine Cancer; Laparoscopic Surgery; **Hospital:** Meml Sloan-Kettering Canc Ctr (page 114); **Address:** 1275 York Ave, rm H1311, New York, NY 10065; **Phone:** 212-639-7659; **Board Cert:** Obstetrics & Gynecology 2012; Gynecologic Oncology 2012; **Med School:** Columbia P&S 1986; **Resid:** Obstetrics & Gynecology, Hosp Univ Penn 1990; **Fellow:** Gynecologic Oncology, Meml Sloan Kettering Cancer Ctr 1992; Research, Meml Sloan Kettering Cancer Ctr 1994; **Fac Appt:** Asst Prof ObG, Cornell Univ-Weill Med Coll

Caputo, Thomas A MD (GO) - **Spec Exp:** Cervical Cancer; Ovarian Cancer; Uterine Cancer; Vulvar Disease/Cancer; **Hospital:** NY-Presby/Weill Cornell Med Ctr, NY (page 104); **Address:** NY Presby Hosp-Weill Cornell, 525 E 68th St, Ste J-130, New York, NY 10021; **Phone:** 212-746-3179; **Board Cert:** Obstetrics & Gynecology 1993; Gynecologic Oncology 1977; **Med School:** UMDNJ-NJ Med Sch, Newark 1965; **Resid:** Obstetrics & Gynecology, Martland Hosp 1969; **Fellow:** Gynecologic Oncology, Emory Univ Hosp 1975; **Fac Appt:** Clin Prof ObG, Cornell Univ-Weill Med Coll

Chi, Dennis S MD (GO) - **Spec Exp:** Ovarian Cancer; Uterine Cancer; Cervical Cancer; Gynecologic Surgery-Complex; **Hospital:** Meml Sloan-Kettering Canc Ctr (page 114); **Address:** 1275 York Ave, New York, NY 10065; **Phone:** 212-639-5016; **Board Cert:** Obstetrics & Gynecology 2012; Gynecologic Oncology 2012; **Med School:** NYU Sch Med 1990; **Resid:** Obstetrics & Gynecology, NYU Med Ctr 1994; **Fellow:** Gynecologic Oncology, Meml Sloan Kettering Cancer Ctr 1997; **Fac Appt:** Prof ObG, NYU Sch Med

Chuang, Linus T MD (GO) - **Spec Exp:** Laparoscopic Surgery; Ovarian Cancer; Uterine Cancer; Cervical Cancer; **Hospital:** Mt Sinai Med Ctr (page 102), White Plains Hosp (page 640); **Address:** 1176 5th Ave, Box 1173, New York, NY 10029; **Phone:** 212-241-1111; **Board Cert:** Obstetrics & Gynecology 2009; Gynecologic Oncology 2097; **Med School:** Taiwan 1981; **Resid:** Obstetrics & Gynecology, Flushing Hosp 1990; **Fellow:** Gynecologic Oncology, MD Anderson Cancer Ctr 1994; **Fac Appt:** Assoc Prof ObG, Mount Sinai Sch Med

Curtin, John P MD (GO) - **Spec Exp:** Uterine Cancer; Ovarian Cancer; Laparoscopic Surgery; Gestational Trophoblastic Disease; **Hospital:** NYU Langone Med Ctr (page 108); **Address:** NYU Clin Cancer Ctr, 240 E 38th St, Fl 19, New York, NY 10016-6402; **Phone:** 212-731-5345; **Board Cert:** Obstetrics & Gynecology 2012; Gynecologic Oncology 2012; **Med School:** Creighton Univ 1979; **Resid:** Obstetrics & Gynecology, Univ Minn Med Ctr 1984; **Fellow:** Gynecologic Oncology, Meml Sloan-Kettering Cancer Ctr 1988; **Fac Appt:** Prof ObG, NYU Sch Med

Dottino, Peter R MD (GO) - **Spec Exp:** Laparoscopic Surgery; Gynecologic Cancer; Uterine Cancer; Ovarian Cancer; **Hospital:** Mt Sinai Med Ctr (page 102), Maimonides Med Ctr (page 98); **Address:** The Group for Women, 800-A 5th Ave, Ste 405, New York, NY 10065; **Phone:** 212-888-8439; **Board Cert:** Obstetrics & Gynecology 2012; Gynecologic Oncology 2012; **Med School:** Georgetown Univ 1979; **Resid:** Obstetrics & Gynecology, SUNY Downstate Med Ctr 1983; **Fellow:** Gynecologic Oncology, Mt Sinai Hosp 1986; **Fac Appt:** Assoc Clin Prof ObG, Mount Sinai Sch Med

Fishman, David A MD (GO) - **Spec Exp:** Gynecologic Cancer; Ovarian Cancer-Early Detection; Minimally Invasive Surgery; **Hospital:** Mt Sinai Med Ctr (page 102); **Address:** 5 E 98th St, Fl 2, New York, NY 10029; **Phone:** 212-241-7952; **Board Cert:** Obstetrics & Gynecology 2011; Gynecologic Oncology 2011; **Med School:** Texas Tech Univ 1988; **Resid:** Obstetrics & Gynecology, Yale-New Haven Hosp 1992; **Fellow:** Gynecologic Oncology, Yale-New Haven Hosp 1994; **Fac Appt:** Prof ObG, Mount Sinai Sch Med

Herzog, Thomas J MD (GO) - **Spec Exp:** Cervical Cancer; Gynecologic Cancer; Laparoscopic Surgery; Ovarian Cancer; **Hospital:** NY-Presby/Columbia Univ Med Ctr, NY (page 104); **Address:** Herbert Irving Pavilion, 161 Fort Washington Ave, Fl 8, rm 837, New York, NY 10032; **Phone:** 212-305-3410; **Board Cert:** Obstetrics & Gynecology 2012; Gynecologic Oncology 2012; **Med School:** Univ Cincinnati 1986; **Resid:** Obstetrics & Gynecology, Good Samaritan Hosp 1990; **Fellow:** Gynecologic Oncology, Barnes Jewish Hosp/Wash Univ 1993; **Fac Appt:** Prof ObG, Columbia P&S

Holcomb, Kevin M MD (GO) - **Spec Exp:** Robotic Surgery; Laparoscopic Surgery; Ovarian Cancer; **Hospital:** NY-Presby/Weill Cornell Med Ctr, NY (page 104); **Address:** 525 E 68th St, Ste J 130, New York, NY 10021; **Phone:** 212-746-7553; **Board Cert:** Obstetrics & Gynecology 2012; Gynecologic Oncology 2012; **Med School:** NY Med Coll 1992; **Resid:** Obstetrics & Gynecology, NY Hosp-Cornell Med Ctr 1996; **Fellow:** Gynecologic Oncology, Downstate Med Ctr 1999; **Fac Appt:** Assoc Clin Prof ObG, Cornell Univ-Weill Med Coll

Koulos, John P MD (GO) - **Spec Exp:** Uterine Cancer; Ovarian Cancer; Cervical Cancer; Vulvar & Vaginal Cancer; **Hospital:** Beth Israel Med Ctr - Petrie Div (page 94); **Address:** Beth Israel Hosp Cancer Ctr, 10 Union Square E, Ste 4C, New York, NY 10003; **Phone:** 212-844-5729; **Board Cert:** Obstetrics & Gynecology 2012; Gynecologic Oncology 2012; **Med School:** Northwestern Univ 1978; **Resid:** Obstetrics & Gynecology, Northwestern Univ Med Sch 1982; **Fellow:** Gynecologic Oncology, Meml Sloan Kettering Cancer Ctr 1984; **Fac Appt:** Assoc Prof ObG, Albert Einstein Coll Med

Nagarsheth, Nimesh MD (GO) - **Spec Exp:** Cervical Cancer; Ovarian Cancer; Uterine Cancer; Vaginal Cancer; **Hospital:** Mt Sinai Med Ctr (page 102), Englewood Hosp & Med Ctr; **Address:** Ruttenberg Treatment Ctr, 1470 Madison Ave, New York, NY 10029; **Phone:** 212-241-1111; **Board Cert:** Obstetrics & Gynecology 2007; Gynecologic Oncology 2007; **Med School:** Mount Sinai Sch Med 1997; **Resid:** Obstetrics & Gynecology, Duke Univ Med Ctr 1997; **Fellow:** Gynecologic Oncology, Mt Sinai Med Ctr 2004; **Fac Appt:** Assoc Prof ObG, Mount Sinai Sch Med

Pothuri, Bhavana MD (GO) - **Spec Exp:** Gynecologic Cancers; Minimally Invasive Gynecologic Surgery; Fertility Preservation in Cancer; **Hospital:** NYU Langone Med Ctr (page 108); **Address:** 240 E 38th St Fl 19, New York, NY 10016; **Phone:** 212-731-6455; **Board Cert:** Obstetrics & Gynecology 2012; Gynecologic Oncology 2012; **Med School:** Jefferson Med Coll 1995; **Resid:** Obstetrics & Gynecology, Lankenau Hosp 1999; **Fellow:** Gynecologic Oncology, Meml Sloan Kettering Cancer Ctr 2003; **Fac Appt:** Assoc Prof ObG, NYU Sch Med

Poynor, Elizabeth A MD/PhD (GO) - **Spec Exp:** Gynecologic Cancer; Gynecologic Surgery-Complex; Laparoscopic Surgery; Breast Cancer; **Hospital:** Lenox Hill Hosp (page 106); **Address:** 1050 5th Ave, New York, NY 10028; **Phone:** 212-426-2700; **Board Cert:** Obstetrics & Gynecology 2012; Gynecologic Oncology 2012; **Med School:** Columbia P&S 1988; **Resid:** Obstetrics & Gynecology, Hosp Univ Penn 1992; **Fellow:** Gynecologic Oncology, Meml Sloan-Kettering Cancer Ctr 1995

Rahaman, Jamal MD (GO) - **Spec Exp:** Minimally Invasive Surgery; Gynecologic Cancer; Robotic Surgery; Laparoscopic Surgery; **Hospital:** Mt Sinai Med Ctr (page 102); **Address:** 1136 Fifth Ave, Ste 1B, New York, NY 10128-0122; **Phone:** 212-427-1415; **Board Cert:** Obstetrics & Gynecology 2012; Gynecologic Oncology 2012; **Med School:** Jamaica 1984; **Resid:** Obstetrics & Gynecology, Lincoln Med Ctr 1991; Obstetrics & Gynecology, Mt Sinai Med Ctr 1993; **Fellow:** Cardiovascular Surgery, Texas Heart Inst 1990; Gynecologic Oncology, Mt Sinai Med Ctr 1995; **Fac Appt:** Assoc Clin Prof ObG, Mount Sinai Sch Med

Sonoda, Yukio MD (GO) - **Spec Exp:** Laparoscopic Surgery; Fertility Preservation in Cancer; **Hospital:** Meml Sloan-Kettering Canc Ctr (page 114); **Address:** 1275 York Ave, New York, NY 10065; **Phone:** 212-639-6450; **Board Cert:** Obstetrics & Gynecology 2012; Gynecologic Oncology 2012; **Med School:** Geo Wash Univ 1992; **Resid:** Obstetrics & Gynecology, SUNY Buffalo 1997

Wallach, Robert C MD (GO) - **Spec Exp:** Vulvar & Vaginal Cancer; Ovarian Cancer; Cervical Cancer; Peritoneal Carcinomatosis; **Hospital:** NYU Langone Med Ctr (page 108), Bellevue Hosp Ctr; **Address:** 240 E 38th St Fl 19th, New York, NY 10016; **Phone:** 212-731-6450; **Board Cert:** Obstetrics & Gynecology 1967; Gynecologic Oncology 1974; **Med School:** Yale Univ 1960; **Resid:** Obstetrics & Gynecology, Beth Israel Med Ctr 1965; **Fellow:** Gynecologic Oncology, SUNY Downstate Med Ctr 1966; **Fac Appt:** Prof ObG, NYU Sch Med

Zakashansky, Konstantin MD (GO) - **Spec Exp:** HPV-Human Papilloma Virus; Hysterectomy Alternatives; Robotic Surgery; **Hospital:** Mt Sinai Med Ctr (page 102), Lutheran Med Ctr - Brooklyn; **Address:** 1176 5th Ave Fl 9th, New York, NY 10029; **Phone:** 212-241-5034; **Board Cert:** Obstetrics & Gynecology 2012; Gynecologic Oncology 2012; **Med School:** SUNY Stony Brook 2000; **Resid:** Obstetrics & Gynecology, Beth Israel Med Ctr 2004; **Fellow:** Gynecologic Oncology, Mt Sinai 2007; **Fac Appt:** Assoc Prof ObG, Mount Sinai Sch Med

Hand Surgery

Athanasian, Edward A MD (HS) - **Spec Exp:** Bone & Soft Tissue Tumors; Hand & Upper Extremity Tumors; **Hospital:** Hosp For Special Surgery (page 113), Meml Sloan-Kettering Canc Ctr (page 114); **Address:** Hospital for Special Surgery, 523 E 72nd St Fl 4th, New York, NY 10021; **Phone:** 212-606-1962; **Board Cert:** Orthopaedic Surgery 2008; Hand Surgery 2008; **Med School:** Columbia P&S 1988; **Resid:** Surgery, Beth Israel Deaconess Hosp 1989; Orthopaedic Surgery, Hosp Special Surgery 1993; **Fellow:** Hand Surgery, Mayo Clinic 1994; Orthopaedic Oncology, Meml Sloan Kettering Cancer Ctr 1995; **Fac Appt:** Assoc Clin Prof OrS, Cornell Univ-Weill Med Coll

Barron Jr, Otis A MD (HS) - **Spec Exp:** Shoulder Arthroscopic Surgery; Elbow Surgery; Nerve & Tendon Reconstruction; Shoulder Reconstruction; **Hospital:** St. Luke's - Roosevelt Hosp Ctr - Roosevelt Div (page 94); **Address:** CV Starr Hand Surgery Ctr, 1000 10th Ave Fl 3rd, New York, NY 10019; **Phone:** 212-523-7590; **Board Cert:** Orthopaedic Surgery 2009; Hand Surgery 2009; **Med School:** Tulane Univ 1989; **Resid:** Surgery, Tulane Univ Affil Hosps 1994; **Fellow:** Shoulder Surgery, Columbia Presby Hosp 1995; Hand Surgery, St Lukes Roosevelt Hosp 1996; **Fac Appt:** Asst Clin Prof S, Columbia P&S

Beldner, Steven MD (HS) - **Spec Exp:** Elbow Surgery; Hand & Wrist Surgery; Scleroderma; **Hospital:** Beth Israel Med Ctr - Petrie Div (page 94), St. Luke's - Roosevelt Hosp Ctr - St Luke's Hosp (page 94); **Address:** 321 E 34th St, The Hand Ctr, New York, NY 10016; **Phone:** 212-340-0000; **Board Cert:** Orthopaedic Surgery 2010; Hand Surgery 2010; **Med School:** UMDNJ-NJ Med Sch, Newark 1991; **Resid:** Orthopaedic Surgery, Bellevue Hosp 1996; **Fellow:** Hand Surgery, NYU Med Ctr 1997; **Fac Appt:** Asst Prof OrS, Albert Einstein Coll Med

Botwinick, Nelson MD (HS) - **Spec Exp:** Trauma; Carpal Tunnel Syndrome; Arthritis Hand Surgery; **Hospital:** NY-Presby/Lower Manhattan Hosp (page 104); **Address:** 170 William St Fl 8, New York, NY 10038; **Phone:** 212-312-5598; **Board Cert:** Orthopaedic Surgery 2009; Hand Surgery 2009; **Med School:** NYU Sch Med 1980; **Resid:** Orthopaedic Surgery, NYU Med Ctr 1985; **Fellow:** Orthopaedic Surgery, NYU Med Ctr 1986; **Fac Appt:** Assoc Clin Prof OrS, NYU Sch Med

Carlson, Michelle Gerwin MD (HS) - **Spec Exp:** Sports Injuries; Hand & Upper Extremity Surgery; Arthritis; Pediatric Hand Surgery; **Hospital:** Hosp For Special Surgery (page 113), NY-Presby/Weill Cornell Med Ctr, NY (page 104); **Address:** 523 E 72nd St, Fl 4, rm 439, New York, NY 10021; **Phone:** 212-606-1546; **Board Cert:** Orthopaedic Surgery 2007; Hand Surgery 2007; **Med School:** Cornell Univ-Weill Med Coll 1987; **Resid:** Orthopaedic Surgery, Hosp Special Surg 1992; **Fellow:** Hand Surgery, Hosp Special Surg 1993; **Fac Appt:** Assoc Prof OrS, Cornell Univ-Weill Med Coll

Catalano III, Louis W MD (HS) - **Spec Exp:** Hand & Upper Extremity Surgery; Wrist Surgery; Rotator Cuff Surgery; **Hospital:** St. Luke's - Roosevelt Hosp Ctr - Roosevelt Div (page 94); **Address:** 1000 10th Ave, Fl 3rd, New York, NY 10019; **Phone:** 212-523-7590; **Board Cert:** Orthopaedic Surgery 2003; Hand Surgery 2004; **Med School:** NYU Sch Med 1994; **Resid:** Surgery, Barnes Jewish Hosp 1995; Orthopaedic Surgery, Barnes Jewish Hosp 1999; **Fellow:** Hand Surgery, St. Lukes Roosevelt Hosp 2000; **Fac Appt:** Asst Clin Prof OrS, Columbia P&S

Daluiski, Aaron MD (HS) - **Spec Exp:** Pediatric Hand Surgery; Elbow Surgery; Fractures; **Hospital:** Hosp For Special Surgery (page 113); **Address:** East River Professional Bldg, 523 E 72nd St, 4th Fl, New York, NY 10021; **Phone:** 212-606-1284; **Board Cert:** Orthopaedic Surgery ; Hand Surgery ; **Med School:** UCLA 1994; **Resid:** Orthopaedic Surgery, UCLA Med Ctr 2000; **Fellow:** Orthopaedic Research, UCLA School of Med; Hand & Microvascular Surgery, Hosp Special Surgery; **Fac Appt:** Asst Prof OrS, Cornell Univ-Weill Med Coll

Glickel, Steven Z MD (HS) - **Spec Exp:** Hand & Wrist Surgery; Elbow Surgery; Peripheral Nerve Surgery; **Hospital:** St. Luke's - Roosevelt Hosp Ctr - Roosevelt Div (page 94); **Address:** 1000 10th Ave Fl 3, New York, NY 10019-1147; **Phone:** 212-523-7590; **Board Cert:** Orthopaedic Surgery 1985; Hand Surgery 2010; **Med School:** Harvard Med Sch 1976; **Resid:** Surgery, NY-Presby/Columbia Univ Med Ctr 1978; Orthopaedic Surgery, Brigham & Women's Hosp 1981; **Fellow:** Hand Surgery, St. Luke's - Roosevelt Hosp Ctr - Roosevelt Div 1983; Research, NY-Presby/Columbia Univ Med Ctr 1982; **Fac Appt:** Clin Prof OrS, Columbia P&S

Hotchkiss, Robert N MD (HS) - **Spec Exp:** Wrist Surgery; Elbow Reconstruction; Dupuytren's Contracture; **Hospital:** Hosp For Special Surgery (page 113); **Address:** 523 E 72nd St Fl 4, New York, NY 10021-4099; **Phone:** 212-606-1964; **Board Cert:** Orthopaedic Surgery 2010; Hand Surgery 2010; **Med School:** Johns Hopkins Univ 1980; **Resid:** Surgery, Johns Hopkins Hosp 1982; Orthopaedic Surgery, Johns Hopkins Hosp 1985; **Fellow:** Hand Surgery, Union Meml Hosp 1987; **Fac Appt:** Assoc Prof OrS, Cornell Univ-Weill Med Coll

King, William MD (HS) - **Spec Exp:** Carpal Tunnel Syndrome; Hand Reconstruction; Microvascular Surgery; Fractures; **Hospital:** NYU Hosp For Joint Dis (page 108), Lenox Hill Hosp (page 106); **Address:** 424 Madison Ave, Fl 9, New York, NY 10017; **Phone:** 212-813-2104; **Board Cert:** Orthopaedic Surgery 2009; **Med School:** Columbia P&S 1974; **Resid:** Surgery, St Lukes-Roosevelt Hosp Ctr 1976; Orthopaedic Surgery, Columbia-Presby Med Ctr 1979; **Fellow:** Hand & Microvascular Surgery, Univ Colorado Hosp 1980; **Fac Appt:** Asst Prof OrS, NYU Sch Med

Lee, Steve K MD (HS) - **Spec Exp:** Peripheral Nerve Surgery; Tendon Surgery; Wrist/Hand Injuries; Ligament Reconstruction; **Hospital:** Hosp For Special Surgery (page 113), NY-Presby/Weill Cornell Med Ctr, NY (page 104); **Address:** 523 E 72nd St, Fl 4, New York, NY 10021; **Phone:** 212-606-1730; **Board Cert:** Orthopaedic Surgery 2011; Hand Surgery 2011; **Med School:** Duke Univ 1993; **Resid:** Orthopaedic Surgery, Yale-New Haven Hosp 1998; **Fellow:** Hand Surgery, NYU Hosp for Joint Diseases 2003; **Fac Appt:** Assoc Prof OrS, Cornell Univ-Weill Med Coll

Lenzo, Salvatore MD (HS) - **Spec Exp:** Carpal Tunnel Syndrome; Arthritis; Hand Injuries; Congenital Hand Deformities; **Hospital:** NYU Hosp For Joint Dis (page 108), NYU Langone Med Ctr (page 108); **Address:** 955 5th Ave, New York, NY 10075; **Phone:** 212-734-9949; **Board Cert:** Orthopaedic Surgery 2010; Hand Surgery 2010; **Med School:** NYU Sch Med 1981; **Resid:** Orthopaedic Surgery, Bellevue Hosp 1986; **Fellow:** Hand Surgery, Bellevue Hosp 1987; **Fac Appt:** Asst Clin Prof OrS, NYU Sch Med

Melone Jr, Charles P MD (HS) - **Spec Exp:** Wrist Surgery; Fractures; **Hospital:** Beth Israel Med Ctr - Petrie Div (page 94); **Address:** Hand Surgery Ctr, 321 E 34th St, New York, NY 10016; **Phone:** 212-340-0000; **Board Cert:** Orthopaedic Surgery 1976; Hand Surgery 2004; **Med School:** Georgetown Univ 1969; **Resid:** Surgery, Nassau Univ Med Ctr 1971; Orthopaedic Surgery, Nassau Univ Med Ctr 1974; **Fellow:** Hand Surgery, NYU Langone Med Ctr 1975; **Fac Appt:** Prof OrS, Albert Einstein Coll Med

Polatsch, Daniel B MD (HS) - **Spec Exp:** Hand & Elbow Surgery; **Hospital:** Beth Israel Med Ctr - Petrie Div (page 94); **Address:** 321 E 34th St, The Hand Center, New York, NY 10016; **Phone:** 212-340-0000; **Board Cert:** Orthopaedic Surgery 2005; Hand Surgery 2008; **Med School:** NYU Sch Med 1997; **Resid:** Orthopaedic Surgery, Hosp for Joint Dis 2002

Pruzansky, Mark E MD (HS) - **Spec Exp:** Arthritis Hand Surgery; Carpal Tunnel Syndrome; Sports Injuries; Wrist Surgery; **Hospital:** Mt Sinai Med Ctr (page 102), Lenox Hill Hosp (page 106); **Address:** 975 Park Ave, Ste 1B, MS 10028, New York, NY 10028; **Phone:** 212-249-8700; **Board Cert:** Orthopaedic Surgery 1980; Hand Surgery 2013; Orthopaedic Sports Medicine 2007; **Med School:** Mount Sinai Sch Med 1974; **Resid:** Orthopaedic Surgery, Mount Sinai Med Ctr 1978; **Fellow:** Hand Surgery, South Baptist Hosp 1978; Hand Surgery, Pacific Presby Hosp 1979; **Fac Appt:** Asst Prof OrS, Mount Sinai Sch Med

Raskin, Keith B MD (HS) - **Spec Exp:** Wrist/Hand Injuries; Arthritis; Carpal Tunnel Syndrome; Elbow Surgery; **Hospital:** NYU Langone Med Ctr (page 108), NYU Hosp For Joint Dis (page 108); **Address:** 317 E 34th St, Fl 3, New York, NY 10016; **Phone:** 212-263-4263; **Board Cert:** Orthopaedic Surgery 2013; Hand Surgery 2013; **Med School:** Geo Wash Univ 1983; **Resid:** Orthopaedic Surgery, NYU Langone Med Ctr 1988; **Fellow:** Hand Surgery, Union Mem Hosp 1989; **Fac Appt:** Assoc Clin Prof OrS, NYU Sch Med

Rettig, Michael E MD (HS) - **Spec Exp:** Fractures; Arthritis; Nerve Disorders/Surgery; **Hospital:** NYU Langone Med Ctr (page 108), NYU Hosp For Joint Dis (page 108); **Address:** 317 E 34th St Fl 3, New York, NY 10016-4974; **Phone:** 212-889-8600; **Board Cert:** Orthopaedic Surgery 2005; Hand Surgery 2005; **Med School:** SUNY Upstate Med Univ 1986; **Resid:** Orthopaedic Surgery, NYU Med Ctr 1991; **Fellow:** Hand Surgery, Mayo Clinic 1992; **Fac Appt:** Asst Prof OrS, NYU Sch Med

Rosenwasser, Melvin P MD (HS) - **Spec Exp:** Carpal Tunnel Syndrome; Sports Injuries; Elbow Surgery; Trauma; **Hospital:** NY-Presby/Columbia Univ Med Ctr, NY (page 104); **Address:** New York Orthopedic Hosp Assocs, 622 W 168th St, PH 11, rm 1150, New York, NY 10032; **Phone:** 212-305-8036; **Board Cert:** Orthopaedic Surgery 1999; Hand Surgery 2011; **Med School:** Columbia P&S 1976; **Resid:** Surgery, St. Luke's - Roosevelt Hosp Ctr - Roosevelt Div 1979; Orthopaedic Surgery, NY-Presby/Columbia Univ Med Ctr 1982; **Fellow:** Hand Surgery, NY-Presby/Columbia Univ Med Ctr 1983; **Fac Appt:** Prof OrS, Columbia P&S

Strauch, Robert J MD (HS) - **Spec Exp:** Hand Reconstruction; Hand & Elbow Nerve Disorders; Hand & Wrist Surgery; Elbow Surgery; **Hospital:** NY-Presby/Columbia Univ Med Ctr, NY (page 104); **Address:** New York Orthopedic Hosp Assocs, 622 W 168th St, PH 11, rm 1119, New York, NY 10032; **Phone:** 212-305-4272; **Board Cert:** Orthopaedic Surgery 2005; Hand Surgery 2005; **Med School:** Columbia P&S 1986; **Resid:** Orthopaedic Surgery, NY-Presby/Columbia Univ Med Ctr 1991; **Fellow:** Hand Surgery, Indiana Hand Ctr 1992; **Fac Appt:** Prof OrS, Columbia P&S

Wolfe, Scott W MD (HS) - **Spec Exp:** Wrist Surgery; Nerve Disorders/Surgery; Fractures; **Hospital:** Hosp For Special Surgery (page 113); **Address:** Hosp for Special Surgery, 535 E 70 St, New York, NY 10021; **Phone:** 212-606-1529; **Board Cert:** Orthopaedic Surgery 2013; Hand Surgery 2013; **Med School:** Cornell Univ-Weill Med Coll 1984; **Resid:** Surgery, St. Luke's - Roosevelt Hosp Ctr - Roosevelt Div 1986; Orthopaedic Surgery, Hosp Special Surg 1989; **Fellow:** Hand & Microvascular Surgery, Presby/Columbia Univ Med Ctr 1990; **Fac Appt:** Prof OrS, Cornell Univ-Weill Med Coll

Yang, S Steven MD (HS) - **Spec Exp:** Shoulder Surgery; Congenital Hand Deformities; Reconstructive Surgery; Microvascular Surgery; **Hospital:** NYU Langone Med Ctr (page 108), NYU Hosp For Joint Dis (page 108); **Address:** NYU Hand Center, 530 First Ave, Ste 8U, New York, NY 10016; **Phone:** 646-501-0740; **Board Cert:** Orthopaedic Surgery 2009; Hand Surgery 2009; **Med School:** Duke Univ 1988; **Resid:** Orthopaedic Surgery, Lenox Hill Hosp 1994; **Fellow:** Hand Surgery, Hosp for Special Surgery 1995; **Fac Appt:** Assoc Prof OrS, NYU Sch Med

Hematology

Aledort, Louis M MD (Hem) - **Spec Exp:** Bleeding/Coagulation Disorders; Platelet Disorders; Paroxysmal Nocturnal Hemoglobinuria; **Hospital:** Mt Sinai Med Ctr (page 102); **Address:** 1470 Madison Ave Fl 3rd, New York, NY 10029; **Phone:** 212-860-0205; **Board Cert:** Internal Medicine 1966; Hematology 1972; **Med School:** Albert Einstein Coll Med 1959; **Resid:** Internal Medicine, Univ Va Hlth Sci Ctr 1961; Internal Medicine, U Rochester Med Ctr 1964; **Fellow:** Hematology, Strong Meml Hosp 1965; **Fac Appt:** Prof Med, Mount Sinai Sch Med

Amorosi, Edward L MD (Hem) - **Hospital:** NYU Langone Med Ctr (page 108); **Address:** 240 E 38th St Fl 19th, New York, NY 10016; **Phone:** 212-731-5187; **Board Cert:** Internal Medicine 1966; Hematology 1972; Medical Oncology 1977; **Med School:** NYU Sch Med 1959; **Resid:** Internal Medicine, Bellevue Hosp Ctr- NYU 1962; Internal Medicine, Francis Delafield Hosp 1963; **Fellow:** Hematology, NYU Med Ctr 1965; **Fac Appt:** Prof Med, NYU Sch Med

Castro-Malaspina, Hugo MD (Hem) - **Spec Exp:** Myelodysplastic Syndromes; Bone Marrow Failure Disorders; Bone Marrow Transplant; Anemia-Aplastic; **Hospital:** Meml Sloan-Kettering Canc Ctr (page 114); **Address:** 1275 York Ave, New York, NY 10065; **Phone:** 800-525-2225; **Med School:** Peru 1971; **Resid:** Internal Medicine, St Louis Hosp; **Fellow:** Hematology & Oncology, Andean Biology Inst; Pediatric Hematology-Oncology, St Louis Hosp

Cook, Perry MD (Hem) - **Spec Exp:** Bone Marrow Transplant; Leukemia; Lymphoma; **Hospital:** NYU Langone Med Ctr (page 108); **Address:** 240 E 38th St Fl 19th, New York, NY 10016; **Phone:** 212-731-5184; **Board Cert:** Internal Medicine 1980; Hematology 1982; Medical Oncology 1983; **Med School:** Univ Iowa Coll Med 1977; **Resid:** Internal Medicine, St Luke's-Roosevelt Hosp Ctr 1979; Internal Medicine, Columbia-Presby Med Ctr 1980; **Fellow:** Hematology & Oncology, Columbia-Presby Med Ctr 1983; **Fac Appt:** Assoc Clin Prof Med, NYU Sch Med

Diaz, Michael MD (Hem) - **Spec Exp:** Anemia; Bleeding/Coagulation Disorders; Lymphoma; **Hospital:** Mt Sinai Med Ctr (page 102); **Address:** 1112 Park Ave, New York, NY 10128; **Phone:** 212-876-4500; **Board Cert:** Internal Medicine 1979; Hematology 1986; **Med School:** St Louis Univ 1971; **Resid:** Internal Medicine, Lenox Hill Hosp 1974; **Fellow:** Hematology, Elmhurst Hosp 1976; **Fac Appt:** Asst Clin Prof Med, Mount Sinai Sch Med

Diuguid, David L MD (Hem) - **Spec Exp:** Bleeding/Coagulation Disorders; **Hospital:** NY-Presby/Columbia Univ Med Ctr, NY (page 104); **Address:** 161 Ft Washington Ave, Irving Bldg Fl 10, New York, NY 10032; **Phone:** 212-305-0527; **Board Cert:** Internal Medicine 1982; Hematology 1986; Medical Oncology 1985; **Med School:** Cornell Univ-Weill Med Coll 1979; **Resid:** Internal Medicine, Boston Med Ctr 1983; **Fellow:** Hematology & Oncology, New England Bapt Hosp 1986; **Fac Appt:** Assoc Prof Med, Columbia P&S

Fruchtman, Steven M MD (Hem) - **Spec Exp:** Myeloproliferative Disorders; Polycythemia Rubra Vera; **Address:** 1150 Park Ave, Ste Medical, New York, NY 10128; **Phone:** 212-427-7700; **Board Cert:** Internal Medicine 1980; Hematology 1984; **Med School:** NY Med Coll 1977; **Resid:** Internal Medicine, Univ Hosp 1981; **Fellow:** Hematology, Mount Sinai Med Ctr 1984; Hematology, Meml Sloan Kettering Cancer Ctr 1985; **Fac Appt:** Assoc Prof Hem & Onc, NY Med Coll

Goldenberg, Alec S MD (Hem) - **Spec Exp:** Breast Cancer; Lymphoma; Bleeding/Coagulation Disorders; **Hospital:** NYU Langone Med Ctr (page 108); **Address:** 157 E 32nd St Fl 2, New York, NY 10016; **Phone:** 212-689-6791; **Board Cert:** Internal Medicine 1986; Medical Oncology 1987; **Med School:** Johns Hopkins Univ 1980; **Resid:** Internal Medicine, Bellevue Hosp-NYU 1984; **Fellow:** Hematology & Oncology, Meml Sloan Kettering Canc Ctr 1988; **Fac Appt:** Assoc Clin Prof Med, NYU Sch Med

Gruenstein, Steven MD (Hem) - **Spec Exp:** Hematologic Malignancies; Gastrointestinal Cancer; Lung Cancer; **Hospital:** Mt Sinai Med Ctr (page 102); **Address:** 12 E 86th St, Central Park Hematology/Oncology, New York, NY 10028-0506; **Phone:** 212-861-6660; **Board Cert:** Internal Medicine 1988; **Med School:** Italy 1984; **Resid:** Internal Medicine, Metropolitan Hosp Ctr 1987; **Fellow:** Hematology & Oncology, Beth Israel Med Ctr 1990; **Fac Appt:** Assoc Clin Prof Med, Mount Sinai Sch Med

Halperin, Ira MD (Hem) - **Spec Exp:** Leukemia; Myeloproliferative Disorders; **Hospital:** Beth Israel Med Ctr - Petrie Div (page 94); **Address:** 2 Fifth Ave, Ste 9, New York, NY 10011-8855; **Phone:** 212-254-5940; **Board Cert:** Internal Medicine 1970; Hematology 1976; Medical Oncology 1979; **Med School:** NYU Sch Med 1962; **Resid:** Internal Medicine, St Vincents Hosp 1966; **Fellow:** Hematology, Mt Sinai Hosp 1969

Hymes, Kenneth B MD (Hem) - **Spec Exp:** Bleeding/Coagulation Disorders; Leukemia & Lymphoma; Cutaneous T-cell Lymphoma; Mycosis Fungoides; **Hospital:** NYU Langone Med Ctr (page 108); **Address:** NYU Clinical Cancer Center, 240 E 38th St, Fl 19, New York, NY 10016-6402; **Phone:** 212-731-5189; **Board Cert:** Internal Medicine 1978; Hematology 1980; Medical Oncology 1981; **Med School:** SUNY Upstate Med Univ 1975; **Resid:** Internal Medicine, Barnes Hosp 1978; **Fellow:** Hematology, NYU Med Ctr 1980; Medical Oncology, NYU Med Ctr 1981; **Fac Appt:** Assoc Prof Hem & Onc, NYU Sch Med

Isola, Luis M MD (Hem) - **Spec Exp:** Anemia-Aplastic; Hodgkin's Lymphoma; Multiple Myeloma; **Hospital:** Mt Sinai Med Ctr (page 102); **Address:** Ruttenberg Treatment Ctr, 1470 Madison Ave Fl 3rd, New York, NY 10029; **Phone:** 212-824-8709; **Board Cert:** Internal Medicine 1986; Hematology 1988; **Med School:** Argentina 1979; **Resid:** Internal Medicine, Ctr for Med Education 1983; **Fellow:** Hematology, Mt Sinai Med Ctr 1985; **Fac Appt:** Prof Med, Mount Sinai Sch Med

Jurcic, Joseph G MD (Hem) - **Spec Exp:** Leukemia; Myelodysplastic Syndromes; Clinical Trials; **Hospital:** NY-Presby/Columbia Univ Med Ctr, NY (page 104); **Address:** 161 Fort Washington Ave, Garden Level, New York, NY 10032; **Phone:** 646-317-5077; **Board Cert:** Medical Oncology 2005; Hematology 2008; **Med School:** Univ Pennsylvania 1988; **Resid:** Internal Medicine, Barnes Hosp 1991; **Fellow:** Hematology & Oncology, Meml Sloan Kettering Cancer Ctr 1994; **Fac Appt:** Clin Prof Med, Columbia P&S

Kempin, Sanford J MD (Hem) - **Spec Exp:** Bleeding/Coagulation Disorders; Leukemia; Lymphoma; Thrombotic Disorders; **Hospital:** Beth Israel Med Ctr - Petrie Div (page 94); **Address:** 325 W 15th St, New York, NY 10011; **Phone:** 212-604-6010; **Board Cert:** Internal Medicine 1976; Medical Oncology 1977; Hematology 1978; **Med School:** Belgium 1971; **Resid:** Internal Medicine, Lemuel Shattuck Hosp 1972; **Fellow:** Hematology, St Jude Chldns Rsch Hosp 1975; Medical Oncology, Meml Sloan Kettering Cancer Ctr 1976; **Fac Appt:** Asst Prof Hem & Onc, Albert Einstein Coll Med

Leonard, John P MD (Hem) - **Spec Exp:** Lymphoma; Multiple Myeloma; Hematologic Malignancies; Leukemia; **Hospital:** NY-Presby/Weill Cornell Med Ctr, NY (page 104); **Address:** NY Presby Hosp-NY Weill Cornell Med Ctr, 525 E 68th St, Payson Pavilion 3, New York, NY 10065; **Phone:** 646-962-2068; **Board Cert:** Hematology 2006; Medical Oncology 2007; **Med School:** Univ VA Sch Med 1990; **Resid:** Internal Medicine, NY Hosp-Cornell Med Ctr 1993; **Fellow:** Hematology & Oncology, NY Hosp-Cornell Med Ctr 1996; **Fac Appt:** Prof Med, Cornell Univ-Weill Med Coll

Levine, Randy MD (Hem) - **Spec Exp:** Hematologic Malignancies; Bleeding/Coagulation Disorders; **Hospital:** Lenox Hill Hosp (page 106), St. Luke's - Roosevelt Hosp Ctr - Roosevelt Div (page 94); **Address:** 4 E 76th St, New York, NY 10021-2611; **Phone:** 212-717-1020; **Board Cert:** Internal Medicine 1982; Hematology 1984; Blood Banking 1985; **Med School:** SUNY Buffalo 1979; **Resid:** Internal Medicine, Montefiore Med Ctr 1982; **Fellow:** Hematology, Montefiore Med Ctr 1983; Blood Banking, Mt Sinai Hosp 1984; **Fac Appt:** Assoc Clin Prof Med, NYU Sch Med

Maslak, Peter G MD (Hem) - **Spec Exp:** Leukemia; Stem Cell Transplant; Myelodysplastic Syndromes; Clinical Trials; **Hospital:** Meml Sloan-Kettering Canc Ctr (page 114); **Address:** 1275 York Avenue, New York, NY 10065; **Phone:** 212-639-5518; **Board Cert:** Internal Medicine 1987; Hematology 2000; Medical Oncology 1989; **Med School:** Mount Sinai Sch Med 1984; **Resid:** Internal Medicine, Univ Michigan Med Ctr 1987; Internal Medicine, Meml Sloan Kettering Cancer Ctr 1991; **Fellow:** Hematology & Oncology, Meml Sloan Kettering Cancer Ctr 1990; **Fac Appt:** Clin Prof Med, Cornell Univ-Weill Med Coll

Mears, John Gregory MD (Hem) - **Spec Exp:** Lymphoma; Leukemia; Multiple Myeloma; **Hospital:** NY-Presby/Columbia Univ Med Ctr, NY (page 104); **Address:** 161 Ft Washington Ave, Ste 923, New York, NY 10032; **Phone:** 212-305-3506; **Board Cert:** Internal Medicine 1976; Hematology 1978; **Med School:** Columbia P&S 1973; **Resid:** Internal Medicine, Boston Univ Med Ctr 1975; **Fellow:** Hematology & Oncology, Columbia-Presby Med Ctr 1978; **Fac Appt:** Clin Prof Hem & Onc, Columbia P&S

Meyer, Richard MD (Hem) - **Spec Exp:** Lymphoma; Leukemia; Anemia; **Hospital:** Mt Sinai Med Ctr (page 102); **Address:** 1150 Park Ave, New York, NY 10128-1234; **Phone:** 212-427-7700; **Board Cert:** Internal Medicine 1975; Hematology 1978; Medical Oncology 1979; **Med School:** Mount Sinai Sch Med 1972; **Resid:** Internal Medicine, Mt Sinai Hosp 1975; Hematology, Mt Sinai Hosp 1977; **Fellow:** Medical Oncology, Mt Sinai Hosp 1977; **Fac Appt:** Assoc Clin Prof Hem, Mount Sinai Sch Med

Moskovits, Tibor MD (Hem) - **Spec Exp:** Lymphoma; Breast Cancer; Lung Cancer; **Hospital:** NYU Langone Med Ctr (page 108); **Address:** 240 E 38th St Fl 19th, New York, NY 10016; **Phone:** 212-731-5191; **Board Cert:** Internal Medicine 1988; Hematology 2003; Medical Oncology 2004; **Med School:** SUNY Downstate 1985; **Resid:** Internal Medicine, Beth Israel Med Ctr 1989; **Fellow:** Hematology & Oncology, NYU Med Ctr 1992; **Fac Appt:** Asst Clin Prof Med, NYU Sch Med

Ossias, A Lawrence MD (Hem) - **Spec Exp:** Lymphoma; Leukemia; Coagulation/Bleeding Disorders; **Hospital:** Mt Sinai Med Ctr (page 102); **Address:** 1112 Park Ave, New York, NY 10128; **Phone:** 212-427-9333; **Board Cert:** Internal Medicine 1972; Hematology 1972; Medical Oncology 1979; **Med School:** Yale Univ 1965; **Resid:** Internal Medicine, Bronx Municipal Hosp 1970; **Fellow:** Hematology, Mt Sinai Med Ctr 1972; **Fac Appt:** Asst Clin Prof Med, Mount Sinai Sch Med

Raphael, Bruce Gordon MD (Hem) - **Spec Exp:** Lymphoma; Leukemia; Multiple Myeloma; Anemia; **Hospital:** NYU Langone Med Ctr (page 108), Bellevue Hosp Ctr; **Address:** NYU Clinical Cancer Ctr, 240 E 38th St, Fl 19, New York, NY 10016-6402; **Phone:** 212-731-5185; **Board Cert:** Internal Medicine 1978; Hematology 1980; Medical Oncology 1981; **Med School:** McGill Univ 1975; **Resid:** Internal Medicine, Jewish Genl Hosp 1977; **Fellow:** Medical Oncology, Meml Sloan Kettering Cancer Ctr 1978; Hematology, NYU Med Ctr 1980; **Fac Appt:** Clin Prof Med, NYU Sch Med

Savage, David G MD (Hem) - **Spec Exp:** Stem Cell Transplant; Bone Marrow Transplant; Lymphoma; **Hospital:** NY-Presby/Columbia Univ Med Ctr, NY (page 104); **Address:** 177 Fort Washington Ave, Millstein Bldg - Fl 6, rm 435, New York, NY 10032; **Phone:** 212-305-9783; **Board Cert:** Internal Medicine 1977; Hematology 1982; Medical Oncology 1985; **Med School:** Columbia P&S 1974; **Resid:** Internal Medicine, Harlem Hosp/Columbia Presby Med Ctr 1977; **Fellow:** Hematology & Oncology, Harlem Hosp/Columbia Presby Med Ctr 1982; **Fac Appt:** Prof Med, Columbia P&S

Scigliano, Eileen MD (Hem) - **Spec Exp:** Bone Marrow Transplant; **Hospital:** Mt Sinai Med Ctr (page 102); **Address:** 1470 Madison Ave Fl 3rd, New York, NY 10029; **Phone:** 212-241-6021; **Board Cert:** Internal Medicine 1984; Hematology 1988; **Med School:** Israel 1981; **Resid:** Internal Medicine, Kings County Hosp 1984; **Fellow:** Medical Oncology, VA Med Ctr 1985; Hematology, Mount Sinai Hosp 1988; **Fac Appt:** Assoc Prof Med, Mount Sinai Sch Med

Soff, Gerald A MD (Hem) - **Spec Exp:** Bleeding/Coagulation Disorders; Thrombotic Disorders; Hematologic Disorders in Cancer Patients; Anemia; **Hospital:** Meml Sloan-Kettering Canc Ctr (page 114); **Address:** MSKCC Div Hematology, 1275 York Ave Fl 4 - Ste 6, New York, NY 10065; **Phone:** 212-639-2335; **Board Cert:** Internal Medicine 1984; Hematology 1988; **Med School:** Johns Hopkins Univ 1981; **Resid:** Internal Medicine, Med Coll Virginia Affil Hosp 1984; **Fellow:** Hematology & Oncology, Beth Israel Deaconess Med Ctr 1988

Tallman, Martin S MD (Hem) - **Spec Exp:** Leukemia; **Hospital:** Meml Sloan-Kettering Canc Ctr (page 114); **Address:** Meml Hematology Lymphoma Grp, 1275 York Ave, Ste H-719, Box 380, New York, NY 10065; **Phone:** 212-639-3842; **Board Cert:** Internal Medicine 1983; Medical Oncology 1987; Hematology 1988; **Med School:** Ros Franklin Univ/Chicago Med Sch 1980; **Resid:** Internal Medicine, Evanston Hosp 1983; **Fellow:** Medical Oncology, Fred Hutchinson Cancer Ctr 1987; **Fac Appt:** Prof Med, Cornell Univ-Weill Med Coll

Troy, Kevin M MD (Hem) - **Spec Exp:** Leukemia; Lymphoma; Multiple Myeloma; **Hospital:** Mt Sinai Med Ctr (page 102); **Address:** 1735 York Ave, Ste P2, New York, NY 10128; **Phone:** 212-860-9055; **Board Cert:** Internal Medicine 1982; Hematology 1984; **Med School:** Univ Conn 1979; **Resid:** Internal Medicine, Lenox Hill Hosp 1982; **Fellow:** Hematology, Mount Sinai Hosp 1984; **Fac Appt:** Assoc Clin Prof Med, Mount Sinai Sch Med

Van Besien, Koen W MD/PhD (Hem) - **Spec Exp:** Lymphoma; Stem Cell Transplant; **Hospital:** NY-Presby/Weill Cornell Med Ctr, NY (page 104); **Address:** Stem Cell Transplant Program, 520 E 70th St, Starr Bldg, Ste 303, New York, NY 10021; **Phone:** 212-746-2048; **Board Cert:** Internal Medicine 2005; Medical Oncology 2005; Hematology 2006; **Med School:** Belgium 1984; **Resid:** Internal Medicine, Univ Leuven Med Ctr 1987; **Fellow:** Hematology & Oncology, Indiana Univ Med Ctr 1990; **Fac Appt:** Prof Hem & Onc, Cornell Univ-Weill Med Coll

Vogel, James M MD (Hem) - **Spec Exp:** Breast Cancer; Colon Cancer; Leukemia & Lymphoma; Platelet Disorders; **Hospital:** Mt Sinai Med Ctr (page 102), Mount Sinai Hosp of Queens (page 102); **Address:** 1150 Fifth Ave, New York, NY 10128-1243; **Phone:** 212-369-4250; **Board Cert:** Internal Medicine 1969; Hematology 1972; Medical Oncology 1973; **Med School:** Columbia P&S 1962; **Resid:** Hematology, Mount Sinai Hosp 1968; Medical Oncology, Natl Cancer Inst 1966; **Fellow:** Hematology, Mount Sinai Hosp 1968; **Fac Appt:** Assoc Prof Med, Mount Sinai Sch Med

Wisch, Nathaniel MD (Hem) - **Spec Exp:** Lymphoma; Breast Cancer; Leukemia; Anemia-Cancer Related; **Hospital:** Lenox Hill Hosp (page 106), Mt Sinai Med Ctr (page 102); **Address:** Central Park Hematology & Oncology, 12 E 86th St, New York, NY 10028-0506; **Phone:** 212-861-6660; **Board Cert:** Internal Medicine 1965; Hematology 1972; Medical Oncology 1977; **Med School:** Northwestern Univ 1958; **Resid:** Internal Medicine, VA Hosp 1960; Internal Medicine, Montefiore Hosp 1961; **Fellow:** Hematology & Oncology, Mount Sinai Hosp 1964; **Fac Appt:** Clin Prof Med, Mount Sinai Sch Med

Wolf, David J MD (Hem) - **Spec Exp:** Hematologic Malignancies; Hematology-Benign; Solid Tumors; **Hospital:** NY-Presby/Weill Cornell Med Ctr, NY (page 104); **Address:** 115 E 61st St Fl 11, New York, NY 10065; **Phone:** 212-688-7100; **Board Cert:** Internal Medicine 1976; Hematology 1978; Medical Oncology 1979; **Med School:** SUNY Hlth Sci Ctr 1973; **Resid:** Internal Medicine, NY Hosp/Meml Hosp 1976; **Fellow:** Hematology, NY Hosp 1976; **Fac Appt:** Asst Clin Prof Med, Cornell Univ-Weill Med Coll

Hospice & Palliative Medicine

Chai, Emily J MD (H & PM) - **Spec Exp:** Palliative Care; **Hospital:** Mt Sinai Med Ctr (page 102); **Address:** One Gustave L Levy Pl, Box 1070, New York, NY 10029; **Phone:** 212-659-8552; **Board Cert:** Internal Medicine 2011; Geriatric Medicine 2012; Hospice & Palliative Medicine 2008; **Med School:** NYU Sch Med 1998; **Resid:** Internal Medicine, Mt Sinai Hosp 2001; **Fellow:** Geriatric Medicine, Mt Sinai Hosp 2003; **Fac Appt:** Asst Prof Med, Mount Sinai Sch Med

Edwards, Wendy S A MD (H & PM) - **Spec Exp:** Palliative Care; Pain Management; **Hospital:** Lenox Hill Hosp (page 106); **Address:** 100 E 77th St, New York, NY 10075; **Phone:** 212-434-2140; **Board Cert:** Internal Medicine ; Hospice & Palliative Medicine ; **Med School:** Med Coll PA 1976; **Resid:** Internal Medicine, Metrowest Med Ctr 1978; Internal Medicine, Boston Univ Hosp 1979

Glare, Paul MD (H & PM) - **Spec Exp:** Palliative Care; Pain-Cancer; **Hospital:** Meml Sloan-Kettering Canc Ctr (page 114); **Address:** Meml Sloan Kettering Cancer Ctr, 1275 York Ave, Box 492, New York, NY 10065; **Phone:** 646-888-3065; **Med School:** Australia 1981; **Resid:** Internal Medicine, Syndey Hosp; Pain Medicine, Royal Prince Alfred Hosp; **Fellow:** Pain & Palliative Care, Eversleigh Hosp; Hospice & Palliative Medicine, Cleveland Clinic

Portenoy, Russell MD (H & PM) - **Spec Exp:** Pain Management; Palliative Care; **Hospital:** Beth Israel Med Ctr - Petrie Div (page 94); **Address:** Beth Israel Med Ctr, Dept Pain Medicine/Palliative Care, First Ave at 16th St, New York, NY 10003; **Phone:** 212-844-1505; **Board Cert:** Neurology 1985; Hospice & Palliative Medicine 2008; **Med School:** Univ MD Sch Med 1980; **Resid:** Neurology, Montefiore Med Ctr 1984; **Fellow:** Pain Medicine, Meml Sloan-Kettering Cancer Ctr 1985; **Fac Appt:** Prof N, Albert Einstein Coll Med

Tickoo, Roma MD (H & PM) - **Spec Exp:** Palliative Care; Pain-Cancer; Geriatric Care; **Hospital:** Meml Sloan-Kettering Canc Ctr (page 114); **Address:** Meml Sloan Kettering Cancer Ctr, 1275 York Ave, New York, NY 10065; **Phone:** 646-888-2694; **Board Cert:** Internal Medicine ; Geriatric Medicine ; Hospice & Palliative Medicine ; Pain Medicine ; **Med School:** India 1985; **Resid:** Internal Medicine, Flushing Med Ctr 2004; **Fellow:** Geriatric Medicine, NYU Med Ctr 2005

Infectious Disease

Aberg, Judith A MD (Inf) - **Spec Exp:** AIDS/HIV; **Hospital:** Bellevue Hosp Ctr; **Address:** 550 First Ave, Bellevue C&D Bldg, 5th Fl, Rm 558, New York, NY 10016; **Phone:** 212-263-6565; **Board Cert:** Infectious Disease 2006; **Med School:** Penn State Coll Med 1990; **Resid:** Internal Medicine, Cleveland Clinic Fdn 1994; **Fellow:** Infectious Disease, Washington Univ Sch Med Affil Hosp 1996; **Fac Appt:** Prof Med, NYU Sch Med

Brause, Barry MD (Inf) - **Spec Exp:** Bone/Joint Infections; Skin/Soft Tissue Infections; Infections in Prosthetic Devices; **Hospital:** Hosp For Special Surgery (page 113), NY-Presby/Weill Cornell Med Ctr, NY (page 104); **Address:** 535 E 70th St, Ste 657W, New York, NY 10021-5718; **Phone:** 212-774-7411; **Board Cert:** Internal Medicine 1973; Infectious Disease 1976; **Med School:** Univ Pittsburgh 1970; **Resid:** Internal Medicine, NY Presby/Weill Cornell Med Ctr 1973; **Fellow:** Infectious Disease, NY Presby/Weill Cornell Med Ctr 1975; **Fac Appt:** Clin Prof Med, Cornell Univ-Weill Med Coll

Brown, Arthur E MD (Inf) - **Spec Exp:** Infections in Cancer Patients; Fungal Infections; Infections in Immunocompromised Patients; **Hospital:** Meml Sloan-Kettering Canc Ctr (page 114); **Address:** 1275 York Ave, New York, NY 10065; **Phone:** 212-639-8475; **Med School:** Jefferson Med Coll 1971; **Resid:** Internal Medicine, Roosevelt Hosp 1972; Internal Medicine, USPHS Hosp-Staten Island NY & USPHS Hosp 1974; **Fellow:** Internal Medicine, Roosevelt Hosp 1976; Infectious Disease, Mem Sloan Kettering Cancer Ctr 1978; **Fac Appt:** Clin Prof Med, Cornell Univ-Weill Med Coll

Busillo, Christopher P MD (Inf) - **Spec Exp:** AIDS/HIV; Travel Medicine; Lyme Disease; **Hospital:** NY-Presby/Lower Manhattan Hosp (page 104); **Address:** 156 Williams St Fl 7th, New York, NY 10038-2668; **Phone:** 212-312-5920; **Board Cert:** Internal Medicine 2011; Infectious Disease 2012; **Med School:** Italy 1986; **Resid:** Internal Medicine, Cabrini Med Ctr 1989; **Fellow:** Infectious Disease, Cabrini Med Ctr 1991

Caplivski, Daniel Simon MD (Inf) - **Spec Exp:** Travel Medicine; Tropical Diseases; Malaria; AIDS/HIV; **Hospital:** Mt Sinai Med Ctr (page 102); **Address:** 5 E 98th St Fl 8, New York, NY 10029; **Phone:** 212-241-7468; **Board Cert:** Internal Medicine 2003; Infectious Disease 2005; **Med School:** Yale Univ 2000; **Resid:** Internal Medicine, Mt Sinai Med Ctr 2003; **Fellow:** Infectious Disease, Mt Sinai Med Ctr 2005; **Fac Appt:** Asst Prof Med, Mount Sinai Sch Med

El-Sadr, Wafaa M MD (Inf) - **Spec Exp:** AIDS/HIV; Tuberculosis; **Hospital:** Harlem Hosp Ctr; **Address:** Harlem Hosp, Div of Infectious Dis, 506 Lenox Ave MLK Bldg - rm 3101A, New York, NY 10037; **Phone:** 212-939-2936; **Board Cert:** Internal Medicine 1979; Infectious Disease 1982; **Med School:** Egypt 1975; **Resid:** Internal Medicine, Our Lady of Mercy Med Ctr 1977; Internal Medicine, Cabrini Med Ctr 1979; **Fellow:** Infectious Disease, VA Medical Ctr 1982; **Fac Appt:** Prof Epidemiol, Columbia P&S

Flood, Mary T MD/PhD (Inf) - **Spec Exp:** HIV; Hepatitis; Sexually Transmitted Diseases; **Hospital:** NY-Presby/Columbia Univ Med Ctr, NY (page 104); **Address:** 161 Fort Washington Ave, Ste 3-346, New York, NY 10032-3702; **Phone:** 212-305-8039; **Board Cert:** Internal Medicine 2012; Infectious Disease 2004; **Med School:** Columbia P&S 1987; **Resid:** Internal Medicine, NY-Presby Hosp 1991; **Fellow:** Infectious Disease, NY-Presby Hosp 1993; **Fac Appt:** Asst Clin Prof Med, Columbia P&S

Glesby, Marshall J MD/PhD (Inf) - **Spec Exp:** HIV/AIDS; **Hospital:** NY-Presby/Weill Cornell Med Ctr, NY (page 104); **Address:** 525 E 68th St, Baker Bldg - Fl 24, MS 97, New York, NY 10065; **Phone:** 212-746-4177; **Board Cert:** Internal Medicine 2003; Infectious Disease 2004; **Med School:** Johns Hopkins Univ 1989; **Resid:** Internal Medicine, Johns Hopkins Hosp 1992; **Fellow:** Infectious Disease, Johns Hopkins Hosp 1996; **Fac Appt:** Prof Med, Cornell Univ-Weill Med Coll

Greene, Jeffrey B MD (Inf) - **Spec Exp:** AIDS/HIV; Fungal Infections; Bone/Joint Infections; Epstein-Barr Virus; **Hospital:** NYU Langone Med Ctr (page 108); **Address:** 530 First Ave HCC Bldg - Ste 7J, New York, NY 10016; **Phone:** 212-375-2940; **Board Cert:** Internal Medicine 1979; Infectious Disease 1982; **Med School:** NYU Sch Med 1976; **Resid:** Internal Medicine, Bellevue Hosp 1979; **Fellow:** Infectious Disease, Bellevue Hosp 1982; **Fac Appt:** Clin Prof Med, NYU Sch Med

Gumprecht, Jeffrey P MD (Inf) - **Spec Exp:** AIDS/HIV; Travel Medicine; Infections-Surgical; **Hospital:** Mt Sinai Med Ctr (page 102); **Address:** 1100 Park Ave, Ste 1C, New York, NY 10128; **Phone:** 212-427-9550; **Board Cert:** Internal Medicine 1987; Infectious Disease 2003; **Med School:** Albany Med Coll 1983; **Resid:** Internal Medicine, Mt Sinai Hosp 1987; **Fellow:** Infectious Disease, Montefiore Med Ctr 1990; **Fac Appt:** Asst Clin Prof Med, Mount Sinai Sch Med

Hammer, Glenn S MD (Inf) - **Spec Exp:** AIDS/HIV; Hospital Acquired Infections; Infections-Surgical; **Hospital:** Mt Sinai Med Ctr (page 102); **Address:** 1100 Park Ave, Ste 1C, New York, NY 10128-1202; **Phone:** 212-427-9550; **Board Cert:** Infectious Disease 1974; Internal Medicine 1973; **Med School:** NYU Sch Med 1969; **Resid:** Internal Medicine, Mount Sinai Hosp 1972; **Fellow:** Infectious Disease, Mount Sinai Hosp 1974; **Fac Appt:** Asst Clin Prof Med, Mount Sinai Sch Med

Hammer, Scott M MD (Inf) - **Spec Exp:** AIDS/HIV; **Hospital:** NY-Presby/Columbia Univ Med Ctr, NY (page 104); **Address:** 630 W 168th St, P&S Box 82, New York, NY 10032; **Phone:** 212-305-8039; **Board Cert:** Internal Medicine 1975; Infectious Disease 1980; **Med School:** Columbia P&S 1972; **Resid:** Internal Medicine, Columbia-Presby Hosp 1975; Internal Medicine, Stanford Univ Hosp 1975; **Fellow:** Infectious Disease, Mass Genl Hosp 1981; **Fac Appt:** Prof Med, Columbia P&S

Hartman, Barry J MD (Inf) - **Spec Exp:** Endocarditis; Infections-Surgical; Parasitic Infections; **Hospital:** NY-Presby/Weill Cornell Med Ctr, NY (page 104); **Address:** 407 E 70th St, Fl 4, New York, NY 10021-5302; **Phone:** 212-744-4882; **Board Cert:** Internal Medicine 1976; Infectious Disease 1980; **Med School:** Penn State Coll Med 1973; **Resid:** Internal Medicine, NY Hosp/Cornell Med Ctr 1976; **Fellow:** Infectious Disease, NY Hosp/Cornell Med Ctr 1981; **Fac Appt:** Clin Prof Med, Cornell Univ-Weill Med Coll

Helfgott, David C MD (Inf) - **Spec Exp:** Infections in Immunocompromised Patients; **Hospital:** NY-Presby/Weill Cornell Med Ctr, NY (page 104); **Address:** The Travel Med Ctr of Manhattan, 212 E 68th St, New York, NY 10065; **Phone:** 212-879-6004; **Board Cert:** Internal Medicine 1986; Infectious Disease 1988; **Med School:** Yale Univ 1983; **Resid:** Internal Medicine, NY Hosp/Cornell Med Ctr 1986; **Fellow:** Infectious Disease, NY Hosp/Cornell Med Ctr 1988; **Fac Appt:** Asst Clin Prof Med, Cornell Univ-Weill Med Coll

Horowitz, Harold W MD (Inf) - **Spec Exp:** AIDS/HIV; Tick-borne Diseases; Clinical Trials; Fevers of Unknown Origin; **Hospital:** NYU Langone Med Ctr (page 108), Bellevue Hosp Ctr; **Address:** NYU Schl Med, Div of Infectious Dis, 550 First Ave, NBV 16 S 5, New York, NY 10016; **Phone:** 212-263-2115; **Board Cert:** Internal Medicine 1983; Infectious Disease 1988; **Med School:** NYU Sch Med 1979; **Resid:** Internal Medicine, Univ Wisconsin Hosp 1983; **Fellow:** Infectious Disease, New England Med Ctr 1986; **Fac Appt:** Prof Med, NYU Sch Med

Huprikar, Shirish S MD (Inf) - **Spec Exp:** Infections in Transplant Patients; Infections in Immunocompromised Patients; Infections in Transplant Patients w/HIV; **Hospital:** Mt Sinai Med Ctr (page 102); **Address:** Mt Sinai Med Ctr, Div Infectious Dis, 5 E 98th St Fl 12, New York, NY 10029; **Phone:** 212-241-7968; **Board Cert:** Internal Medicine 2010; Infectious Disease 2011; **Med School:** Northwestern Univ 1996; **Resid:** Internal Medicine, Mt Sinai Med Ctr 1999; **Fellow:** Infectious Disease, Mt Sinai Med Ctr 2001; **Fac Appt:** Assoc Prof Med, Mount Sinai Sch Med

Jacobs, Jonathan L MD (Inf) - **Spec Exp:** AIDS/HIV; **Hospital:** NY-Presby/Weill Cornell Med Ctr, NY (page 104); **Address:** 449 E 68th St, Ground Fl, New York, NY 10065; **Phone:** 212-734-1365; **Board Cert:** Internal Medicine 1983; Infectious Disease 1986; **Med School:** Yale Univ 1980; **Resid:** Internal Medicine, NY Hosp/Cornell Med Ctr 1983; **Fellow:** Infectious Disease, NY Hosp/Cornell Med Ctr 1986; **Fac Appt:** Assoc Clin Prof Med, Cornell Univ-Weill Med Coll

Lerner, Chester W MD (Inf) - **Spec Exp:** AIDS/HIV; Travel Medicine; Sexually Transmitted Diseases; **Hospital:** NY-Presby/Lower Manhattan Hosp (page 104); **Address:** Weill Cornell Physician Organization, 156 William St Fl 7, New York, NY 10038-2612; **Phone:** 212-312-5920; **Board Cert:** Internal Medicine 1981; Infectious Disease 1984; **Med School:** Univ Pittsburgh 1978; **Resid:** Internal Medicine, Lenox Hill Hosp 1981; **Fellow:** Infectious Disease, Lenox Hill Hosp 1983; **Fac Appt:** Asst Clin Prof Med, Cornell Univ-Weill Med Coll

Louie, Eddie MD (Inf) - **Spec Exp:** Lyme Disease; AIDS/HIV; Hospital Acquired Infections; **Hospital:** NYU Langone Med Ctr (page 108); **Address:** 5 31st Ave, Ste 7J, New York, NY 10016; **Phone:** 212-682-9202; **Board Cert:** Internal Medicine 1982; Infectious Disease 1986; **Med School:** NYU Sch Med 1979; **Resid:** Internal Medicine, Kings County Hosp 1983; **Fellow:** Infectious Disease, NYU Med Ctr 1985; **Fac Appt:** Assoc Clin Prof Med, NYU Sch Med

McMeeking, Alexander A MD (Inf) - **Spec Exp:** AIDS/HIV; Hepatitis; Lyme Disease; Travel Medicine; **Hospital:** NYU Langone Med Ctr (page 108); **Address:** Chelsea Village Medical, 155 W 19th St Fl 4th, New York, NY 10011; **Phone:** 212-929-2629; **Board Cert:** Internal Medicine 1985; Infectious Disease 1988; **Med School:** UMDNJ-NJ Med Sch, Newark 1982; **Resid:** Internal Medicine, St Luke's-Roosevelt Hosp 1985; **Fellow:** Infectious Disease, Bellvue Hosp/NYU Med Ctr 1987; **Fac Appt:** Assoc Clin Prof Med, NYU Sch Med

Mildvan, Donna MD (Inf) - **Spec Exp:** AIDS/HIV; Clinical Trials; **Hospital:** Beth Israel Med Ctr - Petrie Div (page 94); **Address:** Beth Israel Med Ctr, Div Infectious Dis, 1st Ave at 16th St, 19BH17, New York, NY 10003; **Phone:** 212-420-4005; **Board Cert:** Internal Medicine 1972; Infectious Disease 1972; **Med School:** Johns Hopkins Univ 1967; **Resid:** Internal Medicine, Mt Sinai Med Ctr 1970; **Fellow:** Infectious Disease, Mt Sinai Med Ctr 1972; **Fac Appt:** Prof Med, Albert Einstein Coll Med

Miller, Dennis K MD (Inf) - **Spec Exp:** Lyme Disease; AIDS/HIV; Travel Medicine; **Hospital:** Lenox Hill Hosp (page 106); **Address:** 4 E 76th St, New York, NY 10021-1811; **Phone:** 212-472-1237; **Board Cert:** Internal Medicine 1985; Infectious Disease 1988; **Med School:** Rush Med Coll 1982; **Resid:** Internal Medicine, Lenox Hill Hosp 1985; **Fellow:** Infectious Disease, Lenox Hill Hosp 1987

Mullen, Michael P MD (Inf) - **Spec Exp:** Osteomyelitis; AIDS/HIV; Hospital Acquired Infections; Tuberculosis; **Hospital:** Mt Sinai Med Ctr (page 102); **Address:** Mount Sinai Faculty Practice Assocs, 5 E 98th St Fl 8th, New York, NY 10029; **Phone:** 212-241-3150; **Board Cert:** Internal Medicine 1985; Infectious Disease 1986; **Med School:** Spain 1981; **Resid:** Internal Medicine, Kingsbrook Jewish Med Ctr 1984; **Fellow:** Infectious Disease, Cabrini Med Ctr 1986; **Fac Appt:** Assoc Clin Prof Med, Mount Sinai Sch Med

Murray, Henry W MD (Inf) - **Spec Exp:** Parasitic Infections; Travel Medicine; Tropical Diseases; **Hospital:** NY-Presby/Weill Cornell Med Ctr, NY (page 104); **Address:** NY Presby-Cornell Med Ctr, 525 E 68th St, Box 125, New York, NY 10065; **Phone:** 212-746-6330; **Board Cert:** Internal Medicine 1975; Infectious Disease 1978; **Med School:** Cornell Univ-Weill Med Coll 1972; **Resid:** Internal Medicine, New York Hosp 1974; Internal Medicine, Johns Hopkins Hosp 1975; **Fellow:** Infectious Disease, G Washington Univ Hosp 1978; **Fac Appt:** Prof Med, Cornell Univ-Weill Med Coll

Neibart, Eric P MD (Inf) - **Spec Exp:** Travel Medicine; AIDS/HIV; Fungal Infections; **Hospital:** Mt Sinai Med Ctr (page 102); **Address:** 1100 Park Ave, Ste 1C, New York, NY 10128-1202; **Phone:** 212-427-9550; **Board Cert:** Internal Medicine 1983; Infectious Disease 1986; **Med School:** UMDNJ-NJ Med Sch, Newark 1980; **Resid:** Internal Medicine, Mt Sinai Med Ctr 1983; **Fellow:** Infectious Disease, Mt Sinai Med Ctr 1986; **Fac Appt:** Asst Clin Prof Med, Mount Sinai Sch Med

Perlman, David MD (Inf) - **Spec Exp:** AIDS/HIV; Lyme Disease; Travel Medicine; Tuberculosis; **Hospital:** Beth Israel Med Ctr - Petrie Div (page 94), Lenox Hill Hosp (page 106); **Address:** Beth Israel Med Ctr, 120 E 16th St Fl 12, New York, NY 10003; **Phone:** 212-844-8549; **Board Cert:** Internal Medicine 1986; Infectious Disease 1988; **Med School:** Albert Einstein Coll Med 1983; **Resid:** Internal Medicine, New York Hosp/Meml-Sloan Kettering 1986; **Fellow:** Infectious Disease, Montefiore Hosp 1988; **Fac Appt:** Prof Med, Albert Einstein Coll Med

Pollock, Alan A MD (Inf) - **Spec Exp:** Lyme Disease; Viral Infections; **Hospital:** Lenox Hill Hosp (page 106); **Address:** 184 E 70th St, Ste B1, New York, NY 10021-5110; **Phone:** 212-988-2702; **Board Cert:** Internal Medicine 1975; Infectious Disease 1978; **Med School:** NY Med Coll 1972; **Resid:** Internal Medicine, Lenox Hill Hosp 1975; **Fellow:** Infectious Disease, Manhattan VA Hosp 1977; **Fac Appt:** Asst Clin Prof Med, NYU Sch Med

Polsky, Bruce W MD (Inf) - **Spec Exp:** AIDS/HIV; Viral Infections; Infections in Cancer Patients; AIDS Related Cancers; **Hospital:** St. Luke's - Roosevelt Hosp Ctr - Roosevelt Div (page 94), St. Luke's - Roosevelt Hosp Ctr - St Luke's Hosp (page 94); **Address:** University Medical Practice Associates, 425 W 59th St, Ste 8A, New York, NY 10019; **Phone:** 212-523-7335; **Board Cert:** Internal Medicine 1983; Infectious Disease 1986; **Med School:** Wayne State Univ 1980; **Resid:** Internal Medicine, Montefiore Hosp 1983; **Fellow:** Infectious Disease, Meml Sloan Kettering Cancer Ctr 1986; **Fac Appt:** Prof Med, Columbia P&S

Press, Robert A MD/PhD (Inf) - **Spec Exp:** Infections-Surgical; Hospital Acquired Infections; **Hospital:** NYU Langone Med Ctr (page 108); **Address:** 530 1st Ave, Ste 4G, New York, NY 10016-6402; **Phone:** 212-263-7229; **Board Cert:** Internal Medicine 1976; **Med School:** NYU Sch Med 1973; **Resid:** Internal Medicine, Beth Israel Hosp 1975; Internal Medicine, Bellevue Hosp 1976; **Fellow:** Infectious Disease, Montefiore Hosp Med Ctr 1978; **Fac Appt:** Clin Prof Med, NYU Sch Med

Romagnoli, Mario MD (Inf) - **Spec Exp:** AIDS/HIV; Bone/Joint Infections; **Hospital:** Lenox Hill Hosp (page 106); **Address:** 903 Park Ave, New York, NY 10075; **Phone:** 212-396-3390; **Board Cert:** Internal Medicine 1979; Infectious Disease 1982; **Med School:** Columbia P&S 1976; **Resid:** Internal Medicine, Columbia-Presby Med Ctr 1979; **Fellow:** Infectious Disease, Beth Israel Med Ctr 1981; **Fac Appt:** Assoc Prof Med, Columbia P&S

Rosenberg, Howard MD (Inf) - **Spec Exp:** Travel Medicine; **Hospital:** NY-Presby/Weill Cornell Med Ctr, NY (page 104); **Address:** 235 E 67th St, Ste 205, New York, NY 10065; **Phone:** 212-744-1170; **Board Cert:** Internal Medicine 2005; Infectious Disease 2008; **Med School:** SUNY Downstate 1992; **Resid:** Internal Medicine, NY-Presby/Weill Cornell Med Ctr 1995; Internal Medicine, Meml Sloan-Kettering Cancer Ctr 1996; **Fellow:** Infectious Disease, NY-Presby/Weill Cornell Med Ctr 1998; **Fac Appt:** Assoc Prof Med, Cornell Univ-Weill Med Coll

Scully, Brian E MD (Inf) - **Spec Exp:** Lyme Disease; Infections in Transplant Patients; Hospital Acquired Infections; Infections in Immunocompromised Patients; **Hospital:** NY-Presby/Columbia Univ Med Ctr, NY (page 104); **Address:** 161 Fort Washington Ave, Ste 3-346, New York, NY 10032; **Phone:** 212-305-8039; **Board Cert:** Internal Medicine 1975; Infectious Disease 1982; **Med School:** Ireland 1971; **Resid:** Internal Medicine, St Luke's-Roosevelt Hosp Ctr 1975; **Fellow:** Infectious Disease, Columbia Presby Med Ctr 1982

Sepkowitz, Kent A MD (Inf) - **Spec Exp:** Hospital Acquired Infections; Tuberculosis; Infections in Cancer Patients; **Hospital:** Meml Sloan-Kettering Canc Ctr (page 114), NY-Presby/Weill Cornell Med Ctr, NY (page 104); **Address:** 1275 York Ave, New York, NY 10065; **Phone:** 212-639-2441; **Board Cert:** Internal Medicine 1983; Infectious Disease 2010; **Med School:** Univ Okla Coll Med 1980; **Resid:** Internal Medicine, St Luke's-Roosevelt Hosp 1983; **Fellow:** Infectious Disease, Meml Sloan Kettering Cancer Ctr 1990; **Fac Appt:** Prof Med, Cornell Univ-Weill Med Coll

Simberkoff, Michael S MD (Inf) - **Spec Exp:** AIDS/HIV; Infections-Respiratory; Hospital Acquired Infections; Tuberculosis; **Hospital:** VA NY Harbor Hlthcare Sys-Manhattan Campus; **Address:** 423 E 23rd St, 3 West Executive Office, New York, NY 10010; **Phone:** 212-951-3417; **Board Cert:** Internal Medicine 1980; Infectious Disease 1972; **Med School:** NYU Sch Med 1962; **Resid:** Internal Medicine, Bellevue Hosp Ctr 1964; Internal Medicine, NYU Med Ctr 1967; **Fellow:** Infectious Disease, Bellevue Hosp Ctr 1969; **Fac Appt:** Prof Med, NYU Sch Med

Smith, Paul T MD (Inf) - **Spec Exp:** AIDS/HIV; Skin/Soft Tissue Infections; Infections in Transplant Patients; Travel Medicine; **Hospital:** NY-Presby/Weill Cornell Med Ctr, NY (page 104), Hosp For Special Surgery (page 113); **Address:** 943 Lexington Ave, New York, NY 10021; **Phone:** 212-396-4077; **Board Cert:** Internal Medicine 2005; Infectious Disease 2007; **Med School:** Hahnemann Univ 1992; **Resid:** Internal Medicine, NY Hosp-Cornell Med Ctr 1995; **Fellow:** Infectious Disease, Yale-New Haven Hosp 1997; **Fac Appt:** Asst Clin Prof Med, Cornell Univ-Weill Med Coll

Soave, Rosemary MD (Inf) - **Spec Exp:** Infections in Transplant Patients; Parasitic Infections; Infections in Immunocompromised Patients; AIDS/HIV; **Hospital:** NY-Presby/Weill Cornell Med Ctr, NY (page 104); **Address:** I D Assocs, 450 E 69th St, New York, NY 10021; **Phone:** 646-962-4800; **Board Cert:** Internal Medicine 1979; Infectious Disease 1984; **Med School:** Cornell Univ-Weill Med Coll 1976; **Resid:** Internal Medicine, New York Hosp 1979; Internal Medicine, Meml Sloan Kettering Cancer Ctr 1980; **Fellow:** Infectious Disease, New York Hosp/Cornell Med Ctr 1982; **Fac Appt:** Assoc Prof Med, Cornell Univ-Weill Med Coll

Wallach, Frances MD (Inf) - **Spec Exp:** AIDS/HIV; Infection Control; HIV & Blood Transfusions; **Hospital:** Mt Sinai Med Ctr (page 102); **Address:** 17 E 102nd St Fl 3rd, New York, NY 10029; **Phone:** 212-241-7968; **Board Cert:** Internal Medicine 1989; Infectious Disease 2002; **Med School:** Albany Med Coll 1985; **Resid:** Internal Medicine, Montefiore Med Ctr 1989; **Fellow:** Nuclear Medicine, Montefiore Med Ctr 1990; Infectious Disease, NY Hosp-Cornell Med Ctr 1992; **Fac Appt:** Asst Prof Med, Mount Sinai Sch Med

Yancovitz, Stanley R MD (Inf) - **Spec Exp:** Lyme Disease; Endocarditis; Bone/Joint Infections; Tuberculosis; **Hospital:** Beth Israel Med Ctr - Petrie Div (page 94); **Address:** 10 Union Sq, Ste 3F, New York, NY 10003; **Phone:** 212-420-2600; **Board Cert:** Internal Medicine 1973; Infectious Disease 1976; **Med School:** SUNY Downstate 1967; **Resid:** Internal Medicine, Metropolitan Hosp 1969; Internal Medicine, Beth Israel Med Ctr 1972; **Fellow:** Infectious Disease, Mt Sinai Hosp 1975; **Fac Appt:** Prof Med, Albert Einstein Coll Med

Internal Medicine

Aronne, Louis J MD (IM) - **Spec Exp:** Weight Management; Obesity; Diabetes; **Hospital:** NY-Presby/Weill Cornell Med Ctr, NY (page 104); **Address:** 1165 York Ave, New York, NY 10065; **Phone:** 212-583-1000; **Board Cert:** Internal Medicine 1984; **Med School:** Johns Hopkins Univ 1981; **Resid:** Internal Medicine, Bronx Muni Hosp 1984; **Fellow:** Internal Medicine, New York Hosp 1986; **Fac Appt:** Clin Prof Med, Cornell Univ-Weill Med Coll

Barley, Christopher L MD (IM) *PCP* - **Hospital:** NY-Presby/Weill Cornell Med Ctr, NY (page 104); **Address:** 110 E 55th St Fl 9, New York, NY 10022; **Phone:** 212-758-3590; **Board Cert:** Internal Medicine 2006; **Med School:** Geo Wash Univ 1993; **Resid:** Internal Medicine, New York Hosp 1996; **Fac Appt:** Asst Clin Prof Med, Cornell Univ-Weill Med Coll

Baskin, David H MD (IM) *PCP* - **Spec Exp:** Preventive Medicine; Cholesterol/Lipid Disorders; **Hospital:** St. Luke's - Roosevelt Hosp Ctr - Roosevelt Div (page 94); **Address:** 185 West End Ave, Ste 1M, New York, NY 10023-5540; **Phone:** 212-595-7701; **Board Cert:** Internal Medicine 1985; **Med School:** Boston Univ 1982; **Resid:** Internal Medicine, St Luke's-Roosevelt Hosp 1985; **Fac Appt:** Asst Clin Prof Med, Columbia P&S

Boxer, William P MD (IM) *PCP* - **Spec Exp:** Osteoporosis; **Hospital:** Lenox Hill Hosp (page 106); **Address:** Medical Associates East, 220 E 69th St, New York, NY 10021; **Phone:** 212-570-1800; **Board Cert:** Internal Medicine 2010; **Med School:** SUNY Upstate Med Univ 1997; **Resid:** Internal Medicine, Boston Univ Med Ctr 2000

Bregman, Zachary MD (IM) *PCP* - **Spec Exp:** Pulmonary Disease; Complex Diagnosis; **Hospital:** NYU Langone Med Ctr (page 108), Beth Israel Med Ctr - Petrie Div (page 94); **Address:** 247 3rd Ave, Ste 304, New York, NY 10010; **Phone:** 212-505-6663; **Board Cert:** Internal Medicine 1986; **Med School:** Univ Pennsylvania 1981; **Resid:** Internal Medicine, Beth Israel Med Ctr 1984; **Fellow:** Pulmonary Disease, Beth Israel Med Ctr 1986; **Fac Appt:** Asst Prof Med, NYU Sch Med

Bruno, Peter J MD (IM) *PCP* - **Spec Exp:** Sports Medicine; **Hospital:** Lenox Hill Hosp (page 106), Beth Israel Med Ctr - Petrie Div (page 94); **Address:** 110 E 59th St, Ste 9A, New York, NY 10022; **Phone:** 212-583-2898; **Board Cert:** Internal Medicine 1979; **Med School:** Hahnemann Univ 1975; **Resid:** Internal Medicine, Lenox Hill Hosp 1979; **Fac Appt:** Assoc Prof Med, NYU Sch Med

Bush, Michael N MD (IM) *PCP* - **Spec Exp:** Preventive Medicine; Travel Medicine; **Hospital:** Lenox Hill Hosp (page 106), NYU Langone Med Ctr (page 108); **Address:** 115 E 57th St, Ste 630, New York, NY 10022; **Phone:** 212-583-2990; **Board Cert:** Internal Medicine 1981; **Med School:** SUNY Downstate 1978; **Resid:** Internal Medicine, Lenox Hill Hosp 1981; **Fac Appt:** Assoc Clin Prof Med, NYU Sch Med

Case, David B MD (IM) *PCP* - **Spec Exp:** Hypertension; Preventive Cardiology; **Hospital:** NY-Presby/Columbia Univ Med Ctr, NY (page 104); **Address:** New York Physicians, 635 Madison Ave Fl 7, New York, NY 10022; **Phone:** 212-857-4660; **Board Cert:** Internal Medicine 1974; **Med School:** Columbia P&S 1968; **Resid:** Internal Medicine, Johns Hopkins Hosp 1970; **Fellow:** Cardiovascular Disease, NY-Presby/Columbia Univ Med Ctr 1972; **Fac Appt:** Assoc Clin Prof Med, Cornell Univ-Weill Med Coll

Charap, Mitchell MD (IM) *PCP* - **Hospital:** NYU Langone Med Ctr (page 108); **Address:** 530 1st Ave, Ste 7B, New York, NY 10016; **Phone:** 212-263-7442; **Board Cert:** Internal Medicine 2012; **Med School:** NYU Sch Med 1977; **Resid:** Internal Medicine, NYU Med Ctr 1981; **Fac Appt:** Prof Med, NYU Sch Med

Charap, Peter MD (IM) *PCP* - **Spec Exp:** Preventive Medicine; **Hospital:** Mt Sinai Med Ctr (page 102); **Address:** 234 Central Park West, New York, NY 10024; **Phone:** 212-579-2200; **Board Cert:** Internal Medicine 1987; **Med School:** Mount Sinai Sch Med 1984; **Resid:** Internal Medicine, Mount Sinai Hosp 1987; **Fellow:** Public Health & Genl Preventive Med, Mount Sinai Hosp 1988; **Fac Appt:** Asst Clin Prof Med, Mount Sinai Sch Med

Cohen, Richard P MD (IM) *PCP* - **Spec Exp:** Complex Diagnosis; Preventive Medicine; **Hospital:** NY-Presby/Weill Cornell Med Ctr, NY (page 104); **Address:** 235 E 67th St, New York, NY 10021-6040; **Phone:** 212-734-6464; **Board Cert:** Internal Medicine 1978; **Med School:** Cornell Univ-Weill Med Coll 1975; **Resid:** Internal Medicine, New York Hosp 1978; **Fellow:** Infectious Disease, New York Hosp 1979; **Fac Appt:** Clin Prof Med, Cornell Univ-Weill Med Coll

Cohen, Robert L MD (IM) *PCP* - **Spec Exp:** Preventive Medicine; **Hospital:** NYU Langone Med Ctr (page 108); **Address:** 314 W 14th St, FL 5, New York, NY 10014-5002; **Phone:** 212-620-0144; **Board Cert:** Internal Medicine 1978; **Med School:** Rush Med Coll 1975; **Resid:** Internal Medicine, Cook County Hosp 1978; **Fac Appt:** Asst Clin Prof Med, NYU Sch Med

Cohn, Symra A MD (IM) *PCP* - **Spec Exp:** Women's Health; **Hospital:** NY-Presby/Weill Cornell Med Ctr, NY (page 104); **Address:** 3 E 71st St Fl 1, New York, NY 10021; **Phone:** 212-288-1302; **Board Cert:** Internal Medicine 2005; **Med School:** NY Med Coll 1991; **Resid:** Internal Medicine, NY-Presby/Weill Cornell Med Ctr 1994; **Fac Appt:** Asst Clin Prof Med, Cornell Univ-Weill Med Coll

Constantiner, Arturo MD (IM) *PCP* - **Spec Exp:** Hypertension; Kidney Disease; Kidney Stones; Dialysis Care; **Hospital:** NY-Presby/Lower Manhattan Hosp (page 104); **Address:** 19 Beekman St, Fl 6, New York, NY 10038-1522; **Phone:** 212-349-8455; **Board Cert:** Internal Medicine 1979; Nephrology 2006; **Med School:** Mexico 1975; **Resid:** Internal Medicine, Elmhurst Hosp 1979; **Fellow:** Nephrology, Mt Sinai Hosp 1981; **Fac Appt:** Asst Clin Prof Med, NYU Sch Med

Cunningham-Rundles, Ward MD (IM) *PCP* - **Spec Exp:** Allergy & Immunology; **Hospital:** NY-Presby/Weill Cornell Med Ctr, NY (page 104), Mt Sinai Med Ctr (page 102); **Address:** 240 E 68th St, New York, NY 10065-6001; **Phone:** 212-737-8973; **Board Cert:** Internal Medicine 1976; **Med School:** NYU Sch Med 1971; **Resid:** Internal Medicine, Bellevue Hosp 1973; **Fellow:** Immunology, Meml Sloan-Kettering Cancer Ctr 1975; Medical Oncology, Meml Sloan-Kettering Cancer Ctr 1976; **Fac Appt:** Asst Clin Prof Med, Cornell Univ-Weill Med Coll

Dhalla, Satish MD (IM) *PCP* - **Spec Exp:** Hypertension; Cholesterol/Lipid Disorders; Diabetes; Travel Medicine; **Hospital:** NYU Langone Med Ctr (page 108); **Address:** NYU Langone at Trinity Ctr, 111 Broadway Fl 2, New York, NY 10006; **Phone:** 212-263-9700; **Board Cert:** Internal Medicine 1976; **Med School:** India 1972; **Resid:** Internal Medicine, Beekman Downtown Hosp 1976; **Fac Appt:** Assoc Clin Prof Med, NYU Sch Med

Dolinsky, Jason H MD (IM) *PCP* - **Spec Exp:** Preventive Medicine; **Hospital:** Mt Sinai Med Ctr (page 102), Beth Israel Med Ctr - Petrie Div (page 94); **Address:** 899 Lexington Ave, New York, NY 10065; **Phone:** 212-737-1102; **Board Cert:** Internal Medicine 2007; **Med School:** NYU Sch Med 1994; **Resid:** Internal Medicine, Hosp Univ Penn 1997

Ehrlich, Martin Harvey MD (IM) *PCP* - **Spec Exp:** Complementary Medicine; Preventive Medicine; Acupuncture; **Hospital:** Beth Israel Med Ctr - Petrie Div (page 94); **Address:** Center for Health & Healing, 245 Fifth Ave Fl 2, New York, NY 10016; **Phone:** 646-935-2265; **Board Cert:** Internal Medicine 1988; **Med School:** Columbia P&S 1985; **Resid:** Internal Medicine, Harlem Hosp 1989; **Fac Appt:** Asst Prof Med, Albert Einstein Coll Med

Etingin, Orli MD (IM) *PCP* - **Spec Exp:** Preventive Medicine; Bleeding/Coagulation Disorders; Women's Health; **Hospital:** NY-Presby/Weill Cornell Med Ctr, NY (page 104); **Address:** 425 E 61st St, Fl 11, New York, NY 10065; **Phone:** 212-821-0926; **Board Cert:** Internal Medicine 1984; Hematology 1988; **Med School:** Albert Einstein Coll Med 1980; **Resid:** Internal Medicine, NY Hosp 1983; **Fellow:** Hematology & Oncology, NY Hosp 1986; **Fac Appt:** Clin Prof Med, Cornell Univ-Weill Med Coll

Fafalak, Robert G MD (IM) *PCP* - **Spec Exp:** Rheumatology; **Hospital:** NYU Langone Med Ctr (page 108); **Address:** 36 W 9th St, Ste 1A, New York, NY 10011; **Phone:** 212-933-0072; **Board Cert:** Internal Medicine 2008; **Med School:** NY Med Coll 1987; **Resid:** Internal Medicine, New York Hosp 1990; **Fellow:** Rheumatology, Hosp for Special Surgery 1992

Federman, Alex D MD (IM) *PCP* - **Spec Exp:** Preventive Medicine; Hypertension; **Hospital:** Mt Sinai Med Ctr (page 102); **Address:** Internal Medicine Assocs, 17 E 102 St Fl 7, New York, NY 10029; **Phone:** 212-659-8551; **Board Cert:** Internal Medicine 2009; **Med School:** SUNY Downstate 1996; **Resid:** Internal Medicine, Montefiore Med Ctr 1999; **Fac Appt:** Assoc Prof Med, Mount Sinai Sch Med

Feltheimer, Seth D MD (IM) *PCP* - **Spec Exp:** Preventive Medicine; Perioperative Medical Care; **Hospital:** NY-Presby/Columbia Univ Med Ctr, NY (page 104); **Address:** 161 Ft Washington Ave, Ste 336, New York, NY 10032; **Phone:** 212-305-8669; **Board Cert:** Internal Medicine 1984; **Med School:** Spain 1981; **Resid:** Internal Medicine, Interfaith Med Ctr 1984; **Fellow:** Internal Medicine, Columbia-Presby Med Ctr 1985; **Fac Appt:** Assoc Clin Prof Med, Columbia P&S

Feuer, Martin M MD (IM) *PCP* - **Spec Exp:** Bronchitis; Asthma; Emphysema; Chronic Obstructive Lung Disease (COPD); **Hospital:** Beth Israel Med Ctr - Petrie Div (page 94), Mt Sinai Med Ctr (page 102); **Address:** 899 Lexington Ave, New York, NY 10065; **Phone:** 212-744-5433; **Board Cert:** Internal Medicine 1966; Pulmonary Disease 1972; **Med School:** NYU Sch Med 1959; **Resid:** Internal Medicine, Mount Sinai Hosp 1963; **Fellow:** Pulmonary Disease, Montefiore Med Ctr 1965; **Fac Appt:** Asst Prof Med, Albert Einstein Coll Med

Fiedler, Robert P MD (IM) *PCP* - **Spec Exp:** Thyroid Disorders; Diabetes; **Hospital:** Mt Sinai Med Ctr (page 102); **Address:** 1175 Park Ave, New York, NY 10128-1211; **Phone:** 212-289-6500 x114; **Board Cert:** Internal Medicine 1970; Endocrinology, Diabetes & Metabolism 1972; **Med School:** Albert Einstein Coll Med 1964; **Resid:** Internal Medicine, DC Gen Hosp 1966; Internal Medicine, VA Med Ctr 1967; **Fellow:** Endocrinology, Mount Sinai Med Ctr 1969; **Fac Appt:** Assoc Clin Prof Med, Mount Sinai Sch Med

Fisher, Laura Lani MD (IM) *PCP* - **Spec Exp:** Preventive Medicine; Lyme Disease; Women's Health; **Hospital:** NY-Presby/Weill Cornell Med Ctr, NY (page 104); **Address:** 1385 York Ave, New York, NY 10021; **Phone:** 212-717-5920; **Board Cert:** Internal Medicine 1987; **Med School:** Brown Univ 1984; **Resid:** Internal Medicine, NY Hosp-Cornell Med Ctr 1987; **Fellow:** Infectious Disease, Mass Genl Hosp 1989; **Fac Appt:** Asst Clin Prof Med, Cornell Univ-Weill Med Coll

Fried, Richard P MD (IM) *PCP* - **Spec Exp:** Lyme Disease; Fevers of Unknown Origin; AIDS/HIV; **Hospital:** St. Luke's - Roosevelt Hosp Ctr - Roosevelt Div (page 94); **Address:** 15 W 72nd St, Ste 1N, New York, NY 10023; **Phone:** 212-580-4840; **Board Cert:** Internal Medicine 1972; Infectious Disease 1974; **Med School:** Columbia P&S 1968; **Resid:** Internal Medicine, St Luke's Hosp 1972; **Fellow:** Infectious Disease, Stanford Univ Med Ctr 1974; **Fac Appt:** Assoc Clin Prof Med, Columbia P&S

Friedman, Jeffrey P MD (IM) *PCP* - **Spec Exp:** Preventive Medicine; Travel Medicine; **Hospital:** NYU Langone Med Ctr (page 108); **Address:** 317 E 34th St, Fl 10, New York, NY 10016; **Phone:** 212-726-7440; **Board Cert:** Internal Medicine 1986; **Med School:** NYU Sch Med 1983; **Resid:** Internal Medicine, Bellevue Hosp 1987; **Fac Appt:** Assoc Clin Prof Med, NYU Sch Med

Galland, Leo MD (IM) - **Spec Exp:** Nutrition; Chronic Illness; Complementary Medicine; **Address:** Foundation for Integrated Medicine, 20 Fifth Ave, Ste 1E, New York, NY 10011; **Phone:** 212-989-6733; **Board Cert:** Internal Medicine 1972; **Med School:** NYU Sch Med 1968; **Resid:** Internal Medicine, Bellevue Hosp 1972; **Fellow:** Behavioral Medicine, Univ Conn Hlth Ctr 1981

Gelbard, Sandra N MD (IM) *PCP* - **Spec Exp:** Preventive Medicine; **Hospital:** Lenox Hill Hosp (page 106); **Address:** 993 Park Ave, New York, NY 10028; **Phone:** 212-988-5303; **Board Cert:** Internal Medicine 2003; **Med School:** SUNY Stony Brook 1999; **Resid:** Internal Medicine, NYU Med Ctr 2003

Golden, Flavia A MD (IM) *PCP* - **Spec Exp:** Women's Health; **Hospital:** NY-Presby/Weill Cornell Med Ctr, NY (page 104); **Address:** 310 E 72nd St, New York, NY 10021; **Phone:** 212-396-3016; **Board Cert:** Internal Medicine 2003; **Med School:** NYU Sch Med 1990; **Resid:** Internal Medicine, NY-Presby/Weill Cornell Med Ctr 1993; **Fac Appt:** Asst Prof Med, Cornell Univ-Weill Med Coll

Goldin, Daniel MD (IM) *PCP* - **Hospital:** NY-Presby/Weill Cornell Med Ctr, NY (page 104); **Address:** 646 Park Ave, New York, NY 10065; **Phone:** 212-717-4884; **Board Cert:** Internal Medicine 2004; **Med School:** Cornell Univ-Weill Med Coll 2001; **Resid:** Internal Medicine, NY-Presby/Weill Cornell Med Ctr 2004; **Fac Appt:** Asst Clin Prof Psyc, Cornell Univ-Weill Med Coll

Goldstein, Paul H MD (IM) *PCP* - **Spec Exp:** Preventive Medicine; **Hospital:** NYU Langone Med Ctr (page 108); **Address:** 80 5th Ave, Ste 1601, New York, NY 10011-8002; **Phone:** 212-645-8500; **Board Cert:** Internal Medicine 1985; **Med School:** NY Med Coll 1982; **Resid:** Internal Medicine, St Vincent's Hosp 1985

Greaney, Edward J MD (IM) *PCP* - **Spec Exp:** Preventive Medicine; Nutrition; **Hospital:** NYU Langone Med Ctr (page 108); **Address:** 317 E 34th St, Fl 4, New York, NY 10016; **Phone:** 212-726-7488; **Board Cert:** Internal Medicine 2010; **Med School:** NYU Sch Med 1995; **Resid:** Internal Medicine, NYU Med Ctr-Bellevue Hosp 1999; **Fac Appt:** Asst Clin Prof Med, NYU Sch Med

Haber, Stuart W MD (IM) *PCP* - **Spec Exp:** AIDS/HIV; Travel Medicine; Infectious Disease; **Hospital:** St. Luke's - Roosevelt Hosp Ctr - Roosevelt Div (page 94); **Address:** 12-A Sheridan Square, New York, NY 10014; **Phone:** 212-929-2370; **Board Cert:** Internal Medicine 1986; **Med School:** NYU Sch Med 1983; **Resid:** Internal Medicine, Emory Univ Hosp 1986; **Fellow:** Infectious Disease, Emory Univ Hosp 1989

Hart, Catherine C MD (IM) *PCP* - **Spec Exp:** Infectious Disease; **Hospital:** NY-Presby/Weill Cornell Med Ctr, NY (page 104); **Address:** 310 E 72nd St, Fl 2, New York, NY 10021; **Phone:** 212-396-3272; **Board Cert:** Internal Medicine 1984; Infectious Disease 1986; **Med School:** Univ Pennsylvania 1980; **Resid:** Internal Medicine, New York Hosp 1983; **Fellow:** Infectious Disease, New York Hosp 1985; **Fac Appt:** Asst Clin Prof Med, Cornell Univ-Weill Med Coll

Hauptman, Allen S MD (IM) *PCP* - **Spec Exp:** Preventive Medicine; **Hospital:** NYU Langone Med Ctr (page 108); **Address:** 317 E 34th St Fl 7, New York, NY 10016-4974; **Phone:** 212-726-7494; **Board Cert:** Internal Medicine 1981; **Med School:** NYU Sch Med 1978; **Resid:** Internal Medicine, Bellevue Hosp 1981; **Fac Appt:** Asst Clin Prof Med, NYU Sch Med

Hoffman, Eileen M MD (IM) - **Spec Exp:** Women's Health; **Hospital:** NYU Langone Med Ctr (page 108); **Address:** 35 E 35 St, Ste 1J, New York, NY 10016; **Phone:** 646-424-1530; **Board Cert:** Internal Medicine 1982; **Med School:** SUNY Stony Brook 1979; **Resid:** Internal Medicine, Bellevue Hosp Ctr 1982; **Fellow:** Immunology, Rockefeller Univ 1983; **Fac Appt:** Asst Clin Prof Med, NYU Sch Med

Horbar, Gary M MD (IM) *PCP* - **Spec Exp:** Preventive Medicine; **Hospital:** Lenox Hill Hosp (page 106); **Address:** 6 E 85th St, New York, NY 10028; **Phone:** 212-570-9119; **Board Cert:** Internal Medicine 1979; **Med School:** NY Med Coll 1976; **Resid:** Internal Medicine, Lenox Hill Hosp 1980; **Fac Appt:** Asst Clin Prof Med, NYU Sch Med

Horovitz, Len H MD (IM) *PCP* - **Spec Exp:** Bronchoscopy; Asthma; Emphysema; **Hospital:** Lenox Hill Hosp (page 106), Lenox Hill Hosp (Manh Eye, Ear & Throat Hosp) (page 106); **Address:** 47 E 77th St, Ste 201, New York, NY 10075; **Phone:** 212-744-3001; **Board Cert:** Internal Medicine 1980; Pulmonary Disease 1984; **Med School:** NYU Sch Med 1976; **Resid:** Internal Medicine, Lenox Hill Hosp 1980; **Fellow:** Pulmonary Disease, Lenox Hill Hosp 1982

Kaminsky, Donald L MD (IM) - **Spec Exp:** AIDS/HIV; Tropical Diseases; Travel Medicine; **Hospital:** Beth Israel Med Ctr - Petrie Div (page 94); **Address:** Gramercy Park Physicians, 10 Union Square East, Ste 5M-1, New York, NY 10003-3314; **Phone:** 212-253-6800; **Board Cert:** Internal Medicine 1982; **Med School:** Geo Wash Univ 1979; **Resid:** Internal Medicine, Beth Israel Hosp 1982; **Fellow:** Infectious Disease, Beth Israel Hosp 1984

Kennedy, James T MD (IM) *PCP* - **Spec Exp:** Preventive Medicine; **Hospital:** NYU Langone Med Ctr (page 108); **Address:** 650 1st Ave Fl 3, New York, NY 10016; **Phone:** 212-689-7768; **Board Cert:** Internal Medicine 1978; **Med School:** NYU Sch Med 1972; **Resid:** Internal Medicine, Bellevue Hosp 1977; **Fac Appt:** Clin Prof Med, NYU Sch Med

Kennish, Arthur J MD (IM) - **Spec Exp:** Mitral Valve Disease; Coronary Artery Disease; Cardiovascular Disease; Preventive Cardiology; **Hospital:** Mt Sinai Med Ctr (page 102); **Address:** 108 E 96th St, New York, NY 10128-6217; **Phone:** 212-410-6610; **Board Cert:** Internal Medicine 1980; Cardiovascular Disease 1983; **Med School:** Albert Einstein Coll Med 1977; **Resid:** Internal Medicine, Mt Sinai Hosp 1980; **Fellow:** Cardiovascular Disease, Mt Sinai Hosp 1982; **Fac Appt:** Asst Clin Prof Med, Mount Sinai Sch Med

Kent, Jennifer MD (IM) *PCP* - **Hospital:** Mt Sinai Med Ctr (page 102); **Address:** Mt Sinai Med Ctr, 10 E 102 St Fl 6, New York, NY 10029; **Phone:** 212-241-6585; **Board Cert:** Internal Medicine 2003; **Med School:** Israel 2000; **Resid:** Internal Medicine, Mt Sinai Med Ctr 2003; **Fac Appt:** Asst Prof Med, Mount Sinai Sch Med

Korenstein, Deborah R MD (IM) *PCP* - **Spec Exp:** Women's Health; Eating Disorders; **Hospital:** Mt Sinai Med Ctr (page 102); **Address:** 17 E 102 St Fl 7, New York, NY 10029; **Phone:** 212-659-8551; **Board Cert:** Internal Medicine 2006; **Med School:** Columbia P&S 1993; **Resid:** Internal Medicine, Beth Israel Deaconess Med Ctr 1996

Lamm, Steven MD (IM) *PCP* - **Spec Exp:** Obesity; Sexual Dysfunction; Preventive Medicine; **Hospital:** NYU Langone Med Ctr (page 108), Lenox Hill Hosp (page 106); **Address:** 12 E 86th St, New York, NY 10028-0506; **Phone:** 212-988-1146; **Board Cert:** Internal Medicine 1977; **Med School:** NYU Sch Med 1974; **Resid:** Internal Medicine, NYU Med Ctr 1979; **Fellow:** Rheumatology, NYU Med Ctr 1978; **Fac Appt:** Asst Clin Prof Med, NYU Sch Med

Lee, Roberta A MD (IM) - **Spec Exp:** Complementary Medicine; Acupuncture; Preventive Medicine; **Hospital:** Beth Israel Med Ctr - Petrie Div (page 94); **Address:** Center for Health & Healing, 245 Fifth Ave Fl 2, New York, NY 10016; **Phone:** 646-935-2265; **Board Cert:** Internal Medicine 2012; **Med School:** Geo Wash Univ 1985; **Resid:** Internal Medicine, Washington Hosp Ctr 1988; **Fellow:** Complementary Medicine, Univ Arizona Med Ctr 1999

Legato, Marianne J MD (IM) *PCP* - **Spec Exp:** Cardiovascular Disease; Gender Specific Medicine; **Hospital:** NY-Presby/Columbia Univ Med Ctr, NY (page 104), Lenox Hill Hosp (page 106); **Address:** 903 Park Ave, Ste 2A, New York, NY 10075; **Phone:** 212-737-5663; **Board Cert:** Internal Medicine 2003; **Med School:** NYU Sch Med 1962; **Resid:** Internal Medicine, NY-Presby/Columbia Univ Med Ctr 1965; **Fellow:** Cardiovascular Disease, NY-Presby/Columbia Univ Med Ctr 1968; **Fac Appt:** Prof Emeritus Med, NYU Sch Med

Lewin, Margaret MD (IM) *PCP* - **Spec Exp:** Preventive Medicine; Women's Health; Travel Medicine; **Hospital:** NY-Presby/Weill Cornell Med Ctr, NY (page 104), Hosp For Special Surgery (page 113); **Address:** 635 Madison Ave, Fl 8, New York, NY 10022; **Phone:** 212-857-4505; **Board Cert:** Internal Medicine 1980; Hematology 1982; Medical Oncology 1983; **Med School:** Case West Res Univ 1977; **Resid:** Internal Medicine, NY Hosp/Cornell Med Ctr 1980; **Fellow:** Hematology & Oncology, NY Hosp/Cornell Med Ctr 1983; **Fac Appt:** Assoc Clin Prof Med, Cornell Univ-Weill Med Coll

Lewin, Neal A MD (IM) *PCP* - **Spec Exp:** Preventive Medicine; Headache; Migraine; Complex Diagnosis; **Hospital:** NYU Langone Med Ctr (page 108); **Address:** 120 E 36th St, Ste 1B, New York, NY 10016-3426; **Phone:** 212-889-2813; **Board Cert:** Internal Medicine 1977; Emergency Medicine 2012; **Med School:** SUNY Downstate 1974; **Resid:** Internal Medicine, NYU-Bellevue Hosp 1977; **Fac Appt:** Prof Med, NYU Sch Med

Lewin, Sharon MD (IM) *PCP* - **Spec Exp:** AIDS/HIV; Travel Medicine; Women's Health; Fevers of Unknown Origin; **Hospital:** St. Luke's - Roosevelt Hosp Ctr - Roosevelt Div (page 94); **Address:** 139 W 82nd St, New York, NY 10024-5544; **Phone:** 212-496-7200; **Board Cert:** Internal Medicine 1978; Infectious Disease 1980; **Med School:** Univ Toronto 1975; **Resid:** Internal Medicine, Wadsworth VA Hosp 1978; **Fellow:** Infectious Disease, Bellevue Hosp/NYU Med Ctr 1980; **Fac Appt:** Asst Clin Prof Med, Columbia P&S

Liguori, Michael MD (IM) *PCP* - **Spec Exp:** Geriatric Rehabilitation; AIDS/HIV; Geriatric Care; **Hospital:** NYU Langone Med Ctr (page 108); **Address:** 80 5th Ave, Ste 1601, New York, NY 10011-8002; **Phone:** 212-645-8500; **Board Cert:** Internal Medicine 1985; **Med School:** Mount Sinai Sch Med 1981; **Resid:** Internal Medicine, St Vincent's Hosp 1984

Lipton, Mark S MD (IM) *PCP* - **Spec Exp:** Preventive Cardiology; Coronary Artery Disease; Non-Invasive Cardiology; Cholesterol/Lipid Disorders; **Hospital:** NYU Langone Med Ctr (page 108); **Address:** 635 Madison Ave, Fl 3, New York, NY 10022-1009; **Phone:** 212-570-2077; **Board Cert:** Internal Medicine 1981; Cardiovascular Disease 1985; **Med School:** NYU Sch Med 1978; **Resid:** Internal Medicine, Bellevue Hosp 1981; **Fellow:** Cardiovascular Disease, NYU Med Ctr 1985; **Fac Appt:** Assoc Clin Prof Med, NYU Sch Med

Liu, George C K MD (IM) *PCP* - **Spec Exp:** Endocrinology; Chinese Community Health; Diabetes; **Hospital:** NY-Presby/Weill Cornell Med Ctr, NY (page 104), NYU Langone Med Ctr (page 108); **Address:** 185 Canal St Fl 6, New York, NY 10013-4513; **Phone:** 212-343-7323; **Board Cert:** Internal Medicine 1983; **Med School:** Cornell Univ-Weill Med Coll 1978; **Resid:** Internal Medicine, NYU Med Ctr-Manhattan VA Hosp 1981; **Fellow:** Endocrinology, Stanford Univ Med Ctr 1983; **Fac Appt:** Asst Clin Prof Med, NYU Sch Med

Lodge Jr, Henry S MD (IM) *PCP* - **Spec Exp:** Preventive Medicine; **Hospital:** NY-Presby/Columbia Univ Med Ctr, NY (page 104); **Address:** New York Physicians, 635 Madison Ave Fl 8, New York, NY 10022-1009; **Phone:** 212-857-4555; **Board Cert:** Internal Medicine 1988; **Med School:** Columbia P&S 1985; **Resid:** Internal Medicine, NY-Presby/Columbia Univ Med Ctr 1988; **Fac Appt:** Assoc Clin Prof Med, Columbia P&S

Logan, Bruce D MD (IM) *PCP* - **Spec Exp:** Preventive Medicine; Hypertension; Diabetes; Cholesterol/Lipid Disorders; **Hospital:** NY-Presby/Lower Manhattan Hosp (page 104), NY-Presby/Weill Cornell Med Ctr, NY (page 104); **Address:** 170 William St Fl 1st, Wellness Center, New York, NY 10038; **Phone:** 212-608-6634; **Board Cert:** Internal Medicine 1978; **Med School:** Columbia P&S 1972; **Resid:** Internal Medicine, Harlem Hosp Ctr 1978; **Fac Appt:** Assoc Clin Prof Med, Cornell Univ-Weill Med Coll

Mann, Samuel J MD (IM) - **Spec Exp:** Hypertension; **Hospital:** NY-Presby/Weill Cornell Med Ctr, NY (page 104); **Address:** Hypertension Center, Weill Cornell Med Ctr, 424 E 70th St, New York, NY 10021; **Phone:** 646-962-2606; **Board Cert:** Internal Medicine 1975; **Med School:** SUNY Downstate 1972; **Resid:** Internal Medicine, St Lukes Roosevelt Hosp 1975; **Fellow:** Hypertension, Mt Sinai Hosp 1983; **Fac Appt:** Clin Prof Med, Cornell Univ-Weill Med Coll

Minkowitz, Susan MD (IM) *PCP* - **Spec Exp:** Asthma; Emphysema; Hypertension; Chronic Obstructive Lung Disease (COPD); **Hospital:** NYU Langone Med Ctr (page 108); **Address:** 355 W 52nd St Fl 7, New York, NY 10019; **Phone:** 646-778-5555; **Board Cert:** Internal Medicine 1988; **Med School:** NY Med Coll 1984; **Resid:** Internal Medicine, Metropolitan Hosp Ctr 1987; **Fellow:** Pulmonary Disease, Montefiore Med Ctr 1989; **Fac Appt:** Asst Prof Med, NY Med Coll

Morledge, Louis J MD (IM) *PCP* - **Spec Exp:** Travel Medicine; **Hospital:** Lenox Hill Hosp (page 106), Winthrop Univ Hosp (page 524); **Address:** 150 E 58th St, Fl 18, New York, NY 10155; **Phone:** 212-583-2830; **Board Cert:** Internal Medicine 2007; **Med School:** NY Med Coll 1990; **Resid:** Internal Medicine, Lenox Hill Hosp 1993; **Fellow:** Community Medicine, St Vincent Hosp 1994; **Fac Appt:** Clin Prof Med, NY Med Coll

Mulvehill, Joseph MD (IM) *PCP* - **Spec Exp:** Concierge Medicine; House Calls; **Hospital:** Lenox Hill Hosp (page 106), Mt Sinai Med Ctr (page 102); **Address:** Park Avenue Concierge Med, 10 E 78th St, Ste 1B, New York, NY 10075; **Phone:** 212-737-3136; **Board Cert:** Internal Medicine 2001; **Med School:** SUNY Stony Brook 1997; **Resid:** Internal Medicine, A Einstein Coll Med Affil Hosp 2000

Nelson, Deena J MD (IM) *PCP* - **Spec Exp:** Cancer Survivors-Late Effects of Therapy; Cancer Prevention; **Hospital:** NY-Presby/Weill Cornell Med Ctr, NY (page 104); **Address:** 635 Madison Ave Fl 8, New York, NY 10022-1009; **Phone:** 212-857-4670; **Board Cert:** Internal Medicine 1980; **Med School:** Albert Einstein Coll Med 1977; **Resid:** Internal Medicine, New York Hosp 1979; Internal Medicine, Barnes Hosp 1980; **Fac Appt:** Asst Clin Prof Med, Cornell Univ-Weill Med Coll

Olichney, John J MD (IM) *PCP* - **Hospital:** St. Luke's - Roosevelt Hosp Ctr - Roosevelt Div (page 94); **Address:** 350 W 58th St, Ground Fl, New York, NY 10019-1804; **Phone:** 212-246-9101; **Board Cert:** Internal Medicine 1974; **Med School:** Albany Med Coll 1969; **Resid:** Internal Medicine, St Luke's-Roosevelt Hosp 1972; **Fellow:** Hematology, St Luke's-Roosevelt Hosp Ctr 1973; **Fac Appt:** Clin Prof Med, Columbia P&S

Orsher, Stuart I MD (IM) *PCP* - **Spec Exp:** Preventive Medicine; **Hospital:** Lenox Hill Hosp (page 106); **Address:** 9 E 79th St, New York, NY 10075; **Phone:** 212-535-7763; **Board Cert:** Internal Medicine 1983; **Med School:** Hahnemann Univ 1975; **Resid:** Internal Medicine, Lenox Hill Hosp 1978

Pecker, Mark S MD (IM) - **Spec Exp:** Hypertension; **Hospital:** NY-Presby/Weill Cornell Med Ctr, NY (page 104); **Address:** NY-Presby/Weill Cornell Med Ctr, Hypertension Ctr, 424 E 70 St, New York, NY 10021; **Phone:** 212-746-2210; **Board Cert:** Internal Medicine 1980; **Med School:** NYU Sch Med 1977; **Resid:** Internal Medicine, Univ Tex SW Affil Hosps 1980; **Fac Appt:** Clin Prof Med, Cornell Univ-Weill Med Coll

Porder, Joseph B MD (IM) *PCP* - **Spec Exp:** Preventive Cardiology; Nutrition; Echocardiography; Preventive Medicine; **Hospital:** Mt Sinai Med Ctr (page 102); **Address:** Mt Sinai, Cardiology Dept, 1160 5th Ave, Ste 102, New York, NY 10029; **Phone:** 212-860-5500; **Board Cert:** Internal Medicine 1985; Cardiovascular Disease 1987; **Med School:** Columbia P&S 1982; **Resid:** Internal Medicine, Mount Sinai Med Ctr 1985; **Fellow:** Cardiovascular Disease, Mount Sinai Med Ctr 1987

Postley, John E MD (IM) *PCP* - **Spec Exp:** Preventive Medicine; **Hospital:** NY-Presby/Columbia Univ Med Ctr, NY (page 104); **Address:** New York Physicians, 635 Madison Ave Fl 7, New York, NY 10022; **Phone:** 212-857-4646; **Board Cert:** Internal Medicine 1973; **Med School:** Columbia P&S 1968; **Resid:** Internal Medicine, NY-Presby/Columbia Univ Med Ctr 1973; **Fac Appt:** Asst Clin Prof Med, Columbia P&S

Primas, Ronald Alan MD (IM) *PCP* - **Spec Exp:** Preventive Medicine; Travel Medicine; House Calls; Concierge Medicine; **Hospital:** Mt Sinai Med Ctr (page 102); **Address:** 952 5th Ave, Ste 1D, New York, NY 10075; **Phone:** 212-737-1212; **Board Cert:** Internal Medicine 2010; **Med School:** Amer Univ Caribbean 1986; **Resid:** Internal Medicine, Methodist Hosp 1990; **Fellow:** Preventive Medicine, UCSD Med Ctr 1991

Rosen, Nedra J MD (IM) *PCP* - **Spec Exp:** Preventive Medicine; **Hospital:** Lenox Hill Hosp (page 106), NYU Langone Med Ctr (page 108); **Address:** 115 E 57th St, Ste 630, New York, NY 10022; **Phone:** 212-583-2990; **Board Cert:** Internal Medicine 1983; **Med School:** NY Med Coll 1980; **Resid:** Internal Medicine, Lenox Hill Hosp 1983

Salsitz, Edwin A MD (IM) - **Spec Exp:** Addiction/Substance Abuse; Opiate Addiction; **Hospital:** Beth Israel Med Ctr - Petrie Div (page 94); **Address:** Beth Israel Med Ctr, 1st Ave at 16th St, Bernstein Pavilion, Rm 10B45, New York, NY 10003; **Phone:** 212-420-4400; **Board Cert:** Internal Medicine 1977; Pulmonary Disease 1980; **Med School:** SUNY Buffalo 1972; **Resid:** Obstetrics & Gynecology, Beth Israel Med Ctr 1974; Internal Medicine, Beth Israel Med Ctr 1977; **Fellow:** Pulmonary Disease, Beth Israel Med Ctr 1979; **Fac Appt:** Asst Clin Prof Med, Albert Einstein Coll Med

Schneider, Steven J MD (IM) *PCP* - **Spec Exp:** Travel Medicine; Occupational Medicine; Lyme Disease; **Hospital:** NYU Langone Med Ctr (page 108), Lenox Hill Hosp (page 106); **Address:** 115 E 57th St, Ste 630, New York, NY 10022; **Phone:** 212-583-2880; **Board Cert:** Internal Medicine 1979; **Med School:** Johns Hopkins Univ 1976; **Resid:** Internal Medicine, Presby Med Ctr 1979

Sherman, Iris K MD (IM) - **Spec Exp:** Diabetes; Hypertension; Preventive Cardiology; **Hospital:** Mt Sinai Med Ctr (page 102); **Address:** Westside Internal Medicine, 620 Columbus Ave, New York, NY 10024; **Phone:** 212-874-6600; **Board Cert:** Internal Medicine 2006; **Med School:** SUNY Downstate 1993; **Resid:** Internal Medicine, Mt Sinai Med Ctr 1996

Siegel, Marc K MD (IM) *PCP* - **Hospital:** NYU Langone Med Ctr (page 108); **Address:** 650 First Ave Fl 7, New York, NY 10016; **Phone:** 212-532-1214; **Board Cert:** Internal Medicine 2011; **Med School:** SUNY Buffalo 1985; **Resid:** Internal Medicine, NYU/Bellevue Hosp 1988; **Fac Appt:** Assoc Prof Med, NYU Sch Med

Silverman, David MD (IM) *PCP* - **Spec Exp:** Infectious Disease; Preventive Medicine; **Hospital:** NYU Langone Med Ctr (page 108); **Address:** 239 Central Park West, Ste 1A-N, New York, NY 10024; **Phone:** 212-496-1929; **Board Cert:** Internal Medicine 1979; **Med School:** Columbia P&S 1976; **Resid:** Internal Medicine, NYU/Bellevue Hosp 1980; **Fellow:** Infectious Disease, NYU/Bellevue Hosp 1981; **Fac Appt:** Assoc Clin Prof Med, NYU Sch Med

Smith, Sharon E MD (IM) *PCP* - **Spec Exp:** Preventive Medicine; **Hospital:** Lenox Hill Hosp (page 106); **Address:** Manhattan Physician Grp, 215 E 95th St, New York, NY 10128; **Phone:** 212-491-2400; **Board Cert:** Internal Medicine 2009; **Med School:** Howard Univ 1996; **Resid:** Internal Medicine, St. Vincent's Hosp 1999

Solomon, Gregory W MD (IM) *PCP* - **Spec Exp:** Preventive Medicine; Hypertension; Cholesterol/Lipid Disorders; Concierge Medicine; **Hospital:** Mt Sinai Med Ctr (page 102); **Address:** 899 Lexington Ave, New York, NY 10065-6103; **Phone:** 212-717-9205; **Board Cert:** Internal Medicine 2005; **Med School:** NYU Sch Med 1991; **Resid:** Internal Medicine, Montefiore Med Ctr 1994; **Fac Appt:** Assoc Clin Prof Med, Mount Sinai Sch Med

Spero, Marc MD (IM) - **Spec Exp:** Diving Medicine; Asthma; Emphysema; Sarcoidosis; **Hospital:** NYU Langone Med Ctr (page 108), Lenox Hill Hosp (page 106); **Address:** 110 E 55th St Fl 17, New York, NY 10022; **Phone:** 212-355-8315; **Board Cert:** Internal Medicine 1977; Pulmonary Disease 1980; **Med School:** Albert Einstein Coll Med 1973; **Resid:** Internal Medicine, St Luke's Hosp 1977; **Fellow:** Pulmonary Disease, St Luke's Hosp 1979

Steinberg, Charles R MD (IM) *PCP* - **Hospital:** NY-Presby/Weill Cornell Med Ctr, NY (page 104); **Address:** 1305 York Ave Fl 8, New York, NY 10021-4870; **Phone:** 646-962-4100; **Board Cert:** Internal Medicine 1971; Infectious Disease 1974; **Med School:** Cornell Univ-Weill Med Coll 1964; **Resid:** Internal Medicine, New York Hosp 1966; Internal Medicine, New York Hosp 1969; **Fellow:** Infectious Disease, New York Hosp 1971; **Fac Appt:** Prof Med, Cornell Univ-Weill Med Coll

Strauss, Michael L MD (IM) *PCP* - **Spec Exp:** Acupuncture; Preventive Medicine; **Hospital:** Beth Israel Med Ctr - Petrie Div (page 94), New York Eye & Ear Infirm (page 115); **Address:** 310 E 14th St, Fl 3 North, New York, NY 10003; **Phone:** 212-979-4204; **Board Cert:** Internal Medicine 1984; **Med School:** Belgium 1980; **Resid:** Internal Medicine, Cabrini Med Ctr 1983

Tay, Steven I MD (IM) *PCP* - **Spec Exp:** Geriatric Care; Preventive Medicine; **Hospital:** Beth Israel Med Ctr - Petrie Div (page 94); **Address:** Gramercy Park Physicians, 10 Union Square East, Ste 5M-1, New York, NY 10003; **Phone:** 212-253-9322; **Board Cert:** Internal Medicine 1977; Geriatric Medicine 2004; **Med School:** SUNY Downstate 1974; **Resid:** Internal Medicine, Kings Co Hosp 1977

Underberg, James MD (IM) - **Spec Exp:** Cholesterol/Lipid Disorders; Hypertension; Preventive Cardiology; **Hospital:** NYU Langone Med Ctr (page 108); **Address:** Murray Hill Medical Grp, 317 E 34th St Fl 7, New York, NY 10016-4974; **Phone:** 212-726-7430; **Board Cert:** Internal Medicine 1989; **Med School:** Univ Pennsylvania 1986; **Resid:** Internal Medicine, NYU Med Ctr/Bellevue Hosp Ctr 1989; **Fac Appt:** Asst Clin Prof Med, NYU Sch Med

Vega, Aida MD (IM) *PCP* - **Hospital:** Mt Sinai Med Ctr (page 102); **Address:** Primary Care Assocs, 17 E 102 St Fl 5-East, New York, NY 10029; **Phone:** 212-241-6585; **Board Cert:** Internal Medicine 1983; **Med School:** Boston Univ 1980; **Resid:** Internal Medicine, Univ Conn Hlth Ctr 1983

Weinstein, Jay S MD (IM) *PCP* - **Spec Exp:** Preventive Medicine; **Hospital:** Lenox Hill Hosp (page 106); **Address:** 927 Park Ave, New York, NY 10028; **Phone:** 212-584-2619; **Board Cert:** Internal Medicine 2011; **Med School:** Hahnemann Univ 1987; **Resid:** Internal Medicine, St Vincents Hosp 1991

Winchester, James F MD (IM) - **Spec Exp:** Dialysis Care; Polycystic Kidney Disease; Toxicology; Hypertension; **Hospital:** Beth Israel Med Ctr - Petrie Div (page 94); **Address:** 10 Union Square E, Ste 2F, New York, NY 10003; **Phone:** 212-420-4070; **Board Cert:** Internal Medicine 2007; **Med School:** Scotland, UK 1969; **Resid:** Internal Medicine, Royal Infirmiry 1972; **Fellow:** Nephrology, Royal Infirmiry 1974; **Fac Appt:** Clin Prof Med, Scotland, UK

Wiseman, Paul E MD (IM) *PCP* - **Spec Exp:** Preventive Medicine; **Hospital:** St. Luke's - Roosevelt Hosp Ctr - Roosevelt Div (page 94); **Address:** 101 Central Park West, New York, NY 10023-4204; **Phone:** 212-496-5800; **Board Cert:** Internal Medicine 1987; **Med School:** Albert Einstein Coll Med 1981; **Resid:** Internal Medicine, Montefiore Med Ctr 1984

Witt III, Marvin MD (IM) *PCP* - **Spec Exp:** Diabetes; Hypertension; Preventive Medicine; **Hospital:** Lenox Hill Hosp (page 106); **Address:** Manhattan's Physician Grp, 590 5th Ave, New York, NY 10036; **Phone:** 212-582-7117; **Board Cert:** Internal Medicine 1986; **Med School:** Germany 1983; **Resid:** Internal Medicine, Bridgeport Hosp 1986

Yaffe, Bruce H MD (IM) *PCP* - **Spec Exp:** Colonoscopy; Endoscopy; Preventive Medicine; **Hospital:** Lenox Hill Hosp (page 106); **Address:** Yaffe Ruden & Assocs, 201 E 65th St, New York, NY 10065; **Phone:** 212-879-4700; **Board Cert:** Internal Medicine 1979; Gastroenterology 1981; **Med School:** Geo Wash Univ 1976; **Resid:** Internal Medicine, Mount Sinai Hosp 1979; Hepatology, Mount Sinai Hosp 1980; **Fellow:** Gastroenterology, Lenox Hill Hosp 1982

Zaremski, Benjamin MD (IM) - **Spec Exp:** Cardiovascular Disease; Preventive Cardiology; Preventive Medicine; **Hospital:** Beth Israel Med Ctr - Petrie Div (page 94), Lenox Hill Hosp (page 106); **Address:** 510 E 80th St, New York, NY 10075; **Phone:** 212-517-0022; **Board Cert:** Internal Medicine 1986; **Med School:** Dominican Republic 1981; **Resid:** Internal Medicine, Metropolitan Hosp 1984; **Fellow:** Cardiovascular Disease, St Francis Hosp/Metropolitan Hosp 1986

Zeale, Peter J MD (IM) *PCP* - **Spec Exp:** Hypertension; Cholesterol/Lipid Disorders; **Hospital:** NYU Langone Med Ctr (page 108); **Address:** 275 7th Ave Fl 3, New York, NY 10011; **Phone:** 646-660-9998; **Board Cert:** Internal Medicine 1982; **Med School:** Georgetown Univ 1979; **Resid:** Internal Medicine, St Vincent's Hosp 1983

Interventional Cardiology

Attubato, Michael J MD (IC) - **Spec Exp:** Coronary Angioplasty/Stents; Peripheral Vascular Disease; Heart Valve Disease; **Hospital:** NYU Langone Med Ctr (page 108), Bellevue Hosp Ctr; **Address:** NYU Langone Medical Center, 530 First Ave, HCC Bldg - Fl 14, New York, NY 10016; **Phone:** 212-263-5656; **Board Cert:** Internal Medicine 1984; Cardiovascular Disease 1987; Interventional Cardiology 2010; **Med School:** NYU Sch Med 1981; **Resid:** Internal Medicine, NYU Med Ctr 1985; **Fellow:** Cardiovascular Disease, NYU Med Ctr 1987; **Fac Appt:** Assoc Prof Med, NYU Sch Med

Feit, Frederick MD (IC) - **Spec Exp:** Cardiac Catheterization; Angioplasty & Restenosis; **Hospital:** NYU Langone Med Ctr (page 108); **Address:** NYU Cardiac Catheterization Lab, 530 1st Ave, HTC Bldg Fl 14, New York, NY 10016; **Phone:** 212-263-5656; **Board Cert:** Internal Medicine 1976; Cardiovascular Disease 1979; Interventional Cardiology 2010; **Med School:** NYU Sch Med 1972; **Resid:** Internal Medicine, NYU Med Ctr 1976; **Fellow:** Cardiovascular Disease, NYU Med Ctr 1978; **Fac Appt:** Assoc Prof Onc, NYU Sch Med

Fox, John T MD (IC) - **Hospital:** Beth Israel Med Ctr - Petrie Div (page 94); **Address:** Beth Israel Heart Inst, First Ave at 16th St, 11 Dazian, New York, NY 10003; **Phone:** 212-420-2416; **Board Cert:** Cardiovascular Disease 2007; Interventional Cardiology 2011; **Med School:** NY Med Coll 1989; **Resid:** Internal Medicine, Beth Israel Med Ctr 1992; **Fellow:** Cardiovascular Disease, Beth Israel Med Ctr 1996; Interventional Cardiology, Beth Israel Med Ctr 1997; **Fac Appt:** Asst Prof Med, Albert Einstein Coll Med

Gray, William A MD (IC) - **Spec Exp:** Peripheral Vascular Disease; Percutaneous Valve Repair; Coronary Artery Disease; Mitral Valve Surgery; **Hospital:** NY-Presby/Columbia Univ Med Ctr, NY (page 104); **Address:** Ctr for Interventional Vascular Therapy, 161 Fort Washington Ave, Fl 6th, New York, NY 10032; **Phone:** 212-305-7060; **Board Cert:** Internal Medicine 1987; Interventional Cardiology 2011; Vascular Medicine 2004; **Med School:** Temple Univ 1984; **Resid:** Internal Medicine, Rhode Island Hosp/Brown Univ 1988; **Fellow:** Cardiovascular Disease, Brown Univ 1992; **Fac Appt:** Assoc Prof Med, Columbia P&S

Kodali, Susheel K MD (IC) - **Spec Exp:** Cardiac Catheterization; Angioplasty & Stent Placement; Heart Valve Disease; **Hospital:** NY-Presby/Columbia Univ Med Ctr, NY (page 104); **Address:** NY-Presby Interventional Cardiology, 177 Fort Washington Ave, 5C-501, New York, NY 10032; **Phone:** 212-342-0444; **Board Cert:** Interventional Cardiology 2006; Cardiovascular Disease 2005; **Med School:** UCLA-David Geffen Sch Med 1998; **Resid:** Internal Medicine, UCSF Med Ctr 2001; **Fellow:** Cardiovascular Disease, NY-Presby/Columbia Univ Med Ctr 2004; Interventional Cardiology, UCSF Med Ctr 2005; **Fac Appt:** Asst Prof Med, Columbia P&S

Leon, Martin B MD (IC) - **Hospital:** NY-Presby/Columbia Univ Med Ctr, NY (page 104); **Address:** 161 Ft Washington Ave, Irving Pavillion Fl 6 - Ste 607, New York, NY 10032; **Phone:** 212-305-7060; **Board Cert:** Internal Medicine 1979; Cardiovascular Disease 1983; **Med School:** Yale Univ 1975; **Resid:** Internal Medicine, Yale-New Haven Hosp 1978; **Fellow:** Cardiovascular Disease, Yale-New Haven Hosp 1980

Mehran, Roxana MD (IC) - **Spec Exp:** Cardiac Catheterization; Acute Coronary Syndrome; Arrhythmias; **Hospital:** Mt Sinai Med Ctr (page 102); **Address:** Cardiocascular Medicine Associates, 1190 5 Ave S, Guggenheim Pavilion, New York, NY 10029; **Phone:** 212-659-9691; **Board Cert:** Cardiovascular Disease 2011; Interventional Cardiology 2011; **Med School:** Grenada 1987; **Resid:** Internal Medicine, Univ Conn Hlth Ctr 1991; **Fellow:** Cardiovascular Disease, Mount Sinai Med Ctr 1994; Interventional Cardiology, Mount Sinai Med Ctr 1995; **Fac Appt:** Prof Med, Mount Sinai Sch Med

Moreno, Pedro R MD (IC) - **Spec Exp:** Angioplasty & Stent Placement; Cardiac Catheterization; **Hospital:** Mt Sinai Med Ctr (page 102); **Address:** Cardiovascular Medicine Associates, 1190 Fifth Ave, GP1-W, New York, NY 10029; **Phone:** 212-241-3497; **Board Cert:** Cardiovascular Disease 2011; Interventional Cardiology 2011; **Med School:** Colombia 1984; **Resid:** Internal Medicine, Universidad Javeriana Affil Hosp; Internal Medicine, Brigham & Women's Hosp 1997; **Fellow:** Cardiovascular Disease, Brigham & Women's Hosp 2000; Interventional Cardiology, Mass Genl Hosp 2001; **Fac Appt:** Prof Med, Mount Sinai Sch Med

Moses, Jeffrey W MD (IC) - **Spec Exp:** Angiography-Coronary; Angioplasty & Stent Placement; Heart Valve Disease; **Hospital:** NY-Presby/Columbia Univ Med Ctr, NY (page 104); **Address:** 161 Ft Washington Ave, Herbert Irving Pavillion Fl 6th, New York, NY 10032; **Phone:** 212-305-7060; **Board Cert:** Internal Medicine 1977; Cardiovascular Disease 1981; Interventional Cardiology 2009; **Med School:** Univ Pennsylvania 1974; **Resid:** Internal Medicine, Penn Presby Med Ctr 1977; **Fellow:** Cardiovascular Disease, Penn Presby Med Ctr 1980

Parikh, Manish A MD (IC) - **Spec Exp:** Coronary Angioplasty/Stents; **Hospital:** Lenox Hill Hosp (page 106); **Address:** 51 W 51st St, Ste 330, New York, NY 10019; **Phone:** 212-326-8532; **Board Cert:** Cardiovascular Disease 2010; Interventional Cardiology 2010; **Med School:** UMDNJ-NJ Med Sch, Newark 1990; **Resid:** Internal Medicine, New York Hosp 1993; **Fellow:** Cardiovascular Disease, New York Hosp 1997; **Fac Appt:** Asst Prof Med, Cornell Univ-Weill Med Coll

Roubin, Gary MD/PhD (IC) - **Spec Exp:** Coronary Angioplasty/Stents; Carotid Artery Stent Placement; Peripheral Vascular Disease; **Hospital:** St. Luke's - Roosevelt Hosp Ctr - St Luke's Hosp (page 94); **Address:** 425 W 59th St, Ste 94, New York, NY 10019; **Phone:** 212-523-7200; **Med School:** Australia 1975; **Resid:** Internal Medicine, Royal Prince Albert Hosp 1979; Cardiovascular Disease, Hallstrom Inst of Cardiology 1981; **Fellow:** Cardiology Research, Natl Heart Fdn 1983; Interventional Cardiology, Emory Univ 1985; **Fac Appt:** Clin Prof Med, NYU Sch Med

Sharma, Samin K MD (IC) - **Spec Exp:** Angioplasty & Stent Placement; Heart Valve Disease; **Hospital:** Mt Sinai Med Ctr (page 102); **Address:** Mount Sinai Hosp, div Cardiology, 5 E 98th St Fl 1, New York, NY 10029; **Phone:** 212-427-1540; **Board Cert:** Internal Medicine 1986; Cardiovascular Disease 1989; **Med School:** India 1978; **Resid:** Internal Medicine, SMS Hosp 1982; Internal Medicine, NYU Downtown Hosp 1986; **Fellow:** Cardiovascular Disease, City Hosp Ctr at Elmhurst 1988; Interventional Cardiology, Mt Sinai Hosp 2000; **Fac Appt:** Prof Med, Mount Sinai Sch Med

Slater, James N MD (IC) - **Spec Exp:** Coronary Angioplasty/Stents; Heart Valve Disease; **Hospital:** NYU Langone Med Ctr (page 108), St. Luke's - Roosevelt Hosp Ctr - St Luke's Hosp (page 94); **Address:** 426 W 58th St, Fl Ground, New York, NY 10019; **Phone:** 212-247-0790; **Board Cert:** Internal Medicine 1980; Cardiovascular Disease 1985; Interventional Cardiology 2010; **Med School:** Univ Rochester 1977; **Resid:** Internal Medicine, Bellevue Hosp Ctr-NYU 1981; **Fellow:** Cardiovascular Disease, Bellevue Hosp Ctr-NYU 1983; **Fac Appt:** Prof Med, NYU Sch Med

Stone, Gregg W MD (IC) - **Spec Exp:** Angioplasty & Stent Placement; Coronary Artery Disease; **Hospital:** NY-Presby/Columbia Univ Med Ctr, NY (page 104); **Address:** 161 Fort Washington Ave, Irving Pavillion Fl 6 - Ste 607, New York, NY 10032; **Phone:** 212-305-7060; **Board Cert:** Internal Medicine 1985; Cardiovascular Disease 1987; **Med School:** Johns Hopkins Univ 1982; **Resid:** Internal Medicine, NY Hosp-Cornell Medical Ctr 1985; **Fellow:** Cardiovascular Disease, Cedars-Sinai Medical Ctr 1988; Coronary Angioplasty, Mid-America Heart Inst 1989; **Fac Appt:** Prof Med, Columbia P&S

Weinberger, Judah Z MD/PhD (IC) - **Spec Exp:** Cardiac Catheterization; Peripheral Vascular Disease; Coronary Artery Disease; Heart Valve Disease; **Hospital:** NY-Presby/Columbia Univ Med Ctr, NY (page 104), NYU Langone Med Ctr (page 108); **Address:** Heart Ctr, 173 Fort Washington Ave, Ste 4-602, New York, NY 10032; **Phone:** 212-305-1581; **Board Cert:** Internal Medicine 1984; Cardiovascular Disease 1985; Interventional Cardiology 2009; **Med School:** Harvard Med Sch 1980; **Resid:** Internal Medicine, Brigham & Womens Hosp 1982; **Fellow:** Cardiovascular Disease, Brigham & Womens Hosp 1985; **Fac Appt:** Assoc Prof Med, Columbia P&S

Maternal & Fetal Medicine

Berkowitz, Richard L MD (MF) - **Spec Exp:** Fetal Therapy; Multiple Gestation; Pregnancy & Hematologic Abnormalities; **Hospital:** NY-Presby/Columbia Univ Med Ctr, NY (page 104); **Address:** 5939 Broadway, New York, NY 10032; **Phone:** 212-326-8951; **Board Cert:** Obstetrics & Gynecology 2005; Maternal & Fetal Medicine 2005; **Med School:** NYU Sch Med 1965; **Resid:** Obstetrics & Gynecology, NY Hosp-Cornell Med Ctr 1972; **Fac Appt:** Prof ObG, Columbia P&S

Bianco, Angela MD (MF) - **Spec Exp:** Pregnancy-High Risk; Fetal Diagnosis & Therapy; **Hospital:** Mt Sinai Med Ctr (page 102); **Address:** FPA/Maternal Fetal Med, 5 E 98th St, New York, NY 10029; **Phone:** 212-241-5681; **Board Cert:** Obstetrics & Gynecology 2012; Maternal & Fetal Medicine 2012; **Med School:** Penn State Coll Med 1989; **Resid:** Obstetrics & Gynecology, NYU Med Ctr 1993; **Fellow:** Maternal & Fetal Medicine, Mt Sinai Med Ctr 1995; **Fac Appt:** Assoc Prof ObG, Mount Sinai Sch Med

D'Alton, Mary E MD (MF) - **Spec Exp:** Pregnancy-High Risk; Multiple Gestation; Prenatal Diagnosis; **Hospital:** NY-Presby/Columbia Univ Med Ctr, NY (page 104); **Address:** 51 W 51st St, Ste 320, New York, NY 10019; **Phone:** 212-326-8951; **Board Cert:** Obstetrics & Gynecology 2012; Maternal & Fetal Medicine 2012; **Med School:** Ireland 1976; **Resid:** Obstetrics & Gynecology, Ottowa Genl Hosp 1982; **Fellow:** Maternal & Fetal Medicine, Tufts-New Eng Med Ctr 1984; **Fac Appt:** Clin Prof ObG, Columbia P&S

Eddleman, Keith A MD (MF) - **Spec Exp:** Obstetric Ultrasound; Pregnancy-High Risk; Fetal Therapy; Reproductive Genetics; **Hospital:** Mt Sinai Med Ctr (page 102); **Address:** 5 E 98th St, Box 1171, New York, NY 10029; **Phone:** 212-241-5681; **Board Cert:** Obstetrics & Gynecology 2012; Maternal & Fetal Medicine 2012; Clinical Genetics 2010; **Med School:** Wake Forest Univ 1985; **Resid:** Obstetrics & Gynecology, George Washington Univ Med Ctr 1989; **Fellow:** Maternal & Fetal Medicine, Mt Sinai Med Ctr 1991; Genetics, NY Presby Hosp/Weill Cornell 1996; **Fac Appt:** Prof ObG, Mount Sinai Sch Med

Genc, Mehmet R MD/PhD (MF) - **Spec Exp:** Amniocentesis; Hypertension in Pregnancy; Pregnancy-High Risk; Fetal Abnormalities; **Hospital:** NY-Presby/Weill Cornell Med Ctr, NY (page 104); **Address:** 525 E 68th St, Ste J-130, New York, NY 10065; **Phone:** 212-746-1604; **Board Cert:** Obstetrics & Gynecology 2012; Maternal & Fetal Medicine 2012; **Med School:** Turkey 1994; **Resid:** Obstetrics & Gynecology, NY-Presby/Weill Cornell Med Ctr 2000; **Fellow:** Maternal & Fetal Medicine, NY-Presby/Weill Cornell Med Ctr 2001; Maternal & Fetal Medicine, Brigham & Women's Hosp 2003; **Fac Appt:** Asst Prof ObG, Cornell Univ-Weill Med Coll

Grunebaum, Amos MD (MF) - **Spec Exp:** Pregnancy-High Risk; Amniocentesis; **Hospital:** NY-Presby/Weill Cornell Med Ctr, NY (page 104); **Address:** Dept Obstetrics & Gynecology, 525 E 68th St, Ste J-130, New York, NY 10065; **Phone:** 212-746-0714; **Board Cert:** Obstetrics & Gynecology 2012; Maternal & Fetal Medicine 2012; **Med School:** Germany 1974; **Resid:** Anesthesiology, Maimonides Med Ctr 1978; Obstetrics & Gynecology, Downstate Med Ctr 1982; **Fellow:** Maternal & Fetal Medicine, Downstate Med Ctr 1984; **Fac Appt:** Assoc Prof ObG, Columbia P&S

Hutson, J. Milton MD (MF) - **Spec Exp:** Multiple Gestation; Pregnancy After Age 35; Amniocentesis; **Hospital:** NY-Presby/Weill Cornell Med Ctr, NY (page 104); **Address:** 523 E 72nd St Fl 9, New York, NY 10021-4099; **Phone:** 212-472-5340; **Board Cert:** Obstetrics & Gynecology 1997; Maternal & Fetal Medicine 1997; **Med School:** UAB Sch Med 1975; **Resid:** Obstetrics & Gynecology, Univ Hosp 1979; **Fellow:** Maternal & Fetal Medicine, NY-Presby/Columbia Univ Med Ctr 1982; **Fac Appt:** Asst Clin Prof ObG, Cornell Univ-Weill Med Coll

Kalish, Robin MD (MF) - **Spec Exp:** Pregnancy-High Risk; **Hospital:** NY-Presby/Weill Cornell Med Ctr, NY (page 104); **Address:** NY-Presby/Weill Cornell Med Ctr, 525 E 68th St, Ste J130, New York, NY 10065; **Phone:** 212-746-3146; **Board Cert:** Obstetrics & Gynecology 2012; Maternal & Fetal Medicine 2012; **Med School:** Univ Tenn Coll Med 1996; **Resid:** Obstetrics & Gynecology, Winthrop Univ Hosp 2000; **Fellow:** Maternal & Fetal Medicine, NY-Presby/Weill Cornell Med Ctr 2003; **Fac Appt:** Asst Prof ObG, Cornell Univ-Weill Med Coll

Patrick, Sharon MD (MF) - **Spec Exp:** Pregnancy-High Risk; Premature Labor; **Hospital:** St. Luke's - Roosevelt Hosp Ctr - Roosevelt Div (page 94); **Address:** 800-A Fifth Ave, Ste 503, New York, NY 10065; **Phone:** 212-230-1785; **Board Cert:** Obstetrics & Gynecology 2012; Maternal & Fetal Medicine 2012; **Med School:** Case West Res Univ 1986; **Resid:** Obstetrics & Gynecology, NY-Presby/Columbia Univ Med Ctr 1990; **Fellow:** Maternal & Fetal Medicine, NY-Presby/Columbia Univ Med Ctr 1992

Rebarber, Andrei MD (MF) - **Spec Exp:** Pregnancy-High Risk; Ultrasound; Clotting Disorders in Pregnancy; **Hospital:** Mt Sinai Med Ctr (page 102), Valley Hosp (page 721); **Address:** 70 E 90th St, New York, NY 10128; **Phone:** 212-722-7409; **Board Cert:** Obstetrics & Gynecology 2012; Maternal & Fetal Medicine 2012; **Med School:** SUNY Upstate Med Univ 1991; **Resid:** Obstetrics & Gynecology, Beth Israel Med Ctr 1995; **Fellow:** Maternal & Fetal Medicine, Yale-New Haven Hosp 1997; **Fac Appt:** Clin Prof ObG, Mount Sinai Sch Med

Roman, Ashley S MD (MF) - **Spec Exp:** Pregnancy-High Risk; Fetal Diagnosis & Therapy; **Hospital:** NYU Langone Med Ctr (page 108); **Address:** NYU Maternal Fetal Care Ctr, 150 E 32nd St, Ste 101, New York, NY 10016; **Phone:** 212-263-7021; **Board Cert:** Obstetrics & Gynecology 2013; Maternal & Fetal Medicine 2013; **Med School:** Tulane Univ 1998; **Resid:** Obstetrics & Gynecology, UCLA Med Ctr 2002; **Fellow:** Maternal & Fetal Medicine, NYU Med Ctr 2005; **Fac Appt:** Asst Clin Prof ObG, NYU Sch Med

Rosenn, Barak MD (MF) - **Spec Exp:** Diabetes in Pregnancy; Obstetric Ultrasound; **Hospital:** St. Luke's - Roosevelt Hosp Ctr - Roosevelt Div (page 94); **Address:** St Lukes-Roosevelt Hosp, Perinatal Med, 1000 10th Ave, Ste 11A61, New York, NY 10019; **Phone:** 212-523-7579; **Board Cert:** Maternal & Fetal Medicine 2012; Obstetrics & Gynecology 2012; **Med School:** Israel 1983; **Resid:** Obstetrics & Gynecology, Hadassah Israel 1989; Obstetrics & Gynecology, Univ Cincinnati Hosp 1997; **Fellow:** Maternal & Fetal Medicine, Univ Cincinnati Hosp 2000; **Fac Appt:** Prof ObG, Columbia P&S

Saltzman, Daniel MD (MF) - **Spec Exp:** Pregnancy-High Risk; Prenatal Diagnosis; Ultrasound; Diabetes in Pregnancy; **Hospital:** Mt Sinai Med Ctr (page 102); **Address:** 70 E 90th St, New York, NY 10128; **Phone:** 212-722-7409; **Board Cert:** Obstetrics & Gynecology 2012; Maternal & Fetal Medicine 2012; **Med School:** SUNY Buffalo 1979; **Resid:** Obstetrics & Gynecology, G Washington Univ Hosp 1983; **Fellow:** Maternal & Fetal Medicine, Brigham and Women's Hosp 1985; **Fac Appt:** Clin Prof ObG, Mount Sinai Sch Med

Simpson, Lynn L MD (MF) - **Spec Exp:** Pregnancy-High Risk; Prenatal Diagnosis; Fetal Echocardiography; Multiple Gestation; **Hospital:** Morgan Stanley Children's Hosp of NY-Presby, NY (page 104), NY-Presby/Columbia Univ Med Ctr, NY (page 104); **Address:** Center for Prenatal Pediatrics, 3959 Broadway Fl 12, New York, NY 10032; **Phone:** 212-305-3151; **Board Cert:** Obstetrics & Gynecology 2012; Maternal & Fetal Medicine 2012; **Med School:** Queens Univ 1988; **Resid:** Obstetrics & Gynecology, Kingston Genl Hosp 1993; **Fellow:** Maternal & Fetal Medicine, Beth Israel Deaconess Med Ctr 1995; **Fac Appt:** Prof ObG, Columbia P&S

Stone, Joanne L MD (MF) - **Spec Exp:** Prenatal Ultrasound; Twin to Twin Transfusion Syndrome (TTTS); Diabetes in Pregnancy; Genetic Disorders; **Hospital:** Mt Sinai Med Ctr (page 102); **Address:** Mount Sinai Medical Ctr, 5 E 98th St, Box 1171, New York, NY 10029; **Phone:** 212-241-5681; **Board Cert:** Obstetrics & Gynecology 2012; Maternal & Fetal Medicine 2012; **Med School:** Columbia P&S 1987; **Resid:** Obstetrics & Gynecology, Mt Sinai Med Ctr 1991; **Fellow:** Maternal & Fetal Medicine, Mt Sinai Med Ctr 1993; **Fac Appt:** Prof ObG, Mount Sinai Sch Med

Wapner, Ronald J MD (MF) - **Spec Exp:** Perinatal Medicine; Genetic Disorders; Multiple Gestation; Vomiting-Cyclic; **Hospital:** NY-Presby/Columbia Univ Med Ctr, NY (page 104); **Address:** Div Maternal/Fetal Medicine, 51 W 51st St, Ste 320, New York, NY 10019; **Phone:** 212-326-8951; **Board Cert:** Obstetrics & Gynecology 2000; Maternal & Fetal Medicine 2000; Clinical Genetics 2010; **Med School:** Jefferson Med Coll 1972; **Resid:** Obstetrics & Gynecology, Jefferson Univ Hosp 1976; **Fellow:** Maternal & Fetal Medicine, Jefferson Med Coll 1978; **Fac Appt:** Prof ObG, Columbia P&S

Medical Oncology

Aghajanian, Carol A MD (Onc) - **Spec Exp:** Ovarian Cancer; Gynecologic Cancer; Trophoblastic Tumors; **Hospital:** Meml Sloan-Kettering Canc Ctr (page 114); **Address:** 300 E 66th St, New York, NY 10065; **Phone:** 646-888-4217; **Board Cert:** Internal Medicine 2012; Medical Oncology 2005; **Med School:** SUNY Downstate 1989; **Resid:** Internal Medicine, Mt Sinai Med Ctr 1992; **Fellow:** Medical Oncology, Meml Sloan Kettering Cancer Ctr 1995; **Fac Appt:** Prof Med, Cornell Univ-Weill Med Coll

Bajorin, Dean F MD (Onc) - **Spec Exp:** Genitourinary Cancer; Bladder Cancer; Testicular Cancer; Clinical Trials; **Hospital:** Meml Sloan-Kettering Canc Ctr (page 114); **Address:** 1275 York Avenue, New York, NY 10065; **Phone:** 646-422-4333; **Board Cert:** Internal Medicine 1981; Medical Oncology 1985; **Med School:** NY Med Coll 1978; **Resid:** Internal Medicine, Hartford Hosp 1981; **Fellow:** Medical Oncology, Meml Sloan Kettering Ctr 1985; **Fac Appt:** Prof Med, Cornell Univ-Weill Med Coll

Barbasch, Avi MD (Onc) - **Spec Exp:** Breast Cancer; Colon & Rectal Cancer; Lung Cancer; Gastrointestinal Cancer; **Hospital:** Mt Sinai Med Ctr (page 102), Lenox Hill Hosp (page 106); **Address:** 1050 Park Ave, New York, NY 10028-1031; **Phone:** 212-860-3292; **Board Cert:** Medical Oncology 2010; **Med School:** Mexico 1975; **Resid:** Internal Medicine, Elmhurst Hosp Ctr 1980; **Fellow:** Medical Oncology, Roswell Park Cancer Inst 1982; **Fac Appt:** Assoc Clin Prof Med, Mount Sinai Sch Med

Baselga, Jose T MD/PhD (Onc) - **Spec Exp:** Breast Cancer; Drug Development; **Hospital:** Meml Sloan-Kettering Canc Ctr (page 114); **Address:** MSKCC, Breast Cancer Med, 300 E 66TH St, New York, NY 10021; **Phone:** 646-497-9064; **Board Cert:** Internal Medicine 1989; Medical Oncology 2011; **Med School:** Spain 1983; **Resid:** Internal Medicine, SUNY Hlth Sci Ctr 1989; **Fellow:** Medical Oncology, Meml Sloan-Kettering Cancer Ctr 1992

Belenkov, Elliot Michael MD (Onc) - **Spec Exp:** Solid Tumors; **Hospital:** Mt Sinai Med Ctr (page 102), Lenox Hill Hosp (page 106); **Address:** 178 E 85th St, Fl 4, New York, NY 10028; **Phone:** 212-472-5500; **Board Cert:** Internal Medicine 1987; Medical Oncology 2011; **Med School:** Russia 1976; **Resid:** Psychiatry, Metro Hospital 1983; Internal Medicine, Metro Hospital 1986; **Fellow:** Hematology, Lenox Hill Hosp 1988; **Fac Appt:** Asst Clin Prof Onc, Cornell Univ-Weill Med Coll

Berman, Ellin MD (Onc) - **Spec Exp:** Leukemia; Lymphoma; **Hospital:** Meml Sloan-Kettering Canc Ctr (page 114); **Address:** 1275 York Ave, New York, NY 10065; **Phone:** 212-639-7762; **Board Cert:** Internal Medicine 1980; Medical Oncology 1985; Hematology 1984; **Med School:** Harvard Med Sch 1977; **Resid:** Internal Medicine, Boston Univ Med Ctr 1980; **Fellow:** Medical Oncology, Meml Sloan-Kettering Cancer Ctr 1983; **Fac Appt:** Prof Med, Cornell Univ-Weill Med Coll

Blum, Ronald MD (Onc) - **Spec Exp:** Melanoma; Sarcoma; Lung Cancer; Breast Cancer; **Hospital:** Beth Israel Med Ctr - Petrie Div (page 94); **Address:** 10 Union Square East, Ste 4C, New York, NY 10003-3314; **Phone:** 212-844-8282; **Board Cert:** Internal Medicine 1975; Medical Oncology 1975; **Med School:** SUNY Buffalo 1970; **Resid:** Internal Medicine, Boston City Hosp 1974; **Fellow:** Medical Oncology, Dana-Farber Cancer Inst 1975; **Fac Appt:** Prof Med, Albert Einstein Coll Med

Bosl, George J MD (Onc) - **Spec Exp:** Testicular Cancer; **Hospital:** Meml Sloan-Kettering Canc Ctr (page 114); **Address:** 1275 York Avenue, New York, NY 10065; **Phone:** 212-639-8473; **Board Cert:** Internal Medicine 1976; Medical Oncology 1979; **Med School:** Creighton Univ 1973; **Resid:** Internal Medicine, NY Hosp 1975; Internal Medicine, Meml Sloan-Kettering Cancer Ctr 1977; **Fellow:** Medical Oncology, Univ Minn Hosps 1979; **Fac Appt:** Prof Med, Cornell Univ-Weill Med Coll

Brentjens, Renier J MD (Onc) - **Spec Exp:** Leukemia; Leukemia-Chronic Lymphocytic; T cell Immune Therapy; Cancer Immune Therapy; **Hospital:** Meml Sloan-Kettering Canc Ctr (page 114); **Address:** Meml Sloan Kettering Cancer Ctr, 1275 York Ave Fl 4 - Ste 3, New York, NY 10021; **Phone:** 212-639-5279; **Board Cert:** Medical Oncology 2002; **Med School:** SUNY Buffalo 1996; **Resid:** Internal Medicine, Yale-New Haven Hosp 1999; **Fellow:** Medical Oncology, Meml Sloan Kettering Cancer Ctr 2001; **Fac Appt:** Assoc Prof Med, Cornell Univ-Weill Med Coll

Brunckhorst, Keith R MD (Onc) - **Hospital:** Lenox Hill Hosp (page 106); **Address:** 110 E 59th St, Ste 1B, New York, NY 10022-1304; **Phone:** 212-583-2858; **Board Cert:** Internal Medicine 1979; Hematology 1982; Medical Oncology 1983; **Med School:** NY Med Coll 1976; **Resid:** Internal Medicine, Stamford Hosp 1979; **Fellow:** Hematology & Oncology, Lenox Hill Hosp 1983

Chachoua, Abraham MD (Onc) - **Spec Exp:** Lung Cancer; Thoracic Cancers; Solid Tumors; **Hospital:** NYU Langone Med Ctr (page 108); **Address:** NYU Clinical Cancer Ctr, 160 E 34th St Fl 2, New York, NY 10016; **Phone:** 212-731-5388; **Med School:** Australia 1978; **Resid:** Internal Medicine, Alfred Hosp 1982; **Fellow:** Hematology & Oncology, Alfred Hosp 1985; Hematology & Oncology, NYU Med Ctr 1988; **Fac Appt:** Assoc Prof Med, NYU Sch Med

Chapman, Paul B MD (Onc) - **Spec Exp:** Melanoma; Immunotherapy; Clinical Trials; Vaccine Therapy; **Hospital:** Meml Sloan-Kettering Canc Ctr (page 114); **Address:** 300 E 66th St, New York, NY 10065; **Phone:** 646-888-4162; **Board Cert:** Internal Medicine 1984; Medical Oncology 1987; **Med School:** Cornell Univ-Weill Med Coll 1981; **Resid:** Internal Medicine, Univ Chicago Hosps 1984; **Fellow:** Medical Oncology, Meml Sloan-Kettering Cancer Ctr 1987; **Fac Appt:** Prof Med, Cornell Univ-Weill Med Coll

Cohen, Seymour M MD (Onc) - **Spec Exp:** Breast Cancer; Melanoma; Lung Cancer; Lymphoma; **Hospital:** Mt Sinai Med Ctr (page 102); **Address:** 1150 5th Ave, New York, NY 10128; **Phone:** 212-249-9141; **Board Cert:** Internal Medicine 1971; Medical Oncology 1973; **Med School:** Univ Pittsburgh 1962; **Resid:** Internal Medicine, Montefiore Med Ctr 1964; Internal Medicine, Mount Sinai Med Ctr 1965; **Fellow:** Hematology, Mount Sinai Med Ctr 1966; Hematology & Oncology, LI Jewish Hosp 1969; **Fac Appt:** Assoc Clin Prof Onc, Mount Sinai Sch Med

Coleman, Morton MD (Onc) - **Spec Exp:** Leukemia & Lymphoma; Hodgkin's Lymphoma; Multiple Myeloma; Waldenstrom's Macroglobulinemia; **Hospital:** NY-Presby/Weill Cornell Med Ctr, NY (page 104); **Address:** 407 E 70th St, Fl 3, New York, NY 10021-5302; **Phone:** 212-517-5900; **Board Cert:** Internal Medicine 1971; Hematology 1972; Medical Oncology 1973; **Med School:** Med Coll VA 1963; **Resid:** Internal Medicine, Grady Meml Hosp-Emory 1965; Internal Medicine, NY-Presby/Cornell Univ Med Ctr 1968; **Fellow:** Hematology & Oncology, NY-Presby/Cornell Univ Med Ctr 1970; **Fac Appt:** Clin Prof Hem & Onc, Cornell Univ-Weill Med Coll

Decter, Julian A MD (Onc) - **Spec Exp:** Leukemia & Lymphoma; Multiple Myeloma; Myelodysplastic Syndromes; Hodgkin's Lymphoma; **Hospital:** NY-Presby/Weill Cornell Med Ctr, NY (page 104); **Address:** NY-Presby/Weill Cornell Med Ctr, Div Hem/Onc, 407 E 70th St, New York, NY 10021; **Phone:** 212-517-5900; **Board Cert:** Internal Medicine 1972; Hematology 1974; Medical Oncology 1975; **Med School:** NYU Sch Med 1966; **Resid:** Internal Medicine, Ohio State Hosps 1968; **Fellow:** Hematology, NYU Med Ctr 1970; Medical Oncology, Natl Cancer Inst 1974; **Fac Appt:** Assoc Clin Prof Onc, Cornell Univ-Weill Med Coll

Dickler, Maura N MD (Onc) - **Spec Exp:** Breast Cancer; Clinical Trials; **Hospital:** Meml Sloan-Kettering Canc Ctr (page 114); **Address:** 300 E 66th St, New York, NY 10065; **Phone:** 646-888-5456; **Board Cert:** Medical Oncology 2008; **Med School:** Univ Chicago-Pritzker Sch Med 1991; **Resid:** Internal Medicine, Univ Chicago Hosps 1994; **Fellow:** Medical Oncology, Meml Sloan Kettering Cancer Ctr 1998; **Fac Appt:** Assoc Prof Med, Cornell Univ-Weill Med Coll

Feldman, Darren MD (Onc) - **Spec Exp:** Genitourinary Cancer; Testicular Cancer; Kidney Cancer; **Hospital:** Meml Sloan-Kettering Canc Ctr (page 114); **Address:** MSKCC, Genitourinary Oncology Svc, 1275 York Ave, New York, NY 10065; **Phone:** 646-422-4491; **Board Cert:** Medical Oncology 2008; Hematology 2009; Internal Medicine 2004; **Med School:** Univ MD Sch Med 2001; **Resid:** Internal Medicine, NYU Med Ctr 2004; **Fellow:** Hematology & Oncology, Meml Sloan-Kettering Cancer Ctr 2008

Feldman, Eric MD (Onc) - **Spec Exp:** Leukemia; Stem Cell Transplant; Bone Marrow Transplant; Hematologic Malignancies; **Hospital:** NY-Presby/Weill Cornell Med Ctr, NY (page 104); **Address:** Weill Cornell Med Ctr, Oncology HO, 520 E 70th St Fl 3, New York, NY 10021; **Phone:** 646-962-2700; **Board Cert:** Internal Medicine 1984; Medical Oncology 1987; **Med School:** NY Med Coll 1981; **Resid:** Internal Medicine, Westchester Co Med Ctr 1984; **Fellow:** Medical Oncology, Westchester Co Med Ctr 1986; Medical Oncology, Fred Hutchinson Cancer Rsch Ctr 1987; **Fac Appt:** Prof Med, Cornell Univ-Weill Med Coll

Fine, Howard A MD (Onc) - **Spec Exp:** Brain Tumors; Neuro-Oncology; **Hospital:** NYU Langone Med Ctr (page 108); **Address:** NYU Cancer Institute, 160 E 34th St, New York, NY 10016; **Phone:** 212-731-5089; **Board Cert:** Internal Medicine 1987; Medical Oncology 1989; **Med School:** Mount Sinai Sch Med 1984; **Resid:** Internal Medicine, Hosp Univ Penn 1987; **Fellow:** Medical Oncology, Dana Farber Cancer Ctr 1989; **Fac Appt:** Prof Onc, NYU Sch Med

Fine, Robert Lance MD (Onc) - **Spec Exp:** Pancreatic Cancer; Drug Development; Pituitary Tumors; Clinical Trials; **Hospital:** NY-Presby/Columbia Univ Med Ctr, NY (page 104); **Address:** 650 W 168th St Black Bldg, Fl 20 - Ste 20-05, New York, NY 10032; **Phone:** 212-305-1168; **Board Cert:** Internal Medicine 1983; Medical Oncology 1985; **Med School:** Univ Chicago-Pritzker Sch Med 1979; **Resid:** Internal Medicine, Stanford Univ Med Ctr 1982; **Fellow:** Medical Oncology, National Cancer Inst 1985; **Fac Appt:** Assoc Prof Med, Columbia P&S

Fornier, Monica N MD (Onc) - **Spec Exp:** Breast Cancer; **Hospital:** Meml Sloan-Kettering Canc Ctr (page 114); **Address:** Meml Sloan-Kettering Cancer Ctr, 300 E 66th St, New York, NY 10065; **Phone:** 646-888-5240; **Med School:** Italy 1992; **Resid:** Internal Medicine, Univ Hosp; **Fellow:** Medical Oncology, Natl Cancer Inst; Medical Oncology, Meml Sloan-Kettering Cancer Ctr 2002

Gabrilove, Janice L MD (Onc) - **Spec Exp:** Myelodysplastic Syndromes; Leukemia; Hematologic Malignancies; Myeloproliferative Disorders; **Hospital:** Mt Sinai Med Ctr (page 102); **Address:** Mount Sinai Med Ctr-Dept Hem/Onc, One Gustave L Levy Pl, Box 1079, New York, NY 10029-6574; **Phone:** 212-241-9650; **Board Cert:** Internal Medicine 1980; Medical Oncology 1983; **Med School:** Mount Sinai Sch Med 1977; **Resid:** Internal Medicine, Columbia-Presby Med Ctr 1980; **Fellow:** Hematology & Oncology, Meml Sloan-Kettering Cancer Ctr 1983; **Fac Appt:** Prof Med, Mount Sinai Sch Med

Gaynor, Mitchell MD (Onc) - **Spec Exp:** Breast Cancer; Lung Cancer; Nutrition & Cancer; Complementary Medicine; **Hospital:** NY-Presby/Weill Cornell Med Ctr, NY (page 104); **Address:** 215 E 72nd St, New York, NY 10021; **Phone:** 212-472-2828; **Board Cert:** Internal Medicine 1985; Medical Oncology 1987; Hematology 1988; **Med School:** Univ Tex SW, Dallas 1982; **Resid:** Internal Medicine, New York Hosp 1985; **Fellow:** Hematology & Oncology, New York Hosp 1988; **Fac Appt:** Asst Clin Prof Med, Cornell Univ-Weill Med Coll

Gelmann, Edward P MD (Onc) - **Spec Exp:** Prostate Cancer; Bladder Cancer; Kidney Cancer; **Hospital:** NY-Presby/Columbia Univ Med Ctr, NY (page 104); **Address:** Columbia Univ Med Ctr, Milstein Hosp Bldg 6-435, 177 Fort Washington Ave, New York, NY 10032; **Phone:** 212-305-8610; **Board Cert:** Internal Medicine 1979; Medical Oncology 1981; **Med School:** Stanford Univ 1976; **Resid:** Internal Medicine, Univ Chicago Hosps 1979; **Fellow:** Medical Oncology, National Cancer Inst 1981; **Fac Appt:** Prof Med, Columbia P&S

Goldberg, Arthur I MD (Onc) - **Spec Exp:** Breast Cancer; Prostate Cancer; Colon & Rectal Cancer; Anal Cancer; **Hospital:** Lenox Hill Hosp (page 106), Mt Sinai Med Ctr (page 102); **Address:** 121 E 79th St, New York, NY 10075; **Phone:** 212-249-0030; **Board Cert:** Internal Medicine 1974; Medical Oncology 1975; **Med School:** SUNY Hlth Sci Ctr 1969; **Resid:** Internal Medicine, New York Hosp-Cornell 1970; Internal Medicine, Bellevue Hosp 1973; **Fellow:** Cancer Immunology, Natl Cancer Inst 1972; Medical Oncology, Meml Sloan Kettering Cancer Ctr 1975

Grace, William MD (Onc) - **Spec Exp:** Breast Cancer; Liver Cancer; Pancreatic Cancer; Lung Cancer; **Hospital:** Lenox Hill Hosp (page 106); **Address:** 1384 Broadway, New York, NY 10018; **Phone:** 212-675-6826; **Board Cert:** Internal Medicine 1976; Medical Oncology 1977; **Med School:** Boston Univ 1969; **Resid:** Internal Medicine, St Vincent's Hosp & Med Ctr 1971; **Fellow:** Hematology & Oncology, Dartmouth-Hitchcock Med Ctr 1976; **Fac Appt:** Assoc Clin Prof Med, NY Med Coll

Grossbard, Michael L MD (Onc) - **Spec Exp:** Lymphoma; Gastrointestinal Cancer; Breast Cancer; **Hospital:** St. Luke's - Roosevelt Hosp Ctr - Roosevelt Div (page 94), Beth Israel Med Ctr - Petrie Div (page 94); **Address:** 1000 10th Ave, Fl 11, Ste C02, St Luke's-Roosevelt Hospital, New York, NY 10019; **Phone:** 212-523-5419; **Board Cert:** Internal Medicine 1989; Medical Oncology 2011; **Med School:** Yale Univ 1986; **Resid:** Internal Medicine, Mass Genl Hosp 1989; **Fellow:** Medical Oncology, Dana Farber Cancer Inst 1991; **Fac Appt:** Clin Prof Hem & Onc, Columbia P&S

Gulati, Subhash C MD/PhD (Onc) - **Spec Exp:** Breast Cancer; Lymphoma; Lung Cancer; **Hospital:** NY-Presby/Weill Cornell Med Ctr, NY (page 104), Montefiore New Rochelle Hosp; **Address:** 331 E 65th St, New York, NY 10065; **Phone:** 212-535-1514; **Board Cert:** Internal Medicine 1980; Medical Oncology 1983; Hematology 1986; **Med School:** Univ Miami Sch Med 1976; **Resid:** Internal Medicine, Buffalo Genl Hosp 1978; **Fellow:** Hematology & Oncology, Meml Sloan-Kettering Cancer Ctr 1980; **Fac Appt:** Clin Prof Med, Cornell Univ-Weill Med Coll

Hassoun, Hani MD (Onc) - **Spec Exp:** Hematologic Malignancies; Multiple Myeloma; Lymphoma; Stem Cell Transplant; **Hospital:** Meml Sloan-Kettering Canc Ctr (page 114); **Address:** 1275 York Ave, New York, NY 10065; **Phone:** 212-639-3228; **Board Cert:** Internal Medicine 1986; Medical Oncology 1989; **Med School:** France 1983; **Resid:** Internal Medicine, Brigham & Womens Hosp 1986; **Fellow:** Hematology & Oncology, Tufts-St Elizabeth Hosp 1989; **Fac Appt:** Assoc Prof Med, Cornell Univ-Weill Med Coll

Hershman, Dawn L MD (Onc) - **Spec Exp:** Breast Cancer; Cancer Survivors-Late Effects of Therapy; Clinical Trials; **Hospital:** NY-Presby/Columbia Univ Med Ctr, NY (page 104); **Address:** Columbia Univ Med Ctr, Hem/Onc, 161 Fort Washington Ave Fl 10, New York, NY 10032; **Phone:** 212-305-5098; **Board Cert:** Internal Medicine 2007; Medical Oncology 2011; **Med School:** Albert Einstein Coll Med 1994; **Resid:** Internal Medicine, NY-Presby/Columbia Univ Med Ctr 1998; **Fellow:** Medical Oncology, NY-Presby/Columbia Univ Med Ctr 2001; **Fac Appt:** Asst Prof Med, Columbia P&S

Hirschman, Richard J MD (Onc) - **Spec Exp:** Breast Cancer; Colon Cancer; Lung Cancer; **Hospital:** Beth Israel Med Ctr - Petrie Div (page 94); **Address:** 247 3rd Ave, Ste 401, New York, NY 10010-7455; **Phone:** 212-228-0471; **Board Cert:** Internal Medicine 1971; Hematology 1972; Medical Oncology 1973; **Med School:** Johns Hopkins Univ 1965; **Resid:** Internal Medicine, Bellevue Hosp Ctr 1967; Internal Medicine, NY-Presby/Columbia Univ Med Ctr 1970; **Fellow:** Hematology & Oncology, NY-Presby/Columbia Univ Med Ctr 1971; **Fac Appt:** Assoc Clin Prof Med, Mount Sinai Sch Med

Hirshaut, Yashar MD (Onc) - **Spec Exp:** Breast Cancer; Lung Cancer; Colon Cancer; **Hospital:** Lenox Hill Hosp (page 106), NY-Presby/Weill Cornell Med Ctr, NY (page 104); **Address:** 860 5th Ave, New York, NY 10065; **Phone:** 212-861-1799; **Board Cert:** Internal Medicine 1972; Medical Oncology 1975; **Med School:** Albert Einstein Coll Med 1963; **Resid:** Internal Medicine, Montefiore Med Ctr 1965; **Fellow:** Medical Oncology, Natl Cancer Inst 1968; Medical Oncology, Meml Sloan-Kettering Cancer Ctr 1970; **Fac Appt:** Assoc Clin Prof Med, Cornell Univ-Weill Med Coll

Holcombe, Randall F MD (Onc) - **Spec Exp:** Gastrointestinal Cancer; Liver Cancer; Clinical Trials; Pancreatic Cancer; **Hospital:** Mt Sinai Med Ctr (page 102); **Address:** The Ruttenberg Treatment Ctr, 1470 Madison Ave, New York, NY 10029; **Phone:** 212-241-6756; **Board Cert:** Internal Medicine 1986; Medical Oncology 2003; Hematology 2012; **Med School:** UMDNJ-NJ Med Sch, Newark 1983; **Resid:** Internal Medicine, Brigham & Womens Hosp 1986; **Fellow:** Hematology, Brigham & Women's Hosp 1989; Medical Oncology, Brigham & Women's Hosp 1989; **Fac Appt:** Prof Onc, Mount Sinai Sch Med

Holland, James F MD (Onc) - **Spec Exp:** Breast Cancer; Pancreatic Cancer; **Hospital:** Mt Sinai Med Ctr (page 102); **Address:** Mount Sinai Med Ctr, 1 Gustave Levy Pl, Box 1079, New York, NY 10029; **Phone:** 212-241-4495; **Board Cert:** Internal Medicine 1955; **Med School:** Columbia P&S 1947; **Resid:** Internal Medicine, Columbia-Presby Hosp 1949; Internal Medicine, Francis Delafield Hosp 1952; **Fellow:** Medical Oncology, Francis Delafield Hosp 1953; **Fac Appt:** Prof Med, Mount Sinai Sch Med

Horwitz, Steven M MD (Onc) - **Spec Exp:** Cutaneous T-cell Lymphoma; Hodgkin's Lymphoma; Lymphoma, Non-Hodgkin's; Clinical Trials; **Hospital:** Meml Sloan-Kettering Canc Ctr (page 114); **Address:** Meml Sloan-Kettering Cancer Ctr, 1275 York Ave, New York, NY 10065; **Phone:** 212-639-3045; **Board Cert:** Medical Oncology 2011; **Med School:** Case West Res Univ 1993; **Resid:** Internal Medicine, Strong Memorial Hosp 1996; **Fellow:** Medical Oncology, Stanford Univ Med Ctr 1999

Hudis, Clifford A MD (Onc) - **Spec Exp:** Breast Cancer; **Hospital:** Meml Sloan-Kettering Canc Ctr (page 114); **Address:** 300 E 66th St, BAIC Bldg, New York, NY 10065; **Phone:** 646-888-5449; **Board Cert:** Internal Medicine 1986; Medical Oncology 2011; **Med School:** Med Coll PA Hahnemann 1983; **Resid:** Internal Medicine, Hosp Univ Penn 1987; **Fellow:** Medical Oncology, Meml Sloan Kettering Cancer Ctr 1991; **Fac Appt:** Prof Med, Cornell Univ-Weill Med Coll

Ilson, David H MD/PhD (Onc) - **Spec Exp:** Esophageal Cancer; Colon & Rectal Cancer; Mesothelioma; Unknown Primary Cancer; **Hospital:** Meml Sloan-Kettering Canc Ctr (page 114); **Address:** 300 E 66th St, New York, NY 10065; **Phone:** 646-888-4183; **Board Cert:** Internal Medicine 1989; Medical Oncology 2012; **Med School:** NYU Sch Med 1986; **Resid:** Internal Medicine, Bellevue-NYU Sch Med 1989; **Fellow:** Medical Oncology, Meml Sloan Kettering Hosp 1992; **Fac Appt:** Assoc Prof Med, Cornell Univ-Weill Med Coll

Jagannath, Sundar MD (Onc) - **Spec Exp:** Multiple Myeloma; **Hospital:** Mt Sinai Med Ctr (page 102); **Address:** The Ruttenberg Treatment Ctr, 1470 Madison Ave, New York, NY 10029; **Phone:** 212-241-6756; **Board Cert:** Internal Medicine 1980; Medical Oncology 1985; **Med School:** India 1976; **Resid:** Internal Medicine, Bronx Lebanon Hosp 1979; Internal Medicine, Harper-Grace Hosp 1980; **Fellow:** Medical Oncology, Univ Tex-MD Anderson Cancer Ctr 1982; **Fac Appt:** Prof Onc, Mount Sinai Sch Med

Jakubowski, Ann MD (Onc) - **Spec Exp:** Leukemia; Bone Marrow Transplant; **Hospital:** Meml Sloan-Kettering Canc Ctr (page 114); **Address:** 1275 York Ave, New York, NY 10065; **Phone:** 212-639-5013; **Board Cert:** Internal Medicine 1984; Medical Oncology 1987; Hematology 1986; **Med School:** Univ Conn 1981; **Resid:** Internal Medicine, Mt Sinai Hosp 1984; **Fellow:** Hematology, Montefiore Hosp 1985; Medical Oncology, Meml Sloan-Kettering Cancer Ctr 1988

Jarowski, Charles MD (Onc) - **Spec Exp:** Breast Cancer; Lung Cancer; Colon Cancer; **Hospital:** NY-Presby/Weill Cornell Med Ctr, NY (page 104), Hosp For Special Surgery (page 113); **Address:** 407 E 70th St Fl 4, New York, NY 10021; **Phone:** 212-794-9500; **Board Cert:** Internal Medicine 1975; Medical Oncology 1977; Hematology 1978; **Med School:** Cornell Univ-Weill Med Coll 1972; **Resid:** Internal Medicine, New York Hosp 1975; **Fellow:** Hematology & Oncology, New York Hosp 1978; **Fac Appt:** Asst Clin Prof Med, Cornell Univ-Weill Med Coll

Kelsen, David Paul MD (Onc) - **Spec Exp:** Gastrointestinal Cancer; Neuroendocrine Tumors; Unknown Primary Cancer; Merkel Cell Carcinoma; **Hospital:** Meml Sloan-Kettering Canc Ctr (page 114); **Address:** 300 E 66th St Fl 10, New York, NY 10065; **Phone:** 646-888-4179; **Board Cert:** Internal Medicine 1976; Medical Oncology 1979; **Med School:** Hahnemann Univ 1972; **Resid:** Internal Medicine, Temple Univ Hosp 1976; **Fellow:** Medical Oncology, Meml Sloan Kettering Cancer Ctr 1978; **Fac Appt:** Prof Med, Cornell Univ-Weill Med Coll

Kemeny, Nancy E MD (Onc) - **Spec Exp:** Colon Cancer; Rectal Cancer; Liver Cancer; **Hospital:** Meml Sloan-Kettering Canc Ctr (page 114); **Address:** 300 E 66th St Fl 10, New York, NY 10065; **Phone:** 646-888-4180; **Board Cert:** Internal Medicine 1974; Medical Oncology 1981; **Med School:** UMDNJ-NJ Med Sch, Newark 1971; **Resid:** Internal Medicine, St Luke's Hosp 1974; **Fellow:** Medical Oncology, Mem Sloan Kettering Cancer Ctr 1976; **Fac Appt:** Prof Med, Cornell Univ-Weill Med Coll

Klafter, Robert MD (Onc) - **Spec Exp:** Lymphoma; Leukemia; Breast Cancer; **Hospital:** Mt Sinai Med Ctr (page 102); **Address:** 12 E 86th St, New York, NY 10028; **Phone:** 212-861-6660; **Board Cert:** Hematology 2011; Medical Oncology 2011; **Med School:** NYU Sch Med 1994; **Resid:** Internal Medicine, NYU Med Ctr 1997; **Fellow:** Hematology & Oncology, Emory Univ Hosp 2001; **Fac Appt:** Asst Clin Prof Med, Mount Sinai Sch Med

Klein, Paula MD (Onc) - **Spec Exp:** Breast Cancer; **Hospital:** Beth Israel Med Ctr - Petrie Div (page 94); **Address:** BIMC, Cancer Ctr, 325 W 15th St, Ste J, New York, NY 10011; **Phone:** 212-604-6021; **Board Cert:** Internal Medicine 1989; Medical Oncology 2009; **Med School:** SUNY Downstate 1986; **Resid:** Internal Medicine, NYU-Bellevue Hosp 1989; **Fellow:** Hematology & Oncology, NYU-Bellevue Hosp 1998; **Fac Appt:** Asst Prof Med, NY Med Coll

Kozuch, Peter S MD (Onc) - **Spec Exp:** Gastrointestinal Cancer; Esophageal Cancer; Pancreatic Cancer; **Hospital:** Beth Israel Med Ctr - Petrie Div (page 94), St. Luke's - Roosevelt Hosp Ctr - St Luke's Hosp (page 94); **Address:** 10 Union Square E Fl 4 - Ste 4C, New York, NY 10003; **Phone:** 212-844-8070; **Board Cert:** Medical Oncology 2010; Hematology 2004; **Med School:** Hahnemann Univ 1994; **Resid:** Internal Medicine, Boston Med Ctr 1997; **Fellow:** Medical Oncology, UT-MD Anderson Cancer Ctr 2000; **Fac Appt:** Assoc Clin Prof Med, Albert Einstein Coll Med

Kris, Mark G MD (Onc) - **Spec Exp:** Lung Cancer; Mediastinal Tumors; Thymoma; Thoracic Cancers; **Hospital:** Meml Sloan-Kettering Canc Ctr (page 114); **Address:** 300 E 66th St, New York, NY 10065; **Phone:** 646-888-4197; **Board Cert:** Internal Medicine 1980; Medical Oncology 1983; **Med School:** Cornell Univ-Weill Med Coll 1977; **Resid:** Internal Medicine, New York Hosp 1980; **Fellow:** Medical Oncology, Meml Sloan Kettering Cancer Ctr 1983; **Fac Appt:** Prof Med, Cornell Univ-Weill Med Coll

Krug, Lee M MD (Onc) - **Spec Exp:** Small Cell Lung Cancer; Mesothelioma; Clinical Trials; **Hospital:** Meml Sloan-Kettering Canc Ctr (page 114); **Address:** Meml Sloan-Kettering Cancer Ctr, Dept Thoracic Oncology, 300 E 66th St, New York, NY 10065; **Phone:** 646-888-4201; **Board Cert:** Internal Medicine 2007; Medical Oncology 2009; **Med School:** Washington Univ, St Louis 1994; **Resid:** Internal Medicine, Johns Hopkins Hosp 1997; **Fellow:** Medical Oncology, Meml Sloan-Kettering Canc Ctr 1999

Kruger, Bernard M MD (Onc) - **Spec Exp:** Breast Cancer; **Hospital:** Lenox Hill Hosp (page 106); **Address:** 170 E 78th St, New York, NY 10075; **Phone:** 212-772-9222; **Board Cert:** Internal Medicine 1974; Medical Oncology 1979; **Med School:** Univ Colorado 1968; **Resid:** Internal Medicine, Boston City Hosp 1972; Internal Medicine, Georgetown Hosp 1974; **Fellow:** Medical Oncology, Mt Sinai Hosp 1976

Lamanna, Nicole MD (Onc) - **Spec Exp:** Leukemia-Chronic Lymphocytic; Hematologic Malignancies; Leukemia; **Hospital:** NY-Presby/Columbia Univ Med Ctr, NY (page 104); **Address:** 161 Fort Washington Ave, Herbert Irving Pavilion, Garden Level, New York, NY 10032; **Phone:** 212-305-5098; **Board Cert:** Medical Oncology 2004; **Med School:** Albert Einstein Coll Med 1997; **Resid:** Internal Medicine, NYU Langone Med Ctr 2000; **Fellow:** Hematology & Oncology, Meml Sloan-Kettering Cancer Ctr 2004; **Fac Appt:** Assoc Clin Prof Med, Columbia P&S

Maki, Robert G MD/PhD (Onc) - **Spec Exp:** Sarcoma; Gastrointestinal Stromal Tumors; Desmoid Tumors; **Hospital:** Mt Sinai Med Ctr (page 102); **Address:** The Ruttenberg Treatment Ctr, 1470 Madison Ave, New York, NY 10029-6574; **Phone:** 212-241-6756; **Board Cert:** Internal Medicine 2005; Medical Oncology 2007; **Med School:** Cornell Univ-Weill Med Coll 1992; **Resid:** Internal Medicine, Brigham & Womens Hosp 1995; **Fellow:** Medical Oncology, Dana-Farber Cancer Inst 1998; **Fac Appt:** Prof Onc, Mount Sinai Sch Med

Malamud, Stephen C MD (Onc) - **Spec Exp:** Breast Cancer; Gastrointestinal Cancer; Lung Cancer; **Hospital:** Beth Israel Med Ctr - Petrie Div (page 94), St. Luke's - Roosevelt Hosp Ctr - Roosevelt Div (page 94); **Address:** 325 W 15th St W, Fl Ground, New York, NY 10011; **Phone:** 212-604-6011; **Board Cert:** Internal Medicine 1981; Medical Oncology 1983; **Med School:** Albert Einstein Coll Med 1978; **Resid:** Internal Medicine, Beth Israel Med Ctr 1981; **Fellow:** Medical Oncology, Mt Sinai Hosp 1983; **Fac Appt:** Assoc Clin Prof Onc, Albert Einstein Coll Med

Moore, Anne MD (Onc) - **Spec Exp:** Breast Cancer; **Hospital:** NY-Presby/Weill Cornell Med Ctr, NY (page 104); **Address:** Weill Cornell Breast Ctr, 425 E 61st St Fl 8, New York, NY 10065; **Phone:** 212-821-0550; **Board Cert:** Internal Medicine 1973; Hematology 1976; Medical Oncology 2008; **Med School:** Columbia P&S 1969; **Resid:** Internal Medicine, Cornell Univ Med Ctr 1973; **Fellow:** Medical Oncology, Rockefeller Univ 1976; **Fac Appt:** Prof Med, Cornell Univ-Weill Med Coll

Morris, Michael J MD (Onc) - **Spec Exp:** Prostate Cancer; Genitourinary Cancer; **Hospital:** Meml Sloan-Kettering Canc Ctr (page 114); **Address:** MSKCC, Genitourinary Oncology Svc, 1275 York Ave, New York, NY 10065; **Phone:** 646-422-4469; **Board Cert:** Medical Oncology 2009; **Med School:** Mount Sinai Sch Med 1994; **Resid:** Internal Medicine, NY-Presby/Columbia Univ Med Ctr 1997; **Fellow:** Hematology & Oncology, Meml Sloan-Kettering Cancer Ctr 1999

Moskowitz, Craig H MD (Onc) - **Spec Exp:** Hodgkin's Lymphoma; Lymphoma, Non-Hodgkin's; Bone Marrow Transplant; **Hospital:** Meml Sloan-Kettering Canc Ctr (page 114); **Address:** 1275 York Ave, New York, NY 10065; **Phone:** 646-497-9137; **Board Cert:** Hematology 2002; Medical Oncology 2005; **Med School:** Wayne State Univ 1988; **Resid:** Internal Medicine, Bronx Muni Hosp 1992; **Fellow:** Hematology & Oncology, Meml Sloan-Kettering Cancer Ctr 1994

Motzer, Robert J MD (Onc) - **Spec Exp:** Kidney Cancer; Testicular Cancer; **Hospital:** Meml Sloan-Kettering Canc Ctr (page 114); **Address:** 1275 York Avenue, New York, NY 10065; **Phone:** 646-422-4312; **Board Cert:** Internal Medicine 1984; Medical Oncology 1987; **Med School:** Univ Mich Med Sch 1981; **Resid:** Internal Medicine, Meml Sloan Kettering Cancer Ctr 1984; **Fellow:** Medical Oncology, Meml Sloan Kettering Cancer Ctr 1987; **Fac Appt:** Assoc Prof Med, Cornell Univ-Weill Med Coll

Muggia, Franco M MD (Onc) - **Spec Exp:** Gynecologic Cancer; **Hospital:** NYU Langone Med Ctr (page 108); **Address:** NYU Clinical Cancer Ctr, 160 E 34th St Fl 4, New York, NY 10016; **Phone:** 212-731-5433; **Board Cert:** Internal Medicine 1968; Medical Oncology 1973; Hematology 1974; **Med School:** Cornell Univ-Weill Med Coll 1961; **Resid:** Internal Medicine, Hartford Hosp 1964; **Fellow:** Hematology & Oncology, Francis A Delafield Hosp 1967; **Fac Appt:** Prof Med, NYU Sch Med

Nanus, David M MD (Onc) - **Spec Exp:** Prostate Cancer; Bladder Cancer; Testicular Cancer; Genitourinary Cancer; **Hospital:** NY-Presby/Weill Cornell Med Ctr, NY (page 104); **Address:** NY Hosp-Cornell Med Ctr,Payson Pavillion, 525 E 68th St, Fl 3, Ste 341, New York, NY 10021; **Phone:** 646-962-2072; **Board Cert:** Internal Medicine 1985; Medical Oncology 1987; **Med School:** Univ Hlth Scis, Chicago Med Sch 1982; **Resid:** Internal Medicine, Bronx Muni Hosp 1985; **Fellow:** Medical Oncology, Meml Sloan Kettering Canc Ctr 1989; **Fac Appt:** Prof Onc, Cornell Univ-Weill Med Coll

Norton, Larry MD (Onc) - **Spec Exp:** Breast Cancer; **Hospital:** Meml Sloan-Kettering Canc Ctr (page 114); **Address:** 300 E 66th St, BAIC Bldg Fl 9 - Ste 933, New York, NY 10065; **Phone:** 646-888-5438; **Board Cert:** Internal Medicine 1975; Medical Oncology 1977; **Med School:** Columbia P&S 1972; **Resid:** Internal Medicine, Bronx Muni Hosp 1975; **Fellow:** Medical Oncology, Natl Cancer Inst 1977; **Fac Appt:** Prof Med, Cornell Univ-Weill Med Coll

O'Connor, Owen A MD/PhD (Onc) - **Spec Exp:** Hodgkin's Lymphoma; Lymphoma, Non-Hodgkin's; Drug Development; Clinical Trials; **Hospital:** NY-Presby/Columbia Univ Med Ctr, NY (page 104); **Address:** Columbia Doctors Midtown, 51 W 51st St, Ste 200, New York, NY 10019; **Phone:** 212-326-5720; **Board Cert:** Internal Medicine 2004; Medical Oncology 2005; **Med School:** UMDNJ-RW Johnson Med Sch 1994; **Resid:** Internal Medicine, NY-Presby/Weill Cornell Univ Med Ctr 1996; **Fellow:** Medical Oncology, Memorial Sloan-Kettering Cancer Ctr 2000; **Fac Appt:** Asst Clin Prof Med, Columbia P&S

O'Reilly, Eileen M MD (Onc) - **Spec Exp:** Pancreatic Cancer; Neuroendocrine Tumors; Colon & Rectal Cancer; **Hospital:** Meml Sloan-Kettering Canc Ctr (page 114), NY-Presby/Weill Cornell Med Ctr, NY (page 104); **Address:** Meml Sloan-Kettering Cancer Ctr, 300 E 66th St, rm 1021, New York, NY 10065; **Phone:** 646-888-4182; **Med School:** Ireland 1990; **Resid:** Internal Medicine, St Vincent's Hosp 1994; **Fellow:** Hematology & Oncology, St Vincent's Hosp 1995; Medical Oncology, Memorial Sloan-Kettering Cancer Ctr 1997; **Fac Appt:** Assoc Prof Onc, Cornell Univ-Weill Med Coll

Offit, Kenneth MD (Onc) - **Spec Exp:** Cancer Genetics; Breast Cancer; Lymphoma; Hodgkin's Disease Consultation; **Hospital:** Meml Sloan-Kettering Canc Ctr (page 114); **Address:** Meml Sloan-Kettering Cancer Ctr, 1275 York Ave, Box 192, New York, NY 10065; **Phone:** 646-888-4050; **Board Cert:** Internal Medicine 1985; Medical Oncology 1987; **Med School:** Harvard Med Sch 1982; **Resid:** Internal Medicine, Lenox Hill Hosp 1985; **Fellow:** Medical Oncology, Meml Sloan Kettering Cancer Ctr 1987; Hematology, Meml Sloan Kettering Cancer Ctr 1988; **Fac Appt:** Prof Med, Cornell Univ-Weill Med Coll

Oh, William K MD (Onc) - **Spec Exp:** Genitourinary Cancer; Prostate Cancer; Testicular Cancer; Adrenal Cancer; **Hospital:** Mt Sinai Med Ctr (page 102); **Address:** Ruttenberg Treatment Center, 1470 Madison Ave, New York, NY 10029; **Phone:** 212-659-5429; **Board Cert:** Medical Oncology 2009; **Med School:** NYU Sch Med 1992; **Resid:** Internal Medicine, Brigham & Womens Hosp 1995; **Fellow:** Medical Oncology, Dana-Farber Cancer Inst 1997; **Fac Appt:** Prof Onc, Mount Sinai Sch Med

Oratz, Ruth MD (Onc) - **Spec Exp:** Breast Cancer; **Hospital:** NYU Langone Med Ctr (page 108), Lenox Hill Hosp (page 106); **Address:** The Women's Oncology & Wellness Practice, 345 E 37th St, Ste 202, New York, NY 10016; **Phone:** 212-400-4904; **Board Cert:** Internal Medicine 1985; Medical Oncology 1989; **Med School:** Albert Einstein Coll Med 1982; **Resid:** Internal Medicine, Bellevue Hosp 1985; **Fellow:** Medical Oncology, Bellevue Hosp 1988; **Fac Appt:** Assoc Clin Prof Med, NYU Sch Med

Oster, Martin W MD (Onc) - **Spec Exp:** Breast Cancer; Gastrointestinal Cancer; Head & Neck Cancer; Lung Cancer; **Hospital:** NY-Presby/Columbia Univ Med Ctr, NY (page 104); **Address:** NY Presby Hosp-Columbia University Med Ctr, 161 Fort Washington Ave, New York, NY 10032-3713; **Phone:** 212-305-8231; **Board Cert:** Internal Medicine 1974; Medical Oncology 1975; **Med School:** Columbia P&S 1971; **Resid:** Internal Medicine, Mass Genl Hosp 1973; **Fellow:** Medical Oncology, Natl Cancer Inst/NIH 1976; **Fac Appt:** Assoc Clin Prof Onc, Columbia P&S

Pasmantier, Mark W MD (Onc) - **Spec Exp:** Lung Cancer; Ovarian Cancer; Breast Cancer; Lymphoma; **Hospital:** NY-Presby/Weill Cornell Med Ctr, NY (page 104); **Address:** 407 E 70th St, Fl 3, New York, NY 10021-5302; **Phone:** 212-517-5900; **Board Cert:** Internal Medicine 1972; Hematology 1974; Medical Oncology 1975; **Med School:** NYU Sch Med 1966; **Resid:** Internal Medicine, Harlem Hosp 1970; **Fellow:** Hematology, Montefiore Med Ctr 1971; Medical Oncology, NY Hosp 1972; **Fac Appt:** Clin Prof Med, Cornell Univ-Weill Med Coll

Pavlick, Anna C DO (Onc) - **Spec Exp:** Melanoma; Skin Cancer; Sarcoma; **Hospital:** NYU Langone Med Ctr (page 108), Bellevue Hosp Ctr; **Address:** NYU Cancer Inst, 160 E 34th St Fl 9, New York, NY 10016; **Phone:** 212-731-5431; **Board Cert:** Medical Oncology 2008; **Med School:** UMDNJ Sch Osteo Med 1990; **Resid:** Internal Medicine, Hackensack Med Ctr 1993; **Fellow:** Hematology & Oncology, Meml Sloan Kettering Cancer Ctr 1996; **Fac Appt:** Assoc Prof Med, NYU Sch Med

Pfister, David G MD (Onc) - **Spec Exp:** Head & Neck Cancer; Laryngeal Cancer; Thyroid Cancer; Immunotherapy; **Hospital:** Meml Sloan-Kettering Canc Ctr (page 114); **Address:** 300 E 66th St Fl 14, New York, NY 10065; **Phone:** 646-888-4232; **Board Cert:** Internal Medicine 1985; Medical Oncology 1989; **Med School:** Univ Pennsylvania 1982; **Resid:** Internal Medicine, Hosp Univ Penn 1985; **Fellow:** Epidemiology, Yale-New Haven Hosp 1987; Hematology & Oncology, Meml Sloan Kettering Cancer Ctr 1989; **Fac Appt:** Assoc Prof Med, Cornell Univ-Weill Med Coll

Pietanza, Maria Catherine MD (Onc) - **Spec Exp:** Lung Cancer; Carcinoid Tumors; Neuroendocrine Tumors; **Hospital:** Meml Sloan-Kettering Canc Ctr (page 114); **Address:** MSKCC, Thoracic Oncology Svc, 300 E 66th St, New York, NY 10065; **Phone:** 646-497-9163; **Board Cert:** Internal Medicine 2004; Medical Oncology 2007; **Med School:** SUNY Downstate 2001; **Resid:** Internal Medicine, NY-Presby/Weill Cornell Med Ctr 2004; **Fellow:** Hematology & Oncology, Mt Sinai Med Ctr 2007

Portlock, Carol S MD (Onc) - **Spec Exp:** Lymphoma; Hodgkin's Lymphoma; **Hospital:** Meml Sloan-Kettering Canc Ctr (page 114); **Address:** 1275 York Ave, New York, NY 10065; **Phone:** 212-639-8109; **Board Cert:** Internal Medicine 1976; Medical Oncology 1977; **Med School:** Stanford Univ 1971; **Resid:** Internal Medicine, Stanford Univ Med Ctr 1974; **Fellow:** Medical Oncology, Stanford Univ Med Ctr 1976; **Fac Appt:** Clin Prof Med, Cornell Univ-Weill Med Coll

Posner, Marshall R MD (Onc) - **Spec Exp:** Head & Neck Cancer; Skin Cancer-Head & Neck; **Hospital:** Mt Sinai Med Ctr (page 102); **Address:** The Ruttenberg Treatment Ctr, 1470 Madison Ave, New York, NY 10029; **Phone:** 212-659-5461; **Board Cert:** Internal Medicine 1978; Medical Oncology 1981; **Med School:** Tufts Univ 1975; **Resid:** Internal Medicine, Boston City Hosp 1978; **Fellow:** Oncology, Dana-Farber Cancer Inst 1981; **Fac Appt:** Prof Onc, Mount Sinai Sch Med

Ratner, Lynn H MD (Onc) - **Spec Exp:** Breast Cancer; Carcinoid Tumors; Neuroendocrine Tumors; Gliomas; **Hospital:** Mt Sinai Med Ctr (page 102), Lenox Hill Hosp (page 106); **Address:** 112 E 83rd St, New York, NY 10028-0506; **Phone:** 212-396-0400; **Board Cert:** Internal Medicine 1977; Medical Oncology 1973; **Med School:** Albert Einstein Coll Med 1964; **Resid:** Internal Medicine, Bellevue Hosp 1966; Internal Medicine, Bellevue Hosp 1970; **Fellow:** Medical Oncology, Meml Sloan-Kettering Cancer Ctr 1970

Raza, Azra MD (Onc) - **Spec Exp:** Myelodysplastic Syndromes; Leukemia; Clinical Trials; **Hospital:** NY-Presby/Columbia Univ Med Ctr, NY (page 104); **Address:** 161 Ft Washington Ave Fl 9, New York, NY 10032; **Phone:** 212-305-5098; **Board Cert:** Internal Medicine 1980; Medical Oncology 1985; **Med School:** Pakistan 1976; **Resid:** Internal Medicine, Franklin Sq Hosp 1979; Internal Medicine, Georgetown Univ/VA Med Ctr 1980; **Fellow:** Medical Oncology, Roswell Park Cancer Inst 1982

Rizvi, Naiyer A MD (Onc) - **Spec Exp:** Thoracic Cancers; Thymoma; Lung Cancer; Clinical Trials; **Hospital:** Meml Sloan-Kettering Canc Ctr (page 114); **Address:** 300 E 66 St, New York, NY 10065; **Phone:** 646-888-4204; **Board Cert:** Medical Oncology 2003; **Med School:** Canada 1987; **Resid:** Internal Medicine, University of Manitoba Med Ctr 1992; **Fellow:** Medical Oncology, Beth Israel Med Ctr 1994

Roboz, Gail J MD (Onc) - **Spec Exp:** Leukemia; Myelodysplastic Syndromes; Myeloproliferative Disorders; **Hospital:** NY-Presby/Weill Cornell Med Ctr, NY (page 104); **Address:** 520 E 70th St, New York, NY 10021; **Phone:** 646-962-2700; **Board Cert:** Medical Oncology 2010; Hematology 2010; **Med School:** Mount Sinai Sch Med 1994; **Resid:** Internal Medicine, NY-Presby/Weill Cornell Med Ctr 1997; **Fellow:** Hematology & Oncology, NY-Presby/Weill Cornell Med Ctr 2000; **Fac Appt:** Assoc Prof Med, Cornell Univ-Weill Med Coll

Robson, Mark Emerson MD (Onc) - **Spec Exp:** Breast Cancer; Cancer Genetics; **Hospital:** Meml Sloan-Kettering Canc Ctr (page 114); **Address:** 300 E 66th St, New York, NY 10065; **Phone:** 646-888-5434; **Board Cert:** Internal Medicine 1989; Medical Oncology 2012; Hematology 2002; **Med School:** Univ VA Sch Med 1986; **Resid:** Internal Medicine, Walter Reed Army Med Ctr 1989; **Fellow:** Hematology & Oncology, Walter Reed Army Med Ctr 1991

Ruggiero, Joseph T MD (Onc) - **Spec Exp:** Gastrointestinal Cancer; **Hospital:** NY-Presby/Weill Cornell Med Ctr, NY (page 104); **Address:** 1305 York Ave, Fl 12, New York, NY 10021-4635; **Phone:** 646-962-6200; **Board Cert:** Internal Medicine 1980; Hematology 1982; Medical Oncology 1983; **Med School:** NYU Sch Med 1977; **Resid:** Internal Medicine, New York Hosp 1980; **Fellow:** Hematology & Oncology, New York Hosp/Cornell 1983; **Fac Appt:** Assoc Clin Prof Onc, Cornell Univ-Weill Med Coll

Sabbatini, Paul J MD (Onc) - **Spec Exp:** Gynecologic Cancer; Uterine Cancer; Ovarian Cancer; **Hospital:** Meml Sloan-Kettering Canc Ctr (page 114); **Address:** Meml Sloan-Kettering Cancer Ctr, 300 E 66 St, New York, NY 10065; **Phone:** 646-888-4218; **Board Cert:** Internal Medicine 2012; Medical Oncology 2008; **Med School:** Univ Miss 1989; **Resid:** Internal Medicine, Vanderbilt Univ Med Ctr 1992; **Fellow:** Medical Oncology, Meml Sloan-Kettering Cancer Ctr 1996; **Fac Appt:** Asst Prof Med, Cornell Univ-Weill Med Coll

Saltz, Leonard B MD (Onc) - **Spec Exp:** Colon & Rectal Cancer; Gastrointestinal Cancer & Rare Tumors; Neuroendocrine Tumors; Unknown Primary Cancer; **Hospital:** Meml Sloan-Kettering Canc Ctr (page 114); **Address:** Memorial Sloan Kettering Cancer Center, 300 E 66th St, rm 1049, New York, NY 10065; **Phone:** 646-888-4181; **Board Cert:** Internal Medicine 1986; Hematology 1988; Medical Oncology 1989; **Med School:** Yale Univ 1983; **Resid:** Internal Medicine, New York Hosp 1986; **Fellow:** Hematology, New York Hosp-Cornell/Rockefeller Univ 1988; Oncology, New York Hosp-Cornell/Rockefeller Univ 1989; **Fac Appt:** Assoc Prof Med, Cornell Univ-Weill Med Coll

Sara, Gabriel MD (Onc) - **Spec Exp:** Breast Cancer; Lung Cancer; Lymphoma; Gastrointestinal Cancer; **Hospital:** St. Luke's - Roosevelt Hosp Ctr - Roosevelt Div (page 94); **Address:** 1000 10th Ave, Fl 11, New York, NY 10019; **Phone:** 212-523-7580; **Board Cert:** Internal Medicine 1984; Hematology 1986; Medical Oncology 1987; **Med School:** Lebanon 1980; **Resid:** Internal Medicine, SUNY Downstate Med Ctr 1984; **Fellow:** Hematology & Oncology, St Luke's-Roosevelt Med Ctr 1986; Hematology & Oncology, Columbia-Presby Med Ctr 1987; **Fac Appt:** Asst Clin Prof Med, Columbia P&S

Scheinberg, David A MD/PhD (Onc) - **Spec Exp:** Leukemia; Immunotherapy; Vaccine Therapy; **Hospital:** Meml Sloan-Kettering Canc Ctr (page 114); **Address:** 1275 York Avenue, New York, NY 10065; **Phone:** 646-888-2190; **Board Cert:** Internal Medicine 1986; Medical Oncology 2005; **Med School:** Johns Hopkins Univ 1983; **Resid:** Internal Medicine, NY Hosp-Cornell Med Ctr 1986; **Fellow:** Medical Oncology, Meml Sloan Kettering Cancer Ctr 1989; **Fac Appt:** Prof Med, Cornell Univ-Weill Med Coll

Scher, Howard I MD (Onc) - **Spec Exp:** Genitourinary Cancer; Prostate Cancer; Bladder Cancer; Immunotherapy; **Hospital:** Meml Sloan-Kettering Canc Ctr (page 114); **Address:** 1275 York Avenue, New York, NY 10065; **Phone:** 646-422-4330; **Board Cert:** Internal Medicine 1979; Medical Oncology 1985; **Med School:** NYU Sch Med 1976; **Resid:** Internal Medicine, Bellevue Hosp 1980; **Fellow:** Medical Oncology, Meml Sloan Kettering Cancer Ctr 1983; **Fac Appt:** Prof Med, Cornell Univ-Weill Med Coll

Sherman, William H MD (Onc) - **Spec Exp:** Pancreatic Cancer; Multiple Myeloma; Melanoma; **Hospital:** NY-Presby/Columbia Univ Med Ctr, NY (page 104); **Address:** 161 Fort Washington Ave, Ste 809, New York, NY 10032-3729; **Phone:** 212-305-3856; **Board Cert:** Internal Medicine 1975; Medical Oncology 1979; **Med School:** Jefferson Med Coll 1969; **Resid:** Internal Medicine, Univ Illinois Hosp 1971; **Fellow:** Medical Oncology, Columbia-Presby Hosp 1977; **Fac Appt:** Assoc Clin Prof Med, Columbia P&S

Silverman, Lewis R MD (Onc) - **Spec Exp:** Myelodysplastic Syndromes; Leukemia & Lymphoma; Multiple Myeloma; **Hospital:** Mt Sinai Med Ctr (page 102); **Address:** Ruttenberg Treatment Ctr, 1470 Madison Ave Fl 3, New York, NY 10029; **Phone:** 212-241-6756; **Board Cert:** Internal Medicine 1981; Hematology 1986; Medical Oncology 1987; **Med School:** Belgium 1978; **Resid:** Internal Medicine, Metropolitan Hosp Ctr 1980; Internal Medicine, Montefiore Med Ctr 1981; **Fellow:** Hematology, Montefiore Med Ctr 1982; Medical Oncology, Mt Sinai Med Ctr 1984; **Fac Appt:** Assoc Prof Med, Mount Sinai Sch Med

Sklarin, Nancy T MD (Onc) - **Spec Exp:** Breast Cancer; **Hospital:** Meml Sloan-Kettering Canc Ctr (page 114); **Address:** 300 E 66th St, New York, NY 10065; **Phone:** 646-888-5488; **Board Cert:** Internal Medicine 1984; Medical Oncology 1987; Hematology 1988; **Med School:** Albert Einstein Coll Med 1981; **Resid:** Internal Medicine, LI Jewish Med Ctr 1984; **Fellow:** Hematology & Oncology, Mount Sinai Med Ctr 1987; **Fac Appt:** Assoc Prof Med, Cornell Univ-Weill Med Coll

Slovin, Susan F MD/PhD (Onc) - **Spec Exp:** Prostate Cancer; Genitourinary Cancer; Immunotherapy; **Hospital:** Meml Sloan-Kettering Canc Ctr (page 114); **Address:** 1275 York Ave, New York, NY 10065; **Phone:** 646-422-4470; **Board Cert:** Internal Medicine 2005; Medical Oncology 2009; **Med School:** Jefferson Med Coll 1990; **Resid:** Internal Medicine, Mt Sinai Hosp 1993; **Fellow:** Medical Oncology, Meml Sloan-Kettering Cancer Ctr 1996; **Fac Appt:** Assoc Prof Med, Cornell Univ-Weill Med Coll

Smith, Julia A MD/PhD (Onc) - **Spec Exp:** Breast Cancer; Cancer Risk Assessment; **Hospital:** NYU Langone Med Ctr (page 108), Bellevue Hosp Ctr; **Address:** 221 Lexington Ave Fl 1, New York, NY 10016; **Phone:** 212-731-5452; **Board Cert:** Internal Medicine 1985; Medical Oncology 1989; **Med School:** NYU Sch Med 1980; **Resid:** Internal Medicine, Brigham & Women's Hosp 1983; **Fellow:** Hematology & Oncology, Meml Sloan-Kettering Cancer Ctr 1986; **Fac Appt:** Asst Clin Prof Med, NYU Sch Med

Speyer, James L MD (Onc) - **Spec Exp:** Ovarian Cancer; Breast Cancer; **Hospital:** NYU Langone Med Ctr (page 108), Bellevue Hosp Ctr; **Address:** 160 E 34th St Fl 4, New York, NY 10016-4750; **Phone:** 212-731-5432; **Board Cert:** Internal Medicine 1977; Hematology 1978; Medical Oncology 1979; **Med School:** Johns Hopkins Univ 1974; **Resid:** Internal Medicine, Columbia-Presby Med Ctr 1976; Hematology, Columbia-Presby Med Ctr 1977; **Fellow:** Medical Oncology, Natl Cancer Inst 1979; **Fac Appt:** Prof Med, NYU Sch Med

Spriggs, David R MD (Onc) - **Spec Exp:** Ovarian Cancer; Drug Development; Uterine Cancer; Gynecologic Cancer; **Hospital:** Meml Sloan-Kettering Canc Ctr (page 114); **Address:** 300 E 66th St, New York, NY 10021; **Phone:** 646-888-4223; **Board Cert:** Internal Medicine 1981; Medical Oncology 2006; **Med School:** Univ Wisc 1977; **Resid:** Internal Medicine, Columbia-Presby Hosp 1981; **Fellow:** Medical Oncology, Dana-Farber Cancer Inst 1985; **Fac Appt:** Prof Med, Cornell Univ-Weill Med Coll

Stoopler, Mark Benjamin MD (Onc) - **Spec Exp:** Lung Cancer; Esophageal Cancer; Unknown Primary Cancer; **Hospital:** NY-Presby/Columbia Univ Med Ctr, NY (page 104); **Address:** 161 Fort Washington Ave, Ste 936, New York, NY 10032-3713; **Phone:** 212-305-8230; **Board Cert:** Internal Medicine 1978; Medical Oncology 1981; **Med School:** Cornell Univ-Weill Med Coll 1975; **Resid:** Internal Medicine, North Shore Univ Hosp 1978; Internal Medicine, NY Meml Hosp 1978; **Fellow:** Medical Oncology, Meml-Sloan Kettering Cancer Ctr 1980; **Fac Appt:** Assoc Clin Prof Onc, Columbia P&S

Straus, David J MD (Onc) - **Spec Exp:** Lymphoma; Multiple Myeloma; Hodgkin's Lymphoma; **Hospital:** Meml Sloan-Kettering Canc Ctr (page 114); **Address:** 1275 York Ave, Box 406, New York, NY 10065; **Phone:** 212-639-8365; **Board Cert:** Internal Medicine 1972; Hematology 1976; Medical Oncology 1977; **Med School:** Marquette Sch Med 1969; **Resid:** Internal Medicine, Montefiore Med Ctr 1972; **Fellow:** Hematology, Beth Israel Hosp/Brigham Hosp 1974; Medical Oncology, Meml Sloan Kettering Cancer Ctr 1976; **Fac Appt:** Prof Onc, Cornell Univ-Weill Med Coll

Tagawa, Scott T MD (Onc) - **Spec Exp:** Prostate Cancer; Bladder Cancer; Kidney Cancer; Urologic Cancer; **Hospital:** NY-Presby/Weill Cornell Med Ctr, NY (page 104); **Address:** NY Presby-Weill Cornell Med Ctr, 525 E 68th St, Box 403, New York, NY 10065; **Phone:** 646-962-2072; **Board Cert:** Medical Oncology 2005; Hematology 2006; **Med School:** USC-Keck School of Medicine 1998; **Resid:** Internal Medicine, USC Med Ctr 2002; **Fellow:** Hematology & Oncology, USC Med Ctr 2005; **Fac Appt:** Assoc Clin Prof Onc, Cornell Univ-Weill Med Coll

Tap, William D MD (Onc) - **Spec Exp:** Sarcoma; Sarcoma-Soft Tissue; Ewing's Sarcoma; Bone Tumors; **Hospital:** Meml Sloan-Kettering Canc Ctr (page 114); **Address:** 300 E 66th St Fl 10, New York, NY 10065; **Phone:** 646-888-4163; **Board Cert:** Internal Medicine 2003; Hematology 2006; Medical Oncology 2006; **Med School:** Thomas Jefferson Univ 2000; **Resid:** Internal Medicine, Vanderbilt Univ Med Ctr 2003; **Fellow:** Hematology & Oncology, UCLA Med Ctr 2006

Vahdat, Linda T MD (Onc) - **Spec Exp:** Breast Cancer; Breast Cancer-Novel Therapies; Clinical Trials; **Hospital:** NY-Presby/Weill Cornell Med Ctr, NY (page 104); **Address:** 425 E 61st St Fl 8, New York, NY 10065; **Phone:** 212-821-0644; **Board Cert:** Medical Oncology 2005; **Med School:** Mount Sinai Sch Med 1987; **Resid:** Internal Medicine, Mt Sinai Hosp 1990; **Fellow:** Hematology & Oncology, Meml Sloan Kettering Cancer Ctr 1994; **Fac Appt:** Prof Med, Cornell Univ-Weill Med Coll

Volm, Matthew MD (Onc) - **Spec Exp:** Breast Cancer; **Hospital:** NYU Langone Med Ctr (page 108); **Address:** NYU Cancer Ctr, 160 E 34th St Fl 4, New York, NY 10016; **Phone:** 212-731-5346; **Board Cert:** Medical Oncology 2009; **Med School:** Univ Minn 1989; **Resid:** Internal Medicine, Bellevue Med Ctr 1992; **Fellow:** Hematology & Oncology, VA Med Ctr-Lakeside 1996

Wolchok, Jedd D MD/PhD (Onc) - **Spec Exp:** Melanoma; Immunotherapy; Clinical Trials; Vaccine Therapy; **Hospital:** Meml Sloan-Kettering Canc Ctr (page 114); **Address:** Meml Sloan Kettering Cancer Ctr, 1275 York Ave, New York, NY 10065; **Phone:** 646-888-2395; **Board Cert:** Medical Oncology 2011; **Med School:** NYU Sch Med 1994; **Resid:** Internal Medicine, NYU Med Ctr 1997; **Fellow:** Medical Oncology, Meml Sloan-Kettering Canc Ctr 2000

Zelenetz, Andrew D MD/PhD (Onc) - **Spec Exp:** Lymphoma; **Hospital:** Meml Sloan-Kettering Canc Ctr (page 114); **Address:** 205 E 64th St, New York, NY 10065; **Phone:** 212-639-2656; **Board Cert:** Medical Oncology 2009; **Med School:** Harvard Med Sch 1984; **Resid:** Internal Medicine, Stanford Univ Med Ctr 1988; **Fellow:** Medical Oncology, Stanford Univ Med Ctr 1991; **Fac Appt:** Asst Prof Med, Cornell Univ-Weill Med Coll

Neonatal-Perinatal Medicine

Caprio, Martha C MD (NP) - **Spec Exp:** Prematurity/Low Birth Weight Infants; **Hospital:** NYU Langone Med Ctr (page 108); **Address:** NYU Neonatology Assocs, 530 1st Ave, rm 7A, New York, NY 10016; **Phone:** 212-263-7950; **Board Cert:** Pediatrics 2010; Neonatal-Perinatal Medicine 2012; **Med School:** Mexico 1985; **Resid:** Pediatrics, NYU Med Ctr 1992; **Fellow:** Neonatal-Perinatal Medicine, NYU Med Ctr 1993; **Fac Appt:** Assoc Prof Med, NYU Sch Med

Holzman, Ian R MD (NP) - **Spec Exp:** Neonatal Nutrition; Necrotizing Enterocolitis; Ethics; Prematurity/Low Birth Weight Infants; **Hospital:** Mt Sinai Med Ctr (page 102); **Address:** Newborn Assocs, 1 Gustave L Levy Pl, Box 1508, New York, NY 10029-6500; **Phone:** 212-241-5446; **Board Cert:** Pediatrics 1974; Neonatal-Perinatal Medicine 1977; **Med School:** Univ Pittsburgh 1971; **Resid:** Pediatrics, Chldns Hosp 1975; **Fellow:** Neonatal-Perinatal Medicine, Univ Colorado 1977; **Fac Appt:** Prof Ped, Mount Sinai Sch Med

Klein, Janice F MD (NP) - **Hospital:** St. Luke's - Roosevelt Hosp Ctr - Roosevelt Div (page 94); **Address:** St Luke's-Roosevelt Hosp Ctr, 1000 10th Ave, New York, NY 10019; **Phone:** 212-523-5710; **Board Cert:** Pediatrics 1985; Neonatal-Perinatal Medicine 1985; **Med School:** Albert Einstein Coll Med 1980; **Resid:** Pediatrics, Montefiore Med Ctr 1983; **Fellow:** Neonatal-Perinatal Medicine, Montefiore Med Ctr 1985; **Fac Appt:** Asst Clin Prof Ped, Columbia P&S

Mally, Pradeep MD (NP) - **Hospital:** NYU Langone Med Ctr (page 108); **Address:** NYU Neonatology Assocs, 530 1st Ave, rm 7A, New York, NY 10016; **Phone:** 212-263-7950; **Board Cert:** Neonatal-Perinatal Medicine 2011; **Med School:** India 1988; **Resid:** Pediatrics, Maimonides Med Ctr 1999; **Fellow:** Neonatal-Perinatal Medicine, Westchester Co Med Ctr 2002; **Fac Appt:** Asst Prof Ped, NYU Sch Med

Marron-Corwin, Mary MD (NP) - **Spec Exp:** Neonatal Respiratory Care; Critical Care; Neonatal Liver Disease; **Hospital:** Harlem Hosp Ctr; **Address:** 506 Lenox Ave, MLK Pavilion, Ste 4417, New York, NY 10037; **Phone:** 212-939-8457; **Board Cert:** Neonatal-Perinatal Medicine 2008; **Med School:** Philippines 1985; **Resid:** Pediatrics, St Vincents Hosp Med Ctr 1988; **Fellow:** Neonatal-Perinatal Medicine, Babies Hosp/Colum-Presby Med Ctr 1990; **Fac Appt:** Prof Ped, Columbia P&S

Perlman, Jeffrey M MD (NP) - **Spec Exp:** Neonatal Critical Care; Prematurity/Low Birth Weight Infants; Neonatal Neurology; Lung Disease in Newborns; **Hospital:** NY-Presby/Weill Cornell Med Ctr, NY (page 104); **Address:** 525 E 68th St, Ste N 506, New York, NY 10065; **Phone:** 212-746-3530; **Board Cert:** Pediatrics 1983; Neonatal-Perinatal Medicine 1983; **Med School:** South Africa 1974; **Resid:** Pediatrics, Johannesburg Chldns Hosp 1979; Pediatrics, St Louis Chldns Hosp 1981; **Fellow:** Neonatology, St Louis Chldns Hosp 1983; **Fac Appt:** Prof Ped, Cornell Univ-Weill Med Coll

Polin, Richard A MD (NP) - **Spec Exp:** Neonatal Infections; **Hospital:** Morgan Stanley Children's Hosp of NY-Presby, NY (page 104); **Address:** 3959 Broadway CHN-1201, New York, NY 10032; **Phone:** 212-305-5827; **Board Cert:** Pediatrics 1975; Neonatal-Perinatal Medicine 2010; **Med School:** Temple Univ 1970; **Resid:** Pediatrics, Chldns Meml Hosp 1972; Pediatrics, Babies Hosp 1973; **Fellow:** Neonatal-Perinatal Medicine, Babies Hosp-Columbia 1974; **Fac Appt:** Prof Ped, Columbia P&S

Rosen, Tove S MD (NP) - **Spec Exp:** Neonatal Care; Substance Abuse Effects in Newborn; **Hospital:** Morgan Stanley Children's Hosp of NY-Presby, NY (page 104); **Address:** Morgan Stanley Chldns Hosp of NY-Presby, 3959 Broadway, rm CHN 1214, New York, NY 10032-1559; **Phone:** 212-305-8500; **Board Cert:** Pediatrics 1971; Neonatal-Perinatal Medicine 1975; **Med School:** SUNY Hlth Sci Ctr 1965; **Resid:** Pediatrics, St Luke's Hosp 1970; **Fellow:** Neonatal-Perinatal Medicine, NY-Presby/Columbia Univ Med Ctr 1974; **Fac Appt:** Clin Prof Ped, Columbia P&S

Shahrivar, Farrokh MD (NP) - **Spec Exp:** Neonatology; Prematurity/Low Birth Weight Infants; **Hospital:** St. Luke's - Roosevelt Hosp Ctr - Roosevelt Div (page 94), Beth Israel Med Ctr - Petrie Div (page 94); **Address:** 1000 10th Ave, NICU, Fl 12, New York, NY 10019-1192; **Phone:** 212-523-3760; **Board Cert:** Pediatrics 1974; Neonatal-Perinatal Medicine 1975; **Med School:** Iran 1966; **Resid:** Pediatrics, St Luke's-Roosevelt Hosp Ctr 1971; Pediatrics, St Luke's-Roosevelt Hosp Ctr 1972; **Fellow:** Neonatal-Perinatal Medicine, St Christopher's Hosp 1973; Neonatal-Perinatal Medicine, Montefiore Med Ctr 1973; **Fac Appt:** Assoc Clin Prof Ped, Columbia P&S

Nephrology

Ames, Richard P MD (Nep) - **Spec Exp:** Hypertension; Kidney Disease; Dialysis Care; **Hospital:** St. Luke's - Roosevelt Hosp Ctr - Roosevelt Div (page 94); **Address:** 200 W 57th St Fl 15, New York, NY 10019; **Phone:** 917-224-4270; **Board Cert:** Internal Medicine 1974; Nephrology 1972; Medical Oncology 1973; Hematology 1974; **Med School:** Columbia P&S 1958; **Resid:** Internal Medicine, Boston Med Ctr 1961; **Fellow:** Nephrology, Columbia-Presby Hosp 1963; **Fac Appt:** Clin Prof Med, Columbia P&S

Appel, Gerald B MD/PhD (Nep) - **Spec Exp:** Glomerulonephritis; Lupus Nephritis; Nephrotic Syndrome; **Hospital:** NY-Presby/Columbia Univ Med Ctr, NY (page 104); **Address:** 161 Fort Washington Ave Fl 2 - Ste 202, New York, NY 10032-3720; **Phone:** 212-305-0320 x3; **Board Cert:** Internal Medicine 1975; Nephrology 1978; **Med School:** Albert Einstein Coll Med 1972; **Resid:** Internal Medicine, Columbia Presby Hosp 1975; **Fellow:** Nephrology, Columbia Presby Hosp 1976; Nephrology, Yale-New Haven Hosp 1978; **Fac Appt:** Clin Prof Med, Columbia P&S

August, Phyllis MD (Nep) - **Spec Exp:** Hypertension; Hypertension in Pregnancy; Kidney Disease; **Hospital:** NY-Presby/Weill Cornell Med Ctr, NY (page 104); **Address:** NY Presby/Weill Cornell Med Ctr, Hypertension Center, 424 E 70th St, New York, NY 10021-4870; **Phone:** 646-962-2605; **Board Cert:** Internal Medicine 1980; Nephrology 1982; **Med School:** Yale Univ 1977; **Resid:** Internal Medicine, NY Hosp-Cornell Med Ctr 1980; **Fellow:** Nephrology, NY Hosp-Cornell Med Ctr 1983; **Fac Appt:** Prof Med, Cornell Univ-Weill Med Coll

Blumenfeld, Jon D MD (Nep) - **Spec Exp:** Polycystic Kidney Disease; Hypertension; Adrenal Disorders; **Hospital:** NY-Presby/Weill Cornell Med Ctr, NY (page 104), Rockefeller Univ; **Address:** The Rogosin Institute, 505 E 70th St, Fl 2, New York, NY 10021; **Phone:** 212-746-1495; **Board Cert:** Internal Medicine 1984; Nephrology 1986; **Med School:** Yale Univ 1981; **Resid:** Internal Medicine, New York Hosp 1984; **Fellow:** Nephrology, Brigham & Womens Hosp 1988; **Fac Appt:** Prof Med, Cornell Univ-Weill Med Coll

Cohen, David J MD (Nep) - **Spec Exp:** Transplant Medicine-Kidney; Glomerulonephritis; **Hospital:** NY-Presby/Columbia Univ Med Ctr, NY (page 104); **Address:** Columbia Univ Med Ctr, 622 W 168th St, rm PH 4-124, New York, NY 10032-3720; **Phone:** 212-305-0320 x4; **Board Cert:** Internal Medicine 1980; Nephrology 1984; **Med School:** Albert Einstein Coll Med 1977; **Resid:** Internal Medicine, Mount Sinai Hosp 1980; **Fellow:** Nephrology, Columbia-Presby Hosp 1981; Transplant Immunobiology, Brigham & Womens Hosp 1983; **Fac Appt:** Clin Prof Med, Columbia P&S

DeFabritus, Albert Michael MD (Nep) - **Spec Exp:** Kidney Disease-Chronic; Hypertension; Anemia in Chronic Kidney Disease; Kidney Stones; **Hospital:** Beth Israel Med Ctr - Petrie Div (page 94); **Address:** 352 7th Ave, Ste 1003, New York, NY 10001; **Phone:** 212-807-8817; **Board Cert:** Internal Medicine 1976; Nephrology 1978; **Med School:** NY Med Coll 1973; **Resid:** Internal Medicine, St Vincent's Hosp & Med Ctr 1976; **Fellow:** Nephrology, New York Hosp 1978; **Fac Appt:** Asst Clin Prof Med, NY Med Coll

DeVita, Maria V MD (Nep) - **Spec Exp:** Glomerulonephritis; Dialysis Care; Hypertension; Kidney Disease-Chronic; **Hospital:** Lenox Hill Hosp (page 106); **Address:** 130 E 77th St Fl 5, New York, NY 10075; **Phone:** 212-439-9251; **Board Cert:** Internal Medicine 1988; Nephrology 2012; **Med School:** Georgetown Univ 1984; **Resid:** Internal Medicine, Lenox Hill Hosp 1987; **Fellow:** Nephrology, Lenox Hill Hosp 1989; **Fac Appt:** Clin Prof Med, NYU Sch Med

Gardenswartz, Mark MD (Nep) - **Spec Exp:** Hypertension; Hypertension in Pregnancy; Polycystic Kidney Disease; **Hospital:** Lenox Hill Hosp (page 106), Mt Sinai Med Ctr (page 102); **Address:** 110 E 59th St, Ste 10B, New York, NY 10022; **Phone:** 212-583-2930; **Board Cert:** Internal Medicine 1978; Nephrology 1980; Critical Care Medicine 2002; **Med School:** Univ Colorado 1975; **Resid:** Internal Medicine, NY-Presby/Columbia Univ Med Ctr 1978; **Fellow:** Nephrology, Univ Colorado Hosp 1980; **Fac Appt:** Asst Clin Prof Med, NY Med Coll

Garvey, Michael MD (Nep) - **Spec Exp:** Dialysis Care; **Hospital:** Beth Israel Med Ctr - Petrie Div (page 94); **Address:** 510-526 6th Ave, Ste S-C, New York, NY 10011; **Phone:** 212-807-7920; **Board Cert:** Internal Medicine 1979; Nephrology 1982; **Med School:** NY Med Coll 1975; **Resid:** Internal Medicine, St Vincent's Hosp & Med Ctr 1979; **Fellow:** Nephrology, NYU Med Ctr 1981

Liu, David T MD (Nep) - **Spec Exp:** Glomerulonephritis; Nephrotic Syndrome; Kidney Failure; Hypertension; **Hospital:** NYU Langone Med Ctr (page 108); **Address:** 530 1st Ave, Ste 4B, New York, NY 10016-6402; **Phone:** 212-263-0705; **Board Cert:** Internal Medicine 1980; Nephrology 1984; **Med School:** SUNY Buffalo 1977; **Resid:** Internal Medicine, Univ Miami Hosps 1980; **Fellow:** Nephrology, NYU Med Ctr 1984; **Fac Appt:** Asst Clin Prof Med, NYU Sch Med

Matalon, Robert MD (Nep) - **Spec Exp:** Dialysis Care; Kidney Failure; **Hospital:** NYU Langone Med Ctr (page 108), NY-Presby/Lower Manhattan Hosp (page 104); **Address:** 530 1st Ave, Ste 4A, New York, NY 10016-6402; **Phone:** 212-263-7239; **Board Cert:** Internal Medicine 1970; Nephrology 1974; **Med School:** NYU Sch Med 1964; **Resid:** Internal Medicine, Bellevue Hosp 1967; **Fellow:** Nephrology, NYU Med Ctr 1969; **Fac Appt:** Assoc Prof Med, NYU Sch Med

Michelis, Michael F MD (Nep) - **Spec Exp:** Kidney Disease; Hypertension; Dialysis Care; **Hospital:** Lenox Hill Hosp (page 106); **Address:** 130 E 77th St, FL 5 Bldg, New York, NY 10075-1851; **Phone:** 212-988-3506; **Board Cert:** Internal Medicine 1969; **Med School:** Geo Wash Univ 1963; **Resid:** Internal Medicine, Lenox Hill Hosp 1965; Internal Medicine, Hosp Med Coll Penn 1967; **Fellow:** Renal Disease, Univ Pittsburgh 1970; **Fac Appt:** Clin Prof Med, NYU Sch Med

Radhakrishnan, Jai MD (Nep) - **Spec Exp:** Kidney Disease-Chronic; Glomerulonephritis; Lupus Nephritis; **Hospital:** NY-Presby/Columbia Univ Med Ctr, NY (page 104); **Address:** NY Presby Hosp/Columbia-Nephrology, 622 W 168 St, PH 4-124, New York, NY 10032; **Phone:** 212-305-5020; **Board Cert:** Internal Medicine 2013; Nephrology 2013; **Med School:** India 1984; **Resid:** Internal Medicine, Jawaharal Institute 1987; Internal Medicine, Lincoln Hosp 1990; **Fellow:** Nephrology, Mass Genl Hosp 1991; Nephrology, Columbia Univ Med Ctr 1993; **Fac Appt:** Prof Med, Columbia P&S

Saal, Stuart MD (Nep) - **Spec Exp:** Transplant Medicine-Kidney; **Hospital:** NY-Presby/Weill Cornell Med Ctr, NY (page 104); **Address:** 505 E 70th St, Ste 230, New York, NY 10021-4872; **Phone:** 212-746-1553; **Board Cert:** Internal Medicine 1974; Nephrology 1978; **Med School:** NY Med Coll 1971; **Resid:** Internal Medicine, St Luke's-Roosevelt Hosp Ctr 1974; **Fellow:** Nephrology, NY Hosp 1976; **Fac Appt:** Assoc Clin Prof Med, Cornell Univ-Weill Med Coll

Sherman, Raymond L MD (Nep) - **Spec Exp:** Glomerulonephritis; Hypertension; Kidney Failure-Chronic; **Hospital:** NY-Presby/Weill Cornell Med Ctr, NY (page 104); **Address:** 407 E 70th St Fl 4, New York, NY 10021-5302; **Phone:** 212-879-8245; **Board Cert:** Internal Medicine 1969; Nephrology 1974; **Med School:** SUNY Hlth Sci Ctr 1961; **Resid:** Internal Medicine, St Luke's-Roosevelt Hosp Ctr 1965; Nephrology, Strong Meml Hosp 1965; **Fellow:** Nephrology, NY Hosp/Cornell Med Ctr 1969; **Fac Appt:** Clin Prof Med, Cornell Univ-Weill Med Coll

Stern, Leonard MD (Nep) - **Spec Exp:** Kidney Failure-Chronic; Transplant Medicine-Kidney; Bone Disorders-Metabolic; Dialysis Care; **Hospital:** NY-Presby/Columbia Univ Med Ctr, NY (page 104); **Address:** 622 W 168th St, Room PH4-4124, New York, NY 10032-3702; **Phone:** 212-305-3273; **Board Cert:** Internal Medicine 1978; Nephrology 1980; **Med School:** NY Med Coll 1975; **Resid:** Internal Medicine, Jacobi Med Ctr 1978; **Fellow:** Nephrology, Montefiore Med Ctr 1979; Nephrology, Yale-New Haven Hosp 1981; **Fac Appt:** Assoc Prof Med, Columbia P&S

Wang, John C MD/PhD (Nep) - **Spec Exp:** Hypertension; **Hospital:** NY-Presby/Weill Cornell Med Ctr, NY (page 104); **Address:** 505 E 70th St, rm 213, New York, NY 10021; **Phone:** 212-746-3097; **Board Cert:** Internal Medicine 1985; Nephrology 1986; **Med School:** Cornell Univ-Weill Med Coll 1979; **Resid:** Internal Medicine, Laguardia Hosp 1982; **Fellow:** Nephrology, New York Hosp 1984; **Fac Appt:** Assoc Clin Prof Med, Cornell Univ-Weill Med Coll

Weisstuch, Joseph M MD (Nep) - **Hospital:** NYU Langone Med Ctr (page 108); **Address:** 530 1st Ave, Ste 4B, New York, NY 10016-6402; **Phone:** 212-263-0705; **Board Cert:** Internal Medicine 1988; Nephrology 2012; **Med School:** NYU Sch Med 1985; **Resid:** Internal Medicine, NYU Med Ctr 1989; **Fellow:** Nephrology, Bellevue Hosp 1991; **Fac Appt:** Asst Clin Prof Med, NYU Sch Med

Williams, Gail S MD (Nep) - **Spec Exp:** Kidney Failure-Chronic; Transplant Medicine-Kidney; Hypertension; **Hospital:** NY-Presby/Columbia Univ Med Ctr, NY (page 104); **Address:** NY-Presby, Neurology Dept, 161 Fort Washington Ave, Ste 351, New York, NY 10032; **Phone:** 212-305-5376; **Board Cert:** Internal Medicine 1972; Nephrology 1974; **Med School:** Columbia P&S 1968; **Resid:** Internal Medicine, NY-Presby/Columbia Univ Med Ctr 1973; **Fellow:** Nephrology, NY-Presby/Columbia Univ Med Ctr 1974; **Fac Appt:** Assoc Clin Prof Med, Columbia P&S

Winston, Jonathan MD (Nep) - **Spec Exp:** Kidney Disease-Chronic; Kidney Failure; HIV Related Kidney Disease; Glomerulonephritis; **Hospital:** Mt Sinai Med Ctr (page 102); **Address:** 5 E 98th St Fl 11, New York, NY 10029-6501; **Phone:** 212-241-4060; **Board Cert:** Internal Medicine 1980; Nephrology 1984; **Med School:** Geo Wash Univ 1977; **Resid:** Internal Medicine, LI Jewish Med Ctr 1980; **Fellow:** Nephrology, Mt Sinai Hosp 1982; **Fac Appt:** Assoc Prof Med, Mount Sinai Sch Med

Neurological Surgery

Anderson, Richard CE MD (NS) - **Spec Exp:** Spinal Disorders; Spina Bifida; Peripheral Nerve Surgery; Pediatric Neurosurgery; **Hospital:** Morgan Stanley Children's Hosp of NY-Presby, NY (page 104), St. Joseph's Regl Med Ctr - Paterson; **Address:** Morgan Stanley Children's Hosp, The Neurological Institute, 710 W 168th St, rm 213, New York, NY 10032; **Phone:** 212-305-0219; **Board Cert:** Neurological Surgery 2007; Pediatric Neurological Surgery 2008; **Med School:** Johns Hopkins Univ 1997; **Resid:** Neurological Surgery, Columbia Neuro Inst 2004; **Fellow:** Pediatric Neurological Surgery, Univ Utah Med Ctr 2005; **Fac Appt:** Prof NS, Columbia P&S

Angevine, Peter D MD (NS) - **Spec Exp:** Spinal Surgery; Pediatric Neurosurgery; Scoliosis; Spinal Deformity; **Hospital:** NY-Presby/Columbia Univ Med Ctr, NY (page 104), Morgan Stanley Children's Hosp of NY-Presby, NY (page 104); **Address:** Columbia Neurological Surgery, Neurological Institute, 710 W 168th St, rm 502, New York, NY 10032; **Phone:** 212-305-1550; **Board Cert:** Neurological Surgery 2008; **Med School:** Columbia P&S 1998; **Resid:** Neurological Surgery, Columbia Presby Med Ctr 2004; **Fellow:** Spine Surgery, Barnes Jewish Hosp 2005; **Fac Appt:** Asst Prof NS, Columbia P&S

Bederson, Joshua B MD (NS) - **Spec Exp:** Brain & Spinal Cord Tumors; Aneurysm-Cerebral; Meningioma; Cerebrovascular Surgery; **Hospital:** Mt Sinai Med Ctr (page 102); **Address:** Mount Sinai Med Ctr, 1 Gustave Levy Pl, Box 1136, New York, NY 10029; **Phone:** 212-241-2377; **Board Cert:** Neurological Surgery 1993; **Med School:** UCSF 1984; **Resid:** Neurological Surgery, UCSF Med Ctr 1990; **Fellow:** Neurovascular Surgery, Barrow Neur Inst 1990; Neurovascular Surgery, Univ Hosp Zurich 1990; **Fac Appt:** Prof NS, Mount Sinai Sch Med

Bilsky, Mark H MD (NS) - **Spec Exp:** Brain & Spinal Cord Tumors; Skull Base Tumors; Spinal Cord Tumors; Spinal Surgery; **Hospital:** Meml Sloan-Kettering Canc Ctr (page 114), NY-Presby/Weill Cornell Med Ctr, NY (page 104); **Address:** Meml Sloan Kettering Cancer Ctr-Neurosurgery, 1275 York Ave, Ste C705, New York, NY 10065; **Phone:** 212-639-8526; **Board Cert:** Neurological Surgery 2010; **Med School:** Emory Univ 1988; **Resid:** Neurological Surgery, NY Hosp-Cornell Med Ctr 1994; **Fellow:** Neurological Surgery, Louisville Univ Med Ctr 1995; Spine Surgery, Louisville Univ Med Ctr 1995; **Fac Appt:** Prof NS, Cornell Univ-Weill Med Coll

Boockvar, John A MD (NS) - **Spec Exp:** Brain & Spinal Surgery; Meningioma; Metastatic Cancer; Minimally Invasive Surgery; **Hospital:** NY-Presby/Weill Cornell Med Ctr, NY (page 104); **Address:** 525 E 68 St, Box 99, New York, NY 10065; **Phone:** 212-746-1996; **Board Cert:** Neurological Surgery 2007; **Med School:** SUNY Downstate 1997; **Resid:** Neurological Surgery, Hosp Univ Penn 2003; **Fellow:** Neuro-Oncology, Univ Penn Cancer Ctr 2004; **Fac Appt:** Prof NS, Cornell Univ-Weill Med Coll

Bruce, Jeffrey N MD (NS) - **Spec Exp:** Brain Tumors-Complex; Pituitary Tumors; Skull Base Surgery; Meningioma; **Hospital:** NY-Presby/Columbia Univ Med Ctr, NY (page 104); **Address:** Neurological Inst, 710 W 168th St N1 Bldg Fl 4 - rm 434, New York, NY 10032; **Phone:** 212-305-7346; **Board Cert:** Neurological Surgery 1993; **Med School:** UMDNJ-RW Johnson Med Sch 1983; **Resid:** Neurological Surgery, Columbia-Presby Med Ctr 1990; **Fellow:** Neurological Surgery, Nat Inst Hlth 1985; **Fac Appt:** Prof NS, Columbia P&S

Chen, Chun Siang MD (NS) - **Spec Exp:** Skull Base Tumors; Skull Base Surgery; Microsurgery; Brain & Spinal Cord Tumors; **Hospital:** Mt Sinai Med Ctr (page 102); **Address:** Mount Sinai Med Ctr, Annenberg Bldg, One Gustave L Levy Pl, Fl 8, rm 10, New York, NY 10029; **Phone:** 212-241-8480; **Med School:** Brazil 1978; **Resid:** Neurological Surgery, Santa Casa de Misericordia of Sao Paulo Med Sch 1983; Neurological Surgery, Mt Sinai Med Ctr 2005; **Fellow:** Skull Base Surgery, St Lukes Roosevelt Hosp 2006; **Fac Appt:** Asst Prof NS, Mount Sinai Sch Med

Choudhri, Tanvir F MD (NS) - **Spec Exp:** Spinal Surgery; Minimally Invasive Surgery; Spinal Tumors; Spinal Disorders-Degenerative; **Hospital:** Mt Sinai Med Ctr (page 102); **Address:** Mt Sinai, Neurological Surgery, 5 E 98th St Fl 7, Box 1136, New York, NY 10029; **Phone:** 212-241-8560; **Board Cert:** Neurological Surgery 2007; **Med School:** Columbia P&S 1994; **Resid:** Neurological Surgery, NY-Presby/Columbia Univ Med Ctr 2001; **Fellow:** Spine Surgery, Barrow Neurological Inst 2002; **Fac Appt:** Asst Prof NS, Mount Sinai Sch Med

Di Giacinto, George V MD (NS) - **Spec Exp:** Spinal Surgery; Pain Management; **Hospital:** St. Luke's - Roosevelt Hosp Ctr - Roosevelt Div (page 94); **Address:** 425 W 59th St, Ste 4E, New York, NY 10019; **Phone:** 212-523-8500; **Board Cert:** Neurological Surgery 1981; **Med School:** Harvard Med Sch 1970; **Resid:** Surgery, St Luke's-Roosevelt Hosp Ctr 1972; Neurological Surgery, Columbia-Presby Hosp 1978

Doyle, Werner K MD (NS) - **Spec Exp:** Epilepsy; **Hospital:** NYU Langone Med Ctr (page 108); **Address:** NYU Comprehensive Epilepsy Ctr, 223 E 34th St, New York, NY 10016; **Phone:** 646-558-0804; **Board Cert:** Neurological Surgery 1995; **Med School:** Columbia P&S 1982; **Resid:** Surgery, Roosevelt Hosp Ctr 1985; Neurological Surgery, NYU Med Ctr 1991; **Fellow:** Epilepsy, Yale Med Sch 1992; **Fac Appt:** Assoc Prof NS, NYU Sch Med

Feldstein, Neil A MD (NS) - **Spec Exp:** Brain & Spinal Tumors-Pediatric; MoyaMoya Disease; Chiari's Deformity; Hydrocephalus; **Hospital:** Morgan Stanley Children's Hosp of NY-Presby, NY (page 104), NY-Presby/Columbia Univ Med Ctr, NY (page 104); **Address:** Neurological Inst, 710 W 168th St, Fl 2, rm 213, New York, NY 10032; **Phone:** 212-305-1396; **Board Cert:** Neurological Surgery 1995; **Med School:** NYU Sch Med 1984; **Resid:** Neurological Surgery, Baylor Coll Med 1990; **Fellow:** Pediatric Neurological Surgery, NYU Med Ctr 1991; **Fac Appt:** Assoc Prof NS, Columbia P&S

Frempong-Boadu, Anthony K MD (NS) - **Spec Exp:** Minimally Invasive Spinal Surgery; Spinal Reconstructive Surgery; Spinal Cord Tumors; Spinal Reconstructive Surgery; **Hospital:** NYU Langone Med Ctr (page 108); **Address:** 530 1st Ave, Skirball Bldg - Fl 8 - Ste S, New York, NY 10016; **Phone:** 212-263-6514; **Board Cert:** Neurological Surgery 2004; **Med School:** Temple Univ 1992; **Resid:** Neurological Surgery, NYU Med Ctr 1999; **Fellow:** Spine Surgery, NYU Med Ctr 1997; Minimally Invasive Surgery, Univ Florida/Shands Hosp 2000; **Fac Appt:** Assoc Prof NS, NYU Sch Med

Gamache Jr, Francis W MD (NS) - **Spec Exp:** Brain & Spinal Cord Tumors; Spinal Surgery-Neck; **Hospital:** NY-Presby/Weill Cornell Med Ctr, NY (page 104), Hosp For Special Surgery (page 113); **Address:** 523 E 72nd St Fl 8, New York, NY 10021-4099; **Phone:** 212-988-5200; **Board Cert:** Neurological Surgery 1982; **Med School:** Cornell Univ-Weill Med Coll 1971; **Resid:** Surgery, NY Hosp-Cornell Med Ctr 1975; Neurological Surgery, NY Hosp-Cornell Med Ctr 1979; **Fellow:** Trauma, MD Inst Emerg Med Serv 1979; Neurovascular Surgery, Univ West Ontario 1980; **Fac Appt:** Clin Prof NS, Cornell Univ-Weill Med Coll

Ghatan, Saadi MD (NS) - **Spec Exp:** Pediatric Neurosurgery; Epilepsy; Neuro-Endoscopy; Cerebrovascular Disease; **Hospital:** Beth Israel Med Ctr - Petrie Div (page 94); **Address:** 1000 Tenth Ave, Ste 5G-49, New York, NY 10019; **Phone:** 212-636-3204; **Board Cert:** Neurological Surgery 2007; **Med School:** Univ Wash 1993; **Resid:** Surgery, Univ Washington Med Ctr 1994; Neurological Surgery, Univ Washington Med Ctr 2001; **Fellow:** Pediatric Neurological Surgery, Chldn's Hosp 2002; Pediatric Neurological Surgery, Great Ormond Street Hosp 2003

Golfinos, John G MD (NS) - **Spec Exp:** Brain Tumors; Skull Base Tumors; **Hospital:** NYU Langone Med Ctr (page 108), Bellevue Hosp Ctr; **Address:** 530 First Ave, Ste 8R, New York, NY 10016; **Phone:** 212-263-2950; **Board Cert:** Neurological Surgery 1998; **Med School:** Columbia P&S 1988; **Resid:** Neurological Surgery, Barrow Neuro Inst 1995; **Fac Appt:** Assoc Prof NS, NYU Sch Med

Goodman, Robert R MD/PhD (NS) - **Spec Exp:** Parkinson's Disease/Movement Disorders; Epilepsy; Trigeminal Neuralgia; Hydrocephalus-Adult; **Hospital:** St. Luke's - Roosevelt Hosp Ctr - Roosevelt Div (page 94), Beth Israel Med Ctr - Petrie Div (page 94); **Address:** 1000 Tenth Ave, Ste 5G-80, New York, NY 10019; **Phone:** 212-636-3666; **Board Cert:** Neurological Surgery 1993; **Med School:** Johns Hopkins Univ 1982; **Resid:** Neurological Surgery, Columbia-Presby Med Ctr 1989; **Fac Appt:** Assoc Prof NS, Columbia P&S

Gutin, Philip H MD (NS) - **Spec Exp:** Brain Tumors; Meningioma; Acoustic Neuroma; **Hospital:** Meml Sloan-Kettering Canc Ctr (page 114), NY-Presby/Weill Cornell Med Ctr, NY (page 104); **Address:** 1275 York Ave, rm C703, New York, NY 10065; **Phone:** 212-639-8556; **Board Cert:** Neurological Surgery 1981; **Med School:** Univ Pennsylvania 1971; **Resid:** Neurological Surgery, UCSF Med Ctr 1979; **Fellow:** Neurological Surgery, Natl Cancer Inst 1976; **Fac Appt:** Prof NS, Cornell Univ-Weill Med Coll

Hartl, Roger MD (NS) - **Spec Exp:** Spinal Surgery-Complex; Minimally Invasive Spinal Surgery; Spinal Disc Replacement; Spinal Trauma; **Hospital:** NY-Presby/Weill Cornell Med Ctr, NY (page 104); **Address:** Cornell Neurosurgery, 520 E 70th St, Starr Pavillion Fl 6 - rm 651, New York, NY 10065; **Phone:** 212-746-2152; **Board Cert:** Neurological Surgery 2008; **Med School:** Germany 1993; **Resid:** Neurological Surgery, NY Presby-Cornell Med Ctr 2003; **Fellow:** Spine Surgery, Barrow Neurological Inst 2004; **Fac Appt:** Assoc Prof NS, Cornell Univ-Weill Med Coll

Jafar, Jafar J MD (NS) - **Spec Exp:** Aneurysm-Cerebral; Brain Tumors; Skull Base Tumors; Acoustic Neuroma; **Hospital:** NYU Langone Med Ctr (page 108), Lenox Hill Hosp (page 106); **Address:** 530 1st Ave, Ste 7W, New York, NY 10016-6402; **Phone:** 212-263-6312; **Board Cert:** Neurological Surgery 1984; **Med School:** Iran 1976; **Resid:** Neurological Surgery, Univ Chicago Hosps 1982; Neurological Surgery, Natl Hosp for Nervous Disease; **Fac Appt:** Prof NS, NYU Sch Med

Jenkins III, Arthur L MD (NS) - **Spec Exp:** Spinal Surgery; Minimally Invasive Spinal Surgery; Scoliosis; Spinal Tumors; **Hospital:** Mt Sinai Med Ctr (page 102); **Address:** Faculty Practice Assocs, 5 E 98th St, Fl 7, Box 1136, New York, NY 10029; **Phone:** 212-241-8175; **Board Cert:** Neurological Surgery 2005; **Med School:** Univ Pennsylvania 1993; **Resid:** Neurological Surgery, Mtount Sinai Med Ctr 2000; **Fellow:** Spine Surgery, Brigham & Women's Hosp 2001; **Fac Appt:** Assoc Prof NS, Mount Sinai Sch Med

Kaiser, Michael G MD (NS) - **Spec Exp:** Spinal Surgery-Complex; Minimally Invasive Spinal Surgery; Spinal Disc Replacement; Spinal Cord Tumors; **Hospital:** NY-Presby/Columbia Univ Med Ctr, NY (page 104); **Address:** Neurological Institute, Dept Neurological Surgery, 710 W 168th St, New York, NY 10032; **Phone:** 212-305-0378; **Board Cert:** Neurological Surgery 2004; **Med School:** Yale Univ 1994; **Resid:** Neurological Surgery, Columbia Neuro Inst 2000; **Fellow:** Spine Surgery, Emory Univ 2001; **Fac Appt:** Assoc Prof NS, Columbia P&S

Kondziolka, Douglas MD (NS) - **Spec Exp:** Brain Tumors-Adult & Pediatric; Brain Tumors-Metastatic; Stereotactic Radiosurgery; Movement Disorders; **Hospital:** NYU Langone Med Ctr (page 108); **Address:** 530 First Ave, Ste 8R, New York, NY 10016; **Phone:** 646-501-2360; **Board Cert:** Neurological Surgery 1994; **Med School:** Univ Toronto 1985; **Resid:** Neurological Surgery, Univ Toronto Affil Hosp 1989; **Fellow:** Stereotactic Neurological Surgery, Univ Pittsburgh Med Ctr 1991

Langer, David J MD (NS) - **Spec Exp:** Neurovascular Surgery; Arteriovenous Malformations; Aneurysm-Cerebral; Carotid Artery Surgery; **Hospital:** Lenox Hill Hosp (page 106), N Shore Univ Hosp (page 106); **Address:** Lenox Hill Hosp, 100 E 77th St, New York, NY 10075; **Phone:** 212-434-3900; **Board Cert:** Neurological Surgery 2003; **Med School:** Univ Pennsylvania 1991; **Resid:** Neurological Surgery, Hosp Univ Penn 1998; **Fellow:** Neurovascular Surgery, Beth Israel Med Ctr 1999; **Fac Appt:** Asst Prof NS, Albert Einstein Coll Med

Lavyne, Michael H MD (NS) - **Spec Exp:** Spinal Cord Tumors; **Hospital:** NY-Presby/Weill Cornell Med Ctr, NY (page 104), Hosp For Special Surgery (page 113); **Address:** 110 E 55th St Fl 9, MS 10022, New York, NY 10022; **Phone:** 212-486-9100; **Board Cert:** Neurological Surgery 1982; **Med School:** Cornell Univ-Weill Med Coll 1972; **Resid:** Neurological Surgery, Mass Genl Hosp 1979; **Fellow:** Neurology, Beth Israel Hosp 1974; **Fac Appt:** Clin Prof NS, Cornell Univ-Weill Med Coll

McCormick, Paul C MD (NS) - **Spec Exp:** Spinal Surgery; Spinal Tumors; Arteriovenous Malformations; **Hospital:** NY-Presby/Columbia Univ Med Ctr, NY (page 104); **Address:** 710 W 168th St, Ste 506, New York, NY 10032-2603; **Phone:** 212-305-7976; **Board Cert:** Neurological Surgery 1993; **Med School:** Columbia P&S 1982; **Resid:** Neurological Surgery, Columbia Presby Med Ctr 1989; **Fellow:** Neurological Surgery, Natl Inst Hlth 1984; Spine Surgery, John Doyne Hosp 1990; **Fac Appt:** Prof NS, Columbia P&S

McKhann II, Guy M MD (NS) - **Spec Exp:** Brain Tumors; Epilepsy; **Hospital:** NY-Presby/Columbia Univ Med Ctr, NY (page 104); **Address:** 710 W 168th St, Ste 411, New York, NY 10032; **Phone:** 212-305-0052; **Board Cert:** Neurological Surgery 2004; **Med School:** Yale Univ 1990; **Resid:** Neurological Surgery, Univ Wash Med Ctr 1998; Neurological Surgery, Atkinson Morley's Hosp 1995; **Fellow:** Epilepsy, Univ Wash Med Ctr 1999; **Fac Appt:** Assoc Prof NS, Columbia P&S

Patel, Aman B MD (NS) - **Spec Exp:** Interventional Neuroradiology; Endovascular Neurosurgery; Aneurysm-Cerebral; Arteriovenous Malformations; **Hospital:** Mt Sinai Med Ctr (page 102); **Address:** 14668 Madison Ave Fl 8th - rm 40, New York, NY 10029; **Phone:** 212-241-3457; **Board Cert:** Neurological Surgery 2004; **Med School:** UCLA 1993; **Resid:** Neurological Surgery, UCLA Med Ctr 1999; **Fellow:** Interventional Neuroradiology, UCLA Med Ctr 2001; **Fac Appt:** Assoc Prof NS, Mount Sinai Sch Med

Perin, Noel I MD (NS) - **Spec Exp:** Spinal Surgery-Minimally Invasive; Spinal Tumors; **Hospital:** NYU Langone Med Ctr (page 108); **Address:** NYU Langone Med Ctr, Neurosurgery, 530 First Ave, Ste 8S, New York, NY 10016; **Phone:** 212-263-5732; **Board Cert:** Neurological Surgery 1995; **Med School:** Sri Lanka 1973; **Resid:** Neurological Surgery, NYU Med Ctr 1990; **Fellow:** Spine Surgery, NYU Med Ctr 1991; **Fac Appt:** Asst Prof NS, NYU Sch Med

Post, Kalmon D MD (NS) - **Spec Exp:** Pituitary Tumors; Acoustic Neuroma; Meningioma; **Hospital:** Mt Sinai Med Ctr (page 102); **Address:** 5 E 98th St, Fl 7, New York, NY 10029-6501; **Phone:** 212-241-0933; **Board Cert:** Neurological Surgery 1978; **Med School:** NYU Sch Med 1967; **Resid:** Surgery, Bellevue Hosp 1969; Neurological Surgery, Bellevue Hosp-NYU 1975; **Fac Appt:** Prof NS, Mount Sinai Sch Med

Quest, Donald O MD (NS) - **Spec Exp:** Spinal Surgery; Neurovascular Surgery; Carotid Artery Surgery; **Hospital:** NY-Presby/Columbia Univ Med Ctr, NY (page 104), Valley Hosp (page 721); **Address:** 710 W 168th St, Ste 440, New York, NY 10032; **Phone:** 212-305-5582; **Board Cert:** Neurological Surgery 1978; **Med School:** Columbia P&S 1970; **Resid:** Surgery, Mass Genl Hosp 1972; Neurological Surgery, Columbia-Presby Hosp 1976; **Fac Appt:** Clin Prof NS, Columbia P&S

Riina, Howard A MD (NS) - **Spec Exp:** Neuroradiology; Aneurysm-Cerebral; Cerebrovascular Malformations; Stroke; **Hospital:** NYU Langone Med Ctr (page 108); **Address:** NYU Langone Med Ctr, 530 First Ave, SK1, Ste 8R, New York, NY 10016; **Phone:** 212-263-5382; **Board Cert:** Neurological Surgery 2004; **Med School:** Temple Univ 1993; **Resid:** Neurological Surgery, Hosp Univ Penn 2000; **Fellow:** Interventional Neuroradiology, Beth Israel Med Ctr 1997; Skull Base Surgery, Barrow Neuro Inst 2001; **Fac Appt:** Prof NS, NYU Sch Med

Schwartz, Theodore H MD (NS) - **Spec Exp:** Brain Tumors; Pituitary Tumors; Minimally Invasive Surgery; **Hospital:** NY-Presby/Weill Cornell Med Ctr, NY (page 104); **Address:** Weill Cornell Med Ctr-Neurosurgery Dept, 525 E 68th St, rm 651, Starr Pavilion, Box 99, New York, NY 10065; **Phone:** 212-746-5620; **Board Cert:** Neurological Surgery 2013; **Med School:** Harvard Med Sch 1993; **Resid:** Neurological Surgery, Columbia-Presby Med Ctr 1999; **Fellow:** Neurological Surgery, Yale-New Haven Med Ctr 2000; **Fac Appt:** Prof NS, Cornell Univ-Weill Med Coll

Sen, Chandranath MD (NS) - **Spec Exp:** Brain Tumors; Skull Base Tumors; Meningioma; **Hospital:** NYU Langone Med Ctr (page 108); **Address:** NYU Langone Med Ctr-Dept Neurosurgery, 530 First Ave, Ste 8R, New York, NY 10016; **Phone:** 212-263-5333; **Board Cert:** Neurological Surgery 1989; **Med School:** India 1976; **Resid:** Surgery, Univ Wisconsin Hosps 1980; Neurological Surgery, Univ Wisconsin Hosps 1985; **Fellow:** Neurological Surgery, Univ Pittsburgh Med Ctr 1986; **Fac Appt:** Prof NS, Mount Sinai Sch Med

Sisti, Michael B MD (NS) - **Spec Exp:** Brain Tumors-Complex; Meningioma; Arteriovenous Malformations; **Hospital:** NY-Presby/Columbia Univ Med Ctr, NY (page 104); **Address:** Neurological Inst, 710 W 168th St, Ste 413, New York, NY 10032-2603; **Phone:** 212-305-1728; **Board Cert:** Neurological Surgery 1991; **Med School:** Columbia P&S 1981; **Resid:** Neurological Surgery, NY-Presby/Columbia Med Ctr 1988; **Fellow:** Neurological Surgery, Natl Inst Hlth 1983; **Fac Appt:** Assoc Prof NS, Columbia P&S

Snow, Robert B MD (NS) - **Spec Exp:** Spinal Surgery; Spinal Cord Tumors; Minimally Invasive Surgery; **Hospital:** NY-Presby/Weill Cornell Med Ctr, NY (page 104); **Address:** 55 E 72nd St Fl 1st, New York, NY 10021-4099; **Phone:** 212-717-0256; **Board Cert:** Neurological Surgery 1989; **Med School:** Stanford Univ 1981; **Resid:** Neurological Surgery, New York Hosp 1986; **Fac Appt:** Prof NS, Cornell Univ-Weill Med Coll

Solomon, Robert A MD (NS) - **Spec Exp:** Aneurysm-Cerebral; Arteriovenous Malformations; **Hospital:** NY-Presby/Columbia Univ Med Ctr, NY (page 104); **Address:** 710 W 168th St, Ste 439, New York, NY 10032; **Phone:** 212-305-4118; **Board Cert:** Neurological Surgery 1988; **Med School:** Johns Hopkins Univ 1980; **Resid:** Neurological Surgery, Neuro Inst-Columbia 1986; **Fac Appt:** Prof NS, Columbia P&S

Souweidane, Mark M MD (NS) - **Spec Exp:** Pediatric Neurosurgery; Minimally Invasive Surgery; Endoscopic Surgery; Brain Tumors-Pediatric; **Hospital:** NY-Presby/Weill Cornell Med Ctr, NY (page 104), Meml Sloan-Kettering Canc Ctr (page 114); **Address:** Weill Cornell Med Ctr-Neurosurgery Dept, 525 E 68th St, Ste 651, Starr Pavilion, Box 99, New York, NY 10065-4870; **Phone:** 212-746-2363; **Board Cert:** Neurological Surgery 2010; **Med School:** Wayne State Univ 1988; **Resid:** Neurological Surgery, NYU Med Ctr 1994; **Fellow:** Pediatric Neurological Surgery, Hosp Sick Chldn 1995; **Fac Appt:** Prof NS, Cornell Univ-Weill Med Coll

Stieg, Philip E MD/PhD (NS) - **Spec Exp:** Aneurysm-Cerebral; Stroke; Meningioma; Arteriovenous Malformations; **Hospital:** NY-Presby/Weill Cornell Med Ctr, NY (page 104); **Address:** Weill Cornell Med Ctr-Neurosurgery Dept, 525 E 68th St, Ste 651, Starr Pavilion, Box 99, New York, NY 10065; **Phone:** 212-746-1349; **Board Cert:** Neurological Surgery 1992; **Med School:** Med Coll Wisc 1983; **Resid:** Neurological Surgery, Parkland Meml Hosp/Dallas Chldns Hosp 1989; **Fellow:** Neurological Biology, Karolinska Inst 1988; **Fac Appt:** Prof NS, Cornell Univ-Weill Med Coll

Sundaresan, Narayan MD (NS) - **Spec Exp:** Spinal Surgery; Brain Tumors; Neuro-Oncology; **Hospital:** Mt Sinai Med Ctr (page 102), Bronx Lebanon Hosp Ctr; **Address:** Central Park Neurosurgery, 1148 5th Ave, New York, NY 10128; **Phone:** 212-876-7575; **Board Cert:** Neurological Surgery 1980; **Med School:** India 1969; **Resid:** Neurological Surgery, Northwestern Meml Hosp 1976; **Fellow:** Neuro-Oncology, Meml Sloan Kettering Cancer Ctr 1977; **Fac Appt:** Prof NS, Mount Sinai Sch Med

Tabar, Viviane MD (NS) - **Spec Exp:** Brain Tumors; **Hospital:** Meml Sloan-Kettering Canc Ctr (page 114); **Address:** 1275 York Ave, rm C711, New York, NY 10065; **Phone:** 212-639-3006; **Board Cert:** Neurological Surgery 2006; **Med School:** Amer Univ Beirut 1989; **Resid:** Neurological Surgery, Univ Mass Med Ctr 1998

Weiner, Howard L MD (NS) - **Spec Exp:** Pediatric Neurosurgery; Epilepsy; Tuberous Sclerosis; **Hospital:** NYU Langone Med Ctr (page 108); **Address:** NYU Med Ctr, Div Pediatric Neurosurgery, 317 E 34th St, Ste 1002, New York, NY 10016; **Phone:** 212-263-6419; **Board Cert:** Neurological Surgery 2012; **Med School:** Cornell Univ 1989; **Resid:** Neurological Surgery, NYU Med Ctr 1996; **Fellow:** Pediatric Neurological Surgery, NYU Med Ctr 1997; **Fac Appt:** Prof NS, NYU Sch Med

Winfree, Christopher J MD (NS) - **Spec Exp:** Peripheral Nerve Surgery; Pain-Chronic; Microsurgery; **Hospital:** NY-Presby/Columbia Univ Med Ctr, NY (page 104); **Address:** Neurological Institute, Dept Neurological Surgery, 710 W 168th St, Fl 4, New York, NY 10032; **Phone:** 212-342-2776; **Board Cert:** Neurological Surgery 2007; **Med School:** Columbia P&S 1996; **Resid:** Neurological Surgery, Neurological Inst 2003; **Fellow:** Peripheral Nerve Surgery, LSU Med Ctr 2004; Stereotactic Neurological Surgery, Oregon Hlth & Science Univ 2005; **Fac Appt:** Asst Prof NS, Columbia P&S

Wisoff, Jeffrey H MD (NS) - **Spec Exp:** Pediatric Neurosurgery; Brain Tumors-Pediatric; Arteriovenous Malformations; **Hospital:** NYU Langone Med Ctr (page 108), Maimonides Med Ctr (page 98); **Address:** 317 E 34th St, Ste 1002, New York, NY 10016-4974; **Phone:** 212-263-6419; **Board Cert:** Neurological Surgery 1990; Pediatric Neurological Surgery 2008; **Med School:** Geo Wash Univ 1978; **Resid:** Neurological Surgery, NYU/Bellevue Hosp 1984; **Fellow:** Pediatric Neurological Surgery, NYU Med Ctr 1985; **Fac Appt:** Assoc Prof NS, NYU Sch Med

Neurology

Apatoff, Brian R MD/PhD (N) - **Spec Exp:** Multiple Sclerosis; Neuro-Immunology; **Hospital:** NY-Presby/Weill Cornell Med Ctr, NY (page 104); **Address:** Multiple Sclerosis Institute, 401 E 55th St, New York, NY 10022; **Phone:** 212-593-6262; **Board Cert:** Neurology 1991; **Med School:** Univ Chicago-Pritzker Sch Med 1984; **Resid:** Neurology, Columbia Presby Med Ctr 1990; **Fellow:** Multiple Sclerosis, Neuro Inst-Columbia Univ 1992; **Fac Appt:** Assoc Prof N, Cornell Univ-Weill Med Coll

Balcer, Laura J MD (N) - **Spec Exp:** Neuro-Ophthalmology; Multiple Sclerosis/Visual Disorders; Parkinson's Disease/Visual Disorders; **Hospital:** NYU Langone Med Ctr (page 108); **Address:** NYU Dept Neurology, 240 E 38th St Fl 15, New York, NY 10016; **Phone:** 646-501-7681; **Board Cert:** Neurology 2006; **Med School:** Johns Hopkins Univ 1991; **Resid:** Neurology, Hosp Univ Penn 1995; **Fellow:** Neuro-Ophthalmology, Hosp Univ Penn/Scheie Inst 1995; **Fac Appt:** Prof N, NYU Sch Med

Belok, Lennart C MD (N) - **Spec Exp:** Carpal Tunnel Syndrome; **Hospital:** Beth Israel Med Ctr - Petrie Div (page 94); **Address:** 410 E 20th St, New York, NY 10009-8113; **Phone:** 212-254-9716; **Board Cert:** Internal Medicine 1977; Neurology 1983; **Med School:** NY Med Coll 1973; **Resid:** Internal Medicine, Beth Israel Med Ctr 1976; Neurology, NYU Med Ctr 1979

Brannagan III, Thomas H MD (N) - **Spec Exp:** Peripheral Neuropathy; Diabetic Neuropathy; **Hospital:** NY-Presby/Columbia Univ Med Ctr, NY (page 104); **Address:** Ciolumbia Univ Dept Neurology, 710 W 168th St, New York, NY 10032; **Phone:** 212-305-0405; **Board Cert:** Neurology 2005; Clinical Neurophysiology 2009; **Med School:** Univ VA Sch Med 1990; **Resid:** Neurology, Columbia-Presby Med Ctr 1994; **Fac Appt:** Prof N, Columbia P&S

Bressman, Susan MD (N) - **Spec Exp:** Parkinson's Disease; Movement Disorders; Dystonia; **Hospital:** Beth Israel Med Ctr - Petrie Div (page 94); **Address:** 10 Union Square East, Ste 5H, New York, NY 10003-3314; **Phone:** 212-844-8379; **Board Cert:** Neurology 1983; **Med School:** Columbia P&S 1977; **Resid:** Neurology, Columbia-Presby Med Ctr 1981; **Fellow:** Movement Disorders, Columbia-Presby Med Ctr 1983; **Fac Appt:** Prof N, Albert Einstein Coll Med

Britton, Carolyn B MD (N) - **Spec Exp:** Neurologic Complications-HIV/Infections; Lyme Disease; Multiple Sclerosis; **Hospital:** NY-Presby/Columbia Univ Med Ctr, NY (page 104); **Address:** 710 W 168th St, Ste 232, New York, NY 10032-2603; **Phone:** 212-305-5220; **Board Cert:** Internal Medicine 1979; Neurology 1982; **Med School:** NYU Sch Med 1975; **Resid:** Internal Medicine, Harlem Hosp 1977; Neurology, Columbia-Presby Hosp 1980; **Fellow:** Neurology, Columbia-Presby Hosp 1983; **Fac Appt:** Assoc Prof N, Columbia P&S

Bronster, David J MD (N) - **Spec Exp:** Headache; Dizziness; Seizure Disorders; **Hospital:** Mt Sinai Med Ctr (page 102); **Address:** 3 E 83rd St, New York, NY 10028-0459; **Phone:** 212-772-0008; **Board Cert:** Neurology 1984; **Med School:** Mount Sinai Sch Med 1979; **Resid:** Neurology, Mount Sinai Hosp 1983; **Fac Appt:** Assoc Clin Prof N, Mount Sinai Sch Med

Cafferty, Maureen S MD (N) - **Hospital:** St. Luke's - Roosevelt Hosp Ctr - Roosevelt Div (page 94); **Address:** St Lukes-Roosevelt Hosp-Neuro Clinic, 440 W 114th St, New York, NY 10025-1737; **Phone:** 212-523-4480; **Board Cert:** Internal Medicine 1982; Neurology 1987; **Med School:** Columbia P&S 1979; **Resid:** Internal Medicine, St Luke's-Roosevelt Hosp Ctr 1982; Neurology, Columbia-Presby Hosp 1985; **Fac Appt:** Asst Prof N, Columbia P&S

Carver, Alan C MD (N) - **Spec Exp:** Palliative Care; Pain-Cancer; Headache; Pain Management; **Hospital:** Meml Sloan-Kettering Canc Ctr (page 114); **Address:** Meml Sloan Kettering Cancer Ctr, 1275 York Ave, New York, NY 10065; **Phone:** 212-639-4851; **Board Cert:** Neurology 2011; Hospice & Palliative Medicine ; **Med School:** Boston Univ 1995; **Resid:** Neurology, NY Hosp Cornell Med Ctr 1999; **Fellow:** Pain & Palliative Care, Meml Sloan Kettering Cancer Ctr 2000

Charney, Jonathan Z MD (N) - **Spec Exp:** Headache; Stroke; **Hospital:** Mt Sinai Med Ctr (page 102); **Address:** 1111 Park Ave, Ste 1H, New York, NY 10128-1234; **Phone:** 212-831-2886; **Board Cert:** Neurology 1977; **Med School:** NY Med Coll 1969; **Resid:** Neurology, Methodist Hosp-Baylor 1971; Neurology, Columbia-Presby Med Ctr 1973; **Fac Appt:** Asst Prof N, Mount Sinai Sch Med

Coll, Raymond MD (N) - **Spec Exp:** Multiple Sclerosis; Headache; Stroke; **Hospital:** NY-Presby/Weill Cornell Med Ctr, NY (page 104); **Address:** 1365 York Ave, New York, NY 10021-4035; **Phone:** 212-249-0840; **Board Cert:** Neurology 1974; **Med School:** South Africa 1961; **Resid:** Neurology, NY Hosp 1971; **Fac Appt:** Assoc Clin Prof N, Cornell Univ-Weill Med Coll

Daras, Michael MD (N) - **Spec Exp:** Neuromuscular Disorders; **Hospital:** NY-Presby/Columbia Univ Med Ctr, NY (page 104); **Address:** 710 W 168 St, rm 246, New York, NY 10032; **Phone:** 212-305-6876; **Board Cert:** Neurology 1980; **Med School:** Greece 1969; **Resid:** Psychiatry, Elmhurst City Hosp 1976; Neurology, Metropolitan Hosp 1979; **Fellow:** Clinical Neurophysiology, Albert Einstein 1980; **Fac Appt:** Prof N, Columbia P&S

DeAngelis, Lisa M MD (N) - **Spec Exp:** Neuro-Oncology; Brain Tumors; Clinical Trials; **Hospital:** Meml Sloan-Kettering Canc Ctr (page 114); **Address:** Meml Sloan Kettering Cancer Ctr, Neurology Dept, 1275 York Ave, New York, NY 10065; **Phone:** 212-639-7123; **Board Cert:** Neurology 1986; **Med School:** Columbia P&S 1980; **Resid:** Neurology, Neuro Inst-Presby Hosp 1984; **Fellow:** Neuro-Oncology, Neuro Inst-Presby Hosp 1985; Neuro-Oncology, Meml Sloan-Kettering Cancer Ctr 1986; **Fac Appt:** Prof N, Cornell Univ-Weill Med Coll

Devinsky, Orrin MD (N) - **Spec Exp:** Epilepsy; Tuberous Sclerosis; Behavioral Neurology; **Hospital:** NYU Langone Med Ctr (page 108), Saint Barnabas Med Ctr; **Address:** 223 E 34th St Fl Ground, New York, NY 10016-4972; **Phone:** 646-558-0803; **Board Cert:** Neurology 1987; **Med School:** Harvard Med Sch 1982; **Resid:** Neurology, NY Hosp-Cornell Med Ctr 1986; **Fellow:** Epilepsy, Natl Inst Health 1988; **Fac Appt:** Prof N, NYU Sch Med

Dinkin, Marc J MD (N) - **Spec Exp:** Neuro-Ophthalmology; Optic Nerve Disorders; Neuromyelitis Optica; **Hospital:** NY-Presby/Weill Cornell Med Ctr, NY (page 104); **Address:** Weill-Cornell Eye Assocs, 1305 York Ave, 11th Fl, Nw York, NY 10021; **Phone:** 646-962-2020; **Board Cert:** Neurology 2007; **Med School:** Cornell Univ-Weill Med Coll 2002; **Resid:** Ophthalmology, Weill Cornell Med Ctr 2006; **Fellow:** Neuro-Ophthalmology, Mass Eye & Ear Infirm 2007; **Fac Appt:** Asst Prof Oph, Cornell Univ-Weill Med Coll

Elkind, Mitchell MD (N) - **Spec Exp:** Stroke; Cerebrovascular Disease; Dizziness/Vertigo; **Hospital:** NY-Presby/Columbia Univ Med Ctr, NY (page 104); **Address:** 710 W 168th St Neurologic Bldg Fl 2, Neurological Inst-Stroke Div, rm 640, New York, NY 10032; **Phone:** 212-305-1710; **Board Cert:** Neurotology 2007; Vascular Neurology 2008; **Med School:** Harvard Med Sch 1992; **Resid:** Internal Medicine, Brigham & Women's Hosp 1993; Neurology, Mass General Hosp 1996; **Fac Appt:** Asst Prof N, Columbia P&S

Fahn, Stanley MD (N) - **Spec Exp:** Movement Disorders; Parkinson's Disease; **Hospital:** NY-Presby/Columbia Univ Med Ctr, NY (page 104); **Address:** Neurological Institute, 710 W 168th St Fl 3 - rm 350, New York, NY 10032; **Phone:** 212-305-1303; **Board Cert:** Neurology 1968; **Med School:** UCSF 1958; **Resid:** Neurology, Neuro Inst-Columbia 1962; **Fellow:** Neurological Chemistry, Natl Inst Hlth 1968; **Fac Appt:** Prof N, Columbia P&S

Feinberg, Todd E MD (N) - **Spec Exp:** Alzheimer's Disease; Dementia; **Hospital:** Beth Israel Med Ctr - Petrie Div (page 94); **Address:** Yarmon Neurobehavior Ctr, 1st Ave at 16th St, Bernstein Pavilion Fl 10th, New York, NY 10003; **Phone:** 212-420-4111; **Board Cert:** Psychiatry 1984; Neurology 1987; **Med School:** Mount Sinai Sch Med 1978; **Resid:** Psychiatry, Mt Sinai Med Ctr 1982; Neurology, Mt Sinai Med Ctr 1984; **Fellow:** Behavioral Neurology, Univ Florida 1986; **Fac Appt:** Clin Prof N, Albert Einstein Coll Med

Fink, Matthew E MD (N) - **Spec Exp:** Cerebrovascular Disease; Stroke; Critical Care; **Hospital:** NY-Presby/Weill Cornell Med Ctr, NY (page 104); **Address:** Presby/Weill Cornell, Neurology Dept, 525 E 68 St F Bldg - Ste 610, New York, NY 10065; **Phone:** 212-746-4564; **Board Cert:** Internal Medicine 1980; Neurology 1983; Vascular Neurology 2005; Neurocritical Care 2010; **Med School:** Univ Pittsburgh 1976; **Resid:** Internal Medicine, Boston Med Ctr 1978; Neurology, NY-Presby/Columbia Univ Med Ctr 1982; **Fac Appt:** Prof N, Cornell Univ

Foo, Sun-Hoo MD (N) - **Spec Exp:** Stroke; Headache; Parkinson's Disease; Dementia; **Hospital:** NYU Langone Med Ctr (page 108), NY-Presby/Lower Manhattan Hosp (page 104); **Address:** 650 1st Ave, Fl 4 Floor, New York, NY 10016-3240; **Phone:** 212-213-0270; **Board Cert:** Internal Medicine 1976; Neurology 1980; **Med School:** Taiwan 1972; **Resid:** Internal Medicine, St Vincent's Hosp 1976; Neurology, NYU Med Ctr 1979; **Fac Appt:** Prof N, NYU Sch Med

French, Jacqueline MD (N) - **Spec Exp:** Epilepsy/Seizure Disorders; **Hospital:** NYU Langone Med Ctr (page 108); **Address:** 223 E 34th St, New York, NY 10016; **Phone:** 646-558-0802; **Board Cert:** Neurology 1987; **Med School:** Brown Univ 1982; **Resid:** Neurology, Mount Sinai Hosp 1986; **Fellow:** Epilepsy, Mount Sinai Hosp 1988; Epilepsy, Yale-New Haven Hosp 1989; **Fac Appt:** Prof N, NYU Sch Med

Galetta, Steven MD (N) - **Spec Exp:** Neuro-Ophthalmology; Optic Nerve Disorders; Multiple Sclerosis; **Hospital:** NYU Langone Med Ctr (page 108); **Address:** NYU Med Ctr, Neurology Dept, 240 E 38 St, Fl 15, New York, NY 10016; **Phone:** 646-501-7680; **Board Cert:** Neurology 1988; **Med School:** Cornell Univ-Weill Med Coll 1983; **Resid:** Neurology, Hosp Univ Penn 1987; **Fellow:** Neuro-Ophthalmology, Bascom Palmer Eye Inst 1988; **Fac Appt:** Prof N, NYU Sch Med

Gendelman, Seymour MD (N) - **Spec Exp:** Parkinson's Disease; Dementia; Headache; **Hospital:** Mt Sinai Med Ctr (page 102); **Address:** 5 E 98th St, Fl 7, Box 1139, New York, NY 10029-6501; **Phone:** 212-241-8172; **Board Cert:** Neurology 1971; **Med School:** Geo Wash Univ 1964; **Resid:** Neurology, Mt Sinai Hosp 1968; **Fac Appt:** Clin Prof N, Mount Sinai Sch Med

Goldstein, Jonathan M MD (N) - **Spec Exp:** Myasthenia Gravis; Peripheral Neuropathy; Parkinson's Disease; **Hospital:** Hosp For Special Surgery (page 113); **Address:** HSS, Neurology Dept, 525 E 71st St Fl 5, New York, NY 10021; **Phone:** 646-714-6053; **Board Cert:** Neurology 1991; Neuromuscular Medicine 2011; **Med School:** Brown Univ 1986; **Resid:** Neurology, Yale-New Haven Hosp 1990; **Fellow:** Clinical Neurophysiology, Yale-New Haven Hosp 1991; Neurological Immunology, Yale-New Haven Hosp 1992

Green, Mark W MD (N) - **Spec Exp:** Headache; Pain-Facial; **Hospital:** Mt Sinai Med Ctr (page 102); **Address:** Mount Sinai Sch Med, 5 E 98th St Fl 7, New York, NY 10029; **Phone:** 212-241-7076; **Board Cert:** Neurology 1979; **Med School:** Albert Einstein Coll Med 1974; **Resid:** Neurology, Albert Einstein Affil Hosp 1979; **Fac Appt:** Prof N, Mount Sinai Sch Med

Gruber, Michael L MD (N) - **Spec Exp:** Neuro-Oncology; Headache; Pain-Back & Neck; **Hospital:** NYU Langone Med Ctr (page 108), Overlook Med Ctr (page 92); **Address:** NYU Clinical Cancer Ctr, 160 E 34th St, Fl 9, New York, NY 10016; **Phone:** 212-731-5577; **Board Cert:** Neurology 1975; **Med School:** Temple Univ 1966; **Resid:** Pediatrics, Columbia-Presby Med Ctr 1968; Neurology, Columbia-Presby Med Ctr 1973; **Fellow:** Neuro-Oncology, Mass Genl Hosp 1990; **Fac Appt:** Prof N, NYU Sch Med

Herbert, Joseph MD (N) - **Spec Exp:** Multiple Sclerosis; Neuromuscular Disorders; Neuro-Rehabilitation; **Hospital:** NYU Hosp For Joint Dis (page 108), Saint Barnabas Behavioral Hlth Ctr; **Address:** Multiple Sclerosis Comp Care Ctr, 240 E 38th St Fl 18, New York, NY 10016; **Phone:** 212-598-6305; **Board Cert:** Neurology 1987; **Med School:** Israel 1974; **Resid:** Neurology, Harvard Med Sch Affil Hosp 1983; Neuropathology, Chldns Hosp 1984; **Fellow:** Clinical Genetics, NY-Presby/Columbia Univ Med Ctr 1986; **Fac Appt:** Assoc Prof N, NYU Sch Med

Herbstein, Diego J MD (N) - **Spec Exp:** Parkinson's Disease; Cerebrovascular Disease; **Hospital:** Lenox Hill Hosp (page 106), NY Hosp Queens (page 488); **Address:** 162 E 78th St, New York, NY 10075; **Phone:** 212-794-2281; **Board Cert:** Neurology 1976; **Med School:** Argentina 1968; **Resid:** Internal Medicine, Fernandez 1970; Neurology, Albert Einstein 1973; **Fellow:** Neurology, Jacobi Med Ctr 1974; **Fac Appt:** Asst Clin Prof N, Cornell Univ-Weill Med Coll

Heublum, Michael MD (N) - **Spec Exp:** Neuromuscular Disorders; Electrodiagnosis; **Hospital:** Mt Sinai Med Ctr (page 102), Beth Israel Med Ctr - Petrie Div (page 94); **Address:** 247 3rd Ave, Ste 203, New York, NY 10010; **Phone:** 212-505-9800; **Board Cert:** Internal Medicine 1989; Neurology 1993; **Med School:** SUNY Downstate 1986; **Resid:** Internal Medicine, Staten Island Univ Hosp 1989; Neurology, Mt Sinai Med Ctr 1992; **Fellow:** Neuromuscular Disease, Univ Michigan Med Ctr 1993

Hiesiger, Emile M MD (N) - **Spec Exp:** Pain-Spine; Pain-Cancer, Spine; Pain-Back; **Hospital:** NYU Langone Med Ctr (page 108), VA NY Harbor Hlthcare Sys-Manhattan Campus; **Address:** 345 E 37th St, Ste 320, New York, NY 10016; **Phone:** 212-263-6123; **Board Cert:** Neurology 1983; **Med School:** NY Med Coll 1978; **Resid:** Neurology, NYU Med Ctr 1982; **Fellow:** Neurology, Meml Sloan-Kettering Cancer Ctr 1983; **Fac Appt:** Assoc Clin Prof N, NYU Sch Med

Horvath, Susanna E MD (N) - **Spec Exp:** Stroke; Cerebrovascular Disease; Dizziness; **Hospital:** NY-Presby/Columbia Univ Med Ctr, NY (page 104), NY-Presby Hosp/The Allen Hosp (page 104); **Address:** 710 W 168th St Neurologic Bldg Fl 2, Neurological Inst-Stroke Div, rm 640, New York, NY 10032; **Phone:** 212-305-1710; **Board Cert:** Neurology 2003; Vascular Neurology 2005; **Med School:** Hungary 1990; **Resid:** Internal Medicine, Kaleida/Millard Fillmore Hosp 1994; Neurology, SUNY-Buffalo Med Ctr 1998; **Fac Appt:** Asst Clin Prof N, Columbia P&S

Koppel, Barbara Sue MD (N) - **Spec Exp:** Epilepsy; Headache; Stroke; AIDS/HIV; **Hospital:** Metropolitan Hosp Ctr - NY; **Address:** Metropolitan Hosp, 1901 First Ave, rm 7C5, New York, NY 10029; **Phone:** 212-423-6676; **Board Cert:** Neurology 1983; **Med School:** Columbia P&S 1978; **Resid:** Internal Medicine, Montefiore Med Ctr 1979; Neurology, Columbia-Presby Hosp 1982; **Fac Appt:** Prof N, NY Med Coll

Kuzniecky, Ruben MD (N) - **Spec Exp:** Epilepsy/Seizure Disorders; MRI; Developmental Disorders; Brain Malformations; **Hospital:** NYU Langone Med Ctr (page 108); **Address:** 223 E 34th St Fl Ground, New York, NY 10016; **Phone:** 646-558-0806; **Board Cert:** Neurology 1990; **Med School:** Argentina 1980; **Resid:** Neurology, McGill Univ 1986; **Fellow:** Epilepsy, McGill Univ 1988; **Fac Appt:** Prof N, NYU Sch Med

Labar, Douglas R MD/PhD (N) - **Spec Exp:** Epilepsy/Seizure Disorders; **Hospital:** NY-Presby/Weill Cornell Med Ctr, NY (page 104); **Address:** Weill Cornell Epilepsy Center, 525 E 68th St, rm K-619, New York, NY 10065; **Phone:** 212-746-2359; **Board Cert:** Neurology 1987; **Med School:** Med Coll PA 1982; **Resid:** Neurology, Columbia Presby Med Ctr 1986; **Fellow:** Epilepsy, Columbia Presby Med Ctr 1988; **Fac Appt:** Prof N, Cornell Univ-Weill Med Coll

Lange, Dale J MD (N) - **Spec Exp:** Neuromuscular Disorders; Amyotrophic Lateral Sclerosis (ALS); Electromyography; **Hospital:** Hosp For Special Surgery (page 113), NY-Presby/Weill Cornell Med Ctr, NY (page 104); **Address:** Hosp For Special Surgery, 535 E 70th St, New York, NY 10021; **Phone:** 646-797-8917; **Board Cert:** Neurology 1985; Neuromuscular Medicine 2008; **Med School:** NY Med Coll 1978; **Resid:** Neurology, New England Med Ctr 1982; **Fellow:** Neuromuscular Medicine, Columbia-Presby Med Ctr 1983; **Fac Appt:** Prof N, Cornell Univ-Weill Med Coll

Lassman, Andrew B MD (N) - **Spec Exp:** Neuro-Oncology; Gliomas; Brain Tumors; Brain Tumors-Metastatic; **Hospital:** NY-Presby/Columbia Univ Med Ctr, NY (page 104); **Address:** NY Presbyterian-Columbia Medical Ctr, Div Neuro-Oncology, 622 W 168th St Fl 2, New York, NY 10032; **Phone:** 212-342-0571; **Board Cert:** Neurology 2012; **Med School:** Columbia P&S 1997; **Resid:** Neurology, NY-Presby/Columbia Univ Med Ctr 2001; **Fellow:** Neuro-Oncology, Meml Sloan-Kettering Cancer Ctr 2001; **Fac Appt:** Assoc Prof N, Columbia P&S

Latov, Norman MD/PhD (N) - **Spec Exp:** Peripheral Neuropathy; Neuro-Immunology; **Hospital:** NY-Presby/Weill Cornell Med Ctr, NY (page 104); **Address:** 1305 York Ave Fl 2 - Ste 217, New York, NY 10021; **Phone:** 646-962-3320; **Board Cert:** Neurology 1989; **Med School:** Univ Pennsylvania 1975; **Resid:** Internal Medicine, Boston City Hosp 1976; Neurology, Columbia-Presby Med Ctr 1979; **Fellow:** Immunology, Columbia-Presby Med Ctr 1981; **Fac Appt:** Prof N, Cornell Univ-Weill Med Coll

Levine, David N MD (N) - **Spec Exp:** Dementia; Stroke; Spinal Cord Disorders; Syringomyelia & Spinal Cord Diseases; **Hospital:** NYU Langone Med Ctr (page 108); **Address:** 240 E 38th St Fl 15th, New York, NY 10016-4901; **Phone:** 212-263-7744; **Board Cert:** Neurology 1976; **Med School:** Harvard Med Sch 1968; **Resid:** Neurology, Mass Genl Hosp 1974; **Fellow:** Neurology, Mass Genl Hosp 1976; **Fac Appt:** Prof N, NYU Sch Med

Lin, Michael Tai-Ju MD (N) - **Spec Exp:** Memory Disorders; Neurodegenerative Disorders; **Hospital:** NY-Presby/Weill Cornell Med Ctr, NY (page 104); **Address:** 428 E 72nd St Ground Bldg, New York, NY 10021; **Phone:** 212-746-2441; **Board Cert:** Neurology 2007; **Med School:** UCSF 1992; **Resid:** Neurology, Mass General Hosp 1996; **Fellow:** Memory Disorders, Mass General Hosp 1997; **Fac Appt:** Assoc Prof N, Cornell Univ-Weill Med Coll

Louis, Elan D MD (N) - **Spec Exp:** Tremor & Dystonia; Huntington's Disease; Parkinson's Disease/Movement Disorders; **Hospital:** NY-Presby/Columbia Univ Med Ctr, NY (page 104); **Address:** Neurological Inst of New York, 710 W 168th St, Ste 350, New York, NY 10032; **Phone:** 212-305-1303; **Board Cert:** Neurology 2004; **Med School:** Yale Univ 1989; **Resid:** Neurology, NY-Presby/Columbia Univ Med Ctr 1993; **Fellow:** Movement Disorders, Neurol Inst of New York 1995; Epidemiology, Neurol Inst of New York 1995; **Fac Appt:** Prof N, Columbia P&S

Lublin, Fred D MD (N) - **Spec Exp:** Multiple Sclerosis; **Hospital:** Mt Sinai Med Ctr (page 102); **Address:** Mount Sinai Med Ctr, Corinne Goldsmith Dickinson Ctr for MS, 5 E 98th St, Box 1138, New York, NY 10029-6574; **Phone:** 212-241-6854; **Board Cert:** Neurology 1977; **Med School:** Jefferson Med Coll 1972; **Resid:** Neurology, NY Hosp/Cornell Med Ctr 1976; **Fac Appt:** Prof N, Mount Sinai Sch Med

Luciano, Daniel J MD (N) - **Spec Exp:** Epilepsy/Seizure Disorders; **Hospital:** NYU Langone Med Ctr (page 108); **Address:** NYU Comprehensive Epilepsy Center, 223 E 34th St, New York, NY 10016; **Phone:** 646-558-0805; **Board Cert:** Neurology 1992; Clinical Neurophysiology 2004; **Med School:** UMDNJ-NJ Med Sch, Newark 1984; **Resid:** Neurology, Mt Sinai Med Ctr 1988; **Fellow:** Epilepsy, Mt Sinai Med Ctr 1990; **Fac Appt:** Asst Prof N, NYU Sch Med

Marder, Karen S MD (N) - **Spec Exp:** Huntington's Disease; Alzheimer's Disease; Dementia; **Hospital:** NY-Presby/Columbia Univ Med Ctr, NY (page 104); **Address:** Neurological Institute, 710 W 168th St, Ste 104, New York, NY 10032-2603; **Phone:** 212-305-6939; **Board Cert:** Neurology 1989; **Med School:** Cornell Univ-Weill Med Coll 1983; **Resid:** Neurology, Columbia Presby Med Ctr 1987; **Fellow:** Behavioral Neurology, Columbia Presby Med Ctr 1989; **Fac Appt:** Assoc Prof N, Columbia P&S

Marshall, Randolph S MD (N) - **Spec Exp:** Stroke; Cerebrovascular Disease; Dizziness/Vertigo; Behavioral Neurology; **Hospital:** NY-Presby/Columbia Univ Med Ctr, NY (page 104); **Address:** CUMC/Neurological Inst-Stroke Div, 710 W 168th St Neurologic Bldg, Fl 2nd - rm 640, New York, NY 10032; **Phone:** 212-305-8389; **Board Cert:** Neurology 2004; Vascular Neurology 2008; **Med School:** UCSF 1988; **Resid:** Internal Medicine, NY Presby-Cornell Med Ctr 1989; Neurology, NY Presby-Columbia Med Ctr 1992; **Fellow:** Cerebrovascular Disease, Neurological Inst/Columbia Med Ctr 1994; **Fac Appt:** Prof N, Columbia P&S

Mauskop, Alexander MD (N) - **Spec Exp:** Headache; Migraine; Botox Therapy; Pain Management; **Hospital:** Beth Israel Med Ctr - Petrie Div (page 94); **Address:** New York Headache Ctr, 30 E 76th St, New York, NY 10021; **Phone:** 212-794-3550; **Board Cert:** Neurology 1987; Headache Medicine 2006; **Med School:** Ukraine 1979; **Resid:** Internal Medicine, Brookdale Hosp 1981; Neurology, Univ Hosp 1984; **Fellow:** Pain Management, Meml Sloan Kettering Cancer Ctr 1986; **Fac Appt:** Assoc Clin Prof N, SUNY Downstate

Mayer, Stephan A MD (N) - **Spec Exp:** Neurologic Critical Care; Stroke; Coma; **Hospital:** NY-Presby/Columbia Univ Med Ctr, NY (page 104); **Address:** 177 Fort Washington Ave, Ste A-300, New York, NY 10032-2603; **Phone:** 212-305-7236; **Board Cert:** Neurology 1993; **Med School:** Cornell Univ-Weill Med Coll 1988; **Resid:** Neurology, Columbia-Presby Med Ctr 1992; **Fellow:** Critical Care Neurology, Columbia-Presby Med Ctr 1993; **Fac Appt:** Assoc Prof N, Columbia P&S

Mayeux, Richard MD (N) - **Spec Exp:** Alzheimer's Disease; Dementia; **Hospital:** NY-Presby/Columbia Univ Med Ctr, NY (page 104); **Address:** 630 W 168th St, PH 19, New York, NY 10032; **Phone:** 212-305-6939; **Board Cert:** Neurology 1978; **Med School:** Univ Okla Coll Med 1972; **Resid:** Internal Medicine, Boston City Hosp 1974; Neurology, Columbia Presby Med Ctr 1977; **Fellow:** Neurology, Boston Univ 1978; **Fac Appt:** Prof N, Columbia P&S

Miller, Aaron E MD (N) - **Spec Exp:** Multiple Sclerosis; Autoimmune Disease; Optic Nerve Disorders; **Hospital:** Mt Sinai Med Ctr (page 102); **Address:** 5 E 98th St, Fl 1st, Box 1138, New York, NY 10029; **Phone:** 212-241-6854; **Board Cert:** Internal Medicine 1972; Neurology 1977; **Med School:** NYU Sch Med 1968; **Resid:** Internal Medicine, Jacobi Med Ctr 1970; Neurology, Montefiore Med Ctr 1975; **Fellow:** Neurovirology, Johns Hopkins Hosp 1977; **Fac Appt:** Prof N, Mount Sinai Sch Med

Mitsumoto, Hiroshi MD (N) - **Spec Exp:** Amyotrophic Lateral Sclerosis (ALS); Neuromuscular Disorders; Clinical Trials; **Hospital:** NY-Presby/Columbia Univ Med Ctr, NY (page 104); **Address:** Neurological Institute, 710 W 168th St Fl 9, New York, NY 10032; **Phone:** 212-305-1319; **Board Cert:** Neurology 1978; **Med School:** Japan 1968; **Resid:** Internal Medicine, Toho Univ Hosps 1972; Neurology, Univ Hosps 1976; **Fellow:** Neurological Pathology, Cleveland Clinic 1978; Neuromuscular Medicine, New England Med Ctr 1981; **Fac Appt:** Prof N, Columbia P&S

Mohr, JP MD (N) - **Spec Exp:** Stroke; Arteriovenous Malformations; Aphasia; MoyaMoya Disease; **Hospital:** NY-Presby/Columbia Univ Med Ctr, NY (page 104); **Address:** 710 W 168th St, Fl 6, rm 616, New York, NY 10032-2603; **Phone:** 212-305-8033; **Board Cert:** Neurology 1971; Vascular Neurology 2005; **Med School:** Univ VA Sch Med 1963; **Resid:** Neurology, Columbia Presby Med Ctr 1966; Neurology, Mass Genl Hosp 1968; **Fellow:** Neurology, Mass Genl Hosp 1969; **Fac Appt:** Prof N, Columbia P&S

Motiwala, Rajeev S MD (N) - **Hospital:** Mt Sinai Med Ctr (page 102); **Address:** Mount Sinai Neurology, 5 E 98 St Fl 7, New York, NY 10029; **Phone:** 212-241-7076; **Board Cert:** Neurology 1990; **Med School:** India 1979; **Resid:** Neurology, UMDMNJ Med Ctr 1988; **Fac Appt:** Asst Prof N, Mount Sinai Sch Med

Nealon, Nancy M MD (N) - **Spec Exp:** Multiple Sclerosis; **Hospital:** NY-Presby/Weill Cornell Med Ctr, NY (page 104); **Address:** 1305 York Ave Fl 2nd, New York, NY 10021; **Phone:** 646-962-9800; **Board Cert:** Internal Medicine 1978; Neurology 1984; **Med School:** Penn State Coll Med 1975; **Resid:** Neurology, NY Hosp 1981; **Fellow:** Neuromuscular Disease, Columbia-Presby Med Ctr 1982; Neuromuscular Medicine, Meml Sloan Kettering Cancer Ctr 1983; **Fac Appt:** Asst Prof N, Cornell Univ-Weill Med Coll

Neophytides, Andreas MD (N) - **Spec Exp:** Spinal Disorders; Stroke; **Hospital:** NYU Langone Med Ctr (page 108); **Address:** 650 1st Ave, New York, NY 10016; **Phone:** 212-213-9580; **Board Cert:** Neurology 1978; **Med School:** Greece 1970; **Resid:** Surgery, LIJ Med Ctr 1973; Neurology, NYU Med Ctr 1976; **Fellow:** Neurological Pharmacology, Natl Inst Hlth 1978; **Fac Appt:** Clin Prof N, NYU Sch Med

Newman, Lawrence C MD (N) - **Spec Exp:** Headache; Pain-Facial; **Hospital:** St. Luke's - Roosevelt Hosp Ctr - Roosevelt Div (page 94); **Address:** St Luke's-Roosevelt Hosp-Headache Inst, 425 W 59th St Fl 4 - Ste A, New York, NY 10019; **Phone:** 212-523-5869; **Board Cert:** Neurology 2005; Headache Medicine 2006; **Med School:** Mexico 1983; **Resid:** Internal Medicine, Elmhurst Hosp 1986; Neurology, Montefiore Med Ctr 1989; **Fellow:** Headache, Montefiore Med Ctr 1990; **Fac Appt:** Prof N, Albert Einstein Coll Med

Olanow, C Warren MD (N) - **Spec Exp:** Parkinson's Disease; Movement Disorders; **Hospital:** Mt Sinai Med Ctr (page 102); **Address:** 5 E 98 St, New York, NY 10029; **Phone:** 212-241-8435; **Med School:** Univ Toronto 1965; **Resid:** Neurology, Toronto Genl Hosp 1968; Neurology, Columbia Presby Hosp 1970; **Fellow:** Neurological Anatomy, Columbia Presby Hosp 1971; **Fac Appt:** Prof N, Mount Sinai Sch Med

Olarte, Marcelo R MD (N) - **Spec Exp:** Myasthenia Gravis; Electrodiagnosis; Headache; Neuromuscular Disorders; **Hospital:** St. Luke's - Roosevelt Hosp Ctr - Roosevelt Div (page 94), Lenox Hill Hosp (page 106); **Address:** 903 Park Ave, New York, NY 10075; **Phone:** 212-988-9100; **Board Cert:** Neurology 1976; **Med School:** Argentina 1970; **Resid:** Neurology, St Vincent's Hosp 1974; **Fellow:** Neuromuscular Medicine, Columbia-Presby Hosp 1975

Pacia, Steven V MD (N) - **Spec Exp:** Epilepsy/Seizure Disorders; **Hospital:** NYU Langone Med Ctr (page 108), Lenox Hill Hosp (page 106); **Address:** NYU Comprehensive Epilepsy Center, 223 E 34th St, New York, NY 10016; **Phone:** 646-558-0867; **Board Cert:** Neurology 1992; Clinical Neurophysiology 2007; **Med School:** Yale Univ 1987; **Resid:** Neurology, Yale-New Haven Hosp 1991; **Fellow:** Epilepsy, Yale-New Haven Hosp 1992; **Fac Appt:** Assoc Prof N, NYU Sch Med

Petito, Frank A MD (N) - **Spec Exp:** Multiple Sclerosis; Headache; Lyme Disease; **Hospital:** NY-Presby/Weill Cornell Med Ctr, NY (page 104); **Address:** 525 E 68th St, Ste 607, New York, NY 10065; **Phone:** 212-746-2309; **Board Cert:** Neurology 1974; **Med School:** Columbia P&S 1967; **Resid:** Neurology, New York Hosp 1971; **Fac Appt:** Prof N, Cornell Univ-Weill Med Coll

Posner, Jerome B MD (N) - **Spec Exp:** Neuro-Oncology; Brain Tumors; Paraneoplastic Syndromes; **Hospital:** Meml Sloan-Kettering Canc Ctr (page 114); **Address:** 1275 York Ave, rm C731, New York, NY 10065; **Phone:** 212-639-7047; **Board Cert:** Neurology 1962; **Med School:** Univ Wash 1955; **Resid:** Neurology, Univ WA Affil Hosp 1959; **Fellow:** Biochemistry, Univ WA Affil Hosp 1963; **Fac Appt:** Prof N, Cornell Univ-Weill Med Coll

Rapoport, Samuel MD/PhD (N) - **Spec Exp:** Peripheral Neuropathy; Pain-Back & Neck; Electromyography; **Hospital:** NY-Presby/Weill Cornell Med Ctr, NY (page 104), Lenox Hill Hosp (page 106); **Address:** 354 E 76th St, New York, NY 10021-2505; **Phone:** 212-570-0642; **Board Cert:** Neurology 1986; **Med School:** Cornell Univ-Weill Med Coll 1976; **Resid:** Neurology, New York Hosp-Cornell 1982; **Fac Appt:** Assoc Prof N, Cornell Univ-Weill Med Coll

Relkin, Norman R MD/PhD (N) - **Spec Exp:** Alzheimer's Disease; Dementia; Memory Disorders; **Hospital:** NY-Presby/Weill Cornell Med Ctr, NY (page 104); **Address:** Weill Cornell Memory Disorders Program, 428 E 72nd St, Ste 500, New York, NY 10021; **Phone:** 212-746-2441; **Board Cert:** Neurology 1992; **Med School:** Albert Einstein Coll Med 1987; **Resid:** Neurology, New York Hosp 1991; **Fellow:** Behavioral Neurology, New York Hosp-Cornell 1992; **Fac Appt:** Asst Prof N, Cornell Univ-Weill Med Coll

Roberts, J Kirk MD (N) - **Spec Exp:** Stroke; Dizziness; Vascular Neurology; **Hospital:** NY-Presby/Columbia Univ Med Ctr, NY (page 104); **Address:** Columbia University Medical Center, New York Presbyterian Hospital, 710 W 168th St, Ste 246, New York, NY 10032; **Phone:** 212-305-6876; **Board Cert:** Neurology 2006; Vascular Neurology 2008; **Med School:** Cornell Univ-Weill Med Coll 1989; **Resid:** Internal Medicine, Columbia-Presby Med Ctr 1992; Neurology, Columbia-Presby Med Ctr 1995; **Fellow:** Stroke, Columbia-Presby Med Ctr 1997; **Fac Appt:** Assoc Clin Prof N, Columbia P&S

Sadiq, Saud MD (N) - **Spec Exp:** Multiple Sclerosis; **Hospital:** St. Luke's - Roosevelt Hosp Ctr - Roosevelt Div (page 94); **Address:** International MS Management Practice, 521 W 57th St Fl 4, New York, NY 10019; **Phone:** 212-265-8070; **Board Cert:** Neurology 2009; **Med School:** Africa 1979; **Resid:** Neurology, Univ TX Med Branch 1988; **Fellow:** Neurological Immunology, Ny Presby-Columbia Med Ctr 1991; **Fac Appt:** , Albert Einstein Coll Med

Safdieh, Joseph E MD (N) - **Spec Exp:** Headache; Migraine; Stroke; Dizziness; **Hospital:** NY-Presby/Weill Cornell Med Ctr, NY (page 104); **Address:** 520 E 70th St, Starr Pavilion, rm 607, New York, NY 10021; **Phone:** 212-746-3113; **Board Cert:** Neurology 2007; **Med School:** NYU Sch Med 2002; **Resid:** Neurology, NY Hosp-Cornell Med Ctr 2006; **Fac Appt:** Assoc Prof N, Cornell Univ-Weill Med Coll

Sander, Howard W MD (N) - **Spec Exp:** Electromyography; Peripheral Neuropathy; Neuromuscular Disorders; Nerve Conduction Studies; **Hospital:** NYU Langone Med Ctr (page 108); **Address:** NYU Neurology Assocs, 240 E 38th St Fl 15, New York, NY 10016; **Phone:** 212-263-3895; **Board Cert:** Neuromuscular Medicine 2009; Clinical Neurophysiology 2005; Pain Medicine 2010; Vascular Neurology 2008; **Med School:** SUNY Downstate 1988; **Resid:** Neurology, Albert Einstein Coll Med Affil Hosp 1992; **Fellow:** Electromyography, Mass Genl Hosp 1993; **Fac Appt:** Prof N, NYU Sch Med

Saunders-Pullman, Rachel MD (N) - **Spec Exp:** Movement Disorders; Parkinson's Disease; **Hospital:** Beth Israel Med Ctr - Petrie Div (page 94); **Address:** 10 Union Square E, Ste 5H, New York, NY 10003; **Phone:** 212-844-8719; **Board Cert:** Neurology 2010; **Med School:** Columbia P&S 1992; **Resid:** Neurology, Ny Presby-Columbia Med Ctr 1996

Sheinart, Kara F MD (N) - **Spec Exp:** Cerebrovascular Disease; Stroke; **Hospital:** Mt Sinai Med Ctr (page 102); **Address:** 5 E 98th St Fl 7th, New York, NY 10029; **Phone:** 212-241-7076; **Board Cert:** Neurology 2005; **Med School:** SUNY Downstate 1989; **Resid:** Internal Medicine, Mt Sinai Med Ctr 1990; Neurology, Mt Sinai Med Ctr 1993; **Fellow:** Cerebrovascular Disease, Mt Sinai Med Ctr 1995; **Fac Appt:** Asst Prof N, Mount Sinai Sch Med

Shulman, Melanie MD (N) - **Spec Exp:** Memory Disorders; Epilepsy; **Hospital:** NYU Langone Med Ctr (page 108); **Address:** Barlow Center, 145 E 32 St Fl 2, New York, NY 10016; **Phone:** 212-263-3210; **Board Cert:** Neurology 2007; **Med School:** Univ Pennsylvania 1991; **Resid:** Neurology, Brigham & Women's Hosp 1995; **Fac Appt:** Asst Clin Prof N, NYU Sch Med

Simpson, David M MD (N) - **Spec Exp:** Infections-CNS; AIDS-Neurologic Complications; Peripheral Neuropathy; Neuromuscular Disorders; **Hospital:** Mt Sinai Med Ctr (page 102); **Address:** Mt Sinai Med Ctr, Dept Neurology, 1 Gustave L Levy Pl, Box 1052, Annenberg, 2nd Flr, New York, NY 10029; **Phone:** 212-241-8748; **Board Cert:** Neurology 1984; Clinical Neurophysiology 2005; Neuromuscular Medicine 2008; **Med School:** SUNY Buffalo 1979; **Resid:** Neurology, NY Hosp-Cornell Med Ctr 1983; **Fellow:** Clinical Neurophysiology, Mass Genl Hosp 1984; **Fac Appt:** Prof N, Mount Sinai Sch Med

Sivak, Mark A MD (N) - **Spec Exp:** Myasthenia Gravis; Amyotrophic Lateral Sclerosis (ALS); Neuromuscular Disorders; **Hospital:** Mt Sinai Med Ctr (page 102); **Address:** 1468 Madison Ave Fl 2nd, Annenberg Bldg, New York, NY 10029-6501; **Phone:** 212-241-8747; **Board Cert:** Neurology 1978; Neuromuscular Medicine 2008; **Med School:** Univ Louisville Sch Med 1971; **Resid:** Neurology, Mt Sinai Med Ctr 1975; **Fellow:** Electromyography, Mt Sinai Med Ctr 1976; Clinical Neurophysiology, Uppsala Univ 1986; **Fac Appt:** Asst Prof N, Mount Sinai Sch Med

Smallberg, Gerald J MD (N) - **Spec Exp:** Spinal Disorders; **Hospital:** Lenox Hill Hosp (page 106), Hosp For Special Surgery (page 113); **Address:** 1010 5th Ave, New York, NY 10028-0130; **Phone:** 212-535-5348; **Board Cert:** Neurology 1977; **Med School:** Yale Univ 1969; **Resid:** Internal Medicine, Univ Mich Med Ctr 1971; Neurology, Hosp Univ Penn 1975; **Fellow:** Neurology, Columbia-Presby Med Ctr 1976

Snyder, David H MD (N) - **Spec Exp:** Multiple Sclerosis; **Hospital:** NY Hosp Queens (page 488), Lenox Hill Hosp (page 106); **Address:** 162 E 78th St, New York, NY 10075; **Phone:** 212-794-2281; **Board Cert:** Neurology 1975; **Med School:** Univ MD Sch Med 1969; **Resid:** Neurology, Univ Maryland Hosp 1973; **Fellow:** Neuropathology, Albert Einstein Med Ctr 1975; **Fac Appt:** Asst Clin Prof N, Cornell Univ-Weill Med Coll

Stuebgen, Joerg-Patrick MD (N) - **Spec Exp:** Amyotrophic Lateral Sclerosis (ALS); Peripheral Neuropathy; Neuromuscular Disorders; **Hospital:** NY-Presby/Weill Cornell Med Ctr, NY (page 104), Hosp For Special Surgery (page 113); **Address:** Dept Neur Starr 607, 520 E 70th St, New York, NY 10021; **Phone:** 212-746-2334; **Board Cert:** Neurology 2006; Clinical Neurophysiology 2009; **Med School:** South Africa 1983; **Resid:** Neurology, Univ Pretoria Med Ctr 1989; Neurology, New York Hosp 1995; **Fellow:** Clinical Neurophysiology, Menl Sloan Kettering Cancer Ctr 1995; **Fac Appt:** Prof N, Cornell Univ-Weill Med Coll

Tuchman, Alan J MD (N) - **Spec Exp:** Epilepsy; Multiple Sclerosis; **Hospital:** Montefiore Med Ctr-Wakefield Campus (page 100); **Address:** 975 Park Ave, New York, NY 10028; **Phone:** 212-772-9305; **Board Cert:** Neurology 1979; **Med School:** Univ Cincinnati 1972; **Resid:** Neurology, Mt Sinai Med Ctr 1976; **Fellow:** Multiple Sclerosis, Albert Einstein Med Ctr 1979; **Fac Appt:** Clin Prof N, NY Med Coll

Tuhrim, Stanley MD (N) - **Spec Exp:** Stroke; Cerebrovascular Disease; Fibromuscular Dysplasia; **Hospital:** Mt Sinai Med Ctr (page 102); **Address:** 5 E 98th St, Box 1139, New York, NY 10029-6501; **Phone:** 212-241-7076; **Board Cert:** Neurology 1984; Vascular Neurology 2005; **Med School:** Mount Sinai Sch Med 1979; **Resid:** Neurology, Mt Sinai Med Ctr 1983; **Fellow:** Cerebrovascular Disease, Univ MD Sch Med 1984; **Fac Appt:** Prof N, Mount Sinai Sch Med

Waters, Cheryl H MD (N) - **Spec Exp:** Parkinson's Disease; Movement Disorders; **Hospital:** NY-Presby/Columbia Univ Med Ctr, NY (page 104); **Address:** NY-Presby, Neurological Inst, 710 W 168th St Fl 3, New York, NY 10032; **Phone:** 212-305-1303; **Board Cert:** Neurology 1986; **Med School:** Univ Toronto 1980; **Resid:** Internal Medicine, Univ Toronto Med Ctr 1982; Neurology, Univ Toronto Med Ctr 1985; **Fellow:** Clinical Pharmacology, Univ Toronto Med Ctr 1987; **Fac Appt:** Prof N, Columbia P&S

Weinberg, Harold J MD (N) - **Spec Exp:** Headache; Spinal Disorders; Neuromuscular Disorders; Memory Disorders; **Hospital:** NYU Langone Med Ctr (page 108); **Address:** Neurology Consultants of NY, 650 1st Ave Fl 4, New York, NY 10016-3240; **Phone:** 212-213-9339; **Board Cert:** Neurology 1983; Electrodiagnostic Medicine 1989; **Med School:** Albert Einstein Coll Med 1978; **Resid:** Neurology, Columbia-Presby Med Ctr 1982; **Fellow:** Neuromuscular Medicine, Columbia-Presby Med Ctr 1982; **Fac Appt:** Clin Prof N, NYU Sch Med

Weinberger, Jesse MD (N) - **Spec Exp:** Stroke; **Hospital:** Mt Sinai Med Ctr (page 102); **Address:** 1468 Madison Ave Fl 2nd, Annenberg Blgd, New York, NY 10029-6501; **Phone:** 212-241-5621; **Board Cert:** Neurology 1976; Vascular Neurology 2005; **Med School:** Johns Hopkins Univ 1971; **Resid:** Neurology, Mt Sinai Med Ctr 1975; **Fellow:** Cerebrovascular Disease, Univ Penn 1978; **Fac Appt:** Prof N, Mount Sinai Sch Med

Neuroradiology

Berenstein, Alejandro MD (NRad) - **Spec Exp:** Interventional Neuroradiology; Aneurysm-Cerebral; Endovascular Surgery; Vascular Malformations; **Hospital:** St. Luke's - Roosevelt Hosp Ctr - Roosevelt Div (page 94); **Address:** Center for Endovascular Surgery, 1000 10th Ave, 10th Fl, Ste 10G - INN, New York, NY 10019; **Phone:** 212-636-3400; **Board Cert:** Diagnostic Radiology 1976; **Med School:** Mexico 1970; **Resid:** Diagnostic Radiology, Mt Sinai Med Ctr 1976; **Fellow:** Neuroradiology, NYU Med Ctr 1978; **Fac Appt:** Prof Rad, Albert Einstein Coll Med

Drayer, Burton P MD (NRad) - **Spec Exp:** Parkinson's Disease/Aging Brain; Alzheimer's Disease; Vascular Neurology; MRI & CT of Brain & Spine; **Hospital:** Mt Sinai Med Ctr (page 102); **Address:** 1176 Fifth Ave, New York, NY 10029; **Phone:** 212-241-8333; **Board Cert:** Neurology 1976; Diagnostic Radiology 1978; Neuroradiology 2006; **Med School:** Ros Franklin Univ/Chicago Med Sch 1971; **Resid:** Neurology, Univ Vt Med Ctr 1975; Diagnostic Radiology, Univ Pitt Hlth Ctr 1978; **Fellow:** Neuroradiology, Univ Pitt Hlth Ctr 1978; **Fac Appt:** Prof Rad, Mount Sinai Sch Med

Gobin, Y Pierre MD (NRad) - **Spec Exp:** Aneurysm-Cerebral; Cerebrovascular Disease; Endovascular Surgery; Interventional Neuroradiology; **Hospital:** NY-Presby/Weill Cornell Med Ctr, NY (page 104); **Address:** NY Presby/Weill Cornell Med Ctr, Neuroradiology Dept, 525 E 68th St, New York, NY 10065; **Phone:** 212-746-4998; **Med School:** France 1988; **Resid:** Diagnostic Radiology, Univ Paris Affil Hosp; **Fellow:** Interventional Neuroradiology, Hosp Lariboisiere; **Fac Appt:** Prof Rad, Cornell Univ-Weill Med Coll

Holodny, Andrei I MD (NRad) - **Spec Exp:** MRI; Brain Tumors; **Hospital:** Meml Sloan-Kettering Canc Ctr (page 114); **Address:** Meml Sloan Kettering Cancer Ctr, 1275 York Ave, Box 29, New York, NY 10065; **Phone:** 212-639-3182; **Board Cert:** Diagnostic Radiology ; Neuroradiology 2009; **Med School:** UMDNJ-NJ Med Sch, Newark 1989; **Resid:** Diagnostic Radiology, Bellevue Hosp 1994; **Fellow:** Neurological Radiology, NYU School of Med 1995

Jahre, Caren MD (NRad) - **Spec Exp:** Cardiac CT Angiography; **Address:** Lenox Hill Radiology & Med Assocs, 61 E 77th St, New York, NY 10075; **Phone:** 212-772-3111; **Board Cert:** Diagnostic Radiology 1988; Neuroradiology 2005; **Med School:** Cornell Univ-Weill Med Coll 1982; **Resid:** Pathology, New York Hosp 1984; Diagnostic Radiology, New York Hosp 1988; **Fellow:** Neuroradiology, New York Hosp 1990; **Fac Appt:** Asst Prof Rad, NYU Sch Med

Kelly, Anna B MD (NRad) - **Hospital:** NY-Presby/Columbia Univ Med Ctr, NY (page 104); **Address:** Columbia Presby Eastside Radiology, 16 E 60th St, New York, NY 10022; **Phone:** 212-326-8518; **Board Cert:** Diagnostic Radiology 1986; Neuroradiology 2005; **Med School:** Univ Cincinnati 1982; **Resid:** Diagnostic Radiology, NY Hosp-Cornell Med Ctr 1986; **Fellow:** Neurological Radiology, NY Hosp-Cornell Med Ctr 1989; **Fac Appt:** Asst Prof Rad, Columbia P&S

Khandji, Alexander G MD (NRad) - **Spec Exp:** Pituitary Disorders; Spine Imaging & Intervention; MRI; Headache; **Hospital:** NY-Presby/Columbia Univ Med Ctr, NY (page 104); **Address:** 177 Ft Washington Ave, Ste 3-113, New York, NY 10032-3173; **Phone:** 212-305-7669; **Board Cert:** Diagnostic Radiology 1985; Neuroradiology 2006; **Med School:** SUNY Downstate 1980; **Resid:** Surgery, MS Hershey Med Ctr 1982; Diagnostic Radiology, Columbia-Presby Med Ctr 1985; **Fellow:** Neuroradiology, Columbia-Presby Med Ctr 1987; **Fac Appt:** Prof Rad, Columbia P&S

Knopp, Edmond A MD (NRad) - **Spec Exp:** MRI; Brain Imaging; Spinal Imaging & Intervention; Brain Tumors; **Address:** Zwanger-Pesiri Radiology, 150 E Sunrise Hwy Fl 2, Lindenhurst, NY 11757; **Phone:** 631-225-7200 x4071; **Board Cert:** Diagnostic Radiology 1992; Neuroradiology 2005; **Med School:** SUNY Downstate 1986; **Resid:** Surgery, Maimonides Med Ctr 1988; Diagnostic Radiology, St Lukes/Roosevelt Hosp 1992; **Fellow:** Neuroradiology, NYU Med Ctr 1994

Lefton, Daniel R MD (NRad) - **Spec Exp:** Pediatric Neuroradiology; MRI; **Hospital:** Beth Israel Med Ctr - Petrie Div (page 94), St. Luke's - Roosevelt Hosp Ctr - Roosevelt Div (page 94); **Address:** BIMC, Radiology Dept, 1000 10th Ave, New York, NY 10019; **Phone:** 212-523-8320; **Board Cert:** Diagnostic Radiology 1993; Neuroradiology 2005; **Med School:** Boston Univ 1988; **Resid:** Diagnostic Radiology, SUNY Downstate Med Ctr 1993; **Fellow:** Neurological Radiology, NYU Med Ctr 1995; Pediatric Neuroradiology, Chldns Hosp 1996; **Fac Appt:** Assoc Prof Rad, Albert Einstein Coll Med

Lis, Eric MD (NRad) - **Spec Exp:** Spinal Cord Tumors; Brain Tumors; Pain-Spine; MRI; **Hospital:** Meml Sloan-Kettering Canc Ctr (page 114); **Address:** Meml Sloan Kettering Cancer Ctr, 1275 York Ave, Ste MRI 1158, New York, NY 10065; **Phone:** 212-639-8330; **Board Cert:** Diagnostic Radiology 1995; Neuroradiology 2008; **Med School:** UMDNJ-NJ Med Sch, Newark 1990; **Resid:** Internal Medicine, Mountainside Hosp 1991; Diagnostic Radiology, UMDNJ-RW Johnson Med Sch 1995; **Fellow:** Neuroradiology, NY-Presby-Weill Cornell Med Ctr 1997

Meyers, Philip M MD (NRad) - **Spec Exp:** Interventional Neuroradiology; Endovascular Surgery; Aneurysm-Cerebral; Arteriovenous Malformations; **Hospital:** NY-Presby/Columbia Univ Med Ctr, NY (page 104), Valley Hosp (page 721); **Address:** 710 W 168 St, Ste 428, New York, NY 10032; **Phone:** 212-305-6384; **Board Cert:** Diagnostic Radiology 1997; Neuroradiology 2012; **Med School:** Case West Res Univ 1989; **Resid:** Neurological Surgery, Univ Cincinnati Med Ctr 1990; Diagnostic Radiology, Univ Cincinnati Med Ctr 1997; **Fellow:** Neurological Radiology, Univ Cincinnati Med Ctr 1998; Neurovascular Surgery, UCSF Med Ctr 2001; **Fac Appt:** Assoc Prof Rad, Columbia P&S

Naidich, Thomas MD (NRad) - **Spec Exp:** Brain Tumors; Stroke; **Hospital:** Mt Sinai Med Ctr (page 102); **Address:** Mt Sinai, Radiology Dept, 1176 5th Ave, New York, NY 10029; **Phone:** 212-241-3423; **Board Cert:** Diagnostic Radiology 1974; Neuroradiology 2005; **Med School:** NYU Sch Med 1969; **Resid:** Diagnostic Radiology, Montefiore Med Ctr 1973; **Fellow:** Neuroradiology, NYU Med Ctr 1975; **Fac Appt:** Prof Rad, Mount Sinai Sch Med

Sanelli, Pina MD (NRad) - **Spec Exp:** Spine Imaging & Intervention; MRI & CT of Brain & Spine; MRI; **Hospital:** NY-Presby/Weill Cornell Med Ctr, NY (page 104); **Address:** Weill Cornell Imaging at NY Presby Hosp, 1305 York Ave Fl 3, New York, NY 10021; **Phone:** 212-746-2577; **Board Cert:** Diagnostic Radiology ; Neuroradiology 2011; **Med School:** SUNY Buffalo 1994; **Resid:** Diagnostic Radiology, Albany Med Ctr 1997; Diagnostic Radiology, N Shore Univ Hosp 1999; **Fellow:** Neurological Radiology, Mass Genl Hosp 2001; **Fac Appt:** Assoc Prof Rad, Cornell Univ-Weill Med Coll

Stambuk, Hilda MD (NRad) - **Spec Exp:** Head & Neck Cancer; Head & Neck Imaging; **Hospital:** Meml Sloan-Kettering Canc Ctr (page 114); **Address:** Meml Sloan Kettering Cancer Ctr, 1275 York Ave, Box 29, New York, NY 10065; **Phone:** 212-639-2728; **Board Cert:** Diagnostic Radiology ; Neuroradiology 2010; **Med School:** Med Coll GA 1990; **Resid:** Diagnostic Radiology, Univ FL Coll Of Med 1994; **Fellow:** Neuroradiology, Univ FL Coll of Med 1996

Nuclear Medicine

Carrasquillo, Jorge A MD (NuM) - **Spec Exp:** Radioimmunotherapy of Cancer; PET Imaging; Nuclear Endocrinology; **Hospital:** Meml Sloan-Kettering Canc Ctr (page 114); **Address:** 1275 York Ave, Nuclear Medicine Svc, Box 77, New York, NY 10065; **Phone:** 212-639-2459; **Board Cert:** Internal Medicine 1977; Nuclear Medicine 1982; **Med School:** Univ Puerto Rico 1974; **Resid:** Internal Medicine, Univ Dist Hosp 1977; Nuclear Medicine, Univ Wash Hosp 1982; **Fac Appt:** Prof NuM, SUNY Upstate Med Univ

Divgi, Chaitanya MD (NuM) - **Spec Exp:** Nuclear Oncology; **Hospital:** NY-Presby/Columbia Univ Med Ctr, NY (page 104); **Address:** 722 W 168th St, New York, NY 10032; **Phone:** 212-342-2899; **Board Cert:** Nuclear Medicine ; **Med School:** India 1976; **Resid:** Nuclear Medicine, Meml Sloan Kettering Cancer Ctr 1987; **Fellow:** Immunology, Meml Sloan Kettering Cancer Ctr 1988; **Fac Appt:** Prof Rad, Columbia P&S

Friedman, Kent MD (NuM) - **Spec Exp:** PET Imaging; Cancer Detection & Staging; **Hospital:** NYU Langone Med Ctr (page 108); **Address:** NYU Med Ctr, Radiology Dept, 560 1 Ave Fl 2, New York, NY 10016; **Phone:** 212-263-7410; **Board Cert:** Nuclear Medicine 2004; **Med School:** Univ Conn 2001; **Resid:** Internal Medicine, Univ Conn Hlth Ctr 2002; **Fellow:** Nuclear Medicine, Johns Hopkins Hosp 2003; **Fac Appt:** Asst Prof NuM, NYU Sch Med

Ghesani, Munir MD (NuM) - **Spec Exp:** PET Imaging; Nuclear Cardiology; **Hospital:** St. Luke's - Roosevelt Hosp Ctr - Roosevelt Div (page 94); **Address:** St Lukes-Roosevelt Hosp, Radiology, 1000 10 Ave Fl 4th, New York, NY 10019; **Phone:** 212-523-7171; **Board Cert:** Nuclear Medicine 2011; Diagnostic Radiology 2010; **Med School:** India 1986; **Resid:** Internal Medicine, Jersey City Med Ctr 1993; **Fellow:** Nuclear Medicine, St Lukes-Roosevelt Hosp Ctr 1996; **Fac Appt:** Asst Prof Rad, Columbia P&S

Goldfarb, C. Richard MD (NuM) - **Spec Exp:** Thyroid Cancer; Thyroid Disorders; **Hospital:** Beth Israel Med Ctr - Petrie Div (page 94); **Address:** Beth Israel Med Ctr, Dept Radiology, 1st Ave at 16th St, New York, NY 10003; **Phone:** 212-252-6070; **Board Cert:** Nuclear Medicine 1974; Diagnostic Radiology 1975; **Med School:** NY Med Coll 1970; **Resid:** Diagnostic Radiology, St Lukes Hosp 1974; **Fellow:** Nuclear Medicine, St Lukes Hosp 1975; **Fac Appt:** Assoc Prof NuM, Albert Einstein Coll Med

Goldsmith, Stanley J MD (NuM) - **Spec Exp:** Thyroid Cancer; Thyroid Disorders; Nuclear Cardiology; PET Imaging; **Hospital:** NY-Presby/Weill Cornell Med Ctr, NY (page 104); **Address:** 520 E 70th St Starr Bldg - rm 2-21, New York, NY 10021-9800; **Phone:** 212-746-4588; **Board Cert:** Internal Medicine 1969; Nuclear Medicine 1972; Endocrinology, Diabetes & Metabolism 1972; **Med School:** SUNY Downstate 1962; **Resid:** Internal Medicine, Kings Co Hosp 1968; **Fellow:** Endocrinology, Diabetes & Metabolism, Mt Sinai Hosp 1970; Nuclear Medicine, Bronx VA Hosp 1972; **Fac Appt:** Prof Rad, Cornell Univ-Weill Med Coll

Pandit-Taskar, Neeta MD (NuM) - **Spec Exp:** Radioimmunotherapy of Cancer; Thyroid Cancer; PET Imaging; **Hospital:** Meml Sloan-Kettering Canc Ctr (page 114); **Address:** Memorial Sloan Kettering Cancer Ctr, 1275 York Ave, New York, NY 10065; **Phone:** 212-639-7372; **Board Cert:** Nuclear Medicine 2008; **Med School:** India 1990; **Resid:** Nuclear Medicine, Mt Sinai Med Ctr 1995; **Fellow:** Nuclear Medicine, Meml Sloan Kettering Cancer Ctr 2001

Sanger, Joseph J MD (NuM) - **Spec Exp:** Nuclear Cardiology; Nuclear Oncology; **Hospital:** NYU Langone Med Ctr (page 108), Bellevue Hosp Ctr; **Address:** Department of Radiology, 560 First Ave Fl 2nd, New York, NY 10016-6402; **Phone:** 212-263-7410; **Board Cert:** Nuclear Medicine 1981; **Med School:** NYU Sch Med 1977; **Resid:** Diagnostic Radiology, NYU Med Ctr 1979; **Fellow:** Nuclear Medicine, NYU Med Ctr 1981; **Fac Appt:** Assoc Prof Rad, NYU Sch Med

Santos, Elmer B MD/PhD (NuM) - **Spec Exp:** Thyroid Cancer; PET Imaging; **Hospital:** Meml Sloan-Kettering Canc Ctr (page 114); **Address:** 1275 York Ave, New York, NY 10065; **Phone:** 212-639-7373; **Board Cert:** Nuclear Medicine 2007; **Med School:** Philippines 1991; **Resid:** Internal Medicine, Hosp St Raphael 1995; Nuclear Medicine, Meml Sloan Kettering Cancer Ctr 1997; **Fellow:** Cancer Immunology, Cambridge Univ 2001; Radiotracer Imaging, Meml Sloan Kettering Cancer Inst 2002; **Fac Appt:** Asst Prof Rad, Cornell Univ-Weill Med Coll

Scharf, Stephen MD (NuM) - **Spec Exp:** Thyroid & Parathyroid Imaging; Bone Imaging; CT Scan; **Hospital:** Lenox Hill Hosp (page 106); **Address:** Lenox Hill Hospital, Dept Nuclear Medicine, 100 E 77th St, Fl 3, New York, NY 10075; **Phone:** 212-434-2630; **Board Cert:** Internal Medicine 1977; Nuclear Medicine 1979; **Med School:** Albert Einstein Coll Med 1974; **Resid:** Internal Medicine, Bronx Municipal Hosp 1976; Nuclear Medicine, Montefiore Med Ctr 1978; **Fellow:** Nephrology, Montefiore Med Ctr 1979; **Fac Appt:** Asst Clin Prof NuM, Albert Einstein Coll Med

Obstetrics & Gynecology

Ascher-Walsh, Charles J MD (ObG) - **Spec Exp:** Uro-Gynecology; Gynecologic Surgery; Pelvic Surgery; Robotic Surgery; **Hospital:** Mt Sinai Med Ctr (page 102); **Address:** 5 E 98th St Fl 2, New York, NY 10029; **Phone:** 212-241-7952; **Board Cert:** Obstetrics & Gynecology 2013; **Med School:** SUNY Hlth Sci Ctr 1995; **Resid:** Obstetrics & Gynecology, Columbia Univ Med Ctr 1999; **Fellow:** Uro-Gynecology, Columbia Univ 2000; **Fac Appt:** Assoc Prof ObG, Mount Sinai Sch Med

Bacall, Charles J MD (ObG) - **Hospital:** Mt Sinai Med Ctr (page 102); **Address:** 1150 5th Ave, Ste 1B, New York, NY 10128-2920; **Phone:** 212-996-9100; **Board Cert:** Obstetrics & Gynecology 1981; **Med School:** NY Med Coll 1975; **Resid:** Obstetrics & Gynecology, Mt Sinai Hosp 1979; **Fac Appt:** Asst Clin Prof ObG, Mount Sinai Sch Med

Berman, Alvin MD (ObG) - **Spec Exp:** Menopause Problems; Osteoporosis; Sexual Dysfunction; Women's Health over age 40; **Hospital:** Mt Sinai Med Ctr (page 102); **Address:** 111B E 88th St, New York, NY 10128; **Phone:** 212-722-5757; **Board Cert:** Obstetrics & Gynecology 1978; **Med School:** South Africa 1969; **Resid:** Obstetrics & Gynecology, Mount Sinai Hosp 1976; **Fellow:** Neonatal-Perinatal Medicine, Mount Sinai Hosp 1977; **Fac Appt:** Asst Clin Prof ObG, Mount Sinai Sch Med

Blanco, Jody MD (ObG) - **Spec Exp:** Uro-Gynecology; Uterine Fibroids; Colposcopy; **Hospital:** NY-Presby/Columbia Univ Med Ctr, NY (page 104); **Address:** 161 Ft Washington Ave Fl 4 - rm 442, New York, NY 10032-3713; **Phone:** 212-305-1107; **Board Cert:** Obstetrics & Gynecology 2012; **Med School:** SUNY Hlth Sci Ctr 1981; **Resid:** Obstetrics & Gynecology, Columbia-Presby Med Ctr 1985; **Fellow:** Uro-Gynecology, UC Irvine 1986; **Fac Appt:** Asst Clin Prof ObG, Columbia P&S

Brightman, Rebecca C MD (ObG) - **Spec Exp:** Preconception Planning; Menopause Problems; Pregnancy-High Risk; **Hospital:** Mt Sinai Med Ctr (page 102); **Address:** 134 E 93rd St Fl 2nd, New York, NY 10128; **Phone:** 212-348-7800; **Board Cert:** Obstetrics & Gynecology 2012; **Med School:** Mount Sinai Sch Med 1986; **Resid:** Obstetrics & Gynecology, Mt Sinai Med Ctr 1990

Brodman, Michael L MD (ObG) - **Spec Exp:** Incontinence; Laparoscopic Surgery; Pelvic Organ Prolapse Repair; Uro-Gynecology; **Hospital:** Mt Sinai Med Ctr (page 102); **Address:** Dept Gynecology/Urogynecology, 5 E 98th St Fl 2, New York, NY 10029; **Phone:** 212-241-7952; **Board Cert:** Obstetrics & Gynecology 2012; **Med School:** Mount Sinai Sch Med 1982; **Resid:** Obstetrics & Gynecology, Mt Sinai Hosp 1986; **Fellow:** Pelvic Surgery, Mt Sinai Hosp 1987; **Fac Appt:** Assoc Prof ObG, Mount Sinai Sch Med

Brustman, Lois E MD (ObG) - **Spec Exp:** Prematurity/Low Birth Weight Infants; Diabetes in Pregnancy; Preconception Planning; Maternal & Fetal Medicine; **Hospital:** St. Luke's - Roosevelt Hosp Ctr - Roosevelt Div (page 94); **Address:** 1000 Tenth Ave, Ste 11A-61, New York, NY 10019-1147; **Phone:** 212-523-7579; **Board Cert:** Obstetrics & Gynecology 2012; Maternal & Fetal Medicine 2012; **Med School:** NY Med Coll 1979; **Resid:** Obstetrics & Gynecology, Montefiore Med Ctr 1984; **Fellow:** Maternal & Fetal Medicine, Montefiore Med Ctr 1988; **Fac Appt:** Assoc Prof ObG, NY Med Coll

Buchman, Myron I MD (ObG) - **Spec Exp:** Gynecology Only; **Hospital:** NY-Presby/Weill Cornell Med Ctr, NY (page 104); **Address:** 117 E 72nd St, New York, NY 10021-4249; **Phone:** 212-861-1950; **Board Cert:** Obstetrics & Gynecology 2004; **Med School:** Johns Hopkins Univ 1946; **Resid:** Obstetrics & Gynecology, Johns Hopkins Hosp 1947; Obstetrics & Gynecology, New York Lying-In Hosp 1952; **Fac Appt:** Assoc Clin Prof ObG, Cornell Univ-Weill Med Coll

Buterman, Irving MD (ObG) - **Spec Exp:** Women's Health; Pregnancy-High Risk; **Hospital:** Lenox Hill Hosp (page 106), Beth Israel Med Ctr - Petrie Div (page 94); **Address:** 950 Park Ave, New York, NY 10028-0320; **Phone:** 212-472-8200; **Board Cert:** Obstetrics & Gynecology 1983; **Med School:** Netherlands 1971; **Resid:** Obstetrics & Gynecology, Lenox Hill Hosp 1976; **Fellow:** Gyne cologic Oncology, Lenox Hill Hosp 1977; **Fac Appt:** Asst Clin Prof ObG, NY Med Coll

Chin, Jean M MD (ObG) *PCP* - **Spec Exp:** Menopause Problems; **Hospital:** Mt Sinai Med Ctr (page 102); **Address:** 785 Park Ave, New York, NY 10021; **Phone:** 212-249-7800; **Board Cert:** Obstetrics & Gynecology 1982; **Med School:** Columbia P&S 1976; **Resid:** Obstetrics & Gynecology, Mt Sinai Hosp 1980; **Fac Appt:** Asst Clin Prof ObG, Columbia P&S

Cox, Kathryn A MD (ObG) - **Spec Exp:** Gynecology Only; Menopause Problems; Gynecologic Surgery; **Hospital:** NY-Presby/Weill Cornell Med Ctr, NY (page 104); **Address:** 330 E 63rd St, Ste 1J, New York, NY 10065; **Phone:** 212-535-2600; **Board Cert:** Obstetrics & Gynecology 1981; **Med School:** Univ Mich Med Sch 1975; **Resid:** Obstetrics & Gynecology, New York Hosp/Cornell 1979

Dabney, Lisa MD (ObG) - **Spec Exp:** Uro-Gynecology; Minimally Invasive Surgery; Incontinence; **Hospital:** St. Luke's - Roosevelt Hosp Ctr - St Luke's Hosp (page 94); **Address:** 425 W 59th St Fl 5 - Ste D, New York, NY 10019; **Phone:** 212-523-7570; **Board Cert:** Obstetrics & Gynecology 2012; **Med School:** UCLA 1995; **Resid:** Obstetrics & Gynecology, Beth Israel Deaconess Med Ctr 1999; **Fellow:** Uro-Gynecology, Bellvue Med Ctr 2000

Diamond, Sharon MD (ObG) *PCP* - **Spec Exp:** Menopause Problems; Pap Smear Abnormalities; Gynecology Only; **Hospital:** Mt Sinai Med Ctr (page 102); **Address:** 61 E 86th St, Ste 1, New York, NY 10028-1003; **Phone:** 212-876-2200; **Board Cert:** Obstetrics & Gynecology 2012; **Med School:** Mount Sinai Sch Med 1979; **Resid:** Obstetrics & Gynecology, Mt Sinai Med Ctr 1983; **Fac Appt:** Asst Clin Prof ObG, Mount Sinai Sch Med

Evanko, John C MD (ObG) - **Spec Exp:** Pelvic Reconstruction; Minimally Invasive Surgery; Robotic Surgery; Gynecologic Surgery-Complex; **Hospital:** NY-Presby/Columbia Univ Med Ctr, NY (page 104); **Address:** 161 Fort Washington Ave, Ste 447, New York, NY 10032; **Phone:** 212-305-1107 x6; **Board Cert:** Obstetrics & Gynecology 2008; **Med School:** NY Med Coll 1995; **Resid:** Obstetrics & Gynecology, Columbia-Presby Med Ctr 1999Meml Sloan Kettering Cancer Ctr 1998; **Fac Appt:** Assoc Clin Prof ObG, Columbia P&S

Evans, Mark I MD (ObG) - **Spec Exp:** Reproductive Genetics; Fetal Diagnosis & Therapy; Multiple Gestation; Ultrasound; **Hospital:** Mt Sinai Med Ctr (page 102); **Address:** Comprehensive Genetics, 131 E 65th St, New York, NY 10065; **Phone:** 212-288-1422; **Board Cert:** Obstetrics & Gynecology 2012; Clinical Genetics 1984; **Med School:** SUNY Downstate 1978; **Resid:** Obstetrics & Gynecology, Lying-In Hosp 1982; **Fellow:** Clinical Genetics, Natl Inst Hlth 1984; **Fac Appt:** Prof ObG, Mount Sinai Sch Med

Fishbane-Mayer, Jill MD (ObG) - **Spec Exp:** Gynecology Only; **Hospital:** Mt Sinai Med Ctr (page 102); **Address:** 4 E 95th St, Ste 1A Bldg, New York, NY 10128-0705; **Phone:** 212-348-1111; **Board Cert:** Obstetrics & Gynecology 1982; **Med School:** Mount Sinai Sch Med 1976; **Resid:** Obstetrics & Gynecology, Mount Sinai Med Ctr 1980; **Fac Appt:** Assoc Clin Prof ObG, Mount Sinai Sch Med

Francis, Michelle MD (ObG) - **Hospital:** St. Luke's - Roosevelt Hosp Ctr - St Luke's Hosp (page 94); **Address:** 425 W 59th St, Ste 5D, New York, NY 10019; **Phone:** 212-523-6333; **Board Cert:** Obstetrics & Gynecology 2012; **Med School:** SUNY Hlth Sci Ctr 1999; **Resid:** Obstetrics & Gynecology, SUNY Hlth Sci Ctr 2003

Friedman Jr, Frederick MD (ObG) *PCP* - **Spec Exp:** Women's Health; Pap Smear Abnormalities; **Hospital:** Mt Sinai Med Ctr (page 102); **Address:** 47 E 88th St. Ground Fl, New York, NY 10128; **Phone:** 212-534-0200; **Board Cert:** Obstetrics & Gynecology 2012; **Med School:** SUNY Hlth Sci Ctr 1985; **Resid:** Obstetrics & Gynecology, Mount Sinai Hosp 1989; **Fac Appt:** Assoc Prof ObG, Mount Sinai Sch Med

Friedman, Lynn S MD (ObG) - **Spec Exp:** Miscarriage-Recurrent; Infertility; Pregnancy After Age 35; Pap Smear Abnormalities; **Hospital:** Mt Sinai Med Ctr (page 102); **Address:** 885 Park Ave, Ste 1-D, New York, NY 10075; **Phone:** 212-737-3282; **Board Cert:** Obstetrics & Gynecology 2012; **Med School:** NYU Sch Med 1984; **Resid:** Obstetrics & Gynecology, Mt Sinai Med Ctr 1988; **Fac Appt:** Asst Clin Prof ObG, Mount Sinai Sch Med

Goldman, Gary MD (ObG) - **Spec Exp:** Endometriosis; Laparoscopic Surgery-Complex; Hysterectomy Alternatives; **Hospital:** NY-Presby/Weill Cornell Med Ctr, NY (page 104); **Address:** 715 Park Ave, New York, NY 10021; **Phone:** 212-535-6100; **Board Cert:** Obstetrics & Gynecology 2012; **Med School:** SUNY Stony Brook 1986; **Resid:** Obstetrics & Gynecology, New York Hosp 1990; **Fac Appt:** Asst Clin Prof ObG, Cornell Univ-Weill Med Coll

Goldstein, Martin S MD (ObG) - **Spec Exp:** Uterine Fibroids; Laparoscopic Surgery; Pelvic Organ Prolapse Repair; Endometriosis; **Hospital:** Mt Sinai Med Ctr (page 102); **Address:** 40 E 84th St, New York, NY 10028-1314; **Phone:** 212-472-6500; **Board Cert:** Obstetrics & Gynecology 1980; **Med School:** SUNY Hlth Sci Ctr 1966; **Resid:** Obstetrics & Gynecology, Mount Sinai Hosp 1971; **Fac Appt:** Assoc Clin Prof ObG, Mount Sinai Sch Med

Goldstein, Steven R MD (ObG) - **Spec Exp:** Gynecologic Ultrasound; Menopause Problems; Uterine Fibroids; **Hospital:** NYU Langone Med Ctr (page 108); **Address:** 530 1st Av, Ste 10N, New York, NY 10016-6402; **Phone:** 212-263-7416; **Board Cert:** Obstetrics & Gynecology 2011; **Med School:** NYU Sch Med 1975; **Resid:** Obstetrics & Gynecology, NYU Affil Hosps 1980; **Fac Appt:** Prof ObG, NYU Sch Med

Gruss, Leslie MD (ObG) *PCP* - **Spec Exp:** HPV-Human Papilloma Virus; Pap Smear Abnormalities; **Hospital:** NYU Langone Med Ctr (page 108); **Address:** Downtown Women Ob-Gyn Assocs, 568 Broadway, Ste 304, New York, NY 10012; **Phone:** 212-966-7600; **Board Cert:** Obstetrics & Gynecology 2012; **Med School:** Med Coll PA Hahnemann 1983; **Resid:** Obstetrics & Gynecology, Montefiore Hosp Med Ctr 1987

Gubernick, Martin MD (ObG) - **Spec Exp:** Pregnancy-High Risk; **Hospital:** NY-Presby/Weill Cornell Med Ctr, NY (page 104); **Address:** 131 E 65th St, New York, NY 10065; **Phone:** 212-288-1422; **Board Cert:** Obstetrics & Gynecology 2013; **Med School:** Northwestern Univ 1982; **Resid:** Obstetrics & Gynecology, New York Hosp 1986

Hardart, Anne MD (ObG) *PCP* - **Spec Exp:** Uro-Gynecology; Incontinence; Laparoscopic Surgery; **Hospital:** St. Luke's - Roosevelt Hosp Ctr - St Luke's Hosp (page 94); **Address:** 425 W 59th St, Ste 5D, New York, NY 10019; **Phone:** 212-523-7570; **Board Cert:** Obstetrics & Gynecology 2013; Female Pelvic Medicine & Reconstuctive Surgery ; **Med School:** SUNY Stony Brook 1995; **Resid:** Obstetrics & Gynecology, SUNY Stony Brook 1999; **Fellow:** Uro-Gynecology, UCLA 2002; **Fac Appt:** Asst Clin Prof ObG, Columbia P&S

Harris, Dena E MD (ObG) *PCP* - **Spec Exp:** Gynecology Only; Menopause Problems; Vulvar Disease; **Hospital:** NYU Langone Med Ctr (page 108); **Address:** 430 W Broadway, Ste 2A, New York, NY 10012; **Phone:** 212-941-0011; **Board Cert:** Obstetrics & Gynecology 2012; **Med School:** Hahnemann Univ 1976; **Resid:** Obstetrics & Gynecology, NYU Med Ctr 1980; **Fac Appt:** Asst Clin Prof ObG, NYU Sch Med

Hirsch, Lissa B MD (ObG) - **Spec Exp:** Menopause Problems; **Hospital:** Lenox Hill Hosp (page 106); **Address:** 755 Park Ave, New York, NY 10021-4255; **Phone:** 212-570-2222; **Board Cert:** Obstetrics & Gynecology 1985; **Med School:** UMDNJ-NJ Med Sch, Newark 1979; **Resid:** Obstetrics & Gynecology, NYU Med Ctr 1985

Hockstein, Steven MD (ObG) - **Spec Exp:** Uterine Fibroids; **Hospital:** NY-Presby/Weill Cornell Med Ctr, NY (page 104); **Address:** 425 E 61st St Fl 11, New York, NY 10021; **Phone:** 212-821-0810; **Board Cert:** Obstetrics & Gynecology 2012; **Med School:** Univ MD Sch Med 1993; **Resid:** Obstetrics & Gynecology, McGaw Med Ctr 1997; **Fac Appt:** Asst Clin Prof ObG, Cornell Univ-Weill Med Coll

Holland, Claudia MD (ObG) *PCP* - **Hospital:** St. Luke's - Roosevelt Hosp Ctr - Roosevelt Div (page 94); **Address:** 800A 5th Ave, Ste 503, New York, NY 10065; **Phone:** 212-230-1760; **Board Cert:** Obstetrics & Gynecology 2012; **Med School:** Mount Sinai Sch Med 1981; **Resid:** Obstetrics & Gynecology, NYU Med Ctr 1985

Karamitsos, Harry MD (ObG) - **Hospital:** Lenox Hill Hosp (page 106); **Address:** Manhattan's Physician Group, 215 E 95th St, 590 5th Ave, Fl 7th, New York, NY 10128; **Phone:** 212-996-8000; **Board Cert:** Obstetrics & Gynecology 2012; **Med School:** NY Med Coll 1993; **Resid:** Obstetrics & Gynecology, Montefiore Med Ctr 1997

Kent, Joan L MD (ObG) - **Spec Exp:** Gynecology Only; **Hospital:** NY-Presby/Weill Cornell Med Ctr, NY (page 104); **Address:** 235 E 67th St, Ste 204, New York, NY 10065; **Phone:** 212-772-2900; **Board Cert:** Obstetrics & Gynecology 2012; **Med School:** Cornell Univ-Weill Med Coll 1984; **Resid:** Obstetrics & Gynecology, New York Hosp 1988; **Fac Appt:** Assoc Prof ObG, Cornell Univ-Weill Med Coll

Kessler, Alan A MD (ObG) - **Spec Exp:** Multiple Gestation; Pregnancy-High Risk; **Hospital:** NY-Presby/Weill Cornell Med Ctr, NY (page 104); **Address:** 131 E 65th St, MS 10065, New York, NY 10065; **Phone:** 212-288-1422; **Board Cert:** Obstetrics & Gynecology 2012; **Med School:** Mexico 1978; **Resid:** Obstetrics & Gynecology, New York Hosp 1983; **Fac Appt:** Assoc Prof ObG, Cornell Univ-Weill Med Coll

Kim, Joyce M MD (ObG) *PCP* - **Spec Exp:** Pregnancy-High Risk; **Hospital:** Mt Sinai Med Ctr (page 102); **Address:** 885 Park Ave St, Ste 1D, New York, NY 10021; **Phone:** 212-737-3282; **Board Cert:** Obstetrics & Gynecology 2012; **Med School:** Mount Sinai Sch Med 1986; **Resid:** Obstetrics & Gynecology, Mount Sinai Hosp 1990; **Fac Appt:** Asst Clin Prof ObG, Mount Sinai Sch Med

Krause, Cynthia L MD (ObG) *PCP* - **Spec Exp:** Menopause Problems; Pap Smear Abnormalities; Ovarian Cancer Genetics; Breast Cancer Genetics; **Hospital:** Mt Sinai Med Ctr (page 102); **Address:** 1185 Park Ave, Ste 1L, New York, NY 10128; **Phone:** 212-369-0602; **Board Cert:** Obstetrics & Gynecology 2012; **Med School:** Duke Univ 1980; **Resid:** Internal Medicine, Baltimore City Hosp 1982; Obstetrics & Gynecology, Mount Sinai Med Ctr 1986; **Fac Appt:** Asst Clin Prof ObG, Mount Sinai Sch Med

Leiter, Gila MD (ObG) - **Spec Exp:** Osteoporosis; Multiple Gestation; Menopause Problems; Uterine Fibroids; **Hospital:** Mt Sinai Med Ctr (page 102), Beth Israel Med Ctr - Petrie Div (page 94); **Address:** Park Ave Womens Center, 1160 Park Ave, New York, NY 10028; **Phone:** 212-860-2600; **Board Cert:** Obstetrics & Gynecology 2012; **Med School:** Albert Einstein Coll Med 1983; **Resid:** Obstetrics & Gynecology, Mt Sinai Hosp 1987; **Fac Appt:** Assoc Clin Prof ObG, Mount Sinai Sch Med

Levey, Kenneth A MD (ObG) - **Spec Exp:** Pain-Chronic Pelvic; Endometriosis; Uterine Fibroids; Robotic Surgery; **Hospital:** NYU Langone Med Ctr (page 108); **Address:** NY Pelvic Pain, 90 Maiden Lane, Ste 300, New York, NY 10038; **Phone:** 646-290-9560; **Board Cert:** Obstetrics & Gynecology 2012; **Med School:** SUNY Buffalo 1997; **Resid:** Obstetrics & Gynecology, G Washington Univ Med Ctr 2001; **Fac Appt:** Asst Clin Prof ObG, NYU Sch Med

Levine, Richard U MD (ObG) - **Spec Exp:** HPV-Human Papilloma Virus; Pap Smear Abnormalities; Gynecology Only; **Hospital:** NY-Presby/Columbia Univ Med Ctr, NY (page 104); **Address:** 51 W 51st St Fl 3, New York, NY 10019; **Phone:** 212-326-8491; **Board Cert:** Obstetrics & Gynecology 1994; **Med School:** Cornell Univ-Weill Med Coll 1966; **Resid:** Obstetrics & Gynecology, Columbia-Presby Med Ctr 1975; **Fellow:** Minimally Invasive Gynecologic Surgery, Karolinska Inst 1970; **Fac Appt:** Clin Prof ObG, Columbia P&S

Melnick, Hugh D MD (ObG) - **Spec Exp:** Infertility-IVF; Infertility-Male; Impotence; **Hospital:** Lenox Hill Hosp (page 106); **Address:** Advanced Fertility Services, 1625 Third Ave, Ground Fl, New York, NY 10128-3603; **Phone:** 212-369-8700; **Board Cert:** Obstetrics & Gynecology 1978; **Med School:** Temple Univ 1972; **Resid:** Obstetrics & Gynecology, Lenox Hill Hosp 1976

Michel, Ketly MD (ObG) - **Hospital:** Lenox Hill Hosp (page 106); **Address:** 261 E 78th St, New York, NY 10075; **Phone:** 212-249-4501; **Board Cert:** Obstetrics & Gynecology 2012; **Med School:** SUNY Upstate Med Univ 1984; **Resid:** Obstetrics & Gynecology, Metropolitan Hosp 1988

Moritz, Jacques MD (ObG) - **Hospital:** St. Luke's - Roosevelt Hosp Ctr - Roosevelt Div (page 94); **Address:** 315 W 57th St, Ste 204, Ob/Gyn Assocs at 57th St, New York, NY 10019; **Phone:** 212-603-4160; **Board Cert:** Obstetrics & Gynecology 2012; **Med School:** Univ Miami Sch Med 1988; **Resid:** Obstetrics & Gynecology, NY Presby-Columbia Med Ctr 1992; **Fac Appt:** Asst Clin Prof ObG, Columbia P&S

Ordorica, Steven Anthony MD (ObG) - **Spec Exp:** Pregnancy-High Risk; Miscarriage-Recurrent; Maternal & Fetal Medicine; **Hospital:** NYU Langone Med Ctr (page 108); **Address:** NYU Med Ctr, Dept OB/GYN, 530 1st Ave, Ste 10Q, New York, NY 10016-6402; **Phone:** 212-263-5982; **Board Cert:** Obstetrics & Gynecology 2013; Maternal & Fetal Medicine 2012; **Med School:** SUNY Stony Brook 1983; **Resid:** Obstetrics & Gynecology, NYU Med Ctr 1987; **Fellow:** Maternal & Fetal Medicine, NYU Med Ctr 1989; **Fac Appt:** Assoc Prof ObG, NYU Sch Med

Phillips, Robin N MD (ObG) *PCP* - **Spec Exp:** Gynecology Only; Menopause Problems; Women's Health over age 40; **Hospital:** Mt Sinai Med Ctr (page 102); **Address:** 1126 Park Ave, New York, NY 10128; **Phone:** 212-534-5300; **Board Cert:** Obstetrics & Gynecology 2000; **Med School:** Mount Sinai Sch Med 1977; **Resid:** Obstetrics & Gynecology, Mount Sinai Med Ctr 1982; **Fac Appt:** Asst Clin Prof ObG, Mount Sinai Sch Med

Rodke, Gae MD (ObG) *PCP* - **Spec Exp:** Vulvar Disease; Gynecologic Surgery; **Hospital:** St. Luke's - Roosevelt Hosp Ctr - Roosevelt Div (page 94); **Address:** 185 West End Ave, Ste 1D, New York, NY 10023-2005; **Phone:** 212-496-9800; **Board Cert:** Obstetrics & Gynecology ; **Med School:** Albert Einstein Coll Med 1981; **Resid:** Family Medicine, Univ Hosp 1982; Obstetrics & Gynecology, Univ Hosp 1986; **Fac Appt:** Asst Clin Prof ObG, Columbia P&S

Russell, Shereen H MD (ObG) - **Hospital:** Lenox Hill Hosp (page 106); **Address:** 755 Park Ave, New York, NY 10021; **Phone:** 212-570-2222; **Board Cert:** Obstetrics & Gynecology 2012; **Med School:** Univ Conn 1997; **Resid:** Obstetrics & Gynecology, Lenox Hill Hosp 2001

Rutenberg, Kathryn MD (ObG) - **Hospital:** St. Luke's - Roosevelt Hosp Ctr - St Luke's Hosp (page 94); **Address:** 30 W 60th St, Ste 1S, New York, NY 10023; **Phone:** 212-636-8900; **Board Cert:** Obstetrics & Gynecology 2012; **Med School:** SUNY Stony Brook 1998; **Resid:** Obstetrics & Gynecology, NYU Med Ctr 2002; **Fac Appt:** Asst Clin Prof ObG, Columbia P&S

Sadarangani, Balvinder Roy MD (ObG) - **Spec Exp:** Women's Health; Infertility; Menopause Problems; Ultrasound; **Hospital:** Beth Israel Med Ctr - Petrie Div (page 94); **Address:** 247 3rd Ave, Ste 503, New York, NY 10010; **Phone:** 212-982-4100; **Board Cert:** Obstetrics & Gynecology 1980; **Med School:** India 1968; **Resid:** Obstetrics & Gynecology, St Vincent's Hosp & Med Ctr 1978

Sandler, Benjamin MD (ObG) - **Spec Exp:** Infertility-IVF; Reproductive Endocrinology; **Hospital:** Mt Sinai Med Ctr (page 102); **Address:** Reproductive Medicine Associates of NY, 635 Madison Ave, Fl 10, New York, NY 10022-1009; **Phone:** 212-756-5777; **Board Cert:** Obstetrics & Gynecology 2012; **Med School:** Mexico 1982; **Resid:** Obstetrics & Gynecology, Michael Reese Hosp 1987; **Fellow:** Reproductive Endocrinology, Mt Sinai Hosp 1989; **Fac Appt:** Asst Clin Prof ObG, Mount Sinai Sch Med

Sassoon, Robert I MD (ObG) - **Spec Exp:** Laparoscopic Surgery; Pregnancy-High Risk; Gynecologic Surgery; **Hospital:** NY-Presby/Weill Cornell Med Ctr, NY (page 104); **Address:** 449 E 68th St Fl 2, Starr Pavilion, New York, NY 10021; **Phone:** 212-628-1500; **Board Cert:** Obstetrics & Gynecology 2012; **Med School:** Cornell Univ-Weill Med Coll 1981; **Resid:** Obstetrics & Gynecology, New York Hosp 1985; **Fac Appt:** Clin Prof ObG, Cornell Univ-Weill Med Coll

Scher, Jonathan MD (ObG) - **Spec Exp:** Gynecology Only; **Hospital:** Mt Sinai Med Ctr (page 102); **Address:** 1126 Park Ave, New York, NY 10128-1203; **Phone:** 212-427-7400; **Board Cert:** Obstetrics & Gynecology 1981; **Med School:** South Africa 1964; **Resid:** Obstetrics & Gynecology, Groote Schuur Hosp 1970; Obstetrics & Gynecology, Kings College Hosp 1972; **Fac Appt:** Asst Clin Prof ObG, Mount Sinai Sch Med

Schwartz, Judith W MD (ObG) - **Spec Exp:** Gynecologic Surgery; Menopause Problems; **Hospital:** Mt Sinai Med Ctr (page 102); **Address:** 45 E 82nd St Fl 1, New York, NY 10028; **Phone:** 212-879-5959; **Board Cert:** Obstetrics & Gynecology 2012; **Med School:** Mount Sinai Sch Med 1982; **Resid:** Obstetrics & Gynecology, Mount Sinai Hosp 1986; **Fac Appt:** Asst Clin Prof ObG, Mount Sinai Sch Med

Schweizer III, William E MD (ObG) - **Spec Exp:** Minimally Invasive Surgery; Gynecologic Surgery; **Hospital:** NYU Langone Med Ctr (page 108); **Address:** 150 E 32nd St, Ste 101, New York, NY 10016; **Phone:** 212-263-7021; **Board Cert:** Obstetrics & Gynecology 2009; **Med School:** SUNY Stony Brook 1983; **Resid:** Obstetrics & Gynecology, NYU Med Ctr 1987; **Fac Appt:** Assoc Clin Prof ObG, NYU Sch Med

Simon, Beth J MD (ObG) - **Spec Exp:** Gynecologic Surgery; Laparoscopic Surgery; **Hospital:** St. Luke's - Roosevelt Hosp Ctr - St Luke's Hosp (page 94); **Address:** 1090 Amsterdam Ave, Ste 6A, New York, NY 10025; **Phone:** 212-523-5179; **Board Cert:** Obstetrics & Gynecology 2013; **Med School:** Albert Einstein Coll Med 1998; **Resid:** Obstetrics & Gynecology, Montefiore Med Ctr 2002; **Fac Appt:** Asst Clin Prof ObG, Colombia

Smilen, Scott W MD (ObG) - **Spec Exp:** Uro-Gynecology; Pelvic Organ Prolapse Repair; Minimally Invasive Surgery; Incontinence; **Hospital:** NYU Langone Med Ctr (page 108), Valley Hosp (page 721); **Address:** NYU Med Ctr, Urogynecology, 150 E 32nd St Fl 2, New York, NY 10016-6497; **Phone:** 212-263-0395; **Board Cert:** Obstetrics & Gynecology 2012; **Med School:** NYU Sch Med 1988; **Resid:** Obstetrics & Gynecology, NYU Med Ctr 1992; **Fellow:** Uro-Gynecology, NYU Med Ctr 1993; **Fac Appt:** Assoc Prof ObG, NYU Sch Med

Sullum, Stanford N MD (ObG) *PCP* - **Spec Exp:** Gynecology Only; **Hospital:** Mt Sinai Med Ctr (page 102); **Address:** 1136 5th Ave, New York, NY 10128-0122; **Phone:** 212-876-4630; **Board Cert:** Obstetrics & Gynecology 1979; **Med School:** Jefferson Med Coll 1973; **Resid:** Obstetrics & Gynecology, Mount Sinai Hosp 1977; **Fac Appt:** Asst Clin Prof ObG, Mount Sinai Sch Med

Tyagi, Renuka MD (ObG) - **Spec Exp:** Uro-Gynecology; Urology-Female; Incontinence; Interstitial Cystitis; **Hospital:** NY-Presby/Weill Cornell Med Ctr, NY (page 104); **Address:** Iris Cantor Women's Ctr, 425 E 61st St Fl 11, New York, NY 10021; **Phone:** 212-821-0710; **Board Cert:** Obstetrics & Gynecology 2012; **Med School:** Wayne State Univ 2000; **Resid:** Obstetrics & Gynecology, NY Presby-Cornell Med Ctr 2004; **Fellow:** Female Urology, NY Presby-Cornell Med Ctr 2005; **Fac Appt:** Asst Prof U, Cornell Univ-Weill Med Coll

Waterstone, Melissa B MD (ObG) - **Hospital:** NY-Presby/Weill Cornell Med Ctr, NY (page 104); **Address:** Weill Cornell Med Assocs-East Side, 211 E 80th St Fl 2, New York, NY 10021; **Phone:** 646-962-7300; **Board Cert:** Obstetrics & Gynecology 2012; **Med School:** Cornell Univ-Weill Med Coll 1998; **Resid:** Obstetrics & Gynecology, George Washington Univ Hosp 2002

Yale, Suzanne I MD (ObG) - **Hospital:** Lenox Hill Hosp (page 106); **Address:** 16 E 82nd St, New York, NY 10028; **Phone:** 212-744-9300; **Board Cert:** Obstetrics & Gynecology 1984; **Med School:** UMDNJ-RW Johnson Med Sch 1977; **Resid:** Obstetrics & Gynecology, Lenox Hill Hosp 1981

Yarberry-Allen, Patricia MD (ObG) - **Spec Exp:** Gynecology Only; Menopause Problems; Women's Health; Vulvar & Vaginal Disorders; **Hospital:** NY-Presby/Weill Cornell Med Ctr, NY (page 104); **Address:** 509 Madison Ave, Ste 1212, New York, NY 10022; **Phone:** 212-410-4280; **Board Cert:** Obstetrics & Gynecology 1985; **Med School:** Univ Louisville Sch Med 1976; **Resid:** Obstetrics & Gynecology, New York Hosp 1982; **Fellow:** Infectious Disease, New York Hosp 1980; Gynecology, New York Hosp 1980

Young, Bruce Kenneth MD (ObG) - **Spec Exp:** Infertility; Minimally Invasive Surgery; Miscarriage-Recurrent; Pelvic Reconstruction; **Hospital:** NYU Langone Med Ctr (page 108), Bellevue Hosp Ctr; **Address:** 530 1st Ave, HCC-5th Fl, Ste 5G, NYU-Langone Medical Center, New York, NY 10016; **Phone:** 212-263-6359; **Board Cert:** Obstetrics & Gynecology 1970; Maternal & Fetal Medicine 1975; **Med School:** NYU Sch Med 1963; **Resid:** Obstetrics & Gynecology, NYU Med Ctr 1968; **Fellow:** Reproductive Endocrinology, NYU Med Ctr 1968; **Fac Appt:** Prof ObG, NYU Sch Med

Occupational Medicine

Landrigan, Philip MD (OM) - **Spec Exp:** Environmental Health in Children; **Hospital:** Mt Sinai Med Ctr (page 102); **Address:** Dept Preventive Med, One Gustave L Levy Pl, Box 1057, New York, NY 10029-6500; **Phone:** 212-824-7018; **Board Cert:** Pediatrics 1973; Public Health & Genl Preventive Med 1979; Occupational Medicine 1983; **Med School:** Harvard Med Sch 1967; **Resid:** Internal Medicine, Metro Genl Hosp 1968; Pediatrics, Chldns Hosp 1970; **Fellow:** Epidemiology, Ctrs for Disease Control 1973; Occupational Medicine, Univ London 1977; **Fac Appt:** Prof Ped, Mount Sinai Sch Med

Ophthalmology

Abramson, David H MD (Oph) - **Spec Exp:** Eye Tumors/Cancer; Orbital Tumors/Cancer; Retinoblastoma; Melanoma-Choroidal (eye); **Hospital:** Meml Sloan-Kettering Canc Ctr (page 114), NY-Presby/Weill Cornell Med Ctr, NY (page 104); **Address:** 70 E 66th St, New York, NY 10065; **Phone:** 212-744-1700; **Board Cert:** Ophthalmology 1975; **Med School:** Albert Einstein Coll Med 1969; **Resid:** Ophthalmology, Harkness Eye Inst 1974; **Fellow:** Ocular Oncology, Columbia-Presby Med Ctr 1975; **Fac Appt:** Prof Oph, Cornell Univ-Weill Med Coll

Accardi, Frank E MD (Oph) - **Spec Exp:** Cataract Surgery; Refractive Surgery; **Hospital:** New York Eye & Ear Infirm (page 115); **Address:** 114 E 27th St, New York, NY 10016; **Phone:** 212-481-4000; **Board Cert:** Ophthalmology 1987; **Med School:** Italy 1979; **Resid:** Internal Medicine, Cabrini Med Ctr 1982; Ophthalmology, SUNY-Downstate Med Ctr 1985; **Fellow:** Cornea, SUNY-Downstate Med Ctr 1986; **Fac Appt:** Asst Clin Prof Oph, NY Med Coll

Al-Aswad, Lama MD (Oph) - **Spec Exp:** Glaucoma; **Hospital:** NY-Presby/Columbia Univ Med Ctr, NY (page 104); **Address:** Columbia Ophthalmology Consultants, 635 W 165th St Fl 1, New York, NY 10032; **Phone:** 212-342-0943; **Board Cert:** Ophthalmology 2005; **Med School:** Syria 1993; **Resid:** Ophthalmology, SUNY Downstate Med Ctr 2001; **Fellow:** Research, Mass E&E Infirmary 1998; Glaucoma, Univ Tennessee Hlth Sci Ctr 2003; **Fac Appt:** Assoc Prof Oph, Columbia P&S

Angioletti Jr, Louis V MD (Oph) - **Spec Exp:** Retinal Disorders; Diabetic Eye Disease/Retinopathy; Macular Degeneration; **Hospital:** New York Eye & Ear Infirm (page 115); **Address:** Angioletti Retina Assocs, 7 Gramercy Park, New York, NY 10003-1759; **Phone:** 212-505-8510; **Board Cert:** Ophthalmology 1975; **Med School:** NY Med Coll 1966; **Resid:** Internal Medicine, St Vincents Hosp 1967; Ophthalmology, NY Eye & Ear Infirm 1973; **Fellow:** Retina, NY Eye & Ear Infirm 1974; **Fac Appt:** Clin Prof Oph, NY Med Coll

Asbell, Penny A MD (Oph) - **Spec Exp:** Corneal Disease & Transplant; LASIK-Refractive Surgery; Cataract Surgery; Keratoconus; **Hospital:** Mt Sinai Med Ctr (page 102); **Address:** 17 E 102nd St Fl 8, New York, NY 10029; **Phone:** 212-241-7977; **Board Cert:** Ophthalmology 1980; **Med School:** SUNY Buffalo 1975; **Resid:** Ophthalmology, NYU Med Ctr 1979; **Fellow:** Immunology, NYU Med Ctr 1980; Cornea & Ext Eye Disease, LSU Eye Ctr 1982; **Fac Appt:** Prof Oph, Mount Sinai Sch Med

Auran, James D MD (Oph) - **Spec Exp:** Cataract Surgery; Cornea & External Eye Disease; Acanthamoeba Keratitis; Dry Eye Syndrome; **Hospital:** NY-Presby/Columbia Univ Med Ctr, NY (page 104); **Address:** Edward S Harkness Eye Inst, 635 W 165th St Fl 5th, New York, NY 10032-3701; **Phone:** 212-305-9535; **Board Cert:** Ophthalmology 1989; **Med School:** Cornell Univ-Weill Med Coll 1983; **Resid:** Ophthalmology, Manhattan EET Hosp 1987; **Fellow:** Ophthalmology, Manhattan EET Hosp 1988; **Fac Appt:** Assoc Clin Prof Oph, Columbia P&S

Bansal, Rajendra K MD (Oph) - **Spec Exp:** Glaucoma; Cataract Surgery; **Hospital:** NY-Presby/Columbia Univ Med Ctr, NY (page 104); **Address:** Harkness Eye Inst, 635 W 165th St, New York, NY 10032; **Phone:** 212-350-2241; **Board Cert:** Ophthalmology 1977; **Med School:** India 1967; **Resid:** Ophthalmology, Univ Delhi Hosp 1973; **Fellow:** Glaucoma, Columbia Presby Med Ctr 1979; **Fac Appt:** Assoc Clin Prof Oph, Columbia P&S

Barile, Gaetano R MD (Oph) - **Spec Exp:** Macular Disease/Degeneration; Retinal Disorders; Diabetic Eye Disease/Retinopathy; Retina/Vitreous Consultation; **Hospital:** Lenox Hill Hosp (Manh Eye, Ear & Throat Hosp) (page 106); **Address:** 210 E 64 St, Fl 7, New York, NY 10065; **Phone:** 212-702-7400; **Board Cert:** Ophthalmology 2008; **Med School:** Cornell Univ 1991; **Resid:** Ophthalmology, Manhattan EET Hosp 1995; **Fellow:** Retina/Vitreous Surgery, Roosevelt Hosp/Harkness Eye Inst 1997; Retina, Moorfields Eye Hosp 1997

Barker, Barbara Ann MD (Oph) - **Spec Exp:** Glaucoma; Corneal Disease; Laser Surgery; **Hospital:** New York Eye & Ear Infirm (page 115), Mt Sinai Med Ctr (page 102); **Address:** 70 E 96th St, Ste 1B, New York, NY 10028; **Phone:** 212-289-2244; **Board Cert:** Ophthalmology 1981; **Med School:** Mount Sinai Sch Med 1976; **Resid:** Ophthalmology, Mt Sinai Med Ctr 1980; **Fellow:** Glaucoma, Beth Israel Med Ctr 1981; Cornea, Beth Israel Med Ctr 1983; **Fac Appt:** Assoc Clin Prof Oph, Mount Sinai Sch Med

Braunstein, Richard E MD (Oph) - **Spec Exp:** LASIK-Refractive Surgery; Corneal Disease & Transplant; Cataract Surgery; **Hospital:** Lenox Hill Hosp (Manh Eye, Ear & Throat Hosp) (page 106); **Address:** MEETH Ophthalmology, 210 E 64th St, New York, NY 10065; **Phone:** 212-702-7300; **Board Cert:** Ophthalmology 2006; **Med School:** Columbia P&S 1989; **Resid:** Ophthalmology, Harkness Eye Inst 1993; **Fellow:** Cornea & Ext Eye Disease, Wilmer Inst/Johns Hopkins Hosp 1994

Buxton, Douglas F MD (Oph) - **Spec Exp:** Corneal Disease & Transplant; LASIK-Refractive Surgery; Cataract Surgery-Lens Implant; Glaucoma-Pediatric; **Hospital:** New York Eye & Ear Infirm (page 115), Lenox Hill Hosp (Manh Eye, Ear & Throat Hosp) (page 106); **Address:** 310 E 14th St, Ste 403, New York, NY 10003-4201; **Phone:** 212-979-4410; **Board Cert:** Ophthalmology 2008; Penetrating Keratoplasty 2007; Cataract/Implant Surgery 2002; Refractive Surgery(LASIK) 2002; **Med School:** Cornell Univ-Weill Med Coll 1982; **Resid:** Ophthalmology, New York Eye & Ear Infirm 1986; **Fellow:** Cornea & Ext Eye Disease, New York Eye & Ear Infirm 1988; **Fac Appt:** Assoc Clin Prof Oph, NY Med Coll

Campolattaro, Brian N MD (Oph) - **Spec Exp:** Pediatric Ophthalmology; Strabismus; Tear Duct Problems; Eye Muscle Disorders; **Hospital:** New York Eye & Ear Infirm (page 115), Lenox Hill Hosp (Manh Eye, Ear & Throat Hosp) (page 106); **Address:** Ped Ophthalmology of NY, 30 E 40th St, Ste 405, New York, NY 10016-3507; **Phone:** 212-684-3980; **Board Cert:** Ophthalmology 2006; **Med School:** UMDNJ-NJ Med Sch, Newark 1990; **Resid:** Ophthalmology, New York Eye & Ear Infirm 1994; **Fellow:** Pediatric Ophthalmology, St Louis Chldns Hosp 1995; **Fac Appt:** Asst Clin Prof Oph, NY Med Coll

Casper, Daniel S MD/PhD (Oph) - **Spec Exp:** Diabetic Eye Disease; Diabetic Eye Disease/Retinopathy; **Hospital:** NY-Presby/Columbia Univ Med Ctr, NY (page 104); **Address:** 635 W 165th St, Flanzer Suite, New York, NY 10032-3822; **Phone:** 212-305-9535; **Board Cert:** Ophthalmology 1991; **Med School:** Albany Med Coll 1985; **Resid:** Ophthalmology, Harkness Eye Inst-Columbia 1989; **Fellow:** Oculoplastic Surgery, Harkness Eye Inst-Columbia 1990; **Fac Appt:** Asst Clin Prof Oph, Columbia P&S

Ceisler, Emily J MD (Oph) - **Spec Exp:** Pediatric Ophthalmology; Strabismus; Eye Muscle Disorders-Child & Adult; **Hospital:** NYU Langone Med Ctr (page 108), New York Eye & Ear Infirm (page 115); **Address:** Pediatric Ophthalmic Consultants, 40 W 72nd St, New York, NY 10023; **Phone:** 212-981-9800; **Board Cert:** Ophthalmology 2008; **Med School:** Harvard Med Sch 1991; **Resid:** Ophthalmology, Mass Eye & Ear Infirmary 1995; **Fellow:** Pediatric Ophthalmology, Manhattan Eye & Ear Infirmary 1996; **Fac Appt:** Asst Clin Prof Oph, NYU Sch Med

Chaiken, Barry G MD (Oph) - **Spec Exp:** Cataract Surgery; LASIK-Refractive Surgery; **Hospital:** New York Eye & Ear Infirm (page 115), St. Luke's - Roosevelt Hosp Ctr - Roosevelt Div (page 94); **Address:** 625 Park Ave, New York, NY 10065; **Phone:** 212-249-1976; **Board Cert:** Ophthalmology 1981; **Med School:** Columbia P&S 1976; **Resid:** Ophthalmology, Mt Sinai Hosp 1980

Chang, Stanley MD (Oph) - **Spec Exp:** Retina/Vitreous Surgery; Diabetic Eye Disease/Retinopathy; Macular Disease/Degeneration; Retinal Disorders; **Hospital:** NY-Presby/Columbia Univ Med Ctr, NY (page 104); **Address:** 635 W 165th St, Box 92, New York, NY 10032; **Phone:** 212-305-9535; **Board Cert:** Ophthalmology 1979; **Med School:** Columbia P&S 1974; **Resid:** Ophthalmology, Mass Eye & Ear Infirm 1978; **Fellow:** Vitreoretinal Surgery, Bascom Palmer Eye Inst 1979; **Fac Appt:** Prof Oph, Columbia P&S

Charles, Norman C MD (Oph) - **Spec Exp:** Contact Lenses; Cornea & External Eye Disease; Ophthalmic Pathology; Cataract Surgery; **Hospital:** NYU Langone Med Ctr (page 108); **Address:** 620 Park Ave, New York, NY 10065-6561; **Phone:** 212-772-6920; **Board Cert:** Ophthalmology 1971; **Med School:** NYU Sch Med 1963; **Resid:** Ophthalmology, NYU Med Ctr 1970; **Fellow:** Ophthalmic Pathology, NYU Med Ctr 1971; **Fac Appt:** Clin Prof Oph, NYU Sch Med

Chern, Relly D MD (Oph) - **Spec Exp:** Cataract Surgery; Ophthalmic Plastic Surgery; **Hospital:** Lenox Hill Hosp (Manh Eye, Ear & Throat Hosp) (page 106), New York Eye & Ear Infirm (page 115); **Address:** 923 5th Ave, Ste 1B, New York, NY 10021; **Phone:** 212-628-0160; **Board Cert:** Ophthalmology 1983; **Med School:** Albert Einstein Coll Med 1976; **Resid:** Ophthalmology, Montefiore Hosp Med Ctr 1980; **Fac Appt:** Asst Clin Prof Oph, Albert Einstein Coll Med

Cioffi, George MD (Oph) - **Spec Exp:** Glaucoma; Cataract Surgery; Anterior Segment Surgery; **Hospital:** NY-Presby/Columbia Univ Med Ctr, NY (page 104); **Address:** 635 W 165th St, Columbia Ophthalmic Consultants, Flazner Ste, New York, NY 10032; **Phone:** 212-305-9535; **Board Cert:** Ophthalmology 2004; **Med School:** Univ SC Sch Med 1987; **Resid:** Ophthalmology, Univ Maryland Affil Hosp 1991; **Fellow:** Glaucoma, Devers Eye Inst 1992; **Fac Appt:** Prof Oph, Columbia P&S

Cohen, Ben Z MD (Oph) - **Spec Exp:** Retina/Vitreous Surgery; Macular Degeneration; Diabetic Eye Disease/Retinopathy; **Hospital:** New York Eye & Ear Infirm (page 115), Mt Sinai Med Ctr (page 102); **Address:** Retina Assocs of NY, 140 E 80th St Fl 1, New York, NY 10075; **Phone:** 212-772-0600; **Board Cert:** Ophthalmology 1981; **Med School:** NY Med Coll 1976; **Resid:** Ophthalmology, Univ Chicago Hosps 1980; **Fellow:** Macular Disease, Manhattan Eye & Ear Infirmary 1981; Retina/Vitreous Surgery, Mass Eye & Ear Infirmary 1983; **Fac Appt:** Asst Prof Oph, Mount Sinai Sch Med

Cohen, Leeber MD (Oph) - **Spec Exp:** Cataract Surgery; AIDS Related Eye Diseases; Botox Therapy; **Hospital:** New York Eye & Ear Infirm (page 115); **Address:** 11 5th Ave, Ste B Bldg, New York, NY 10003-4342; **Phone:** 212-777-1644; **Board Cert:** Ophthalmology 1989; **Med School:** SUNY Hlth Sci Ctr 1983; **Resid:** Ophthalmology, Kings Co Hosp/SUNY Downstate 1987; **Fac Appt:** Asst Clin Prof Med, SUNY Downstate

Coleman, Donald Jackson MD (Oph) - **Spec Exp:** Retina/Vitreous Surgery; Ultrasound-Eye; Melanoma-Choroidal (eye); **Hospital:** NY-Presby/Columbia Univ Med Ctr, NY (page 104); **Address:** Columbia Ophthalmology Consultants, Edward S Harkness Eye Inst, 635 W 165th St Fl 1st, Box 92, New York, NY 10032; **Phone:** 212-305-9535; **Board Cert:** Ophthalmology 1969; **Med School:** SUNY Buffalo 1960; **Resid:** Ophthalmology, Columbia-Presby Med Ctr 1967; **Fellow:** Research, Natl Inst Hlth 1968; **Fac Appt:** Prof Oph, Cornell Univ-Weill Med Coll

Cykiert, Robert MD (Oph) - **Spec Exp:** LASIK-Refractive Surgery; Cataract Surgery; Corneal Disease & Transplant; Keratoconus; **Hospital:** NYU Langone Med Ctr (page 108), New York Eye & Ear Infirm (page 115); **Address:** 345 E 37th St, Ste 210, New York, NY 10016-3217; **Phone:** 212-922-1430; **Board Cert:** Ophthalmology 1981; **Med School:** NY Med Coll 1976; **Resid:** Ophthalmology, Montefiore Med Ctr 1980; **Fellow:** Cornea & Ext Eye Disease, Wills Eye Hosp 1981; **Fac Appt:** Assoc Clin Prof Oph, NYU Sch Med

D'Amico, Donald J MD (Oph) - **Spec Exp:** Diabetic Eye Disease/Retinopathy; Retinal Detachment; Retinal Disorders; **Hospital:** NY-Presby/Weill Cornell Med Ctr, NY (page 104); **Address:** Weill Cornell Eye Associates, Dept of Ophthalmology, 1305 York Ave, Fl 11th, New York, NY 10021; **Phone:** 646-962-2020; **Board Cert:** Ophthalmology 1982; **Med School:** Univ IL Coll Med 1977; **Resid:** Ophthalmology, Mass Eye & Ear Infirm 1981; **Fellow:** Vitreoretinal Surgery, Bascom Palmer Eye Inst 1982; **Fac Appt:** Prof Oph, Cornell Univ-Weill Med Coll

Dayan, Alan R MD (Oph) - **Spec Exp:** Retinal Disorders; Retina/Vitreous Surgery; Macular Degeneration; Retinal Detachment; **Hospital:** New York Eye & Ear Infirm (page 115); **Address:** 310 E 14th St South Bldg - Ste 419, New York, NY 10003; **Phone:** 212-677-2000; **Board Cert:** Ophthalmology 2009; **Med School:** Mount Sinai Sch Med 1992; **Resid:** Ophthalmology, NY Eye & Ear Infirm 1996; **Fellow:** Vitreoretinal Disease, Vitreoretinal Fdn 1998

Delerme, Milton MD (Oph) - **Spec Exp:** Anterior Segment Surgery; **Hospital:** Harlem Hosp Ctr; **Address:** 75 E 116th St, New York, NY 10029; **Phone:** 212-828-7700; **Board Cert:** Ophthalmology 1987; **Med School:** UMDNJ-NJ Med Sch, Newark 1978; **Resid:** Surgery, UMDNJ-Univ Hosp 1980; Ophthalmology, Harlem Hosp 1984; **Fellow:** Anterior Segment - External Disease, St Francis Hosp 1985

Della Rocca, Robert C MD (Oph) - **Spec Exp:** Orbital Tumors/Cancer; Eyelid Tumors/Cancer; Oculoplastic Surgery; Eyelid Cancer & Reconstruction; **Hospital:** New York Eye & Ear Infirm (page 115), Montefiore New Rochelle Hosp; **Address:** 310 E 14th St, South Bldg, rm 319, New York, NY 10003; **Phone:** 212-979-4575; **Board Cert:** Ophthalmology 1975; **Med School:** Creighton Univ 1967; **Resid:** Ophthalmology, NY Eye & Ear Infirm 1973; **Fellow:** Oculoplastic Surgery, Albany Med Coll/NY Eye & Ear Infirm 1975

Dodick, Jack M MD (Oph) - **Spec Exp:** Cataract Surgery-Lens Implant; Laser Vision Surgery; **Hospital:** NYU Langone Med Ctr (page 108), Lenox Hill Hosp (Manh Eye, Ear & Throat Hosp) (page 106); **Address:** 535 Park Ave, New York, NY 10065; **Phone:** 212-288-7638; **Board Cert:** Ophthalmology 1969; **Med School:** Univ Toronto 1963; **Resid:** Ophthalmology, Manhattan EE&T Hosp 1967; **Fellow:** Anterior Segment - External Disease, Westchester Co Med Ctr 1968; **Fac Appt:** Prof Oph, NYU Sch Med

Eggers, Howard M MD (Oph) - **Spec Exp:** Pediatric Ophthalmology; Strabismus-Adult & Pediatric; **Hospital:** NY-Presby/Columbia Univ Med Ctr, NY (page 104); **Address:** Harkness Eye Institute, 635 W 165th St, New York, NY 10032-3724; **Phone:** 212-305-5409; **Board Cert:** Ophthalmology 1978; **Med School:** Columbia P&S 1971; **Resid:** Ophthalmology, Harkness Inst-Presby Hosp 1975; **Fac Appt:** Prof Oph, Columbia P&S

Eichenbaum, Joseph W MD (Oph) - **Spec Exp:** Uveitis; Glaucoma; Toxicology; Eye Infections; **Hospital:** Mt Sinai Med Ctr (page 102); **Address:** 1050 Park Ave, New York, NY 10028; **Phone:** 212-289-7200; **Board Cert:** Ophthalmology 1980; **Med School:** Yale Univ 1973; **Resid:** Ophthalmology, NYU Med Ctr 1977; **Fellow:** Oculoplastic & Reconstructive Surgery, Mount Sinai Hosp 1980; **Fac Appt:** Assoc Clin Prof Oph, Mount Sinai Sch Med

Elahi, Ebrahim MD (Oph) - **Spec Exp:** Cosmetic & Reconstructive Surgery; Oculoplastic & Orbital Surgery; Eyelid Tumors/Cancer; Facial Plastic Surgery; **Hospital:** Mt Sinai Med Ctr (page 102), Beth Israel Med Ctr - Petrie Div (page 94); **Address:** 1034 Fifth Ave, MS 10028, New York, NY 10028; **Phone:** 212-570-0707; **Board Cert:** Ophthalmology 2012; **Med School:** Mount Sinai Sch Med 1996; **Resid:** Ophthalmology, Mt Sinai Hosp 2000; **Fellow:** Ophthalmic Plastic & Reconstructive Surgery, Manhattan EE&T Infirmary 2001; **Fac Appt:** Assoc Clin Prof Oph, Mount Sinai Sch Med

Engel, Harry M MD (Oph) - **Spec Exp:** Retinal Disorders; **Hospital:** Montefiore Med Ctr-Moses Campus (page 100), New York Eye & Ear Infirm (page 115); **Address:** West Side Retina, 40 W 72nd St, New York, NY 10023; **Phone:** 212-724-2555; **Board Cert:** Ophthalmology 1981; **Med School:** NY Med Coll 1976; **Resid:** Ophthalmology, U Michigan Med Ctr 1980; **Fellow:** Eye Pathology, Wilmer Inst 1981; Retina/Vitreous Surgery, Barnes Jewish Hosp 1982; **Fac Appt:** Clin Prof Oph, Albert Einstein Coll Med

Esposito, Donna A MD (Oph) - **Spec Exp:** Glaucoma; Cataract Surgery; **Hospital:** New York Eye & Ear Infirm (page 115); **Address:** 49 W 23rd St Fl 12th, New York, NY 10010; **Phone:** 212-255-4373; **Board Cert:** Ophthalmology 1991; **Med School:** NY Med Coll 1983; **Resid:** Surgery, St Vincent's Hosp 1985; Ophthalmology, St Vincent's Hosp 1989; **Fellow:** Glaucoma, NY Hosp 1990

Finger, Paul T MD (Oph) - **Spec Exp:** Eye Tumors/Cancer; Melanoma-Choroidal (eye); Retinoblastoma; Orbital Tumors/Cancer; **Hospital:** New York Eye & Ear Infirm (page 115), Lenox Hill Hosp (Manh Eye, Ear & Throat Hosp) (page 106); **Address:** 115 E 61st St, Fl 5, Ste B, New York, NY 10065; **Phone:** 212-832-8170; **Board Cert:** Ophthalmology 1990; **Med School:** Tulane Univ 1982; **Resid:** Ophthalmology, Manhattan EET Hosp 1986; **Fellow:** Ocular Oncology, N Shore Univ Hosp 1987; **Fac Appt:** Clin Prof Oph, NYU Sch Med

Fisher, Yale L MD (Oph) - **Spec Exp:** Retina/Vitreous Consultation; Diabetic Eye Disease; Ocular Ultrasound; **Hospital:** Lenox Hill Hosp (Manh Eye, Ear & Throat Hosp) (page 106), NY-Presby/Weill Cornell Med Ctr, NY (page 104); **Address:** Vitreous-Retina-Macula Consults of NY, 460 Park Ave Fl 5, New York, NY 10022; **Phone:** 212-861-9797; **Board Cert:** Ophthalmology 1973; **Med School:** Cornell Univ-Weill Med Coll 1967; **Resid:** Internal Medicine, Cornell Med Ctr 1968; Ophthalmology, Manhattan EE&T Hosp 1971; **Fac Appt:** Clin Prof Oph, Cornell Univ-Weill Med Coll

Florakis, George J MD (Oph) - **Spec Exp:** Cornea Transplant; Corneal Disease; Keratoconus; Anterior Segment Trauma/Reconstruction; **Hospital:** NY-Presby/Columbia Univ Med Ctr, NY (page 104), White Plains Hosp (page 640); **Address:** Edward S Harkness Eye Inst, Columbia Univ Med Ctr/NY Presby Hosp, 635 W 165th St, Ste 303, New York, NY 10032; **Phone:** 212-927-2394; **Board Cert:** Ophthalmology 1989; **Med School:** Columbia P&S 1983; **Resid:** Ophthalmology, Harkness Eye Inst 1987; **Fellow:** Cornea & Ext Eye Disease, Univ Iowa Hosps & Clins 1988; **Fac Appt:** Clin Prof Oph, Columbia P&S

Fong, Raymond MD (Oph) - **Spec Exp:** Cataract Surgery; LASIK-Refractive Surgery; Glaucoma; **Hospital:** Lenox Hill Hosp (Manh Eye, Ear & Throat Hosp) (page 106), NY-Presby/Lower Manhattan Hosp (page 104); **Address:** Raymond Fong Eye Care, 109 Lafayette St Fl 4, New York, NY 10013-4154; **Phone:** 212-274-1900; **Board Cert:** Ophthalmology 1987; **Med School:** Cornell Univ 1981; **Resid:** Internal Medicine, Beth Israel Med Ctr 1982; Ophthalmology, Manhattan EE&T Hosp 1985

Fox, Martin L MD (Oph) - **Spec Exp:** LASIK-Refractive Surgery; Cornea Transplant; Corneal Ring Implants; **Hospital:** New York Eye & Ear Infirm (page 115); **Address:** 425 Madison Ave, Ste 1501, New York, NY 10017; **Phone:** 212-838-1053; **Board Cert:** Ophthalmology 1981; **Med School:** Hahnemann Univ 1976; **Resid:** Ophthalmology, Boston Univ Med Ctr 1980; **Fellow:** Cornea, NY Eye & Ear Infirmary 1981

Friedman, Alan H MD (Oph) - **Spec Exp:** Uveitis; Eye Tumors/Cancer; Retinal Disorders; Ophthalmic Pathology; **Hospital:** Mt Sinai Med Ctr (page 102), Lenox Hill Hosp (page 106); **Address:** 888 Park Ave, Ste 1A, New York, NY 10075; **Phone:** 212-794-2277; **Board Cert:** Ophthalmology 1971; **Med School:** NYU Sch Med 1963; **Resid:** Ophthalmology, NYU Med Ctr 1969; **Fellow:** Ocular Pathology, NYU Langone Med Ctr 1970; Pathology, Hammersmith Hosp 1972; **Fac Appt:** Clin Prof Oph, Mount Sinai Sch Med

Friedman, Robert MD (Oph) - **Spec Exp:** Laser-Refractive Surgery; Cataract Surgery; Retina/Vitreous Surgery; Macular Disease/Degeneration; **Hospital:** Lenox Hill Hosp (page 106), Mt Sinai Med Ctr (page 102); **Address:** 1001 Park Ave, New York, NY 10028-0935; **Phone:** 212-772-6202; **Board Cert:** Ophthalmology 1989; **Med School:** Albert Einstein Coll Med 1983; **Resid:** Internal Medicine, St Lukes-Roosevelt Hosp 1984; Ophthalmology, Lenox Hill Hosp 1987; **Fellow:** Vitreoretinal Surgery, Manhattan EE&T Hosp 1988; **Fac Appt:** Asst Clin Prof Oph, Mount Sinai Sch Med

Fromer, Mark D MD (Oph) - **Spec Exp:** Retinal Disorders; Laser Vision Surgery; Cataract Surgery; Diabetic Eye Disease/Retinopathy; **Hospital:** New York Eye & Ear Infirm (page 115), Lenox Hill Hosp (Manh Eye, Ear & Throat Hosp) (page 106); **Address:** Fromer Eye Centers, 550 Park Ave, New York, NY 10065; **Phone:** 212-832-9228; **Board Cert:** Ophthalmology 1989; **Med School:** UMDNJ-Rutgers Med Sch 1984; **Resid:** Ophthalmology, St Vincents Hosp 1988; **Fellow:** Vitreoretinal Surgery, Manhattan EE&T Hosp 1989; **Fac Appt:** Asst Clin Prof Oph, NY Med Coll

Fuchs, Wayne MD (Oph) - **Spec Exp:** Diabetic Eye Disease/Retinopathy; Macular Disease/Degeneration; Retinal Disorders; Pseudoxanthoma Elasticum; **Hospital:** Mt Sinai Med Ctr (page 102), Lenox Hill Hosp (Manh Eye, Ear & Throat Hosp) (page 106); **Address:** 121 E 60th St, Ste 5B, New York, NY 10022-1186; **Phone:** 212-319-8205; **Board Cert:** Ophthalmology 1985; **Med School:** Mount Sinai Sch Med 1979; **Resid:** Ophthalmology, Mt Sinai Hosp 1983; **Fellow:** Vitreoretinal Surgery & Disease, NY Hosp-Cornell Med Ctr 1984; **Fac Appt:** Clin Prof Oph, Mount Sinai Sch Med

Gallin, Pamela F MD (Oph) - **Spec Exp:** Pediatric Ophthalmology; Amblyopia; Strabismus; Lacrimal Gland Disorders; **Hospital:** NY-Presby/Columbia Univ Med Ctr, NY (page 104), Lenox Hill Hosp (Manh Eye, Ear & Throat Hosp) (page 106); **Address:** NY Presbyterian-Columbia Univ Med Ctr, 635 W 165th St, Ste 224, New York, NY 10032-3701; **Phone:** 212-305-5407; **Board Cert:** Ophthalmology 1983; **Med School:** Washington Univ, St Louis 1978; **Resid:** Ophthalmology, Mount Sinai Med Ctr 1982; **Fellow:** Pediatric Ophthalmology, Chldns Natl Med Ctr 1983; Strabismus, Columbia-Presby Med Ctr 1983; **Fac Appt:** Prof Oph, Columbia P&S

Gentile, Ronald C MD (Oph) - **Spec Exp:** Retina/Vitreous Surgery; Diabetic Eye Disease/Retinopathy; Macular Degeneration; Retinal Disorders; **Hospital:** New York Eye & Ear Infirm (page 115), Winthrop Univ Hosp (page 524); **Address:** 310 E 14th St, South Bldg, Ste 319S, New York, NY 10003-4201; **Phone:** 212-979-4120; **Board Cert:** Ophthalmology 2008; **Med School:** SUNY Downstate 1991; **Resid:** Ophthalmology, NY Eye & Ear Infirm 1995; **Fellow:** Ocular Pathology, NY Eye & Ear Infirm 1996; Retina/Vitreous Surgery, Kresge Eye Inst 1998; **Fac Appt:** Prof Oph, NY Med Coll

Gibralter, Richard P MD (Oph) - **Spec Exp:** Cataract Surgery; Laser Vision Surgery; Cornea Transplant; Corneal Disease & Surgery; **Hospital:** Lenox Hill Hosp (Manh Eye, Ear & Throat Hosp) (page 106), New York Eye & Ear Infirm (page 115); **Address:** 154 E 71st St, New York, NY 10021-5123; **Phone:** 212-628-2202; **Board Cert:** Ophthalmology 1981; **Med School:** Mount Sinai Sch Med 1976; **Resid:** Ophthalmology, Manhattan EE&T Hosp 1980; **Fellow:** Cornea, Manhattan EE&T Hosp 1981; **Fac Appt:** Assoc Clin Prof Oph, NYU Sch Med

Goldstein, Michael T MD (Oph) - **Spec Exp:** Corneal Disease; Keratoconus; LASIK-Refractive Surgery; **Hospital:** New York Eye & Ear Infirm (page 115), Lenox Hill Hosp (Manh Eye, Ear & Throat Hosp) (page 106); **Address:** 115 E 61st St, Ste 3A, New York, NY 10065; **Phone:** 212-371-6209; **Board Cert:** Ophthalmology 1980; **Med School:** SUNY Downstate 1974; **Resid:** Ophthalmology, Brookdale Hosp Med Ctr 1979; **Fellow:** Cornea, Manhattan Eye, Ear & Throat Hosp 1980

Grayson, Douglas K MD (Oph) - **Spec Exp:** Cataract Surgery; Glaucoma; **Hospital:** New York Eye & Ear Infirm (page 115); **Address:** Omni Eye Services, 36 E 36th St, New York, NY 10016-3463; **Phone:** 212-353-0030; **Board Cert:** Ophthalmology 2006; **Med School:** Brown Univ 1989; **Resid:** Ophthalmology, NY Eye & Ear Infirm 1993; **Fellow:** Glaucoma, NY Eye & Ear Infirm 1994; **Fac Appt:** Asst Prof Oph, NY Med Coll

Guillory, Samuel L MD (Oph) - **Spec Exp:** LASIK-Refractive Surgery; PRK-Refractive Surgery; Pediatric Ophthalmology; Cataract Surgery; **Hospital:** Mt Sinai Med Ctr (page 102); **Address:** 1103 Park Ave, New York, NY 10128-1236; **Phone:** 212-860-5400; **Board Cert:** Ophthalmology 1980; **Med School:** Mount Sinai Sch Med 1975; **Resid:** Ophthalmology, Mount Sinai Med Ctr 1979; **Fellow:** Ocular Ultrasound, Cornell Med Ctr 1981; **Fac Appt:** Assoc Clin Prof Oph, Mount Sinai Sch Med

Haight, David H MD (Oph) - **Spec Exp:** Laser Vision Surgery; Cornea Transplant; Cataract Surgery; **Hospital:** Lenox Hill Hosp (page 106), NY-Presby/Weill Cornell Med Ctr, NY (page 104); **Address:** 155 E 72nd St, New York, NY 10021-4371; **Phone:** 212-772-9474; **Board Cert:** Ophthalmology 1985; **Med School:** Johns Hopkins Univ 1980; **Resid:** Internal Medicine, Hartford Hosp 1981; Ophthalmology, Manhattan EE&T Hosp 1984; **Fellow:** Cornea, Manhattan EE&T Hosp 1985; **Fac Appt:** Clin Prof Oph, NYU Sch Med

Hall, Lisabeth S MD (Oph) - **Spec Exp:** Pediatric Ophthalmology; Strabismus-Adult & Pediatric; Eye Muscle Disorders; Cataract-Pediatric; **Hospital:** New York Eye & Ear Infirm (page 115); **Address:** 40 W 72nd St, New York, NY 10023; **Phone:** 212-979-4614; **Board Cert:** Ophthalmology 2009; **Med School:** SUNY Stony Brook 1992; **Resid:** Ophthalmology, Manhattan Eye & Ear Infirm 1996; **Fellow:** Pediatric Ophthalmology, Jules Stein Eye Inst 1997; **Fac Appt:** Assoc Prof Oph, NY Med Coll

Harmon, Gregory K MD (Oph) - **Spec Exp:** Cataract Surgery; Glaucoma; **Hospital:** NY-Presby/Weill Cornell Med Ctr, NY (page 104); **Address:** 205 E 64th St, Ste 101, New York, NY 10065; **Phone:** 212-888-4100; **Board Cert:** Ophthalmology 1991; **Med School:** Mount Sinai Sch Med 1982; **Resid:** Ophthalmology, NY-Presby/Weill Cornell Med Ctr 1986; **Fellow:** Glaucoma, NY-Presby/Weill Cornell Med Ctr 1987; **Fac Appt:** Assoc Prof Oph, Cornell Univ-Weill Med Coll

Heinemann, Murk Hein MD (Oph) - **Spec Exp:** Ocular Ultrasound; Diagnostic Problems; Eye Tumors/Cancer; **Hospital:** Meml Sloan-Kettering Canc Ctr (page 114), NY-Presby/Weill Cornell Med Ctr, NY (page 104); **Address:** 1275 York Ave, rm A330, New York, NY 10065; **Phone:** 212-639-7237; **Board Cert:** Ophthalmology 1982; **Med School:** Cornell Univ-Weill Med Coll 1976; **Resid:** Internal Medicine, New York Hosp/Cornell Med Ctr 1977; Ophthalmology, Yale New Haven Hosp 1980; **Fellow:** Ophthalmology, New York Hosp/Cornell Med Ctr 1982; **Fac Appt:** Assoc Prof Oph, Cornell Univ-Weill Med Coll

Jabs, Douglas A MD (Oph) - **Spec Exp:** Uveitis; **Hospital:** Mt Sinai Med Ctr (page 102); **Address:** 17 E 102nd St, New York, NY 10029; **Phone:** 212-241-0939; **Board Cert:** Ophthalmology 1982; Internal Medicine 1983; **Med School:** Johns Hopkins Univ 1977; **Resid:** Ophthalmology, Wilmer Eye Inst 1981; Internal Medicine, Johns Hopkins Hosp 1983; **Fellow:** Rheumatology, Johns Hopkins Hosp 1984; **Fac Appt:** Prof Oph, Mount Sinai Sch Med

Kazim, Michael MD (Oph) - **Spec Exp:** Thyroid Eye Disease; Oculoplastic Surgery; Orbital Tumors/Cancer; Eyelid Tumors/Cancer; **Hospital:** NY-Presby/Columbia Univ Med Ctr, NY (page 104), New York Eye & Ear Infirm (page 115); **Address:** 635 W 165th St, Ste 207, New York, NY 10032-3701; **Phone:** 212-305-5477; **Board Cert:** Ophthalmology 1989; **Med School:** Columbia P&S 1984; **Resid:** Ophthalmology, Columbia-Presby Hosp 1988; **Fellow:** Oculoplastic Surgery, Univ Penn-Childrens Hosp 1989; Orbital Surgery, Allegheny Genl Hosp 1990; **Fac Appt:** Clin Prof Oph, Columbia P&S

Kelly, Stephen E MD (Oph) - **Spec Exp:** LASIK-Refractive Surgery; Cataract Surgery; Corneal Disease; **Hospital:** New York Eye & Ear Infirm (page 115), Lenox Hill Hosp (Manh Eye, Ear & Throat Hosp) (page 106); **Address:** 154 E 71st St, New York, NY 10021-5125; **Phone:** 212-628-2202; **Board Cert:** Ophthalmology 1976; **Med School:** Washington Univ, St Louis 1970; **Resid:** Ophthalmology, NY Eye & Ear Infirmary 1975; **Fellow:** Cornea, Manhattan EET Hosp 1976

Klapper, Daniel MD (Oph) - **Spec Exp:** Laser-Refractive Surgery; Glaucoma; Cataract Surgery; **Hospital:** Lenox Hill Hosp (Manh Eye, Ear & Throat Hosp) (page 106), Montefiore Med Ctr-Einstein Campus (page 100); **Address:** 7 W 81st St, Ste 1A, New York, NY 10024; **Phone:** 212-874-2726; **Board Cert:** Ophthalmology 1991; **Med School:** Albert Einstein Coll Med 1984; **Resid:** Ophthalmology, Brookdale Univ Hosp 1988

Koplin, Richard Steven MD (Oph) - **Spec Exp:** Cataract Surgery; Laser-Refractive Surgery; Eye Trauma; Eye Infections; **Hospital:** New York Eye & Ear Infirm (page 115); **Address:** Ophthalmic Consultants, 310 E 14th St South Bldg, Fl 2nd, MS 10003, New York, NY 10003-4201; **Phone:** 212-505-6550; **Board Cert:** Ophthalmology 1975; **Med School:** NY Med Coll 1969; **Resid:** Ophthalmology, NY Eye & Ear Infirm 1973; **Fac Appt:** Assoc Clin Prof Oph, NY Med Coll

Kupersmith, Mark J MD (Oph) - **Spec Exp:** Neuro-Ophthalmology; **Hospital:** St. Luke's - Roosevelt Hosp Ctr - Roosevelt Div (page 94); **Address:** Roosevelt Hosp, 1000 10th Ave, 10 INN Bldg, New York, NY 10019; **Phone:** 212-636-3200 x1; **Board Cert:** Ophthalmology 1981; Neurology 1981; **Med School:** Northwestern Univ 1974; **Resid:** Neurology, NYU Med Ctr 1978; Ophthalmology, NYU Med Ctr 1980; **Fac Appt:** Prof Oph, Albert Einstein Coll Med

Lauer, Simeon A MD (Oph) - **Spec Exp:** Oculoplastic Surgery; Ophthalmic Plastic Surgery; Lacrimal Gland Disorders; Orbital Surgery; **Hospital:** Hackensack Univ Med Ctr (page 718), New York Eye & Ear Infirm (page 115); **Address:** 130 E 67th St, New York, NY 10065; **Phone:** 212-879-6824; **Board Cert:** Ophthalmology 1991; **Med School:** SUNY Downstate 1984; **Resid:** Internal Medicine, Montefiore Med Ctr 1986; Ophthalmology, Montefiore Med Ctr 1989; **Fellow:** Oculoplastic & Reconstructive Surgery, LSU Eye Ctr 1990; **Fac Appt:** Assoc Clin Prof Oph, Albert Einstein Coll Med

Lee, Carol M MD (Oph) - **Spec Exp:** Retina/Vitreous Surgery; Diabetic Eye Disease/Retinopathy; Macular Disease/Degeneration; **Hospital:** NYU Langone Med Ctr (page 108); **Address:** 161 Madison Ave, Ste 5NE, New York, NY 10016-5405; **Phone:** 212-684-2424; **Board Cert:** Ophthalmology 1991; **Med School:** SUNY Downstate 1984; **Resid:** Research, Univ Illinois E&E Inst 1986; Ophthalmology, NYU Med Ctr 1989; **Fellow:** Vitreoretinal Surgery & Disease, Barnes Jewish Hosp 1991; **Fac Appt:** Clin Prof Oph, NYU Sch Med

Leib, Martin L MD (Oph) - **Spec Exp:** Cataract Surgery; Laser Refractive Surgery; Oculoplastic & Orbital Surgery; Laser Surgery; **Hospital:** NY-Presby/Columbia Univ Med Ctr, NY (page 104), St. Luke's - Roosevelt Hosp Ctr - Roosevelt Div (page 94); **Address:** 635 W 165th St, Ste 230, New York, NY 10032; **Phone:** 212-305-2303; **Board Cert:** Ophthalmology 1982; **Med School:** NY Med Coll 1974; **Resid:** Surgery, Mount Sinai Med Ctr 1976; Ophthalmology, McGill Univ Affil Hosp 1979; **Fellow:** Ophthalmic Plastic Surgery, Columbia-Presby Med Ctr 1980; Orbital Surgery, Columbia-Presby Med Ctr 1980; **Fac Appt:** Clin Prof Oph, Columbia P&S

Liebmann, Jeffrey M MD (Oph) - **Spec Exp:** Glaucoma; Cataract Surgery; **Hospital:** New York Eye & Ear Infirm (page 115), Lenox Hill Hosp (Manh Eye, Ear & Throat Hosp) (page 106); **Address:** Glaucoma Associates of New York, 121 E 60th St Fl 8, New York, NY 10022; **Phone:** 212-477-7540; **Board Cert:** Ophthalmology 1989; **Med School:** Boston Univ 1983; **Resid:** Ophthalmology, SUNY Downstate Med Ctr 1987; **Fellow:** Glaucoma, New York EE Infirmary 1988; **Fac Appt:** Clin Prof Oph, NYU Sch Med

Lisman, Richard D MD (Oph) - **Spec Exp:** Oculoplastic Surgery; Eyelid/Tear Duct Reconstruction; Eyelid Cosmetic & Reconstructive Surgery; Orbital & Eyelid Tumors/Cancer; **Hospital:** NYU Langone Med Ctr (page 108), Lenox Hill Hosp (Manh Eye, Ear & Throat Hosp) (page 106); **Address:** 635 Park Ave, New York, NY 10065-6546; **Phone:** 212-585-1405; **Board Cert:** Ophthalmology 1981; **Med School:** NYU Sch Med 1976; **Resid:** Ophthalmology, Manhattan EE Hosp 1980; **Fellow:** Ophthalmic Plastic Surgery, NY Eye & Ear Infirmary 1981; Plastic Surgery, Manhattan EE&T Hosp 1982; **Fac Appt:** Prof Oph, NYU Sch Med

MacKay, Cynthia J MD (Oph) - **Spec Exp:** Diabetic Eye Disease/Retinopathy; Macular Degeneration; Laser Surgery; Retinitis Pigmentosa; **Hospital:** NY-Presby/Columbia Univ Med Ctr, NY (page 104), Lenox Hill Hosp (Manh Eye, Ear & Throat Hosp) (page 106); **Address:** 315 Central Park West, Ste 1B, New York, NY 10025; **Phone:** 212-772-6050; **Board Cert:** Ophthalmology 1982; **Med School:** SUNY Hlth Sci Ctr 1977; **Resid:** Ophthalmology, Columbia-Presby Med Ctr 1981; **Fellow:** Retina, NYU Med Ctr 1982; **Fac Appt:** Clin Prof Oph, Columbia P&S

Magramm, Irene MD (Oph) - **Spec Exp:** Pediatric Ophthalmology; Strabismus; Cataract Surgery; Diplopia; **Hospital:** Lenox Hill Hosp (Manh Eye, Ear & Throat Hosp) (page 106); **Address:** 220 E 63rd St, Ste LM, New York, NY 10055; **Phone:** 212-644-5100; **Board Cert:** Ophthalmology 1987; **Med School:** Cornell Univ-Weill Med Coll 1981; **Resid:** Ophthalmology, North Shore Univ Hosp 1985; **Fellow:** Pediatric Ophthalmology, Manhattan EE&T Hosp 1986; **Fac Appt:** Asst Clin Prof Oph, Cornell Univ-Weill Med Coll

Maher, Elizabeth A MD (Oph) - **Spec Exp:** Orbital Surgery; Oculoplastic Surgery; **Hospital:** New York Eye & Ear Infirm (page 115); **Address:** OMNI Eye Services, 36 E 36th St, New York, NY 10016; **Phone:** 212-353-0030; **Board Cert:** Ophthalmology 1989; **Med School:** Harvard Med Sch 1984; **Resid:** Internal Medicine, St Lukes-Roosevelt Hosp 1985; Ophthalmology, Manhattan EE&T Hosp 1988; **Fellow:** Ophthalmic Plastic & Reconstructive Surgery, Manhattan EE&T Hosp 1989

Mandel, Eric R MD (Oph) - **Spec Exp:** LASIK-Refractive Surgery; PRK-Refractive Surgery; Corneal Disease; **Hospital:** Lenox Hill Hosp (page 106); **Address:** 211 E 70th St, New York, NY 10021; **Phone:** 212-734-0111; **Board Cert:** Ophthalmology 1988; **Med School:** SUNY Stony Brook 1982; **Resid:** Ophthalmology, Lenox Hill Hosp 1986; **Fellow:** Cornea & Ext Eye Disease, Mass EE Infirm 1987

Mandelbaum, Sidney H MD (Oph) - **Spec Exp:** Cataract Surgery; Cornea Transplant; Corneal Disease & Surgery; **Hospital:** New York Eye & Ear Infirm (page 115), Lenox Hill Hosp (Manh Eye, Ear & Throat Hosp) (page 106); **Address:** East Side Eye Surgeons, 178 E 71st St, New York, NY 10021; **Phone:** 212-650-0400; **Board Cert:** Ophthalmology 1982; **Med School:** Yale Univ 1976; **Resid:** Internal Medicine, NY Hosp 1978; Ophthalmology, LAC-USC Med Ctr 1981; **Fellow:** Cornea, Bascom Palmer Eye Inst 1982; **Fac Appt:** Assoc Clin Prof Oph, Albert Einstein Coll Med

Marr, Brian MD (Oph) - **Spec Exp:** Eye Tumors/Cancer; **Hospital:** Meml Sloan-Kettering Canc Ctr (page 114); **Address:** 70 E 66th St, New York, NY 10065; **Phone:** 212-744-1700; **Board Cert:** Ophthalmology 2012; **Med School:** Temple Univ 1995; **Resid:** Ophthalmology, NY Eye & Ear Infirmary 1999; **Fellow:** Ophthalmic Oncology, Wills Eye Hosp 2001

McDermott, John A MD (Oph) - **Spec Exp:** Glaucoma; Laser Vision Surgery; **Hospital:** New York Eye & Ear Infirm (page 115); **Address:** 310 E 14th St, New York, NY 10003; **Phone:** 212-979-4446; **Board Cert:** Ophthalmology 1982; **Med School:** NY Med Coll 1976; **Resid:** Internal Medicine, LI Jewish Med Ctr 1978; Ophthalmology, NY Eye & Ear Infirm 1981; **Fellow:** Glaucoma, Mass Eye & Ear Infirm 1983; **Fac Appt:** Asst Clin Prof Oph, NY Med Coll

Melton, Roberta Christine MD (Oph) - **Spec Exp:** Glaucoma; Diabetic Eye Disease; **Hospital:** NY-Presby/Weill Cornell Med Ctr, NY (page 104); **Address:** 247 3rd Ave, Ste 202, New York, NY 10010-7454; **Phone:** 212-475-3791; **Board Cert:** Ophthalmology 1982; **Med School:** Canada 1977; **Resid:** Ophthalmology, St Vincent's Hosp & Med Ctr 1981; **Fac Appt:** Asst Clin Prof Oph, Cornell Univ-Weill Med Coll

Merhige, Kenneth E MD (Oph) - **Spec Exp:** Cataract Surgery; **Hospital:** St. Luke's - Roosevelt Hosp Ctr - Roosevelt Div (page 94); **Address:** St Luke's-Roosevelt Hosp Ctr, 1111 Amsterdam Ave, New York, NY 10025; **Phone:** 212-523-2562; **Board Cert:** Ophthalmology 1985; **Med School:** Cornell Univ-Weill Med Coll 1980; **Resid:** Ophthalmology, St Luke's Hosp 1984; **Fellow:** Vitreoretinal Surgery, NY Hosp-Cornell 1985

Merriam, John C MD (Oph) - **Spec Exp:** Cataract Surgery; Reconstructive Surgery; Ophthalmic Plastic Surgery; **Hospital:** NY-Presby/Columbia Univ Med Ctr, NY (page 104); **Address:** Edward S Harkness Eye Inst, 635 W 165th St, Ste 3-305, New York, NY 10032-3724; **Phone:** 212-305-5402; **Board Cert:** Ophthalmology 1983; **Med School:** Harvard Med Sch 1977; **Resid:** Plastic Surgery, Brigham-Boston Chldns Hosp 1979; Ophthalmology, Mass Eye & Ear Infirm 1982; **Fellow:** Ophthalmology, UCSF Med Ctr 1983; **Fac Appt:** Clin Prof Oph, Columbia P&S

Mindel, Joel S MD/PhD (Oph) - **Spec Exp:** Neuro-Ophthalmology; Myasthenia Gravis; Temporal Arteritis; **Hospital:** Mt Sinai Med Ctr (page 102), James J. Peters VA Med Ctr-Bronx; **Address:** 17 E 102nd St Fl 8, New York, NY 10029; **Phone:** 212-241-0939; **Board Cert:** Ophthalmology 1970; **Med School:** Univ MD Sch Med 1964; **Resid:** Ophthalmology, Univ Michigan Med Ctr 1969; **Fellow:** Neuro-Ophthalmology, Columbia-Presby Med Ctr 1966; Ocular Pharmacology, Mount Sinai Med Ctr 1973; **Fac Appt:** Prof Oph, Mount Sinai Sch Med

Mitchell, John P MD (Oph) - **Spec Exp:** Neuro-Ophthalmology; Cataract Surgery; Glaucoma; **Hospital:** NY-Presby/Columbia Univ Med Ctr, NY (page 104); **Address:** Macula Care, 147 W 142 St, New York, NY 10030; **Phone:** 212-281-8400; **Board Cert:** Ophthalmology 1978; **Med School:** Cornell Univ-Weill Med Coll 1973; **Resid:** Ophthalmology, Harlem Hosp 1977; **Fellow:** Neuro-Ophthalmology, Columbia-Presby Med Ctr 1978

Moazed, Kambiz T MD (Oph) - **Spec Exp:** Cataract Surgery; Eyelid/Tear Duct Reconstruction; Ophthalmic Plastic Surgery; **Hospital:** St. Luke's - Roosevelt Hosp Ctr - Roosevelt Div (page 94); **Address:** Manhattan's Physician Group, 4337 Broadway, New York, NY 10033; **Phone:** 212-568-6300; **Board Cert:** Ophthalmology 1983; **Med School:** Iran 1973; **Resid:** Ophthalmology, Mass EE Infirm 1982; **Fellow:** Eye Pathology, Stanford Univ Med Ctr 1977; Oculoplastic Surgery, Edward Harkness Eye Inst 1983; **Fac Appt:** Asst Clin Prof Oph, Columbia P&S

Moskowitz, Bruce K MD (Oph) - **Spec Exp:** Oculoplastic Surgery; Reconstructive Surgery; **Hospital:** New York Eye & Ear Infirm (page 115); **Address:** 310 E 14th St, Ste 401, New York, NY 10003; **Phone:** 212-979-4586; **Board Cert:** Ophthalmology 2013; **Med School:** SUNY Downstate 1987; **Resid:** Ophthalmology, SUNY Downstate Med Ctr 1991; **Fellow:** Ophthalmology, Kingsbrook Jewish Med Ctr 1992; **Fac Appt:** Asst Clin Prof Oph, NY Med Coll

Muchnick, Richard S MD (Oph) - **Spec Exp:** Pediatric Ophthalmology; Strabismus; **Hospital:** NY-Presby/Weill Cornell Med Ctr, NY (page 104), Lenox Hill Hosp (page 106); **Address:** 69 E 71st St, New York, NY 10021-4213; **Phone:** 212-744-1726; **Board Cert:** Ophthalmology 1975; **Med School:** Cornell Univ-Weill Med Coll 1967; **Resid:** Ophthalmology, New York Hosp 1973; **Fellow:** Ophthalmic Plastic Surgery, UCSF Med Ctr 1974; Pediatric Ophthalmology, Manhattan EE&T Hosp 1975; **Fac Appt:** Clin Prof Oph, Cornell Univ-Weill Med Coll

Muldoon, Thomas O MD (Oph) - **Spec Exp:** Retina/Vitreous Surgery; Macular Disease/Degeneration; Diabetic Eye Disease/Retinopathy; **Hospital:** New York Eye & Ear Infirm (page 115); **Address:** 310 E 14th St, Ste 402, New York, NY 10003-4201; **Phone:** 212-979-4595; **Board Cert:** Ophthalmology 1971; **Med School:** Univ Rochester 1962; **Resid:** Surgery, St Lukes Hosp 1966; Ophthalmology, NY EE Infirm 1969; **Fellow:** Retinal Surgery, NY EE Infirm 1970; **Fac Appt:** Assoc Clin Prof Oph, NY Med Coll

Newton, Michael J MD (Oph) - **Spec Exp:** Cornea & Cataract Surgery; Refractive Surgery; Eye Infections; Corneal Disease; **Hospital:** New York Eye & Ear Infirm (page 115), Mt Sinai Med Ctr (page 102); **Address:** 799 Park Ave, New York, NY 10021-3275; **Phone:** 212-861-0146; **Board Cert:** Ophthalmology 1978; **Med School:** Tufts Univ 1971; **Resid:** Ophthalmology, Mount Sinai Hosp 1977; **Fellow:** Cornea & Ext Eye Disease, AB Nesburn MD/Doheny Eye Inst 1978; **Fac Appt:** Assoc Clin Prof Oph, Mount Sinai Sch Med

Nightingale, Jeffrey MD (Oph) - **Spec Exp:** LASIK-Refractive Surgery; Cataract Surgery; **Hospital:** New York Eye & Ear Infirm (page 115); **Address:** 211 Central Park West, New York, NY 10024-6020; **Phone:** 212-877-7188; **Board Cert:** Ophthalmology 1977; **Med School:** SUNY Hlth Sci Ctr 1972; **Resid:** Ophthalmology, Bronx Lebanon Hosp 1976; **Fellow:** Oculoplastic Surgery, NY Eye & Ear Infirmary 1977

Obstbaum, Stephen A MD (Oph) - **Spec Exp:** Cataract Surgery; Glaucoma; **Hospital:** Lenox Hill Hosp (page 106), Lenox Hill Hosp (Manh Eye, Ear & Throat Hosp) (page 106); **Address:** 210 E 64th St Fl 7th, New York, NY 10065; **Phone:** 212-702-7620; **Board Cert:** Ophthalmology 1974; **Med School:** NY Med Coll 1967; **Resid:** Ophthalmology, Flower Fifth Ave Hosp 1972; **Fellow:** Glaucoma, Washington Univ Affil Hosp 1973; **Fac Appt:** Prof Oph, NYU Sch Med

Odel, Jeffrey G MD (Oph) - **Spec Exp:** Neuro-Ophthalmology; Retinal Disorders; Optic Nerve Disorders; **Hospital:** NY-Presby/Columbia Univ Med Ctr, NY (page 104); **Address:** Harkness Eye Institute, 635 W 165th St, rm 316, New York, NY 10032-3701; **Phone:** 212-305-5415; **Board Cert:** Ophthalmology 1981; **Med School:** Univ Rochester 1975; **Resid:** Ophthalmology, Mt Sinai Hosp 1981; **Fellow:** Ophthalmology, Bascom-Palmer Eye Inst 1977; Ophthalmology, Columbia Presby Med Ctr 1982; **Fac Appt:** Assoc Clin Prof Oph, Columbia P&S

Paccione, Jeffrey C MD (Oph) - **Spec Exp:** Retinal Disorders; Macular Degeneration; **Hospital:** Lenox Hill Hosp (Manh Eye, Ear & Throat Hosp) (page 106), New York Eye & Ear Infirm (page 115); **Address:** Retina Associates of New York, 140 E 80th St, New York, NY 10075; **Phone:** 212-772-0600; **Board Cert:** Ophthalmology 2010; **Med School:** Columbia P&S 1989; **Resid:** Ophthalmology, Manhattan EE&T Hosp 1994; **Fellow:** Vitreoretinal Disease, Mt Sinai Med Ctr 1998; **Fac Appt:** Assoc Clin Prof Oph, Mount Sinai Sch Med

Palu, Richard N MD (Oph) - **Spec Exp:** Oculoplastic & Reconstructive Surgery; **Hospital:** NYU Langone Med Ctr (page 108), Valley Hosp (page 721); **Address:** 161 Madison Ave Fl 6, New York, NY 10016; **Phone:** 212-213-9783; **Board Cert:** Ophthalmology 1990; **Med School:** NYU Sch Med 1984; **Resid:** Ophthalmology, NYU Med Ctr 1988; **Fellow:** Ophthalmic Plastic & Reconstructive Surgery, Mass EE Infirm 1989; **Fac Appt:** Assoc Clin Prof Oph, NYU Sch Med

Prince, Andrew M MD (Oph) - **Spec Exp:** Glaucoma; Cataract Surgery; **Hospital:** New York Eye & Ear Infirm (page 115), Lenox Hill Hosp (Manh Eye, Ear & Throat Hosp) (page 106); **Address:** Glaucoma Consultants of Greater NY & NJ, 178 E 71st St, New York, NY 10021-5119; **Phone:** 212-717-2200; **Board Cert:** Ophthalmology 1987; **Med School:** SUNY Downstate 1981; **Resid:** Internal Medicine, Kings Co Hosp Ctr 1982; Ophthalmology, SUNY Downstate Med Ctr 1985; **Fellow:** Glaucoma, NY Eye & Ear Infirmary 1986; **Fac Appt:** Assoc Prof Oph, NYU Sch Med

Raab, Edward L MD (Oph) - **Spec Exp:** Pediatric Ophthalmology; Strabismus-Adult & Pediatric; Glaucoma-Pediatric; **Hospital:** Mt Sinai Med Ctr (page 102); **Address:** 17 E 102nd St Fl 8th, New York, NY 10029-6501; **Phone:** 212-369-0988; **Board Cert:** Ophthalmology 1966; **Med School:** NYU Sch Med 1958; **Resid:** Ophthalmology, Mount Sinai 1964; **Fellow:** Pediatric Ophthalmology, Chldns Natl Med Ctr 1967; **Fac Appt:** Prof Oph, Mount Sinai Sch Med

Relland, Maureen A MD (Oph) - **Spec Exp:** Oculoplastic Surgery; Eyelid Cosmetic Surgery; Botox Therapy; **Hospital:** New York Eye & Ear Infirm (page 115), Richmond Univ Med Ctr; **Address:** 352 7th Ave, Ste 805, New York, NY 10001; **Phone:** 212-645-7771; **Board Cert:** Ophthalmology 1971; **Med School:** NY Med Coll 1964; **Resid:** Ophthalmology, St Vincent's Hosp Med Ctr 1968; **Fac Appt:** Asst Clin Prof Oph, NY Med Coll

Ritch, Robert MD (Oph) - **Spec Exp:** Glaucoma; Complementary Medicine; **Hospital:** New York Eye & Ear Infirm (page 115); **Address:** 310 E 14th St, South Bldg - Fl 3, New York, NY 10003-4201; **Phone:** 212-477-7540; **Board Cert:** Ophthalmology 1977; **Med School:** Albert Einstein Coll Med 1972; **Resid:** Ophthalmology, Mt Sinai Med Ctr 1976; **Fellow:** Glaucoma, Mt Sinai Med Ctr 1978; **Fac Appt:** Prof Oph, NY Med Coll

Ritterband, David MD (Oph) - **Spec Exp:** Cataract Surgery; Cornea Transplant; Refractive Surgery; Corneal Disease; **Hospital:** New York Eye & Ear Infirm (page 115); **Address:** Ophthalmic Consultants, 310 E 14th St, South Bldg - Fl 2, The New York Eye & Ear Infirmary, New York, NY 10003-4201; **Phone:** 212-979-4428; **Board Cert:** Ophthalmology 2006; **Med School:** NY Med Coll 1990; **Resid:** Ophthalmology, NY Med Coll 1994; **Fellow:** Cornea & Ext Eye Disease, Eye & Ear Inst 1995; **Fac Appt:** Clin Prof Oph, NY Med Coll

Rodgers, I Rand MD (Oph) - **Spec Exp:** Oculoplastic Surgery; Eyelid Cosmetic & Reconstructive Surgery; Eyelid/Tear Duct Disorders; **Hospital:** Mt Sinai Med Ctr (page 102), N Shore Univ Hosp (page 106); **Address:** 229 E 79 St, New York, NY 10075; **Phone:** 212-249-7600; **Board Cert:** Ophthalmology 1989; **Med School:** Mount Sinai Sch Med 1983; **Resid:** Surgery, Mt Sinai Med Ctr 1984; Ophthalmology, Mt Sinai Med Ctr 1987; **Fellow:** Ocular Oncology, Manhattan EE&T Hosp 1988; Ophthalmic Plastic Surgery, Mass E&E Infirm 1990; **Fac Appt:** Asst Clin Prof Oph, Mount Sinai Sch Med

Rodriguez-Sains, Rene S MD (Oph) - **Spec Exp:** Eyelid Cosmetic & Reconstructive Surgery; Eyelid Tumors/Cancer; Melanoma; Eye Tumors/Cancer; **Hospital:** New York Eye & Ear Infirm (page 115), NYU Langone Med Ctr (page 108); **Address:** 799 Park Ave, New York, NY 10021-3275; **Phone:** 212-535-0315; **Board Cert:** Ophthalmology 1982; **Med School:** NYU Sch Med 1977; **Resid:** Internal Medicine, NYU Med Ctr 1988; Ophthalmology, Manhattan EET Hosp 1981; **Fellow:** Ophthalmic Plastic Surgery, Manhattan EET Hosp 1982; **Fac Appt:** Asst Clin Prof Oph, NYU Sch Med

Rosenthal, Jeanne L MD (Oph) - **Spec Exp:** Retina/Vitreous Surgery; Macular Degeneration; Diabetic Eye Disease/Retinopathy; **Hospital:** New York Eye & Ear Infirm (page 115); **Address:** 20 E 9th St, New York, NY 10003-5944; **Phone:** 212-674-2970; **Board Cert:** Ophthalmology 1985; **Med School:** SUNY Downstate 1979; **Resid:** Ophthalmology, NY Eye & Ear Infirm 1983; **Fellow:** Retina/Vitreous Surgery, NY Eye & Ear Infirm 1985; **Fac Appt:** Clin Prof Oph, NY Med Coll

Rudick Jr, Albert Joseph MD (Oph) - **Spec Exp:** LASIK-Refractive Surgery; Glaucoma; **Hospital:** New York Eye & Ear Infirm (page 115), NY-Presby/Lower Manhattan Hosp (page 104); **Address:** Assoc Ophthalmologists of NY, 150 Broadway Fl 14 - Ste 1401, MS 10038, New York, NY 10038; **Phone:** 212-233-2344; **Board Cert:** Ophthalmology 1989; **Med School:** Univ Pennsylvania 1983; **Resid:** Ophthalmology, Manhattan EE&T Hosp 1989

Samson, C Michael MD (Oph) - **Spec Exp:** Uveitis; Immunotherapy; Eye Infections; **Hospital:** New York Eye & Ear Infirm (page 115); **Address:** 310 E 14th St, Ste 319 S, New York, NY 10003; **Phone:** 212-979-4515; **Board Cert:** Ophthalmology 2011; **Med School:** SUNY Downstate 1994; **Resid:** Ophthalmology, NY Eye & Ear Infirm 1998; **Fellow:** Ophthalmology, Mass Eye & Ear Infirm 2000; **Fac Appt:** Assoc Prof Oph, NY Med Coll

Schiff, William M MD (Oph) - **Spec Exp:** Macular Disease/Degeneration; Diabetic Eye Disease/Retinopathy; Retinal Detachment; **Hospital:** Lenox Hill Hosp (Manh Eye, Ear & Throat Hosp) (page 106), St. Luke's - Roosevelt Hosp Ctr - Roosevelt Div (page 94); **Address:** 210 E 64th St, Fl 7, New York, NY 10068; **Phone:** 212-702-7400; **Board Cert:** Ophthalmology 2006; **Med School:** NYU Sch Med 1988; **Resid:** Ophthalmology, New York Eye & Ear Infirm 1994; **Fellow:** Retina/Vitreous Surgery, NY Hosp-Harkness Eye Inst 1996; **Fac Appt:** Prof Oph, Hofstra N Shore-LIJ Sch Med

Schrier, Amilia MD (Oph) - **Spec Exp:** Corneal Disease & Surgery; Corneal & External Eye Disease; Cataract Surgery; **Hospital:** Lenox Hill Hosp (Manh Eye, Ear & Throat Hosp) (page 106), NY-Presby/Columbia Univ Med Ctr, NY (page 104); **Address:** 210 E 64th St Fl 7, New York, NY 10065; **Phone:** 212-702-7300; **Board Cert:** Ophthalmology 2013; **Med School:** SUNY Downstate 1987; **Resid:** Ophthalmology, SUNY Downstate 1991; **Fellow:** Cornea & Ext Eye Disease, North Shore Univ Hosp 1992; **Fac Appt:** Prof Oph, Hofstra N Shore-LIJ Sch Med

Schubert, Hermann D MD (Oph) - **Spec Exp:** Diabetic Eye Disease/Retinopathy; Macular Degeneration; Retinal Disorders; Retinal Detachment; **Hospital:** NY-Presby/Columbia Univ Med Ctr, NY (page 104); **Address:** 635 W 165th St, Rm 206, New York, NY 10032-3701; **Phone:** 212-305-6534; **Board Cert:** Ophthalmology 1987; Anatomic Pathology 1981; **Med School:** Germany 1974; **Resid:** Pathology, Columbia-Presby Hosp 1979; Ophthalmology, Columbia-Presby Hosp 1985; **Fellow:** Retina/Vitreous Surgery, Wills Eye Hosp 1987; **Fac Appt:** Prof Oph, Columbia P&S

Schwarcz, Robert M MD (Oph) - **Spec Exp:** Oculoplastic Surgery; Cosmetic Surgery-Face; Reconstructive Surgery-Face; Eyelid Surgery; **Hospital:** Montefiore Med Ctr-Wakefield Campus (page 100), New York Eye & Ear Infirm (page 115); **Address:** 135 E 71st St, New York, NY 10021; **Phone:** 212-396-4400; **Board Cert:** Ophthalmology 2006; **Med School:** Howard Univ 1999; **Resid:** Internal Medicine, St Lukes-Roosevelt Hosp Ctr 2000; Ophthalmology, SUNY Downstate Med Ctr 2003; **Fellow:** Facial Plastic & Reconstr Surgery, Jules Stein Eye Inst 2004; Oculoplastic Surgery, Jules Stein Eye Inst 2005; **Fac Appt:** Assoc Prof Oph, Albert Einstein Coll Med

Seedor, John A MD (Oph) - **Spec Exp:** Cornea & External Eye Disease; Laser Vision Surgery; Laser Refractive Surgery; **Hospital:** New York Eye & Ear Infirm (page 115); **Address:** Ophthalmic Consultants, 310 E 14th St, Ste 219, New York, NY 10003-4201; **Phone:** 212-505-6550; **Board Cert:** Ophthalmology 1987; **Med School:** Hahnemann Univ 1981; **Resid:** Ophthalmology, NY Eye & Ear Infirm 1985; **Fellow:** Cornea, Emory Univ Hosp 1987; **Fac Appt:** Assoc Clin Prof Oph, NY Med Coll

Serle, Janet B MD (Oph) - **Spec Exp:** Glaucoma; **Hospital:** Mt Sinai Med Ctr (page 102), Syosset Hosp (page 106); **Address:** 17 E 102 St, 8th Fl, Box 1183, New York, NY 10029; **Phone:** 212-241-0939; **Board Cert:** Ophthalmology 1987; **Med School:** Harvard Med Sch 1980; **Resid:** Ophthalmology, Mount Sinai Hosp 1985; **Fellow:** Glaucoma, Mount Sinai Hosp 1986; **Fac Appt:** Prof Oph, Mount Sinai Sch Med

Shabto, Uri MD (Oph) - **Spec Exp:** Retinopathy of Prematurity; Macular Disease/Degeneration; Diabetic Eye Disease/Retinopathy; Retinal Detachment; **Hospital:** New York Eye & Ear Infirm (page 115); **Address:** 310 E 14th St, South Bldg, Ste 419, New York, NY 10003-4201; **Phone:** 212-677-2000; **Board Cert:** Ophthalmology 1991; **Med School:** Harvard Med Sch 1986; **Resid:** Ophthalmology, NY Eye & Ear Infirm 1990; **Fellow:** Vitreoretinal Surgery, Montefiore Hosp 1991; **Fac Appt:** Asst Clin Prof Oph, NY Med Coll

Sherman, Spencer E MD (Oph) - **Spec Exp:** Cataract Surgery; Glaucoma; Contact Lenses; Refractive Surgery; **Hospital:** Lenox Hill Hosp (Manh Eye, Ear & Throat Hosp) (page 106), Mt Sinai Med Ctr (page 102); **Address:** 166 E 63rd St, New York, NY 10065; **Phone:** 212-753-8300; **Board Cert:** Ophthalmology 1970; **Med School:** Columbia P&S 1962; **Resid:** Ophthalmology, Mt Sinai Hosp 1968; **Fac Appt:** Asst Clin Prof Oph, Mount Sinai Sch Med

Shulman, Julius MD (Oph) - **Spec Exp:** Cataract Surgery; LASIK-Refractive Surgery; Contact Lenses; Glaucoma; **Hospital:** Mt Sinai Med Ctr (page 102); **Address:** Eastside Eye Assocs, 229 E 79th St, New York, NY 10075; **Phone:** 212-861-6200; **Board Cert:** Ophthalmology 2006; **Med School:** SUNY Downstate 1969; **Resid:** Ophthalmology, Mt Sinai Med Ctr 1975; **Fac Appt:** Asst Clin Prof Oph, Mount Sinai Sch Med

Sidoti, Paul A MD (Oph) - **Spec Exp:** Glaucoma; **Hospital:** New York Eye & Ear Infirm (page 115), Beth Israel Med Ctr - Petrie Div (page 94); **Address:** New York Eye & Ear Infirmary, 310 E 14th St, Ste 319, New York, NY 10003-4201; **Phone:** 212-979-4590; **Board Cert:** Ophthalmology 2005; **Med School:** Albert Einstein Coll Med 1988; **Resid:** Ophthalmology, NY Eye & Ear Infirm 1992; **Fellow:** Glaucoma, Doheny Eye Inst-USC 1994; **Fac Appt:** Prof Oph, NY Med Coll

Slakter, Jason S MD (Oph) - **Spec Exp:** Retinal Disorders; Macular Degeneration; **Hospital:** Lenox Hill Hosp (Manh Eye, Ear & Throat Hosp) (page 106); **Address:** Vitreous-Retina-Macula Consultants of NY, 460 Park Ave Fl 5, New York, NY 10022; **Phone:** 212-861-9797; **Board Cert:** Ophthalmology 1989; **Med School:** Albert Einstein Coll Med 1983; **Resid:** Internal Medicine, Winthrop Univ Hosp 1984; Ophthalmology, Manhattan Eye & Ear Infirm 1987; **Fellow:** Retina/Vitreous Surgery, Manhattan Eye & Ear Infirm 1988; **Fac Appt:** Clin Prof Oph, NYU Sch Med

Solomon, Joel M MD (Oph) - **Spec Exp:** Cornea & Cataract Surgery; Refractive Surgery; Glaucoma; Contact Lenses; **Hospital:** NYU Langone Med Ctr (page 108), Bellevue Hosp Ctr; **Address:** 614 2nd Ave, Ste C, New York, NY 10016; **Phone:** 212-689-5080; **Board Cert:** Ophthalmology 1987; **Med School:** Cornell Univ-Weill Med Coll 1981; **Resid:** Internal Medicine, Albany Med Ctr 1983; Ophthalmology, NYU Med Ctr 1986; **Fellow:** Cornea & Ext Eye Disease, Med Coll Wisc/Eye Inst 1987; **Fac Appt:** Clin Prof Oph, NYU Sch Med

Spaide, Richard F MD (Oph) - **Spec Exp:** Retinal Disorders; Macular Degeneration; Diabetic Eye Disease/Retinopathy; Retina/Vitreous Surgery; **Hospital:** Lenox Hill Hosp (Manh Eye, Ear & Throat Hosp) (page 106); **Address:** Vitreous-Retina-Macula Consultants of NY, 460 Park Ave Fl 5, New York, NY 10022; **Phone:** 212-861-9797; **Board Cert:** Ophthalmology 1987; **Med School:** Jefferson Med Coll 1981; **Resid:** Ophthalmology, St Vincent's Hosp & Med Ctr 1985; **Fellow:** Vitreoretinal Surgery & Disease, Manhattan EET Hosp 1990; **Fac Appt:** Assoc Clin Prof Oph, NY Med Coll

Sperber, Laurence TD MD (Oph) - **Spec Exp:** LASIK-Refractive Surgery; Cornea Transplant; Corneal Ring Implants; Cataract Surgery; **Hospital:** Lenox Hill Hosp (Manh Eye, Ear & Throat Hosp) (page 106); **Address:** Refractive Laser Specialists of NY, 166 E 63rd St, New York, NY 10021-7636; **Phone:** 212-753-8300; **Board Cert:** Ophthalmology 2013; **Med School:** Boston Univ 1987; **Resid:** Ophthalmology, Lenox Hill Hosp (Manh Eye, Ear & Throat Hosp) 1991; **Fellow:** Cornea & Ext Eye Disease, Wills Eye Inst 1992; **Fac Appt:** Clin Prof Oph, NYU Sch Med

Starr, Christopher E MD (Oph) - **Spec Exp:** Corneal Disease & Surgery; Cornea Transplant; Cataract Surgery-Lens Implant; LASIK-Refractive Surgery; **Hospital:** NY-Presby/Weill Cornell Med Ctr, NY (page 104); **Address:** Weill Cornell Eye Assocs, Weill Greenberg Ctr, 1305 York Ave, Fl 12, New York, NY 10021; **Phone:** 646-962-2020; **Board Cert:** Ophthalmology 2003; **Med School:** Cornell Univ-Weill Med Coll 1998; **Resid:** Ophthalmology, Harvard/Mass Eye & Ear Infirm 2002; **Fellow:** Cornea & Refractive Surgery, Johns Hopkins Hosp/Wilmer Eye Inst 2003; **Fac Appt:** Assoc Prof Oph, Cornell Univ-Weill Med Coll

Starr, Michael B MD (Oph) - **Spec Exp:** Cataract Surgery; Corneal Disease & Surgery; Eye Infections; **Hospital:** Lenox Hill Hosp (Manh Eye, Ear & Throat Hosp) (page 106), NY-Presby/Weill Cornell Med Ctr, NY (page 104); **Address:** 67 E 78th St, New York, NY 10075; **Phone:** 212-717-0222; **Board Cert:** Ophthalmology 1978; **Med School:** Mount Sinai Sch Med 1972; **Resid:** Neurology, Mount Sinai 1974; Ophthalmology, Lenox Hill Hosp 1977; **Fellow:** Cornea, UCSF Med Ctr/ Francis Proctor Fdn 1979; **Fac Appt:** Assoc Clin Prof Oph, Mount Sinai Sch Med

Steele, Mark MD (Oph) - **Spec Exp:** Pediatric Ophthalmology; Strabismus; Eye Muscle Disorders; **Hospital:** NYU Langone Med Ctr (page 108), New York Eye & Ear Infirm (page 115); **Address:** 40 W 72nd St, New York, NY 10023; **Phone:** 212-981-9800; **Board Cert:** Ophthalmology 1991; **Med School:** NYU Sch Med 1986; **Resid:** Ophthalmology, NYU Med Ctr 1990; **Fellow:** Pediatric Ophthalmology, Wills Eye Hosp 1991; **Fac Appt:** Assoc Clin Prof Oph, NYU Sch Med

Suh, Leejee H MD (Oph) - **Spec Exp:** Cornea Transplant; Laser Vision Surgery; Cataract Surgery; **Hospital:** NY-Presby/Columbia Univ Med Ctr, NY (page 104); **Address:** Columbia Dept Ophthalmology, 635 W 165th St, New York, NY 10032; **Phone:** 212-305-9535; **Board Cert:** Ophthalmology 2009; **Med School:** NYU Sch Med 2002; **Resid:** Ophthalmology, Johns Hopkins Hosp 2006; **Fellow:** Cornea & Refractive Surgery, Bascom Palmer Eye Inst 2007; **Fac Appt:** Assoc Prof Oph, Columbia P&S

Tello, Celso MD (Oph) - **Spec Exp:** Glaucoma; Cataract Surgery; **Hospital:** New York Eye & Ear Infirm (page 115); **Address:** Glaucoma Assocs of NY, 310 E 14th St, Ste 304, South Bldg, New York, NY 10003; **Phone:** 212-477-7540; **Board Cert:** Ophthalmology 2011; **Med School:** Ecuador 1988; **Resid:** Ophthalmology, NY Eye & Ear Infirm 1998; **Fellow:** Glaucoma, NY Eye & Ear Infirm 2000; **Fac Appt:** Asst Prof Oph, NYU Sch Med

Walsh, Joseph B MD (Oph) - **Spec Exp:** Diabetic Eye Disease/Retinopathy; Macular Degeneration; Retinal Disorders; **Hospital:** New York Eye & Ear Infirm (page 115); **Address:** 310 E 14th St, S Bldg Fl 3 - Ste 319, New York, NY 10003-4201; **Phone:** 212-979-4282; **Board Cert:** Ophthalmology 2005; **Med School:** Georgetown Univ 1966; **Resid:** Internal Medicine, Univ Hosp 1968; Ophthalmology, NY Eye & Ear Infirmary 1973; **Fellow:** Retina, Montefiore Med Ctr 1974; **Fac Appt:** Prof Oph, NY Med Coll

Wang, Frederick Mark MD (Oph) - **Spec Exp:** Pediatric Ophthalmology; Strabismus; Eye Muscle Disorders; **Hospital:** Lenox Hill Hosp (Manh Eye, Ear & Throat Hosp) (page 106), Montefiore Med Ctr-Moses Campus (page 100); **Address:** 30 E 40th St, Ste 405, New York, NY 10016-1201; **Phone:** 212-684-3980; **Board Cert:** Pediatrics 1978; Ophthalmology 1980; **Med School:** Albert Einstein Coll Med 1972; **Resid:** Pediatrics, Jacobi Med Ctr 1974; Ophthalmology, Albert Einstein 1979; **Fellow:** Pediatric Ophthalmology, Children's Hosp Natl Med Ctr 1980; **Fac Appt:** Clin Prof Oph, Albert Einstein Coll Med

Warren, Floyd A MD (Oph) - **Spec Exp:** Neuro-Ophthalmology; Optic Nerve Disorders; Orbital Diseases; Diplopia; **Hospital:** NYU Langone Med Ctr (page 108), Lenox Hill Hosp (Manh Eye, Ear & Throat Hosp) (page 106); **Address:** NYU Langone Med Ctr-Dept of Ophthalmology, 530 First Ave, Ste 3B, New York, NY 10016; **Phone:** 212-263-7030; **Board Cert:** Ophthalmology 1985; **Med School:** NYU Sch Med 1979; **Resid:** Ophthalmology, St Vincents Hosp 1983; **Fellow:** Neuro-Ophthalmology, NYU Med Ctr 1984; Neuro-Ophthalmology, Eye & Ear Hosp 1985; **Fac Appt:** Clin Prof Oph, NYU Sch Med

Weiss, Michael J MD/PhD (Oph) - **Spec Exp:** Uveitis; Retinal Disorders; Cataract Surgery; Diabetic Eye Disease; **Hospital:** NY-Presby/Columbia Univ Med Ctr, NY (page 104); **Address:** 635 W 165th St, Ste 101, New York, NY 10032-3701; **Phone:** 212-305-9925; **Board Cert:** Ophthalmology 1987; **Med School:** Columbia P&S 1981; **Resid:** Ophthalmology, Columbia-Presby Med Ctr 1985; **Fac Appt:** Clin Prof Oph, Columbia P&S

Weseley, Peter E MD (Oph) - **Spec Exp:** Retina/Vitreous Surgery; Macular Degeneration; Diabetic Eye Disease/Retinopathy; **Hospital:** New York Eye & Ear Infirm (page 115); **Address:** 310 E 14th St, Ste 419, New York, NY 10003; **Phone:** 212-979-4286; **Board Cert:** Ophthalmology 2013; **Med School:** Tulane Univ 1987; **Resid:** Ophthalmology, NY E&E Infirm 1991; **Fellow:** Retina/Vitreous Surgery, Devers Eye Inst 1993

Whitmore, Wayne G MD (Oph) - **Spec Exp:** Cataract Surgery; Glaucoma; Corneal Disease; **Hospital:** NY-Presby/Weill Cornell Med Ctr, NY (page 104), Lenox Hill Hosp (Manh Eye, Ear & Throat Hosp) (page 106); **Address:** 116 E 68th St, New York, NY 10065; **Phone:** 212-249-3030; **Board Cert:** Ophthalmology 1982; **Med School:** Dartmouth Med Sch 1977; **Resid:** Ophthalmology, NY Hosp 1981; **Fellow:** Ophthalmic Oncology, NY Hosp 1982; **Fac Appt:** Asst Clin Prof Oph, Cornell Univ-Weill Med Coll

Wisnicki, H Jay MD (Oph) - **Spec Exp:** Strabismus; Eye Muscle Disorders; Pediatric Ophthalmology; **Hospital:** Beth Israel Med Ctr - Petrie Div (page 94), New York Eye & Ear Infirm (page 115); **Address:** Union Square Eye Care, 235 Park Ave S Fl 2, New York, NY 10003; **Phone:** 212-844-2020; **Board Cert:** Ophthalmology 1987; **Med School:** SUNY Hlth Sci Ctr 1981; **Resid:** Ophthalmology, Mount Sinai Med Ctr 1985; **Fellow:** Strabismus, Johns Hopkins Hosp 1986; **Fac Appt:** Prof Oph, Albert Einstein Coll Med

Wong, Raymond F MD (Oph) - **Spec Exp:** Diabetic Eye Disease/Retinopathy; Retinal Detachment; Macular Disease/Degeneration; **Hospital:** New York Eye & Ear Infirm (page 115); **Address:** 139 Centre St, Ste PH 105, New York, NY 10013; **Phone:** 212-227-5451; **Board Cert:** Ophthalmology 1990; **Med School:** SUNY Hlth Sci Ctr 1984; **Resid:** Ophthalmology, Yale-New Haven Hosp 1988; **Fellow:** Retina/Vitreous Surgery, USC-Doheny Eye Inst 1990; **Fac Appt:** Asst Prof Oph, NY Med Coll

Yagoda, Arnold D MD (Oph) - **Spec Exp:** Macular Degeneration; Laser Vision Surgery; Diabetic Eye Disease/Retinopathy; Retinal Disorders; **Hospital:** New York Eye & Ear Infirm (page 115); **Address:** 67 E 78th St, New York, NY 10075; **Phone:** 212-744-2513; **Board Cert:** Ophthalmology 1980; **Med School:** Cornell Univ-Weill Med Coll 1975; **Resid:** Ophthalmology, Lenox Hill Hosp 1979; **Fellow:** Vitreoretinal Disease, Montefiore Hosp Med Ctr 1980; **Fac Appt:** Asst Clin Prof Oph, Albert Einstein Coll Med

Yannuzzi, Lawrence A MD (Oph) - **Spec Exp:** Retina/Vitreous Surgery; Macular Disease/Degeneration; Diabetic Eye Disease/Retinopathy; **Hospital:** NY-Presby/Columbia Univ Med Ctr, NY (page 104), Lenox Hill Hosp (Manh Eye, Ear & Throat Hosp) (page 106); **Address:** Vitreous-Retina-Macula Consultants of NY, 460 Park Ave Fl 5, New York, NY 10022; **Phone:** 212-861-9797; **Board Cert:** Ophthalmology 1970; **Med School:** Boston Univ 1964; **Resid:** Ophthalmology, Manhattan EE&T Hosp 1968; **Fellow:** Ophthalmology, Manhattan EE&T Hosp 1971; **Fac Appt:** Clin Prof Oph, Columbia P&S

Young, Joshua A MD (Oph) - **Spec Exp:** Glaucoma; Corneal Disease; **Hospital:** NYU Langone Med Ctr (page 108), Lenox Hill Hosp (Manh Eye, Ear & Throat Hosp) (page 106); **Address:** Madison Ophthalmology, 161 Madison Ave, Ste 5 SE, New York, NY 10016; **Phone:** 212-448-0101; **Board Cert:** Ophthalmology 2008; **Med School:** NYU Sch Med 1990; **Resid:** Ophthalmology, NYU Med Ctr 1994; **Fellow:** Cornea & Ext Eye Disease, Mass Eye & Ear Infirm/Harvard 1996; **Fac Appt:** Clin Prof Oph, NYU Sch Med

Zweifach, Philip H MD (Oph) - **Spec Exp:** Cataract Surgery; Neuro-Ophthalmology; **Hospital:** NY-Presby/Weill Cornell Med Ctr, NY (page 104); **Address:** 131 E 69th St, New York, NY 10021-5158; **Phone:** 212-535-1508; **Board Cert:** Ophthalmology 1968; **Med School:** Cornell Univ-Weill Med Coll 1961; **Resid:** Neurology, Boston City Hosp 1963; Ophthalmology, New York Hosp 1966; **Fellow:** Neuro-Ophthalmology, Mass Eye & Ear Infirmary 1967; **Fac Appt:** Clin Prof Oph, Cornell Univ-Weill Med Coll

Orthopaedic Surgery

Adler, Edward M MD (OrS) - **Spec Exp:** Hip Surgery; Knee Surgery; Joint Replacement; Shoulder Surgery; **Hospital:** NYU Hosp For Joint Dis (page 108), NYU Langone Med Ctr (page 108); **Address:** Madison Ave Ortho Assocs, 145 E 32nd St Fl 4th, New York, NY 10016; **Phone:** 212-427-3986; **Board Cert:** Orthopaedic Surgery 2013; **Med School:** UMDNJ-NJ Med Sch, Newark 1984; **Resid:** Orthopaedic Surgery, University Hosp 1989; **Fellow:** Joint Replacement Surgery, Hosp for Joint Diseases 1990; **Fac Appt:** Assoc Clin Prof OrS, NYU Sch Med

Ahmad, Christopher S MD (OrS) - **Spec Exp:** Sports Medicine; Knee Injuries/ACL; Pediatric Orthopaedic Surgery; Shoulder & Elbow Surgery; **Hospital:** NY-Presby/Columbia Univ Med Ctr, NY (page 104); **Address:** 161 Fort Washington Ave, Fl 2, New York, NY 10032; **Phone:** 212-305-4565; **Board Cert:** Orthopaedic Surgery 2003; Orthopaedic Sports Medicine 2007; **Med School:** NYU Sch Med 1994; **Resid:** Orthopaedic Surgery, NY Orthopaedic Hosp/Columbia 2000; **Fellow:** Sports Medicine, Kerlan-Jobe Orthopaedic Clinic 2001; **Fac Appt:** Assoc Prof OrS, Columbia P&S

Alexiades, Michael M MD (OrS) - **Spec Exp:** Hip Replacement; Knee Replacement; Arthroscopic Surgery; Minimally Invasive Surgery; **Hospital:** Hosp For Special Surgery (page 113), Lenox Hill Hosp (page 106); **Address:** 523 E 72nd St Fl 7, East River Professional Bldg, New York, NY 10021; **Phone:** 212-774-7557; **Board Cert:** Orthopaedic Surgery 2012; **Med School:** Cornell Univ-Weill Med Coll 1983; **Resid:** Surgery, Lenox Hill Hosp 1984; Orthopaedic Surgery, Lenox Hill Hosp 1988; **Fellow:** Arthritis Surgery, Hosp for Special Surgery 1989; **Fac Appt:** Asst Clin Prof OrS, Cornell Univ-Weill Med Coll

Allen, Answorth A MD (OrS) - **Spec Exp:** Shoulder & Elbow Surgery; Knee Surgery; Shoulder & Knee Reconstruction; Sports Medicine; **Hospital:** Hosp For Special Surgery (page 113); **Address:** Hosp for Special Surgery, 525 E 71st St, Belaire Bldg Fl 1, New York, NY 10021; **Phone:** 212-606-1447; **Board Cert:** Orthopaedic Surgery 2007; Orthopaedic Sports Medicine 2009; **Med School:** Cornell Univ 1988; **Resid:** Orthopaedic Surgery, NY-Presby/Columbia Univ Med Ctr 1993; **Fellow:** Sports Medicine, Univ Pittsburgh 1994; **Fac Appt:** Assoc Prof OrS, Cornell Univ-Weill Med Coll

Bauman, Phillip A MD (OrS) - **Spec Exp:** Foot & Ankle Surgery; Knee Surgery; Dance/Sports Medicine; Arthroscopic Surgery; **Hospital:** St. Luke's - Roosevelt Hosp Ctr - Roosevelt Div (page 94); **Address:** Orthopaedic Associates of NY, 343 W 58th St, Ste 1, New York, NY 10019; **Phone:** 212-506-0228; **Board Cert:** Orthopaedic Surgery 2011; **Med School:** Columbia P&S 1981; **Resid:** Surgery, St Lukes-Roosevelt Hosp Ctr 1983; Orthopaedic Surgery, Columbia-Presby Med Ctr 1987; **Fac Appt:** Asst Prof OrS, Columbia P&S

Bendo, John A MD (OrS) - **Spec Exp:** Spinal Surgery-Minimally Invasive; Scoliosis; Spinal Disc Replacement; **Hospital:** NYU Hosp For Joint Dis (page 108), NYU Langone Med Ctr (page 108); **Address:** Center For Musculoskeletal Care, 301 E 17th St, Ste 400, New York, NY 10003; **Phone:** 212-598-6625; **Board Cert:** Orthopaedic Surgery 2008; **Med School:** Mount Sinai Sch Med 1989; **Resid:** Orthopaedic Surgery, Mt Sinai Hosp 1994; **Fellow:** Spine Surgery, Hosp Joint Diseases 1995; **Fac Appt:** Assoc Prof OrS, NYU Sch Med

Bigliani, Louis U MD (OrS) - **Spec Exp:** Shoulder Surgery; Sports Medicine; Arthroscopic Surgery; Rotator Cuff Surgery; **Hospital:** NY-Presby/Columbia Univ Med Ctr, NY (page 104); **Address:** Presby/Columbia Univ Med Ctr-Dept Ortho Surg, 622 W 168 St, rm 1130, New York, NY 10032-3720; **Phone:** 212-305-0998; **Board Cert:** Orthopaedic Surgery 1979; **Med School:** Loyola Univ-Stritch Sch Med 1973; **Resid:** Surgery, St Luke's-Roosevelt Hosp Ctr 1974; Orthopaedic Surgery, NY-Presby/Columbia Univ Med Ctr 1978; **Fac Appt:** Prof OrS, Columbia P&S

Bitan, Fabien D MD (OrS) - **Spec Exp:** Spinal Surgery-Pediatric & Adult; Spinal Disc Replacement; Spinal Deformity; Spinal Disorders-Degenerative; **Hospital:** Lenox Hill Hosp (page 106), Beth Israel Med Ctr - Petrie Div (page 94); **Address:** Manhattan Orthopaedics, 130 E 77th St Fl 7, New York, NY 10075; **Phone:** 212-744-8114; **Med School:** France 1981; **Resid:** Orthopaedic Surgery, Hospital Beaujon 1987; Pediatric Orthopaedic Surgery, Hosp des Enfants Malades 1996; **Fellow:** Pediatric Orthopaedic Surgery, Hosp Special Surgery 1997; Spine Surgery, Beth Israel Med Ctr 1998

Boachie-Adjei, Oheneba MD (OrS) - **Spec Exp:** Spinal Surgery; Scoliosis; Spinal Reconstructive Surgery; **Hospital:** Hosp For Special Surgery (page 113); **Address:** Hosp for Special Surgery, 535 E 70th St, New York, NY 10021; **Phone:** 212-606-1948; **Board Cert:** Orthopaedic Surgery 2010; **Med School:** Columbia P&S 1980; **Resid:** Surgery, St Vincents Hosp 1982; Orthopaedic Surgery, Hosp Spec Surg 1986; **Fellow:** Orthopaedic Pathology, Hosp Spec Surg 1983; Spine Surgery, Twin Cities Scoliosis Ctr/Minn Spine Ctr 1987; **Fac Appt:** Prof OrS, Cornell Univ-Weill Med Coll

Boland, Patrick MD (OrS) - **Spec Exp:** Bone Cancer; Spinal Tumors; Bone & Soft Tissue Tumors; Limb Sparing Surgery; **Hospital:** Meml Sloan-Kettering Canc Ctr (page 114); **Address:** Meml Sloan-Kettering Cancer Ctr, 1275 York Avenue, New York, NY 10065; **Phone:** 212-639-8684; **Board Cert:** Orthopaedic Surgery 2009; **Med School:** Ireland 1967; **Resid:** Surgery, Brigham & Women's Hosp 1973; Orthopaedic Surgery, Middlesex/Hammersmith Hosp 1981; **Fellow:** Orthopaedic Oncology, Meml Sloan-Kettering Cancer Ctr 1982

Bosco III, Joseph A MD (OrS) - **Spec Exp:** Sports Medicine; Knee Surgery; Shoulder Surgery; **Hospital:** NYU Hosp For Joint Dis (page 108), Jamaica Hosp Med Ctr; **Address:** Ctr for Musculoskeletal Care, 333 E 38th St, New York, NY 10016; **Phone:** 646-501-7223; **Board Cert:** Orthopaedic Surgery 2006; **Med School:** Univ VT Coll Med 1986; **Resid:** Orthopaedic Surgery, Univ NC Med Ctr 1991; **Fellow:** Reconstructive Surgery, Univ Ariz Coll Med Affil Hosp 1992; **Fac Appt:** Asst Clin Prof OrS, NYU Sch Med

Bostrom, Mathias P MD (OrS) - **Spec Exp:** Knee Replacement & Revision; Hip Replacement & Revision; Hip & Knee Reconstruction; Musculoskeletal Infections; **Hospital:** Hosp For Special Surgery (page 113), NY-Presby/Weill Cornell Med Ctr, NY (page 104); **Address:** 535 E 70th St Fl 3, New York, NY 10021; **Phone:** 212-606-1674; **Board Cert:** Orthopaedic Surgery 2009; **Med School:** Johns Hopkins Univ 1989; **Resid:** Orthopaedic Surgery, Hosp for Special Surg 1995; **Fellow:** Reconstructive Surgery, Hosp for Special Surg 1996; **Fac Appt:** Prof OrS, Cornell Univ-Weill Med Coll

Brisson, Paul M MD (OrS) - **Spec Exp:** Spinal Surgery; **Hospital:** NY-Presby/Lower Manhattan Hosp (page 104), NY-Presby/Weill Cornell Med Ctr, NY (page 104); **Address:** NY Spine Care, 51 E 25th St Fl 6, New York, NY 10010; **Phone:** 212-813-3632; **Board Cert:** Orthopaedic Surgery 2014; **Med School:** Univ Montreal 1979; **Resid:** Orthopaedic Surgery, McGill Med Ctr 1987; **Fellow:** Spine Surgery, Hosp Joint Diseases 1988; Spine Surgery, Buffalo Genl Hosp 1989

Bronson, Michael J MD (OrS) - **Spec Exp:** Joint Replacement; Knee Replacement; Hip Replacement; Arthritis; **Hospital:** Mt Sinai Med Ctr (page 102); **Address:** Mt Sinai Med Ctr, Dept Orthopedic Surg, 5 E 98th St, Box 1188, New York, NY 10029; **Phone:** 212-241-1640; **Board Cert:** Orthopaedic Surgery 1984; **Med School:** NY Med Coll 1976; **Resid:** Orthopaedic Surgery, Lenox Hill Hosp 1980; **Fellow:** Joint Replacement Surgery, NY Presby/Columbia Med Ctr 1981; Hip & Knee Surgery, NY Presby/Columbia Med Ctr 1981; **Fac Appt:** Assoc Prof OrS, Mount Sinai Sch Med

Buly, Robert L MD (OrS) - **Spec Exp:** Hip Replacement & Revision; Arthroscopic Surgery-Hip; Knee Replacement; Arthritis; **Hospital:** Hosp For Special Surgery (page 113), NY-Presby/Weill Cornell Med Ctr, NY (page 104); **Address:** Hospital for Special Surgery, 535 E 70th St, New York, NY 10021; **Phone:** 212-606-1971; **Board Cert:** Orthopaedic Surgery 2004; **Med School:** Cornell Univ-Weill Med Coll 1985; **Resid:** Orthopaedic Surgery, Hosp for Special Surg 1990; **Fellow:** Hip Surgery, Mueller Fdn 1991; Joint Reconstruction, Case Western Res/Univ Hosp 1992; **Fac Appt:** Assoc Clin Prof OrS, Cornell Univ-Weill Med Coll

Cammisa Jr, Frank P MD (OrS) - **Spec Exp:** Spinal Surgery; Spinal Disc Replacement; Minimally Invasive Spinal Surgery; Scoliosis; **Hospital:** Hosp For Special Surgery (page 113); **Address:** 523 E 72nd St, Fl 3, New York, NY 10021; **Phone:** 212-606-1946; **Board Cert:** Orthopaedic Surgery 2011; **Med School:** Columbia P&S 1982; **Resid:** Surgery, Columbia-Presby Hosp 1983; Orthopaedic Surgery, Hosp for Special Surgery 1987; **Fellow:** Spine Surgery, Jackson Meml Hosp 1988; **Fac Appt:** Assoc Prof OrS, Cornell Univ-Weill Med Coll

Casden, Andrew M MD (OrS) - **Spec Exp:** Spinal Surgery; Spinal Disc Replacement; Minimally Invasive Spinal Surgery; Scoliosis; **Hospital:** Mt Sinai Med Ctr (page 102); **Address:** Mount Sinai Med Ctr, Dept Orth Surg, 5 E 98th St Fl 9, Box 1188, New York, NY 10029; **Phone:** 212-241-8947; **Board Cert:** Orthopaedic Surgery 2012; **Med School:** Cornell Univ-Weill Med Coll 1983; **Resid:** Orthopaedic Surgery, Hosp Joint Diseases 1988; **Fellow:** Spine Surgery, Rush-Presby Med Ctr 1989; **Fac Appt:** Assoc Prof OrS, Mount Sinai Sch Med

Compito, Catherine A MD (OrS) - **Spec Exp:** Shoulder Surgery; Elbow Surgery; Sports Medicine; Arthroscopic Surgery; **Hospital:** Beth Israel Med Ctr - Petrie Div (page 94); **Address:** Beth Israel Orthopedics and Sports Med, 10 Union Square E, Ste 3K, New York, NY 10003; **Phone:** 212-844-8544; **Board Cert:** Orthopaedic Surgery 2009; Orthopaedic Sports Medicine 2011; **Med School:** Albert Einstein Coll Med 1986; **Resid:** Orthopaedic Surgery, Montefiore Med Ctr 1991; **Fellow:** Sports Medicine, Staten Island Univ Hosp 1992; Shoulder Surgery, NY-Presby/Columbia Univ Med Ctr 1993

Cordasco, Frank A MD (OrS) - **Spec Exp:** Sports Medicine; Arthroscopic Surgery-Shoulder; Rotator Cuff Surgery; Shoulder Replacement; **Hospital:** Hosp For Special Surgery (page 113); **Address:** Hospital for Special Surgery, 525 E 71 St Fl 2nd, Belaire Bldg, New York, NY 10021; **Phone:** 212-606-1636; **Board Cert:** Orthopaedic Surgery 2013; Orthopaedic Sports Medicine 2009; **Med School:** UMDNJ-NJ Med Sch, Newark 1985; **Resid:** Surgery, NY Univ Med Ctr 1996; Orthopaedic Surgery, Columbia-Presby Hosp 1990; **Fellow:** Elbow & Shoulder Surgery, Columbia-Presby Hosp 1991; **Fac Appt:** Assoc Prof OrS, Cornell Univ-Weill Med Coll

Cornell, Charles N MD (OrS) - **Spec Exp:** Hip Replacement; Knee Replacement; **Hospital:** Hosp For Special Surgery (page 113); **Address:** 535 E 70th St, Ste 306, New York, NY 10021; **Phone:** 212-606-1414; **Board Cert:** Orthopaedic Surgery 2009; **Med School:** Cornell Univ-Weill Med Coll 1980; **Resid:** Surgery, Presby Hosp 1982; Orthopaedic Surgery, Hosp For Special Surgery 1985; **Fellow:** Orthopaedic Trauma Surgery, Univ Washington Med Ctr 1986; **Fac Appt:** Clin Prof OrS, Cornell Univ-Weill Med Coll

Craig, Edward V MD (OrS) - **Spec Exp:** Shoulder Arthroscopic Surgery; Shoulder Replacement; Sports Medicine; Elbow Surgery; **Hospital:** Hosp For Special Surgery (page 113), NY-Presby/Weill Cornell Med Ctr, NY (page 104); **Address:** 535 E 70th St, New York, NY 10021; **Phone:** 212-606-1966; **Board Cert:** Orthopaedic Surgery 1984; **Med School:** Columbia P&S 1972; **Resid:** Surgery, St Lukes-Roosevelt Hosp 1976; Orthopaedic Surgery, Columbia-Presby Hosp 1980; **Fellow:** Shoulder Surgery, Columbia-Presby Hosp 1981; Hand Surgery, Columbia-Presby Hosp 1982; **Fac Appt:** Clin Prof OrS, Cornell Univ-Weill Med Coll

Cuomo, Frances MD (OrS) - **Spec Exp:** Shoulder Surgery; Elbow Surgery; Arthroscopic Surgery; **Hospital:** Beth Israel Med Ctr - Petrie Div (page 94); **Address:** Beth Israel Orthpaedics & Sports Med, 10 Union Square E, Ste 3M, New York, NY 10003; **Phone:** 212-844-6938; **Board Cert:** Orthopaedic Surgery 2012; **Med School:** NYU Sch Med 1983; **Resid:** Surgery, Beth Israel Med Ctr 1984; Orthopaedic Surgery, Lenox Hill Hosp 1988; **Fellow:** Shoulder Surgery, Columbia-Presby Med Ctr 1989; **Fac Appt:** Asst Prof OrS, Albert Einstein Coll Med

Cushner, Fred D MD (OrS) - **Spec Exp:** Knee Reconstruction; Knee Injuries/Ligament Surgery; Cartilage Damage; Sports Medicine; **Hospital:** Lenox Hill Hosp (page 106), Southside Hosp (page 106); **Address:** ISK-Inst for Ortho & Sports Med, 210 E 64th St Fl 4, New York, NY 10065; **Phone:** 212-434-4312; **Board Cert:** Orthopaedic Surgery 2007; **Med School:** Med Univ SC 1988; **Resid:** Orthopaedic Surgery, Univ SC Med Ctr 1993; **Fellow:** Knee Reconstruction, Beth Israel Med Ctr 1994; Orthopaedic Sports Medicine, ISK-Inst for Ortho & Sports Med 1995

Deland, Jonathan T MD (OrS) - **Spec Exp:** Foot & Ankle Surgery; Sports Medicine; Arthritis; **Hospital:** Hosp For Special Surgery (page 113); **Address:** Hosp Spec Surg-Dept Foot & Ankle Service, 535 E 70th St, New York, NY 10021-4099; **Phone:** 212-606-1665; **Board Cert:** Orthopaedic Surgery 2013; **Med School:** Columbia P&S 1980; **Resid:** Surgery, St Luke's-Roosevelt Hosp Ctr 1982; Orthopaedic Surgery, Mass Genl Hosp 1987; **Fellow:** Foot & Ankle Surgery, St Luke's-Roosevelt Hosp 1988; Trauma, Mass Genl Hosp 1989; **Fac Appt:** Clin Prof S, Cornell Univ-Weill Med Coll

Egol, Kenneth A MD (OrS) - **Spec Exp:** Trauma; Reconstructive Surgery; Limb Lengthening (Ilizarov Procedure); Fractures-Non Union; **Hospital:** NYU Hosp For Joint Dis (page 108), Jamaica Hosp Med Ctr; **Address:** 301 E 17th St, New York, NY 10003; **Phone:** 212-598-3889; **Board Cert:** Orthopaedic Surgery 2012; **Med School:** SUNY Upstate Med Univ 1993; **Resid:** Orthopaedic Surgery, Hosp For Joint Diseases 1998; **Fellow:** Trauma, Carolinas Med Ctr 1999; **Fac Appt:** Assoc Prof OrS, NYU Sch Med

Elliott, Andrew J MD (OrS) - **Spec Exp:** Foot & Ankle Surgery; Arthroscopic Surgery; Sports Injuries; **Hospital:** Hosp For Special Surgery (page 113); **Address:** HSS, Orthopaedic Surgery Dept, 420 E 72 St, Ste 1B, New York, NY 10021; **Phone:** 212-203-0740; **Board Cert:** Orthopaedic Surgery 2010; **Med School:** Harvard Med Sch 1991; **Resid:** Surgery, Yale-New Haven Hosp 1996; **Fellow:** Orthopaedic Surgery, Hosp Special Surgery 1997; **Fac Appt:** Asst Clin Prof OrS, Cornell Univ-Weill Med Coll

Errico, Thomas J MD (OrS) - **Spec Exp:** Spinal Surgery; Pediatric Orthopaedic Surgery; Scoliosis; **Hospital:** NYU Langone Med Ctr (page 108), NYU Hosp For Joint Dis (page 108); **Address:** Ctr for Musculoskeletal Care, 333 E 38th St Fl 6, MS 10016, New York, NY 10016-6402; **Phone:** 646-501-7200; **Board Cert:** Orthopaedic Surgery 2007; **Med School:** UMDNJ-NJ Med Sch, Newark 1978; **Resid:** Orthopaedic Surgery, NYU Med Ctr 1983; **Fellow:** Spine Surgery, Toronto Genl Hosp 1984; **Fac Appt:** Prof OrS, NYU Sch Med

Farmer, James C MD (OrS) - **Spec Exp:** Spinal Disorders-Degenerative; Trauma; Spinal Surgery; **Hospital:** Hosp For Special Surgery (page 113); **Address:** Hosp for Special Surgery, 523 E 72nd St Fl 3, East River Professional Bldg, New York, NY 10021; **Phone:** 212-606-1591; **Board Cert:** Orthopaedic Surgery 2007; **Med School:** Georgetown Univ 1988; **Resid:** Orthopaedic Surgery, Hosp Univ Penn 1993; **Fellow:** Spine Surgery, Thos Jefferson Univ Hosp 1994; **Fac Appt:** Assoc Prof OrS, Cornell Univ-Weill Med Coll

Fealy, Stephen MD (OrS) - **Spec Exp:** Sports Medicine; Shoulder Arthroscopic Surgery; Shoulder Replacement; Knee Replacement; **Hospital:** Hosp For Special Surgery (page 113); **Address:** Hospital for Special Surgery, 523 E 72nd St Fl 2nd, New York, NY 10021; **Phone:** 212-606-1894; **Board Cert:** Orthopaedic Surgery 2004; **Med School:** Columbia P&S 1995; **Resid:** Orthopaedic Surgery, Hosp for Special Surg 2000; **Fellow:** Sports Medicine, Hosp for Special Surg 2001; **Fac Appt:** Asst Prof OrS, Cornell Univ-Weill Med Coll

Feldman, David S MD (OrS) - **Spec Exp:** Limb Deformities; Spinal Surgery; Pediatric Orthopaedic Surgery; Scoliosis; **Hospital:** NYU Hosp For Joint Dis (page 108), NYU Langone Med Ctr (page 108); **Address:** 67 Irving Pl Fl 8, New York, NY 10003; **Phone:** 212-533-5310; **Board Cert:** Orthopaedic Surgery 2007; **Med School:** Albert Einstein Coll Med 1988; **Resid:** Surgery, NYU Med Ctr 1989; Orthopaedic Surgery, Hosp for Joint Diseases 1993; **Fellow:** Pediatric Surgery, Hosp For Sick Chldn 1994; **Fac Appt:** Prof OrS, NYU Sch Med

Figgie, Mark P MD (OrS) - **Spec Exp:** Joint Replacement; Minimally Invasive Surgery; Hip Surgery; Knee Surgery; **Hospital:** Hosp For Special Surgery (page 113), NY-Presby/Weill Cornell Med Ctr, NY (page 104); **Address:** 535 E 70th St, Ste 305, New York, NY 10021; **Phone:** 212-606-1932; **Board Cert:** Orthopaedic Surgery 2011; **Med School:** Case West Res Univ 1981; **Resid:** Orthopaedic Surgery, Univ Hosp-Case Western Reserve 1986; **Fellow:** Biomedical Engineering, Hosp For Special Surgery 1987; Arthritis Surgery, Hosp For Special Surgery 1988; **Fac Appt:** Clin Prof OrS, Cornell Univ-Weill Med Coll

Flatow, Evan L MD (OrS) - **Spec Exp:** Rotator Cuff Surgery; Shoulder Injuries; Shoulder Replacement; Shoulder Arthroscopic Surgery; **Hospital:** Mt Sinai Med Ctr (page 102); **Address:** 5 E 98th St, Fl 9, Box 1188, New York, NY 10029; **Phone:** 212-241-1663; **Board Cert:** Orthopaedic Surgery 2010; **Med School:** Columbia P&S 1981; **Resid:** Surgery, Roosevelt Hosp 1983; Orthopaedic Surgery, Columbia-Presby Med Ctr 1986; **Fellow:** Shoulder Surgery, Columbia-Presby Med Ctr 1987; **Fac Appt:** Prof OrS, Mount Sinai Sch Med

Fragomen, Austin T MD (OrS) - **Spec Exp:** Limb Deformities; Limb Lengthening; Bone Infections; Blount's Disease; **Hospital:** Hosp For Special Surgery (page 113); **Address:** Inst for Limb Lengthening, 519 E 72nd St, Ste 204, River Terrace, New York, NY 10021; **Phone:** 212-606-1550; **Board Cert:** Orthopaedic Surgery 2007; **Med School:** SUNY Downstate 1997; **Resid:** Surgery, Montefiore Med Ctr 1998; Orthopaedic Surgery, Westchester Med Ctr 2003; **Fac Appt:** Asst Prof OrS, Cornell Univ-Weill Med Coll

Gladstone, James N MD (OrS) - **Spec Exp:** Shoulder & Knee Surgery; Cartilage Damage; Knee-Patella Problems; Arthritis; **Hospital:** Mt Sinai Med Ctr (page 102); **Address:** Mt Sinai Med Ctr, 5 E 98th St Fl 9, Box 1188, New York, NY 10029; **Phone:** 212-241-1645; **Board Cert:** Orthopaedic Surgery 2009; Orthopaedic Sports Medicine 2007; **Med School:** Tufts Univ 1990; **Resid:** Orthopaedic Surgery, Columbia-Presby Med Ctr 1995; **Fellow:** Sports Medicine, American Sports Med Inst 1996; **Fac Appt:** Assoc Prof OrS, Mount Sinai Sch Med

Glashow, Jonathan L MD (OrS) - **Spec Exp:** Sports Medicine; Shoulder Surgery; Knee Surgery; Arthroscopic Surgery; **Hospital:** Mt Sinai Med Ctr (page 102); **Address:** 737 Park Ave, Ste 1C, New York, NY 10021; **Phone:** 212-794-5096; **Board Cert:** Orthopaedic Surgery 2004; **Med School:** Cornell Univ-Weill Med Coll 1984; **Resid:** Surgery, Mt Sinai Hosp 1985; Orthopaedic Surgery, Lenox Hill Hosp 1989; **Fellow:** Arthroscopic Surgery, S CA Ortho Inst/UCLA Med Ctr 1990; Shoulder Surgery, Univ Texas Med Ctr 1990; **Fac Appt:** Assoc Clin Prof OrS, Mount Sinai Sch Med

Goldstein, Jeffrey A MD (OrS) - **Spec Exp:** Spinal Surgery; Minimally Invasive Spinal Surgery; Spinal Disc Replacement; Scoliosis; **Hospital:** NYU Hosp For Joint Dis (page 108), NYU Langone Med Ctr (page 108); **Address:** NYU Hospital for Joint Diseases, 19 Beekman St, New York, NY 10038; **Phone:** 212-513-7711; **Board Cert:** Orthopaedic Surgery 2009; **Med School:** SUNY Downstate 1990; **Resid:** Orthopaedic Surgery, Case West Univ Med Ctr 1995; **Fellow:** Spine Surgery, Maryland Spine Ctr 1996; **Fac Appt:** Clin Prof OrS, NYU Sch Med

Goodwin, Charles B MD (OrS) - **Spec Exp:** Spinal Reconstructive Surgery; Shoulder Arthroscopic Surgery; Minimally Invasive Spinal Surgery; Arthroscopic Surgery-Knee; **Hospital:** Hosp For Special Surgery (page 113), St. Luke's - Roosevelt Hosp Ctr - Roosevelt Div (page 94); **Address:** 635 Madison Ave Fl 7, New York, NY 10022-1009; **Phone:** 212-317-4600; **Board Cert:** Orthopaedic Surgery 1985; **Med School:** Univ Cincinnati 1976; **Resid:** Surgery, St Luke's Roosevelt Hosp Ctr 1979; Orthopaedic Surgery, NY Presby Hosp/ Columbia 1982; **Fellow:** Spine Surgery, Univ Toronto Affil Hosp 1983; **Fac Appt:** Asst Prof OrS, Cornell Univ-Weill Med Coll

Green, Steven M MD (OrS) - **Spec Exp:** Hand & Wrist Surgery; Carpal Tunnel Syndrome; Hand Surgery; **Hospital:** Mt Sinai Med Ctr (page 102), NYU Hosp For Joint Dis (page 108); **Address:** 2 E 88th St, New York, NY 10128-0555; **Phone:** 212-348-6644; **Board Cert:** Orthopaedic Surgery 1977; **Med School:** Albert Einstein Coll Med 1970; **Resid:** Surgery, Georgia Bapt Hosp 1972; Orthopaedic Surgery, Mt Sinai Hosp 1975; **Fellow:** Hand Surgery, Thomas Jefferson Univ Hosp 1978; **Fac Appt:** Assoc Clin Prof OrS, NYU Sch Med

Greisberg, Justin K MD (OrS) - **Spec Exp:** Foot & Ankle Surgery-Complex; Ankle Replacement & Revision; Reconstructive Surgery; Trauma; **Hospital:** NY-Presby/Columbia Univ Med Ctr, NY (page 104); **Address:** Presby/Columbia Univ Med Ctr-Dept Ortho Surg, 622 W 168 St Fl PH 11 - rm 1153, New York, NY 10032; **Phone:** 212-305-5604; **Board Cert:** Orthopaedic Surgery 2004; **Med School:** Albert Einstein Coll Med 1995; **Resid:** Surgery, Brown Univ Affil Hosp 1996; Orthopaedic Surgery, Rhode Island Hosp 2000; **Fellow:** Orthopaedic Trauma Surgery, Rhode Island Hosp 2001; Foot & Ankle Surgery, Harborview Med Ctr 2002; **Fac Appt:** Assoc Clin Prof OrS, Columbia P&S

Grelsamer, Ronald P MD (OrS) - **Spec Exp:** Knee-Patella Problems Consult; Arthritis-Hip & Knee; **Hospital:** Mt Sinai Med Ctr (page 102); **Address:** 303 2nd Ave, Ste 19, Ground Floor, New York, NY 10003; **Phone:** 646-704-4158; **Board Cert:** Orthopaedic Surgery 2008; **Med School:** Columbia P&S 1979; **Resid:** Orthopaedic Surgery, Columbia Presby Med Ctr 1984; **Fellow:** Hip & Knee Surgery, Columbia Presby Med Ctr 1985; **Fac Appt:** Assoc Prof OrS, Mount Sinai Sch Med

Haas, Steven B MD (OrS) - **Spec Exp:** Knee Surgery; Knee Replacement; Minimally Invasive Knee Replacement; **Hospital:** Hosp For Special Surgery (page 113); **Address:** Hosp for Special Surgery, 535 E 70th St, Fl 3, New York, NY 10021; **Phone:** 212-606-1852; **Board Cert:** Orthopaedic Surgery 2004; **Med School:** Univ Rochester 1985; **Resid:** Orthopaedic Surgery, Hosp Special Surgery 1990; **Fellow:** Knee Surgery, Hosp Special Surgery 1991; **Fac Appt:** Clin Prof OrS, Cornell Univ-Weill Med Coll

Hamilton, William G MD (OrS) - **Spec Exp:** Dance Medicine; Sports Medicine; **Hospital:** St. Luke's - Roosevelt Hosp Ctr - Roosevelt Div (page 94), Hosp For Special Surgery (page 113); **Address:** 343 W 58th St, New York, NY 10019-1173; **Phone:** 212-765-2260; **Board Cert:** Orthopaedic Surgery 1971; **Med School:** Columbia P&S 1964; **Resid:** Surgery, St Luke's-Roosevelt Hosp Ctr 1966; Orthopaedic Surgery, Columbia-Presby Hosp 1970; **Fellow:** Pediatric Orthopaedic Surgery, Newington Chldrn's Hosp 1971; **Fac Appt:** Clin Prof OrS, Columbia P&S

Hannafin, Jo Ann MD/PhD (OrS) - **Spec Exp:** Sports Medicine-Women; Shoulder Arthroscopic Surgery; Knee Injuries/Ligament Surgery; Ligament Reconstruction; **Hospital:** Hosp For Special Surgery (page 113), NY-Presby/Weill Cornell Med Ctr, NY (page 104); **Address:** 523 E 72nd St, Fl 6, New York, NY 10021-4872; **Phone:** 212-606-1469; **Board Cert:** Orthopaedic Surgery 2005; Orthopaedic Sports Medicine 2009; **Med School:** Albert Einstein Coll Med 1985; **Resid:** Orthopaedic Surgery, Montefiore Med Ctr 1990; **Fellow:** Sports Medicine, Hosp Special Surgery 1992; **Fac Appt:** Prof OrS, Cornell Univ-Weill Med Coll

Harwin, Steven F MD (OrS) - **Spec Exp:** Hip & Knee Replacement; Minimally Invasive Surgery; Transfusion Free Surgery; Osteonecrosis; **Hospital:** Beth Israel Med Ctr - Petrie Div (page 94); **Address:** Ctr for Reconstructive Joint Surgery, 910 Park Ave, New York, NY 10075; **Phone:** 212-861-9800; **Board Cert:** Orthopaedic Surgery 1976; **Med School:** SUNY Upstate Med Univ 1971; **Resid:** Orthopaedic Surgery, Einstein Affil Hosp 1975; **Fellow:** Joint Replacement Surgery, Traveling Fellowship 1978; **Fac Appt:** Assoc Prof OrS, Albert Einstein Coll Med

Hausman, Michael R MD (OrS) - **Spec Exp:** Hand Reconstruction; Elbow Reconstruction; Reconstructive Microvascular Surgery; Arthroscopic Surgery; **Hospital:** Mt Sinai Med Ctr (page 102); **Address:** 5 E 98th St, Fl 9, Box 1188, New York, NY 10029-6501; **Phone:** 212-241-1658; **Board Cert:** Orthopaedic Surgery 2010; Hand Surgery 2010; **Med School:** Yale Univ 1979; **Resid:** Surgery, Yale-New Haven Hosp 1981; Orthopaedic Surgery, Yale-New Haven Hosp 1985; **Fellow:** Hand Surgery, Roosevelt Hosp 1987; **Fac Appt:** Assoc Clin Prof OrS, Mount Sinai Sch Med

Healey, John H MD (OrS) - **Spec Exp:** Bone Tumors; Hip & Knee Replacement in Bone Tumors; Sarcoma; Sarcoma-Soft Tissue; **Hospital:** Meml Sloan-Kettering Canc Ctr (page 114), Hosp For Special Surgery (page 113); **Address:** 1275 York Ave, Ste A342, New York, NY 10065; **Phone:** 212-639-7610; **Board Cert:** Orthopaedic Surgery 2007; **Med School:** Univ VT Coll Med 1978; **Resid:** Orthopaedic Surgery, Hosp Special Surg 1983; **Fellow:** Musculoskeletal Oncology, Meml Sloan Kettering Cancer Ctr 1984; Orthopaedic Surgery, Hosp Special Surgery 1984; **Fac Appt:** Prof OrS, Cornell Univ-Weill Med Coll

Hecht, Andrew MD (OrS) - **Spec Exp:** Spinal Surgery; Minimally Invasive Spinal Surgery; Spinal Surgery-Neck; Spinal Cord Injury; **Hospital:** Mt Sinai Med Ctr (page 102); **Address:** Mount Sinai Med Ctr, Dept Orthopaedic Surg, 5 E 98th St, Fl 9, Box 1188, New York, NY 10029; **Phone:** 212-241-0735; **Board Cert:** Orthopaedic Surgery 2013; **Med School:** Harvard Med Sch 1994; **Resid:** Orthopaedic Surgery, Mass Genl Hosp 1999; **Fellow:** Spine Surgery, Emory Univ Spine Ctr 2001; **Fac Appt:** Assoc Prof OrS, Mount Sinai Sch Med

Helfet, David L MD (OrS) - **Spec Exp:** Fractures-Complex & Non Union; Deformity Reconstruction; Pelvic & Acetabular Fractures; Fractures-Stress; **Hospital:** Hosp For Special Surgery (page 113), NY-Presby/Weill Cornell Med Ctr, NY (page 104); **Address:** 525 E 71st St Belaire Bldg Fl 2, New York, NY 10021; **Phone:** 212-606-1888; **Board Cert:** Orthopaedic Surgery 1984; **Med School:** South Africa 1975; **Resid:** Surgery, Edendale Hosp 1977; Orthopaedic Surgery, Johns Hopkins Hosp 1981; **Fellow:** Orthopaedic Surgery, Insel Hosp 1981; Orthopaedic Sports Medicine, UCLA Med Ctr 1982; **Fac Appt:** Prof OrS, Cornell Univ-Weill Med Coll

Huang, Russel C MD (OrS) - **Spec Exp:** Minimally Invasive Spinal Surgery; Spinal Disc Replacement; Spinal Cord Injury; Scoliosis; **Hospital:** Hosp For Special Surgery (page 113); **Address:** Hosp for Special Surgery, East River Profl Bldg Fl 3, 523 E 72nd St, New York, NY 10021; **Phone:** 212-606-1634; **Board Cert:** Orthopaedic Surgery 2006; **Med School:** Yale Univ 1998; **Resid:** Orthopaedic Surgery, Hosp for Special Surgery 2003; **Fellow:** Spine Surgery, Case Western Reserve Univ 2004; **Fac Appt:** Asst Prof OrS, Cornell Univ-Weill Med Coll

Hubbard, Christopher E MD (OrS) - **Spec Exp:** Foot & Ankle Surgery; Sports Medicine; Arthroscopic Surgery; Ligament Reconstruction; **Hospital:** Beth Israel Med Ctr - Petrie Div (page 94); **Address:** BIMC, Orthopaedics & Sports Med, 10 Union Square E, Ste 3M, New York, NY 10003; **Phone:** 212-844-6940; **Board Cert:** Orthopaedic Surgery 2012; **Med School:** UMDNJ-NJ Med Sch, Newark 1994; **Resid:** Orthopaedic Surgery, NY-Presby/Columbia Univ Med Ctr 1999; **Fellow:** Foot & Ankle Surgery, Hosp Special Surgery 2000; **Fac Appt:** Asst Prof OrS, Albert Einstein Coll Med

Hyman, Joshua E MD (OrS) - **Spec Exp:** Pediatric Orthopaedic Surgery; Fractures-Pediatric; Scoliosis; Clubfoot/Foot Deformities in Children; **Hospital:** Morgan Stanley Children's Hosp of NY-Presby, NY (page 104), NY-Presby/Columbia Univ Med Ctr, NY (page 104); **Address:** Columbia Orthopedics, 3959 Broadway, Ste 8 North, New York, NY 10032-3784; **Phone:** 212-305-5475; **Board Cert:** Orthopaedic Surgery 2013; **Med School:** Columbia P&S 1990; **Resid:** Surgery, Beth Israel Hosp 1993; Orthopaedic Surgery, Mass Genl Hosp/Beth Israel Hosp 1998; **Fellow:** Pediatric Orthopaedic Surgery, Hosp for Sick Children 1999; **Fac Appt:** Assoc Prof OrS, Columbia P&S

Iorio, Richard MD (OrS) - **Spec Exp:** Joint Replacement; **Hospital:** NYU Langone Med Ctr (page 108); **Address:** NYU Langone Med Ctr, 333 E 38th St, New York, NY 10016; **Phone:** 646-501-7300; **Board Cert:** Orthopaedic Surgery 2015; **Med School:** Boston Univ 1986; **Resid:** Orthopaedic Surgery, Hahnemann Univ Hosp 1991; **Fellow:** Columbia-Presby Med Ctr 1992; **Fac Appt:** Prof OrS, NYU Sch Med

Jaffe, Fredrick F MD (OrS) - **Spec Exp:** Hip Replacement; Knee Replacement; Hip & Knee Reconstruction; Joint Replacement; **Hospital:** NYU Hosp For Joint Dis (page 108); **Address:** Ctr for Musculoskeletal Care, 333 E 38th St, New York, NY 10016; **Phone:** 212-598-7605; **Board Cert:** Orthopaedic Surgery 1974; **Med School:** Tufts Univ 1968; **Resid:** Surgery, New York Hosp 1970; Orthopaedic Surgery, Hosp for Joint Diseases 1973; **Fellow:** Reconstructive Surgery, Hosp for Joint Diseases 1974; **Fac Appt:** Clin Prof OrS, NYU Sch Med

Jazrawi, Laith M MD (OrS) - **Spec Exp:** Sports Medicine; Arthroscopic Surgery; Cartilage Damage & Transplant; Knee Surgery; **Hospital:** NYU Langone Med Ctr (page 108); **Address:** NYU Ctr for Musculoskeletal Care, 333 E 38th St, New York, NY 10016; **Phone:** 646-501-7223; **Board Cert:** Orthopaedic Surgery 2004; Orthopaedic Sports Medicine 2010; **Med School:** Mount Sinai Sch Med 1995; **Resid:** Orthopaedic Surgery, Hosp for Joint Diseases 2001; **Fellow:** Sports Medicine, Amer Sports Med Inst 2002

Kelly, Bryan T MD (OrS) - **Spec Exp:** Hip Surgery; Arthroscopic Surgery; Sports Medicine; **Hospital:** Hosp For Special Surgery (page 113); **Address:** Ctr for Hip Pain & Preservation, 541 E 71 St Caspary Bldg Fl Ground, New York, NY 10021; **Phone:** 212-606-1159; **Board Cert:** Orthopaedic Surgery 2006; **Med School:** Duke Univ 1996; **Resid:** Surgery, NY-Presby/ Weill Cornell Med Ctr 1997; Orthopaedic Surgery, Hosp Special Surg 2001; **Fellow:** Orthopaedic Sports Medicine, Hosp Special Surg 2003; Hip Sports Injuries/Arthroscopy, Univ Pittsburgh Med Ctr 2004; **Fac Appt:** Assoc Prof OrS, Cornell Univ-Weill Med Coll

Kiernan, Howard A MD (OrS) - **Spec Exp:** Hip Disorders & Dysplasia; Knee Injuries; **Hospital:** NY-Presby/Columbia Univ Med Ctr, NY (page 104); **Address:** 903 Park Ave Fl 1st, New York, NY 10075; **Phone:** 212-602-1800; **Board Cert:** Orthopaedic Surgery 1975; **Med School:** NYU Sch Med 1966; **Resid:** Surgery, Bellevue Hosp Ctr-NYU 1970; Orthopaedic Surgery, Columbia-Presby Med Ctr/NY Ortho Hosp 1973; **Fellow:** Hip Surgery, NY Ortho Hosp 1974; **Fac Appt:** Clin Prof OrS, Columbia P&S

Kuflik, Paul L MD (OrS) - **Spec Exp:** Spinal Surgery; Minimally Invasive Spinal Surgery; Spinal Deformity; Spinal Disc Replacement; **Hospital:** Mt Sinai Med Ctr (page 102); **Address:** Mt Sinai Med Ctr, Orthopaedics, 17 E 102 St Fl 5, New York, NY 10029; **Phone:** 212-241-8947; **Board Cert:** Orthopaedic Surgery 2010; **Med School:** SUNY Hlth Sci Ctr 1981; **Resid:** Orthopaedic Surgery, NYU Hosp For Joint Diseases 1986; **Fellow:** Spine Surgery, Toronto Genl Hosp 1986; **Fac Appt:** Assoc Prof OrS, Albert Einstein Coll Med

Lane, Joseph M MD (OrS) - **Spec Exp:** Bone Tumors-Benign; Bone Tumors-Metastatic; Bone Tumors; Bone Disorders-Metabolic; **Hospital:** Hosp For Special Surgery (page 113), NY-Presby/Weill Cornell Med Ctr, NY (page 104); **Address:** Hosp for Special Surgery-Ortho Surg Dept, 535 E 70th St, New York, NY 10021; **Phone:** 212-606-1172; **Board Cert:** Orthopaedic Surgery 1998; **Med School:** Harvard Med Sch 1965; **Resid:** Surgery, Hosp Univ Penn 1967; Orthopaedic Surgery, Hosp Univ Penn 1973; **Fellow:** Research, NIH 19691970; **Fac Appt:** Prof OrS, Cornell Univ-Weill Med Coll

Lee, Francis Y MD/PhD (OrS) - **Spec Exp:** Bone & Soft Tissue Tumors; Pediatric Orthopaedic Surgery; Bone Tumors-Metastatic; Bone Tumors-Benign; **Hospital:** Morgan Stanley Children's Hosp of NY-Presby, NY (page 104), NY-Presby/Columbia Univ Med Ctr, NY (page 104); **Address:** Columbia Univ Med Ctr, 3959 Broadway, Ste 800 N, New York, NY 10032; **Phone:** 212-305-3293; **Board Cert:** Orthopaedic Surgery 2012; **Med School:** South Korea 1986; **Resid:** Orthopaedic Surgery, NJ Med Ctr 1997; **Fellow:** Orthopaedic Oncology, Mass Genl Hosp/Chldns Hosp 1998; Pediatric Orthopaedic Surgery, Hosp for Sick Chldn/Univ Toronto 1999; **Fac Appt:** Prof OrS, Columbia P&S

Levine, David S MD (OrS) - **Spec Exp:** Foot & Ankle Surgery; Ankle Reconstruction; **Hospital:** Hosp For Special Surgery (page 113); **Address:** Hospital for Special Surgery, 523 E 72 St Fl 5, East River Professional Bldg, New York, NY 10021; **Phone:** 212-606-1940; **Board Cert:** Orthopaedic Surgery 2011; **Med School:** Cornell Univ-Weill Med Coll 1992; **Resid:** Surgery, UCSD Med Ctr 1993; Orthopaedic Surgery, Hosp for Special Surgery 1997; **Fellow:** Foot & Ankle Surgery, Harborview Med Ctr 1998; **Fac Appt:** Asst Prof OrS, Cornell Univ-Weill Med Coll

Lonner, Baron S MD (OrS) - **Spec Exp:** Scoliosis; Minimally Invasive Surgery; Spinal Deformity; Spinal Surgery; **Hospital:** NYU Hosp For Joint Dis (page 108), NYU Langone Med Ctr (page 108); **Address:** 820 2nd Ave, Ste 7A, New York, NY 10017; **Phone:** 212-986-0140; **Board Cert:** Orthopaedic Surgery 2008; **Med School:** Boston Univ 1989; **Resid:** Orthopaedic Surgery, Montefiore Med Ctr 1994; **Fellow:** Orthopaedic Surgery, Hosp Special Surgery 1995; **Fac Appt:** Clin Prof OrS, NYU Sch Med

Lorich, Dean G MD (OrS) - **Spec Exp:** Trauma; Fractures-Complex & Non Union; **Hospital:** Hosp For Special Surgery (page 113), NY-Presby/Weill Cornell Med Ctr, NY (page 104); **Address:** Hospital for Special Surgery, 535 E 70th St, New York, NY 10021; **Phone:** 212-746-4509; **Board Cert:** Orthopaedic Surgery 2010; **Med School:** Univ Pennsylvania 1990; **Resid:** Orthopaedic Surgery, Hosp Univ Penn 1995; **Fellow:** Orthopaedic Surgery, Hosp Special Surg 1996; **Fac Appt:** Assoc Prof OrS, Cornell Univ-Weill Med Coll

Lubliner, Jerry A MD (OrS) - **Spec Exp:** Arthroscopic Surgery; Shoulder Surgery; Knee Surgery; Rotator Cuff Surgery; **Hospital:** Beth Israel Med Ctr - Petrie Div (page 94), NYU Hosp For Joint Dis (page 108); **Address:** New York Orthopaedics and Sports Med, 215 E 73rd St, Ste 1C, New York, NY 10021-3653; **Phone:** 212-249-8200; **Board Cert:** Orthopaedic Surgery 2009; Orthopaedic Sports Medicine 2008; **Med School:** SUNY Hlth Sci Ctr 1980; **Resid:** Orthopaedic Surgery, Hosp Joint Diseases 1985; **Fellow:** Sports Medicine, Univ West Ontario Affil Hosps 1986; **Fac Appt:** Assoc Clin Prof S, NYU Sch Med

Lyden, John P MD (OrS) - **Spec Exp:** Joint Replacement; Trauma; Arthroscopic Surgery; Fractures; **Hospital:** Hosp For Special Surgery (page 113), NY-Presby/Weill Cornell Med Ctr, NY (page 104); **Address:** 535 E 70th St, rm 355, New York, NY 10021-4872; **Phone:** 212-606-1126; **Board Cert:** Orthopaedic Surgery 1973; **Med School:** Columbia P&S 1965; **Resid:** Surgery, Roosevelt Hosp 1967; Orthopaedic Surgery, Hosp Special Surg 1972; **Fellow:** Hand Surgery, Hosp Special Surg 1973; **Fac Appt:** Assoc Prof OrS, NY Med Coll

Macaulay, William B MD (OrS) - **Spec Exp:** Hip Replacement; Knee Replacement; Minimally Invasive Surgery; Reconstructive Surgery; **Hospital:** NY-Presby/Columbia Univ Med Ctr, NY (page 104); **Address:** Columbia-Orthopaedics Dept, 161 Fort Washington Ave, Irving Pavilion Fl 2, New York, NY 10032; **Phone:** 212-305-6959; **Board Cert:** Orthopaedic Surgery 2012; **Med School:** Columbia P&S 1992; **Resid:** Surgery, Univ Pittsburgh Med Ctr 1993; Orthopaedic Surgery, Univ Pittsburgh Med Ctr 1997; **Fellow:** Adult Reconstructive Surgery, Hosp for Special Surgery 1999; **Fac Appt:** Prof OrS, Columbia P&S

Marx, Robert G MD (OrS) - **Spec Exp:** Shoulder Surgery; Knee Injuries/Ligament Surgery; Knee Replacement; Sports Medicine; **Hospital:** Hosp For Special Surgery (page 113); **Address:** 519 E 72nd St, Ste 206, New York, NY 10021; **Phone:** 212-606-1645; **Board Cert:** Orthopaedic Surgery 2003; **Med School:** McGill Univ 1991; **Resid:** Orthopaedic Surgery, Univ Toronto Affil Hosp 1996; **Fellow:** Sports Medicine, Hosp Special Surgery 1998; **Fac Appt:** Prof OrS, Cornell Univ-Weill Med Coll

McCance, Sean E MD (OrS) - **Spec Exp:** Spinal Surgery; Scoliosis; **Hospital:** Mt Sinai Med Ctr (page 102), Lenox Hill Hosp (page 106); **Address:** Spine Assocs, 1155 Park Ave Fl Ground - Ste E, New York, NY 10128; **Phone:** 212-360-6500; **Board Cert:** Orthopaedic Surgery 2010; **Med School:** Columbia P&S 1991; **Resid:** Surgery, Strong Meml Hosp 1992; Orthopaedic Surgery, Strong Meml Hosp 1996; **Fellow:** Spine Surgery, Twin Cities Spine Ctr 1997; **Fac Appt:** Asst Clin Prof OrS, Mount Sinai Sch Med

McCann, Peter D MD (OrS) - **Spec Exp:** Shoulder Surgery; Elbow Surgery; **Hospital:** Beth Israel Med Ctr - Petrie Div (page 94); **Address:** Beth Israel Orthopedics & Sports Med, 10 Union Square E, Ste 3M, New York, NY 10003; **Phone:** 212-844-6735; **Board Cert:** Orthopaedic Surgery 2009; **Med School:** Columbia P&S 1980; **Resid:** Surgery, St Vincent's Hosp 1982; Orthopaedic Surgery, Columbia-Presby Med Ctr 1985; **Fellow:** Shoulder Surgery, Columbia-Presby Med Ctr 1986; **Fac Appt:** Clin Prof OrS, Albert Einstein Coll Med

McClelland, Shearwood J MD (OrS) - **Spec Exp:** Musculoskeletal Injuries; Joint Replacement; **Hospital:** Harlem Hosp Ctr; **Address:** Harlem Hosp Ctr, Dept Ortho Surgery, 506 Lenox Ave, MLK Bldg - Fl 9, rm 9122, New York, NY 10037-1889; **Phone:** 212-939-3510; **Board Cert:** Orthopaedic Surgery 2007; **Med School:** Columbia P&S 1974; **Resid:** Surgery, St. Lukes Hosp 1976; Orthopaedic Surgery, NY Ortho Hosp-Columbia 1979; **Fellow:** Joint Arthroplasty, Ohio State Univ Med Ctr 1982; **Fac Appt:** Assoc Prof OrS, Columbia P&S

Meere, Patrick MD (OrS) - **Spec Exp:** Hip Replacement & Revision; Knee Replacement & Revision; Knee Injuries/ACL/Meniscus Tears; Joint Infections; **Hospital:** NYU Hosp For Joint Dis (page 108), NYU Langone Med Ctr (page 108); **Address:** 530 1st Ave FPO Bldg - Ste 5J, New York, NY 10016; **Phone:** 212-263-2366; **Board Cert:** Orthopaedic Surgery 2008; **Med School:** McGill Univ 1988; **Resid:** Orthopaedic Surgery, McGill Univ Affil Hosp 1993; **Fellow:** Reconstructive Surgery, Hosp for Joint Diseases 1995; **Fac Appt:** Assoc Prof OrS, NYU Sch Med

Mendoza, Francis X MD (OrS) - **Spec Exp:** Shoulder & Elbow Surgery; Sports Medicine; **Hospital:** Lenox Hill Hosp (page 106); **Address:** FXM Shoulders, 333 E 56th St, New York, NY 10022; **Phone:** 212-628-9600; **Board Cert:** Orthopaedic Surgery 1984; **Med School:** Columbia P&S 1976; **Resid:** Surgery, Roosevelt Hosp 1978; Orthopaedic Surgery, Columbia-Presby Hosp 1981; **Fellow:** Shoulder Surgery, Columbia-Presby Hosp 1982

Morris, Carol D MD (OrS) - **Spec Exp:** Bone Cancer; Bone & Soft Tissue Tumors; Musculoskeletal Tumors; Pediatric Orthopaedic Cancers; **Hospital:** Meml Sloan-Kettering Canc Ctr (page 114); **Address:** Meml Sloan Kettering Cancer Ctr, 1275 York Ave, rm A342, New York, NY 10065; **Phone:** 212-639-2893; **Board Cert:** Orthopaedic Surgery 2013; **Med School:** Boston Univ 1994; **Resid:** Orthopaedic Surgery, Boston Univ Med Ctr 1999; **Fellow:** Orthopaedic Oncology, Meml Sloan Kettering Cancer Ctr 2001

Moskovich, Ronald MD (OrS) - **Spec Exp:** Scoliosis; Spinal Surgery; Spondylitis; Microsurgery; **Hospital:** NYU Hosp For Joint Dis (page 108), NYU Langone Med Ctr (page 108); **Address:** 240 E 18th St, New York, NY 10003; **Phone:** 212-598-6622; **Board Cert:** Orthopaedic Surgery 2012; **Med School:** South Africa 1978; **Resid:** Surgery, St George's Hosp 1984; Orthopaedic Surgery, NYU Hosp Joint Diseases 1988; **Fellow:** Spine Surgery, UC Davis Med Ctr 1989; Neurological Surgery, Natl Hosp 1989; **Fac Appt:** Asst Prof OrS, NYU Sch Med

Moucha, Calin Stefan MD (OrS) - **Spec Exp:** Hip Replacement & Revision; Knee Reconstruction & Revision; Knee Replacement & Revision; Infections in Prosthetic Devices; **Hospital:** Mt Sinai Med Ctr (page 102); **Address:** Mount Sinai Medical Center, 5 E 98th St, Fl 7, New York, NY 10029; **Phone:** 212-241-1461; **Board Cert:** Orthopaedic Surgery 2005; **Med School:** Mount Sinai Sch Med 1997; **Resid:** Orthopaedic Surgery, St Lukes-Roosevelt Hosp 2002; **Fellow:** Hip/Knee Reconstruction, Rush Univ Med Ctr 2003; **Fac Appt:** Asst Prof OrS, Mount Sinai Sch Med

Neuwirth, Michael G MD (OrS) - **Spec Exp:** Scoliosis; Spinal Deformity; Spinal Surgery; **Hospital:** Mt Sinai Med Ctr (page 102); **Address:** 17 E 102nd St Fl 5, New York, NY 10029; **Phone:** 212-241-1071; **Board Cert:** Orthopaedic Surgery 1980; **Med School:** SUNY Hlth Sci Ctr 1974; **Resid:** Orthopaedic Surgery, Hosp for Joint Diseases 1979; **Fellow:** Spine Surgery, Rush-Presby Med Ctr 1980; **Fac Appt:** Prof OrS, Mount Sinai Sch Med

Nicholas, Stephen J MD (OrS) - **Spec Exp:** Sports Medicine; Shoulder & Knee Surgery; Arthroscopic Surgery; **Hospital:** Lenox Hill Hosp (page 106); **Address:** NY Orthopedics, 130 E 77th St Fl 5, New York, NY 10075; **Phone:** 212-737-3301; **Board Cert:** Orthopaedic Surgery 2005; **Med School:** NY Med Coll 1986; **Resid:** Orthopaedic Surgery, Hosp for Special Surgery 1991; **Fellow:** Sports Medicine, Lenox Hill Hosp 1992

O'Leary, Patrick F MD (OrS) - **Spec Exp:** Spinal Surgery; **Hospital:** Hosp For Special Surgery (page 113); **Address:** 1015 Madison Ave, Fl 4, New York, NY 10075; **Phone:** 212-249-8100; **Board Cert:** Orthopaedic Surgery 1983; **Med School:** Ireland 1968; **Resid:** Surgery, Roosevelt Hosp 1972; Orthopaedic Surgery, Hosp Spec Surg 1975; **Fellow:** Spine Surgery, Univ Toronto Genl Ortho Hosp 1976; **Fac Appt:** Assoc Clin Prof OrS, Cornell Univ-Weill Med Coll

O'Malley, Martin J MD (OrS) - **Spec Exp:** Foot & Ankle Surgery; Sports Medicine; Ankle Replacement & Revision; Arthroscopic Surgery; **Hospital:** Hosp For Special Surgery (page 113), NY-Presby/Weill Cornell Med Ctr, NY (page 104); **Address:** Foot & Ankle Orthopedic Surgery, 420 E 72nd St, Ste 1B, New York, NY 10021; **Phone:** 212-203-0740; **Board Cert:** Orthopaedic Surgery 2006; **Med School:** Case West Res Univ 1986; **Resid:** Orthopaedic Surgery, Tufts-New Eng Med Ctr 1992; **Fellow:** Foot & Ankle Surgery, Hosp for Special Surg 1993; **Fac Appt:** Asst Prof OrS, Cornell Univ-Weill Med Coll

Otsuka, Norman Y MD (OrS) - **Spec Exp:** Pediatric Orthopaedic Surgery; Trauma; Neuromuscular Disorders; Cerebral Palsy; **Hospital:** NYU Hosp For Joint Dis (page 108); **Address:** NYU Hosp for Joint Diseases, Center for Children, 301 E 17th St, Ste 301/303, New York, NY 10003; **Phone:** 212-598-6286; **Board Cert:** Orthopaedic Surgery 2009; **Med School:** McMaster Univ 1988; **Resid:** Orthopaedic Surgery, Univ Toronto Affil Hosps 1994; **Fellow:** Pediatric Orthopaedic Surgery, Childrens Hosp 1995; **Fac Appt:** Prof OrS, NYU Sch Med

Padgett, Douglas E MD (OrS) - **Spec Exp:** Hip & Knee Replacement; Arthroscopic Surgery-Hip; Arthroscopic Surgery-Knee; Dance Medicine; **Hospital:** Hosp For Special Surgery (page 113); **Address:** Hosp for Special Surgery, 535 E 70 St Fl 3, New York, NY 10021; **Phone:** 212-606-1642; **Board Cert:** Orthopaedic Surgery 2013; **Med School:** NY Med Coll 1982; **Resid:** Surgery, St Luke's-Roosevelt Hosp Ctr 1983; Orthopaedic Surgery, Hosp Spec Surg 1989; **Fellow:** Hip & Knee Surgery, Rush Presby Med Ctr 1990; **Fac Appt:** Assoc Prof OrS, Cornell Univ-Weill Med Coll

Parks, Michael MD (OrS) - **Spec Exp:** Hip & Knee Replacement; Joint Replacement; Reconstructive Surgery; Arthritis; **Hospital:** Hosp For Special Surgery (page 113); **Address:** 535 E 70th St Fl 6, New York, NY 10021; **Phone:** 646-797-8995; **Board Cert:** Orthopaedic Surgery 2010; **Med School:** Med Univ SC 1990; **Resid:** Orthopaedic Surgery, Duke Univ Med Ctr 1997; **Fellow:** Hip & Knee Surgery, Hosp for Spec Surgery 1998; **Fac Appt:** Asst Prof OrS, Cornell Univ-Weill Med Coll

Pearle, Andrew D MD (OrS) - **Spec Exp:** Knee Replacement; Robotic Surgery; Knee Injuries/ACL; Sports Medicine; **Hospital:** Hosp For Special Surgery (page 113); **Address:** Hosp for Special Surgery, 523 E 72nd St Fl 7, New York, NY 10021; **Phone:** 212-774-2878; **Board Cert:** Orthopaedic Surgery 2009; **Med School:** Stanford Univ 1998; **Resid:** Orthopaedic Surgery, Hosp For Special Surgery 2004; **Fellow:** Sports Medicine, Hosp For Special Surgery 2005; **Fac Appt:** Assoc Prof OrS, Columbia P&S

Pellicci, Paul M MD (OrS) - **Spec Exp:** Hip Replacement-Young Adults; Knee Replacement; Joint Replacement; Hip Replacement; **Hospital:** Hosp For Special Surgery (page 113), NY-Presby/Weill Cornell Med Ctr, NY (page 104); **Address:** Hosp for Spec Surgery, 535 E 70th St, New York, NY 10021-4872; **Phone:** 212-606-1010; **Board Cert:** Orthopaedic Surgery 1982; **Med School:** Cornell Univ-Weill Med Coll 1975; **Resid:** Surgery, NY Hosp 1977; Orthopaedic Surgery, Hosp Spec Surg 1981; **Fellow:** Adult Reconstructive Surgery, Brigham & Womens Hosp 1982; **Fac Appt:** Clin Prof OrS, Cornell Univ-Weill Med Coll

Plancher, Kevin D MD (OrS) - **Spec Exp:** Shoulder Surgery; Elbow Surgery; Cartilage Damage & Transplant; Shoulder Replacement; **Hospital:** Beth Israel Med Ctr - Petrie Div (page 94), Lenox Hill Hosp (page 106); **Address:** Plancher Orthopaedics & Sports Medicine, 1160 Park Ave, New York, NY 10128; **Phone:** 212-876-5200; **Board Cert:** Orthopaedic Surgery 2007; Hand Surgery 2008; Orthopaedic Sports Medicine 2009; **Med School:** Georgetown Univ 1986; **Resid:** Orthopaedic Surgery, Mass Genl Hosp/Brigham & Womens Hosp 1991; **Fellow:** Hand Surgery, Indiana Hand Ctr 1993; Sports Medicine, Steadman-Hawkins Clinic 1994; **Fac Appt:** Assoc Clin Prof OrS, Albert Einstein Coll Med

Price, Andrew E MD (OrS) - **Spec Exp:** Erbs Palsy/Brachial Plexus Injuries; Neuromuscular Disorders; Fractures-Pediatric; Trauma-Pediatric; **Hospital:** NYU Langone Med Ctr (page 108), St. Luke's - Roosevelt Hosp Ctr - Roosevelt Div (page 94); **Address:** 129A W 20th St, New York, NY 10011; **Phone:** 212-974-7242; **Board Cert:** Orthopaedic Surgery 2011; **Med School:** NYU Sch Med 1980; **Resid:** Surgery, St Luke's Roosevelt Hosp 1981; Orthopaedic Surgery, NYU Med Ctr 1985; **Fellow:** Pediatric Orthopaedic Surgery, Newington Chldns Hosp 1986; **Fac Appt:** Assoc Clin Prof OrS, NYU Sch Med

Qureshi, Sheeraz A MD (OrS) - **Spec Exp:** Spinal Surgery; Spinal Disc Replacement; Spinal Tumors; Minimally Invasive Spinal Surgery; **Hospital:** Mt Sinai Med Ctr (page 102), Elmhurst Hosp Ctr; **Address:** 5 E 98th St Fl 9, Box 1188, New York, NY 10029; **Phone:** 212-241-3909; **Board Cert:** Orthopaedic Surgery 2010; **Med School:** Tufts Univ 2002; **Resid:** Orthopaedic Surgery, Mt Siani Med Ctr 2007; **Fellow:** Spine Surgery, Case Western Reserve Univ Med Ctr 2009; **Fac Appt:** Assoc Prof OrS, Mount Sinai Sch Med

Ranawat, Amar S MD (OrS) - **Spec Exp:** Knee Replacement & Revision; Hip Replacement & Revision; **Hospital:** Hosp For Special Surgery (page 113); **Address:** Hospital for Special Surgery, Ranawat Orthopaedics, 535 E 70th St Fl 6, New York, NY 10021; **Phone:** 646-797-8700; **Board Cert:** Orthopaedic Surgery 2004; **Med School:** Cornell Univ-Weill Med Coll 1996; **Resid:** Orthopaedic Surgery, Hosp Special Surgey 2001; **Fellow:** Orthopaedic Surgery, Lenox Hill Hosp 2002

Rawlins, Bernard A MD (OrS) - **Spec Exp:** Scoliosis; Spinal Surgery; Minimally Invasive Spinal Surgery; **Hospital:** Hosp For Special Surgery (page 113); **Address:** 523 E 72nd St Fl 2nd, East River Professional Bldg, New York, NY 10021; **Phone:** 212-606-1632; **Board Cert:** Orthopaedic Surgery 2006; **Med School:** Cornell Univ 1987; **Resid:** Orthopaedic Surgery, Columbia-Presby Hosp 1992; **Fellow:** Spine Surgery, Minnesota Spine Ctr 1993; **Fac Appt:** Clin Prof OrS, Cornell Univ-Weill Med Coll

Roberts, Matthew M MD (OrS) - **Spec Exp:** Foot & Ankle Surgery; Arthritis; Foot Deformities; Sports Medicine; **Hospital:** Hosp For Special Surgery (page 113); **Address:** HSS, Orthopaedic Surgery, 535 E 70 St, New York, NY 10021; **Phone:** 212-606-1181; **Board Cert:** Orthopaedic Surgery 2005; **Med School:** Univ Tex, Houston 1997; **Resid:** Orthopaedic Surgery, Hosp Special Surg 2003; **Fellow:** Foot & Ankle Surgery, Hosp Special Surg 2004; **Fac Appt:** Assoc Prof OrS, Cornell Univ-Weill Med Coll

Rodriguez, Jose A MD (OrS) - **Spec Exp:** Hip & Knee Replacement; Arthroscopic Surgery-Hip; Arthroscopic Surgery-Knee; Fractures-Complex; **Hospital:** Lenox Hill Hosp (page 106); **Address:** NY Orthopedics, 130 E 77th St Fl 11, New York, NY 10021; **Phone:** 212-434-4799; **Board Cert:** Orthopaedic Surgery 2009; **Med School:** Columbia P&S 1989; **Resid:** Surgery, NY Presby-Colombia Med Ctr 1990; Orthopaedic Surgery, Hosp fpr Special Surgery 1994; **Fellow:** Arthritis Surgery, Lenox Hill Hosp 1995

Rose, Donald Joseph MD (OrS) - **Spec Exp:** Dance/Ballet Injuries; Arthroscopic Surgery; Sports Injuries; Hip Surgery; **Hospital:** NYU Hosp For Joint Dis (page 108), NYU Langone Med Ctr (page 108); **Address:** 1095 Park Ave, New York, NY 10128-1154; **Phone:** 212-427-7750; **Board Cert:** Orthopaedic Surgery 2009; **Med School:** UMDNJ-RW Johnson Med Sch 1980; **Resid:** Surgery, Beth Israel Med Ctr 1981; Orthopaedic Surgery, Hosp for Joint Diseases 1985; **Fellow:** Sports Medicine, Temple Univ Hosp 1986; **Fac Appt:** Assoc Clin Prof OrS, NYU Sch Med

Rose, Howard A MD (OrS) - **Spec Exp:** Sports Medicine; Joint Replacement; Arthroscopic Surgery; **Hospital:** Hosp For Special Surgery (page 113), NY-Presby/Weill Cornell Med Ctr, NY (page 104); **Address:** 535 E 70th St, New York, NY 10021; **Phone:** 212-606-1278; **Board Cert:** Orthopaedic Surgery 1985; **Med School:** Geo Wash Univ 1977; **Resid:** Orthopaedic Surgery, Hosp Special Surg 1982; **Fellow:** Sports Medicine, Brigham & Womens Hosp 1983; Joint Replacement Surgery, Brigham & Womens Hosp 1983; **Fac Appt:** Asst Prof OrS, Cornell Univ-Weill Med Coll

Roye Jr, David P MD (OrS) - **Spec Exp:** Pediatric Orthopaedic Surgery; Scoliosis; Hip Disorders-Pediatric; Neuromuscular Disorders; **Hospital:** Morgan Stanley Children's Hosp of NY-Presby, NY (page 104), NY-Presby/Columbia Univ Med Ctr, NY (page 104); **Address:** Columbia Orthopaedics, 3959 Broadway, rm 800-North, New York, NY 10032-1559; **Phone:** 212-305-5475; **Board Cert:** Orthopaedic Surgery 1981; **Med School:** Columbia P&S 1975; **Resid:** Orthopaedic Surgery, Columbia-Presby Med Ctr 1980; **Fellow:** Pediatric Orthopaedic Surgery, Hosp for Sick Chldn 1981; **Fac Appt:** Prof OrS, Columbia P&S

Rozbruch, Jacob D MD (OrS) - **Spec Exp:** Spinal Surgery; Shoulder Surgery; Knee Surgery; **Hospital:** Beth Israel Med Ctr - Petrie Div (page 94); **Address:** 420 E 72nd St, Ste 1J, New York, NY 10021; **Phone:** 212-744-9857; **Board Cert:** Orthopaedic Surgery 1980; Pediatrics 1979; **Med School:** SUNY Buffalo 1973; **Resid:** Surgery, NY Hosp 1976; Orthopaedic Surgery, Hosp Special Surg 1979; **Fac Appt:** Asst Clin Prof OrS, Albert Einstein Coll Med

Rozbruch, S Robert MD (OrS) - **Spec Exp:** Limb Lengthening; Limb Deformities; Limb Surgery/Reconstruction; Fractures-Complex & Non Union; **Hospital:** Hosp For Special Surgery (page 113), NY-Presby/Weill Cornell Med Ctr, NY (page 104); **Address:** Hospital for Special Surgery, 535 E 70th St, River Terr Bldg Fl 2 - Ste 204, New York, NY 10021; **Phone:** 212-606-1415; **Board Cert:** Orthopaedic Surgery 2009; **Med School:** Cornell Univ-Weill Med Coll 1990; **Resid:** Orthopaedic Surgery, Hosp Special Surgery 1995; **Fellow:** Trauma, Univ Bern Hosp 1997; Limb Lengthening, Intl Ctr Limb Length/Univ MD 1999; **Fac Appt:** Prof OrS, Cornell Univ-Weill Med Coll

Salvati, Eduardo A MD (OrS) - **Spec Exp:** Hip Replacement; Knee Replacement; **Hospital:** Hosp For Special Surgery (page 113); **Address:** 535 E 71st St Belaire Bldg, New York, NY 10021; **Phone:** 212-606-1472; **Board Cert:** Orthopaedic Surgery 1972; **Med School:** Argentina 1963; **Resid:** Orthopaedic Surgery, Univ Florence Ortho Clinic 1965; Orthopaedic Surgery, Hosp Buenos Aires 1969; **Fellow:** Hip & Knee Surgery, Hosp For Spec Surg 1972; **Fac Appt:** Clin Prof OrS, Cornell Univ-Weill Med Coll

Sama, Andrew A MD (OrS) - **Spec Exp:** Spinal Surgery; Spinal Trauma; Spinal Disorders-Degenerative; Spinal Deformity; **Hospital:** Hosp For Special Surgery (page 113), NY-Presby/Weill Cornell Med Ctr, NY (page 104); **Address:** Hosp for Special Surgery, East River Profl Bldg, 523 E 72nd St, New York, NY 10021; **Phone:** 212-606-1946; **Board Cert:** Orthopaedic Surgery 2014; **Med School:** Univ Miami Sch Med 1995; **Resid:** Surgery, Jackson Meml Hosp 2000; **Fellow:** Spine Surgery, Hosp for Special Surg 2001; **Fac Appt:** Assoc Prof OrS, Cornell Univ-Weill Med Coll

Sandhu, Harvinder S MD (OrS) - **Spec Exp:** Minimally Invasive Spinal Surgery; Spinal Surgery; **Hospital:** Hosp For Special Surgery (page 113); **Address:** Hosp for Special Surgery, 523 E 72nd St, East River Professional Bldg, New York, NY 10021; **Phone:** 212-606-1798; **Board Cert:** Orthopaedic Surgery 2007; **Med School:** Northwestern Univ 1987; **Resid:** Orthopaedic Surgery, Univ Hosp-SUNY Hlth Sci Ctr 1992; **Fellow:** Spine Surgery, UCLA Med Ctr 1993; **Fac Appt:** Assoc Prof OrS, Cornell Univ-Weill Med Coll

Sands, Andrew K MD (OrS) - **Spec Exp:** Foot & Ankle Surgery; Ankle Replacement & Revision; Arthroscopic Surgery; Sports Medicine; **Hospital:** Beth Israel Med Ctr - Petrie Div (page 94), Kingsbrook Jewish Med Ctr; **Address:** NY Downtown Ortho Assocs, 170 William St Fl 8, New York, NY 10038; **Phone:** 212-312-5966; **Board Cert:** Orthopaedic Surgery 2013; **Med School:** NY Med Coll 1985; **Resid:** Orthopaedic Surgery, Lenox Hill Hosp 1990; **Fellow:** Foot & Ankle Surgery, Harborview Med Ctr 1994

Scher, David M MD (OrS) - **Spec Exp:** Pediatric Orthopaedic Surgery; Musculoskeletal Disorders; Trauma; Gait Disorders; **Hospital:** Hosp For Special Surgery (page 113); **Address:** Hosp for Special Surgery, 535 E 70th St Fl 5, New York, NY 10021; **Phone:** 212-606-1253; **Board Cert:** Orthopaedic Surgery 2013; **Med School:** Duke Univ 1993; **Resid:** Orthopaedic Surgery, Hosp Joint Diseases 1999; **Fellow:** Pediatric Orthopaedic Surgery, Childrens Hosp 2000; **Fac Appt:** Assoc Prof OrS, Cornell Univ-Weill Med Coll

Schwab, Frank J MD (OrS) - **Spec Exp:** Spinal Surgery; Pain-Back; Spinal Deformity; Scoliosis; **Hospital:** NYU Hosp For Joint Dis (page 108), New York Methodist Hosp (page 440); **Address:** 333 E 38th St, Fl 6th, New York, NY 10003; **Phone:** 212-598-2781; **Board Cert:** Orthopaedic Surgery 2010; **Med School:** Columbia P&S 1990; **Resid:** Surgery, NY Presby-Columbia Med Ctr 1992; Orthopaedic Surgery, NY Presby-Columbia Med Ctr 1996; **Fellow:** Orthopaedic Surgery, Hospital Lariboisiere 1991; Spine Surgery, Maimonides Med Ctr 1997; **Fac Appt:** Clin Prof OrS, NYU Sch Med

Schwartz, Jeffrey M MD (OrS) - **Spec Exp:** Arthroscopic Surgery; Fractures; **Hospital:** Lenox Hill Hosp (page 106), NS-LIJ Hlth Sys (page 106); **Address:** 73 E 71st St, New York, NY 10021; **Phone:** 212-535-6600; **Board Cert:** Orthopaedic Surgery 1978; **Med School:** NY Med Coll 1972; **Resid:** Surgery, Mount Sinai Med Ctr 1973; Orthopaedic Surgery, Lenox Hill Hosp 1978; **Fac Appt:** Asst Clin Prof OrS, Mount Sinai Sch Med

Scott, W Norman MD (OrS) - **Spec Exp:** Knee Injuries; Knee Replacement; Sports Medicine; Knee Surgery; **Hospital:** Lenox Hill Hosp (page 106); **Address:** ISK-Inst for Ortho & Sports Med, 210 E 64th St Fl 4, New York, NY 10065; **Phone:** 646-293-7501; **Board Cert:** Orthopaedic Surgery 1978; **Med School:** Cornell Univ-Weill Med Coll 1972; **Resid:** Surgery, St Lukes-Roosevelt Hosp Ctr 1974; Orthopaedic Surgery, Hosp Special Surg 1978; **Fac Appt:** Clin Prof OrS, Cornell Univ-Weill Med Coll

Scuderi, Giles R MD (OrS) - **Spec Exp:** Knee Replacement; Knee Reconstruction; Knee Injuries/Ligament Surgery; Sports Medicine; **Hospital:** Lenox Hill Hosp (page 106), Franklin Hosp (page 106); **Address:** 210 E 64th St, Fl 4, New York, NY 10065; **Phone:** 212-434-4310; **Board Cert:** Orthopaedic Surgery 2011; **Med School:** SUNY Downstate 1982; **Resid:** Orthopaedic Surgery, Lenox Hill Hosp 1987; **Fellow:** Knee Surgery, Hosp Special Surgery 1988; **Fac Appt:** Asst Clin Prof OrS, Albert Einstein Coll Med

Sculco, Thomas P MD (OrS) - **Spec Exp:** Hip Replacement; Knee Replacement; Minimally Invasive Surgery; Joint Replacement; **Hospital:** Hosp For Special Surgery (page 113); **Address:** 535 E 70th St, New York, NY 10021-4872; **Phone:** 212-606-1475; **Board Cert:** Orthopaedic Surgery 1976; **Med School:** Columbia P&S 1969; **Resid:** Surgery, Roosevelt Hosp 1971; Orthopaedic Surgery, Hosp For Special Surgery 1974; **Fellow:** Orthopaedic Surgery, The London Hosp 1975; **Fac Appt:** Prof OrS, Cornell Univ-Weill Med Coll

Simon, Sheldon R MD (OrS) - **Spec Exp:** Foot & Ankle Surgery; Pediatric Orthopaedic Surgery; **Hospital:** Beth Israel Med Ctr - Petrie Div (page 94); **Address:** Beth Israel Orthopedics and Sports Med, 10 Union Square E, Ste 3K, New York, NY 10003; **Phone:** 212-844-6756; **Board Cert:** Orthopaedic Surgery 1976; **Med School:** NYU Sch Med 1966; **Resid:** Surgery, NYU Med Ctr 1968; Orthopaedic Surgery, Mass Genl Hosp 1973; **Fac Appt:** Clin Prof OrS, Albert Einstein Coll Med

Sink, Ernest L MD (OrS) - **Spec Exp:** Hip Surgery; Pediatric Orthopaedic Surgery; Trauma; **Hospital:** Hosp For Special Surgery (page 113), NY-Presby/Weill Cornell Med Ctr, NY (page 104); **Address:** 541 E 71 St, Ground Fl, New York, NY 10021; **Phone:** 212-606-1268; **Board Cert:** Orthopaedic Surgery 2013; **Med School:** Univ Tex SW, Dallas 1994; **Resid:** Orthopaedic Surgery, Univ Tex SW Med Ctr 1999; **Fellow:** Pediatric Orthopaedic Surgery, Rady Chldn's Hosp 2000

Spivak, Jeffrey M MD (OrS) - **Spec Exp:** Spinal Surgery; Scoliosis; Sports Medicine Back Injuries; **Hospital:** NYU Hosp For Joint Dis (page 108), NYU Langone Med Ctr (page 108); **Address:** Hosp for Joint Diseases, Spine Ctr, 301 E 17th St, Ste 400, New York, NY 10003-3804; **Phone:** 212-598-6696; **Board Cert:** Orthopaedic Surgery 2006; **Med School:** Cornell Univ-Weill Med Coll 1986; **Resid:** Orthopaedic Surgery, Hosp for Joint Diseases 1992; **Fellow:** Spine Surgery, Thos Jefferson Univ Hosp 1993; **Fac Appt:** Asst Prof OrS, NYU Sch Med

Stuchin, Steven A MD (OrS) - **Spec Exp:** Hand Surgery; Arthritis; Hip & Knee Replacement; Hip Resurfacing; **Hospital:** NYU Hosp For Joint Dis (page 108); **Address:** 333 E 38th St, New York, NY 10016; **Phone:** 212-598-6708; **Board Cert:** Orthopaedic Surgery 1984; **Med School:** Columbia P&S 1976; **Resid:** Surgery, St Luke's-Roosevelt Hosp 1978; Orthopaedic Surgery, Hosp for Special Surg 1982; **Fellow:** Hand Surgery, Thos Jefferson Univ Hosp 1983; **Fac Appt:** Assoc Prof OrS, NYU Sch Med

Su, Edwin P MD (OrS) - **Spec Exp:** Hip Resurfacing; Hip Replacement; Reconstructive Surgery; **Hospital:** Hosp For Special Surgery (page 113); **Address:** Hosp for Special Surgery, 541 E 71st St, Fl Ground, New York, NY 10021; **Phone:** 212-606-1128; **Board Cert:** Orthopaedic Surgery 2006; **Med School:** Cornell Univ-Weill Med Coll 1997; **Resid:** Orthopaedic Surgery, Hosp for Special Surgery 2002; **Fellow:** Reconstructive Surgery, Hosp for Special Surgery 2003; **Fac Appt:** Asst Prof OrS, Cornell Univ-Weill Med Coll

Tindel, Nathaniel L MD (OrS) - **Spec Exp:** Spinal Surgery; Scoliosis; Minimally Invasive Surgery; Spinal Reconstructive Surgery; **Hospital:** Lenox Hill Hosp (page 106); **Address:** NY Ctr for Spinal Disorders, 425 E 79th St, Ste 1H, New York, NY 10075; **Phone:** 212-249-3840; **Board Cert:** Orthopaedic Surgery 2009; **Med School:** Univ Pennsylvania 1989; **Resid:** Orthopaedic Surgery, Lenox Hill Hosp 1994; **Fellow:** Spine Surgery, Univ Miami Affil Hosp 1995; **Fac Appt:** Asst Prof OrS, Albert Einstein Coll Med

Turtel, Andrew H MD (OrS) - **Spec Exp:** Knee Surgery; Shoulder Surgery; Sports Medicine; Arthroscopic Surgery; **Hospital:** Lenox Hill Hosp (page 106), Beth Israel Med Ctr - Petrie Div (page 94); **Address:** 333 E 56th St, New York, NY 10022-3758; **Phone:** 212-319-6500; **Board Cert:** Orthopaedic Surgery 2005; **Med School:** SUNY Upstate Med Univ 1985; **Resid:** Surgery, SUNY Upstate Med Ctr 1987; Orthopaedic Surgery, LI Jewish Med Ctr 1991; **Fellow:** Sports Medicine, NYU Med Ctr 1992; **Fac Appt:** Assoc Clin Prof OrS, Albert Einstein Coll Med

Unis, George L MD (OrS) - **Spec Exp:** Sports Medicine; **Hospital:** St. Luke's - Roosevelt Hosp Ctr - Roosevelt Div (page 94), St. Luke's - Roosevelt Hosp Ctr - St Luke's Hosp (page 94); **Address:** 115 E 61st St Fl 8, New York, NY 10065; **Phone:** 212-688-3710; **Board Cert:** Orthopaedic Surgery 1973; **Med School:** UMDNJ-NJ Med Sch, Newark 1965; **Resid:** Surgery, St Lukes Roosevelt Hosp 1967; Orthopaedic Surgery, St Lukes Roosevelt Hosp 1971; **Fac Appt:** Asst Clin Prof OrS, Columbia P&S

Vitale, Michael Guy MD (OrS) - **Spec Exp:** Spinal Surgery-Pediatric; Scoliosis; Limb Lengthening (Ilizarov Procedure); Clubfoot/Foot Deformities in Children; **Hospital:** Morgan Stanley Children's Hosp of NY-Presby, NY (page 104), NY-Presby/Columbia Univ Med Ctr, NY (page 104); **Address:** Morgan Stanley Chldn's Hosp, 3959 Broadway, Ste 800N, New York, NY 10032; **Phone:** 212-305-5475; **Board Cert:** Orthopaedic Surgery 2014; **Med School:** Columbia P&S 1995; **Resid:** Orthopaedic Surgery, Columbia Presby Med Ctr 2000; **Fellow:** Pediatric Orthopaedic Surgery, Chldn's Hosp of Los Angeles 2001

Warren, Russell MD (OrS) - **Spec Exp:** Knee Injuries/Ligament Surgery; Shoulder Surgery; Shoulder Replacement; Rotator Cuff Surgery; **Hospital:** Hosp For Special Surgery (page 113); **Address:** 525 E 71st St Belaire Bldg, New York, NY 10021-4892; **Phone:** 212-606-1178; **Board Cert:** Orthopaedic Surgery 1974; **Med School:** SUNY Upstate Med Univ 1966; **Resid:** Surgery, St Lukes Hosp 1968; Orthopaedic Surgery, Hosp For Special Surgery 1973; **Fellow:** Shoulder Surgery, Columbia-Presby Med Ctr 1977; **Fac Appt:** Prof OrS, Cornell Univ-Weill Med Coll

Weiland, Andrew J MD (OrS) - **Spec Exp:** Hand Surgery; Hand Reconstruction; Wrist/Hand Injuries; **Hospital:** Hosp For Special Surgery (page 113), NY-Presby/Weill Cornell Med Ctr, NY (page 104); **Address:** Hosp for Special Surgery, 535 E 70th St, New York, NY 10021-4872; **Phone:** 212-606-1575; **Board Cert:** Orthopaedic Surgery 1977; **Med School:** Wake Forest Univ 1968; **Resid:** Surgery, Univ Michigan Med Ctr 1970; Orthopaedic Surgery, Johns Hopkins Hosp 1975; **Fellow:** Hand Surgery, Univ Louisville Hosp 1975; **Fac Appt:** Prof OrS, Cornell Univ-Weill Med Coll

Weiner, Lon S MD (OrS) - **Spec Exp:** Trauma; Fractures; Fractures-Complex & Non Union; **Hospital:** Lenox Hill Hosp (page 106), Riverview Med Ctr; **Address:** 130 E 77th St, Black Hall, Fl 12, New York, NY 10075; **Phone:** 212-434-4880; **Board Cert:** Orthopaedic Surgery 2011; **Med School:** Mount Sinai Sch Med 1982; **Resid:** Orthopaedic Surgery, Mount Sinai Hosp 1987; **Fellow:** Pediatric Orthopaedic Surgery, Hosp Special Surg 1988

Weinfeld, Steven B MD (OrS) - **Spec Exp:** Foot & Ankle Surgery; Diabetic Leg/Foot; Foot Deformities; **Hospital:** Mt Sinai Med Ctr (page 102), Hackensack Univ Med Ctr (page 718); **Address:** Mt Sinai Hosp-Dept Ortho Surgery, 5 E 98th St Fl 9, Box 1188, New York, NY 10029; **Phone:** 212-241-1634; **Board Cert:** Orthopaedic Surgery 2009; **Med School:** Albany Med Coll 1990; **Resid:** Orthopaedic Surgery, Albany Med Ctr 1995; **Fellow:** Ankle and Foot Surgery, Union Meml Hosp 1996; **Fac Appt:** Assoc Prof OrS, Mount Sinai Sch Med

Westrich, Geoffrey H MD (OrS) - **Spec Exp:** Hip Replacement & Revision; Knee Replacement & Revision; Arthroscopic Surgery-Hip; Arthroscopic Surgery-Knee; **Hospital:** Hosp For Special Surgery (page 113), NY-Presby/Weill Cornell Med Ctr, NY (page 104); **Address:** Hospital for Special Surgery, 535 E 70th St Fl 3, New York, NY 10021; **Phone:** 212-606-1510; **Board Cert:** Orthopaedic Surgery 2009; **Med School:** Tufts Univ 1990; **Resid:** Surgery, North Shore Hosp 1991; Orthopaedic Surgery, Hosp for Spec Surg 1995; **Fellow:** Orthopaedic Trauma Surgery, Inselspital 1996; Hip/Knee Reconstruction, Hosp for Special Surg 1998; **Fac Appt:** Assoc Prof OrS, Cornell Univ-Weill Med Coll

Wickiewicz, Thomas L MD (OrS) - **Spec Exp:** Knee Injuries/ACL; Sports Medicine; Shoulder Surgery; Rotator Cuff Surgery; **Hospital:** Hosp For Special Surgery (page 113), NY-Presby/Weill Cornell Med Ctr, NY (page 104); **Address:** Hosp for Spec Surg, 525 E 71st St Belaire Bldg Fl 1, New York, NY 10021; **Phone:** 212-606-1450; **Board Cert:** Orthopaedic Surgery 1984; **Med School:** UMDNJ-NJ Med Sch, Newark 1976; **Resid:** Orthopaedic Surgery, Hosp for Special Surg 1981; **Fellow:** Sports Medicine, UCLA Med Ctr 1982; **Fac Appt:** Clin Prof OrS, Cornell Univ-Weill Med Coll

Widmann, Roger F MD (OrS) - **Spec Exp:** Pediatric Orthopaedic Surgery; Scoliosis; Limb Lengthening; Limb Deformities; **Hospital:** Hosp For Special Surgery (page 113); **Address:** 535 E 70th St, New York, NY 10021; **Phone:** 212-606-1325; **Board Cert:** Orthopaedic Surgery 2008; **Med School:** Yale Univ 1989; **Resid:** Orthopaedic Surgery, Mass General Hosp 1994; **Fellow:** Pediatric Orthopaedic Surgery, Children's Hosp 1995; **Fac Appt:** Clin Prof OrS, Cornell Univ-Weill Med Coll

Windsor, Russell E MD (OrS) - **Spec Exp:** Knee Replacement; Hip Replacement; Knee Injuries/Ligament Surgery; **Hospital:** Hosp For Special Surgery (page 113), NY-Presby/Weill Cornell Med Ctr, NY (page 104); **Address:** Hosp for Special Surgery, 535 E 70th St, New York, NY 10021; **Phone:** 212-606-1166; **Board Cert:** Orthopaedic Surgery 2007; **Med School:** Georgetown Univ 1978; **Resid:** Orthopaedic Surgery, Hosp Univ Penn 1983; **Fellow:** Knee Surgery, Hosp For Special Surg 1984; **Fac Appt:** Prof OrS, Cornell Univ-Weill Med Coll

Wittig, James C MD (OrS) - **Spec Exp:** Bone Tumors; Sarcoma-Soft Tissue; Reconstructive Surgery; Pediatric Orthopaedic Cancers; **Hospital:** Mt Sinai Med Ctr (page 102), Hackensack Univ Med Ctr (page 718); **Address:** 5 E 98th St, Fl 9, New York, NY 10029; **Phone:** 212-241-1807; **Board Cert:** Orthopaedic Surgery 2003; **Med School:** NYU Sch Med 1994; **Resid:** Orthopaedic Surgery, Columbia Presby Med Ctr 1999; **Fellow:** Orthopaedic Oncology, Washington Cancer Inst 2001; Orthopaedic Oncology, NIH 2001; **Fac Appt:** Assoc Prof OrS, Mount Sinai Sch Med

Zambetti Jr, George J MD (OrS) - **Spec Exp:** Knee Reconstruction; Shoulder Surgery; Sports Medicine; Arthroscopic Surgery; **Hospital:** St. Luke's - Roosevelt Hosp Ctr - Roosevelt Div (page 94); **Address:** Columbus Circle Orthopaedics, 343 W 58th St, Ste 7, New York, NY 10019-1173; **Phone:** 212-506-0236; **Board Cert:** Orthopaedic Surgery 1983; **Med School:** Albany Med Coll 1976; **Resid:** Surgery, St Luke's-Roosevelt Hosp 1978; Orthopaedic Surgery, Columbia-Presby Med Ctr 1981

Zuckerman, Joseph D MD (OrS) - **Spec Exp:** Shoulder Surgery; Hip Replacement; Knee Replacement; Rotator Cuff Surgery; **Hospital:** NYU Hosp For Joint Dis (page 108), NYU Langone Med Ctr (page 108); **Address:** NYU Hosp for Joint Diseases, Dept Ortho Surg, 301 E 17th St, Fl 14, Ste 1402, New York, NY 10003; **Phone:** 212-598-6674; **Board Cert:** Orthopaedic Surgery 2007; **Med School:** Med Coll Wisc 1978; **Resid:** Orthopaedic Surgery, Univ WA Med Ctr 1983; **Fellow:** Arthritis Surgery, Brigham & Womans Hosp 1984; Shoulder Surgery, Mayo Clinic 1984; **Fac Appt:** Prof OrS, NYU Sch Med

Otolaryngology

Amin, Milan R MD (Oto) - **Spec Exp:** Swallowing Disorders; Voice Disorders; Vocal Cord Disorders; Laser Surgery; **Hospital:** NYU Langone Med Ctr (page 108); **Address:** 345 E 37 St, Ste 306, New York, NY 10016; **Phone:** 646-754-1207; **Board Cert:** Otolaryngology 2000; **Med School:** Northwestern Univ 1994; **Resid:** Otolaryngology, Temple Univ Med Ctr 1999; **Fellow:** Otolaryngology, Wake Forest Univ Med Ctr 2000; **Fac Appt:** Assoc Prof Oto, NYU Sch Med

Aviv, Jonathan MD (Oto) - **Spec Exp:** Voice Disorders; Swallowing Disorders; Cough; Endoscopy; **Hospital:** Mt Sinai Med Ctr (page 102); **Address:** ENT & Allergy Assocs, 210 E 86th St Fl 9, New York, NY 10028; **Phone:** 212-722-5570; **Board Cert:** Otolaryngology 1990; **Med School:** Columbia P&S 1985; **Resid:** Surgery, Mt Sinai Med Ctr 1987; Otolaryngology, Mt Sinai Med Ctr 1990; **Fellow:** Head and Neck Surgery, Mt Sinai Med Ctr 1991; **Fac Appt:** Prof Oto, Mount Sinai Sch Med

Blitzer, Andrew MD/DDS (Oto) - **Spec Exp:** Voice Disorders; Swallowing Disorders; Nasal & Sinus Surgery; Botox Therapy; **Hospital:** St. Luke's - Roosevelt Hosp Ctr - Roosevelt Div (page 94); **Address:** 425 W 59th St Fl 10, New York, NY 10019-1104; **Phone:** 212-262-9500; **Board Cert:** Otolaryngology 1977; **Med School:** Mount Sinai Sch Med 1973; **Resid:** Surgery, Beth Israel Med Ctr 1974; Otolaryngology, Mt Sinai Hosp 1977; **Fac Appt:** Clin Prof Oto, Columbia P&S

Boyle, Jay O MD (Oto) - **Spec Exp:** Oral Cancers; Melanoma-Head & Neck; Thyroid Cancer; **Hospital:** Meml Sloan-Kettering Canc Ctr (page 114); **Address:** Memorial Sloan Kettering Cancer Ctr, 1275 York Ave, New York, NY 10065; **Phone:** 212-639-2906; **Board Cert:** Otolaryngology 1997; **Med School:** Univ Ariz Coll Med 1990; **Resid:** Surgery, Johns Hopkins Hosp 1992; Otolaryngology, Johns Hopkins Bayview Med Ctr 1996; **Fellow:** Head and Neck Surgery, Meml Sloan Kettering Cancer Ctr 1998; **Fac Appt:** Assoc Prof Oto, Cornell Univ-Weill Med Coll

Brown, Kevin D MD/PhD (Oto) - **Spec Exp:** Neuro-Otology; Cochlear Implant; Hearing Loss; Acoustic Neuroma; **Hospital:** NY-Presby/Weill Cornell Med Ctr, NY (page 104); **Address:** 1305 York Ave at 70th St Fl 5, New York, NY 10021; **Phone:** 646-962-2032; **Board Cert:** Otolaryngology 2009; Neurotology 2010; **Med School:** Univ Iowa Coll Med 2002; **Resid:** Otolaryngology, Univ Iowa Hosps & Clinics 2007; **Fellow:** Neurotology, Jackson Meml Hosp 2009; **Fac Appt:** Asst Prof Oto, Cornell Univ-Weill Med Coll

Carew, John F MD (Oto) - **Spec Exp:** Head & Neck Surgery; Head & Neck Cancer; **Hospital:** Lenox Hill Hosp (page 106), Mt Sinai Med Ctr (page 102); **Address:** 785 Park Ave, Ste 1A, New York, NY 10021; **Phone:** 212-744-1941; **Board Cert:** Otolaryngology 1998; **Med School:** Cornell Univ-Weill Med Coll 1991; **Resid:** Otolaryngology, Manhattan EE&T 1997; **Fellow:** Head & Neck Oncology, Meml Sloan Kettering Cancer Ctr 1998

Caruana, Salvatore M MD (Oto) - **Spec Exp:** Head & Neck Cancer; Thyroid & Parathyroid Cancer & Surgery; Laser Surgery; Robotic Surgery; **Hospital:** NY-Presby/Columbia Univ Med Ctr, NY (page 104); **Address:** 180 Fort Washington Ave, Harkness Bldg - Fl 7, New York, NY 10032; **Phone:** 212-305-5335; **Board Cert:** Otolaryngology 1996; **Med School:** Mount Sinai Sch Med 1989; **Resid:** Otolaryngology, NY EE Infirm 1995; **Fellow:** Head & Neck Surgical Oncology, Meml Sloan-Kettering Canc Ctr 1997; **Fac Appt:** Asst Prof Oto, Columbia P&S

Chandrasekhar, Sujana S MD (Oto) - **Spec Exp:** Hearing & Balance Disorders; Cochlear Implants; Acoustic Neuroma; Meniere's Disease; **Hospital:** Mt Sinai Med Ctr (page 102), New York Eye & Ear Infirm (page 115); **Address:** 210 E 64th St Fl 3, New York, NY 10021; **Phone:** 212-249-3232; **Board Cert:** Otolaryngology 1993; Neurotology 2011; **Med School:** Mount Sinai Sch Med 1986; **Resid:** Surgery, NYU Med Ctr 1988; Otolaryngology, NYU Med Ctr 1992; **Fellow:** Neurotology, House Ear Clinic 1993; **Fac Appt:** Assoc Clin Prof Oto, Mount Sinai Sch Med

Close, Lanny Garth MD (Oto) - **Spec Exp:** Sinus Disorders/Surgery; Endoscopic Sinus Surgery; **Hospital:** NY-Presby/Columbia Univ Med Ctr, NY (page 104); **Address:** 51 W 51st St, Fl 3rd, New York, NY 10022; **Phone:** 212-326-8475; **Board Cert:** Otolaryngology 1977; **Med School:** Baylor Coll Med 1972; **Resid:** Surgery, Johns Hopkins Hosp 1974; Otolaryngology, Baylor Affil Hosps 1977; **Fellow:** Head and Neck Surgery, MD Anderson Cancer Ctr 1979; **Fac Appt:** Prof Oto, Columbia P&S

Constantinides, Minas MD (Oto) - **Spec Exp:** Rhinoplasty; Rhinoplasty Revision; Facial Rejuvenation; **Hospital:** Lenox Hill Hosp (Manh Eye, Ear & Throat Hosp) (page 106), NYU Langone Med Ctr (page 108); **Address:** 74 E 79th St, Ste 1B, New York, NY 10075; **Phone:** 212-861-0200; **Board Cert:** Otolaryngology 1994; Facial Plastic & Reconstr Surgery 1997; **Med School:** Columbia P&S 1987; **Resid:** Surgery, Harvard Surg Svcs 1989; Otolaryngology, NYU Medical Center 1993; **Fellow:** Facial Plastic Surgery, Univ Toronto 1994; **Fac Appt:** Asst Prof Oto, NYU Sch Med

Costantino, Peter D MD (Oto) - **Spec Exp:** Skull Base Tumors; Head & Neck Cancer; Craniofacial Surgery/Reconstruction; **Hospital:** Lenox Hill Hosp (page 106); **Address:** 130 E 77th St Fl 10, New York, NY 10075; **Phone:** 212-434-4500; **Board Cert:** Otolaryngology 1990; Facial Plastic & Reconstr Surgery 2000; **Med School:** Northwestern Univ 1984; **Resid:** Surgery, Northwestern Meml Hosp 1986; Otolaryngology, Northwestern Meml Hosp 1989; **Fellow:** Head and Neck Surgery, Northwestern Meml Hosp 1990; Skull Base Surgery, Univ Pittsburgh 1991; **Fac Appt:** Prof Oto, Columbia P&S

DeLacure, Mark D MD (Oto) - **Spec Exp:** Head & Neck Cancer; Head & Neck Cancer Reconstruction; Reconstructive Microsurgery; **Hospital:** NYU Langone Med Ctr (page 108), VA NY Harbor Hlthcare Sys-Manhattan Campus; **Address:** 160 E 34th St Fl 9, New York, NY 10016; **Phone:** 212-731-5329; **Board Cert:** Otolaryngology 1992; Plastic Surgery 2012; **Med School:** Univ Fla Coll Med 1986; **Resid:** Otolaryngology, Yale Univ Sch Med 1991; Plastic/Reconstructive Surgery, UCLA Med Ctr 1993; **Fellow:** Head & Neck Oncology, Meml Sloan-Kettering Cancer Ctr 1992; **Fac Appt:** Assoc Clin Prof Oto, NYU Sch Med

Dropkin, Lloyd R MD (Oto) - **Hospital:** NY-Presby/Weill Cornell Med Ctr, NY (page 104); **Address:** 30 E End Ave, 1F, New York, NY 10028; **Phone:** 212-535-9191; **Board Cert:** Otolaryngology 1976; **Med School:** Cornell Univ-Weill Med Coll 1970; **Resid:** Surgery, NY Presby/Weill Cornell Med Ctr 1972; Otolaryngology, NY Presby/Weill Cornell Med Ctr 1976; **Fac Appt:** Assoc Prof Oto, Cornell Univ-Weill Med Coll

Edelstein, David R MD (Oto) - **Spec Exp:** Endoscopic Sinus Surgery; Nasal Reconstruction; Sleep Disorders/Apnea; Sleep Disorders/Apnea; **Hospital:** Lenox Hill Hosp (Manh Eye, Ear & Throat Hosp) (page 106), Mt Sinai Med Ctr (page 102); **Address:** Manhattan Otolaryngology Head & Neck Surg, 1421 3rd Ave Fl 4, New York, NY 10028; **Phone:** 212-452-1500; **Board Cert:** Otolaryngology 1985; **Med School:** Boston Univ 1980; **Resid:** Surgery, Mount Sinai Hosp 1981; Otolaryngology, Mount Sinai Hosp 1984; **Fac Appt:** Clin Prof Oto, Cornell Univ-Weill Med Coll

Genden Sr, Eric M MD (Oto) - **Spec Exp:** Head & Neck Cancer & Surgery; Head & Neck Cancer Reconstruction; Airway Reconstruction; Thyroid & Parathyroid Cancer & Surgery; **Hospital:** Mt Sinai Med Ctr (page 102); **Address:** Mt Sinai Dept Otolaryngology, 1 Gustave L Levy Pl, Box 1191, New York, NY 10029; **Phone:** 212-241-9410; **Board Cert:** Otolaryngology 1999; Facial Plastic & Reconstr Surgery 2000; **Med School:** Mount Sinai Sch Med 1992; **Resid:** Otolaryngology, Barnes Jewish Hosp 1998; **Fellow:** Head and Neck Surgery, Mt Sinai Med Ctr 1999; **Fac Appt:** Prof Oto, Mount Sinai Sch Med

Godin, David A MD (Oto) - **Spec Exp:** Laryngeal & Voice Disorders; Sinus Disorders/Surgery; Pediatric Otolaryngology; Thyroid & Parathyroid Surgery; **Hospital:** New York Eye & Ear Infirm (page 115), Beth Israel Med Ctr - Petrie Div (page 94); **Address:** 261 5th Ave, Fl 9th, Ste 901, New York, NY 10016; **Phone:** 212-679-3499; **Board Cert:** Otolaryngology 2001; **Med School:** SUNY Upstate Med Univ 1995; **Resid:** Surgery, Tulane Univ 1996; Otolaryngology, Tulane Univ 2000; **Fac Appt:** Asst Prof Oto, NY Med Coll

Gold, Scott D MD (Oto) - **Spec Exp:** Endoscopic Sinus Surgery; Sinus Disorders/Surgery; **Hospital:** Beth Israel Med Ctr - Petrie Div (page 94), Mt Sinai Med Ctr (page 102); **Address:** NY Otolaryngology Group, 36A E 36th St, Ste 200, New York, NY 10016-3401; **Phone:** 212-889-8575; **Board Cert:** Otolaryngology 1983; **Med School:** Mount Sinai Sch Med 1979; **Resid:** Surgery, Mt Sinai Med Ctr 1980; Otolaryngology, Mt Sinai Med Ctr 1983; **Fac Appt:** Asst Clin Prof Oto, Mount Sinai Sch Med

Green, Robert P MD (Oto) - **Spec Exp:** Sinus Disorders; Hearing Loss/Tinnitus; Throat Disorders; **Hospital:** Mt Sinai Med Ctr (page 102); **Address:** 210 E 86th St Fl 9, New York, NY 10028; **Phone:** 212-722-5570; **Board Cert:** Otolaryngology 1981; **Med School:** Harvard Med Sch 1977; **Resid:** Otolaryngology, Mount Sinai Hosp 1981

Grunstein, Eli MD (Oto) - **Spec Exp:** Pediatric Otolaryngology; **Hospital:** NY-Presby/Columbia Univ Med Ctr, NY (page 104); **Address:** Morgan Stanley Chldns Hosp of NY, 3959 Broadway, rm 510N, New York, NY 10032; **Phone:** 212-305-8933; **Board Cert:** Otolaryngology 2006; **Med School:** Albert Einstein Coll Med 2000; **Resid:** Otolaryngology, NY Presby Hosp 2005

Guida, Robert A MD (Oto) - **Spec Exp:** Rhinoplasty; Nasal Surgery; Cosmetic Surgery-Face; Skin Laser Surgery; **Hospital:** NY-Presby/Weill Cornell Med Ctr, NY (page 104), Lenox Hill Hosp (Manh Eye, Ear & Throat Hosp) (page 106); **Address:** 1175 Park Ave, Ste 1B, New York, NY 10128; **Phone:** 212-871-0900; **Board Cert:** Otolaryngology 1989; Facial Plastic & Reconstr Surgery 1994; **Med School:** Hahnemann Univ 1983; **Resid:** Surgery, Graduate Hosp 1985; Otolaryngology, NY Eye & Ear Infirm 1989; **Fellow:** Facial Plastic Surgery, Oregon Hlth Sci Ctr 1990; **Fac Appt:** Assoc Prof Oto, Cornell Univ-Weill Med Coll

Hammerschlag, Paul E MD (Oto) - **Spec Exp:** Cochlear Implants; Hearing Loss; Meniere's Disease; Balance Disorders; **Hospital:** NYU Langone Med Ctr (page 108), New York Eye & Ear Infirm (page 115); **Address:** 650 First Ave, New York, NY 10016-3240; **Phone:** 212-889-2600; **Board Cert:** Otolaryngology 1978; **Med School:** Albert Einstein Coll Med 1972; **Resid:** Surgery, Virginia Mason Hosp 1974; Otolaryngology, Mass Eye & Ear Infirm 1978; **Fellow:** Otolaryngology, Mass Eye & Ear Infirm 1978; **Fac Appt:** Assoc Clin Prof Oto, NYU Sch Med

Har-El, Gady MD (Oto) - **Spec Exp:** Head & Neck Cancer; Thyroid & Parathyroid Surgery; Sinus Tumors; Skull Base Tumors; **Hospital:** Lenox Hill Hosp (page 106), Lenox Hill Hosp (Manh Eye, Ear & Throat Hosp) (page 106); **Address:** 186 E 76th St E, Fl 2, New York, NY 10021; **Phone:** 212-744-4368; **Board Cert:** Otolaryngology 1992; **Med School:** Israel 1982; **Resid:** Otolaryngology, SUNY Downstate Med Ctr 1991; **Fellow:** Head and Neck Surgery, Long Island Coll Hosp 1987; **Fac Appt:** Prof Oto, SUNY Hlth Sci Ctr

Hoffman, Ronald A MD (Oto) - **Spec Exp:** Cochlear Implants; Balance Disorders; Ear Disorders/Surgery; **Hospital:** New York Eye & Ear Infirm (page 115), Beth Israel Med Ctr - Petrie Div (page 94); **Address:** 380 2nd Ave Fl 9, New York, NY 10010; **Phone:** 212-614-8388; **Board Cert:** Otolaryngology 1976; **Med School:** Jefferson Med Coll 1971; **Resid:** Surgery, Lenox Hill Hosp 1973; Otolaryngology, NYU Med Ctr 1976; **Fac Appt:** Prof Oto, Albert Einstein Coll Med

Horn, Corinne E MD (Oto) - **Spec Exp:** Cosmetic Surgery-Face; Plastic & Reconstructive Surgery; **Hospital:** Beth Israel Med Ctr - Petrie Div (page 94), New York Eye & Ear Infirm (page 115); **Address:** NY Eye & Ear Infirmary, 36A E 36th St, Ste 200, New York, NY 10016; **Phone:** 212-889-8575; **Board Cert:** Otolaryngology 2006; **Med School:** Columbia P&S 2000; **Resid:** Otolaryngology, Columbia-Presby Hosp 2005; **Fellow:** Facial Plastic & Reconstr Surgery, Univ Illinois Med Ctr 2006

Jacobs, Joseph B MD (Oto) - **Spec Exp:** Endoscopic Sinus Surgery; Sinus Disorders/Surgery; Sinus Surgery-Revision; **Hospital:** NYU Langone Med Ctr (page 108); **Address:** 345 E 37 St, Ste 306, MS 10016, New York, NY 10016-6402; **Phone:** 646-754-1203; **Board Cert:** Otolaryngology 1978; **Med School:** Albert Einstein Coll Med 1974; **Resid:** Surgery, Montefiore Med Ctr 1975; Otolaryngology, NYU Med Ctr 1978; **Fellow:** Plastic/Reconstructive Surgery, UCLA Med Ctr 1979; **Fac Appt:** Prof Oto, NYU Sch Med

Jahn, Anthony F MD (Oto) - **Spec Exp:** Voice Disorders/Professional Voice Care; Hearing Loss; Otology & Neuro-Otology; **Hospital:** St. Luke's - Roosevelt Hosp Ctr - Roosevelt Div (page 94); **Address:** Head & Neck Surgical Group, 425 W 59th St Fl 10, New York, NY 10019; **Phone:** 212-262-4400; **Board Cert:** Otolaryngology 1979; **Med School:** Canada 1974; **Resid:** Otolaryngology, Toronto Genl Hosp 1979

Jones, Jacqueline E MD (Oto) - **Spec Exp:** Pediatric Otolaryngology; Sinus Disorders/Surgery; Ear Infections; **Hospital:** NY-Presby/Weill Cornell Med Ctr, NY (page 104), Lenox Hill Hosp (page 106); **Address:** 1175 Park Ave, Ste 1A, New York, NY 10128; **Phone:** 212-996-2559; **Board Cert:** Otolaryngology 1989; **Med School:** Cornell Univ 1984; **Resid:** Otolaryngology, Hosp Univ Penn 1989; **Fellow:** Pediatric Otolaryngology, Chldns Hosp 1990; **Fac Appt:** Assoc Prof Oto, Cornell Univ-Weill Med Coll

Josephson, Jordan S MD (Oto) - **Spec Exp:** Rhinoplasty Revision; Endoscopic Sinus Surgery; Nasal & Sinus Disorders; Sleep Apnea; **Hospital:** Lenox Hill Hosp (Manh Eye, Ear & Throat Hosp) (page 106); **Address:** 205 E 76th St, Ste M1, New York, NY 10021; **Phone:** 212-717-1773; **Board Cert:** Otolaryngology 1988; **Med School:** SUNY Downstate 1983; **Resid:** Surgery, LI Jewish Med Ctr 1984; Otolaryngology, LI Jewish Med Ctr 1988; **Fellow:** Sinus Surgery, Johns Hopkins Hosp 1989

Kacker, Ashutosh MD (Oto) - **Spec Exp:** Sinus Surgery; **Hospital:** NY-Presby/Weill Cornell Med Ctr, NY (page 104); **Address:** 1305 York Ave Fl 5, New York, NY 10021; **Phone:** 646-962-5097; **Board Cert:** Otolaryngology 2012; **Med School:** India 1989; **Resid:** Surgery, Lenox Hill Hosp 1997; **Fellow:** Otolaryngology, Manhattan Eye, Ear & Throat 2001; **Fac Appt:** Assoc Prof Oto, Cornell Univ

Khosh, Maurice M MD (Oto) - **Spec Exp:** Cosmetic Surgery-Face; Reconstructive Surgery-Face; Rhinoplasty; **Hospital:** St. Luke's - Roosevelt Hosp Ctr - Roosevelt Div (page 94); **Address:** Head & Neck Surgical Group, 425 W 59th St Fl 10, New York, NY 10022; **Phone:** 212-262-0056; **Board Cert:** Otolaryngology 1997; **Med School:** Albert Einstein Coll Med 1990; **Resid:** Surgery, Columbia Presby Hosp 1992; Otolaryngology, Columbia Presby Hosp 1996; **Fellow:** Facial Plastic Surgery, Univ Washington 1997; **Fac Appt:** Asst Prof Oto, Columbia P&S

Kohan, Darius MD (Oto) - **Spec Exp:** Cochlear Implants; Acoustic Neuroma; Hearing Disorders; Ear Tumors; **Hospital:** Lenox Hill Hosp (Manh Eye, Ear & Throat Hosp) (page 106), NYU Langone Med Ctr (page 108); **Address:** 863 Park Ave, Ste 1E, New York, NY 10021; **Phone:** 212-472-1300; **Board Cert:** Otolaryngology 1990; Neurotology 2012; **Med School:** NYU Sch Med 1984; **Resid:** Surgery, Beth Israel Med Ctr 1986; Otolaryngology, NYU Med Ctr 1990; **Fellow:** Otology, NYU Med Ctr 1991; **Fac Appt:** Assoc Prof Oto, NYU Sch Med

Komisar, Arnold MD/DDS (Oto) - **Spec Exp:** Thyroid & Parathyroid Surgery; Salivary Gland Tumors; Nasal & Sinus Surgery; **Hospital:** Lenox Hill Hosp (page 106), Lenox Hill Hosp (Manh Eye, Ear & Throat Hosp) (page 106); **Address:** 130 E 77 St, Lenox Hill Hospital, Black Hall, Fl 10th, New York, NY 10075; **Phone:** 212-861-8888; **Board Cert:** Otolaryngology 1979; **Med School:** Hahnemann Univ 1975; **Resid:** Surgery, Beth Israel Hosp 1976; Otolaryngology, Mt Sinai Med Ctr 1979; **Fac Appt:** Clin Prof Oto, NYU Sch Med

Korovin, Gwen S MD (Oto) - **Spec Exp:** Voice Disorders; Throat Disorders; Laryngeal Disorders; Vocal Cord Disorders; **Hospital:** Lenox Hill Hosp (page 106), Lenox Hill Hosp (Manh Eye, Ear & Throat Hosp) (page 106); **Address:** 70 E 77th St, Ste 1B, New York, NY 10075; **Phone:** 212-879-6630; **Board Cert:** Otolaryngology 1989; **Med School:** SUNY Upstate Med Univ 1984; **Resid:** Otolaryngology, NY Eye & Ear Infirm 1989; **Fac Appt:** Asst Clin Prof Oto, NYU Sch Med

Koufman, Jamie A MD (Oto) - **Spec Exp:** Voice Disorders; Laryngeal Disorders; **Hospital:** New York Eye & Ear Infirm (page 115); **Address:** 200 W 57th St, Ste 1203, New York, NY 10019; **Phone:** 212-463-8014; **Board Cert:** Otolaryngology 1978; **Med School:** Boston Univ 1973; **Resid:** Surgery, Hartford Hosp 1975; Otolaryngology, Boston Univ Med Ctr 1978

Kraus, Dennis H MD (Oto) - **Spec Exp:** Head & Neck Cancer; Skull Base Tumors; Thyroid & Parathyroid Surgery; Sarcoma; **Hospital:** Lenox Hill Hosp (page 106); **Address:** 130 E 77th St, Fl 10, New York, NY 10075-1851; **Phone:** 212-434-4500; **Board Cert:** Otolaryngology 1990; **Med School:** Univ Rochester 1985; **Resid:** Surgery, Cleveland Clinic 1987; Otolaryngology, Cleveland Clinic 1990; **Fellow:** Head and Neck Surgery, Meml Sloan Kettering Cancer Ctr 1991; **Fac Appt:** Prof Oto, Cornell Univ-Weill Med Coll

Krespi, Yosef P MD (Oto) - **Spec Exp:** Sleep Disorders/Apnea/Snoring; Nasal & Sinus Surgery; Head & Neck Cancer & Surgery; Thyroid Cancer; **Hospital:** Lenox Hill Hosp (Manh Eye, Ear & Throat Hosp) (page 106); **Address:** 110 E 59th St, Ste 10A, New York, NY 10022; **Phone:** 212-434-4500; **Board Cert:** Otolaryngology 1981; **Med School:** Israel 1973; **Resid:** Surgery, Mt Sinai Hosp 1976; Otolaryngology, Mt Sinai Hosp 1980; **Fellow:** Surgery, Northwestern Meml Hosp 1981; **Fac Appt:** Clin Prof Oto, Columbia P&S

Krevitt, Lane David MD (Oto) - **Spec Exp:** Thyroid & Parathyroid Surgery; Endoscopic Sinus Surgery; Head & Neck Cancer & Surgery; Sleep Apnea; **Hospital:** Beth Israel Med Ctr - Petrie Div (page 94); **Address:** New York Otolaryngology Group, 36A E 36th St, Ste 200, New York, NY 10016-3453; **Phone:** 212-889-8575; **Board Cert:** Otolaryngology 1999; **Med School:** Hahnemann Univ 1993; **Resid:** Surgery, Albert Einstein Affil Hosps 1994; Otolaryngology, Albert Einstein Uni Affil Hosps 1998; **Fellow:** Head & Neck Surgical Oncology, Montefiore Med Ctr 1999

Kuhel, William I MD (Oto) - **Spec Exp:** Head & Neck Cancer & Surgery; Thyroid Cancer; Parathyroid Cancer; **Hospital:** NY-Presby/Weill Cornell Med Ctr, NY (page 104); **Address:** 1305 York Ave Fl 5, Weill-Greenberg Ctr, New York, NY 10021; **Phone:** 646-962-6325; **Board Cert:** Otolaryngology 1988; **Med School:** Univ Mich Med Sch 1983; **Resid:** Surgery, St Vincent's Hosp 1985; Otolaryngology, Indiana Univ 1988; **Fellow:** Head and Neck Surgery, MD Anderson Cancer Ctr 1989; **Fac Appt:** Assoc Clin Prof Oto, Cornell Univ-Weill Med Coll

Kuriloff, Daniel B MD (Oto) - **Spec Exp:** Thyroid Surgery; Parathyroid Surgery; Minimally Invasive Surgery; Head & Neck Surgery; **Hospital:** Lenox Hill Hosp (page 106); **Address:** NY Head & Neck Inst, 110 E 59th St Fl 10 - Ste 10A, New York, NY 10022; **Phone:** 212-262-5555; **Board Cert:** Otolaryngology 1988; **Med School:** Mount Sinai Sch Med 1982; **Resid:** Surgery, Beth Israel Hosp 1984; Otolaryngology, NY Eye & Ear Infirmary 1988; **Fellow:** Head & Neck Surgical Oncology, Univ Mich Med Ctr 1990; **Fac Appt:** Assoc Clin Prof Oto, Columbia P&S

Lalwani, Anil K MD (Oto) - **Spec Exp:** Ear Disorders/Surgery; Facial Nerve Disorders; Cochlear Implants; Skull Base Surgery; **Hospital:** NY-Presby/Columbia Univ Med Ctr, NY (page 104), Morgan Stanley Children's Hosp of NY-Presby, NY (page 104); **Address:** 180 Fort Washington Ave, Harkness Pavilion Fl 7, New York, NY 10032; **Phone:** 212-305-1696; **Board Cert:** Otolaryngology 1992; Neurotology 2010; **Med School:** Univ Mich Med Sch 1985; **Resid:** Surgery, Duke Univ Med Ctr 1987; Otolaryngology, UCSF Med Ctr 1991; **Fellow:** Skull Base Surgery, UCSF Med Ctr 1992; Molecular Genetics, Natl Inst Hlth 1994; **Fac Appt:** Prof Oto, Columbia P&S

Lawson, William MD (Oto) - **Spec Exp:** Sinus Disorders/Surgery; Endoscopic Sinus Surgery; **Hospital:** Mt Sinai Med Ctr (page 102); **Address:** 5 E 98th St Fl 8, Box 1191, New York, NY 10029-6501; **Phone:** 212-241-9410; **Board Cert:** Otolaryngology 1974; **Med School:** NYU Sch Med 1965; **Resid:** Surgery, Bronx VA Hosp 1967; Otolaryngology, Mt Sinai Hosp 1974; **Fac Appt:** Prof Oto, Mount Sinai Sch Med

Lebovics, Robert S MD (Oto) - **Spec Exp:** Head & Neck Inflammatory Disorders; Head & Neck Autoimmune Disease; Head & Neck Infectious Disease; Wegener's Granulomatosis; **Hospital:** St. Luke's - Roosevelt Hosp Ctr - Roosevelt Div (page 94); **Address:** 425 W 59th St, Fl 10, New York, NY 10019; **Phone:** 212-262-2002; **Board Cert:** Otolaryngology 1988; **Med School:** SUNY Downstate 1982; **Resid:** Surgery, Montefiore-Weiler Einstein Div 1983; Otolaryngology, Montefiore-Weiler Einstein Div 1987

Lim, Jessica W MD (Oto) - **Spec Exp:** Head & Neck Cancer; Sinus Disorders; Sleep Disorders; Swallowing Disorders; **Hospital:** Lenox Hill Hosp (page 106), Lenox Hill Hosp (Manh Eye, Ear & Throat Hosp) (page 106); **Address:** Lenox Otolaryngology Head & Neck Surgery, 186 E 76th St Fl 2, New York, NY 10021; **Phone:** 212-434-2323; **Board Cert:** Otolaryngology 1998; **Med School:** W VA Univ 1991; **Resid:** Surgery, NYU Med Ctr 1993; Otolaryngology, NYU Med Ctr 1996; **Fellow:** Head and Neck Surgery, Rush Univ Med Ctr 1998; **Fac Appt:** Asst Prof Oto, SUNY Downstate

Linstrom, Christopher J MD (Oto) - **Spec Exp:** Cochlear Implants; Acoustic Neuroma; Encephalocele; Cholesteatoma; **Hospital:** New York Eye & Ear Infirm (page 115); **Address:** NY Eye & Ear Infirmary, Dept Otolaryngology, 310 E 14th St, New York, NY 10003-4201; **Phone:** 212-979-4200; **Board Cert:** Otolaryngology 1987; Neurotology 2004; **Med School:** McGill Univ 1982; **Resid:** Surgery, Geo Wash Med Ctr 1984; Otolaryngology, Cornell Univ Med Ctr 1987; **Fellow:** Otology & Neurotology, Michigan Ear Inst 1989; **Fac Appt:** Prof Oto, Albert Einstein Coll Med

Markowitz, Arlene H MD (Oto) - **Spec Exp:** Sinus Disorders/Surgery; Endoscopic Sinus Surgery; **Hospital:** NY-Presby/Columbia Univ Med Ctr, NY (page 104), Lenox Hill Hosp (page 106); **Address:** 903 Park Ave, New York, NY 10075; **Phone:** 212-794-3999; **Board Cert:** Otolaryngology 1990; **Med School:** Columbia P&S 1984; **Resid:** Surgery, Columbia-Presby Med Ctr 1986; Otolaryngology, Columbia-Presby Med Ctr 1990; **Fac Appt:** Asst Clin Prof Oto, Columbia P&S

McMenomey, Sean O'Leary MD (Oto) - **Spec Exp:** Otology & Neuro-Otology; Hearing Loss; Dizziness/Vertigo; Cochlear Implants; **Hospital:** NYU Langone Med Ctr (page 108), Bellevue Hosp Ctr; **Address:** NYU Otology Assocs, 550 First Ave, Ste 7Q, MC PV-01, New York, NY 10016; **Phone:** 212-263-5565; **Board Cert:** Otolaryngology 1993; Neurotology 2004; **Med School:** St Louis Univ 1987; **Resid:** Otolaryngology, Oregon Hlth Sci Ctr 1992; **Fellow:** Otology & Neurotology, Vanderbilt Univ Hosp 1993; **Fac Appt:** Prof Oto, NYU Sch Med

Miller, Philip J MD (Oto) - **Spec Exp:** Rhinoplasty; Cosmetic Surgery-Face; Facial Nerve Disorders; Facial Rejuvenation; **Hospital:** Lenox Hill Hosp (Manh Eye, Ear & Throat Hosp) (page 106), NYU Langone Med Ctr (page 108); **Address:** 60 E 56 St Fl 3rd, New York, NY 10022; **Phone:** 212-750-7100; **Board Cert:** Otolaryngology 1996; Facial Plastic & Reconstr Surgery 1999; **Med School:** Univ Mass Sch Med 1989; **Resid:** Surgery, NYU Med Ctr 1991; Otolaryngology, NYU Med Ctr 1995; **Fellow:** Facial Plastic Surgery, Oregon Health Sci Ctr 1996; **Fac Appt:** Asst Prof Oto, NYU Sch Med

Myssiorek, David MD (Oto) - **Spec Exp:** Thyroid & Parathyroid Surgery; Head & Neck Cancer; Salivary Gland Surgery; Paragangliomas; **Hospital:** NYU Langone Med Ctr (page 108), Bellevue Hosp Ctr; **Address:** 160 E 34th St, Fl 9, New York, NY 10016; **Phone:** 212-731-6085; **Board Cert:** Otolaryngology 1985; **Med School:** NYU Sch Med 1980; **Resid:** Otolaryngology, Bellevue/NYU/VA Med Ctr 1984; **Fellow:** Head & Neck Oncology, Montefiore Med Ctr 1985; **Fac Appt:** Prof Oto, NYU Sch Med

Nass, Richard L MD (Oto) - **Spec Exp:** Allergy; Sinus Disorders/Surgery; Nasal Surgery; **Hospital:** NYU Langone Med Ctr (page 108), Lenox Hill Hosp (page 106); **Address:** 1430 2nd Ave, Ste 108, New York, NY 10021; **Phone:** 212-734-4515; **Board Cert:** Otolaryngology 1979; **Med School:** NYU Sch Med 1975; **Resid:** Otolaryngology, NYU-Bellevue Hosp 1979; **Fac Appt:** Assoc Clin Prof Oto, NYU Sch Med

Pastorek, Norman MD (Oto) - **Spec Exp:** Rhinoplasty; Eyelid Surgery; Cosmetic Surgery-Face; **Hospital:** Lenox Hill Hosp (Manh Eye, Ear & Throat Hosp) (page 106), NY-Presby/Weill Cornell Med Ctr, NY (page 104); **Address:** 12 E 88 St, New York, NY 10128; **Phone:** 212-987-4700; **Board Cert:** Otolaryngology 1970; Facial Plastic & Reconstr Surgery 2008; **Med School:** Univ IL Coll Med 1964; **Resid:** Surgery, Hines VA Hosp 1967; Otolaryngology, Univ IL Med Ctr 1969; **Fac Appt:** Clin Prof Oto, Cornell Univ-Weill Med Coll

Persky, Mark S MD (Oto) - **Spec Exp:** Head & Neck Cancer; Skull Base Tumors; Thyroid Cancer; Vascular Lesions-Head & Neck; **Hospital:** Beth Israel Med Ctr - Petrie Div (page 94), New York Eye & Ear Infirm (page 115); **Address:** 10 Union Square East, Ste 4J, New York, NY 10003; **Phone:** 212-844-8648; **Board Cert:** Otolaryngology 1976; **Med School:** SUNY Upstate Med Univ 1972; **Resid:** Otolaryngology, Bellevue Hosp 1976; **Fellow:** Head and Neck Surgery, Beth Israel Med Ctr 1977; **Fac Appt:** Clin Prof Oto, Albert Einstein Coll Med

Pincus, Robert L MD (Oto) - **Spec Exp:** Sinus Disorders; Voice Disorders; Endoscopic Sinus Surgery; Facial Plastic & Reconstructive Surgery; **Hospital:** Beth Israel Med Ctr - Petrie Div (page 94), Lenox Hill Hosp (page 106); **Address:** 36A E 36th St, Ste 200, New York, NY 10016-3401; **Phone:** 212-889-8575; **Board Cert:** Otolaryngology 1983; **Med School:** Univ Mich Med Sch 1978; **Resid:** Surgery, Lenox Hill Hosp 1980; Otolaryngology, Mt Sinai Med Ctr 1983; **Fac Appt:** Assoc Prof Oto, NY Med Coll

Pollack, Geoffrey MD (Oto) - **Spec Exp:** Head & Neck Surgery; **Hospital:** St. Luke's - Roosevelt Hosp Ctr - St Luke's Hosp (page 94); **Address:** 211 Central Park West, New York, NY 10024; **Phone:** 212-873-6175; **Board Cert:** Otolaryngology 1984; **Med School:** Columbia P&S 1979; **Resid:** Otolaryngology, Columbia-Presby Med Ctr 1984

Portnoy, William M MD (Oto) - **Spec Exp:** Head & Neck Cancer & Surgery; Head & Neck Cancer Reconstruction; Facial Plastic & Reconstructive Surgery; Rhinoplasty; **Hospital:** Beth Israel Med Ctr - Petrie Div (page 94), New York Eye & Ear Infirm (page 115); **Address:** Manhattan Rhinoplasty Surgeon, 160 W 18th St, New York, NY 10011; **Phone:** 212-366-0848 x201; **Board Cert:** Otolaryngology 1993; Facial Plastic & Reconstr Surgery 1996; **Med School:** Geo Wash Univ 1987; **Resid:** Surgery, North Shore Univ Hosp 1988; Otolaryngology, NY E&E Infirm 1992; **Fellow:** Microvascular Surgery, UPMC Mercy Hosp 1993

Rizk, Samieh S MD (Oto) - **Spec Exp:** Facial Plastic & Reconstructive Surgery; Rhinoplasty Revision; Nasal Surgery; **Hospital:** Lenox Hill Hosp (page 106), Lenox Hill Hosp (Manh Eye, Ear & Throat Hosp) (page 106); **Address:** Manhattan Facial Plastic Surgery, 1040 Park Ave, New York, NY 10028; **Phone:** 212-452-3362; **Board Cert:** Facial Plastic & Reconstr Surgery 2000; Otolaryngology 2004; **Med School:** Univ Mich Med Sch 1993; **Resid:** Surgery, Lenox Hill Hosp 1995; Otolaryngology, Manhattan EE&T Hosp 1998; **Fellow:** Facial Plastic Surgery, Facial Surgery Center 1999

Roland Jr, J Thomas MD (Oto) - **Spec Exp:** Acoustic Neuroma; Cochlear Implants; Neuro-Otology; Facial Nerve Disorders; **Hospital:** NYU Langone Med Ctr (page 108), Bellevue Hosp Ctr; **Address:** NYU Otology Assocs, 550 First Ave, Ste 7Q, New York, NY 10016; **Phone:** 212-263-5565; **Board Cert:** Otolaryngology 1993; Neurotology 2004; **Med School:** Temple Univ 1983; **Resid:** Otolaryngology, NYU Med Ctr 1992; **Fellow:** Neurotology, NYU Med Ctr 1993; **Fac Appt:** Prof Oto, NYU Sch Med

Romo III, Thomas MD (Oto) - **Spec Exp:** Facial Plastic & Reconstructive Surgery; Cosmetic Surgery-Face; Rhinoplasty Revision; Ear Reconstruction/Microtia; **Hospital:** Lenox Hill Hosp (page 106), Lenox Hill Hosp (Manh Eye, Ear & Throat Hosp) (page 106); **Address:** 135 E 74th St, New York, NY 10021; **Phone:** 212-288-1500; **Board Cert:** Otolaryngology 1985; Facial Plastic & Reconstr Surgery 1992; **Med School:** Baylor Coll Med 1979; **Resid:** Otolaryngology, Baylor Hosps 1982; Otolaryngology, New York Eye & Ear Infirm 1984; **Fellow:** Facial Plastic Surgery, New York Eye & Ear Infirm 1985; Facial Plastic Surgery, Tampa General Hosp 1987; **Fac Appt:** Asst Clin Prof Oto, NY Med Coll

Rosenberg, David B MD (Oto) - **Spec Exp:** Rhinoplasty Revision; Cosmetic Surgery-Face; Reconstructive Plastic Surgery; **Hospital:** Lenox Hill Hosp (Manh Eye, Ear & Throat Hosp) (page 106); **Address:** 115 E 61st St Fl 1, New York, NY 10065; **Phone:** 212-832-8595; **Board Cert:** Otolaryngology 2000; Facial Plastic & Reconstr Surgery 2012; **Med School:** Cornell Univ-Weill Med Coll 1993; **Resid:** Surgery, Lenox Hill 1995; Otolaryngology, Manhattan EE&T Hosp 1999; **Fellow:** Facial Plastic Surgery, RWJohnson Univ Hosp 2000

Rothstein, Stephen G MD (Oto) - **Spec Exp:** Voice Disorders; Swallowing Disorders; Laser Surgery; **Hospital:** NYU Langone Med Ctr (page 108); **Address:** 240 E 38th St Fl 14, New York, NY 10016; **Phone:** 212-263-7165; **Board Cert:** Otolaryngology 1988; **Med School:** Ros Franklin Univ/Chicago Med Sch 1982; **Resid:** Surgery, NYU Med Ctr 1984; Otolaryngology, NYU Med Ctr 1987; **Fellow:** Head and Neck Surgery, NYU Med Ctr 1988; **Fac Appt:** Assoc Clin Prof Oto, NYU Sch Med

Sacks, Steven H MD (Oto) - **Spec Exp:** Sinus Disorders/Surgery; Thyroid & Parathyroid Surgery; Salivary Gland Tumors & Surgery; **Hospital:** Mt Sinai Med Ctr (page 102); **Address:** 210 E 86th St, Fl 9th, ENT and Allergy Associates St, New York, NY 10028; **Phone:** 212-722-5570; **Board Cert:** Otolaryngology 1981; **Med School:** Washington Univ, St Louis 1977; **Resid:** Otolaryngology, Mt Sinai Hosp 1981; **Fac Appt:** Asst Clin Prof Oto, Mount Sinai Sch Med

Schaefer, Steven D MD (Oto) - **Spec Exp:** Sinus Disorders/Surgery; Head & Neck Surgery; Endoscopic Sinus Surgery; **Hospital:** Lenox Hill Hosp (Manh Eye, Ear & Throat Hosp) (page 106); **Address:** NY Head & Neck Inst, 110 W 59th St Fl 10 - Ste 10A, New York, NY 10022; **Phone:** 212-434-4500 x3; **Board Cert:** Otolaryngology 1978; **Med School:** UC Irvine 1972; **Resid:** Surgery, UCLA Med Ctr 1974; Otolaryngology, Stanford Med Ctr 1977; **Fac Appt:** Prof Oto, NY Med Coll

Schantz, Stimson P MD (Oto) - **Spec Exp:** Head & Neck Surgery; Head & Neck Cancer; Thyroid Cancer; **Hospital:** New York Eye & Ear Infirm (page 115), Beth Israel Med Ctr - Petrie Div (page 94); **Address:** 310 E 14th St Fl 6, New York, NY 10003; **Phone:** 212-979-4535; **Board Cert:** Surgery 2005; **Med School:** Univ Cincinnati 1975; **Resid:** Surgery, Georgetown Univ Med Ctr 1982; Otolaryngology, Univ Illinois Eye & Ear Infirm 1980; **Fellow:** Surgical Oncology, MD Anderson Cancer Ctr 1984; **Fac Appt:** Prof Oto, NY Med Coll

Schley, W Shain MD (Oto) - **Spec Exp:** Nasal & Sinus Disorders; Throat Disorders; Voice Disorders; Gastroesophageal Reflux Disease (GERD); **Hospital:** NY-Presby/Weill Cornell Med Ctr, NY (page 104); **Address:** 1305 York Ave Fl 5, New York, NY 10021; **Phone:** 646-962-2221; **Board Cert:** Otolaryngology 1973; **Med School:** Emory Univ 1966; **Resid:** Surgery, St Lukes-Roosevelt Hosp 1968; Otolaryngology, New York Presby Hosp 1973; **Fac Appt:** Assoc Clin Prof Oto, Cornell Univ-Weill Med Coll

Schneider, Kenneth L MD (Oto) - **Spec Exp:** Snoring/Sleep Apnea; Nasal & Sinus Disorders; Sleep Disorders/Apnea; **Hospital:** NYU Langone Med Ctr (page 108); **Address:** 240 E 38th St Fl 14, New York, NY 10016; **Phone:** 212-263-7165; **Board Cert:** Otolaryngology 1982; **Med School:** SUNY Downstate 1978; **Resid:** Otolaryngology, NYU Med Ctr 1982; **Fellow:** Head and Neck Surgery, Montefiore Med Ctr 1983; **Fac Appt:** Assoc Prof Oto, NYU Sch Med

Sclafani, Anthony P MD (Oto) - **Spec Exp:** Cosmetic Surgery-Face; Rhinoplasty; Botox Therapy; Facial Rejuvenation; **Hospital:** New York Eye & Ear Infirm (page 115), Northern Westchester Hosp (page 639); **Address:** 310 E 14th St, Fl 6, New York, NY 10003; **Phone:** 212-979-4534; **Board Cert:** Otolaryngology 1996; Facial Plastic & Reconstr Surgery 1999; **Med School:** Univ Pennsylvania 1989; **Resid:** Surgery, Beth Israel Med Ctr 1991; Otolaryngology, NY Eye & Ear Infirm 1995; **Fellow:** Facial Plastic Surgery, St Louis Univ 1996; **Fac Appt:** Prof Oto, NY Med Coll

Selesnick, Samuel H MD (Oto) - **Spec Exp:** Acoustic Neuroma; Cholesteatoma; Otosclerosis; **Hospital:** NY-Presby/Weill Cornell Med Ctr, NY (page 104), Meml Sloan-Kettering Canc Ctr (page 114); **Address:** 1305 York Ave, Fl 5, New York, NY 10021; **Phone:** 646-962-3277; **Board Cert:** Otolaryngology 1990; Neurotology 2008; **Med School:** NYU Sch Med 1985; **Resid:** Surgery, St Vincent's Med Ctr 1987; Otolaryngology, Manhattan EE&T Hosp 1990; **Fellow:** Skull Base Surgery, UCSF Med Ctr 1991; **Fac Appt:** Prof Oto, Cornell Univ-Weill Med Coll

Shemen, Larry J MD (Oto) - **Spec Exp:** Head & Neck Cancer; Thyroid Cancer; Parathyroid Cancer; Snoring/Sleep Apnea; **Hospital:** NY Hosp Queens (page 488), Lenox Hill Hosp (page 106); **Address:** 233 E 69th St, Ste 1D, New York, NY 10021; **Phone:** 212-472-8882; **Board Cert:** Otolaryngology 1983; **Med School:** Univ Toronto 1978; **Resid:** Surgery, Cedar-Sinai Med Ctr 1982; Otolaryngology, Toronto Genl Hosp 1983; **Fellow:** Head and Neck Surgery, Meml Sloan-Kettering Cancer Ctr 1984; **Fac Appt:** Assoc Clin Prof Oto, Cornell Univ-Weill Med Coll

Shugar, Joel MD (Oto) - **Spec Exp:** Facial Plastic Surgery; Head & Neck Surgery; Nasal & Sinus Disorders; **Hospital:** Mt Sinai Med Ctr (page 102); **Address:** 55 E 87th St, Ste 1K, New York, NY 10128-1043; **Phone:** 212-289-1731; **Board Cert:** Otolaryngology 1978; **Med School:** McGill Univ 1972; **Resid:** Surgery, Jewish Genl Hosp 1974; Otolaryngology, Mount Sinai Med Ctr 1978; **Fellow:** Otolaryngology, Mount Sinai Med Ctr 1975; **Fac Appt:** Assoc Clin Prof Oto, Mount Sinai Sch Med

Singh, Bhuvanesh MD/PhD (Oto) - **Spec Exp:** Head & Neck Cancer & Surgery; Thyroid Cancer; **Hospital:** Meml Sloan-Kettering Canc Ctr (page 114); **Address:** 1275 York Ave, MC C1073, New York, NY 10065; **Phone:** 212-639-2024; **Board Cert:** Otolaryngology 1998; **Med School:** SUNY Downstate 1991; **Resid:** Otolaryngology, SUNY Downstate Med Ctr 1997; **Fellow:** Head and Neck Surgery, Meml Sloan-Kettering Canc Ctr 1999; **Fac Appt:** Assoc Prof Oto, Cornell Univ-Weill Med Coll

Slavit, David H MD (Oto) - **Spec Exp:** Voice Disorders; Nasal & Sinus Disorders; Head & Neck Surgery; Thyroid Surgery; **Hospital:** Lenox Hill Hosp (page 106), Lenox Hill Hosp (Manh Eye, Ear & Throat Hosp) (page 106); **Address:** 787 Park Ave, New York, NY 10021-3552; **Phone:** 212-517-9177; **Board Cert:** Otolaryngology 1992; **Med School:** Mount Sinai Sch Med 1986; **Resid:** Otolaryngology, Mayo Clinic 1991; **Fac Appt:** Asst Prof Oto, SUNY Hlth Sci Ctr

Slupchynskyj, Oleh S MD (Oto) - **Spec Exp:** Facial Plastic & Reconstructive Surgery; Eyelid Surgery/Blepharoplasty; Facial Surgery-Chin & Lip; Rhinoplasty; **Hospital:** New York Eye & Ear Infirm (page 115), Lenox Hill Hosp (Manh Eye, Ear & Throat Hosp) (page 106); **Address:** The Aesthetic Institute of NY, 44 E 65th St, Ste 1a, New York, NY 10065; **Phone:** 212-628-6464; **Board Cert:** Otolaryngology 1998; Facial Plastic & Reconstr Surgery 2000; **Med School:** NY Med Coll 1991; **Resid:** Surgery, St. Vincent's Midtown 1993; Otolaryngology, New York Eye & Ear Infirm 1997; **Fellow:** Facial Plastic Surgery, Univ of Rochester Strong Meml Hosp 1998

Sperling, Neil M MD (Oto) - **Spec Exp:** Otosclerosis; Hearing Loss; Meniere's Disease; **Hospital:** New York Eye & Ear Infirm (page 115), SUNY Downstate Med Ctr (Univ Hosp Brooklyn) (page 441); **Address:** New York Otolaryngology Group, 36A E 36th St Fl 2, New York, NY 10016; **Phone:** 718-780-1498; **Board Cert:** Otolaryngology 1990; **Med School:** NY Med Coll 1985; **Resid:** Surgery, Beth Israel Med Ctr 1986; Otolaryngology, NY Eye & Ear Infirm 1990; **Fellow:** Otology, Minnesota Ear Clinic 1991; **Fac Appt:** Assoc Prof Oto, SUNY Downstate

Stewart, Michael G MD (Oto) - **Spec Exp:** Nasal & Sinus Disorders; Sleep Disorders/Apnea; Head & Neck Surgery; Vocal Cord Disorders; **Hospital:** NY-Presby/Weill Cornell Med Ctr, NY (page 104); **Address:** Weill Greenberg Center, 1305 York Ave Fl 5, New York, NY 10021; **Phone:** 646-962-6673; **Board Cert:** Otolaryngology 1995; **Med School:** Johns Hopkins Univ 1988; **Resid:** Surgery, Baylor Coll Med Affil Hosp 1990; Otolaryngology, Baylor Coll Med Affil Hosp 1994; **Fac Appt:** Prof Oto, Cornell Univ-Weill Med Coll

Storper, Ian S MD (Oto) - **Spec Exp:** Skull Base Surgery; Cochlear Implants; Acoustic Neuroma; Meniere's Disease; **Hospital:** Lenox Hill Hosp (Manh Eye, Ear & Throat Hosp) (page 106), Lenox Hill Hosp (page 106); **Address:** NY Head & Neck Inst, 110 E 59th St, Ste 10A, New York, NY 10022; **Phone:** 212-434-4500 x3; **Board Cert:** Otolaryngology 1995; **Med School:** Univ Pennsylvania 1988; **Resid:** Otolaryngology, UCLA Med Ctr 1994; **Fellow:** Otology & Neurotology, Ear Foundation 1995

Strome, Marshall MD (Oto) - **Spec Exp:** Voice Disorders; Swallowing Disorders; Head & Neck Cancer Reconstruction; Head & Neck Cancer & Surgery; **Hospital:** St. Luke's - Roosevelt Hosp Ctr - St Luke's Hosp (page 94), Mt Sinai Med Ctr (page 102); **Address:** 425 W 59th St, Fl 10, New York, NY 10019; **Phone:** 212-262-4444; **Board Cert:** Otolaryngology 1970; **Med School:** Univ Mich Med Sch 1964; **Resid:** Surgery, Harper Hosp 1966; Otolaryngology, Univ Michigan Hosp 1970; **Fac Appt:** Prof Oto, Univ Mich Med Sch

Sulica, Radu Lucian MD (Oto) - **Spec Exp:** Laryngeal Disorders; Voice Disorders; Vocal Cord Disorders; Botox Therapy; **Hospital:** NY-Presby/Weill Cornell Med Ctr, NY (page 104); **Address:** 1305 York Ave, Fl 5th Floor, New York, NY 10021; **Phone:** 646-962-4734; **Board Cert:** Otolaryngology 2000; **Med School:** Georgetown Univ 1993; **Resid:** Surgery, Georgetown Univ Hosp 1995; Otolaryngology, Georgetown Univ Hosp 1999; **Fellow:** Laryngology, St Lukes Roosevelt Hosp 2000; **Fac Appt:** Assoc Prof Oto, Cornell Univ-Weill Med Coll

Urken, Mark MD (Oto) - **Spec Exp:** Head & Neck Cancer & Surgery; Head & Neck Cancer Reconstruction; Thyroid & Parathyroid Cancer & Surgery; Salivary Gland Tumors; **Hospital:** Beth Israel Med Ctr - Petrie Div (page 94); **Address:** Inst for Head, Neck & Thyroid Cancer, 10 Union Square E, Ste 5B, New York, NY 10003-3314; **Phone:** 212-844-8775; **Board Cert:** Otolaryngology 1986; **Med School:** Univ VA Sch Med 1981; **Resid:** Otolaryngology, Mt Sinai Hosp 1986; **Fellow:** Microvascular Surgery, Mercy Hosp 1987; **Fac Appt:** Prof Oto, Albert Einstein Coll Med

Volpi, David O MD (Oto) - **Spec Exp:** Sinus Disorders; Sleep Disorders; Snoring/Sleep Apnea; **Hospital:** Lenox Hill Hosp (page 106), New York Eye & Ear Infirm (page 115); **Address:** eOs Sleep, 262 Central Park West, Ste 1H, New York, NY 10024; **Phone:** 212-873-6036; **Board Cert:** Otolaryngology 1988; **Med School:** Hahnemann Univ 1982; **Resid:** Surgery, Hosp Univ Penn 1984; Otolaryngology, NY Eye & Ear Infirm 1988

Waner, Milton MD (Oto) - **Spec Exp:** Pediatric Facial Plastic Surgery; Birthmarks/Hemangiomas; Vascular Malformations; **Hospital:** Lenox Hill Hosp (Manh Eye, Ear & Throat Hosp) (page 106); **Address:** The Center for Vascular Birthmarks, 210 E 64th St Fl 7, New York, NY 10065; **Phone:** 212-434-4050; **Med School:** South Africa 1977; **Resid:** Surgery, Univ of Witwatersrand 1980; Otolaryngology, Univ of Witwatersrand 1984; **Fellow:** Otolaryngology, Univ Cincinnatti Med Ctr 1985

Wong, Richard J MD (Oto) - **Spec Exp:** Head & Neck Cancer; Thyroid Cancer; **Hospital:** Meml Sloan-Kettering Canc Ctr (page 114); **Address:** 1275 York Ave, C-1069, New York, NY 10065; **Phone:** 212-639-7638; **Board Cert:** Otolaryngology 2000; **Med School:** Harvard Med Sch 1994; **Resid:** Otolaryngology, Mass General Hosp 1999; **Fellow:** Head & Neck Surgical Oncology, Meml Sloan Kettering Cancer Ctr 2000

Woo, Peak MD (Oto) - **Spec Exp:** Voice Disorders; Laryngeal Disorders; Laryngeal Cancer; **Hospital:** Mt Sinai Med Ctr (page 102); **Address:** 300 Central Park West, Ste 1-H, New York, NY 10024; **Phone:** 212-580-1004; **Board Cert:** Otolaryngology 1983; **Med School:** Boston Univ 1978; **Resid:** Otolaryngology, Boston Univ Med Ctr 1983; **Fac Appt:** Clin Prof Oto, Mount Sinai Sch Med

Zimbler, Marc S MD (Oto) - **Spec Exp:** Cosmetic Surgery-Face; Blepharoplasty; Rhinoplasty; Reconstructive Surgery-Face; **Hospital:** Beth Israel Med Ctr - Petrie Div (page 94), Lenox Hill Hosp (Manh Eye, Ear & Throat Hosp) (page 106); **Address:** 990 Fifth Ave, New York, NY 10075; **Phone:** 212-570-9900; **Board Cert:** Otolaryngology 2001; Facial Plastic & Reconstr Surgery 2012; **Med School:** Mount Sinai Sch Med 1993; **Resid:** Surgery, NYU Med Ctr 1995; Otolaryngology, NYU Med Ctr 1999; **Fellow:** Facial Plastic Surgery, Washington Univ 2000; **Fac Appt:** Asst Prof Oto, Albert Einstein Coll Med

Pain Medicine

Ahmed Hosny, M Amr MD (PM) - **Spec Exp:** Pain-Spine; Pain-Neuropathic; Pain-Chronic; **Address:** NY Pain Care, 95 University Pl Fl 8, New York, NY 10003; **Phone:** 212-604-1300; **Board Cert:** Anesthesiology 2003; Pain Medicine 2004; Hospice & Palliative Medicine 2008; **Med School:** Egypt 1995; **Resid:** Anesthesiology, St Lukes-Roosevelt Hosp Ctr 2002; **Fellow:** Pain Management, Beth Israel Deaconess Med Ctr 2003; **Fac Appt:** Assoc Prof Anes, NY Med Coll

Bakshi, Sanjay MD (PM) - **Spec Exp:** Pain-Spine; Pain-Back & Neck; **Hospital:** Lenox Hill Hosp (page 106), Bayshore Community Hosp; **Address:** Manhattan Spine & Pain Medicine, 115 E 57th St, Ste 610, New York, NY 10022; **Phone:** 212-535-3505; **Board Cert:** Anesthesiology 1995; Pain Medicine 2007; **Med School:** India 1989; **Resid:** Anesthesiology, Brookdale Hosp Med Ctr 1994; **Fellow:** Pain Medicine, Johns Hopkins Hosp 1995

Diwan, Sudhir MD (PM) - **Spec Exp:** Pain-after Spinal Intervention; Pain-Musculoskeletal; Pain-Neuropathic; Pain-Cancer; **Hospital:** Lenox Hill Hosp (page 106); **Address:** Manhattan Spine & Pain Med, 115 E 57th St, Ste 610, New York, NY 10022; **Phone:** 212-535-3505; **Board Cert:** Anesthesiology 2012; Pain Medicine 2013; **Med School:** India 1983; **Resid:** Surgery, St Lukes-Roosevelt Hosp Ctr 1994; Anesthesiology, St Lukes-Roosevelt Hosp Ctr 1997; **Fellow:** Pain Medicine, NY-Presby/Weill Cornell Med Ctr 1998

Epstein, Lawrence J MD (PM) - **Spec Exp:** Pain-Spine; Pain-Neck; Sciatica; **Hospital:** Mt Sinai Med Ctr (page 102); **Address:** Mount Sinai Medical Ctr, Pain Management, 5 E 98th St Fl 6, New York, NY 10029; **Phone:** 212-241-6372; **Board Cert:** Anesthesiology 1987; Pain Medicine 2004; **Med School:** Israel 1983; **Resid:** Anesthesiology, SUNY Brooklyn Med Ctr 1986; **Fellow:** Obstetrics & Anesthesiology, SUNY Brooklyn Med Ctr 1987; **Fac Appt:** Asst Prof Anes, Mount Sinai Sch Med

Freedman, Gordon MD (PM) - **Spec Exp:** Pain-Back & Neck; Reflex Sympathetic Dystrophy (RSD); Pain-Neuropathic; Pain-Cancer; **Hospital:** Mt Sinai Med Ctr (page 102), Mount Sinai Hosp of Queens (page 102); **Address:** 1540 York Ave, New York, NY 10028; **Phone:** 212-288-2180; **Board Cert:** Anesthesiology 1992; Pain Medicine 2004; **Med School:** Israel 1985; **Resid:** Anesthesiology, Mt Sinai Hosp 1991; **Fellow:** Pain Medicine, Mt Sinai Hosp 1991; **Fac Appt:** Assoc Prof Anes, Mount Sinai Sch Med

Gharibo, Christopher G MD (PM) - **Spec Exp:** Pain-Back & Neck; Pain-Neuropathic; Pain-Chronic; Complex Regional Pain Syndromes; **Hospital:** NYU Langone Med Ctr (page 108), NYU Hosp For Joint Dis (page 108); **Address:** Ctr for Musculoskeletal Care, 333 E 38th St N Fl 6, New York, NY 10016; **Phone:** 646-501-7246; **Board Cert:** Anesthesiology 1997; Pain Medicine 2009; **Med School:** UMDNJ-NJ Med Sch, Newark 1992; **Resid:** Internal Medicine, UMDNJ-RW Johnson Univ Hosp 1993; Anesthesiology, NYU Med Ctr 1996; **Fellow:** Pain Medicine, Jefferson Univ Hosp 1997; **Fac Appt:** Assoc Prof Anes, NYU Sch Med

Gusmorino, Paul MD (PM) - **Spec Exp:** Pain-Chronic; Pain Rehabilitation & Psychiatry; **Hospital:** NYU Hosp For Joint Dis (page 108); **Address:** 246 E 20th St, New York, NY 10003; **Phone:** 212-598-6606; **Board Cert:** Psychiatry 1980; Child & Adolescent Psychiatry 1982; Pain Medicine 2006; **Med School:** Italy 1974; **Resid:** Psychiatry, Kings County Hosp 1978; **Fellow:** Child & Adolescent Psychiatry, NY Hosp 1980; **Fac Appt:** Asst Clin Prof Psyc, NYU Sch Med

Jain, Subhash MD (PM) - **Spec Exp:** Pain-Cancer; Pain-Pelvic; Reflex Sympathetic Dystrophy (RSD); Complex Regional Pain Syndromes; **Hospital:** Beth Israel Med Ctr - Petrie Div (page 94); **Address:** 360 E 72nd St, Ste C, New York, NY 10021; **Phone:** 212-439-6100; **Board Cert:** Anesthesiology 1994; **Med School:** India 1968; **Resid:** Surgery, St Vincent Med Ctr 1977; Anesthesiology, New York Hosp 1979; **Fellow:** Pain Medicine, New York Hosp/Meml Sloan Kettering Cancer Ctr 1980; **Fac Appt:** Assoc Prof Anes, Cornell Univ-Weill Med Coll

Kahn, Stuart B MD (PM) - **Spec Exp:** Pain Management; Pain-Spine; Acupuncture; **Hospital:** Mt Sinai Med Ctr (page 102); **Address:** 17 E 102nd St Fl 5, New York, NY 10029; **Phone:** 212-241-1075; **Board Cert:** Physical Medicine & Rehabilitation 2003; Pain Medicine 2011; **Med School:** SUNY Stony Brook 1988; **Resid:** Physical Medicine & Rehabilitation, Columbia-Presby Med Ctr 1992; **Fellow:** Medical Acupuncture, UCLA Sch Med 1995; **Fac Appt:** Assoc Prof PMR, Mount Sinai Sch Med

Kaplan, Ronald MD (PM) - **Spec Exp:** Pain-Chronic; **Hospital:** Beth Israel Med Ctr - Petrie Div (page 94); **Address:** Pain Medicine & Palliative Care, 10 Union Square E, Ste 2R, New York, NY 10003; **Phone:** 212-844-8930; **Board Cert:** Anesthesiology 2009; Pain Medicine 2014; **Med School:** Univ MD Sch Med 1974; **Resid:** Anesthesiology, Univ Maryland Hosp 1978; **Fellow:** Pediatric Anesthesiology, Chldns Hosp 1979; **Fac Appt:** Clin Prof Anes, Albert Einstein Coll Med

Kotkes, Herschel MD (PM) - **Spec Exp:** Pain-Interventional Techniques; Pain-Back & Neck; Pain-Neuropathic; Reflex Sympathetic Dystrophy (RSD); **Hospital:** Beth Israel Med Ctr - Petrie Div (page 94); **Address:** Manhattan Spine & Sports Medicine, 305 E 55th St, Ste 206, New York, NY 10022; **Phone:** 212-319-1339; **Board Cert:** Anesthesiology 2004; Pain Medicine 2005; **Med School:** Israel 1998; **Resid:** Anesthesiology, Hosp Univ Penn 2002; **Fellow:** Pain Medicine, Hosp Univ Penn 2004

Kreitzer, Joel M MD (PM) - **Spec Exp:** Pain-Back; Pain-Cancer; Pain-Neuropathic; **Hospital:** Mt Sinai Med Ctr (page 102), Mount Sinai Hosp of Queens (page 102); **Address:** Upper East Side Pain Medicine, 1540 York Ave, New York, NY 10028; **Phone:** 212-288-2180; **Board Cert:** Anesthesiology 1990; Pain Medicine 2004; **Med School:** Albert Einstein Coll Med 1985; **Resid:** Anesthesiology, Mt Sinai Hosp 1989; **Fellow:** Pain Medicine, Mt Sinai Hosp 1989; **Fac Appt:** Assoc Clin Prof Anes, Mount Sinai Sch Med

Marcus, Norman J MD (PM) - **Spec Exp:** Pain-Back & Neck; Headache; Pain-Musculoskeletal; Reflex Sympathetic Dystrophy (RSD); **Hospital:** NYU Langone Med Ctr (page 108), Lenox Hill Hosp (page 106); **Address:** 30 E 40th St, Ste 1100, New York, NY 10016-1201; **Phone:** 212-532-7999; **Board Cert:** Psychiatry 1974; Pain Medicine 1993; **Med School:** SUNY Upstate Med Univ 1967; **Resid:** Psychiatry, Montefiore Med Ctr 1971; **Fellow:** Psychosomatic Medicine, Montefiore Med Ctr 1973; Pain Medicine, Lenox Hill Hosp 1995; **Fac Appt:** Assoc Clin Prof Anes, NYU Sch Med

Moqtaderi, Farideh MD (PM) - **Spec Exp:** Acupuncture; Pain-Musculoskeletal; Herpetic Neuralgia (Shingles); Fibromyalgia; **Hospital:** Mt Sinai Med Ctr (page 102); **Address:** One Belmont Drive, Ste 1, Irvington, NY 10533-4850; **Phone:** 917-916-6869; **Board Cert:** Anesthesiology 1973; **Med School:** Iran 1966; **Resid:** Anesthesiology, Mount Sinai Hosp 1969; Anesthesiology, Meml Sloan Kettering Hosp 1971; **Fellow:** Pain Medicine, Westchester Co Med Ctr 1973; Critical Care Anesthesiology, Meml Sloan Ketting Hosp 1973; **Fac Appt:** Asst Clin Prof Anes, Mount Sinai Sch Med

Ngeow, Jeffrey Y MD (PM) - **Spec Exp:** Pain-Musculoskeletal-Spine & Neck; Reflex Sympathetic Dystrophy (RSD); Acupuncture; Pain-Neuropathic; **Hospital:** Hosp For Special Surgery (page 113); **Address:** Hosp Spec Surg-Integrative Care Ctr, 635 Madison Ave Fl 5, New York, NY 10022; **Phone:** 212-224-7918; **Board Cert:** Anesthesiology 1980; Pain Medicine 2005; **Med School:** England, UK 1971; **Resid:** Anesthesiology, Peter Bent Brigham Hosp 1977; **Fellow:** Pain Medicine, Tufts New England Med Ctr 1978; **Fac Appt:** Assoc Clin Prof Anes, Cornell Univ-Weill Med Coll

Richman, Daniel MD (PM) - **Spec Exp:** Pain-Back & Neck; Complex Regional Pain Syndromes; Reflex Sympathetic Dystrophy (RSD); Pain-Neuropathic; **Hospital:** Hosp For Special Surgery (page 113); **Address:** Hosp Special Surgery, Pain Mgmt Ctr, 429 E 75th St Fl 5, New York, NY 10021; **Phone:** 212-606-1768; **Board Cert:** Anesthesiology 1991; Pain Medicine 2005; **Med School:** UMDNJ-NJ Med Sch, Newark 1986; **Resid:** Anesthesiology, Hartford Hosp 1990; **Fellow:** Pain Medicine, Hosp Special Surgery 1991; **Fac Appt:** Asst Clin Prof Anes, Cornell Univ-Weill Med Coll

Schottenstein, Douglas C MD (PM) - **Spec Exp:** Pain-Spine; Pain-Musculoskeletal; Arthritis; Regenokine Therapy (PRP); **Hospital:** NY-Presby/Columbia Univ Med Ctr, NY (page 104); **Address:** 18 E 48th St, Ste 901, New York, NY 10017; **Phone:** 212-750-1155; **Board Cert:** Neurology 2005; Pain Medicine 2006; **Med School:** Ohio State Univ 2000; **Resid:** Neurology, Emory Univ Hosps 2004; **Fellow:** Pain Medicine, NY Presby-Columbia Med Ctr 2005

Thomas, Gary P MD (PM) - **Spec Exp:** Pain-Neuropathic; Fibromyalgia; Headache; Pain-after Spinal Intervention; **Hospital:** Beth Israel Med Ctr - Petrie Div (page 94), New York Methodist Hosp (page 440); **Address:** Comprehensive Pain Mngmt, 10 Union Square E, Ste 4K, New York, NY 10003; **Phone:** 212-995-6495; **Board Cert:** Pain Medicine 2007; Anesthesiology 1996; **Med School:** Mount Sinai Sch Med 1991; **Resid:** Anesthesiology, Mount Sinai Med Ctr 1995; **Fellow:** Pain Medicine, Mount Sinai Med Ctr 1996

Waldman, Seth MD (PM) - **Spec Exp:** Pain-Spine; Pain-Neuropathic; Sciatica; **Hospital:** Hosp For Special Surgery (page 113), Burke Rehab Hosp; **Address:** Hosp For Special Surgery, 535 E 70th St, New York, NY 10021-4872; **Phone:** 212-606-1686; **Board Cert:** Anesthesiology 1994; Pain Medicine 2005; **Med School:** Albany Med Coll 1988; **Resid:** Internal Medicine, Beth Israel Med Ctr 1990; Anesthesiology, Beth Israel Deaconess Hosp 1993; **Fellow:** Pain Medicine, Beth Israel Hosp/Mass Genl Hosp 1994; **Fac Appt:** Asst Clin Prof Anes, Cornell Univ-Weill Med Coll

Weinberger, Michael L MD (PM) - **Spec Exp:** Pain-Cancer; Pain-Back; Palliative Care; **Hospital:** NY-Presby/Columbia Univ Med Ctr, NY (page 104); **Address:** 630 W 168th St, PH5, rm 500, New York, NY 10032-3720; **Phone:** 212-305-7114; **Board Cert:** Internal Medicine 1986; Anesthesiology 1990; Pain Medicine 2004; Hospice & Palliative Medicine 2006; **Med School:** Columbia P&S 1983; **Resid:** Internal Medicine, St Vincent's Hosp 1986; Anesthesiology, Columbia-Presby Med Ctr 1989; **Fellow:** Pain Medicine, Meml Sloan Kettering Cancer Ctr 1990; **Fac Appt:** Assoc Prof Anes, Columbia P&S

Zou, Shengping MD (PM) - **Spec Exp:** Pain-Chronic; Pain-Back; Pain-Neuropathic; Pain-Cancer; **Hospital:** NYU Langone Med Ctr (page 108); **Address:** 240 E 38th St Fl 14, New York, NY 10016; **Phone:** 212-201-1004; **Board Cert:** Anesthesiology 1999; Pain Medicine 2012; **Med School:** China 1986; **Resid:** Anesthesiology, UMDNJ Med Ctr 1998; **Fellow:** Pain Medicine, UMDNJ Med Ctr 1999; **Fac Appt:** Asst Clin Prof Anes, NYU Sch Med

Pathology

Antonescu, Cristina R MD (Path) - **Spec Exp:** Bone Pathology; Sarcoma-Soft Tissue; Ewing's Sarcoma; **Hospital:** Meml Sloan-Kettering Canc Ctr (page 114); **Address:** Meml Sloan Kettering Cancer Ctr, Dept Pathology, 1275 York Ave, New York, NY 10021; **Phone:** 212-639-5905; **Board Cert:** Anatomic Pathology 1998; **Med School:** Romania 1992; **Resid:** Anatomic Pathology, Lenox Hill Hosp 1996; **Fellow:** Pathology-Oncology, Meml Sloan-Kettering Canc Ctr 1997; **Fac Appt:** Assoc Prof Path, Cornell Univ-Weill Med Coll

Bleiweiss, Ira J MD (Path) - **Spec Exp:** Breast Pathology; Breast Cancer; **Hospital:** Mt Sinai Med Ctr (page 102); **Address:** Mt Sinai Med Ctr, Dept Pathology, 1 Gustave Levy Pl, Box 1194, New York, NY 10029-6504; **Phone:** 212-241-9159; **Board Cert:** Anatomic & Clinical Pathology 1988; **Med School:** West Indies 1984; **Resid:** Pathology, Mt Sinai Med Ctr 1988; **Fellow:** Surgical Pathology, Mt Sinai Med Ctr 1989; Surgical Pathology, Meml-Sloan Kettering Cancer Ctr 1990; **Fac Appt:** Prof Path, Mount Sinai Sch Med

Cohen, Jean-Marc MD (Path) - **Spec Exp:** Breast Pathology; Thyroid Disorders; **Hospital:** Beth Israel Med Ctr - Petrie Div (page 94); **Address:** 10 Union Square East, PACC Bldg, Ste 4H, New York, NY 10003; **Phone:** 212-844-8962; **Board Cert:** Anatomic Pathology 1997; Cytopathology 1997; **Med School:** France 1985; **Resid:** Pathology, Mount Sinai Med Ctr 1991; **Fellow:** Cytopathology, Montefiore Med Ctr-Moses Campus 1992

Ellenson, Lora Hendrick MD (Path) - **Spec Exp:** Gynecologic Pathology; Endometrial Cancer; Cervical Cancer; Ovarian Cancer; **Hospital:** NY-Presby/Weill Cornell Med Ctr, NY (page 104); **Address:** NY-Presby/Weill Cornell, Pathology Dept, 525 E 68th St, Starr Pavilion, 10th Fl, New York, NY 10021; **Phone:** 212-746-2700; **Board Cert:** Anatomic Pathology 1990; **Med School:** Stanford Univ 1986; **Resid:** Anatomic Pathology, Johns Hopkins Univ 1990; **Fac Appt:** Prof Path, Cornell Univ-Weill Med Coll

Harpaz, Noam MD/PhD (Path) - **Spec Exp:** Gastrointestinal Pathology; **Hospital:** Mt Sinai Med Ctr (page 102); **Address:** 1468 Madison Ave, Annenberg Bldg Fl 15 - rm 38, New York, NY 10029; **Phone:** 212-241-9115; **Board Cert:** Anatomic & Clinical Pathology 1986; **Med School:** Univ Miami Sch Med 1981; **Resid:** Anatomic & Clinical Pathology, Mt Sinai Med Ctr 1985; **Fac Appt:** Prof Path, Mount Sinai Sch Med

Hoda, Syed A MD (Path) - **Spec Exp:** Breast Cancer; Surgical Pathology; **Hospital:** NY-Presby/Weill Cornell Med Ctr, NY (page 104); **Address:** 525 E 68th St, 1028 Starr, New York, NY 10021-4870; **Phone:** 212-746-2700; **Board Cert:** Anatomic & Clinical Pathology 2012; Cytopathology 1991; **Med School:** Pakistan 1984; **Resid:** Anatomic & Clinical Pathology, Tulane Univ Affil Hosps 1990; **Fellow:** Cytopathology, Meml Sloan Kettering Cancer Ctr 1991; Pathology, Meml Sloan Kettering Cancer Ctr 1992; **Fac Appt:** Clin Prof Path, Cornell Univ-Weill Med Coll

Jessurun, Jose MD (Path) - **Spec Exp:** Gastrointestinal Pathology; **Hospital:** NY-Presby/Weill Cornell Med Ctr, NY (page 104); **Address:** 525 E 68th St, New York, NY 10065; **Phone:** 212-746-2700; **Board Cert:** Anatomic Pathology 1985; **Med School:** Mexico 1978; **Resid:** Internal Medicine, Genl Hosp 1982; Pathology, Jackson Meml Hosp 1983; **Fellow:** Pathology, Mass Genl Hosp 1984; Gastrointestinal Pathology, Johns Hopkins Hosp 1986; **Fac Appt:** Prof Path, Univ Minn

Klimstra, David MD (Path) - **Spec Exp:** Gastrointestinal Pathology; Pulmonary Pathology; **Hospital:** Meml Sloan-Kettering Canc Ctr (page 114); **Address:** Meml Sloan Kettering Canc Ctr, Dept Pathology, 1275 York Ave, New York, NY 10065; **Phone:** 212-639-5905; **Board Cert:** Anatomic Pathology 1992; **Med School:** Yale Univ 1988; **Resid:** Pathology, Yale New Haven Hosp 1991; **Fellow:** Pathology, Meml Sloan Kettering Canc Ctr 1992; **Fac Appt:** Asst Prof Path, Cornell Univ

Magro, Cynthia M MD (Path) - **Spec Exp:** Cutaneous Lymphoma; **Hospital:** NY-Presby/Weill Cornell Med Ctr, NY (page 104); **Address:** 1300 York Ave, Ste F310, New York, NY 10065; **Phone:** 212-746-6434; **Board Cert:** Anatomic Pathology 1988; Dermatopathology 1990; Cytopathology 1991; **Med School:** Univ Manitoba 1984; **Resid:** Anatomic Pathology, Mass Genl Hosp 1988; **Fellow:** Cytopathology, Mass Genl Hosp 1989; Dermatology, Mass Genl Hosp 1991

Melamed, Jonathan MD (Path) - **Spec Exp:** Prostate Cancer; Tumor Banking-Prostate; **Hospital:** NYU Langone Med Ctr (page 108); **Address:** NYU Medical Ctr, Dept Pathology, TH-461, 560 First Ave, New York, NY 10016; **Phone:** 212-263-8927; **Board Cert:** Anatomic & Clinical Pathology 1992; **Med School:** South Africa 1985; **Resid:** Pathology, Lenox Hill Hosp 1991; **Fellow:** Pathology, Meml Sloan Kettering Cancer Ctr 1992; Urologic Pathology, Meml Sloan Kettering Cancer Ctr 1993; **Fac Appt:** Prof Path, NYU Sch Med

Orazi, Attilio MD (Path) - **Spec Exp:** Hematopathology; Bone Marrow Pathology; Lymph Node Pathology; Spleen Pathology; **Hospital:** NY-Presby/Weill Cornell Med Ctr, NY (page 104); **Address:** NY Presby-Cornell Medical Ctr, 525 E 68th St, Starr Pavilion, rm 715, New York, NY 10065; **Phone:** 212-746-2050; **Board Cert:** Anatomic Pathology 1997; Hematology 1998; **Med School:** Italy 1979; **Resid:** Internal Medicine, Leicester Royal Infirmary 1982; Histopathology, Northampton Genl Hosp 1983; **Fellow:** Anatomic Pathology, Natl Cancer Inst 1985; **Fac Appt:** Prof Path, Cornell Univ-Weill Med Coll

Reuter, Victor E MD (Path) - **Spec Exp:** Prostate Cancer; Genitourinary Pathology; Bladder Cancer; Testicular Cancer; **Hospital:** Meml Sloan-Kettering Canc Ctr (page 114); **Address:** Memorial Sloan Kettering Cancer Ctr, Dept Pathology, 1275 York Ave, New York, NY 10021; **Phone:** 212-639-6780; **Board Cert:** Anatomic & Clinical Pathology 1983; **Med School:** Dominican Republic 1978; **Resid:** Anatomic Pathology, Thos Jefferson Univ Hosp 1981; Clinical Pathology, Thos Jefferson Univ Hosp 1983; **Fellow:** Surgical Pathology, Meml Sloan Kettering Cancer Ctr 1985; **Fac Appt:** Prof Path, Cornell Univ-Weill Med Coll

Rosenblum, Marc K MD (Path) - **Spec Exp:** Neuro-Pathology; Brain Tumors; **Hospital:** Meml Sloan-Kettering Canc Ctr (page 114); **Address:** Meml Sloan-Kettering Cancer Ctr, 1275 York Ave, New York, NY 10065; **Phone:** 212-639-3844; **Board Cert:** Anatomic Pathology 1984; Neuropathology 1988; **Med School:** Univ Miami Sch Med 1979; **Resid:** Anatomic Pathology, Mt Sinai Med Ctr 1984; **Fellow:** Pathology, Meml Sloan-Kettering Cancer Ctr 1985; Neurological Pathology, Bellevue-NYU Med Ctr 1987; **Fac Appt:** Prof Path, Cornell Univ-Weill Med Coll

Soslow, Robert A MD (Path) - **Spec Exp:** Gynecologic Pathology; **Hospital:** Meml Sloan-Kettering Canc Ctr (page 114); **Address:** 1275 York Avenue, Pathology Department, New York, NY 10065; **Phone:** 212-639-5905; **Board Cert:** Anatomic Pathology 1995; **Med School:** Univ Pennsylvania 1991; **Resid:** Anatomic Pathology, Stanford Univ Med Ctr 1994; **Fellow:** Immunopathology, Stanford Univ Med Ctr 1995; **Fac Appt:** Assoc Prof Path, Cornell Univ

Thung, Swan N MD (Path) - **Spec Exp:** Liver Pathology; Immunopathology; Liver Tumors; **Hospital:** Mt Sinai Med Ctr (page 102); **Address:** Mount Sinai Med Ctr-Pathology Dept, 1 Gustave L Levy Plaza, New York, NY 10029; **Phone:** 212-241-9139; **Board Cert:** Anatomic & Clinical Pathology 1977; Immunopathology 1983; **Med School:** Indonesia 1970; **Resid:** Anatomic & Clinical Pathology, James J. Peters VA Med Ctr 1977; **Fac Appt:** Prof Path, Mount Sinai Sch Med

Travis, William D MD (Path) - **Spec Exp:** Pulmonary Pathology; Lung Cancer; **Hospital:** Meml Sloan-Kettering Canc Ctr (page 114); **Address:** Meml Sloan Kettering Cancer Ctr-Dept Path, 1275 York Ave, New York, NY 10065; **Phone:** 212-639-6364; **Board Cert:** Anatomic & Clinical Pathology 1985; **Med School:** Univ Fla Coll Med 1981; **Resid:** Anatomic Pathology, New England Deaconess Hosp 1983; Clinical Pathology, Mayo Clinic 1985; **Fellow:** Surgical Pathology, Mayo Clinic 1986

Wang, Beverly Y MD (Path) - **Spec Exp:** Head & Neck Pathology; **Hospital:** Beth Israel Med Ctr - Petrie Div (page 94); **Address:** Beth Israel Medical Ctr, Dept Pathology, First Avenue at 16th St, Silver Bldg Fl 11, New York, NY 10003; **Phone:** 212-844-1959; **Board Cert:** Anatomic Pathology 1998; Cytopathology 1999; **Med School:** China 1982; **Resid:** Pathology, Mount Sinai Med Ctr 1998; **Fellow:** Cytopathology, Mount Sinai Med Ctr 1999; **Fac Appt:** Prof Path, Albert Einstein Coll Med

Wenig, Bruce M MD (Path) - **Spec Exp:** Head & Neck Pathology; Surgical Pathology; Endocrine Pathology; **Hospital:** Beth Israel Med Ctr - Petrie Div (page 94), St. Luke's - Roosevelt Hosp Ctr - St Luke's Hosp (page 94); **Address:** Beth Israel Med Ctr, Dept Pathology, First Ave at 16th St, 11 Silver, Rm 34, New York, NY 10003; **Phone:** 212-420-4031; **Board Cert:** Anatomic & Clinical Pathology 1985; **Med School:** Israel 1981; **Resid:** Pathology, Mt Sinai Med Ctr 1985; Surgical Pathology, Cedars-Sinai Med Ctr 1986; **Fellow:** Head and Neck Pathology, AFIP 1987; **Fac Appt:** Prof Path, Albert Einstein Coll Med

Zagzag, David MD/PhD (Path) - **Spec Exp:** Neuro-Pathology; Brain Tumors; Tumor Banking-Brain; **Hospital:** NYU Langone Med Ctr (page 108), Bellevue Hosp Ctr; **Address:** NYU Med Ctr, Dept Pathology, 550 First Ave, Div Neuropathology, NB-4N30, New York, NY 10016; **Phone:** 212-263-6449; **Board Cert:** Anatomic Pathology 1993; Neuropathology 1993; **Med School:** France 1984; **Resid:** Surgical Pathology, NYU Med Ctr 1990; **Fellow:** Neurological Pathology, NYU Med Ctr 1992; **Fac Appt:** Assoc Prof Path, NYU Sch Med

Pediatric Allergy & Immunology

Ehrlich, Paul M MD (PA&I) - **Spec Exp:** Asthma; Food Allergy; **Hospital:** NYU Langone Med Ctr (page 108), New York Eye & Ear Infirm (page 115); **Address:** Allergy & Asthma Assocs of Murray Hill, 35 E 35th St, Ste 202, New York, NY 10016-3823; **Phone:** 212-685-4225; **Board Cert:** Pediatrics 1975; Allergy & Immunology 1977; **Med School:** NYU Sch Med 1970; **Resid:** Pediatrics, Bellevue Hosp Ctr 1973; **Fellow:** Allergy & Immunology, Walter Reed Army Med Ctr 1976; **Fac Appt:** Asst Clin Prof Ped, NYU Sch Med

Herzog, Ronit MD (PA&I) - **Spec Exp:** Asthma & Allergy; Sinusitis; Food Allergy; **Hospital:** NY-Presby/Weill Cornell Med Ctr, NY (page 104); **Address:** NY-Presby, Ped Allergy & Immunology, 505 E 70 St Fl 3, Helmsley Tower, New York, NY 10021; **Phone:** 646-962-3410; **Board Cert:** Pediatrics 2006; Allergy & Immunology 2013; **Med School:** Israel 1991; **Resid:** Pediatrics, Long Island Jewish Med Ctr 1998; **Fellow:** Pediatric Pulmonology, Mount Sinai Med Ctr 2004; Allergy & Immunology, Albert Einstein Coll Med 2006; **Fac Appt:** Asst Prof Ped, Cornell Univ-Weill Med Coll

Nowak-Wegrzyn, Anna MD (PA&I) - **Spec Exp:** Food Allergy; **Hospital:** Mt Sinai Med Ctr (page 102); **Address:** Mount Sinai, Ped Allergy & Immun, 5 E 98 St Fl 10, New York, NY 10029; **Phone:** 212-241-5548; **Board Cert:** Pediatrics 2012; Allergy & Immunology 2012; **Med School:** Poland 1990; **Resid:** Pediatrics, Univ MD Med Ctr 1997; **Fellow:** Allergy & Immunology, Johns Hopkins Hosp 2000; **Fac Appt:** Assoc Prof Ped, Mount Sinai Sch Med

Sampson Jr, Hugh A MD (PA&I) - **Spec Exp:** Food Allergy; Eczema; Atopic Dermatitis; **Hospital:** Mt Sinai Med Ctr (page 102); **Address:** Faculty Practice Assocs, 5 E 98th St Fl 10, New York, NY 10029; **Phone:** 212-241-5548; **Board Cert:** Pediatrics 1980; Allergy & Immunology 1981; **Med School:** SUNY Buffalo 1975; **Resid:** Pediatrics, Chldns Meml Hosp 1979; **Fellow:** Allergy & Immunology, Duke Univ Med Ctr 1980; **Fac Appt:** Prof Ped, Mount Sinai Sch Med

Sicherer, Scott H MD (PA&I) - **Spec Exp:** Food Allergy; Drug Sensitivity; Eczema; Asthma; **Hospital:** Mt Sinai Med Ctr (page 102); **Address:** Faculty Practice Assocs, 5 E 98th St Fl 10, New York, NY 10029-6500; **Phone:** 212-241-5548; **Board Cert:** Pediatrics 2008; Allergy & Immunology 2007; **Med School:** Johns Hopkins Univ 1990; **Resid:** Pediatrics, Mt Sinai Hosp 1994; **Fellow:** Allergy & Immunology, Johns Hopkins Hosp 1997; **Fac Appt:** Prof Ped, Mount Sinai Sch Med

Wang, Julie MD (PA&I) - **Spec Exp:** Food Allery; Anaphylaxis; Immunotherapy; **Hospital:** Mt Sinai Med Ctr (page 102); **Address:** Mount Sinai, Ped Allergy & Immun, 5 E 98 St Fl 10, New York, NY 10029; **Phone:** 212-241-5548; **Board Cert:** Pediatrics 2011; Allergy & Immunology 2005; **Med School:** Cornell Univ-Weill Med Coll 2000; **Resid:** Pediatrics, NY-Presby/Weill Cornell Med Ctr 2003; **Fellow:** Allergy & Immunology, Mount Sinai Med Ctr 2005; **Fac Appt:** Asst Prof Ped, Mount Sinai Sch Med

Pediatric Cardiology

Addonizio, Linda J MD (PCd) - **Spec Exp:** Transplant Medicine-Heart; Heart Failure; Hypertrophic Cardiomyopathy; **Hospital:** Morgan Stanley Children's Hosp of NY-Presby, NY (page 104); **Address:** NY-Presby/Morgan Stanley Chldns Hosp, 3953 Broadway N, Ste 229, New York, NY 10032; **Phone:** 212-305-6575; **Board Cert:** Pediatrics 1983; Pediatric Cardiology 1985; **Med School:** Columbia P&S 1978; **Resid:** Pediatrics, NY-Presby/Columbia Univ Med Ctr 1981; **Fellow:** Pediatric Cardiology, NY-Presby/Columbia Univ Med Ctr 1984; **Fac Appt:** Prof Ped, Columbia P&S

Altmann, Karen MD (PCd) - **Spec Exp:** Congenital Heart Disease; Echocardiography; **Hospital:** NY-Presby/Columbia Univ Med Ctr, NY (page 104); **Address:** 3959 Broadway, 2 North, New York, NY 10032; **Phone:** 212-305-4320; **Board Cert:** Pediatrics 2007; Pediatric Cardiology 2011; **Med School:** Univ Pennsylvania 1988; **Resid:** Pediatrics, Morgan Stanley Chldn's Hosp 1991; **Fellow:** Pediatric Cardiology, Morgan Stanley Chldn's Hosp 1996; Pediatric Cardiology, Chldn's Hosp 1997; **Fac Appt:** Assoc Prof Ped, Columbia P&S

Argilla, Michael MD (PCd) - **Spec Exp:** Cardiac Catheterization; Heart Failure; Critical Care; **Hospital:** NYU Langone Med Ctr (page 108); **Address:** NYU Pediatric Cardiology Assocs, 160 E 32 St Fl 2, New York, NY 10016; **Phone:** 212-263-5940; **Board Cert:** Pediatrics 2011; Pediatric Cardiology 2008; **Med School:** Univ Colorado 1992; **Resid:** Pediatrics, NYU Langone Med Ctr 1997; **Fellow:** Pediatric Cardiology, NYU Langone Med Ctr 2002; **Fac Appt:** Asst Prof Ped, NYU Sch Med

Arnon, Rica G MD (PCd) - **Spec Exp:** Congenital Heart Disease; **Hospital:** Mt Sinai Med Ctr (page 102), Elmhurst Hosp Ctr; **Address:** 1468 Madison Ave, Ste 3-50, New York, NY 10029-6504; **Phone:** 212-241-7672; **Board Cert:** Pediatrics 1970; Pediatric Cardiology 1973; **Med School:** SUNY Hlth Sci Ctr 1967; **Resid:** Pediatrics, Kings County Hosp 1970; **Fellow:** Pediatric Cardiology, Kings County Hosp 1973; **Fac Appt:** Assoc Prof Ped, Mount Sinai Sch Med

Borg, Morton D MD (PCd) - **Spec Exp:** Fetal Echocardiography; **Hospital:** Beth Israel Med Ctr - Petrie Div (page 94), Mt Sinai Med Ctr (page 102); **Address:** Phillips Amb Care Ctr, Dept Peds, 10 Union Square E, Ste 2J, New York, NY 10003-3314; **Phone:** 212-844-8313; **Board Cert:** Pediatrics 1986; Pediatric Cardiology 2010; **Med School:** Albert Einstein Coll Med 1981; **Resid:** Pediatrics, Brookdale Hosp 1984; **Fellow:** Pediatric Cardiology, New York Hosp 1986; **Fac Appt:** Asst Prof Ped, Albert Einstein Coll Med

Brick, David H MD (PCd) - **Spec Exp:** Fetal Echocardiography; Congenital Heart Disease; **Hospital:** NYU Langone Med Ctr (page 108); **Address:** Village Pediatric Cardiology, 154 W 14th St, Fl 4, New York, NY 10011; **Phone:** 212-604-7880; **Board Cert:** Pediatrics 2011; Pediatric Cardiology 2008; **Med School:** Ohio State Univ 1993; **Resid:** Pediatrics, Univ Hosp Cleveland 1996; **Fellow:** Pediatric Cardiology, NY-Presby Hosp 2000; **Fac Appt:** Asst Clin Prof Ped, NYU Sch Med

Flynn, Patrick A MD (PCd) - **Spec Exp:** Congenital Heart Disease; Echocardiography; Kawasaki Disease; Marfan's Syndrome; **Hospital:** NY-Presby/Weill Cornell Med Ctr, NY (page 104); **Address:** Weill Cornell, Pediatric Cardiology, 525 E 68 St, Ste F666, New York, NY 10065; **Phone:** 212-746-3561; **Board Cert:** Pediatric Cardiology 2006; **Med School:** Univ MD Sch Med 1986; **Resid:** Pediatrics, NY-Presby/Weill Cornell Med Ctr 1990; **Fellow:** Pediatric Cardiology, NY-Presby/Weill Cornell Med Ctr 1993; **Fac Appt:** Assoc Clin Prof Ped, Cornell Univ-Weill Med Coll

Gelb, Bruce D MD (PCd) - **Spec Exp:** Noonan Syndrome; Marfan's Syndrome; **Hospital:** Mt Sinai Med Ctr (page 102); **Address:** 1 Gustave Levy Pl, Box 1201, New York, NY 10029; **Phone:** 212-241-8592; **Board Cert:** Pediatric Cardiology 2013; **Med School:** Univ Rochester 1984; **Resid:** Pediatrics, NYPresby-Columbia Univ Med Ctr 1987; **Fellow:** Pediatric Cardiology, Baylor College Med 1991; **Fac Appt:** Prof Ped, Mount Sinai Sch Med

Love, Barry A MD (PCd) - **Spec Exp:** Patent Foramen Ovale(PFO) Closure; Cardiac Catheterization; Interventional Cardiology; Atrial Septal Defect; **Hospital:** Mt Sinai Med Ctr (page 102); **Address:** Mt Sinai Med Ctr, Div Ped Cardiology, 1468 Madison Ave, Ste 3-50, New York, NY 10029; **Phone:** 212-241-9516; **Board Cert:** Pediatrics 2011; Pediatric Cardiology 2008; **Med School:** Univ Western Ontario 1993; **Resid:** Pediatrics, Chldns Hosp Montreal 1996; **Fellow:** Pediatric Cardiology, Chldns Hosp 2000; **Fac Appt:** Asst Prof Ped, Mount Sinai Sch Med

Parness, Ira A MD (PCd) - **Spec Exp:** Echocardiography; Congenital Heart Disease; Fetal Echocardiography; **Hospital:** Mt Sinai Med Ctr (page 102), Englewood Hosp & Med Ctr; **Address:** 1 Gustave L Levy Pl, Anbg Bldg, rm 3-40, Box 1201, New York, NY 10029-6574; **Phone:** 212-241-6640; **Board Cert:** Pediatrics 1984; Pediatric Cardiology 1985; **Med School:** SUNY Downstate 1979; **Resid:** Pediatrics, Brookdale Hosp 1982; **Fellow:** Pediatric Cardiology, Chldns Hosp 1985; **Fac Appt:** Prof Ped, Mount Sinai Sch Med

Presti, Salvatore MD (PCd) - **Spec Exp:** Fetal Echocardiography; Congenital Heart Disease; Kawasaki Disease; **Hospital:** Lenox Hill Hosp (page 106), NYU Langone Med Ctr (page 108); **Address:** 110 E 59th St, New York, NY 10022; **Phone:** 212-838-9880; **Board Cert:** Pediatrics 1984; Pediatric Cardiology 2010; **Med School:** Italy 1978; **Resid:** Pediatrics, Lenox Hill Hosp 1982; **Fellow:** Pediatric Cardiology, NYU Med Ctr 1984; **Fac Appt:** Assoc Clin Prof Ped, NYU Sch Med

Sommer, Robert J MD (PCd) - **Spec Exp:** Congenital Heart Disease; Atrial Septal Defect; Cardiac Catheterization; **Hospital:** NY-Presby/Columbia Univ Med Ctr, NY (page 104), St. Joseph's Regl Med Ctr - Paterson; **Address:** 161 Fort Washington Ave Fl 6, Herbert Irving Pavilion, New York, NY 10032; **Phone:** 212-342-0886; **Board Cert:** Pediatric Cardiology 2013; **Med School:** NYU Sch Med 1985; **Resid:** Pediatrics, Mt Sinai Med Ctr 1988; **Fellow:** Pediatric Cardiology, Mt Sinai Med Ctr 1991; Interventional Cardiology, Childrens Hosp 1991; **Fac Appt:** Asst Clin Prof Ped, Columbia P&S

Starc, Thomas J MD (PCd) - **Spec Exp:** Cholesterol/Lipid Disorders; **Hospital:** Morgan Stanley Children's Hosp of NY-Presby, NY (page 104); **Address:** NY-Presby/Morgan Stanley Chdns Hosp, 3959 Broadway N, Ste 255, New York, NY 10032-1537; **Phone:** 212-305-4432; **Board Cert:** Pediatrics 1981; Pediatric Cardiology 1983; **Med School:** Mount Sinai Sch Med 1976; **Resid:** Pediatrics, UCSD Med Ctr 1980; **Fellow:** Pediatric Cardiology, NY-Presby/Columbia Univ Med Ctr 1984; **Fac Appt:** Clin Prof Ped, Columbia P&S

Steinberg, L Gary MD (PCd) - **Spec Exp:** Echocardiography; Congenital Heart Disease; **Hospital:** NY-Presby/Weill Cornell Med Ctr, NY (page 104); **Address:** Pediatric Cardiovascular Services, NY Presby Hosp/ Weill Cornell, 525 E 68 St, Ste F666, New York, NY 10065; **Phone:** 212-746-3561; **Board Cert:** Pediatrics 2013; Pediatric Cardiology 2013; **Med School:** Philippines 1985; **Resid:** Pediatrics, Elmhurst Hosp 1989; **Fellow:** Pediatric Cardiology, Mount Sinai Hosp 1992; **Fac Appt:** Asst Prof Ped, Cornell Univ-Weill Med Coll

Steinherz, Laurel J MD (PCd) - **Spec Exp:** Cardiac Effects of Cancer/Cancer Therapy; **Hospital:** Meml Sloan-Kettering Canc Ctr (page 114), NY-Presby/Weill Cornell Med Ctr, NY (page 104); **Address:** 1275 York Ave, New York, NY 10021; **Phone:** 212-639-8103; **Board Cert:** Pediatrics 1976; Pediatric Cardiology 1978; **Med School:** Albert Einstein Coll Med 1970; **Resid:** Pediatrics, NY Hosp-Cornell Med Ctr 1971; Pediatrics, Chldns Hosp 1972; **Fellow:** Pediatric Cardiology, NY Hosp-Cornell Med Ctr 1975; **Fac Appt:** Prof Ped, Cornell Univ-Weill Med Coll

Vincent, Julie A MD (PCd) - **Spec Exp:** Interventional Cardiology; Congenital Heart Disease; Cardiac Catheterization; **Hospital:** NY-Presby/Columbia Univ Med Ctr, NY (page 104); **Address:** 3959 Broadway Fl 2 - Ste 253, New York, NY 10032; **Phone:** 212-305-6069; **Board Cert:** Pediatrics 2013; Pediatric Cardiology 2011; **Med School:** Wayne State Univ 1988; **Resid:** Pediatrics, Chldn's Hosp of MI 1991; **Fellow:** Pediatric Cardiology, Chldn's Hosp of MI 1994; Pediatric Cardiology, TX Chldns Hosp 1995; **Fac Appt:** Assoc Prof Ped, Columbia P&S

Pediatric Critical Care Medicine

Conway Jr, Edward E MD (PCCM) - **Spec Exp:** Neurologic Critical Care; Respiratory Failure; Head Injury; **Hospital:** Beth Israel Med Ctr - Petrie Div (page 94); **Address:** Beth Israel Med Ctr, Dept Peds, 350 E 17th St, New York, NY 10003; **Phone:** 212-420-4018; **Board Cert:** Pediatrics 2008; Pediatric Critical Care Medicine 2010; **Med School:** SUNY Hlth Sci Ctr 1984; **Resid:** Pediatrics, Montefiore Med Ctr 1988; **Fellow:** Pediatric Critical Care Medicine, Montefiore Med Ctr-Albert Einstein 1990; **Fac Appt:** Prof Ped, Albert Einstein Coll Med

Greenwald, Bruce M MD (PCCM) - **Spec Exp:** Respiratory Failure; Sepsis & Septic Shock; Asthma; Diabetes Ketoacidosis; **Hospital:** NY-Presby/Weill Cornell Med Ctr, NY (page 104), Meml Sloan-Kettering Canc Ctr (page 114); **Address:** Div Pediatric Critical Care Med, 525 E 68th St, Ste M-508, New York, NY 10065; **Phone:** 212-746-3056; **Board Cert:** Pediatrics 1987; Pediatric Critical Care Medicine 2012; **Med School:** NYU Sch Med 1982; **Resid:** Pediatrics, NYU-Bellevue Hosp Ctr 1986; **Fellow:** Pediatric Critical Care Medicine, NY Hosp-Cornell 1988; **Fac Appt:** Clin Prof Ped, Cornell Univ-Weill Med Coll

Sagy, Mayer MD (PCCM) - **Hospital:** NYU Langone Med Ctr (page 108); **Address:** NYU Langone Medical Ctr, Pediatric Critical Care, 550 First Ave, New York, NY 10016; **Phone:** 212-263-2377; **Board Cert:** Pediatrics 2007; Pediatric Critical Care Medicine 2007; **Med School:** Israel 1972; **Resid:** Pediatrics, Chaim Sheba Med Ctr 1982; **Fellow:** Pediatric Critical Care Medicine, Children's Hosp 1984

Pediatric Endocrinology

Fennoy, Ilene MD (PEn) - **Spec Exp:** Growth/Development Disorders; Diabetes; Klinefelter's Syndrome; Obesity; **Hospital:** Morgan Stanley Children's Hosp of NY-Presby, NY (page 104), Harlem Hosp Ctr; **Address:** 3959 Broadway, rm 106, New York, NY 10032; **Phone:** 212-305-6559; **Board Cert:** Pediatrics 1979; Pediatric Endocrinology 1980; **Med School:** UCSF 1973; **Resid:** Pediatrics, Montefiore Med Ctr 1975; **Fellow:** Nutrition, Columbia-Presby Med Ctr 1977; Endocrinology, Natl Inst Hlth 1979; **Fac Appt:** Assoc Clin Prof Ped, Columbia P&S

Franklin, Bonita H MD (PEn) - **Spec Exp:** Diabetes; Growth Disorders; Thyroid Disorders; **Hospital:** NYU Langone Med Ctr (page 108); **Address:** 160 E 32nd St, L3 Medical, New York, NY 10016; **Phone:** 212-263-5940 x6; **Board Cert:** Pediatrics 1982; Pediatric Endocrinology 2009; **Med School:** SUNY Hlth Sci Ctr 1976; **Resid:** Pediatrics, Bronx Muni Hosp 1978; Pediatrics, Mt Sinai Hosp 1979; **Fellow:** Pediatric Endocrinology, Mt Sinai Hosp 1981; **Fac Appt:** Assoc Clin Prof Ped, NYU Sch Med

Gallagher, Mary P MD (PEn) - **Spec Exp:** Diabetes; **Hospital:** Morgan Stanley Children's Hosp of NY-Presby, NY (page 104); **Address:** 1150 St Nicholas Ave Fl 2, New York, NY 10032; **Phone:** 212-851-5494; **Board Cert:** Pediatrics 2006; Pediatric Endocrinology 2011; **Med School:** UMDNJ-NJ Med Sch, Newark 1995; **Resid:** Pediatrics, NY Presby-Columbia Med Ctr 1998; **Fellow:** Pediatric Endocrinology, NY Presby-Columbia Med Ctr 2002; **Fac Appt:** Asst Prof Ped, Columbia P&S

Kohn, Brenda MD (PEn) - **Spec Exp:** Growth Disorders; Pituitary Disorders; Thyroid Disorders; Adrenal Disorders; **Hospital:** NYU Langone Med Ctr (page 108); **Address:** 160 E 32nd St, Ste L3, New York, NY 10016-6402; **Phone:** 212-263-5940 x6; **Board Cert:** Pediatrics 1981; Pediatric Endocrinology 1983; **Med School:** Albert Einstein Coll Med 1976; **Resid:** Pediatrics, NYU Med Ctr 1979; **Fellow:** Endocrinology, Diabetes & Metabolism, NY-Cornell Med Ctr 1983; **Fac Appt:** Assoc Prof Ped, NYU Sch Med

New, Maria I MD (PEn) - **Spec Exp:** Adrenal Disorders; Growth/Development Disorders; **Hospital:** Mt Sinai Med Ctr (page 102); **Address:** Mount Sinai Medical Ctr, Ped Adrenal Steroid Disorders Program, 5 E 98th St Fl 10, New York, NY 10029; **Phone:** 212-241-8210; **Board Cert:** Pediatrics 1960; **Med School:** Univ Pennsylvania 1954; **Resid:** Pediatrics, New York Hosp 1957; **Fellow:** Pediatric Endocrinology, New York Hosp 1958; Endocrinology, Diabetes & Metabolism, New York Hosp 1964; **Fac Appt:** Prof Ped, Cornell Univ-Weill Med Coll

Oberfield, Sharon E MD (PEn) - **Spec Exp:** Adrenal Disorders; Neuroendocrine Disorders; Growth Disorders; **Hospital:** Morgan Stanley Children's Hosp of NY-Presby, NY (page 104); **Address:** 630 W 168th St, PH East Bldg - Fl 5 East - Ste 522, New York, NY 10032; **Phone:** 212-305-6559; **Board Cert:** Pediatrics 1979; Pediatric Endocrinology 2000; **Med School:** Cornell Univ 1974; **Resid:** Pediatrics, New York Hosp 1976; **Fellow:** Pediatric Endocrinology, New York Hosp-Cornell 1979; **Fac Appt:** Prof Ped, Columbia P&S

Rapaport, Robert MD (PEn) - **Spec Exp:** Growth Disorders; Thyroid Disorders; Diabetes; **Hospital:** Mt Sinai Med Ctr (page 102); **Address:** 1468 Madison Ave Fl 4 - Ste 4-81, New York, NY 10029; **Phone:** 212-241-8487; **Board Cert:** Pediatrics 1980; Pediatric Endocrinology 1983; **Med School:** SUNY Downstate 1974; **Resid:** Pediatrics, LIJ-Hillside Med Ctr 1977; **Fellow:** Pediatric Endocrinology, St Christopher's Hosp 1978; Pediatric Endocrinology, New York Hosp 1980; **Fac Appt:** Prof Ped, Mount Sinai Sch Med

Sklar, Charles A MD (PEn) - **Spec Exp:** Cancer Survivors-Late Effects of Therapy; Growth Disorders in Childhood Cancer; **Hospital:** Meml Sloan-Kettering Canc Ctr (page 114); **Address:** 1275 York Avenue, New York, NY 10065; **Phone:** 212-639-8138; **Board Cert:** Pediatrics 1979; Pediatric Endocrinology 1980; **Med School:** USC Sch Med 1974; **Resid:** Pediatrics, Childrens Hosp 1976; **Fellow:** Pediatric Endocrinology, UCSF Med Ctr 1979; **Fac Appt:** Assoc Prof Ped, Cornell Univ-Weill Med Coll

Vargas-Rodriguez, Ileana MD (PEn) - **Spec Exp:** Diabetes; **Hospital:** NY-Presby/Columbia Univ Med Ctr, NY (page 104); **Address:** 1150 St Nicholas Ave, Fl 2, New York, NY 10032; **Phone:** 212-851-5494; **Board Cert:** Pediatric Endocrinology 2010; **Med School:** Albert Einstein Coll Med 1986; **Resid:** Pediatrics, Babies Hosp 1989; **Fellow:** Pediatric Endocrinology, Mt Sinai Hosp 1990

Vogiatzi, Maria G MD (PEn) - **Spec Exp:** Growth Disorders; Pubertal Disorders; Adrenal Disorders; Bone Disorders-Metabolic; **Hospital:** NY-Presby/Weill Cornell Med Ctr, NY (page 104); **Address:** 505 E 70th St, Helmsley Tower Fl 3, New York, NY 10065; **Phone:** 212-746-3462; **Board Cert:** Pediatrics 2007; Pediatric Endocrinology 2012; **Med School:** Greece 1987; **Resid:** Pediatrics, Univ Hosp 1991; **Fellow:** Pediatric Endocrinology, New York Hosp 1993; Pediatric Endocrinology, Baylor Coll Med 1995; **Fac Appt:** Assoc Clin Prof Ped, Cornell Univ-Weill Med Coll

Pediatric Gastroenterology

Bangaru, Babu S MD (PGe) - **Spec Exp:** Ulcerative Colitis/Crohn's; Liver Disease; Nutrition; Endoscopy; **Hospital:** NYU Langone Med Ctr (page 108), Flushing Hosp Med Ctr; **Address:** NYU Medical Center, 530 First Ave, Ste 3A, New York, NY 10016; **Phone:** 212-263-7868; **Board Cert:** Pediatrics 1978; Pediatric Gastroenterology 2013; **Med School:** India 1970; **Resid:** Pediatrics, St Lukes Hosp 1976; **Fellow:** Hepatology, Albert Einstein Coll Med 1978; Gastroenterology & Nutrition, Emory Univ Sch Med 1979; **Fac Appt:** Assoc Clin Prof Ped, NYU Sch Med

Benkov, Keith J MD (PGe) - **Spec Exp:** Inflammatory Bowel Disease/Crohn's; Liver Disease; Celiac Disease; **Hospital:** Mt Sinai Med Ctr (page 102), Englewood Hosp & Med Ctr; **Address:** Mt Sinai Div Ped Gastroenterology, 5 E 98th St, Fl 10, New York, NY 10029; **Phone:** 212-241-5415; **Board Cert:** Pediatrics 1984; Pediatric Gastroenterology 2012; **Med School:** Mount Sinai Sch Med 1979; **Resid:** Pediatrics, Mt Sinai Hosp 1982; **Fellow:** Pediatric Gastroenterology, Mt Sinai Hosp 1984; **Fac Appt:** Assoc Prof Ped, Mount Sinai Sch Med

Breglio, Keith J MD (PGe) - **Spec Exp:** Crohn's Disease; Ulcerative Colitis; Gastroesophageal Reflux Disease (GERD); **Hospital:** Mt Sinai Med Ctr (page 102); **Address:** Mount Sinai, Div Ped Gastroenterology, 5 E 98th St, Fl 10, New York, NY 10029; **Phone:** 212-241-5415; **Board Cert:** Pediatrics 2006; Pediatric Gastroenterology 2009; **Med School:** SUNY Upstate Med Univ 2002; **Resid:** Pediatrics, Schneider Chldns Hosp 2006; **Fellow:** Pediatric Gastroenterology, Mount Sinai Med Ctr 2009; **Fac Appt:** Asst Prof Ped, Mount Sinai Sch Med

Chehade, Mirna A MD (PGe) - **Spec Exp:** Endoscopy; Food Allergy; Esophageal Disorders; **Hospital:** Mt Sinai Med Ctr (page 102); **Address:** Mount Sinai, Ped Gastroenterology, 5 E 98 St Fl 10, New York, NY 10029; **Phone:** 212-241-4880; **Board Cert:** Pediatric Gastroenterology 2011; **Med School:** Amer Univ Beirut 1996; **Resid:** Pediatrics, Chldns Hosp 2000; **Fellow:** Pediatric Gastroenterology, Mount Sinai Med Ctr 2003; **Fac Appt:** Asst Prof Ped, Mount Sinai Sch Med

Kazlow, Philip G MD (PGe) - **Spec Exp:** Inflammatory Bowel Disease; Celiac Disease; Nutrition; **Hospital:** Morgan Stanley Children's Hosp of NY-Presby, NY (page 104), Valley Hosp (page 721); **Address:** Morgan Stanley Children's Hosp, 3959 Broadway, 7 Central, New York, NY 10032; **Phone:** 212-305-5903; **Board Cert:** Pediatrics 1985; Pediatric Gastroenterology 2005; **Med School:** Mount Sinai Sch Med 1980; **Resid:** Pediatrics, Mt Sinai Hosp 1984; **Fellow:** Pediatric Gastroenterology, Mt Sinai Hosp 1986; **Fac Appt:** Prof Ped, Columbia P&S

Lavine, Joel E MD/PhD (PGe) - **Spec Exp:** Celiac Disease; Liver Disease; Short Bowel Syndrome; Nutrition; **Hospital:** Morgan Stanley Children's Hosp of NY-Presby, NY (page 104); **Address:** Morgan Stanley Childns Hosp, Pediatric Gastroenterology Dept, 21 W 86th St, New York, NY 10024; **Phone:** 212-305-5903; **Board Cert:** Pediatric Gastroenterology 2012; Pediatric Transplant Hepatology 2008; **Med School:** UCSD 1984; **Resid:** Pediatrics, UCSF Med Ctr 1986; **Fellow:** Pediatric Gastroenterology, UCSF Med Ctr 1989; **Fac Appt:** Prof Ped

Levine, Jeremiah J MD (PGe) - **Spec Exp:** Inflammatory Bowel Disease; Crohn's Disease; Liver Disease; **Hospital:** NYU Langone Med Ctr (page 108); **Address:** 160 E 32nd St, Medical Level, L3, NY, NY 10016; **Phone:** 212-263-5407; **Board Cert:** Pediatrics 1985; Pediatric Gastroenterology 2012; **Med School:** Harvard Med Sch 1980; **Resid:** Pediatrics, Montefiore Med Ctr 1983; **Fellow:** Pediatric Gastroenterology, Children's Hosp 1985; **Fac Appt:** Prof Ped, Albert Einstein Coll Med

Levy, Joseph MD (PGe) - **Spec Exp:** Celiac Disease; Gastroesophageal Reflux Disease (GERD); Nutrition in Autism; Inflammatory Bowel Disease/Crohn's; **Hospital:** NYU Langone Med Ctr (page 108); **Address:** 160 E 32nd St, Medical Suite L-3, New York, NY 10016; **Phone:** 212-263-5407; **Board Cert:** Pediatrics 1981; Pediatric Gastroenterology 2012; **Med School:** Israel 1973; **Resid:** Pediatrics, Beth Israel Med Ctr 1977; **Fellow:** Research, Columbia-Presby Med Ctr 1975; Pediatric Gastroenterology, Columbia-Presby Med Ctr 1979; **Fac Appt:** Prof Ped, NYU Sch Med

Lobritto, Steven MD (PGe) - **Spec Exp:** Hepatitis; Liver Disease; Transplant Medicine-Liver; **Hospital:** Morgan Stanley Children's Hosp of NY-Presby, NY (page 104); **Address:** Morgan Stanley Chldns Hosp of NY-Presby, 3959 Broadway, rm 726, New York, NY 10032; **Phone:** 212-305-3000; **Board Cert:** Pediatric Gastroenterology 2007; Pediatric Transplant Hepatology 2008; **Med School:** NY Med Coll 1988; **Resid:** Internal Medicine & Pediatrics, New York Hosp 1992; **Fellow:** Pediatric Gastroenterology, Columbia-Presby Med Ctr 1996

Sockolow, Robbyn E MD (PGe) - **Spec Exp:** Celiac Disease; Crohn's Disease; **Hospital:** NY-Presby/Weill Cornell Med Ctr, NY (page 104); **Address:** Ny Presby-Cornell Med Ctr, Ped Gastroenterology, 505 E 70th St, Helmsley Tower, Fl 3, New York, NY 10021; **Phone:** 646-962-3869; **Board Cert:** Pediatrics 2012; Pediatric Gastroenterology 2010; **Med School:** NY Med Coll 1986; **Resid:** Pediatrics, Montefiore Med Ctr 1989; **Fellow:** Pediatric Gastroenterology, Mt Sinai Med Ctr 1990; Pediatric Gastroenterology, Montefiore Med Ctr 1992; **Fac Appt:** Assoc Clin Prof Ped, Cornell Univ-Weill Med Coll

Spivak, William MD (PGe) - **Spec Exp:** Ulcerative Colitis; Crohn's Disease; Nutrition; Esophageal Disorders; **Hospital:** NY-Presby/Weill Cornell Med Ctr, NY (page 104), Lenox Hill Hosp (page 106); **Address:** 177 E 87th St, Ste 305, New York, NY 10128; **Phone:** 212-369-7700; **Board Cert:** Pediatrics 1981; Pediatric Gastroenterology 2012; **Med School:** Albert Einstein Coll Med 1976; **Resid:** Pediatrics, Jacobi Med Ctr/Albert Einstein Med Sch 1979; **Fellow:** Gastroenterology, Childrens Hosp 1982; Research, Brigham & Womens Hosp 1982; **Fac Appt:** Clin Prof Ped, Cornell Univ-Weill Med Coll

Pediatric Hematology-Oncology

Aledo, Alexander MD (PHO) - **Spec Exp:** Leukemia; Lymphoma; Bone Tumors; **Hospital:** NY-Presby/Weill Cornell Med Ctr, NY (page 104), NY Hosp Queens (page 488); **Address:** 525 E 68th St, rm P695, New York, NY 10021-4870; **Phone:** 212-746-3400; **Board Cert:** Pediatric Hematology-Oncology 2004; **Med School:** NYU Sch Med 1984; **Resid:** Pediatrics, NYPresby/Weill Cornell Med Ctr 1987; **Fellow:** Pediatric Hematology-Oncology, Meml Sloan Kettering Cancer Ctr 1990; **Fac Appt:** Assoc Clin Prof Ped, Cornell Univ-Weill Med Coll

Blei, Francine MD (PHO) - **Spec Exp:** Vascular Malformations/Birthmarks; Hemangiomas; Lymphedema; **Hospital:** St. Luke's - Roosevelt Hosp Ctr - Roosevelt Div (page 94); **Address:** Vascular Birthmark Inst of New York, 1000 10th Ave, 10G INN, New York, NY 10023; **Phone:** 212-523-8931; **Board Cert:** Pediatrics 1987; Pediatric Hematology-Oncology 1987; **Med School:** Israel 1982; **Resid:** Pediatrics, NYU-Bellevue 1985; **Fellow:** Pediatric Hematology-Oncology, Babies Hosp-Columbia Presby 1987

Bussel, James MD (PHO) - **Spec Exp:** Bleeding/Coagulation Disorders; Platelet Disorders; Wiskott-Aldrich Syndrome; **Hospital:** NY-Presby/Weill Cornell Med Ctr, NY (page 104), Lenox Hill Hosp (page 106); **Address:** 525 E 68th St, rm P-695, New York, NY 10065; **Phone:** 212-746-3400; **Board Cert:** Pediatrics 1979; Pediatric Hematology-Oncology 1980; **Med School:** Columbia P&S 1975; **Resid:** Pediatrics, Chldns Hosp 1978; **Fellow:** Pediatric Hematology-Oncology, NY Presby Hosp/Cornell 1981; **Fac Appt:** Prof Ped, Cornell Univ-Weill Med Coll

Carroll, William L MD (PHO) - **Spec Exp:** Leukemia; Hematologic Malignancies; **Hospital:** NYU Langone Med Ctr (page 108); **Address:** NYU Med Ctr, Div Ped Hem/Onc, 160 E 32nd Level L3 St, New York, NY 10016; **Phone:** 212-263-8400; **Board Cert:** Pediatrics 1984; Pediatric Hematology-Oncology 1987; **Med School:** UC Irvine 1978; **Resid:** Pediatrics, Chldns Hosp Med Ctr 1981; **Fellow:** Pediatric Hematology-Oncology, Stanford Univ Med Ctr 1987; **Fac Appt:** Prof Ped, NYU Sch Med

Cheung, Nai-Kong V MD/PhD (PHO) - **Spec Exp:** Neuroblastoma; Pediatric Cancers; Clinical Trials; **Hospital:** Meml Sloan-Kettering Canc Ctr (page 114); **Address:** 1275 York Ave, New York, NY 10065; **Phone:** 646-888-2313; **Board Cert:** Pediatrics 1987; Pediatric Hematology-Oncology 2012; **Med School:** Harvard Med Sch 1978; **Resid:** Pediatrics, Stanford Univ Hosp 1981; **Fellow:** Pediatric Hematology-Oncology, Stanford Univ Hosp 1984; **Fac Appt:** Assoc Prof Ped, Cornell Univ-Weill Med Coll

Dunkel, Ira J MD (PHO) - **Spec Exp:** Retinoblastoma; Brain & Spinal Cord Tumors; Brain Tumors; Pediatric Cancers; **Hospital:** Meml Sloan-Kettering Canc Ctr (page 114); **Address:** 1275 York Ave, New York, NY 10065; **Phone:** 212-639-2153; **Board Cert:** Pediatric Hematology-Oncology 2007; **Med School:** Duke Univ 1985; **Resid:** Pediatrics, Duke Univ Med Ctr 1988; **Fellow:** Pediatric Hematology-Oncology, Memorial-Sloan Kettering 1992; Pediatric Infectious Disease, Duke Univ Med Ctr 1989; **Fac Appt:** Assoc Prof Ped, Cornell Univ-Weill Med Coll

Gardner, Sharon L MD (PHO) - **Spec Exp:** Neuro-Oncology; **Hospital:** NYU Langone Med Ctr (page 108); **Address:** Steven B Hassenfeld Childrns Ctr, 160 E 32nd St Fl 2, New York, NY 10016; **Phone:** 212-263-8400; **Board Cert:** Pediatrics 2000; Pediatric Hematology-Oncology 2000; **Med School:** Hahnemann Univ 1986; **Resid:** Pediatrics, St Christophers Hosp Chldn 1989; **Fellow:** Pediatric Hematology-Oncology, Sloan Kettering Canc Ctr 1993; **Fac Appt:** Assoc Prof Ped, NYU Sch Med

Garvin Jr, James H MD/PhD (PHO) - **Spec Exp:** Brain Tumors; Pediatric Cancers; Bone Marrow Transplant; **Hospital:** Morgan Stanley Children's Hosp of NY-Presby, NY (page 104); **Address:** 161 Fort Washington Ave, Fl 7, rm 708, New York, NY 10032-3729; **Phone:** 212-305-5808; **Board Cert:** Pediatrics 1982; Pediatric Hematology-Oncology 1984; **Med School:** Jefferson Med Coll 1976; **Resid:** Pediatrics, Chldns Hosp 1978; Pediatrics, Middlesex Hosp 1979; **Fellow:** Pediatric Hematology-Oncology, Dana Farber Cancer Inst/Childrens Hosp 1982; **Fac Appt:** Clin Prof Ped, Columbia P&S

Giardina, Patricia J V MD (PHO) - **Spec Exp:** Thalassemia; Sickle Cell Disease; Hemophilia; **Hospital:** NY-Presby/Weill Cornell Med Ctr, NY (page 104); **Address:** 525 E 68th St, Payson Pavilion, Ste 695, New York, NY 10065; **Phone:** 212-746-3400; **Board Cert:** Pediatrics 1973; Pediatric Hematology-Oncology 1974; **Med School:** NY Med Coll 1968; **Resid:** Pediatrics, New York Hosp-Cornell 1971; **Fellow:** Pediatric Hematology-Oncology, New York Hosp-Cornell 1974; **Fac Appt:** Clin Prof Ped, Cornell Univ-Weill Med Coll

Granowetter, Linda MD (PHO) - **Spec Exp:** Bone Tumors; Lymphoma; Sarcoma-Soft Tissue; Ewing's Sarcoma; **Hospital:** NYU Langone Med Ctr (page 108); **Address:** NYU, Hassenfeld Chldns Ctr, 160 E 32 St, New York, NY 10016; **Phone:** 212-263-9660; **Board Cert:** Pediatric Hematology-Oncology 1984; Pediatrics 1983; Hospice & Palliative Medicine 2012; **Med School:** SUNY Stony Brook 1978; **Resid:** Pediatrics, St Christophers Chldns Hosp 1981; **Fellow:** Pediatric Oncology, Chldns Hosp 1984; **Fac Appt:** Prof Ped, NYU Sch Med

Kernan, Nancy A MD (PHO) - **Spec Exp:** Bone Marrow Transplant; Stem Cell Transplant; Leukemia; Immune Deficiency; **Hospital:** Meml Sloan-Kettering Canc Ctr (page 114); **Address:** 1275 York Ave, New York, NY 10065; **Phone:** 212-639-7250; **Board Cert:** Pediatrics 1983; Pediatric Hematology-Oncology 1984; **Med School:** Cornell Univ-Weill Med Coll 1978; **Resid:** Pediatrics, Chldns Hosp Natl Med Ctr 1981; **Fellow:** Pediatric Hematology-Oncology, Meml Sloan Kettering Cancer Ctr 1984

Kramer, Kim MD (PHO) - **Spec Exp:** Neuroblastoma; Brain & Spinal Cord Tumors; **Hospital:** Meml Sloan-Kettering Canc Ctr (page 114); **Address:** 1275 York, Box 429, New York, NY 10021; **Phone:** 212-639-6410; **Board Cert:** Pediatric Hematology-Oncology 2011; **Med School:** SUNY Upstate Med Univ 1989; **Resid:** Pediatrics, Strong Meml Hosp 1992; **Fellow:** Pediatric Hematology-Oncology, Meml Sloan Kettering Cancer Ctr 1994

Kushner, Brian H MD (PHO) - **Spec Exp:** Neuroblastoma; Bone Marrow Transplant; Immunotherapy; **Hospital:** Meml Sloan-Kettering Canc Ctr (page 114); **Address:** 1275 York Avenue, New York, NY 10065; **Phone:** 212-639-6793; **Board Cert:** Pediatrics 1983; Pediatric Hematology-Oncology 1987; **Med School:** Johns Hopkins Univ 1976; **Resid:** Pediatrics, Columbia-Presby Med Ctr 1978; Pediatrics, NY Hosp 1979; **Fellow:** Pediatric Hematology-Oncology, Boston Chldns Hosp 1980; Pediatric Hematology-Oncology, Meml Sloan Kettering Cancer Ctr 1986; **Fac Appt:** Prof Ped, Cornell Univ-Weill Med Coll

Marcus, Judith R MD (PHO) - **Spec Exp:** Leukemia; Lymphoma; Bleeding/Coagulation Disorders; Solid Tumors; **Hospital:** Morgan Stanley Children's Hosp of NY-Presby, NY (page 104), White Plains Hosp (page 640); **Address:** 161 Ft Wasthington Ave, Ste 7l, New York, NY 10032; **Phone:** 212-305-5808; **Board Cert:** Pediatrics 1997; Pediatric Hematology-Oncology 1997; **Med School:** NYU Sch Med 1971; **Resid:** Pediatrics, Bronx Muni Hosp-Albert Einstein 1974; **Fellow:** Pediatric Hematology-Oncology, Meml Sloan Kettering Cancer Ctr 1979; **Fac Appt:** Clin Prof Ped, Columbia P&S

Meyers, Paul A MD (PHO) - **Spec Exp:** Pediatric Cancers; Bone Tumors; Sarcoma; **Hospital:** Meml Sloan-Kettering Canc Ctr (page 114); **Address:** 1275 York Ave, New York, NY 10065; **Phone:** 212-639-5952; **Board Cert:** Pediatrics 1978; Pediatric Hematology-Oncology 1978; **Med School:** Mount Sinai Sch Med 1973; **Resid:** Pediatrics, Mt Sinai Hosp 1976; **Fellow:** Pediatric Hematology-Oncology, NY Hosp-Cornell Med Ctr 1979; **Fac Appt:** Prof Ped, Cornell Univ-Weill Med Coll

O'Reilly, Richard MD (PHO) - **Spec Exp:** Bone Marrow Transplant; Stem Cell Transplant; Hematologic Disorders in Cancer Patients; Hematologic Malignancies; **Hospital:** Meml Sloan-Kettering Canc Ctr (page 114); **Address:** 1275 York Avenue, New York, NY 10065; **Phone:** 212-639-5957; **Board Cert:** Pediatrics 1974; **Med School:** Univ Rochester 1968; **Resid:** Pediatrics, Chldrns Hosp 1972; **Fellow:** Hematology, Chldrns Hosp 1973; **Fac Appt:** Prof Ped, Cornell Univ-Weill Med Coll

Sheth, Sujit MD (PHO) - **Spec Exp:** Sickle Cell Disease; Hemophilia; Thalassemia; **Hospital:** NY-Presby/Weill Cornell Med Ctr, NY (page 104); **Address:** NY Presby, Payson Pav, Ped Hem/Onc, 525 E 68 St Fl 6, New York, NY 10065; **Phone:** 212-746-3400; **Board Cert:** Pediatric Hematology-Oncology 2010; **Med School:** India 1988; **Resid:** Pediatrics, NY-Presby/Columbia Univ Med Ctr 1996; **Fellow:** Pediatric Hematology-Oncology, NY-Presby/Columbia Univ Med Ctr 1995; **Fac Appt:** Assoc Clin Prof Ped, Columbia P&S

Steinherz, Peter G MD (PHO) - **Spec Exp:** Leukemia & Lymphoma; Pediatric Cancers; Wilms' Tumor; Kidney Cancer; **Hospital:** Meml Sloan-Kettering Canc Ctr (page 114); **Address:** 1275 York Avenue, New York, NY 10065; **Phone:** 212-639-7951; **Board Cert:** Pediatrics 1973; Pediatric Hematology-Oncology 1978; **Med School:** Albert Einstein Coll Med 1968; **Resid:** Pediatrics, NYPresby/Weill Cornell Med Ctr 1971; **Fellow:** Pediatric Hematology-Oncology, NYPresby/Weill Cornell Med Ctr 1975; **Fac Appt:** Prof Ped, Cornell Univ-Weill Med Coll

Trippett, Tanya M MD (PHO) - **Spec Exp:** Hodgkin's Lymphoma; Pediatric Cancers; **Hospital:** Meml Sloan-Kettering Canc Ctr (page 114); **Address:** Dept Pediatric Hem/Oncology, 1275 York Ave, New York, NY 10065; **Phone:** 212-639-8267; **Board Cert:** Pediatric Hematology-Oncology 2009; **Med School:** Duke Univ 1985; **Resid:** Pediatrics, Duke Univ Med Ctr 1988; **Fellow:** Pediatric Hematology-Oncology, Meml Sloan-Kettering Cancer Ctr 1990

Weiner, Michael A MD (PHO) - **Spec Exp:** Lymphoma; Lymphoma, Non-Hodgkin's; Leukemia; **Hospital:** Morgan Stanley Children's Hosp of NY-Presby, NY (page 104); **Address:** 161 Fort Washington Ave, Herbert Irving Pavilion, FL 7, New York, NY 10032-3710; **Phone:** 212-305-9770; **Board Cert:** Pediatrics 1980; Pediatric Hematology-Oncology 1980; **Med School:** SUNY Hlth Sci Ctr 1972; **Resid:** Pediatrics, Montefiore Hosp 1973; Pediatrics, Thos Jefferson Univ Hosp 1974; **Fellow:** Pediatric Hematology-Oncology, NYU Med Ctr 1976; Pediatric Hematology-Oncology, Johns Hopkins Hosp 1977; **Fac Appt:** Prof Ped, Columbia P&S

Wexler, Leonard MD (PHO) - **Spec Exp:** Rhabdomyosarcoma; Bone Cancer; Gastrointestinal Stromal Tumors; Sarcoma-Soft Tissue; **Hospital:** Meml Sloan-Kettering Canc Ctr (page 114); **Address:** 1275 York Avenue, New York, NY 10065; **Phone:** 212-639-7990; **Board Cert:** Pediatrics 2007; Pediatric Hematology-Oncology 2007; **Med School:** Boston Univ 1985; **Resid:** Pediatrics, Montefiore Med Ctr 1988; **Fellow:** Pediatric Hematology-Oncology, National Cancer Inst 1991; **Fac Appt:** Assoc Prof Ped, Columbia P&S

Wistinghausen, Birte MD (PHO) - **Spec Exp:** Sarcoma; Leukemia & Lymphoma; **Hospital:** Mt Sinai Med Ctr (page 102); **Address:** 1468 Madison Ave Fl 4, New York, NY 10029; **Phone:** 212-241-7022; **Board Cert:** Pediatrics 2007; Pediatric Hematology-Oncology 2010; **Med School:** Germany 1993; **Resid:** Pediatrics, NYU Med Ctr 1999; **Fellow:** Pediatric Hematology-Oncology, NYU Med Ctr 2001; **Fac Appt:** Asst Prof Med, NYU Sch Med

Pediatric Infectious Disease

Borkowsky, William MD (PInf) - **Spec Exp:** AIDS/HIV; Congenital Infections; Immune Deficiency; **Hospital:** NYU Langone Med Ctr (page 108), Bellevue Hosp Ctr; **Address:** 550 1st Ave, Dept Pediatrics, New York, NY 10016; **Phone:** 212-263-5680; **Board Cert:** Pediatrics 1979; Pediatric Infectious Disease 2009; **Med School:** NYU Sch Med 1972; **Resid:** Pediatrics, Bellevue Hosp Ctr 1975; **Fellow:** Infectious Disease, Bellevue Hosp Ctr-NYU 1978; **Fac Appt:** Prof Ped, NYU Sch Med

Gershon, Anne A MD (PInf) - **Spec Exp:** HIV; Vaccines; Hepatitis; **Hospital:** Morgan Stanley Children's Hosp of NY-Presby, NY (page 104); **Address:** 3959 Broadway St, Ste BNH 106, New York, NY 10032; **Phone:** 212-305-9445; **Board Cert:** Pediatrics 1992; Pediatric Infectious Disease 2010; **Med School:** Cornell Univ-Weill Med Coll 1964; **Resid:** Pediatrics, New York Hosp 1968; **Fellow:** Infectious Disease, NYU Langone Med Ctr 1971; Infectious Disease, Oxford Univ 1972; **Fac Appt:** Prof Ped, Columbia P&S

Larsen, John G MD (PInf) - **Hospital:** Mt Sinai Med Ctr (page 102); **Address:** 1245 Park Ave, New York, NY 10128-1211; **Phone:** 212-427-0540; **Board Cert:** Pediatrics 1979; Pediatric Infectious Disease 2012; **Med School:** SUNY Hlth Sci Ctr 1974; **Resid:** Pediatrics, Mount Sinai Med Ctr 1977; **Fellow:** Pediatric Infectious Disease, Mount Sinai Med Ctr 1978; **Fac Appt:** Assoc Clin Prof Ped, Mount Sinai Sch Med

Neu, Natalie M MD (PInf) - **Spec Exp:** AIDS/HIV; Sexually Transmitted Diseases; **Hospital:** NY-Presby/Columbia Univ Med Ctr, NY (page 104); **Address:** 3959 Broadway, rm 106, New York, NY 10032; **Phone:** 212-305-0635; **Board Cert:** Pediatrics 2009; Pediatric Infectious Disease 2012; **Med School:** Columbia P&S 1991; **Resid:** Pediatrics, Michigan State Med Ctr 1994; **Fellow:** Pediatric Infectious Disease, Columbia Presby Med Ctr 1997; **Fac Appt:** Assoc Clin Prof Ped, Columbia P&S

Posada, Roberto MD (PInf) - **Spec Exp:** HIV; Lyme Disease; **Hospital:** Mt Sinai Med Ctr (page 102); **Address:** Mount Sinai, Ped Infectious Disease, 5 E 98 St Fl 8, New York, NY 10029; **Phone:** 212-241-7968; **Board Cert:** Pediatrics 2012; Pediatric Infectious Disease 2009; **Med School:** Colombia 1993; **Resid:** Pediatrics, Montefiore Med Ctr 1997; **Fellow:** Pediatric Infectious Disease, Montefiore Med Ctr 2000; **Fac Appt:** Assoc Prof Ped, Mount Sinai Sch Med

Prince, Alice S MD (PInf) - **Hospital:** Morgan Stanley Children's Hosp of NY-Presby, NY (page 104); **Address:** 650 W 168th St, New York, NY 10032-3702; **Phone:** 212-305-4558; **Board Cert:** Pediatrics 1979; Pediatric Infectious Disease 2009; **Med School:** Columbia P&S 1975; **Resid:** Pediatrics, NY Presby-Columbia Med Ctr 1978; **Fellow:** Infectious Disease, NY Presby-Columbia Med Ctr 1981; **Fac Appt:** Prof Ped, Columbia P&S

Saiman, Lisa R MD (PInf) - **Spec Exp:** Cystic Fibrosis Infection; Fungal Infections; Tick-borne Diseases; Tuberculosis; **Hospital:** Morgan Stanley Children's Hosp of NY-Presby, NY (page 104); **Address:** 3959 Broadway, rm 106, New York, NY 10032; **Phone:** 212-305-0635; **Board Cert:** Pediatrics 1987; Pediatric Infectious Disease 2009; **Med School:** Albert Einstein Coll Med 1983; **Resid:** Pediatrics, Babies Hosp/NY Presby 1986; **Fellow:** Infectious Disease, Babies Hosp/NY Presby 1989; **Fac Appt:** Clin Prof Ped, Columbia P&S

Pediatric Nephrology

Benchimol, Corinne MD (PNep) - **Spec Exp:** Dialysis Care; Hemolytic Uremic Syndrome; Glomerulonephritis; **Hospital:** Mt Sinai Med Ctr (page 102); **Address:** 5 E 98 St Fl 10, New York, NY 10029; **Phone:** 212-241-6187; **Board Cert:** Pediatric Nephrology 2009; **Med School:** Southeastern Univ Coll Osteo Med 1990; **Resid:** Pediatrics, Miami Chldns Hosp 1993; **Fellow:** Pediatric Nephrology, Jacobi Med Ctr 1996; **Fac Appt:** Asst Prof Ped, Mount Sinai Sch Med

Johnson, Valerie L MD/PhD (PNep) - **Spec Exp:** Nephrotic Syndrome; Glomerulonephritis; Hypertension; Transplant Medicine-Kidney; **Hospital:** NY-Presby/Weill Cornell Med Ctr, NY (page 104), Valley Hosp (page 721); **Address:** 505 E 70th St, Helmsley Tower Fl 3, New York, NY 10021; **Phone:** 646-962-4324; **Board Cert:** Pediatrics 1984; Pediatric Nephrology 1985; **Med School:** Cornell Univ-Weill Med Coll 1977; **Resid:** Pediatrics, Mt Sinai Hosp 1979; **Fellow:** Nephrology, Montefiore Med Ctr 1982; **Fac Appt:** Assoc Clin Prof Ped, Cornell Univ-Weill Med Coll

Lin, Fangming MD/PhD (PNep) - **Spec Exp:** Kidney Disease; Hypertension in Children; **Hospital:** Morgan Stanley Children's Hosp of NY-Presby, NY (page 104), NY-Presby/Columbia Univ Med Ctr, NY (page 104); **Address:** Columbia-Ped Nephrology, 630 W 168th St, PH 17, New York, NY 10032; **Phone:** 212-305-5825; **Board Cert:** Pediatrics 2013; Pediatric Nephrology 2011; **Med School:** China 1984; **Resid:** Pediatrics, NYU Med Ctr 1998; **Fellow:** Pediatric Nephrology, Univ Washington Med Ctr 2001; **Fac Appt:** Assoc Prof Ped, Columbia P&S

Perelstein, Eduardo M MD (PNep) - **Spec Exp:** Kidney Failure; Glomerulonephritis; Hypertension; **Hospital:** NY-Presby/Weill Cornell Med Ctr, NY (page 104), NY Hosp Queens (page 488); **Address:** 505 E 70th St Fl 3, New York, NY 10021; **Phone:** 646-962-4324; **Board Cert:** Pediatrics 2011; Pediatric Nephrology 2012; **Med School:** Argentina 1974; **Resid:** Pediatrics, Chldn's Hosp 1978; **Fellow:** Pediatric Nephrology, St Christopher's Hosp for Chldn 1985; Pediatric Nephrology, NY Hosp-Cornell Med Ctr 1987; **Fac Appt:** Assoc Clin Prof Ped, Cornell Univ-Weill Med Coll

Saland, Jeffrey M MD (PNep) - **Spec Exp:** Transplant Medicine-Kidney; Kidney Disease; Hypertension in Children; Hemolytic Uremic Syndrome; **Hospital:** Mt Sinai Med Ctr (page 102); **Address:** Mount Sinai Medical Center, 5 E 98th St, Fl 10, New York, NY 10029; **Phone:** 212-241-6187; **Board Cert:** Pediatric Nephrology 2011; **Med School:** Univ New Mexico 1995; **Resid:** Pediatrics, Chldns Hosp Med Ctr 1998; **Fellow:** Pediatric Nephrology, Univ TX-SW Med Ctr 2000; Pediatric Nephrology, Mt Sinai Med Ctr 2002; **Fac Appt:** Asst Prof Ped, Mount Sinai Sch Med

Trachtman, Howard MD (PNep) - **Spec Exp:** Electrolyte Disorders; Hypertension; Hemolytic Uremic Syndrome; Nephrotic Syndrome; **Hospital:** NYU Langone Med Ctr (page 108); **Address:** 160 E 32nd St, Level 3 Medical, New York, NY 10016; **Phone:** 212-263-5940; **Board Cert:** Pediatrics 1983; Nephrology 2003; **Med School:** Univ Pennsylvania 1978; **Resid:** Pediatrics, New England Med Ctr 1980; Pediatrics, Bronx Muni Hosp Ctr 1981; **Fellow:** Pediatric Nephrology, Montefiore Med Ctr 1983; **Fac Appt:** Prof Ped, Albert Einstein Coll Med

Pediatric Otolaryngology

April, Max M MD (PO) - **Spec Exp:** Sinus Disorders; Neck Masses; Laryngeal Disorders; Sleep Apnea; **Hospital:** NYU Langone Med Ctr (page 108); **Address:** NYU ENT Center, 240 E 38th St, Fl 14, New York, NY 10016; **Phone:** 646-501-7890; **Board Cert:** Otolaryngology 1990; **Med School:** Boston Univ 1985; **Resid:** Otolaryngology, Boston Univ Med Ctr 1990; **Fellow:** Pediatric Otolaryngology, Johns Hopkins 1991; **Fac Appt:** Clin Prof Oto, NYU Sch Med

Dolitsky, Jay N MD (PO) - **Spec Exp:** Ear Infections; Neck Masses; Tonsil/Adenoid Disorders; Sleep Disorders; **Hospital:** New York Eye & Ear Infirm (page 115); **Address:** ENT & Allergy Assocs, 261 Fifth Ave Fl 9 - Ste 901, MS 10016, New York, NY 10016; **Phone:** 212-679-3499; **Board Cert:** Otolaryngology 1990; **Med School:** SUNY Downstate 1984; **Resid:** Surgery, NYU/Bellevue Hosp 1987; Otolaryngology, Manhattan EET Hosp 1990; **Fellow:** Pediatric Otolaryngology, Children's Hosp 1992; **Fac Appt:** Assoc Clin Prof, NY Med Coll

Haddad Jr, Joseph MD (PO) - **Spec Exp:** Ear Infections; Sinus Disorders; Cleft Palate/Lip; **Hospital:** Morgan Stanley Children's Hosp of NY-Presby, NY (page 104); **Address:** Morgan Stanley Chldns Hosp of NY-Presby, 3959 Broadway, Ste 501N, New York, NY 10032-1559; **Phone:** 212-305-8933; **Board Cert:** Otolaryngology 1988; **Med School:** NYU Sch Med 1983; **Resid:** Surgery, Columbia-Presby Hosp 1985; Otolaryngology, Columbia-Presby Hosp 1988; **Fellow:** Pediatric Otolaryngology, Chldns Hosp 1990; **Fac Appt:** Prof Oto, Columbia P&S

Modi, Vikash K MD (PO) - **Spec Exp:** Airway Disorders; Airway Reconstruction; Tonsil/Adenoid Disorders; Cleft Palate/Lip; **Hospital:** NY-Presby/Weill Cornell Med Ctr, NY (page 104); **Address:** 428 E 72nd St, Oxford Bldg, Ste 100, New York, NY 10021; **Phone:** 646-962-3017; **Board Cert:** Otolaryngology 2008; **Med School:** UMDNJ-Univ Med Dent NJ 2002; **Resid:** Otolaryngology, USC Univ Hosp 2007; **Fellow:** Pediatric Otolaryngology, Northwestern Univ/Chldns Meml Hosp 2008; **Fac Appt:** Asst Prof Oto, Cornell Univ-Weill Med Coll

Rothschild, Michael A MD (PO) - **Spec Exp:** Ear Disorders; Sleep Apnea; Sinusitis; **Hospital:** Mt Sinai Med Ctr (page 102); **Address:** 1175 Park Ave, Ste 1A, New York, NY 10128; **Phone:** 212-996-2995; **Board Cert:** Otolaryngology 1994; **Med School:** Yale Univ 1988; **Resid:** Surgery, Mt Sinai Med Ctr 1990; Otolaryngology, Mt Sinai Med Ctr 1993; **Fellow:** Pediatric Otolaryngology, Chldn's Hosp 1994; **Fac Appt:** Clin Prof Oto, Mount Sinai Sch Med

Ward, Robert F MD (PO) - **Spec Exp:** Airway Disorders; Sinus Disorders/Surgery; Choanal Atresia; Cleft Palate/Lip; **Hospital:** NYU Langone Med Ctr (page 108); **Address:** NYU Langone Med Ctr-Dept Ped Otolaryngology, 240 E 38th St Fl 14, New York, NY 10016; **Phone:** 646-501-7890; **Board Cert:** Otolaryngology 1986; **Med School:** Cornell Univ-Weill Med Coll 1981; **Resid:** Surgery, NY Hosp 1983; Otolaryngology, NY Hosp 1986; **Fellow:** Pediatric Otolaryngology, Chldns Hosp 1987; **Fac Appt:** Clin Prof Ped, NYU Sch Med

Pediatric Pulmonology

Constantinescu, Andrei E MD/PhD (PPul) - **Spec Exp:** Cystic Fibrosis; Pulmonary Complications-Neurodisability; Pulmonary Infections; Asthma; **Hospital:** Morgan Stanley Children's Hosp of NY-Presby, NY (page 104); **Address:** Morgan Stanley Chldns Hosp-NYP, Dept Pediatric Pulmonology, 3959 Broadway, Ste 7C, New York, NY 10032; **Phone:** 212-305-5122; **Board Cert:** Pediatrics 2010; Pediatric Pulmonology 2006; **Med School:** Johns Hopkins Univ 1997; **Resid:** Pediatrics, NY-Presby/Weill Cornell Med Ctr 2002; **Fellow:** Pediatric Pulmonology, Morgan Stanley Children's Hosp of NY-Presby 2005; **Fac Appt:** Asst Prof Ped, Columbia P&S

Dimaio, Mary MD (PPul) - **Spec Exp:** Cystic Fibrosis; Asthma; Allergy; **Hospital:** NY-Presby/Weill Cornell Med Ctr, NY (page 104); **Address:** 1440 York Ave, Ste P5, New York, NY 10075; **Phone:** 212-988-5008; **Board Cert:** Pediatrics 1987; Pediatric Pulmonology 2007; Allergy & Immunology 2009; **Med School:** SUNY Hlth Sci Ctr 1981; **Resid:** Pediatrics, Kings Co Hosp/Downstate 1983; Pediatrics, N Shore Univ Hosp 1985; **Fellow:** Pediatric Pulmonology, Mt Sinai Hosp 1988

Kattan, Meyer MD (PPul) - **Spec Exp:** Asthma; Cystic Fibrosis; Chronic Lung Disease; **Hospital:** Morgan Stanley Children's Hosp of NY-Presby, NY (page 104), Englewood Hosp & Med Ctr; **Address:** Morgan Stanley Chldns Hosp of NY-Presby, 3959 Broadway, CHC 7-701, New York, NY 10032; **Phone:** 212-305-5122; **Board Cert:** Pediatrics 1980; Pediatric Pulmonology 2010; **Med School:** McGill Univ 1973; **Resid:** Pediatrics, Chldns Hosp 1975; Pediatrics, Hosp for Sick Chldn 1976; **Fellow:** Pulmonary Disease, Hosp for Sick Chldn 1978; **Fac Appt:** Prof Ped, Columbia P&S

Lamm, Carin I MD (PPul) - **Spec Exp:** Sleep Disorders/Apnea; Asthma; Cystic Fibrosis; **Hospital:** Morgan Stanley Children's Hosp of NY-Presby, NY (page 104); **Address:** NY-Presby, Pediatric Pulmonology Dept, 3959 Broadway Fl 7, New York, NY 10032; **Phone:** 212-305-5122; **Board Cert:** Pediatrics 1980; Pediatric Pulmonology 2010; Sleep Medicine 2011; **Med School:** NYU Sch Med 1975; **Resid:** Pediatrics, Mount Sinai Med Ctr 1979; **Fellow:** Pediatric Pulmonology, Mount Sinai Med Ctr 1981; **Fac Appt:** Assoc Prof Ped, Columbia P&S

Loughlin, Gerald M MD (PPul) - **Spec Exp:** Sleep Disorders/Apnea; Swallowing Disorders; Asthma & Chronic Lung Disease; Breathing Disorders; **Hospital:** NY-Presby/Weill Cornell Med Ctr, NY (page 104); **Address:** Cornell Med Coll, Dept Peds, 525 E 68th St, rm M-622, New York, NY 10021-4870; **Phone:** 646-962-3410; **Board Cert:** Pediatrics 1993; Pediatric Pulmonology 2010; **Med School:** Univ Rochester 1973; **Resid:** Pediatrics, Univ Ariz Med Ctr 1976; **Fellow:** Pediatric Pulmonology, Univ Ariz Med Ctr 1979; **Fac Appt:** Prof Ped, Cornell Univ-Weill Med Coll

Quittell, Lynne M MD (PPul) - **Spec Exp:** Cystic Fibrosis; Asthma; **Hospital:** Morgan Stanley Children's Hosp of NY-Presby, NY (page 104), NY-Presby/Columbia Univ Med Ctr, NY (page 104); **Address:** Morgan Stanley Children's Hosp of NY, 3959 Broadway, CHONY Bldg - Fl 7, New York, NY 10032; **Phone:** 212-305-5122; **Board Cert:** Pediatrics 1986; Pediatric Pulmonology 2011; **Med School:** Israel 1981; **Resid:** Pediatrics, Schneider Chldns Hosp 1984; **Fellow:** Pediatric Pulmonology, St Christopher's Hosp 1988

Ting, Andrew S MD (PPul) - **Spec Exp:** Asthma; Cystic Fibrosis; Bronchoscopy; Cough; **Hospital:** Mt Sinai Med Ctr (page 102); **Address:** 5 E 98th St, Fl 10, New York, NY 10029; **Phone:** 212-241-7788; **Board Cert:** Pediatric Pulmonology 2009; **Med School:** NYU Sch Med 1987; **Resid:** Pediatrics, Mt Sinai Med Ctr 1991; **Fellow:** Pediatric Pulmonology, Mt Sinai Med Ctr 1994; **Fac Appt:** Asst Prof Ped, Mount Sinai Sch Med

Vicencio, Alfin G MD (PPul) - **Spec Exp:** Asthma; Bronchoscopy; Interventional Pulmonology; **Hospital:** Mt Sinai Med Ctr (page 102); **Address:** Mount Sinai Pediatric Pulmonology, 5 E 98th St Fl 10, New York, NY 10029; **Phone:** 212-241-7788; **Board Cert:** Pediatric Pulmonology 2012; **Med School:** Univ Toledo, Med Univ OH 1996; **Resid:** Pediatrics, Columbia Presby Med Ctr 1999; **Fellow:** Pediatric Pulmonology, Yale-New Haven Hosp 2002; **Fac Appt:** Assoc Prof Ped, Mount Sinai Sch Med

Pediatric Rheumatology

Eichenfield, Andrew H MD (PRhu) - **Spec Exp:** Juvenile Arthritis; Lyme Disease; Lupus/SLE; **Hospital:** Morgan Stanley Children's Hosp of NY-Presby, NY (page 104), Nyack Hosp; **Address:** Morgan Stanley Chldns Hosp, 3959 Broadway, CHN-106, Ped Rheumatology, New York, NY 10032; **Phone:** 212-305-9304; **Board Cert:** Pediatrics 1983; Pediatric Rheumatology 2007; **Med School:** Ros Franklin Univ/Chicago Med Sch 1978; **Resid:** Pediatrics, Mt Sinai Hosp 1982; **Fellow:** Pediatric Rheumatology, Chldns Hosp 1984; **Fac Appt:** Asst Prof Ped, Columbia P&S

Imundo, Lisa F MD (PRhu) - **Spec Exp:** Lupus/SLE; Juvenile Arthritis; **Hospital:** Morgan Stanley Children's Hosp of NY-Presby, NY (page 104); **Address:** Morgan Stanley Children's Hospital, 3959 Broadway, rm 106, New York, NY 10023-3448; **Phone:** 212-305-9304; **Board Cert:** Pediatric Rheumatology 2011; **Med School:** SUNY Hlth Sci Ctr 1988; **Resid:** Pediatrics, NY-Presby Columbia Univ Med Ctr 1992; **Fellow:** Pediatric Rheumatology, NY-Presby Columbia Univ Med Ctr 1995; **Fac Appt:** Asst Clin Prof Ped, Columbia P&S

Lazarus, Herbert M MD (PRhu) - **Spec Exp:** Juvenile Arthritis; Lyme Disease; Pain-Musculoskeletal; **Hospital:** NYU Langone Med Ctr (page 108), Lenox Hill Hosp (page 106); **Address:** 390 West End Ave, Ste 1E, New York, NY 10024; **Phone:** 212-787-1444; **Board Cert:** Pediatrics 1987; Pediatric Rheumatology 2007; **Med School:** UMDNJ-NJ Med Sch, Newark 1983; **Resid:** Pediatrics, NYU Med Ctr 1986; **Fellow:** Pediatric Rheumatology, Hosp for Joint Diseases 1987; **Fac Appt:** Assoc Clin Prof Ped, NYU Sch Med

Lehman, Thomas J A MD (PRhu) - **Spec Exp:** Arthritis; Scleroderma; Lupus/SLE; Rheumatoid Arthritis; **Hospital:** Hosp For Special Surgery (page 113), NY-Presby/Weill Cornell Med Ctr, NY (page 104); **Address:** Hospital for Special Surgery, 535 E 70 St, Ste 714, New York, NY 10021-4872; **Phone:** 212-606-1151; **Board Cert:** Pediatrics 1979; Pediatric Rheumatology 2007; **Med School:** Jefferson Med Coll 1974; **Resid:** Pediatrics, Chldns Hosp 1976; Pediatrics, UCSF Med Ctr 1977; **Fellow:** Pediatric Rheumatology, Chldns Hosp 1979; Rheumatology, Natl Inst Hlth 1983; **Fac Appt:** Prof Ped, Cornell Univ-Weill Med Coll

Starr, Amy J MD (PRhu) - **Hospital:** Morgan Stanley Children's Hosp of NY-Presby, NY (page 104); **Address:** 3959 Broadway, CHN 106, New York, NY 10032; **Phone:** 212-305-9304; **Board Cert:** Pediatrics ; Pediatric Rheumatology 2010; **Med School:** Yale Univ 1974; **Resid:** Pediatrics, Albany Med Coll Affil Hosp 1978; **Fac Appt:** Asst Prof Ped, Columbia P&S

Pediatric Surgery

Bodenstein, Lawrence E MD/PhD (PS) - **Spec Exp:** Neonatal Surgery; Tumor Surgery; **Hospital:** Morgan Stanley Children's Hosp of NY-Presby, NY (page 104); **Address:** 3959 Broadway, CHN-215 Fl 2 North, New York, NY 10032; **Phone:** 212-342-8586; **Board Cert:** Surgery 2012; Pediatric Surgery 2005; **Med School:** Harvard Med Sch 1986; **Resid:** Surgery, Beth Israel Deaconess Hosp 1991; **Fellow:** Critical Care Medicine, Beth Israel Deaconess Hosp 1992; Pediatric Surgery, Chldns Hosp-Presbyterian Hosp 1994; **Fac Appt:** Asst Prof S, Columbia P&S

Cooper, Arthur MD (PS) - **Spec Exp:** Endoscopy; Trauma; Disaster Preparedness; Child Abuse; **Hospital:** Harlem Hosp Ctr, Metropolitan Hosp Ctr - NY; **Address:** Harlem Hospital, Dept Surgery, 506 Lenox Ave, Ste 11-153, New York, NY 10037; **Phone:** 212-939-4003; **Board Cert:** Surgery 2012; Pediatric Surgery 2003; Surgical Critical Care 2004; **Med School:** Univ Pennsylvania 1975; **Resid:** Surgery, Hosp Univ Penn 1981; Pediatric Surgery, Childrens Hosp 1984; **Fellow:** Pediatric Nutrition, Columbia P&S-Inst Human Nutrition 1982; **Fac Appt:** Prof S, Columbia P&S

Ginsburg, Howard B MD (PS) - **Spec Exp:** Neonatal Surgery; Tumor Surgery; Pediatric Urology; Gastrointestinal Surgery; **Hospital:** NYU Langone Med Ctr (page 108), Bellevue Hosp Ctr; **Address:** 530 First Ave, Ste 10W, New York, NY 10016-6402; **Phone:** 212-263-7391; **Board Cert:** Pediatric Surgery 2012; **Med School:** Univ Cincinnati 1972; **Resid:** Surgery, NYU-Bellvue Hosp 1977; Pediatric Surgery, Columbia-Presby Med Ctr 1979; **Fellow:** Pediatric Surgery, Mass Genl Hosp 1980; **Fac Appt:** Assoc Prof PS, NYU Sch Med

La Quaglia, Michael MD (PS) - **Spec Exp:** Cancer Surgery; Neuroblastoma; Liver Cancer; Wilms' Tumor; **Hospital:** Meml Sloan-Kettering Canc Ctr (page 114), NY-Presby/Weill Cornell Med Ctr, NY (page 104); **Address:** 1275 York Ave, Ste H1315, New York, NY 10065; **Phone:** 212-639-7002; **Board Cert:** Surgery 2003; Pediatric Surgery 2007; **Med School:** UMDNJ-NJ Med Sch, Newark 1976; **Resid:** Surgery, Mass Genl Hosp 1983; **Fellow:** Cardiothoracic Surgery, Broadgreen Ctr 1984; Pediatric Surgery, Chldns Hosp 1985; **Fac Appt:** Prof S, Cornell Univ-Weill Med Coll

Middlesworth, William MD (PS) - **Spec Exp:** Cancer Surgery; Neonatal Surgery; **Hospital:** Morgan Stanley Children's Hosp of NY-Presby, NY (page 104); **Address:** Morgan Stanley Children's Hospital, Div Pediatric Surgery, 3959 Broadway, CHN 216B, New York, NY 10032-1537; **Phone:** 212-342-8585; **Board Cert:** Surgery 2007; Pediatric Surgery 2007; **Med School:** UMDNJ-RW Johnson Med Sch 1989; **Resid:** Surgery, Univ Maryland Hosps 1995; **Fellow:** Pediatric Surgery, Columbia Presby Med Ctr 1997; **Fac Appt:** Asst Prof S, Columbia P&S

Midulla, Peter MD (PS) - **Spec Exp:** Hernia; Gastrointestinal Surgery; Minimally Invasive Surgery; Neonatal Surgery; **Hospital:** Mt Sinai Med Ctr (page 102); **Address:** Mount Sinai, Pediatric Surgery Dept, 5 E 98 St Fl 10, New York, NY 10029; **Phone:** 212-241-1608; **Board Cert:** Surgery 2007; Pediatric Surgery 2009; **Med School:** Albert Einstein Coll Med 1990; **Resid:** Surgery, Mount Sinai Med Ctr 1997; **Fellow:** Pediatric Surgery, Chldns Natl Med Ctr 1999; **Fac Appt:** Asst Prof Ped, Mount Sinai Sch Med

Quaegebeur, Jan M MD/PhD (PS) - **Spec Exp:** Arterial Switch; Heart Valve Surgery; Pediatric Cardiac Surgery; **Hospital:** Morgan Stanley Children's Hosp of NY-Presby, NY (page 104); **Address:** Morgan Stanley Chldns Hosp of NY-Presby, 3959 Broadway, Ste BHN276, New York, NY 10032; **Phone:** 212-305-5975; **Med School:** Belgium 1969; **Resid:** Surgery, St Michel Clinic 1973; **Fellow:** Thoracic Surgery, Baylor Coll Med 1974; Cardiothoracic Surgery, Univ Hosp 1978; **Fac Appt:** Prof S, Columbia P&S

Spigland, Nitsana A MD (PS) - **Spec Exp:** Pediatric Cancers; Minimally Invasive Surgery; Pediatric Thoracic Surgery; Neonatal Surgery; **Hospital:** NY-Presby/Weill Cornell Med Ctr, NY (page 104); **Address:** NY Hosp-Cornell Med Ctr, 520 E 70th St, Ste Starr-7, New York, NY 10065; **Phone:** 212-746-5648; **Board Cert:** Pediatric Surgery 2003; **Med School:** NY Med Coll 1982; **Resid:** Surgery, Lenox Hill Hosp 1987; **Fellow:** Pediatric Surgery, St Justine Chldn's Hosp 1989; **Fac Appt:** Prof S, Cornell Univ-Weill Med Coll

Stylianos, Steven MD (PS) - **Spec Exp:** Trauma; Neonatal Surgery; Chest Wall Deformities; Congenital Anomalies; **Hospital:** Morgan Stanley Children's Hosp of NY-Presby, NY (page 104); **Address:** Morgan Stanley Chldn's Hosp, 3959 Broadway Fl 205-N, New York, NY 10032; **Phone:** 212-342-8586; **Board Cert:** Surgery 2002; Pediatric Surgery 2003; **Med School:** NYU Sch Med 1983; **Resid:** Surgery, Columbia-Presby Med Ctr 1988; Pediatric Surgery, Chldns Hosp 1992; **Fellow:** Pediatric Surgical Critical Care, New England Med Ctr 1990; **Fac Appt:** Prof S, Columbia P&S

Tomita, Sandra MD (PS) - **Hospital:** NYU Langone Med Ctr (page 108), Hackensack Univ Med Ctr (page 718); **Address:** 530 1st Ave, Ste 10W, New York, NY 10016; **Phone:** 212-263-7391; **Board Cert:** Surgery 2001; Pediatric Surgery 2007; **Med School:** Northwestern Univ 1988; **Resid:** Surgery, Vanderbilt Univ Hosp 1993; **Fellow:** Pediatric Surgery, St Louis Univ Hosp 1998; **Fac Appt:** Asst Prof S, NYU Sch Med

Velcek, Francisca T MD (PS) - **Spec Exp:** Anorectal Malformations; Pediatric Gynecology; Neonatal Surgery; Hernia; **Hospital:** Lenox Hill Hosp (page 106); **Address:** Ped Surg, 965 5th Ave, New York, NY 10075; **Phone:** 212-744-9396; **Board Cert:** Surgery 1974; Pediatric Surgery 2007; **Med School:** Philippines 1966; **Resid:** Surgery, St Clares Hosp 1971; Pediatric Surgery, SUNY Downstate Med Ctr 1975; **Fac Appt:** Clin Prof S, SUNY Hlth Sci Ctr

Pediatric Urology

Casale, Pasquale MD (Ped Uro) - **Spec Exp:** Genitourinary Reconstruction; Minimally Invasive Surgery-Pediatric; Genital Reconstruction-Pediatric; Robotic Surgery-Pediatric; **Hospital:** Morgan Stanley Children's Hosp of NY-Presby, NY (page 104), NY-Presby/Columbia Univ Med Ctr, NY (page 104); **Address:** Columbia Pediatric Urology, 3959 Broadway Fl 11N, New York, NY 10032; **Phone:** 212-305-9918; **Board Cert:** Urology 2008; Pediatric Urology ; **Med School:** Albert Einstein Coll Med 1996; **Resid:** Urology, Thomas Jefferson Univ Hosp 2002; **Fellow:** Pediatric Urology, Seattle Chldn's Hosp 2004; **Fac Appt:** Prof U, Columbia P&S

Hyun, Grace S MD (Ped Uro) - **Spec Exp:** Hypospadias; Varicocele; Undescended Testis; Minimally Invasive Surgery; **Hospital:** Mt Sinai Med Ctr (page 102), Lenox Hill Hosp (page 106); **Address:** Mount Sinai, Ped Urology Dept, 5 E 98 St, Fl 6, New York, NY 10029; **Phone:** 212-241-4812; **Board Cert:** Urology 2009; Pediatric Urology 2009; **Med School:** Cornell Univ-Weill Med Coll 1997; **Resid:** Urology, NY-Presby/Columbia Univ Med Ctr 2002; **Fellow:** Pediatric Urology, Chldns Hosp 2005; **Fac Appt:** Asst Prof U, Mount Sinai Sch Med

Poppas, Dix P MD (Ped Uro) - **Spec Exp:** Genital Reconstruction-Pediatric; Robotic Surgery-Pediatric; Minimally Invasive Surgery-Pediatric; **Hospital:** NY-Presby/Weill Cornell Med Ctr, NY (page 104); **Address:** Inst for Pediatric Urology, NY Presby Hosp-Weill Cornell, 525 E 68th St, rm F931, Box 94, New York, NY 10065; **Phone:** 212-746-5337; **Board Cert:** Urology 2008; Pediatric Urology 2008; **Med School:** Eastern VA Med Sch 1988; **Resid:** Surgery, Eastern VA Med Schl Affil Hosp 1990; Urology, NY Hosp-Cornell Med Ctr 1994; **Fellow:** Pediatric Urology, Boston Children's Hosp 1996; **Fac Appt:** Prof U, Cornell Univ-Weill Med Coll

Schlussel, Richard N MD (Ped Uro) - **Spec Exp:** Hypospadias; Robotic Surgery; Reconstructive Surgery; Pyeloplasty; **Hospital:** NY-Presby/Weill Cornell Med Ctr, NY (page 104), Englewood Hosp & Med Ctr; **Address:** Pediatric Urology Assocs, 65 E 96th St, Ste 1B, New York, NY 10128; **Phone:** 212-987-9500; **Board Cert:** Urology 2010; Pediatric Urology 2010; **Med School:** Albert Einstein Coll Med 1986; **Resid:** Urology, Mt Sinai Med Ctr 1992; **Fellow:** Pediatric Urology, Boston Children's Hosp 1994

Shapiro, Ellen MD (Ped Uro) - **Spec Exp:** Genitourinary Congenital Anomalies; Fetal Urology; Genital Reconstruction-Pediatric; **Hospital:** NYU Langone Med Ctr (page 108), Hackensack Univ Med Ctr (page 718); **Address:** NYU Urology Assocs, 150 E 32nd St Fl 2, New York, NY 10016; **Phone:** 646-825-6326; **Board Cert:** Urology 2008; Pediatric Urology 2008; **Med School:** Univ Nebr Coll Med 1978; **Resid:** Surgery, Johns Hopkins Hosp 1980; Urology, Johns Hopkins Hosp 1986; **Fellow:** Pediatric Urology, Chldns Hosp Michigan 1987; **Fac Appt:** Prof U, NYU Sch Med

Pediatrics

Allendorf, Dennis MD (Ped) *PCP* - **Hospital:** Morgan Stanley Children's Hosp of NY-Presby, NY (page 104), St. Luke's - Roosevelt Hosp Ctr - Roosevelt Div (page 94); **Address:** 401 W 118th St, Ste 2, New York, NY 10027-7216; **Phone:** 212-666-4610; **Board Cert:** Pediatrics 1987; **Med School:** NY Med Coll 1970; **Resid:** Pediatrics, St Luke's-Roosevelt Hosp Ctr 1972; Pediatrics, NY-Presby/Columbia Univ Med Ctr 1973

Arpadi, Stephen MD (Ped) *PCP* - **Spec Exp:** AIDS/HIV; **Hospital:** St. Luke's - Roosevelt Hosp Ctr - St Luke's Hosp (page 94), NY-Presby/Columbia Univ Med Ctr, NY (page 104); **Address:** St Luke's-Spencer Cox Ctr for Hlth, 1111 Amsterdam Ave/West 114th St, New York, NY 10025; **Phone:** 212-523-3847; **Board Cert:** Pediatrics 2009; **Med School:** Geo Wash Univ 1982; **Resid:** Pediatrics, Chldns Hosp Natl Med Ctr 1985; **Fac Appt:** Assoc Prof Ped, Columbia P&S

Axelrod, Felicia B MD (Ped) - **Spec Exp:** Dysautonomia; **Hospital:** NYU Langone Med Ctr (page 108); **Address:** NYU Langone Med Ctr, 530 1st Ave, Ste 9Q, New York, NY 10016-6402; **Phone:** 212-263-7225; **Board Cert:** Pediatrics 1971; **Med School:** NYU Sch Med 1966; **Resid:** Pediatrics, Bellevue/NYU Med Ctr 1969; **Fellow:** Clinical Genetics, Mt Sinai Med Ctr 1976; **Fac Appt:** Prof Ped, NYU Sch Med

Bodner, Staci M MD/PhD (Ped) *PCP* - **Spec Exp:** Neonatology; **Hospital:** NY-Presby/Weill Cornell Med Ctr, NY (page 104), Morgan Stanley Children's Hosp of NY-Presby, NY (page 104); **Address:** Manhattan Pediatrics, 125 E 72nd St, Ste 1A, New York, NY 10021; **Phone:** 212-988-6500; **Board Cert:** Pediatrics 2011; **Med School:** Albert Einstein Coll Med 2000; **Resid:** Pediatrics, Mount Sinai Med Ctr 2003

Brovender, Bruce J MD (Ped) *PCP* - **Hospital:** NY-Presby/Weill Cornell Med Ctr, NY (page 104), Lenox Hill Hosp (page 106); **Address:** 1559 York Ave, New York, NY 10028; **Phone:** 212-585-3329; **Board Cert:** Pediatrics 2011; **Med School:** Italy 1984; **Resid:** Pediatrics, Lenox Hill Hosp 1987; **Fellow:** Pediatric Hematology-Oncology, NYU/Bellvue Hosp 1988; **Fac Appt:** Asst Clin Prof Ped, Cornell Univ-Weill Med Coll

Brown, Jocelyn MD (Ped) - **Spec Exp:** Child Abuse; **Hospital:** Morgan Stanley Children's Hosp of NY-Presby, NY (page 104); **Address:** Child Advocacy Center, 922 W 168th St Fl 8, New York, NY 10032; **Phone:** 212-305-2393; **Board Cert:** Pediatrics 1987; **Med School:** France 1981; **Resid:** Pediatrics, St Luke's-Roosevelt Hosp 1984; **Fellow:** Ambulatory Pediatrics, NY Presby Hosp/Columbia 1986; **Fac Appt:** Prof Ped, Columbia P&S

Burstin, Harris E MD (Ped) *PCP* - **Hospital:** NYU Langone Med Ctr (page 108); **Address:** 317 E 34th St Fl 3, New York, NY 10016-4974; **Phone:** 212-725-6300; **Board Cert:** Pediatrics 1983; **Med School:** Mexico 1977; **Resid:** Pediatrics, Bellevue Hosp Ctr 1982; **Fac Appt:** Assoc Prof Ped, NYU Sch Med

Cohen, Michel A MD (Ped) *PCP* - **Spec Exp:** Child Development; Sleep Disorders; **Hospital:** NY-Presby/Weill Cornell Med Ctr, NY (page 104); **Address:** Tribeca Pediatrics, 46 Warren St, New York, NY 10007; **Phone:** 212-226-7666; **Board Cert:** Pediatrics 2010; **Med School:** France 1989; **Resid:** Pediatrics, NYU Med Ctr 1991; Pediatrics, Long Island Coll Hosp 1993

Cross, Jennifer MD (Ped) *PCP* - **Spec Exp:** Learning Disorders; Child Development; Behavioral Disorders; **Hospital:** NY-Presby/Weill Cornell Med Ctr, NY (page 104); **Address:** 525 E 68th St Fl 3, New York, NY 10065; **Phone:** 646-962-4303; **Board Cert:** Pediatrics 2005; Developmental-Behavioral Pediatrics 2002; **Med School:** England, UK 1983; **Resid:** Pediatrics, Lenox Hill Hosp 1988; **Fellow:** Neonatal-Perinatal Medicine, NY Hosp 1991; Developmental-Behavioral Pediatrics, Westchester Co Med Ctr 1994; **Fac Appt:** Asst Prof Ped, Cornell Univ-Weill Med Coll

Edelstein, Gary S MD (Ped) *PCP* - **Hospital:** Morgan Stanley Children's Hosp of NY-Presby, NY (page 104), NY-Presby/Weill Cornell Med Ctr, NY (page 104); **Address:** Manhattan Pediatrics, 125 E 72nd St, Ste 1A, New York, NY 10021; **Phone:** 212-988-6500; **Board Cert:** Pediatrics 2008; **Med School:** NYU Sch Med 1990; **Resid:** Pediatrics, Columbia Presby Babies Hosp 1993; **Fellow:** Ambulatory Pediatrics, Columbia Presby Babies Hosp 1995; **Fac Appt:** Asst Clin Prof Ped, Columbia P&S

Ferrier, Genevieve E MD (Ped) *PCP* - **Hospital:** NYU Langone Med Ctr (page 108); **Address:** 46 W 11th St, New York, NY 10011-8602; **Phone:** 212-529-4330; **Board Cert:** Pediatrics 2013; **Med School:** Mount Sinai Sch Med 1988; **Resid:** Pediatrics, Chldn's Hosp of Los Angeles 1991; **Fac Appt:** Asst Prof Ped, NY Med Coll

Freilich, Stephanie B MD (Ped) *PCP* - **Hospital:** Mt Sinai Med Ctr (page 102); **Address:** 1125 Park Ave, Ste A, New York, NY 10128-2322; **Phone:** 212-289-1400; **Board Cert:** Pediatrics 2009; **Med School:** Mount Sinai Sch Med 1991; **Resid:** Pediatrics, Mount Sinai Med Ctr 1994; **Fac Appt:** Asst Clin Prof Ped, Mount Sinai Sch Med

Goldstein, Judith MD (Ped) *PCP* - **Spec Exp:** Infectious Disease; **Hospital:** NY-Presby/Weill Cornell Med Ctr, NY (page 104), Lenox Hill Hosp (page 106); **Address:** 1559 York Ave SW, Fl ground, none, New York, NY 10028; **Phone:** 212-585-3329; **Board Cert:** Pediatrics 1977; **Med School:** SUNY Downstate 1972; **Resid:** Pediatrics, Lenox Hill Hosp 1975; **Fac Appt:** Asst Clin Prof Ped, Cornell Univ-Weill Med Coll

Hes, Dyan S MD (Ped) *PCP* - **Spec Exp:** Obesity; Weight Management; **Hospital:** NY-Presby/Weill Cornell Med Ctr, NY (page 104); **Address:** Gramercy Pediatrics, 67 Irving Pl Fl 3 South, New York, NY 10003; **Phone:** 212-473-4200; **Board Cert:** Pediatrics 2009; **Med School:** Israel 1997; **Resid:** Pediatrics, Montefiore Med Ctr 2000; **Fac Appt:** Asst Clin Prof Ped, Cornell Univ-Weill Med Coll

Hiltebeitel, Carolyn B MD (Ped) *PCP* - **Hospital:** NY-Presby/Weill Cornell Med Ctr, NY (page 104); **Address:** Weill Cornell Medical Associates, 12 W 72nd St, New York, NY 10023; **Phone:** 646-962-7800; **Board Cert:** Pediatrics 2012; **Med School:** Albert Einstein Coll Med 1994; **Resid:** Pediatrics, Mt Sinai Hosp 1997; **Fac Appt:** Asst Clin Prof Ped, Cornell Univ-Weill Med Coll

Ho, Sharon H MD (Ped) *PCP* - **Hospital:** Morgan Stanley Children's Hosp of NY-Presby, NY (page 104); **Address:** Manhattan Pediatrics, 125 E 72nd St, Ste 1A, New York, NY 10021; **Phone:** 212-988-6500; **Board Cert:** Pediatrics 2010; **Med School:** SUNY Upstate Med Univ 1999; **Resid:** Pediatrics, Wash Univ/St Louis Chldn's Hosp 2002

Inamdar, Sarla MD (Ped) *PCP* - **Spec Exp:** Rheumatology; **Hospital:** Metropolitan Hosp Ctr - NY; **Address:** 1901 1st Ave, rm 523, New York, NY 10029-7404; **Phone:** 212-423-6228; **Board Cert:** Pediatrics 1974; **Med School:** India 1969; **Resid:** Pediatrics, Metropolitan Hosp Ctr 1972; **Fac Appt:** Clin Prof Ped, NY Med Coll

Kahn, Max A MD (Ped) *PCP* - **Hospital:** NYU Langone Med Ctr (page 108), Lenox Hill Hosp (page 106); **Address:** 390 West End Ave, Ste 1E, New York, NY 10024; **Phone:** 212-787-1444; **Board Cert:** Pediatrics 1980; **Med School:** Columbia P&S 1975; **Resid:** Pediatrics, Bronx Muni Hosp 1978; **Fac Appt:** Assoc Clin Prof Ped, NYU Sch Med

Karlsrud, Katherine MD (Ped) *PCP* - **Spec Exp:** Adolescent Medicine; **Hospital:** NY-Presby/Columbia Univ Med Ctr, NY (page 104); **Address:** 56 E 76th St, New York, NY 10021; **Phone:** 212-249-5544; **Board Cert:** Pediatrics 2012; **Med School:** Albany Med Coll 1980; **Resid:** Pediatrics, New York Hosp 1983

Keith, Marie B MD (Ped) *PCP* - **Hospital:** NYU Langone Med Ctr (page 108); **Address:** 552 Broadway Fl 5, New York, NY 10012; **Phone:** 212-334-3366; **Board Cert:** Pediatrics 1979; **Med School:** Mount Sinai Sch Med 1974; **Resid:** Pediatrics, NY-Presby/Columbia Univ Med Ctr 1977

Kon, Shulamite MD (Ped) *PCP* - **Hospital:** Mt Sinai Med Ctr (page 102); **Address:** 240 W 98th St, Ste 1C, New York, NY 10025; **Phone:** 212-662-1212; **Board Cert:** Pediatrics 2008; **Med School:** SUNY Downstate 1985; **Resid:** Pediatrics, Mt Sinai Med Ctr 1988

Kotin, Neal M MD (Ped) *PCP* - **Spec Exp:** Asthma; Bronchitis; Sleep Disorders; Pulmonary Disease; **Hospital:** Mt Sinai Med Ctr (page 102), Lenox Hill Hosp (page 106); **Address:** Carnegie Hill Pediatrics, 1125 Park Ave, New York, NY 10128-1243; **Phone:** 212-289-1400; **Board Cert:** Pediatrics 2010; Pediatric Pulmonology 2011; **Med School:** Albany Med Coll 1982; **Resid:** Pediatrics, Johns Hopkins Hosp 1985; **Fellow:** Pediatric Pulmonology, Mt Sinai Med Ctr 1988; **Fac Appt:** Asst Clin Prof Ped, Mount Sinai Sch Med

Larson, Signe S MD (Ped) *PCP* - **Spec Exp:** Pediatric Endocrinology; **Hospital:** Mt Sinai Med Ctr (page 102); **Address:** Uptown Padiatrics, 1245 Park Ave, New York, NY 10128; **Phone:** 212-427-0540; **Board Cert:** Pediatrics 1984; Pediatric Endocrinology 2011; **Med School:** SUNY Stony Brook 1978; **Resid:** Family Medicine, Vancouver Genl Hosp 1979; Pediatrics, St Lukes Med Ctr 1982; **Fellow:** Pediatric Endocrinology, Mount Sinai Med Ctr 1984

Lazarus, George M MD (Ped) *PCP* - **Hospital:** Morgan Stanley Children's Hosp of NY-Presby, NY (page 104), NY-Presby/Weill Cornell Med Ctr, NY (page 104); **Address:** 106 E 78th, New York, NY 10075-0302; **Phone:** 212-744-0840; **Board Cert:** Pediatrics 1976; **Med School:** Columbia P&S 1971; **Resid:** Pediatrics, NY Presby-Columbia Med Ctr 1974; **Fac Appt:** Assoc Clin Prof Ped, Columbia P&S

Licata, Joseph C MD (Ped) *PCP* - **Hospital:** Lenox Hill Hosp (page 106), NY-Presby/Weill Cornell Med Ctr, NY (page 104); **Address:** Global Pediatrics, 1559 York Ave, New York, NY 10028; **Phone:** 212-585-3329; **Board Cert:** Pediatrics 1984; **Med School:** Italy 1978; **Resid:** Pediatrics, Lenox Hill Hosp 1982

Lipper, Evelyn G MD (Ped) *PCP* - **Spec Exp:** Learning Disorders; Behavioral Disorders; Child Development; **Hospital:** NY-Presby/Weill Cornell Med Ctr, NY (page 104); **Address:** 525 E 68th St Fl 3, New York, NY 10065; **Phone:** 646-962-4303; **Board Cert:** Pediatrics 1976; **Med School:** Albert Einstein Coll Med 1971; **Resid:** Pediatrics, Babies Hosp 1973; Pediatrics, Jacobi Med Ctr 1975; **Fac Appt:** Assoc Clin Prof Ped, Cornell Univ-Weill Med Coll

McCarton, Cecelia MD (Ped) - **Spec Exp:** Autism; Learning Disorders; ADD/ADHD; Developmental Disorders; **Address:** McCarton Ctr for Developmental Peds, 350 E 82nd St, New York, NY 10028; **Phone:** 212-996-9019; **Board Cert:** Pediatrics 1988; **Med School:** Albert Einstein Coll Med 1970; **Resid:** Pediatrics, Bronx Muni Hosp 1974; **Fellow:** Developmental-Behavioral Pediatrics, Montefiore Med Ctr-Weiler Einstein Div 1977; **Fac Appt:** Clin Prof Ped, Albert Einstein Coll Med

McHugh, Margaret T MD (Ped) - **Spec Exp:** Child Abuse; Adolescent Medicine; **Hospital:** Bellevue Hosp Ctr, NYU Langone Med Ctr (page 108); **Address:** Bellevue Hosp Child Protection Ctr, 462 First Ave, rm GC65, New York, NY 10016; **Phone:** 212-562-6073; **Board Cert:** Pediatrics 1975; Child Abuse Pediatrics 2009; **Med School:** Georgetown Univ 1970; **Resid:** Pediatrics, Metropolitan Hosp 1973; **Fellow:** Ambulatory Pediatrics, Columbia-Presby Med Ctr 1975; **Fac Appt:** Assoc Prof Ped, NYU Sch Med

Meyer, Dodi D MD (Ped) *PCP* - **Hospital:** NY-Presby/Columbia Univ Med Ctr, NY (page 104); **Address:** Washington Heights Family Ctr, 575 W 181st St, New York, NY 10033; **Phone:** 212-342-3060; **Board Cert:** Pediatrics 2013; **Med School:** Argentina 1986; **Resid:** Pediatrics, Bronx-Lebanon Hosp 1991; **Fac Appt:** Assoc Prof Ped, Columbia P&S

Monti, Louis G MD (Ped) *PCP* - **Spec Exp:** Infectious Disease; **Hospital:** Mt Sinai Med Ctr (page 102); **Address:** 55 E 87th St, Ste 1G, New York, NY 10128-1049; **Phone:** 212-722-0707; **Board Cert:** Pediatrics 2009; **Med School:** Mount Sinai Sch Med 1980; **Resid:** Pediatrics, Mount Sinai Hosp 1983; **Fellow:** Infectious Disease, Childrens Hosp 1984; **Fac Appt:** Asst Clin Prof Ped, Mount Sinai Sch Med

Murphy, Ramon J C MD (Ped) *PCP* - **Hospital:** Mt Sinai Med Ctr (page 102); **Address:** Uptown Pediatrics, 1245 Park Ave, New York, NY 10128; **Phone:** 212-427-0540; **Board Cert:** Pediatrics 2009; **Med School:** Northwestern Univ 1969; **Resid:** Internal Medicine, Cook Co Hosp 1970; Pediatrics, Chldns Meml Hosp 1971; **Fellow:** Pediatrics, Babies Hosp 1973; Community Medicine, Mt Sinai Med Ctr 1974; **Fac Appt:** Clin Prof Ped, Mount Sinai Sch Med

Newman-Cedar, Meryl MD (Ped) *PCP* - **Spec Exp:** Child Development; **Hospital:** NY-Presby/Weill Cornell Med Ctr, NY (page 104), Lenox Hill Hosp (page 106); **Address:** Upper East Side Pediatrics, 215 E 79th St, Ste 1C, New York, NY 10075; **Phone:** 212-737-7800; **Board Cert:** Pediatrics 1987; **Med School:** SUNY Downstate 1981; **Resid:** Pediatrics, NY Hosp 1984; **Fellow:** Developmental-Behavioral Pediatrics, NY Hosp 1987

Oeffinger, Kevin C MD (Ped) - **Spec Exp:** Cancer Survivors-Late Effects of Therapy; **Hospital:** Meml Sloan-Kettering Canc Ctr (page 114); **Address:** 300 E 66th St, New York, NY 10065; **Phone:** 646-888-4730; **Board Cert:** Family Medicine 2006; **Med School:** Univ Tex, San Antonio 1984; **Resid:** Family Medicine, Baylor Coll Med 1987; **Fellow:** Family Medicine, Fam Practice Faculty Dev Ctr 1999; Research, Natl Cancer Inst 2000

Orbe, Jessica MD (Ped) *PCP* - **Hospital:** St. Luke's - Roosevelt Hosp Ctr - St Luke's Hosp (page 94), St. Luke's - Roosevelt Hosp Ctr - Roosevelt Div (page 94); **Address:** West Care Medical, 50 W 77th St, New York, NY 10024; **Phone:** 212-579-5001; **Board Cert:** Pediatrics 2011; **Med School:** SUNY Downstate 1993; **Resid:** Pediatrics, NY-Presby/Columbia Univ Med Ctr 1996

Pasquariello, Palmo J MD (Ped) *PCP* - **Hospital:** Lenox Hill Hosp (page 106), NY-Presby/Weill Cornell Med Ctr, NY (page 104); **Address:** Global Pediatrics, 1559 York Ave, New York, NY 10028; **Phone:** 212-585-3329; **Board Cert:** Pediatrics 2010; **Med School:** NY Med Coll 1985; **Resid:** Pediatrics, Lenox Hill Hosp 1988

Poon, Eric Sin-Kam MD (Ped) *PCP* - **Spec Exp:** Asthma; Pediatric Cardiology; Developmental Disorders; **Hospital:** NY-Presby/Lower Manhattan Hosp (page 104), NY-Presby/Weill Cornell Med Ctr, NY (page 104); **Address:** 28 E Broadway St, Fl 4, MS 10002, New York, NY 10038-2612; **Phone:** 212-312-5350; **Board Cert:** Pediatrics 1988; **Med School:** Mexico 1982; **Resid:** Pediatrics, LI Coll Hosp 1986; **Fellow:** Pediatric Cardiology, NY Hosp-Cornell Med Ctr 1988; **Fac Appt:** Asst Clin Prof Ped, Cornell Univ-Weill Med Coll

Popper, Laura MD (Ped) *PCP* - **Hospital:** Mt Sinai Med Ctr (page 102); **Address:** 116 E 66th St, Ste 1C, New York, NY 10065; **Phone:** 212-794-2136; **Board Cert:** Pediatrics 1981; **Med School:** Columbia P&S 1974; **Resid:** Pediatrics, Babies Hosp 1976; **Fellow:** Pediatrics, Babies Hosp 1977; **Fac Appt:** Asst Clin Prof Ped, NY Coll Osteo Med

Prezioso, Paula J MD (Ped) *PCP* - **Hospital:** NYU Langone Med Ctr (page 108); **Address:** 317 E 34th St, Fl 3, New York, NY 10016-4974; **Phone:** 212-725-6300; **Board Cert:** Pediatrics 2013; **Med School:** SUNY Downstate 1987; **Resid:** Pediatrics, NYU Med Ctr 1991; **Fac Appt:** Assoc Clin Prof Ped, NYU Sch Med

Raucher, Harold S MD (Ped) *PCP* - **Spec Exp:** Infectious Disease; Travel Medicine; **Hospital:** Mt Sinai Med Ctr (page 102), Lenox Hill Hosp (page 106); **Address:** Carnegie Hill Pediatrics, 1125 Park Ave, New York, NY 10128-1243; **Phone:** 212-289-1400; **Board Cert:** Pediatrics 2006; Pediatric Infectious Disease 2009; **Med School:** Mount Sinai Sch Med 1978; **Resid:** Pediatrics, Mt Sinai Med Ctr 1980; **Fellow:** Pediatric Infectious Disease, Mt Sinai Med Ctr 1982; **Fac Appt:** Assoc Clin Prof Ped, Mount Sinai Sch Med

Rosello, Lori J MD (Ped) *PCP* - **Hospital:** NYU Langone Med Ctr (page 108); **Address:** 46 W 11th St, New York, NY 10011-8602; **Phone:** 212-529-4330; **Board Cert:** Pediatrics 2012; **Med School:** Albert Einstein Coll Med 1987; **Resid:** Pediatrics, Babies Hosp/Columbia 1990; **Fac Appt:** Asst Clin Prof Ped, NYU Sch Med

Rosenbaum, Michael MD (Ped) *PCP* - **Hospital:** NY-Presby/Weill Cornell Med Ctr, NY (page 104), Lenox Hill Hosp (page 106); **Address:** West End Pediatrics, 450 West End Ave, New York, NY 10024-5307; **Phone:** 212-769-3070; **Board Cert:** Pediatrics 1988; **Med School:** Cornell Univ-Weill Med Coll 1982; **Resid:** Pediatrics, NY-Presby/Columbia Univ Med Ctr 1985; **Fellow:** Pediatric Endocrinology, NY-Presby/Weill Cornell Med Ctr 1988; **Fac Appt:** Prof Ped, Columbia P&S

Rosenfeld, Suzanne MD (Ped) *PCP* - **Spec Exp:** Adolescent Medicine; **Hospital:** NY-Presby/Weill Cornell Med Ctr, NY (page 104), Lenox Hill Hosp (page 106); **Address:** West End Pediatrics, 450 West End Ave, New York, NY 10024-5393; **Phone:** 212-769-3070; **Board Cert:** Pediatrics 1986; **Med School:** Columbia P&S 1980; **Resid:** Pediatrics, Columbia-Presby Med Ctr 1983

Sacker, Ira M MD (Ped) - **Spec Exp:** Eating Disorders; Obesity; **Hospital:** NYU Langone Med Ctr (page 108); **Address:** 19 W 34th St, Fl PH, New York, NY 10011; **Phone:** 212-268-4440; **Board Cert:** Pediatrics 1982; **Med School:** UCLA 1968; **Resid:** Pediatrics, Bellevue Hosp/NYU Med Ctr 1971; **Fellow:** Adolescent Medicine, Chldns Hosp 1972; **Fac Appt:** Asst Clin Prof Ped, NYU Sch Med

Saha, Prantik MD (Ped) *PCP* - **Hospital:** St. Luke's - Roosevelt Hosp Ctr - Roosevelt Div (page 94); **Address:** West Care Pediatrics, 241 Central Park W, Ste 1G, New York, NY 10024; **Phone:** 212-787-1788; **Board Cert:** Pediatrics 2011; **Med School:** Case West Res Univ 1993; **Resid:** Pediatrics, Johns Hopkins Hosp 1996; **Fac Appt:** Asst Clin Prof Ped, Columbia P&S

Sanford, Marie V MD (Ped) *PCP* - **Hospital:** NY-Presby/Weill Cornell Med Ctr, NY (page 104); **Address:** Weill Cornell Medical Associates, 12 W 72nd St, New York, NY 10023; **Phone:** 646-962-7800; **Board Cert:** Pediatrics 2009; **Med School:** Mount Sinai Sch Med 1991; **Resid:** Pediatrics, Mount Sinai Med Ctr 1995; **Fac Appt:** Asst Clin Prof Ped, Mount Sinai Sch Med

Similon, Philippe L MD/PhD (Ped) *PCP* - **Hospital:** Lenox Hill Hosp (page 106), NY-Presby/Columbia Univ Med Ctr, NY (page 104); **Address:** Park Avenue Pediatrics, 1111 Park Ave, New York, NY 10128; **Phone:** 212-534-3000; **Board Cert:** Pediatrics 2009; **Med School:** Columbia P&S 1997; **Resid:** Pediatrics, NY Presby Hosp/Columbia 2001

Softness, Barney MD (Ped) *PCP* - **Spec Exp:** Diabetes; **Hospital:** NY-Presby/Weill Cornell Med Ctr, NY (page 104), Lenox Hill Hosp (page 106); **Address:** West End Pediatrics, 450 West End Ave, New York, NY 10024-5307; **Phone:** 212-769-3070; **Board Cert:** Pediatrics 1986; Pediatric Endocrinology 1986; **Med School:** Columbia P&S 1980; **Resid:** Pediatrics, NY-Presby/Columbia Univ Med Ctr 1983; **Fellow:** Pediatric Endocrinology, NY-Presby/Weill Cornell Med Ctr 1985; **Fac Appt:** Assoc Clin Prof Ped, Columbia P&S

Stein, Barry B MD (Ped) *PCP* - **Spec Exp:** Developmental & Behavioral Disorders; **Hospital:** Mt Sinai Med Ctr (page 102), Lenox Hill Hosp (page 106); **Address:** Carnegie Hill Pediatrics, 1125 Park Ave, New York, NY 10128-1243; **Phone:** 212-289-1400; **Board Cert:** Pediatrics 1987; **Med School:** South Africa 1980; **Resid:** Pediatrics, Mt Sinai Hosp 1986; **Fac Appt:** Asst Clin Prof Ped, Mount Sinai Sch Med

Trachtenberg, Jennifer MD (Ped) *PCP* - **Spec Exp:** Parenting Issues; Weight Management; **Hospital:** Mt Sinai Med Ctr (page 102), Lenox Hill Hosp (page 106); **Address:** Carnegie Hill Pediatrics, 1125 Park Ave, New York, NY 10128; **Phone:** 212-289-1400; **Board Cert:** Pediatrics 2004; **Med School:** Mount Sinai Sch Med 1993; **Resid:** Pediatrics, Mount Sinai Med Ctr 1996; **Fac Appt:** Asst Clin Prof Ped, Mount Sinai Sch Med

Traister, Michael R MD (Ped) *PCP* - **Spec Exp:** Adoption & Foster Care; **Hospital:** NYU Langone Med Ctr (page 108), Lenox Hill Hosp (page 106); **Address:** 390 West End Ave, Ste 1E, New York, NY 10024; **Phone:** 212-787-1444; **Board Cert:** Pediatrics 1980; **Med School:** NY Med Coll 1975; **Resid:** Pediatrics, Bronx Muni Hosp 1978; **Fellow:** Ambulatory Pediatrics, Bellevue Hosp 1979; **Fac Appt:** Assoc Clin Prof Ped, NYU Sch Med

van Gilder, Max F MD (Ped) *PCP* - **Hospital:** St. Luke's - Roosevelt Hosp Ctr - Roosevelt Div (page 94); **Address:** West Care Pediatrics, 241 Central Park W, Ste 1G, New York, NY 10024; **Phone:** 212-787-1788; **Board Cert:** Pediatrics 1976; **Med School:** Tulane Univ 1971; **Resid:** Pediatrics, Montefiore Med Ctr 1974; **Fac Appt:** Asst Clin Prof Ped, Columbia P&S

Weinberger, Sylvain M MD (Ped) *PCP* - **Spec Exp:** Prematurity/Low Birth Weight Infants; **Hospital:** NYU Langone Med Ctr (page 108), Beth Israel Med Ctr - Petrie Div (page 94); **Address:** Premier Pediatrics, 51 E 25 St Fl 3, New York, NY 10010; **Phone:** 212-598-0331; **Board Cert:** Pediatrics 1982; Neonatal-Perinatal Medicine 1983; **Med School:** Belgium 1977; **Resid:** Pediatrics, LI Jewish Med Ctr 1979; **Fellow:** Neonatal-Perinatal Medicine, LI Jewish Med Ctr 1981; **Fac Appt:** Asst Clin Prof Ped, NYU Sch Med

Weiss, Jona MD (Ped) *PCP* - **Spec Exp:** Adolescent Medicine; **Hospital:** NY-Presby/Weill Cornell Med Ctr, NY (page 104), Lenox Hill Hosp (page 106); **Address:** 114 E 72nd St, New York, NY 10021; **Phone:** 212-988-6060; **Board Cert:** Pediatrics 2010; **Med School:** SUNY Downstate 1986; **Resid:** Pediatrics, Bellevue Hosp Ctr 1989; **Fac Appt:** Asst Clin Prof Ped, Cornell Univ-Weill Med Coll

Yaker, Michael MD (Ped) *PCP* - **Hospital:** Mt Sinai Med Ctr (page 102); **Address:** Westside Pediatrics, 620 Columbus Ave, Ste 1, New York, NY 10024; **Phone:** 212-874-4500; **Board Cert:** Pediatrics 2010; **Med School:** Mount Sinai Sch Med 1992; **Resid:** Pediatrics, Mt Sinai Med Ctr 1995; **Fac Appt:** Asst Clin Prof Ped, Mount Sinai Sch Med

Zimmerman, Sol S MD (Ped) *PCP* - **Spec Exp:** Growth/Development Disorders; Behavioral Disorders; Cough-Tic Syndrome; **Hospital:** NYU Langone Med Ctr (page 108); **Address:** Pediatric Associates of NYC, 317 E 34th St, New York, NY 10016-4974; **Phone:** 212-725-6300; **Board Cert:** Pediatrics 1977; **Med School:** NYU Sch Med 1972; **Resid:** Pediatrics, Bellevue Hosp Ctr 1975; Pediatrics, Bellevue Hosp/NYU 1978; **Fac Appt:** Assoc Prof Ped, NYU Sch Med

Physical Medicine & Rehabilitation

Ahn, Jung Hwan MD (PMR) - **Spec Exp:** Spinal Cord Injury; Stroke Rehabilitation; Neurologic Rehabilitation; **Hospital:** NYU Langone Med Ctr (page 108); **Address:** Ambulatory Care Ctr, 240 E 38th St Fl 15, New York, NY 10016; **Phone:** 212-263-6122; **Board Cert:** Physical Medicine & Rehabilitation 1980; Spinal Cord Injury Medicine 2008; **Med School:** South Korea 1970; **Resid:** Obstetrics & Gynecology, Elmhurst City Hosp 1976; Physical Medicine & Rehabilitation, NYU Med Ctr 1979; **Fellow:** Spinal Cord Injury Medicine, NYU Med Ctr 1980; **Fac Appt:** Clin Prof PMR, NYU Sch Med

Birnbaum, Henry P MD (PMR) - **Spec Exp:** Pain-Chronic; Sports Medicine; **Hospital:** NYU Langone Med Ctr (page 108); **Address:** 48 E 43rd St Fl 5, New York, NY 10017; **Phone:** 212-627-0593; **Board Cert:** Physical Medicine & Rehabilitation ; **Med School:** NYU Sch Med 1991; **Resid:** Physical Medicine & Rehabilitation, NYU-Rusk Inst 1995

Brown, Andrew MD (PMR) - **Spec Exp:** Electromyography; **Hospital:** NY-Presby/Lower Manhattan Hosp (page 104); **Address:** 19 Beekman St Fl 6, New York, NY 10038; **Phone:** 212-513-7711; **Board Cert:** Physical Medicine & Rehabilitation 1988; **Med School:** Grenada 1982; **Resid:** Pediatrics, Univ MD Hosp 1984; Physical Medicine & Rehabilitation, Mt Sinai Med Ctr 1987

Bryce, Thomas MD (PMR) - **Spec Exp:** Spinal Cord Injury; Pain-Neuropathic; **Hospital:** Mt Sinai Med Ctr (page 102); **Address:** Rehabilitation Medicine Assocs, 5 E 98th St, Box 1240B, New York, NY 10029; **Phone:** 212-241-6321; **Board Cert:** Physical Medicine & Rehabilitation 2008; Spinal Cord Injury Medicine 2010; Pain Medicine 2013; **Med School:** Albany Med Coll 1993; **Resid:** Physical Medicine & Rehabilitation, Thomas Jefferson Univ Hosp 1997; **Fac Appt:** Assoc Prof PMR, Mount Sinai Sch Med

Dillard, James N MD (PMR) - **Spec Exp:** Pain Management; Acupuncture; Complementary Medicine; Nutrition; **Address:** 161 Madison Ave, Ste 11E, New York, NY 10016; **Phone:** 212-265-4038; **Board Cert:** Physical Medicine & Rehabilitation 2005; **Med School:** Rush Med Coll 1990; **Resid:** Physical Medicine & Rehabilitation, Columbia-Presby Med Ctr 1994; **Fac Appt:** Asst Clin Prof PMR, Columbia P&S

Feinberg, Joseph H MD (PMR) - **Spec Exp:** Peripheral Neuropathy; Spinal Rehabilitation; Electrodiagnosis; Sports Medicine; **Hospital:** Hosp For Special Surgery (page 113), Kessler Inst for Rehab - W Orange; **Address:** 429 E 75th St Fl 3, New York, NY 10021; **Phone:** 212-606-1568; **Board Cert:** Physical Medicine & Rehabilitation 1991; Sports Medicine 2009; **Med School:** Albany Med Coll 1983; **Resid:** Surgery, Mt Sinai Hosp 1985; Physical Medicine & Rehabilitation, Rusk Inst Rehab 1990; **Fellow:** Orthopaedic Pathology, Hosp Spec Surg 1986; Orthopaedic Biomechanics, Univ Iowa Hosp & Clins 1987; **Fac Appt:** Assoc Prof PMR, Cornell Univ-Weill Med Coll

Flanagan, Steven R MD (PMR) - **Spec Exp:** Brain Injury Rehabilitation; Stroke Rehabilitation; **Hospital:** NYU Langone Med Ctr (page 108), NYU Rusk Inst (page 108); **Address:** Ambulatory Care Ctr, 240 E 38th St Fl 15, New York, NY 10016; **Phone:** 212-263-6037; **Board Cert:** Physical Medicine & Rehabilitation 2013; **Med School:** UMDNJ-NJ Med Sch, Newark 1988; **Resid:** Physical Medicine & Rehabilitation, Mt Sinai Hosp 1992; **Fac Appt:** Prof PMR, NYU Sch Med

Frieden, Richard A MD (PMR) - **Spec Exp:** Amputee Rehabilitation; Stroke; **Hospital:** Mt Sinai Med Ctr (page 102); **Address:** Mount Sinai, Rehab Med Assocs, 5 E 98th St Fl 6, New York, NY 10029; **Phone:** 212-241-6335; **Board Cert:** Physical Medicine & Rehabilitation 1988; **Med School:** NY Med Coll 1984; **Resid:** Physical Medicine & Rehabilitation, Rusk Inst Rehab Med 1987; **Fac Appt:** Asst Prof PMR, Mount Sinai Sch Med

Gold, Joan T MD (PMR) - **Spec Exp:** Cerebral Palsy; Spina Bifida; Pediatric Rehabilitation; **Hospital:** NYU Langone Med Ctr (page 108), NYU Hosp For Joint Dis (page 108); **Address:** NYU Hosp for Joint Dis, 301 E 17th St, Ste 452, New York, NY 10003; **Phone:** 212-598-7671; **Board Cert:** Pediatrics 1979; Physical Medicine & Rehabilitation 1981; Pediatric Rehabilitation Medicine 2008; **Med School:** SUNY Downstate 1974; **Resid:** Pediatrics, Beth Israel Med Ctr 1977; Physical Medicine & Rehabilitation, NYU Rusk Inst 1979; **Fac Appt:** Clin Prof PMR, NYU Sch Med

Gotlin, Robert S DO (PMR) - **Spec Exp:** Sports Medicine; Running Injuries; Pain-Coccyx; Pain-Knee & Shoulder; **Hospital:** Beth Israel Med Ctr - Petrie Div (page 94); **Address:** 245 Fifth Ave, Fl 3, New York, NY 10016; **Phone:** 646-935-2255; **Board Cert:** Physical Medicine & Rehabilitation 1992; **Med School:** Southeastern Univ Coll Osteo Med 1987; **Resid:** Physical Medicine & Rehabilitation, Mount Sinai Hosp 1991; **Fac Appt:** Assoc Prof PMR, Albert Einstein Coll Med

Kim, Heakyung MD (PMR) - **Spec Exp:** Pediatric Rehabilitation; Neuromuscular Disorders; Stroke Rehabilitation; Musculoskeletal Disorders; **Hospital:** Morgan Stanley Children's Hosp of NY-Presby, NY (page 104), NY-Presby/Columbia Univ Med Ctr, NY (page 104); **Address:** 180 Fort Washington Ave, Harkness Pavilion, Ste 199, New York, NY 10032; **Phone:** 212-305-3535; **Board Cert:** Physical Medicine & Rehabilitation 2009; Pediatric Rehabilitation Medicine 2003; **Med School:** South Korea 1984; **Resid:** Physical Medicine & Rehabilitation, UMDNJ Univ Hosp 1998; **Fellow:** Physical Medicine & Rehabilitation, UMDNJ Univ Hosp 1993; **Fac Appt:** Prof PMR, Columbia P&S

Lachmann, Elisabeth A MD (PMR) - **Spec Exp:** Pain-Back; Sports Medicine; **Hospital:** NY-Presby/Weill Cornell Med Ctr, NY (page 104); **Address:** 117 1/2 E 62nd St, New York, NY 10065; **Phone:** 212-535-3005; **Board Cert:** Physical Medicine & Rehabilitation 1992; **Med School:** Med Coll PA Hahnemann 1987; **Resid:** Physical Medicine & Rehabilitation, NY-Cornell Med Ctr 1991; **Fac Appt:** Assoc Prof PMR, Cornell Univ-Weill Med Coll

Lee, Alexander J MD (PMR) - **Spec Exp:** Pain Management; Pain-Neck; Pain-Low Back; Spinal Rehabilitation; **Hospital:** Mt Sinai Med Ctr (page 102); **Address:** 17 E 102nd St, Fl 5, New York, NY 10029; **Phone:** 212-241-1076; **Board Cert:** Physical Medicine & Rehabilitation 2009; Pain Medicine 2003; **Med School:** Wayne State Univ 1994; **Resid:** Physical Medicine & Rehabilitation, UMDNJ/Kessler Inst for Rehab 1998; **Fellow:** Pain Medicine, Beth Israel Med Ctr 1999; **Fac Appt:** Asst Prof PMR, Mount Sinai Sch Med

Lutz, Christopher MD (PMR) - **Spec Exp:** Pain-Spine; Pain-Low Back; Sports Medicine; **Hospital:** Hosp For Special Surgery (page 113); **Address:** Hosp for Special Surgery, 75th Street Campus, 429 E 75th St Fl 3, New York, NY 10021; **Phone:** 212-606-1494; **Board Cert:** Physical Medicine & Rehabilitation 2012; **Med School:** Georgetown Univ 1996; **Resid:** Physical Medicine & Rehabilitation, UMDNJ-Kessler Inst for Rehab 2000; **Fellow:** Sports Medicine, Hosp for Special Surgery 2001

Lutz, Gregory MD (PMR) - **Spec Exp:** Spinal Rehabilitation; Sports Medicine; Pain-Low Back; **Hospital:** Hosp For Special Surgery (page 113), Univ Med Ctr Princeton at Plainsboro; **Address:** 429 E 75 St Fl 3, New York, NY 10021; **Phone:** 212-606-1648; **Board Cert:** Physical Medicine & Rehabilitation 2013; **Med School:** Georgetown Univ 1988; **Resid:** Physical Medicine & Rehabilitation, Mayo Clinic 1992; **Fellow:** Sports Medicine, Hosp For Spec Surg 1993; **Fac Appt:** Assoc Prof PMR, Cornell Univ-Weill Med Coll

Ma, Dong M MD (PMR) - **Spec Exp:** Electromyography; Musculoskeletal Disorders; **Hospital:** NYU Rusk Inst (page 108), NYU Langone Med Ctr (page 108); **Address:** NYU Ctr for Musculoskeletal Care, 333 E 38th St Fl 5, New York, NY 10016; **Phone:** 646-501-7277; **Board Cert:** Physical Medicine & Rehabilitation 1979; **Med School:** South Korea 1968; **Resid:** Physical Medicine & Rehabilitation, NYU Med Ctr 1976; **Fellow:** Neuromuscular Disease, NYU Med Ctr 1977; **Fac Appt:** Clin Prof PMR, NYU Sch Med

Moldover, Jonathan MD (PMR) - **Spec Exp:** Spinal Rehabilitation; Pain-Chronic; Post Polio Syndrome/Rehabilitation; **Hospital:** Beth Israel Med Ctr - Petrie Div (page 94); **Address:** 200 W 57th St, Ste 608, New York, NY 10019-3211; **Phone:** 212-581-4488; **Board Cert:** Physical Medicine & Rehabilitation 1979; Pain Medicine 2013; **Med School:** Columbia P&S 1974; **Resid:** Internal Medicine, Strong Meml Hosp 1976; Physical Medicine & Rehabilitation, NY-Presby/Columbia Univ Med Ctr 1978; **Fac Appt:** Assoc Clin Prof PMR, Albert Einstein Coll Med

Neely, Michael J DO (PMR) - **Spec Exp:** Sports Medicine; Spinal Rehabilitation; Pain-Knee & Shoulder; Osteoarthritis; **Hospital:** NYU Rusk Inst (page 108), NY-Presby/Lower Manhattan Hosp (page 104); **Address:** NY Sports Med & Physical Therapy, 18 E 48th St, Ste 802, New York, NY 10017; **Phone:** 212-750-1110; **Board Cert:** Physical Medicine & Rehabilitation 2012; Sports Medicine 2010; **Med School:** Ohio Univ, Coll Osteo Med 1997; **Resid:** Physical Medicine & Rehabilitation, Metro Hlth Med Ctr 2001

O'Dell, Michael Wayne MD (PMR) - **Spec Exp:** Brain Injury Rehabilitation; Stroke Rehabilitation; Multiple Sclerosis; **Hospital:** NY-Presby/Weill Cornell Med Ctr, NY (page 104); **Address:** NY-Presby, Physical Med & Rehab, 525 E 68 St Fl 16, New York, NY 10065; **Phone:** 212-746-1504; **Board Cert:** Physical Medicine & Rehabilitation 1990; **Med School:** Indiana Univ 1985; **Resid:** Physical Medicine & Rehabilitation, Pennsylvania Hosp-UPHS 1989; **Fellow:** Brain Injury, Mediplex-Rehab 1991; **Fac Appt:** Prof PMR, Cornell Univ-Weill Med Coll

Ragnarsson, Kristjan T MD (PMR) - **Spec Exp:** Spinal Cord Injury; Brain Injury Rehabilitation; Pain-Back & Neck; **Hospital:** Mt Sinai Med Ctr (page 102); **Address:** Faculty Practice Assocs, 5 E 98th St Fl 6, New York, NY 10029-6501; **Phone:** 212-824-8380; **Board Cert:** Physical Medicine & Rehabilitation 1976; **Med School:** Iceland 1969; **Resid:** Physical Medicine & Rehabilitation, NYU Med Ctr 1974; **Fellow:** Spinal Cord & Brain Injury Rehab, NYU Med Ctr 1975; **Fac Appt:** Prof PMR, Mount Sinai Sch Med

Rashbaum, Ira G MD (PMR) - **Spec Exp:** Stroke Rehabilitation; Pain-Back; **Hospital:** NYU Langone Med Ctr (page 108), NYU Rusk Inst (page 108); **Address:** NYU Med Ctr, Phys Rehab Ctr, 240 E 38 St Fl 15, New York, NY 10016; **Phone:** 212-263-6477; **Board Cert:** Physical Medicine & Rehabilitation 2004; **Med School:** SUNY Upstate Med Univ 1989; **Resid:** Physical Medicine & Rehabilitation, NYU Rusk Inst 1993; **Fac Appt:** Clin Prof PMR, NYU Sch Med

Reid, Malcolm D MD (PMR) - **Hospital:** St. Luke's - Roosevelt Hosp Ctr - Roosevelt Div (page 94); **Address:** 1000 Tenth Ave, Ste 3B-20, New York, NY 10019; **Phone:** 212-523-6595; **Board Cert:** Physical Medicine & Rehabilitation 1992; **Med School:** Harvard Med Sch 1987; **Resid:** Internal Medicine, Winthrop Univ Hosp 1988; **Fellow:** Physical Medicine & Rehabilitation, NY-Presby/Columbia Univ Med Ctr 1991; **Fac Appt:** Asst Clin Prof PMR, Columbia P&S

Rho, Dae Sik MD (PMR) - **Spec Exp:** Sports Medicine; Pain Management; **Hospital:** Lenox Hill Hosp (page 106); **Address:** 159 E 74th St, New York, NY 10021; **Phone:** 212-434-2465; **Board Cert:** Physical Medicine & Rehabilitation 1980; **Med School:** South Korea 1962; **Resid:** Physical Medicine & Rehabilitation, NYU Med Ctr 1975; **Fac Appt:** Asst Clin Prof PMR, Cornell Univ-Weill Med Coll

Sheth, Parag MD (PMR) - **Spec Exp:** Musculoskeletal Disorders; **Hospital:** Mt Sinai Med Ctr (page 102); **Address:** Mt Sinai Dept Rehabilitation Med, 5 E 98th St Fl 6, Box 1240B, New York, NY 10029; **Phone:** 212-241-6321; **Board Cert:** Physical Medicine & Rehabilitation 2004; Pain Medicine 2002; **Med School:** SUNY Stony Brook 1987; **Resid:** Physical Medicine & Rehabilitation, St Vincent Hosp Med Ctr 1993; **Fellow:** Physical Medicine & Rehabilitation, Mayo Clin 1994; **Fac Appt:** Asst Prof PMR, Mount Sinai Sch Med

Simotas, Alexander C MD (PMR) - **Spec Exp:** Spinal Rehabilitation; **Hospital:** Hosp For Special Surgery (page 113); **Address:** 429 E 75th St Fl 4, New York, NY 10021; **Phone:** 212-606-1879; **Board Cert:** Physical Medicine & Rehabilitation 2003; **Med School:** Columbia P&S 1986; **Resid:** Physical Medicine & Rehabilitation, Rusk Inst-NYU 1991; **Fellow:** Pain Medicine, Hosp Special Surgery 1992

Solomon, Jennifer L MD (PMR) - **Spec Exp:** Spinal Rehabilitation; Sports Medicine; **Hospital:** Hosp For Special Surgery (page 113); **Address:** 429 E 75th St Fl 4, New York, NY 10021; **Phone:** 212-606-1720; **Board Cert:** Physical Medicine & Rehabilitation 2004; Sports Medicine 2012; **Med School:** SUNY Downstate 1999; **Resid:** Physical Medicine & Rehabilitation, UMDNJ/Kessler Rehab Inst 2003; **Fellow:** Sports Medicine, Hosp Special Surg 2004

Stein, Joel MD (PMR) - **Spec Exp:** Stroke Rehabilitation; Neurologic Rehabilitation; **Hospital:** NY-Presby/Columbia Univ Med Ctr, NY (page 104); **Address:** 180 Fort Washington Ave, Ste 199, Harkness Pavilion, New York, NY 10032; **Phone:** 212-305-3535; **Board Cert:** Internal Medicine 1989; Physical Medicine & Rehabilitation 2013; **Med School:** Albert Einstein Coll Med 1986; **Resid:** Internal Medicine, Montefiore Med Ctr 1989; Physical Medicine & Rehabilitation, NY-Presby/Columbia Univ Med Ctr 1992

Stubblefield, Michael Dean MD (PMR) - **Spec Exp:** Cancer Rehabilitation; Pain-Cancer; Pain-Neuropathic; Spasticity Management; **Hospital:** Meml Sloan-Kettering Canc Ctr (page 114); **Address:** Meml Sloan Kettering Cancer Ctr, Sillerman Ctr for Rehabilitation, 515 Madison Ave Fl 5, New York, NY 10022; **Phone:** 646-888-1936; **Board Cert:** Internal Medicine 2011; Physical Medicine & Rehabilitation 2012; Electrodiagnostic Medicine 2003; **Med School:** Columbia P&S 1996; **Resid:** Internal Medicine, Columbia Presby Med Ctr 1999; **Fellow:** Physical Medicine & Rehabilitation, Columbia Presby Med Ctr 2002; **Fac Appt:** Assoc Prof PMR, Cornell Univ-Weill Med Coll

Thomas, David C MD (PMR) - **Hospital:** Mt Sinai Med Ctr (page 102); **Address:** Mount Sinai Med Ctr, 17 E 102nd St Fl 7, New York, NY 10029; **Phone:** 212-824-7210; **Board Cert:** Internal Medicine 2007; Physical Medicine & Rehabilitation 2008; **Med School:** Hahnemann Univ 1991; **Resid:** Internal Medicine, St Vincent Hosp Med Ctr 1994; Physical Medicine & Rehabilitation, Mt Sinai Med Ctr 1998; **Fac Appt:** Prof Med, Mount Sinai Sch Med

Vad, Vijay B MD (PMR) - **Spec Exp:** Pain-Back; Pain-Knee & Shoulder; Sports Medicine-Golf & Tennis Injuries; Joint Pain-Minimally Invasive Therapy; **Hospital:** Hosp For Special Surgery (page 113); **Address:** 519 E 72 St, Ste 203, New York, NY 10021; **Phone:** 212-606-1306; **Board Cert:** Physical Medicine & Rehabilitation 2007; Sports Medicine 2007; **Med School:** Univ Okla Coll Med 1992; **Resid:** Physical Medicine & Rehabilitation, NY-Presby/Weill Cornell Med Ctr 1996; **Fellow:** Sports Medicine, Hosp Special Surg 1997; **Fac Appt:** Asst Prof PMR, Cornell Univ-Weill Med Coll

Varlotta, Gerard P DO (PMR) - **Spec Exp:** Sports Medicine; Pain-Musculoskeletal; Spinal Rehabilitation; Pain-Spine; **Hospital:** NYU Langone Med Ctr (page 108); **Address:** NYU Ctr for Musculoskeletal Care, 333 E 38th St Fl 6, New York, NY 10016; **Phone:** 646-501-7200; **Board Cert:** Physical Medicine & Rehabilitation 1992; **Med School:** NY Coll Osteo Med 1983; **Resid:** Orthopaedic Surgery, Maimonides Med Ctr 1988; Physical Medicine & Rehabilitation, Rusk Inst-NYU 1991; **Fac Appt:** Assoc Clin Prof PMR, NYU Sch Med

Whiteson, Johnathan H MD (PMR) - **Spec Exp:** Cardiac Rehabilitation; Pulmonary Rehabilitation; Geriatric Rehabilitation; Neuro-Rehabilitation; **Hospital:** NYU Rusk Inst (page 108); **Address:** NYU Cardiac Rehab Assocs, 530 1st Ave Fl 9, Schwartz Heath Care Ctr, New York, NY 10016; **Phone:** 212-263-6125; **Board Cert:** Physical Medicine & Rehabilitation 1999; **Med School:** England, UK 1989; **Resid:** Rehabilitation, NYU Rusk Inst 1998; **Fellow:** Cardiac Rehabilitation, NYU Rusk Inst 1999; **Fac Appt:** Asst Prof PMR, NYU Sch Med

Plastic Surgery

Ahn, Christina Y MD (PlS) - **Spec Exp:** Breast Reconstruction; Cosmetic Surgery-Face & Body; Cosmetic Surgery-Breast; **Hospital:** NYU Langone Med Ctr (page 108); **Address:** 630 Third Ave Fl 6 - Ste 601, New York, NY 10017; **Phone:** 212-717-8860; **Board Cert:** Plastic Surgery 1994; **Med School:** NYU Sch Med 1983; **Resid:** Surgery, Mt Sinai Med Ctr 1988; Plastic Surgery, Univ Pittsburgh Med Ctr 1990; **Fellow:** Microvascular Surgery, UCLA Med Ctr 1991; **Fac Appt:** Assoc Prof S, NYU Sch Med

Allen, Robert J MD (PlS) - **Spec Exp:** Breast Reconstruction; Microsurgery; **Hospital:** NYU Langone Med Ctr (page 108), New York Eye & Ear Infirm (page 115); **Address:** The Ctr for Microsurgucal Breast Recon, 630 3rd Ave, Ste 601, New York, NY 10017; **Phone:** 888-890-3437; **Board Cert:** Plastic Surgery 1985; **Med School:** Med Univ SC 1976; **Resid:** Surgery, LSU Med Ctr 1982; Plastic Surgery, LSU Med Ctr 1981; **Fellow:** Microsurgery, NYU Med Ctr 1983

Almeyda, Elizabeth MD (PlS) - **Spec Exp:** Abdominoplasty; Cosmetic Surgery-Breast; Liposuction; **Hospital:** St. Luke's - Roosevelt Hosp Ctr - Roosevelt Div (page 94); **Address:** 75 Central Park West, New York, NY 10023-6011; **Phone:** 212-501-0600; **Board Cert:** Plastic Surgery 1988; **Med School:** Univ Rochester 1978; **Resid:** Surgery, Roosevelt Hosp 1983; **Fellow:** Plastic Surgery, New York Hosp 1985

Ascherman, Jeffrey MD (PlS) - **Spec Exp:** Breast Cosmetic & Reconstructive Surgery; Craniofacial Surgery; Cleft Palate/Lip; Cosmetic Surgery; **Hospital:** NY-Presby/Columbia Univ Med Ctr, NY (page 104), New York Eye & Ear Infirm (page 115); **Address:** 161 Ft Washington Ave, Ste 509, New York, NY 10032-3713; **Phone:** 212-305-9612; **Board Cert:** Plastic Surgery 2007; **Med School:** Columbia P&S 1988; **Resid:** Surgery, Columbia-Presby Med Ctr 1991; Plastic Surgery, Columbia-Presby Med Ctr 1994; **Fellow:** Craniofacial Surgery, Hosp Necke-Enfants Malades 1995; **Fac Appt:** Prof S, Columbia P&S

Aston, Sherrell MD (PlS) - **Spec Exp:** Cosmetic Surgery-Face & Body; Rhinoplasty; Cosmetic Surgery-Breast; Liposuction & Body Contouring; **Hospital:** Lenox Hill Hosp (page 106), NYU Langone Med Ctr (page 108); **Address:** 728 Park Ave, New York, NY 10021; **Phone:** 212-249-6000; **Board Cert:** Surgery 1974; Plastic Surgery 1978; **Med School:** Univ VA Sch Med 1968; **Resid:** Surgery, UCLA Med Ctr 1973; Plastic Surgery, NY Hosp 1975; **Fellow:** Surgery, Johns Hopkins Hosp 1970; **Fac Appt:** Prof PlS, NYU Sch Med

Baker III, Daniel C MD (PlS) - **Spec Exp:** Cosmetic Surgery-Face; Reconstructive Surgery-Face; Cancer Reconstruction; Facial Paralysis Reconstruction; **Hospital:** Lenox Hill Hosp (Manh Eye, Ear & Throat Hosp) (page 106); **Address:** 65 E 66th St, New York, NY 10065; **Phone:** 212-734-9695; **Board Cert:** Plastic Surgery 1978; **Med School:** Columbia P&S 1968; **Resid:** Surgery, UCSF Med Ctr 1975; Plastic Surgery, NYU Med Ctr 1977; **Fellow:** Head and Neck Surgery, Columbia Presby Med Ctr 1978; **Fac Appt:** Prof PlS, NYU Sch Med

Bromley, Gary S MD (PlS) - **Spec Exp:** Cosmetic Surgery; **Hospital:** NY-Presby/Weill Cornell Med Ctr, NY (page 104), Jamaica Hosp Med Ctr; **Address:** 5 E 84th St, New York, NY 10028-0407; **Phone:** 212-570-5443; **Board Cert:** Plastic Surgery 1986; **Med School:** Cornell Univ-Weill Med Coll 1978; **Resid:** Surgery, New York Hosp 1981; Plastic Surgery, New York Hosp 1983; **Fellow:** Hand Surgery, NYU Med Ctr 1984

Broumand, Stafford MD (PlS) - **Spec Exp:** Eyelid Surgery; Breast Surgery; Liposuction & Body Contouring; Craniofacial Surgery/Reconstruction; **Hospital:** Mt Sinai Med Ctr (page 102); **Address:** 740 Park Ave, New York, NY 10021-4251; **Phone:** 212-879-7900; **Board Cert:** Plastic Surgery 2006; **Med School:** Yale Univ 1985; **Resid:** Surgery, Mt Sinai Med Ctr 1990; **Fellow:** Plastic Surgery, Mass Genl Hosp 1992; Cosmetic Plastic Surgery, Cran Hosp Necker 1993; **Fac Appt:** Assoc Clin Prof PlS, Mount Sinai Sch Med

Chen, Constance MD (PlS) - **Spec Exp:** Breast Cosmetic & Reconstructive Surgery; Microsurgery; Breast Cancer & Surgery; **Hospital:** Lenox Hill Hosp (page 106), New York Eye & Ear Infirm (page 115); **Address:** 875 Park Ave, Ste 1F, New York, NY 10075; **Phone:** 212-792-6378; **Board Cert:** Plastic Surgery 2010; **Med School:** Stanford Univ 2001; **Resid:** Surgery, Univ WA Med Ctr 2004; Plastic Surgery, Univ WA Med Ctr 2005; **Fellow:** Plastic/Reconstructive Surgery, NY Presby-Columbia Med Ctr 2008

Chiu, David T.W. MD (PlS) - **Spec Exp:** Hand & Microvascular Surgery; Reconstructive Surgery; Peripheral Nerve Surgery; **Hospital:** NYU Langone Med Ctr (page 108), Lenox Hill Hosp (page 106); **Address:** 900 Park Ave, New York, NY 10075; **Phone:** 212-879-8880; **Board Cert:** Plastic Surgery 1982; Hand Surgery 2010; **Med School:** Columbia P&S 1973; **Resid:** Surgery, Barnes-Jewish Hosp 1977; Plastic Surgery, NY-Presby/Columbia Univ Med Ctr 1979; **Fellow:** Hand Surgery, NYU Med Ctr 1980; **Fac Appt:** Prof PlS, NYU Sch Med

Choi, Mihye MD (PlS) - **Spec Exp:** Breast Reconstruction; Liposuction & Body Contouring; Cosmetic Surgery-Breast; Cosmetic Surgery-Face; **Hospital:** NYU Langone Med Ctr (page 108); **Address:** KCNY Plastic Surgery, 305 E 47th St, Ste 1A, New York, NY 10017; **Phone:** 212-355-5779; **Board Cert:** Plastic Surgery 2008; Hand Surgery 2010; **Med School:** Univ Rochester 1987; **Resid:** Surgery, Beth Israel Hosp 1990; Plastic Surgery, Mt Sinai Med Ctr 1995; **Fellow:** Hand Surgery, NYU Med Ctr 1996; Research, Mass Genl Hosp 1992; **Fac Appt:** Assoc Prof S, NYU Sch Med

Colen, Helen S MD (PlS) - **Spec Exp:** Cosmetic Surgery-Face & Breast; Liposuction & Body Contouring; Vaginal Reconstruction; Tuberous Breasts; **Hospital:** NYU Langone Med Ctr (page 108), Lenox Hill Hosp (Manh Eye, Ear & Throat Hosp) (page 106); **Address:** 742 Park Ave, New York, NY 10021-4251; **Phone:** 212-772-1300; **Board Cert:** Plastic Surgery 1983; **Med School:** NYU Sch Med 1972; **Resid:** Surgery, Univ Colorado Med Ctr 1979; Plastic Surgery, St Lukes Hosp 1981; **Fellow:** Microsurgery, NYU Med Ctr 1982; **Fac Appt:** Assoc Clin Prof PlS, NYU Sch Med

Cordeiro, Peter G MD (PlS) - **Spec Exp:** Reconstructive Surgery; Breast Reconstruction; Facial Plastic & Reconstructive Surgery; **Hospital:** Meml Sloan-Kettering Canc Ctr (page 114), Lenox Hill Hosp (Manh Eye, Ear & Throat Hosp) (page 106); **Address:** 1275 York Ave, New York, NY 10065; **Phone:** 212-639-2521; **Board Cert:** Surgery 2008; Plastic Surgery 2007; **Med School:** Harvard Med Sch 1983; **Resid:** Surgery, New Engl Deaconess Hosp-Harvard 1989; Plastic Surgery, NYU Med Ctr 1991; **Fellow:** Microsurgery, Meml Sloan-Kettering Cancer Ctr. 1992; Craniofacial Surgery, Univ Miami Affil Hosp 1992; **Fac Appt:** Prof S, Cornell Univ-Weill Med Coll

Diktaban, Theodore MD (PlS) - **Spec Exp:** Liposuction & Body Contouring; Rhinoplasty; Breast Augmentation; Facial Rejuvenation; **Hospital:** Lenox Hill Hosp (page 106), Lenox Hill Hosp (Manh Eye, Ear & Throat Hosp) (page 106); **Address:** 635 Madison Ave, Fl 4th, New York, NY 10022; **Phone:** 212-206-0023; **Board Cert:** Otolaryngology 1981; Plastic Surgery 1988; **Med School:** NY Med Coll 1976; **Resid:** Otolaryngology, Mt Sinai Hosp 1981; Plastic Surgery, Lenox Hill Hosp 1983; **Fellow:** Reconstructive Microsurgery, Univ Louisville Hosp 1984

Disa, Joseph J MD (PlS) - **Spec Exp:** Cancer Reconstruction; Breast Reconstruction; Head & Neck Reconstruction; Microsurgery; **Hospital:** Meml Sloan-Kettering Canc Ctr (page 114); **Address:** 1275 York Ave, New York, NY 10065; **Phone:** 212-639-5022; **Board Cert:** Surgery 2005; Plastic Surgery 2009; **Med School:** Univ Mass Sch Med 1988; **Resid:** Surgery, Univ Md Med Ctr 1994; Plastic Surgery, Johns Hopkins Univ 1996; **Fellow:** Reconstructive Microsurgery, Meml Sloan-Kettering Cancer Ctr.; **Fac Appt:** Prof PlS, Cornell Univ-Weill Med Coll

Forley, Bryan G MD (PlS) - **Spec Exp:** Cosmetic Surgery; Reconstructive Surgery; **Hospital:** Beth Israel Med Ctr - Petrie Div (page 94), New York Eye & Ear Infirm (page 115); **Address:** 5 E 82nd St, New York, NY 10028-0342; **Phone:** 212-861-3757; **Board Cert:** Plastic Surgery 2008; **Med School:** Mount Sinai Sch Med 1984; **Resid:** Surgery, NYU Med Ctr & Mt Sinai Med Ctr 1989; Plastic Surgery, Saint Francis Meml Hosp 1992; **Fellow:** Craniofacial Surgery, Hosp for Sick Children, Great Ormond St 1993

Foster, Craig A MD (PlS) - **Spec Exp:** Cosmetic Surgery-Face & Nose; Cosmetic Surgery-Breast; Rhinoplasty Revision; Head & Neck Surgery; **Hospital:** Lenox Hill Hosp (page 106); **Address:** 850 Park Ave, Ste 1A, New York, NY 10075; **Phone:** 212-744-5746; **Board Cert:** Otolaryngology 1980; Plastic Surgery 1984; **Med School:** Univ Minn 1974; **Resid:** Otolaryngology, Univ Minn Hosp 1980; Plastic Surgery, NYU Med Ctr 1982

Freund, Robert M MD (PlS) - **Spec Exp:** Cosmetic Surgery-Face & Neck; Cosmetic Surgery-Breast; Rhinoplasty Revision; **Hospital:** Lenox Hill Hosp (page 106), Long Is Jewish Med Ctr (page 106); **Address:** 170 East End Ave, Ste CS, New York, NY 10128; **Phone:** 212-583-1200; **Board Cert:** Plastic Surgery 2008; **Med School:** Cornell Univ 1987; **Resid:** Surgery, NYU Med Ctr 1993; Plastic Surgery, NYU Med Ctr 1995; **Fellow:** Microvascular Surgery, NYU Med Ctr 1991

Friedman, David J MD (PlS) - **Spec Exp:** Cosmetic Surgery-Face; Liposuction & Body Contouring; Abdominoplasty; Breast Reconstruction; **Hospital:** Beth Israel Med Ctr - Petrie Div (page 94), Lenox Hill Hosp (page 106); **Address:** 630 Park Ave, New York, NY 10065; **Phone:** 212-439-1600; **Board Cert:** Plastic Surgery 2008; **Med School:** Albany Med Coll 1988; **Resid:** Surgery, Beth Israel Med Ctr 1993; Plastic Surgery, Mt Sinai Med Ctr 1994

Gayle, Lloyd MD (PlS) - **Spec Exp:** Breast Reconstruction & Augmentation; Hand Surgery; Cosmetic Surgery-Body; **Hospital:** NY-Presby/Weill Cornell Med Ctr, NY (page 104), Maimonides Med Ctr (page 98); **Address:** 50 E 69th St, New York, NY 10021; **Phone:** 212-452-5121; **Board Cert:** Plastic Surgery 1993; **Med School:** NYU Sch Med 1983; **Resid:** Surgery, NYU Med Ctr 1988; Plastic Surgery, NY Hosp-Cornell Univ 1990; **Fellow:** Hand & Microvascular Surgery, Davies Med Ctr 1991; **Fac Appt:** Assoc Prof S, Cornell Univ-Weill Med Coll

Ginsberg, Gerald D MD (PlS) - **Spec Exp:** Cosmetic Surgery; Reconstructive Plastic Surgery; **Hospital:** NY-Presby/Lower Manhattan Hosp (page 104); **Address:** Dept of Surgery, 170 William St Fl 5, New York, NY 10038; **Phone:** 212-452-3421; **Board Cert:** Plastic Surgery 1984; **Med School:** Northwestern Univ 1974; **Resid:** Surgery, NYU Med Ctr 1980; Plastic Surgery, NYU Med Ctr 1982; **Fellow:** Hand Surgery, NYU Med Ctr 1983; **Fac Appt:** Assoc Clin Prof PlS, NYU Sch Med

Godfrey, Norman V MD (PlS) - **Spec Exp:** Rhinoplasty; Nasal Reconstruction; Nasal Surgery; **Hospital:** NY-Presby/Weill Cornell Med Ctr, NY (page 104), NY Hosp Queens (page 488); **Address:** 1158 5th Ave, New York, NY 10029; **Phone:** 212-628-6600; **Board Cert:** Plastic Surgery 1984; **Med School:** Harvard Med Sch 1973; **Resid:** Surgery, Bellevue Hosp 1978; Plastic Surgery, Bellevue Hosp 1980; **Fellow:** Microvascular Surgery, Bellevue Hosp 1981; **Fac Appt:** Asst Clin Prof S, Cornell Univ-Weill Med Coll

Godfrey, Philip M MD/DMD (PlS) - **Spec Exp:** Breast Cosmetic & Reconstructive Surgery; Liposuction & Body Contouring; Abdominoplasty; Congenital Breast Anomalies; **Hospital:** NY-Presby/Weill Cornell Med Ctr, NY (page 104); **Address:** 1158 5th Ave, New York, NY 10029; **Phone:** 212-628-6600; **Board Cert:** Plastic Surgery 1988; **Med School:** Med Coll PA 1981; **Resid:** Surgery, Hartford Hosp 1984; Plastic Surgery, New York Hosp 1986; **Fellow:** Plastic Surgery, Meml Sloan-Kettering Cancer Ctr 1987; **Fac Appt:** Asst Clin Prof S, Cornell Univ-Weill Med Coll

Grant, Robert T MD (PlS) - **Spec Exp:** Cosmetic Surgery-Face & Eyes; Cosmetic Surgery-Breast; Breast Reconstruction; Reconstructive Plastic Surgery; **Hospital:** NY-Presby/Columbia Univ Med Ctr, NY (page 104), NY-Presby/Weill Cornell Med Ctr, NY (page 104); **Address:** 161 Fort Washington Ave, rm 511, 50 E 69th St, New York, NY 10032; **Phone:** 212-305-3103; **Board Cert:** Surgery 2011; Plastic Surgery 2013; **Med School:** Albany Med Coll 1983; **Resid:** Surgery, New York Hosp 1988; Plastic Surgery, NY-Presby/Weill Cornell Med Ctr 1990; **Fellow:** Microvascular Surgery, NYU Med Ctr/Bellevue Hosp 1991; **Fac Appt:** Prof PlS, Columbia P&S

Hidalgo, David A MD (PlS) - **Spec Exp:** Cosmetic Surgery-Face; Cosmetic Surgery-Breast; Rhinoplasty; **Hospital:** NY-Presby/Weill Cornell Med Ctr, NY (page 104), Lenox Hill Hosp (page 106); **Address:** 655 Park Ave, New York, NY 10065; **Phone:** 212-517-9777; **Board Cert:** Plastic Surgery 1987; **Med School:** Georgetown Univ 1978; **Resid:** Surgery, NYU Med Ctr 1983; Plastic Surgery, NYU Med Ctr 1985; **Fellow:** Microsurgery, NYU Med Ctr 1986; **Fac Appt:** Clin Prof S, Cornell Univ-Weill Med Coll

Hirmand, Haideh MD (PlS) - **Spec Exp:** Eyelid Surgery/Blepharoplasty; Facial Rejuvenation; Cosmetic Surgery-Face & Eyes; Cosmetic Surgery-Breast; **Hospital:** NY-Presby/Weill Cornell Med Ctr, NY (page 104), Lenox Hill Hosp (Manh Eye, Ear & Throat Hosp) (page 106); **Address:** Haideh Hirmand M.D., 1040 Park Ave, Ste 1D-1E, New York, NY 10026; **Phone:** 212-744-4400; **Board Cert:** Plastic Surgery 2010; **Med School:** Harvard Med Sch 1990; **Resid:** Plastic Surgery, NY Presby/Weill-Cornell Med Ctr 1997; **Fellow:** Oculoplastic Surgery, Paces Plastic Surgery/Emory University 1998; Craniofacial Surgery, Necker Children's Hospital 1999; **Fac Appt:** Asst Clin Prof S, Cornell Univ-Weill Med Coll

Hoffman, Lloyd A MD (PlS) - **Spec Exp:** Cosmetic Surgery-Face; Liposuction & Body Contouring; Breast Reconstruction; Facial Rejuvenation; **Hospital:** NY-Presby/Weill Cornell Med Ctr, NY (page 104), Lenox Hill Hosp (page 106); **Address:** 12 E 68th St, New York, NY 10021; **Phone:** 212-861-1640; **Board Cert:** Plastic Surgery 1989; **Med School:** Northwestern Univ 1978; **Resid:** Surgery, New York Hosp 1983; Plastic Surgery, NYU Med Ctr 1986; **Fellow:** Hand Surgery, NYU Med Ctr 1987; **Fac Appt:** Assoc Prof PlS, Cornell Univ-Weill Med Coll

Hunter, John G MD (PlS) - **Spec Exp:** Female Genital Cosmetic Surgery; Cosmetic Surgery-Breast; Cosmetic Surgery-Body; **Hospital:** NY-Presby/Weill Cornell Med Ctr, NY (page 104), New York Methodist Hosp (page 440); **Address:** 47 E 63rd St, Fl Ground, New York, NY 10065; **Phone:** 212-751-4444; **Board Cert:** Plastic Surgery 1991; **Med School:** SUNY Downstate 1983; **Resid:** Surgery, Mount Sinai Hosp 1986; **Fellow:** Plastic Surgery, Univ Hosp-SUNY Downstate 1988; **Fac Appt:** Assoc Clin Prof S, Cornell Univ-Weill Med Coll

Imber, Gerald MD (PlS) - **Spec Exp:** Cosmetic Surgery-Breast; Eyelid Surgery; Mohs' Surgery; Cosmetic Surgery-Face; **Hospital:** NY-Presby/Weill Cornell Med Ctr, NY (page 104); **Address:** 121A E 83rd St, New York, NY 10028; **Phone:** 212-472-1800; **Board Cert:** Plastic Surgery 1976; **Med School:** SUNY Downstate 1966; **Resid:** Surgery, LIJ Med Ctr 1972; Plastic Surgery, NY Hosp 1974; **Fac Appt:** Asst Clin Prof S, Cornell Univ-Weill Med Coll

Jacobs, Elliot W MD (PlS) - **Spec Exp:** Cosmetic Surgery-Face & Breast; Gynecomastia; Body Contouring; Rhinoplasty; **Hospital:** New York Eye & Ear Infirm (page 115), Beth Israel Med Ctr - Petrie Div (page 94); **Address:** 815 Park Ave, New York, NY 10021-3276; **Phone:** 212-570-6080; **Board Cert:** Plastic Surgery 1982; **Med School:** Mount Sinai Sch Med 1970; **Resid:** Surgery, Mt Sinai Med Ctr 1974; Plastic Surgery, Mt Sinai Med Ctr 1977

Karp, Nolan MD (PlS) - **Spec Exp:** Breast Cosmetic & Reconstructive Surgery; Liposuction & Body Contouring; Skin Cancer; **Hospital:** NYU Langone Med Ctr (page 108); **Address:** KCNY Plastic Surgery, 305 E 47th St, Ste 1A, New York, NY 10017; **Phone:** 212-355-5779; **Board Cert:** Plastic Surgery 1994; **Med School:** Northwestern Univ 1983; **Resid:** Surgery, NYU Med Ctr 1988; **Fellow:** Plastic Surgery, NYU Med Ctr 1991; **Fac Appt:** Assoc Prof PlS, NYU Sch Med

Kolker, Adam R MD (PlS) - **Spec Exp:** Cosmetic Surgery-Breast; Breast Reconstruction; Abdominoplasty; Body Contouring after Weight Loss; **Hospital:** Mt Sinai Med Ctr (page 102), Lenox Hill Hosp (page 106); **Address:** 710 Park Ave, New York, NY 10021; **Phone:** 212-744-6500; **Board Cert:** Plastic Surgery 2011; Surgery 2005; **Med School:** Albany Med Coll 1990; **Resid:** Surgery, St Vincent's Hosp 1995; Plastic/Reconstructive Surgery, Beth Israel Deaconess Med Ctr 1998; **Fellow:** Microsurgery, NYU Med Ctr 1996; Craniofacial Surgery, Univ Melbourne Chldns Hosp 2000; **Fac Appt:** Assoc Clin Prof S, Mount Sinai Sch Med

LaBruna, Anthony N MD (PlS) - **Spec Exp:** Cosmetic Surgery-Face; Facial Plastic & Reconstructive Surgery; Rhinoplasty Revision; Facial Deformities/Reconstruction; **Hospital:** NY-Presby/Weill Cornell Med Ctr, NY (page 104), Mt Sinai Med Ctr (page 102); **Address:** 45 E 85th St, rm 1A, New York, NY 10028; **Phone:** 212-584-7001; **Board Cert:** Otolaryngology 1997; Plastic Surgery 2012; **Med School:** Cornell Univ-Weill Med Coll 1990; **Resid:** Surgery, Lenox Hill Hosp 1992; Otolaryngology, Manhattan EE&T Hosp 1996; **Fellow:** Plastic Surgery, Mt Sinai Med Ctr 2000; **Fac Appt:** Assoc Clin Prof PlS, Cornell Univ-Weill Med Coll

Levine, Joshua L MD (PlS) - **Spec Exp:** Breast Reconstruction; Microsurgery; **Hospital:** New York Eye & Ear Infirm (page 115), Montefiore Med Ctr-Einstein Campus (page 100); **Address:** 3 Columbus Cir, Ste 1410, New York, NY 10019; **Phone:** 212-245-8140; **Board Cert:** Plastic Surgery 2005; **Med School:** Med Coll GA 1994; **Resid:** Plastic Surgery, Montefiore Med Ctr 2001; Plastic Surgery, Montefiore Med Ctr 2003; **Fellow:** Cosmetic Plastic Surgery, NY Eye & Ear Infirm 2003; Reconstructive Microsurgery, Louisiana State Univ Affil Hosp 2004

Matarasso, Alan MD (PlS) - **Spec Exp:** Cosmetic Surgery-Face & Eyes; Rhinoplasty; Liposuction; Abdominoplasty; **Hospital:** Lenox Hill Hosp (Manh Eye, Ear & Throat Hosp) (page 106); **Address:** 1009 Park Ave, New York, NY 10028-0936; **Phone:** 212-249-7500; **Board Cert:** Plastic Surgery 1986; **Med School:** Univ Miami Sch Med 1979; **Resid:** Surgery, Montefiore Med Ctr 1983; Plastic Surgery, Montefiore Med Ctr 1985; **Fellow:** Plastic Surgery, Manhattan EET Hosp/NYU 1985; **Fac Appt:** Clin Prof PlS, Albert Einstein Coll Med

Mehrara, Babak J MD (PlS) - **Spec Exp:** Breast Reconstruction; Cancer Reconstruction; Microsurgery; Reconstructive Surgery-Face; **Hospital:** Meml Sloan-Kettering Canc Ctr (page 114); **Address:** 160 E 63rd St Fl 10, New York, NY 10022; **Phone:** 212-639-8639; **Board Cert:** Plastic Surgery 2003; **Med School:** Columbia P&S 1993; **Resid:** Surgery, NYU Med Ctr 1996; Plastic Surgery, NYU Med Ctr 2001; **Fellow:** Microsurgery, UCLA Med Ctr 2002; **Fac Appt:** Assoc Prof S, Cornell Univ-Weill Med Coll

Monasebian, Douglas M MD/DMD (PlS) - **Spec Exp:** Cosmetic Surgery-Face; Facial Plastic & Reconstructive Surgery; **Hospital:** Mt Sinai Med Ctr (page 102), St. Luke's - Roosevelt Hosp Ctr - St Luke's Hosp (page 94); **Address:** 784 Park Ave, New York, NY 10021; **Phone:** 212-472-8700; **Board Cert:** Plastic Surgery 2009; **Med School:** Univ Nebr Coll Med 1992; **Resid:** Surgery, Univ Nebraska Med Ctr 1995; **Fellow:** Plastic Surgery, Montefiore Med Ctr 1997; **Fac Appt:** Asst Clin Prof PlS, Mount Sinai Sch Med

Perrotti, John A MD (PlS) - **Spec Exp:** Liposuction & Body Contouring; Cosmetic Surgery-Face & Breast; Abdominoplasty; **Hospital:** Lenox Hill Hosp (Manh Eye, Ear & Throat Hosp) (page 106), Lenox Hill Hosp (page 106); **Address:** 330 E 63rd St, New York, NY 10065; **Phone:** 212-861-6363; **Board Cert:** Plastic Surgery 2010; **Med School:** NY Med Coll 1991; **Resid:** Surgery, Westchester Medical Ctr 1996; Plastic Surgery, Cleveland Clinic 1998; **Fac Appt:** Asst Clin Prof S, NY Med Coll

Pfeifer, Tracy M MD (PlS) - **Spec Exp:** Cosmetic Surgery-Breast; Body Contouring; Cosmetic Surgery-Face; **Hospital:** Lenox Hill Hosp (page 106), Lenox Hill Hosp (Manh Eye, Ear & Throat Hosp) (page 106); **Address:** Pfeifer Plastic Surgery, 969 Park Ave, New York, NY 10028; **Phone:** 212-860-0670; **Board Cert:** Surgery 2008; Plastic Surgery 2011; **Med School:** UMDNJ-RW Johnson Med Sch 1991; **Resid:** Surgery, NY-Presby/Weill Cornell Med Ctr 1996; Plastic Surgery, NYU Langone Med Ctr 1998; **Fellow:** Breast Surgery, Inst Reconstructive Breast Surgery 1999

Pitman, Gerald H MD (PlS) - **Spec Exp:** Cosmetic Surgery-Face; Liposuction & Body Contouring; Abdominoplasty; Cosmetic Surgery-Breast; **Hospital:** Lenox Hill Hosp (Manh Eye, Ear & Throat Hosp) (page 106); **Address:** Ctr Specialty Care, Plastic Surgery, 50 E 69th St Fl 5, New York, NY 10021; **Phone:** 212-517-2600; **Board Cert:** Plastic Surgery 1978; **Med School:** Univ Pennsylvania 1968; **Resid:** Surgery, NY-Presby/Columbia Univ Med Ctr 1975; Plastic Surgery, NYU Med Ctr 1977; **Fellow:** Microsurgery, NYU Med Ctr 1981; **Fac Appt:** Clin Prof PlS, NYU Sch Med

Razaboni, Rosa M MD (PlS) - **Spec Exp:** Cosmetic Surgery; Breast Reconstruction; Body Contouring after Weight Loss; **Hospital:** Lenox Hill Hosp (page 106), Mt Sinai Med Ctr (page 102); **Address:** 14-A E 68th St, New York, NY 10065; **Phone:** 212-772-0200; **Board Cert:** Plastic Surgery 1993; **Med School:** Brazil 1975; **Resid:** Surgery, St Vincent Hosp 1985; Plastic Surgery, NYU Med Ctr 1988; **Fellow:** Microsurgery, Hosp Trousseau 1986; **Fac Appt:** Asst Clin Prof S, Mount Sinai Sch Med

Romita, Mauro C MD (PlS) - **Spec Exp:** Cosmetic Surgery-Face; Liposuction & Body Contouring; Reconstructive Plastic Surgery; **Hospital:** Lenox Hill Hosp (page 106); **Address:** 853 5th Ave, New York, NY 10065; **Phone:** 212-772-3220; **Board Cert:** Plastic Surgery 1983; **Med School:** Univ Miami Sch Med 1973; **Resid:** Surgery, NYU Med Ctr 1978; Plastic Surgery, NYU Med Ctr 1980; **Fellow:** Craniofacial Surgery, NYU Med Ctr 1981; Microsurgery, NYU Med Ctr 1982

Rose, Elliott H MD (PlS) - **Spec Exp:** Facial Plastic & Reconstructive Surgery; Cosmetic Surgery-Face & Body; Facial Paralysis Reconstruction; Burns-Reconstructive Plastic Surgery; **Hospital:** Mt Sinai Med Ctr (page 102); **Address:** The Aesthetic Surgery Center, 895 Park Ave, New York, NY 10029; **Phone:** 212-639-1346; **Board Cert:** Plastic Surgery 1979; **Med School:** Univ Tex Med Br, Galveston 1970; **Resid:** Surgery, Johns Hopkins Hosp 1973; Plastic Surgery, Stanford Univ Med Ctr 1977; **Fellow:** Hand & Microvascular Surgery, UCSF Med Ctr 1978; **Fac Appt:** Assoc Clin Prof PlS, Mount Sinai Sch Med

Rosenblatt, William B MD (PlS) - **Spec Exp:** Nasal Surgery; Cosmetic Surgery-Face & Body; Cosmetic Surgery-Breast; Rhinoplasty; **Hospital:** Lenox Hill Hosp (page 106), Lenox Hill Hosp (Manh Eye, Ear & Throat Hosp) (page 106); **Address:** 308 E 79th St, Ste 1D, New York, NY 10075; **Phone:** 212-570-6100; **Board Cert:** Otolaryngology 1977; Plastic Surgery 1980; **Med School:** NY Med Coll 1973; **Resid:** Otolaryngology, Metropolitan Hosp 1977; Plastic Surgery, Lenox Hill Hosp 1979; **Fac Appt:** Asst Clin Prof PlS, Touro Coll Osteopathic Med-NY

Sabry, M. Zakir MD (PlS) - **Spec Exp:** Cosmetic Surgery; Breast Reconstruction; Craniofacial Surgery; Cleft Palate/Lip; **Hospital:** Lenox Hill Hosp (page 106); **Address:** 936 5th Ave, Office 2, New York, NY 10021; **Phone:** 212-737-1308; **Board Cert:** Plastic Surgery 2004; **Med School:** NY Med Coll 1993; **Resid:** Surgery, St Vincent Hosp 1999; Plastic Surgery, VA Commonwealth Univ Med Ctr 2001; **Fellow:** Craniofacial Surgery, Barnes-Jewish Hosp 2002; **Fac Appt:** Asst Prof S, NY Med Coll

Schulman, Matthew R MD (PlS) - **Spec Exp:** Cosmetic Surgery-Face; Cosmetic Surgery-Breast; Liposuction; Body Contouring; **Hospital:** Mt Sinai Med Ctr (page 102), Westchester Med Ctr; **Address:** 950 Park Ave, New York, NY 10028; **Phone:** 212-289-1851; **Board Cert:** Plastic Surgery 2007; **Med School:** Jefferson Med Coll 2000; **Resid:** Surgery, Mt Sinai Med Ctr 2003; **Fellow:** Plastic Surgery, Mt Sinai Med Ctr 2006; **Fac Appt:** Assoc Prof PlS, Mount Sinai Sch Med

Schulman, Norman H MD (PlS) - **Spec Exp:** Cosmetic Surgery-Face & Body; Breast Cosmetic & Reconstructive Surgery; Nasal Surgery; Tuberous Breasts; **Hospital:** Lenox Hill Hosp (page 106), Lenox Hill Hosp (Manh Eye, Ear & Throat Hosp) (page 106); **Address:** 308 E 79th St, New York, NY 10075; **Phone:** 212-861-5004; **Board Cert:** Surgery 1973; Plastic Surgery 1976; **Med School:** Tufts Univ 1965; **Resid:** Surgery, Bronx Muni Hosp 1972; Plastic Surgery, Lenox Hill Hosp 1974; **Fellow:** Head and Neck Surgery, Roswell Park Cancer Inst 1975; **Fac Appt:** Clin Prof PlS, Cornell Univ-Weill Med Coll

Scott, Susan Craig MD (PlS) - **Spec Exp:** Cosmetic Surgery-Face; Hand Surgery; **Hospital:** NYU Hosp For Joint Dis (page 108), Lenox Hill Hosp (page 106); **Address:** 150 E 77th St, New York, NY 10075; **Phone:** 212-288-9922; **Board Cert:** Plastic Surgery 1987; Hand Surgery 2005; **Med School:** Columbia P&S 1974; **Resid:** Surgery, St Luke's-Roosevelt Hosp Ctr 1979; Plastic Surgery, NYU Med Ctr 1981; **Fellow:** Hand Surgery, St Luke's-Roosevelt Hosp Ctr 1982; **Fac Appt:** Asst Clin Prof PlS, Columbia P&S

Sherman, John E MD (PlS) - **Spec Exp:** Cosmetic Surgery-Face; Liposuction & Body Contouring; Facial Plastic & Reconstructive Surgery; Breast Cosmetic & Reconstructive Surgery; **Hospital:** NY-Presby/Weill Cornell Med Ctr, NY (page 104), Lenox Hill Hosp (page 106); **Address:** 1016 Fifth Ave, New York, NY 10028-0132; **Phone:** 212-535-2300; **Board Cert:** Plastic Surgery 1984; **Med School:** NY Med Coll 1975; **Resid:** Surgery, Montefiore Med Ctr 1978; Plastic Surgery, NY Hosp/Meml Sloan Kettering Cancer Ctr 1980; **Fac Appt:** Asst Clin Prof S, Cornell Univ-Weill Med Coll

Silich, Robert C MD (PlS) - **Spec Exp:** Cosmetic Surgery-Face & Eyes; Blepharoplasty; Rhinoplasty; **Hospital:** NY-Presby/Weill Cornell Med Ctr, NY (page 104), Lenox Hill Hosp (page 106); **Address:** 121 E 83rd St, Ste A, MS 10028, New York, NY 10028; **Phone:** 212-628-6800; **Board Cert:** Plastic Surgery 2011; **Med School:** Georgetown Univ 1993; **Resid:** Surgery, Cornell Med Ctr 1997; Plastic Surgery, Cornell Med Ctr 1999; **Fac Appt:** Asst Clin Prof PlS, Cornell Univ-Weill Med Coll

Silver, Lester MD (PlS) **Spec Exp:** Cleft Palate/Lip; Pediatric Plastic Surgery; Reconstructive Surgery; **Hospital:** Mt Sinai Med Ctr (page 102); **Address:** 5 E 98th St, Box 1259, New York, NY 10029-6574; **Phone:** 212-241-1968; **Board Cert:** Plastic Surgery 1978; **Med School:** Ros Franklin Univ/Chicago Med Sch 1960; **Resid:** Surgery, Montefiore Med Ctr 1966; Plastic Surgery, Mt Sinai Med Ctr 1969; **Fac Appt:** Prof PlS, Mount Sinai Sch Med

Skolnik, Richard A MD (PlS) - **Spec Exp:** Cosmetic Surgery-Face; Cosmetic Surgery-Breast; Liposuction & Body Contouring; **Hospital:** Mt Sinai Med Ctr (page 102); **Address:** 21 E 87th St, Ste 1A, New York, NY 10128-0506; **Phone:** 212-722-1977; **Board Cert:** Plastic Surgery 1983; **Med School:** Cornell Univ-Weill Med Coll 1976; **Resid:** Surgery, Mt Sinai Hosp 1979; Plastic Surgery, Mt Sinai Hosp 1982; **Fac Appt:** Assoc Clin Prof PlS, Mount Sinai Sch Med

Smith, Mark MD (PlS) - **Spec Exp:** Breast Reconstruction; Head & Neck Reconstruction; Craniofacial Surgery-Pediatric; Cleft Palate/Lip; **Hospital:** Beth Israel Med Ctr - Petrie Div (page 94); **Address:** 10 Union Square E, Ste 2L, New York, NY 10003; **Phone:** 212-844-8796; **Board Cert:** Plastic Surgery 2010; **Med School:** Albert Einstein Coll Med 1991; **Resid:** Surgery, NY-Presby/Columbia Univ Med Ctr 1994; Plastic Surgery, NY-Presby/Columbia Univ Med Ctr 1996; **Fellow:** Microsurgery, UT MD Anderson Cancer Ctr 1997; Craniofacial Surgery, Univ Wash Med Ctr 1998; **Fac Appt:** Asst Prof PlS, Albert Einstein Coll Med

Spector, Jason A MD (PlS) - **Spec Exp:** Cosmetic Surgery; **Hospital:** NY-Presby/Weill Cornell Med Ctr, NY (page 104); **Address:** NY-Presby/Weill Cornell Med Ctr, 520 E 70th St, Star Pavilion, 8th Fl, New York, NY 10065-4870; **Phone:** 212-746-4532; **Board Cert:** Plastic Surgery 2007; **Med School:** NYU Sch Med 1996; **Resid:** Surgery, NYU Med Ctr 2002; Plastic Surgery, NYU Med Ctr 2005; **Fellow:** Plastic Surgery, NYU Med Ctr 2006; Microsurgery, NYU Med Ctr 2006; **Fac Appt:** Asst Prof S, Cornell Univ-Weill Med Coll

Spinelli, Henry M MD (PlS) - **Spec Exp:** Cosmetic Surgery-Face; Craniofacial Surgery/Reconstruction; Oculoplastic & Orbital Surgery; Eyelid Surgery/Blepharoplasty; **Hospital:** NY-Presby/Weill Cornell Med Ctr, NY (page 104), Lenox Hill Hosp (Manh Eye, Ear & Throat Hosp) (page 106); **Address:** 875 5th Ave, New York, NY 10021; **Phone:** 212-570-6235; **Board Cert:** Ophthalmology 1987; Plastic Surgery 1993; **Med School:** NYU Sch Med 1981; **Resid:** Ophthalmology, Manhattan EE&T Hosp 1985; Plastic/Reconstructive Surgery, NYU Med Ctr 1990; **Fellow:** Craniofacial Surgery, NYU Med Ctr 1991; **Fac Appt:** Clin Prof S, Cornell Univ-Weill Med Coll

Staffenberg, David A MD (PlS) - **Spec Exp:** Maxillofacial & Craniofacial Surgery; Pediatric Plastic Surgery; Cleft Palate/Lip; Cosmetic & Reconstructive Surgery; **Hospital:** NYU Langone Med Ctr (page 108); **Address:** NYU Plastic Surgery Assocs, 305 E 33rd St, New York, NY 10016; **Phone:** 212-263-8065; **Board Cert:** Plastic Surgery 2009; **Med School:** NY Med Coll 1989; **Resid:** Surgery, Maimonides Med Ctr 1995; Plastic Surgery, Emory Univ Hosp 1997; **Fellow:** Craniofacial & Maxillofacial Surgery, UCLA Med Ctr 1998; **Fac Appt:** Clin Prof PlS, NYU Sch Med

Sultan, Mark R MD (PlS) - **Spec Exp:** Cosmetic Surgery-Face; Cosmetic Surgery-Breast; Breast Reconstruction; Liposuction & Body Contouring; **Hospital:** St. Luke's - Roosevelt Hosp Ctr - Roosevelt Div (page 94), Beth Israel Med Ctr - Petrie Div (page 94); **Address:** 1100 Park Ave, New York, NY 10128; **Phone:** 212-360-0700; **Board Cert:** Plastic Surgery 1992; **Med School:** Columbia P&S 1982; **Resid:** Surgery, Columbia-Presby Hosp 1987; Plastic Surgery, Columbia-Presby Hosp 1990; **Fellow:** Head and Neck Surgery, Emory Univ Hosp 1989; **Fac Appt:** Prof S, Columbia P&S

Swift Jr, Richard W MD (PlS) - **Spec Exp:** Cosmetic Surgery-Face; Cosmetic Surgery-Breast; Liposuction & Body Contouring; **Hospital:** Lenox Hill Hosp (Manh Eye, Ear & Throat Hosp) (page 106); **Address:** 110 E 87th St, Ste 1C, New York, NY 10128; **Phone:** 212-828-9906; **Board Cert:** Plastic Surgery 2009; **Med School:** Brown Univ 1988; **Resid:** Surgery, SUNY Hlth Sci Ctr 1992; Surgery, St Barnabas Med Ctr 1994; **Fellow:** Plastic Surgery, Oregon Hlth Sci Ctr 1996

Tabbal, Nicolas MD (PlS) - **Spec Exp:** Rhinoplasty; Cosmetic Surgery-Face; Eyelid Surgery; **Hospital:** Lenox Hill Hosp (Manh Eye, Ear & Throat Hosp) (page 106), NYU Langone Med Ctr (page 108); **Address:** 521 Park Ave, New York, NY 10065; **Phone:** 212-644-5800; **Board Cert:** Plastic Surgery 1980; **Med School:** Lebanon 1972; **Resid:** Surgery, Ameri Univ Med Ctr 1976; Plastic Surgery, Akron City Hosp 1979; **Fellow:** Surgery, SUNY Upstate Med Univ Hosp 1977; Plastic/Reconstructive Surgery, NYU Med Ctr 1980; **Fac Appt:** Assoc Clin Prof PlS, NYU Sch Med

Talmor, Mia MD (PlS) - **Spec Exp:** Breast Reconstruction; Reconstructive Surgery; Cosmetic Surgery-Breast; Nipple Sparing Mastectomy; **Hospital:** NY-Presby/Weill Cornell Med Ctr, NY (page 104); **Address:** 425 E 61st St Fl 10, New York, NY 10065; **Phone:** 212-821-0933; **Board Cert:** Plastic Surgery 2012; Surgery 2011; **Med School:** Cornell Univ 1993; **Resid:** Surgery, NY Hosp-Cornell Med Ctr 1999; Plastic Surgery, NY Hosp-Cornell Med Ctr 2001; **Fac Appt:** Assoc Clin Prof PlS, Cornell Univ-Weill Med Coll

Taub, Peter J MD (PlS) - **Spec Exp:** Pediatric Plastic Surgery; Craniofacial Surgery; Maxillofacial Surgery; Cleft Palate/Lip; **Hospital:** Mt Sinai Med Ctr (page 102), Westchester Med Ctr; **Address:** 5 E 98th St Fl 14 - Ste B, New York, NY 10029-6574; **Phone:** 212-241-4178; **Board Cert:** Surgery 2009; Plastic Surgery 2013; **Med School:** Albert Einstein Coll Med 1993; **Resid:** Surgery, Mt Sinai Med Ctr 1999; Plastic Surgery, UCLA Med Ctr 2001; **Fellow:** Craniofacial Surgery, UCLA Med Ctr 2002; **Fac Appt:** Prof S, Mount Sinai Sch Med

Thorne, Charles H MD (PlS) - **Spec Exp:** Cosmetic Surgery-Face; Ear Reconstruction/Microtia; Ear Reshaping (Otoplasty); Craniofacial Surgery; **Hospital:** NYU Langone Med Ctr (page 108); **Address:** 812 Park Ave, New York, NY 10021; **Phone:** 212-794-0044; **Board Cert:** Plastic Surgery 2007; **Med School:** UCLA 1981; **Resid:** Surgery, Mass Genl Hosp 1986; Plastic Surgery, NYU Med Ctr 1988; **Fellow:** Craniofacial Surgery, NYU Med Ctr 1989; **Fac Appt:** Assoc Prof PlS, NYU Sch Med

Ting, Jess MD (PlS) - **Spec Exp:** Breast Reconstruction; Cosmetic Surgery; **Hospital:** Mt Sinai Med Ctr (page 102), Mount Sinai Hosp of Queens (page 102); **Address:** 5 E 98th St, Fl 14, Ste B, Box 1259, New York, NY 10029; **Phone:** 212-241-4410; **Board Cert:** Plastic Surgery 2012; Hand Surgery 2012; **Med School:** Columbia P&S 1995; **Resid:** Surgery, Columbia Presby Med Ctr 1998; Plastic Surgery, Univ Pittsburgh Med Ctr 2000; **Fellow:** Hand Surgery, Hosp Special Surgery 2001; **Fac Appt:** Asst Prof S, Mount Sinai Sch Med

Verga, Michele MD (PlS) - **Spec Exp:** Cosmetic Surgery-Face; Liposuction; Body Contouring; Reconstructive Surgery; **Hospital:** Mt Sinai Med Ctr (page 102); **Address:** 1010 5th Ave, New York, NY 10028-0130; **Phone:** 212-535-0470; **Board Cert:** Plastic Surgery 1984; **Med School:** Italy 1974; **Resid:** Surgery, Mt Sinai Hosp 1978; Surgery, Lutheran Med Ctr 1980; **Fellow:** Plastic Surgery, Mt Sinai Hosp 1983; **Fac Appt:** Asst Clin Prof S, Mount Sinai Sch Med

Vickery, Carlin MD (PlS) - **Spec Exp:** Breast Cosmetic & Reconstructive Surgery; Cosmetic Surgery-Body; Cosmetic Surgery-Face; **Hospital:** Mt Sinai Med Ctr (page 102); **Address:** 1125 5th Ave, New York, NY 10128; **Phone:** 212-288-9800; **Board Cert:** Plastic Surgery 1987; **Med School:** NYU Sch Med 1977; **Resid:** Surgery, New York Univ Med Ctr 1982; **Fellow:** Microsurgery, New York Univ Med Ctr 1985; **Fac Appt:** Assoc Clin Prof S, Mount Sinai Sch Med

Weiss, Paul R MD (PlS) - **Spec Exp:** Breast Cosmetic & Reconstructive Surgery; Cosmetic Surgery-Face; Cosmetic Surgery-Body; **Hospital:** Montefiore Med Ctr-Moses Campus (page 100), Lawrence Hosp Ctr; **Address:** 1049 5th Ave, Ste 2D, New York, NY 10028-0115; **Phone:** 212-861-8000; **Board Cert:** Surgery 1975; Plastic Surgery 2010; **Med School:** Tulane Univ 1969; **Resid:** Surgery, Montefiore Med Ctr/Bronx Muni Hosp 1974; Plastic Surgery, Montefiore Med Ctr 1976; **Fac Appt:** Clin Prof S, Albert Einstein Coll Med

Wells, Scott B MD (PlS) - **Spec Exp:** Cosmetic Surgery-Face; Abdominoplasty; Breast Augmentation; Eyelid Surgery; **Hospital:** Winthrop Univ Hosp (page 524); **Address:** 655 Park Ave, New York, NY 10065; **Phone:** 212-794-3900; **Board Cert:** Plastic Surgery 2005; **Med School:** NY Med Coll 1985; **Resid:** Surgery, Beth Israel Med Ctr 1990; Plastic/Reconstructive Surgery, SUNY Hlth Sci Ctr 1992

Zevon, Scott J MD (PlS) - **Spec Exp:** Breast Augmentation; Breast Cosmetic & Reconstructive Surgery; Body Contouring; Liposuction; **Hospital:** St. Luke's - Roosevelt Hosp Ctr - Roosevelt Div (page 94); **Address:** 75 Central Park W, Ste 1AB, New York, NY 10023; **Phone:** 212-496-6600; **Board Cert:** Plastic Surgery 1989; **Med School:** Boston Univ 1979; **Resid:** Surgery, St Luke's-Roosevelt Hosp Ctr 1984; Plastic Surgery, Nassau Co Med Ctr 1986; **Fellow:** Craniofacial Surgery, Mayo Clinic 1987

Zide, Barry M MD/DMD (PlS) - **Spec Exp:** Facial Surgery-Chin & Lip; Birthmarks/Hemangiomas; Reconstructive Plastic Surgery; Melanoma; **Hospital:** NYU Langone Med Ctr (page 108), Lenox Hill Hosp (page 106); **Address:** 420 E 55th St, Ste 1D, New York, NY 10022; **Phone:** 212-421-2424; **Board Cert:** Plastic Surgery 1981; **Med School:** Tufts Univ 1973; **Resid:** Surgery, Stanford Univ Hosp & Clins 1976; Plastic Surgery, Univ NC Hosp 1978; **Fellow:** Head & Neck Oncology, Roswell Park Cancer Inst 1979; Craniofacial Surgery, NYU Med Ctr 1980; **Fac Appt:** Prof PlS, NYU Sch Med

Preventive Medicine

Cahill, John MD (PrM) - **Spec Exp:** Tropical Diseases; Travel Medicine; Parasitic Infections; International Health; **Hospital:** St. Luke's - Roosevelt Hosp Ctr - Roosevelt Div (page 94); **Address:** Univ Med Practice Assocs, 36 W 60th St, New York, NY 10023; **Phone:** 212-523-8672; **Board Cert:** Emergency Medicine 2011; **Med School:** Mount Sinai Sch Med 1996; **Resid:** Emergency Medicine, Rhode Island Hosp 1997; Emergency Medicine, Rhode Island Hosp 2000; **Fellow:** Tropical Medicine, Royal Coll Surgeons 1998; **Fac Appt:** Asst Clin Prof Med, Columbia P&S

Crane, Michael MD (PrM) - **Spec Exp:** Poison Control; **Hospital:** Mt Sinai Med Ctr (page 102); **Address:** Mount Sinai, WTC Treatment Ctr, 1468 Madison Ave Fl 3, New York, NY 10029; **Phone:** 212-241-0659; **Board Cert:** Internal Medicine 1980; Occupational Medicine 1989; **Med School:** Univ Rochester 1977; **Resid:** Internal Medicine, Montefiore Med Ctr 1980; **Fellow:** Preventive Medicine, NY-Presby/Columbia Univ Med Ctr 1985; **Fac Appt:** Asst Prof PrM, Mount Sinai Sch Med

Hoffman, Robert S MD (PrM) - **Spec Exp:** Poison Control; Disaster Preparedness; **Hospital:** NYU Langone Med Ctr (page 108), Bellevue Hosp Ctr; **Address:** NY Poison Control Ctr, 455 1st Ave, rm 123, New York, NY 10016; **Phone:** 212-340-4494; **Board Cert:** Internal Medicine 1987; Emergency Medicine 2005; Medical Toxicology 2008; **Med School:** NYU Sch Med 1984; **Resid:** Internal Medicine, NYU Med Ctr 1987; **Fellow:** Medical Toxicology, NYU Med Ctr 1989; **Fac Appt:** Prof EM, NYU Sch Med

Psychiatry

Adler, Lenard A MD (Psyc) - **Spec Exp:** ADD/ADHD; Psychopharmacology; **Hospital:** NYU Langone Med Ctr (page 108); **Address:** 1 Park Ave Fl 8, New York, NY 10016; **Phone:** 212-263-3580; **Board Cert:** Psychiatry 1987; **Med School:** Emory Univ 1982; **Resid:** Psychiatry, NYU Med Ctr 1986; **Fac Appt:** Prof Psyc, NYU Sch Med

Almeleh, Jack MD (Psyc) - **Spec Exp:** Cognitive Psychotherapy; Anxiety & Depression; **Hospital:** Mt Sinai Med Ctr (page 102); **Address:** 340 E 52nd St, Ste 1F, New York, NY 10022; **Phone:** 212-355-4250; **Board Cert:** Psychiatry 1977; **Med School:** SUNY Buffalo 1969; **Resid:** Psychiatry, Temple Univ Hosp 1973; **Fac Appt:** Asst Clin Prof Psyc, Mount Sinai Sch Med

Alper, Kenneth R MD (Psyc) - **Spec Exp:** Psychopharmacology; **Hospital:** NYU Langone Med Ctr (page 108); **Address:** 150 E 58th St, Fl 25, New York, NY 10155; **Phone:** 212-966-3506; **Board Cert:** Psychiatry 1989; **Med School:** Univ Tex, San Antonio 1984; **Resid:** Psychiatry, NYU Med Ctr 1988; **Fellow:** Clinical Neurophysiology, NYU Med Ctr 1990; **Fac Appt:** Assoc Prof Psyc, NYU Sch Med

Appelbaum, Paul S MD (Psyc) - **Spec Exp:** Forensic Psychiatry; Depression; Anxiety & Mood Disorders; **Hospital:** NY-Presby/Columbia Univ Med Ctr, NY (page 104); **Address:** Columbia University Medical Center, 1051 Riverside Drive, Unit 122, New York, NY 10032; **Phone:** 212-543-4184; **Board Cert:** Psychiatry 1981; Forensic Psychiatry 2013; **Med School:** Harvard Med Sch 1976; **Resid:** Psychiatry, Mass Mental Health Ctr 1980; **Fac Appt:** Prof Psyc, Columbia P&S

Arkow, Stan D MD (Psyc) - **Spec Exp:** Psychotherapy; Psychopharmacology; **Hospital:** NY-Presby/Columbia Univ Med Ctr, NY (page 104); **Address:** 740 W End Ave, Ste 5A, New York, NY 10025; **Phone:** 212-663-5185; **Board Cert:** Psychiatry 1985; **Med School:** Columbia P&S 1977; **Resid:** Psychiatry, NY State Psych Inst 1981; **Fac Appt:** Assoc Clin Prof Psyc, Columbia P&S

Aronoff, Michael S MD (Psyc) - **Spec Exp:** Stress Management; Anxiety & Depression; Sleep Disorders; Family & Couples Therapy; **Hospital:** Lenox Hill Hosp (page 106), NYU Langone Med Ctr (page 108); **Address:** 60 Riverside Drive, Ste 16E, New York, NY 10024-6171; **Phone:** 212-799-8257; **Board Cert:** Psychiatry 1977; **Med School:** Univ Pennsylvania 1966; **Resid:** Psychiatry, NY State Psych Inst/Columbia Univ 1972; **Fellow:** Psychoanalysis, Columbia-Presby Hosp 1976; **Fac Appt:** Clin Prof Psyc, NYU Sch Med

Attia, Evelyn MD (Psyc) - **Spec Exp:** Eating Disorders; Obesity; Mood Disorders; **Hospital:** NY-Presby/Columbia Univ Med Ctr, NY (page 104), NY-Presby/Weill Cornell Med Ctr, NY (page 104); **Address:** NY State Psychiatric Inst, 1051 Riverside Drive, Box 98, New York, NY 10032; **Phone:** 212-543-5923; **Board Cert:** Psychiatry 1992; **Med School:** Columbia P&S 1986; **Resid:** Psychiatry, Hosp Univ Penn 1987; Psychiatry, NY State Psych Inst 1990; **Fac Appt:** Clin Prof Psyc, Columbia P&S

Barbuto, Joseph MD (Psyc) - **Spec Exp:** Psychiatry in Cancer; Anxiety & Mood Disorders; Personality Disorders; **Hospital:** NY-Presby/Weill Cornell Med Ctr, NY (page 104), Meml Sloan-Kettering Canc Ctr (page 114); **Address:** 945 Fifth Ave Ave, Ste 5, New York, NY 10021; **Phone:** 212-724-7366; **Board Cert:** Psychiatry 1983; **Med School:** Albert Einstein Coll Med 1978; **Resid:** Psychiatry, NY Hosp 1982; **Fellow:** Psychiatric Oncology, Meml Sloan-Kettering Cancer Ctr 1986; **Fac Appt:** Assoc Clin Prof Psyc, Cornell Univ-Weill Med Coll

Basch, Samuel H MD (Psyc) - **Spec Exp:** Psychotherapy; Psychopharmacology; Psychoanalysis; Psychiatry in Physical Illness; **Hospital:** Mt Sinai Med Ctr (page 102); **Address:** 10 E 85th St, Ste 1B, New York, NY 10028; **Phone:** 212-427-0344; **Board Cert:** Psychiatry 1970; **Med School:** Hahnemann Univ 1961; **Resid:** Psychiatry, Mount Sinai Hosp 1965; **Fellow:** Psychoanalysis, Columbia Presby Hosp 1976; **Fac Appt:** Prof Psyc, Mount Sinai Sch Med

Bialer, Philip MD (Psyc) - **Spec Exp:** Psychiatry in Physical Illness; Psychiatry in Head & Neck Cancer; **Hospital:** Meml Sloan-Kettering Canc Ctr (page 114); **Address:** 641 Lexington Ave, at E 54th St, Fl 7, New York, NY 10022; **Phone:** 646-888-0009; **Board Cert:** Psychiatry 1989; Psychosomatic Medicine 2005; **Med School:** Ohio State Univ 1977; **Resid:** Internal Medicine, Mt Sinai Med Ctr 1978; Psychiatry, SUNY Hlth Sci Ctr 1988; **Fellow:** Psychosomatic Medicine, Beth Israel Med Ctr 1989; **Fac Appt:** Assoc Clin Prof Psyc, Cornell Univ-Weill Med Coll

Blatter, Brett L MD (Psyc) - **Spec Exp:** Mood Disorders; Forensic Psychiatry; Psychopharmacology; **Hospital:** NY-Presby/Columbia Univ Med Ctr, NY (page 104), NY State Psychiatric Inst; **Address:** 160 W 73rd St, Ste 1B, New York, NY 10023; **Phone:** 212-769-4128; **Board Cert:** Psychiatry 2013; **Med School:** Johns Hopkins Univ 1997; **Resid:** Psychiatry, NY State Psychiatric Inst 2001; Forensic Psychiatry, NY State Psychiatric Inst 2002; **Fellow:** Emergency Psychiatry, Columbia Univ Med Ctr 2003; **Fac Appt:** Asst Clin Prof Psyc, Columbia P&S

Bone, Stanley MD (Psyc) - **Spec Exp:** Psychotherapy; Psychoanalysis; **Hospital:** NY-Presby/Columbia Univ Med Ctr, NY (page 104); **Address:** 1155 Park Ave, New York, NY 10128; **Phone:** 212-831-0917; **Board Cert:** Psychiatry 1979; **Med School:** Mount Sinai Sch Med 1974; **Resid:** Psychiatry, NY-Presby/Columbia Univ Med Ctr 1978; **Fellow:** Psychoanalysis, NY-Presby/Columbia Univ Med Ctr 1983; **Fac Appt:** Clin Prof Psyc, Columbia P&S

Borbely, Antal MD (Psyc) - **Spec Exp:** Career Related Problems; Relationship Problems; Creativity Enhancement; Psychopharmacology; **Address:** 675 W End Ave, Ste 1A, New York, NY 10025; **Phone:** 212-222-1678; **Board Cert:** Psychiatry 1976; **Med School:** Switzerland 1968; **Resid:** Psychiatry, NY State Psyc Inst 1972; Psychiatry, Albert Einstein Affil Hosp 1973; **Fellow:** Community Psychiatry, Albert Einstein Affil Hosp 1975

Breitbart, William S MD (Psyc) - **Spec Exp:** Psychiatry in Cancer; AIDS Related Cancers; Pain-Cancer; Palliative Care; **Hospital:** Meml Sloan-Kettering Canc Ctr (page 114); **Address:** 1275 York Ave, New York, NY 10065; **Phone:** 646-888-0020; **Board Cert:** Internal Medicine 1982; Psychiatry 1986; Psychosomatic Medicine 2005; **Med School:** Albert Einstein Coll Med 1978; **Resid:** Internal Medicine, Bronx Muni Hosp Ctr 1982; Internal Medicine, Bronx Muni Hosp Ctr 1984; **Fellow:** Psychiatric Oncology, Meml Sloan Kettering Cancer Ctr 1986; **Fac Appt:** Prof Psyc, Cornell Univ-Weill Med Coll

Brenner, Ronald L MD (Psyc) - **Spec Exp:** Depression; Dementia; Panic Disorder; **Hospital:** St. John's Episcopal Hosp - Queens, Mercy Med Ctr - Rockville Centre; **Address:** 740 Park Ave, New York, NY 10021; **Phone:** 718-869-7248; **Board Cert:** Psychiatry 1979; Geriatric Psychiatry 2006; **Med School:** Spain 1974; **Resid:** Psychiatry, St Luke's Hosp 1978; **Fellow:** Pharmacology, New York Univ Med Ctr 1979; **Fac Appt:** Clin Prof Psyc, SUNY Hlth Sci Ctr

Brodie, Jonathan D MD (Psyc) - **Spec Exp:** Psychopharmacology; Anxiety & Depression; Neuro-Psychiatry; **Hospital:** NYU Langone Med Ctr (page 108); **Address:** 155 E 38th St, Ste 3L, New York, NY 10016; **Phone:** 212-986-6693; **Board Cert:** Psychiatry 1979; **Med School:** NYU Sch Med 1975; **Resid:** Psychiatry, NYU Med Ctr/Bellevue Hosp 1978; **Fac Appt:** Prof Psyc, NYU Sch Med

Bronheim, Harold E MD (Psyc) - **Spec Exp:** Body Image Issues; Relationship Problems; Psychiatry in Physical Illness; Anxiety & Depression; **Hospital:** Mt Sinai Med Ctr (page 102); **Address:** 1155 Park Ave, New York, NY 10128; **Phone:** 212-996-5777; **Board Cert:** Psychiatry 1985; Internal Medicine 1986; Psychosomatic Medicine 2005; Geriatric Psychiatry 2011; **Med School:** SUNY Downstate 1980; **Resid:** Psychiatry, Mount Sinai Med Ctr 1986; Internal Medicine, Beth Israel Med Ctr 1985; **Fac Appt:** Clin Prof Psyc, Mount Sinai Sch Med

Brown, Richard P MD (Psyc) - **Spec Exp:** Psychopharmacology; Complementary Medicine; **Hospital:** NY-Presby/Columbia Univ Med Ctr, NY (page 104); **Address:** 30 East End Ave, Ste 1C, New York, NY 10028-7053; **Phone:** 212-737-0821; **Board Cert:** Psychiatry 1983; **Med School:** Columbia P&S 1977; **Resid:** Psychiatry, NY Hosp 1982; **Fellow:** Psychopharmacology, NY Hosp 1984; **Fac Appt:** Assoc Prof Psyc, Columbia P&S

Bukberg, Judith MD (Psyc) - **Spec Exp:** Psychotherapy; Psychoanalysis; **Address:** 88 University Pl, Ste 701A, New York, NY 10003; **Phone:** 212-614-0312; **Board Cert:** Psychiatry 1979; **Med School:** Mount Sinai Sch Med 1974; **Resid:** Psychiatry, Mt Sinai Hosp 1978; **Fellow:** Liaison Psychiatry, Meml Sloan-Kettering Cancer Ctr 1980; Psychoanalysis, NY Psychiatric Inst 1996; **Fac Appt:** Assoc Clin Prof Psyc, NY Med Coll

Bulgarelli, Christopher G MD (Psyc) - **Spec Exp:** Psychoanalysis; Depression; Anxiety Disorders; **Hospital:** Lenox Hill Hosp (page 106); **Address:** 455 W 23rd St, Ste 1BB, New York, NY 10011-2148; **Phone:** 212-807-1054; **Board Cert:** Psychiatry 1991; **Med School:** Tufts Univ 1986; **Resid:** Psychiatry, NYU/Bellevue Hosp 1990; **Fac Appt:** Asst Clin Prof Psyc, NYU Sch Med

Cabaniss, Deborah L MD (Psyc) - **Spec Exp:** Psychoanalysis; Psychodynamic Psychotherapy; **Hospital:** NY State Psychiatric Inst; **Address:** NY State Psychiatric Inst, 1051 Riverside Dr, Unit 63 rm 1300E, New York, NY 10032; **Phone:** 212-543-5666; **Board Cert:** Psychiatry 1993; **Med School:** Columbia P&S 1988; **Resid:** Psychiatry, NY State Psychiatric Inst 1992; **Fellow:** Psychoanalysis, Columbia Univ-Ctr Psychoanalytic Training 1996; **Fac Appt:** Clin Prof Psyc, Columbia P&S

Caligor, Eve MD (Psyc) - **Spec Exp:** Psychoanalysis; Personality Disorders; **Hospital:** NYU Langone Med Ctr (page 108); **Address:** 19 E 88th St, Ste 1D, MS 10128, New York, NY 10128; **Phone:** 212-996-5285; **Board Cert:** Psychiatry 1987; **Med School:** Harvard Med Sch 1982; **Resid:** Psychiatry, NY Presby/Columbia Univ Med Ctr 1986; **Fellow:** Psychiatry, NY Presby/Columbia Univ Med Ctr 1987; **Fac Appt:** Clin Prof Psyc, NYU Sch Med

Cherry, Sabrina MD (Psyc) - **Spec Exp:** Psychoanalysis; Psychotherapy; **Hospital:** NY State Psychiatric Inst; **Address:** 285 Central Park W, New York, NY 10024; **Phone:** 212-721-2869; **Board Cert:** Psychiatry 1992; **Med School:** Harvard Med Sch 1987; **Resid:** Psychiatry, NY State Psychiatric Inst 1991; **Fellow:** Psychoanalysis, Columbia Univ-Ctr Psychoanalytic Training 1998; **Fac Appt:** Assoc Clin Prof Psyc, Columbia P&S

Chung, Henry MD (Psyc) - **Spec Exp:** Anxiety & Depression; **Hospital:** Montefiore Med Ctr-Moses Campus (page 100); **Address:** 85 5th Ave, Ste 907, New York, NY 10003; **Phone:** 917-533-6908; **Board Cert:** Psychiatry 2004; **Med School:** SUNY Buffalo 1989; **Resid:** Psychiatry, NY-Presby/Weschester Div 1994; **Fac Appt:** Assoc Clin Prof Psyc, Albert Einstein Coll Med

Cohen, Arnold R MD (Psyc) - **Spec Exp:** Psychotherapy; ADD/ADHD; Autism; **Hospital:** Mt Sinai Med Ctr (page 102); **Address:** 64 E 94th St, Ste 1A, New York, NY 10128; **Phone:** 212-289-6800; **Board Cert:** Psychiatry 1969; **Med School:** SUNY Hlth Sci Ctr 1963; **Resid:** Psychiatry, Mount Sinai Med Ctr 1966; **Fellow:** Child & Adolescent Psychiatry, Mount Sinai Med Ctr 1970; **Fac Appt:** Asst Clin Prof Psyc, Mount Sinai Sch Med

Douglas, Carolyn Jory MD (Psyc) - **Spec Exp:** Depression; Anxiety Disorders; Relationship Problems; **Hospital:** NY-Presby/Columbia Univ Med Ctr, NY (page 104), NY-Presby/Weill Cornell Med Ctr, NY (page 104); **Address:** 345 E 84th St, New York, NY 10028-4434; **Phone:** 212-396-9808; **Board Cert:** Psychiatry 1985; **Med School:** Harvard Med Sch 1980; **Resid:** Psychiatry, Payne Whitney Clin 1984; **Fac Appt:** Assoc Clin Prof Psyc, Columbia P&S

Drooker, Martin A MD (Psyc) - **Spec Exp:** Anxiety & Depression; Bipolar/Mood Disorders; Memory Disorders; Psychopharmacology; **Hospital:** Mt Sinai Med Ctr (page 102); **Address:** 1158 5th Ave, New York, NY 10029; **Phone:** 212-876-6820; **Board Cert:** Psychiatry 1993; Psychosomatic Medicine 2005; Geriatric Psychiatry 2005; **Med School:** SUNY Downstate 1988; **Resid:** Psychiatry, Yale-New Haven Hosp 1992; **Fellow:** Psychosomatic Medicine, Yale-New Haven Hosp 1993; **Fac Appt:** Assoc Clin Prof Psyc, Mount Sinai Sch Med

Fallon, Brian A MD (Psyc) - **Spec Exp:** Lyme Disease-Neuro Complications; Psychosomatic Disorders; Obsessive-Compulsive Disorder; Psychiatry in Physical Illness; **Hospital:** NY State Psychiatric Inst, NY-Presby/Columbia Univ Med Ctr, NY (page 104); **Address:** NY State Psychiatric Inst, 1051 Riverside Drive, rm 3724, Box 69, New York, NY 10032; **Phone:** 212-543-5487; **Board Cert:** Psychiatry 1991; **Med School:** Columbia P&S 1985; **Resid:** Psychiatry, NYS Psychiatric Inst 1989; **Fellow:** Psychiatric Research, NYS Psychiatric Inst 1992; Psychodynamic Psychotherapy, NYS Psychiatric Inst 1990; **Fac Appt:** Prof Psyc, Columbia P&S

Ferran Jr, Ernesto MD (Psyc) - **Spec Exp:** Cultural Psychiatry; Child & Adolescent Psychiatry; Mood Disorders; Couples Therapy; **Hospital:** NYU Langone Med Ctr (page 108); **Address:** 15 Charles St, Ste 6H, New York, NY 10014-3011; **Phone:** 212-924-2673; **Board Cert:** Psychiatry 1983; Child & Adolescent Psychiatry 1986; **Med School:** Albert Einstein Coll Med 1976; **Resid:** Psychiatry, Bellevue Hosp/NYU Med Ctr 1979; **Fellow:** Child & Adolescent Psychiatry, Bellevue Hosp/NYU Med Ctr 1981; **Fac Appt:** Clin Prof Psyc, NYU Sch Med

Finkel, Jay MD (Psyc) - **Spec Exp:** Anxiety Disorders; Mood Disorders; **Hospital:** Mt Sinai Med Ctr (page 102); **Address:** 108 E 91st St, New York, NY 10128-1657; **Phone:** 212-289-2077; **Board Cert:** Psychiatry 1985; **Med School:** NY Med Coll 1980; **Resid:** Psychiatry, Mount Sinai Hosp 1984; **Fac Appt:** Asst Clin Prof Psyc, Mount Sinai Sch Med

First, Michael B MD (Psyc) - **Spec Exp:** Psychotherapy; Psychopharmacology; Sexual Addiction; Sexual Behavior-Compulsive; **Hospital:** NY State Psychiatric Inst, NY-Presby/Columbia Univ Med Ctr, NY (page 104); **Address:** NY State Psychiatric Inst, 1051 Riverside Drive, Box 60, New York, NY 10032; **Phone:** 212-543-5531; **Board Cert:** Psychiatry 1989; **Med School:** Univ Pittsburgh 1983; **Resid:** Psychiatry, NYS Psychiatric Inst 1987; **Fellow:** Psychiatric Research, NYS Psychiatric Inst 1988; **Fac Appt:** Prof Psyc, Columbia P&S

Fox, Herbert A MD (Psyc) - **Spec Exp:** Electroconvulsive Therapy (ECT); Psychotherapy; Psychopharmacology; **Hospital:** Lenox Hill Hosp (page 106), Gracie Square Hosp; **Address:** 416 E 76th St, New York, NY 10021-4032; **Phone:** 212-674-8622; **Board Cert:** Psychiatry 1976; **Med School:** Albert Einstein Coll Med 1969; **Resid:** Psychiatry, Montefiore Med Ctr 1973; **Fac Appt:** Assoc Prof Psyc, Cornell Univ-Weill Med Coll

Friedman, Richard Alan MD (Psyc) - **Spec Exp:** Psychopharmacology; Anxiety & Mood Disorders; Depression; **Hospital:** NY-Presby/Weill Cornell Med Ctr, NY (page 104); **Address:** 525 E 68th St, Box 140, New York, NY 10065; **Phone:** 212-746-5775; **Board Cert:** Psychiatry 1989; **Med School:** UMDNJ-RW Johnson Med Sch 1982; **Resid:** Psychiatry, Mt Sinai Med Ctr 1987; **Fellow:** Psychiatry, Baylor Coll Med Affil Hosps 1989; **Fac Appt:** Clin Prof Psyc, Cornell Univ-Weill Med Coll

Fyer, Abby J MD (Psyc) - **Spec Exp:** Anxiety Disorders; Panic Disorder; **Hospital:** NY State Psychiatric Inst, NY-Presby/Columbia Univ Med Ctr, NY (page 104); **Address:** NY State Psychiatric Inst, 1051 Riverside Drive, Ste 5814, New York, NY 10032; **Phone:** 212-543-5372; **Board Cert:** Psychiatry 1980; **Med School:** NYU Sch Med 1973; **Resid:** Psychiatry, Montefiore Med Ctr 1978; **Fac Appt:** Prof Psyc, Columbia P&S

Fyer, Minna R MD (Psyc) - **Spec Exp:** Anxiety Disorders; Mood Disorders; Menopause Problems; **Hospital:** NY-Presby/Weill Cornell Med Ctr, NY (page 104); **Address:** 242 E 72nd St, New York, NY 10021-4574; **Phone:** 212-861-2586; **Board Cert:** Psychiatry 1985; **Med School:** SUNY Hlth Sci Ctr 1980; **Resid:** Psychiatry, NY Hosp/Payne Whitney Clin 1984; **Fellow:** Psychopharmacology, NY State Psych Inst 1986; **Fac Appt:** Asst Clin Prof Psyc, Cornell Univ-Weill Med Coll

Ginsberg, David Lloyd MD (Psyc) - **Spec Exp:** Depression; Bipolar/Mood Disorders; Anxiety Disorders; Psychopharmacology; **Hospital:** NYU Langone Med Ctr (page 108); **Address:** NYU Med Ctr, Behavioral Hlth Prog, 1 Park Ave Fl 8, New York, NY 10016; **Phone:** 212-263-7419; **Board Cert:** Psychiatry 2005; Psychosomatic Medicine 2009; **Med School:** Brown Univ 1990; **Resid:** Psychiatry, NYU Med Ctr 1994; **Fac Appt:** Assoc Clin Prof Psyc, NYU Sch Med

Goff, Donald C MD (Psyc) - **Spec Exp:** Schizophrenia; Psychopharmacology; **Hospital:** NYU Langone Med Ctr (page 108); **Address:** 1 Park Ave Fl 8 - rm 8-212, New York, NY 10016; **Phone:** 646-754-4843; **Board Cert:** Psychiatry 1986; **Med School:** UCLA 1980; **Resid:** Psychiatry, Mass Genl Hosp 1984; **Fellow:** Psychopharmacology, Tufts-New England Med Ctr 1985; **Fac Appt:** Prof Psyc, NYU Sch Med

Goldenberg, David B MD (Psyc) - **Spec Exp:** HIV Psychiatry; Psychoanalysis; Gender Issues; Psychiatry in Cancer; **Hospital:** NY-Presby/Weill Cornell Med Ctr, NY (page 104); **Address:** 35 E 85th St, New York, NY 10028; **Phone:** 212-717-4834; **Board Cert:** Psychiatry 2007; Psychosomatic Medicine 2005; **Med School:** Univ MD Sch Med 1991; **Resid:** Psychiatry, Yale-New Haven Hosp 1996; **Fellow:** Psychiatry, Meml Sloan-Kettering Cancer Ctr 1997

Goldman, Neil S MD (Psyc) - **Spec Exp:** Mood Disorders; Anxiety Disorders; Addiction/Substance Abuse; **Hospital:** N Shore Univ Hosp (page 106); **Address:** 235 W 48th St, Apt 26-H, New York, NY 10036; **Phone:** 212-929-4395; **Board Cert:** Psychiatry 1981; **Med School:** Ros Franklin Univ/Chicago Med Sch 1970; **Resid:** Psychiatry, Brookdale Hosp 1974; **Fellow:** Addiction Psychiatry, St Vincents Hosp 1979; **Fac Appt:** Asst Prof Psyc, NY Med Coll

Goldstein, Susanna K MD (Psyc) - **Spec Exp:** Psychopharmacology; Anxiety & Depression; Clinical Trials; **Hospital:** Lenox Hill Hosp (page 106); **Address:** 65 Central Park West, Ste 1BR, New York, NY 10023; **Phone:** 212-362-6657; **Board Cert:** Psychiatry 1985; **Med School:** Israel 1975; **Resid:** Psychiatry, Rambam Med Ctr 1980; Neurology, Rambam Med Ctr 1981; **Fellow:** Biological Psychiatry, Montefiore Med Ctr 1983; **Fac Appt:** Asst Clin Prof Psyc, NYU Sch Med

Goodman, Wayne K MD (Psyc) - **Spec Exp:** Obsessive-Compulsive Disorder; Tourette's Syndrome; Anxiety Disorders; **Hospital:** Mt Sinai Med Ctr (page 102); **Address:** Mount Sinai,, 1 Gustave Levy Pl, Box 1230, New York, NY 10029; **Phone:** 212-659-8860; **Board Cert:** Psychiatry 1988; **Med School:** Boston Univ 1981; **Resid:** Psychiatry, Yale-New Haven Hosp 1985; **Fellow:** Psychiatric Research, Yale-New Haven Hosp 1986; **Fac Appt:** Prof Psyc, Mount Sinai Sch Med

Gorman, Lauren K MD (Psyc) - **Spec Exp:** Psychopharmacology; Anxiety & Mood Disorders; **Hospital:** Mt Sinai Med Ctr (page 102); **Address:** 685 West End Ave, Ste 1AF, New York, NY 10025; **Phone:** 212-580-7713; **Board Cert:** Psychiatry 1983; **Med School:** Columbia P&S 1977; **Resid:** Ophthalmology, Bellevue Hosp 1979; Psychiatry, Mt Sinai Hosp 1982; **Fellow:** Biological Psychiatry, Montefiore Med Ctr 1984; **Fac Appt:** Asst Clin Prof Psyc, Mount Sinai Sch Med

Heller, Stanley S MD (Psyc) - **Spec Exp:** Panic Disorder; Depression; Psychiatry in Physical Illness; **Address:** 1136 Fifth Ave, New York, NY 10128; **Phone:** 212-831-5919; **Board Cert:** Psychiatry 1975; **Med School:** Columbia P&S 1960; **Resid:** Psychiatry, NY State Psychiatric Inst 1966; **Fac Appt:** Assoc Clin Prof Psyc, Columbia P&S

Hoffman, Joel MD (Psyc) - **Spec Exp:** Psychopharmacology; Depression; Treatment Resistant Mental Illness; **Hospital:** Lenox Hill Hosp (page 106), NY-Presby/Weill Cornell Med Ctr, NY (page 104); **Address:** 1236 Park Ave, New York, NY 10128-1717; **Phone:** 212-722-3004; **Board Cert:** Psychiatry 1977; **Med School:** Columbia P&S 1963; **Resid:** Internal Medicine, Univ Michigan Med Ctr 1967; Psychiatry, NY State Psychiatric Inst 1972; **Fac Appt:** Asst Clin Prof Psyc, Columbia P&S

Hollander, Eric MD (Psyc) - **Spec Exp:** Obsessive-Compulsive Disorder; Anxiety Disorders; Autism; Body Dysmorphic Disorder (BDD); **Hospital:** Montefiore Med Ctr-Moses Campus (page 100), Lenox Hill Hosp (page 106); **Address:** 901 5th Ave, New York, NY 10021; **Phone:** 212-873-4051; **Board Cert:** Psychiatry 1987; **Med School:** SUNY Hlth Sci Ctr 1982; **Resid:** Internal Medicine, Mount Sinai Med Ctr 1983; Psychiatry, Mount Sinai Med Ctr 1986; **Fellow:** Psychopharmacology, Columbia Univ-Psych Inst 1988; **Fac Appt:** Prof Psyc, Albert Einstein Coll Med

Kahn, David A MD (Psyc) - **Spec Exp:** Anxiety & Mood Disorders; Psychopharmacology; Psychotherapy; Schizophrenia; **Hospital:** NY-Presby/Columbia Univ Med Ctr, NY (page 104); **Address:** 35 E 85th St, New York, NY 10028; **Phone:** 212-472-0100; **Board Cert:** Psychiatry 1984; **Med School:** Columbia P&S 1979; **Resid:** Psychiatry, NY State Psych Inst 1983; **Fellow:** Biological Psychiatry, NY State Psych Inst 1984; **Fac Appt:** Prof Emeritus Psyc, Columbia P&S

Kalinich, Lila J MD (Psyc) - **Spec Exp:** Psychoanalysis; Psychotherapy; Adolescent Psychiatry; **Hospital:** NY-Presby/Columbia Univ Med Ctr, NY (page 104), NY State Psychiatric Inst; **Address:** 333 Central Park W, Ste 12, New York, NY 10025; **Phone:** 212-866-0200; **Board Cert:** Psychiatry 1975; **Med School:** Northwestern Univ 1969; **Resid:** Psychiatry, NY-Presby/Columbia Univ Med Ctr 1973; **Fac Appt:** Clin Prof Psyc, Columbia P&S

Karasu, Sylvia R MD (Psyc) - **Spec Exp:** Weight Management; Eating Disorders; **Hospital:** NY-Presby/Weill Cornell Med Ctr, NY (page 104); **Address:** 2 E 88th St, New York, NY 10128; **Phone:** 212-534-7822; **Board Cert:** Psychiatry 1981; Child & Adolescent Psychiatry 1982; **Med School:** Albert Einstein Coll Med 1976; **Resid:** Psychiatry, Payne Whitney Clin 1979; **Fellow:** Child Psychiatry, Payne Whitney Clin 1981; **Fac Appt:** Assoc Clin Prof Psyc, Cornell Univ-Weill Med Coll

Karasu, T Byram MD (Psyc) - **Spec Exp:** Depression; Personality Disorders; Psychotherapy; **Hospital:** Montefiore Med Ctr-Moses Campus (page 100), Montefiore Med Ctr-Einstein Campus (page 100); **Address:** 2 E 88th St, New York, NY 10128-0555; **Phone:** 212-426-5208; **Board Cert:** Psychiatry 1972; **Med School:** Turkey 1959; **Resid:** Psychiatry, Yale Univ Affil Hosp 1969; **Fac Appt:** Prof Psyc, Albert Einstein Coll Med

Kaufmann, Charles A MD (Psyc) - **Spec Exp:** Schizophrenia; Bipolar/Mood Disorders; Alcohol Abuse; **Hospital:** NY-Presby/Columbia Univ Med Ctr, NY (page 104), NY State Psychiatric Inst; **Address:** NY-Presby, Psychiatry Dept, 161 Fort Washington Ave, Ste 348, New York, NY 10032; **Phone:** 914-238-7909; **Board Cert:** Psychiatry 1982; **Med School:** Columbia P&S 1977; **Resid:** Psychiatry, NY-Presby/Weill Cornell Med Ctr 1981; **Fellow:** Research, Natl Inst Hlth 1985; Research, Ctr for Neurobio & Behavior 1988; **Fac Appt:** Assoc Prof Psyc, Columbia P&S

Kellner, Charles H MD (Psyc) - **Spec Exp:** Electroconvulsive Therapy (ECT); Depression; Geriatric Psychiatry; **Hospital:** Mt Sinai Med Ctr (page 102); **Address:** 1425 Madison Ave, Box 1230, New York, NY 10029; **Phone:** 212-659-8285; **Board Cert:** Psychiatry ; Geriatric Psychiatry 2011; **Med School:** Cornell Univ-Weill Med Coll 1978; **Resid:** Psychiatry, Cedars-Sinai Med Ctr 1981; **Fellow:** Biological Psychiatry, NIH Clinical Ctr 1984; **Fac Appt:** Prof Psyc, Mount Sinai Sch Med

Kocsis, James MD (Psyc) - **Spec Exp:** Psychopharmacology; Mood Disorders; Anxiety Disorders; **Hospital:** NY-Presby/Weill Cornell Med Ctr, NY (page 104); **Address:** 525 E 68th St, Box 140, New York, NY 10021-4885; **Phone:** 212-746-5913; **Board Cert:** Psychiatry 1977; **Med School:** Cornell Univ-Weill Med Coll 1968; **Resid:** Psychiatry, NY Hosp 1975; **Fac Appt:** Prof Psyc, Cornell Univ-Weill Med Coll

Kowallis, George MD (Psyc) - **Spec Exp:** Depression; Anxiety Disorders; ADD/ADHD; **Address:** 162 W 56th St, Ste 407, New York, NY 10019-3831; **Phone:** 212-757-0324; **Board Cert:** Psychiatry 1977; Child & Adolescent Psychiatry 1978; **Med School:** Univ Pennsylvania 1969; **Resid:** Psychiatry, St Luke's-Roosevelt Hosp Ctr 1974; **Fac Appt:** Asst Clin Prof Psyc, NY Med Coll

Kranzler, Elliot MD (Psyc) - **Spec Exp:** Anxiety & Depression; Bereavement/Traumatic Grief; ADD/ADHD; **Hospital:** NY-Presby/Columbia Univ Med Ctr, NY (page 104); **Address:** 451 West End Ave, New York, NY 10024-5329; **Phone:** 212-580-9758; **Board Cert:** Psychiatry 1984; Child & Adolescent Psychiatry 1986; **Med School:** Albert Einstein Coll Med 1978; **Resid:** Psychiatry, Payne-Whitney Clin 1982; **Fellow:** Child & Adolescent Psychiatry, NY-Presby/Columbia Univ Med Ctr 1984; Research, NY-Presby/Columbia-NIMH; **Fac Appt:** Asst Prof Psyc, Columbia P&S

Kremberg, M Roy MD (Psyc) - **Spec Exp:** Mood Disorders; Anxiety Disorders; ADD/ADHD; **Hospital:** St. Luke's - Roosevelt Hosp Ctr - St Luke's Hosp (page 94); **Address:** 2109 Broadway, Ste 8144, New York, NY 10023-2106; **Phone:** 212-875-8568; **Board Cert:** Psychiatry 1980; Child & Adolescent Psychiatry 1982; **Med School:** Columbia P&S 1976; **Resid:** Psychiatry, St Luke's Hosp 1978; **Fellow:** Child & Adolescent Psychiatry, St Luke's Hosp 1980

Krueger, Richard B MD (Psyc) - **Spec Exp:** Sexual Behavior-Compulsive; **Hospital:** NY State Psychiatric Inst, NY-Presby/Columbia Univ Med Ctr, NY (page 104); **Address:** NY State Psychiatric Inst, 1051 Riverside Drive, Box 45, New York, NY 10032; **Phone:** 212-740-7330; **Board Cert:** Psychiatry 1984; Internal Medicine 1980; Addiction Psychiatry 2007; Forensic Psychiatry 2006; **Med School:** Harvard Med Sch 1977; **Resid:** Internal Medicine, Boston VA Hosp 1980; **Fellow:** Psychiatry, Boston Med Ctr 1983; **Fac Appt:** Assoc Clin Prof Psyc, Columbia P&S

Levitan, Stephan MD (Psyc) - **Spec Exp:** Psychotherapy; Psychopharmacology; Couples Therapy; Psychoanalysis; **Hospital:** NY-Presby/Columbia Univ Med Ctr, NY (page 104); **Address:** 185 E 85th St, Ste 29J, New York, NY 10028-2143; **Phone:** 212-722-4311; **Board Cert:** Psychiatry 1974; **Med School:** SUNY Buffalo 1965; **Resid:** Psychiatry, Hillside Hosp 1969; **Fellow:** Psychoanalysis, Columbia Psychoanalysis Training Ctr 1973; **Fac Appt:** Clin Prof Psyc, Columbia P&S

Lindenmayer, Jean-Pierre MD (Psyc) - **Spec Exp:** Psychopharmacology; Schizophrenia; Bipolar/Mood Disorders; **Address:** 18 E 77th St, Ste B, New York, NY 10021-1700; **Phone:** 212-249-2720; **Board Cert:** Psychiatry 1975; **Med School:** Switzerland 1967; **Resid:** Psychiatry, Univ Hosp-Geneva Med Sch 1969; Psychiatry, SUNY Downstate Med Ctr 1973; **Fellow:** Research, SUNY Downstate Med Ctr 1975; **Fac Appt:** Clin Prof Psyc, NYU Sch Med

Lipton, Brian P MD (Psyc) - **Spec Exp:** Psychotherapy; Psychopharmacology; Anxiety & Mood Disorders; Psychosomatic Disorders; **Hospital:** Lenox Hill Hosp (page 106); **Address:** 1111 Park Ave, Ste 1A, New York, NY 10128-1234; **Phone:** 212-427-4499; **Board Cert:** Psychiatry 1970; **Med School:** SUNY Downstate 1964; **Resid:** Psychiatry, Hillside Hosp 1968; **Fac Appt:** Asst Clin Prof Psyc, NYU Sch Med

Malaspina, Dolores MD (Psyc) - **Spec Exp:** Anxiety Disorders; Depression; Trauma Psychiatry; **Hospital:** NYU Langone Med Ctr (page 108); **Address:** 136 E 57th St, Ste 1201, New York, NY 10022; **Phone:** 718-877-5708; **Board Cert:** Psychiatry 1989; **Med School:** UMDNJ-NJ Med Sch, Newark 1983; **Resid:** Psychiatry, NY-Presby/Columbia Univ Med Ctr 1987; **Fellow:** Psychiatry, NY State Psych Inst 1989; **Fac Appt:** Prof Psyc, NYU Sch Med

Manevitz, Alan MD (Psyc) - **Spec Exp:** Marital/Family/Sex Therapy; Depression-TMS Therapy; ADD/PTSD; Frbromyalgia Syndrome (FMS); **Hospital:** NY-Presby/Weill Cornell Med Ctr, NY (page 104), Lenox Hill Hosp (page 106); **Address:** 60 Sutton Place South, Ste 1CN, New York, NY 10022; **Phone:** 212-751-5072; **Board Cert:** Psychiatry 1987; **Med School:** Columbia P&S 1980; **Resid:** Psychiatry, NY Hosp 1984; **Fellow:** Psychopharmacology, NY Hosp 1985; **Fac Appt:** Assoc Clin Prof Psyc, Cornell Univ-Weill Med Coll

Mann, J. John MD/PhD (Psyc) - **Spec Exp:** Mood Disorders; Clinical Trials; Suicide; **Hospital:** NY-Presby/Columbia Univ Med Ctr, NY (page 104); **Address:** 161 Fort Washington Ave, Irving Bldg, Fl 2 - Ste 209, New York, NY 10032; **Phone:** 212-543-5571; **Board Cert:** Psychiatry 1980; **Med School:** Australia 1971; **Resid:** Internal Medicine, Royal Melbourne Hosp 1974; Psychiatry, Royal Melbourne Hosp 1976; **Fac Appt:** Prof Psyc, Columbia P&S

Marin, Deborah B MD (Psyc) - **Spec Exp:** Memory Disorders; Depression; Depression in the Elderly; Geriatric Psychiatry; **Hospital:** Mt Sinai Med Ctr (page 102); **Address:** Mount Sinai Med Ctr, Psychiatry Dept, 1425 Madison Ave Fl 5, New York, NY 10029; **Phone:** 212-659-8092; **Board Cert:** Psychiatry 1990; **Med School:** Mount Sinai Sch Med 1984; **Resid:** Psychiatry, Mount Sinai Med Ctr 1988; **Fellow:** Psychiatry, NY-Presby/Weill Cornell Med Ctr 1991; **Fac Appt:** Prof Psyc, Mount Sinai Sch Med

Markowitz, John C MD (Psyc) - **Spec Exp:** Depression; Post Traumatic Stress Disorder; Cognitive Psychotherapy; Psychopharmacology; **Hospital:** NY-Presby/Columbia Univ Med Ctr, NY (page 104), NY State Psychiatric Inst; **Address:** 40 E 83rd St, New York, NY 10028; **Phone:** 212-288-3070; **Board Cert:** Psychiatry 1987; **Med School:** Columbia P&S 1982; **Resid:** Psychiatry, Payne Whitney Clin/New York Hosp 1987; **Fac Appt:** Prof Psyc, Columbia P&S

Massie, Mary Jane MD (Psyc) - **Spec Exp:** Psychiatry in Cancer; Depression; **Hospital:** Meml Sloan-Kettering Canc Ctr (page 114); **Address:** MSKCC, Psychiatry Dept, 1275 York Ave, New York, NY 10065; **Phone:** 646-888-0181; **Board Cert:** Psychiatry 1978; Psychosomatic Medicine 2005; **Med School:** SUNY Buffalo 1984; **Resid:** Psychiatry, Montefiore Med Ctr 1987; **Fellow:** Psychosomatic Medicine, Meml Sloan-Kettering Cancer Ctr 1987

McGrath, Patrick J MD (Psyc) - **Spec Exp:** Psychopharmacology-Consultation; Depression-Consultation; **Hospital:** NY-Presby/Columbia Univ Med Ctr, NY (page 104), NY State Psychiatric Inst; **Address:** 710 W 168th St, New York, NY 10032; **Phone:** 212-543-5764; **Board Cert:** Psychiatry 1979; **Med School:** Columbia P&S 1974; **Resid:** Psychiatry, NY State Psych Inst 1978; **Fac Appt:** Clin Prof Psyc, Columbia P&S

McMullen Jr, Robert MD (Psyc) - **Spec Exp:** Psychopharmacology; Anxiety Disorders; Bipolar/Mood Disorders; **Address:** 171 W 79th St, Ste 2, New York, NY 10024-6449; **Phone:** 212-362-9635; **Board Cert:** Psychiatry 1982; **Med School:** Georgetown Univ 1976; **Resid:** Psychiatry, NY State Psychiatric Inst 1980; **Fac Appt:** Asst Prof Psyc, Columbia P&S

Mellman, Lisa A MD (Psyc) - **Spec Exp:** Anxiety & Depression; Relationship Problems; **Hospital:** NY-Presby/Columbia Univ Med Ctr, NY (page 104), NY State Psychiatric Inst; **Address:** NY-Presby, Psychiatry Dept, 630 W 168th St, rm 3-401, New York, NY 10032; **Phone:** 917-620-6010; **Board Cert:** Psychiatry 1986; **Med School:** Case West Res Univ 1981; **Resid:** Psychiatry, NY-Presby/Columbia Univ Med Ctr 1985; **Fellow:** Psychoanalysis, NY-Presby/Columbia Univ Med Ctr 1991; **Fac Appt:** Clin Prof Psyc, Columbia P&S

Michels, Robert MD (Psyc) - **Spec Exp:** Psychoanalysis; **Hospital:** NY-Presby/Weill Cornell Med Ctr, NY (page 104); **Address:** 418 E 71st St, New York, NY 10021-4894; **Phone:** 212-746-6001; **Board Cert:** Psychiatry 1964; **Med School:** Northwestern Univ 1958; **Resid:** Psychiatry, Columbia-Presby/NY Psych Inst 1962; **Fac Appt:** Prof Psyc, Cornell Univ-Weill Med Coll

Moore, Joanne MD (Psyc) - **Spec Exp:** Eating Disorders; Anxiety & Depression; Addiction/Substance Abuse; Geriatric Psychiatry; **Hospital:** NY-Presby/Columbia Univ Med Ctr, NY (page 104); **Address:** NY-Presby, Psychiatry Dept, 635 W 165th St, Ste 303, New York, NY 10032; **Phone:** 212-305-9499; **Board Cert:** Psychiatry 1988; Addiction Psychiatry 2006; **Med School:** Harvard Med Sch 1982; **Resid:** Psychiatry, NY-Presby/Columbia Univ Med Ctr 1987; **Fellow:** Geriatric Psychiatry, NY-Presby/Columbia Univ Med Ctr 1984; **Fac Appt:** Assoc Prof Psyc, Columbia P&S

Muskin, Philip R MD (Psyc) - **Spec Exp:** Psychopharmacology; Anxiety & Depression; Psychiatry in Physical Illness; Psychoanalysis; **Hospital:** NY-Presby/Columbia Univ Med Ctr, NY (page 104); **Address:** 1700 York Ave, New York, NY 10128-7820; **Phone:** 212-722-8438; **Board Cert:** Psychiatry 1979; Geriatric Psychiatry 2011; Psychosomatic Medicine 2005; **Med School:** NY Med Coll 1974; **Resid:** Psychiatry, NYS Psych Inst 1978; **Fellow:** Psychosomatic Medicine, Columbia-Presby Hosp 1979; Psychopharmacology, NY State Psych Inst 1979; **Fac Appt:** Prof Psyc, Columbia P&S

Nininger, James MD (Psyc) - **Spec Exp:** Psychotherapy; Psychopharmacology; Geriatric Psychiatry; **Hospital:** NY-Presby/Weill Cornell Med Ctr, NY (page 104); **Address:** 10 E 78th St, Ste 5A, New York, NY 10075; **Phone:** 212-879-8338; **Board Cert:** Psychiatry 1978; **Med School:** Univ Cincinnati 1974; **Resid:** Psychiatry, Mount Sinai Hosp 1977; **Fac Appt:** Assoc Clin Prof Psyc, Cornell Univ-Weill Med Coll

Nunes, Edward MD (Psyc) - **Spec Exp:** Depression; Substance Abuse; **Hospital:** NY State Psychiatric Inst, NY-Presby/Columbia Univ Med Ctr, NY (page 104); **Address:** 617 West End Ave, Ste 1B, New York, NY 10032; **Phone:** 212-579-0339; **Board Cert:** Psychiatry 1986; Addiction Psychiatry 2002; **Med School:** Univ Conn 1981; **Resid:** Psychiatry, Columbia-Presby/NYS Psyc Inst 1985; **Fellow:** Psychopharmacology, Columbia-Presby/NYS Psyc Inst 1988; **Fac Appt:** Prof Psyc, Columbia P&S

Oberfield, Richard MD (Psyc) - **Spec Exp:** Child & Adolescent Psychiatry; Divorce/Family Issues; ADD/ADHD; **Hospital:** NYU Langone Med Ctr (page 108); **Address:** 200 E 33rd St, Ste 2J, New York, NY 10016-4874; **Phone:** 212-684-0148; **Board Cert:** Psychiatry 1979; Child & Adolescent Psychiatry 1980; **Med School:** Mount Sinai Sch Med 1974; **Resid:** Psychiatry, Bellevue Hosp 1976; **Fellow:** Child & Adolescent Psychiatry, Bellevue Hosp 1978; **Fac Appt:** Clin Prof Psyc, NYU Sch Med

Olds, David D MD (Psyc) - **Spec Exp:** Psychoanalysis; Psychotherapy; **Hospital:** NY-Presby/Columbia Univ Med Ctr, NY (page 104); **Address:** 108 E 96th St, Ste 6F, New York, NY 10128; **Phone:** 212-427-9688; **Board Cert:** Psychiatry 1975; **Med School:** Columbia P&S 1967; **Resid:** Psychiatry, NY State Psych Inst 1971; **Fellow:** Psychoanalysis, NY-Presby/Columbia Univ Med Ctr 1978; **Fac Appt:** Clin Prof Psyc, Columbia P&S

Papp, Laszlo A MD (Psyc) - **Spec Exp:** Anxiety & Mood Disorders; Depression; Panic Disorder; Psychopharmacology; **Hospital:** NY-Presby/Columbia Univ Med Ctr, NY (page 104); **Address:** 124 E 84th St, Ste 1B, New York, NY 10028; **Phone:** 212-360-5750; **Board Cert:** Psychiatry 1993; **Med School:** Hungary 1978; **Resid:** Internal Medicine, Natl Inst Rheumatology 1981; Psychiatry, Beth Israel Med Ctr 1986; **Fellow:** Psychopharmacology, NY-Presby/Columbia Univ Med Ctr 1989; **Fac Appt:** Assoc Clin Prof Psyc, Columbia P&S

Pawel, Michael A MD (Psyc) - **Spec Exp:** Adolescent Psychiatry; **Hospital:** St. Luke's - Roosevelt Hosp Ctr - St Luke's Hosp (page 94); **Address:** 15 W 72nd St, Ste 1J, New York, NY 10023; **Phone:** 212-873-9170; **Board Cert:** Psychiatry 1977; **Med School:** Albert Einstein Coll Med 1971; **Resid:** Psychiatry, Montefiore Hosp Med Ctr 1974; **Fac Appt:** Asst Prof Psyc, Columbia P&S

Pfeffer, Cynthia R MD (Psyc) - **Spec Exp:** Child & Adolescent Psychiatry; Bereavement/Traumatic Grief; Anxiety & Depression; ADD/ADHD; **Hospital:** NY-Presby/Weill Cornell Med Ctr, NY (page 104), NYU Langone Med Ctr (page 108); **Address:** 1100 Park Ave, Ste 1B, New York, NY 10128; **Phone:** 212-717-2334; **Board Cert:** Psychiatry 1975; Child & Adolescent Psychiatry 1976; **Med School:** NYU Sch Med 1968; **Resid:** Psychiatry, Montefiore Med Ctr 1973; **Fellow:** Child & Adolescent Psychiatry, Montefiore Med Ctr 1973; **Fac Appt:** Prof Psyc, Cornell Univ-Weill Med Coll

Pines, Jeffrey M MD (Psyc) - **Spec Exp:** Substance Abuse; **Hospital:** NY-Presby/Columbia Univ Med Ctr, NY (page 104); **Address:** 295 Central Park W, Ste 2, New York, NY 10024; **Phone:** 212-579-1913; **Board Cert:** Psychiatry 1982; **Med School:** Columbia P&S 1973; **Resid:** Internal Medicine, NY-Presby/Columbia Univ Med Ctr 1976; Psychiatry, NY State Psych Inst 1980; **Fellow:** Rheumatology, Hosp Special Surgery 1977; Liaison Psychiatry, NY-Presby/Columbia Univ Med Ctr 1981; **Fac Appt:** Assoc Clin Prof Psyc, Columbia P&S

Preven, David W MD (Psyc) - **Spec Exp:** Anxiety & Mood Disorders; Psychopharmacology; Psychotherapy; Forensic Psychiatry; **Hospital:** Montefiore Med Ctr-Moses Campus (page 100); **Address:** 451 West End Ave, Ste 2H, New York, NY 10024; **Phone:** 212-799-4907; **Board Cert:** Psychiatry 1969; Forensic Psychiatry 2005; **Med School:** Harvard Med Sch 1963; **Resid:** Psychiatry, Jacobi Hosp/Albert Einstein 1967; **Fellow:** Psychiatry, NIMH-Albert Einstein Affil Hosp 1971; **Fac Appt:** Clin Prof Psyc, Albert Einstein Coll Med

Rees, Ellen MD (Psyc) - **Spec Exp:** Psychoanalysis; Psychotherapy; **Hospital:** NY-Presby/Weill Cornell Med Ctr, NY (page 104); **Address:** 108 E 96th St Fl 7 - Ste F, New York, NY 10128-6217; **Phone:** 212-722-5988; **Board Cert:** Psychiatry 1979; **Med School:** Albert Einstein Coll Med 1974; **Resid:** Psychiatry, Mt Sinai Hosp 1977; **Fellow:** Psychiatry, NY Hosp-Cornell 1978; Psychoanalysis, Columbia Univ Ctr Psych Trng 1991; **Fac Appt:** Assoc Clin Prof Psyc, Cornell Univ-Weill Med Coll

Roose, Steven MD (Psyc) - **Spec Exp:** Depression in the Elderly; Psychoanalysis; **Hospital:** NY State Psychiatric Inst; **Address:** NY State Psychiatric Inst, 1051 Riverside Drive, rm 2211, Box 98, New York, NY 10032; **Phone:** 212-831-8644; **Board Cert:** Psychiatry 1979; **Med School:** Mount Sinai Sch Med 1974; **Resid:** Psychiatry, NY State Psych Inst 1978; **Fellow:** Research, NY-Presby/Columbia Univ Med Ctr 1981; **Fac Appt:** Prof Psyc, Columbia P&S

Rosen, Arnold M MD (Psyc) - **Spec Exp:** Depression; Psychopharmacology; **Address:** 200 E 78th St, New York, NY 10075; **Phone:** 212-288-6380; **Board Cert:** Psychiatry 1976; **Med School:** Univ Tex SW, Dallas 1968; **Resid:** Psychiatry, Metropolitan Hosp Ctr 1970; Psychiatry, Metropolitan Hosp Ctr 1974; **Fellow:** Psychiatry, Metropolitan Hosp Ctr 1975

Rosenthal, Jesse S MD (Psyc) - **Spec Exp:** ADD/ADHD; Anxiety Disorders; Depression; **Hospital:** Beth Israel Med Ctr - Petrie Div (page 94); **Address:** 21 E 93rd St, New York, NY 10128-0609; **Phone:** 212-876-3080; **Board Cert:** Psychiatry 1978; **Med School:** Geo Wash Univ 1973; **Resid:** Psychiatry, Mount Sinai Hosp 1976; **Fac Appt:** Asst Clin Prof Psyc, Mount Sinai Sch Med

Rosenthal, Richard N MD (Psyc) - **Spec Exp:** Anxiety & Mood Disorders; Addiction/Substance Abuse; **Hospital:** St. Luke's - Roosevelt Hosp Ctr - Roosevelt Div (page 94), Beth Israel Med Ctr - Petrie Div (page 94); **Address:** 1090 Amerstdam Ave, Ste 16G, New York, NY 10025; **Phone:** 212-523-5366; **Board Cert:** Psychiatry 1985; Addiction Psychiatry 2012; **Med School:** SUNY Hlth Sci Ctr 1980; **Resid:** Psychiatry, Mount Sinai Med Ctr 1984; **Fac Appt:** Prof Psyc, Columbia P&S

Rosner, Richard MD (Psyc) - **Spec Exp:** Adolescent Psychiatry; Forensic Psychiatry; Addiction/Substance Abuse; **Hospital:** NYU Langone Med Ctr (page 108), Bellevue Hosp Ctr; **Address:** 140 E 83rd St, Ste 6A, New York, NY 10028-1928; **Phone:** 212-988-6014; **Board Cert:** Psychiatry 1974; Forensic Psychiatry 2004; Addiction Medicine 2004; **Med School:** NYU Sch Med 1966; **Resid:** Psychiatry, Mount Sinai Hosp 1970; **Fac Appt:** Clin Prof Psyc, NYU Sch Med

Ross, Steven G MD (Psyc) - **Spec Exp:** Addiction/Substance Abuse; Alcohol Abuse; Adolescent Psychiatry; Psychiatry in Cancer; **Hospital:** NYU Langone Med Ctr (page 108), Bellevue Hosp Ctr; **Address:** 462 1st Ave, rm NBV 10E-7, New York, NY 10016; **Phone:** 212-562-4097; **Board Cert:** Psychiatry 2009; **Med School:** Mexico 1980; **Resid:** Psychiatry, Maimonides Med Ctr 1986; **Fac Appt:** Asst Prof Psyc, NYU Sch Med

Roth, Andrew J MD (Psyc) - **Spec Exp:** Psychiatry of Prostate Cancer; Geriatric Psychiatry; **Hospital:** Meml Sloan-Kettering Canc Ctr (page 114); **Address:** 641 Lexington Ave, Fl 7, New York, NY 10022; **Phone:** 646-888-0024; **Board Cert:** Psychiatry 1993; Geriatric Psychiatry 2007; Psychosomatic Medicine 2005; **Med School:** NY Med Coll 1988; **Resid:** Psychiatry, Mt Sinai Med Ctr 1992; **Fellow:** Liaison Psychiatry, Meml Sloan-Kettering Canc Ctr 1994; **Fac Appt:** Clin Prof Psyc, Cornell Univ-Weill Med Coll

Rubinstein, Morton E MD (Psyc) - **Spec Exp:** Psychopharmacology; **Hospital:** VA NY Harbor Hlthcare Sys-Manhattan Campus; **Address:** 423 E 23rd St, New York, NY 10010-5013; **Phone:** 212-686-7500 x7991; **Board Cert:** Psychiatry 1988; **Med School:** NY Med Coll 1976; **Resid:** Psychiatry, Bellevue Hosp 1979; **Fellow:** Psychiatry, Mount Sinai Med Ctr 1980; **Fac Appt:** Assoc Clin Prof Psyc, NYU Sch Med

Sacks, Michael MD (Psyc) - **Spec Exp:** Personality Disorders; Relationship Problems; Anxiety & Depression; **Hospital:** NY-Presby/Weill Cornell Med Ctr, NY (page 104); **Address:** 525 E 68th St, Box 140, New York, NY 10021-4870; **Phone:** 212-746-3710; **Board Cert:** Psychiatry 1973; **Med School:** NYU Sch Med 1967; **Resid:** Psychiatry, NY State Psych Inst 1971; **Fellow:** Psychiatry, Natl Inst Mental Hlth 1973; **Fac Appt:** Prof Psyc, Cornell Univ-Weill Med Coll

Sadock, Virginia MD (Psyc) - **Spec Exp:** Psychotherapy; Sexual Dysfunction; Anxiety & Depression; Marital/Family/Sex Therapy; **Hospital:** NYU Langone Med Ctr (page 108); **Address:** 4 E 89th St, Ste 1E, New York, NY 10128; **Phone:** 212-427-0885; **Board Cert:** Psychiatry 1975; **Med School:** NY Med Coll 1970; **Resid:** Psychiatry, Metropolitan Hosp Ctr 1973; **Fac Appt:** Clin Prof Psyc, NYU Sch Med

Samberg, Eslee MD (Psyc) - **Spec Exp:** Psychoanalysis; Personality Disorders; Psychotherapy; **Hospital:** NY-Presby/Weill Cornell Med Ctr, NY (page 104); **Address:** 165 W End Ave, Ste 1M, New York, NY 10024; **Phone:** 212-874-7725; **Board Cert:** Psychiatry 1983; **Med School:** Cornell Univ-Weill Med Coll 1978; **Resid:** Psychiatry, NY-Presby/Weill Cornell Med Ctr 1982; **Fac Appt:** Assoc Clin Prof Psyc, Cornell Univ-Weill Med Coll

Sawyer, David MD (Psyc) - **Spec Exp:** Psychoanalysis; Child & Adolescent Psychiatry; Psychosomatic Disorders; Anxiety & Mood Disorders; **Address:** 1 W 64th St, Ste 1C, New York, NY 10023; **Phone:** 212-787-8260; **Board Cert:** Psychiatry 1982; Child & Adolescent Psychiatry 1984; **Med School:** NY Med Coll 1977; **Resid:** Psychiatry, NY Hosp-Cornell/Westchester 1980; **Fellow:** Child & Adolescent Psychiatry, NY Hosp-Cornell/Westchester 1982

Scharf, Robert D MD (Psyc) - **Spec Exp:** Psychotherapy; Psychopharmacology; Psychoanalysis; **Hospital:** St. Luke's - Roosevelt Hosp Ctr - Roosevelt Div (page 94), St. Luke's - Roosevelt Hosp Ctr - St Luke's Hosp (page 94); **Address:** 207 E 74th St, Ste 1L, New York, NY 10021-3341; **Phone:** 212-988-4145; **Board Cert:** Psychiatry 1976; **Med School:** Albert Einstein Coll Med 1960; **Resid:** Internal Medicine, Barnes Hosp 1961; Psychiatry, Kings Co Hosp 1964; **Fellow:** Psychoanalysis, NY Psychoanalytic Inst 1973

Schein, Jonah MD (Psyc) - **Spec Exp:** Depression; Anxiety Disorders; **Hospital:** NY-Presby/Weill Cornell Med Ctr, NY (page 104); **Address:** 1349 Lexington Ave, Ste 1E, New York, NY 10128-1514; **Phone:** 212-876-2324; **Board Cert:** Psychiatry 1975; **Med School:** NYU Sch Med 1969; **Resid:** Psychiatry, NY State Psych Inst 1973; **Fac Appt:** Assoc Clin Prof Psyc, Cornell Univ-Weill Med Coll

Seaman, Cheryl MD (Psyc) - **Spec Exp:** Psychotherapy; Anxiety Disorders; Depression; Psychopharmacology; **Address:** 286 Madison Ave, PH, New York, NY 10017; **Phone:** 917-687-8901; **Board Cert:** Psychiatry 1986; **Med School:** Columbia P&S 1979; **Resid:** Psychiatry, NY Hosp-Westchester Div 1983

Shapiro, Peter A MD (Psyc) - **Spec Exp:** Depression; Psychiatry in Physical Illness; Liaison Psychiatry; **Hospital:** NY-Presby/Columbia Univ Med Ctr, NY (page 104); **Address:** 239 Central Park West, Ste 1-BW, New York, NY 10024-6038; **Phone:** 212-874-6030; **Board Cert:** Psychiatry 1985; Psychosomatic Medicine 2005; **Med School:** Columbia P&S 1980; **Resid:** Psychiatry, NY State Psych Inst 1984; **Fellow:** Liaison Psychiatry, NY-Presby/Columbia Univ Med Ctr 1986; **Fac Appt:** Clin Prof Psyc, Columbia P&S

Shaw, Ronda R MD (Psyc) - **Spec Exp:** Psychoanalysis; Psychotherapy; **Hospital:** Mt Sinai Med Ctr (page 102); **Address:** 35 E 85th St, Ste 2, New York, NY 10028; **Phone:** 212-772-0321; **Board Cert:** Psychiatry 1977; **Med School:** Wayne State Univ 1966; **Resid:** Psychiatry, Jacobi Med Ctr 1970; **Fac Appt:** Assoc Clin Prof Psyc, Mount Sinai Sch Med

Shinbach, Kent MD (Psyc) - **Spec Exp:** Depression; Psychopharmacology; Geriatric Psychiatry; **Hospital:** Gracie Square Hosp, NY-Presby/Lower Manhattan Hosp (page 104); **Address:** 14 EAST 75 E 75th St, Ste 1A, MS 10021, New York, NY 10021; **Phone:** 212-744-7100; **Board Cert:** Psychiatry 1970; **Med School:** Jefferson Med Coll 1963; **Resid:** Psychiatry, NY Med Coll 1968; **Fac Appt:** Asst Clin Prof Psyc, Cornell Univ-Weill Med Coll

Siever, Larry J MD (Psyc) - **Spec Exp:** Psychopharmacology; Depression; Personality Disorders; **Hospital:** Mt Sinai Med Ctr (page 102), James J. Peters VA Med Ctr-Bronx; **Address:** 1 Gustave L Levy Pl, Box 1230, New York, NY 10029-6500; **Phone:** 212-774-1722; **Board Cert:** Psychiatry 1980; **Med School:** Stanford Univ 1975; **Resid:** Psychiatry, McLean Hosp 1978; **Fellow:** Biological Psychiatry, Natl Inst Mental Hlth 1982; **Fac Appt:** Prof Psyc, Mount Sinai Sch Med

Silver, Jonathan M MD (Psyc) - **Spec Exp:** Neuro-Psychiatry; Psychopharmacology; Brain Injury; **Address:** 40 E 83rd St, Ste 1E, New York, NY 10028; **Phone:** 212-874-6453; **Board Cert:** Psychiatry 1984; Behavioral Neurology & Neuropsychiatry 2006; **Med School:** Albert Einstein Coll Med 1979; **Resid:** Psychiatry, NY State Psych Inst 1983; **Fellow:** Research, NY State Psych Inst 1985; **Fac Appt:** Clin Prof Psyc, NYU Sch Med

Snyder, Stephen L MD (Psyc) - **Spec Exp:** Sexual Dysfunction; Relationship Problems; Couples Therapy; **Hospital:** Mt Sinai Med Ctr (page 102); **Address:** 115 Central Park W, Ste 15, New York, NY 10023; **Phone:** 212-875-9800; **Board Cert:** Psychiatry 1989; **Med School:** UCSF 1983; **Resid:** Psychiatry, Payne Whitney Psych Clin 1987; **Fellow:** Behavioral Medicine, Mt Sinai Med Ctr 1989; **Fac Appt:** Assoc Clin Prof Psyc, Mount Sinai Sch Med

Spitz, Henry MD (Psyc) - **Spec Exp:** Family & Couples Therapy; Addiction/Substance Abuse; Anxiety & Depression; **Hospital:** NY-Presby/Columbia Univ Med Ctr, NY (page 104); **Address:** 101 Central Park W, Ste 1C, New York, NY 10023; **Phone:** 212-873-1415; **Board Cert:** Psychiatry 1973; **Med School:** NY Med Coll 1965; **Resid:** Psychiatry, NY Med Coll Hosp 1969; **Fellow:** Psychiatry, NY Med Coll Hosp 1971; **Fac Appt:** Clin Prof Psyc, Columbia P&S

Stein, Stefan MD (Psyc) - **Spec Exp:** Couples Therapy; Psychotherapy & Psychopharmacology; **Hospital:** NY-Presby/Weill Cornell Med Ctr, NY (page 104); **Address:** 850 Park Ave, Ste 1E, New York, NY 10075; **Phone:** 212-249-0200; **Board Cert:** Psychiatry 1970; **Med School:** NYU Sch Med 1963; **Resid:** Internal Medicine, Boston City Hosp 1964; Psychiatry, Albert Einstein Coll Med 1968; **Fellow:** Psychiatry, Mass Genl Hosp 1965; Psychoanalysis, NY Psychoan Inst 1974; **Fac Appt:** Prof Psyc, Cornell Univ-Weill Med Coll

Stone, Michael H MD (Psyc) - **Spec Exp:** Personality Disorders; Psychoanalysis; Forensic Psychiatry; Addiction/Substance Abuse; **Address:** 225 Central Park West, Ste 114, New York, NY 10024-6027; **Phone:** 212-758-2000; **Board Cert:** Psychiatry 1971; **Med School:** Cornell Univ-Weill Med Coll 1958; **Resid:** Internal Medicine, Bellevue Hosp 1961; Psychiatry, NY State Psychiatric Inst 1966; **Fellow:** Hematology, Meml Sloan-Kettering Cancer Ctr 1962; Medical Oncology, Meml Sloan-Kettering Cancer Ctr 1963; **Fac Appt:** Prof Emeritus Psyc, Columbia P&S

Strain, James J MD (Psyc) - **Spec Exp:** Psychiatry in Physical Illness; Psychoanalysis; **Hospital:** Mt Sinai Med Ctr (page 102); **Address:** 1425 Madison Ave, Ste 6-24, New York, NY 10029; **Phone:** 212-659-8728; **Board Cert:** Psychiatry ; **Med School:** Case West Res Univ 1962; **Resid:** Psychiatry, Univ Hosps 1966; **Fellow:** Psychiatric Research, Univ Hosps 1967; Psychoanalysis, NY Psychoanalytic Inst 1972; **Fac Appt:** Prof Psyc, Mount Sinai Sch Med

Sussman, Norman MD (Psyc) - **Spec Exp:** Psychopharmacology; Anxiety & Mood Disorders; Bipolar/Mood Disorders; **Hospital:** NYU Langone Med Ctr (page 108); **Address:** 150 E 58th St,, Fl 27, New York, NY 10155; **Phone:** 212-588-9722; **Board Cert:** Psychiatry 1980; **Med School:** NY Med Coll 1975; **Resid:** Psychiatry, Metropolitan Hosp Ctr 1977; Psychiatry, Westchester Med Ctr 1978; **Fac Appt:** Prof Psyc, NYU Sch Med

Swiller, Hillel MD (Psyc) - **Spec Exp:** Psychotherapy; Couples Therapy; **Hospital:** Mt Sinai Med Ctr (page 102); **Address:** 108 E 96th St, Ste 9F, New York, NY 10128; **Phone:** 212-534-5588; **Board Cert:** Psychiatry 1972; **Med School:** Cornell Univ-Weill Med Coll 1965; **Resid:** Psychiatry, Jacobi Med Ctr 1969; **Fac Appt:** Clin Prof Psyc, Mount Sinai Sch Med

Tancredi, Laurence R MD (Psyc) - **Spec Exp:** Forensic Psychiatry; Anxiety & Depression; **Hospital:** Lenox Hill Hosp (page 106); **Address:** 129-B E 71st St, New York, NY 10021-4201; **Phone:** 212-288-5197; **Board Cert:** Psychiatry 1979; **Med School:** Univ Pennsylvania 1966; **Resid:** Psychiatry, NY State Psychiatric Inst 1975; Psychiatry, Yale-New Haven Hosp 1977; **Fac Appt:** Clin Prof Psyc, NYU Sch Med

Taylor, Noel MD (Psyc) - **Spec Exp:** Anxiety Disorders; Mood Disorders; **Address:** 150 E 58 St, Fl 27, New York, NY 10155; **Phone:** 212-888-9038; **Board Cert:** Psychiatry 1985; **Med School:** Johns Hopkins Univ 1980; **Resid:** Psychiatry, Johns Hopkins Hosp 1984; **Fellow:** Psychiatry, Beth Israel Med Ctr 1986; **Fac Appt:** Asst Prof Psyc, Albert Einstein Coll Med

Teusink, J. Paul MD (Psyc) - **Spec Exp:** Geriatric Psychiatry; Depression; Dementia; **Hospital:** Beth Israel Med Ctr - Petrie Div (page 94); **Address:** 88 University Pl, Ste 705, New York, NY 10003; **Phone:** 347-466-2521; **Board Cert:** Psychiatry 1976; **Med School:** Univ Mich Med Sch 1969; **Resid:** Psychiatry, Topeka State Hosp 1971; Psychiatry, CF Menninger Meml Hosp 1973; **Fac Appt:** Asst Clin Prof Psyc, Albert Einstein Coll Med

Tolchin, Joan MD (Psyc) - **Spec Exp:** Child & Adolescent Psychiatry; Psychotherapy; Anxiety & Depression; **Hospital:** NY-Presby/Weill Cornell Med Ctr, NY (page 104); **Address:** 35 E 84th St, New York, NY 10028-0871; **Phone:** 212-744-1446; **Board Cert:** Psychiatry 1979; Child & Adolescent Psychiatry 1982; **Med School:** NYU Sch Med 1972; **Resid:** Psychiatry, Bronx Muni Hosp 1975; **Fellow:** Child & Adolescent Psychiatry, NY Hosp/Cornell 1977; **Fac Appt:** Assoc Clin Prof Psyc, Cornell Univ-Weill Med Coll

Wachtel, Alan B MD (Psyc) - **Spec Exp:** ADD/ADHD; Mood Disorders; Learning Disorders; **Hospital:** NYU Langone Med Ctr (page 108); **Address:** 201 E 87th St, Ste 16J, New York, NY 10128; **Phone:** 212-348-0175; **Board Cert:** Psychiatry 1977; **Med School:** Mount Sinai Sch Med 1972; **Resid:** Psychiatry, Mt Sinai Hosp 1976; **Fellow:** Liaison Psychiatry, NY Hosp-Cornell Med Ctr 1977; **Fac Appt:** Assoc Clin Prof Psyc, NYU Sch Med

Wager, Steven G MD (Psyc) - **Spec Exp:** Psychopharmacology; Depression; Anxiety Disorders; **Address:** 145 W 86th St, Ste 1B, New York, NY 10024-3421; **Phone:** 212-769-9620; **Board Cert:** Psychiatry 1986; **Med School:** Case West Res Univ 1980; **Resid:** Psychiatry, NY-Presby/Columbia Univ Med Ctr 1984; **Fellow:** Psychopharmacology, NY-Presby/Columbia Univ Med Ctr 1986

Wallack, Joel J MD (Psyc) - **Spec Exp:** Psychopharmacology; Psychiatry in Physical Illness; Anxiety & Depression; **Hospital:** Beth Israel Med Ctr - Petrie Div (page 94), Mt Sinai Med Ctr (page 102); **Address:** Beth Israel Med Ctr, 10 Union Square E, New York, NY 10003; **Phone:** 212-420-2398; **Board Cert:** Psychiatry 1979; Psychosomatic Medicine 2005; **Med School:** UMDNJ-NJ Med Sch, Newark 1974; **Resid:** Psychiatry, St Lukes Hosp 1978; **Fellow:** Consultation Psychiatry, Montefiore Med Ctr 1979; Psychosomatic Medicine, Mt Sinai Hosp 1980; **Fac Appt:** Prof Psyc, Mount Sinai Sch Med

Walsh, B. Timothy MD (Psyc) - **Spec Exp:** Eating Disorders; Obesity; **Hospital:** NY State Psychiatric Inst, NY-Presby/Columbia Univ Med Ctr, NY (page 104); **Address:** NY State Psychiatric Inst, 1051 Riverside Drive, rm 2306, Box 98, New York, NY 10032; **Phone:** 212-543-5739; **Board Cert:** Psychiatry 1978; **Med School:** Harvard Med Sch 1972; **Resid:** Psychiatry, Bronx Muni Hosp Ctr 1977; **Fac Appt:** Prof Psyc, Columbia P&S

Weill, Terry L MD (Psyc) - **Spec Exp:** Bipolar/Mood Disorders; Psychiatry in Physical Illness; **Hospital:** Mt Sinai Med Ctr (page 102), Beth Israel Med Ctr - Petrie Div (page 94); **Address:** 350 Central Park West, New York, NY 10023-6547; **Phone:** 212-316-5818; **Board Cert:** Psychiatry 1985; **Med School:** Hahnemann Univ 1980; **Resid:** Psychiatry, Mount Sinai Med Ctr 1984; **Fellow:** Psychoanalysis, NYS Psyc Inst 1991; **Fac Appt:** Asst Prof Psyc, Mount Sinai Sch Med

Welsh, Howard K MD (Psyc) - **Spec Exp:** Psychotherapy; Psychoanalysis; **Hospital:** NYU Langone Med Ctr (page 108); **Address:** 27 W 86th St, Ste 1C, New York, NY 10024-3615; **Phone:** 212-362-5846; **Board Cert:** Psychiatry 1976; **Med School:** Albert Einstein Coll Med 1971; **Resid:** Psychiatry, Kings County Hosp 1974; **Fac Appt:** Clin Prof Psyc, NYU Sch Med

Wilner, Philip MD (Psyc) - **Hospital:** NY-Presby/Weill Cornell Med Ctr, NY (page 104); **Address:** 525 E 68th St, Box 140, New York, NY 10065; **Phone:** 212-746-3705; **Board Cert:** Psychiatry 1989; **Med School:** Columbia P&S 1983; **Resid:** Psychiatry, Payne Whitney Clin 1987; **Fellow:** Psychopharmacology, Payne Whitney Clin 1991; **Fac Appt:** Clin Prof Psyc, Cornell Univ-Weill Med Coll

Winters, Richard A MD (Psyc) - **Spec Exp:** Psychopharmacology; Crisis Intervention; Psychodynamic Psychotherapy; **Address:** 201 E 87th St, Ste 12-B, New York, NY 10128; **Phone:** 212-744-1346; **Board Cert:** Psychiatry 1977; **Med School:** NY Med Coll 1972; **Resid:** Psychiatry, Metropolitan Hosp Ctr 1975; **Fac Appt:** Asst Prof Psyc, NY Med Coll

Zimberg, Sheldon MD (Psyc) - **Spec Exp:** Addiction Psychiatry; Hypnosis; Geriatric Psychiatry; **Address:** 245-A E 61st St, New York, NY 10065; **Phone:** 212-988-5139; **Board Cert:** Psychiatry 1969; Addiction Psychiatry 2004; **Med School:** SUNY Hlth Sci Ctr 1961; **Resid:** Psychiatry, NYS Psych Inst 1965; **Fellow:** Community Psychiatry, Columbia Univ Sch Pub Hlth 1966; **Fac Appt:** Clin Prof Psyc, Columbia P&S

Pulmonary Disease

Acquista, Angelo J MD (Pul) - **Spec Exp:** Asthma; Disaster Preparedness; **Hospital:** Lenox Hill Hosp (page 106); **Address:** Madison Medical, 110 E 59th St, Ste 9C, New York, NY 10022; **Phone:** 212-583-2850; **Board Cert:** Internal Medicine 1984; Pulmonary Disease 1986; **Med School:** NYU Sch Med 1981; **Resid:** Internal Medicine, Lenox Hill Hosp 1984; **Fellow:** Pulmonary Disease, Lenox Hill Hosp 1986

Adams, Francis V MD (Pul) - **Spec Exp:** Asthma; Chronic Obstructive Lung Disease (COPD); Pulmonary Fibrosis; Sarcoidosis; **Hospital:** NYU Langone Med Ctr (page 108); **Address:** 650 First Ave, New York, NY 10016-3240; **Phone:** 212-447-0088; **Board Cert:** Internal Medicine 1974; Pulmonary Disease 1976; **Med School:** Cornell Univ-Weill Med Coll 1971; **Resid:** Internal Medicine, Georgetown Univ Hosp 1973; **Fellow:** Pulmonary Disease, Bellevue Hosp 1975; **Fac Appt:** Asst Prof Med, NYU Sch Med

Addrizzo-Harris, Doreen MD (Pul) - **Spec Exp:** Bronchoscopy; Tuberculosis; Lung Cancer; Interstitial Lung Disease; **Hospital:** NYU Langone Med Ctr (page 108), Bellevue Hosp Ctr; **Address:** 530 First Ave, Ste 5E, New York, NY 10016; **Phone:** 212-263-7951; **Board Cert:** Pulmonary Disease 2006; Critical Care Medicine 2007; **Med School:** NYU Sch Med 1989; **Resid:** Internal Medicine, Bellevue Hosp/NYU Med Ctr 1992; **Fellow:** Pulmonary Critical Care Medicine, Bellevue Hosp/NYU Med Ctr 1996; **Fac Appt:** Assoc Prof Med, NYU Sch Med

Adler, Jack MD (Pul) - **Spec Exp:** Asthma; Chronic Obstructive Lung Disease (COPD); Tuberculosis; **Hospital:** Mt Sinai Med Ctr (page 102), Lenox Hill Hosp (page 106); **Address:** 210 E 86th St, New York, NY 10028; **Phone:** 212-535-3622; **Board Cert:** Internal Medicine 1970; Pulmonary Disease 1971; **Med School:** Univ Chicago-Pritzker Sch Med 1962; **Resid:** Internal Medicine, Philadelphia Genl Hosp 1967; Internal Medicine, Michael Reese Hosp Med Ctr 1968; **Fellow:** Pulmonary Disease, Bronx Municipal Hosp Ctr 1971; **Fac Appt:** Assoc Prof Med, Mount Sinai Sch Med

Arcasoy, Selim M MD (Pul) - **Spec Exp:** Transplant Medicine-Lung; Interstitial Lung Disease; Chronic Obstructive Lung Disease (COPD); Pulmonary Embolism; **Hospital:** NY-Presby/Columbia Univ Med Ctr, NY (page 104); **Address:** Ctr for Advanced Lung Dis/Transp, 622 W 168th St, PH Bldg - Fl 14E, rm 104, New York, NY 10032-3720; **Phone:** 212-305-6589; **Board Cert:** Internal Medicine 2003; Pulmonary Disease 2006; Critical Care Medicine 2007; **Med School:** Turkey 1990; **Resid:** Internal Medicine, SUNY Downstate Med Ctr 1994; **Fellow:** Pulmonary Critical Care Medicine, Univ Pittsburgh Med Ctr 1998; **Fac Appt:** Prof Med, Columbia P&S

Baskin, Martin MD (Pul) - **Spec Exp:** Asthma; Pneumonia; Emphysema; **Hospital:** St. Luke's - Roosevelt Hosp Ctr - Roosevelt Div (page 94); **Address:** 185 W End Ave, Ste 1M, New York, NY 10023-5567; **Phone:** 212-595-7701; **Board Cert:** Internal Medicine 1985; Pulmonary Disease 1988; **Med School:** Mount Sinai Sch Med 1981; **Resid:** Internal Medicine, Beth Israel Med Ctr 1984; **Fellow:** Pulmonary Disease, St Luke's Roosevelt Hosp Ctr 1988; Critical Care Medicine, St Luke's Roosevelt Hosp Ctr 1989; **Fac Appt:** Asst Clin Prof Med, Columbia P&S

Basner, Robert C MD (Pul) - **Spec Exp:** Sleep Disorders/Apnea; **Hospital:** NY-Presby/Columbia Univ Med Ctr, NY (page 104); **Address:** 622 W 168th, Ste 859, Columbia University Medical Center, New York, NY 10032; **Phone:** 212-305-7591; **Board Cert:** Internal Medicine 1986; Pulmonary Disease 1988; Sleep Medicine 2009; **Med School:** Columbia P&S 1983; **Resid:** Internal Medicine, Beth Israel Hosp 1986; **Fellow:** Pulmonary Disease, Brigham & Women's Hosp 1989; **Fac Appt:** Assoc Clin Prof Med, Columbia P&S

Bevelaqua, Frederick MD (Pul) - **Spec Exp:** Asthma; Lung Cancer; Chronic Obstructive Lung Disease (COPD); Sarcoidosis; **Hospital:** NYU Langone Med Ctr (page 108); **Address:** 35A E 35th St, Ste 204, New York, NY 10016; **Phone:** 212-213-6796; **Board Cert:** Internal Medicine 1978; Pulmonary Disease 1980; **Med School:** NYU Sch Med 1974; **Resid:** Internal Medicine, NYU Med Ctr 1978; **Fellow:** Pulmonary Disease, NYU Med Ctr 1980; **Fac Appt:** Asst Clin Prof Med, NYU Sch Med

Blair, Lester W MD (Pul) - **Spec Exp:** Asthma; Sarcoidosis; Bronchitis; Chronic Obstructive Lung Disease (COPD); **Hospital:** NY-Presby/Weill Cornell Med Ctr, NY (page 104); **Address:** 156 William St, Fl 7, New York, NY 10038; **Phone:** 646-588-2500; **Board Cert:** Internal Medicine 1987; Pulmonary Disease 1980; Critical Care Medicine 2009; **Med School:** Columbia P&S 1974; **Resid:** Internal Medicine, Columbia-Presby Med Ctr 1977; **Fellow:** Pulmonary Disease, Bellevue Hosp 1979; **Fac Appt:** Assoc Clin Prof Med, Cornell Univ-Weill Med Coll

Burschtin, Omar E MD (Pul) - **Spec Exp:** Sleep Medicine; Sleep Disorders/Apnea; **Hospital:** NYU Langone Med Ctr (page 108); **Address:** Sleep Med Assocs, 11 E 26th St Fl 13, New York, NY 10010; **Phone:** 212-481-1818; **Board Cert:** Pulmonary Disease 2008; Sleep Medicine 2009; **Med School:** Uruguay 1988; **Resid:** Internal Medicine, NYU Med Ctr 1994; **Fellow:** Pulmonary Critical Care Medicine, NYU Med Ctr 1997; Sleep Medicine, Bellevue Hosp 1998; **Fac Appt:** Asst Clin Prof Med, NYU Sch Med

DePalo, Louis R MD (Pul) - **Spec Exp:** Critical Care; Lung Cancer; **Hospital:** Mt Sinai Med Ctr (page 102); **Address:** 1130 Park Ave, Ste 3, New York, NY 10128; **Phone:** 212-289-3627; **Board Cert:** Internal Medicine 1985; Pulmonary Disease 1988; Critical Care Medicine 2009; **Med School:** NY Med Coll 1982; **Resid:** Internal Medicine, Mt Sinai Med Ctr 1985; **Fellow:** Pulmonary Disease, Univ Penn Hosps 1988; **Fac Appt:** Asst Clin Prof Med, Mount Sinai Sch Med

DiFabrizio, Larry MD (Pul) - **Hospital:** Mt Sinai Med Ctr (page 102); **Address:** Mt Sinai, Pulmonary Dept, 5 E 98 St Fl 8, New York, NY 10029; **Phone:** 212-241-5656; **Board Cert:** Internal Medicine 1987; Critical Care Medicine 2012; Pulmonary Disease 2012; Sleep Medicine 2009; **Med School:** Washington Univ, St Louis 1984; **Resid:** Internal Medicine, Brigham & Womens Hosp 1987; **Fellow:** Pulmonary Critical Care Medicine, Brigham & Womens Hosp 1988; Rheumatology, NY-Presby/Columbia Univ Med Ctr 1990

DiMango, Angela MD (Pul) - **Spec Exp:** Chronic Obstructive Lung Disease (COPD); Asthma; **Hospital:** NY-Presby/Columbia Univ Med Ctr, NY (page 104); **Address:** 161 Ft Washington Ave, Ste 338, New York, NY 10032; **Phone:** 212-305-5730; **Board Cert:** Internal Medicine 2003; Pulmonary Disease 2006; **Med School:** SUNY Downstate 1989; **Resid:** Internal Medicine, NY Presby-Columbia Med Ctr 1992; **Fellow:** Pulmonary Disease, NY Presby-Columbia Med Ctr 1995; Critical Care Medicine, NY Presby-Columbia Med Ctr 1996; **Fac Appt:** Assoc Clin Prof Med, Columbia P&S

Dimango, Emily MD (Pul) - **Spec Exp:** Cystic Fibrosis; Asthma; Chronic Obstructive Lung Disease (COPD); Bronchiectasis; **Hospital:** NY-Presby/Columbia Univ Med Ctr, NY (page 104); **Address:** NY-Presbyterian, Pulmonary Dept, 622 W 168 St, rm 859, New York, NY 10032; **Phone:** 212-305-0631; **Board Cert:** Internal Medicine 2006; Pulmonary Disease 2005; **Med School:** NYU Sch Med 1989; **Resid:** Internal Medicine, NY-Presby/Columbia Univ Med Ctr 1992; **Fellow:** Pulmonary Disease, NY-Presby/Columbia Univ Med Ctr 1995; **Fac Appt:** Assoc Prof Med, Columbia P&S

Eden, Edward MD (Pul) - **Spec Exp:** Emphysema; Asthma; Sarcoidosis; Emphysema/Alpha-1 Antitrypsin Deficiency; **Hospital:** St. Luke's - Roosevelt Hosp Ctr - Roosevelt Div (page 94); **Address:** 425 W 59th St, Ste 8A, New York, NY 10019-1104; **Phone:** 212-492-5500; **Board Cert:** Internal Medicine 1980; Pulmonary Disease 1982; Critical Care Medicine 2007; **Med School:** England, UK 1975; **Resid:** Internal Medicine, Wayne State Univ Affil Hosp 1978; Internal Medicine, Univ Hosp 1980; **Fellow:** Pulmonary Disease, Mount Sinai Hosp 1982; Pulmonary Disease, Columbia-Presby Med Ctr 1985; **Fac Appt:** Assoc Prof Med, Columbia P&S

Fishman, Donald MD (Pul) - **Spec Exp:** Asthma; Chronic Obstructive Lung Disease (COPD); Bronchoscopy; Interstitial Lung Disease; **Hospital:** St. Luke's - Roosevelt Hosp Ctr - Roosevelt Div (page 94), Lenox Hill Hosp (page 106); **Address:** 200 W 57th St, Ste 1201, New York, NY 10019; **Phone:** 212-765-5151; **Board Cert:** Internal Medicine 1976; Pulmonary Disease 1978; **Med School:** Univ Pennsylvania 1973; **Resid:** Internal Medicine, Univ Mich Med Ctr 1976; **Fellow:** Pulmonary Disease, NYU Med Ctr 1978; **Fac Appt:** Asst Clin Prof Med, Columbia P&S

Garay, Stuart M MD (Pul) - **Spec Exp:** Asthma; Chronic Obstructive Lung Disease (COPD); Sleep Apnea; **Hospital:** NYU Langone Med Ctr (page 108); **Address:** New York Pulmonary Associates, 463 Third Ave Fl 2, New York, NY 10016-6025; **Phone:** 212-685-6001; **Board Cert:** Internal Medicine 1977; Pulmonary Disease 1980; **Med School:** Harvard Med Sch 1974; **Resid:** Internal Medicine, Mt Sinai Hosp 1977; **Fellow:** Pulmonary Disease, Bellevue Hosp 1979; **Fac Appt:** Clin Prof Med, NYU Sch Med

Gelbman, Brian D MD (Pul) - **Spec Exp:** Asthma; Chronic Obstructive Lung Disease (COPD); Lung Cancer; **Hospital:** NY-Presby/Weill Cornell Med Ctr, NY (page 104), Hosp For Special Surgery (page 113); **Address:** Pulmonary Consultants of NY, 635 Madison Ave, Ste 1101, New York, NY 10022; **Phone:** 212-628-6611; **Board Cert:** Internal Medicine 2003; Pulmonary Disease 2005; Critical Care Medicine 2006; **Med School:** Vanderbilt Univ 2000; **Resid:** Internal Medicine, NY-Presby/Weill Cornell Univ Med Ctr 2003; **Fellow:** Pulmonary Critical Care Medicine, NY-Presby/Weill Cornell Univ Med Ctr 2006; **Fac Appt:** Assoc Clin Prof Med, Cornell Univ-Weill Med Coll

Kaplan, Rana MD (Pul) - **Spec Exp:** Asthma; Cystic Fibrosis; **Hospital:** Meml Sloan-Kettering Canc Ctr (page 114), NY-Presby/Weill Cornell Med Ctr, NY (page 104); **Address:** 1275 York Ave, Ste A3, New York, NY 10065; **Phone:** 212-639-8025; **Board Cert:** Critical Care Medicine 2004; **Med School:** Cornell Univ-Weill Med Coll 1996; **Resid:** Internal Medicine, New Eng Med Ctr 1999; **Fellow:** Pulmonary Critical Care Medicine, NY Presby Hosp 2003

Klapholz, Ari MD (Pul) - **Spec Exp:** Lung Cancer; Sleep Disorders/Apnea; Emphysema; Asthma; **Hospital:** Beth Israel Med Ctr - Petrie Div (page 94); **Address:** 275 7th Ave Fl 3, New York, NY 10001; **Phone:** 646-660-9999; **Board Cert:** Internal Medicine 1987; Pulmonary Disease 2010; Critical Care Medicine 2011; Sleep Medicine 2007; **Med School:** NY Med Coll 1984; **Resid:** Internal Medicine, Beth Israel Med Ctr 1987; **Fellow:** Pulmonary Disease, Beth Israel Med Ctr 1989; Critical Care Medicine, Mount Sinai Med Ctr 1990; **Fac Appt:** Asst Prof Med, Mount Sinai Sch Med

Kolodny, Erwin MD (Pul) - **Spec Exp:** Asthma; Emphysema; Bronchitis; **Hospital:** NYU Langone Med Ctr (page 108); **Address:** 650 1st Ave, New York, NY 10016-3240; **Phone:** 212-213-0090; **Board Cert:** Internal Medicine 1977; Pulmonary Disease 1978; **Med School:** NYU Sch Med 1973; **Resid:** Internal Medicine, Bellevue Hosp 1976; **Fellow:** Pulmonary Disease, NYU Med Ctr 1978; **Fac Appt:** Asst Clin Prof Med, NYU Sch Med

Krieger, Ana C MD (Pul) - **Spec Exp:** Sleep Disorders/Apnea; Narcolepsy; Pulmonary Hypertension; **Hospital:** NY-Presby/Weill Cornell Med Ctr, NY (page 104); **Address:** Weill Cornell Center for Sleep Medicine, 425 E 61st St, Fl 5, New York, NY 10065; **Phone:** 646-962-7378; **Board Cert:** Internal Medicine 2011; Pulmonary Disease 2011; Sleep Medicine 2000; **Med School:** Brazil 1992; **Resid:** Internal Medicine, Univ Chicago Hosps 1996; **Fellow:** Critical Care Medicine, Finch/Chicago Med Sch 1998; Pulmonary Disease, NYU 2000; **Fac Appt:** Assoc Prof Med, Cornell Univ-Weill Med Coll

Lederer, David MD (Pul) - **Spec Exp:** Transplant-Lung; Pulmonary Fibrosis; Interstitial Lung Disease; **Hospital:** NY-Presby/Columbia Univ Med Ctr, NY (page 104); **Address:** 622 W 168th St, rm 104, PH-14, New York, NY 10032; **Phone:** 212-305-7771; **Board Cert:** Pulmonary Disease 2005; Internal Medicine 2012; Critical Care Medicine 2006; **Med School:** SUNY Downstate 1999; **Resid:** Internal Medicine, NY Presby/Columbia Med Ctr 2003; **Fellow:** Pulmonary Critical Care Medicine, NY Presby/Columbia Med Ctr 2006; **Fac Appt:** Asst Prof Med, Columbia P&S

Lee, Marjorie MD (Pul) - **Spec Exp:** Emphysema & Asthma; Sarcoidosis; **Hospital:** Beth Israel Med Ctr - Petrie Div (page 94); **Address:** 247 3rd Ave, Ste 403, New York, NY 10010-7455; **Phone:** 212-533-1185; **Board Cert:** Internal Medicine 1976; Pulmonary Disease 1978; **Med School:** SUNY Hlth Sci Ctr 1973; **Resid:** Internal Medicine, Kaiser Hosp 1976; Pulmonary Disease, Cabrini Hosp 1977; **Fellow:** Pulmonary Disease, Yale-New Haven Hosp 1979

Libby, Daniel M MD (Pul) - **Spec Exp:** Asthma; Lung Cancer; Interstitial Lung Disease; Chronic Obstructive Lung Disease (COPD); **Hospital:** NY-Presby/Weill Cornell Med Ctr, NY (page 104); **Address:** 635 Madison Ave, Ste 1101, New York, NY 10022; **Phone:** 212-628-6611; **Board Cert:** Internal Medicine 1977; Pulmonary Disease 1980; **Med School:** Baylor Coll Med 1974; **Resid:** Internal Medicine, NY Hosp 1977; **Fellow:** Pulmonary Disease, NY Hosp 1979; **Fac Appt:** Clin Prof Med, Cornell Univ-Weill Med Coll

Lowy, Joseph MD (Pul) - **Spec Exp:** Lung Cancer; Palliative Care; Chronic Obstructive Lung Disease (COPD); Pulmonary Fibrosis; **Hospital:** NYU Langone Med Ctr (page 108); **Address:** 530 First Ave, HCC-Suite 5D, New York, NY 10016; **Phone:** 212-263-6202; **Board Cert:** Internal Medicine 1983; Pulmonary Disease 1986; Hospice & Palliative Medicine 2008; **Med School:** Univ Rochester 1980; **Resid:** Internal Medicine, Bellevue Hosp 1983; **Fellow:** Pulmonary Disease, UCSD Med Ctr 1986; **Fac Appt:** Assoc Clin Prof Med, NYU Sch Med

Maxfield, Roger A MD (Pul) - **Spec Exp:** Emphysema & Asthma; Occupational Lung Disease; Lung Cancer; Bronchoscopy; **Hospital:** NY-Presby/Columbia Univ Med Ctr, NY (page 104); **Address:** 51 W 51st St, Ste 360, New York, NY 10019; **Phone:** 212-326-8415; **Board Cert:** Internal Medicine 1980; Pulmonary Disease 1986; **Med School:** Brown Univ 1977; **Resid:** Internal Medicine, Georgetown Univ Hosp 1980; **Fellow:** Pulmonary Disease, Bellevue Hosp 1985; **Fac Appt:** Clin Prof Med, Columbia P&S

Miller, Rachel L MD (Pul) - **Spec Exp:** Asthma; **Hospital:** NY-Presby/Columbia Univ Med Ctr, NY (page 104); **Address:** 622 W 168th St - PH8, New York, NY 10032; **Phone:** 212-305-0631; **Board Cert:** Internal Medicine 2003; Pulmonary Disease 2006; Critical Care Medicine 2007; Allergy & Immunology 2009; **Med School:** NYU Sch Med 1990; **Resid:** Internal Medicine, NY Presby/Columbia Med Ctr 1993; **Fellow:** Pulmonary Critical Care Medicine, NY Presby/Columbia Med Ctr 1995

Nash, Thomas MD (Pul) - **Spec Exp:** Asthma; Cough; Pneumonia; **Hospital:** NY-Presby/Weill Cornell Med Ctr, NY (page 104), Hosp For Special Surgery (page 113); **Address:** 310 E 72nd St, New York, NY 10021; **Phone:** 212-734-6612; **Board Cert:** Internal Medicine 1981; Infectious Disease 1984; Pulmonary Disease 1988; **Med School:** NYU Sch Med 1978; **Resid:** Internal Medicine, NY-Presby/Weill Cornell Med Ctr 1981; **Fellow:** Infectious Disease, NY-Presby/Weill Cornell Med Ctr 1983; Pulmonary Disease, Meml Sloan-Kettering Cancer Ctr 1985; **Fac Appt:** Assoc Clin Prof Med, NYU Sch Med

Nelson, Judith E MD (Pul) - **Spec Exp:** Palliative Care; **Hospital:** Mt Sinai Med Ctr (page 102); **Address:** Mt Sinai Medical Ctr, One Gustave Levy Pl, Box 1232, New York, NY 10029; **Phone:** 212-241-2587; **Board Cert:** Internal Medicine 1989; Pulmonary Disease 2012; Critical Care Medicine 2003; Hospice & Palliative Medicine 2012; **Med School:** NYU Sch Med 1986; **Resid:** Internal Medicine, Mt Sinai Med Ctr 1989; **Fellow:** Pulmonary Critical Care Medicine, Mt Sinai Med Ctr 1992; **Fac Appt:** Prof Med, Mount Sinai Sch Med

Padilla, Maria L MD (Pul) - **Spec Exp:** Transplant Medicine-Lung; Sarcoidosis; Pulmonary Hypertension; Cystic Fibrosis; **Hospital:** Mt Sinai Med Ctr (page 102); **Address:** Mount Sinai Med Ctr, Pulmonary Assocs, 5 E 98th St Fl 8, New York, NY 10029; **Phone:** 212-241-5656; **Board Cert:** Internal Medicine 1978; Pulmonary Disease 1980; **Med School:** Mount Sinai Sch Med 1975; **Resid:** Internal Medicine, Mount Sinai Med Ctr 1978; **Fellow:** Pulmonary Disease, Mount Sinai Med Ctr 1980; Critical Care Medicine, Mount Sinai Med Ctr 1991; **Fac Appt:** Prof Med, Mount Sinai Sch Med

Posner, David H MD (Pul) - **Spec Exp:** Interstitial Lung Disease; Lung Cancer; Sarcoidosis; Pulmonary Fibrosis; **Hospital:** Lenox Hill Hosp (page 106), NY-Presby/Weill Cornell Med Ctr, NY (page 104); **Address:** 178 E 85th St, Fl 3, New York, NY 10028-2119; **Phone:** 212-737-0470; **Board Cert:** Internal Medicine 1984; Pulmonary Disease 1988; **Med School:** NY Med Coll 1981; **Resid:** Internal Medicine, Lenox Hill Hosp 1985; **Fellow:** Pulmonary Disease, LI Jewish Med Ctr 1987; **Fac Appt:** Assoc Clin Prof Med, NYU Sch Med

Powell, Charles A MD (Pul) - **Spec Exp:** Lung Cancer; Bronchoscopy; **Hospital:** Mt Sinai Med Ctr (page 102); **Address:** Mount Sinai, Pulmonary Dept, 5 E 98 St Fl 8, New York, NY 10029; **Phone:** 212-241-5656; **Board Cert:** Internal Medicine 2012; Pulmonary Disease 2006; Critical Care Medicine 2010; **Med School:** Univ Chicago-Pritzker Sch Med 1989; **Resid:** Internal Medicine, NY-Presby/Columbia Univ Med Ctr 1993; **Fellow:** Pulmonary Critical Care Medicine, Bostom Med Ctr 1996; **Fac Appt:** Prof Med, Mount Sinai Sch Med

Prager, Kenneth MD (Pul) - **Spec Exp:** Lung Disease; Asthma; Ethics; **Hospital:** NY-Presby/Columbia Univ Med Ctr, NY (page 104); **Address:** 161 Ft Washington Ave, Ste 310, New York, NY 10032; **Phone:** 212-305-5535; **Board Cert:** Internal Medicine 1973; **Med School:** Harvard Med Sch 1968; **Resid:** Internal Medicine, Columbia-Presby Med Ctr 1972; Internal Medicine, Billings Hosp 1973; **Fac Appt:** Clin Prof Med, Columbia P&S

Raskin, Jonathan MD (Pul) - **Spec Exp:** Asthma; Chronic Obstructive Lung Disease (COPD); Pulmonary Rehabilitation; **Hospital:** Beth Israel Med Ctr - Petrie Div (page 94), Lenox Hill Hosp (page 106); **Address:** 1000 Park Ave, New York, NY 10028-0934; **Phone:** 212-288-4600; **Board Cert:** Internal Medicine 1982; Pulmonary Disease 1984; **Med School:** Mexico 1978; **Resid:** Internal Medicine, Beth Israel Med Ctr 1982; **Fellow:** Pulmonary Disease, Mount Sinai Hosp 1985; **Fac Appt:** Asst Clin Prof Med, Albert Einstein Coll Med

Sanders, Abraham MD (Pul) - **Hospital:** NY-Presby/Weill Cornell Med Ctr, NY (page 104), Hosp For Special Surgery (page 113); **Address:** 425 E 61st St Fl 4, New York, NY 10021; **Phone:** 646-962-2333; **Board Cert:** Internal Medicine 1979; Pulmonary Disease 1982; Critical Care Medicine 2008; **Med School:** SUNY Downstate 1976; **Resid:** Internal Medicine, Univ Hosp/Kings County Hosp 1980; **Fellow:** Pulmonary Disease, Kings County Hosp 1980; Pulmonary Disease, Royal Postgraduate Sch Med 1981; **Fac Appt:** Assoc Prof Med, Cornell Univ-Weill Med Coll

Schluger, Neil MD (Pul) - **Spec Exp:** Tuberculosis; **Hospital:** NY-Presby/Columbia Univ Med Ctr, NY (page 104); **Address:** NY-Presby, Pulmonology Dept, 161 Fort Washington Ave, rm 338, New York, NY 10032; **Phone:** 212-305-1544; **Board Cert:** Internal Medicine 1988; Pulmonary Disease 2003; **Med School:** Univ Pennsylvania 1985; **Resid:** Internal Medicine, St Lukes Hosp 1989; **Fellow:** Pulmonary Critical Care Medicine, NY-Presby/Weill Cornell Med Ctr 1992; **Fac Appt:** Prof Med, Columbia P&S

Schultz, Barbara L MD (Pul) - **Hospital:** Mt Sinai Med Ctr (page 102); **Address:** 1120 Park Ave, New York, NY 10028-0250; **Phone:** 212-517-8680; **Board Cert:** Internal Medicine 1986; Pulmonary Disease 1988; **Med School:** Mount Sinai Sch Med 1983; **Resid:** Internal Medicine, Mount Sinai Med Ctr 1986; **Fellow:** Pulmonary Disease, Mount Sinai Med Ctr 1988; **Fac Appt:** Asst Clin Prof Med, Mount Sinai Sch Med

Steiger, David MD (Pul) - **Spec Exp:** Rheumatologic Diseases of the Lung; Thromboembolic Disorders; Pulmonary Hypertension; Critical Care; **Hospital:** NYU Hosp For Joint Dis (page 108), NYU Langone Med Ctr (page 108); **Address:** 305 2nd Ave, Ste 16, New York, NY 10003; **Phone:** 212-598-6422; **Board Cert:** Internal Medicine 1987; Critical Care Medicine 2005; **Med School:** England, UK 1981; **Resid:** Internal Medicine, St Thomas's Hosp 1984; Internal Medicine, St Lukes Hosp 1989; **Fellow:** Pulmonary Disease, UCSF Med Ctr 1994; **Fac Appt:** Asst Prof Med, NYU Sch Med

Stein, Sidney MD (Pul) - **Spec Exp:** Asthma; Bronchitis; Emphysema; Hiccups-Chronic; **Hospital:** Beth Israel Med Ctr - Petrie Div (page 94); **Address:** 55 E 34th St Fl 6, New York, NY 10016-4337; **Phone:** 212-879-7777; **Board Cert:** Internal Medicine 1982; Pulmonary Disease 1988; **Med School:** SUNY Hlth Sci Ctr 1979; **Resid:** Internal Medicine, Beth Israel Med Ctr 1982; **Fellow:** Pulmonary Disease, Beth Israel Med Ctr 1984; **Fac Appt:** Asst Clin Prof Med, Albert Einstein Coll Med

Stover-Pepe, Diane E MD (Pul) - **Spec Exp:** Interstitial Lung Disease; Pulmonary Infections; Pulmonary Disease/Immunocompromised; Bronchiolitis Oblitorans; **Hospital:** Meml Sloan-Kettering Canc Ctr (page 114); **Address:** 1275 York Ave, New York, NY 10065; **Phone:** 212-639-8380; **Board Cert:** Internal Medicine 1975; Pulmonary Disease 1978; **Med School:** Albert Einstein Coll Med 1970; **Resid:** Internal Medicine, Harlem Hosp Ctr 1972; Internal Medicine, NY Hosp-Cornell Med Ctr 1975; **Fellow:** Pulmonary Disease, Montefiore Med Ctr 1977; **Fac Appt:** Prof Med, Cornell Univ-Weill Med Coll

Sukumaran, Muthiah MD (Pul) - **Spec Exp:** Asthma; Chronic Obstructive Lung Disease (COPD); Lung Cancer; Tuberculosis; **Hospital:** NY-Presby/Lower Manhattan Hosp (page 104), NYU Langone Med Ctr (page 108); **Address:** Trinty Medical Centre, 111 Broadway Fl 2, New York, NY 10006; **Phone:** 212-263-9700; **Board Cert:** Internal Medicine 1976; Pulmonary Disease 1980; **Med School:** India 1973; **Resid:** Internal Medicine, Elmhurst City Hosp 1976; **Fellow:** Pulmonary Disease, Elmhurst City Hosp 1977; **Fac Appt:** Assoc Clin Prof Med, NY Med Coll

Thomashow, Byron MD (Pul) - **Spec Exp:** Emphysema & Asthma; Respiratory Failure; Chronic Obstructive Lung Disease (COPD); Interstitial Lung Disease; **Hospital:** NY-Presby/Columbia Univ Med Ctr, NY (page 104); **Address:** NY-Presby, Pulmonology Dept, 161 Fort Washington Ave, Ste 311, New York, NY 10032; **Phone:** 212-305-5261; **Board Cert:** Internal Medicine 1977; Pulmonary Disease 1980; **Med School:** Columbia P&S 1974; **Resid:** Internal Medicine, St Lukes Hosp 1977; Pulmonary Disease, St Lukes Hosp 1978; **Fellow:** Pulmonary Disease, Harlem Hosp Ctr 1979; **Fac Appt:** Clin Prof Med, Columbia P&S

Villamena, Patricia C MD (Pul) - **Spec Exp:** Lung Cancer; Chronic Obstructive Lung Disease (COPD); Critical Care; **Hospital:** Beth Israel Med Ctr - Petrie Div (page 94); **Address:** Beth Israel Med Ctr, 1st Ave & 16th St, Dazian Bldg, 7th Fl, Pulm Div, New York, NY 10003; **Phone:** 212-420-2377; **Board Cert:** Internal Medicine 1989; Pulmonary Disease 2006; **Med School:** NY Med Coll 1977; **Resid:** Internal Medicine, Metropolitan Hosp 1980; **Fellow:** Pulmonary Disease, Beth Israel Med Ctr 1986; **Fac Appt:** Asst Prof Med, Albert Einstein Coll Med

Yip, Chun MD (Pul) - **Spec Exp:** Asthma; Emphysema; Chronic Obstructive Lung Disease (COPD); **Hospital:** NY-Presby/Columbia Univ Med Ctr, NY (page 104); **Address:** 67 Hudson St, Ste 1A, New York, NY 10013; **Phone:** 212-305-8548; **Board Cert:** Internal Medicine 1979; Pulmonary Disease 1984; **Med School:** Albert Einstein Coll Med 1976; **Resid:** Internal Medicine, Columbia-Presby Med Ctr 1979; **Fellow:** Pulmonary Disease, Bellevue Hosp Ctr 1981; **Fac Appt:** Clin Prof Med, Columbia P&S

Radiation Oncology

Chadha, Manjeet MD (RadRO) - **Spec Exp:** Breast Cancer; Gynecologic Cancer; **Hospital:** Beth Israel Med Ctr - Petrie Div (page 94), St. Luke's - Roosevelt Hosp Ctr - St Luke's Hosp (page 94); **Address:** Charles & Bernice Blitman Dept, Div of Radiation Oncology, 10 Union Square E, Ste 4G, New York, NY 10003; **Phone:** 212-844-8022; **Board Cert:** Therapeutic Radiology 1985; **Med School:** India 1980; **Resid:** Radiation Oncology, Columbia Presby Med Ctr 1983; Radiation Oncology, Meml Sloan Kettering Cancer Ctr 1985; **Fac Appt:** Assoc Prof RadRO, Albert Einstein Coll Med

Chao, K.S. Clifford MD (RadRO) - **Spec Exp:** Intensity Modulated Radiotherapy (IMRT); **Hospital:** NY-Presby/Weill Cornell Med Ctr, NY (page 104); **Address:** 622 W 168th St, New York, NY 10032; **Phone:** 212-305-9987; **Board Cert:** Radiation Oncology 2010; **Med School:** Taiwan 1982; **Resid:** Radiation Oncology, Mallinckrodt Inst Rad-Wash Med Ctr 1993; **Fellow:** Radiation Oncology, Mallinckrodt Inst Rad-Wash Med Ctr 1994; **Fac Appt:** Prof RadRO, Cornell Univ-Weill Med Coll

Ennis, Ronald D MD (RadRO) - **Spec Exp:** Prostate Cancer; Brachytherapy; Breast Cancer; Stereotactic Radiosurgery; **Hospital:** St. Luke's - Roosevelt Hosp Ctr - Roosevelt Div (page 94), Beth Israel Med Ctr - Petrie Div (page 94); **Address:** 1000 10th Ave, Lower Level, Dept Radiation Oncology, Roosevelt Hospital, New York, NY 10019; **Phone:** 212-523-7165; **Board Cert:** Radiation Oncology 2004; **Med School:** Yale Univ 1990; **Resid:** Therapeutic Radiology, Yale-New Haven Hosp 1994; **Fac Appt:** Assoc Prof RadRO, Albert Einstein Coll Med

Evans, Andrew MD (RadRO) - **Spec Exp:** Breast Cancer; Lung Cancer; Thoracic Cancers; **Hospital:** St. Luke's - Roosevelt Hosp Ctr - Roosevelt Div (page 94); **Address:** Roosevelt Hosp, Rad Onc Dept, 1000 10th Ave, New York, NY 10019; **Phone:** 212-523-7170; **Board Cert:** Radiation Oncology 2011; **Med School:** South Africa 1988; **Resid:** Radiation Oncology, Montefiore Med Ctr 1993; **Fellow:** Radiation Oncology, Cross Cancer Inst 1994; Radiation Oncology, Montefiore Med Ctr 1996; **Fac Appt:** Asst Clin Prof RadRO, Albert Einstein Coll Med

Formenti, Silvia C MD (RadRO) - **Spec Exp:** Breast Cancer; Chemo-Radiation Combined Therapy; **Hospital:** NYU Langone Med Ctr (page 108); **Address:** NYU Med Ctr, Dept Radiation Oncology, 160 E 34th St, New York, NY 10016; **Phone:** 212-263-2601; **Board Cert:** Radiation Oncology 1991; **Med School:** Italy 1980; **Resid:** Internal Medicine, San Carlo Borromeo Hosp 1983; Medical Oncology, Univ of Pavia Med Ctr 1985; **Fellow:** Radiation Oncology, USC Med Ctr 1990; **Fac Appt:** Prof RadRO, NYU Sch Med

Goodman, Karyn MD (RadRO) - **Spec Exp:** Gastrointestinal Cancer; Stereotactic Radiosurgery; Chemo-Radiation Combined Therapy; Brachytherapy; **Hospital:** Meml Sloan-Kettering Canc Ctr (page 114); **Address:** MSKCC, Radiation Oncology, 1275 York Ave, Box 22, New York, NY 10065; **Phone:** 212-639-3983; **Board Cert:** Radiation Oncology 2005; **Med School:** Stanford Univ 1999; **Resid:** Radiation Oncology, Meml Sloan-Kettering Cancer Ctr 2004

Harrison, Louis B MD (RadRO) - **Spec Exp:** Brachytherapy; Head & Neck Cancer; Radiation Therapy-Intraoperative; **Hospital:** Beth Israel Med Ctr - Petrie Div (page 94); **Address:** Beth Israel Med Ctr, Dept Rad Onc, 10 Union Square East, Ste 4G, New York, NY 10003-3314; **Phone:** 212-844-8087; **Board Cert:** Therapeutic Radiology 1986; **Med School:** SUNY Downstate 1982; **Resid:** Therapeutic Radiology, Yale-New Haven Hosp 1986; **Fac Appt:** Prof RadRO, Albert Einstein Coll Med

Hu, Kenneth MD (RadRO) - **Spec Exp:** Head & Neck Cancer; Gastrointestinal Cancer; Brachytherapy; **Hospital:** Beth Israel Med Ctr - Petrie Div (page 94); **Address:** BIMC, Radiation Onc Dept, 10 Union Square E, Ste 4F, New York, NY 10003; **Phone:** 212-844-6550; **Board Cert:** Radiation Oncology 1999; **Med School:** Harvard Med Sch 1994; **Resid:** Radiation Oncology, Meml Sloan-Kettering Cancer Ctr 1998; **Fellow:** Brachytherapy, Meml Sloan-Kettering Cancer Ctr 1999; **Fac Appt:** Assoc Prof RadRO, Albert Einstein Coll Med

Isaacson, Steven R MD (RadRO) - **Spec Exp:** Brain Tumors; Neuro-Oncology; Stereotactic Radiosurgery; Gliomas; **Hospital:** NY-Presby/Columbia Univ Med Ctr, NY (page 104); **Address:** NY Presbyterian-Columbia Med Ctr, Dept Radiation Oncology, 622 W 168th St BHN Bldg - rm B-11, New York, NY 10032-3720; **Phone:** 212-305-2611; **Board Cert:** Radiation Oncology 1988; Otolaryngology 1978; **Med School:** Jefferson Med Coll 1973; **Resid:** Otolaryngology, Hosp Univ Penn 1978; Radiation Oncology, SUNY Hlth Sci Ctr 1988; **Fac Appt:** Clin Prof RadRO, Columbia P&S

Lee, Nancy MD (RadRO) - **Spec Exp:** Intensity Modulated Radiotherapy (IMRT); Head & Neck Cancer; Thyroid Cancer; Nasopharyngeal Cancer; **Hospital:** Meml Sloan Kettering Canc Ctr (page 114); **Address:** MSKCC, Dept Radiation Oncology, 1275 York Ave, New York, NY 10065; **Phone:** 212-639-3341; **Board Cert:** Radiation Oncology 2010; **Med School:** UMDNJ-NJ Med Sch, Newark 1995; **Resid:** Radiation Oncology, Columbia Presby Med Ctr 2000

McCormick, Beryl MD (RadRO) - **Spec Exp:** Breast Cancer; Eye Tumors/Cancer; **Hospital:** Meml Sloan-Kettering Canc Ctr (page 114); **Address:** 1275 York Avenue, New York, NY 10065; **Phone:** 212-639-6828; **Board Cert:** Therapeutic Radiology 1977; **Med School:** UMDNJ-NJ Med Sch, Newark 1973; **Resid:** Therapeutic Radiology, Meml Sloan Kettering Cancer Ctr 1977; **Fac Appt:** Prof RadRO, Cornell Univ-Weill Med Coll

Ng, John Paul Tracy MD (RadRO) - **Spec Exp:** Prostate Cancer; Head & Neck Cancer; **Address:** Tribeca Radiation, 408 Broadway, New York, NY 10013; **Phone:** 212-925-8882; **Board Cert:** Radiation Oncology 1993; **Med School:** Albert Einstein Coll Med 1988; **Resid:** Radiation Oncology, Meml Sloan Kettering Cancer Ctr 1992

Nori, Dattatreyudu MD (RadRO) - **Spec Exp:** Prostate Cancer; Brachytherapy; Lung Cancer; Breast Cancer; **Hospital:** NY-Presby/Weill Cornell Med Ctr, NY (page 104), NY Hosp Queens (page 488); **Address:** 525 E 68th St, Box 575, New York, NY 10065; **Phone:** 212-746-3679; **Board Cert:** Therapeutic Radiology 1979; **Med School:** India 1970; **Resid:** Radiation Oncology, Meml Sloan Kettering Cancer Ctr 1975; **Fellow:** Radiation Oncology, Meml Sloan Kettering Cancer Ctr 1978; **Fac Appt:** Prof RadRO, Cornell Univ-Weill Med Coll

Parashar, Bhupesh MD (RadRO) - **Spec Exp:** Head & Neck Cancer; Lung Cancer; Breast Cancer; Gastrointestinal Cancer; **Hospital:** NY-Presby/Weill Cornell Med Ctr, NY (page 104); **Address:** NY Presbyterian-Cornell Med Ctr, 525 E 68th St, rm N-046, New York, NY 10065; **Phone:** 212-746-3612; **Board Cert:** Radiation Oncology 2006; **Med School:** India 1995; **Resid:** Radiation Oncology, Montefiore Med Ctr 2005; **Fac Appt:** Assoc Clin Prof RadRO, Cornell Univ-Weill Med Coll

Rosenbaum, Alfred MD (RadRO) - **Spec Exp:** Breast Cancer; Prostate Cancer; Intensity Modulated Radiotherapy (IMRT); **Hospital:** Mt Sinai Med Ctr (page 102), Lenox Hill Hosp (page 106); **Address:** Rosetta Radiology, 1421 Third Ave, New York, NY 10028; **Phone:** 212-744-5538; **Board Cert:** Diagnostic Radiology 1973; **Med School:** Germany 1966; **Resid:** Diagnostic Radiology, Maimonides Med Ctr 1970; Radiation Oncology, Mount Sinai Hosp 1972; **Fellow:** Diagnostic Radiology, Montefiore Med Ctr 1973; **Fac Appt:** Asst Clin Prof Rad, Mount Sinai Sch Med

Schiff, Peter B MD/PhD (RadRO) - **Spec Exp:** Prostate Cancer; Gynecologic Cancer; Lung Cancer; **Hospital:** NYU Langone Med Ctr (page 108); **Address:** NYU Clinical Cancer Ctr, 160 E 34th St Fl 1, New York, NY 10016; **Phone:** 212-731-5003; **Board Cert:** Radiation Oncology 1990; **Med School:** Albert Einstein Coll Med 1984; **Resid:** Radiation Oncology, Meml Sloan Kettering Cancer Ctr 1988; **Fac Appt:** Prof RadRO, NYU Sch Med

Sherr, David L MD (RadRO) - **Spec Exp:** Intensity Modulated Radiotherapy (IMRT); Stereotactic Radiosurgery; Image Guided Radiotherapy (IGRT); **Address:** Rosetta Radiology, 1421 Third Ave, New York, NY 10028; **Phone:** 212-744-5538; **Board Cert:** Radiation Oncology 1987; **Med School:** Albert Einstein Coll Med 1981; **Resid:** Internal Medicine, Brookdale Hosp Med Ctr 1983; Radiation Oncology, Columbia-Presby Med Ctr 1986

Stock, Richard MD (RadRO) - **Spec Exp:** Prostate Cancer; Urologic Cancer; **Hospital:** Mt Sinai Med Ctr (page 102); **Address:** 61 E 77th St, level C, New York, NY 10075; **Phone:** 212-772-2130; **Board Cert:** Radiation Oncology 1993; **Med School:** Mount Sinai Sch Med 1988; **Resid:** Radiation Oncology, Meml Sloan Kettering Cancer Ctr 1992; **Fac Appt:** Prof RadRO, Mount Sinai Sch Med

Yahalom, Joachim MD (RadRO) - **Spec Exp:** Lymphoma; Hodgkin's Lymphoma; Multiple Myeloma; **Hospital:** Meml Sloan-Kettering Canc Ctr (page 114); **Address:** 1275 York Ave, SM03, Dept Radiation Onc, New York, NY 10065; **Phone:** 212-639-5999; **Board Cert:** Radiation Oncology 1988; **Med School:** Israel 1976; **Resid:** Internal Medicine, Hadassah Hosp 1979; Radiation Oncology, Hadassah Hosp 1984; **Fellow:** Radiation Oncology, Meml Sloan Kettering Canc Ctr 1986; **Fac Appt:** Prof RadRO, Cornell Univ-Weill Med Coll

Zelefsky, Michael J MD (RadRO) - **Spec Exp:** Prostate Cancer; Brachytherapy; Head & Neck Cancer; **Hospital:** Meml Sloan-Kettering Canc Ctr (page 114); **Address:** 1275 York Ave, New York, NY 10065; **Phone:** 212-639-6802; **Board Cert:** Radiation Oncology 1991; **Med School:** Albert Einstein Coll Med 1986; **Resid:** Radiation Oncology, Meml Sloan Kettering Cancer Ctr 1990; **Fac Appt:** Prof RadRO, Cornell Univ-Weill Med Coll

Reproductive Endocrinology

Brown, Jessica Rosenberg MD (RE) - **Spec Exp:** Infertility-IVF; Polycystic Ovarian Syndrome; Menopause Problems; **Hospital:** NYU Langone Med Ctr (page 108); **Address:** Madison Womens Hlth & Fertility, 50 E 77 St, New York, NY 10075; **Phone:** 212-639-9122; **Board Cert:** Obstetrics & Gynecology 2012; Reproductive Endocrinology 2012; **Med School:** NYU Sch Med 1987; **Resid:** Obstetrics & Gynecology, NY-Presby/Weill Cornell Med Ctr 1991; **Fellow:** Reproductive Endocrinology, Univ Hosp-UMDNJ 1993; **Fac Appt:** Asst Clin Prof ObG, NYU Sch Med

Chang, Peter L MD (RE) - **Spec Exp:** Infertility-IVF; Polycystic Ovarian Syndrome; Ovarian Failure; **Hospital:** Beth Israel Med Ctr - Petrie Div (page 94); **Address:** Center Infertility/Reproductive Health, 10 Union Square East, Ste 2E, New York, NY 10003; **Phone:** 212-844-8587; **Board Cert:** Obstetrics & Gynecology 2012; Reproductive Endocrinology/Infertility 2012; **Med School:** Univ Tex, San Antonio 1992; **Resid:** Obstetrics & Gynecology, Univ Hosp 1996; **Fellow:** Reproductive Endocrinology, Columbia P&S 1998; **Fac Appt:** Asst Prof ObG, Albert Einstein Coll Med

Choi, Janet M K MD (RE) - **Spec Exp:** Infertility-IVF; Fertility Preservation; Infertility-Advanced Maternal Age; Pregnancy Loss-Recurrent; **Hospital:** NY-Presby/Columbia Univ Med Ctr, NY (page 104); **Address:** Center for Women's Reproductive Care, 1970 Broadway Fl 2, New York, NY 10019; **Phone:** 646-756-8282; **Board Cert:** Obstetrics & Gynecology 2012; Reproductive Endocrinology/Infertility 2012; **Med School:** Columbia P&S 1996; **Resid:** Obstetrics & Gynecology, NY Presby Hosp/Columbia 2000; **Fellow:** Reproductive Endocrinology, NY Presby Hosp/Weill Cornel 2003; **Fac Appt:** Asst Prof ObG, Columbia P&S

Cholst, Ina N MD (RE) - **Spec Exp:** Laparoscopic Surgery; Infertility-IVF; **Hospital:** NY-Presby/Weill Cornell Med Ctr, NY (page 104); **Address:** Ctr for Reproductive Med & Infertility, 1305 York Ave Fl 6, New York, NY 10021; **Phone:** 646-962-3025; **Board Cert:** Obstetrics & Gynecology 1984; Reproductive Endocrinology 1985; **Med School:** NYU Sch Med 1977; **Resid:** Obstetrics & Gynecology, Yale-New Haven Hosp 1981; **Fellow:** Reproductive Endocrinology, Columbia-Presby Med Ctr 1983; **Fac Appt:** Assoc Prof ObG, Cornell Univ-Weill Med Coll

Copperman, Alan B MD (RE) - **Spec Exp:** Infertility-IVF; Fertility Preservation in Cancer; Hysteroscopic Surgery; **Hospital:** Mt Sinai Med Ctr (page 102); **Address:** Reproductive Med Assocs, 635 Madison Ave Fl 10, New York, NY 10022; **Phone:** 212-756-5777; **Board Cert:** Obstetrics & Gynecology 2012; Reproductive Endocrinology 2012; **Med School:** NY Med Coll 1989; **Resid:** Obstetrics & Gynecology, Yale-New Haven Hosp 1993; **Fellow:** Reproductive Endocrinology, Mount Sinai Med Ctr 1995; **Fac Appt:** Clin Prof ObG, Mount Sinai Sch Med

David, Sami MD (RE) - **Spec Exp:** Infertility; Miscarriage-Recurrent; Endometriosis; Uterine Fibroids; **Hospital:** Mt Sinai Med Ctr (page 102); **Address:** 1045 Fifth Ave, Ste 1A, New York, NY 10028-1002; **Phone:** 212-831-0430; **Board Cert:** Obstetrics & Gynecology 1980; **Med School:** Columbia P&S 1971; **Resid:** Obstetrics & Gynecology, New York Hosp 1976; **Fellow:** Reproductive Endocrinology, Hosp Univ Penn 1978; **Fac Appt:** Prof ObG, Mount Sinai Sch Med

Davis, Owen K MD (RE) - **Spec Exp:** Infertility-IVF; Reproductive Surgery; **Hospital:** NY-Presby/Weill Cornell Med Ctr, NY (page 104); **Address:** 1305 York Ave, Fl 6, New York, NY 10021-4872; **Phone:** 646-962-3765; **Board Cert:** Obstetrics & Gynecology 2012; Reproductive Endocrinology/Infertility 2012; **Med School:** Wake Forest Univ 1982; **Resid:** Obstetrics & Gynecology, NY Hosp 1986; **Fellow:** Reproductive Endocrinology, Brigham & Women's Hosp 1988; **Fac Appt:** Prof ObG, Cornell Univ-Weill Med Coll

Fateh, Majid MD (RE) - **Spec Exp:** Infertility-IVF; Laparoscopic Surgery; Endometriosis; **Hospital:** Lenox Hill Hosp (page 106); **Address:** 1016 5th Ave, New York, NY 10028-0132; **Phone:** 212-734-5555; **Board Cert:** Obstetrics & Gynecology 2012; **Med School:** West Indies 1980; **Resid:** Obstetrics & Gynecology, Lenox Hill Hosp 1984; **Fellow:** Reproductive Endocrinology, Univ Penn 1986

Gleicher, Norbert MD (RE) - **Spec Exp:** Infertility-IVF; **Address:** Ctr Human Reproduction, 21 E 69 St, New York, NY 10021; **Phone:** 212-994-4400; **Board Cert:** Obstetrics & Gynecology 1981; **Med School:** Israel 1973; **Resid:** Obstetrics & Gynecology, Mount Sinai Med Ctr 1978; **Fellow:** Reproductive Immunology, Mount Sinai Med Ctr 1975

Grifo, James A MD/PhD (RE) - **Spec Exp:** Preimplantation Genetic Diagnosis; Fertility Preservation in Cancer; Hysteroscopic Surgery; Laparoscopic Surgery; **Hospital:** NYU Langone Med Ctr (page 108); **Address:** NYU Med Ctr, Reproductive Endocrinology, 660 1st Ave Fl 5, New York, NY 10016; **Phone:** 212-263-7978; **Board Cert:** Obstetrics & Gynecology 2012; Reproductive Endocrinology 2012; **Med School:** Case West Res Univ 1984; **Resid:** Obstetrics & Gynecology, NY-Presby/Weill Cornell Med Ctr 1988; **Fellow:** Reproductive Endocrinology, Yale-New Haven Hosp 1990; **Fac Appt:** Prof ObG, NYU Sch Med

Grunfeld, Lawrence MD (RE) - **Spec Exp:** Infertility-IVF; Hysteroscopic Surgery; **Hospital:** Mt Sinai Med Ctr (page 102); **Address:** Reproductive Medicine Associates of NY, 635 Madison Ave, Fl 10th, New York, NY 10022-1009; **Phone:** 212-756-5777; **Board Cert:** Obstetrics & Gynecology 2011; Reproductive Endocrinology 2011; **Med School:** Mount Sinai Sch Med 1979; **Resid:** Obstetrics & Gynecology, Montefiore Med Ctr 1984; **Fellow:** Reproductive Endocrinology, Montefiore Med Ctr 1987; **Fac Appt:** Assoc Clin Prof ObG, Mount Sinai Sch Med

Keefe, David L MD (RE) - **Spec Exp:** Infertility-IVF; Infertility-Advanced Maternal Age; **Hospital:** NYU Langone Med Ctr (page 108); **Address:** NYU Fertility Center, 660 First Ave Fl 5, New York, NY 10016; **Phone:** 212-263-3360; **Board Cert:** Obstetrics & Gynecology 2012; Reproductive Endocrinology 2012; **Med School:** Georgetown Univ 1980; **Resid:** Psychiatry, Cambridge Hosp 1983; Obstetrics & Gynecology, Yale New Haven Hosp 1989; **Fellow:** Neuroendocrinology, Northwestern Univ 1985; Reproductive Endocrinology, Yale New Haven Hosp 1992; **Fac Appt:** Prof ObG, NYU Sch Med

Keltz, Martin D MD (RE) - **Spec Exp:** Infertility-IVF; Pregnancy Loss-Recurrent; **Hospital:** St. Luke's - Roosevelt Hosp Ctr - Roosevelt Div (page 94); **Address:** 425 W 59th St, Ste 5A, New York, NY 10019; **Phone:** 212-523-7751; **Board Cert:** Obstetrics & Gynecology 2012; Reproductive Endocrinology 2012; **Med School:** NYU Sch Med 1989; **Resid:** Obstetrics & Gynecology, Bellevue Hosp 1993; **Fellow:** Reproductive Endocrinology, Yale-New Haven Hosp 1996; **Fac Appt:** Assoc Clin Prof ObG, Columbia P&S

Licciardi, Frederick L MD (RE) - **Spec Exp:** Fertility Preservation in Cancer; Reproductive Surgery; Infertility; Infertility-IVF; **Hospital:** NYU Langone Med Ctr (page 108); **Address:** NYU Fertility Ctr, 660 First Ave, 5th Fl, New York, NY 10016; **Phone:** 212-263-7754; **Board Cert:** Obstetrics & Gynecology 2012; Reproductive Endocrinology 2012; **Med School:** UMDNJ-Rutgers Med Sch 1986; **Resid:** Obstetrics & Gynecology, St Barnabas Med Ctr 1990; **Fellow:** Reproductive Endocrinology, NY Hosp-Cornell Med Ctr 1992; **Fac Appt:** Assoc Prof ObG, NYU Sch Med

Matera, Cristina MD (RE) - **Spec Exp:** Infertility; Miscarriage-Recurrent; Laparoscopic Surgery; Endometriosis; **Hospital:** NY-Presby/Columbia Univ Med Ctr, NY (page 104); **Address:** 50 E 77th St, New York, NY 10075; **Phone:** 212-639-9122; **Board Cert:** Obstetrics & Gynecology 2012; Reproductive Endocrinology 2012; **Med School:** NYU Sch Med 1986; **Resid:** Obstetrics & Gynecology, Columbia-Presby Hosp 1990; **Fellow:** Reproductive Endocrinology, Columbia-Presby Hosp 1992; **Fac Appt:** Asst Clin Prof ObG, Columbia P&S

Mukherjee, Tanmoy MD (RE) - **Spec Exp:** Infertility-IVF; Endometriosis; Uterine Fibroids; **Hospital:** Mt Sinai Med Ctr (page 102); **Address:** Reproductive Medicine Assocs, 635 Madison Ave, Fl 10, New York, NY 10022; **Phone:** 212-756-5777; **Board Cert:** Obstetrics & Gynecology 2012; Reproductive Endocrinology 2012; **Med School:** Albert Einstein Coll Med 1990; **Resid:** Obstetrics & Gynecology, Montefiore Med Ctr 1994; **Fellow:** Reproductive Endocrinology, Mount Sinai Med Ctr 1996; **Fac Appt:** Clin Prof ObG, Mount Sinai Sch Med

Noyes, Nicole MD (RE) - **Spec Exp:** Fertility Preservation in Cancer; Infertility-IVF; Infertility; **Hospital:** NYU Langone Med Ctr (page 108), Bellevue Hosp Ctr; **Address:** NYU Fertility Ctr, 660 First Ave, 5th FL, New York, NY 10016; **Phone:** 212-263-7981; **Board Cert:** Obstetrics & Gynecology 2012; Reproductive Endocrinology 2012; **Med School:** Univ VT Coll Med 1986; **Resid:** Obstetrics & Gynecology, NY Hosp-Cornell Med Ctr 1990; **Fellow:** Reproductive Endocrinology, NY Hosp-Cornell Med Ctr 1992; **Fac Appt:** Assoc Prof ObG, NYU Sch Med

Quagliarello, John R MD (RE) - **Spec Exp:** Infertility; Gynecologic Surgery; Uterine Fibroids; Menopause Problems; **Hospital:** NYU Langone Med Ctr (page 108), Bellevue Hosp Ctr; **Address:** 530 1st Ave, Ste 10-Q, New York, NY 10016-6402; **Phone:** 212-263-6358; **Board Cert:** Obstetrics & Gynecology 1979; Reproductive Endocrinology 1981; **Med School:** McGill Univ 1970; **Resid:** Obstetrics & Gynecology, NYU Med Ctr 1977; **Fellow:** Reproductive Endocrinology, NYU Med Ctr 1979; **Fac Appt:** Assoc Prof ObG, NYU Sch Med

Rosenwaks, Zev MD (RE) - **Spec Exp:** Infertility-IVF; Genetic Disorders; Fertility Preservation in Cancer; **Hospital:** NY-Presby/Weill Cornell Med Ctr, NY (page 104); **Address:** Ctr For Reproductive Medicine & Infertility, 1305 York Ave Fl 6, New York, NY 10021-4872; **Phone:** 646-962-3743; **Board Cert:** Obstetrics & Gynecology 1978; Reproductive Endocrinology 1981; **Med School:** SUNY Downstate 1972; **Resid:** Obstetrics & Gynecology, LI Jewish Med Ctr 1976; **Fellow:** Reproductive Endocrinology, Johns Hopkins Hosp 1978; **Fac Appt:** Prof ObG, Cornell Univ-Weill Med Coll

Sauer, Mark V MD (RE) - **Spec Exp:** Infertility-IVF; Fertility Preservation in Cancer; **Hospital:** NY-Presby/Columbia Univ Med Ctr, NY (page 104); **Address:** 1790 Broadway, Fl 2, New York, NY 10019; **Phone:** 646-756-8282; **Board Cert:** Obstetrics & Gynecology 2012; Reproductive Endocrinology 2012; **Med School:** Univ IL Coll Med 1980; **Resid:** Obstetrics & Gynecology, Univ Illinois Med Ctr 1984; **Fellow:** Reproductive Endocrinology, Harbor-UCLA Med Ctr 1986; **Fac Appt:** Prof ObG, Columbia P&S

Schattman, Glenn L MD (RE) - **Spec Exp:** Infertility; Robotic Assisted Laparoscopic Surgery; Minimally Invasive Surgery; Congenital Anomalies-Gynecologic; **Hospital:** NY-Presby/Weill Cornell Med Ctr, NY (page 104); **Address:** Ctr for Reproductive Med & Infertility, 1305 York Ave Fl 6, New York, NY 10021; **Phone:** 646-962-3836; **Board Cert:** Obstetrics & Gynecology 2012; Reproductive Endocrinology 2012; **Med School:** SUNY Downstate 1987; **Resid:** Obstetrics & Gynecology, Geo Wash Univ Med Ctr 1991; **Fellow:** Reproductive Endocrinology, New York Hosp/Cornell 1993; **Fac Appt:** Assoc Prof ObG, Cornell Univ-Weill Med Coll

Schmidt-Sarosi, Cecilia MD (RE) - **Spec Exp:** Infertility-IVF; Menopause Problems; Polycystic Ovarian Syndrome; Uterine Fibroids; **Hospital:** NYU Langone Med Ctr (page 108); **Address:** 51 E 67th St, New York, NY 10065; **Phone:** 212-535-5350; **Board Cert:** Obstetrics & Gynecology 2009; Reproductive Endocrinology/Infertility 2009; **Med School:** NYU Sch Med 1976; **Resid:** Obstetrics & Gynecology, NYU Med Ctr 1980; **Fellow:** Reproductive Endocrinology, NYU Med Ctr 1982; **Fac Appt:** Prof ObG, NYU Sch Med

Spandorfer, Steven MD (RE) - **Spec Exp:** Infertility-IVF; Laparoscopic Surgery; **Hospital:** NY-Presby/Weill Cornell Med Ctr, NY (page 104); **Address:** Ctr for Reproductive Med & Infertility, 1305 York Ave Fl 6, New York, NY 10021; **Phone:** 646-962-3638; **Board Cert:** Obstetrics & Gynecology 2012; Reproductive Endocrinology 2012; **Med School:** Emory Univ 1988; **Resid:** Obstetrics & Gynecology, Univ Penn Affil HOsp 1996; **Fellow:** Reproductive Endocrinology, New York Hosp 1998; **Fac Appt:** Asst Prof ObG, Cornell Univ-Weill Med Coll

Stein, Daniel E MD (RE) - **Spec Exp:** Infertility-IVF; Polycystic Ovarian Syndrome; Laparoscopic Surgery; Hormonal Disorders; **Hospital:** St. Luke's - Roosevelt Hosp Ctr - Roosevelt Div (page 94); **Address:** 425 W 59th St, Ste 5A, New York, NY 10019; **Phone:** 212-523-7751; **Board Cert:** Obstetrics & Gynecology 2012; Reproductive Endocrinology/Infertility 2012; **Med School:** NY Med Coll 1989; **Resid:** Obstetrics & Gynecology, Thomas Jefferson Univ Hosp 1995; **Fellow:** Reproductive Endocrinology, UMDNJ-New Jersey Med Sch 1997

Sultan, Khalid M MD (RE) - **Spec Exp:** Infertility-IVF; Laparoscopic Surgery; **Hospital:** Lenox Hill Hosp (page 106); **Address:** New York Fertility Inst, 1016 5th Ave, New York, NY 10028-0132; **Phone:** 212-734-5555; **Board Cert:** Obstetrics & Gynecology 2012; Reproductive Endocrinology 2012; **Med School:** NY Med Coll 1988; **Resid:** Obstetrics & Gynecology, Lenox Hill Hosp 1992; **Fellow:** Reproductive Endocrinology, New York Hosp 1994; **Fac Appt:** Asst Clin Prof ObG, NYU Sch Med

Tortoriello, Drew MD (RE) - **Spec Exp:** Infertility-IVF; Polycystic Ovarian Syndrome; **Hospital:** St. Luke's - Roosevelt Hosp Ctr - Roosevelt Div (page 94); **Address:** 425 5th Ave, Fl 3, New York, NY 10016; **Phone:** 646-792-7476; **Board Cert:** Obstetrics & Gynecology 2007; Reproductive Endocrinology 2007; **Med School:** SUNY Downstate 1992; **Resid:** Obstetrics & Gynecology, NY Presby Hosp/Cornell 1996; **Fellow:** Reproductive Endocrinology, UMDNJ Affil Hosp 1998; Reproductive Endocrinology, Mass Genl Hosp

Warren, Michelle P MD (RE) - **Spec Exp:** Menopause Problems; Infertility; Menstrual Disorders; Women's Health; **Hospital:** NY-Presby/Columbia Univ Med Ctr, NY (page 104); **Address:** Center for Menopause,, Hormonal Disorders & Women's Health, 134 E 73rd St, New York, NY 10021; **Phone:** 212-737-4664; **Board Cert:** Internal Medicine 1972; Endocrinology 1973; **Med School:** Cornell Univ 1965; **Resid:** Internal Medicine, Bellevue Hosp Ctr 1968; Internal Medicine, Meml Hosp Cancer Ctr 1968; **Fellow:** Endocrinology, Columbia Presby Med Ctr 1971; **Fac Appt:** Prof ObG, Columbia P&S

Rheumatology

Adlersberg, Jay B MD (Rhu) - **Spec Exp:** Rheumatoid Arthritis; Psoriatic Arthritis; Osteoarthritis; Pain-Back; **Hospital:** Lenox Hill Hosp (page 106); **Address:** 220 E 69th St, Ground Fl, New York, NY 10021-5737; **Phone:** 212-570-1800; **Board Cert:** Internal Medicine 1972; Rheumatology 1980; **Med School:** Univ Pennsylvania 1969; **Resid:** Internal Medicine, Bellevue Hosp 1972; **Fellow:** Rheumatology, Bellevue Hosp 1974; **Fac Appt:** Asst Clin Prof Med, NYU Sch Med

Agus, Bertrand MD (Rhu) - **Spec Exp:** Lupus/SLE; Rheumatoid Arthritis; Sarcoidosis; Gout; **Hospital:** NYU Langone Med Ctr (page 108); **Address:** 251 E 33rd St, Fl 4, New York, NY 10016-4804; **Phone:** 212-779-8421; **Board Cert:** Internal Medicine 1972; Rheumatology 1972; **Med School:** NYU Sch Med 1965; **Resid:** Internal Medicine, NYU Med Ctr 1970; **Fellow:** Rheumatology, NYU Med Ctr 1972; **Fac Appt:** Assoc Clin Prof Med, NYU Sch Med

Ali, Yousaf MD (Rhu) - **Spec Exp:** Gout; Osteoporosis; Behcet's Syndrome; **Hospital:** Mt Sinai Med Ctr (page 102); **Address:** Mount Sinai Faculty Practice Assocs, 5 E 98th St, Fl 11, New York, NY 10029; **Phone:** 212-241-1671; **Board Cert:** Internal Medicine 2008; Rheumatology 2009; **Med School:** England, UK 1992; **Resid:** Internal Medicine, OR Hlth & Sci Univ Hosp 1997; **Fellow:** Rheumatology, Yale-New Haven Hosp 1999; **Fac Appt:** Asst Prof Med, Mount Sinai Sch Med

Ashany, Dalit MD (Rhu) - **Spec Exp:** Lupus/SLE; Rheumatoid Arthritis; Osteoarthritis; **Hospital:** Hosp For Special Surgery (page 113); **Address:** Hosp for Special Surg-Rheum Div, 535 E 70th St, New York, NY 10021; **Phone:** 212-606-1671; **Board Cert:** Internal Medicine 1988; Rheumatology 2003; **Med School:** Albert Einstein Coll Med 1985; **Resid:** Internal Medicine, NY-Presby/Columbia Univ Med Ctr 1988; **Fellow:** Rheumatology, Hosp For Special Surgery 1991; **Fac Appt:** Asst Prof Med, Cornell Univ-Weill Med Coll

Belmont, H. Michael MD (Rhu) - **Spec Exp:** Lupus/SLE; Antiphospholipid Syndrome (APS); Wegener's Granulomatosis; Rheumatoid Arthritis; **Hospital:** NYU Hosp For Joint Dis (page 108), NYU Langone Med Ctr (page 108); **Address:** NYU, Ctr Musculoskeletal Care, 333 E 38th St Fl 4, New York, NY 10016; **Phone:** 646-501-7400; **Board Cert:** Internal Medicine 1983; Rheumatology 1986; **Med School:** Univ Pittsburgh 1980; **Resid:** Internal Medicine, Mount Sinai Med Ctr 1983; **Fellow:** Rheumatology, Bellevue Hosp Ctr 1985; **Fac Appt:** Assoc Prof Med, NYU Sch Med

Belostotsky, Olga MD/PhD (Rhu) - **Spec Exp:** Autoimmune Disorders; Asthma; Food & Drug Allergy; Immunodeficiency Disorders; **Hospital:** Lenox Hill Hosp (page 106), NS-LIJ Hlth Sys (page 106); **Address:** Manhattan Allergy, Immunology & Rheum, 47 E 77th St, Ste 201, New York, NY 10075; **Phone:** 646-688-3443; **Board Cert:** Internal Medicine 2005; Rheumatology 2010; **Med School:** Russia 1983; **Resid:** Allergy & Immunology, Brigham & Womens Hosp 1999; Internal Medicine, Lenox Hill Hosp 2002; **Fellow:** Rheumatology, N Shore Univ Hosp 2005; Allergy & Immunology, N Shore-LIJ Hlth Sys 2005; **Fac Appt:** Asst Clin Prof A&I, NYU Sch Med

Blume, Ralph S MD (Rhu) - **Spec Exp:** Vasculitis; Lupus/SLE; Rheumatoid Arthritis; **Hospital:** NY-Presby/Columbia Univ Med Ctr, NY (page 104); **Address:** NY-Presby, Rheumatology Dept, 161 Fort Washington Ave, Ste 638, New York, NY 10032; **Phone:** 212-305-5512; **Board Cert:** Internal Medicine 1972; Rheumatology 1974; **Med School:** Columbia P&S 1964; **Resid:** Internal Medicine, NY-Presby/Columbia Univ Med Ctr 1968; **Fellow:** Rheumatology, NY-Presby/Columbia Univ Med Ctr 1970; **Fac Appt:** Prof Med, Columbia P&S

Buyon, Jill P MD (Rhu) - **Spec Exp:** Lupus/SLE in Pregnancy; Lupus/SLE in Menopause; **Hospital:** NYU Hosp For Joint Dis (page 108), NYU Langone Med Ctr (page 108); **Address:** NYU, Ctr Musculoskeletal Care, 333 E 38th St Fl 4, New York, NY 10016; **Phone:** 646-501-7400; **Board Cert:** Internal Medicine 1981; Rheumatology 1984; **Med School:** Albert Einstein Coll Med 1978; **Resid:** Internal Medicine, Montefiore Med Ctr 1981; **Fellow:** Rheumatology, NYU Med Ctr 1983; **Fac Appt:** Prof Med, NYU Sch Med

Crane, Richard P MD (Rhu) - **Spec Exp:** Rheumatoid Arthritis; Gout; Osteoarthritis; Arthritis; **Hospital:** Mt Sinai Med Ctr (page 102); **Address:** 1088 Park Ave, New York, NY 10128-1132; **Phone:** 212-860-4000; **Board Cert:** Internal Medicine 1984; Rheumatology 1986; **Med School:** Mount Sinai Sch Med 1981; **Resid:** Internal Medicine, Mt Sinai Hosp 1984; **Fellow:** Rheumatology, Mt Sinai Hosp 1986

Faller, Jason MD (Rhu) - **Spec Exp:** Gout; Rheumatoid Arthritis; Lyme Disease; Lupus/SLE; **Hospital:** St. Luke's - Roosevelt Hosp Ctr - Roosevelt Div (page 94), Lenox Hill Hosp (page 106); **Address:** 333 W 57th St, Ste 104, New York, NY 10019-3115; **Phone:** 212-307-6880; **Board Cert:** Internal Medicine 1980; Rheumatology 1982; **Med School:** Univ Pennsylvania 1977; **Resid:** Internal Medicine, Rush Presby St Lukes Med Ctr 1980; **Fellow:** Rheumatology, Univ Michigan 1982; **Fac Appt:** Asst Clin Prof Med, Columbia P&S

Fields, Theodore R MD (Rhu) - **Spec Exp:** Gout; Rheumatoid Arthritis; Osteoarthritis; **Hospital:** Hosp For Special Surgery (page 113), NY-Presby/Weill Cornell Med Ctr, NY (page 104); **Address:** 535 E 70th St, Fl 8, Ste 848F, New York, NY 10021-4872; **Phone:** 212-606-1286; **Board Cert:** Internal Medicine 1979; Rheumatology 1982; **Med School:** SUNY Downstate 1976; **Resid:** Internal Medicine, Nassau Co Med Ctr 1979; **Fellow:** Rheumatology, Univ Hosp 1982; **Fac Appt:** Clin Prof Med, Cornell Univ-Weill Med Coll

Fischer, Harry D MD (Rhu) - **Spec Exp:** Lupus/SLE; Rheumatoid Arthritis; Vasculitis; **Hospital:** Beth Israel Med Ctr - Petrie Div (page 94); **Address:** 10 Union Square East, Ste 3D, New York, NY 10003-3314; **Phone:** 212-844-8101; **Board Cert:** Internal Medicine 1983; Rheumatology 2010; **Med School:** Mount Sinai Sch Med 1979; **Resid:** Internal Medicine, Beth Israel Med Ctr 1983; **Fellow:** Rheumatology, Hosp Joint Diseases 1985; **Fac Appt:** Assoc Clin Prof Med, Albert Einstein Coll Med

Gibofsky, Allan MD (Rhu) - **Spec Exp:** Rheumatic Fever; Rheumatoid Arthritis; Inflammatory Arthritis; Behcet's Syndrome; **Hospital:** Hosp For Special Surgery (page 113), NY-Presby/Weill Cornell Med Ctr, NY (page 104); **Address:** 535 E 70th St, New York, NY 10021-4872; **Phone:** 212-606-1423; **Board Cert:** Internal Medicine 1977; Rheumatology 1980; **Med School:** Cornell Univ 1973; **Resid:** Internal Medicine, New York Hosp 1977; **Fellow:** Rheumatology/Immunology, Hosp for Special Surgery 1979; **Fac Appt:** Prof Med, Cornell Univ-Weill Med Coll

Goodman, Susan M MD (Rhu) - **Spec Exp:** Lupus Nephritis; Rheumatoid Arthritis; Psoriatic Arthritis; **Hospital:** Hosp For Special Surgery (page 113), NY-Presby/Weill Cornell Med Ctr, NY (page 104); **Address:** Hosp for Special Surgery, 535 E 70th St, New York, NY 10021; **Phone:** 212-606-1163; **Board Cert:** Internal Medicine 1980; Rheumatology 1982; **Med School:** Univ Cincinnati 1977; **Resid:** Internal Medicine, Lenox Hill Hosp 1980; **Fellow:** Rheumatology, Columbia Presby Hosp 1983; **Fac Appt:** Assoc Prof Med, Cornell Univ-Weill Med Coll

Gorevic, Peter D MD (Rhu) - **Spec Exp:** Autoimmune Disease; Amyloidosis/Joint Disease; Cryoglobulinemia; **Hospital:** Mt Sinai Med Ctr (page 102); **Address:** Mount Sinai Med Ctr, Rheumatology Dept, 5 E 98th St Fl 11, New York, NY 10029; **Phone:** 212-241-1671; **Board Cert:** Internal Medicine 1973; Rheumatology 1976; Allergy & Immunology 1977; Diagnostic Lab Immunology 1986; **Med School:** NYU Sch Med 1970; **Resid:** Internal Medicine, NYU Med Ctr 1973; **Fellow:** Rheumatology, NYU Med Ctr 1975; Allergy & Immunology, NYU Med Ctr 1977; **Fac Appt:** Prof Med, Mount Sinai Sch Med

Greisman, Stewart G MD (Rhu) - **Spec Exp:** Lupus/SLE; Rheumatoid Arthritis; **Hospital:** St. Luke's - Roosevelt Hosp Ctr - Roosevelt Div (page 94), Hosp For Special Surgery (page 113); **Address:** 457 W 57th St, Ste 106, New York, NY 10019-1701; **Phone:** 212-265-1471; **Board Cert:** Internal Medicine 1984; Rheumatology 1986; **Med School:** Yale Univ 1981; **Resid:** Internal Medicine, Yale-New Haven Hosp 1984; **Fellow:** Rheumatology, Hosp Special Surg 1986; **Fac Appt:** Assoc Clin Prof Med, Columbia P&S

Honig, Stephen MD (Rhu) - **Spec Exp:** Osteoporosis; Rheumatoid Arthritis; Osteoarthritis; Lupus/SLE; **Hospital:** NYU Hosp For Joint Dis (page 108), NYU Langone Med Ctr (page 108); **Address:** 301 E 17th St, Ste 1100, New York, NY 10003-3804; **Phone:** 212-598-6367; **Board Cert:** Internal Medicine 1975; Rheumatology 1978; **Med School:** Univ Tenn Coll Med 1972; **Resid:** Internal Medicine, St Vincent's Hosp Med Ctr 1975; **Fellow:** Rheumatology, NYU Med Ctr 1977; **Fac Appt:** Assoc Clin Prof Med, NYU Sch Med

Horowitz, Mark D MD (Rhu) - **Spec Exp:** Lupus/SLE; Rheumatoid Arthritis; Fibromyalgia; **Hospital:** Mt Sinai Med Ctr (page 102); **Address:** 21 E 90th St, Ground Fl, New York, NY 10128-0654; **Phone:** 212-860-3077; **Board Cert:** Internal Medicine 1986; **Med School:** NE Ohio Univ 1983; **Resid:** Internal Medicine, Mt Sinai Med Ctr 1986; **Fellow:** Rheumatology, Mt Sinai Med Ctr 1989

Kerr, Leslie D MD (Rhu) - **Spec Exp:** Connective Tissue Disorders; Geriatric Rheumatology; Gout; Rheumatoid Arthritis; **Hospital:** Mt Sinai Med Ctr (page 102); **Address:** Mount Sinai Med Ctr, 5 E 98th St, 11th Fl, New York, NY 10029; **Phone:** 212-241-1671; **Board Cert:** Internal Medicine 1983; Rheumatology 1986; **Med School:** Columbia P&S 1980; **Resid:** Internal Medicine, Mt Sinai Hosp 1983; **Fellow:** Rheumatology, Mt Sinai Hosp 1985; **Fac Appt:** Assoc Prof Med, Mount Sinai Sch Med

Lee, Sicy H MD (Rhu) - **Spec Exp:** Rheumatoid Arthritis; Psoriatic Arthritis; Lupus/SLE; **Hospital:** NYU Hosp For Joint Dis (page 108), NYU Langone Med Ctr (page 108); **Address:** 333 E 38th St, Fl 4, New York, NY 10016; **Phone:** 646-501-7400; **Board Cert:** Internal Medicine 1982; Rheumatology 1984; **Med School:** Univ Cincinnati 1979; **Resid:** Internal Medicine, Good Samaritan 1982; **Fellow:** Rheumatology, Hosp for Joint Diseases 1984; **Fac Appt:** Asst Clin Prof Med, NYU Sch Med

MacKenzie, C Ronald MD (Rhu) - **Spec Exp:** Complementary Medicine; **Hospital:** Hosp For Special Surgery (page 113), NY-Presby/Weill Cornell Med Ctr, NY (page 104); **Address:** 535 E 70th St, New York, NY 10021; **Phone:** 212-606-1669; **Board Cert:** Internal Medicine ; Rheumatology 2002; **Med School:** Univ Calgary 1977; **Resid:** Family Medicine, Calgary Gen Hosp 1978; **Internal** Medicine, Univ Manitoba Hosp 1981; **Fellow:** Internal Medicine, New York Hosp/Cornell 1983; Rheumatology, Hosp For Spec Surg 1992; **Fac Appt:** Assoc Clin Prof Med, Cornell Univ-Weill Med Coll

Magid, Steven K MD (Rhu) - **Spec Exp:** Rheumatoid Arthritis; Osteoarthritis; Lyme Disease; Polymyalgia Rheumatica; **Hospital:** Hosp For Special Surgery (page 113); **Address:** HSS, Rheumatology Dept, 535 E 70th St, Fl 7, New York, NY 10021; **Phone:** 212-606-1060; **Board Cert:** Internal Medicine 1979; Rheumatology 1984; **Med School:** Cornell Univ 1976; **Resid:** Internal Medicine, New York Hosp 1979; **Fellow:** Rheumatology, Hosp For Special Surgery 1981; **Fac Appt:** Clin Prof Med, Cornell Univ-Weill Med Coll

Marchetta, Paula MD (Rhu) - **Spec Exp:** Rheumatoid Arthritis; Psoriatic Arthritis; Sjogren's Syndrome; Osteoarthritis; **Hospital:** NYU Langone Med Ctr (page 108); **Address:** Concorde Medical Group, 40 Park Ave, New York, NY 10016-3467; **Phone:** 212-696-5415; **Board Cert:** Internal Medicine 1986; Rheumatology 2010; **Med School:** NYU Sch Med 1983; **Resid:** Internal Medicine, Bellevue Hosp-NYU Med Ctr 1986; **Fellow:** Rheumatology, NYU Med Ctr 1989; **Fac Appt:** Assoc Clin Prof Med, NYU Sch Med

Markenson, Joseph A MD (Rhu) - **Spec Exp:** Rheumatoid Arthritis; Lupus/SLE; Osteoarthritis; **Hospital:** Hosp For Special Surgery (page 113), NY-Presby/Weill Cornell Med Ctr, NY (page 104); **Address:** Hosp for Special Surgery, 535 E 70th St, Ste 659W, New York, NY 10021-4892; **Phone:** 212-606-1261; **Board Cert:** Internal Medicine 1976; Rheumatology 1978; **Med School:** SUNY Downstate 1970; **Resid:** Internal Medicine, New York Hosp 1975; **Fellow:** Rheumatology, Hosp For Special Surg 1976; **Fac Appt:** Clin Prof Med, Cornell Univ-Weill Med Coll

Meed, Steven D MD (Rhu) - **Spec Exp:** Lyme Disease; Chronic Fatigue Syndrome; Acupuncture; Fibromyalgia; **Hospital:** Lenox Hill Hosp (page 106), St. Luke's - Roosevelt Hosp Ctr - Roosevelt Div (page 94); **Address:** 150 E 58th St Fl 18, New York, NY 10155; **Phone:** 212-583-2960; **Board Cert:** Internal Medicine 1978; Rheumatology 1986; **Med School:** NYU Sch Med 1975; **Resid:** Internal Medicine, Brookdale Hosp 1977; **Fellow:** Rheumatology, Barnes Hosp-Wash Univ 1979; **Fac Appt:** Asst Clin Prof Med, NYU Sch Med

Mitnick, Hal J MD (Rhu) - **Spec Exp:** Rheumatoid Arthritis; Psoriatic Arthritis; Osteoporosis; Dermatomyositis; **Hospital:** NYU Langone Med Ctr (page 108); **Address:** 333 E 34th St, Ste 1C, New York, NY 10016-4977; **Phone:** 212-889-7217; **Board Cert:** Internal Medicine 1976; Rheumatology 1978; **Med School:** NYU Sch Med 1972; **Resid:** Internal Medicine, Bellevue Hosp 1976; **Fellow:** Rheumatology, NYU Med Ctr 1978; **Fac Appt:** Clin Prof Med, NYU Sch Med

Nickerson, Katherine G MD (Rhu) - **Spec Exp:** Lupus/SLE; Rheumatoid Arthritis; **Hospital:** NY-Presby/Columbia Univ Med Ctr, NY (page 104); **Address:** 161 Ft Washington Ave, Fl 2, New York, NY 10032; **Phone:** 212-305-4308; **Board Cert:** Internal Medicine 1984; Rheumatology 1986; **Med School:** UCSF 1981; **Resid:** Internal Medicine, Beth Israel Hosp 1984; **Fellow:** Rheumatology, Columbia-Presby Med Ctr 1986; **Fac Appt:** Clin Prof Med, Columbia P&S

Ornstein, Matthew MD (Rhu) - **Spec Exp:** Arthritis; **Hospital:** Mt Sinai Med Ctr (page 102); **Address:** 65 E 96th St, Ste 1B, New York, NY 10128-1307; **Phone:** 212-722-7157; **Board Cert:** Rheumatology 2004; **Med School:** SUNY Stony Brook 1988; **Resid:** Internal Medicine, Mt Sinai Med Ctr 1991; **Fellow:** Rheumatology, Mt Sinai Med Ctr 1993

Paget, Stephen MD (Rhu) - **Spec Exp:** Rheumatoid Arthritis; Lupus/SLE; Vasculitis; Connective Tissue Disorders; **Hospital:** Hosp For Special Surgery (page 113); **Address:** HSS, Rheumatology Dept, 535 E 70th St Fl 7, New York, NY 10021; **Phone:** 212-606-1845; **Board Cert:** Internal Medicine 1974; Rheumatology 2009; **Med School:** SUNY Downstate 1971; **Resid:** Internal Medicine, Johns Hopkins Hosp 1973; **Fellow:** Rheumatology, Hosp Special Surgery 1975; **Fac Appt:** Prof Med, Cornell Univ-Weill Med Coll

Parrish, Edward MD (Rhu) - **Spec Exp:** Musculoskeletal Disorders in HIV/AIDS; Autoimmune Disease; **Hospital:** Hosp For Special Surgery (page 113), NY-Presby/Weill Cornell Med Ctr, NY (page 104); **Address:** 525 E 71th St Fl 7, New York, NY 10021; **Phone:** 212-606-1743; **Board Cert:** Internal Medicine 1983; Rheumatology 1986; **Med School:** Wake Forest Univ 1980; **Resid:** Internal Medicine, Columbia-Presby Med Ctr 1983; **Fellow:** Rheumatology/Immunology, Columbia-Presby Med Ctr 1985; **Fac Appt:** Asst Prof Med, Cornell Univ-Weill Med Coll

Rackoff, Paula J MD (Rhu) - **Spec Exp:** Osteoporosis; Sjogren's Syndrome; Arthritis; Lupus/SLE; **Hospital:** NYU Langone Med Ctr (page 108); **Address:** NYU Langone Med Ctr, Ctr for Musculoskeletal Care, 333 E 38th St Fl 4, New York, NY 10028; **Phone:** 646-501-7400; **Board Cert:** Internal Medicine 1989; Rheumatology 2004; **Med School:** Yale Univ 1986; **Resid:** Internal Medicine, Yale-New Haven Hosp 1989; **Fellow:** Rheumatology, Yale-New Haven Hosp 1992; **Fac Appt:** Assoc Prof Med, Albert Einstein Coll Med

Russell, Linda MD (Rhu) - **Spec Exp:** Arthritis; Osteoporosis; **Hospital:** Hosp For Special Surgery (page 113); **Address:** HSS, Rheumatology Dept, 535 E 70 St, New York, NY 10021; **Phone:** 212-606-1305; **Board Cert:** Internal Medicine 2012; Rheumatology 2004; **Med School:** Tufts Univ 1989; **Resid:** Internal Medicine, NY-Presby/Weill Cornell Med Ctr 1992; **Fellow:** Rheumatology, Hosp Special Surgery 1995; **Fac Appt:** Asst Prof Med, Cornell Univ-Weill Med Coll

Salmon, Jane E MD (Rhu) - **Spec Exp:** Lupus/SLE; Antiphospholipid Syndrome (APS); Rheumatoid Arthritis; **Hospital:** Hosp For Special Surgery (page 113); **Address:** 535 E 70th St, New York, NY 10021-4872; **Phone:** 212-606-1728; **Board Cert:** Internal Medicine 1981; Rheumatology 1984; **Med School:** Columbia P&S 1978; **Resid:** Internal Medicine, New York Hosp 1981; **Fellow:** Rheumatology, Hosp Special Surgery 1983; **Fac Appt:** Prof Med, Cornell Univ-Weill Med Coll

Samuels, Jonathan MD (Rhu) - **Spec Exp:** Rheumatoid Arthritis; Osteoarthritis; Musculoskeletal Disorders; Musculoskeletal Ultrasound; **Hospital:** NYU Langone Med Ctr (page 108); **Address:** Center for Musculoskeletal Care, 333 E 38th St, Fl 4, New York, NY 10016; **Phone:** 646-501-7400; **Board Cert:** Internal Medicine 2002; Rheumatology 2004; **Med School:** Cornell Univ 1999; **Resid:** Internal Medicine, University Hosp 2002; **Fellow:** Rheumatology, Weill-Cornell Med Ctr 2005; **Fac Appt:** Asst Prof Med, NYU Sch Med

Schwartzfarb, Lanny S MD (Rhu) - **Spec Exp:** Rheumatoid Arthritis; Psoriatic Arthritis; Sapho Syndrome; **Hospital:** Beth Israel Med Ctr - Petrie Div (page 94), NYU Langone Med Ctr (page 108); **Address:** 315 E 69th St, Lobby, Ste J, New York, NY 10021; **Phone:** 212-734-5670; **Board Cert:** Internal Medicine 1975; Rheumatology 1978; **Med School:** NYU Sch Med 1972; **Resid:** Internal Medicine, Beth Israel Med Ctr 1975; **Fellow:** Rheumatology, Columbia-Presby Med Ctr 1977

Schwartzman, Sergio MD (Rhu) - **Spec Exp:** Lupus/SLE; Raynaud's Disease; Uveitis; Vasculitis; **Hospital:** Hosp For Special Surgery (page 113); **Address:** Hosp for Special Surgery, 535 E 70th St Fl 7, New York, NY 10021-4892; **Phone:** 212-606-1557; **Board Cert:** Internal Medicine 1985; Rheumatology 1988; **Med School:** Mount Sinai Sch Med 1982; **Resid:** Internal Medicine, LI Jewish Med Ctr 1985; **Fellow:** Rheumatology, Hosp Special Surgery 1987; **Fac Appt:** Assoc Prof Med, Cornell Univ-Weill Med Coll

Smiles, Stephen A MD (Rhu) - **Spec Exp:** Arthritis; Osteoporosis; Lupus/SLE; Gout; **Hospital:** NYU Langone Med Ctr (page 108); **Address:** Ctr for Arthritis & Autoimmunity, 333 E 38th St Fl 4, New York, NY 10016; **Phone:** 646-501-7400; **Board Cert:** Internal Medicine 1977; Rheumatology 1980; **Med School:** SUNY Buffalo 1973; **Resid:** Internal Medicine, Bellevue Hosp Ctr 1977; **Fellow:** Rheumatology, Bellevue Hosp Ctr 1979; **Fac Appt:** Assoc Clin Prof Med, NYU Sch Med

Solitar, Bruce M MD (Rhu) - **Spec Exp:** Arthritis; Fibromyalgia; Reiter's Syndrome; Retroperitoneal Fibrosis; **Hospital:** NYU Langone Med Ctr (page 108), NYU Hosp For Joint Dis (page 108); **Address:** NYU Med Ctr, Rheumatology Dept, 333 E 34th St, Ste 1C, New York, NY 10016; **Phone:** 212-889-7217; **Board Cert:** Internal Medicine 2012; Rheumatology 2004; **Med School:** NYU Sch Med 1988; **Resid:** Internal Medicine, Bellevue Hosp 1992; **Fellow:** Rheumatology, Bellevue Hosp 1994; **Fac Appt:** Assoc Clin Prof Med, NYU Sch Med

Solomon, Gary MD (Rhu) - **Spec Exp:** Psoriatic Arthritis; Rheumatoid Arthritis; Autoimmune Disease; **Hospital:** NYU Hosp For Joint Dis (page 108), NYU Langone Med Ctr (page 108); **Address:** Ctr for Musculoskeletal Care, 333 E 38th St, New York, NY 10016; **Phone:** 646-501-7400; **Board Cert:** Internal Medicine 1980; Rheumatology 1982; **Med School:** Mount Sinai Sch Med 1977; **Resid:** Internal Medicine, Mt Sinai Med Ctr 1980; **Fellow:** Rheumatology, Montefiore Med Ctr 1982; **Fac Appt:** Assoc Clin Prof Med, NYU Sch Med

Spiera, Harry MD (Rhu) - **Spec Exp:** Lupus/SLE; Scleroderma; Vasculitis; Behcet's Syndrome; **Hospital:** Mt Sinai Med Ctr (page 102); **Address:** Rheumatology Assocs, 1088 Park Ave, New York, NY 10128-1132; **Phone:** 212-860-4000 x2; **Board Cert:** Internal Medicine 1965; Rheumatology 1972; **Med School:** NYU Sch Med 1958; **Resid:** Internal Medicine, VA Med Ctr 1960; Internal Medicine, Mt Sinai Hosp 1961; **Fellow:** Rheumatology, Columbia-Presby Med Ctr 1963; **Fac Appt:** Clin Prof Med, Mount Sinai Sch Med

Spiera, Robert MD (Rhu) - **Spec Exp:** Vasculitis; Lupus/SLE; Scleroderma; **Hospital:** Hosp For Special Surgery (page 113); **Address:** Rheumatology Assocs, 1088 Park Ave, New York, NY 10128-1132; **Phone:** 212-860-2100; **Board Cert:** Internal Medicine 2002; Rheumatology 2004; **Med School:** Yale Univ 1989; **Resid:** Internal Medicine, New York Hosp 1992; **Fellow:** Rheumatology, Hosp Special Surg 1995; **Fac Appt:** Clin Prof Med, Cornell Univ-Weill Med Coll

Stern, Richard MD (Rhu) - **Spec Exp:** Rheumatoid Arthritis; Osteoporosis; Osteoarthritis; Polymyalgia Rheumatica; **Hospital:** Hosp For Special Surgery (page 113), NY-Presby/Weill Cornell Med Ctr, NY (page 104); **Address:** 475 E 72nd St, New York, NY 10021-4458; **Phone:** 212-879-2282; **Board Cert:** Internal Medicine 1973; Rheumatology 1976; **Med School:** Tufts Univ 1970; **Resid:** Internal Medicine, New York Hosp 1973; **Fellow:** Immunology, Rockefeller Univ Hosp 1975; Rheumatology, Hosp Special Surgery 1975; **Fac Appt:** Assoc Clin Prof Med, Cornell Univ-Weill Med Coll

Whitman III, Hendricks H MD (Rhu) - **Spec Exp:** Rheumatoid Arthritis; Scleroderma; Osteoarthritis; **Hospital:** Hosp For Special Surgery (page 113); **Address:** Hospital for Special Surgery, 525 E 71st St Fl 7, New York, NY 10021; **Phone:** 212-774-2802; **Board Cert:** Internal Medicine 1978; Rheumatology 1980; **Med School:** Univ NC Sch Med 1975; **Resid:** Internal Medicine, New York Hosp 1978; **Fellow:** Rheumatology, Hosp for Special Surg 1980; **Fac Appt:** Asst Clin Prof Med, Cornell Univ-Weill Med Coll

Yee, Arthur M F MD/PhD (Rhu) - **Spec Exp:** Sarcoidosis; Gout; Rheumatoid Arthritis; Psoriatic Arthritis; **Hospital:** Hosp For Special Surgery (page 113), NY-Presby/Weill Cornell Med Ctr, NY (page 104); **Address:** Hosp for Special Surgery, 535 E 70th St, New York, NY 10021; **Phone:** 212-606-1171; **Board Cert:** Internal Medicine 2004; Rheumatology 2006; **Med School:** NYU Sch Med 1991; **Resid:** Internal Medicine, New York Hosp 1994; **Fellow:** Rheumatology, Hosp Special Surg 1996; **Fac Appt:** Asst Prof Med, Cornell Univ-Weill Med Coll

Sports Medicine

Altchek, David MD (SM) - **Spec Exp:** Shoulder Surgery; Elbow Surgery; Knee Surgery; Arthroscopic Surgery; **Hospital:** Hosp For Special Surgery (page 113); **Address:** HSS, Sports Med Dept, 535 E 70th St, New York, NY 10021; **Phone:** 212-606-1909; **Board Cert:** Orthopaedic Surgery 2011; **Med School:** Cornell Univ-Weill Med Coll 1982; **Resid:** Orthopaedic Surgery, Hosp Special Surgery 1987; **Fellow:** Sports Medicine, Hosp Special Surgery 1988; **Fac Appt:** Prof OrS, Cornell Univ-Weill Med Coll

Callahan, Lisa MD (SM) - **Spec Exp:** Primary Care Sports Medicine; Sports Medicine-Women; Fractures-Stress; **Hospital:** Hosp For Special Surgery (page 113), NY-Presby/Weill Cornell Med Ctr, NY (page 104); **Address:** Hospital for Special Surgery, 535 E 70th St, New York, NY 10021; **Phone:** 212-606-1532; **Board Cert:** Family Medicine 2004; Sports Medicine 2003; **Med School:** E Carolina Univ 1987; **Resid:** Family Medicine, San Jose Med Ctr 1990; **Fellow:** Sports Medicine, San Jose Med Ctr 1991; **Fac Appt:** Assoc Prof FMed, Cornell Univ-Weill Med Coll

Halpern, Brian MD (SM) - **Spec Exp:** Primary Care Sports Medicine; Knee Injuries; Shoulder Injuries; Overuse Injuries; **Hospital:** Hosp For Special Surgery (page 113); **Address:** 525 E 71st St, New York, NY 10021; **Phone:** 212-606-1329; **Board Cert:** Family Medicine 2008; Sports Medicine 2004; **Med School:** Cornell Univ 1981; **Resid:** Family Medicine, Univ Md Med Ctr 1984; **Fellow:** Sports Medicine, Hughston Ortho Clinic 1985; **Fac Appt:** Assoc Clin Prof Med, Cornell Univ-Weill Med Coll

Hamner, Daniel MD (SM) - **Spec Exp:** Running Injuries; Acupuncture; Primary Care Sports Medicine; **Address:** 80 E 11th St, Ste 619, New York, NY 10003; **Phone:** 212-260-5999; **Board Cert:** Physical Medicine & Rehabilitation 1986; **Med School:** NY Med Coll 1976; **Resid:** Physical Medicine & Rehabilitation, New York Hosp-Cornell Med Ctr 1983; **Fellow:** Cardiac Rehabilitation, Emory Univ 1986

Hershman, Elliott B MD (SM) - **Spec Exp:** Knee Injuries; Knee Surgery; Arthroscopic Surgery; Ligament Reconstruction; **Hospital:** Lenox Hill Hosp (page 106); **Address:** 130 E 77th St, Fl 7, New York, NY 10075; **Phone:** 212-744-8114; **Board Cert:** Orthopaedic Surgery 2008; **Med School:** Univ Rochester 1979; **Resid:** Orthopaedic Surgery, Lenox Hill Hosp 1984; **Fellow:** Sports Medicine, Cleveland Clinic 1985; **Fac Appt:** Asst Clin Prof OrS, Mount Sinai Sch Med

Krinick, Ronald M MD (SM) - **Spec Exp:** Knee Injuries; Shoulder Injuries; **Hospital:** NY-Presby/Lower Manhattan Hosp (page 104), NYU Hosp For Joint Dis (page 108); **Address:** Seacoast Orthopaedic Associates, 19 Beekman St Fl 5, New York, NY 10038; **Phone:** 212-513-7711; **Board Cert:** Orthopaedic Surgery 2008; **Med School:** NYU Sch Med 1979; **Resid:** Orthopaedic Surgery, NYU/Bellvue Med Ctr 1984; **Fellow:** Sports Medicine, NYU Med Ctr 1985; **Fac Appt:** Assoc Clin Prof OrS, NYU Sch Med

Levine, William N MD (SM) - **Spec Exp:** Arthroscopic Surgery; Shoulder & Elbow Surgery; Knee Injuries; **Hospital:** NY-Presby/Columbia Univ Med Ctr, NY (page 104); **Address:** 622 W 168th St, PH-11, rm 1117, New York, NY 10032; **Phone:** 212-305-0762; **Board Cert:** Orthopaedic Surgery 2010; Orthopaedic Sports Medicine 2008; **Med School:** Case West Res Univ 1990; **Resid:** Surgery, Beth Israel Hosp 1991; Orthopaedic Surgery, New Eng Med Ctr Hosps 1995; **Fellow:** Shoulder Surgery, Columbia-Presby Med Ctr 1996; Sports Medicine, Univ MD Med Ctr 1998; **Fac Appt:** Clin Prof OrS, Columbia P&S

Maharam, Lewis G MD (SM) - **Spec Exp:** Primary Care Sports Medicine; Running Injuries; Pain-Back; **Hospital:** Mt Sinai Med Ctr (page 102); **Address:** 24 W 57th St, Ste 509, New York, NY 10019-3918; **Phone:** 212-765-5763; **Board Cert:** Sports Medicine 1991; **Med School:** Emory Univ 1985; **Resid:** Internal Medicine, Danbury Hosp 1987; Internal Medicine, NY Infirm/Beekman Downtown 1989; **Fellow:** Sports Medicine, Pascack Valley Hosp 1990; **Fac Appt:** Asst Clin Prof Med, Mount Sinai Sch Med

Metzl, Jordan D MD (SM) - **Spec Exp:** Adolescent Sports Medicine; Running Injuries; Dance/Ballet Injuries; **Hospital:** Hosp For Special Surgery (page 113); **Address:** 519 E 72nd St, Ste 206, New York, NY 10021; **Phone:** 212-606-1678; **Board Cert:** Sports Medicine 2012; **Med School:** Univ MO-Columbia Sch Med 1993; **Resid:** Pediatrics, Tufts-New Engl Med Ctr 1996; **Fellow:** Sports Medicine, Vanderbilt Univ Med Ctr 1997; Sports Medicine, Harvard Med Sch 1998; **Fac Appt:** Assoc Prof Ped, Cornell Univ-Weill Med Coll

Nisonson, Barton MD (SM) - **Spec Exp:** Shoulder & Knee Surgery; Arthroscopic Surgery; Knee Replacement; **Hospital:** Lenox Hill Hosp (page 106); **Address:** Lenox Hill Hosp, Orthopaedics, 130 E 77th St Fl 8, New York, NY 10021; **Phone:** 212-570-9120; **Board Cert:** Orthopaedic Surgery 1974; **Med School:** Columbia P&S 1966; **Resid:** Surgery, NY-Presby/Columbia Univ Med Ctr 1968; Orthopaedic Surgery, NY-Presby/Columbia Univ Med Ctr 1973

Noy, Ron MD (SM) - **Spec Exp:** Knee Ligament Reconstruction; Knee Injuries/ACL/Meniscus Tears; Arthroscopic Surgery; Rotator Cuff Surgery; **Hospital:** Beth Israel Med Ctr - Petrie Div (page 94); **Address:** Prestige Orthopaedics/Sports Medicine, 424 Madison Ave Fl 9, New York, NY 10017; **Phone:** 646-862-0180; **Board Cert:** Orthopaedic Surgery 2003; Orthopaedic Sports Medicine 2008; **Med School:** UMDNJ-NJ Med Sch, Newark 1991; **Resid:** Orthopaedic Surgery, Kingsbrook Jewish Med Ctr 2000; **Fellow:** Orthopaedic Sports Medicine, Indiana Univ 2001

Rodeo, Scott A MD (SM) - **Spec Exp:** Knee Injuries; Cartilage Damage; Shoulder Surgery; **Hospital:** Hosp For Special Surgery (page 113); **Address:** HSS, Sports Med Dept, 535 E 70th St, New York, NY 10021; **Phone:** 212-606-1513; **Board Cert:** Orthopaedic Surgery 2009; Orthopaedic Sports Medicine 2007; **Med School:** Cornell Univ-Weill Med Coll 1989; **Resid:** Orthopaedic Surgery, Hosp Special Surgery 1994; **Fellow:** Sports Medicine, Hosp Special Surgery 1996; **Fac Appt:** Prof OrS, Cornell Univ-Weill Med Coll

Rokito, Andrew MD (SM) - **Spec Exp:** Shoulder & Elbow Surgery; Rotator Cuff Surgery; Knee Injuries/ACL; **Hospital:** NYU Hosp For Joint Dis (page 108); **Address:** NYU, Musculoskeletal Care, 333 E 38 St Fl 4, New York, NY 10016; **Phone:** 646-501-7223; **Board Cert:** Orthopaedic Surgery 2007; **Med School:** Boston Univ 1988; **Resid:** Orthopaedic Surgery, NYU Hosp Joint Diseases 1993; **Fellow:** Sports Medicine, Kerlan-Jobe Orthopaedic Clin 1994; **Fac Appt:** Assoc Prof OrS, NYU Sch Med

Roth, Neil S MD (SM) - **Spec Exp:** Shoulder Surgery; Rotator Cuff Surgery; Knee Surgery; Fractures; **Hospital:** Lenox Hill Hosp (page 106), White Plains Hosp (page 640); **Address:** Lenox Hill Hospital, 130 E 77th St, 8th Fl - Black Hall, New York, NY 10075; **Phone:** 212-861-2300; **Board Cert:** Orthopaedic Surgery 2001; Orthopaedic Sports Medicine 2008; **Med School:** Duke Univ 1991; **Resid:** Orthopaedic Surgery, Columbia Presby Med Ctr 1997; **Fellow:** Sports Medicine, Kerlan-Jobe Ortho Clin 1999

Seneviratne, Aruna M MD (SM) - **Spec Exp:** Shoulder Surgery; Rotator Cuff Surgery; Elbow Surgery; Knee Surgery; **Hospital:** Lenox Hill Hosp (page 106); **Address:** 800A Fifth Ave at 61st St, Ste 300, New York, NY 10075; **Phone:** 212-960-8887; **Board Cert:** Orthopaedic Surgery 2007; Orthopaedic Sports Medicine 2008; **Med School:** NY Med Coll 1995; **Resid:** Surgery, Lenox Hill Hosp 1997; Orthopaedic Surgery, Hosp for Special Surgery 2003; **Fellow:** Orthopaedic Sports Medicine, Lenox Hill Hosp 2004

Wickiewicz, Thomas MD (SM) - **Spec Exp:** Knee Injuries/ACL; Shoulder Surgery; **Hospital:** Hosp For Special Surgery (page 113); **Address:** HSS, Orthopaedic Surgery, 535 E 70 St, New York, NY 10021; **Phone:** 212-606-1450; **Board Cert:** Orthopaedic Surgery 1984; **Med School:** UMDNJ-NJ Med Sch, Newark 1976; **Resid:** Surgery, NY-Presby/Weill Cornell Med Ctr 1978; Orthopaedic Surgery, Hosp Special Surgery 1982

Williams III, Riley J MD (SM) - **Spec Exp:** Cartilage Damage & Transplant; Shoulder Arthroscopic Surgery; Knee Injuries/ACL; Knee Surgery; **Hospital:** Hosp For Special Surgery (page 113), NY-Presby/Weill Cornell Med Ctr, NY (page 104); **Address:** HSS, Rheumatology Dept, 535 E 70th St, New York, NY 10021; **Phone:** 212-606-1855; **Board Cert:** Orthopaedic Sports Medicine 2012; Orthopaedic Surgery 2012; **Med School:** Stanford Univ 1992; **Resid:** Orthopaedic Surgery, Hosp Special Surgery 1997; **Fellow:** Sports Medicine & Shoulder Surgery, Hosp Special Surgery 1998; **Fac Appt:** Assoc Prof OrS, Cornell Univ-Weill Med Coll

Surgery

Allen, Peter J MD (S) - **Spec Exp:** Pancreatic Cancer; Pancreatic Surgery; Liver Cancer; Gastrointestinal Cancer; **Hospital:** Meml Sloan-Kettering Canc Ctr (page 114); **Address:** Meml Sloan-Kettering Cancer Ctr, 1275 York Ave, New York, NY 10065; **Phone:** 212-639-5132; **Board Cert:** Surgery 2012; **Med School:** Dartmouth Med Sch 1993; **Resid:** Surgery, Walter Reed Army Med Ctr 1999; **Fellow:** Surgical Oncology, Meml Sloan Kettering Cancer Ctr 2004

Amory, Spencer E MD (S) - **Spec Exp:** Laparoscopic Surgery; Gastrointestinal Surgery; Hernia; **Hospital:** NY-Presby Hosp/The Allen Hosp (page 104); **Address:** 5141 Broadway, Ste 3-178, New York, NY 10034; **Phone:** 212-305-5221; **Board Cert:** Surgery 2010; **Med School:** Johns Hopkins Univ 1983; **Resid:** Surgery, NY-Presby/Columbia Univ Med Ctr 1989; **Fellow:** Emergency Medicine, Peninsula Hosp 1990; **Fac Appt:** Assoc Clin Prof S, Columbia P&S

Attiyeh, Fadi F MD (S) - **Spec Exp:** Colon & Rectal Cancer; Hepatobiliary Surgery; Pancreatic Surgery; **Hospital:** St. Luke's - Roosevelt Hosp Ctr - Roosevelt Div (page 94); **Address:** 425 W 59th St, Ste 8B-1, New York, NY 10019; **Phone:** 212-307-1144; **Board Cert:** Surgery 1975; Colon & Rectal Surgery 1982; **Med School:** Amer Univ Beirut 1969; **Resid:** Surgery, Amer Univ Hosp 1973; **Fellow:** Surgical Oncology, Meml Sloan Kettering Canc Ctr 1976; **Fac Appt:** Clin Prof S, Columbia P&S

Axelrod, Deborah MD (S) - **Spec Exp:** Breast Cancer & Surgery; **Hospital:** NYU Langone Med Ctr (page 108); **Address:** NYU, Cancer Ctr, 160 E 34th St Fl 3, New York, NY 10016; **Phone:** 212-731-5366; **Board Cert:** Surgery 2008; **Med School:** Israel 1982; **Resid:** Surgery, Beth Israel Med Ctr 1988; **Fellow:** Surgical Oncology, Meml Sloan-Kettering Cancer Ctr 1986; **Fac Appt:** Assoc Prof S, NYU Sch Med

Barie, Philip MD (S) - **Spec Exp:** Trauma; Critical Care; Hernia; Gastrointestinal Surgery; **Hospital:** NY-Presby/Weill Cornell Med Ctr, NY (page 104); **Address:** NY-Presby, Surgery Dept, 525 E 68th St, Box 116, New York, NY 10065; **Phone:** 212-746-5401; **Board Cert:** Surgery 2004; Surgical Critical Care 2005; **Med School:** Boston Univ 1977; **Resid:** Surgery, NY-Presby/Weill Cornell Med Ctr 1984; **Fellow:** Trauma, Albany Med Coll Affil Hosp 1981; **Fac Appt:** Prof S, Cornell Univ-Weill Med Coll

Berman, Russell S MD (S) - **Spec Exp:** Melanoma; **Hospital:** NYU Langone Med Ctr (page 108); **Address:** NYU Clin Canc Ctr, 160 E 34th St Fl 9, New York, NY 10016; **Phone:** 212-731-5415; **Board Cert:** Surgery 2007; **Med School:** NYU Sch Med 1990; **Resid:** Surgery, NYU Med Ctr/Bellevue Hosp 1997; **Fellow:** Surgical Oncology, Meml Sloan Kettering Canc Ctr 1994; Surgical Oncology, UT MD Anderson Canc Ctr 2000; **Fac Appt:** Asst Prof S, NYU Sch Med

Bernik, Stephanie F MD (S) - **Spec Exp:** Breast Cancer & Surgery; Breast Disease; Phyllodes Tumors; Angiosarcoma; **Hospital:** Lenox Hill Hosp (page 106); **Address:** Lenox Hill Hosp - Dept Surgery, 100 E 77th St Wollman Bldg Fl 3, New York, NY 10075; **Phone:** 212-434-6900; **Board Cert:** Surgery 2011; **Med School:** Yale Univ 1993; **Resid:** Surgery, St Vincents Hosp 1999; **Fellow:** Breast Surgery, Meml Sloan Kettering Canc Ctr 2000

Bessey, Palmer Q MD (S) - **Spec Exp:** Burn Care; Wound Healing/Care; Trauma; **Hospital:** NY-Presby/Weill Cornell Med Ctr, NY (page 104); **Address:** NY-Presby, Burn Ctr, 525 E 68th St Fl 7, New York, NY 10065; **Phone:** 212-746-0242; **Board Cert:** Surgery 2011; Surgical Critical Care 2005; **Med School:** Univ VT Coll Med 1975; **Resid:** Surgery, UAB Hosp 1981; **Fellow:** Nutrition & Metabolism, Brigham & Womens Hosp 1983; **Fac Appt:** Prof S, Cornell Univ-Weill Med Coll

Bessler, Marc MD (S) - **Spec Exp:** Obesity/Bariatric Surgery; Laparoscopic Surgery; Gastrointestinal Metabolic Surgery; Natural Orifice Surgery (NOTES); **Hospital:** NY-Presby/Columbia Univ Med Ctr, NY (page 104), Valley Hosp (page 721); **Address:** NY-Presby, Surgery Dept, 161 Fort Washington Ave, rm 524, New York, NY 10032; **Phone:** 212-305-9506; **Board Cert:** Surgery 2007; **Med School:** NYU Sch Med 1989; **Resid:** Surgery, NY-Presby/Columbia Univ Med Ctr 1995; **Fac Appt:** Clin Prof S, Columbia P&S

Bloom, Norman D MD (S) - **Spec Exp:** Breast Cancer; Sarcoma; Cancer Surgery; **Hospital:** Beth Israel Med Ctr - Petrie Div (page 94), NYU Langone Med Ctr (page 108); **Address:** The Gramercy, 61 Irving Place, Ste LL-B, New York, NY 10003; **Phone:** 212-505-6167; **Board Cert:** Surgery 2010; **Med School:** SUNY Downstate 1974; **Resid:** Surgery, Maimonides Med Ctr 1978; **Fellow:** Surgical Oncology, Meml Sloan Kettering Canc Ctr 1979; **Fac Appt:** Clin Prof S, NYU Sch Med

Boolbol, Susan K MD (S) - **Spec Exp:** Breast Cancer; Breast Surgery; Sentinel Node Surgery; **Hospital:** Beth Israel Med Ctr - Petrie Div (page 94); **Address:** 10 Union Square East, Ste 4E, New York, NY 10003; **Phone:** 212-844-6231; **Board Cert:** Surgery 2011; **Med School:** Geo Wash Univ 1994; **Resid:** Surgery, New York Hosp 2000; **Fellow:** Breast Surgery, Meml Sloan Kettering Cancer Ctr 2001

Brady, Mary Sue MD (S) - **Spec Exp:** Melanoma; Merkel Cell Carcinoma; Sarcoma-Soft Tissue; **Hospital:** Meml Sloan-Kettering Canc Ctr (page 114); **Address:** 1275 York Ave, rm H1211, New York, NY 10065; **Phone:** 212-639-8347; **Board Cert:** Surgery 2009; **Med School:** Univ Miami Sch Med 1983; **Resid:** Surgery, NY Hosp-Cornell Med Ctr 1988; **Fellow:** Surgical Oncology, Meml Sloan-Kettering Cancer Ctr 1990; Immunology, Meml Sloan-Kettering Cancer Ctr 1992; **Fac Appt:** Assoc Prof S, Cornell Univ-Weill Med Coll

Cassell, Lauren S MD (S) - **Spec Exp:** Breast Surgery; Breast Cancer; Nipple Sparing Mastectomy; **Hospital:** Lenox Hill Hosp (page 106); **Address:** 114A E 78th St, New York, NY 10075; **Phone:** 212-535-4040; **Board Cert:** Surgery 2003; **Med School:** NY Med Coll 1977; **Resid:** Surgery, Lenox Hill Hosp 1982

Chabot, John A MD (S) - **Spec Exp:** Liver & Biliary Surgery; Pancreatic Cancer; Pancreatic Surgery; Thyroid & Parathyroid Surgery; **Hospital:** NY-Presby/Columbia Univ Med Ctr, NY (page 104); **Address:** NY Presby-Columbia Medical Ctr, 161 Ft Washington Ave Fl 8 - Ste 819, New York, NY 10032; **Phone:** 212-305-9468; **Board Cert:** Surgery 2010; **Med School:** Dartmouth Med Sch 1983; **Resid:** Surgery, Columbia-Presby Med Ctr 1990; **Fac Appt:** Prof S, Columbia P&S

Cioroiu, Michael G MD (S) - **Spec Exp:** Breast Disease; Wound Healing/Care; Endoscopy; **Hospital:** Mount Sinai Hosp of Queens (page 102), Beth Israel Med Ctr - Petrie Div (page 94); **Address:** 247 3rd Ave, Ste L 3, New York, NY 10010-7453; **Phone:** 212-995-8099; **Board Cert:** Surgery 2004; **Med School:** Romania 1971; **Resid:** Surgery, Cabrini Med Ctr 1985; **Fac Appt:** Assoc Clin Prof S, Mount Sinai Sch Med

Coit, Daniel G MD (S) - **Spec Exp:** Melanoma; Pancreatic Cancer; Stomach Cancer; **Hospital:** Meml Sloan-Kettering Canc Ctr (page 114); **Address:** 1275 York Avenue, Dept Surgery, New York, NY 10065; **Phone:** 212-639-8411; **Board Cert:** Surgery 2004; **Med School:** Univ Cincinnati 1976; **Resid:** Internal Medicine, New Eng Deaconess Hosp 1978; Surgery, New Eng Deaconess Hosp 1983; **Fellow:** Surgical Oncology, Meml Sloan Kettering Canc Ctr 1985; **Fac Appt:** Prof S, Cornell Univ-Weill Med Coll

DeMatteo, Ronald P MD (S) - **Spec Exp:** Liver Cancer; Gallbladder & Biliary Cancer; Pancreatic Cancer; Pancreatic Surgery; **Hospital:** Meml Sloan-Kettering Canc Ctr (page 114); **Address:** MSKCC, Surgery Dept, 1275 York Ave, rm C896, New York, NY 10065; **Phone:** 212-639-5726; **Board Cert:** Surgery 2008; **Med School:** Cornell Univ-Weill Med Coll 1990; **Resid:** Surgery, Hosp U Penn 1997; **Fellow:** Surgical Oncology, Meml Sloan-Kettering Cancer Ctr 1999; **Fac Appt:** Prof S, Cornell Univ-Weill Med Coll

El-Tamer, Mahmoud B MD (S) - **Spec Exp:** Breast Cancer; **Hospital:** Meml Sloan-Kettering Canc Ctr (page 114); **Address:** Meml Sloan Kettering Canc Ctr, 300 E 66th St, New York, NY 10065; **Phone:** 646-888-4753; **Board Cert:** Surgery 2001; **Med School:** Amer Univ Beirut 1981; **Resid:** Surgery, American Univ Hosp 1985; Surgery, SUNY Downstate Med Ctr 1992; **Fellow:** Surgical Oncology, Meml Sloan Kettering Canc Ctr 1989; **Fac Appt:** Assoc Prof S, Columbia P&S

Emond, Jean C MD (S) - **Spec Exp:** Transplant-Liver; Liver Cancer; Liver & Biliary Cancer; Hepatobiliary Surgery; **Hospital:** NY-Presby/Columbia Univ Med Ctr, NY (page 104); **Address:** 622 W 168th St, PH - Fl 14, New York, NY 10032; **Phone:** 212-305-9691; **Board Cert:** Surgery 2006; **Med School:** Univ Chicago-Pritzker Sch Med 1979; **Resid:** Surgery, Cook Cty Hosp 1984; **Fellow:** Surgery, Hopital P Brousse/Univ de Paris Sud 1985; Transplant Surgery, Univ Chicago Hosps 1987; **Fac Appt:** Prof S, Columbia P&S

Estabrook, Alison MD (S) - **Spec Exp:** Breast Cancer; Breast Surgery; Breast Cancer-High Risk Women; **Hospital:** St. Luke's - Roosevelt Hosp Ctr - Roosevelt Div (page 94); **Address:** Comprehensive Breast Center, 425 W 59th St Fl 7 - Ste 7A, New York, NY 10019-1104; **Phone:** 212-523-7500; **Board Cert:** Surgery 2004; **Med School:** NYU Sch Med 1978; **Resid:** Surgery, Columbia Presby Med Ctr 1984; **Fellow:** Surgical Oncology, Columbia Presby Med Ctr 1982; **Fac Appt:** Prof S, Columbia P&S

Fahey III, Thomas J MD (S) - **Spec Exp:** Endocrine Surgery; Pheochromocytoma; Pancreatic Cancer; Minimally Invasive Surgery; **Hospital:** NY-Presby/Weill Cornell Med Ctr, NY (page 104); **Address:** NY Presby Cornell Med Ctr, Dept Surgery, 525 E 68 St, rm Starr 8, Box 249, New York, NY 10065; **Phone:** 212-746-5130; **Board Cert:** Surgery 2002; **Med School:** Cornell Univ-Weill Med Coll 1986; **Resid:** Surgery, New York Hosp 1992; **Fellow:** Endocrine Surgery, Royal North Shore Hosp 1993; **Fac Appt:** Prof S, Cornell Univ-Weill Med Coll

Feldman, Sheldon M MD (S) - **Spec Exp:** Breast Surgery; Breast Cancer; Complementary Medicine; **Hospital:** NY-Presby/Columbia Univ Med Ctr, NY (page 104); **Address:** NY-Presby-Columbia Univ Med Ctr, Div Surgical Oncology, 161 Fort Washington Ave, Fl 10, Ste 1005, New York, NY 10032; **Phone:** 212-305-9676; **Board Cert:** Surgery 2011; **Med School:** NYU Sch Med 1975; **Resid:** Surgery, Bellevue Hosp Ctr 1980; **Fellow:** Peripheral Vascular Surgery, Beth Israel Med Ctr 1981; **Fac Appt:** Assoc Clin Prof S, Columbia P&S

Fong, Yuman MD (S) - **Spec Exp:** Pancreatic Cancer; Liver & Biliary Cancer; Stomach Cancer; **Hospital:** Meml Sloan-Kettering Canc Ctr (page 114); **Address:** 1275 York Ave, rm C887, New York, NY 10065; **Phone:** 212-639-2016; **Board Cert:** Surgery 2002; **Med School:** Cornell Univ-Weill Med Coll 1984; **Resid:** Surgery, NY Hosp-Cornell Med Ctr 1992; **Fellow:** Surgical Oncology, Meml Sloan-Kettering Cancer Ctr 1994; **Fac Appt:** Prof S, Cornell Univ-Weill Med Coll

Geller, Peter MD (S) - **Spec Exp:** Gastrointestinal Surgery; Hernia; **Hospital:** NY-Presby/Columbia Univ Med Ctr, NY (page 104); **Address:** Columbia Doctors Midtown, 51 W 51st St, #380, New York, NY 10019; **Phone:** 212-326-5547; **Board Cert:** Surgery 2011; **Med School:** Columbia P&S 1980; **Resid:** Surgery, Columbia-Presby Med Ctr 1985; **Fellow:** Vascular Surgery, Columbia-Presby Med Ctr 1986; **Fac Appt:** Assoc Prof S, Columbia P&S

Goldfarb, Alisan B MD (S) - **Spec Exp:** Breast Surgery; Breast Cancer; Sentinel Node Surgery; **Hospital:** Mt Sinai Med Ctr (page 102); **Address:** 1185 Park Ave, Ste 1A, New York, NY 10128; **Phone:** 212-987-5000; **Board Cert:** Surgery 2011; **Med School:** Mount Sinai Sch Med 1975; **Resid:** Surgery, Mt Sinai Med Ctr 1980; **Fac Appt:** Asst Clin Prof S, Mount Sinai Sch Med

Gouge, Thomas H MD (S) - **Spec Exp:** Esophageal Cancer; Pancreatic Cancer; Gastroesophageal Reflux Disease (GERD); **Hospital:** VA NY Harbor Hlthcare Sys-Manhattan Campus, NYU Langone Med Ctr (page 108); **Address:** 423 E 23rd St Fl 6, New York, NY 10010; **Phone:** 212-951-3366; **Board Cert:** Surgery 2007; **Med School:** Yale Univ 1970; **Resid:** Surgery, NYU Med Ctr 1975; **Fac Appt:** Prof S, NYU Sch Med

Heerdt, Alexandra S MD (S) - **Spec Exp:** Breast Cancer; **Hospital:** Meml Sloan-Kettering Canc Ctr (page 114); **Address:** Meml Sloan-Kettering Canc Ctr, 300 E 66th St, New York, NY 10065; **Phone:** 646-888-5253; **Board Cert:** Surgery 2012; **Med School:** Jefferson Med Coll 1987; **Resid:** Surgery, NY Hosp-Cornell Med Ctr 1992; **Fellow:** Surgical Oncology, Meml Sloan Kettering Canc Ctr 1993

Heller, Keith S MD (S) - **Spec Exp:** Thyroid & Parathyroid Surgery; Minimally Invasive Surgery; Endocrine Surgery; **Hospital:** NYU Langone Med Ctr (page 108); **Address:** NYU Langone Med Ctr, Dept Surgery, 530 First Ave, Ste 6H, New York, NY 10016; **Phone:** 212-263-7710; **Board Cert:** Surgery 2006; **Med School:** NYU Sch Med 1971; **Resid:** Surgery, NYU Langone Med Ctr-Bellevue Hosp 1976; **Fellow:** Surgical Oncology, Meml Sloan Kettering Canc Ctr 1977; **Fac Appt:** Prof S, NYU Sch Med

Herron, Daniel M MD (S) - **Spec Exp:** Obesity/Bariatric Surgery; Laparoscopic Surgery; Endoscopic Surgery; **Hospital:** Mt Sinai Med Ctr (page 102); **Address:** 17 E 102nd St, CAM Bldg - Fl 5, New York, NY 10029; **Phone:** 212-824-7891; **Board Cert:** Surgery 2008; **Med School:** Univ Pennsylvania 1992; **Resid:** Surgery, New England Med Ctr 1998; **Fellow:** Laparoscopic Surgery, Oregon Univ Hlth Sci Ctr 1999; **Fac Appt:** Prof S, Mount Sinai Sch Med

Hiotis, Spiros P MD/PhD (S) - **Spec Exp:** Liver Cancer; Gallbladder & Biliary Cancer; Pancreatic Cancer; Stomach Cancer; **Hospital:** Mt Sinai Med Ctr (page 102); **Address:** Surgical Oncology Assocs, 1470 Madison Ave Fl 3rd, New York, NY 10029; **Phone:** 212-241-2891; **Board Cert:** Surgery 2010; **Med School:** Univ MD Sch Med 1992; **Resid:** Surgery, USF Med Ctr 1998; **Fellow:** Surgical Oncology, Meml Sloan Kettering Cancer Ctr 2000; **Fac Appt:** Assoc Prof S, Mount Sinai Sch Med

Inabnet, William B MD (S) - **Spec Exp:** Thyroid Surgery; Adrenal Surgery; Pancreatic Surgery; Minimally Invasive Surgery; **Hospital:** Mt Sinai Med Ctr (page 102); **Address:** 5 E 98th St Fl 15, Box 1259, New York, NY 10029; **Phone:** 212-241-6918; **Board Cert:** Surgery 2007; **Med School:** Univ NC Sch Med 1991; **Resid:** Surgery, Rush Univ Med Ctr 1996; **Fellow:** Endocrine Surgery, Cochin Hosp 1997; **Fac Appt:** Prof S, Columbia P&S

Jacob, Brian P MD (S) - **Spec Exp:** Hernia; Obesity/Bariatric Surgery; Laparoscopic Surgery; **Hospital:** Mt Sinai Med Ctr (page 102); **Address:** 1010 Fifth Ave, New York, NY 10028; **Phone:** 212-879-6677; **Board Cert:** Surgery 2005; **Med School:** Wayne State Univ 1998; **Resid:** Surgery, Mt Sinai Sch Med 2004; **Fellow:** Minimally Invasive Surgery, NY Presby/Columbia Med Ctr 2005; **Fac Appt:** Assoc Clin Prof S, Mount Sinai Sch Med

Jarnagin, William MD (S) - **Spec Exp:** Hepatobiliary Surgery; Liver Cancer; Pancreatic Cancer; Gallbladder & Biliary Cancer; **Hospital:** Meml Sloan-Kettering Canc Ctr (page 114); **Address:** 1275 York Ave, Dept Surgery, New York, NY 10065; **Phone:** 212-639-7601; **Board Cert:** Surgery 2006; **Med School:** Rush Med Coll 1988; **Resid:** Surgery, UCSF Med Ctr 1996; **Fellow:** Hepatopancreatobiliary Surgery, Meml Sloan-Kettering Cancer Ctr 1997; **Fac Appt:** Prof S, Cornell Univ

Kapur, Sandip MD (S) - **Spec Exp:** Transplant-Kidney; Transplant-Pancreas; **Hospital:** NY-Presby/Weill Cornell Med Ctr, NY (page 104); **Address:** 525 E 68th St, Baker Bldg Fl 19 - Ste F1919, Box 98, New York, NY 10065; **Phone:** 212-746-5330; **Board Cert:** Surgery 2007; **Med School:** Cornell Univ-Weill Med Coll 1990; **Resid:** Surgery, Cornell Univ Med Ctr 1996; **Fellow:** Research, The Rogosin Inst 1994; Transplant Surgery, Thomas E Starzl Transplant Inst 1998; **Fac Appt:** Assoc Prof S, Cornell Univ-Weill Med Coll

Karpeh Jr, Martin S MD (S) - **Spec Exp:** Gastrointestinal Cancer; Esophageal Cancer; Pancreatic Cancer; Liver Cancer; **Hospital:** Beth Israel Med Ctr - Petrie Div (page 94); **Address:** Beth Israel Medical Center, Philips Ambulatory Care Center, 10 Union Square E, Ste 4D, New York, NY 10003; **Phone:** 212-420-4041; **Board Cert:** Surgery 2006; **Med School:** Penn State Coll Med 1983; **Resid:** Surgery, Hosp Univ Penn 1989; **Fellow:** Surgical Oncology, Meml Sloan Kettering Cancer Ctr 1991; **Fac Appt:** Prof S, Mount Sinai Sch Med

Kato, Tomoaki MD (S) - **Spec Exp:** Transplant-Liver; Transplant Surgery-Pediatric; Transplant-Multi Organ; Transplant-Auto Transplantation; **Hospital:** NY-Presby/Columbia Univ Med Ctr, NY (page 104); **Address:** Columbia Univ Med Ctr, 622 W 168th St PH 14 Bldg - rm 105, New York, NY 10032; **Phone:** 212-305-5101; **Med School:** Japan 1991; **Resid:** Surgery, Itami City Hospital 1995; **Fellow:** Transplant Surgery, Jackson Meml Hosp 1997; **Fac Appt:** Prof S, Columbia P&S

Katz, Lester Brian MD (S) - **Spec Exp:** Laparoscopic Abdominal Surgery; Esophageal Surgery; Hernia; **Hospital:** Mt Sinai Med Ctr (page 102); **Address:** 1010 Fifth Ave, New York, NY 10028; **Phone:** 212-879-6677; **Board Cert:** Surgery 2001; **Med School:** South Africa 1975; **Resid:** Surgery, Mount Sinai Hosp 1982; **Fac Appt:** Assoc Clin Prof S, Mount Sinai Sch Med

Kimmelstiel, Fred M MD (S) - **Spec Exp:** Laparoscopic Surgery; Breast Surgery; Cancer Surgery; Hernia; **Hospital:** St. Luke's - Roosevelt Hosp Ctr - Roosevelt Div (page 94); **Address:** 225 W 71st St, New York, NY 10023; **Phone:** 212-362-6060; **Board Cert:** Surgery 2006; **Med School:** NY Med Coll 1980; **Resid:** Surgery, St. Luke's - Roosevelt Hosp Ctr - St Luke's Hosp 1985; **Fellow:** Transplant Surgery, Stony Brook Univ Med Ctr 1986; **Fac Appt:** Asst Clin Prof S, Columbia P&S

Kini, Subhash U MD (S) - **Spec Exp:** Obesity/Bariatric Surgery; Laparoscopic Surgery; **Hospital:** Mt Sinai Med Ctr (page 102); **Address:** Mount Sinai, Bariatric Surgery, 17 E 102 St Fl 5, New York, NY 10029; **Phone:** 212-241-8958; **Board Cert:** Surgery 2004; **Med School:** India 1986; **Resid:** Surgery, Our Lady Mercy Med Ctr 2003; **Fellow:** Bariatric Surgery, NY Med Coll 2004; **Fac Appt:** Asst Prof S, Mount Sinai Sch Med

Labow, Daniel M MD (S) - **Spec Exp:** Pancreatic Cancer; Gastrointestinal Cancer; Liver Cancer; **Hospital:** Mt Sinai Med Ctr (page 102); **Address:** 1 Gustave L Levy Pl, Box 1259, New York, NY 10029; **Phone:** 212-241-2891; **Board Cert:** Surgery 2003; **Med School:** Brown Univ 1995; **Resid:** Surgery, Univ Chicago Affil Hosps 1997; Research, NY-Presby/Weill Cornell Med Ctr 1999; **Fellow:** Surgical Oncology, Sloan Kettering Canc Ctr 2004; **Fac Appt:** Asst Prof S, Mount Sinai Sch Med

Lee, James A MD (S) - **Spec Exp:** Adrenal Surgery; Endocrine Cancers; Thyroid & Parathyroid Cancer & Surgery; Pancreatic Surgery; **Hospital:** NY-Presby/Columbia Univ Med Ctr, NY (page 104); **Address:** Columbia Univ Med Ctr, Irving Pavilion, 161 Fort Washington Ave, rm 808, New York, NY 10032; **Phone:** 212-305-0444; **Board Cert:** Surgery 2005; **Med School:** Columbia P&S 1999; **Resid:** Surgery, NY Presby Hosp 2005; Research, NY Presby Hosp 2003; **Fellow:** Endocrine Surgery, UCSF Med Ctr 2006; **Fac Appt:** Assoc Prof S, Columbia P&S

Leitman, I Michael MD (S) - **Spec Exp:** Hernia; Obesity/Bariatric Surgery; Laparoscopic Surgery; **Hospital:** Beth Israel Med Ctr - Petrie Div (page 94), Lenox Hill Hosp (page 106); **Address:** BIMC, Surgery Dept, 10 Union Square E, Ste 2M, New York, NY 10003; **Phone:** 212-844-8570; **Board Cert:** Surgery 2009; Surgical Critical Care 2010; **Med School:** Boston Univ 1985; **Resid:** Surgery, NY-Presby/Weill Cornell Med Ctr 1990; **Fellow:** Surgical Critical Care, N Shore Univ Hosp 1991; **Fac Appt:** Prof S, Albert Einstein Coll Med

Lieberman, Michael D MD (S) - **Spec Exp:** Gastrointestinal Cancer; Colon & Rectal Cancer & Surgery; Hepatobiliary Surgery; Pancreatic Cancer; **Hospital:** NY-Presby/Weill Cornell Med Ctr, NY (page 104); **Address:** 1315 York Ave, Box 216, New York, NY 10021; **Phone:** 212-746-5434; **Board Cert:** Surgery 2003; **Med School:** UMDNJ-NJ Med Sch, Newark 1985; **Resid:** Surgery, Hosp Univ Penn 1992; **Fellow:** Surgical Oncology, Hosp Univ Penn 1990; Surgical Oncology, Meml Sloan Kettering Cancer Ctr 1994; **Fac Appt:** Assoc Prof S, Cornell Univ-Weill Med Coll

McGinty Jr, James J MD (S) - **Spec Exp:** Laparoscopic Surgery; Minimally Invasive Surgery; Obesity/Bariatric Surgery; **Hospital:** St. Luke's - Roosevelt Hosp Ctr - Roosevelt Div (page 94), St. Luke's - Roosevelt Hosp Ctr - St Luke's Hosp (page 94); **Address:** 1111 Amsterdam Ave Fl 4 - Ste 4W, New York, NY 10025; **Phone:** 212-636-1000; **Board Cert:** Surgery ; **Med School:** Drexel Univ Coll Med 1997; **Resid:** Surgery, Allegheny Genl Hosp 2003; **Fellow:** Minimally Invasive Surgery, NY-Presby/Columbia Univ Med Ctr 2006; **Fac Appt:** Asst Clin Prof S, Columbia P&S

Michelassi, Fabrizio MD (S) - **Spec Exp:** Gastrointestinal Cancer; Crohn's Disease; Ulcerative Colitis; Colon Cancer; **Hospital:** NY-Presby/Weill Cornell Med Ctr, NY (page 104); **Address:** 525 E 68th St, Fl 7, rm F-739, Box 129, New York, NY 10065; **Phone:** 212-746-6006; **Board Cert:** Surgery 2002; **Med School:** Italy 1975; **Resid:** Surgery, NYU Med Ctr 1981; **Fellow:** Research, Mass Genl Hosp 1983; **Fac Appt:** Prof S, Cornell Univ-Weill Med Coll

Mills, Christopher B MD (S) - **Spec Exp:** Breast Cancer; Breast Surgery; **Hospital:** Beth Israel Med Ctr - Petrie Div (page 94); **Address:** 325 W 15th St, New York, NY 10011; **Phone:** 212-604-6006; **Board Cert:** Surgery 2009; **Med School:** UMDNJ-NJ Med Sch, Newark 1973; **Resid:** Surgery, St Vincent's Hosp 1978; **Fellow:** Nutrition & Metabolism, Ravenswood Hosp Med Ctr 1979

Morrow, Monica MD (S) - **Spec Exp:** Breast Cancer; **Hospital:** Meml Sloan-Kettering Canc Ctr (page 114); **Address:** 300 E 66th St, Fl 4, New York, NY 10065; **Phone:** 646-888-5354; **Board Cert:** Surgery 2011; **Med School:** Jefferson Med Coll 1976; **Resid:** Surgery, Med Ctr Hosp Vermont 1981; **Fellow:** Surgical Oncology, Meml Sloan Kettering Cancer Ctr 1983; **Fac Appt:** Prof S, Cornell Univ-Weill Med Coll

Newman, Elliot MD (S) - **Spec Exp:** Gastrointestinal Cancer; Robotic Surgery; Liver & Biliary Cancer; Colon & Rectal Cancer; **Hospital:** NYU Langone Med Ctr (page 108); **Address:** NYU Clinical Cancer Ctr, 160 E 34th St Fl 9, New York, NY 10016; **Phone:** 212-731-5466; **Board Cert:** Surgery 2004; **Med School:** NYU Sch Med 1986; **Resid:** Surgery, NYU Langone Med Ctr 1993; **Fellow:** Research, Meml Sloan-Kettering Cancer Ctr 1991; Surgical Oncology, Meml Sloan-Kettering Cancer Ctr 1995; **Fac Appt:** Assoc Prof S, NYU Sch Med

Nowak, Eugene J MD (S) - **Spec Exp:** Breast Cancer; Hernia; Sentinel Node Surgery; Gastrointestinal Surgery; **Hospital:** NY-Presby/Weill Cornell Med Ctr, NY (page 104); **Address:** 325 E 79th St, Ground Fl, New York, NY 10075-0954; **Phone:** 212-517-6693; **Board Cert:** Surgery 2012; **Med School:** UMDNJ-NJ Med Sch, Newark 1975; **Resid:** Surgery, New York Hosp 1980; **Fac Appt:** Asst Clin Prof S, Cornell Univ-Weill Med Coll

Pachter, H Leon MD (S) - **Spec Exp:** Gastrointestinal Surgery; Pancreatic Cancer; Colon Cancer; Minimally Invasive Surgery; **Hospital:** NYU Langone Med Ctr (page 108); **Address:** 530 1st Ave, Ste 6C, New York, NY 10016; **Phone:** 212-263-7302; **Board Cert:** Surgery 2009; **Med School:** NYU Sch Med 1971; **Resid:** Surgery, NYU Med Ctr 1976; **Fac Appt:** Prof S, NYU Sch Med

Paty, Philip B MD (S) - **Spec Exp:** Colon & Rectal Cancer; Gastrointestinal Cancer; Pelvic Tumors; **Hospital:** Meml Sloan-Kettering Canc Ctr (page 114); **Address:** 1275 York Avenue, Dept Surgery, New York, NY 10065; **Phone:** 212-639-6703; **Board Cert:** Surgery 2011; **Med School:** Stanford Univ 1983; **Resid:** Surgery, UCSF Med Ctr 1990; **Fellow:** Surgical Oncology, Meml Sloan Kettering Cancer Ctr 1992; **Fac Appt:** Prof S, Cornell Univ-Weill Med Coll

Pomp, Alfons MD (S) - **Spec Exp:** Obesity/Bariatric Surgery; Laparoscopic Abdominal Surgery; Hernia; **Hospital:** NY-Presby/Weill Cornell Med Ctr, NY (page 104); **Address:** NY-Presby, Surgery Dept, 525 E 68th St, Box 294, New York, NY 10065; **Phone:** 212-746-5294; **Board Cert:** Surgery 2010; **Med School:** Univ Sherbrooke 1980; **Resid:** Surgery, Univ Montreal Med Ctr 1985; **Fellow:** Nutrition, Rhode Island Hosp 1988; **Fac Appt:** Prof S, Cornell Univ-Weill Med Coll

Port, Elisa R MD (S) - **Spec Exp:** Breast Cancer & Surgery; Sentinel Node Surgery; Nipple Sparing Mastectomy; Breast Cancer-Male; **Hospital:** Mt Sinai Med Ctr (page 102); **Address:** 1176 5th Ave, Fl 1, Dubin Breast Ctr, New York, NY 10029; **Phone:** 212-241-3806; **Board Cert:** Surgery 2011; **Med School:** Mount Sinai Sch Med 1992; **Resid:** Surgery, Cedars Sinai Med Ctr 1995; Surgery, LIJ Med Ctr 1997; **Fac Appt:** Assoc Prof S, Mount Sinai Sch Med

Ratner, Lloyd E MD (S) - **Spec Exp:** Transplant-Kidney; Transplant-Pancreas; Pancreatic Surgery; **Hospital:** NY-Presby/Columbia Univ Med Ctr, NY (page 104); **Address:** NY-Presby/Columbia Univ Med Ctr, 622 W 168th St PH Bldg - rm 14-408, New York, NY 10032; **Phone:** 212-305-6469; **Board Cert:** Surgery 2009; **Med School:** Hahnemann Univ 1983; **Resid:** Surgery, Long Is Jewish Med Ctr 1988; **Fellow:** Transplant Surgery, Barnes-Jewish Hosp 1990; **Fac Appt:** Assoc Prof S, Columbia P&S

Reiner, Mark A MD (S) - **Spec Exp:** Laparoscopic Surgery; Hernia; Esophageal Surgery; Pancreatic Surgery; **Hospital:** Mt Sinai Med Ctr (page 102); **Address:** Laparoscopic Surgical Ctr, 1010 5th Ave, New York, NY 10028; **Phone:** 212-879-6677; **Board Cert:** Surgery 2011; **Med School:** SUNY Downstate 1974; **Resid:** Surgery, Mount Sinai Med Ctr 1979; **Fac Appt:** Assoc Clin Prof S, Mount Sinai Sch Med

Rosenberg, Vladimiro MD (S) - **Spec Exp:** Breast Cancer; Melanoma; Thyroid & Parathyroid Surgery; Sarcoma-Soft Tissue; **Hospital:** Mt Sinai Med Ctr (page 102), Lenox Hill Hosp (page 106); **Address:** 1440 York Ave, Ste P-10, New York, NY 10075; **Phone:** 212-772-0010; **Med School:** Argentina 1965; **Resid:** Surgery, Mt Sinai Hosp 1977; **Fellow:** Surgical Oncology, MD Anderson Cancer Ctr 1978; **Fac Appt:** Asst Clin Prof S, Mount Sinai Sch Med

Roses, Daniel F MD (S) - **Spec Exp:** Breast Cancer; Melanoma; Thyroid & Parathyroid Surgery; **Hospital:** NYU Langone Med Ctr (page 108); **Address:** NYU, Surgery Dept, 530 1 Ave, Ste 6B, New York, NY 10016; **Phone:** 212-263-7329; **Board Cert:** Surgery 1975; **Med School:** NYU Sch Med 1969; **Resid:** Surgery, NYU-Bellevue Hosp 1974; **Fellow:** Surgical Oncology, NYU-Bellevue Hosp 1978; **Fac Appt:** Prof S, NYU Sch Med

Salky, Barry A MD (S) - **Spec Exp:** Laparoscopic Abdominal Surgery; Gastroesophageal Reflux Disease (GERD); Colon Cancer; Ulcerative Colitis; **Hospital:** Mt Sinai Med Ctr (page 102); **Address:** Mount Sinai Med Ctr, Surgery Dept, 5 E 98th St Fl 14 - Ste C, Box 1259, New York, NY 10029; **Phone:** 212-241-6156; **Board Cert:** Surgery 2010; **Med School:** Univ Tenn Coll Med 1970; **Resid:** Surgery, Mount Sinai Med Ctr 1973; Surgery, Mount Sinai Med Ctr 1978; **Fac Appt:** Prof S, Mount Sinai Sch Med

Schnabel, Freya MD (S) - **Spec Exp:** Breast Cancer; Breast Cancer-High Risk Women; **Hospital:** NYU Langone Med Ctr (page 108); **Address:** 160 E 34th St Fl 3, NYU Clinical Cancer Ctr, New York, NY 10016; **Phone:** 212-731-5367; **Board Cert:** Surgery 2008; **Med School:** NYU Sch Med 1982; **Resid:** Surgery, NYU Med Ctr 1987; **Fellow:** Research, SUNY Hlth Sci Ctr 1988; **Fac Appt:** Prof S, NYU Sch Med

Schwartz, Myron E MD (S) - **Spec Exp:** Gastrointestinal Cancer; Liver Cancer; Hepatobiliary Surgery; Transplant-Liver; **Hospital:** Mt Sinai Med Ctr (page 102); **Address:** Mount Sinai Med Ctr, 5 E 98th St Fl 12, Box 1104, New York, NY 10029; **Phone:** 212-659-8084; **Board Cert:** Surgery 2009; **Med School:** Jefferson Med Coll 1976; **Resid:** Surgery, Mt Sinai Hosp 1986; Vascular Surgery, Mt Sinai Hosp 1987; **Fac Appt:** Prof S, Mount Sinai Sch Med

Shah, Jatin P MD/PhD (S) - **Spec Exp:** Head & Neck Cancer & Surgery; Thyroid Cancer; Skull Base Tumors; Salivary Gland Tumors & Surgery; **Hospital:** Meml Sloan-Kettering Canc Ctr (page 114); **Address:** 1275 York Ave, New York, NY 10065; **Phone:** 646-497-9161; **Board Cert:** Surgery 1975; **Med School:** India 1964; **Resid:** Surgery, SSG Hosp 1967; Surgery, NY Eye & Ear Infirm 1974; **Fellow:** Head & Neck Surgical Oncology, Meml Sloan-Kettering Hosp 1972; **Fac Appt:** Prof S, Cornell Univ-Weill Med Coll

Shah, Paresh C MD (S) - **Spec Exp:** Laparoscopic Surgery; Obesity/Bariatric Surgery; Minimally Invasive Surgery; **Hospital:** NYU Langone Med Ctr (page 108); **Address:** NYU Langone Med Ctr - Dept Surgery, 530 First Ave, Ste 6C, New York, NY 10016; **Phone:** 212-263-7302; **Board Cert:** Surgery 2010; **Med School:** SUNY Downstate 1991; **Resid:** Surgery, SUNY- Downstate Med Ctr 1993; Surgery, Mass Genl Hosp 1995; **Fellow:** Laparoscopic Surgery, Lahey Clin 1999

Shapiro, Richard L MD (S) - **Spec Exp:** Breast Cancer; Melanoma; Thyroid & Parathyroid Surgery; Cancer Surgery; **Hospital:** NYU Langone Med Ctr (page 108); **Address:** NYU Medical Clinical Cancer Center, 160 E 34th St Fl 4, New York, NY 10016; **Phone:** 212-731-5347; **Board Cert:** Surgery 2004; **Med School:** NYU Sch Med 1988; **Resid:** Surgery, NYU Langone Med Ctr 1993; **Fellow:** Surgical Oncology, NYU Langone Med Ctr 1995; **Fac Appt:** Assoc Prof S, NYU Sch Med

Simmons, Rache M MD (S) - **Spec Exp:** Breast Cancer; Breast Surgery; **Hospital:** NY-Presby/Weill Cornell Med Ctr, NY (page 104); **Address:** Weill Cornell Breast Ctr, 425 E 61st St Fl 10, New York, NY 10065; **Phone:** 212-821-0853; **Board Cert:** Surgery 2005; **Med School:** Duke Univ 1988; **Resid:** Surgery, Univ NC Hosp 1993; **Fellow:** Surgical Oncology, NY Hosp-Cornell Hosp 1994; **Fac Appt:** Assoc Prof S, Cornell Univ-Weill Med Coll

Singer, Samuel MD (S) - **Spec Exp:** Sarcoma-Soft Tissue; Gastrointestinal Stromal Tumors; **Hospital:** Meml Sloan-Kettering Canc Ctr (page 114); **Address:** MSCC, GMT Surgery Dept, 1275 York Ave, Ste H1210, New York, NY 10065; **Phone:** 646-497-9072; **Board Cert:** Surgery 2010; **Med School:** Harvard Med Sch 1982; **Resid:** Surgery, Brigham & Womens Hosp 1988; **Fellow:** Surgical Oncology, Dana Farber Cancer Inst 1990; **Fac Appt:** Assoc Prof S, Cornell Univ-Weill Med Coll

Slater, Gary I MD (S) - **Spec Exp:** Vascular Surgery; **Hospital:** Mt Sinai Med Ctr (page 102); **Address:** 5 E 98th St Fl 3, New York, NY 10029-6501; **Phone:** 212-241-9281; **Board Cert:** Surgery 1975; **Med School:** NYU Sch Med 1968; **Resid:** Surgery, Mt Sinai Med Ctr 1974; **Fac Appt:** Prof S, Mount Sinai Sch Med

Swistel, Alexander J MD (S) - **Spec Exp:** Breast Cancer & Surgery; Cancer Reconstruction; Nipple Sparing Mastectomy; **Hospital:** NY-Presby/Weill Cornell Med Ctr, NY (page 104), St. Luke's - Roosevelt Hosp Ctr - Roosevelt Div (page 94); **Address:** 425 E 61st St, Fl 10, New York, NY 10065; **Phone:** 212-821-0602; **Board Cert:** Surgery 2005; **Med School:** Brown Univ 1975; **Resid:** Surgery, St Luke's Roosevelt Hosp Ctr 1981; **Fellow:** Surgical Oncology, Meml Sloan Kettering Canc Ctr 1983; **Fac Appt:** Assoc Clin Prof S, Cornell Univ-Weill Med Coll

Tartter, Paul I MD (S) - **Spec Exp:** Breast Cancer; Breast Cancer in Elderly; Sentinel Node Surgery; **Hospital:** St. Luke's - Roosevelt Hosp Ctr - Roosevelt Div (page 94); **Address:** Comprehensive Breast Center, 425 W 59th St, Ste 7A, New York, NY 10019-1104; **Phone:** 212-523-7500; **Board Cert:** Surgery 2011; **Med School:** Brown Univ 1977; **Resid:** Surgery, Mt Sinai Hosp 1982; **Fac Appt:** Assoc Prof S, Columbia P&S

Teperman, Lewis W MD (S) - **Spec Exp:** Transplant-Liver; Transplant-Kidney; Liver Cancer; Hepatobiliary Surgery; **Hospital:** NYU Langone Med Ctr (page 108); **Address:** NYU Transplant Associates, 403 E 34th St Fl 3, New York, NY 10016; **Phone:** 212-263-8134; **Board Cert:** Surgery 2007; **Med School:** Mount Sinai Sch Med 1981; **Resid:** Surgery, Columbia Presby Med Ctr 1984; Surgery, LI Jewish Med Ctr 1986; **Fellow:** Transplant Surgery, Univ Pittsburgh Med Ctr 1988; **Fac Appt:** Assoc Prof S, NYU Sch Med

Van Zee, Kimberly J MD (S) - **Spec Exp:** Breast Cancer; **Hospital:** Meml Sloan-Kettering Canc Ctr (page 114); **Address:** Meml Sloan Kettering Cancer Ctr, Evelyn H Lauder Breast Center, 300 E 66th St, New York, NY 10065; **Phone:** 646-888-5241; **Board Cert:** Surgery 2003; **Med School:** Harvard Med Sch 1987; **Resid:** Surgery, NY Hosp-Cornell Univ Med Ctr 1990; Surgery, NY Hosp-Cornell Univ Med Ctr 1994; **Fellow:** Research, NY Hosp-Cornell Univ Med Ctr 1993; **Fac Appt:** Prof S, Cornell Univ-Weill Med Coll

Vine, Anthony J MD (S) - **Spec Exp:** Laparoscopic Abdominal Surgery; Gastroesophageal Reflux Disease (GERD); Colon & Rectal Surgery; **Hospital:** Mt Sinai Med Ctr (page 102); **Address:** 1010 5th Ave, New York, NY 10028-0130; **Phone:** 212-879-6677; **Board Cert:** Surgery 2009; **Med School:** Vanderbilt Univ 1989; **Resid:** Surgery, Mt Sinai Med Ctr 1996; **Fellow:** Colon & Rectal Surgery, Mass Genl Hosp 1994; **Fac Appt:** Asst Clin Prof S, Mount Sinai Sch Med

Wallack, Marc MD (S) - **Spec Exp:** Melanoma; Breast Surgery; **Hospital:** Metropolitan Hosp Ctr - NY; **Address:** 1901 1st Ave, rm 12A-1, New York, NY 10029; **Phone:** 212-423-6614; **Board Cert:** Surgery 2011; **Med School:** Univ Pittsburgh 1970; **Resid:** Surgery, Hosp Univ Penn - UPHS 1976; **Fellow:** Medical Oncology, Wistar Inst Anatomy & Biology 1977; **Fac Appt:** Prof S, NY Med Coll

Wedderburn, Raymond V MD (S) - **Spec Exp:** Trauma; **Hospital:** St. Luke's - Roosevelt Hosp Ctr - Roosevelt Div (page 94); **Address:** 1111 Amsterdam Ave Muhlenberg Bldg, Fl 2 - Ste M2 Section D, New York, NY 10025; **Phone:** 212-523-5295; **Board Cert:** Surgery 2012; Surgical Critical Care 2003; **Med School:** Cornell Univ-Weill Med Coll 1986; **Resid:** Surgery, St Luke's - Roosevelt Hosp Ctr 1991; **Fellow:** Surgical Critical Care, Jackson Meml Hosp 1993; **Fac Appt:** Asst Clin Prof S, Columbia P&S

Yurt, Roger W MD (S) - **Spec Exp:** Burn Care; Wound Healing/Care; Hyperbaric Medicine; Critical Care; **Hospital:** NY-Presby/Weill Cornell Med Ctr, NY (page 104); **Address:** NY-Presby, Burn Ctr, 525 E 68th St, rm L706, New York, NY 10021; **Phone:** 212-746-5410; **Board Cert:** Surgery 2008; **Med School:** Univ Miami Sch Med 1972; **Resid:** Surgery, Parkland Meml Hosp 1974; Surgery, NY-Presby/Weill Cornell Med Ctr 1980; **Fellow:** Internal Medicine, Brigham & Womens Hosp 1978; **Fac Appt:** Prof S, Cornell Univ-Weill Med Coll

Zarnegar, Rasa MD (S) - **Spec Exp:** Minimally Invasive Surgery; Endocrine Surgery; Gallbladder & Biliary Disease; Stomach Cancer; **Hospital:** NY-Presby/Weill Cornell Med Ctr, NY (page 104); **Address:** 525 E 68th St, Starr Bldg Fl 8, New York, NY 10065; **Phone:** 212-746-5130; **Board Cert:** Surgery 2006; **Med School:** Univ Chicago-Pritzker Sch Med 1999; **Resid:** Surgery, Univ Chicago Affil Hosps 2003; Surgery, Case West Res Univ Affil Hosps 2005; **Fellow:** Endocrine Surgery, UCSF Med Ctr 2006; Minimally Invasive Surgery, UCSF Med Ctr 2006; **Fac Appt:** Asst Prof S, Cornell Univ-Weill Med Coll

Thoracic & Cardiac Surgery

Adams, David H MD (T&CS) - **Spec Exp:** Mitral Valve Surgery; Heart Valve Surgery; Minimally Invasive Cardiac Surgery; Aortic Surgery; **Hospital:** Mt Sinai Med Ctr (page 102); **Address:** Mount Sinai, Cardiothoracic Surgery, 1190 5th Ave, New York, NY 10029; **Phone:** 212-659-6820; **Board Cert:** Thoracic & Cardiac Surgery 2003; **Med School:** Duke Univ 1983; **Resid:** Surgery, Brigham & Women's Hosp 1990; Thoracic & Cardiac Surgery, Brigham & Women's Hosp/Chldn's Hosp 1992; **Fellow:** Research, Harvard Med Sch 1988; Surgery, Brigham & Women's Hosp 1992; **Fac Appt:** Prof T&CS, Mount Sinai Sch Med

Altorki, Nasser K MD (T&CS) - **Spec Exp:** Esophageal Cancer; Lung Cancer; Thoracic Cancers; **Hospital:** NY-Presby/Weill Cornell Med Ctr, NY (page 104); **Address:** 525 E 68th St, M-404, New York, NY 10065; **Phone:** 212-746-5156; **Board Cert:** Surgery 2006; Thoracic Surgery 2007; **Med School:** Egypt 1978; **Resid:** Surgery, Univ Chicago Hosps 1985; **Fellow:** Cardiothoracic Surgery, Univ Chicago Hosps 1987; **Fac Appt:** Prof S, Cornell Univ-Weill Med Coll

Argenziano, Michael MD (T&CS) - **Spec Exp:** Robotic Cardiac Surgery; Coronary Artery Surgery; Maze Procedure for Atrial Fibrillation; **Hospital:** NY-Presby/Columbia Univ Med Ctr, NY (page 104); **Address:** NY Presby Med Ctr, Milstein Bldg, 177 Fort Washington Ave, rm 7-435, New York, NY 10032; **Phone:** 212-305-5888; **Board Cert:** Thoracic & Cardiac Surgery 2013; **Med School:** Columbia P&S 1992; **Resid:** Surgery, Columbia Presby Med Ctr 1998; **Fellow:** Cardiothoracic Surgery, Columbia Presby Med Ctr 1999; **Fac Appt:** Asst Prof S, Columbia P&S

Bacha, Emile A MD (T&CS) - **Spec Exp:** Pediatric Cardiac Surgery; Congenital Heart Disease; Neonatal & Infant Cardiac Surgery; Minimally Invasive Cardiac Surgery; **Hospital:** NY-Presby/Columbia Univ Med Ctr, NY (page 104), Morgan Stanley Children's Hosp of NY-Presby, NY (page 104); **Address:** NY-Presby, Ped Cardiothoracic Surgery, 3959 Broadway, rm 276, New York, NY 10032; **Phone:** 212-305-2688; **Board Cert:** Thoracic & Cardiac Surgery 2009; Congenital Cardiac Surgery 2009; **Med School:** Germany 1989; **Resid:** Thoracic Surgery, Mass Genl Hosp 1993; Surgery, Emory Univ Med Ctr 1995; **Fellow:** Pediatric Cardiac Surgery, Hosp Marie Lanne Longe 1996; Pediatric Cardiac Surgery, Mass Genl Hosp 1998; **Fac Appt:** Prof S, Columbia P&S

Bains, Manjit MD (T&CS) - **Spec Exp:** Cardiothoracic Surgery; Esophageal Cancer; Lung Cancer; **Hospital:** Meml Sloan-Kettering Canc Ctr (page 114); **Address:** 1275 York Ave, rm C861, New York, NY 10065; **Phone:** 212-639-7450; **Board Cert:** Surgery 1971; Thoracic Surgery 1972; **Med School:** India 1963; **Resid:** Surgery, Rochester Genl Hosp 1970; **Fellow:** Thoracic Surgery, Sloan Kettering Cancer Ctr 1972; **Fac Appt:** Clin Prof S, Cornell Univ-Weill Med Coll

Bhora, Faiz Y MD (T&CS) - **Spec Exp:** Lung Cancer; Esophageal Cancer; Thoracic Cancers; Robotic Surgery; **Hospital:** St. Luke's - Roosevelt Hosp Ctr - Roosevelt Div (page 94); **Address:** 325 W 15th St, New York, NY 10011; **Phone:** 212-523-7475; **Board Cert:** Thoracic Surgery 2004; **Med School:** Pakistan 1992; **Resid:** Surgery, George Washington Univ Med Ctr 2000; Cardiothoracic Surgery, UCLA Med Ctr 2002; **Fellow:** Transplant Surgery, UCLA Med Ctr 2004; Thoracic Oncology, Hosp U Penn 2005; **Fac Appt:** Assoc Clin Prof S, Columbia P&S

Chen, Jonathan M MD (T&CS) - **Spec Exp:** Pediatric Cardiothoracic Surgery; Arrhythmias; Congenital Heart Disease-Adult & Child; **Hospital:** Morgan Stanley Children's Hosp of NY-Presby, NY (page 104), NY-Presby/Weill Cornell Med Ctr, NY (page 104); **Address:** NY-Presby, Cardiothoracic Surgery, 525 E 68th St, Ste M404, New York, NY 10065; **Phone:** 212-746-5014; **Board Cert:** Thoracic & Cardiac Surgery 2011; Congenital Cardiac Surgery 2010; **Med School:** Columbia P&S 1994; **Resid:** Surgery, NY-Presby/Columbia Univ Med Ctr 2000; **Fellow:** Cardiothoracic Surgery, NY-Presby/Columbia Univ Med Ctr 2001; **Fac Appt:** Prof Ped, Columbia P&S

Connery, Cliff MD (T&CS) - **Spec Exp:** Thoracic Cancers; Mediastinal Tumors; Minimally Invasive Surgery; Lung Cancer; **Hospital:** St. Luke's - Roosevelt Hosp Ctr - Roosevelt Div (page 94), Beth Israel Med Ctr - Petrie Div (page 94); **Address:** 325 W 15th St, Main Floor, Area J, New York, NY 10011; **Phone:** 212-523-7475; **Board Cert:** Surgery 2010; Thoracic & Cardiac Surgery 2013; Surgical Critical Care 2003; **Med School:** Eastern VA Med Sch 1984; **Resid:** Surgery, Stony Brook Univ Med Ctr 1989; Thoracic Surgery, Strong Meml Hosp 1992; **Fac Appt:** Asst Prof S, Columbia P&S

Crawford, Bernard MD (T&CS) - **Spec Exp:** Lung Cancer; Minimally Invasive Surgery; Esophageal Cancer; **Hospital:** NYU Langone Med Ctr (page 108); **Address:** 160 E 34th St, Fl 8, New York, NY 10016; **Phone:** 212-731-5580; **Board Cert:** Thoracic & Cardiac Surgery 2009; **Med School:** Geo Wash Univ 1980; **Resid:** Surgery, NYU Langone Med Ctr 1985; **Fellow:** Cardiothoracic Surgery, NYU Langone Med Ctr 1987; **Fac Appt:** Asst Prof TS, NYU Sch Med

Culliford III, Alfred T MD (T&CS) - **Spec Exp:** Mitral Valve Minimally Invasive Surgery; Coronary Artery Surgery; **Hospital:** NYU Langone Med Ctr (page 108); **Address:** NYU Langone Med Ctr, 530 1st Ave, Ste 9V, New York, NY 10016; **Phone:** 212-263-7288; **Board Cert:** Surgery 1975; Thoracic & Cardiac Surgery 2007; **Med School:** NY Med Coll 1969; **Resid:** Surgery, NYU Langone Med Ctr 1974; **Fellow:** Thoracic Surgery, NYU Langone Med Ctr 1976; **Fac Appt:** Prof TS, NYU Sch Med

DeAnda Jr, Abelardo MD (T&CS) - **Spec Exp:** Aneurysm-Aortic; Heart Valve Surgery; Cardiothoracic Surgery; Marfan's Syndrome; **Hospital:** NYU Langone Med Ctr (page 108), Bellevue Hosp Ctr; **Address:** NYU Medical Ctr, Cardiothoracic Surgery, 530 First Ave, Ste 9V, New York, NY 10016; **Phone:** 212-263-6516; **Board Cert:** Thoracic Surgery 2011; **Med School:** Stanford Univ 1990; **Resid:** Surgery, Stanford Med Ctr 1997; **Fellow:** Cardiothoracic Surgery, Stanford Med Ctr 2000; Cardiothoracic Research, Stanford Med Ctr 1994; **Fac Appt:** Assoc Prof TS, NYU Sch Med

Downey, Robert J MD (T&CS) - **Spec Exp:** Lung Cancer; Thoracic Cancers; **Hospital:** Meml Sloan-Kettering Canc Ctr (page 114); **Address:** 1275 York Avenue, New York, NY 10065; **Phone:** 212-639-8124; **Board Cert:** Surgery 2002; Surgical Critical Care 2006; Thoracic & Cardiac Surgery 2005; **Med School:** Columbia P&S 1985; **Resid:** Surgery, Columbia-Presby Med Ctr 1991; **Fellow:** Thoracic Surgery, Mayo Clinic 1992; Thoracic Surgery, Columbia-Presby Med Ctr 1994

Filsoufi, Farzan MD (T&CS) - **Spec Exp:** Mitral Valve Surgery; Minimally Invasive Heart Valve Surgery; Heart Valve Surgery; Robotic Cardiac Surgery; **Hospital:** Mt Sinai Med Ctr (page 102); **Address:** Mount Sinai, Cardiothoracic Surgery, 1190 5th Ave Fl 2, Box 1028, New York, NY 10029; **Phone:** 212-659-6813; **Med School:** France 1991; **Resid:** Surgery, Univ Paris Hosps 1994; Thoracic Surgery, Hosp Broussais/Univ Paris 1995; **Fellow:** Cardiothoracic Surgery, Hosp Broussais/Univ Paris 1996; Heart Valve Surgery, Brigham & Womens Hosp 2000; **Fac Appt:** Prof TS, Mount Sinai Sch Med

Flores, Raja M MD (T&CS) - **Spec Exp:** Mesothelioma; Lung Cancer; Video Assisted Thoracic Surgery (VATS); Esophageal Cancer; **Hospital:** Mt Sinai Med Ctr (page 102); **Address:** Mt Sinai Medical Ctr, 1190 Fifth Ave, Box 1028, New York, NY 10029; **Phone:** 212-241-9466; **Board Cert:** Surgery 2009; Thoracic & Cardiac Surgery 2010; **Med School:** Albert Einstein Coll Med 1992; **Resid:** Surgery, Columbia Presby Med Ctr 1997; **Fellow:** Thoracic Surgery, Brigham & Womens Hosp/Dana Faber Cancer Inst 2000; **Fac Appt:** Assoc Prof TS, Cornell Univ-Weill Med Coll

Fontana, Gregory MD (T&CS) - **Spec Exp:** Minimally Invasive Surgery; Pediatric Cardiac Surgery; Mitral Valve Surgery; Coronary Artery Surgery; **Hospital:** Lenox Hill Hosp (page 106); **Address:** Lenox Hill Hosp, Cardiothoracic Dept, 130 E 77th St Fl 4, New York, NY 10075; **Phone:** 212-434-3792; **Board Cert:** Thoracic & Cardiac Surgery 2004; **Med School:** UCLA 1984; **Resid:** Surgery, Duke Univ Med Ctr 1989; Thoracic Surgery, Duke Univ Med Ctr 1993; **Fellow:** Pediatric Cardiac Surgery, UCLA Med Ctr 1994; Pediatric Cardiac Surgery, Chldns Hosp 1994

Galloway, Aubrey MD (T&CS) - **Spec Exp:** Minimally Invasive Heart Valve Surgery; Mitral Valve Surgery; Coronary Artery Surgery; Robotic Surgery; **Hospital:** NYU Langone Med Ctr (page 108); **Address:** NYU Med Ctr, Cardiothoracic Surgery, 560 1st Ave, Ste 9V, New York, NY 10016; **Phone:** 212-263-7185; **Board Cert:** Thoracic Surgery 2006; **Med School:** Tulane Univ 1978; **Resid:** Surgery, Univ CO Hlth Sci Ctr 1983; Cardiovascular Surgery, NYU Med Ctr 1985; **Fellow:** Research, Chldns Hosp 1981; Cardiothoracic Surgery, NYU Med Ctr 1985; **Fac Appt:** Prof TS, NYU Sch Med

Ginsburg, Mark E MD (T&CS) - **Spec Exp:** Lung Cancer; Transplant-Lung; Emphysema-Lung Volume Reduction; **Hospital:** NY-Presby/Columbia Univ Med Ctr, NY (page 104), Good Samaritan Regional Med Ctr; **Address:** NY-Presby, Cardiothoracic Surgery, 161 Fort Washington Ave, Ste 301, New York, NY 10032; **Phone:** 212-305-3408; **Board Cert:** Surgery 2005; Thoracic & Cardiac Surgery 2006; **Med School:** Tufts Univ 1980; **Resid:** Surgery, Univ Rochester-Strong Meml Hosp 1985; **Fellow:** Thoracic & Cardiac Surgery, Univ Rochester-Strong Meml Hosp 1987; **Fac Appt:** Assoc Clin Prof S, Columbia P&S

Girardi, Leonard N MD (T&CS) - **Spec Exp:** Aneurysm-Aortic; Cardiac Surgery; Marfan's Syndrome; Aneurysm; **Hospital:** NY-Presby/Weill Cornell Med Ctr, NY (page 104); **Address:** NY-Presby, Cardiothoracic Surgery, 525 E 68th St, Ste M404, New York, NY 10065; **Phone:** 212-746-5194; **Board Cert:** Surgery 2005; Thoracic & Cardiac Surgery 2007; **Med School:** Cornell Univ-Weill Med Coll 1989; **Resid:** Surgery, NY-Presby/Weill Cornell Med Ctr 1994; **Fellow:** Cardiothoracic Surgery, NY-Presby/Weill Cornell Med Ctr 1996; Cardiothoracic Surgery, Baylor Med Ctr 1997; **Fac Appt:** Prof TS, Cornell Univ-Weill Med Coll

Gorenstein, Lyall A MD (T&CS) - **Spec Exp:** Esophageal Surgery; Minimally Invasive Thoracic Surgery; Thoracic Cancers; Hyperhidrosis-Palmar; **Hospital:** NY-Presby/Columbia Univ Med Ctr, NY (page 104), Nyack Hosp; **Address:** Rockland Thoracic & Vascular Assocs, 161 Fort Washington Ave, Irving Pavilion, rm 301, New York, NY 10032; **Phone:** 212-305-3408; **Board Cert:** Surgery 2009; Thoracic Surgery 2013; **Med School:** Univ Toronto 1983; **Resid:** Radiation Therapy, Univ Toronto Affil Hosps 1988; Thoracic Surgery, Univ Toronto Affil Hosps 1992; **Fellow:** Thoracic Surgery, MD Anderson Canc Ctr 1990; **Fac Appt:** Asst Clin Prof S, Columbia P&S

Grossi, Eugene A MD (T&CS) - **Spec Exp:** Minimally Invasive Cardiac Surgery; Mitral Valve Surgery; Cardiac Tumors, Myxomas; **Hospital:** NYU Langone Med Ctr (page 108); **Address:** NYU Med Ctr, Cardiothoracic Surgery, 530 1st Ave, Ste 9V, New York, NY 10016; **Phone:** 212-263-7452; **Board Cert:** Thoracic & Cardiac Surgery 2011; **Med School:** Columbia P&S 1981; **Resid:** Surgery, NYU Med Ctr 1987; Thoracic Surgery, NYU Med Ctr 1991; **Fac Appt:** Prof S, NYU Sch Med

Hoffman, Darryl M MD (T&CS) - **Spec Exp:** Coronary Artery Surgery; Heart Valve Surgery; Atrial Fibrillation; Pacemakers; **Hospital:** Beth Israel Med Ctr - Petrie Div (page 94), St. Luke's - Roosevelt Hosp Ctr - Roosevelt Div (page 94); **Address:** Division of Cardiac Surgery, 317 E 17th St, Fierman Hall, 11th Fl, New York, NY 10003; **Phone:** 212-420-2584; **Med School:** South Africa 1983; **Resid:** Surgery 1989Edinburgh Royal Infirm 1989; **Fellow:** Cardiac Surgery, Allegheny Genl Hosp 1993; Cardiac Surgery, Mayo Clinic 1994; **Fac Appt:** Asst Prof S, Albert Einstein Coll Med

Isom, O. Wayne MD (T&CS) - **Spec Exp:** Cardiac Surgery; Coronary Artery Surgery; Heart Valve Surgery; **Hospital:** NY-Presby/Weill Cornell Med Ctr, NY (page 104), NY Hosp Queens (page 488); **Address:** NY-Presby, Cardiothoracic Surgery, 525 E 68th St, Ste M404, New York, NY 10065; **Phone:** 212-746-5151; **Board Cert:** Surgery 1971; Thoracic Surgery 1972; **Med School:** Univ Tex, Houston 1965; **Resid:** Surgery, Parkland Meml Hosp 1970; **Fellow:** Thoracic Surgery, NYU Med Ctr 1972; **Fac Appt:** Prof TS, Cornell Univ-Weill Med Coll

Jones, David R MD (T&CS) - **Spec Exp:** Lung Cancer; Esophageal Cancer; Minimally Invasive Thoracic Surgery; **Hospital:** Meml Sloan-Kettering Canc Ctr (page 114); **Address:** Meml Sloan-Kettering Canc Ctr, 1275 York Ave, Box 7, New York, NY 10065; **Phone:** 646-497-9163; **Board Cert:** Surgery 2005; Thoracic Surgery 2007; **Med School:** W VA Univ 1989; **Resid:** Surgery, W VA Univ Affil Hosp 1995; **Fellow:** Thoracic Surgery, Univ NC Affil Hosp 1998; **Fac Appt:** Prof S, Cornell Univ-Weill Med Coll

Krellenstein, Daniel J MD/PhD (T&CS) - **Spec Exp:** Lung Cancer; Minimally Invasive Thoracic Surgery; Asbestos-related Lung Disease; **Hospital:** Mt Sinai Med Ctr (page 102), Lenox Hill Hosp (page 106); **Address:** 16 E 98th St, Ste 1F, New York, NY 10029-6545; **Phone:** 212-423-9311; **Board Cert:** Surgery 1974; Thoracic & Cardiac Surgery 2006; **Med School:** SUNY Buffalo 1964; **Resid:** Surgery, SUNY Downstate Med Ctr 1971; **Fellow:** Thoracic & Cardiac Surgery, Kings County Hosp Ctr 1972; **Fac Appt:** Assoc Clin Prof TS, Mount Sinai Sch Med

Krieger, Karl H MD (T&CS) - **Spec Exp:** Heart Valve Surgery; Coronary Artery Surgery; Cardiac Surgery-Adult; **Hospital:** NY-Presby/Weill Cornell Med Ctr, NY (page 104); **Address:** NY-Presby, Cardiothoracic Surgery, 525 E 68th St, Ste M404, New York, NY 10065; **Phone:** 212-746-5152; **Board Cert:** Thoracic & Cardiac Surgery 2004; **Med School:** Johns Hopkins Univ 1975; **Resid:** Surgery, Johns Hopkins Hosp 1976Bellevue Hosp 1979; **Fellow:** Thoracic Surgery, NYU Med Ctr 1981; **Fac Appt:** Prof S, Cornell Univ-Weill Med Coll

Lazzaro, Richard S MD (T&CS) - **Spec Exp:** Thoracic Surgery; Robotic Surgery; Minimally Invasive Surgery; Thoracic Surgery; **Hospital:** Lenox Hill Hosp (page 106), N Shore Univ Hosp (page 106); **Address:** Lenox Hill Hosp, Cardiothoracic Surgery, 130 E 77th St Fl 4, New York, NY 10075; **Phone:** 212-434-3000; **Board Cert:** Surgery 2006; Thoracic & Cardiac Surgery 2007; **Med School:** Albany Med Coll 1988; **Resid:** Surgery, N Shore Univ Hosp 1994; **Fellow:** Cardiothoracic Surgery, Maimonides Med Ctr 1997; Thoracic Surgery, UPMC 1998

Loulmet, Didier F MD (T&CS) - **Spec Exp:** Heart Valve Surgery; Robotic Cardiac Surgery; Minimally Invasive Cardiac Surgery; Aneurysm-Aortic; **Hospital:** NYU Langone Med Ctr (page 108); **Address:** NYU Med Ctr, Cardiothoracic Surgery, 530 1st Ave, Ste 9V, New York, NY 10016; **Phone:** 212-263-2329; **Med School:** France 1984; **Resid:** Cardiothoracic Surgery, Paris Univ Hosp 1990; Cardiothoracic Surgery, Brigham & Womens Hosp 1991; **Fellow:** Pediatric Cardiac Surgery, Chdns Hosp 1992; **Fac Appt:** Assoc Prof TS, NYU Sch Med

Mosca, Ralph S MD (T&CS) - **Spec Exp:** Congenital Heart Disease-Adult & Child; Pediatric Cardiac Surgery; **Hospital:** NYU Langone Med Ctr (page 108); **Address:** 530 1st Ave, Ste 9V, New York, NY 10016; **Phone:** 212-263-5989; **Board Cert:** Thoracic Surgery 2011; **Med School:** SUNY Upstate Med Univ 1985; **Resid:** Surgery, SUNY Hlth Sci Ctr 1990; **Fellow:** Cardiothoracic Surgery, Columbia-Presby Med Ctr 1992; Pediatric Cardiac Surgery, Univ Mich Med Ctr 1993; **Fac Appt:** Prof TS, NYU Sch Med

Naka, Yoshifumi MD/PhD (T&CS) - **Spec Exp:** Transplant-Heart; Ventricular Assist Device (LVAD); Heart Failure & Ventricular Containment; Mitral Valve Surgery; **Hospital:** NY-Presby/Columbia Univ Med Ctr, NY (page 104); **Address:** NY-Presby, Cardiothoracic Surgery, 177 Fort Washington Ave, Ste 7-435, New York, NY 10032; **Phone:** 212-305-0828; **Med School:** Japan 1984; **Resid:** Surgery, Osaka Police Hosp 1991; **Fellow:** Cardiovascular Surgery, Osaka Police Hosp 1993; Cardiothoracic Surgery, NY-Presby/Columbia Univ Med Ctr 1998; **Fac Appt:** Prof S, Columbia P&S

Nguyen, Khanh H MD (T&CS) - **Spec Exp:** Pediatric Cardiac Surgery; Congenital Heart Disease-Adult & Child; **Hospital:** Mt Sinai Med Ctr (page 102); **Address:** Mt Sinai Med Ctr, 1190 5th Ave, Box 1028, New York, NY 10029; **Phone:** 212-659-9472; **Board Cert:** Thoracic Surgery 2006; **Med School:** UC Irvine 1985; **Resid:** Surgery, Flushing Hosp 1992; Thoracic Surgery, Mt Sinai Med Ctr 1995

Oz, Mehmet C MD (T&CS) - **Spec Exp:** Transplant-Heart; Heart Valve Surgery; Minimally Invasive Cardiac Surgery; **Hospital:** NY-Presby/Columbia Univ Med Ctr, NY (page 104); **Address:** NY-Presby, Cardiothoracic Surgery, 177 Fort Washington Ave, Ste 7-435, New York, NY 10032; **Phone:** 212-305-4434; **Board Cert:** Thoracic Surgery 2003; **Med School:** Univ Pennsylvania 1986; **Resid:** Surgery, NY-Presby/Columbia Univ Med Ctr 1991; **Fellow:** Cardiothoracic Surgery, NY-Presby/Columbia Univ Med Ctr 1993; **Fac Appt:** Prof S, Columbia P&S

Pass, Harvey I MD (T&CS) - **Spec Exp:** Lung Cancer; Mesothelioma; Clinical Trials; Robotic Surgery; **Hospital:** NYU Langone Med Ctr (page 108); **Address:** NYU Cancer Ctr, 160 E 34th St, Fl 8, New York, NY 10016; **Phone:** 212-731-5414; **Board Cert:** Thoracic & Cardiac Surgery 2001; **Med School:** Duke Univ 1973; **Resid:** Surgery, Duke Univ Med Ctr 1975; Surgery, Univ Miss Med Ctr 1980; **Fellow:** Cardiothoracic Surgery, MUSC Med Ctr 1982; Thoracic Oncology, Natl Cancer Inst 1985; **Fac Appt:** Prof T&CS, NYU Sch Med

Plestis, Konstadinos MD (T&CS) - **Spec Exp:** Aortic Surgery; Heart Valve Surgery; Aneurysm-Aortic; Aneurysm-Abdominal Aortic; **Hospital:** Lenox Hill Hosp (page 106); **Address:** Lenox Hill, Aortic Wellness Ctr, 130 E 77th St, Fl 4th, New York, NY 10075; **Phone:** 212-434-6030; **Board Cert:** Surgery 2003; Vascular Surgery 2005; Thoracic Surgery 2008; **Med School:** Greece 1987; **Resid:** Surgery, Brooklyn Hosp Ctr 1993; Vascular Surgery, Baylor Univ Med Ctr 1995; **Fellow:** Cardiothoracic Surgery, Montefiore Med Ctr 1999; **Fac Appt:** Asst Prof S, Mount Sinai Sch Med

Port, Jeffrey L MD (T&CS) - **Spec Exp:** Lung Cancer; Esophageal Cancer; **Hospital:** NY-Presby/Weill Cornell Med Ctr, NY (page 104); **Address:** 525 E 68th St, Ste M404, New York, NY 10065; **Phone:** 212-746-5197; **Board Cert:** Surgery 2009; Thoracic & Cardiac Surgery 2009; **Med School:** NYU Sch Med 1991; **Resid:** Surgery, NYU Med Ctr 1998; **Fellow:** Thoracic Surgery, NY Presby Hosp 2000; **Fac Appt:** Assoc Prof TS, Cornell Univ-Weill Med Coll

Rizk, Nabil P MD (T&CS) - **Spec Exp:** Esophageal Cancer; Lung Cancer; Thoracic Cancers; Minimally Invasive Surgery; **Hospital:** Meml Sloan-Kettering Canc Ctr (page 114); **Address:** Meml Sloan-Kettering Cancer Ctr, 1275 York Ave, New York, NY 10021; **Phone:** 212-639-8357; **Board Cert:** Surgery 2009; Thoracic Surgery 2005; **Med School:** Yale Univ 1992; **Resid:** Surgery, Univ PA Hlth Systm 1999; **Fellow:** Thoracic Surgery, NY-Presby Hosp 2004; Thoracic Surgery, Meml Sloan-Kettering Canc Ctr 2005

Rusch, Valerie MD (T&CS) - **Spec Exp:** Mesothelioma; Lung Cancer; Esophageal Cancer; Thoracic Cancers; **Hospital:** Meml Sloan-Kettering Canc Ctr (page 114); **Address:** 1275 York Ave, New York, NY 10021-6094; **Phone:** 212-639-5873; **Board Cert:** Surgery 2011; Thoracic Surgery 2003; **Med School:** Columbia P&S 1975; **Resid:** Surgery, Univ Washington Med Ctr 1980; Cardiothoracic Surgery, Univ Washington Med Ctr 1982; **Fac Appt:** Prof TS, Cornell Univ-Weill Med Coll

Smith Jr, Craig R MD (T&CS) - **Spec Exp:** Mitral Valve Surgery; Minimally Invasive Cardiac Surgery; Robotic Cardiac Surgery; Coronary Artery Surgery; **Hospital:** NY-Presby/Columbia Univ Med Ctr, NY (page 104); **Address:** NY-Presby, Cardiothoracic Surgery, 177 Fort Washington Ave, Ste 7-435, New York, NY 10032; **Phone:** 212-305-8312; **Board Cert:** Thoracic Surgery 2004; **Med School:** Case West Res Univ 1977; **Resid:** Surgery, Univ Rochester-Strong Meml Hosp 1982; **Fellow:** Cardiothoracic Surgery, NY-Presby/Columbia Univ Med Ctr 1984; **Fac Appt:** Prof S, Columbia P&S

Sonett, Joshua R MD (T&CS) - **Spec Exp:** Minimally Invasive Thoracic Surgery; Transplant-Lung; Thoracic Cancers; Emphysema-Lung Volume Reduction; **Hospital:** NY-Presby/Columbia Univ Med Ctr, NY (page 104); **Address:** 161 Fort Washington Ave, Ste 301, New York, NY 10032; **Phone:** 212-305-8086; **Board Cert:** Surgery 2004; Thoracic Surgery 2007; **Med School:** E Carolina Univ 1988; **Resid:** Surgery, Univ Mass Med Ctr 1993; **Fellow:** Cardiothoracic Surgery, Univ Pittsburgh Med Ctr 1994; Thoracic Surgery, Meml Sloan Kettering Cancer Ctr; **Fac Appt:** Prof S, Columbia P&S

Stelzer, Paul MD (T&CS) - **Spec Exp:** Heart Valve Surgery; Aneurysm-Thoracic Aortic; Ross Procedure/Aortic Valve Disease; **Hospital:** Mt Sinai Med Ctr (page 102); **Address:** 1190 5th Ave, Box 1028, New York, NY 10029; **Phone:** 212-659-6871; **Board Cert:** Thoracic Surgery 2013; **Med School:** Columbia P&S 1972; **Resid:** Surgery, St Luke's Roosevelt Hosp 1977; Thoracic Surgery, NY Hosp 1981; **Fac Appt:** Prof T&CS, Mount Sinai Sch Med

Stewart, Allan MD (T&CS) - **Spec Exp:** Heart Valve Surgery-Aortic; Aneurysm-Aortic; Aortic Surgery; **Hospital:** Mt Sinai Med Ctr (page 102); **Address:** Mt Sinai Med Ctr, Guggenheim Pavilion, 1190 5th Ave Fl 2, Cardiothoracic Surgery, New York, NY 10029; **Phone:** 212-659-6800; **Board Cert:** Surgery 2003; Thoracic Surgery 2006; **Med School:** UMDNJ-NJ Med Sch, Newark 1995; **Resid:** Surgery, Hosp Univ Penn 2002; **Fellow:** Thoracic Surgery, NY-Presby/Columbia Univ Med Ctr 2004; **Fac Appt:** Asst Prof TS, Mount Sinai Sch Med

Swistel, Daniel MD (T&CS) - **Spec Exp:** Coronary Artery Surgery; Minimally Invasive Surgery; Heart Valve Surgery; Hypertrophic Cardiomyopathy; **Hospital:** St. Luke's - Roosevelt Hosp Ctr - St Luke's Hosp (page 94); **Address:** St Lukes Hosp, Cardiothoracic Surgery, 111 Amsterdam Ave, Ste A, New York, NY 10025; **Phone:** 212-523-4088; **Board Cert:** Thoracic & Cardiac Surgery 2006; **Med School:** UMDNJ-RW Johnson Med Sch 1979; **Resid:** Surgery, St Lukes Hosp 1984; Cardiothoracic Surgery, Montefiore Med Ctr 1986; **Fac Appt:** Assoc Clin Prof TS, Columbia P&S

Tranbaugh, Robert F MD (T&CS) - **Spec Exp:** Coronary Artery Surgery; Heart Valve Surgery; Aneurysm-Thoracic Aortic; **Hospital:** Beth Israel Med Ctr - Petrie Div (page 94), St. Luke's - Roosevelt Hosp Ctr - Roosevelt Div (page 94); **Address:** Beth Israel Med Ctr, Division of Cardiac Surgery, 317 E 17th St, Fl 11, New York, NY 10003; **Phone:** 212-420-2584; **Board Cert:** Thoracic & Cardiac Surgery 2004; **Med School:** Univ Pennsylvania 1976; **Resid:** Surgery, UCSF Med Ctr 1983; Cardiothoracic Surgery, UCSF Med Ctr 1985; **Fac Appt:** Assoc Clin Prof T&CS, Albert Einstein Coll Med

Williams, Mathew R MD (T&CS) - **Spec Exp:** Interventional Cardiology; Heart Valve Surgery; **Hospital:** NY-Presby/Columbia Univ Med Ctr, NY (page 104); **Address:** NY-Presby, Thoracic & Cardiac Surgery, 177 Fort Washington Ave, 5C-501, New York, NY 10032; **Phone:** 212-342-0444; **Board Cert:** Thoracic Surgery 2007; **Med School:** Columbia P&S 1996; **Resid:** Surgery, Columbia Univ Med Ctr 2003; Cardiothoracic Surgery, Columbia Univ Med Ctr 2005; **Fellow:** Research, Columbia Univ 2001; Interventional Cardiology, Columbia Univ 2006; **Fac Appt:** Asst Prof S, Columbia P&S

Urology

Armenakas, Noel A MD (U) - **Spec Exp:** Genitourinary Reconstruction; Erectile Dysfunction; **Hospital:** Lenox Hill Hosp (page 106), NY-Presby/Weill Cornell Med Ctr, NY (page 104); **Address:** NY Urological Assocs, 880 5th Ave, New York, NY 10021-4951; **Phone:** 212-535-1950; **Board Cert:** Urology 2012; **Med School:** Greece 1985; **Resid:** Urology, Monmouth Med Ctr 1987; Urology, Lenox Hill Hosp 1991; **Fellow:** Trauma, UCSF Med Ctr 1992; Reconstructive Surgery, UCSF Med Ctr 1992; **Fac Appt:** Assoc Clin Prof U, Cornell Univ-Weill Med Coll

Badani, Ketan MD (U) - **Spec Exp:** Robotic Surgery; Prostate Cancer/Robotic Surgery; Minimally Invasive Urologic Surgery; **Hospital:** NY-Presby/Columbia Univ Med Ctr, NY (page 104); **Address:** Herbert Irving Pavillion, 161 Fort Washington Ave Fl 11, New York, NY 10032; **Phone:** 212-305-9722; **Board Cert:** Urology 2009; **Med School:** Case West Res Univ 2001; **Resid:** Urology, Henry Ford Hosp 2005; **Fellow:** Robotic Surgery, Vattikuti Urology Inst 2006; **Fac Appt:** Assoc Prof U, Columbia P&S

Bar-Chama, Natan MD (U) - **Spec Exp:** Infertility-Male; Erectile Dysfunction; Vasectomy Reversal; Varicocele Microsurgery; **Hospital:** Mt Sinai Med Ctr (page 102); **Address:** RMA, Ctr Male Reproductive Hlth, 635 Madison Ave Fl 10, New York, NY 10022; **Phone:** 212-756-5777; **Board Cert:** Urology 2006; **Med School:** Albert Einstein Coll Med 1987; **Resid:** Urology, Montefiore Med Ctr 1993; **Fellow:** Male Infertility, Baylor Med Ctr 1994; **Fac Appt:** Assoc Prof U, Mount Sinai Sch Med

Benson, Mitchell C MD (U) - **Spec Exp:** Prostate Cancer/Robotic Surgery; Bladder Cancer; Kidney Cancer; Continent Urinary Diversions; **Hospital:** NY-Presby/Columbia Univ Med Ctr, NY (page 104); **Address:** 161 Fort Washington Ave, Ste 1102, New York, NY 10032-3713; **Phone:** 212-305-5201; **Board Cert:** Urology 1984; **Med School:** Columbia P&S 1977; **Resid:** Surgery, Mount Sinai Med Ctr 1979; Urology, Columbia-Presby Hosp 1982; **Fellow:** Oncology, Johns Hopkins Hosp 1984; **Fac Appt:** Prof U, Columbia P&S

Berman, Steven M MD (U) - **Spec Exp:** Prostate Cancer; Kidney Stones; **Hospital:** Beth Israel Med Ctr - Petrie Div (page 94); **Address:** Advanced Urology Ctr, 201 E 19th St, New York, NY 10003; **Phone:** 212-673-7300; **Board Cert:** Urology 2006; **Med School:** SUNY Downstate 1981; **Resid:** Surgery, Montefiore Med Ctr 1983; Urology, Montefiore Med Ctr 1986

Birns, Douglas R MD (U) - **Spec Exp:** Prostate Cancer; Kidney Cancer; Bladder Cancer; **Hospital:** Mt Sinai Med Ctr (page 102), Beth Israel Med Ctr - Petrie Div (page 94); **Address:** 157 E 72nd St, Ground Fl, New York, NY 10021-4331; **Phone:** 212-744-8700; **Board Cert:** Urology 2006; **Med School:** SUNY Downstate 1981; **Resid:** Surgery, Mt Sinai Med Ctr 1982; Urology, Mt Sinai Med Ctr 1988; **Fac Appt:** Asst Clin Prof U, Mount Sinai Sch Med

Blaivas, Jerry G MD (U) - **Spec Exp:** Uro-Gynecology; Urology-Female; Neurogenic Bladder; Incontinence after Prostate Cancer; **Hospital:** NY-Presby/Weill Cornell Med Ctr, NY (page 104), Lenox Hill Hosp (page 106); **Address:** UroCenter, 445 E 77th St, New York, NY 10075; **Phone:** 212-772-3900; **Board Cert:** Urology 1978; **Med School:** Tufts Univ 1968; **Resid:** Surgery, Boston Med Ctr 1971; Urology, Tufts Med Ctr 1976; **Fac Appt:** Clin Prof U, Cornell Univ-Weill Med Coll

Bochner, Bernard H MD (U) - **Spec Exp:** Bladder Cancer; Urinary Reconstruction; **Hospital:** Meml Sloan-Kettering Canc Ctr (page 114); **Address:** MSKCC, Dept Urology, 353 E 68 St, New York, NY 10065; **Phone:** 646-422-4387; **Board Cert:** Urology 2011; **Med School:** UCLA 1990; **Resid:** Surgery, LAC & USC Med Ctr 1992; Urology, LAC & USC Med Ctr 1996; **Fellow:** Urologic Oncology, USC/Norris Comp Canc Ctr 1999

Boczko, Stanley MD (U) - **Spec Exp:** Prostate Cancer; Impotence; Prostate Disease; **Hospital:** Montefiore Med Ctr-Moses Campus (page 100), Lenox Hill Hosp (page 106); **Address:** 23 E 79th St, New York, NY 10021; **Phone:** 212-628-1800; **Board Cert:** Urology 1981; **Med School:** Albert Einstein Coll Med 1973; **Resid:** Surgery, Montefiore Med Ctr 1975; Urology, Montefiore Med Ctr 1979; **Fellow:** Transplant Surgery, Montefiore Med Ctr 1975

Brodherson, Michael S MD (U) - **Spec Exp:** Urologic Cancer; Kidney Stones; Concierge Medicine; **Hospital:** Lenox Hill Hosp (page 106); **Address:** 4 E 76th St, New York, NY 10021-2611; **Phone:** 212-794-2749; **Board Cert:** Urology 1981; **Med School:** SUNY Downstate 1973; **Resid:** Internal Medicine, Lenox Hill Hosp 1976; Urology, Lenox Hill Hosp 1979

Coleman, Jonathan A MD (U) - **Spec Exp:** Prostate Cancer; Kidney Cancer; Adrenal Cancer; Minimally Invasive Surgery; **Hospital:** Meml Sloan-Kettering Canc Ctr (page 114); **Address:** 1275 York Ave, New York, NY 10065; **Phone:** 646-422-4432; **Board Cert:** Urology 2006; **Med School:** Cornell Univ-Weill Med Coll 1996; **Resid:** Surgery, NY Presby-Cornell Med Ctr 1998; **Fellow:** Urology, NY Presby-Cornell Med Ctr 2002; Urology, NIH/Natl Cancer Inst 2003

Cooper, Kimberly L MD (U) - **Spec Exp:** Urology-Female; Incontinence-Female; Neuro-Urology; Voiding Dysfunction; **Hospital:** NY-Presby/Columbia Univ Med Ctr, NY (page 104); **Address:** New York Presby/Columbia Univ Med Ctr, Urology Dept, Irving Pavilion, 161 Fort Washington Ave Fl 11, New York, NY 10032; **Phone:** 212-305-0114; **Board Cert:** Urology 2005; **Med School:** Columbia P&S 1997; **Resid:** Urology, NY-Presby/Columbia Univ Med Ctr 2002; **Fellow:** Female Urology, NY-Presby/Columbia Univ Med Ctr 2005; Neurourology, NY-Presby/Columbia Univ Med Ctr 2005; **Fac Appt:** Asst Prof U, Columbia P&S

Del Pizzo, Joseph J MD (U) - **Spec Exp:** Laparoscopic Kidney Surgery; Robotic Surgery; Minimally Invasive Surgery; Kidney Stones; **Hospital:** NY-Presby/Weill Cornell Med Ctr, NY (page 104); **Address:** NY Presby/Cornell Med Ctr, Dept Urology, 525 E 68th St Fl 9 - rm 900, New York, NY 10021; **Phone:** 212-746-5250; **Board Cert:** Urology 2013; **Med School:** Albert Einstein Coll Med 1994; **Resid:** Surgery, Mercy Med Ctr 1996; Urology, Univ of MD Med Ctr 2002; **Fac Appt:** Assoc Prof U, Cornell Univ-Weill Med Coll

Dillon, Robert W MD (U) - **Spec Exp:** Kidney Stones; Urologic Cancer; Urology-Female; **Hospital:** Mt Sinai Med Ctr (page 102); **Address:** 1120 Park Ave, New York, NY 10128; **Phone:** 212-794-9000; **Board Cert:** Urology 1980; **Med School:** NY Med Coll 1973; **Resid:** Surgery, Mt Sinai Hosp 1975; Urology, Mt Sinai Hosp 1978; **Fac Appt:** Asst Clin Prof U, Mount Sinai Sch Med

Dinlenc, Caner Z MD (U) - **Spec Exp:** Kidney Stones; Kidney Cancer; Bladder Cancer; Prostate Cancer; **Hospital:** Beth Israel Med Ctr - Petrie Div (page 94); **Address:** 10 Union Square E, Ste 3A, New York, NY 10003; **Phone:** 212-844-8900; **Board Cert:** Urology 2002; **Med School:** Boston Univ 1993; **Resid:** Urology, Boston Univ Med Ctr 1999; **Fellow:** Endourology, LIJ Med Ctr 2000; **Fac Appt:** Assoc Prof U, Albert Einstein Coll Med

Droller, Michael J MD (U) - **Spec Exp:** Urologic Cancer; Bladder Cancer; Prostate Cancer; Kidney Cancer; **Hospital:** Mt Sinai Med Ctr (page 102); **Address:** 5 E 98th St, Fl 6, Box 1272, New York, NY 10029-6501; **Phone:** 212-241-3868; **Board Cert:** Urology 2001; **Med School:** Harvard Med Sch 1968; **Resid:** Surgery, Peter Bent Brigham Hosp 1970; Urology, Stanford Univ Med Ctr 1976; **Fellow:** Research, Univ Stockholm 1977; **Fac Appt:** Prof U, Mount Sinai Sch Med

Eastham, James A MD (U) - **Spec Exp:** Prostate Cancer; Prostate Cancer/Robotic Surgery; **Hospital:** Meml Sloan-Kettering Canc Ctr (page 114); **Address:** 1275 York Ave, New York, NY 10065; **Phone:** 646-422-4390; **Board Cert:** Urology 2005; **Med School:** USC Sch Med 1987; **Resid:** Urology, LAC & USC Med Ctr 1993

Fine, Eugene M MD (U) - **Spec Exp:** Prostate Cancer; Prostate Disease; Erectile Dysfunction; Kidney Stones; **Hospital:** Mt Sinai Med Ctr (page 102), Lenox Hill Hosp (page 106); **Address:** 12 E 86th St, New York, NY 10028; **Phone:** 212-517-9555; **Board Cert:** Urology 2005; **Med School:** Mexico 1978; **Resid:** Surgery, Downstate Med Ctr Univ Hosp 1981; Urology, Mount Sinai Hosp 1985; **Fac Appt:** Asst Clin Prof U, Mount Sinai Sch Med

Fisch, Harry MD (U) - **Spec Exp:** Infertility-Male; Microsurgery; Vasectomy Reversal; **Hospital:** NY-Presby/Weill Cornell Med Ctr, NY (page 104), Lenox Hill Hosp (page 106); **Address:** 944 Park Ave, Ste 1C, New York, NY 10028; **Phone:** 212-879-0800; **Board Cert:** Urology 2010; **Med School:** Mount Sinai Sch Med 1983; **Resid:** Surgery, Montefiore Med Ctr 1985; Urology, Montefiore Med Ctr 1989; **Fac Appt:** Prof U, Columbia P&S

Fracchia, John MD (U) - **Spec Exp:** Urologic Cancer; **Hospital:** Lenox Hill Hosp (page 106), NY-Presby/Weill Cornell Med Ctr, NY (page 104); **Address:** NY Urological Assocs, 245 E 54th St Fl 2 - Ste 2N, New York, NY 10022; **Phone:** 212-570-6800 x185; **Board Cert:** Urology 1981; **Med School:** UMDNJ-NJ Med Sch, Newark 1973; **Resid:** Urology, NY-Presby/Weill Cornell Med Ctr 1980; **Fac Appt:** Assoc Clin Prof S, Cornell Univ-Weill Med Coll

Goldstein, Marc MD (U) - **Spec Exp:** Infertility-Male; Varicocele Microsurgery; Vasectomy & Vasectomy Reversal; Erectile Dysfunction; **Hospital:** NY-Presby/Weill Cornell Med Ctr, NY (page 104); **Address:** NY-Presby, Reproductive Med, 525 E 68th St, Box 269, New York, NY 10065; **Phone:** 212-746-5470; **Board Cert:** Urology 1982; **Med School:** SUNY Downstate 1972; **Resid:** Surgery, NY-Presby/Columbus Univ Med Ctr 1974; Urology, SUNY Downstate Med Ctr 1980; **Fellow:** Microsurgery, Rockefeller Univ 1982; Reproductive Medicine, Rockefeller Univ 1982; **Fac Appt:** Prof U, Cornell Univ-Weill Med Coll

Grasso III, Michael MD (U) - **Spec Exp:** Urologic Cancer; Laparoscopic Surgery; Kidney Stones; Testicular Cancer; **Hospital:** Lenox Hill Hosp (page 106), Westchester Med Ctr; **Address:** 100 E 77 th St, East Bldg - Fl 4th, New York, NY 10075; **Phone:** 212-434-6300; **Board Cert:** Urology 2013; **Med School:** Jefferson Med Coll 1986; **Resid:** Surgery, Jefferson Univ Hosp 1988; Urology, Jefferson Univ Hosp 1992; **Fac Appt:** Prof U, NY Med Coll

Gribetz, Michael Elliot MD (U) - **Spec Exp:** Prostate Disease; Urology-Female; Sexual Dysfunction; Bladder Cancer; **Hospital:** Mt Sinai Med Ctr (page 102); **Address:** 1155 Park Ave, New York, NY 10128-1209; **Phone:** 212-831-1300; **Board Cert:** Urology 1980; **Med School:** Albert Einstein Coll Med 1973; **Resid:** Surgery, Montefiore Med Ctr 1975; Urology, Mt Sinai Hosp 1978; **Fac Appt:** Asst Clin Prof U, Mount Sinai Sch Med

Gupta, Mantu MD (U) - **Spec Exp:** Kidney Stones; **Hospital:** NY-Presby/Columbia Univ Med Ctr, NY (page 104); **Address:** Columbia Univ Med Ctr - Urology, 161 Fort Washington Ave Fl 11, New York, NY 10032; **Phone:** 212-305-0114; **Board Cert:** Urology 2007; **Med School:** Northwestern Univ 1989; **Resid:** Urology, UCSF Med Ctr 1995; **Fellow:** Endourology, Long Is Jewish Med Ctr 1996; **Fac Appt:** Assoc Prof U, Columbia P&S

Hall, Simon J MD (U) - **Spec Exp:** Urologic Cancer; Minimally Invasive Urologic Surgery; Continent Urinary Diversions; Prostate Cancer; **Hospital:** Mt Sinai Med Ctr (page 102); **Address:** 5 E 98th St, Box 1272, New York, NY 10029; **Phone:** 212-241-4812; **Board Cert:** Urology 2009; **Med School:** Columbia P&S 1988; **Resid:** Surgery, Mt Sinai Med Ctr 1990; Urology, Boston Univ 1994; **Fellow:** Urology, Baylor Coll Med 1996; **Fac Appt:** Assoc Prof U, Mount Sinai Sch Med

Herr, Harry W MD (U) - **Spec Exp:** Bladder Cancer; Prostate Cancer; Testicular Cancer; **Hospital:** Meml Sloan-Kettering Canc Ctr (page 114), NY-Presby/Weill Cornell Med Ctr, NY (page 104); **Address:** 1275 York Avenue, New York, NY 10021; **Phone:** 646-422-4411; **Board Cert:** Urology 1976; **Med School:** UCSF 1969; **Resid:** Urology, UC Irvine Med Ctr 1974; **Fellow:** Urology, Meml Sloan Kettering Cancer Ctr 1976; **Fac Appt:** Assoc Prof S, Cornell Univ-Weill Med Coll

Kaminetsky, Jed C MD (U) - **Spec Exp:** Sexual Dysfunction; Prostate Cancer; Kidney Stones; Prostate Disease; **Hospital:** NYU Langone Med Ctr (page 108); **Address:** Univ Urology, 215 Lexington Ave Fl 20, New York, NY 10016; **Phone:** 212-686-9015; **Board Cert:** Urology 2010; **Med School:** NYU Sch Med 1984; **Resid:** Urology, NYU Langone Med Ctr 1990; **Fac Appt:** Asst Clin Prof U, NYU Sch Med

Kaplan, Steven A MD (U) - **Spec Exp:** Prostate Disease; Voiding Dysfunction; Incontinence after Prostate Cancer; Incontinence; **Hospital:** NY-Presby/Weill Cornell Med Ctr, NY (page 104); **Address:** 425 E 61 St, Fl 12, New York, NY 10065; **Phone:** 646-962-4811; **Board Cert:** Urology 2011; **Med School:** Mount Sinai Sch Med 1982; **Resid:** Surgery, Mount Sinai Hosp 1984; Urology, Columbia Presby Med Ctr 1988; **Fellow:** Urology, Columbia Presby Med Ctr 1990; **Fac Appt:** Prof U, Cornell Univ-Weill Med Coll

Kavaler, Elizabeth MD (U) - **Spec Exp:** Urology-Female; Incontinence; Uro-Gynecology; Pelvic Organ Prolapse Repair; **Hospital:** NY-Presby/Weill Cornell Med Ctr, NY (page 104), Lenox Hill Hosp (page 106); **Address:** NY Urological Assocs, 245 E 54th St, Ste 2N, New York, NY 10022; **Phone:** 212-570-6800; **Board Cert:** Urology 2010; Female Pelvic Medicine & Reconstuctive Surgery ; **Med School:** SUNY Downstate 1992; **Resid:** Urology, Mt Sinai Med Ctr 1998; **Fellow:** Female Urology, UCLA Med Ctr 2000

Kirschenbaum, Alexander M MD (U) - **Spec Exp:** Prostate Cancer; Bladder Cancer; Kidney Cancer; **Hospital:** Mt Sinai Med Ctr (page 102); **Address:** 229 E 79th St, Ste 1A, New York, NY 10075; **Phone:** 646-422-0926; **Board Cert:** Urology 2006; **Med School:** Mount Sinai Sch Med 1980; **Resid:** Surgery, Mt Sinai Hosp 1982; Urology, Mt Sinai Hosp 1985; **Fellow:** Urologic Oncology, Mt Sinai Hosp 1987; **Fac Appt:** Assoc Prof U, Mount Sinai Sch Med

Klein, George MD (U) - **Spec Exp:** Kidney Stones; Sexual Dysfunction; Prostate Cancer; **Hospital:** Mt Sinai Med Ctr (page 102), Lenox Hill Hosp (page 106); **Address:** 157 E 72nd St, Ground Fl, New York, NY 10021; **Phone:** 212-744-8700; **Board Cert:** Urology 1983; **Med School:** Cornell Univ-Weill Med Coll 1976; **Resid:** Surgery, N Shore Univ Hosp 1978; Urology, Mount Sinai Med Ctr 1983; **Fac Appt:** Asst Prof U, Mount Sinai Sch Med

Laudone, Vincent P MD (U) - **Spec Exp:** Robotic Surgery; Prostate Cancer; Bladder Cancer; Genitourinary Cancer; **Hospital:** Meml Sloan-Kettering Canc Ctr (page 114); **Address:** Meml Sloan-Kettering, Urology Dept, 1275 York Ave, New York, NY 10065; **Phone:** 646-497-9068; **Board Cert:** Urology 2009; **Med School:** Georgetown Univ 1981; **Resid:** Urology, Univ Virginia Health Sys 1986; **Fellow:** Urologic Oncology, Meml Sloan-Kettering Cancer Ctr 1988

Lepor, Herbert MD (U) - **Spec Exp:** Prostate Cancer; **Hospital:** NYU Langone Med Ctr (page 108); **Address:** 150 E 32nd St, Fl 2, NYU Urology Assocaites, New York, NY 10016; **Phone:** 646-825-6327; **Board Cert:** Urology 2006; **Med School:** Johns Hopkins Univ 1975; **Resid:** Urology, Johns Hopkins Hosp 1986; **Fac Appt:** Prof U, NYU Sch Med

Lizza, Eli F MD (U) - **Spec Exp:** Impotence; Infertility-Male; **Hospital:** Lenox Hill Hosp (page 106), NY-Presby/Weill Cornell Med Ctr, NY (page 104); **Address:** New York Urological Assocs, 245 E 54th St Fl 2 - Ste 2N, New York, NY 10022; **Phone:** 212-570-6800 x180; **Board Cert:** Urology 2006; **Med School:** UMDNJ-NJ Med Sch, Newark 1979; **Resid:** Surgery, Lenox Hill Hosp 1981; Urology, W VA Med Ctr 1984; **Fellow:** Infertility, NY-Presby/Columbia Univ Med Ctr 1985

Loo, Marcus Hsieu-Hong MD (U) - **Spec Exp:** Prostate Disease; Kidney Stones; Voiding Dysfunction; Prostate Cancer; **Hospital:** NY-Presby/Weill Cornell Med Ctr, NY (page 104); **Address:** 254 Canal St, Ste 3001, New York, NY 10013-3501; **Phone:** 212-925-8388; **Board Cert:** Urology 2008; **Med School:** Cornell Univ-Weill Med Coll 1981; **Resid:** Surgery, NY Hosp-Cornell Med Ctr 1983; Urology, NY Hosp-Cornell Med Ctr 1988; **Fellow:** Urology, NY Hosp-Cornell Med Ctr 1984; **Fac Appt:** Clin Prof U, Cornell Univ-Weill Med Coll

Lowe, Franklin Charles MD (U) - **Spec Exp:** Prostate Disease; Complementary Medicine; Prostate Cancer; Kidney Stones; **Hospital:** St. Luke's - Roosevelt Hosp Ctr - Roosevelt Div (page 94), NY-Presby/Columbia Univ Med Ctr, NY (page 104); **Address:** 425 W 59th St, Ste 3A, New York, NY 10019-1104; **Phone:** 212-523-7790; **Board Cert:** Urology 2006; **Med School:** Columbia P&S 1979; **Resid:** Surgery, Johns Hopkins Hosp 1981; Urology, Johns Hopkins Hosp 1984; **Fac Appt:** Clin Prof U, Columbia P&S

Marks, Jon O MD (U) - **Spec Exp:** Kidney Stones; Interstitial Cystitis; **Hospital:** Beth Israel Med Ctr - Petrie Div (page 94); **Address:** Advanced Urology Ctr, 201 E 19th St, New York, NY 10003; **Phone:** 212-673-7300; **Board Cert:** Urology 1983; **Med School:** NY Med Coll 1976; **Resid:** Surgery, Lenox Hill Hosp 1978; Urology, Lenox Hill Hosp 1981

McGovern, Thomas P MD (U) - **Spec Exp:** Bladder Cancer; Prostate Cancer; **Hospital:** NY-Presby/Weill Cornell Med Ctr, NY (page 104); **Address:** 525 E 68 St, Fl 9, rm F9W, New York, NY 10065-6310; **Phone:** 212-772-7411; **Board Cert:** Urology 1983; **Med School:** Cornell Univ-Weill Med Coll 1974; **Resid:** Surgery, Mass Genl Hosp 1976; Urology, New York Hosp 1980; **Fac Appt:** Asst Clin Prof U, Cornell Univ-Weill Med Coll

McKiernan, James M MD (U) - **Spec Exp:** Kidney Cancer; Bladder Cancer; Prostate Cancer; Testicular Cancer; **Hospital:** NY-Presby/Columbia Univ Med Ctr, NY (page 104); **Address:** Columbia Univ Med Ctr - Dept Urology, 161 Ft Washington Ave Fl 11, New York, NY 10032; **Phone:** 212-305-5526; **Board Cert:** Urology 2012; **Med School:** Columbia P&S 1993; **Resid:** Surgery, NY-Presby/Columbia Univ Med Ctr 1995; Urology, NY-Presby/Columbia Univ Med Ctr 1999; **Fellow:** Urologic Oncology, Meml Sloan-Kettering Canc Ctr 2001; **Fac Appt:** Prof U, Columbia P&S

Mulhall, John P MD (U) - **Spec Exp:** Erectile Dysfunction; Peyronie's Disease; Penile Prostheses; Infertility-Male; **Hospital:** Meml Sloan-Kettering Canc Ctr (page 114); **Address:** MSKCC, Urology Dept, 353 E 68th St, Fl 5, New York, NY 10021; **Phone:** 646-422-4359; **Board Cert:** Urology 2008; **Med School:** Ireland 1985; **Resid:** Urology, Univ Conn Hlth Ctr 1995; **Fellow:** Urology, Boston Med Ctr 1996; **Fac Appt:** Assoc Prof U, Cornell Univ-Weill Med Coll

Nagler, Harris M MD (U) - **Spec Exp:** Vasectomy Reversal; Infertility-Male; Varicocele Microsurgery; Erectile Dysfunction; **Hospital:** Beth Israel Med Ctr - Petrie Div (page 94); **Address:** Beth Israel Med Ctr, Dept Urology, 10 Union Square E, Ste 3A, New York, NY 10003-3314; **Phone:** 212-844-8700; **Board Cert:** Urology 1982; **Med School:** Temple Univ 1975; **Resid:** Urology, Columbia Presby Med Ctr 1980; **Fellow:** Reproductive Medicine, Columbia Presby Med Ctr 1981; **Fac Appt:** Prof U, Albert Einstein Coll Med

Nitti, Victor MD (U) - **Spec Exp:** Urology-Female; Incontinence-Male & Female; Urodynamics; Voiding Dysfunction; **Hospital:** NYU Langone Med Ctr (page 108); **Address:** NYU Urology Assocs, 150 E 32nd St Fl 2, New York, NY 10016; **Phone:** 646-825-6324; **Board Cert:** Urology 2002; **Med School:** UMDNJ-NJ Med Sch, Newark 1985; **Resid:** Surgery, Univ Hosp 1987; Urology, Univ Hosp 1991; **Fellow:** Female Urology, UCLA Med Ctr 1992; **Fac Appt:** Prof U, NYU Sch Med

Nobert, Craig MD (U) - **Spec Exp:** Laparoscopic Surgery; Robotic Surgery; **Hospital:** St. Luke's - Roosevelt Hosp Ctr - Roosevelt Div (page 94); **Address:** St Lukes-Roosevelt Hosp, Urology Dept, 425 W 59 St, Ste 3A, New York, NY 10019; **Phone:** 212-523-7586; **Board Cert:** Urology ; **Med School:** Tufts Univ 1998; **Resid:** Urology, NY Presby Hosp 2004

Palese, Michael A MD (U) - **Spec Exp:** Kidney Cancer; Laparoscopic Surgery; Robotic Surgery; Kidney Stones; **Hospital:** Mt Sinai Med Ctr (page 102); **Address:** 5 E 98th St Fl 6, New York, NY 10029; **Phone:** 212-241-3868; **Board Cert:** Urology 2006; **Med School:** Mount Sinai Sch Med 1997; **Resid:** Surgery, Univ MD Med Ctr 1999; Urology, Univ MD Med Ctr 2003; **Fellow:** Urologic Oncology, NY Presby-Cornell Med Ctr 2004; Robotic Surgery, NY Presby-Cornell Med Ctr 2004; **Fac Appt:** Assoc Prof U, Mount Sinai Sch Med

Peng, Benjamin C.H. MD (U) - **Spec Exp:** Prostate Disease; Kidney Stones; Urologic Cancer; **Hospital:** NY-Presby/Lower Manhattan Hosp (page 104), NYU Langone Med Ctr (page 108); **Address:** 168 Canal St, Ste 510, New York, NY 10013-4503; **Phone:** 212-226-2200; **Board Cert:** Urology 2011; **Med School:** Columbia P&S 1984; **Resid:** Surgery, Mount Sinai Med Ctr 1986; Urology, NY-Presby/Columbia Univ Med Ctr 1992; **Fac Appt:** Asst Clin Prof U, NYU Sch Med

Provet, John A MD (U) - **Spec Exp:** Urologic Cancer; Kidney Stones; Prostate Disease; **Hospital:** NYU Langone Med Ctr (page 108); **Address:** Univ Urology, 215 Lexington Ave Fl 20, New York, NY 10016; **Phone:** 212-686-9015; **Board Cert:** Urology 2009; **Med School:** NYU Sch Med 1983; **Resid:** Surgery, NYU Langone Med Ctr 1985; Urology, NYU Langone Med Ctr 1989; **Fac Appt:** Assoc Clin Prof U, NYU Sch Med

Reckler, Jon M MD (U) - **Spec Exp:** Urologic Cancer; Adrenal Surgery; **Hospital:** NY-Presby/Weill Cornell Med Ctr, NY (page 104), Lenox Hill Hosp (page 106); **Address:** NY Urological Assocs, 880 5th Ave, New York, NY 10021; **Phone:** 212-535-1950; **Board Cert:** Urology 1976; **Med School:** Harvard Med Sch 1966; **Resid:** Surgery, Univ Hosp 1968; Urology, Brigham & Women's Hosp 1976; **Fac Appt:** Assoc Clin Prof U, Cornell Univ-Weill Med Coll

Romas, Nicholas A MD (U) - **Spec Exp:** Prostate Disease; Prostate Cancer; Erectile Dysfunction; **Hospital:** St. Luke's - Roosevelt Hosp Ctr - Roosevelt Div (page 94), NY-Presby/Columbia Univ Med Ctr, NY (page 104); **Address:** 425 W 59th St, Ste 3A, New York, NY 10019-1104; **Phone:** 212-523-7788; **Board Cert:** Urology 1974; **Med School:** Columbia P&S 1962; **Resid:** Surgery, NY-Presby/Weill Cornell Med Ctr 1964; Urology, NY-Presby/Columbia Univ Med Ctr 1969; **Fac Appt:** Clin Prof U, Columbia P&S

Russo, Paul MD (U) - **Spec Exp:** Kidney Cancer; Prostate Cancer; Penile Cancer; **Hospital:** Meml Sloan-Kettering Canc Ctr (page 114); **Address:** 1275 York Ave, New York, NY 10065; **Phone:** 800-525-2225; **Board Cert:** Urology 2004; **Med School:** Columbia P&S 1979; **Resid:** Urology, Barnes-Jewish Hosp 1984; **Fellow:** Urologic Oncology, Mem Sloan Kettering Canc Ctr 1988; **Fac Appt:** Assoc Prof U, Cornell Univ-Weill Med Coll

Samadi, David B MD (U) - **Spec Exp:** Prostate Cancer/Robotic Surgery; Kidney Cancer; Bladder Cancer; Urologic Cancer; **Hospital:** Lenox Hill Hosp (page 106); **Address:** 485 Madison Ave Fl 21, New York, NY 10022; **Phone:** 212-365-5000; **Board Cert:** Urology 2013; **Med School:** SUNY Stony Brook 1994; **Resid:** Surgery, Montefiore Med Ctr 1996; Urology, Montefiore Med Ctr 2000; **Fellow:** Urologic Oncology, Meml Sloan Kettering Cancer Ctr 2001; Laparoscopic Surgery, Henri Mondor Hosp 2003; **Fac Appt:** Prof U, Hofstra N Shore-LIJ Sch Med

Scardino, Peter T MD (U) - **Spec Exp:** Prostate Cancer; Bladder Cancer; Urologic Cancer; Urinary Reconstruction; **Hospital:** Meml Sloan-Kettering Canc Ctr (page 114); **Address:** 1275 York Avenue, New York, NY 10065; **Phone:** 646-422-4329; **Board Cert:** Urology 1981; **Med School:** Duke Univ 1971; **Resid:** Surgery, Mass Genl Hosp 1973; Urology, UCLA Med Ctr 1979; **Fellow:** Urology, Natl Cancer Inst 1976; **Fac Appt:** Prof U, Cornell Univ-Weill Med Coll

Scherr, Douglas S MD (U) - **Spec Exp:** Prostate Cancer/Robotic Surgery; Bladder Cancer; Robotic Surgery; Testicular Cancer; **Hospital:** NY-Presby/Weill Cornell Med Ctr, NY (page 104); **Address:** Brady Urologic Health Ctr, 525 E 68th St Starr 900, New York, NY 10021; **Phone:** 212-746-5788; **Board Cert:** Urology 2013; **Med School:** Geo Wash Univ 1994; **Resid:** Urology, NY Hosp-Cornell Med Ctr 2000; **Fellow:** Urologic Oncology, Meml Sloan-Kettering Canc Ctr 2002; **Fac Appt:** Asst Prof U, Cornell Univ-Weill Med Coll

Schiff, Howard I MD (U) - **Spec Exp:** Prostate Benign Disease; Infertility-Male; Prostate Cancer; Lupus Cystitis; **Hospital:** Mt Sinai Med Ctr (page 102), NY-Presby/Weill Cornell Med Ctr, NY (page 104); **Address:** 1120 Park Ave, Ste 1E, New York, NY 10128-1242; **Phone:** 212-996-6660; **Board Cert:** Urology 1982; **Med School:** W VA Univ 1975; **Resid:** Surgery, Montefiore Med Ctr 1977; Urology, Mt Sinai Med Ctr 1982; **Fac Appt:** Asst Clin Prof U, Mount Sinai Sch Med

Schlegel, Peter N MD (U) - **Spec Exp:** Prostate Cancer; Fertility Preservation in Cancer; Infertility-Male; Testicular Cancer; **Hospital:** NY-Presby/Weill Cornell Med Ctr, NY (page 104), Hosp For Special Surgery (page 113); **Address:** Brady Urologic Health Ctr, 525 E 68th St, Starr Bldg - Fl 9 - Ste 900, New York, NY 10065-4870; **Phone:** 212-746-5491; **Board Cert:** Urology 2011; **Med School:** Univ Mass Sch Med 1983; **Resid:** Surgery, Johns Hopkins Hosp 1985; Urology, Johns Hopkins Hosp 1989; **Fellow:** Medical Oncology, Johns Hopkins Hosp 1987; Male Reproduction, NY Hosp-Cornell Med Ctr 1991; **Fac Appt:** Prof U, Cornell Univ-Weill Med Coll

Sheinfeld, Joel MD (U) - **Spec Exp:** Testicular Cancer; Fertility Preservation in Cancer; **Hospital:** Meml Sloan-Kettering Canc Ctr (page 114); **Address:** 353 E 68th St, New York, NY 10065; **Phone:** 646-422-4311; **Board Cert:** Urology 2009; **Med School:** Univ Fla Coll Med 1981; **Resid:** Urology, Strong Meml Hosp 1986; **Fellow:** Urologic Oncology, Meml Sloan Kettering Cancer Ctr 1989; **Fac Appt:** Assoc Prof U, Cornell Univ-Weill Med Coll

Shemtov, Menachem MD (U) - **Spec Exp:** Prostate Cancer; Bladder Cancer; Kidney Cancer; Testicular Cancer; **Hospital:** NY-Presby/Weill Cornell Med Ctr, NY (page 104); **Address:** NY-Presby, Urology Dept, 525 E 68 St, Starr Pav Rm 900, New York, NY 10065; **Phone:** 212-746-5449; **Board Cert:** Urology 2010; **Med School:** Univ Pennsylvania 1989; **Resid:** Surgery, Mount Sinai Med Ctr 1991; Urology, Mount Sinai Med Ctr 1995; **Fellow:** Urologic Oncology, NY-Presby/Weill Cornell Med Ctr 1997; **Fac Appt:** Assoc Prof U, Cornell Univ-Weill Med Coll

Sogani, Pramod C MD (U) - **Spec Exp:** Prostate Cancer; Testicular Cancer; Bladder Cancer; Kidney Cancer; **Hospital:** Meml Sloan-Kettering Canc Ctr (page 114); **Address:** 1275 York Ave, New York, NY 10065; **Phone:** 646-422-4395; **Board Cert:** Urology 1976; **Med School:** India 1960; **Resid:** Urology, NYU Med Ctr 1969; Urology, Geo Wash Univ Med Ctr 1971; **Fellow:** Surgical Oncology, Meml Sloan Kettering Cancer Ctr 1973; **Fac Appt:** Prof U, Cornell Univ-Weill Med Coll

Stifelman, Michael D MD (U) - **Spec Exp:** Robotic Surgery; Reconstructive Surgery; Minimally Invasive Urologic Surgery; **Hospital:** NYU Langone Med Ctr (page 108), Englewood Hosp & Med Ctr; **Address:** 150 E 32nd St, Fl 2, New York, NY 10016-6024; **Phone:** 646-825-6325; **Board Cert:** Urology 2011; **Med School:** Albert Einstein Coll Med 1993; **Resid:** Surgery, NY Presbyterian/Columbia Med Ctr 1995; Urology, NY Presbyterian/Columbia Med Ctr 1999; **Fellow:** Minimally Invasive Surgery, NY Presbyterian/Weill Cornell Med Ctr 2000; **Fac Appt:** Assoc Prof U, NYU Sch Med

Taneja, Samir S MD (U) - **Spec Exp:** Prostate Cancer; Kidney Cancer; Bladder Cancer; **Hospital:** NYU Langone Med Ctr (page 108); **Address:** NYU Urology Associates, 150 E 32nd St, Fl 2, New York, NY 10016-6024; **Phone:** 646-825-6321; **Board Cert:** Urology 2009; **Med School:** Northwestern Univ 1990; **Resid:** Urology, UCLA Med Ctr 1996; **Fac Appt:** Prof U, NYU Sch Med

Te, Alexis E MD (U) - **Spec Exp:** Prostate Benign Disease; Prostate Surgery; Incontinence; **Hospital:** NY-Presby/Weill Cornell Med Ctr, NY (page 104); **Address:** NY-Presby/Weill Cornell Med Ctr, Brady Prostate Ctr, 425 E 61st St, New York, NY 10065; **Phone:** 212-746-4811; **Board Cert:** Urology 2006; **Med School:** Cornell Univ-Weill Med Coll 1988; **Resid:** Urology, NY Presbyterian-Columbia Presby Med Ctr 1994; **Fellow:** Urodynamics, NY Presbyterian-Columbia Presby Med Ctr 1995; **Fac Appt:** Assoc Prof U, Cornell Univ-Weill Med Coll

Tewari, Ashutosh K MD (U) - **Spec Exp:** Prostate Cancer/Robotic Surgery; **Hospital:** Mt Sinai Med Ctr (page 102); **Address:** 625 Madison Ave Fl 2, New York, NY 10019; **Phone:** 212-241-9955; **Board Cert:** Urology 2006; **Med School:** India 1984; **Resid:** Surgery, GSVM Medical College 1990; Urology, Henry Ford Hosp 2003; **Fellow:** Transplant Surgery, Liverpool Univ Med Ctr 1993; Urologic Oncology, Shands Healthcare 1995; **Fac Appt:** Assoc Prof U, Mount Sinai Sch Med

Vapnek, Jonathan M MD (U) - **Spec Exp:** Incontinence; Urology-Female; Neurogenic Bladder; Urodynamics; **Hospital:** Mt Sinai Med Ctr (page 102); **Address:** 229 E 79th St, Ste 1A, New York, NY 10075; **Phone:** 212-717-9500; **Board Cert:** Urology 2005; **Med School:** UCSD 1986; **Resid:** Surgery, UCSD Med Ctr 1988; Urology, UCSF Med Ctr 1992; **Fellow:** Neurourology, UC Davis Med Ctr 1993; **Fac Appt:** Assoc Clin Prof U, Mount Sinai Sch Med

Weiner, David M MD (U) - **Spec Exp:** Prostate Cancer; **Hospital:** St. Luke's - Roosevelt Hosp Ctr - Roosevelt Div (page 94); **Address:** 425 W 59th St, Ste 3A, New York, NY 10019; **Phone:** 212-523-7016; **Board Cert:** Urology 2012; **Med School:** UMDNJ-NJ Med Sch, Newark 1994; **Resid:** Surgery, St Lukes-Roosevelt Hosp 1996; Urology, NY Presby-Columbia Med Ctr 2000

Williams, John J MD (U) - **Spec Exp:** Genitourinary Cancer; Prostate Disease; Kidney Stones; **Hospital:** NY-Presby/Weill Cornell Med Ctr, NY (page 104), Lenox Hill Hosp (page 106); **Address:** 820 Park Ave, New York, NY 10021-2758; **Phone:** 212-861-1100; **Board Cert:** Urology 1976; **Med School:** Georgetown Univ 1966; **Resid:** Surgery, Univ Rochester Strong Meml Hosp 1968; Urology, NY-Presby/Weill Cornell Med Ctr 1975

Young, George P H MD (U) - **Spec Exp:** Incontinence-Female; Urologic Cancer; Urology-Female; Voiding Dysfunction; **Hospital:** Lenox Hill Hosp (page 106), NY Hosp Queens (page 488); **Address:** 1060 5th Ave, Fl 1EF, New York, NY 10128; **Phone:** 212-876-9811; **Board Cert:** Urology 2006; **Med School:** Brazil 1983; **Resid:** Surgery, Staten Island Univ Hosp 1989; Urology, New York Hosp 1993; **Fellow:** Microsurgery, Population Council, Rockefeller Univ 1985; Female Urology, UCLA Med Ctr 1994; **Fac Appt:** Assoc Prof U, Cornell Univ-Weill Med Coll

Vascular & Interventional Radiology

Brown, Karen T MD (VIR) - **Spec Exp:** Liver Cancer; Radiofrequency Tumor Ablation; **Hospital:** Meml Sloan-Kettering Canc Ctr (page 114); **Address:** 1275 York Ave, New York, NY 10065; **Phone:** 212-639-5882; **Board Cert:** Diagnostic Radiology 1984; Vascular & Interventional Radiology 2004; **Med School:** Boston Univ 1979; **Resid:** Diagnostic Radiology, Mass Genl Hosp 1984; **Fellow:** Vascular & Interventional Radiology, Mass Genl Hosp 1985; **Fac Appt:** Clin Prof Rad, Cornell Univ-Weill Med Coll

Covey, Anne M MD (VIR) - **Spec Exp:** Liver Tumors; Chemoembolization & Tumor Ablation; Biliary Surgery; **Hospital:** Meml Sloan-Kettering Canc Ctr (page 114); **Address:** MSKCC, Interventional Radiology, 1275 York Ave, New York, NY 10065; **Phone:** 212-639-6746; **Board Cert:** Diagnostic Radiology 1999; Vascular & Interventional Radiology 2011; **Med School:** Columbia P&S 1994; **Resid:** Diagnostic Radiology, Yale-New Haven Hosp 1998; **Fellow:** Vascular & Interventional Radiology, Yale-New Haven Hosp 2001

Dreifuss, Ronald MD (VIR) - **Spec Exp:** Interventional Radiology; **Hospital:** St. Luke's - Roosevelt Hosp Ctr - St Luke's Hosp (page 94), Beth Israel Med Ctr - Petrie Div (page 94); **Address:** St Lukes Hosp, Interventional Radiology, 1000 10th Ave, New York, NY 10019; **Phone:** 212-523-4446; **Board Cert:** Diagnostic Radiology ; **Med School:** Mount Sinai Sch Med 1987; **Resid:** Diagnostic Radiology, Mount Sinai Med Ctr 1993; **Fellow:** Vascular & Interventional Radiology, NY-Presby/Weill Cornell Med Ctr 1994; **Fac Appt:** Asst Clin Prof Rad, Columbia P&S

Getrajdman, George I MD (VIR) - **Hospital:** Meml Sloan-Kettering Canc Ctr (page 114); **Address:** Meml Sloan Kettering Canc Ctr, 1275 York Ave, New York, NY 10021; **Phone:** 212-639-2598; **Board Cert:** Diagnostic Radiology 1988; **Med School:** Johns Hopkins Univ 1980; **Resid:** Surgery, NY Presby/Columbia Med Ctr 1985; Diagnostic Radiology, NY Presby/Columbia Med Ctr 1988; **Fellow:** Vascular & Interventional Radiology, NY Presby/Columbia Med Ctr 1989

Javit, Daniel J MD (VIR) - **Hospital:** Lenox Hill Hosp (page 106); **Address:** Lenox Hill Hosp, Dept Radiology, 100 E 77th St, New York, NY 10021; **Phone:** 212-434-2908; **Board Cert:** Diagnostic Radiology 1993; Vascular & Interventional Radiology 2005; **Med School:** Cornell Univ-Weill Med Coll 1988; **Resid:** Diagnostic Radiology, Mt Sinai Med Ctr 1993; **Fellow:** Interventional Radiology, NY-Presby/Weill Cornell Med Ctr 1994

Khilnani, Neil M MD (VIR) - **Spec Exp:** Varicose Veins; Vein Disorders; Iliac Vein Obstruction; **Hospital:** NY-Presby/Weill Cornell Med Ctr, NY (page 104); **Address:** Weill Cornell Vascular Assocs, 2315 Broadway at 84th ST, Fl 4, New York, NY 10024; **Phone:** 646-962-9179; **Board Cert:** Diagnostic Radiology 1991; Vascular & Interventional Radiology 2008; **Med School:** Mount Sinai Sch Med 1986; **Resid:** Diagnostic Radiology, Columbia Presby Med Ctr 1991; **Fellow:** Vascular & Interventional Radiology, Columbia Presby Med Ctr 1992; **Fac Appt:** Assoc Prof Rad, Cornell Univ-Weill Med Coll

Lookstein, Robert A MD (VIR) - **Spec Exp:** Peripheral Vascular Disease; Renovascular Disease; Vein Disorders; Radiofrequency Tumor Ablation; **Hospital:** Mt Sinai Med Ctr (page 102); **Address:** Mt Sinai Med Ctr, Dept Radiology, 1176 Fifth Ave, New York, NY 10029; **Phone:** 212-241-3666; **Board Cert:** Diagnostic Radiology 2001; Vascular & Interventional Radiology 2003; **Med School:** SUNY Downstate 1995; **Resid:** Diagnostic Radiology, Mt Sinai Med Ctr 2001; **Fellow:** Vascular & Interventional Radiology, Mt Sinai Med Ctr 2002; **Fac Appt:** Assoc Prof Rad, Mount Sinai Sch Med

Rosen, Robert J MD (VIR) - **Spec Exp:** Vascular Malformations; Aneurysm-Aortic; Chemoembolization & Tumor Ablation; **Hospital:** Lenox Hill Hosp (page 106); **Address:** Lenox Hill Heart & Vascular Inst, 130 E 77th St Fl 9, New York, NY 10075; **Phone:** 212-434-2606; **Board Cert:** Diagnostic Radiology 1980; **Med School:** Hahnemann Univ 1976; **Resid:** Diagnostic Radiology, Hahnemann Univ Hosp 1979; **Fellow:** Vascular & Interventional Radiology, Hosp Univ Penn - UPHS 1980; **Fac Appt:** Assoc Prof Rad, NYU Sch Med

Saboeiro, Gregory R MD (VIR) - **Spec Exp:** Musculoskeletal Imaging; Ultrasound; Spinal Imaging & Intervention; **Hospital:** Hosp For Special Surgery (page 113); **Address:** Hosp for Special Surgery, 535 E 70th St Fl 3, New York, NY 10021; **Phone:** 212-606-1566; **Board Cert:** Diagnostic Radiology 1993; **Med School:** St Louis Univ 1989; **Resid:** Radiology, St Louis Univ Hosp 1993; **Fellow:** Interventional Radiology, Mallinckrodt Inst 1994; Musculoskeletal Imaging, Hosp Special Surgery 2005; **Fac Appt:** Asst Prof Rad, Cornell Univ-Weill Med Coll

Shams, Joseph N MD (VIR) - **Spec Exp:** Peripheral Vascular Disease; Uterine Fibroid Embolization; Liver Tumors; Vascular Disease; **Hospital:** Beth Israel Med Ctr - Petrie Div (page 94), St. Luke's - Roosevelt Hosp Ctr - Roosevelt Div (page 94); **Address:** 144 4th Ave, New York, NY 10003; **Phone:** 212-420-2509; **Board Cert:** Diagnostic Radiology 1993; Vascular & Interventional Radiology 2006; **Med School:** SUNY Downstate 1988; **Resid:** Diagnostic Radiology, Beth Israel Med Ctr - Petrie Div 1993; **Fellow:** Vascular & Interventional Radiology, Yale-New Haven Hosp 1994; **Fac Appt:** Asst Prof Rad, Albert Einstein Coll Med

Sofocleous, Constantinos T MD/PhD (VIR) - **Spec Exp:** Interventional Oncology; Chemoembolization & Tumor Ablation; Liver Cancer; Lung Cancer; **Hospital:** Meml Sloan-Kettering Canc Ctr (page 114); **Address:** Meml Sloan-Kettering Cancer Ctr, 1275 York Ave, New York, NY 10065; **Phone:** 212-639-3379; **Board Cert:** Diagnostic Radiology ; Vascular & Interventional Radiology 2012; **Med School:** Greece 1991; **Resid:** Diagnostic Radiology, St Luke's-Roosevelt Hosp/Columbia 1998; **Fellow:** Vascular & Interventional Radiology, NYU Med Ctr 1999

Solomon, Stephen B MD (VIR) - **Spec Exp:** Radiofrequency Tumor Ablation; Kidney Cancer; Liver Cancer; Lung Cancer; **Hospital:** Meml Sloan-Kettering Canc Ctr (page 114); **Address:** Meml Sloan-Kettering Cancer Ctr, Ctr for Image Guided Intervention, 1275 York Ave, rm H118, New York, NY 10021; **Phone:** 212-639-5012; **Board Cert:** Diagnostic Radiology 1998; **Med School:** Yale Univ 1993; **Resid:** Diagnostic Radiology, Johns Hopkins Hosp 1998

Sperling, David C MD (VIR) - **Spec Exp:** Liver Cancer; Varicose Veins; Uterine Fibroid Embolization; Pelvic Congestion Syndrome; **Hospital:** NY-Presby/Columbia Univ Med Ctr, NY (page 104); **Address:** Columbia Endovascular Assocs Midtown, 51 W 51st St, Ste 301, New York, NY 10019; **Phone:** 212-326-8874; **Board Cert:** Diagnostic Radiology 1998; Vascular & Interventional Radiology 2010; **Med School:** SUNY Downstate 1993; **Resid:** Diagnostic Radiology, Thomas Jefferson Univ Hosp 1998; **Fellow:** Vascular & Interventional Radiology, Thomas Jefferson Univ Hosp 1999; **Fac Appt:** Assoc Clin Prof Rad, Columbia P&S

Susman, Jonathan MD (VIR) - **Spec Exp:** Chemoembolization & Tumor Ablation; Uterine Fibroid Embolization; **Hospital:** NY-Presby/Columbia Univ Med Ctr, NY (page 104); **Address:** NY Presby-Columbia Univ Med Ctr, Dept Radiology, 177 Fort Washington Ave, 4th Fl, Ste 100, New York, NY 10032; **Phone:** 212-305-7094; **Board Cert:** Diagnostic Radiology 1996; Vascular & Interventional Radiology 2011; **Med School:** Albert Einstein Coll Med 1991; **Resid:** Diagnostic Radiology, LIJ Med Ctr 1996; **Fellow:** Vascular & Interventional Radiology, NYU Med Ctr 1997

Thornton, Raymond H MD (VIR) - **Spec Exp:** Chemoembolization & Tumor Ablation; Liver Cancer; Kidney Cancer; **Hospital:** Meml Sloan-Kettering Canc Ctr (page 114); **Address:** Ctr for Image Guided Intervention, 1275 York Ave, rm H118, New York, NY 10021; **Phone:** 212-639-2463; **Board Cert:** Diagnostic Radiology 2003; Vascular & Interventional Radiology 2005; **Med School:** Univ Pittsburgh 1998; **Resid:** Diagnostic Radiology, UCSF Med Ctr 2003; **Fellow:** Vascular & Interventional Radiology, UCSF Med Ctr 2005

Weintraub, Joshua L MD (VIR) - **Spec Exp:** Gastrointestinal Cancer; Chemoembolization & Tumor Ablation; Uterine Fibroid Embolization; Vascular Malformations; **Hospital:** NY-Presby/Columbia Univ Med Ctr, NY (page 104); **Address:** NY Presbyterian-Columbia Med Ctr, Dept Radiology, 622 W 168th St, New York, NY 10032; **Phone:** 212-305-7094; **Board Cert:** Diagnostic Radiology 1996; Vascular & Interventional Radiology 2009; **Med School:** Wayne State Univ 1991; **Resid:** Diagnostic Radiology, Beth Israel Hosp 1996; **Fellow:** Vascular & Interventional Radiology, Hosp Univ Penn 1997; **Fac Appt:** Assoc Prof Rad, Columbia P&S

Westcott, Mark A MD (VIR) - **Spec Exp:** Interventional Radiology; **Hospital:** Lenox Hill Hosp (page 106); **Address:** 100 E 77th St, New York, NY 10075; **Phone:** 212-434-2908; **Board Cert:** Diagnostic Radiology ; Vascular & Interventional Radiology 2006; **Med School:** Georgetown Univ 1988; **Resid:** Diagnostic Radiology, Northwestern Meml Hosp 1993; **Fellow:** Vascular & Interventional Radiology, Thomas Jefferson Univ Hosp 1995

Vascular Surgery

Adelman, Mark Alan MD (VascS) - **Spec Exp:** Carotid Artery Surgery; Aneurysm-Abdominal Aortic; Vein Disorders; Endovascular Surgery; **Hospital:** NYU Langone Med Ctr (page 108), Bellevue Hosp Ctr; **Address:** NYU Vascular Assocs, 530 1st Ave, Ste 6F, New York, NY 10016; **Phone:** 212-263-7311; **Board Cert:** Vascular Surgery 2012; **Med School:** NYU Sch Med 1985; **Resid:** Surgery, NYU Med Ctr 1990; **Fellow:** Vascular Surgery, NYU Med Ctr 1991; **Fac Appt:** Prof VascS, NYU Sch Med

Benvenisty, Alan I MD (VascS) - **Spec Exp:** Renovascular Disease; Aneurysm-Aortic; Endovascular Surgery; Minimally Invasive Vascular Surgery; **Hospital:** St. Luke's - Roosevelt Hosp Ctr - St Luke's Hosp (page 94), St. Luke's - Roosevelt Hosp Ctr - Roosevelt Div (page 94); **Address:** 1090 Amsterdam Ave Fl 12, New York, NY 10025; **Phone:** 212-523-4706; **Board Cert:** Surgery 2004; Vascular Surgery 2009; **Med School:** Columbia P&S 1978; **Resid:** Surgery, NY-Presby/Columbia Univ Med Ctr 1983; **Fellow:** Vascular Surgery, NY-Presby/Columbia Univ Med Ctr 1984; Transplant Surgery, NY-Presby/Columbia Univ Med Ctr 1984; **Fac Appt:** Prof S, Columbia P&S

Bernik, Thomas R MD (VascS) - **Spec Exp:** Carotid Artery Surgery; Aortic Surgery; Peripheral Vascular Disease; Endovascular Surgery; **Hospital:** Beth Israel Med Ctr - Petrie Div (page 94); **Address:** Beth Israel Med Ctr, Div Vasc Surg, 1st Ave at 16th St, 12 Fierman Hall, New York, NY 10003; **Phone:** 212-844-5555; **Board Cert:** Surgery 2012; Vascular Surgery 2005; **Med School:** Geo Wash Univ 1994; **Resid:** Surgery, St Vincent's Hosp 2000; **Fellow:** Vascular Surgery, N Shore Univ Hosp 2002; Endovascular Surgery, Univ Rochester Strong Meml Hosp 2002; **Fac Appt:** Asst Prof VascS, NY Med Coll

Carroccio, Alfio MD (VascS) - **Spec Exp:** Aneurysm-Aortic; Minimally Invasive Surgery; Endovascular Surgery; **Hospital:** Lenox Hill Hosp (page 106); **Address:** 130 E 77 St Fl 13, New York, NY 10075; **Phone:** 212-434-3420; **Board Cert:** Surgery 2010; Vascular Surgery 2005; **Med School:** Mount Sinai Sch Med 1996; **Resid:** Surgery, Mt Sinai Med Ctr 2001; **Fellow:** Vascular Surgery, Mt Sinai Med Ctr 2003

Cayne, Neal S MD (VascS) - **Spec Exp:** Endovascular Surgery; Aneurysm-Abdominal & Thoracic Aortic; Carotid Artery Surgery; Endovascular Stent Grafts; **Hospital:** NYU Langone Med Ctr (page 108); **Address:** 530 First Ave, Ste 6F, MS 10016, New York, NY 10016-6402; **Phone:** 212-263-5626; **Board Cert:** Surgery 2010; Vascular Surgery 2003; **Med School:** NY Med Coll 1995; **Resid:** Surgery, Montefiore Med Ctr 2000; **Fellow:** Vascular Surgery, Montefiore Med Ctr 2002; **Fac Appt:** Asst Prof VascS, NYU Sch Med

Chideckel, Norman MD (VascS) - **Spec Exp:** Vein Disorders; Wound Healing/Care; Laser Surgery; **Hospital:** Beth Israel Med Ctr - Petrie Div (page 94); **Address:** 380 2nd Ave, Ste 1004, New York, NY 10010; **Phone:** 212-473-1877; **Board Cert:** Surgery 2007; **Med School:** SUNY Downstate 1979; **Resid:** Surgery, Beth Israel Med Ctr 1984; **Fellow:** Vascular Surgery, Lutheran Med Ctr 1985; **Fac Appt:** Asst Clin Prof S, Albert Einstein Coll Med

Ellozy, Sharif Hamed MD (VascS) - **Spec Exp:** Endovascular Surgery; Aneurysm-Aortic; **Hospital:** Mt Sinai Med Ctr (page 102); **Address:** 5 E 98th St Fl 3, New York, NY 10029; **Phone:** 212-241-5315; **Board Cert:** Surgery 2004; Vascular Surgery 2005; **Med School:** NYU Sch Med 1996; **Resid:** Surgery, Mt Sinai Med Ctr 2002; **Fellow:** Vascular Surgery, Mt Sinai Med Ctr 2003; **Fac Appt:** Assoc Prof S, Mount Sinai Sch Med

Faries, Peter L MD (VascS) - **Spec Exp:** Aneurysm-Abdominal Aortic; Carotid Artery Surgery; Renovascular Disease; Peripheral Vascular Disease; **Hospital:** Mt Sinai Med Ctr (page 102); **Address:** 1425 Madison Ave, Box 1273, New York, NY 10029; **Phone:** 212-241-5386; **Board Cert:** Surgery 2008; Vascular Surgery 2009; **Med School:** Univ Pennsylvania 1992; **Resid:** Surgery, Montefiore Med Ctr 1998; **Fellow:** Vascular Surgery, Beth Israel Deaconess Med Ctr 2000; **Fac Appt:** Prof S, Mount Sinai Sch Med

Giangola, Gary MD (VascS) - **Spec Exp:** Carotid Artery Surgery; Aneurysm-Aortic; Diabetic Leg/Foot; Vein Disorders; **Hospital:** Lenox Hill Hosp (page 106), NS-LIJ Hlth Sys (page 106); **Address:** Lenox Hill-Dept Vascular Surgery, 130 E 77th St Fl 13, New York, NY 10075; **Phone:** 212-434-3420; **Board Cert:** Vascular Surgery 2008; **Med School:** NYU Sch Med 1980; **Resid:** Surgery, NYU Langone Med Ctr 1986; **Fellow:** Vascular Surgery, NYU Langone Med Ctr 1988; **Fac Appt:** Assoc Prof S, NYU Sch Med

Green, Richard M MD (VascS) - **Spec Exp:** Aneurysm-Abdominal Aortic; Carotid Artery Surgery; Percutaneous Vascular Interventions; **Hospital:** NY-Presby/Columbia Univ Med Ctr, NY (page 104); **Address:** NY-Presby, Vascular Surgery Dept, 161 Fort Washington Ave, rm 532, New York, NY 10032; **Phone:** 212-305-1165; **Board Cert:** Vascular Surgery 2003; **Med School:** Univ Rochester 1970; **Resid:** Surgery, Strong Meml Hosp 1976

Grossi, Robert J MD (VascS) - **Spec Exp:** Carotid Artery Surgery; Aneurysm-Abdominal Aortic; Wound Healing/Care; **Hospital:** Beth Israel Med Ctr - Petrie Div (page 94), NY-Presby/Lower Manhattan Hosp (page 104); **Address:** Beth Israel Med Ctr, Div Vasc Surg, 1st Ave at 16th St, 12 Fierman Hall, New York, NY 10003; **Phone:** 212-844-5559; **Board Cert:** Surgery 2006; Vascular Surgery 2008; **Med School:** UMDNJ-NJ Med Sch, Newark 1981; **Resid:** Surgery, St Vincent's Hosp 1986; **Fellow:** Vascular Surgery, Temple Univ Hosp 1987

Harrington, Elizabeth MD (VascS) - **Spec Exp:** Carotid Artery Surgery; Aneurysm-Aortic; Arterial Bypass Surgery-Leg; **Hospital:** Mt Sinai Med Ctr (page 102); **Address:** 2 E 93rd St, New York, NY 10128; **Phone:** 212-876-7400; **Board Cert:** Surgery 2009; Vascular Surgery 2006; **Med School:** NY Med Coll 1975; **Resid:** Surgery, Mount Sinai Med Ctr 1980; **Fellow:** Vascular Surgery, Mount Sinai Med Ctr 1981; **Fac Appt:** Assoc Prof VascS, Mount Sinai Sch Med

Harrington, Martin E MD (VascS) - **Spec Exp:** Carotid Artery Surgery; Aneurysm-Aortic; Arterial Bypass Surgery-Leg; **Hospital:** Mt Sinai Med Ctr (page 102); **Address:** 2 E 93rd St, New York, NY 10128; **Phone:** 212-876-7400; **Board Cert:** Internal Medicine 1978; Hematology 1980; Surgery 2003; Vascular Surgery 2007; **Med School:** Harvard Med Sch 1975; **Resid:** Internal Medicine, St Luke's Roosevelt Hosp Ctr 1979; Surgery, Mt Sinai Med Ctr 1984; **Fellow:** Surgical Oncology, Meml Sloan Kettering Canc Ctr 1986; Vascular Surgery, Mt Sinai Med Ctr 1989

Jacobowitz, Glenn R MD (VascS) - **Spec Exp:** Vein Disorders; Minimally Invasive Vascular Surgery; Aneurysm-Abdominal Aortic; Carotid Artery Surgery; **Hospital:** NYU Langone Med Ctr (page 108), Bellevue Hosp Ctr; **Address:** Schwartz Hlth Care Ctr, 530 First Ave, Ste 6F, New York, NY 10016; **Phone:** 212-263-7311; **Board Cert:** Surgery 2006; Vascular Surgery 2005; **Med School:** NYU Sch Med 1989; **Resid:** Surgery, NYU Langone Med Ctr 1995; **Fellow:** Vascular Surgery, NYU Langone Med Ctr 1996; **Fac Appt:** Assoc Prof VascS, NYU Sch Med

Lantis II, John C MD (VascS) - **Spec Exp:** Limb Sparing Surgery; Wound Healing/Care; Endovascular Surgery; Carotid Artery Stent Placement; **Hospital:** St. Luke's - Roosevelt Hosp Ctr - Roosevelt Div (page 94), St. Luke's - Roosevelt Hosp Ctr - St Luke's Hosp (page 94); **Address:** St Lukes-Roosevelt Hosp, Surgery Dept, 1090 Amsterdam Ave, Ste 7A, New York, NY 10025; **Phone:** 212-523-4797; **Board Cert:** Surgery 2009; Vascular Surgery 2010; **Med School:** Albany Med Coll 1993; **Resid:** Surgery, Tufts Med Ctr 1999; **Fellow:** Vascular Surgery, Brigham & Womens Hosp 2000; **Fac Appt:** Asst Prof S, Columbia P&S

Maldonado, Thomas MD (VascS) - **Spec Exp:** Aortic Stent Grafts; Endovascular Surgery; Aneurysm-Aortic; **Hospital:** NYU Langone Med Ctr (page 108); **Address:** NYU Med Ctr, Univ Vascular Assocs, 530 First Ave, Ste 6F, New York, NY 10016; **Phone:** 212-263-5626; **Board Cert:** Surgery 2003; Vascular Surgery 2005; **Med School:** NYU Sch Med 1995; **Resid:** Surgery, NYU Langone Med Ctr 1998; Surgery, NYU Langone Med Ctr 2002; **Fellow:** Research, NYU Langone Med Ctr 2000; Vascular Surgery, NYU Langone Med Ctr 2003; **Fac Appt:** Assoc Prof S, NYU Sch Med

Marin, Michael L MD (VascS) - **Spec Exp:** Aneurysm-Aortic; Peripheral Vascular Disease; Limb Sparing Surgery; Endovascular Surgery; **Hospital:** Mt Sinai Med Ctr (page 102); **Address:** Mount Sinai Med Ctr, Vascular Surgery, 5 E 98th St Fl 3, Box 1273, New York, NY 10029; **Phone:** 212-241-5315; **Board Cert:** Surgery 2011; **Med School:** Mount Sinai Sch Med 1984; **Resid:** Surgery, NY-Presby/Columbia Univ Med Ctr 1990; **Fellow:** Transplant Surgery, NY-Presby/Columbia Univ Med Ctr 1988; Vascular Surgery, Montefiore Med Ctr 1992; **Fac Appt:** Prof S, Mount Sinai Sch Med

McKinsey, James F MD (VascS) - **Spec Exp:** Aneurysm-Abdominal Aortic; Endovascular Surgery; Carotid Artery Surgery; **Hospital:** NY-Presby/Columbia Univ Med Ctr, NY (page 104); **Address:** NY-Presby, Vascular Surgery Dept, 161 Fort Washington Ave, rm 535, New York, NY 10032; **Phone:** 212-342-3255; **Board Cert:** Surgery 2001; Vascular Surgery 2003; **Med School:** Univ Fla Coll Med 1987; **Resid:** Surgery, Georgia Baptist Med Ctr 1992; **Fellow:** Vascular Surgery, Univ Chicago Hosps 1993; **Fac Appt:** Assoc Prof S, Columbia P&S

Mendes, Donna M MD (VascS) - **Spec Exp:** Varicose Veins; Aneurysm-Aortic; Limb Sparing Surgery; **Hospital:** St. Luke's - Roosevelt Hosp Ctr - Roosevelt Div (page 94), Lenox Hill Hosp (page 106); **Address:** 10 W 66th St, New York, NY 10023; **Phone:** 212-636-4990; **Board Cert:** Surgery 2004; Vascular Surgery 2011; **Med School:** Columbia P&S 1977; **Resid:** Surgery, St Luke's-Roosevelt Hosp Ctr 1982; **Fellow:** Vascular Surgery, Englewood Hosp & Med Ctr 1984; **Fac Appt:** Assoc Prof S, Columbia P&S

Morrissey, Nicholas J MD (VascS) - **Spec Exp:** Endovascular Surgery; Aneurysm-Abdominal & Thoracic Aortic; Carotid Artery Surgery; **Hospital:** NY-Presby/Columbia Univ Med Ctr, NY (page 104); **Address:** 161 Fort Washington Ave, Herbert Irving Pavilion, rm 538, New York, NY 10032; **Phone:** 212-342-2929; **Board Cert:** Surgery 2009; Vascular Surgery 2012; **Med School:** Univ Rochester 1992; **Resid:** Surgery, Strong Meml Hosp 1999; **Fellow:** Vascular Surgery, Mount Sinai Hosp 2001; **Fac Appt:** Assoc Prof S, Columbia P&S

Nalbandian, Matthew M MD (VascS) - **Spec Exp:** Spinal Access Surgery; Endovascular Surgery; Varicose Veins; Vein Disorders; **Hospital:** NYU Langone Med Ctr (page 108), Holy Name Med Ctr (page 720); **Address:** 247 Third Ave, Ste 504, New York, NY 10010; **Phone:** 212-254-6882; **Board Cert:** Surgery 2009; Vascular Surgery 2008; **Med School:** UMDNJ-NJ Med Sch, Newark 1993; **Resid:** Surgery, Boston Med Ctr 1998; **Fellow:** Vascular Surgery, NYU Langone Med Ctr 2000; **Fac Appt:** Asst Prof VascS, NYU Sch Med

Rockman, Caron B MD (VascS) - **Spec Exp:** Carotid Artery Surgery; Aneurysm-Abdominal Aortic; Peripheral Vascular Disease; Vein Disorders; **Hospital:** NYU Langone Med Ctr (page 108); **Address:** 530 1st Ave, Fl 6, Ste F, New York, NY 10016; **Phone:** 212-263-7311; **Board Cert:** Surgery 2006; Vascular Surgery 2007; **Med School:** NYU Sch Med 1990; **Resid:** Surgery, NYU Med Ctr 1995; **Fellow:** Vascular Surgery, NYU Med Ctr 1997; **Fac Appt:** Assoc Prof S, NYU Sch Med

Schanzer, Harry MD (VascS) - **Spec Exp:** Vein Disorders; Carotid Artery Surgery; Aneurysm-Aortic; **Hospital:** Mt Sinai Med Ctr (page 102), Lenox Hill Hosp (page 106); **Address:** 993 Park Ave, New York, NY 10028-0809; **Phone:** 212-396-1254; **Board Cert:** Vascular Surgery 2007; **Med School:** Chile 1968; **Resid:** Surgery, Mount Sinai Med Ctr 1976; **Fellow:** Transplant Surgery, Mount Sinai Med Ctr 1974; **Fac Appt:** Clin Prof S, Mount Sinai Sch Med

Schneider, Darren B MD (VascS) - **Spec Exp:** Endovascular Surgery; Minimally Invasive Vascular Surgery; Aneurysm-Aortic; Peripheral Vascular Disease; **Hospital:** NY-Presby/Weill Cornell Med Ctr, NY (page 104); **Address:** NY-Presby, Vascular Surgery Dept, 525 E 68th St Starr Bldg Fl 8, New York, NY 10065; **Phone:** 212-746-5192; **Med School:** UCSD 1992; **Resid:** Surgery, UCSF Med Ctr 2000; **Fellow:** Interventional Radiology, UCSF Med Ctr 2001; Vascular Surgery, UCSF Med Ctr 2002; **Fac Appt:** Assoc Prof S, Cornell Univ-Weill Med Coll

Stein, Jeffrey S MD (VascS) - **Spec Exp:** Aneurysm-Aortic; Arterial Disease; Varicose Veins; **Hospital:** Mt Sinai Med Ctr (page 102), Lenox Hill Hosp (page 106); **Address:** 12 E 97th St, Ste 1C, New York, NY 10029; **Phone:** 212-396-0500; **Board Cert:** Surgery 2009; Vascular Surgery 2002; **Med School:** Washington Univ, St Louis 1982; **Resid:** Surgery, Mt Sinai Med Ctr 1988; **Fellow:** Surgical Critical Care, Mt Sinai Med Ctr 1989; Vascular Surgery, Mt Sinai Med Ctr 1990; **Fac Appt:** Asst Clin Prof S, Mount Sinai Sch Med

Teodorescu, Victoria J MD (VascS) - **Spec Exp:** Endovascular Surgery; Aneurysm; Diabetic Leg/Foot; Peripheral Vascular Disease; **Hospital:** Mt Sinai Med Ctr (page 102); **Address:** 5 E 98th St, Fl 3, New York, NY 10029; **Phone:** 212-241-5315; **Board Cert:** Surgery 2011; Vascular Surgery 2003; **Med School:** NYU Sch Med 1985; **Resid:** Surgery, Mt Sinai Hosp 1991; **Fellow:** Vascular Surgery, Mt Sinai Hosp 1992; **Fac Appt:** Assoc Prof S, Mount Sinai Sch Med

Todd, George MD (VascS) - **Spec Exp:** Minimally Invasive Vascular Surgery; Aneurysm-Abdominal Aortic; Carotid Artery Surgery; **Hospital:** St. Luke's - Roosevelt Hosp Ctr - Roosevelt Div (page 94); **Address:** St Lukes Hosp, Vascular Surgery Dept, 1000 10th Ave, rm 5G77, New York, NY 10019; **Phone:** 212-523-7481; **Board Cert:** Surgery 2010; Vascular Surgery 2006; **Med School:** Penn State Coll Med 1974; **Resid:** Surgery, NY-Presby/Columbia Univ Med Ctr 1979; **Fellow:** Vascular Surgery, NY-Presby/Columbia Univ Med Ctr 1980; **Fac Appt:** Prof S, Columbia P&S

Bronx

Bronx

Adolescent Medicine

Alderman, Elizabeth MD (AM) - **Spec Exp:** Adolescent Gynecology; Eating Disorders; Parenting Issues; **Hospital:** Chldns Hosp at Montefiore; **Address:** Chldns Hosp Montefiore, Adolescent Med, 3415 Bainbridge Rd, Bronx, NY 10467; **Phone:** 718-741-2450; **Board Cert:** Pediatrics 2012; Adolescent Medicine 2009; **Med School:** SUNY Stony Brook 1987; **Resid:** Pediatrics, Montefiore Med Ctr 1990; **Fellow:** Adolescent Medicine, Montefiore Med Ctr 1992; **Fac Appt:** Prof Ped, Albert Einstein Coll Med

Coupey, Susan MD (AM) - **Spec Exp:** Adolescent Gynecology; Menstrual Disorders; Reproductive Endocrinology; Uterine/Vaginal Agenisis; **Hospital:** Chldns Hosp at Montefiore; **Address:** Chldns Hosp Montefiore, Adolescent Med, 3415 Bainbridge Rd Fl 4, Bronx, NY 10467; **Phone:** 718-920-6781; **Board Cert:** Pediatrics 1979; Adolescent Medicine 2009; **Med School:** Canada 1975; **Resid:** Pediatrics, Chldns Hosp 1978; **Fellow:** Adolescent Medicine, Montefiore Med Ctr 1979; **Fac Appt:** Prof Ped, Albert Einstein Coll Med

Rieder, Jessica MD (AM) - **Spec Exp:** Obesity; Vaccines; Eating Disorders; **Hospital:** Chldns Hosp at Montefiore; **Address:** Chldns Hosp Montefiore, Adolescent Med, 3415 Bainbridge Ave, Bronx, NY 10467; **Phone:** 718-741-2450; **Board Cert:** Pediatrics 2013; Adolescent Medicine 2009; **Med School:** Univ Alberta 1994; **Resid:** Pediatrics, Montefiore Med Ctr 1998; **Fellow:** Adolescent Medicine, Montefiore Med Ctr 2001; **Fac Appt:** Assoc Clin Prof Ped, Albert Einstein Coll Med

Allergy & Immunology

Bernstein, Larry J MD (A&I) - **Spec Exp:** Asthma; Immune Deficiency; Sinus Disorders; Food Allergy; **Hospital:** Montefiore Med Ctr-Moses Campus (page 100), NY Hosp Queens (page 488); **Address:** 72-35 112th St, Ste pr-5, forest hills, NY 10461; **Phone:** 718-544-6641; **Board Cert:** Pediatrics 1981; Allergy & Immunology 1985; **Med School:** Albert Einstein Coll Med 1977; **Resid:** Pediatrics, Jacobi Med Ctr 1981; **Fellow:** Allergy & Immunology, Albert Einstein Coll Med 1983; **Fac Appt:** Assoc Clin Prof Ped, Albert Einstein Coll Med

Kaufman, Alan MD (A&I) - **Spec Exp:** Asthma; Sinus Disorders; Urticaria; Immunodeficiency Disorders; **Hospital:** Montefiore Med Ctr-Moses Campus (page 100), Lawrence Hosp Ctr; **Address:** 3626 E Tremont Ave, Ste 202, Bronx, NY 10465-2030; **Phone:** 718-597-9000; **Board Cert:** Internal Medicine 1988; Allergy & Immunology 2009; **Med School:** West Indies 1984; **Resid:** Internal Medicine, Metropolitan Hosp Ctr 1987; **Fellow:** Allergy & Immunology, Albert Einstein Coll Med 1989

Lehach, Joan G MD (A&I) - **Spec Exp:** Asthma; **Hospital:** St. Barnabas Hosp - Bronx, Montefiore Med Ctr-Einstein Campus (page 100); **Address:** 1488 Metropolitan Ave, Ste 12, Bronx, NY 10462; **Phone:** 718-918-1991; **Board Cert:** Internal Medicine 2010; **Med School:** Dominican Republic 1985; **Resid:** Internal Medicine, St Barnabas Hosp 1988; **Fellow:** Allergy & Immunology, Jacobi Med Ctr 1990

Rosenstreich, David L MD (A&I) - **Spec Exp:** Urticaria; Sinusitis; Atopic Dermatitis; **Hospital:** Montefiore Med Ctr-Moses Campus (page 100), Jacobi Med Ctr; **Address:** 1515 Blondell Ave, Fl 2, Ste 220, Bronx, NY 10461; **Phone:** 866-633-8255; **Board Cert:** Internal Medicine 1972; Allergy & Immunology 1975; Clinical & Laboratory Immunology 1990; **Med School:** NYU Sch Med 1967; **Resid:** Internal Medicine, Albert Einstein Med Ctr 1969; **Fellow:** Allergy & Immunology, Natl Inst Hlth 1972; **Fac Appt:** Prof Med, Albert Einstein Coll Med

Rubinstein, Arye MD/PhD (A&I) - **Spec Exp:** Immune Deficiency; Asthma; Drug Sensitivity; **Hospital:** Montefiore Med Ctr-Moses Campus (page 100), Montefiore Med Ctr-Einstein Campus (page 100); **Address:** Montefiore, Allergy & Immunology, 1180 Morris Park Ave Fl 3, Bronx, NY 10461; **Phone:** 347-498-2410; **Board Cert:** Pediatrics 1976; Allergy & Immunology 1977; **Med School:** Switzerland 1962; **Resid:** Pediatrics, Tel Aviv Univ Hosp 1967; **Fellow:** Allergy & Immunology, Univ Bern 1969; Allergy & Immunology, Harvard Med Sch 1973; **Fac Appt:** Prof Ped, Albert Einstein Coll Med

Cardiac Electrophysiology

Ferrick, Kevin J MD (CE) - **Spec Exp:** Arrhythmias; Sudden Death Prevention; Pacemakers; **Hospital:** Montefiore Med Ctr-Moses Campus (page 100), Stamford Hosp (page 939); **Address:** Montefiore Medical Center, Arrhythmia Service, 111 E 210th St, Bronx, NY 10467; **Phone:** 718-920-4148; **Board Cert:** Internal Medicine 1981; Cardiovascular Disease 1983; Cardiac Electrophysiology 2013; **Med School:** Med Coll Wisc 1977; **Resid:** Internal Medicine, Montefiore Hosp 1980; **Fellow:** Cardiovascular Disease, Columbia-Presby Med Ctr 1981; Cardiac Electrophysiology, Columbia-Presby Med Ctr 1983; **Fac Appt:** Prof Med, Albert Einstein Coll Med

Gross, Jay MD (CE) - **Spec Exp:** Pacemakers; **Hospital:** Montefiore Med Ctr-Moses Campus (page 100); **Address:** Montefiore, Arrhythmia Svc, 111 E 210th St Fl 2, Bronx, NY 10467; **Phone:** 718-920-6190; **Board Cert:** Internal Medicine 1986; Cardiovascular Disease 1989; Cardiac Electrophysiology 2013; **Med School:** Albert Einstein Coll Med 1983; **Resid:** Internal Medicine, Montefiore Med Ctr 1986; **Fellow:** Cardiovascular Disease, Montrfiore Med Ctr 1988; **Fac Appt:** Prof Med, Albert Einstein Coll Med

Krumerman, Andrew K MD (CE) - **Spec Exp:** Atrial Fibrillation; Arrhythmias; Catheter Ablation; **Hospital:** Montefiore Med Ctr-Moses Campus (page 100); **Address:** Montefiore, Arrhythmia Svc, 111 E 210th St Fl 2, Bronx, NY 10467; **Phone:** 718-920-4776; **Board Cert:** Cardiovascular Disease 2003; Cardiac Electrophysiology 2004; **Med School:** Israel 1996; **Resid:** Internal Medicine, Montefiore Med Ctr 1999; **Fellow:** Cardiovascular Disease, N Shore Univ Hosp 2001; Cardiac Electrophysiology, Montefiore Med Ctr 2002; **Fac Appt:** Asst Prof Med, Albert Einstein Coll Med

Palma, Eugen C MD (CE) - **Spec Exp:** Arrhythmias; Atrial Fibrillation; Catheter Ablation; **Hospital:** Montefiore Med Ctr-Einstein Campus (page 100), Montefiore Med Ctr-Moses Campus (page 100); **Address:** 1825 Eastchester Rd, Weiler Bldg - Fl 2ND - Ste RAU, Bronx, NY 10461; **Phone:** 718-904-2588; **Board Cert:** Cardiovascular Disease 2007; Cardiac Electrophysiology 2010; **Med School:** Philippines 1989; **Resid:** Internal Medicine, SUNY Hlth Sci Ctr 1993; **Fellow:** Cardiovascular Disease, Montefiore Med Ctr-Moses Div 1997; Cardiac Electrophysiology, UCSF Med Ctr 1999; **Fac Appt:** Assoc Clin Prof Med, Albert Einstein Coll Med

Cardiovascular Disease

Cohen, Martin N MD (Cv) - **Spec Exp:** Preventive Cardiology; **Hospital:** Montefiore Med Ctr-Einstein Campus (page 100); **Address:** 1628 Eastchester Road, Bronx, NY 10461; **Phone:** 718-904-2927; **Board Cert:** Internal Medicine 1968; Cardiovascular Disease 1972; **Med School:** Columbia P&S 1961; **Resid:** Internal Medicine, Peter Bent Brigham Hosp 1965; **Fellow:** Cardiovascular Disease, Peter Bent Brigham Hosp 1968; **Fac Appt:** Prof Med, Albert Einstein Coll Med

Forman, Robert MD (Cv) - **Spec Exp:** Heart Valve Disease; Coronary Artery Disease; **Hospital:** Montefiore Med Ctr-Einstein Campus (page 100); **Address:** 1628 Eastchester Rd, Div Cardiology, Bronx, NY 10461-2301; **Phone:** 646-670-5120; **Med School:** Africa 1961; **Fellow:** Cardiovascular Disease, Peter Bent Brigham Hosp 1970; **Fac Appt:** Prof Med, Albert Einstein Coll Med

Garcia, Mario J MD (Cv) - **Spec Exp:** Echocardiography-Transesophageal; Echocardiography; **Hospital:** Montefiore Med Ctr-Moses Campus (page 100); **Address:** Montefiore Einstein Heart/Cardiovascular Care, 111 E 210th St, Bronx, NY 10467; **Phone:** 718-920-4172; **Board Cert:** Internal Medicine 2003; Cardiovascular Disease 2003; **Med School:** Dominican Republic 1986; **Resid:** Internal Medicine, St Vincent's Med Ctr 1990; **Fellow:** Nuclear Cardiology, Mass Genl Hosp 1994; Cardiovascular Disease, Cleveland Clinic 1996; **Fac Appt:** Prof Med, Albert Einstein Coll Med

Greenberg, Mark A MD (Cv) - **Spec Exp:** Interventional Cardiology; Cardiac Catheterization; Heart Valve Disease; **Hospital:** Montefiore Med Ctr-Moses Campus (page 100); **Address:** 111 E 210th St, Division of Cardiology, Bronx, NY 10467; **Phone:** 718-920-4212; **Board Cert:** Internal Medicine 1976; Cardiovascular Disease 1979; **Med School:** Univ IL Coll Med 1973; **Resid:** Internal Medicine, Montefiore Med Ctr 1976; **Fellow:** Cardiovascular Disease, Montefiore Med Ctr 1979; **Fac Appt:** Clin Prof Med, Albert Einstein Coll Med

Kaufman, David B MD (Cv) - **Spec Exp:** Nuclear Cardiology; **Hospital:** Montefiore Med Ctr-Einstein Campus (page 100); **Address:** Riverdale Heart Ctr, 2600 Netherland Ave, Ste 121, Riverdale, NY 10463; **Phone:** 718-548-1590; **Board Cert:** Internal Medicine 1980; Cardiovascular Disease 1983; **Med School:** Cornell Univ-Weill Med Coll 1977; **Resid:** Internal Medicine, Montefiore Med Ctr 1980; **Fellow:** Cardiovascular Disease, Montefiore Med Ctr 1983

Keller, Peter Karl MD (Cv) - **Spec Exp:** Congestive Heart Failure; Coronary Artery Disease; Arrhythmias; **Hospital:** Montefiore Med Ctr-Einstein Campus (page 100), Montefiore Westchester Sq; **Address:** Montefiore, Cardiology Dept, 1578 Williamsbridge Rd Fl 1, Bronx, NY 10461; **Phone:** 718-892-7817; **Board Cert:** Internal Medicine 1988; Cardiovascular Disease 2011; **Med School:** Mount Sinai Sch Med 1985; **Resid:** Internal Medicine, Jacobi Med Ctr 1988; **Fellow:** Cardiovascular Disease, Jacobi Med Ctr 1991; **Fac Appt:** Assoc Clin Prof Med, Albert Einstein Coll Med

Lucariello, Richard MD (Cv) - **Spec Exp:** Congestive Heart Failure; Angina; Hypertension; **Hospital:** Montefiore Med Ctr-Wakefield Campus (page 100); **Address:** Montefiore, Cardiovascular Disease, 4256 Bronx Blvd, Bronx, NY 10466; **Phone:** 646-329-8200; **Board Cert:** Internal Medicine 1987; Cardiovascular Disease 2011; **Med School:** NY Med Coll 1984; **Resid:** Internal Medicine, Westchester Med Ctr 1987; **Fellow:** Cardiovascular Disease, St Vincents Hosp 1989; Cardiovascular Disease, Westchester Med Ctr 1990

Menegus, Mark A MD (Cv) - **Spec Exp:** Acute Coronary Syndromes; Cardiac Catheterization; Interventional Cardiology; Heart Valve Disease; **Hospital:** Montefiore Med Ctr-Moses Campus (page 100), St Barnabas Hosp - Bronx; **Address:** Montefiore Medical Center-Div Cardiology, 111 E 210th St, Bronx, NY 10467-2401; **Phone:** 718-920-5528; **Board Cert:** Internal Medicine 1984; Cardiovascular Disease 1987; **Med School:** UMDNJ-RW Johnson Med Sch 1981; **Resid:** Internal Medicine, Montefiore Med Ctr 1984; **Fellow:** Cardiovascular Disease, Montefiore Med Ctr 1987; **Fac Appt:** Clin Prof Med, Albert Einstein Coll Med

Monrad, E. Scott MD (Cv) - **Spec Exp:** Coronary Artery Disease; Heart Valve Disease; Cardiac Catheterization; **Hospital:** Montefiore Med Ctr-Einstein Campus (page 100), Jacobi Med Ctr; **Address:** Montefiore, Cardiovascular Disease, 1628 Eastchester Rd, Bronx, NY 10461; **Phone:** 646-670-5120; **Board Cert:** Internal Medicine 1982; Cardiovascular Disease 1985; **Med School:** McGill Univ 1979; **Resid:** Internal Medicine, New England Med Ctr 1982; **Fellow:** Cardiovascular Disease, Beth Israel Deaconess Med Ctr 1985; **Fac Appt:** Prof Med, Albert Einstein Coll Med

Neuberg, Gerald W MD (Cv) - **Spec Exp:** Congestive Heart Failure; Preventive Cardiology; **Hospital:** NY-Presby/Columbia Univ Med Ctr, NY (page 104), NY-Presby Hosp/The Allen Hosp (page 104); **Address:** 3050 Corlear Ave, Ste 204, Bronx, NY 10463; **Phone:** 718-601-8720; **Board Cert:** Internal Medicine 1986; Cardiovascular Disease 1989; **Med School:** Columbia P&S 1983; **Resid:** Internal Medicine, NY Presby Hosp 1986; **Fellow:** Cardiovascular Disease, Westchester Med Ctr 1988; Cardiovascular Disease, Mt Sinai Med Ctr 1989; **Fac Appt:** Clin Prof Med, Columbia P&S

Phillips, Malcolm C MD (Cv) - **Spec Exp:** Preventive Cardiology; Echocardiography; Cardiac Stress Testing; **Hospital:** St. Barnabas Hosp - Bronx; **Address:** 4422 3rd Ave, Bronx, NY 10457-2545; **Phone:** 718-960-6205; **Board Cert:** Internal Medicine 1979; Cardiovascular Disease 1981; **Med School:** Columbia P&S 1976; **Resid:** Internal Medicine, New York Hosp 1978; **Fellow:** Cardiovascular Disease, New York Hosp 1980; **Fac Appt:** Asst Clin Prof Med, Cornell Univ-Weill Med Coll

Sahar, David I MD (Cv) - **Spec Exp:** Arrhythmias; Atrial Fibrillation; Heart Valve Disease; Coronary Artery Disease; **Hospital:** NY-Presby/Columbia Univ Med Ctr, NY (page 104); **Address:** 3050 Corlear Ave, Ste 204, Bronx, NY 10463; **Phone:** 212-305-4567; **Board Cert:** Internal Medicine 1983; Cardiovascular Disease 1987; **Med School:** Columbia P&S 1980; **Resid:** Internal Medicine, Ohio State Univ Hosp 1983; **Fellow:** Cardiovascular Disease, St Lukes-Roosevelt Hosp 1985; Cardiac Electrophysiology, NY-Presby/Columbia Univ Med Ctr 1987; **Fac Appt:** Assoc Prof Med, Columbia P&S

Silverman, Rubin MD (Cv) - **Spec Exp:** Echocardiography; **Hospital:** St. Barnabas Hosp - Bronx, Montefiore Med Ctr-Einstein Campus (page 100); **Address:** 1250 Waters Pl, Ste 1207, Bronx, NY 10461; **Phone:** 718-409-3335; **Board Cert:** Internal Medicine 1981; Cardiovascular Disease 1983; **Med School:** Albert Einstein Coll Med 1978; **Resid:** Internal Medicine, Jacobi Med Ctr 1981; **Fellow:** Cardiovascular Disease, Montefiore Med Ctr 1983; **Fac Appt:** Asst Prof Med, Albert Einstein Coll Med

Child Neurology

Moshe, Solomon L MD (ChiN) - **Spec Exp:** Epilepsy/Seizure Disorders; **Hospital:** Montefiore Med Ctr-Moses Campus (page 100); **Address:** 3415 Bainbridge Ave Fl 4, Bronx, NY 10467; **Phone:** 718-920-4378; **Board Cert:** Pediatrics 1978; Child Neurology 1979; Clinical Neurophysiology 2006; **Med School:** Greece 1972; **Resid:** Pediatrics, Univ MD Hosp 1975; **Fellow:** Pediatric Neurology, Jacobi Med Ctr 1978; **Fac Appt:** Prof N, Albert Einstein Coll Med

Shinnar, Shlomo MD/PhD (ChiN) - **Spec Exp:** Epilepsy/Seizure Disorders; Infantile Spasms-West Syndrome; **Hospital:** Montefiore Med Ctr-Moses Campus (page 100); **Address:** Montefiore Med Ctr, Pediatric Neurology and Epilepsy, 111 E 210th St, Fl 4, Bronx, NY 10467; **Phone:** 718-920-4378; **Board Cert:** Neurology 1984; Pediatrics 1984; Clinical Neurophysiology 2005; **Med School:** Albert Einstein Coll Med 1978; **Resid:** Pediatrics, Johns Hopkins Hosp 1980; Neurology, Johns Hopkins Hosp 1983; **Fac Appt:** Prof N, Albert Einstein Coll Med

Clinical Genetics

Marion, Robert W MD (CG) - **Spec Exp:** Spina Bifida; Williams Syndrome; Marfan's Syndrome; Down Syndrome; **Hospital:** Montefiore Med Ctr-Moses Campus (page 100), Blythedale Children's Hosp; **Address:** 3415 Bainbridge Ave, Bronx, NY 10467; **Phone:** 718-741-2323; **Board Cert:** Pediatrics 1985; Clinical Genetics 1987; **Med School:** Albert Einstein Coll Med 1979; **Resid:** Pediatrics, Einstein Affil Hosp 1982; **Fellow:** Clinical Genetics, Einstein Affil Hosp 1984; **Fac Appt:** Prof Ped, Albert Einstein Coll Med

Ostrer, Harry MD (CG) - **Spec Exp:** Genetic Disorders; Hereditary Cancer; **Hospital:** Montefiore Med Ctr-Wakefield Campus (page 100); **Address:** Albert Einstein College of Medicine, 1300 Morris Park Ave, Ullman Blg, rm 819, Bronx, NY 10461; **Phone:** 718-430-8605; **Board Cert:** Clinical Genetics 1984; Pediatrics 1985; Clinical Cytogenetics 1990; Clinical Molecular Genetics 2010; **Med School:** Columbia P&S 1976; **Resid:** Pediatrics, Johns Hopkins Hosp 1978; Clinical Genetics, Johns Hopkins Hosp 1984; **Fellow:** Molecular Genetics, Natl Inst Health 1981; **Fac Appt:** Prof Path, Albert Einstein Coll Med

Critical Care Medicine

Siegel, Robert MD (CCM) - **Spec Exp:** Pneumonia; Infectious Disease; **Hospital:** James J. Peters VA Med Ctr-Bronx, Mt Sinai Med Ctr (page 102); **Address:** 130 W Kingsbridge Rd, Ste 8C-100, Bronx, NY 10468-3992; **Phone:** 718-584-9000 x6723; **Board Cert:** Internal Medicine 1982; Pulmonary Disease 1986; Critical Care Medicine 2009; **Med School:** Columbia P&S 1979; **Resid:** Internal Medicine, St Luke's Hosp 1982; Internal Medicine, Booth Meml Hosp 1983; **Fellow:** Pulmonary Disease, Bronx Municipal Hosp 1985; **Fac Appt:** Assoc Prof Med, Mount Sinai Sch Med

Dermatology

Cohen, Steven R MD (D) - **Spec Exp:** Occupational Dermatology; Contact Dermatitis; Psoriasis; **Hospital:** Montefiore Med Ctr-Moses Campus (page 100); **Address:** 3514 Bainbridge Ave Fl 1, Bronx, NY 10467; **Phone:** 866-633-8255; **Board Cert:** Dermatology 2009; **Med School:** Univ Pennsylvania 1971; **Resid:** Dermatology, Yale-New Haven Hosp 1977; **Fac Appt:** Prof D, Albert Einstein Coll Med

Lerman, Jay S MD (D) - **Spec Exp:** Acne; Eczema; **Hospital:** Montefiore Med Ctr-Einstein Campus (page 100), Montefiore Med Ctr-Moses Campus (page 100); **Address:** 2426 Eastchester Rd, Bronx, NY 10469; **Phone:** 718-865-8733; **Board Cert:** Dermatology 1974; **Med School:** SUNY Downstate 1969; **Resid:** Dermatology, Jacobi Med Ctr 1973; **Fac Appt:** Asst Clin Prof D, Albert Einstein Coll Med

Liteplo, Ronald R MD (D) - **Spec Exp:** Melanoma; Skin Diseases-Immunologic; **Hospital:** Montefiore Med Ctr-Moses Campus (page 100); **Address:** 3176 Bainbridge Ave, Bronx, NY 10467; **Phone:** 718-515-0200; **Board Cert:** Internal Medicine 1975; Dermatology 1978; **Med School:** NYU Sch Med 1972; **Resid:** Internal Medicine, SUNY Buffalo Affil Hosp 1975; Dermatology, SUNY Buffalo Affil Hosp 1978; **Fellow:** Immunology, SUNY Buffalo Affil Hosp 1976; **Fac Appt:** Asst Clin Prof Med, Albert Einstein Coll Med

Rosen, Douglas MD (D) - **Spec Exp:** Skin Cancer; Hair Removal-Laser; Acne; **Hospital:** Montefiore Westchester Sq; **Address:** 3620 E Tremont Ave, FL 2, Bronx, NY 10465; **Phone:** 718-792-4700; **Board Cert:** Dermatology 1984; **Med School:** Albert Einstein Coll Med 1980; **Resid:** Dermatology, Montefiore Hosp Med Ctr 1984; **Fac Appt:** Assoc Prof D, Albert Einstein Coll Med

Rudikoff, Donald MD (D) - **Spec Exp:** AIDS Related Skin Disorders; Skin Infections; Smallpox; **Hospital:** Bronx Lebanon Hosp Ctr; **Address:** 2739 3rd Ave, Bronx, NY 10451; **Phone:** 718-838-1066; **Board Cert:** Internal Medicine 1980; Dermatology 2009; **Med School:** NY Med Coll 1973; **Resid:** Internal Medicine, Beth Israel Med Ctr 1980; Dermatology, Mount Sinai Med Ctr 1982; **Fac Appt:** Assoc Clin Prof D, Albert Einstein Coll Med

Diagnostic Radiology

Amis Jr, E Stephen MD (DR) - **Spec Exp:** Urologic Imaging; **Hospital:** Montefiore Med Ctr-Moses Campus (page 100); **Address:** Montefiore Med Ctr, Dept Radiology, 111 E 210th St, Bronx, NY 10467; **Phone:** 718-920-5113; **Board Cert:** Urology 1975; Diagnostic Radiology 1979; **Med School:** Northwestern Univ 1967; **Resid:** Urology, US Naval Hosp 1972; Diagnostic Radiology, US Naval Hosp 1978; **Fellow:** Urologic Radiology, Mass General Hosp 1981; **Fac Appt:** Prof Rad, Albert Einstein Coll Med

Friedman, Stanley N MD (DR) - **Hospital:** Montefiore Westchester Sq; **Address:** NY Westchester Sq Med Ctr, Dept Rad, 2475 St Raymond Ave, Bronx, NY 10461-3124; **Phone:** 718-430-7321; **Board Cert:** Diagnostic Radiology 1974; **Med School:** NY Med Coll 1968; **Resid:** Diagnostic Radiology, Mt Sinai Hosp 1970; Radiation Oncology, Albert Einstein 1972; **Fellow:** Diagnostic Radiology, Mt Sinai Hosp 1973

Haramati, Linda B MD (DR) - **Spec Exp:** AIDS/HIV; Lung Cancer; **Hospital:** Montefiore Med Ctr-Moses Campus (page 100), Jacobi Med Ctr; **Address:** Montefiore Med Ctr, Dept Radiology, 111 E 210th St, Bronx, NY 10467-2401; **Phone:** 718-920-7458; **Board Cert:** Diagnostic Radiology 1990; **Med School:** Albert Einstein Coll Med 1985; **Resid:** Diagnostic Radiology, Montefiore Med Ctr 1990; **Fellow:** Thoracic Radiology, Columbia-Presby Med Ctr 1991; **Fac Appt:** Clin Prof Rad, Albert Einstein Coll Med

Haramati, Nogah MD (DR) - **Spec Exp:** Orthopaedic Imaging; Rheumatology; Musculoskeletal Imaging; **Hospital:** Montefiore Med Ctr-Moses Campus (page 100), Jacobi Med Ctr; **Address:** 1825 Eastchester Rd, rm 3-006, Bronx, NY 10461; **Phone:** 718-904-2965; **Board Cert:** Diagnostic Radiology 1990; **Med School:** SUNY Hlth Sci Ctr 1985; **Resid:** Diagnostic Radiology, Montefiore Hosp Med Ctr 1990; **Fellow:** Musculoskeletal Imaging, Columbia-Presby Med Ctr 1991; **Fac Appt:** Clin Prof Rad, Albert Einstein Coll Med

Laks, Mitchell P MD/PhD (DR) - **Spec Exp:** MRI; Ultrasound; CT Body Scan; **Hospital:** Montefiore Med Ctr-Moses Campus (page 100); **Address:** Montefiore Med Ctr, Dept Rad, 111 E 210th St, Bronx, NY 10467; **Phone:** 718-920-4396; **Board Cert:** Diagnostic Radiology 1990; **Med School:** Harvard Med Sch 1985; **Resid:** Diagnostic Radiology, Einstein Affil Hosp 1990; **Fellow:** Magnetic Resonance Imaging, Brigham & Womens Hosp 1991; **Fac Appt:** Asst Prof Rad, Albert Einstein Coll Med

Rozenblit, Alla MD (DR) - **Spec Exp:** CT Scan; MRI; **Hospital:** Montefiore Med Ctr-Moses Campus (page 100); **Address:** 111 E 210th St, Bronx, NY 10467-2401; **Phone:** 718-920-4396; **Board Cert:** Diagnostic Radiology 1984; **Med School:** Russia 1971; **Resid:** Diagnostic Radiology, Queens Hosp Ctr 1984; **Fellow:** Ultrasound/CT, LI Jewish Med Ctr 1985; **Fac Appt:** Clin Prof Rad, Albert Einstein Coll Med

Spindola-Franco, Hugo MD (DR) - **Spec Exp:** Thoracic Radiology; Cardiac Imaging; Congenital Heart Disease; **Hospital:** Montefiore Med Ctr-Moses Campus (page 100); **Address:** 111 E 210th St, Bronx, NY 10467-2401; **Phone:** 718-920-4872; **Board Cert:** Diagnostic Radiology 1970; **Med School:** Mexico 1966; **Resid:** Diagnostic Radiology, Montefiore Hosp Med Ctr 1970; **Fellow:** Cardiovascular Radiology, Peter Bent Brigham Hosp/Harvard Med Sch 1971; **Fac Appt:** Prof Rad, Albert Einstein Coll Med

Stern, Harvey MD (DR) - **Spec Exp:** Nuclear Medicine; **Hospital:** Bronx Lebanon Hosp Ctr; **Address:** Bronx-Lebanon Hosp, Dept Radiology, 1650 Grand Concourse, Bronx, NY 10457-7606; **Phone:** 718-960-4522; **Board Cert:** Diagnostic Radiology 1975; Nuclear Radiology 1978; **Med School:** Albert Einstein Coll Med 1971; **Resid:** Diagnostic Radiology, Bronx Muni Hosp 1975; **Fac Appt:** Asst Prof Rad, Albert Einstein Coll Med

Wolf, Ellen L MD (DR) - **Spec Exp:** Gastrointestinal Imaging; Abdominal Imaging; **Hospital:** Montefiore Med Ctr-Moses Campus (page 100); **Address:** 111 E 210th St, Bronx, NY 10467; **Phone:** 718-920-4851; **Board Cert:** Diagnostic Radiology 1976; **Med School:** Mount Sinai Sch Med 1972; **Resid:** Diagnostic Radiology, Columbia-Presby 1974; Diagnostic Radiology, Johns Hopkins 1976; **Fellow:** Pediatric Radiology, Columbia-Presby 1977; **Fac Appt:** Clin Prof Rad, Albert Einstein Coll Med

Endocrinology, Diabetes & Metabolism

Cohen, Charmian D MD (EDM) - **Spec Exp:** Diabetes; Thyroid Disorders; Obesity; **Hospital:** Montefiore Med Ctr-Einstein Campus (page 100); **Address:** 1200 Waters Pl, Ste M105, Bronx, NY 10461; **Phone:** 718-892-7033; **Board Cert:** Internal Medicine 1987; Endocrinology, Diabetes & Metabolism 1989; **Med School:** South Africa 1977; **Resid:** Internal Medicine, G Schuer Hosp 1984; **Fellow:** Endocrinology, Diabetes & Metabolism, Albert Einstein 1986

Grajower, Martin M MD (EDM) - **Spec Exp:** Diabetes; Osteoporosis; Thyroid Disorders; Metabolic Disorders; **Hospital:** Montefiore Med Ctr-Moses Campus (page 100); **Address:** 3736 Henry Hudson Pkwy E, Riverdale, NY 10463; **Phone:** 718-549-6268; **Board Cert:** Internal Medicine 1987; Endocrinology, Diabetes & Metabolism 1981; **Med School:** Albert Einstein Coll Med 1973; **Resid:** Internal Medicine, Montefiore Hosp Med Ctr 1975; Internal Medicine, Boston Med Ctr 1976; **Fellow:** Endocrinology, Diabetes & Metabolism, Montefiore Hosp Med Ctr 1978; **Fac Appt:** Assoc Clin Prof Med, Albert Einstein Coll Med

Guzman, Rodolfo MD (EDM) - **Spec Exp:** Endocrinology; Diabetes; Thyroid Disorders; **Hospital:** Bronx Lebanon Hosp Ctr; **Address:** 860 Grand Concourse, Ste 1K, Bronx, NY 10451; **Phone:** 718-585-5060; **Board Cert:** Internal Medicine 2013; Endocrinology, Diabetes & Metabolism 2000; **Med School:** Dominican Republic 1979; **Resid:** Internal Medicine, Bronx-Lebanon Hosp 1990; **Fellow:** Endocrinology, Diabetes & Metabolism, Lincoln Med Ctr 1992

Shamoon, Harry MD (EDM) - **Hospital:** Montefiore Med Ctr-Einstein Campus (page 100); **Address:** 1575 Blondell Ave, Ste 200, Bronx, NY 10461-2601; **Phone:** 718-405-8260; **Board Cert:** Internal Medicine 1977; Endocrinology, Diabetes & Metabolism 1979; **Med School:** Yale Univ 1974; **Resid:** Internal Medicine, Jacobi Med Ctr 1977; **Fellow:** Endocrinology, Diabetes & Metabolism, Yale-New Haven Hosp 1979; **Fac Appt:** Prof Med, Albert Einstein Coll Med

Surks, Martin I MD (EDM) - **Spec Exp:** Thyroid Disorders; **Hospital:** Montefiore Med Ctr-Moses Campus (page 100), N Central Bronx Hosp; **Address:** 3400 Bainbridge Ave Fl 2, Bronx, NY 10467; **Phone:** 866-633-8255; **Board Cert:** Internal Medicine 1967; Endocrinology, Diabetes & Metabolism 1977; **Med School:** NYU Sch Med 1960; **Resid:** Internal Medicine, Montefiore Med Ctr 1962; Internal Medicine, VA Hosp 1964; **Fellow:** Research, Natl Inst Arthritis-Metabolic Disease 1966; **Fac Appt:** Prof Med, Albert Einstein Coll Med

Zonszein, Joel MD (EDM) - **Spec Exp:** Diabetes; Throid Disorders; Heart Disease in Diabetes Patients; **Hospital:** Montefiore Med Ctr-Moses Campus (page 100); **Address:** 1575 Blondell Ave, Ste 200, Bronx, NY 10461; **Phone:** 866-633-8255; **Board Cert:** Nuclear Medicine 1976; Internal Medicine 1977; Endocrinology 1977; **Med School:** Mexico 1969; **Resid:** Internal Medicine, Maimonides Med Ctr 1972; Internal Medicine, Jacobi Med Ctr 1973; **Fellow:** Endocrinology, Northwestern Univ 1974; Endocrinology, Georgetown Univ 1975; **Fac Appt:** Prof Med, Albert Einstein Coll Med

Family Medicine

Biagiotti, Wendy L MD (FMed) *PCP* - **Hospital:** Montefiore Med Ctr-Moses Campus (page 100); **Address:** 3101 E Tremont Ave, Bronx, NY 10461; **Phone:** 718-863-7925; **Board Cert:** Family Medicine 2009; **Med School:** Mexico 1988; **Resid:** Family Medicine, St Joseph's Hosp&Med Ctr 1994; **Fac Appt:** Asst Clin Prof FMed, Albert Einstein Coll Med

Coloka-Kump, Rodika DO (FMed) *PCP* - **Spec Exp:** Preventive Medicine; **Hospital:** Saint Joseph's Med Ctr - Yonkers, St. John's Riverside Hosp-Andrus Pavil; **Address:** 530 W 236th St, rm #1D, Bronx, NY 10463; **Phone:** 718-548-4560; **Board Cert:** Family Medicine 2004; **Med School:** NY Coll Osteo Med 1988; **Resid:** Family Medicine, St Joseph's Med Ctr 1991

Cordero, Evelyn MD (FMed) *PCP* - **Hospital:** Montefiore Med Ctr-Wakefield Campus (page 100), Montefiore Westchester Sq; **Address:** 941 Castle Hill Ave, Bronx, NY 10473; **Phone:** 718-792-3117; **Board Cert:** Family Medicine 2003; **Med School:** SUNY Hlth Sci Ctr 1979; **Resid:** Family Medicine, St Joseph's Med Ctr 1982

Delaney, Brian MD (FMed) *PCP* - **Spec Exp:** Geriatric Care; **Hospital:** Montefiore Med Ctr-Moses Campus (page 100), St. Barnabas Hosp - Bronx; **Address:** 2371 Arthur Ave, Bronx, NY 10458; **Phone:** 718-364-6199; **Board Cert:** Family Medicine 2007; Geriatric Medicine 2012; **Med School:** Albert Einstein Coll Med 1983; **Resid:** Family Medicine, Montefiore Med Ctr 1986; **Fac Appt:** Asst Prof FMed, Albert Einstein Coll Med

Franzetti, Carl J DO (FMed) *PCP* - **Spec Exp:** Diabetes; **Hospital:** Saint Joseph's Med Ctr - Yonkers, NY-Presby/Columbia Univ Med Ctr, NY (page 104); **Address:** 3050 Corlear Ave, Ste 201, Bronx, NY 10463; **Phone:** 718-543-2700; **Board Cert:** Family Medicine 2005; **Med School:** NY Coll Osteo Med 1984; **Resid:** Family Medicine, Warren Hosp 1987

Gold, Marji MD (FMed) *PCP* - **Hospital:** Montefiore Med Ctr-Moses Campus (page 100); **Address:** Montefiore Medical Group, Family Health Ctr, 360 E 193rd St, Bronx, NY 10458; **Phone:** 718-933-2400; **Board Cert:** Family Medicine 2010; **Med School:** NYU Sch Med 1973; **Resid:** Family Medicine, Montefiore Med Ctr 1976

Maselli, Frank J MD (FMed) *PCP* - **Spec Exp:** Diving Medicine; Hyperbaric Medicine; **Hospital:** Saint Joseph's Med Ctr - Yonkers, NY-Presby/Columbia Univ Med Ctr, NY (page 104); **Address:** 3050 Corlear Ave, Ste 201, Bronx, NY 10463; **Phone:** 718-543-2700; **Board Cert:** Family Medicine 2004; **Med School:** Israel 1983; **Resid:** Family Medicine, Univ Hosp 1986

Morrow, Robert MD (FMed) *PCP* - **Spec Exp:** Preventive Medicine; Geriatric Medicine; Autism; **Hospital:** Montefiore Med Ctr-Moses Campus (page 100), Saint Joseph's Med Ctr - Yonkers; **Address:** 5997 Riverdale Ave, Bronx, NY 10471-1602; **Phone:** 718-884-9803; **Board Cert:** Family Medicine 2009; **Med School:** Mount Sinai Sch Med 1974; **Resid:** Family Medicine, Montefiore Med Ctr 1977; **Fac Appt:** Assoc Clin Prof FMed, Albert Einstein Coll Med

Soloway, Bruce H MD (FMed) *PCP* - **Spec Exp:** AIDS/HIV; **Hospital:** Montefiore Med Ctr-Moses Campus (page 100); **Address:** Montefiore Medical Center, 360 E 193 St, Bronx, NY 10458; **Phone:** 718-933-2400; **Board Cert:** Family Medicine 2007; **Med School:** Albert Einstein Coll Med 1985; **Resid:** Family Medicine, Montefiore Med Ctr 1988; **Fac Appt:** Assoc Prof FMed, Albert Einstein Coll Med

Gastroenterology

Abelow, Arthur MD (Ge) - **Spec Exp:** Endoscopy; Nutrition; **Hospital:** Montefiore Med Ctr-Einstein Campus (page 100), Montefiore Westchester Sq; **Address:** New York Associates in Gastroenterology, 1250 Waters Pl Fl 12 - Ste 1201, Bronx, NY 10461; **Phone:** 718-863-7397; **Board Cert:** Internal Medicine 1983; Gastroenterology 1985; **Med School:** Albert Einstein Coll Med 1980; **Resid:** Internal Medicine, Bronx Muni Hosp Ctr 1983; **Fellow:** Gastroenterology, Montefiore Med Ctr 1985; **Fac Appt:** Asst Clin Prof Med, Albert Einstein Coll Med

Antony, Michael A MD (Ge) - **Spec Exp:** Colonoscopy; Endoscopy; Liver Disease; **Hospital:** Montefiore Med Ctr-Einstein Campus (page 100), Montefiore Westchester Sq; **Address:** 1842 Williamsbridge Rd, Bronx, NY 10461; **Phone:** 718-828-0100; **Board Cert:** Internal Medicine 1985; Gastroenterology 1989; **Med School:** SUNY Stony Brook 1982; **Resid:** Internal Medicine, Bronx Muni Hosp 1985; **Fellow:** Gastroenterology, Montefiore Med Ctr 1988

Brandt, Lawrence MD (Ge) - **Spec Exp:** Inflammatory Bowel Disease; Clostridium Difficile Disease; **Hospital:** Montefiore Med Ctr-Moses Campus (page 100); **Address:** 3400 Bainbridge Ave Fl 2, Bronx, NY 10467-2401; **Phone:** 866-633-8255; **Board Cert:** Internal Medicine 1972; Gastroenterology 2006; **Med School:** SUNY Downstate 1968; **Resid:** Internal Medicine, Mt Sinai Med Ctr 1972; **Fellow:** Gastroenterology, Mt Sinai Med Ctr 1972; **Fac Appt:** Prof Emeritus Med, Albert Einstein Coll Med

Frager, Joseph D MD (Ge) - **Spec Exp:** Colon Cancer; Endoscopy; Laser Surgery; **Hospital:** Montefiore Med Ctr-Moses Campus (page 100), NY Hosp Queens (page 488); **Address:** 277 Van Cortlandt Ave E, Bronx, NY 10467-3011; **Phone:** 718-798-8867; **Board Cert:** Internal Medicine 1983; Gastroenterology 1985; **Med School:** Univ Pennsylvania 1980; **Resid:** Internal Medicine, Montefiore Med Ctr 1983; **Fellow:** Gastroenterology, Montefiore Med Ctr 1985; **Fac Appt:** Asst Clin Prof Med, Albert Einstein Coll Med

Gaglio, Paul J MD (Ge) - **Spec Exp:** Transplant Medicine-Liver; Liver Disease; Hepatitis B & C; **Hospital:** Montefiore Med Ctr-Moses Campus (page 100); **Address:** Montefiore Einstein Liver Ctr, 111 E 210th St, Rosenthal Bldg, Fl 2, Bronx, NY 10467; **Phone:** 718-920-6240; **Board Cert:** Internal Medicine 2011; Gastroenterology 2003; Transplant Hepatology 2006; **Med School:** UMDNJ-NJ Med Sch, Newark 1988; **Resid:** Internal Medicine, Mt Sinai Med Ctr 1991; **Fellow:** Gastroenterology, UMDNJ-NJ Med Sch 1993; **Fac Appt:** Prof Med, Albert Einstein Coll Med

Greenwald, David A MD (Ge) - **Spec Exp:** Endoscopy; Gastroesophageal Reflux Disease (GERD); Peptic Ulcer Disease; **Hospital:** Montefiore Med Ctr-Moses Campus (page 100), Montefiore Med Ctr-Einstein Campus (page 100); **Address:** Montefiore Med Ctr, Div Gastroenterology, 111 E 210th St, Bronx, NY 10467; **Phone:** 718-920-4846; **Board Cert:** Internal Medicine 1989; Gastroenterology 2003; **Med School:** Albert Einstein Coll Med 1986; **Resid:** Internal Medicine, Columbia Presby Med Ctr 1989; **Fellow:** Gastroenterology, Columbia Presby Med Ctr 1993; **Fac Appt:** Clin Prof Med, Albert Einstein Coll Med

Gupta, Sanjeev MD (Ge) - **Spec Exp:** Hepatitis; Liver Failure; Liver Disease; **Hospital:** Montefiore Med Ctr-Einstein Campus (page 100); **Address:** 1515 Blondell Ave, Ste 220, Montefiore Medical Park, Bronx, NY 10461-2601; **Phone:** 866-633-8255 x4802; **Board Cert:** Internal Medicine 1989; **Med School:** India 1976; **Resid:** Internal Medicine, PGIMER 1980; Internal Medicine, Hammersmith Hosp 1982; **Fellow:** Gastroenterology, Hammersmith Hosp 1985; Hepatology, LAC-USC Med Ctr 1987; **Fac Appt:** Prof Med, Albert Einstein Coll Med

Gutwein, Isadore P MD (Ge) - **Spec Exp:** Pancreatic/Biliary Endoscopy (ERCP); Colonoscopy; Hepatitis; Inflammatory Bowel Disease/Crohn's; **Hospital:** Montefiore Med Ctr-Moses Campus (page 100); **Address:** 3765 Riverdale Ave, Ste 7, Bronx, NY 10463-1845; **Phone:** 718-543-3636; **Board Cert:** Internal Medicine 1976; Gastroenterology 1979; **Med School:** Albert Einstein Coll Med 1973; **Resid:** Internal Medicine, Montefiore Hosp Med Ctr 1976; **Fellow:** Gastroenterology, St Luke's Hosp 1978; **Fac Appt:** Asst Clin Prof Med, Albert Einstein Coll Med

Hertan, Hilary I MD (Ge) - **Spec Exp:** Endoscopic Ultrasound; **Hospital:** Montefiore Med Ctr-Wakefield Campus (page 100); **Address:** Dept Gastroenterology, 600 E 233rd St Fl 4, Bronx, NY 10466; **Phone:** 718-920-9887; **Board Cert:** Internal Medicine 1986; Gastroenterology 1989; **Med School:** NY Med Coll 1982; **Resid:** Internal Medicine, North Shore Univ Hosp 1985; **Fellow:** Gastroenterology, Our Lady of Mercy Med Ctr 1990; **Fac Appt:** Asst Prof Med, NY Med Coll

Ho, Sammy MD (Ge) - **Spec Exp:** Pancreatic/Biliary Endoscopy (ERCP); Endoscopic Ultrasound; Endoscopy; **Hospital:** Montefiore Med Ctr-Moses Campus (page 100); **Address:** 111 E 210th St, Bronx, NY 10467; **Phone:** 718-920-4846; **Board Cert:** Gastroenterology 2005; **Med School:** SUNY Stony Brook 1998; **Resid:** Internal Medicine, Kaiser Fdn Hosp 2001; **Fellow:** Gastroenterology, Winthrop Univ Hosp 2004; **Fac Appt:** Asst Prof Med, Albert Einstein Coll Med

Korsten, Mark A MD (Ge) - **Spec Exp:** Constipation; Gastrointestinal Motility Disorders; Spinal Cord Injury & Colonic Motility; Liver Disease; **Hospital:** James J. Peters VA Med Ctr-Bronx; **Address:** 130 W Kingsbridge Rd, Ste 3H, Bronx, NY 10468; **Phone:** 718-584-9000 x6753; **Board Cert:** Internal Medicine 1973; Gastroenterology 1975; **Med School:** Yale Univ 1970; **Resid:** Internal Medicine, Mt Sinai Med Ctr 1973; **Fellow:** Gastroenterology, Mt Sinai Med Ctr 1975; **Fac Appt:** Prof Med, Mount Sinai Sch Med

Remy, Prospere MD (Ge) - **Spec Exp:** Liver Disease; **Hospital:** Bronx Lebanon Hosp Ctr; **Address:** 860 Grand Concourse, Ste 1K, Bronx, NY 10451-2815; **Phone:** 718-585-5060; **Board Cert:** Internal Medicine 2004; Gastroenterology 2004; **Med School:** Mexico 1984; **Resid:** Internal Medicine, Bronx-Lebanon Hosp 1990; **Fellow:** Gastroenterology, Bronx-Lebanon Hosp 1992; **Fac Appt:** Asst Prof Med, Albert Einstein Coll Med

Sable, Robert A MD (Ge) - **Spec Exp:** Hepatitis B & C; Gastroesophageal Reflux Disease (GERD); Inflammatory Bowel Disease; Irritable Bowel Syndrome; **Hospital:** Montefiore Med Ctr-Moses Campus (page 100), St. Barnabas Hosp - Bronx; **Address:** 3765 Riverdale Ave, Ste 7, Bronx, NY 10463-1845; **Phone:** 718-543-3636; **Board Cert:** Internal Medicine 1987; Gastroenterology 2000; **Med School:** Albert Einstein Coll Med 1973; **Resid:** Internal Medicine, Montefiore Hosp Med Ctr 1976; **Fellow:** Gastroenterology, NY Med Coll 1978; **Fac Appt:** Asst Clin Prof Med, Albert Einstein Coll Med

Schweitzer, Philip E MD (Ge) - **Spec Exp:** Liver Disease; Gastrointestinal Disorders; Esophageal Disorders; **Hospital:** Montefiore Med Ctr-Moses Campus (page 100), Montefiore Med Ctr-Wakefield Campus (page 100); **Address:** 3184 Grand Concourse, Ste 2D, Bronx, NY 10458-1007; **Phone:** 718-584-0404; **Board Cert:** Internal Medicine 1972; Gastroenterology 1977; **Med School:** Cornell Univ-Weill Med Coll 1967; **Resid:** Internal Medicine, St Lukes-Roosevelt Hosp 1972; **Fellow:** Gastroenterology, Mount Sinai Hosp 1974

Sherman, Howard I MD (Ge) - **Spec Exp:** Colonoscopy; **Hospital:** Montefiore Med Ctr-Einstein Campus (page 100), Montefiore Westchester Sq; **Address:** NY Assocs in Gastroenterology, 1250 Waters Pl Fl 12, Bronx, NY 10461-3000; **Phone:** 718-863-7397; **Board Cert:** Internal Medicine 1976; Gastroenterology 1979; **Med School:** Albert Einstein Coll Med 1973; **Resid:** Internal Medicine, Emory Univ Hosp 1976; **Fellow:** Gastroenterology, Emory Univ 1978; **Fac Appt:** Assoc Clin Prof Med, Albert Einstein Coll Med

Stein, David F MD (Ge) - **Spec Exp:** Liver Disease; Hepatitis B & C; AIDS/HIV-Gastrointestinal Complication; Crohn's Disease; **Hospital:** Montefiore Med Ctr-Moses Campus (page 100), St. Barnabas Hosp - Bronx; **Address:** Riverdale Gastro & Liver Diseases, 3765 Riverdale Ave, Ste 7, Bronx, NY 10463; **Phone:** 718-543-3636; **Board Cert:** Gastroenterology 2008; **Med School:** SUNY Downstate 1990; **Resid:** Internal Medicine, NYU Med Ctr 1994; **Fellow:** Gastroenterology, NYU Med Ctr 1996; **Fac Appt:** Asst Clin Prof Med, Albert Einstein Coll Med

Geriatric Medicine

Dharmarajan, Thiruvinvamvalai S MD (Ger) - **Spec Exp:** Kidney Disease; Kidney Failure; Preventive Medicine; **Hospital:** Montefiore Med Ctr-Wakefield Campus (page 100); **Address:** YDR Geriatrics & Nephrology, 4141 Carpenter Ave, Bronx, NY 10466; **Phone:** 718-518-9304; **Board Cert:** Internal Medicine 1977; Geriatric Medicine 2010; Nephrology 1980; **Med School:** India 1967; **Resid:** Internal Medicine, Misericordia Hosp 1977; **Fellow:** Nephrology, Misericordia Hosp 1979; **Fac Appt:** Prof Med, NY Med Coll

Ehrlich, Amy R MD (Ger) - **Spec Exp:** Preventive Medicine; **Hospital:** Montefiore Med Ctr-Moses Campus (page 100); **Address:** Montefiore Med Ctr-Dept Geriatric Med, 111 E 210th St, Bronx, NY 10467; **Phone:** 866-633-8255; **Board Cert:** Internal Medicine 1988; Geriatric Medicine 2004; Hospice & Palliative Medicine 2012; **Med School:** Harvard Med Sch 1985; **Resid:** Internal Medicine, Beth Israel Hosp 1988; **Fac Appt:** Assoc Clin Prof Med, Albert Einstein Coll Med

Goldberg, Roy J MD (Ger) *PCP* - **Spec Exp:** Long Term Care; Medications in the Elderly; Palliative Care; **Hospital:** Montefiore Med Ctr-Einstein Campus (page 100), Montefiore New Rochelle Hosp; **Address:** Director-Kings Harbor Multicare Ctr, 2000 E Gunhill Rd, Bronx, NY 10469; **Phone:** 718-405-3535; **Board Cert:** Internal Medicine 1985; Geriatric Medicine 2012; **Med School:** Albert Einstein Coll Med 1982; **Resid:** Internal Medicine, Montefiore Med Ctr 1985; **Fac Appt:** Assoc Clin Prof Med, Albert Einstein Coll Med

Jacobs, Laurie G MD (Ger) *PCP* - **Spec Exp:** Abuse/Neglect; Frail Elderly; **Hospital:** Montefiore Med Ctr-Moses Campus (page 100); **Address:** Montefiore Med Ctr, Dept Geriatrics, 111 E 210th St, Centennial Bldg, Bronx, NY 10467; **Phone:** 718-920-6471; **Board Cert:** Internal Medicine 1988; Geriatric Medicine 2012; **Med School:** Columbia P&S 1985; **Resid:** Internal Medicine, Montefiore Med Ctr 1988; **Fellow:** Geriatric Medicine, Montefiore Med Ctr 1990; **Fac Appt:** Prof Med, Albert Einstein Coll Med

Malik, Rubina A MD (Ger) *PCP* - **Spec Exp:** Osteoporosis; Falls in the Elderly; Frail Elderly; **Hospital:** Montefiore Med Ctr-Moses Campus (page 100); **Address:** Montefiore Med Ctr-Div of Geriatric Med, 3411 Wayne Ave, Centennial Bldg, Bronx, NY 10467; **Phone:** 718-920-6723; **Board Cert:** Internal Medicine 2006; Geriatric Medicine 2009; Hospice & Palliative Medicine 2012; **Med School:** SUNY Stony Brook 1992; **Resid:** Internal Medicine, Univ Hosp 1993; **Fellow:** Geriatric Medicine, Univ Hosp 1996; **Fac Appt:** Asst Prof Med, Albert Einstein Coll Med

Russell, Robin O MD (Ger) - **Spec Exp:** Kidney Failure; Kidney Disease; Preventive Medicine; **Hospital:** Montefiore Med Ctr-Wakefield Campus (page 100); **Address:** YDR Geriatrics & Nephrology, 4234 Bronx Blvd, Bronx, NY 10466; **Phone:** 347-341-4340; **Board Cert:** Internal Medicine 1974; Nephrology 1980; **Med School:** Univ New Mexico 1971; **Resid:** Internal Medicine, Harlem Hosp 1974; **Fellow:** Nephrology, Harlem Hosp 1976; **Fac Appt:** Asst Prof Med, NY Med Coll

Geriatric Psychiatry

Kennedy, Gary J MD (GerPsy) - **Spec Exp:** Alzheimer's Disease; Dementia; Depression; **Hospital:** Montefiore Med Ctr-Moses Campus (page 100); **Address:** Dept of Psychiatry & Behavioral Sciences, Montefiore Medical Center, 111 E 210th St, Bronx, NY 10467-2490; **Phone:** 718-920-6270; **Board Cert:** Psychiatry 1980; Geriatric Psychiatry 2010; Psychosomatic Medicine 2005; **Med School:** Univ Tex, San Antonio 1975; **Resid:** Psychiatry, VA Hosp-Univ Texas 1979; **Fellow:** Geriatric Psychiatry, Montefiore Med Ctr 1981; Psychosomatic Medicine, Montefiore Med Ctr 1983; **Fac Appt:** Prof Psyc, Albert Einstein Coll Med

Gynecologic Oncology

Einstein, Mark H MD (GO) - **Spec Exp:** Cervical Cancer; HPV-Human Papilloma Virus; Vulvar & Vaginal Cancer; **Hospital:** Montefiore Med Ctr-Moses Campus (page 100); **Address:** 1695 Eastchester Rd, rm 601, Bronx, NY 10461; **Phone:** 718-405-8082; **Board Cert:** Obstetrics & Gynecology 2012; Gynecologic Oncology 2012; **Med School:** Univ Miami Sch Med 1995; **Resid:** Obstetrics & Gynecology, St Barnabas Med Ctr 1999; **Fellow:** Gynecologic Oncology, Albert Einstein Affil Hosp 2002; **Fac Appt:** Prof ObG, Albert Einstein Coll Med

Goldberg, Gary L MD (GO) - **Spec Exp:** Ovarian Cancer; Uterine Cancer; **Hospital:** Montefiore Med Ctr-Moses Campus (page 100); **Address:** 1695 Eastchester Rd, Ste L2, Bronx, NY 10461; **Phone:** 718-405-8082; **Board Cert:** Obstetrics & Gynecology 2012; Gynecologic Oncology 2012; **Med School:** South Africa 1975; **Resid:** Obstetrics & Gynecology, Groote Schuur Hosp 1982; **Fellow:** Gynecologic Oncology, Groote Schuur Hosp 1983; **Fac Appt:** Assoc Prof ObG, Albert Einstein Coll Med

Smith, Harriet O MD (GO) - **Spec Exp:** Uterine Cancer; Pelvic Reconstruction; Ovarian Cancer; **Hospital:** Montefiore Med Ctr-Moses Campus (page 100), Jacobi Med Ctr; **Address:** 1695 Eastchester Rd, Ste 601, Bronx, NY 10461; **Phone:** 718-405-8082; **Board Cert:** Obstetrics & Gynecology 2012; Gynecologic Oncology 2012; **Med School:** Med Coll GA 1980; **Resid:** Obstetrics & Gynecology, Emory Univ Hosp 1986; Gynecologic Oncology, MD Anderson Cancer Ctr 1988; **Fellow:** Reconstructive Pelvic Surgery, Emory Univ 1989; Gynecologic Oncology, Montefiore Med Ctr 1990; **Fac Appt:** Prof ObG, Albert Einstein Coll Med

Smotkin, David MD (GO) - **Spec Exp:** Gynecologic Cancer; Gynecologic Cancer-Rare; **Hospital:** Montefiore Med Ctr-Moses Campus (page 100); **Address:** Montefiore Women's Ctr, 3332 Rochambeau Ave, Bronx, NY 10467; **Phone:** 718-920-4794; **Board Cert:** Obstetrics & Gynecology 2012; Gynecologic Oncology 2012; **Med School:** Yale Univ 1980; **Resid:** Obstetrics & Gynecology, Univ Colorado Hosp 1984; **Fellow:** Gynecologic Oncology, UCLA Med Ctr 1987; **Fac Appt:** Asst Prof ObG, Albert Einstein Coll Med

Hand Surgery

Kulick, Roy G MD (HS) - **Spec Exp:** Carpal Tunnel Syndrome; Arthritis; Tendon Surgery; Hand & Upper Extremity Surgery; **Hospital:** Montefiore Med Ctr-Einstein Campus (page 100); **Address:** Dept Orthopaedic Surgery, 1250 Waters Pl Fl 11, Bronx, NY 10461; **Phone:** 718-920-2060; **Board Cert:** Orthopaedic Surgery 1980; Hand Surgery 2011; **Med School:** Cornell Univ-Weill Med Coll 1973; **Resid:** Surgery, St. Luke's - Roosevelt Hosp Ctr - Roosevelt Div 1975; Orthopaedic Surgery, NY-Presby/Columbia Univ Med Ctr 1978; **Fellow:** Hand Surgery, Hosp for Special Surgery 1979; **Fac Appt:** Assoc Prof OrS, Albert Einstein Coll Med

Hematology

Billett, Henny H MD (Hem) - **Spec Exp:** Bleeding/Coagulation Disorders; Thrombotic Disorders; Platelet Disorders; Sickle Cell Disease; **Hospital:** Montefiore Med Ctr-Einstein Campus (page 100), Montefiore Med Ctr-Moses Campus (page 100); **Address:** 1515 Blondell Ave, Ste 220, Bronx, NY 10461-2601; **Phone:** 718-405-8323; **Board Cert:** Internal Medicine 1979; Hematology 1982; **Med School:** Mount Sinai Sch Med 1974; **Resid:** Internal Medicine, Montefiore Hosp Med Ctr 1979; **Fellow:** Tropical Medicine, London Sch Hygiene/Trop Med 1977; Hematology, Montefiore Hosp Med Ctr 1981; **Fac Appt:** Prof Med, Albert Einstein Coll Med

Landau, Leon C MD (Hem) - **Hospital:** Montefiore Med Ctr-Moses Campus (page 100), St. John's Riverside Hosp-Dobbs Ferry Pavil; **Address:** 75 E Gun Hill Rd, Bronx, NY 10467-2103; **Phone:** 718-655-3932; **Board Cert:** Internal Medicine 1977; Hematology 1978; Medical Oncology 1981; **Med School:** Albert Einstein Coll Med 1971; **Resid:** Internal Medicine, Montefiore Med Ctr 1973; Internal Medicine, Metropolitan Hosp Ctr 1974; **Fellow:** Hematology, Montefiore Med Ctr 1978; Medical Oncology, Montefiore Med Ctr 1978; **Fac Appt:** Asst Prof Med, Albert Einstein Coll Med

Infectious Disease

Berger, Judith J MD (Inf) - **Spec Exp:** AIDS/HIV; Travel Medicine; **Hospital:** St. Barnabas Hosp - Bronx; **Address:** St Barnabas Hosp, Dept Med, 4422 Third Ave, Bronx, NY 10457; **Phone:** 718-960-6205; **Board Cert:** Internal Medicine 1984; Infectious Disease 1986; **Med School:** Mount Sinai Sch Med 1980; **Resid:** Internal Medicine, Brookdale Hosp 1984; **Fellow:** Infectious Disease, SUNY Downstate Med Ctr 1986; **Fac Appt:** Assoc Clin Prof Med, Albert Einstein Coll Med

Berman, Daniel S MD (Inf) - **Spec Exp:** Infectious Disease; **Hospital:** Montefiore Med Ctr-Einstein Campus (page 100); **Address:** 340 City Island Ave, Bronx, NY 10464; **Phone:** 914-524-8138; **Board Cert:** Internal Medicine 1985; Infectious Disease 1988; **Med School:** NYU Sch Med 1982; **Resid:** Internal Medicine, VA Hosp/NYU Med Ctr 1983; Internal Medicine, NYU Med Ctr 1985; **Fellow:** Infectious Disease, NYU Med Ctr 1987

Corpuz, Marilou O MD (Inf) - **Spec Exp:** Hospital Acquired Infections; **Hospital:** Montefiore Med Ctr-Wakefield Campus (page 100); **Address:** Montefiore Med Grp, 4234 Bronx Blvd, Bronx, NY 10466-2604; **Phone:** 347-341-4340; **Board Cert:** Internal Medicine 1988; Infectious Disease 2012; **Med School:** Philippines 1985; **Resid:** Internal Medicine, Griffin Hosp 1988; **Fellow:** Infectious Disease, LI Jewish Med Ctr 1991; **Fac Appt:** Assoc Prof Med, NY Med Coll

Robbins, Noah MD (Inf) - **Spec Exp:** AIDS/HIV; Sexually Transmitted Diseases; **Hospital:** Montefiore Med Ctr-Moses Campus (page 100); **Address:** Montefiore Med Grp, 3400 Bainbridge Ave Fl 8th, Bronx, NY 10467-2490; **Phone:** 718-920-8888; **Board Cert:** Internal Medicine 1974; Infectious Disease 1980; **Med School:** McGill Univ 1969; **Resid:** Internal Medicine, Albany Meml Hosp 1974; **Fellow:** Infectious Disease, Montefiore Hosp Med Ctr 1980; **Fac Appt:** Clin Prof Med, Albert Einstein Coll Med

Telzak, Edward E MD (Inf) - **Spec Exp:** AIDS/HIV; Tuberculosis; Infections-Opportunistic; Clinical Trials; **Hospital:** Bronx Lebanon Hosp Ctr; **Address:** 1650 Selwyn Ave, Milstein Bldg, Ste 10C, Bronx, NY 10457-7606; **Phone:** 718-960-1212; **Board Cert:** Internal Medicine 1983; Infectious Disease 1988; **Med School:** Albert Einstein Coll Med 1980; **Resid:** Internal Medicine, Tufts-New England Med Ctr 1983; **Fellow:** Infectious Disease, Brigham & Womens Hosp 1985; Tropical Medicine, Tufts-New England Med Ctr 1986; **Fac Appt:** Prof Med, Albert Einstein Coll Med

Weiss, Louis M MD (Inf) - **Spec Exp:** Parasitic Infections; AIDS/HIV; **Hospital:** Montefiore Med Ctr-Einstein Campus (page 100); **Address:** 1575 Blondell Ave, Ste 200, Bronx, NY 10461; **Phone:** 718-405-8311; **Board Cert:** Internal Medicine 1985; Infectious Disease 1988; **Med School:** Johns Hopkins Univ 1982; **Resid:** Internal Medicine, Univ Chicago Affil Hosp 1985; **Fellow:** Infectious Disease, Montefiore Med Ctr 1987; **Fac Appt:** Prof Med, Albert Einstein Coll Med

Internal Medicine

Ernst, Jerome A MD (IM) - **Spec Exp:** Asthma; Emphysema; Chronic Obstructive Lung Disease (COPD); AIDS/HIV; **Hospital:** Bronx Lebanon Hosp Ctr; **Address:** BronxCare-Avalon Med Ctr, 1770 Grand Concourse Fl 2, Bronx, NY 10457; **Phone:** 718-518-5581; **Board Cert:** Internal Medicine 1978; Pulmonary Disease 1982; **Med School:** Israel 1969; **Resid:** Internal Medicine, Tel Hashomer Hosp 1970; Internal Medicine, Montefiore Med Ctr 1972; **Fellow:** Pulmonary Disease, Montefiore Med Ctr 1977; **Fac Appt:** Assoc Prof Med, Albert Einstein Coll Med

Fojas Jr, Antonio C MD (IM) *PCP* - **Spec Exp:** Preventive Medicine; **Hospital:** Montefiore Med Ctr-Wakefield Campus (page 100); **Address:** Montefiore Medical Group-Wakefield, 4234 Bronx Blvd, Bronx, NY 10466; **Phone:** 347-341-4300; **Board Cert:** Internal Medicine 2003; **Med School:** Philippines 1984; **Resid:** Internal Medicine, Our Lady of Mercy Med Ctr 1987; **Fellow:** Internal Medicine, Our Lady of Mercy Med Ctr 1988; **Fac Appt:** Asst Prof Med, NY Med Coll

Mojtabai, Shaparak MD (IM) *PCP* - **Spec Exp:** Women's Health-Geriatric; Diabetes; Hypertension; **Hospital:** St. Barnabas Hosp - Bronx; **Address:** 2016 Bronxdale Ave, Ste 302, Bronx Park Medical Pavilion, Bronx, NY 10462-3389; **Phone:** 718-822-1515; **Board Cert:** Internal Medicine 1989; Geriatric Medicine 2004; **Med School:** Iran 1982; **Resid:** Internal Medicine, St Barnabas Hosp-Cornell 1988; **Fellow:** Internal Medicine, St Barnabas Hosp-Cornell 1989

Sander Jr, Norbert W MD (IM) *PCP* - **Spec Exp:** Preventive Medicine; Sports Medicine; **Hospital:** Montefiore New Rochelle Hosp; **Address:** 340 City Island Ave, Bronx, NY 10464; **Phone:** 718-885-0333; **Board Cert:** Internal Medicine 1981; **Med School:** Albert Einstein Coll Med 1971; **Resid:** Internal Medicine, Metropolitan Hosp Ctr 1973; Internal Medicine, Lincoln Med & Mental Hlth Ctr 1974

Selwyn, Peter MD (IM) - **Spec Exp:** AIDS/HIV; Palliative Care; Addiction/Substance Abuse; **Hospital:** Montefiore Med Ctr-Moses Campus (page 100); **Address:** Montfiore Family Hlth Ctr, 360 E 193rd St Fl 2, Bronx, NY 10458; **Phone:** 718-933-2400; **Board Cert:** Family Medicine 2005; Hospice & Palliative Medicine 2012; **Med School:** Harvard Med Sch 1981; **Resid:** Family Medicine, Montefiore Med Ctr 1984; **Fac Appt:** Prof Med, Albert Einstein Coll Med

Swiderski, Deborah M MD (IM) *PCP* - **Spec Exp:** Preventive Medicine; **Hospital:** Montefiore Med Ctr-Moses Campus (page 100); **Address:** MMG-Comprehensive Heath Care Ctr, 305 E 161 St, Bronx, NY 10451; **Phone:** 718-579-2500; **Board Cert:** Internal Medicine 1986; **Med School:** Columbia P&S 1980; **Resid:** Internal Medicine, Montefiore Hosp 1983; **Fac Appt:** Assoc Clin Prof Med, Albert Einstein Coll Med

Teffera, Fassil MD (IM) *PCP* - **Spec Exp:** Diabetes; Hypertension; Preventive Medicine; **Hospital:** Montefiore Med Ctr-Wakefield Campus (page 100), Montefiore Med Ctr-Moses Campus (page 100); **Address:** 2426 Eastchester Rd, Ste 101, Bronx, NY 10469; **Phone:** 718-708-4726; **Board Cert:** Internal Medicine 2003; **Med School:** Ethiopia 1976; **Resid:** Internal Medicine, Our Lady of Mercy Med Ctr 1993; **Fac Appt:** Asst Clin Prof Med, NY Med Coll

Walker, Yvette L MD (IM) *PCP* - **Spec Exp:** Diabetes; Hypertension; Preventive Medicine; **Hospital:** Bronx Lebanon Hosp Ctr, Montefiore Med Ctr-Einstein Campus (page 100); **Address:** Morris Heights Hlth Ctr, 85 W Burnside Ave, Bronx, NY 10453; **Phone:** 718-716-4400; **Board Cert:** Internal Medicine 1986; **Med School:** SUNY Downstate 1983; **Resid:** Internal Medicine, Kings Co Hosp 1986; **Fac Appt:** Asst Prof Med, Albert Einstein Coll Med

Maternal & Fetal Medicine

Chazotte, Cynthia MD (MF) - **Spec Exp:** Pregnancy-High Risk; Asthma in Pregnancy; **Hospital:** Montefiore Med Ctr-Einstein Campus (page 100); **Address:** 1695 Eastchester Rd, Ste L2, Bronx, NY 10461; **Phone:** 718-405-8200; **Board Cert:** Obstetrics & Gynecology 2012; Maternal & Fetal Medicine 2012; **Med School:** NY Med Coll 1981; **Resid:** Obstetrics & Gynecology, Montefiore Med Ctr 1985; **Fellow:** Maternal & Fetal Medicine, Montefiore Med Ctr 1987; **Fac Appt:** Prof ObG, Albert Einstein Coll Med

Dayal, Ashlesha MD (MF) - **Spec Exp:** Pregnancy-High Risk; **Hospital:** Montefiore Med Ctr-Einstein Campus (page 100); **Address:** 1695 Eastchester Rd, Bronx, NY 10462; **Phone:** 718-405-8200; **Board Cert:** Obstetrics & Gynecology 2012; Maternal & Fetal Medicine 2012; **Med School:** Boston Univ 1993; **Resid:** Obstetrics & Gynecology, LI Jewish Med Ctr 1997; **Fellow:** Maternal & Fetal Medicine, NY Presby Hosp/ Columbia 1999; **Fac Appt:** Assoc Clin Prof ObG, Albert Einstein Coll Med

Henderson, Cassandra E MD (MF) - **Spec Exp:** Pregnancy-High Risk; Diabetes in Pregnancy; **Hospital:** Montefiore Med Ctr-Wakefield Campus (page 100); **Address:** 2604 Third Ave, Bronx, NY 10451; **Phone:** 718-579-5513; **Board Cert:** Obstetrics & Gynecology 2012; Maternal & Fetal Medicine 2012; **Med School:** Loyola Univ-Stritch Sch Med 1980; **Resid:** Obstetrics & Gynecology, Univ Chicago Hosp 1984; **Fellow:** Maternal & Fetal Medicine, Montefiore Med Ctr-Einstein Div 1986; **Fac Appt:** Assoc Prof ObG, Albert Einstein Coll Med

Medical Oncology

Bruckner, Howard W MD (Onc) - **Spec Exp:** Pancreatic Cancer; **Hospital:** NY-Presby/Lower Manhattan Hosp (page 104); **Address:** 2330 Eastchester Rd, Bronx, NY 10469; **Phone:** 718-732-4050; **Board Cert:** Internal Medicine 1972; Medical Oncology 1973; **Med School:** Albert Einstein Coll Med 1966; **Resid:** Internal Medicine, Montefiore Med Ctr 1971; **Fellow:** Medical Oncology, Yale-New Haven Hosp 1971

Camacho, Fernando J MD (Onc) - **Spec Exp:** Breast Cancer; Lymphoma; Bladder Cancer; **Hospital:** Montefiore Med Ctr-Moses Campus (page 100), Saint Joseph's Med Ctr - Yonkers; **Address:** 60 E 208th St, Bronx, NY 10467-2702; **Phone:** 718-405-1700; **Board Cert:** Internal Medicine 1976; Hematology 1978; Medical Oncology 1981; **Med School:** SUNY Buffalo 1973; **Resid:** Internal Medicine, Montefiore Med Ctr 1976; Hematology, Montefiore Med Ctr 1977; **Fellow:** Medical Oncology, Meml Sloan-Kettering Cancer Ctr 1979; **Fac Appt:** Asst Clin Prof Med, Albert Einstein Coll Med

Fuks, Joachim MD (Onc) - **Spec Exp:** Lung Cancer; Breast Cancer; Colon Cancer; **Hospital:** Montefiore Westchester Sq, Montefiore Med Ctr-Einstein Campus (page 100); **Address:** 1578 Williamsbridge Rd Fl 2, Bronx, NY 10461-6265; **Phone:** 718-931-2290; **Board Cert:** Internal Medicine 1981; Medical Oncology 1983; **Med School:** Spain 1975; **Resid:** Internal Medicine, Mt Sinai Hosp 1978; **Fellow:** Medical Oncology, Natl Cancer Inst 1981

Perez-Soler, Roman MD (Onc) - **Spec Exp:** Lung Cancer; Mesothelioma; Drug Development; **Hospital:** Montefiore Med Ctr-Einstein Campus (page 100), Montefiore Med Ctr-Moses Campus (page 100); **Address:** Montefiore Med Ctr, Dept Oncology, 111 E 210th St, Hoffheimer Main-Rm 100, Bronx, NY 10467; **Phone:** 718-920-4001; **Board Cert:** Internal Medicine 1987; Medical Oncology 1989; **Med School:** Spain 1977; **Resid:** Internal Medicine, Univ Autonoma Med Ctr 1982; **Fellow:** Medical Oncology, Univ Tex-MD Anderson Cancer Ctr 1985; **Fac Appt:** Prof Med, Albert Einstein Coll Med

Ramirez, Mark Anthony MD (Onc) - **Spec Exp:** Lymphoma, Non-Hodgkin's; Breast Cancer; Lung Cancer; **Hospital:** Montefiore Med Ctr-Moses Campus (page 100), Saint Joseph's Med Ctr - Yonkers; **Address:** 60 E 208th St, Bronx, NY 10467; **Phone:** 718-405-1700; **Board Cert:** Internal Medicine 1985; Medical Oncology 1989; Hematology 2005; **Med School:** Cornell Univ-Weill Med Coll 1982; **Resid:** Internal Medicine, Montefiore Med Ctr 1985; **Fellow:** Hematology & Oncology, Montefiore Med Ctr 1988; **Fac Appt:** Asst Clin Prof Med, Albert Einstein Coll Med

Sparano, Joseph A MD (Onc) - **Spec Exp:** Breast Cancer; Lymphoma; **Hospital:** Montefiore Med Ctr-Einstein Campus (page 100); **Address:** 1825 Eastchester Rd Fl 2 - Ste 2S-48, Bronx, NY 10461; **Phone:** 718-904-2555; **Board Cert:** Internal Medicine 1986; Medical Oncology 1989; **Med School:** NY Med Coll 1982; **Resid:** Internal Medicine, St Vincents Hosp 1986; **Fellow:** Medical Oncology, Montefiore Med Ctr 1988; **Fac Appt:** Prof Med, Albert Einstein Coll Med

Vogl, Steven E MD (Onc) - **Spec Exp:** Breast Cancer; Lung Cancer; **Hospital:** Montefiore Med Ctr-Einstein Campus (page 100), White Plains Hosp (page 640); **Address:** 2220 Tiemann Ave, Bronx, NY 10469; **Phone:** 718-519-7774; **Board Cert:** Internal Medicine 1975; Medical Oncology 1975; **Med School:** Cornell Univ-Weill Med Coll 1970; **Resid:** Internal Medicine, Jacobi Med Ctr 1972; **Fellow:** Medical Oncology, Mt Sinai Med Ctr 1975

Neonatal-Perinatal Medicine

Campbell, Deborah E MD (NP) - **Spec Exp:** Prematurity/Low Birth Weight Infants; Neurodevelopmental Disabilities; Neonatal Nutrition; Ethics; **Hospital:** Montefiore Med Ctr-Einstein Campus (page 100), Montefiore Med Ctr-Wakefield Campus (page 100); **Address:** 1825 Eastchester Rd, Bronx, NY 10461-2301; **Phone:** 718-904-4105; **Board Cert:** Pediatrics 1983; Neonatal-Perinatal Medicine 1985; **Med School:** SUNY Buffalo 1978; **Resid:** Pediatrics, Montefiore Med Ctr 1981; **Fellow:** Neonatal-Perinatal Medicine, Montefiore Med Ctr 1983; **Fac Appt:** Clin Prof Ped, Albert Einstein Coll Med

Nephrology

Charytan, Chaim MD (Nep) - **Spec Exp:** Hypertension; Diabetic Kidney Disease; Kidney Stones; Nephrotic Syndrome; **Hospital:** NY Hosp Queens (page 488); **Address:** 1874 Pelham Pkwy S, Bronx, NY 10461-3733; **Phone:** 718-931-5800; **Board Cert:** Internal Medicine 1969; Nephrology 1974; **Med School:** Albert Einstein Coll Med 1964; **Resid:** Internal Medicine, Bronx Muni Hosp 1967; **Fellow:** Nephrology, Boston Univ Hosp 1968; **Fac Appt:** Clin Prof Med, Cornell Univ-Weill Med Coll

Coco, Maria MD (Nep) - **Spec Exp:** Hypertension; Kidney Disease; **Hospital:** Montefiore Med Ctr-Moses Campus (page 100); **Address:** 111 E 210th St, Bronx, NY 10467-2401; **Phone:** 718-920-4136; **Board Cert:** Internal Medicine 1985; Nephrology 1988; **Med School:** Italy 1982; **Resid:** Internal Medicine, Bronx Lebanon Hosp 1985; **Fellow:** Nephrology, Montefiore Med Ctr 1988; **Fac Appt:** Prof Med, Albert Einstein Coll Med

Croll, James E MD (Nep) - **Spec Exp:** Dialysis Care; Hypertension; Kidney Failure-Chronic; **Hospital:** St. Barnabas Hosp - Bronx; **Address:** 4422 3rd Ave, Bronx, NY 10457; **Phone:** 718-960-6295; **Board Cert:** Internal Medicine 1978; Nephrology 1982; **Med School:** Belgium 1975; **Resid:** Internal Medicine, Genesee Hosp 1978; **Fellow:** Nephrology, VA Med Ctr 1981

Gorkin, Janet U MD (Nep) - **Spec Exp:** Hypertension; Diabetic Kidney Disease; Kidney Failure; **Hospital:** Montefiore Med Ctr-Moses Campus (page 100); **Address:** 3327 Bainbridge Ave, Bronx, NY 10467; **Phone:** 718-881-7100; **Board Cert:** Internal Medicine 1976; Nephrology 1980; **Med School:** Mount Sinai Sch Med 1973; **Resid:** Internal Medicine, Mt Sinai Hosp 1976; **Fellow:** Nephrology, Mt Sinai Hosp 1978; **Fac Appt:** Prof Med, Albert Einstein Coll Med

Laitman, Robert MD (Nep) - **Spec Exp:** Diabetic Kidney Disease; Cholesterol/Lipid Disorders; **Hospital:** Montefiore Med Ctr-Einstein Campus (page 100); **Address:** 2510 Westchester Ave, Ste 106, Bronx, NY 10461-2606; **Phone:** 718-518-1276; **Board Cert:** Internal Medicine 1986; Nephrology 1988; Geriatric Medicine 2010; **Med School:** Washington Univ, St Louis 1983; **Resid:** Internal Medicine, Jacobi Med Ctr 1986; **Fellow:** Nephrology, Montefiore Med Ctr 1988

Lynn, Robert I MD (Nep) - **Spec Exp:** Hypertension; Dialysis Care; **Hospital:** Montefiore Med Ctr-Einstein Campus (page 100); **Address:** 1200 Waters Pl, Ste M104, Bronx, NY 10461; **Phone:** 718-794-1200; **Board Cert:** Internal Medicine 1977; Nephrology 1980; **Med School:** Columbia P&S 1974; **Resid:** Internal Medicine, NY-Presby/Columbia Univ Med Ctr 1977; **Fellow:** Nephrology, Yale-New Haven Hosp 1979; **Fac Appt:** Assoc Prof Med, Albert Einstein Coll Med

Neugarten, Joel MD (Nep) - **Hospital:** Montefiore Med Ctr-Moses Campus (page 100), Montefiore Med Ctr-Einstein Campus (page 100); **Address:** Montefiore Med Ctr, dept Nephrology, 111 E 210th St, rm 605, Bronx, NY 10467; **Phone:** 718-920-5442; **Board Cert:** Internal Medicine 1978; Nephrology 1980; **Med School:** Albert Einstein Coll Med 1975; **Resid:** Internal Medicine, Mt Sinai Med Ctr 1978; **Fellow:** Nephrology, NYU Med Ct 1980; **Fac Appt:** Prof Med, Albert Einstein Coll Med

Uday, Kalpana MD (Nep) - **Spec Exp:** Hypertension; Kidney Disease-Chronic; **Hospital:** Bronx Lebanon Hosp Ctr; **Address:** 1650 Grand Concourse, Fl 2, Bronx, NY 10457-7606; **Phone:** 718-992-7669; **Board Cert:** Internal Medicine 1989; Nephrology 2003; **Med School:** India 1980; **Resid:** Internal Medicine, Jamaica Med Ctr 1989; **Fellow:** Nephrology, Montefiore Med Ctr 1991; **Fac Appt:** Asst Prof Med, Albert Einstein Coll Med

Yoo, Jinil MD (Nep) - **Spec Exp:** Kidney Disease; Hypertension; Diabetes; **Hospital:** Montefiore Med Ctr-Wakefield Campus (page 100); **Address:** 4234 Bronx Blvd Fl 2, Medical Village, Montefiore N, Bronx, NY 10466; **Phone:** 347-341-4340; **Board Cert:** Internal Medicine 1974; Nephrology 1976; **Med School:** South Korea 1967; **Resid:** Internal Medicine, Lahey Clinic 1973; Internal Medicine, Metropolitan Hosp Ctr 1974; **Fellow:** Nephrology, NY Med Coll 1976; **Fac Appt:** Prof Med, NY Med Coll

Neurological Surgery

Flamm, Eugene S MD (NS) - **Spec Exp:** Aneurysm-Cerebral; Brain Tumors; Cerebrovascular Neurosurgery; **Hospital:** Montefiore Med Ctr-Moses Campus (page 100); **Address:** 3316 Rochambeau Ave, Bronx, NY 10467-2841; **Phone:** 718-920-2339; **Board Cert:** Neurological Surgery 1973; **Med School:** SUNY Buffalo 1962; **Resid:** Surgery, New York Hosp 1964; Neurological Surgery, NYU Med Ctr 1970; **Fellow:** Neurological Surgery, Univ Zurich 1971; **Fac Appt:** Prof NS, Albert Einstein Coll Med

LaSala, Patrick A MD (NS) - **Spec Exp:** Brain Tumors; Epilepsy; Stereotactic Radiosurgery; **Hospital:** Montefiore Med Ctr-Moses Campus (page 100); **Address:** Dept Neurosurgery, 3316 Rochambeau Ave, Bronx, NY 10467-2803; **Phone:** 718-920-7466; **Board Cert:** Neurological Surgery 1991; **Med School:** Columbia P&S 1980; **Resid:** Neurological Surgery, Columbia-Presby Med Ctr 1987; **Fac Appt:** Assoc Prof NS, Albert Einstein Coll Med

Neurology

Cohen, Joel S MD (N) - **Spec Exp:** Epilepsy; Headache; Stroke; Parkinson's Disease; **Hospital:** Montefiore Med Ctr-Moses Campus (page 100), Montefiore Med Ctr-Einstein Campus (page 100); **Address:** 1610 Williamsbridge Rd Fl 3rd, Bronx, NY 10461-2601; **Phone:** 718-597-8000; **Board Cert:** Neurology 1992; **Med School:** Albert Einstein Coll Med 1983; **Resid:** Neurology, Montefiore Med Ctr 1987; **Fellow:** Neurology, Montefiore Med Ctr 1988; **Fac Appt:** Assoc Prof N, Albert Einstein Coll Med

Freddo, Lorenza MD (N) - **Spec Exp:** Pain Management; Multiple Sclerosis; Peripheral Neuropathy; **Hospital:** St. Barnabas Hosp - Bronx; **Address:** Belmont Medical Associates, 2371 Arthur Ave, Bronx, NY 10458; **Phone:** 718-364-6199; **Board Cert:** Neurology 1992; **Med School:** Italy 1980; **Resid:** Neurology, Columbia Presby Hosp 1990; Neurology; **Fac Appt:** Asst Prof NPath, Albert Einstein Coll Med

Grenell, Steven L MD (N) - **Spec Exp:** Pain Management; Headache; **Hospital:** Montefiore Med Ctr-Moses Campus (page 100), Lawrence Hosp Ctr; **Address:** 3975 Sedgewick Ave, Ste 1-F, Bronx, NY 10463; **Phone:** 718-796-6055; **Board Cert:** Neurology 1989; **Med School:** UMDNJ-Rutgers Med Sch 1977; **Resid:** Internal Medicine, Montefiore Hosp 1979; Neurology, Montefiore Hosp 1982; **Fellow:** Internal Medicine, Montefiore Hosp 1982; **Fac Appt:** Asst Prof N, Albert Einstein Coll Med

Herskovitz, Steven MD (N) - **Spec Exp:** Electromyography; Neuromuscular Disorders; Peripheral Neuropathy; **Hospital:** Montefiore Med Ctr-Moses Campus (page 100); **Address:** 111 E 210th St, Bronx, NY 10467-2401; **Phone:** 718-920-4930; **Board Cert:** Internal Medicine 1983; Neurology 1987; Neuromuscular Medicine 2008; **Med School:** Cornell Univ-Weill Med Coll 1980; **Resid:** Internal Medicine, Montefiore Med Ctr 1983; Neurology, Montefiore Med Ctr 1986; **Fellow:** Electromyography, Montefiore Med Ctr 1987; **Fac Appt:** Prof N, Albert Einstein Coll Med

Kaufman, David Myland MD (N) - **Spec Exp:** Movement Disorders; **Hospital:** Montefiore Med Ctr-Moses Campus (page 100); **Address:** 3400 Bainbridge Ave, Main Fl, Bronx, NY 10467; **Phone:** 718-920-4730; **Board Cert:** Internal Medicine 1972; Neurology 1976; **Med School:** Univ Chicago-Pritzker Sch Med 1968; **Resid:** Internal Medicine, Montefiore Med Ctr 1971; Neurology, Montefiore Med Ctr 1974; **Fac Appt:** Prof N, Albert Einstein Coll Med

Kirchoff, Kathryn MD (N) - **Spec Exp:** Stroke; **Hospital:** Montefiore Med Ctr-Moses Campus (page 100); **Address:** Stern Stroke Ctr, 111 E 210th St, Bronx, NY 10467; **Phone:** 718-920-6444; **Board Cert:** Neurology 2008; Vascular Neurology 2011; **Med School:** SUNY Stony Brook 2004; **Resid:** Neurology, Mount Sinai Hosp 2008; **Fac Appt:** Asst Prof N, Albert Einstein Coll Med

Lipton, Richard MD (N) - **Spec Exp:** Headache; Clinical Trials; **Hospital:** Montefiore Med Ctr-Einstein Campus (page 100); **Address:** Montefiore at AECOM, 1300 Morris Park Ave, Bronx, NY 10461-1900; **Phone:** 718-430-3886; **Board Cert:** Neurology 1985; **Med School:** Univ Chicago-Pritzker Sch Med 1980; **Resid:** Neurology, Montefiore Med Ctr 1984; **Fellow:** Neurophysiology, Montefiore Med Ctr 1985; NeuroEpidemiology, Columbia Univ 1990; **Fac Appt:** Prof N, Albert Einstein Coll Med

Sparr, Steven MD (N) - **Hospital:** Montefiore Med Ctr-Moses Campus (page 100); **Address:** Montefiore Med Ctr, 111 E 210th St, Bronx, NY 10467; **Phone:** 718-920-6402; **Board Cert:** Internal Medicine 1984; Neurology 1987; Vascular Neurology 2008; **Med School:** SUNY Buffalo 1980; **Resid:** Internal Medicine, Boston City Hosp 1983; Neurology, Albert Einstein 1986; **Fellow:** Neurological Rehabilitation, Burke Rehabilitation Hosp 1987; **Fac Appt:** Assoc Prof N, Albert Einstein Coll Med

Swerdlow, Michael L MD (N) - **Spec Exp:** Myasthenia Gravis; Spinal Disorders; Multiple Sclerosis; **Hospital:** Montefiore Med Ctr-Moses Campus (page 100); **Address:** 3400 Bainbridge Ave, Bronx, NY 10467-2401; **Phone:** 718-920-4178; **Board Cert:** Neurology 1975; **Med School:** Univ Pennsylvania 1967; **Resid:** Internal Medicine, Mount Sinai Hosp 1969; Neurology, Montefiore Med Ctr 1972; **Fellow:** Neurology, Natl Inst Hlth 1974; **Fac Appt:** Prof N, Albert Einstein Coll Med

Neuroradiology

Bello, Jacqueline A MD (NRad) - **Spec Exp:** Aneurysm-Cerebral; Pain-Back; **Hospital:** Montefiore Med Ctr-Moses Campus (page 100); **Address:** Montefiore Med Ctr, 111 E 210th St, Red Zone, Bronx, NY 10467; **Phone:** 718-920-4030; **Board Cert:** Diagnostic Radiology 1984; Neuroradiology 2010; **Med School:** Columbia P&S 1980; **Resid:** Diagnostic Radiology, Columbia-PresbyMed Ctr 1984; **Fellow:** Neuroradiology, Neuro Inst/Columbia-Presby Med Ctr 1986; **Fac Appt:** Prof Rad, Albert Einstein Coll Med

Nuclear Medicine

Freeman, Leonard M MD (NuM) - **Spec Exp:** Nuclear Oncology; Gastrointestinal Disorders; PET Imaging; CT Scan; **Hospital:** Montefiore Med Ctr-Moses Campus (page 100); **Address:** 111 E 210th St Foreman Bldg Fl 4, Bronx, NY 10467-2401; **Phone:** 718-920-6060; **Board Cert:** Diagnostic Radiology 1966; Nuclear Medicine 1972; Nuclear Radiology 1974; **Med School:** Ros Franklin Univ/Chicago Med Sch 1961; **Resid:** Diagnostic Radiology, Bronx Municipal Hosp 1965; **Fac Appt:** Prof NuM, Albert Einstein Coll Med

Milstein, David M MD (NuM) - **Hospital:** Montefiore Med Ctr-Einstein Campus (page 100), Montefiore Med Ctr-Moses Campus (page 100); **Address:** Montefiore Medical Park, 1695A Eastchester Rd, Bronx, NY 10461; **Phone:** 718-405-8455; **Board Cert:** Nuclear Medicine 1972; Diagnostic Radiology 1972; **Med School:** Albert Einstein Coll Med 1967; **Resid:** Diagnostic Radiology, Bronx Muni Hosp Ctr 1972; **Fellow:** Nuclear Medicine, Bronx Muni Hosp Ctr 1972; **Fac Appt:** Prof NuM, Albert Einstein Coll Med

Obstetrics & Gynecology

Dar, Pe'er MD (ObG) - **Spec Exp:** Prenatal Diagnosis; Fetal Ultrasound/Obstetrical Imaging; Fetal Diagnosis & Therapy; Pregnancy-High Risk; **Hospital:** Montefiore Med Ctr-Einstein Campus (page 100); **Address:** Montefiore Medical Park, 1695 Eastchester Rd, Ste L4, Bronx, NY 10461; **Phone:** 718-405-8218; **Board Cert:** Clinical Genetics 2013; Obstetrics & Gynecology ; **Med School:** Israel 1987; **Resid:** Obstetrics & Gynecology, Assaf Harofeh Hosp 1992; Obstetrics & Gynecology, Montefiore Med Ctr 2005; **Fellow:** Clinical Genetics, Albert Einstein/Montefiore Med Ctr 2000; **Fac Appt:** Assoc Prof ObG, Albert Einstein Coll Med

Levy, Judith MD (ObG) *PCP* - **Hospital:** Montefiore Med Ctr-Einstein Campus (page 100); **Address:** 1695 Eastchester Rd, Ste L2, Bronx, NY 10461; **Phone:** 718-405-8200; **Board Cert:** Obstetrics & Gynecology 2012; **Med School:** Albert Einstein Coll Med 1981; **Resid:** Obstetrics & Gynecology, Bronx Muni Hosp 1985; **Fac Appt:** Asst Prof ObG, Albert Einstein Coll Med

Young, Constance A MD (ObG) - **Spec Exp:** Gynecology Only; Pelvic Surgery; Menopause Problems; **Hospital:** Jacobi Med Ctr; **Address:** Jacobi Med Ctr, 1400 Pelham Pkwy S Bldg 1 - rm 3W6, Bronx, NY 10461; **Phone:** 718-918-5700; **Board Cert:** Obstetrics & Gynecology 2012; **Med School:** Cornell Univ-Weill Med Coll 1983; **Resid:** Obstetrics & Gynecology, North Shore Univ Hosp 1987; **Fac Appt:** Asst Prof ObG, Albert Einstein Coll Med

Ophthalmology

Chess, Jeremy MD (Oph) - **Spec Exp:** Retina/Vitreous Surgery; **Hospital:** Montefiore Med Ctr-Moses Campus (page 100); **Address:** Retina Grp, 2221 Boston Rd, Bronx, NY 10467; **Phone:** 718-798-3030; **Board Cert:** Ophthalmology 1977; **Med School:** Boston Univ 1970; **Resid:** Ophthalmology, Boston Univ Med Ctr 1974; **Fellow:** Vitreoretinal Surgery, Boston Univ Med Ctr 1983; **Fac Appt:** Assoc Clin Prof Oph, Albert Einstein Coll Med

Hayworth, Robin S MD (Oph) - **Spec Exp:** Glaucoma; **Hospital:** Lenox Hill Hosp (Manh Eye, Ear & Throat Hosp) (page 106); **Address:** 787 Lydig Ave, Bronx, NY 10462-2144; **Phone:** 718-863-7774; **Board Cert:** Ophthalmology 1985; **Med School:** Cornell Univ-Weill Med Coll 1978; **Resid:** Surgery, NY Hosp 1980; Ophthalmology, Manhattan EET Hosp 1983

Mayers, Martin MD (Oph) - **Spec Exp:** Cataract Surgery; Cornea Transplant; Eye Infections; **Hospital:** Bronx Lebanon Hosp Ctr, Montefiore Med Ctr-Wakefield Campus (page 100); **Address:** Bronx-Lebanon Hosp Ctr, 1650 Grand Concourse, Milstein Bldg - rm 1C, Bronx, NY 10456; **Phone:** 718-518-8008; **Board Cert:** Ophthalmology 1985; **Med School:** Albert Einstein Coll Med 1979; **Resid:** Ophthalmology, SUNY Downstate Med Ctr 1983; **Fellow:** Cornea, Proctor Fdn-UCSF 1984; **Fac Appt:** Assoc Prof Oph, Albert Einstein Coll Med

Medow, Norman B MD (Oph) - **Spec Exp:** Cataract-Pediatric; Glaucoma-Pediatric; Corneal Disease-Pediatric; **Hospital:** Montefiore Med Ctr-Moses Campus (page 100); **Address:** Montefiore Hosp Ctr, Dept Ophthalmology, 3400 Bainbridge Ave, Bronx, NY 10467; **Phone:** 718-920-2020; **Board Cert:** Ophthalmology 1975; **Med School:** SUNY Hlth Sci Ctr 1966; **Resid:** Ophthalmology, Manhattan EE&T Hosp 1972; **Fellow:** Cataract/Lens Implant Surgery, Charles Kelman, MD 1973; **Fac Appt:** Clin Prof Oph, Cornell Univ-Weill Med Coll

Rosenbaum, Pearl S MD (Oph) - **Spec Exp:** Cataract Surgery; Glaucoma; Eye Tumors/Cancer; Ophthalmic Pathology; **Hospital:** Montefiore Med Ctr-Moses Campus (page 100), Bronx Lebanon Hosp Ctr; **Address:** 1250 Waters Pl, Ste 502, Bronx, NY 10463; **Phone:** 718-518-0060; **Board Cert:** Ophthalmology 1988; **Med School:** Albert Einstein Coll Med 1982; **Resid:** Ophthalmology, Albert Einstein 1986; **Fellow:** Ophthalmic Pathology, Baylor Coll of Med Affil Hosp 1988; Ophthalmic Oncology, Baylor Coll of Med Affil Hosp 1988; **Fac Appt:** Prof Oph, Albert Einstein Coll Med

Slamovits, Thomas L MD (Oph) - **Spec Exp:** Neuro-Ophthalmology; Optic Nerve Disorders; Vision Loss-Unexplained Loss; Diabetic Eye Disease/Retinopathy; **Hospital:** Montefiore Med Ctr-Moses Campus (page 100), Hackensack Univ Med Ctr (page 718); **Address:** 1250 Pelham Pkwy S, Bronx, NY 10461; **Phone:** 718-794-1500; **Board Cert:** Ophthalmology 1980; **Med School:** Ohio State Univ 1975; **Resid:** Internal Medicine, Ohio State Univ Hosp 1976; Ophthalmology, Univ Pitts Eye & Ear Hosp 1979; **Fellow:** Neuro-Ophthalmology, Washington Univ-Barnes Hosp 1980; **Fac Appt:** Clin Prof Oph, Albert Einstein Coll Med

Tiwari, Ram P MD (Oph) - **Spec Exp:** Diabetic Eye Disease/Retinopathy; Glaucoma; Cataract Surgery; Dry Eye Syndrome; **Hospital:** Montefiore Med Ctr-Wakefield Campus (page 100), NY-Presby/Columbia Univ Med Ctr, NY (page 104); **Address:** 1739 Williamsbridge Rd, Bronx, NY 10461-6203; **Phone:** 718-824-1560; **Board Cert:** Ophthalmology 1977; **Med School:** India 1966; **Resid:** Ophthalmology, Maulana Azad Med Coll Affil Hosp 1971; **Fellow:** Retina, Columbia-Presby Med Ctr 1978; **Fac Appt:** Asst Clin Prof Oph, Columbia P&S

Wolf, Kenneth J MD (Oph) - **Spec Exp:** Diabetic Eye Disease/Retinopathy; Cataract Surgery; **Address:** 1180 Morris Park Ave Fl 2, Bronx, NY 10461-1925; **Phone:** 718-892-6110; **Board Cert:** Ophthalmology 1980; **Med School:** Albert Einstein Coll Med 1974; **Resid:** Ophthalmology, Montefiore Hosp Med Ctr 1978; **Fac Appt:** Asst Clin Prof Oph, Albert Einstein Coll Med

Orthopaedic Surgery

Cobelli, Neil MD (OrS) - **Spec Exp:** Knee Replacement; Hip Replacement; Reconstructive Surgery; **Hospital:** Montefiore Med Ctr-Wakefield Campus (page 100); **Address:** 1250 Waters Pl Fl 11, Bronx, NY 10461; **Phone:** 718-920-2060; **Board Cert:** Orthopaedic Surgery 1985; **Med School:** Dartmouth Med Sch 1976; **Resid:** Orthopaedic Surgery, Montefiore Med Ctr 1983; **Fac Appt:** Prof OrS, Albert Einstein Coll Med

Geller, David S MD (OrS) - **Spec Exp:** Bone Cancer; Sarcoma; Sarcoma-Soft Tissue; Musculoskeletal Tumors; **Hospital:** Montefiore Med Ctr-Moses Campus (page 100); **Address:** MMC Medical Arts Pavilion, 3400 Bainbridge Ave Fl 6, Bronx, NY 10467; **Phone:** 718-920-5722; **Board Cert:** Orthopaedic Surgery 2008; **Med School:** Israel 2000; **Resid:** Orthopaedic Surgery, Montefiore Med Ctr 2005; **Fellow:** Orthopaedic Oncology, Mass General Hosp 2006; **Fac Appt:** Asst Prof OrS, Albert Einstein Coll Med

Kleinman, Paul G MD (OrS) - **Spec Exp:** Pediatric Orthopaedic Surgery; Hand Surgery; Trauma; Sports Medicine; **Hospital:** St. Barnabas Hosp - Bronx; **Address:** 2016 Bronxdale Ave, Ste 202, Bronx, NY 10462-3365; **Phone:** 718-863-8695; **Board Cert:** Orthopaedic Surgery 2009; **Med School:** Stanford Univ 1979; **Resid:** Surgery, St Lukes Hosp 1981; Orthopaedic Surgery, Columbia-Presby Hosp 1985; **Fellow:** Hand Surgery, Allegheny Genl Hosp 1986; Pediatric Orthopaedic Surgery, Hosp Joint Diseases 1990

Kulsakdinun, Chaiyaporn MD (OrS) - **Spec Exp:** Foot & Ankle Surgery; Foot & Ankle Deformities; Sports Injuries; **Hospital:** Montefiore Med Ctr-Einstein Campus (page 100); **Address:** 1250 Waters Pl Fl 11 - Ste C, Bronx, NY 10461; **Phone:** 718-920-2060; **Board Cert:** Orthopaedic Surgery 2003; **Med School:** Yale Univ 1993; **Resid:** Orthopaedic Surgery, Yale-New Haven Hosp 1998; **Fellow:** Foot & Ankle Surgery, Hosp Special Surgery 1999; **Fac Appt:** Asst Prof OrS, Albert Einstein Coll Med

Levy, I Martin MD (OrS) - **Spec Exp:** Sports Medicine; Arthroscopic Surgery; Knee Meniscal Repair; Knee Injuries/ACL; **Hospital:** Montefiore Med Ctr-Einstein Campus (page 100); **Address:** 1250 Waters Pl Fl 11, Bronx, NY 10461; **Phone:** 347-577-4411; **Board Cert:** Orthopaedic Surgery 1982; **Med School:** NY Med Coll 1976; **Resid:** Orthopaedic Surgery, Bronx Municipal Hosps 1981; **Fellow:** Sports Medicine, Hosp for Special Surg 1982; **Fac Appt:** Clin Prof OrS, Albert Einstein Coll Med

Olsewski, John M MD (OrS) - **Spec Exp:** Spinal Reconstructive Surgery; Scoliosis; Spinal Surgery-Neck; Cervical Myelopathy; **Hospital:** Montefiore Med Ctr-Einstein Campus (page 100), Montefiore New Rochelle Hosp; **Address:** 2157 Tomlinson Ave, Bronx, NY 10461; **Phone:** 718-794-2501; **Board Cert:** Orthopaedic Surgery 2007; **Med School:** SUNY Buffalo 1986; **Resid:** Orthopaedic Surgery, SUNY Buffalo Affil Hosp 1992; **Fellow:** Spine Surgery, Twin Cities Scoliosis/Spine Ctr 1994; **Fac Appt:** Clin Prof OrS, Albert Einstein Coll Med

Sharan, Alok D MD (OrS) - **Spec Exp:** Spinal Tumors; Spinal Surgery; **Hospital:** Montefiore Med Ctr-Moses Campus (page 100); **Address:** 1250 Waters Pl Fl 11, Bronx, NY 10467; **Phone:** 718-920-2060; **Board Cert:** Orthopaedic Surgery 2008; **Med School:** UMDNJ-NJ Med Sch, Newark 2000; **Resid:** Orthopaedic Surgery, Albany Med Ctr 2005; **Fellow:** Spine Surgery, NYU Med Ctr 2006; **Fac Appt:** Asst Prof OrS, Albert Einstein Coll Med

Wilson, Arnold B MD (OrS) - **Spec Exp:** Hip Replacement; Knee Replacement; Knee Injuries/Ligament Surgery; Sports Medicine; **Hospital:** Montefiore Med Ctr-Moses Campus (page 100), NYU Hosp For Joint Dis (page 108); **Address:** Wilson Orthopaedics, 75 E Gun Hill Rd, Bronx, NY 10467-2103; **Phone:** 718-798-1000; **Board Cert:** Orthopaedic Surgery 2007; **Med School:** UMDNJ-Univ Med Dent NJ 1987; **Resid:** Orthopaedic Surgery, Catholic Med Ctr of Brooklyn & Queens 1993; **Fellow:** Sports Medicine/Knee Surgery, Insall Scott Kelly Inst 1994

Otolaryngology

Feghali, Joseph G MD (Oto) - **Spec Exp:** Ear Disorders/Surgery; Acoustic Neuroma; Hearing Disorders; Cholesteatoma; **Hospital:** Montefiore Med Ctr-Moses Campus (page 100); **Address:** 182 E 210th St, Bronx, NY 10467; **Phone:** 718-881-3277; **Board Cert:** Otolaryngology 1990; **Med School:** Lebanon 1978; **Resid:** Surgery, meml Sloan Kettering Cancer Ctr 1986; Otolaryngology, Montefiore Med Ctr 1990; **Fellow:** Otology & Neurotology, House Ear Inst 1983; Neurological Surgery, Meml Sloan Kettering Cancer Ctr 1985; **Fac Appt:** Clin Prof Oto, Albert Einstein Coll Med

Fried, Marvin P MD (Oto) - **Spec Exp:** Endoscopic Sinus Surgery; Head & Neck Tumors; Laryngeal & Voice Disorders; Sinus Disorders/Surgery; **Hospital:** Montefiore Med Ctr-Moses Campus (page 100), Montefiore Med Ctr-Einstein Campus (page 100); **Address:** 3400 Bainbridge Ave, Fl 3, Bronx, NY 10467; **Phone:** 718-920-4646; **Board Cert:** Otolaryngology 1975; **Med School:** Tufts Univ 1969; **Resid:** Surgery, Barnes-Jewish Hosp 1971; Otolaryngology, Barnes-Jewish Hosp 1975; **Fellow:** Washington Univ 1976; **Fac Appt:** Prof Oto, Albert Einstein Coll Med

Goldstein, Steven I MD (Oto) - **Spec Exp:** Sinus Surgery; Nasal Surgery; **Hospital:** Montefiore Westchester Sq, Montefiore Med Ctr-Einstein Campus (page 100); **Address:** 1200 Waters Pl, Bronx, NY 10461; **Phone:** 718-863-4366; **Board Cert:** Otolaryngology 1987; **Med School:** SUNY Buffalo 1982; **Resid:** Surgery, NYU Med Ctr 1984; Otolaryngology, NYU Med Ctr 1987; **Fellow:** Facial Plastic Surgery, Mt Sinai Hosp 1988

Smith, Richard V MD (Oto) - **Spec Exp:** Head & Neck Cancer; Thyroid & Parathyroid Surgery; Salivary Gland Tumors; Robotic Surgery; **Hospital:** Montefiore Med Ctr-Moses Campus (page 100), Montefiore Med Ctr-Einstein Campus (page 100); **Address:** Medical Arts Pavilion, 3400 Bainbridge Ave, Fl 3, Bronx, NY 10467; **Phone:** 718-920-4646; **Board Cert:** Otolaryngology 1996; **Med School:** Univ VT Coll Med 1990; **Resid:** Otolaryngology, Georgetown Univ Hosp 1995; **Fac Appt:** Clin Prof Oto, Albert Einstein Coll Med

Yankelowitz, Stanley M MD (Oto) - **Spec Exp:** Nasal & Sinus Surgery; Pediatric Otolaryngology; **Hospital:** Montefiore Med Ctr-Moses Campus (page 100), Montefiore Westchester Sq; **Address:** 1200 Waters Pl, Ste 110, Bronx, NY 10461; **Phone:** 718-863-4366; **Med School:** South Africa 1974; **Resid:** Otolaryngology, Univ Stellenbosch 1985; Otolaryngology, Univ Cape Town 1987; **Fellow:** Pediatric Otolaryngology, Montefiore Med Ctr-Weiler Div 1988

Pediatric Allergy & Immunology

Wiznia, Andrew A MD (PA&I) - **Hospital:** Jacobi Med Ctr, N Central Bronx Hosp; **Address:** Jacobi Medical Ctr, Bldg 1, 1400 Pelham Pkwy S, Bronx, NY 10461; **Phone:** 718-918-5222; **Board Cert:** Pediatrics 1986; **Med School:** Columbia P&S 1980; **Resid:** Pediatrics, Bronx Muni Hosp Ctr 1983; Pediatrics, Bronx-Lebanon Hosp Ctr 1984; **Fellow:** Allergy & Immunology, Montefiore-Weiler Einstein Div 1986; **Fac Appt:** Prof Ped, Albert Einstein Coll Med

Pediatric Cardiology

Hsu, Daphne T MD (PCd) - **Spec Exp:** Interventional Cardiology; Heart Failure; Transplant Medicine-Heart; **Hospital:** Montefiore Med Ctr-Moses Campus (page 100); **Address:** Children's Hosp at Montefiore, 3415 Bainbridge Ave, Bronx, NY 10467; **Phone:** 718-741-2343; **Board Cert:** Pediatrics 1988; Pediatric Cardiology 2010; **Med School:** Yale Univ 1982; **Resid:** Pediatrics, Columbia Babies & Chldn's Hosp 1985; **Fellow:** Pediatric Cardiology, Columbia Babies & Chldn's Hosp 1988; **Fac Appt:** Prof Ped, Albert Einstein Coll Med

Pass, Robert H MD (PCd) - **Spec Exp:** Arrhythmias; Cardiac Electrophysiology; Cardiac Catheterization; **Hospital:** Montefiore Med Ctr-Moses Campus (page 100); **Address:** Chldn's Hosp at Montefiore, 3415 Bainbridge Ave, Bronx, NY 10467; **Phone:** 718-741-2183; **Board Cert:** Pediatric Cardiology 2013; **Med School:** Boston Univ 1991; **Resid:** Pediatrics, NY Presby/Cornell Med Ctr 1994; **Fellow:** Cardiovascular Disease, Chldn's Hosp 1998; **Fac Appt:** Assoc Prof Ped, Albert Einstein Coll Med

Schiller, Myles S MD (PCd) - **Spec Exp:** Congenital Heart Disease & Acquired; Exercise Physiology; **Hospital:** Montefiore Med Ctr-Moses Campus (page 100), St. Barnabas Hosp - Bronx; **Address:** Children's Hosp Montefiore, 3415 Bainbridge Ave, Bronx, NY 10467; **Phone:** 718-741-2254; **Board Cert:** Pediatrics 1978; Pediatric Cardiology 1979; **Med School:** Ros Franklin Univ/Chicago Med Sch 1973; **Resid:** Pediatrics, New York Hosp-Cornell 1975; **Fellow:** Pediatric Cardiology, New York Hosp-Cornell 1977; **Fac Appt:** Assoc Clin Prof Ped, Albert Einstein Coll Med

Shenoy, Rajesh U MD (PCd) - **Spec Exp:** Echocardiography; Fetal Echocardiography; Congenital Heart Disease; **Hospital:** Mt Sinai Med Ctr (page 102), Queens Hosp Ctr - Jamaica; **Address:** 1 Gustave L. Levy Pl, Annenberg Bldg - Fl 3, MS 1201, Ave, Kravis Children's Hospital at Mount Sinai Medical Center, New York, NY 10029; **Phone:** 212-241-0424; **Board Cert:** Pediatric Cardiology 2008; **Med School:** India 1995; **Resid:** Pediatrics, Univ Illinois Affil Hosp 1996; **Fellow:** Pediatric Cardiology, N Shore Hosp 2000; **Fac Appt:** Asst Prof Ped, Mount Sinai Sch Med

Walsh, Christine A MD (PCd) - **Spec Exp:** Arrhythmias; Congenital Heart Disease; Sudden Infant Death Syndrome (SIDS); Syncope; **Hospital:** Montefiore Med Ctr-Moses Campus (page 100); **Address:** 3415 Bainbridge Ave Fl 5, Bronx, NY 10467-2401; **Phone:** 718-741-2343; **Board Cert:** Pediatrics 1978; Pediatric Cardiology 1983; **Med School:** Yale Univ 1973; **Resid:** Pediatrics, Columbia-Presby Med Ctr 1976; **Fellow:** Pediatric Cardiology, Columbia-Presby Med Ctr 1980; **Fac Appt:** Prof Ped, Albert Einstein Coll Med

Pediatric Critical Care Medicine

Singer, Lewis P MD (PCCM) - **Spec Exp:** Respiratory Failure; Airway Disorders; **Hospital:** Montefiore Med Ctr-Moses Campus (page 100); **Address:** 111 E 210th St, Rosenthal Pavilion Fl 4, Bronx, NY 10467; **Phone:** 718-741-2440; **Board Cert:** Pediatrics 1981; Neonatal-Perinatal Medicine 1983; Pediatric Critical Care Medicine 2012; **Med School:** UMDNJ-NJ Med Sch, Newark 1977; **Resid:** Pediatrics, Montefiore Hosp Med Ctr 1980; **Fellow:** Neonatology, Montefiore Hosp Med Ctr 1983; **Fac Appt:** Clin Prof Ped, Albert Einstein Coll Med

Ushay, H Michael MD/PhD (PCCM) - **Spec Exp:** Respiratory Failure; Sepsis & Septic Shock; Cardiac Critical Care; **Hospital:** Montefiore Med Ctr-Moses Campus (page 100); **Address:** 111 E 210th St, Rosenthal Pavilion Fl 4, Bronx, NY 10467; **Phone:** 718-741-2440; **Board Cert:** Pediatrics 2012; Pediatric Critical Care Medicine 2009; **Med School:** UMDNJ-NJ Med Sch, Newark 1986; **Resid:** Pediatrics, Montefiore/Bronx Muni Hosp 1990; **Fellow:** Pediatric Pulmonology, Montefiore Med Ctr 1991; Pediatric Critical Care Medicine, NY Hosp-Cornell Univ Med Ctr 1993; **Fac Appt:** Clin Prof Ped, Albert Einstein Coll Med

Weingarten-Arams, Jacqueline S MD (PCCM) - **Spec Exp:** Heart Disease; Lung Disease; Nutrition; **Hospital:** Montefiore Med Ctr-Moses Campus (page 100); **Address:** 111 E 210th St, Children's Hospital at Montefiore, Rosenthal Bldg - Fl 4, Bronx, NY 10467; **Phone:** 718-741-2440; **Board Cert:** Pediatrics 2011; Pediatric Critical Care Medicine 2011; **Med School:** Cornell Univ-Weill Med Coll 1986; **Resid:** Pediatrics, Columbia-Presby Med Ctr 1990; **Fellow:** Pediatric Critical Care Medicine, Cornell/NY Hosp 1996; **Fac Appt:** Assoc Clin Prof Ped, Albert Einstein Coll Med

Pediatric Endocrinology

Agarwal, Chhavi MD (PEn) - **Spec Exp:** Diabetes; Rett Syndrome; Calcium Disorders; **Hospital:** Montefiore Med Ctr-Moses Campus (page 100); **Address:** Children's Hospital at Montefiore, 3415 Bainbridge Ave, Fl 4, Bronx, NY 10467; **Phone:** 718-920-4664; **Board Cert:** Pediatrics 2011; Pediatric Endocrinology 2007; **Med School:** India 1990; **Resid:** Pediatrics, Flushing Hosp Med Ctr 2004; **Fellow:** Pediatric Endocrinology, NY-Presby/Columbia Med Ctr 2007; **Fac Appt:** Asst Prof Ped, Albert Einstein Coll Med

Heptulla, Rubina A MD (PEn) - **Spec Exp:** Adrenal Disorders; Diabetes; Thyroid Disorders; **Hospital:** Montefiore Med Ctr-Moses Campus (page 100); **Address:** Chldns Hosp Montefiore, Ped Endocrin, 3415 Bainbridge Ave, Bronx, NY 10467; **Phone:** 718-741-2450; **Board Cert:** Pediatrics 2010; Pediatric Endocrinology 2008; **Med School:** India 1989; **Resid:** Pediatrics, Rhode Island Hosp 1994; Pediatrics, Baystate Med Ctr 1995; **Fellow:** Pediatric Endocrinology, Yale-New Haven Hosp 1997; **Fac Appt:** Prof Ped, Albert Einstein Coll Med

Pediatric Gastroenterology

Thompson, John F MD (PGe) - **Spec Exp:** Inflammatory Bowel Disease/Crohn's; Short Bowel Syndrome; Transplant Medicine-Bowel; **Hospital:** Montefiore Med Ctr-Moses Campus (page 100); **Address:** Children's Hosp at Montefiore, 3415 Bainbridge Ave, Bronx, NY 10467; **Phone:** 718-741-2450; **Board Cert:** Pediatrics 1983; Pediatric Gastroenterology 2012; **Med School:** Loyola Univ-Stritch Sch Med 1977; **Resid:** Pediatrics, Wylers Chldns Hosp-Univ Chicago 1980; **Fellow:** Pediatric Gastroenterology, Babies Hosp-Columbia Univ 1985; Nutrition, Babies Hosp-Columbia Univ 1985; **Fac Appt:** Prof Ped, Albert Einstein Coll Med

Pediatric Hematology-Oncology

Dasgupta, Indira K MD (PHO) - **Hospital:** Montefiore Med Ctr-Wakefield Campus (page 100); **Address:** 600 E 233rd St, Fl 4, Bronx, NY 10466-2697; **Phone:** 718-920-9014; **Board Cert:** Pediatrics 1981; Pediatric Hematology-Oncology 1984; **Med School:** India 1967; **Resid:** Pediatrics, New York Methodist Hosp 1974; **Fellow:** Pediatric Hematology-Oncology, Meml Sloan Kettering Cancer Ctr 1979; Pediatric Hematology-Oncology, Mount Sinai Hosp 1980

Gorlick, Richard MD (PHO) - **Spec Exp:** Bone Tumors; Sarcoma; Solid Tumors; **Hospital:** Montefiore Med Ctr-Moses Campus (page 100); **Address:** 3415 Bainbridge Ave, Rosenthal Pavilion, Room 300, Bronx, NY 10467; **Phone:** 718-741-2342; **Board Cert:** Pediatrics 2008; Pediatric Hematology-Oncology 2011; **Med School:** SUNY Downstate 1990; **Resid:** Pediatrics, Columbia-Presby Med Ctr 1993; **Fellow:** Pediatric Hematology-Oncology, Meml Sloan Kettering Cancer Ctr 1995; **Fac Appt:** Prof Ped, Albert Einstein Coll Med

Levy, Adam S MD (PHO) - **Spec Exp:** Brain Tumors; Spinal Cord Tumors; Neuro-Oncology; **Hospital:** Montefiore Med Ctr-Moses Campus (page 100); **Address:** Chldns Hosp at Montefiore, 3415 Bainbridge Ave, Bronx, NY 10467; **Phone:** 718-741-2342; **Board Cert:** Pediatrics 2012; Pediatric Hematology-Oncology 2010; **Med School:** NYU Sch Med 1994; **Resid:** Pediatrics, Mt Sinai Hosp 1998; **Fellow:** Pediatric Hematology-Oncology, Meml Sloan Kettering Cancer Ctr 2001; **Fac Appt:** Assoc Clin Prof Ped, Albert Einstein Coll Med

Moulton, Thomas A MD (PHO) - **Spec Exp:** Sickle Cell Disease; **Hospital:** Bronx Lebanon Hosp Ctr; **Address:** 2432 Grand Concourse, Bronx, NY 10458; **Phone:** 718-579-7337; **Board Cert:** Pediatric Hematology-Oncology 2012; **Med School:** Loyola Univ-Stritch Sch Med 1984; **Resid:** Pediatrics, Rainbow Babies-Chldns Hosp 1987; **Fellow:** Pediatric Hematology-Oncology, Babies Hosp 1990

Pediatric Infectious Disease

Herold, Betsy C MD (PInf) - **Spec Exp:** AIDS/HIV; HPV-Human Papilloma Virus; **Hospital:** Montefiore Med Ctr-Einstein Campus (page 100); **Address:** 1300 Morris Park Ave, Forchheimer Bldg, Ste 702, Bronx, NY 10461; **Phone:** 718-741-2470; **Board Cert:** Pediatrics 1986; Pediatric Infectious Disease 2012; **Med School:** Univ Pennsylvania 1982; **Resid:** Pediatrics, Northwestern Meml Hosp 1988; **Fellow:** Infectious Disease, Northwestern Meml Hosp 1989; **Fac Appt:** Prof Ped, Albert Einstein Coll Med

Litman, Nathan MD (PInf) - **Spec Exp:** Infections in Immunocompromised Patients; Hospital Acquired Infections; **Hospital:** Montefiore Med Ctr-Moses Campus (page 100); **Address:** Montefiore Med Ctr, Div Ped Infectious Disease, 111 E 210th St Fl 4, Bronx, NY 10467-2401; **Phone:** 718-741-2470; **Board Cert:** Pediatrics 1978; Pediatric Infectious Disease 2009; **Med School:** Albert Einstein Coll Med 1971; **Resid:** Pediatrics, Montefiore Med Ctr 1974; **Fellow:** Infectious Disease, Montefiore Med Ctr 1978; **Fac Appt:** Prof Ped, Albert Einstein Coll Med

Pediatric Nephrology

Kaskel, Frederick J MD/PhD (PNep) - **Spec Exp:** Transplant Medicine-Kidney; Nephrotic Syndrome; Kidney Disease-Chronic; Dialysis Care; **Hospital:** Montefiore Med Ctr-Moses Campus (page 100), St. Barnabas Hosp - Bronx; **Address:** Children's Hospital at Montefiore, 111 E 210th St, Bronx, NY 10467-2401; **Phone:** 718-655-1120; **Board Cert:** Pediatrics 1980; Pediatric Nephrology 1982; **Med School:** Univ Cincinnati 1975; **Resid:** Pediatrics, Montefiore Med Ctr 1977; **Fellow:** Pediatric Nephrology, Montefiore Med Ctr 1981; **Fac Appt:** Prof Ped, Albert Einstein Coll Med

Pediatric Otolaryngology

Bent, John P MD (PO) - **Spec Exp:** Airway Reconstruction; Sinus Disorders/Surgery; Hearing Loss; **Hospital:** Montefiore Med Ctr-Moses Campus (page 100); **Address:** Children's Hospital at Montefiore, Dept Otolaryngology, Head & Neck Surgery, 3400 Bainbridge Ave, Fl 3, Bronx, NY 10467-2490; **Phone:** 718-920-4646; **Board Cert:** Otolaryngology 1995; **Med School:** Wake Forest Univ 1989; **Resid:** Otolaryngology, MCG Hosp & Clinic 1994; **Fellow:** Pediatric Otolaryngology, Univ Iowa 1995; **Fac Appt:** Assoc Prof Oto, Albert Einstein Coll Med

Pediatric Pulmonology

Arens, Raanan MD (PPul) - **Spec Exp:** Sleep Disorders/Apnea; **Hospital:** Montefiore Med Ctr-Einstein Campus (page 100); **Address:** Chldns Hosp at Montefiore, Respiratory & Sleep Medicine, 3415 Bainbridge Ave, Bronx, NY 10467; **Phone:** 718-741-2450; **Board Cert:** Pediatrics 2010; Pediatric Pulmonology 2011; Sleep Medicine 2009; **Med School:** Israel 1986; **Resid:** Pediatrics, Shera Med Ctr 1990; Pediatrics, Chldns Hosp 1995; **Fellow:** Pediatric Pulmonology, Chldns Hosp 1994; **Fac Appt:** Prof Ped, Albert Einstein Coll Med

Pediatric Rheumatology

Ilowite, Norman T MD (PRhu) - **Spec Exp:** Juvenile Arthritis; Lyme Disease; Lupus/SLE; Dermatomyositis; **Hospital:** Montefiore Med Ctr-Moses Campus (page 100), Jacobi Med Ctr; **Address:** Chldns Hosp-Montefiore-Dept Rheumatology, 3415 Bainbridge Ave Fl Rosenthal3, Bronx, NY 10467; **Phone:** 718-741-2450; **Board Cert:** Pediatrics 1985; Clinical & Laboratory Immunology 1990; Pediatric Rheumatology 2007; **Med School:** SUNY Downstate 1979; **Resid:** Pediatrics, Chldns Hosp Natl Med Ctr 1982; **Fellow:** Pediatric Rheumatology, Univ WA Med Ctr 1984; **Fac Appt:** Prof Ped, Albert Einstein Coll Med

Pediatric Surgery

Jan, Dominique M MD/PhD (PS) - **Spec Exp:** Transplant-Bowel; Transplant-Liver; Transplant Surgery-Pediatric; **Hospital:** Montefiore Med Ctr-Moses Campus (page 100); **Address:** 3415 Bainbridge Ave Fl 5, Bronx, NY 10467; **Phone:** 718-920-7200; **Med School:** France 1984; **Resid:** Surgery, Assistance Poblique Hosp 1989; **Fellow:** Pediatric Surgery, Necker Malades Hosp; **Fac Appt:** Prof S, Albert Einstein Coll Med

Weinberg, Gerard MD (PS) - **Spec Exp:** Abdominal Wall Reconstruction; Trauma; Neonatal Surgery; **Hospital:** Montefiore Med Ctr-Moses Campus (page 100); **Address:** 3355 Bainbridge Ave, Bronx, NY 10467; **Phone:** 718-920-7200; **Board Cert:** Surgery 2009; Pediatric Surgery 2009; **Med School:** Albert Einstein Coll Med 1973; **Resid:** Surgery, Albert Einstein Affil Hosps 1976; Pediatric Surgery, Childrens Hosp 1977; **Fellow:** Pediatric Surgery, Univ of Miami Hosps 1979; **Fac Appt:** Prof S, Albert Einstein Coll Med

Pediatrics

Andrade, Joseph MD (Ped) *PCP* - **Hospital:** Montefiore Med Ctr-Wakefield Campus (page 100); **Address:** 1163 Manor Ave, Bronx, NY 10472; **Phone:** 718-589-3501; **Board Cert:** Pediatrics 2007; Internal Medicine 2011; **Med School:** Ecuador 1981; **Resid:** Pediatrics, Our Lady of Mercy Med Ctr 1986; Internal Medicine, Our Lady of Mercy Med Ctr 1988

Arnstein, Ellis J MD (Ped) *PCP* - **Spec Exp:** Developmental Disorders; **Hospital:** Bronx Lebanon Hosp Ctr; **Address:** Bronx Lebanon Hosp Ctr, 2432 Grand Concourse, Bronx, NY 10457; **Phone:** 718-579-7337; **Board Cert:** Pediatrics 1975; Neurodevelopmental Disabilities 2012; **Med School:** SUNY Downstate 1969; **Resid:** Pediatrics, Univ Wash Med Ctr 1973; **Fellow:** Child & Adolescent Psychiatry, Tufts-New England Med Ctr 1974; **Fac Appt:** Asst Prof Ped, NY Med Coll

Balk, Sophie J MD (Ped) *PCP* - **Hospital:** Montefiore Med Ctr-Moses Campus (page 100), Montefiore Med Ctr-Einstein Campus (page 100); **Address:** 1621 Eastchester Rd, Bronx, NY 10461-2604; **Phone:** 718-405-8090; **Board Cert:** Pediatrics 1979; **Med School:** Albert Einstein Coll Med 1974; **Resid:** Pediatrics, Montefiore Med Ctr 1977; **Fac Appt:** Clin Prof Ped, Albert Einstein Coll Med

Belamarich, Peter F MD (Ped) - **Spec Exp:** Cholesterol/Lipid Disorders; **Hospital:** Montefiore Med Ctr-Einstein Campus (page 100); **Address:** Chldn's Hosp at Montefiore, 3415 Bainbridge Ave, Fl 4, Bronx, NY 10467; **Phone:** 718-741-2432; **Board Cert:** Pediatrics 1987; **Med School:** Boston Univ 1983; **Resid:** Pediatrics, Brookdale Univ Hosp 1986; **Fellow:** Pediatric Gastroenterology, NY-Presby/Columbia Univ Med Ctr 1989

Bloomfield, Diane MD (Ped) *PCP* - **Hospital:** Montefiore Med Ctr-Moses Campus (page 100); **Address:** Montefiore Family Care Ctr, 3444 Kossuth Ave, DTC Bldg Fl 1B, Bronx, NY 10467-2461; **Phone:** 718-920-2273; **Board Cert:** Pediatrics 1987; **Med School:** Cornell Univ-Weill Med Coll 1982; **Resid:** Pediatrics, NY Hosp 1985; **Fellow:** Ambulatory Pediatrics, NY Hosp 1986; **Fac Appt:** Asst Prof Ped, Albert Einstein Coll Med

Cahill, Linda T MD (Ped) - **Spec Exp:** Child Abuse; **Hospital:** Montefiore Med Ctr-Moses Campus (page 100); **Address:** Butler Child Advocacy Ctr, Chldns Hosp-Montefiore, 3314 Steuben Ave, Bronx, NY 10467; **Phone:** 718-920-5833; **Board Cert:** Pediatrics 1975; Child Abuse Pediatrics 2009; **Med School:** Med Coll PA 1969; **Resid:** Pediatrics, Beth Israel Med Ctr 1972; **Fellow:** Pediatric Infectious Disease, Mt Sinai Hosp 1974; **Fac Appt:** Assoc Clin Prof Ped, Albert Einstein Coll Med

Esteban-Cruciani, Nora MD (Ped) - **Spec Exp:** Chronic Illness; **Hospital:** Chldns Hosp at Montefiore; **Address:** 3415 Bainbridge Ave, Department of Pediatrics, Rosenthal-3, Bronx, NY 10467; **Phone:** 718-741-2257; **Board Cert:** Pediatrics 2008; **Med School:** Argentina 1980; **Resid:** Pediatrics, Italian Hosp 1983; Pediatrics, Albert Einstein Coll Med 1993; **Fellow:** Research, Nat Inst Hlth 1991; Research, Albert Einstein Coll Med 2005; **Fac Appt:** Prof Ped, Albert Einstein Coll Med

Haber, Patricia MD (Ped) *PCP* - **Hospital:** Montefiore Med Ctr-Moses Campus (page 100); **Address:** 1500 Astor Ave Fl 2, Bronx, NY 10469-5900; **Phone:** 718-881-0100; **Board Cert:** Pediatrics 2009; Pediatric Rheumatology 2011; **Med School:** Johns Hopkins Univ 1976; **Resid:** Pediatrics, Johns Hopkins Hosp 1979; **Fellow:** Immunology, Univ Alabama Hosp 1982; Pediatric Rheumatology, Univ Alabama Hosp 1984; **Fac Appt:** Asst Prof Ped, Albert Einstein Coll Med

Hirschman, Alan MD (Ped) *PCP* - **Hospital:** Montefiore Med Ctr-Moses Campus (page 100); **Address:** 3765 Riverdale Ave, Ste 4, Bronx, NY 10463-1845; **Phone:** 718-548-7300; **Board Cert:** Pediatrics 1981; **Med School:** UMDNJ-NJ Med Sch, Newark 1976; **Resid:** Pediatrics, Montefiore Med Ctr 1980

Igel, Gerard MD (Ped) *PCP* - **Spec Exp:** Chronic Illness; Behavioral Disorders; Developmental Disorders; Foster Care; **Hospital:** Montefiore Med Ctr-Moses Campus (page 100), Jacobi Med Ctr; **Address:** 1613 Tenbroeck Ave, Bronx, NY 10461; **Phone:** 718-828-9060; **Board Cert:** Pediatrics 1986; **Med School:** Israel 1981; **Resid:** Pediatrics, Jacobi Med Ctr 1984; **Fac Appt:** Asst Clin Prof Ped, Albert Einstein Coll Med

Kaminer, Ruth K MD (Ped) - **Spec Exp:** Developmental & Behavioral Disorders; **Hospital:** Montefiore Med Ctr-Moses Campus (page 100); **Address:** Rose F Kennedy Ctr, 1410 Pelham Pkwy S, rm 108, Bronx, NY 10461-1101; **Phone:** 718-839-7070; **Board Cert:** Pediatrics 1971; Developmental-Behavioral Pediatrics 2010; **Med School:** NYU Sch Med 1962; **Resid:** Pediatrics, Chldns Hosp 1964; **Fellow:** Ambulatory Pediatrics, Bronx Muni Hosp 1968; Developmental-Behavioral Pediatrics, Albert Einstein Coll Med Affil Hosp 1974; **Fac Appt:** Prof Ped, Albert Einstein Coll Med

Mayers, Marguerite MD (Ped) *PCP* - **Spec Exp:** Tuberculosis; AIDS/HIV; Travel Medicine; **Hospital:** Montefiore Med Ctr-Moses Campus (page 100); **Address:** Montefiore Family Care Ctr, 3444 Kossuth Ave, Bronx, NY 10467-2401; **Phone:** 718-920-2273; **Board Cert:** Pediatrics 1977; Pediatric Infectious Disease 2009; **Med School:** Albert Einstein Coll Med 1971; **Resid:** Pediatrics, Montefiore Med Ctr 1974; **Fellow:** Infectious Disease, Montefiore Med Ctr 1976; **Fac Appt:** Clin Prof Ped, Albert Einstein Coll Med

Oppedisano, Carlyn Ann MD (Ped) *PCP* - **Hospital:** Morgan Stanley Children's Hosp of NY-Presby, NY (page 104); **Address:** 2600 Netherland Ave, Ste 120, Riverdale, NY 10463-4813; **Phone:** 718-796-3580; **Board Cert:** Pediatrics 2009; **Med School:** Columbia P&S 1981; **Resid:** Pediatrics, Babies Hosp/NY-Presby 1985; **Fac Appt:** Assoc Clin Prof Ped, Columbia P&S

Schechter, Miriam MD (Ped) *PCP* - **Spec Exp:** Asthma; Vaccines; **Hospital:** Montefiore Med Ctr-Moses Campus (page 100); **Address:** 1621 Eastchester Rd, Ste 115, Bronx, NY 10461-2604; **Phone:** 718-405-8090; **Board Cert:** Pediatrics 2007; **Med School:** NYU Sch Med 1989; **Resid:** Pediatrics, Mt Sinai Med Ctr 1992; Pediatrics, Mt Sinai Med Ctr 1993; **Fac Appt:** Asst Prof Ped, Albert Einstein Coll Med

Stein, Ruth E K MD (Ped) - **Spec Exp:** Chronic Illness; Developmental & Behavioral Disorders; **Hospital:** Montefiore Med Ctr-Moses Campus (page 100); **Address:** 1225 Morris Park Ave, Bronx, NY 10461; **Phone:** 718-839-7057; **Board Cert:** Pediatrics 1971; Developmental-Behavioral Pediatrics 2012; **Med School:** Albert Einstein Coll Med 1966; **Resid:** Pediatrics, Bronx Muni Hosp 1968; Pediatrics, Chldns Hosp Natl Med Ctr 1969; **Fellow:** Community Medicine, Chldns Hosp Natl Med Ctr 1969; **Fac Appt:** Prof Ped, Albert Einstein Coll Med

Strassberg, Barbara E MD (Ped) *PCP* - **Spec Exp:** Developmental Disorders; **Hospital:** Morgan Stanley Children's Hosp of NY-Presby, NY (page 104); **Address:** Riverdale Pediatrics, 2600 Netherland Ave, Ste 120, Bronx, NY 10463-4813; **Phone:** 718-796-3580; **Board Cert:** Pediatrics 2009; **Med School:** SUNY Upstate Med Univ 1981; **Resid:** Pediatrics, Columbia-Presby Hosp 1984; **Fac Appt:** Assoc Clin Prof Ped, Columbia P&S

Sullivan, Christina K MD (Ped) *PCP* - **Hospital:** Montefiore Med Ctr-Moses Campus (page 100); **Address:** Montefiore Comprehensive Family Care Ctr, 1621 Eastchester Rd, Bronx, NY 10461-2604; **Phone:** 718-405-8040; **Board Cert:** Pediatrics 2008; **Med School:** Univ Conn 1990; **Resid:** Pediatrics, Mt Sinai Med Ctr 1993; **Fac Appt:** Asst Clin Prof Ped, Albert Einstein Coll Med

Weiner, Richard L MD (Ped) *PCP* - **Spec Exp:** Adolescent Medicine; **Hospital:** Montefiore Med Ctr-Moses Campus (page 100), Montefiore Med Ctr-Einstein Campus (page 100); **Address:** Montefiore Medical Group, 2300 Westchester Ave, Bronx, NY 10462; **Phone:** 718-409-8000; **Board Cert:** Pediatrics 1991; **Med School:** Albert Einstein Coll Med 1975; **Resid:** Pediatrics, Jacobi Med Ctr 1978; **Fac Appt:** Assoc Prof Ped, Albert Einstein Coll Med

Zoltan, Irving MD (Ped) *PCP* - **Spec Exp:** Diagnostic Problems; Asthma; Infectious Disease; **Hospital:** Montefiore Med Ctr-Moses Campus (page 100), Montefiore Med Ctr-Einstein Campus (page 100); **Address:** 1613 Tenbroeck Ave, Bronx, NY 10461; **Phone:** 718-828-9060; **Board Cert:** Pediatrics 1979; **Med School:** Albert Einstein Coll Med 1974; **Resid:** Pediatrics, Bronx Muni Hosp 1978; **Fac Appt:** Asst Clin Prof Ped, Albert Einstein Coll Med

Physical Medicine & Rehabilitation

DeAraujo, Maria MD (PMR) - **Spec Exp:** Arthritis; Pain-Low Back; Electromyography; Pain-Musculoskeletal; **Hospital:** Montefiore Med Ctr-Wakefield Campus (page 100); **Address:** Montefiore Dept Phys Med & Rehab, 600 E 233rd St, Bronx, NY 10466-2604; **Phone:** 718-920-9171; **Board Cert:** Physical Medicine & Rehabilitation 1989; **Med School:** Brazil 1972; **Resid:** Physical Medicine & Rehabilitation, St Vincent Hosp Med Ctr 1981; **Fellow:** Physical Medicine & Rehabilitation, Westchester Med Ctr 1989

Inwald, Gary DO (PMR) - **Spec Exp:** Musculoskeletal Disorders; Pain Management; **Hospital:** Montefiore Med Ctr-Einstein Campus (page 100); **Address:** Montefiore Med Ctr-Dept of Rehab, 1825 Eastchester Rd, Bronx, NY 10461; **Phone:** 718-904-2296; **Board Cert:** Physical Medicine & Rehabilitation 1983; **Med School:** Mich State Univ Coll Osteo Med 1976; **Resid:** Physical Medicine & Rehabilitation, St Vincents Hosp 1982

Levin, Sheryl MD (PMR) - **Spec Exp:** Neuro-Rehabilitation; Pain-Musculoskeletal; Arthritis; **Hospital:** Montefiore Med Ctr-Moses Campus (page 100); **Address:** 3435 Dekalb Ave, Bronx, NY 10467-2301; **Phone:** 718-547-8899; **Board Cert:** Physical Medicine & Rehabilitation ; **Med School:** Cornell Univ-Weill Med Coll 1984; **Resid:** Physical Medicine & Rehabilitation, NY Hosp 1988; **Fac Appt:** Asst Clin Prof PMR, Albert Einstein Coll Med

Thomas, Mark Alvin MD (PMR) - **Hospital:** Montefiore Med Ctr-Moses Campus (page 100); **Address:** 150 E 210th St, Fl 2, Bronx, NY 10467; **Phone:** 718-920-2753; **Board Cert:** Physical Medicine & Rehabilitation 1988; **Med School:** Mexico 1982; **Resid:** Physical Medicine & Rehabilitation, Nassau Co Med Ctr 1986; **Fac Appt:** Assoc Prof PMR, Albert Einstein Coll Med

Plastic Surgery

Garfein, Evan S MD (PlS) - **Spec Exp:** Breast Reconstruction; Head & Neck Reconstruction; Microsurgery; **Hospital:** Montefiore Med Ctr-Moses Campus (page 100); **Address:** Montefiore, Plastic Surgery Dept, 1625 Poplar St, Bronx, NY 10461; **Phone:** 718-405-8444; **Board Cert:** Plastic Surgery 2009; **Med School:** Columbia P&S 1999; **Resid:** Surgery, Brigham & Womens Hosp 2004; **Fellow:** Plastic Surgery, Brigham & Womens Hosp 2007; **Fac Appt:** Asst Prof S, Albert Einstein Coll Med

Goldstein, Robert D MD (PlS) - **Spec Exp:** Breast Surgery; Nasal Surgery; Abdominoplasty; **Hospital:** Montefiore Med Ctr-Einstein Campus (page 100), Montefiore Med Ctr-Moses Campus (page 100); **Address:** Bronx Plastic Surgery, 2425 Eastchester Rd, Bronx, NY 10469; **Phone:** 718-405-7500; **Board Cert:** Plastic Surgery 1985; **Med School:** Penn State Coll Med 1977; **Resid:** Surgery, Montefiore Med Ctr 1981; Plastic Surgery, Montefiore Med Ctr 1984; **Fellow:** Hand Surgery, Montefiore Med Ctr-Einstein Div 1982; **Fac Appt:** Assoc Clin Prof PlS, Albert Einstein Coll Med

Greenstein, Bruce MD (PlS) - **Spec Exp:** Burn Care; Burns-Reconstructive Plastic Surgery; **Hospital:** Jacobi Med Ctr, N Central Bronx Hosp; **Address:** Jacobi Med Ctr, Dept Plastic Surgery, 1400 Pelham Pkwy S, Bldg 1 - rm 209, Bronx, NY 10461; **Phone:** 718-918-5970; **Board Cert:** Plastic Surgery 1984; **Med School:** SUNY Upstate Med Univ 1975; **Resid:** Surgery, Montefiore Med Ctr 1980; Plastic Surgery, Montefiore Med Ctr 1982; **Fellow:** Hand Surgery, Montefiore Med Ctr 1983; **Fac Appt:** Assoc Clin Prof PlS, Albert Einstein Coll Med

Liebling, Ralph W MD (PlS) - **Spec Exp:** Reconstructive Surgery; Microsurgery; Hand Surgery; Burn Care; **Hospital:** Jacobi Med Ctr, N Central Bronx Hosp; **Address:** Jacobi Med Ctr, Dept Plastic & Reconstructive Surg, 1400 Pelham Pkwy S, Bronx, NY 10461; **Phone:** 718-918-7000; **Board Cert:** Plastic Surgery 1988; **Med School:** Albert Einstein Coll Med 1977; **Resid:** Surgery, Montefiore Med Ctr 1981; Plastic Surgery, Montefiore Med Ctr 1983; **Fellow:** Reconstructive Microsurgery, NYU/Bellevue Hosp Ctr 1984; **Fac Appt:** Assoc Clin Prof PlS, Albert Einstein Coll Med

Psychiatry

Asnis, Gregory M MD (Psyc) - **Spec Exp:** Psychopharmacology; Mood Disorders; Anxiety Disorders; Depression; **Hospital:** Montefiore Med Ctr-Moses Campus (page 100), Phelps Meml Hosp Ctr; **Address:** 111 E 210th St, Bronx, NY 10467-2401; **Phone:** 718-920-4287; **Board Cert:** Psychiatry 1978; **Med School:** Hahnemann Univ 1972; **Resid:** Psychiatry, Mt Sinai Hosp 1976; **Fellow:** Psychiatry, Columbia-Presby Med Ctr 1981; **Fac Appt:** Prof Psyc, Albert Einstein Coll Med

Gelfand, Janice MD (Psyc) - **Spec Exp:** Depression; Anxiety Disorders; Psychosomatic Disorders; Personality Disorders; **Hospital:** NY-Presby/Columbia Univ Med Ctr, NY (page 104); **Address:** 3765 Riverdale Ave, Bronx, NY 10463; **Phone:** 718-361-3482; **Board Cert:** Psychiatry 1990; **Med School:** NYU Sch Med 1985; **Resid:** Psychiatry, NYU Med Ctr 1989; **Fellow:** Psychiatry, Beth Israel Med Ctr 1991; **Fac Appt:** Asst Prof Psyc, Columbia P&S

Heiman, Peter L MD (Psyc) - **Spec Exp:** Psychiatry in Physical Illness; **Hospital:** Montefiore Med Ctr-Moses Campus (page 100); **Address:** 4465 Douglas Ave, Ste 1K, Bronx, NY 10471; **Phone:** 212-472-8885; **Board Cert:** Psychiatry 1975; **Med School:** Albert Einstein Coll Med 1968; **Resid:** Psychiatry, Montefiore Med Ctr 1972; **Fac Appt:** Asst Clin Prof Psyc, Albert Einstein Coll Med

Lebinger, Martin B MD (Psyc) - **Spec Exp:** Depression; Anxiety Disorders; Panic Disorder; **Hospital:** Bronx Psych Ctr; **Address:** 1540 Pelham Pkwy S, Ste 1A, Bronx, NY 10461-1130; **Phone:** 718-518-0222; **Board Cert:** Psychiatry 1980; **Med School:** Albert Einstein Coll Med 1976; **Resid:** Psychiatry, Montefiore Med Ctr 1979; **Fellow:** Psychiatry, LI Jewish-Hillside Med Ctr 1981; **Fac Appt:** Asst Clin Prof Psyc, Albert Einstein Coll Med

Osei-Tutu, John MD (Psyc) - **Spec Exp:** Anxiety & Depression; Addiction/Substance Abuse; **Hospital:** Bronx Lebanon Hosp Ctr; **Address:** 1154 Wheeler Ave, Bronx, NY 10472; **Phone:** 718-991-9200; **Board Cert:** Psychiatry 1990; Addiction Psychiatry 2013; **Med School:** Ghana 1976; **Resid:** Psychiatry, Bronx-Lebanon Hosp 1983; **Fac Appt:** Asst Prof Psyc, Albert Einstein Coll Med

Schwartz, Bruce J MD (Psyc) - **Spec Exp:** Depression; Bipolar/Mood Disorders; Schizophrenia; Anxiety & Depression; **Hospital:** Montefiore Med Ctr-Moses Campus (page 100); **Address:** Montefiore Medical Ctr, Dept Psychiatry, 111 E 210th St, Bronx, NY 10467-2490; **Phone:** 718-920-4040; **Board Cert:** Psychiatry 1980; **Med School:** SUNY Downstate 1975; **Resid:** Psychiatry, Bronx Muni Hosp 1979; **Fac Appt:** Clin Prof Psyc, Albert Einstein Coll Med

Wyszynski, Bernard MD (Psyc) - **Hospital:** Montefiore Med Ctr-Moses Campus (page 100); **Address:** Montefore Medical Ctr, KLAU 2, 111 E 210th St, Bronx, NY 10467; **Phone:** 718-920-4737; **Board Cert:** Psychiatry 1987; Neurology 1985; **Med School:** Univ Pennsylvania 1980; **Resid:** Neurology, Mount Sinai Med Ctr 1984; Psychiatry, Mount Sinai Med Ctr 1987; **Fac Appt:** Assoc Prof Psyc, Albert Einstein Coll Med

Pulmonary Disease

Aldrich, Thomas K MD (Pul) - **Spec Exp:** Asthma; Chronic Obstructive Lung Disease (COPD); Sickle Cell Disease-Lung; Sarcoidosis; **Hospital:** Montefiore Med Ctr-Moses Campus (page 100); **Address:** 3400 Bainbridge Ave, Fl 2nd, Bronx, NY 10467-2401; **Phone:** 866-633-8255; **Board Cert:** Internal Medicine 1978; Pulmonary Disease 1980; **Med School:** Univ Minn 1975; **Resid:** Internal Medicine, UC Irvine Med Ctr 1978; **Fellow:** Pulmonary Disease, Univ Virginia Med Ctr 1980; Physiology, Univ Penn 1982; **Fac Appt:** Prof Med, Albert Einstein Coll Med

Appel, David MD (Pul) - **Spec Exp:** Sleep Disorders/Apnea; Asthma; Smoking Cessation; **Hospital:** Montefiore Med Ctr-Moses Campus (page 100); **Address:** 3400 Bainbridge Ave, Bronx, NY 10467; **Phone:** 866-633-8255; **Board Cert:** Internal Medicine 1976; Sleep Medicine 2002; **Med School:** Albert Einstein Coll Med 1973; **Resid:** Internal Medicine, Bronx Municipal Hosp 1976; **Fellow:** Pulmonary Disease, Bronx Municipal Hosp 1978; **Fac Appt:** Assoc Prof Med, Albert Einstein Coll Med

Casper, Theodore MD (Pul) - **Spec Exp:** Critical Care Medicine; **Hospital:** Montefiore Med Ctr-Einstein Campus (page 100), Montefiore Med Ctr-Wakefield Campus (page 100); **Address:** Pulmonary Medicine, 1250 Waters Pl, Ste 506, Bronx, NY 10461; **Phone:** 718-892-1200; **Board Cert:** Internal Medicine 1983; Pulmonary Disease 1986; **Med School:** Columbia P&S 1980; **Resid:** Internal Medicine, St Lukes Hosp 1983; **Fellow:** Pulmonary Disease, St Lukes Hosp 1985; **Fac Appt:** Asst Clin Prof Med, Albert Einstein Coll Med

Karetzky, Monroe MD (Pul) - **Spec Exp:** Asthma; Sleep Disorders; **Hospital:** Hackensack Univ Med Ctr (page 718), Englewood Hosp & Med Ctr; **Address:** Bronx Pulmonary Center, 441 E Tremont Ave, Bronx, NY 10457; **Phone:** 718-583-9240; **Board Cert:** Internal Medicine 1971; Pulmonary Disease 1974; Critical Care Medicine 2011; **Med School:** Cornell Univ-Weill Med Coll 1963; **Resid:** Internal Medicine, Mary I Bassett Hosp 1966; **Fellow:** Cardiopulmonary Disease, Mary I Bassett Hosp 1967; **Fac Appt:** Assoc Clin Prof Med, UMDNJ-NJ Med Sch, Newark

Klapper, Philip MD (Pul) - **Spec Exp:** Asthma; Emphysema; Chronic Obstructive Lung Disease (COPD); **Hospital:** Montefiore Med Ctr-Moses Campus (page 100), Lawrence Hosp Ctr; **Address:** 3322 Bainbridge Ave, Bronx, NY 10467; **Phone:** 718-884-2000; **Board Cert:** Internal Medicine 1986; Pulmonary Disease 2010; Critical Care Medicine 2003; **Med School:** Albert Einstein Coll Med 1983; **Resid:** Internal Medicine, Montefiore Hosp Med Ctr 1986; **Fellow:** Pulmonary Disease, SUNY Downstate Med Ctr 1990; Critical Care Medicine, Montefiore Hosp Med Ctr 1991; **Fac Appt:** Asst Clin Prof Med, Albert Einstein Coll Med

Loganathan, Raghunandan S MD (Pul) - **Spec Exp:** Critical Care; Pneumonia; Asthma; Chronic Obstructive Lung Disease (COPD); **Hospital:** Lincoln Med & Mental Hlth Ctr; **Address:** Lincoln Medical & Mental Health Ctr, 234 E 149th St, Ste 820, Bronx, NY 10451; **Phone:** 914-330-1302; **Board Cert:** Critical Care Medicine 2003; **Med School:** India 1994; **Resid:** Internal Medicine, Bronx-Lebanon Hosp 2000; **Fellow:** Pulmonary Disease, Meml Sloan Kettering Cancer Ctr 2002; Critical Care Medicine, Montefiore Med Ctr 2003

Prezant, David MD (Pul) - **Spec Exp:** Asthma; **Hospital:** Montefiore Med Ctr-Moses Campus (page 100); **Address:** 111 E 210th St, Bronx, NY 10467-2401; **Phone:** 718-920-6095; **Board Cert:** Internal Medicine 1984; Pulmonary Disease 1986; **Med School:** Albert Einstein Coll Med 1981; **Resid:** Internal Medicine, Harlem Hosp 1984; **Fellow:** Pulmonary Disease, Montefiore Hosp Med Ctr 1986; **Fac Appt:** Assoc Prof Med, Albert Einstein Coll Med

Sender, Joel MD (Pul) - **Spec Exp:** Asthma; Sarcoidosis; **Hospital:** St. Barnabas Hosp - Bronx; **Address:** 2016 Bronxdale Ave, Ste 301, Bronx, NY 10462-3300; **Phone:** 718-409-2222; **Board Cert:** Internal Medicine 1978; Pulmonary Disease 1980; Geriatric Medicine 2005; **Med School:** Albany Med Coll 1975; **Resid:** Internal Medicine, Mount Sinai Hosp 1978; **Fellow:** Pulmonary Disease, Mount Sinai Hosp 1980

Radiation Oncology

Bodner, William R MD (RadRO) - **Spec Exp:** Brachytherapy; Stereotactic Radiosurgery; **Hospital:** Montefiore Med Ctr-Einstein Campus (page 100); **Address:** 1625 Poplar St, MS 10461, Bronx, NY 10461; **Phone:** 718-405-8550; **Board Cert:** Radiation Oncology 2005; **Med School:** Wake Forest Univ 1987; **Resid:** Radiation Oncology, NY Med Coll Affil Hosp 1995; **Fac Appt:** Assoc Prof RadRO, Albert Einstein Coll Med

Garg, Madhur MD (RadRO) - **Spec Exp:** Head & Neck Cancer; Genitourinary Cancer; Central Nervous System Cancer; Brain & Spinal Cord Tumors; **Hospital:** Montefiore Med Ctr-Moses Campus (page 100); **Address:** Montefiore Med Ctr, Radiation Oncology, 111 E 210th St, Bronx, NY 10467; **Phone:** 718-920-4140; **Board Cert:** Radiation Oncology 2003; **Med School:** India 1996; **Resid:** Radiation Oncology, Rush Presby St Lukes Med Ctr 1999; Radiation Oncology, Montefiore Med Ctr 2003; **Fac Appt:** Assoc Prof RadRO, Albert Einstein Coll Med

Kalnicki, Shalom MD (RadRO) - **Spec Exp:** Lung Cancer; Head & Neck Cancer; Breast Cancer; Prostate Cancer; **Hospital:** Montefiore Med Ctr-Moses Campus (page 100), Montefiore Med Ctr-Einstein Campus (page 100); **Address:** Montefiore Medical Group, 1625 Poplar St Fl 2, Bronx, NY 10461; **Phone:** 718-920-5280; **Board Cert:** Therapeutic Radiology 1979; **Med School:** Brazil 1974; **Resid:** Radiation Oncology, Montefiore Med Ctr 1979; **Fac Appt:** Prof Rad, Albert Einstein Coll Med

Rheumatology

Efthimiou, Petros MD (Rhu) - **Spec Exp:** Rheumatoid Arthritis; Lupus/SLE; Psoriatic Arthritis; Spondyloarthropathies; **Hospital:** Lincoln Med & Mental Hlth Ctr, Lenox Hill Hosp (page 106); **Address:** 234 E 149 St, Fl 9, Ste 28, Bronx, NY 10451; **Phone:** 646-719-0602; **Board Cert:** Internal Medicine 2011; Rheumatology 2003; **Med School:** Greece 1996; **Resid:** Internal Medicine, Rhode Island Hosp 2001; **Fellow:** Rheumatology, NY-Presby/Weill Cornell Med Ctr 2004; Rheumatology, Hosp for Special Surgery 2004; **Fac Appt:** Assoc Prof Med, Cornell Univ-Weill Med Coll

Fomberstein, Barry MD (Rhu) - **Spec Exp:** Rheumatoid Arthritis; Gout; **Hospital:** Montefiore Med Ctr-Wakefield Campus (page 100); **Address:** Wakefield Medical Village, 4234 Bronx Blvd, Bronx, NY 10466; **Phone:** 347-341-4340; **Board Cert:** Internal Medicine 1979; Rheumatology 1982; **Med School:** Albert Einstein Coll Med 1976; **Resid:** Internal Medicine, LIJ Med Ctr 1979; **Fellow:** Rheumatology, LIJ Med Ctr 1981; **Fac Appt:** Assoc Clin Prof Med, NY Med Coll

Keiser, Harold D MD (Rhu) - **Spec Exp:** Connective Tissue Disorders; Gout; **Hospital:** Montefiore Med Ctr-Einstein Campus (page 100), Jacobi Med Ctr; **Address:** 1575 Blondell Ave, Ste 200, Bronx, NY 10461-2662; **Phone:** 866-633-8255 x4811; **Board Cert:** Internal Medicine 1972; Rheumatology 1972; **Med School:** NYU Sch Med 1964; **Resid:** Internal Medicine, Metro Genl Hosp 1968; **Fellow:** Rheumatology, Albert Einstein Coll Med 1972; **Fac Appt:** Prof Med, Albert Einstein Coll Med

Weinstein, Joshua W MD (Rhu) - **Spec Exp:** Lupus/SLE; Rheumatoid Arthritis; Gout; **Hospital:** Montefiore Med Ctr-Einstein Campus (page 100), NY Hosp Queens (page 488); **Address:** 7235 112 St, Forest Hills, NY 11375; **Phone:** 718-575-0649; **Board Cert:** Internal Medicine 1975; Rheumatology 1978; **Med School:** SUNY Downstate 1972; **Resid:** Internal Medicine, Maimonides Med Ctr 1975; **Fellow:** Rheumatology, Montefiore Med Ctr 1977; **Fac Appt:** Asst Prof Med, Albert Einstein Coll Med

Surgery

Agarwal, Nanakram MD (S) - **Spec Exp:** Breast Surgery; Colon & Rectal Surgery; **Hospital:** Montefiore Med Ctr-Wakefield Campus (page 100); **Address:** 600 E 233rd St, Fl 4, Bronx, NY 10466; **Phone:** 718-920-9143; **Board Cert:** Surgery 2011; Critical Care Medicine 2005; **Med School:** India 1973; **Resid:** Surgery, Our Lady of Mercy Med Ctr 1981; **Fellow:** Critical Care Medicine, Westchester Co Med Ctr 1982; **Fac Appt:** Prof S, NY Med Coll

Bellemare, Sarah MD (S) - **Spec Exp:** Hepatobiliary Surgery; Transplant-Liver; Hepatobiliary Surgery; Laparoscopic Surgery; **Hospital:** Montefiore Med Ctr-Einstein Campus (page 100), Montefiore Med Ctr-Moses Campus (page 100); **Address:** Montefiore Med Ctr - Weiler Div, 111 E 210th St Rosenthal Bldg Fl 2, Bronx, NY 10467; **Phone:** 718-904-2047; **Board Cert:** Surgery 2001; **Med School:** Canada 1996; **Resid:** Surgery, Montreal Univ Med Ctr 2001; **Fellow:** Hepatobiliary Surgery, NY Presby-Columbia Med Ctr 2003; Transplant Surgery, NY Presby-Columbia Med Ctr 2004; **Fac Appt:** Asst Clin Prof S, Albert Einstein Coll Med

Greenstein, Stuart M MD (S) - **Spec Exp:** Laparoscopic Surgery; Dialysis Access Surgery; Transplant-Kidney; **Hospital:** Montefiore Med Ctr-Moses Campus (page 100); **Address:** Montefiore Med Ctr - Dept Surgery, 111 E 210th St, Bronx, NY 10467; **Phone:** 877-287-3536; **Board Cert:** Surgery 2003; **Med School:** Harvard Med Sch 1979; **Resid:** Surgery, UMDNJ, NJ Med Sch Affil Hosp 1984; **Fellow:** Vascular Surgery, Hosp Univ Penn - UPHS 1985; Transplant Surgery, SUNY Downstate Med Ctr 1986; **Fac Appt:** Prof S, Albert Einstein Coll Med

Kennedy, Timothy J MD (S) - **Spec Exp:** Laparoscopic Surgery; Pancreatic Cancer; Stomach Cancer; **Hospital:** Montefiore Med Ctr-Einstein Campus (page 100), Montefiore Med Ctr-Moses Campus (page 100); **Address:** 1575 Blondell Ave Fl 2 - Ste 125, Bronx, NY 10461; **Phone:** 718-405-8240; **Board Cert:** Surgery 2007; **Med School:** Georgetown Univ 1999; **Resid:** Surgery, Northwestern Meml Hosp 2006; **Fellow:** Surgical Oncology, Meml Sloan Kettering Canc Ctr 2007; **Fac Appt:** Asst Prof S, Albert Einstein Coll Med

Kinkhabwala, Milan M MD (S) - **Spec Exp:** Transplant-Liver; Hepatobiliary Surgery; Liver & Biliary Surgery; Liver & Biliary Cancer; **Hospital:** Montefiore Med Ctr-Moses Campus (page 100), Montefiore Med Ctr-Einstein Campus (page 100); **Address:** 111 E 210th St, Bronx, NY 10467; **Phone:** 718-920-6659; **Board Cert:** Surgery 2004; **Med School:** Cornell Univ-Weill Med Coll 1989; **Resid:** Surgery, NY-Presby/Weil Cornell Med Ctr 1994; **Fellow:** Hepatobiliary Surgery, UCLA Med Ctr 1996; **Fac Appt:** Prof S, Albert Einstein Coll Med

Libutti, Steven K MD (S) - **Spec Exp:** Neuroendocrine Tumors; Gastrointestinal Cancer; **Hospital:** Montefiore Med Ctr-Einstein Campus (page 100), Montefiore Med Ctr-Moses Campus (page 100); **Address:** Montefiore-Einstein Ctr for Cancer Care, 1521 Jarret Pl, Bronx, NY 10461; **Phone:** 718-862-8840; **Board Cert:** Surgery 2004; **Med School:** Columbia P&S 1990; **Resid:** Surgery, Columbia Presby Med Ctr 1995; **Fellow:** Surgical Oncology, Natl Cancer Inst 1996; **Fac Appt:** Prof S, Albert Einstein Coll Med

Montgomery, Leslie L MD (S) - **Spec Exp:** Breast Cancer & Surgery; Sentinel Node Surgery; Clinical Trials; **Hospital:** Montefiore Med Ctr-Einstein Campus (page 100); **Address:** Montefiore-Einstein Ctr for Cancer, 1521 Jarret Pl, Bronx, NY 10461; **Phone:** 718-862-8846; **Board Cert:** Surgery 2006; **Med School:** UCSF 1991; **Resid:** Surgery, NY-Presby/Weill Cornell Med Ctr 1996; **Fellow:** Surgical Oncology, Brigham & Womens Hosp; Surgical Oncology, Meml Sloan-Kettering Cancer Ctr

Sas, Norman S MD (S) - **Spec Exp:** Breast Cancer; Laparoscopic Surgery; Hernia; **Hospital:** Montefiore Med Ctr-Moses Campus (page 100), Lawrence Hosp Ctr; **Address:** 3220 Fairfield Ave, Riverdale, NY 10463-3240; **Phone:** 718-549-0700; **Board Cert:** Surgery 2009; **Med School:** NY Med Coll 1974; **Resid:** Surgery, Montefiore Med Ctr 1980; **Fac Appt:** Asst Clin Prof S, Albert Einstein Coll Med

Shamamian, Peter MD (S) - **Spec Exp:** Pancreatic Cancer; **Hospital:** Montefiore Med Ctr-Moses Campus (page 100), Montefiore Med Ctr-Einstein Campus (page 100); **Address:** 3400 Bainbridge St Fl 4, Bronx, NY 10467; **Phone:** 718-920-4089; **Board Cert:** Surgery 2005; **Med School:** UMDNJ-RW Johnson Med Sch 1989; **Resid:** Surgery, NYU Langone Med Ctr 1995; **Fellow:** Surgical Oncology, Natl Inst Hlth 1996; **Fac Appt:** Prof S, Albert Einstein Coll Med

Thoracic & Cardiac Surgery

D'Alessandro, David A MD (T&CS) - **Spec Exp:** Cardiac Surgery; Transplant-Heart; Mechanical Assist Devices; Heart Valve Surgery; **Hospital:** Montefiore Med Ctr-Moses Campus (page 100), Montefiore Med Ctr-Einstein Campus (page 100); **Address:** 3400 Bainbridge Ave MAP Bldg Fl 5, Bronx, NY 10467; **Phone:** 718-920-6515; **Board Cert:** Surgery 2004; Thoracic & Cardiac Surgery 2006; **Med School:** Columbia P&S 1997; **Resid:** Surgery, NY Presby-Columbia Med Ctr 2002; Cardiothoracic Surgery, NY Presby-Columbia Med Ctr 2004; **Fac Appt:** Asst Prof TS, Albert Einstein Coll Med

DeRose Jr, Joseph J MD (T&CS) - **Spec Exp:** Robotic Cardiac Surgery; Aortic Valve Replacement; Mitral Valve Surgery; Minimally Invasive Heart Valve Surgery; **Hospital:** Montefiore Med Ctr-Einstein Campus (page 100), Montefiore Med Ctr-Moses Campus (page 100); **Address:** Montefiore-Weiler Medical Ctr, Dept Cardiothoracic Surgery, 1575 Blondell Ave, Ste 125, Bronx, NY 10461; **Phone:** 718-405-8371; **Board Cert:** Thoracic & Cardiac Surgery 2011; **Med School:** Columbia P&S 1993; **Resid:** Surgery, Columbia Presby Med Ctr 1999; **Fellow:** Cardiothoracic Surgery, Columbia Presby Med Ctr 2001; **Fac Appt:** Assoc Prof TS, Albert Einstein Coll Med

Goldstein, Daniel J MD (T&CS) - **Spec Exp:** Mechanical Assist Devices; Transplant-Heart; Coronary Artery Surgery; Aortic Surgery; **Hospital:** Montefiore Med Ctr-Moses Campus (page 100), Montefiore Med Ctr-Einstein Campus (page 100); **Address:** 3400 Bainbridge Avenue MAP-5, Bronx, NY 10467; **Phone:** 718-920-2144; **Board Cert:** Thoracic Surgery 2010; **Med School:** Mount Sinai Sch Med 1991; **Resid:** Surgery, Columbia Presby Med Ctr 1997; **Fellow:** Cardiothoracic Surgery, Columbia Presby Med Ctr 1999; **Fac Appt:** Prof T&CS, Mount Sinai Sch Med

Keller, Steven M MD (T&CS) - **Spec Exp:** Lung Cancer; Esophageal Cancer; Mediastinal Tumors; Hyperhidrosis-Palmar; **Hospital:** Montefiore Med Ctr-Einstein Campus (page 100); **Address:** Montefiore-Einstein Medical Ctr, 1575 Blondell Ave, Ste 125, Bronx, NY 10461; **Phone:** 718-405-8378; **Board Cert:** Thoracic Surgery 2007; **Med School:** Albany Med Coll 1977; **Resid:** Surgery, Mount Sinai Hosp 1985; Thoracic Surgery, Mem Sloan Kettering Cancer Ctr 1987; **Fellow:** Surgical Oncology, NIH/National Cancer Inst 1983; **Fac Appt:** Prof TS, Albert Einstein Coll Med

Michler, Robert E MD (T&CS) - **Spec Exp:** Heart Valve Surgery; Coronary Artery Surgery; Atrial Fibrillation; Aneurysm-Aortic; **Hospital:** Montefiore Med Ctr-Moses Campus (page 100), Montefiore Med Ctr-Einstein Campus (page 100); **Address:** Montefiore, Dept Cardio/Thoracic Surgery, Green Medical Arts Pavilion, 3400 Bainbridge Ave, Ste 5, New York, NY 10467; **Phone:** 718-920-2100; **Board Cert:** Thoracic & Cardiac Surgery 2010; **Med School:** Dartmouth Med Sch 1981; **Resid:** Surgery, Columbia Presby Med Ctr 1987; **Fellow:** Cardiothoracic Surgery, Columbia Presby Med Ctr 1989; Congenital Heart Surgery, Boston Children's Hosp 1990; **Fac Appt:** Prof T&CS, Albert Einstein Coll Med

Weinstein, Samuel MD (T&CS) - **Spec Exp:** Pediatric Cardiac Surgery; Congenital Heart Disease-Adult; Transplant-Heart; **Hospital:** Montefiore Med Ctr-Moses Campus (page 100), Montefiore Med Ctr-Einstein Campus (page 100); **Address:** Montefiore Med Ctr, Moses Div, Dept Cardiothoracic Surgery, 3400 Bainbridge Ave Fl 5 - Ste 5A, Bronx, NY 10467; **Phone:** 718-920-7745; **Board Cert:** Surgery 2004; Thoracic Surgery 2007; Congenital Cardiac Surgery 2009; **Med School:** SUNY Stony Brook 1989; **Resid:** Surgery, NY-Presby/Columbia Univ Med Ctr 1996; Cardiothoracic Surgery, NY-Presby/Columbia Univ Med Ctr 1998; **Fellow:** Pediatric Cardiothoracic Surgery, Chldns Hosp 1999; **Fac Appt:** Assoc Prof TS, Albert Einstein Coll Med

Urology

Ghavamian, Reza MD (U) - **Spec Exp:** Urologic Cancer; Prostate Cancer/Robotic Surgery; Minimally Invasive Surgery; Kidney Cancer; **Hospital:** Montefiore Med Ctr-Moses Campus (page 100); **Address:** MMC Medical Arts Pavilion, 3400 Bainbridge Ave, Bronx, NY 10467; **Phone:** 718-920-8475; **Board Cert:** Urology 2008; **Med School:** Boston Univ 1991; **Resid:** Urology, Univ Mass Med Ctr 1997; **Fellow:** Urologic Oncology, Mayo Clinic 1998; **Fac Appt:** Clin Prof U, Albert Einstein Coll Med

Stein, Mark MD (U) - **Spec Exp:** Incontinence; Impotence; **Hospital:** Beth Israel Med Ctr - Petrie Div (page 94), NY-Presby/Weill Cornell Med Ctr, NY (page 104); **Address:** 3594 E Tremont Ave, Ste 320, Bronx, NY 10465; **Phone:** 718-518-1108; **Board Cert:** Urology 2011; **Med School:** Yale Univ 1984; **Resid:** Surgery, Montefiore Med Ctr 1985; Urology, Montefiore Med Ctr 1990

Vascular & Interventional Radiology

Cynamon, Jacob MD (VIR) - **Spec Exp:** Peripheral Vascular Disease; Uterine Fibroid Embolization; Liver Cancer; Dialysis Access; **Hospital:** Montefiore Med Ctr-Moses Campus (page 100); **Address:** Montefiore Med Ctr, Dept Interventional Radiology, 111 E 210th St, Bronx, NY 10467; **Phone:** 718-920-5729; **Board Cert:** Diagnostic Radiology 1987; Vascular & Interventional Radiology 2004; **Med School:** Albert Einstein Coll Med 1983; **Resid:** Surgery, Montefiore Med Ctr 1984; Diagnostic Radiology, Montefiore Med Ctr 1987; **Fellow:** Vascular & Interventional Radiology, NY-Presby/Weill Cornell Med Ctr 1988; **Fac Appt:** Clin Prof Rad, Albert Einstein Coll Med

Vascular Surgery

Lipsitz, Evan C MD (VascS) - **Spec Exp:** Aneurysm-Abdominal & Thoracic Aortic; Endovascular Surgery; Limb Sparing Surgery; Carotid Artery Surgery; **Hospital:** Montefiore Med Ctr-Moses Campus (page 100); **Address:** 3400 Bainbridge Ave Fl 4, Bronx, NY 10467; **Phone:** 718-920-2016; **Board Cert:** Vascular Surgery 2008; **Med School:** Columbia P&S 1990; **Resid:** Surgery, NY-Presby/Columbia Univ Med Ctr 1996; **Fellow:** Vascular Surgery, Montefiore Med Ctr 1999; **Fac Appt:** Assoc Prof VascS, Albert Einstein Coll Med

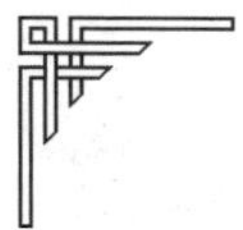

The Best in American Medicine
www.CastleConnolly.com

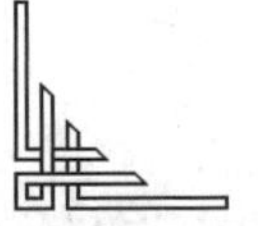
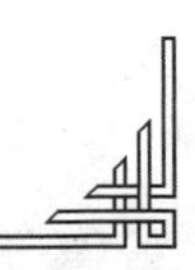

Kings (Brooklyn)

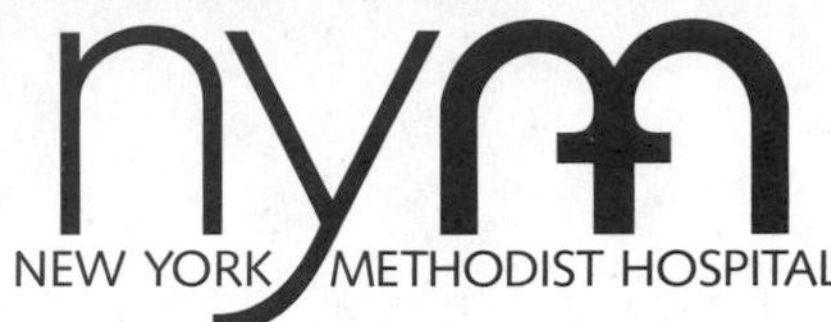

NEW YORK METHODIST HOSPITAL

506 Sixth Street, Brooklyn, N.Y. 11215
Phone (718) 780-3000, Fax (718) 780-3770
http://www.nym.org

Sponsorship	**Voluntary, Not-for-Profit**
Beds	**591; 60 bassinets**
Accreditation	**The Joint Commission, Council on Graduate Medical Education**

GENERAL DESCRIPTION

New York Methodist Hospital (NYM), a member of the NewYork-Presbyterian Healthcare System, has served the neighborhoods of Brooklyn for over 130 years. NYM's medical programs have recently expanded significantly and the Hospital's campus facilities in Park Slope have been extensively renovated. In addition, New York Methodist maintains satellite outpatient health centers throughout Brooklyn.

MEDICAL STAFF

NYM has over 1,000 physicians on staff; 90 percent are board certified or board eligible. Many physicians at NYM are known for the impressive and outstanding work they have done in their individual fields. New York Methodist Hospital offers medical residency programs in internal medicine, surgery, pediatrics, obstetrics/gynecology, radiation oncology, nuclear medicine, anesthesiology, emergency medicine, podiatry and dentistry. The Hospital also offers fellowships in several medical subspecialties.

SPECIAL PROGRAMS

Emergency Medicine: A recently renovated, expanded Emergency Department houses a pediatric emergency room and private rooms for obstetrics/gynecology patients. The Hospital is a State-designated Stroke Center, an AHA Heart Center and EMS 911 Receiving Hospital. 718 780-3148.

Institute for Advanced and Minimally Invasive Surgery: 866 DOCS-14U.

Institute for Asthma and Other Lung Diseases: See Centers of Excellence Section. 866 ASK-LUNG.

Institute for Cancer Care: 866 411-ONCO.

Institute for Cardiology and Cardiac Surgery: See Centers of Excellence Section. 866 84-HEART.

Institute for Diabetes and Other Endocrine Disorders: 866 4-GLAND-2.

Institute for Digestive and Liver Disorders: See Centers of Excellence Section. 866 DIGEST-1.

Institute for Family Care: 866 432-CARE.

Institute for Neurosciences: See Centers of Excellence Section. 866 DO-NEURO.

Institute for Orthopedic Medicine and Surgery: See Centers of Excellence Section. 866 ORTHO-11.

Institute for Vascular Medicine and Surgery: 866 438-VEIN.

Institute for Women's Health: 877 41-WOMAN.

Birthing Center: Spacious, beautifully appointed rooms allow women to experience a "home-like" birth with the reassurance that high-tech medical equipment and specialists are instantly accessible if needed. Full-time lactation services are available for new mothers.

Physician Referral: The Hospital has a free seven-day, 24-hour telephone and computer on-line physician referral service. To find a doctor in any specialty with a convenient office location, area of specialization and insurance and billing policies, call 718 499-CARE or go to http://www.nym.org.

Kings (Brooklyn)

Adolescent Medicine

Birnbaum, Jeffrey MD (AM) - **Spec Exp:** AIDS/HIV in Adolescents; Adolescent Behavior-High Risk; Sexually Transmitted Diseases; **Hospital:** SUNY Downstate Med Ctr (Univ Hosp Brooklyn) (page 441); **Address:** 450 Clarkson Blvd, Brooklyn, NY 11203; **Phone:** 718-282-1199; **Board Cert:** Pediatrics 2013; **Med School:** SUNY Downstate 1986; **Resid:** Pediatrics, SUNY Downstate Med Ctr 1989; **Fac Appt:** Assoc Prof Ped, SUNY Downstate

Hayes, Leslie Allyson MD (AM) - **Spec Exp:** Nutrition; Adolescent Gynecology; **Hospital:** New York Methodist Hosp (page 440); **Address:** 1 Prospect Park W, Brooklyn, NY 11215; **Phone:** 718-636-3960; **Board Cert:** Adolescent Medicine 2012; **Med School:** Mount Sinai Sch Med 1986; **Resid:** Pediatrics, Chldns Hosp Natl Med Ctr 1989; **Fellow:** Adolescent Medicine, Univ Hosp-UMDNJ 1991

Allergy & Immunology

Greeley, Norman H MD (A&I) - **Spec Exp:** Asthma; **Hospital:** Maimonides Med Ctr (page 98), Lenox Hill Hosp (Manh Eye, Ear & Throat Hosp) (page 106); **Address:** 140 Clinton St Fl 1, Brooklyn, NY 11201-4701; **Phone:** 718-624-4465; **Board Cert:** Internal Medicine 1985; Allergy & Immunology 1987; Clinical & Laboratory Immunology 1988; **Med School:** Mexico 1980; **Resid:** Internal Medicine, Long Is Coll Hosp 1985; **Fellow:** Allergy & Immunology, SUNY Downstate Med Ctr 1987

Klein, Norman MD (A&I) - **Spec Exp:** Asthma; Food Allergy; Hay Fever; Immune Deficiency; **Hospital:** Brookdale Univ Hosp Med Ctr, Brooklyn Hosp Ctr; **Address:** 1648 E 14th St, Ste 5, Brooklyn, NY 11229; **Phone:** 718-627-0183; **Board Cert:** Pediatrics 1981; Allergy & Immunology 1983; **Med School:** SUNY Downstate 1976; **Resid:** Pediatrics, Brookdale Univ Hosp 1979; **Fellow:** Allergy & Immunology, Montefiore Med Ctr 1980; **Fac Appt:** Asst Prof Ped, SUNY Downstate

Rao, Yalamanchi K MD (A&I) - **Spec Exp:** Pediatric Allergy & Immunology; **Hospital:** New York Methodist Hosp (page 440); **Address:** Allergy & Asthma Med Care Ctr, 565 Bay Ridge Pkwy, Brooklyn, NY 11209; **Phone:** 718-748-7551; **Board Cert:** Pediatrics 1978; Allergy & Immunology 1989; **Med School:** India 1968; **Resid:** Pediatrics, LI Coll Hosp 1977; Allergy & Immunology, LI Coll Hosp 1979

Silverman, Bernard A MD (A&I) - **Spec Exp:** Eczema; Food Allergy; Urticaria; Atopic Dermatitis; **Hospital:** Mt Sinai Med Ctr (page 102); **Address:** 2044 Ocean Ave, Ste A7, Brooklyn, NY 11230; **Phone:** 718-998-5556; **Board Cert:** Pediatrics 1984; Allergy & Immunology 1985; **Med School:** Wayne State Univ 1979; **Resid:** Pediatrics, Brookdale Univ Hosp Med Ctr 1982; **Fellow:** Allergy & Immunology, Montefiore Med Ctr 1984; **Fac Appt:** Asst Clin Prof Ped, Mount Sinai Sch Med

Cardiac Electrophysiology

Kassotis, John MD (CE) - **Spec Exp:** Arrhythmias; Atrial Fibrillation; Ventricular Tachycardia Ablation; Congenital Heart Disease; **Hospital:** SUNY Downstate Med Ctr (Univ Hosp Brooklyn) (page 441); **Address:** 450 Clarkson Ave, Box 1199, Brooklyn, NY 11203; **Phone:** 718-270-4147; **Board Cert:** Internal Medicine 2007; Cardiovascular Disease 2008; Cardiac Electrophysiology 2009; **Med School:** Columbia P&S 1990; **Resid:** Internal Medicine, Columbia-Presby Med Ctr 1993; **Fellow:** Cardiovascular Disease, Columbia-Presby Med Ctr 1996; Cardiac Electrophysiology, Columbia-Presby Med Ctr 1997; **Fac Appt:** Assoc Prof Med, SUNY Downstate

Turitto, Gioia MD (CE) - **Spec Exp:** Pacemakers; Defibrillators; Arrhythmias; **Hospital:** New York Methodist Hosp (page 440); **Address:** NY Methodist Hosp, Div Cardiology, 506 Sixth St, Fl 2, Brooklyn, NY 11215; **Phone:** 718-780-3626; **Board Cert:** Internal Medicine 2013; Cardiovascular Disease 2003; Cardiac Electrophysiology 2004; **Med School:** Italy 1981; **Resid:** Internal Medicine, SUNY Downstate Med Ctr 1992; **Fellow:** Cardiovascular Disease, SUNY Downstate Med Ctr 1987; **Fac Appt:** Assoc Prof Med, SUNY Downstate

Wilbur, Sabrina L MD (CE) - **Spec Exp:** Arrhythmias; Pacemakers/Defibrillators; **Hospital:** New York Methodist Hosp (page 440), Beth Israel Med Ctr - Petrie Div (page 94); **Address:** 185 Montague St Fl 3, Brooklyn, NY 11201; **Phone:** 718-855-7223; **Board Cert:** Cardiovascular Disease 2005; Cardiac Electrophysiology 2009; **Med School:** Dominican Republic 1987; **Resid:** Internal Medicine, Episcopal Hosp 1991; **Fellow:** Cardiovascular Disease, Episcopal Hosp 1994; Cardiac Electrophysiology, Hosp Univ Penn 1995

Cardiovascular Disease

Borer, Jeffrey S MD (Cv) - **Spec Exp:** Heart Valve Disease; Heart Failure; Nuclear Cardiology; Coronary Artery Disease; **Hospital:** SUNY Downstate Med Ctr (Univ Hosp Brooklyn) (page 441), NY-Presby/Weill Cornell Med Ctr, NY (page 104); **Address:** SUNY Downstate Med Ctr, Div Cardiology, Howard Gilman Institute, 635 Madison Ave Fl 3, New York, NY 10022; **Phone:** 212-289-7777; **Board Cert:** Internal Medicine 1973; Cardiovascular Disease 1975; **Med School:** Cornell Univ-Weill Med Coll 1969; **Resid:** Internal Medicine, Mass Genl Hosp 1971; **Fellow:** Cardiovascular Disease, Natl Heart, Lung & Blood Inst 1974; Cardiovascular Disease, Guy's Hosp 1975; **Fac Appt:** Prof Med, SUNY Downstate

Charnoff, Judah A MD (Cv) - **Spec Exp:** Coronary Artery Disease; Congestive Heart Failure; Cholesterol/Lipid Disorders; **Hospital:** NS-LIJ Hlth Sys (page 106), Lenox Hill Hosp (page 106); **Address:** NSLIJ Med Grp, Heart Surgeons, 1262 Ocean Pkwy, Brooklyn, NY 11230; **Phone:** 718-859-5843; **Board Cert:** Internal Medicine 1987; Cardiovascular Disease 2005; **Med School:** NYU Sch Med 1984; **Resid:** Internal Medicine, Brookdale Hosp 1987; **Fellow:** Cardiovascular Disease, Maimonides Med Ctr 1989; **Fac Appt:** Asst Prof Med, SUNY Downstate

Dilmanian, Hajir E MD (Cv) - **Spec Exp:** Echocardiography; Diagnostic Problems; **Hospital:** New York Methodist Hosp (page 440); **Address:** NY Methodist Hosp, Cardiology Dept, 506 6th St Fl 2, Brooklyn, NY 11215; **Phone:** 718-780-7830; **Board Cert:** Internal Medicine 2004; Cardiovascular Disease 2007; **Med School:** SUNY Downstate 2001; **Resid:** Internal Medicine, NYU Med Ctr 2004; **Fellow:** Cardiovascular Disease, Westchester Med Ctr 2007

Feit, Alan MD (Cv) - **Spec Exp:** Interventional Cardiology; **Hospital:** SUNY Downstate Med Ctr (Univ Hosp Brooklyn) (page 441); **Address:** SUNY, Dept Cardiology, 450 Clarkson Ave, Box 1199, Brooklyn, NY 11203-2012; **Phone:** 718-270-2631; **Board Cert:** Internal Medicine 1978; Cardiovascular Disease 1981; Interventional Cardiology 2009; **Med School:** Columbia P&S 1975; **Resid:** Internal Medicine, Roosevelt Hosp Ctr 1978; **Fellow:** Cardiovascular Disease, Roosevelt Hosp Ctr 1980

Gelbfish, Joseph S MD (Cv) - **Spec Exp:** Preventive Cardiology; Heart Valve Disease; **Hospital:** New York Methodist Hosp (page 440), NY-Presby/Columbia Univ Med Ctr, NY (page 104); **Address:** 2500 Avenue I, Brooklyn, NY 11210; **Phone:** 718-951-0100; **Board Cert:** Internal Medicine 1986; Cardiovascular Disease 1989; **Med School:** NYU Sch Med 1980; **Resid:** Surgery, Maimonides Med Ctr 1984; Internal Medicine, Maimonides Med Ctr 1985; **Fellow:** Cardiovascular Disease, Maimonides Med Ctr 1988; Cardiovascular Disease, Beth Israel Deaconess Med Ctr 1989

Gelles, Jeremiah MD (Cv) - **Spec Exp:** Heart Failure; Hypertension; Arrhythmias; Preventive Cardiology; **Hospital:** New York Methodist Hosp (page 440), Maimonides Med Ctr (page 98); **Address:** 263 7th Ave, Bldg 7186364699, Ste 5H, jeremiah41@mindspring.com, 263 7TH AVE APT 5H, Brooklyn, NY 11215-3690; **Phone:** 718-832-1818; **Board Cert:** Internal Medicine 1972; Cardiovascular Disease 1975; **Med School:** NYU Sch Med 1966; **Resid:** Internal Medicine, Mount Sinai Hosp 1970; Internal Medicine, Montefiore Med Ctr 1969; **Fellow:** Cardiovascular Disease, Mount Sinai Hosp 1971; Cardiac Electrophysiology, Columbia Presby Med Ctr 1973; **Fac Appt:** Asst Clin Prof Med, Cornell Univ-Weill Med Coll

Greengart, Alvin MD (Cv) - **Spec Exp:** Echocardiography; Non-Invasive Cardiology; **Hospital:** Maimonides Med Ctr (page 98); **Address:** Cardiology Assocs, 4802 10th Ave Fl 4, Brooklyn, NY 11219; **Phone:** 718-283-6473; **Board Cert:** Internal Medicine 1977; Cardiovascular Disease 1979; **Med School:** Mount Sinai Sch Med 1974; **Resid:** Internal Medicine, Brookdale Med Ctr 1977; **Fellow:** Cardiovascular Disease, Brookdale Med Ctr 1979

Gupta, Prem MD (Cv) - **Spec Exp:** Heart Valve Disease; Congestive Heart Failure; Atrial Fibrillation; **Hospital:** Maimonides Med Ctr (page 98); **Address:** 4709 Fort Hamilton Pkwy, Brooklyn, NY 11219-2927; **Phone:** 718-633-4244; **Board Cert:** Internal Medicine 1971; Cardiovascular Disease 1973; **Med School:** India 1964; **Resid:** Internal Medicine, VA Med Ctr 1968; Internal Medicine, VA Med Ctr 1969; **Fellow:** Cardiovascular Disease, VA Med Ctr 1971; **Fac Appt:** Clin Prof Med, SUNY Downstate

Hanley, Gerard MD (Cv) - **Hospital:** Beth Israel Med Ctr- Kings Hwy Div (page 94); **Address:** 3131 Kings Hwy, Ste B1, Brooklyn, NY 11234; **Phone:** 718-421-1212; **Board Cert:** Internal Medicine 1989; **Med School:** SUNY Stony Brook 1984; **Resid:** Internal Medicine, SUNY Hlth Sci Ctr 1987; **Fellow:** Cardiovascular Disease, SUNY Hlth Sci Ctr 1990; Cardiovascular Disease, Westchester Med Ctr 1991

Heitner, John F MD (Cv) - **Spec Exp:** Nuclear Cardiology; Cardiac MRI; **Hospital:** New York Methodist Hosp (page 440); **Address:** Div Cardiology, 506 Sixth St, Brooklyn, NY 11215; **Phone:** 718-780-5037; **Board Cert:** Cardiovascular Disease 2004; **Med School:** Albert Einstein Coll Med 1997; **Resid:** Internal Medicine, Duke Univ Hosps 2000; **Fellow:** Cardiovascular Disease, Emory Univ Hosp 2002; Cardiovascular Disease, Duke Univ Hosps 2004

Hollander, Gerald MD (Cv) - **Spec Exp:** Coronary Artery Disease; Heart Failure; Echocardiography; **Hospital:** Maimonides Med Ctr (page 98); **Address:** Cardiology Assocs, 4802 10th Ave Fl 4, Brooklyn, NY 11219; **Phone:** 718-283-7643; **Board Cert:** Internal Medicine 1976; Cardiovascular Disease 1979; **Med School:** SUNY Downstate 1973; **Resid:** Internal Medicine, Brookdale Hosp 1976; **Fellow:** Cardiovascular Disease, Brookdale Hosp 1978; **Fac Appt:** Clin Prof Med, SUNY Hlth Sci Ctr

Kang, Pritpal S MD (Cv) - **Spec Exp:** Nuclear Cardiology; **Hospital:** Lutheran Med Ctr - Brooklyn; **Address:** 705 86th St, Ste M3, Brooklyn, NY 11228; **Phone:** 718-836-0600; **Board Cert:** Internal Medicine 1979; Cardiovascular Disease 1981; **Med School:** India 1972; **Resid:** Internal Medicine, Methodist Hosp 1978; **Fellow:** Cardiovascular Disease, VA Med Ctr 1980

Kerstein, Joshua MD (Cv) - **Spec Exp:** Atrial Fibrillation; Coronary Artery Disease; Brugada Syndrome; Long QT Syndrome; **Hospital:** Maimonides Med Ctr (page 98); **Address:** Maimonides Med Ctr, Cardiology Assocs, 4802 10th Ave Fl 4, Brooklyn, NY 11219; **Phone:** 718-283-8614; **Board Cert:** Cardiovascular Disease 2005; Nuclear Cardiology 2002; **Med School:** SUNY Downstate 1989; **Resid:** Internal Medicine, Maimonides Med Ctr 1992; **Fellow:** Cardiovascular Disease, Maimonides Med Ctr 1995; **Fac Appt:** Asst Prof Med, SUNY Downstate

Kleeman, Harris J MD (Cv) - **Spec Exp:** Hypertension; Coronary Artery Disease; **Hospital:** Maimonides Med Ctr (page 98); **Address:** 1660 E 14th St, Brooklyn, NY 11229; **Phone:** 718-375-6969; **Board Cert:** Internal Medicine 1982; Cardiovascular Disease 1985; **Med School:** SUNY Downstate 1979; **Resid:** Internal Medicine, Staten Island Univ Hosp 1983; **Fellow:** Cardiovascular Disease, Maimonides Med Ctr 1985

Konka, Sudarsanam MD (Cv) - **Hospital:** New York Methodist Hosp (page 440); **Address:** 100 Clinton St, Ste 20, Brooklyn, NY 11201; **Phone:** 718-935-9837; **Board Cert:** Internal Medicine 1974; Cardiovascular Disease 1977; **Med School:** India 1970; **Resid:** Internal Medicine, Long Is Coll Hosp 1974; **Fellow:** Cardiovascular Disease, Nassau Univ Med Ctr 1975; Cardiovascular Disease, Long Is Coll Hosp 1976

Moskovits, Norbert MD (Cv) - **Spec Exp:** Heart Failure; Coronary Artery Disease; Preventive Cardiology; Cholesterol/Lipid Disorders; **Hospital:** Maimonides Med Ctr (page 98); **Address:** Maimonides Med Ctr, Div Cardiology, 4802 10 Ave, Fl 4, Brooklyn, NY 11219; **Phone:** 718-283-7948; **Board Cert:** Advanced Heart Failure & Transplant Cardiology 2012; Cardiovascular Disease 2005; **Med School:** Germany 1986; **Resid:** Internal Medicine, Maimonides Med Ctr 1992; **Fellow:** Cardiovascular Disease, Beth Israel Med Ctr 1995; **Fac Appt:** Asst Prof Med, Albert Einstein Coll Med

Paiusco, Augusto Dino MD (Cv) - **Spec Exp:** Preventive Cardiology; **Hospital:** Beth Israel Med Ctr- Kings Hwy Div (page 94); **Address:** Univ Heart Assocs, 3131 Kings Hwy, Ste A7, Brooklyn, NY 11234; **Phone:** 718-998-2323; **Board Cert:** Internal Medicine 1989; **Med School:** Mexico 1984; **Resid:** Internal Medicine, SUNY Hlth Sci Ctr 1989; **Fellow:** Cardiovascular Disease, SUNY Hlth Sci Ctr 1992

Prabhu, H Sudhakar MD (Cv) - **Spec Exp:** Echocardiography; Nuclear Cardiology; **Hospital:** Lutheran Med Ctr - Brooklyn; **Address:** 699 92nd St, Brooklyn, NY 11228; **Phone:** 718-833-2620; **Board Cert:** Internal Medicine 1978; Cardiovascular Disease 1981; Nuclear Cardiology 2006; Echocardiography 2008; **Med School:** India 1971; **Resid:** Internal Medicine, LI Coll Hosp 1976; **Fellow:** Cardiovascular Disease, LI Coll Hosp 1978; **Fac Appt:** Asst Prof Med, SUNY Downstate

Qadir, Shuja MD (Cv) - **Spec Exp:** Heart Failure; Arrhythmias; Coronary Artery Disease; **Hospital:** NY Hosp Queens (page 488), N Shore Univ Hosp (page 106); **Address:** 934 Manhattan Ave, Brooklyn, NY 11222; **Phone:** 718-275-6061; **Board Cert:** Internal Medicine 1984; Cardiovascular Disease 1987; **Med School:** Pakistan 1977; **Resid:** Internal Medicine, Catholic Med Ctr 1985; **Fellow:** Cardiovascular Disease, Catholic Med Ctr 1987; **Fac Appt:** Asst Prof Med, NY Med Coll

Traube, Charles MD (Cv) - **Spec Exp:** Cholesterol/Lipid Disorders; Hypertension; **Hospital:** Beth Israel Med Ctr- Kings Hwy Div (page 94); **Address:** 2270 Kimball St, Ste 101, Brooklyn, NY 11234; **Phone:** 718-692-2700; **Board Cert:** Internal Medicine 1978; Cardiovascular Disease 1981; **Med School:** Albert Einstein Coll Med 1975; **Resid:** Internal Medicine, Brookdale Univ Hosp Med Ctr 1978; **Fellow:** Cardiovascular Disease, Brookdale Univ Hosp Med Ctr 1980; **Fac Appt:** Asst Clin Prof Med, Albert Einstein Coll Med

Wein, Paul K MD (Cv) - **Spec Exp:** Preventive Cardiology; Hypertension; Cholesterol/Lipid Disorders; Coronary Artery Disease; **Hospital:** Beth Israel Med Ctr- Kings Hwy Div (page 94), Long Is Jewish Med Ctr (page 106); **Address:** BIMC, Cardiology Dept, 3131 Kings Hwy, Ste D6, Brooklyn, NY 11234; **Phone:** 718-338-2283; **Board Cert:** Internal Medicine 1979; Cardiovascular Disease 1983; **Med School:** SUNY Downstate 1976; **Resid:** Internal Medicine, Norwalk Hosp 1979; **Fellow:** Cardiovascular Disease, LI Jewish Med Ctr 1981

Zaloom, Robert MD (Cv) - **Spec Exp:** Cardiac Catheterization; Angiography-Coronary; Nutrition; Cardiac Stress Testing; **Hospital:** Lutheran Med Ctr - Brooklyn, Lenox Hill Hosp (page 106); **Address:** Bay Ridge Hearts, 217 Ovington Ave, Brooklyn, NY 11209; **Phone:** 718-238-0098; **Board Cert:** Internal Medicine 1986; Cardiovascular Disease 1989; **Med School:** France 1983; **Resid:** Internal Medicine, Lutheran Med Ctr 1986; **Fellow:** Cardiovascular Disease, SUNY Downstate Med Ctr 1988; **Fac Appt:** Asst Prof Med, Mount Sinai Sch Med

Child & Adolescent Psychiatry

Engel, Lenore MD (ChAP) - **Hospital:** Kings Co Hosp Ctr, SUNY Downstate Med Ctr (Univ Hosp Brooklyn) (page 441); **Address:** 115 Henry St, Ste 1G, Brooklyn, NY 11201-2562; **Phone:** 718-855-8911; **Board Cert:** Psychiatry 1983; Child & Adolescent Psychiatry 1985; Forensic Psychiatry 2008; **Med School:** SUNY Downstate 1978; **Resid:** Psychiatry, Kings Co Hosp 1982; **Fellow:** Child & Adolescent Psychiatry, SUNY Downstate 1984; **Fac Appt:** Asst Clin Prof Psyc, SUNY Downstate

Holzer, Barry D MD (ChAP) - **Spec Exp:** ADD/ADHD; Behavioral Disorders; Bipolar/Mood Disorders; **Address:** 2350 Ocean Ave, Ste 2J, Brooklyn, NY 11229; **Phone:** 718-743-7600; **Board Cert:** Psychiatry 1990; **Med School:** Albert Einstein Coll Med 1984; **Resid:** Psychiatry, Hillside Hosp-LIJ 1988; **Fellow:** Child & Adolescent Psychiatry, Schneider Chldns Hosp-LIJ 1990

Child Neurology

Cracco, Joan B MD (ChiN) - **Spec Exp:** Spina Bifida; Epilepsy; Neurophysiology; **Hospital:** SUNY Downstate Med Ctr (Univ Hosp Brooklyn) (page 441), Kings Co Hosp Ctr; **Address:** SUNY Downstate Med Ctr, 450 Clarkson Ave, Box 118, Brooklyn, NY 11203-2056; **Phone:** 718-270-2042; **Board Cert:** Pediatrics 1968; Neurology 1972; Clinical Neurophysiology 2011; **Med School:** UMDNJ-NJ Med Sch, Newark 1963; **Resid:** Pediatrics, Mayo Clinic 1966; Neurology, Thomas Jefferson Univ Hosp 1969

Pavlakis, Steven G MD (ChiN) - **Spec Exp:** Cerebrovascular Disease-Pediatric; Stroke; ADD/ADHD; Neurogenetics; **Hospital:** Maimonides Med Ctr (page 98), Mt Sinai Med Ctr (page 102); **Address:** Pediatric Faculty Practice- Neurology, 977 48th St, Brooklyn, NY 11219; **Phone:** 718-283-8260; **Board Cert:** Pediatrics 1985; Child Neurology 1987; Neurodevelopmental Disabilities 2011; **Med School:** Brown Univ 1979; **Resid:** Pediatrics, Columbia-Presby Med Ctr 1981; **Fellow:** Pediatric Neurology, Columbia-Presby Med Ctr 1984; **Fac Appt:** Prof N, Mount Sinai Sch Med

Schubert, Romaine MD (ChiN) - **Spec Exp:** Epilepsy/Seizure Disorders; Developmental Disorders; Tourette's Syndrome; **Hospital:** New York Methodist Hosp (page 440); **Address:** 263 7th Ave, Ste 4A, Brooklyn, NY 11215; **Phone:** 718-246-8590; **Board Cert:** Child Neurology 1991; Clinical Neurophysiology 2010; Neurodevelopmental Disabilities 2012; **Med School:** Germany 1984; **Resid:** Pediatrics, SUNY Downstate/Kings Co Med Ctr 1987; **Fellow:** Child Neurology, SUNY Downstate/Kings Co Med Ctr 1990; **Fac Appt:** Asst Clin Prof Ped, Cornell Univ-Weill Med Coll

Clinical Genetics

Gilbert, Fred MD (CG) - **Spec Exp:** Cancer Genetics; Dysmorphology; **Hospital:** NY-Presby/Weill Cornell Med Ctr, NY (page 104), Brooklyn Hosp Ctr; **Address:** Pediatric Genetics, 240 Willoughby St, Ste 9K, Brooklyn, NY 11201; **Phone:** 718-250-6227; **Board Cert:** Clinical Genetics 1982; Clinical Cytogenetics 1982; **Med School:** Albert Einstein Coll Med 1966; **Resid:** Internal Medicine, Barnes Hosp 1968; Internal Medicine, Natl Inst Hlth 1971; **Fellow:** Clinical Genetics, Yale-New Haven Hosp 1974; **Fac Appt:** Assoc Prof Ped, Cornell Univ-Weill Med Coll

Colon & Rectal Surgery

Asarian, Armand P MD (CRS) - **Spec Exp:** Colon Cancer; Breast Cancer; **Hospital:** Brooklyn Hosp Ctr; **Address:** Brooklyn Hosp Ctr, 121 DeKalb Ave, Dept Surg, Brooklyn, NY 11201; **Phone:** 718-250-6088; **Board Cert:** Surgery 2005; Colon & Rectal Surgery 2009; **Med School:** SUNY Downstate 1991; **Resid:** Surgery, Brooklyn Hosp Ctr 1996; **Fellow:** Colon & Rectal Surgery, Baylor Univ Med Ctr 1997; **Fac Appt:** Asst Clin Prof S, Cornell Univ-Weill Med Coll

Fleischer, Marian MD (CRS) - **Spec Exp:** Colonoscopy; Colon & Rectal Cancer; Pelvic & Perineal Surgery; Pelvic Organ Prolapse Repair; **Hospital:** Maimonides Med Ctr (page 98), New York Methodist Hosp (page 440); **Address:** 9707 4 Ave, Brooklyn, NY 11209-8129; **Phone:** 718-836-3603; **Board Cert:** Colon & Rectal Surgery 1984; **Med School:** Italy 1972; **Resid:** Surgery, Maimonides Med Ctr 1981; Colon & Rectal Surgery, Baltimore Med Ctr 1982

Dermatology

Baldwin, Hilary MD (D) - **Spec Exp:** Acne & Rosacea; Cosmetic Dermatology; **Address:** 142 Joralemon St, Ste 3A, Brooklyn, NY 11201; **Phone:** 718-797-3340; **Board Cert:** Dermatology 1988; **Med School:** Boston Univ 1984; **Resid:** Dermatology, NYU Med Ctr 1988; **Fac Appt:** Assoc Prof D, SUNY Downstate

Berry, Richard MD (D) - **Spec Exp:** Skin Cancer; Laser Hair Removal; Botox Therapy; **Address:** 2820 Ocean Pkwy, Brooklyn, NY 11235-7958; **Phone:** 718-996-3000; **Board Cert:** Dermatology 1978; **Med School:** SUNY Hlth Sci Ctr 1974; **Resid:** Dermatology, SUNY Downstate Med Ctr 1978; **Fac Appt:** Asst Clin Prof D, SUNY Hlth Sci Ctr

Biro, David MD/PhD (D) - **Spec Exp:** Mohs' Surgery; Skin Laser Surgery; Cosmetic Dermatology; **Hospital:** SUNY Downstate Med Ctr (Univ Hosp Brooklyn) (page 441); **Address:** 9921 4th Ave, Fl 1, Brooklyn, NY 11209-8347; **Phone:** 718-833-7616; **Board Cert:** Dermatology 2013; **Med School:** Columbia P&S 1991; **Resid:** Dermatology, SUNY Hlth Sci Ctr 1995; **Fac Appt:** Asst Clin Prof D, SUNY Hlth Sci Ctr

Brancaccio, Ronald R MD (D) - **Spec Exp:** Contact Dermatitis; Skin Laser Surgery; Cosmetic Dermatology; **Hospital:** NYU Langone Med Ctr (page 108); **Address:** Skin Inst NY, 7901 Fourth Ave, Brooklyn, NY 11209-3957; **Phone:** 718-491-5800; **Board Cert:** Dermatology 1977; **Med School:** Geo Wash Univ 1972; **Resid:** Dermatology, Univ Oregon Hlth Sci Ctr 1976; **Fellow:** Tropical Medicine, Univ Sao Paulo 1976; **Fac Appt:** Clin Prof D, NYU Sch Med

Danziger, Stephen MD (D) - **Spec Exp:** Skin Cancer & Moles; Acne & Rosacea; Psoriasis/Eczema; Warts; **Hospital:** New York Methodist Hosp (page 440); **Address:** 20 Plaza St E, Ste A17, Brooklyn, NY 11238; **Phone:** 718-638-3640; **Board Cert:** Dermatology 1975; **Med School:** SUNY Downstate 1968; **Resid:** Internal Medicine, St Luke's - Roosevelt Hosp Ctr 1969; Dermatology, SUNY Downstate Med Ctr/Kings County Med Ctr 1974; **Fac Appt:** Asst Clin Prof D, SUNY Downstate

Deitz, Marcia MD (D) - **Spec Exp:** Acne; Psoriasis; Warts; Eczema; **Hospital:** Coney Island Hosp; **Address:** 1486 Ocean Pkwy, Brooklyn, NY 11230-6453; **Phone:** 718-627-3024; **Board Cert:** Dermatology 1984; **Med School:** SUNY Downstate 1980; **Resid:** Internal Medicine, Brookdale Hosp 1981; Dermatology, NY Med Coll Affil Hosps 1984; **Fac Appt:** Asst Clin Prof Med, NY Coll Osteo Med

Feldman, Philip MD (D) - **Spec Exp:** Acne; Eczema; Psoriasis; **Hospital:** Brooklyn Hosp Ctr; **Address:** 142 Joralemon St, Ste 4B, Brooklyn, NY 11201-4709; **Phone:** 718-237-0404; **Board Cert:** Dermatology 1970; **Med School:** Switzerland 1963; **Resid:** Dermatology, NY Presby Hosp 1967; **Fac Appt:** Asst Clin Prof D, SUNY Downstate

Frankel, David H MD (D) - **Spec Exp:** Skin Cancer; Eczema; Contact Dermatitis; **Hospital:** New York Methodist Hosp (page 440), Maimonides Med Ctr (page 98); **Address:** 263 7th Ave, Ste 5F, Brooklyn, NY 11215; **Phone:** 718-369-3559; **Board Cert:** Internal Medicine 1985; Dermatology 2004; **Med School:** Boston Univ 1982; **Resid:** Internal Medicine, Univ Chicago Hosps 1985; Dermatology, Univ Chicago Hosps 1988; **Fellow:** Mohs Surgery, Amer Coll Mohs Micro Surg 1989; **Fac Appt:** Asst Clin Prof D, Mount Sinai Sch Med

Glick, Sharon A MD (D) - **Spec Exp:** Pediatric Dermatology; **Hospital:** SUNY Downstate Med Ctr (Univ Hosp Brooklyn) (page 441), Kings Co Hosp Ctr; **Address:** SUNY Downstate Med Ctr, Dept Dermatology, 450 Clarkson Ave, Box 46, Brooklyn, NY 11203; **Phone:** 718-270-1230; **Board Cert:** Dermatology 2013; Pediatric Dermatology 2004; **Med School:** Albert Einstein Coll Med 1988; **Resid:** Pediatrics, Yale-New Haven Hosp 1991; Dermatology, Yale-New Haven Hosp 1994; **Fac Appt:** Assoc Prof D, SUNY Downstate

Shapiro, Michael D MD (D) - **Spec Exp:** Mohs' Surgery; Cosmetic Dermatology; Skin Cancer; **Address:** Vanguard Dermatology, 2408 Ocean Ave, Brooklyn, NY 11229; **Phone:** 718-332-2999; **Board Cert:** Dermatology ; **Med School:** Univ Pennsylvania 1999; **Resid:** Dermatology, Hosp Univ Penn-UPHS 2004; **Fellow:** Mohs Surgery, Univ CO Hlth Science Ctr 2005

Simon, Steven I MD (D) - **Spec Exp:** Skin Cancer; Botox Therapy; Laser Hair Removal; **Hospital:** SUNY Downstate Med Ctr (Univ Hosp Brooklyn) (page 441), Franklin Hosp (page 106); **Address:** 2270 Kimball St, Brooklyn, NY 11234-5139; **Phone:** 718-253-4550; **Board Cert:** Dermatology 1981; **Med School:** Mexico 1975; **Resid:** Internal Medicine, Brookdale Hosp 1978; Dermatology, Downstate Med Ctr 1981; **Fac Appt:** Assoc Clin Prof D, SUNY Hlth Sci Ctr

Diagnostic Radiology

Amodio, John B MD (DR) - **Spec Exp:** Pediatric Radiology; **Hospital:** Kings Co Hosp Ctr, SUNY Downstate Med Ctr (Univ Hosp Brooklyn) (page 441); **Address:** SUNY Downstate Med Ctr, Dept Radiology, 450 Clarkson Ave, Box 1198, Brooklyn, NY 11203; **Phone:** 718-270-1603; **Board Cert:** Diagnostic Radiology 1984; Pediatric Radiology 2005; **Med School:** NY Med Coll 1980; **Resid:** Diagnostic Radiology, Montefiore Med Ctr 1984; **Fellow:** Pediatric Radiology, Columbia-Presby Med Ctr 1985

Garner, Steven Charles MD (DR) - **Spec Exp:** Trauma Radiology; **Hospital:** New York Methodist Hosp (page 440); **Address:** 506 6th St, Brooklyn, NY 11215; **Phone:** 718-780-5870; **Board Cert:** Diagnostic Radiology 1984; **Med School:** Ros Franklin Univ/Chicago Med Sch 1976; **Resid:** Diagnostic Radiology, Mt Sinai Hosp 1983

Lerman, Jay E MD (DR) - **Spec Exp:** Urologic Imaging; Musculoskeletal Imaging; **Address:** Lerman Diagnostic Imaging, 6511 Fort Hamilton Pkwy, Brooklyn, NY 11219; **Phone:** 718-491-4545; **Board Cert:** Diagnostic Radiology 1991; **Med School:** Albert Einstein Coll Med 1986; **Resid:** Diagnostic Radiology, Montefiore Med Ctr 1991; **Fellow:** Cross Sectional Imaging, Thom Jefferson Hosp 1992

Endocrinology, Diabetes & Metabolism

Brickman, Alan M MD (EDM) - **Spec Exp:** Diabetes; Thyroid Disorders; Cholesterol/Lipid Disorders; Calcium Disorders; **Hospital:** Maimonides Med Ctr (page 98); **Address:** 1318 52nd St, Brooklyn, NY 11219-3802; **Phone:** 718-436-9898; **Board Cert:** Internal Medicine 1979; Endocrinology, Diabetes & Metabolism 1981; **Med School:** Albert Einstein Coll Med 1976; **Resid:** Internal Medicine, Maimonides Med Ctr 1979; **Fellow:** Endocrinology, Diabetes & Metabolism, Yale-New Haven Hosp 1981

Giegerich, Edmund W MD (EDM) - **Spec Exp:** Thyroid Disorders; Diabetes; **Hospital:** New York Methodist Hosp (page 440); **Address:** 263 7th Ave, Ste 5A, Brooklyn, NY 11215; **Phone:** 718-246-8600; **Board Cert:** Internal Medicine 1980; Endocrinology, Diabetes & Metabolism 1983; **Med School:** SUNY Downstate 1977; **Resid:** Internal Medicine, Rhode Island Hosp 1980; **Fellow:** Endocrinology, Diabetes & Metabolism, Mount Sinai Hosp 1982; **Fac Appt:** Assoc Clin Prof Med, SUNY Hlth Sci Ctr

Goldman, Joel M MD (EDM) - **Spec Exp:** Thyroid Disorders; Diabetes; Calcium Disorders; **Hospital:** Brookdale Univ Hosp Med Ctr, Beth Israel Med Ctr- Kings Hwy Div (page 94); **Address:** 1 Brookdale Plaza, rm 101A-SBSI, Brooklyn, NY 11212-3132; **Phone:** 718-240-5378; **Board Cert:** Internal Medicine 1976; Endocrinology, Diabetes & Metabolism 1979; **Med School:** Univ Ariz Coll Med 1973; **Resid:** Internal Medicine, UMDNJ-Newark Affil Hosps 1975; Internal Medicine, Albert Einstein Coll Med 1976; **Fellow:** Endocrinology, Diabetes & Metabolism, NIAMDD-Natl Inst Hlth 1979; **Fac Appt:** Assoc Prof Med, SUNY Downstate

Resta, Christine MD (EDM) - **Spec Exp:** Diabetes; Thyroid Disorders; Osteoporosis; **Hospital:** Maimonides Med Ctr (page 98); **Address:** 984 50th St, Brooklyn, NY 11219; **Phone:** 718-283-5923; **Board Cert:** Internal Medicine 2012; Endocrinology, Diabetes & Metabolism 2005; **Med School:** Albert Einstein Coll Med 1989; **Resid:** Internal Medicine, Montefiore Med Ctr 1992; **Fellow:** Endocrinology, Diabetes & Metabolism, Montefiore Med Ctr 1994

Silverberg, Arnold MD (EDM) - **Spec Exp:** Thyroid Disorders; Osteoporosis; Diabetes; **Hospital:** Maimonides Med Ctr (page 98); **Address:** 908 48th St, Fl 1, Brooklyn, NY 11219-2918; **Phone:** 718-765-4943; **Board Cert:** Internal Medicine 1968; Endocrinology 1977; **Med School:** Albert Einstein Coll Med 1961; **Resid:** Internal Medicine, Montefiore Hosp Med Ctr 1965; Internal Medicine, Mount Sinai Hosp 1964; **Fellow:** Endocrinology, Diabetes & Metabolism, Mount Sinai Hosp 1968

Warman, Jacob MD (EDM) - **Spec Exp:** Pituitary Disorders; Calcium Disorders; Thyroid Disorders; **Hospital:** Brooklyn Hosp Ctr; **Address:** 240 Willoughby St, Maynard Bldg - Ste 7F, Brooklyn, NY 11201; **Phone:** 718-250-6921; **Board Cert:** Internal Medicine 1976; Endocrinology, Diabetes & Metabolism 1979; **Med School:** SUNY Downstate 1973; **Resid:** Internal Medicine, Maimonides Med Ctr 1976; **Fellow:** Endocrinology, Diabetes & Metabolism, Jewish Hosp 1978

Weinerman, Stuart A MD (EDM) - **Spec Exp:** Osteoporosis; Calcium Disorders; Paget's Disease of Bone; **Hospital:** N Shore Univ Hosp (page 106), Long Is Jewish Med Ctr (page 106); **Address:** 865 Northern Blvd, Ste 203, Great Neck, NY 11201; **Phone:** 516-708-2540; **Board Cert:** Internal Medicine 1987; Endocrinology, Diabetes & Metabolism 1989; **Med School:** Albert Einstein Coll Med 1984; **Resid:** Internal Medicine, N Shore Univ Hosp 1987; **Fellow:** Endocrinology, Diabetes & Metabolism, NY Hosp/Meml Sloan Kettering Cancer Ctr 1989

Family Medicine

Krotowski, Mark MD (FMed) *PCP* - **Spec Exp:** Caribbean Health Care; Hypertension; Diabetes; **Hospital:** Brookdale Univ Hosp Med Ctr, SUNY Downstate Med Ctr (Univ Hosp Brooklyn) (page 441); **Address:** 8923 Avenue A, Brooklyn, NY 11236-1206; **Phone:** 718-385-8181; **Board Cert:** Family Medicine 2008; **Med School:** Israel 1976; **Resid:** Pediatrics, Brookdale Univ Hosp 1977; Family Medicine, Brookdale Univ Hosp 1979; **Fac Appt:** Assoc Clin Prof FMed, SUNY Downstate

Lopez, Clark R MD (FMed) *PCP* - **Spec Exp:** Geriatric Care; **Hospital:** New York Methodist Hosp (page 440), Lutheran Med Ctr - Brooklyn; **Address:** 60 Plaza St E, Brooklyn, NY 11238; **Phone:** 718-783-3919; **Board Cert:** Family Medicine 2003; **Med School:** SUNY Downstate 1972; **Resid:** Family Medicine, Kings County Hosp 1976; **Fellow:** Family Medicine, Kings County Hosp 1977

Moskowitz, George MD (FMed) *PCP* - **Spec Exp:** Geriatric Medicine; Obesity; Preventive Medicine; **Hospital:** Maimonides Med Ctr (page 98), New York Methodist Hosp (page 440); **Address:** 1318 42 St, Brooklyn, NY 11219-1405; **Phone:** 718-436-2496; **Board Cert:** Family Medicine 2005; **Med School:** Belgium 1973; **Resid:** Family Medicine, St Vincents Hosp 1976; Family Medicine, Med Coll S Carolina Hosp 1978

Sadovsky, Richard MD (FMed) *PCP* - **Spec Exp:** Preventive Medicine; Diabetes; Hepatitis; Thyroid Disorders; **Hospital:** SUNY Downstate Med Ctr (Univ Hosp Brooklyn) (page 441); **Address:** 450 Clarkson Ave, Box 67, Brooklyn, NY 11203-2012; **Phone:** 718-270-2697; **Board Cert:** Family Medicine 2008; **Med School:** SUNY Hlth Sci Ctr 1974; **Resid:** Family Medicine, SUNY Hosp 1977; **Fac Appt:** Assoc Prof FMed, SUNY Hlth Sci Ctr

Schiowitz, Emanuel DO (FMed) *PCP* - **Hospital:** Maimonides Med Ctr (page 98); **Address:** 1701 59 St, Brooklyn, NY 11204-2254; **Phone:** 718-259-0222; **Board Cert:** Family Medicine 1968; **Med School:** Philadelphia Coll Osteo Med 1963; **Resid:** Family Medicine, Interboro Med Ctr 1964; **Fac Appt:** Asst Clin Prof FMed, NY Coll Osteo Med

Vincent, Miriam MD/PhD (FMed) *PCP* - **Spec Exp:** Diabetes; Arthritis; Preventive Medicine; **Hospital:** SUNY Downstate Med Ctr (Univ Hosp Brooklyn) (page 441), Kings Co Hosp Ctr; **Address:** 470 Clarkson Ave, Ste B, Brooklyn, NY 11203-2012; **Phone:** 718-270-3260; **Board Cert:** Family Medicine 2008; **Med School:** SUNY Hlth Sci Ctr 1985; **Resid:** Family Medicine, SUNY Downstate Med Ctr 1988; **Fac Appt:** Prof FMed, SUNY Hlth Sci Ctr

Gastroenterology

Erber, William MD (Ge) - **Spec Exp:** Endoscopy; Inflammatory Bowel Disease/Crohn's; Gastrointestinal Cancer; Capsule Endoscopy; **Hospital:** Maimonides Med Ctr (page 98), Beth Israel Med Ctr - Petrie Div (page 94); **Address:** 591 Ocean Pkwy, Brooklyn, NY 11218-5913; **Phone:** 718-972-8500; **Board Cert:** Internal Medicine 1975; Gastroenterology 1979; **Med School:** Ros Franklin Univ/Chicago Med Sch 1967; **Resid:** Internal Medicine, Maimonides Med Ctr 1969; Internal Medicine, Maimonides Med Ctr 1973; **Fellow:** Research, Hadassah Hosp 1972; Gastroenterology, Albert Einstein Coll Med 1975; **Fac Appt:** Asst Clin Prof Med, SUNY Downstate

Gamss, Jeffrey S MD (Ge) - **Spec Exp:** Colonoscopy; **Hospital:** Beth Israel Med Ctr- Kings Hwy Div (page 94); **Address:** 1630 E 14th St, Brooklyn, NY 11229; **Phone:** 718-692-1198; **Board Cert:** Internal Medicine 1986; Gastroenterology 1989; **Med School:** SUNY Downstate 1983; **Resid:** Internal Medicine, Brookdale Hosp 1986; **Fellow:** Gastroenterology, SUNY Downstate 1988

Gettenberg, Gary S MD (Ge) - **Spec Exp:** Gastrointestinal Cancer; Colon Cancer Screening; Gastroesophageal Reflux Disease (GERD); Celiac Disease; **Hospital:** Maimonides Med Ctr (page 98), New York Methodist Hosp (page 440); **Address:** 1630 E 14th St, Brooklyn, NY 11229-1104; **Phone:** 718-339-0391; **Board Cert:** Internal Medicine 1987; Gastroenterology 1989; **Med School:** NY Med Coll 1983; **Resid:** Internal Medicine, Maimonides Med Ctr 1986; **Fellow:** Gastroenterology, Maimonides Med Ctr 1989

Gupta, Jagdish K MD (Ge) - **Spec Exp:** Colon Cancer; Hepatitis; Peptic Ulcer Disease; **Hospital:** SUNY Downstate Med Ctr (Univ Hosp Brooklyn) (page 441); **Address:** 207 Berkeley Pl, Brooklyn, NY 11217; **Phone:** 718-638-3150; **Board Cert:** Internal Medicine 1975; Gastroenterology 1977; **Med School:** India 1970; **Resid:** Internal Medicine, LI Coll Hosp 1975; **Fellow:** Gastroenterology, LI Coll Hosp 1977; **Fac Appt:** Asst Clin Prof Med, SUNY Downstate

Iswara, Kadirawelpillai MD (Ge) - **Spec Exp:** Pancreatic/Biliary Endoscopy (ERCP); Colonoscopy; Endoscopy; Hepatitis; **Hospital:** Maimonides Med Ctr (page 98), Coney Island Hosp; **Address:** 2511 Ocean Ave, Ste 104, Brooklyn, NY 11225; **Phone:** 718-615-0400; **Board Cert:** Internal Medicine 1980; Gastroenterology 1975; **Med School:** Sri Lanka 1968; **Resid:** Internal Medicine, Coney Island Hosp 1972; Internal Medicine, Bronx VA Hosp 1973; **Fellow:** Gastroenterology, Maimonides Med Ctr 1976; **Fac Appt:** Asst Clin Prof Med, Mount Sinai Sch Med

Leb, Alvin D MD (Ge) - **Spec Exp:** Endoscopy; **Hospital:** Beth Israel Med Ctr- Kings Hwy Div (page 94); **Address:** 2985 Quentin Rd, Brooklyn, NY 11229; **Phone:** 718-336-2218; **Board Cert:** Internal Medicine 1985; Gastroenterology 1989; **Med School:** SUNY Downstate 1982; **Resid:** Internal Medicine, Brookdale Univ Hosp 1985; **Fellow:** Gastroenterology, Brookdale Univ Hosp 1988

Maizel, Barry MD (Ge) - **Spec Exp:** Endoscopy; Inflammatory Bowel Disease; Liver Disease; **Hospital:** New York Methodist Hosp (page 440), NY Hosp Queens (page 488); **Address:** 90 8th Ave, Brooklyn, NY 11215-1553; **Phone:** 718-622-8255; **Board Cert:** Internal Medicine 1979; Gastroenterology 1981; **Med School:** Italy 1975; **Resid:** Internal Medicine, Jewish Hosp 1978; **Fellow:** Gastroenterology, NY Med Coll-Metropolitan Hosp 1980

Mayer, Ira E MD (Ge) - **Spec Exp:** Inflammatory Bowel Disease/Crohn's; Gastroesophageal Reflux Disease (GERD); Gastrointestinal Motility Disorders; **Hospital:** Maimonides Med Ctr (page 98); **Address:** 575 Kings Hwy, Brooklyn, NY 11223; **Phone:** 718-891-0100; **Board Cert:** Internal Medicine 1978; Gastroenterology 1981; **Med School:** NY Med Coll 1975; **Resid:** Internal Medicine, Metropolitan Hosp Ctr 1978; **Fellow:** Gastroenterology, Emory Univ Hosp 1980; **Fac Appt:** Asst Clin Prof Med, SUNY Downstate

Notar-Francesco, Vincent J MD (Ge) - **Hospital:** New York Methodist Hosp (page 440); **Address:** 263 7th Ave, Ste 5A, Brooklyn, NY 11215; **Phone:** 718-246-8600; **Board Cert:** Internal Medicine 1989; Gastroenterology 2011; **Med School:** Mount Sinai Sch Med 1986; **Resid:** Internal Medicine, Stony Brook Univ Hosp 1989; **Fellow:** Gastroenterology, SUNY Downstate Med Ctr 1991

Piccione, Paul R MD (Ge) - **Hospital:** Lutheran Med Ctr - Brooklyn; **Address:** 560 Bay Ridge Pkwy, Brooklyn, NY 11209-2702; **Phone:** 718-748-5219; **Board Cert:** Internal Medicine 1985; Gastroenterology 1987; **Med School:** Italy 1981; **Resid:** Internal Medicine, Lutheran Med Ctr 1985; **Fellow:** Gastroenterology, St Luke's-Roosevelt Hosp 1987

Shike, Moshe MD (Ge) - **Spec Exp:** Gastrointestinal Cancer; Nutrition & Cancer Prevention; Endoscopy; **Hospital:** Meml Sloan-Kettering Canc Ctr (page 114), NY-Presby/Weill Cornell Med Ctr, NY (page 104); **Address:** 1275 York Ave, New York, NY 10065; **Phone:** 212-639-7230; **Board Cert:** Internal Medicine 1977; Gastroenterology 1981; **Med School:** Israel 1975; **Resid:** Internal Medicine, Mt Auburn Hosp 1977; **Fellow:** Gastroenterology, Toronto Genl Hosp 1981; **Fac Appt:** Prof Med, Cornell Univ-Weill Med Coll

Sohn, Won MD (Ge) - **Spec Exp:** Endoscopy; Pancreatic/Biliary Endoscopy (ERCP); **Hospital:** New York Methodist Hosp (page 440); **Address:** 213-33 39th Ave, Ste 428, Bayside, NY 11361; **Phone:** 718-428-5333; **Board Cert:** Internal Medicine 2010; Gastroenterology 2010; **Med School:** SUNY Downstate 1994; **Resid:** Internal Medicine, Yale New Haven Hosp 1997; **Fellow:** Gastroenterology, NY Presby Hosp 2000

Sorra, Toomas Mihkel MD (Ge) - **Spec Exp:** Colon & Rectal Cancer; Hepatitis; Gastroesophageal Reflux Disease (GERD); **Hospital:** SUNY Downstate Med Ctr (Univ Hosp Brooklyn) (page 441); **Address:** 166 Clinton St, Brooklyn, NY 11201-4618; **Phone:** 718-834-0100; **Board Cert:** Internal Medicine 1981; Gastroenterology 1983; **Med School:** Mexico 1975; **Resid:** Internal Medicine, LI Coll Hosp 1980; **Fellow:** Gastroenterology, LI Coll Hosp 1982; **Fac Appt:** Asst Prof Med, SUNY Downstate

Zimbalist, Eliot MD (Ge) - **Spec Exp:** Colon Cancer Screening; Hepatitis C; Irritable Bowel Syndrome; Inflammatory Bowel Disease; **Hospital:** Maimonides Med Ctr (page 98), Lutheran Med Ctr - Brooklyn; **Address:** 452 77 St, Brooklyn, NY 11209-3206; **Phone:** 718-921-5548; **Board Cert:** Internal Medicine 1983; Gastroenterology 1985; **Med School:** Mount Sinai Sch Med 1980; **Resid:** Internal Medicine, Maimonides Med Ctr 1983; **Fellow:** Gastroenterology, Meml Sloan Kettering Cancer Ctr 1985

Geriatric Medicine

Baccash Jr, Emil G MD (Ger) *PCP* - **Spec Exp:** Geriatric Care; Preventive Medicine; **Hospital:** New York Methodist Hosp (page 440); **Address:** 20 8th Ave, Brooklyn, NY 11217; **Phone:** 718-622-7000; **Board Cert:** Internal Medicine 1981; Geriatric Medicine 2005; **Med School:** Italy 1978; **Resid:** Internal Medicine, NY Methodist Hosp 1981

Paris, Barbara E MD (Ger) - **Spec Exp:** Preventive Medicine; Frail Elderly; **Hospital:** Maimonides Med Ctr (page 98), Mt Sinai Med Ctr (page 102); **Address:** Maimonides Medical Center, Division of Geriatrics, 4802 10th Ave, Brooklyn, NY 11219; **Phone:** 718-283-7071; **Board Cert:** Internal Medicine 1982; Geriatric Medicine 2008; **Med School:** SUNY Downstate 1977; **Resid:** Internal Medicine, St Vincents Hosp 1980; **Fellow:** Geriatric Medicine, Mt Sinai Hosp 1986; **Fac Appt:** Clin Prof Med, Mount Sinai Sch Med

Geriatric Psychiatry

Amin, Ravindra N MD (GerPsy) - **Spec Exp:** Alzheimer's Disease; Anxiety Disorders; Depression; Memory Disorders; **Hospital:** SUNY Downstate Med Ctr (Univ Hosp Brooklyn) (page 441); **Address:** 161 Atlantic Ave, Brooklyn, NY 11201; **Phone:** 718-313-2994; **Board Cert:** Psychiatry 1993; Geriatric Psychiatry 2004; Addiction Psychiatry 2006; **Med School:** India 1985; **Resid:** Psychiatry, Elmhurst Hosp 1992; **Fellow:** Geriatric Psychiatry, Mt Sinai Med Ctr 1994

Cohen, Carl MD (GerPsy) - **Spec Exp:** Alzheimer's Disease; Schizophrenia; Depression in the Elderly; **Hospital:** SUNY Downstate Med Ctr (Univ Hosp Brooklyn) (page 441); **Address:** SUNY Health Science Center Assocs, 370 Lenox Rd, Brooklyn, NY 11226-2206; **Phone:** 718-287-4806; **Board Cert:** Psychiatry 1977; Geriatric Psychiatry 2009; **Med School:** SUNY Buffalo 1971; **Resid:** Psychiatry, NYU Med Ctr 1974; **Fellow:** Community Psychiatry, NYU Med Ctr 1975; **Fac Appt:** Prof Psyc, SUNY Hlth Sci Ctr

Greenberg, Robert M MD (GerPsy) - **Spec Exp:** Electroconvulsive Therapy (ECT); Neuro-Psychiatry; **Hospital:** Lutheran Med Ctr - Brooklyn, Hoboken Univ Med Ctr - Hoboken; **Address:** Lutheran Med Ctr, Psychiatry Dept, 150 55th St, Brooklyn, NY 11220; **Phone:** 718-630-6079; **Board Cert:** Psychiatry 1986; Geriatric Psychiatry 2011; **Med School:** Mount Sinai Sch Med 1978; **Resid:** Psychiatry, NY-Presby/Westchester Div 1983

Rosen, Evelyn MD (GerPsy) - **Hospital:** New York Methodist Hosp (page 440); **Address:** 583 5th St, Brooklyn, NY 11215-3503; **Phone:** 212-813-9410; **Board Cert:** Psychiatry 1992; **Med School:** Mexico 1986; **Resid:** Psychiatry, Univ Hosp 1991; **Fellow:** Geriatric Psychiatry, Univ Hosp 1992

Gynecologic Oncology

Economos, Katherine MD (GO) - **Spec Exp:** Ovarian Cancer; Cervical Cancer; Uterine Cancer; Vulvar & Vaginal Cancer; **Hospital:** New York Methodist Hosp (page 440); **Address:** 506 6th St, Brooklyn, NY 11215; **Phone:** 718-780-3090; **Board Cert:** Gynecologic Oncology 2012; Obstetrics & Gynecology 2012; **Med School:** SUNY Downstate 1986; **Resid:** Obstetrics & Gynecology, Maimonides Med Ctr 1990; **Fellow:** Gynecologic Oncology, Univ Texas SW Med Ctr 1993; **Fac Appt:** Assoc Clin Prof ObG, Cornell Univ-Weill Med Coll

Khulpateea, Neekianund MD (GO) - **Spec Exp:** Hysterectomy Alternatives; Gynecologic Cancer; **Hospital:** Maimonides Med Ctr (page 98); **Address:** Maimonides Med Ctr, Div Gyn, 953 49th St Fl 2, Brooklyn, NY 11219-2923; **Phone:** 718-283-7370; **Board Cert:** Obstetrics & Gynecology 1981; **Med School:** Israel 1972; **Resid:** Obstetrics & Gynecology, Meth Hosp 1976; **Fellow:** Gynecologic Oncology, Univ Hosp Downstate 1978; **Fac Appt:** Assoc Prof ObG, SUNY Downstate

Serur, Eli MD (GO) - **Spec Exp:** Nutrition & Cancer; Laparoscopic Surgery; Gynecologic Cancer; Minimally Invasive Surgery; **Hospital:** Richmond Univ Med Ctr; **Address:** 240 Willoughby St, Ste 3A, Brooklyn, NY 11201; **Phone:** 718-250-8106; **Board Cert:** Obstetrics & Gynecology 2012; Gynecologic Oncology 2012; **Med School:** NYU Sch Med 1985; **Resid:** Obstetrics & Gynecology, Kings County Hosp 1989; **Fellow:** Gynecologic Oncology, Kings County Hosp 1991; **Fac Appt:** Asst Clin Prof ObG, Cornell Univ-Weill Med Coll

Hand Surgery

Choueka, Jack MD (HS) - **Spec Exp:** Hand & Upper Extremity Surgery; Rotator Cuff Surgery; Wrist Surgery; Shoulder Surgery; **Hospital:** Maimonides Med Ctr (page 98); **Address:** Maimonedes Orthopedics, 1301 57th St, Brooklyn, NY 11219; **Phone:** 718-283-7362; **Board Cert:** Orthopaedic Surgery 2011; Hand Surgery 2011; **Med School:** SUNY Hlth Sci Ctr 1991; **Resid:** Orthopaedic Surgery, Hosp Joint Diseases 1996; Hand Surgery, Univ Chicago Hosps 1998

Hematology

Dosik, Harvey MD (Hem) - **Spec Exp:** Leukemia & Lymphoma; Anemia; Multiple Myeloma; **Hospital:** New York Methodist Hosp (page 440); **Address:** 500 4th Ave, Ste 1, Brooklyn, NY 11215-3609; **Phone:** 718-208-1820; **Board Cert:** Internal Medicine 1970; Hematology 1976; **Med School:** NYU Sch Med 1963; **Resid:** Internal Medicine, Kings County Hosp 1967; **Fellow:** Hematology, Maimonides Med Ctr 1969

Hospice & Palliative Medicine

Popp, Beth MD (H & PM) - **Spec Exp:** Palliative Care; Pain-Cancer; Pain-Chronic; Pain Management; **Hospital:** Maimonides Med Ctr (page 98); **Address:** 6300 Eigth Ave, Brooklyn, NY 11220; **Phone:** 718-765-2600; **Board Cert:** Medical Oncology 2008; Hospice & Palliative Medicine ; **Med School:** Indiana Univ 1988; **Resid:** Internal Medicine, IU Hlth Affil Hosp 1991; **Fellow:** Medical Oncology, IU Hlth Affil Hosp 1993; Hospice & Palliative Medicine, Meml Sloan Kettering Cancer Ctr 1995

Infectious Disease

Augenbraun, Michael H MD (Inf) - **Spec Exp:** AIDS/HIV; Sexually Transmitted Diseases; Infections-Respiratory; Infections-Opportunistic; **Hospital:** SUNY Downstate Med Ctr (Univ Hosp Brooklyn) (page 441), Kings Co Hosp Ctr; **Address:** 450 Clarkson Ave, rm B5-302, Box 56, Brooklyn, NY 11203; **Phone:** 718-270-1432; **Board Cert:** Internal Medicine 1988; Infectious Disease 2010; **Med School:** Univ Rochester 1985; **Resid:** Internal Medicine, North Shore Univ Hosp 1986; Internal Medicine, Meml Sloan Kettering Cancer Ctr 1988; **Fellow:** Infectious Disease, SUNY Downstate Med Ctr 1990; **Fac Appt:** Prof Med, SUNY Hlth Sci Ctr

Berkowitz, Leonard B MD (Inf) - **Spec Exp:** AIDS/HIV; **Hospital:** Brooklyn Hosp Ctr; **Address:** 121 DeKalb Ave, Ste 5H, Brooklyn, NY 11201-5425; **Phone:** 718-250-6922; **Board Cert:** Internal Medicine 1980; Infectious Disease 1984; **Med School:** SUNY Downstate 1977; **Resid:** Internal Medicine, Kings Co Hosp Ctr 1981; **Fellow:** Infectious Disease, Kings Co Hosp Ctr 1983; **Fac Appt:** Asst Clin Prof Med, SUNY Hlth Sci Ctr

Chapnick, Edward K MD (Inf) - **Spec Exp:** AIDS/HIV; Travel Medicine; Antibiotic Resistance; **Hospital:** Maimonides Med Ctr (page 98); **Address:** Maimonides Med Ctr, Div Infectious Dis, 4802 10th Ave, Brooklyn, NY 11219-2844; **Phone:** 718-283-7492; **Board Cert:** Internal Medicine 1988; Infectious Disease 2012; **Med School:** SUNY Downstate 1985; **Resid:** Internal Medicine, Maimonides Med Ctr 1989; **Fellow:** Infectious Disease, Maimonides Med Ctr 1991; **Fac Appt:** Assoc Prof Med, SUNY Downstate

Cofsky, Richard D MD (Inf) - **Spec Exp:** Meningitis; Tuberculosis; AIDS/HIV; **Hospital:** Brookdale Univ Hosp Med Ctr; **Address:** Brookdale Univ Hosp, 1 Brookdale Plaza, rm 596, Brooklyn, NY 11212-3139; **Phone:** 718-240-5096; **Board Cert:** Internal Medicine 1981; Infectious Disease 1984; **Med School:** Univ MD Sch Med 1978; **Resid:** Internal Medicine, Maimonides Med Ctr 1981; **Fellow:** Infectious Disease, Downstate Med Ctr 1984

Landesman, Sheldon H MD (Inf) - **Spec Exp:** AIDS/HIV; Clinical Trials; **Hospital:** SUNY Downstate Med Ctr (Univ Hosp Brooklyn) (page 441); **Address:** SUNY Downstate Med Ctr, 450 Clarkson Ave, MS 97, Brooklyn, NY 11203; **Phone:** 718-270-3034; **Board Cert:** Internal Medicine 1976; **Med School:** SUNY Downstate 1972; **Resid:** Interventional Cardiology, Tufts-New England Med Ctr 1976; **Fellow:** Research, Baltimore Cancer Rsrch Inst/NCI 1977; Infectious Disease, Tufts-New England Med Ctr 1978; **Fac Appt:** Prof Med, SUNY Downstate

Pujol-Morato, Fernando A MD (Inf) - **Spec Exp:** AIDS/HIV; **Hospital:** New York Methodist Hosp (page 440); **Address:** 20 8th Ave, Brooklyn, NY 11217; **Phone:** 718-636-7400; **Board Cert:** Internal Medicine 1986; Infectious Disease 1988; **Med School:** Dominican Republic 1979; **Resid:** Internal Medicine, LI College Hosp 1985; **Fellow:** Infectious Disease, LI College Hosp 1987; **Fac Appt:** Asst Prof Med, Cornell Univ-Weill Med Coll

Stein, Alan J MD (Inf) - **Spec Exp:** AIDS/HIV; Travel Medicine; **Hospital:** New York Methodist Hosp (page 440), Brooklyn Hosp Ctr; **Address:** 348 13th St, Ste 201, Brooklyn, NY 11215; **Phone:** 718-369-4850; **Board Cert:** Internal Medicine 1976; Infectious Disease 1978; **Med School:** NY Med Coll 1972; **Resid:** Internal Medicine, Lenox Hill Hosp 1974; Internal Medicine, Metropolitan Hosp Ctr 1976; **Fellow:** Infectious Disease, NYU Med Ctr 1978; **Fac Appt:** Assoc Clin Prof Med, NYU Sch Med

Internal Medicine

Behm, Dutsi MD (IM) *PCP* - **Hospital:** New York Methodist Hosp (page 440), Maimonides Med Ctr (page 98); **Address:** 421 Ocean Pkwy, Ste 2A, Brooklyn, NY 11218-2408; **Phone:** 718-438-8585; **Med School:** Ukraine 1973; **Resid:** Internal Medicine, NY Methodist Hosp 1983

Bharathan, Thayyullathil MD (IM) *PCP* - **Spec Exp:** Alzheimer's Disease; Dementia; Palliative Care; Pain Management; **Hospital:** New York Methodist Hosp (page 440); **Address:** 263 7th Ave, Ste 4H, Brooklyn, NY 11215-3691; **Phone:** 718-246-8561; **Board Cert:** Internal Medicine 1976; **Med School:** India 1962; **Resid:** Internal Medicine, NY Methodist Hosp 1973; **Fac Appt:** Asst Clin Prof Med, Cornell Univ-Weill Med Coll

Butt, Ahmar A MD (IM) *PCP* - **Spec Exp:** Hypertension; Congestive Heart Failure; Cholesterol/Lipid Disorders; Diabetes; **Hospital:** Brooklyn Hosp Ctr; **Address:** Health Styles Medical, 55 Greene Ave, Ste 1-A, Brooklyn, NY 11238; **Phone:** 718-857-0404; **Board Cert:** Internal Medicine 2005; **Med School:** Pakistan 1983; **Resid:** Internal Medicine, Brooklyn Hosp 1994; **Fac Appt:** Asst Clin Prof Med, Cornell Univ-Weill Med Coll

Cohen, Barry A MD (IM) *PCP* - **Spec Exp:** Preventive Medicine; **Hospital:** Beth Israel Med Ctr- Kings Hwy Div (page 94); **Address:** 151A West End Ave, Brooklyn, NY 11235-4808; **Phone:** 718-934-1222; **Board Cert:** Internal Medicine 1986; **Med School:** Dominican Republic 1982; **Resid:** Internal Medicine, Mt Sinai Serv/City Hosp Ctr 1986

Ditchek, Alan MD (IM) *PCP* - **Spec Exp:** Chronic Fatigue Syndrome; Diabetes; Lyme Disease; Hypertension; **Hospital:** Beth Israel Med Ctr- Kings Hwy Div (page 94), New York Methodist Hosp (page 440); **Address:** 2516 Ocean Ave, Brooklyn, NY 11229-3916; **Phone:** 718-769-0444; **Board Cert:** Internal Medicine 1986; Infectious Disease 2007; **Med School:** Mexico 1981; **Resid:** Internal Medicine, Lutheran Med Ctr 1985; **Fellow:** Infectious Disease, Nassau Co Med Ctr 1986; Infectious Disease, SUNY Downstate 1995; **Fac Appt:** Asst Prof Med, SUNY Downstate

Ellis, Earl A MD (IM) *PCP* - **Spec Exp:** Geriatric Care; Geriatric Medicine; Preventive Medicine; **Hospital:** Brooklyn Hosp Ctr, SUNY Downstate Med Ctr (Univ Hosp Brooklyn) (page 441); **Address:** 66 Rutland Rd, Brooklyn, NY 11225-5313; **Phone:** 718-282-4412; **Board Cert:** Internal Medicine 1984; **Med School:** Howard Univ 1980; **Resid:** Internal Medicine, Elmhurst City Hosp 1983

Gambarin, Boris L MD/PhD (IM) *PCP* - **Spec Exp:** Cardiovascular Disease; Diabetes; **Hospital:** New York Methodist Hosp (page 440); **Address:** 5923 16th Ave, Brooklyn, NY 11204; **Phone:** 718-259-6122; **Board Cert:** Internal Medicine 2005; **Med School:** Russia 1969; **Resid:** Internal Medicine, Interfaith Med Ctr 1995; **Fac Appt:** Asst Prof Med, Cornell Univ-Weill Med Coll

Grunzweig, Milton J MD (IM) *PCP* - **Spec Exp:** Preventive Medicine; **Hospital:** Brookdale Univ Hosp Med Ctr, Beth Israel Med Ctr - Petrie Div (page 94); **Address:** 2000 Ocean Ave, Ste 1, Brooklyn, NY 11230; **Phone:** 718-769-7900; **Board Cert:** Internal Medicine 1989; **Med School:** SUNY Downstate 1986; **Resid:** Internal Medicine, Brookdale Hosp 1989

Hsuih, Terence CH MD (IM) *PCP* - **Spec Exp:** Preventive Medicine; **Hospital:** Lutheran Med Ctr - Brooklyn, Maimonides Med Ctr (page 98); **Address:** 775 57th St, Brooklyn, NY 11220; **Phone:** 718-439-6163; **Board Cert:** Internal Medicine 2008; **Med School:** Mount Sinai Sch Med 1995; **Resid:** Internal Medicine, New York Hosp 1998

Hyman, Jeffrey S MD (IM) *PCP* - **Hospital:** Staten Island Univ Hosp - North (page 106); **Address:** 8012 3rd Ave, Brooklyn, NY 11209; **Phone:** 718-745-5600; **Board Cert:** Internal Medicine 2007; **Med School:** Mexico 1980; **Resid:** Internal Medicine, Maimonides Med Ctr 1984

Joy, Mark MD (IM) *PCP* - **Spec Exp:** Diabetes; Thyroid Disorders; **Hospital:** VA NY Harbor Hlthcr Sys-Brooklyn Campus; **Address:** Dept of Medicine, 800 Poly Pl, Brooklyn, NY 11209; **Phone:** 718-630-3766; **Board Cert:** Internal Medicine 1983; **Med School:** W VA Univ 1979; **Resid:** Internal Medicine, Mercy Hosp 1982; **Fac Appt:** Asst Clin Prof Med, NY Med Coll

Kaiser, Stephen J MD (IM) *PCP* - **Spec Exp:** Diabetes; Hypertension; Preventive Medicine; **Hospital:** Maimonides Med Ctr (page 98); **Address:** 1335 Ocean Pkwy, Brooklyn, NY 11230; **Phone:** 718-382-8900; **Board Cert:** Internal Medicine 1972; **Med School:** SUNY Buffalo 1964; **Resid:** Internal Medicine, Kings County Hosp 1967; **Fellow:** Hematology, Maimonides Med Ctr 1969

Katzenelenbogen, Moshe MD (IM) *PCP* - **Hospital:** Beth Israel Med Ctr- Kings Hwy Div (page 94); **Address:** 3901 Nostrand Ave, Brooklyn, NY 11235; **Phone:** 718-646-1422; **Board Cert:** Internal Medicine 1984; **Med School:** Romania 1980; **Resid:** Internal Medicine, Coney Island Hosp 1984

Levey, Robert L MD (IM) *PCP* - **Spec Exp:** Chronic Obstructive Lung Disease (COPD); Alzheimer's Disease; **Hospital:** SUNY Downstate Med Ctr (Univ Hosp Brooklyn) (page 441); **Address:** 349 Henry St Fl 5th, Brooklyn, NY 11201; **Phone:** 718-780-2838; **Board Cert:** Internal Medicine 1977; **Med School:** Univ Mich Med Sch 1970; **Resid:** Internal Medicine, Long Is Coll Hosp 1977

Lu, Bing MD/PhD (IM) *PCP* - **Spec Exp:** Chinese Community Health; Acupuncture; Sinusitis; Irritable Bowel Syndrome; **Hospital:** Maimonides Med Ctr (page 98), SUNY Downstate Med Ctr (Univ Hosp Brooklyn) (page 441); **Address:** Universal Medical Services, 4506 8th Ave, Brooklyn, NY 11220; **Phone:** 718-972-1233; **Board Cert:** Internal Medicine 2007; **Med School:** China 1982; **Resid:** Internal Medicine, Miriam Hosp 1997; **Fac Appt:** Asst Prof Med, Mount Sinai Sch Med

Malik, Asim R MD (IM) *PCP* - **Spec Exp:** Peptic Acid Disorders; **Hospital:** New York Methodist Hosp (page 440); **Address:** 1224 8th Ave, Brooklyn, NY 11215; **Phone:** 718-788-5588; **Board Cert:** Internal Medicine 2004; Gastroenterology 2007; **Med School:** Pakistan 1976; **Resid:** Surgery, NY Methodist Hosp 1978; Internal Medicine, NY Methodist Hosp 1981; **Fellow:** Gastroenterology, Wayne Cnty Genl Hosp 1983

Mehta, Viplov K MD (IM) *PCP* - **Spec Exp:** Hypertension/Kidney Disease; Dialysis Care; Diabetes; Geriatric Care; **Hospital:** Kingsbrook Jewish Med Ctr, Brooklyn Hosp Ctr; **Address:** 894 Eastern St, Brooklyn, NY 11213-3618; **Phone:** 718-774-6060; **Board Cert:** Internal Medicine 1985; Nephrology 2005; **Med School:** India 1980; **Resid:** Internal Medicine, Kingsbrook Jewish Med Ctr 1985; **Fellow:** Nephrology, SUNY Downstate Med Ctr 1987; **Fac Appt:** Assoc Clin Prof Med, SUNY Downstate

Peterson, Stephen J MD (IM) *PCP* - **Hospital:** New York Methodist Hosp (page 440); **Address:** NY Methodist Hosp, Dept Medicine, 506 Sixth St, Brooklyn, NY 11215; **Phone:** 718-780-5246; **Board Cert:** Internal Medicine 1985; **Med School:** Philippines 1982; **Resid:** Internal Medicine, Metropolitan Hosp Ctr 1985; **Fac Appt:** Prof Med, NY Med Coll

Sherman, Frederic M MD (IM) - **Spec Exp:** Cardiovascular Disease; Alzheimer's Disease; Preventive Medicine; **Hospital:** Lutheran Med Ctr - Brooklyn, Brooklyn Hosp Ctr; **Address:** 8672 Bay Pkwy, Brooklyn, NY 11214-4102; **Phone:** 718-372-2234; **Board Cert:** Internal Medicine 1976; Hospice & Palliative Medicine 2012; **Med School:** NY Med Coll 1972; **Resid:** Internal Medicine, Mount Sinai Hosp 1975Long Island Coll Hosp 1976; **Fellow:** Cardiovascular Disease, Long Island Coll Hosp 1977

Simon, Todd L MD (IM) *PCP* - **Spec Exp:** Preventive Medicine; Asthma; **Hospital:** New York Methodist Hosp (page 440); **Address:** 263 7th Ave, Ste 5A, Brooklyn, NY 11215; **Phone:** 718-246-8561; **Board Cert:** Internal Medicine 2006; **Med School:** NYU Sch Med 1991; **Resid:** Internal Medicine, Mt Sinai Hosp 1994; **Fac Appt:** Assoc Prof Med, Cornell Univ-Weill Med Coll

Tal, Avraham MD (IM) *PCP* - **Spec Exp:** Hypertension; Cholesterol/Lipid Disorders; Diabetes; **Hospital:** Coney Island Hosp; **Address:** 2601 Ocean Pkwy, Ste 4N39, Brooklyn, NY 11235-7745; **Phone:** 718-616-3880; **Board Cert:** Internal Medicine 1983; **Med School:** Italy 1975; **Resid:** Internal Medicine, LI College Hosp 1977; Internal Medicine, Kingsbrook Jewish Med Ctr 1979

Vieira, Jeffrey MD (IM) *PCP* - **Spec Exp:** Infectious Disease; AIDS/HIV; Chronic Fatigue Syndrome; **Hospital:** New York Methodist Hosp (page 440); **Address:** 349 Henry St Fl 5, Brooklyn, NY 11201; **Phone:** 718-780-2838; **Board Cert:** Internal Medicine 1980; **Med School:** NY Med Coll 1977; **Resid:** Internal Medicine, St Elizabeth's Med Ctr 1980; **Fellow:** Infectious Disease, SUNY Hlth Sci Ctr 1982; **Fac Appt:** Assoc Prof Med, SUNY Downstate

Walfish, Jacob S MD (IM) *PCP* - **Spec Exp:** Gastrointestinal Disorders; Irritable Bowel Syndrome; Diagnostic Problems; **Hospital:** NYU Langone Med Ctr (page 108); **Address:** NYU-Williamsburg, 101 Broadway, Ste 301, Brooklyn, NY 11249; **Phone:** 718-384-5179; **Board Cert:** Internal Medicine 1977; Gastroenterology 1979; **Med School:** Harvard Med Sch 1974; **Resid:** Internal Medicine, Mt Sinai Hosp 1977; **Fellow:** Gastroenterology, Mt Sinai Hosp 1979; **Fac Appt:** Asst Clin Prof Med, NYU Sch Med

Interventional Cardiology

Brener, Sorin MD (IC) - **Spec Exp:** Angioplasty & Stent Placement; **Hospital:** New York Methodist Hosp (page 440); **Address:** New York Methodist Hosp, 506 6th St, Brooklyn, NY 11215; **Phone:** 718-780-7830; **Board Cert:** Internal Medicine 2012; Cardiovascular Disease 2005; Interventional Cardiology 2009; **Med School:** Israel 1984; **Resid:** Internal Medicine, Cleveland Clin 1992; **Fellow:** Cardiovascular Disease, Cleveland Clin 1996

Marmur, Jonathan MD (IC) - **Spec Exp:** Coronary Artery Disease; Cardiac Catheterization; **Hospital:** SUNY Downstate Med Ctr (Univ Hosp Brooklyn) (page 441); **Address:** SUNY Hlth Science Ctr, 450 Clarkson Ave, Box 1257, Brooklyn, NY 11203; **Phone:** 718-270-7383; **Board Cert:** Internal Medicine 1986; Cardiovascular Disease 1989; Interventional Cardiology 2010; **Med School:** Laval Univ, Quebec 1982; **Resid:** Internal Medicine, McGill Univ/Montreal Genl Hosp 1986; **Fellow:** Cardiovascular Disease, Univ Toronto/St Michael's Hosp 1988; Interventional Cardiology, Mt Sinai Med Ctr 1992; **Fac Appt:** Prof Med, SUNY Downstate

Shani, Jacob MD (IC) - **Spec Exp:** Cardiac Catheterization; Angioplasty & Stent Placement; Percutaneous Valve Repair; Aortic Valve Replacement; **Hospital:** Maimonides Med Ctr (page 98); **Address:** Maimonides Med Ctr-Cardiology, 4802 10th Ave, Brooklyn, NY 11219-2844; **Phone:** 718-283-7480; **Board Cert:** Internal Medicine 1981; Cardiovascular Disease 1983; Interventional Cardiology 2009; **Med School:** Israel 1977; **Resid:** Internal Medicine, Maimonides Med Ctr 1981; **Fellow:** Cardiovascular Disease, Beth Israel Hosp 1983; **Fac Appt:** Prof Med, NYU Sch Med

Maternal & Fetal Medicine

Bush, Jacqueline MD (MF) - **Spec Exp:** Pregnancy-High Risk; Diabetes in Pregnancy; **Hospital:** New York Methodist Hosp (page 440); **Address:** 263 7th Ave, Ste 3A, Brooklyn, NY 11215; **Phone:** 718-246-8500; **Board Cert:** Obstetrics & Gynecology 2007; **Med School:** SUNY Stony Brook 1989; **Resid:** Obstetrics & Gynecology, SUNY Hlth Sci Ctr 1993; Obstetrics & Gynecology, Kings Co Hosp Ctr 1996

Chandra, Prasanta C MD (MF) - **Spec Exp:** Pregnancy-High Risk; Premature Labor; Pregnancy-Teenage; **Hospital:** Wyckoff Heights Med Ctr; **Address:** 220A Saint Nicholas Ave, Brooklyn, NY 11237; **Phone:** 718-418-8745; **Board Cert:** Obstetrics & Gynecology 1979; Maternal & Fetal Medicine 1980; **Med School:** India 1969; **Resid:** Surgery, Bronx Muni Hosp-Albert Einstein Med Ctr 1972; Obstetrics & Gynecology, Bronx Muni Hosp-Albert Einstein Med Ctr 1976; **Fellow:** Maternal & Fetal Medicine, Bronx Muni Hosp-Albert Einstein Med Ctr 1978

Medical Oncology

Astrow, Alan B MD (Onc) - **Spec Exp:** Ovarian Cancer; Breast Cancer; **Hospital:** Maimonides Med Ctr (page 98); **Address:** Maimonides Cancer Ctr, 6300 8th Ave, Brooklyn, NY 11220; **Phone:** 718-765-2653; **Board Cert:** Internal Medicine 1983; Hematology 1986; Medical Oncology 1987; **Med School:** Yale Univ 1980; **Resid:** Internal Medicine, Boston City Hosp 1983; **Fellow:** Hematology & Oncology, NYU Med Ctr 1986; **Fac Appt:** Assoc Clin Prof Med, NY Med Coll

Bashevkin, Michael L MD (Onc) - **Spec Exp:** Solid Tumors; Hematologic Malignancies; **Hospital:** Maimonides Med Ctr (page 98); **Address:** Hematology Oncology Assocs, 1660 E 14th St, Ste 501, Brooklyn, NY 11229; **Phone:** 718-382-8500 x501; **Board Cert:** Internal Medicine 1976; Hematology 1978; Medical Oncology 1979; **Med School:** SUNY Downstate 1973; **Resid:** Internal Medicine, VA Med Ctr 1976; **Fellow:** Hematology & Oncology, Maimonides Med Ctr 1979

Dosik, David MD (Onc) - **Spec Exp:** Breast Cancer; Lung Cancer; Colon Cancer; **Hospital:** New York Methodist Hosp (page 440), New York Comm Hosp; **Address:** 500 4th Ave, Ste 1, Brooklyn, NY 11215; **Phone:** 718-780-5240; **Board Cert:** Hematology 2006; Medical Oncology 2007; **Med School:** SUNY Downstate 1990; **Resid:** Internal Medicine, Staten Island Univ Hosp 1993; **Fellow:** Hematology & Oncology, NYU Med Ctr 1996

Lebowicz, Joseph MD (Onc) - **Spec Exp:** Lung Cancer; Breast Cancer; Gastrointestinal Cancer; **Hospital:** Maimonides Med Ctr (page 98); **Address:** 1660 E 14th St, Ste 501, Brooklyn, NY 11229; **Phone:** 718-382-8500; **Board Cert:** Internal Medicine 1978; Hematology 1980; Medical Oncology 1981; **Med School:** Albert Einstein Coll Med 1975; **Resid:** Internal Medicine, Maimonides Med Ctr 1978; **Fellow:** Hematology & Oncology, Maimonides Med Ctr 1981

Lichter, Stephen M MD (Onc) - **Spec Exp:** Breast Cancer; Lung Cancer; Gastrointestinal Cancer; Prostate Cancer; **Hospital:** Beth Israel Med Ctr- Kings Hwy Div (page 94), New York Methodist Hosp (page 440); **Address:** 2935 Ave S, Brooklyn, NY 11229; **Phone:** 718-616-0801; **Board Cert:** Internal Medicine 1978; Medical Oncology 1981; **Med School:** Ros Franklin Univ/Chicago Med Sch 1975; **Resid:** Internal Medicine, Brookdale Hosp 1978; **Fellow:** Hematology & Oncology, Brookdale Hosp 1980; **Fac Appt:** Asst Clin Prof Med, SUNY Hlth Sci Ctr

Solomon, William B MD (Onc) - **Spec Exp:** Lung Cancer; Urologic Cancer; Clinical Trials; **Hospital:** Maimonides Med Ctr (page 98); **Address:** Maimonides Med Ctr, Hem/Onc Dept, 6300 8th Ave Fl 2, Brooklyn, NY 11220; **Phone:** 718-765-2613; **Board Cert:** Internal Medicine 1978; Hematology 1982; Medical Oncology 1985; **Med School:** Columbia P&S 1975; **Resid:** Internal Medicine, Montefiore Med Ctr 1978; **Fellow:** Hematology, Beth Israel Deaconess Med Ctr 1981; Molecular Biology, Mass Inst Tech; **Fac Appt:** Prof Med, SUNY Downstate

Neonatal-Perinatal Medicine

Gudavalli, Madhu R MD (NP) - **Spec Exp:** Prematurity/Low Birth Weight Infants; **Hospital:** New York Methodist Hosp (page 440); **Address:** New York Methodist Hosp, NICU, 506 6th St, Brooklyn, NY 11215; **Phone:** 718-780-3727; **Board Cert:** Pediatrics 1980; Neonatal-Perinatal Medicine 2009; **Med School:** India 1972; **Resid:** Pediatrics, NY Infirm 1976; Pediatrics, NY Hosp-Booth Meml 1977; **Fellow:** Neonatal-Perinatal Medicine, Bellevue Hosp 1979

Sokal, Myron MD (NP) - **Spec Exp:** Neonatal Care; **Hospital:** Brookdale Univ Hosp Med Ctr; **Address:** 1 Brookdale Plaza, Strausberg Bldg - rm 244, Brooklyn, NY 11212; **Phone:** 718-240-5629; **Board Cert:** Pediatrics 1972; Neonatal-Perinatal Medicine 1975; **Med School:** Albert Einstein Coll Med 1967; **Resid:** Pediatrics, Yale-New Haven Hosp 1969; **Fellow:** Neonatal-Perinatal Medicine, Columbia-Presby Med Ctr 1971; **Fac Appt:** Prof Ped, SUNY Hlth Sci Ctr

Nephrology

Chou, Shyan-Yih MD (Nep) - **Spec Exp:** Kidney Disease; Hypertension; Dialysis Care; **Hospital:** Brookdale Univ Hosp Med Ctr; **Address:** 1 Brookdale Plaza, rm 169-CHC, Brooklyn, NY 11212-3139; **Phone:** 718-240-5615; **Board Cert:** Internal Medicine 1972; Nephrology 1974; **Med School:** Taiwan 1966; **Resid:** Internal Medicine, Brookdale Hosp 1970; Internal Medicine, Brookdale Hosp 1970; **Fellow:** Nephrology, Brookdale Hosp 1973; **Fac Appt:** Prof Med, SUNY Downstate

Delano, Barbara G MD (Nep) - **Spec Exp:** Dialysis Care; Kidney Failure-Chronic; Kidney Disease-Acute; **Hospital:** SUNY Downstate Med Ctr (Univ Hosp Brooklyn) (page 441), Kings Co Hosp Ctr; **Address:** 450 Clarkson Ave, Box 52, Brooklyn, NY 11203-2056; **Phone:** 718-270-1584; **Board Cert:** Internal Medicine 2010; **Med School:** SUNY Hlth Sci Ctr 1965; **Resid:** Internal Medicine, SUNY Downstate Med Ctr 1967; **Fellow:** Nephrology, SUNY Downstate Med Ctr 1969; **Fac Appt:** Prof Med, SUNY Downstate

Lipner, Henry I MD (Nep) - **Spec Exp:** Kidney Disease; Hypertension; Dialysis Care; **Hospital:** Maimonides Med Ctr (page 98); **Address:** 1435 86th St, Brooklyn, NY 11228; **Phone:** 718-648-0101; **Board Cert:** Internal Medicine 1974; Nephrology 1976; **Med School:** NYU Sch Med 1968; **Resid:** Internal Medicine, Brooklyn Jewish Hosp 1971; **Fellow:** Nephrology, Montefiore Med Ctr 1972

Markell, Mariana S MD (Nep) - **Spec Exp:** Transplant Medicine-Kidney; Complementary Medicine; **Hospital:** SUNY Downstate Med Ctr (Univ Hosp Brooklyn) (page 441), Kings Co Hosp Ctr; **Address:** 450 Clarkson Ave, Box 52, Brooklyn, NY 11203; **Phone:** 718-270-1584; **Board Cert:** Internal Medicine 1984; Nephrology 1986; **Med School:** NY Med Coll 1981; **Resid:** Internal Medicine, Columbia-Presby 1984; **Fellow:** Nephrology, Columbia-Presby 1985UCLA Med Ctr 1986; **Fac Appt:** Assoc Prof Med, SUNY Downstate

Neelakantappa, Kotresha H MD (Nep) - **Spec Exp:** Kidney Disease; Hypertension; **Hospital:** New York Methodist Hosp (page 440); **Address:** 9920 4th Ave, Ste 309, Brooklyn, NY 11209; **Phone:** 718-745-3079; **Board Cert:** Internal Medicine 1977; Nephrology 1978; **Med School:** India 1969; **Resid:** Internal Medicine, NY Methodist Hosp 1974; **Fellow:** Nephrology, NYU Med Ctr 1976; **Fac Appt:** Asst Prof Med, NYU Sch Med

Pannone, John MD (Nep) - **Spec Exp:** Dialysis Care; Kidney Disease-Chronic; Hypertension; **Hospital:** Lutheran Med Ctr - Brooklyn; **Address:** 61 Oliver St, Ste PR-1, Brooklyn, NY 11209; **Phone:** 718-238-4980; **Board Cert:** Internal Medicine 1978; Nephrology 1980; **Med School:** Italy 1974; **Resid:** Internal Medicine, Lutheran Med Ctr 1977; **Fellow:** Nephrology, Brookdale Hosp Med Ctr 1979; Nephrology, New York Hosp-Cornell Med Ctr 1980

Parnes, Eliezer MD (Nep) - **Spec Exp:** Hypertension; Dialysis Care; Diabetic Kidney Disease; **Hospital:** Beth Israel Med Ctr- Kings Hwy Div (page 94); **Address:** 3131 Kings Hwy, rm D-5, Brooklyn, NY 11234-2643; **Phone:** 718-338-2283; **Board Cert:** Internal Medicine 1989; Nephrology 2003; **Med School:** SUNY Downstate 1986; **Resid:** Internal Medicine, Brookdale Hosp Med Ctr 1989; **Fellow:** Nephrology, Brookdale Hosp Med Ctr 1992

Salifu, Moro O MD (Nep) - **Spec Exp:** Kidney Disease; **Hospital:** SUNY Downstate Med Ctr (Univ Hosp Brooklyn) (page 441); **Address:** SUNY Downstate, 450 Clarkson Ave, Box 52, Brooklyn, NY 11203; **Phone:** 718-270-3174; **Board Cert:** Internal Medicine 2009; Nephrology 2010; **Med School:** Turkey 1994; **Resid:** Internal Medicine, SUNY Hlth Sci Ctr 1998; **Fellow:** Nephrology, SUNY Hlth Sci Ctr 2001

Shapiro, Warren B MD (Nep) - **Spec Exp:** Kidney Failure-Chronic; Kidney Failure; Hypertension; Dialysis Care; **Hospital:** Brookdale Univ Hosp Med Ctr; **Address:** 1 Brookdale Plaza, rm 169-CHC, Brooklyn, NY 11212-3139; **Phone:** 718-240-5615; **Board Cert:** Internal Medicine 1972; Nephrology 1974; **Med School:** Ros Franklin Univ/Chicago Med Sch 1966; **Resid:** Internal Medicine, UCSF Med Ctr 1968; Internal Medicine, NY Med Coll 1970; **Fellow:** Nephrology, NY Med Coll 1971; **Fac Appt:** Assoc Clin Prof Med, SUNY Downstate

Shein, Leon MD (Nep) - **Spec Exp:** Hypertension; Diabetic Kidney Disease; Electrolyte Disorders; Nutrition; **Hospital:** New York Methodist Hosp (page 440); **Address:** Prospect Med Grp, 1545 Atlantic Ave, Brooklyn, NY 11213; **Phone:** 718-552-2069; **Board Cert:** Internal Medicine 1989; Nephrology 2003; **Med School:** Philippines 1983; **Resid:** Internal Medicine, Woodhull Med Ctr 1986; **Fellow:** Nephrology, Brookdale Hosp 1988

Spitalewitz, Samuel MD (Nep) - **Spec Exp:** Diabetic Kidney Disease; Hypertension; **Hospital:** Brookdale Univ Hosp Med Ctr; **Address:** 1 Brookdale Plaza, Ste 169-CHC, Brooklyn, NY 11212-3139; **Phone:** 718-240-5615; **Board Cert:** Internal Medicine 1978; Nephrology 1980; **Med School:** NYU Sch Med 1975; **Resid:** Internal Medicine, Brookdale Hosp 1978; **Fellow:** Nephrology, Brookdale Hosp 1981; **Fac Appt:** Assoc Clin Prof Med, SUNY Downstate

Stam, Lawrence MD (Nep) - **Spec Exp:** Dialysis Care; Plasmapheresis; **Hospital:** New York Methodist Hosp (page 440); **Address:** 506 6th St, Ste 5A, Brooklyn, NY 11215-3609; **Phone:** 718-830-7109; **Board Cert:** Internal Medicine 1981; Nephrology 1984; **Med School:** SUNY Stony Brook 1978; **Resid:** Internal Medicine, St Elizabeth Hosp 1981; **Fellow:** Nephrology, Brooklyn Jewish Hosp 1982; **Fac Appt:** Asst Clin Prof Med, Cornell Univ-Weill Med Coll

Neurological Surgery

Cardoso, Erico R MD (NS) - **Spec Exp:** Pituitary Tumors; Spinal Cord Disorders; Hydrocephalus; **Hospital:** Kingsbrook Jewish Med Ctr; **Address:** Kingsbrook Jewish Med Ctr, 585 Schenectady Ave, Brooklyn, NY 11213; **Phone:** 718-604-5500; **Board Cert:** Neurological Surgery 1994; **Med School:** Brazil 1973; **Resid:** Surgery, Ottawa Civic Hosp 1976; Neurological Surgery, Ottawa Civic Hosp 1980; **Fellow:** Neurological Surgery, Clin Rsch Fellowship Univ Hosp 1981; Neurological Surgery, Inst Neurol Scis 1982; **Fac Appt:** Assoc Prof NS, SUNY Downstate

Cohen, Anders DO (NS) - **Spec Exp:** Minimally Invasive Spinal Surgery; Pediatric Neurosurgery; **Hospital:** Brooklyn Hosp Ctr, Long Is Jewish Med Ctr (page 106); **Address:** Brooklyn Hosp Ctr, Neurosurgery Dept, 240 Willoughby St, Ste 4E, Brooklyn, NY 11201; **Phone:** 718-250-8103; **Board Cert:** Neurological Surgery 2009; **Med School:** NY Coll Osteo Med 1997; **Resid:** Neurological Surgery, Long Island Jewish Med Ctr 2002; **Fellow:** Spine Surgery, NY-Presby/Weill Cornell Med Ctr 2003; Pediatric Neurological Surgery, NY-Presby/Weill Cornell Med Ctr 2005; **Fac Appt:** Asst Prof NS, Cornell Univ-Weill Med Coll

Schwartz, Amit Y MD (NS) - **Hospital:** Maimonides Med Ctr (page 98), Mt Sinai Med Ctr (page 102); **Address:** Maimonides Med Ctr, 948 48th St, rm 228, Brooklyn, NY 11219; **Phone:** 718-283-7219; **Board Cert:** Neurological Surgery 2005; **Med School:** Mount Sinai Sch Med 1995; **Resid:** Neurological Surgery, Mt Sinai Med Ctr 2001; **Fellow:** Skull Base Surgery, Jackson Meml Hosp 2002; **Fac Appt:** Asst Clin Prof NS, Mount Sinai Sch Med

Zonenshayn, Martin MD (NS) - **Spec Exp:** Parkinson's Disease; Stereotactic Radiosurgery; Carpal Tunnel Syndrome; Trigeminal Neuralgia; **Hospital:** New York Methodist Hosp (page 440); **Address:** 263 Seventh Ave, Ste 4D, Brooklyn, NY 11215; **Phone:** 718-246-8660; **Board Cert:** Neurological Surgery 2008; **Med School:** NYU Sch Med 1996; **Resid:** Neurological Surgery, NY Presby Cornell Med Ctr/MSKCC 2002; **Fellow:** Stereotactic Neurological Surgery, NYU Hosp Joint Diseases 2003; **Fac Appt:** Assoc Clin Prof NS, Cornell Univ-Weill Med Coll

Neurology

Abou-Fayssal, Nada MD (N) - **Spec Exp:** Multiple Sclerosis; **Hospital:** Lutheran Med Ctr - Brooklyn; **Address:** 8714 Fifth Ave, Brooklyn, NY 11209; **Phone:** 718-630-8600; **Board Cert:** Neurotology 2011; Vascular Neurology ; **Med School:** Lebanon 1991; **Resid:** Neurology, Mt Sinai Med Ctr 1998

Azhar, Salman MD (N) - **Spec Exp:** Stroke; Neuro-Rehabilitation; Dementia; Spasticity Management; **Hospital:** Lutheran Med Ctr - Brooklyn; **Address:** 8714 5th Ave, Brooklyn, NY 11209; **Phone:** 718-630-8600; **Board Cert:** Neurology 2008; Vascular Neurology 2008; **Med School:** Med Coll VA 1993; **Resid:** Neurology, Med Coll Va Hosp 1995; Neurology, Mt Sinai Med Ctr 1997; **Fellow:** Stroke, NINDS/NIH 1999; **Fac Appt:** Asst Prof N, SUNY Downstate

Bodis-Wollner, Ivan G MD (N) - **Spec Exp:** Parkinson's Disease; Neuro-Ophthalmology; Behavioral Neurology; **Hospital:** SUNY Downstate Med Ctr (Univ Hosp Brooklyn) (page 441), Kings Co Hosp Ctr; **Address:** 450 Clarkson Ave, Ste A, Box 35, Brooklyn, NY 11203; **Phone:** 718-270-2734; **Board Cert:** Neurology 1977; **Med School:** Austria 1965; **Resid:** Neurology, Mount Sinai Hosp 1974; **Fellow:** Clinical Neurophysiology, Mass Genl Hosp 1974; **Fac Appt:** Prof N, SUNY Downstate

Buckner, Cary D MD (N) - **Spec Exp:** Neuromuscular Disorders; Clinical Neurophysiology; **Hospital:** New York Methodist Hosp (page 440); **Address:** NYMH Division of Neurology, 263 7th Ave, Ste 4A, Brooklyn, NY 11215; **Phone:** 718-246-8614; **Board Cert:** Neurology 2009; Clinical Neurophysiology 2011; **Med School:** Georgetown Univ 1994; **Resid:** Neurology, Columbia Presby Med Ctr 1998; **Fellow:** Neuromuscular Disease, Columbia Presby Med Ctr 1999

Crystal, Howard A MD (N) - **Spec Exp:** Alzheimer's Disease; Dementia; **Hospital:** SUNY Downstate Med Ctr (Univ Hosp Brooklyn) (page 441), Kings Co Hosp Ctr; **Address:** 450 Clarkson Ave, Box 1274, Brooklyn, NY 11203-2056; **Phone:** 718-221-5188; **Board Cert:** Neurology 1981; **Med School:** Univ Pennsylvania 1976; **Resid:** Neurology, Montefiore Med Ctr 1980; **Fellow:** Neurological Pathology, Montefiore Med Ctr 1982; **Fac Appt:** Prof N, SUNY Downstate

Drexler, Ellen MD (N) - **Spec Exp:** Headache; **Hospital:** Maimonides Med Ctr (page 98); **Address:** 883 65th St, Brooklyn, NY 11210-4737; **Phone:** 718-283-7470; **Board Cert:** Neurology 1983; **Med School:** SUNY Downstate 1978; **Resid:** Neurology, Montefiore Med Ctr 1982; **Fac Appt:** Assoc Prof N, Mount Sinai Sch Med

Kay, Arthur D MD (N) - **Spec Exp:** Alzheimer's Disease; Parkinson's Disease; Dementia; Stroke; **Hospital:** Brookdale Univ Hosp Med Ctr, Flushing Hosp Med Ctr; **Address:** 1 Brookdale Plaza, Ste 475, Brooklyn, NY 11212-3139; **Phone:** 718-240-5622; **Board Cert:** Neurology 1983; **Med School:** SUNY Downstate 1978; **Resid:** Neurology, Brookdale Hosp 1982; **Fellow:** Natl Inst Hlth 1984; **Fac Appt:** Assoc Prof N, SUNY Downstate

Keilson, Marshall MD (N) - **Spec Exp:** Alzheimer's Disease; Epilepsy; **Hospital:** Maimonides Med Ctr (page 98); **Address:** 2044 Ocean Ave, Ste A8, Brooklyn, NY 11230; **Phone:** 718-384-5179; **Board Cert:** Neurology 1982; **Med School:** Albert Einstein Coll Med 1977; **Resid:** Internal Medicine, Montefiore Hosp Med Ctr 1978; Neurology, Albert Einstein 1981; **Fellow:** Clinical Neurophysiology, Univ Hosp 1983

Levine, Steven R MD (N) - **Spec Exp:** Stroke; Cerebrovascular Disease; **Hospital:** SUNY Downstate Med Ctr (Univ Hosp Brooklyn) (page 441); **Address:** SUNY Downstate Medical Center, 450 Clarkson Ave, rm B6-344, MS 1213, Brooklyn, NY 11203; **Phone:** 718-221-5188; **Board Cert:** Neurology 1986; Vascular Neurology 2005; **Med School:** Med Coll Wisc 1981; **Resid:** Neurology, Univ Mich Hosps 1985; **Fellow:** Cerebrovascular Disease, Henry Ford Hosp 1987; **Fac Appt:** Prof N, Mount Sinai Sch Med

Maccabee, Paul J MD (N) - **Spec Exp:** Neuromuscular Disorders; Electromyography; Peripheral Neuropathy; **Hospital:** SUNY Downstate Med Ctr (Univ Hosp Brooklyn) (page 441); **Address:** SUNY Downstate Med Ctr, 450 Clarkson Ave, Box 35, Brooklyn, NY 11203; **Phone:** 718-270-2502; **Board Cert:** Neurology 1977; Clinical Neurophysiology 2003; **Med School:** Boston Univ 1970; **Resid:** Neurology, Boston Univ Med Ctr 1976; **Fellow:** Clinical Neurophysiology, Mass Genl Hosp 1978; Clinical Neurophysiology, Mt Sinai Hosp 1979; **Fac Appt:** Prof N, SUNY Hlth Sci Ctr

Maniscalco, Anthony MD (N) - **Spec Exp:** Movement Disorders; Cerebrovascular Disease; Neuromuscular Disorders; **Hospital:** Beth Israel Med Ctr- Kings Hwy Div (page 94), Lutheran Med Ctr - Brooklyn; **Address:** Brooklyn Neurology, 117 70th St, Brooklyn, NY 11209-1113; **Phone:** 718-836-8800; **Board Cert:** Internal Medicine 1982; Neurology 1988; **Med School:** Italy 1978; **Resid:** Internal Medicine, Maimonides Medical Ctr 1981; Neurology, St Vincent's Hosp & Med Ctr 1984

Nouri, Shahin MD (N) - **Spec Exp:** Epilepsy/Seizure Disorders; **Hospital:** New York Methodist Hosp (page 440); **Address:** NY Methodist Hosp, Dept Neurology, 263 7th Ave, Ste 4A, Brooklyn, NY 11215; **Phone:** 718-246-8614; **Board Cert:** Neurology 2004; Clinical Neurophysiology 2005; **Med School:** Germany 1994; **Resid:** Internal Medicine, Staten Island Univ Hosp 1998; Neurology, Georgetown Univ Med Ctr 2001; **Fellow:** Clinical Neurophysiology, NYU Med Ctr 2002

Rosenbaum, Daniel MD (N) - **Spec Exp:** Stroke; **Hospital:** SUNY Downstate Med Ctr (Univ Hosp Brooklyn) (page 441), Kings Co Hosp Ctr; **Address:** SUNY Downstate, Dept Neurology, 450 Clarkson Ave, Box 1213, Brooklyn, NY 11203; **Phone:** 718-270-2051; **Board Cert:** Neurology 1988; Vascular Neurology 2005; **Med School:** Albert Einstein Coll Med 1982; **Resid:** Internal Medicine, Brookdale Hosp 1983; Neurology, Albert Einstein 1986; **Fellow:** Stroke, Univ Tex Med Sch 1988; **Fac Appt:** Prof N, SUNY Downstate

Rudolph, Steven H MD (N) - **Spec Exp:** Stroke; Neuro-Ophthalmology; Cerebrovascular Disease; **Hospital:** Maimonides Med Ctr (page 98), Mt Sinai Med Ctr (page 102); **Address:** 948 48th St, Brooklyn, NY 11219; **Phone:** 718-283-7670; **Board Cert:** Neurology 1981; Vascular Neurology 2005; **Med School:** SUNY Hlth Sci Ctr 1976; **Resid:** Neurology, Mt Sinai Hosp 1980; **Fellow:** Neuro-Ophthalmology, Mt Sinai Hosp 1982; **Fac Appt:** Asst Clin Prof N, Mount Sinai Sch Med

Salgado, Miran W MD (N) - **Spec Exp:** Movement Disorders; Parkinson's Disease; Botox Therapy; Headache; **Hospital:** New York Methodist Hosp (page 440); **Address:** Center for Neurology, 263 7th Ave, Ste 4A, Brooklyn, NY 11215; **Phone:** 718-246-8614; **Board Cert:** Neurology 2004; Vascular Neurology 2006; **Med School:** Sri Lanka 1990; **Resid:** Neurology, SUNY Downstate Med Ctr 1994; **Fellow:** Movement Disorders, Columbia Presby Med Ctr 1995

Sobol, Norman J MD (N) - **Spec Exp:** Headache; Stroke; Parkinson's Disease; **Hospital:** Beth Israel Med Ctr- Kings Hwy Div (page 94), Maimonides Med Ctr (page 98); **Address:** 3131 Kings Hwy, Ste C7, Brooklyn, NY 11234-2642; **Phone:** 718-677-0009; **Board Cert:** Neurology 1980; Internal Medicine 1977; **Med School:** Univ Chicago-Pritzker Sch Med 1974; **Resid:** Internal Medicine, Kings County Hosp 1976; Neurology, Kings County Hosp 1978; **Fellow:** Clinical Neurophysiology, Kings County Hosp 1980; **Fac Appt:** Asst Prof N, SUNY Downstate

Vas, George A MD (N) - **Spec Exp:** Stroke; Multiple Sclerosis; **Hospital:** SUNY Downstate Med Ctr (Univ Hosp Brooklyn) (page 441), Kings Co Hosp Ctr; **Address:** 450 Clarkson Ave N, Ste A, Brooklyn, NY 11203-2056; **Phone:** 718-270-2502; **Board Cert:** Internal Medicine 1973; Neurology 1977; Clinical Neurophysiology 2002; **Med School:** Univ Pittsburgh 1970; **Resid:** Internal Medicine, New York Hosp 1972; Neurology, New York Hosp 1975; **Fac Appt:** Prof N, SUNY Downstate

Yellin, Joseph C DO (N) - **Spec Exp:** Headache; Memory Disorders; Dementia; **Hospital:** Lenox Hill Hosp (page 106), New York Comm Hosp; **Address:** 1599 E 15 St, Fl 3, Brooklyn, NY 11230; **Phone:** 718-377-2223; **Med School:** Univ Osteo Med & Hlth Sci, Des Moines 1978; **Resid:** Neurology, Kings Co Hosp/Downstate Med Ctr 1982

Nuclear Medicine

Strashun, Arnold M MD (NuM) - **Spec Exp:** Neurological Imaging; Nuclear Cardiology; Thyroid Disorders; PET Imaging-Brain; **Hospital:** SUNY Downstate Med Ctr (Univ Hosp Brooklyn) (page 441), Kings Co Hosp Ctr; **Address:** 450 Clarkson Ave, Box 1210, Dept Radiology, Brooklyn, NY 11203; **Phone:** 718-270-1603; **Board Cert:** Internal Medicine 1977; Nuclear Medicine 1979; **Med School:** Baylor Coll Med 1974; **Resid:** Internal Medicine, Texas Med Ctr 1977; **Fellow:** Nuclear Medicine, VA Med Ctr 1978; Nuclear Medicine, Mount Sinai Hosp 1979; **Fac Appt:** Prof Rad, SUNY Downstate

Obstetrics & Gynecology

Comrie, Millicent A MD (ObG) *PCP* - **Spec Exp:** Menopause Problems; Uterine Fibroids; Prenatal Diagnosis; **Hospital:** SUNY Downstate Med Ctr (Univ Hosp Brooklyn) (page 441); **Address:** 148 Pierrepont St, Brooklyn, NY 11201; **Phone:** 718-852-9180; **Board Cert:** Obstetrics & Gynecology 1983; **Med School:** SUNY Hlth Sci Ctr 1976; **Resid:** Obstetrics & Gynecology, Long Island Coll Hosp 1980; **Fellow:** Public Health, Columbia Univ Affil Hosp 1981; **Fac Appt:** Asst Clin Prof ObG, SUNY Downstate

Dor, Nathan MD (ObG) - **Spec Exp:** Pregnancy-High Risk; **Hospital:** Maimonides Med Ctr (page 98); **Address:** 943 48th St, Brooklyn, NY 11219-2919; **Phone:** 718-853-1535; **Board Cert:** Obstetrics & Gynecology 2012; Maternal & Fetal Medicine 2012; **Med School:** Israel 1973; **Resid:** Obstetrics & Gynecology, Montefiore Med Ctr 1977; **Fellow:** Perinatal Medicine, Westchester Co Med Ctr 1979; **Fac Appt:** Asst Prof ObG, SUNY Downstate

Haratz-Rubinstein, Natan MD (ObG) - **Spec Exp:** Obstetric Ultrasound; Pregnancy-High Risk; **Hospital:** New York Methodist Hosp (page 440); **Address:** NY Methodist Hosp, Dept Ob/Gyn, 506 6th St Fl 4, Brooklyn, NY 11215; **Phone:** 718-780-5799; **Board Cert:** Obstetrics & Gynecology 2012; **Med School:** Venezuela 1989; **Resid:** Obstetrics & Gynecology, Conception Palacio Maternity Hosp 1994; Obstetrics & Gynecology, NY Presby-Columbia Med Ctr 1997; **Fac Appt:** Asst Prof ObG, SUNY Downstate

Lederman, Sanford M MD (ObG) - **Spec Exp:** Pregnancy-High Risk; Ultrasound; Prenatal Diagnosis; **Hospital:** New York Methodist Hosp (page 440); **Address:** 506 6th St, Brooklyn, NY 11215; **Phone:** 718-246-8545; **Board Cert:** Obstetrics & Gynecology 1982; **Med School:** Mexico 1974; **Resid:** Obstetrics & Gynecology, Long Island Coll Hosp 1979; **Fellow:** Maternal & Fetal Medicine, UC-Irvine Mem Hosp 1981; **Fac Appt:** Assoc Clin Prof ObG, SUNY Downstate

Maher, John T MD (ObG) - **Hospital:** New York Methodist Hosp (page 440); **Address:** Brooklyn Women's Healthcare, 110 4th Ave, Brooklyn, NY 11217; **Phone:** 718-852-5810; **Board Cert:** Obstetrics & Gynecology 2012; **Med School:** UMDNJ-NJ Med Sch, Newark 1989; **Resid:** Obstetrics & Gynecology, NY Hosp-Cornell Med Ctr 1993

Minkoff, Howard L MD (ObG) - **Spec Exp:** AIDS/HIV in Pregnancy; Pregnancy-High Risk; **Hospital:** Maimonides Med Ctr (page 98), SUNY Downstate Med Ctr (Univ Hosp Brooklyn) (page 441); **Address:** Maimonides, Womens Primary Care, 4422 9th Ave, Brooklyn, NY 11219; **Phone:** 718-283-8930; **Board Cert:** Obstetrics & Gynecology 1995; Maternal & Fetal Medicine 1995; **Med School:** Penn State Coll Med 1975; **Resid:** Obstetrics & Gynecology, Kings Co Hosp Ctr 1979; **Fellow:** Maternal & Fetal Medicine, Kings Co Hosp Ctr 1981; **Fac Appt:** Prof ObG, SUNY Hlth Sci Ctr

Reizis, Igal MD (ObG) - **Spec Exp:** Gynecology Only; **Hospital:** Maimonides Med Ctr (page 98); **Address:** 5925 15th Ave, Brooklyn, NY 11219-5009; **Phone:** 718-972-2700; **Board Cert:** Obstetrics & Gynecology 1984; **Med School:** Israel 1977; **Resid:** Obstetrics & Gynecology, Maimonides Med Ctr

Ophthalmology

Ackerman, Jacob L MD (Oph) - **Spec Exp:** Glaucoma; Cataract Surgery-Lens Implant; Eyelid Cosmetic Surgery; Macular Degeneration; **Hospital:** Brookdale Univ Hosp Med Ctr, New York Methodist Hosp (page 440); **Address:** Brook Plaza Ophthalmology Assocs, 1987 Utica Ave Fl 1st, Brooklyn, NY 11234-3213; **Phone:** 718-968-8700; **Board Cert:** Ophthalmology 1976; **Med School:** Albert Einstein Coll Med 1971; **Resid:** Ophthalmology, LI Jewish Hillside Med Ctr 1975; **Fac Appt:** Asst Clin Prof Oph, SUNY Downstate

Berman, David H MD (Oph) - **Spec Exp:** Retinal Detachment; Diabetic Eye Disease/Retinopathy; Macular Degeneration; **Hospital:** New York Eye & Ear Infirm (page 115), Brooklyn Hosp Ctr; **Address:** 185 Montague St, Ste PH, Brooklyn, NY 11201; **Phone:** 718-222-3050; **Board Cert:** Ophthalmology 1989; **Med School:** SUNY Downstate 1982; **Resid:** Internal Medicine, Kings Co Hosp 1984; Ophthalmology, Kings Co Hosp 1987; **Fellow:** Ophthalmology, Kings Co Hosp 1988; Retina/Vitreous Surgery, Hermann Eye Ctr 1989; **Fac Appt:** Assoc Clin Prof Oph, SUNY Downstate

Brecher, Rubin MD (Oph) - **Spec Exp:** Diabetic Eye Disease/Retinopathy; Macular Degeneration; **Hospital:** Maimonides Med Ctr (page 98); **Address:** 736 Ocean Pkwy, Brooklyn, NY 11230-1116; **Phone:** 718-851-1186; **Board Cert:** Ophthalmology 1991; **Med School:** Albert Einstein Coll Med 1984; **Resid:** Ophthalmology, Montefiore Med Ctr 1988; **Fellow:** Medical Retina, Moorefields Eye Hosp 1989

Deutsch, James A MD (Oph) - **Spec Exp:** Strabismus; Cataract Surgery; Glaucoma; Pediatric Ophthalmology; **Hospital:** SUNY Downstate Med Ctr (Univ Hosp Brooklyn) (page 441); **Address:** 110 Remsen St, Ste 1B, Brooklyn, NY 11201-4261; **Phone:** 718-855-8700; **Board Cert:** Ophthalmology 1989; **Med School:** NYU Sch Med 1984; **Resid:** Ophthalmology, Mt Sinai Hosp 1988; **Fellow:** Pediatric Ophthalmology, Wills Eye Hosp 1989; **Fac Appt:** Asst Clin Prof Oph, Mount Sinai Sch Med

Douros, Stella MD (Oph) - **Spec Exp:** Diabetic Eye Disease/Retinopathy; Macular Degeneration; Retina/Vitreous Surgery; **Hospital:** New York Eye & Ear Infirm (page 115), Lenox Hill Hosp (Manh Eye, Ear & Throat Hosp) (page 106); **Address:** 7501 6th Ave Fl 1st, Brooklyn, NY 11209; **Phone:** 718-238-2336; **Board Cert:** Ophthalmology 2009; **Med School:** Albert Einstein Coll Med 1991; **Resid:** Ophthalmology, Lenox Hill Hosp 1995; **Fellow:** Vitreoretinal Surgery, Joslin Diabetes Ctr 1996

Dweck, Monica M MD (Oph) - **Spec Exp:** Eyelid Surgery; Tear Duct Problems; Orbital Diseases; **Hospital:** Mt Sinai Med Ctr (page 102); **Address:** Mt Sinai Doctors Brooklyn Heights, 300 Cadman Plaza W, Fl 17, Brooklyn, NY 11201; **Phone:** 929-210-6200; **Board Cert:** Ophthalmology 2008; **Med School:** SUNY Downstate 1986; **Resid:** Ophthalmology, NY Eye & Ear Infirm 1990; **Fellow:** Oculoplastic Surgery, The Cleveland Clinic 1991

Feinstein, Neil C MD (Oph) - **Spec Exp:** Cataract Surgery; Glaucoma; Diabetic Eye Disease/Retinopathy; Macular Degeneration; **Hospital:** Maimonides Med Ctr (page 98), Lenox Hill Hosp (Manh Eye, Ear & Throat Hosp) (page 106); **Address:** 919 48th St, Brooklyn, NY 11219-2919; **Phone:** 718-435-1800; **Board Cert:** Ophthalmology 1979; **Med School:** Albert Einstein Coll Med 1974; **Resid:** Internal Medicine, Maimonides Med Ctr 1975; Ophthalmology, SUNY Downstate Med Ctr 1978

Freedman, Jeffrey MD/PhD (Oph) - **Spec Exp:** Glaucoma; Uveitis; Retinal Disorders; **Hospital:** Kingsbrook Jewish Med Ctr; **Address:** 161 Atlantic Ave, Ste 203, Brooklyn, NY 11201-6720; **Phone:** 718-596-9086; **Board Cert:** Ophthalmology 1975; **Med School:** South Africa 1964; **Resid:** Internal Medicine, Baragwanat Genl Hosp 1966; Ophthalmology, Transvaal General Hosp 1967; **Fellow:** Ophthalmology, SUNY Downstate Med Ctr 1970; **Fac Appt:** Prof Oph, SUNY Downstate

Hyman, George F MD (Oph) - **Spec Exp:** Corneal Disease; Glaucoma; **Hospital:** Brookdale Univ Hosp Med Ctr; **Address:** Brooklyn Eye Inst, 2460 Flatbush Ave, Ste 4, Brooklyn, NY 11234-5000; **Phone:** 718-252-1200; **Board Cert:** Ophthalmology 1976; **Med School:** Univ MD Sch Med 1968; **Resid:** Ophthalmology, Univ Hosp/Downstate Med Ctr 1974; **Fellow:** Anterior Segment - External Disease, Univ Witwatersrand 1975; **Fac Appt:** Asst Clin Prof Oph, SUNY Downstate

Jaffe, Herbert MD (Oph) - **Spec Exp:** Cataract Surgery; Glaucoma; **Hospital:** Beth Israel Med Ctr- Kings Hwy Div (page 94); **Address:** 2128 Ocean Ave, Brooklyn, NY 11229-1406; **Phone:** 718-339-7469; **Board Cert:** Ophthalmology 1983; **Med School:** Belgium 1968; **Resid:** Ophthalmology, SUNY Downstate Med Ctr 1972

Lazzaro, Douglas R MD (Oph) - **Spec Exp:** Corneal Disease & Surgery; Cornea Transplant; Refractive Surgery; **Hospital:** SUNY Downstate Med Ctr (Univ Hosp Brooklyn) (page 441), Lutheran Med Ctr - Brooklyn; **Address:** Lazzaro Eye Ctr, 7901 4th Ave, Brooklyn, NY 11209; **Phone:** 718-748-1334; **Board Cert:** Ophthalmology 2007; **Med School:** SUNY Downstate 1990; **Resid:** Ophthalmology, SUNY Downstate Med Ctr 1994; **Fellow:** Cornea & Refractive Surgery, Manhattan Eye & Ear Infirmary 1995; **Fac Appt:** Prof Oph, SUNY Downstate

Lebowitz, Mark A MD (Oph) - **Spec Exp:** LASIK-Refractive Surgery; Cataract Surgery; Corneal Disease & Surgery; **Hospital:** Lenox Hill Hosp (Manh Eye, Ear & Throat Hosp) (page 106); **Address:** KLM Ophthalmology, 1301 Avenue J, Brooklyn, NY 11230-3605; **Phone:** 718-284-1921; **Board Cert:** Ophthalmology 2006; **Med School:** NYU Sch Med 1982; **Resid:** Internal Medicine, Beth Israel Med Ctr 1983; Ophthalmology, SUNY Downstate Med Ctr 1986; **Fellow:** Cornea & Ext Eye Disease, Manhattan EET Hosp 1987

Lombardo, James J MD (Oph) - **Spec Exp:** Diabetic Eye Disease/Retinopathy; Glaucoma; **Hospital:** New York Eye & Ear Infirm (page 115); **Address:** Lombardo Ophthalmology, 7801 4th Ave, Brooklyn, NY 11209-3701; **Phone:** 718-836-6661; **Board Cert:** Ophthalmology 1982; **Med School:** NYU Sch Med 1976; **Resid:** Internal Medicine, St Vincent's Hosp & Med Ctr 1977; Ophthalmology, NY Eye & Ear Infirmary 1980

Mogil, Laurey G MD (Oph) - **Spec Exp:** Glaucoma; **Hospital:** Mt Sinai Med Ctr (page 102); **Address:** KLM Ophthalmology, 1301 Avenue J, Brooklyn, NY 11230-3605; **Phone:** 718-645-0600; **Board Cert:** Ophthalmology 2006; **Med School:** Albert Einstein Coll Med 1980; **Resid:** Ophthalmology, Mt Sinai Med Ctr 1984; **Fellow:** Glaucoma, Mt Sinai Med Ctr 1985; **Fac Appt:** Asst Clin Prof Oph, Mount Sinai Sch Med

Reich, Raymond MD (Oph) - **Spec Exp:** Cataract Surgery; Ophthalmic Plastic Surgery; Laser Refractive Surgery; **Hospital:** Maimonides Med Ctr (page 98); **Address:** 1575 E 19th St Fl 1, Brooklyn, NY 11230; **Phone:** 718-332-6200; **Board Cert:** Ophthalmology 1978; **Med School:** Albert Einstein Coll Med 1973; **Resid:** Ophthalmology, Univ Hosp 1977; **Fellow:** Ophthalmic Plastic Surgery, Harvard-Mass EE Infirm 1978; **Fac Appt:** Asst Prof Oph, SUNY Hlth Sci Ctr

Saffra, Norman MD (Oph) - **Spec Exp:** Microsurgery; Retinal Disorders; Diabetic Eye Disease/Retinopathy; **Hospital:** Maimonides Med Ctr (page 98); **Address:** 902 49th St, Brooklyn, NY 11219-2922; **Phone:** 718-283-8000; **Board Cert:** Ophthalmology 2005; **Med School:** Albert Einstein Coll Med 1988; **Resid:** Ophthalmology, Montefiore Med Ctr 1992; **Fellow:** Retina/Vitreous Surgery, SUNY Hlth Sci Ctr 1993; **Fac Appt:** Clin Prof Oph, Mount Sinai Sch Med

Sciortino, Patrick J MD (Oph) - **Spec Exp:** LASIK-Refractive Surgery; Cataract Surgery; Laser Vision Surgery; **Hospital:** New York Comm Hosp; **Address:** The Eye Care Ctr, 914 Bay Ridge Pkwy, Brooklyn, NY 11228-2302; **Phone:** 718-748-5700; **Board Cert:** Ophthalmology 2009; **Med School:** NY Med Coll 1978; **Resid:** Ophthalmology, St Vincents Hosp 1980; Ophthalmology, Catholic Med Ctr 1983; **Fellow:** Neuro-Ophthalmology, Univ Hosp 1984

Seidman, Mitchell S DO (Oph) - **Spec Exp:** Cataract Surgery; **Hospital:** New York Methodist Hosp (page 440); **Address:** 2989 Ocean Pkwy, Brooklyn, NY 11235; **Phone:** 718-332-2020; **Board Cert:** Ophthalmology 1979; **Med School:** Philadelphia Coll Osteo Med 1974; **Resid:** Ophthalmology, Temple Univ Hosp 1978; **Fellow:** Anterior Segment - External Disease, Med Ctr Hosp 1979

Sherman, Steven I DO (Oph) - **Spec Exp:** Glaucoma; Anterior Segment Surgery; **Hospital:** New York Methodist Hosp (page 440), Interfaith Med Ctr; **Address:** 2303 Avenue Z Fl 1, Brooklyn, NY 11235-2805; **Phone:** 718-934-6600; **Board Cert:** Ophthalmology 1990; **Med School:** Univ Osteo Med & Hlth Sci, Des Moines 1977; **Resid:** Internal Medicine, Coney Island Hosp 1979; Ophthalmology, UHPHS Hosp 1982; **Fellow:** Glaucoma, Kings Co Hosp Ctr 1983; **Fac Appt:** Asst Clin Prof Oph, Touro Coll Osteopathic Med-NY

Smith, Edward F MD (Oph) - **Spec Exp:** Cataract Surgery; Neuro-Ophthalmology; **Hospital:** SUNY Downstate Med Ctr (Univ Hosp Brooklyn) (page 441), Kingsbrook Jewish Med Ctr; **Address:** Downstate Ophthalmology Assocs, 34 Plaza St East, Brooklyn, NY 11238; **Phone:** 718-638-2020; **Board Cert:** Ophthalmology 1989; **Med School:** SUNY Downstate 1984; **Resid:** Ophthalmology, Univ Hosp 1988; **Fellow:** Neuro-Ophthalmology, Univ Hosp 1989; **Fac Appt:** Assoc Clin Prof Oph, SUNY Downstate

Stein, Arnold Jay MD (Oph) - **Spec Exp:** Retinal Disorders; Glaucoma; Cataract Surgery; Laser Surgery; **Hospital:** Beth Israel Med Ctr- Kings Hwy Div (page 94), Long Is Jewish Med Ctr (page 106); **Address:** 1226 Ocean Pkwy, Lobby Lvl, Ste 1, Brooklyn, NY 11230; **Phone:** 718-692-0400; **Board Cert:** Ophthalmology 1987; **Med School:** SUNY Downstate 1982; **Resid:** Ophthalmology, LI Jewish Med Ctr 1986; **Fac Appt:** Asst Clin Prof Oph, Albert Einstein Coll Med

Unterricht, Sam L MD (Oph) - **Spec Exp:** Macular Disease/Degeneration; Retinal Disorders; Optic Nerve Disorders; Neuro-Ophthalmology; **Hospital:** New York Methodist Hosp (page 440), Kingsbrook Jewish Med Ctr; **Address:** 20 Plaza St E, Brooklyn, NY 11238-4955; **Phone:** 718-622-5800; **Board Cert:** Ophthalmology 1982; **Med School:** SUNY Downstate 1976; **Resid:** Ophthalmology, Univ Hosp 1980; **Fellow:** Neuro-Ophthalmology, Kingsbrook Jewish MC 1981; Retina/Vitreous Surgery, Univ Hosp 1982; **Fac Appt:** Asst Clin Prof Oph, SUNY Downstate

Zellner, James H MD (Oph) - **Spec Exp:** Laser Refractive Surgery; Cataract Surgery; **Hospital:** New York Eye & Ear Infirm (page 115); **Address:** 7817 5th Ave, Brooklyn, NY 11209-2702; **Phone:** 718-748-2020; **Board Cert:** Ophthalmology 1982; **Med School:** Albert Einstein Coll Med 1977; **Resid:** Ophthalmology, SUNY Downstate Med Ctr 1981

Orthopaedic Surgery

Kolker, Dov M MD (OrS) - **Spec Exp:** Foot & Ankle Surgery; Knee Injuries; Trauma; Sports Medicine; **Hospital:** Maimonides Med Ctr (page 98), Mt Sinai Med Ctr (page 102); **Address:** 1301 57th St, Brooklyn, NY 11219; **Phone:** 212-744-2200; **Board Cert:** Orthopaedic Surgery 2008; **Med School:** Tufts Univ 1994; **Resid:** Surgery, Beth Israel Deaconess Hosp 1995; Orthopaedic Surgery, U Mass Med Ctr 1999; **Fellow:** Trauma, AO Trauma Program, Berne 2000; Foot & Ankle Surgery, Mt Sinai Med Ctr 2001

Mani, John Vijay MD (OrS) - **Spec Exp:** Hip Replacement; Knee Replacement; **Hospital:** Lutheran Med Ctr - Brooklyn; **Address:** 161 Atlantic Ave, Brooklyn, NY 11201-6720; **Phone:** 718-855-0088; **Board Cert:** Orthopaedic Surgery 1977; **Med School:** India 1970; **Resid:** Orthopaedic Surgery, Brookdale Hosp 1976; **Fellow:** Arthritis Surgery, Hosp for Special Surgery 1978; **Fac Appt:** Assoc Clin Prof OrS, SUNY Hlth Sci Ctr

Menezes, Placido A MD (OrS) - **Spec Exp:** Knee Replacement; Fractures; Joint Replacement; **Hospital:** New York Methodist Hosp (page 440); **Address:** 543 2nd St, Brooklyn, NY 11215-2607; **Phone:** 718-788-7600; **Board Cert:** Orthopaedic Surgery 1980; **Med School:** India 1970; **Resid:** Surgery, NY Methodist Hosp 1976; Orthopaedic Surgery, Brooklyn Jewish Hosp & Med Ctr 1978

Merola, Andrew A MD (OrS) - **Spec Exp:** Spinal Surgery; Scoliosis; **Hospital:** New York Methodist Hosp (page 440), Mt Sinai Med Ctr (page 102); **Address:** 567 1st St, Brooklyn, NY 11215; **Phone:** 718-783-5542; **Board Cert:** Orthopaedic Surgery 2009; **Med School:** Howard Univ 1990; **Resid:** Orthopaedic Surgery, Kings Co Hosp/SUNY Downstate 1995; **Fellow:** Spine Surgery, Univ Colorado Med Ctr 1996; **Fac Appt:** Assoc Prof OrS, SUNY Downstate

Morgan, Daniel J MD (OrS) - **Spec Exp:** Arthroscopic Surgery; Hip & Knee Replacement; Shoulder Surgery; PRP (Platelet Rich Plasma); **Hospital:** Beth Israel Med Ctr- Kings Hwy Div (page 94); **Address:** Kings Hwy Orthopedic Assocs, 3131 Kings Hwy, Ste C11, Brooklyn, NY 11234-2643; **Phone:** 718-258-2588; **Board Cert:** Orthopaedic Surgery 2011; **Med School:** Univ MD Sch Med 1985; **Resid:** Surgery, Washington Hosp Ctr 1986; Orthopaedic Surgery, Kingsbrook Jewish Med Ctr 1997

Soifer, Todd B MD (OrS) - **Spec Exp:** Arthritis; Knee Injuries; Arthroscopic Surgery; Rotator Cuff Surgery; **Hospital:** Beth Israel Med Ctr- Kings Hwy Div (page 94); **Address:** Kings Hwy Orthopedic Assocs, 3131 Kings Hwy, Ste C11, Brooklyn, NY 11234-2643; **Phone:** 718-258-2588; **Board Cert:** Orthopaedic Surgery 2007; **Med School:** Mount Sinai Sch Med 1989; **Resid:** Orthopaedic Surgery, Beth Israel Med Ctr-Kingsbrook Jewish Med Ctr 1994

Splain, Shepard H DO (OrS) - **Spec Exp:** Arthroscopic Surgery; Shoulder & Knee Reconstruction; Sports Medicine; Joint Replacement; **Hospital:** Brookdale Univ Hosp Med Ctr; **Address:** 1 Brookdale Plaza, Ste 152, Brooklyn, NY 11212; **Phone:** 718-240-5888; **Board Cert:** Orthopaedic Surgery 1980; **Med School:** Mich State Univ Coll Osteo Med 1973; **Resid:** Orthopaedic Surgery, Brookdale Hosp 1978; **Fellow:** Sports Medicine, Oklahoma Hlth Scis Ctr 1979; **Fac Appt:** Assoc Clin Prof OrS, SUNY Downstate

Tepler, Melvin MD (OrS) - **Spec Exp:** Fractures; **Hospital:** Maimonides Med Ctr (page 98); **Address:** 1252 E 9th St, Brooklyn, NY 11230-5180; **Phone:** 718-677-6000; **Board Cert:** Orthopaedic Surgery 2009; **Med School:** NY Med Coll 1980; **Resid:** Surgery, Maimonides Med Ctr 1981; Orthopaedic Surgery, Maimonides Med Ctr 1985

Urban Jr, William P MD (OrS) - **Spec Exp:** Sports Medicine; Arthroscopic Surgery; Shoulder & Knee Surgery; **Hospital:** SUNY Downstate Med Ctr (Univ Hosp Brooklyn) (page 441); **Address:** SUNY Downstate Medical Ctr, Dept Orthopaedic Surgery & Rehab Medicine, 450 Clarkson Ave, Box 30, Brooklyn, NY 11203; **Phone:** 718-270-4673; **Board Cert:** Orthopaedic Surgery 2009; **Med School:** SUNY Downstate 1990; **Resid:** Orthopaedic Surgery, SUNY Downstate Medical Ctr 1994; **Fellow:** Orthopaedic Sports Medicine, Univ Kentucky Med Ctr 1995; **Fac Appt:** Assoc Prof OrS, SUNY Downstate

Walsh, Raymond B MD (OrS) - **Spec Exp:** Hip Replacement; Knee Replacement; **Hospital:** Lutheran Med Ctr - Brooklyn; **Address:** Ovington Orthopedic Assocs, 6900 4th Ave Fl 2nd, Brooklyn, NY 11209-1453; **Phone:** 718-238-6400; **Board Cert:** Orthopaedic Surgery 1981; **Med School:** England, UK 1974; **Resid:** Surgery, Maimonides Med Ctr 1976; Orthopaedic Surgery, Maimonides Med Ctr 1980

Otolaryngology

Branovan, Daniel Igor MD (Oto) - **Spec Exp:** Sinus Disorders/Surgery; Endoscopic Sinus Surgery; Minimally Invasive Surgery; **Address:** NY Ear, Nose & Throat Inst, 1810 Voorhies Ave, Brooklyn, NY 11235; **Phone:** 718-616-1000; **Board Cert:** Otolaryngology 1999; **Med School:** Stanford Univ 1992; **Resid:** Surgery, St Vincent's Hosp 1993; Otolaryngology, NY E&E Infirm 1997

Chaudhry, M Rashid MD (Oto) - **Spec Exp:** Cosmetic Surgery-Face; Sinus Surgery; Head & Neck Cancer Reconstruction; **Hospital:** Brookdale Univ Hosp Med Ctr; **Address:** 1 Brookdale Plaza, Ste 157-CHC, Brooklyn, NY 11212; **Phone:** 718-240-6366; **Board Cert:** Otolaryngology 1978; **Med School:** Pakistan 1969; **Resid:** Surgery, Downstate Med Ctr-Kings Co 1974; Otolaryngology, Downstate Med Ctr-Kings Co 1978; **Fac Appt:** Asst Prof Oto, SUNY Downstate

Hanson, Matthew B MD (Oto) - **Spec Exp:** Otology; **Hospital:** SUNY Downstate Med Ctr (Univ Hosp Brooklyn) (page 441); **Address:** 470 Clarkson Ave, Box 126, Brooklyn, NY 11203; **Phone:** 718-270-4701; **Board Cert:** Otolaryngology 1997; Neurotology 2008; **Med School:** Univ Iowa Coll Med 1989; **Resid:** Otolaryngology, Columbia-Presby Med Ctr 1995; **Fellow:** Neurotology, Baptist Hosp 1997; **Fac Appt:** Asst Prof Oto, SUNY Downstate

Lagmay, Victor M MD (Oto) - **Spec Exp:** Thyroid & Parathyroid Surgery; Head & Neck Cancer & Surgery; Endoscopic Sinus Surgery; **Hospital:** Maimonides Med Ctr (page 98), Lutheran Med Ctr - Brooklyn; **Address:** 919 49th St, Brooklyn, NY 11219; **Phone:** 718-283-6260; **Board Cert:** Otolaryngology 1999; **Med School:** NYU Sch Med 1992; **Resid:** Otolaryngology, NYU Med Ctr 1998; **Fellow:** Head and Neck Surgery, Beth Israel Med Ctr 1999; **Fac Appt:** Asst Clin Prof S, SUNY Downstate

Vastola, A Paul MD (Oto) - **Spec Exp:** Throat Disorders; Pediatric Otolaryngology; Cleft Palate/Lip; **Hospital:** Maimonides Med Ctr (page 98); **Address:** 919 49th St, Brooklyn, NY 11219-2916; **Phone:** 718-283-6260; **Board Cert:** Otolaryngology 1995; **Med School:** Boston Univ 1988; **Resid:** Surgery, NY Hosp-Cornell Med Ctr 1990; Otolaryngology, Manhattan Eye, Ear & Throat Hosp 1993; **Fellow:** Pediatric Otolaryngology, Texas Chldn's Hosp 1994; **Fac Appt:** Asst Clin Prof Oto, SUNY Downstate

Pain Medicine

Lefkowitz, Mathew MD (PM) - **Spec Exp:** Pain-Low Back; Pain-after Spinal Intervention; Sciatica; Pain-Back & Neck; **Hospital:** New York Methodist Hosp (page 440); **Address:** 185 Montague St Fl 6, Brooklyn, NY 11201; **Phone:** 718-625-4244; **Board Cert:** Anesthesiology 1993; Pain Medicine 2005; **Med School:** Belgium 1983; **Resid:** Anesthesiology, Mount Sinai Hosp 1986; **Fellow:** Pain Medicine, Mount Sinai Hosp 1987

Pathology

Mirra, Suzanne S MD (Path) - **Spec Exp:** Neuropathology; Alzheimer's Disease; **Hospital:** SUNY Downstate Med Ctr (Univ Hosp Brooklyn) (page 441), Kings Co Hosp Ctr; **Address:** SUNY Health Science Ctr, Dept Pathology, 450 Clarkson Ave, Box 25, Brooklyn, NY 11203; **Phone:** 718-270-4599; **Board Cert:** Anatomic Pathology 1973; Neuropathology 1973; **Med School:** SUNY Downstate 1967; **Resid:** Anatomic Pathology, Kings Co Hosp 1970; Neuropathology, Montefiore Med Ctr 1971; **Fellow:** Neuropathology, Yale Univ 1973; **Fac Appt:** Prof Path, SUNY Downstate

Vigorita, Vincent J MD (Path) - **Spec Exp:** Bone Pathology; Surgical Pathology; **Hospital:** Maimonides Med Ctr (page 98), SUNY Downstate Med Ctr (Univ Hosp Brooklyn) (page 441); **Address:** 4802 Tenth Ave, Brooklyn, NY 11219; **Phone:** 917-648-5945; **Board Cert:** Anatomic Pathology 1980; **Med School:** NY Med Coll 1976; **Resid:** Pathology, Johns Hopkins Hosp 1978; **Fellow:** Pathology, Meml Sloan Kettering Cancer Ctr 1979; **Fac Appt:** Prof Path, SUNY Downstate

Pediatric Cardiology

Kaplovitz, Harry S MD (PCd) - **Spec Exp:** Syncope; Echocardiography; Heart Failure; **Hospital:** Maimonides Med Ctr (page 98); **Address:** Maimonides Med Ctr, 4802 Tenth Ave, rm K106, Brooklyn, NY 11219; **Phone:** 718-283-7500; **Board Cert:** Pediatrics 1988; Pediatric Cardiology 2007; **Med School:** Albert Einstein Coll Med 1981; **Resid:** Pediatrics, North Shore Univ Hosp 1984; **Fellow:** Pediatric Cardiology, NYU Med Ctr 1986

Ramaswamy, Prema MD (PCd) - **Spec Exp:** Fetal Echocardiography; Congenital Heart Disease; **Hospital:** Maimonides Med Ctr (page 98); **Address:** 4802 10th Ave, rm K106, Brooklyn, NY 11219-2844; **Phone:** 718-283-7500; **Board Cert:** Pediatrics 2009; Pediatric Cardiology 2011; **Med School:** India 1986; **Resid:** Pediatrics, M Y Hosp 1990; Pediatrics, Montefiore Med Ctr 1993; **Fellow:** Pediatric Cardiology, NY Hosp-Cornell 1996; **Fac Appt:** Asst Prof Ped, Mount Sinai Sch Med

Pediatric Endocrinology

Agdere, Levon MD (PEn) - **Spec Exp:** Diabetes; Short Stature in Children; Thyroid Disorders; **Hospital:** New York Methodist Hosp (page 440); **Address:** 263 7th Ave, Ste 3B, Brooklyn, NY 11215; **Phone:** 718-246-8540; **Board Cert:** Pediatric Endocrinology 2013; **Med School:** Turkey 1981; **Resid:** Pediatrics, Lutheran Med Ctr 1986; **Fellow:** Pediatric Endocrinology, NY Hosp-Cornell Med Ctr 1989

Avruskin, Theodore W MD (PEn) - **Spec Exp:** Growth Disorders; Diabetes; Thyroid Disorders; **Hospital:** Brookdale Univ Hosp Med Ctr, SUNY Downstate Med Ctr (Univ Hosp Brooklyn) (page 441); **Address:** 1 Brookdale Plaza, Ste 222, Brooklyn, NY 11212; **Phone:** 718-240-5960; **Board Cert:** Pediatrics 1965; **Med School:** Univ Toronto 1960; **Resid:** Pediatrics, Montreal Chldns Hosp 1962; Pediatrics, Chldns Hosp Med Ctr 1964; **Fellow:** Pediatric Endocrinology, Chldns Hosp Med Ctr 1968

Pediatric Gastroenterology

Jelin, Abraham MD (PGe) - **Spec Exp:** Nutrition; Breast Feeding Problems; Gastroesophageal Reflux Disease (GERD); Constipation; **Hospital:** Brooklyn Hosp Ctr; **Address:** 240 Willoughby St, Brooklyn, NY 11201; **Phone:** 718-250-6277; **Board Cert:** Pediatrics 1977; Pediatric Gastroenterology 2012; **Med School:** NYU Sch Med 1972; **Resid:** Pediatrics, Montefiore Med Ctr 1974; Pediatrics, Brookdale Univ Hosp 1975; **Fellow:** Pediatric Gastroenterology, Emory Univ Hosp 1977; **Fac Appt:** Asst Clin Prof Ped, NYU Sch Med

McFarlane-Ferreira, Yvonne B MD (PGe) - **Spec Exp:** Pain-Abdominal Recurrent; Failure to Thrive; Constipation; Inflammatory Bowel Disease; **Hospital:** New York Methodist Hosp (page 440), Brooklyn Hosp Ctr; **Address:** 263 7th Ave, Ste 3B, Brooklyn, NY 11215; **Phone:** 718-246-8515; **Board Cert:** Pediatrics 2012; Pediatric Gastroenterology 2010; **Med School:** West Indies 1983; **Resid:** Anesthesiology, Princess Margaret Hosp 1986; Pediatrics, Brooklyn Hosp 1989; **Fellow:** Pediatric Gastroenterology, Mt Sinai Hosp 1992; **Fac Appt:** Asst Clin Prof Ped, Cornell Univ-Weill Med Coll

Rabinowitz, Simon S MD/PhD (PGe) - **Spec Exp:** Inflammatory Bowel Disease; Hepatitis; Gastroesophageal Reflux Disease (GERD); Gastrointestinal Disorders; **Hospital:** SUNY Downstate Med Ctr (Univ Hosp Brooklyn) (page 441); **Address:** SUNY Downstate Med Ctr, 445 Lenox Rd, Box 49, Brooklyn, NY 11203; **Phone:** 718-270-4714; **Board Cert:** Pediatrics 2009; Pediatric Gastroenterology 2007; **Med School:** Univ Miami Sch Med 1983; **Resid:** Pediatrics, Mount Sinai Hosp 1985; **Fellow:** Pediatric Gastroenterology, Mount Sinai Hosp 1987

Schwarz, Steven M MD (PGe) - **Spec Exp:** Gastroesophageal Reflux Disease (GERD); Nutrition; Endoscopy; Inflammatory Bowel Disease; **Hospital:** SUNY Downstate Med Ctr (Univ Hosp Brooklyn) (page 441), Beth Israel Med Ctr - Petrie Div (page 94); **Address:** Children's Hosp at SUNY Downstate, 445 Lenox Rd, Box 49, Brooklyn, NY 11203; **Phone:** 718-270-4714; **Board Cert:** Pediatrics 1979; Pediatric Gastroenterology 2012; **Med School:** Columbia P&S 1974; **Resid:** Pediatrics, Columbia-Presby Med Ctr 1977; **Fellow:** Pediatric Gastroenterology, Stanford Univ Med Ctr 1978; Pediatric Gastroenterology, Columbia-Presby Med Ctr 1980; **Fac Appt:** Prof Ped, SUNY Downstate

Wetzler, Graciela MD (PGe) - **Spec Exp:** Gastroesophageal Reflux Disease (GERD); Inflammatory Bowel Disease/Crohn's; Peptic Ulcer Disease; **Hospital:** Maimonides Med Ctr (page 98); **Address:** Maimonides Med Ctr, Dept Peds GE, 948 48th St, Brooklyn, NY 11219; **Phone:** 718-283-7500; **Board Cert:** Pediatric Gastroenterology 2010; **Med School:** Argentina 1984; **Resid:** Pediatrics, Montefiore Med Ctr 1992; **Fellow:** Pediatric Gastroenterology, NY Hosp-Cornell Med Ctr 1995; **Fac Appt:** Assoc Clin Prof Ped, SUNY Downstate

Pediatric Hematology-Oncology

Guarini, Ludovico MD (PHO) - **Spec Exp:** Leukemia; Solid Tumors; **Hospital:** Maimonides Med Ctr (page 98); **Address:** Maimonides Med Ctr-Pediatrics Dept, 6300 Eighth Ave Fl 2, Brooklyn, NY 11220; **Phone:** 718-765-2671; **Board Cert:** Pediatrics 1984; Pediatric Hematology-Oncology 2007; **Med School:** Italy 1974; **Resid:** Pediatrics, Beth Israel Hosp 1981; **Fellow:** Pediatric Hematology-Oncology, Columbia-Presby Med Ctr 1984; **Fac Appt:** Assoc Prof Ped, SUNY Hlth Sci Ctr

Kulpa, Jolanta MD (PHO) - **Spec Exp:** Sickle Cell Disease; Leukemia; Thalassemia; Bleeding/Coagulation Disorders; **Hospital:** New York Methodist Hosp (page 440); **Address:** 502 8th Ave, Brooklyn, NY 11215; **Phone:** 718-780-3066; **Board Cert:** Pediatrics 1983; Pediatric Hematology-Oncology 1984; **Med School:** Med Coll PA 1972; **Resid:** Pediatrics, Lenox Hill Hosp 1975; **Fellow:** Blood Banking Transfusion Medicine, NY Blood Center 1977; Pediatric Hematology-Oncology, NY Hosp/Cornell/Sloan Kettering 1979

Miller, Scott T MD (PHO) - **Spec Exp:** Sickle Cell Disease; **Hospital:** SUNY Downstate Med Ctr (Univ Hosp Brooklyn) (page 441); **Address:** Univ Hosp Brooklyn, 450 Clarkson Ave, Box 49, Brooklyn, NY 11203-2056; **Phone:** 718-270-4714; **Board Cert:** Pediatrics 1981; Pediatric Hematology-Oncology 1982; **Med School:** Albert Einstein Coll Med 1976; **Resid:** Pediatrics, Montefiore Med Ctr 1979; **Fellow:** Pediatric Hematology-Oncology, Meml Sloan Kettering-Cornell Med Ctr 1981

Sadanandan, Swayam MD (PHO) - **Spec Exp:** Sickle Cell Disease; Bleeding/Coagulation Disorders; Anemia; Pediatric Cancers; **Hospital:** Brooklyn Hosp Ctr; **Address:** 121 DeKalb Ave, Brooklyn, NY 11201; **Phone:** 718-250-6074; **Board Cert:** Pediatrics 1980; Pediatric Hematology-Oncology 1984; **Med School:** India 1972; **Resid:** Pediatrics, St Vincent's Hosp & Med Ctr 1979; **Fellow:** Pediatric Hematology-Oncology, NYU Med Ctr 1981

Sundaram, Revathy MD (PHO) - **Spec Exp:** Thalassemia; Sickle Cell Disease; Leukemia; **Hospital:** New York Methodist Hosp (page 440); **Address:** 502 8th Ave, Brooklyn, NY 11215; **Phone:** 718-780-3066; **Board Cert:** Pediatrics 1980; Pediatric Hematology-Oncology 1984; **Med School:** India 1973; **Resid:** Pediatrics, Rutgers Univ Hosp 1978; Pediatrics, Long Island Hosp 1980; **Fellow:** Pediatric Hematology-Oncology, Long Island Hosp 1983; **Fac Appt:** Asst Prof Ped, SUNY Hlth Sci Ctr

Viswanathan, Kusum MD (PHO) - **Spec Exp:** Sickle Cell Disease; Pediatric Cancers; Anemia; **Hospital:** Brookdale Univ Hosp Med Ctr; **Address:** 1 Brookdale Plaza, rm 346-CHC, Brooklyn, NY 11212-3139; **Phone:** 718-240-5904; **Board Cert:** Pediatrics 1986; Pediatric Hematology-Oncology 1987; **Med School:** India 1980; **Resid:** Pediatrics, Long Island Coll Hosp 1984; **Fellow:** Pediatric Hematology-Oncology, Long Island Coll Hosp 1986

Pediatric Infectious Disease

Gesner, Matthew J MD (PInf) - **Spec Exp:** AIDS/HIV; Kawasaki Disease; **Hospital:** Kings Co Hosp Ctr, SUNY Downstate Med Ctr (Univ Hosp Brooklyn) (page 441); **Address:** Kings County Hosp, 451 Clarkson Ave, Box 294, Brooklyn, NY 11203; **Phone:** 718-245-2562; **Board Cert:** Pediatrics 2013; Pediatric Infectious Disease 2009; **Med School:** SUNY Downstate 1988; **Resid:** Pediatrics, Chldns Hosp 1991; **Fellow:** Pediatric Infectious Disease, Bellevue Hosp Ctr 1994; **Fac Appt:** Asst Prof Ped, SUNY Downstate

Pediatric Nephrology

Kaplan, Matthew R MD (PNep) - **Spec Exp:** Hypertension; Glomerulonephritis; **Hospital:** Brooklyn Hosp Ctr, Maimonides Med Ctr (page 98); **Address:** Brooklyn Hosp Ctr, 240 Willoughby St Fl 9, Brooklyn, NY 11201; **Phone:** 718-250-6911; **Board Cert:** Pediatrics 1974; Pediatric Nephrology 1976; **Med School:** SUNY Downstate 1969; **Resid:** Pediatrics, Presby/Weill Cornell Med Ctr 1973; **Fellow:** Pediatric Nephrology, Presby/Weill Cornell Med Ctr 1976; **Fac Appt:** Assoc Clin Prof Ped, SUNY Downstate

Schoeneman, Morris J MD (PNep) - **Spec Exp:** Hypertension; Kidney Failure-Chronic; Urinary Tract Infections; Dialysis Care; **Hospital:** SUNY Downstate Med Ctr (Univ Hosp Brooklyn) (page 441), Maimonides Med Ctr (page 98); **Address:** SUNY Downstate Med Ctr, 470 Clarkson Ave, Box 49, Brooklyn, NY 11203; **Phone:** 718-270-4714; **Board Cert:** Pediatrics 1974; Pediatric Nephrology 1974; **Med School:** Georgetown Univ 1969; **Resid:** Pediatrics, Univ Maryland Med Ctr 1972; **Fellow:** Pediatric Nephrology, Montefiore Med Ctr 1975

Pediatric Otolaryngology

Goldsmith, Ari J MD (PO) - **Spec Exp:** Voice Disorders; Airway Disorders; Hearing Loss; Sleep Apnea; **Hospital:** Maimonides Med Ctr (page 98); **Address:** 921 49th St, Brooklyn, NY 11219; **Phone:** 718-283-6260 x2; **Board Cert:** Otolaryngology 1994; **Med School:** Albert Einstein Coll Med 1988; **Resid:** Otolaryngology, LI Jewish Hosp 1993; **Fellow:** Pediatric Otolaryngology, Chldns Hosp 1994; **Fac Appt:** Assoc Prof Oto, SUNY Hlth Sci Ctr

Rosenfeld, Richard M MD (PO) - **Spec Exp:** Sinus Disorders/Surgery; Head & Neck Surgery; Ear Disorders/Surgery; **Hospital:** SUNY Downstate Med Ctr (Univ Hosp Brooklyn) (page 441); **Address:** Univ Otolaryngologists, 134 Atlantic Ave, Brooklyn, NY 11201; **Phone:** 718-780-1498; **Board Cert:** Otolaryngology 1989; **Med School:** SUNY Buffalo 1984; **Resid:** Surgery, Mount Sinai Med Ctr 1986; Otolaryngology, Mount Sinai Med Ctr 1989; **Fellow:** Pediatric Otolaryngology, Chldn's Hosp 1991; **Fac Appt:** Prof Oto, SUNY Downstate

Pediatric Pulmonology

Giusti, Robert J MD (PPul) - **Spec Exp:** Cystic Fibrosis; Asthma; Cough-Chronic; **Hospital:** NYU Langone Med Ctr (page 108); **Address:** NYU Pediatric Pulmonology, 160 E 32nd St, L-3 Medical, New York, NY 10016; **Phone:** 212-263-5940; **Board Cert:** Pediatrics 1987; Pediatric Pulmonology 2011; **Med School:** SUNY Downstate 1981; **Resid:** Pediatrics, Bellevue Hosp 1985; **Fac Appt:** Assoc Clin Prof Ped, NYU Sch Med

Lee, Haesoon MD (PPul) - **Spec Exp:** Asthma; Sleep Apnea; Tuberculosis; Airway Disorders; **Hospital:** SUNY Downstate Med Ctr (Univ Hosp Brooklyn) (page 441), Kings Co Hosp Ctr; **Address:** SUNY-Downstate Med Ctr, Dept Pediatrics, 450 Clarkson Ave, Box 49, Brooklyn, NY 11203-2056; **Phone:** 718-221-5316; **Board Cert:** Pediatrics 1979; Pediatric Pulmonology 2011; **Med School:** South Korea 1972; **Resid:** Pediatrics, St Francis Hosp 1975; **Fellow:** Pediatric Pulmonology, Albert Einstein Affil Hosp 1977; **Fac Appt:** Assoc Prof Ped, SUNY Downstate

Marcus, Michael MD (PPul) - **Spec Exp:** Asthma; Sleep Apnea; Chronic Lung Disease; Gastroesophageal Reflux Disease (GERD); **Hospital:** Maimonides Med Ctr (page 98), Richmond Univ Med Ctr; **Address:** 948 48th St, brooklyn, NY 11219; **Phone:** 718-980-5864; **Board Cert:** Pediatrics 1984; Allergy & Immunology 1987; Pediatric Pulmonology 2009; **Med School:** SUNY Stony Brook 1980; **Resid:** Pediatrics, Nassau County Med Ctr 1983; **Fellow:** Pediatric Pulmonology, Chldn's Hosp 1985; Allergy & Immunology, Chldn's Hosp 1985; **Fac Appt:** Assoc Clin Prof Ped, NYU Sch Med

Narula, Pramod MD (PPul) - **Spec Exp:** Asthma; Chronic Lung Disease; **Hospital:** New York Methodist Hosp (page 440); **Address:** 502 8th Ave, Brooklyn, NY 11215-3609; **Phone:** 718-780-3066; **Board Cert:** Pediatrics 2012; Pediatric Pulmonology 2009; **Med School:** India 1977; **Resid:** Pediatrics, Winthrop Univ Hosp 1990; **Fellow:** Pediatric Pulmonology, Columbia-Presby Med Ctr 1994; **Fac Appt:** Clin Prof Ped, Cornell Univ-Weill Med Coll

Needleman, Joshua MD (PPul) - **Spec Exp:** Asthma & Chronic Lung Disease; Cystic Fibrosis; Bronchoscopy; Exercise Physiology; **Hospital:** Maimonides Med Ctr (page 98); **Address:** Maimonides Med Ctr - Pediatric Pulmonary, 949 48 St, Brooklyn, NY 11219; **Phone:** 718-283-7500; **Board Cert:** Pediatric Pulmonology 2013; **Med School:** Temple Univ 1991; **Resid:** Pediatrics, Univ MD Med Ctr 1995; **Fellow:** Pediatric Pulmonology, St Christophers Hosp Chldn 1998

Pediatric Surgery

Kessler, Edmund MD (PS) - **Spec Exp:** Neck Masses; Tumor Surgery; Gallbladder Surgery-Pediatric; Neonatal Surgery; **Hospital:** Steven & Alexandra Cohen Chldn's Med Ctr of NY (page 106), New York Methodist Hosp (page 440); **Address:** 1000 Northern Blvd, Bldg 2 - Ste 250, Great Neck, NY 11021; **Phone:** 516-498-9000; **Med School:** South Africa 1968; **Resid:** Surgery, Univ Witwatersrand Affil Hosp 1970; **Fellow:** Pediatric Surgery, Univ Witwatersrand 1977; **Fac Appt:** Asst Clin Prof S, Columbia P&S

Pediatric Urology

Friedman, Steven C MD (Ped Uro) - **Spec Exp:** Urinary Tract Infections; Robotic Urologic Surgery; Urinary Reconstruction; Genital Reconstruction-Pediatric; **Hospital:** Maimonides Med Ctr (page 98); **Address:** 909 49th St, Brooklyn, NY 11219; **Phone:** 718-283-7743; **Board Cert:** Urology 2010; Pediatric Urology 2010; **Med School:** SUNY Downstate 1983; **Resid:** Surgery, Beth Israel 1985; Urology, Maimonides Med Ctr 1988; **Fellow:** Pediatric Urology, Chldns Hosp 1991

Pediatrics

Ajl, Stephen MD (Ped) *PCP* - **Spec Exp:** Child Abuse; **Hospital:** Brooklyn Hosp Ctr; **Address:** 121 DeKalb Ave, Brooklyn, NY 11201; **Phone:** 718-250-8764; **Board Cert:** Pediatrics 1980; Child Abuse Pediatrics 2009; **Med School:** Temple Univ 1975; **Resid:** Pediatrics, NY-Presby Hosp/Cornell 1978; **Fellow:** Ambulatory Pediatrics, Mount Sinai Med Ctr 1979

Fernandes, David R MD (Ped) *PCP* - **Hospital:** New York Methodist Hosp (page 440); **Address:** 126 95th St, Brooklyn, NY 11209-7203; **Phone:** 718-238-7842; **Board Cert:** Pediatrics 1980; **Med School:** SUNY Downstate 1972; **Resid:** Pediatrics, Kings County Hosp 1974; Pediatrics, N Shore Univ Hosp 1976; **Fellow:** Ambulatory Pediatrics, NYU-Bellevue Hosp 1977; **Fac Appt:** Asst Clin Prof Ped, SUNY Downstate

Glaser, Amy L MD (Ped) *PCP* - **Hospital:** NYU Langone Med Ctr (page 108); **Address:** Slope Pediatrics, 60 8th Ave, Brooklyn, NY 11217-3902; **Phone:** 718-636-0019; **Board Cert:** Pediatrics 1985; **Med School:** Mount Sinai Sch Med 1979; **Resid:** Pediatrics, Montefiore Med Ctr 1983; **Fellow:** Adolescent Medicine, Mt Sinai Med Ctr 1985

Jackson, Rosemary M MD (Ped) *PCP* - **Spec Exp:** Diabetes; Obesity; **Hospital:** SUNY Downstate Med Ctr (Univ Hosp Brooklyn) (page 441); **Address:** 86 E 49th St, Ste G, Brooklyn, NY 11203; **Phone:** 718-363-6646; **Board Cert:** Pediatrics 2008; **Med School:** SUNY Upstate Med Univ 1985; **Resid:** Pediatrics, SUNY Downstate Med Ctr 1988; **Fac Appt:** Asst Clin Prof Ped, SUNY Downstate

Laraque, Danielle MD (Ped) *PCP* - **Spec Exp:** Child Abuse; **Hospital:** Maimonides Med Ctr (page 98); **Address:** Maimonides Med Ctr, Dept Pediatrics, 977 48th St, Brooklyn, NY 11219; **Phone:** 718-283-6150; **Board Cert:** Pediatrics 1986; Child Abuse Pediatrics 2009; **Med School:** UCLA 1981; **Resid:** Pediatrics, Chldns Hosp 1984; **Fellow:** Academic Pediatrics, Chldns Hosp 1986

Oghia, Hady MD (Ped) *PCP* - **Hospital:** Richmond Univ Med Ctr; **Address:** 7506 16th Ave, Brooklyn, NY 11214-1064; **Phone:** 718-331-3166; **Med School:** Mexico 1979; **Resid:** Pediatrics, Sisters of Charity Hlth Sys 1983

Oppenheim, Jennifer A MD (Ped) *PCP* - **Spec Exp:** Special Health Care Needs; **Hospital:** NYU Langone Med Ctr (page 108); **Address:** Pediatric Assocs NYC, 20 Plaza St E, Ste A7, Brooklyn, NY 11238; **Phone:** 718-857-5500; **Board Cert:** Pediatrics 2007; **Med School:** Cornell Univ 1996; **Resid:** Pediatrics, Bellevue Hosp/NYU Med Ctr 1999

Preis, Oded MD (Ped) *PCP* - **Spec Exp:** Prematurity/Low Birth Weight Infants; **Hospital:** Maimonides Med Ctr (page 98); **Address:** 1729 E 12th St, Brooklyn, NY 11229; **Phone:** 718-339-4919; **Board Cert:** Pediatrics 1978; Neonatal-Perinatal Medicine 1981; **Med School:** Israel 1971; **Resid:** Pediatrics, Maimonides Med Ctr 1975; **Fellow:** Neonatal-Perinatal Medicine, SUNY Downstate Med Ctr 1977; **Fac Appt:** Assoc Clin Prof Ped, SUNY Downstate

Sergiou, Harry G MD (Ped) *PCP* - **Hospital:** New York Methodist Hosp (page 440); **Address:** 554 Henry St, Brooklyn, NY 11231; **Phone:** 718-625-5591; **Board Cert:** Pediatrics 2011; **Med School:** Greece 1979; **Resid:** Pediatrics, Long Island Coll Hosp 1985

Wu, Jason J MD/PhD (Ped) *PCP* - **Spec Exp:** Chinese Community Health; **Hospital:** Maimonides Med Ctr (page 98); **Address:** 781 47th St, Brooklyn, NY 11220; **Phone:** 718-435-5980; **Board Cert:** Pediatrics 2010; **Med School:** China 1982; **Resid:** Pediatrics, Maimonides Med Ctr 2001; **Fac Appt:** Asst Clin Prof Ped, Mount Sinai Sch Med

Physical Medicine & Rehabilitation

Atakent, Pinar E MD (PMR) - **Spec Exp:** Stroke Rehabilitation; Electrodiagnosis; Acupuncture; **Hospital:** SUNY Downstate Med Ctr (Univ Hosp Brooklyn) (page 441); **Address:** 339 Hicks St, Brooklyn, NY 11201-5509; **Phone:** 718-780-4685; **Board Cert:** Physical Medicine & Rehabilitation 1982; **Med School:** Turkey 1971; **Resid:** Physical Medicine & Rehabilitation, Jacobi Med Ctr 1981

Gifford, Irina MD (PMR) - **Spec Exp:** Musculoskeletal Disorders; Neurologic Rehabilitation; Pediatric Rehabilitation; **Hospital:** Kingsbrook Jewish Med Ctr; **Address:** 585 Schenectady Ave, rm 333, Brooklyn, NY 11203-1822; **Phone:** 718-604-5341; **Board Cert:** Physical Medicine & Rehabilitation 1990; **Med School:** Romania 1960; **Resid:** Physical Medicine & Rehabilitation, Mount Sinai Hosp 1989; **Fellow:** Pediatric Rehabilitation Medicine, Albert Einstein Med Sch 1990

Pipia, Paul A MD (PMR) - **Spec Exp:** Neuromuscular Disorders; Pain-Back; Stroke Rehabilitation; Sports Medicine; **Hospital:** SUNY Downstate Med Ctr (Univ Hosp Brooklyn) (page 441); **Address:** SUNY, Univ Orthopedic Assoc, 710 Parkside Ave, Brooklyn, NY 11226; **Phone:** 718-282-7800; **Board Cert:** Physical Medicine & Rehabilitation 2006; Sports Medicine 2011; **Med School:** SUNY Downstate 1989; **Resid:** Physical Medicine & Rehabilitation, NYU Rusk Inst 1993; **Fac Appt:** Asst Prof PMR, SUNY Downstate

Ross, Marc MD (PMR) - **Spec Exp:** Sports Medicine; Pain-Back; Gait Disorders; **Hospital:** Kingsbrook Jewish Med Ctr, Mt Sinai Med Ctr (page 102); **Address:** Kingsbrook Jewish Med Ctr, Dept Physical Med & Rehab, 585 Schenectady Ave, Brooklyn, NY 11203; **Phone:** 718-604-5341; **Board Cert:** Physical Medicine & Rehabilitation 2004; **Med School:** NY Med Coll 1989; **Resid:** Physical Medicine & Rehabilitation, Mt Sinai Med Ctr 1993; **Fac Appt:** Asst Clin Prof PMR, Mount Sinai Sch Med

Stein, Perry MD (PMR) - **Spec Exp:** Pain Management; Palliative Care; **Hospital:** Mercy Med Ctr - Rockville Centre, Maimonides Med Ctr (page 98); **Address:** 383 Ocean Pkwy, Brooklyn, NY 11218; **Phone:** 718-941-6000; **Board Cert:** Physical Medicine & Rehabilitation 1991; Hospice & Palliative Medicine 2012; **Med School:** Mexico 1985; **Resid:** Physical Medicine & Rehabilitation, SUNY Downstate Med Ctr 1990

Psychiatry

Berkowitz, Howard L MD (Psyc) - **Spec Exp:** Anxiety & Depression; Geriatric Psychiatry; **Hospital:** Maimonides Med Ctr (page 98); **Address:** 910 48th St, Brooklyn, NY 11219; **Phone:** 718-633-2025; **Board Cert:** Psychiatry 1977; Geriatric Psychiatry 2004; **Med School:** Albert Einstein Coll Med 1972; **Resid:** Internal Medicine, Beth Israel Hosp 1973; Psychiatry, Kings Co Hosp 1976; **Fellow:** Liaison Psychiatry, Kings Co Hosp 1977; **Fac Appt:** Assoc Prof Psyc, SUNY Downstate

Coplan, Jeremy MD (Psyc) - **Spec Exp:** Anxiety Disorders; Psychosomatic Disorders; Bipolar/Mood Disorders; **Hospital:** SUNY Downstate Med Ctr (Univ Hosp Brooklyn) (page 441); **Address:** 450 Clarkson Ave, Box 1203, Brooklyn, NY 11203; **Phone:** 718-270-2023; **Board Cert:** Psychiatry 1990; **Med School:** South Africa 1983; **Resid:** Psychiatry, SUNY-Downstate Med Ctr 1989; **Fellow:** Biological Psychiatry, Columbia-Presby Med Ctr 1990; **Fac Appt:** Prof Psyc, SUNY Downstate

Eitan, Noam MD (Psyc) - **Hospital:** Woodhull Med & Mental Hlth Ctr; **Address:** 760 Broadway, Brooklyn, NY 11206; **Phone:** 718-963-8628; **Board Cert:** Psychiatry 2008; **Med School:** Israel 1986; **Resid:** Psychiatry, Shalvata Hosp 1991; **Fellow:** Psychoanalysis, Sackler Sch Med 1995

Goldberg, Jeffrey DO (Psyc) - **Spec Exp:** Geriatric Psychiatry; Anxiety & Depression; Mood Disorders; **Hospital:** Coney Island Hosp; **Address:** 5025 Ft Hamilton Pkwy, Brooklyn, NY 11219; **Phone:** 718-633-8183; **Board Cert:** Psychiatry 2013; Geriatric Psychiatry 2013; **Med School:** NY Coll Osteo Med 1981; **Resid:** Psychiatry, Maimonides Med Ctr 1985; **Fac Appt:** Asst Clin Prof Psyc, SUNY Downstate

Heisman, Alexander MD (Psyc) - **Spec Exp:** Addiction/Substance Abuse; Liaison Psychiatry; Pain-Chronic; Anxiety & Depression; **Hospital:** Beth Israel Med Ctr- Kings Hwy Div (page 94), New York Methodist Hosp (page 440); **Address:** 3045 Ocean Pkwy, Ste 1A, Brooklyn, NY 11235; **Phone:** 718-449-1705; **Board Cert:** Psychiatry 2007; Psychosomatic Medicine 2008; **Med School:** Russia 1976; **Resid:** Psychiatry, Montefiore Med Ctr 1996

Viswanathan, Ramaswamy MD (Psyc) - **Spec Exp:** Depression; Anxiety Disorders; **Hospital:** SUNY Downstate Med Ctr (Univ Hosp Brooklyn) (page 441), Kings Co Hosp Ctr; **Address:** 450 Clarkson Ave, Ste A3-474, Brooklyn, NY 11203-2098; **Phone:** 718-270-2352; **Board Cert:** Psychiatry 1978; Internal Medicine 1989; Psychosomatic Medicine 2005; Forensic Psychiatry 2009; **Med School:** India 1972; **Resid:** Internal Medicine, Queens Hosp Ctr 1974; Psychiatry, SUNY Hlth Sci Ctr 1977; **Fellow:** Psychiatry, SUNY Hlth Sci Ctr 1978; **Fac Appt:** Assoc Prof Psyc, SUNY Hlth Sci Ctr

Pulmonary Disease

Abott, Michael L MD (Pul) - **Spec Exp:** Asthma; Emphysema; **Hospital:** New York Methodist Hosp (page 440), Lutheran Med Ctr - Brooklyn; **Address:** 8714 5th Ave, Brooklyn, NY 11209; **Phone:** 718-630-8600; **Board Cert:** Internal Medicine 1983; Pulmonary Disease 1986; **Med School:** Mexico 1978; **Resid:** Internal Medicine, Coney Island Hosp 1982; **Fellow:** Pulmonary Disease, Montefiore Med Ctr 1984

Amin, Hossam H MD (Pul) - **Spec Exp:** Asthma & Allergy; Critical Care; **Hospital:** Metropolitan Hosp Ctr - NY, New York Methodist Hosp (page 440); **Address:** 6903 4th Ave, Brooklyn, NY 11209; **Phone:** 718-238-6161; **Board Cert:** Internal Medicine 2006; Pulmonary Disease 2008; Critical Care Medicine 2009; **Med School:** Egypt 1988; **Resid:** Internal Medicine, Interfaith Med Ctr 1996; **Fellow:** Pulmonary Disease, Interfaith Med Ctr 1998; Critical Care Medicine, Mt Sinai Med Ctr 1999; **Fac Appt:** Assoc Prof Med, NY Med Coll

Bergman, Michael I MD (Pul) - **Spec Exp:** Asthma; Bronchitis; Respiratory Failure; Pneumonia; **Hospital:** Maimonides Med Ctr (page 98); **Address:** Maimonides Med Ctr, Dept Pulmonary Med, 953 49 St, Ste 511, Brooklyn, NY 11219; **Phone:** 718-283-8380; **Board Cert:** Internal Medicine 1981; Pulmonary Disease 1984; Critical Care Medicine 2007; **Med School:** Albert Einstein Coll Med 1978; **Resid:** Internal Medicine, Brookdale Hosp 1981; **Fellow:** Pulmonary Disease, Mount Sinai Hosp 1984; **Fac Appt:** Asst Prof Med, SUNY Downstate

Bernstein, Chaim MD (Pul) - **Spec Exp:** Asthma; Chronic Obstructive Lung Disease (COPD); Emphysema; **Hospital:** Beth Israel Med Ctr- Kings Hwy Div (page 94); **Address:** 3131 Kings Hwy, Ste D10, Brooklyn, NY 11234-2643; **Phone:** 718-252-3590; **Board Cert:** Internal Medicine 1977; Pulmonary Disease 1982; Critical Care Medicine 2007; **Med School:** NYU Sch Med 1974; **Resid:** Internal Medicine, Brookdale Med Ctr 1977; Pulmonary Disease, Manhattan VA Hosp 1979; **Fellow:** Pulmonary Disease, Bellevue Hosp-NYU 1979

Bondi, Elliott MD (Pul) - **Spec Exp:** Asthma; Tuberculosis; Pneumonia; **Hospital:** Brookdale Univ Hosp Med Ctr; **Address:** Brookdale Hospital, Pulmonary Medicine, 1 Brookdale Plaza, rm A107, Brooklyn, NY 11212; **Phone:** 718-240-5236; **Board Cert:** Internal Medicine 1987; Pulmonary Disease 1982; **Med School:** Univ MD Sch Med 1971; **Resid:** Internal Medicine, Maimonides Medical Ctr 1973; Internal Medicine, Bronx Muni Hosp 1974; **Fellow:** Pulmonary Disease, Bronx Muni Hosp 1976; **Fac Appt:** Assoc Clin Prof Med, SUNY Downstate

Demetis, Spiro MD (Pul) - **Spec Exp:** Sarcoidosis; Lung Cancer; Asthma & Emphysema; Pulmonary Hypertension; **Hospital:** SUNY Downstate Med Ctr (Univ Hosp Brooklyn) (page 441), Lutheran Med Ctr - Brooklyn; **Address:** 9001 Fort Hamilton Pkwy, Brooklyn, NY 11209; **Phone:** 718-748-4446; **Board Cert:** Internal Medicine 1989; Pulmonary Disease 2005; Critical Care Medicine 2005; **Med School:** Mexico 1983; **Resid:** Internal Medicine, Univ Hosp 1988; **Fellow:** Pulmonary Disease, Univ Hosp 1990; Critical Care Medicine, Univ Hosp 1991; **Fac Appt:** Assoc Prof Med, SUNY Hlth Sci Ctr

George, Liziamma MD (Pul) - **Spec Exp:** Sleep Disorders; Smoking Cessation; **Hospital:** New York Methodist Hosp (page 440); **Address:** 506 6th St, Brooklyn, NY 11215; **Phone:** 718-246-8600; **Board Cert:** Internal Medicine 1987; Critical Care Medicine 2011; Pulmonary Disease 2010; Sleep Medicine 2009; **Med School:** India 1980; **Resid:** Internal Medicine, St Joseph's Med Ctr 1987; **Fellow:** Pulmonary Disease, St Joseph's Med Ctr 1989; **Fac Appt:** Assoc Clin Prof Med, Cornell Univ-Weill Med Coll

Gulrajani, Ramesh MD (Pul) - **Spec Exp:** Asthma; Sarcoidosis; Lung Cancer; **Hospital:** Brooklyn Hosp Ctr; **Address:** 121 DeKalb Ave, Dept Internal Med, Ste 7E, Brooklyn, NY 11201-5425; **Phone:** 718-250-6950; **Board Cert:** Internal Medicine 1979; Pulmonary Disease 1984; **Med School:** India 1974; **Resid:** Internal Medicine, Brooklyn Cumberland Med Ctr 1979; **Fellow:** Pulmonary Disease, Brooklyn Cumberland Med Ctr 1981; **Fac Appt:** Assoc Clin Prof Med, Cornell Univ-Weill Med Coll

Hammer, Arthur MD (Pul) - **Spec Exp:** Asthma; Sleep Disorders; Pulmonary Fibrosis; **Hospital:** Beth Israel Med Ctr- Kings Hwy Div (page 94); **Address:** 3131 Kings Hwy, Ste D10, Brooklyn, NY 11234-2643; **Phone:** 718-252-3590; **Board Cert:** Internal Medicine 2006; Pulmonary Disease 2009; **Med School:** Mexico 1970; **Resid:** Internal Medicine, Brookdale Hosp 1974; **Fellow:** Pulmonary Disease, NYU 1976

Kupfer, Yizhak MD (Pul) - **Spec Exp:** Sleep & Snoring Disorders; Cough; Mechanical Ventilation; **Hospital:** Maimonides Med Ctr (page 98); **Address:** Div Pulmonary & Critical Care Medicine, 953 49th St, Ste 511, Brooklyn, NY 11219-2923; **Phone:** 718-283-8380; **Board Cert:** Internal Medicine 1989; Pulmonary Disease 2012; Critical Care Medicine 2013; Sleep Medicine 2007; **Med School:** SUNY Downstate 1986; **Resid:** Internal Medicine, Maimonides Med Ctr 1989; **Fellow:** Pulmonary Disease, Maimonides Med Ctr 1991; Critical Care Medicine, Maimonides Med Ctr 1992; **Fac Appt:** Assoc Clin Prof Med, SUNY Downstate

Lombardo, Gerard T MD (Pul) - **Spec Exp:** Sleep Apnea; Sleep & Snoring Disorders; **Hospital:** New York Methodist Hosp (page 440); **Address:** 808 8th Ave, Brooklyn, NY 11215; **Phone:** 718-369-1818; **Board Cert:** Internal Medicine 1984; Pulmonary Disease 1986; Sleep Medicine 2009; **Med School:** Grenada 1981; **Resid:** Internal Medicine, NY Methodist Hosp 1984; **Fellow:** Pulmonary Disease, NY Methodist Hosp 1986; **Fac Appt:** Asst Clin Prof Med, Cornell Univ-Weill Med Coll

Miarrostami, Rameen M MD (Pul) - **Spec Exp:** Asthma; Chronic Obstructive Lung Disease (COPD); Emphysema; Cough; **Hospital:** New York Methodist Hosp (page 440), Lutheran Med Ctr - Brooklyn; **Address:** 7124 18th Ave, Brooklyn, NY 11204-5203; **Phone:** 718-234-3333; **Board Cert:** Internal Medicine 2011; Pulmonary Disease 2004; **Med School:** Dominican Republic 1985; **Resid:** Internal Medicine, Lincoln Med Ctr 1991; **Fellow:** Pulmonary Disease, LI Coll Hosp 1993

Raoof, Suhail MD (Pul) - **Spec Exp:** Critical Care Medicine; Chronic Obstructive Lung Disease (COPD); Mechanical Ventilation; Lung Disease; **Hospital:** New York Methodist Hosp (page 440); **Address:** 506 6th St, Brooklyn, NY 11215; **Phone:** 718-780-5835; **Board Cert:** Pulmonary Disease 2003; Critical Care Medicine 2004; **Med School:** India 1982; **Resid:** Internal Medicine, LIJ Med Ctr 1989; Internal Medicine, Nassau County Med Ctr 1991; **Fellow:** Pulmonary Critical Care Medicine, Stony Brook Affil Hosps 1992; **Fac Appt:** Prof Med, Cornell Univ-Weill Med Coll

Saleh, Anthony MD (Pul) - **Spec Exp:** Asthma; Interstitial Lung Disease; Chronic Obstructive Lung Disease (COPD); Lung Cancer; **Hospital:** New York Methodist Hosp (page 440); **Address:** 7206 7th Ave, Brooklyn, NY 11209; **Phone:** 718-745-1200; **Board Cert:** Internal Medicine 1988; Pulmonary Disease 2010; **Med School:** Grenada 1985; **Resid:** Internal Medicine, NY Methodist Hosp 1988; **Fellow:** Pulmonary Disease, NY Methodist Hosp 1990; **Fac Appt:** Asst Clin Prof Med, Cornell Univ-Weill Med Coll

Smith, Peter R MD (Pul) - **Spec Exp:** Chronic Obstructive Lung Disease (COPD); Smoking Cessation; Sarcoidosis; Wegener's Granulomatosis; **Hospital:** Brooklyn Hosp Ctr; **Address:** Brooklyn Hosp Ctr, Div Pulmonary Med, 121 DeKalb Ave, rm 14J, Brooklyn, NY 11201; **Phone:** 718-250-6621; **Board Cert:** Internal Medicine 1973; Pulmonary Disease 1974; Critical Care Medicine 2009; **Med School:** Columbia P&S 1968; **Resid:** Internal Medicine, Downstate Med Ctr 1970; Internal Medicine, Jacobi Med Ctr 1971; **Fellow:** Pulmonary Disease, Downstate Med Ctr 1974; **Fac Appt:** Clin Prof Med, SUNY Hlth Sci Ctr

Tessler, Sidney MD (Pul) - **Spec Exp:** Cough; Asthma; Mechanical Ventilation; **Hospital:** Maimonides Med Ctr (page 98); **Address:** 953 49th St, Fl 5, rm 511, Div Pul & Critical Care Med, Brooklyn, NY 11219-2923; **Phone:** 718-283-8380; **Board Cert:** Internal Medicine 1977; Pulmonary Disease 1980; Critical Care Medicine 2007; **Med School:** SUNY Hlth Sci Ctr 1970; **Resid:** Internal Medicine, Coney Island Hosp 1972; Internal Medicine, Maimonides Med Ctr 1976; **Fellow:** Pulmonary Disease, Maimonides Med Ctr 1977; **Fac Appt:** Clin Prof Med, SUNY Hlth Sci Ctr

Radiation Oncology

Ashamalla, Hani MD (RadRO) - **Spec Exp:** Stereotactic Body Radiotherapy; Prostate Cancer; Breast Cancer; **Hospital:** New York Methodist Hosp (page 440); **Address:** NY Methodist Hosp, Dept Rad Oncology, 506 6th St, Brooklyn, NY 11215; **Phone:** 718-780-3677; **Board Cert:** Radiation Oncology 2004; **Med School:** Egypt 1983; **Resid:** Radiation Oncology, NY Methodist Hosp 1994; **Fellow:** Radiation Oncology, NY Methodist Hosp 1995; Radiation Oncology, Chldns Hosp 1995; **Fac Appt:** Clin Prof RadRO, Cornell Univ-Weill Med Coll

Cooper, Jay S MD (RadRO) - **Spec Exp:** Head & Neck Cancer; Skin Cancer; Chemo-Radiation Combined Therapy; Intensity Modulated Radiotherapy (IMRT); **Hospital:** Maimonides Med Ctr (page 98); **Address:** Maimonides Cancer Center, 6300 8th Ave, Brooklyn, NY 11220; **Phone:** 718-765-2700; **Board Cert:** Therapeutic Radiology 1977; **Med School:** NYU Sch Med 1973; **Resid:** Radiation Oncology, NYU Med Ctr 1977; **Fac Appt:** Prof RadRO, Albert Einstein Coll Med

Donahue, Bernadine R MD (RadRO) - **Spec Exp:** Brain Tumors; Gastrointestinal Cancer; Pediatric Cancers; Solid Tumors; **Hospital:** Maimonides Med Ctr (page 98); **Address:** Maimonides Med Ctr, Radiation Onc Dept, 6300 8th Ave, Lower Level, Brooklyn, NY 11220; **Phone:** 718-765-2700; **Board Cert:** Internal Medicine 1987; Radiation Oncology 1991; Hospice & Palliative Medicine 2012; **Med School:** Boston Univ 1984; **Resid:** Internal Medicine, Boston Med Ctr 1987; **Fellow:** Radiation Oncology, NYU Med Ctr 1990

Gliedman, Paul R MD (RadRO) - **Spec Exp:** Breast Cancer; Prostate Cancer; Brain Tumors; Stereotactic Radiosurgery; **Hospital:** St. Luke's - Roosevelt Hosp Ctr - Roosevelt Div (page 94), Beth Israel Med Ctr- Kings Hwy Div (page 94); **Address:** Brooklyn Radiation Oncology, 2101 Avenue X, Brooklyn, NY 11235; **Phone:** 718-512-2160; **Board Cert:** Radiation Oncology 1987; **Med School:** Columbia P&S 1983; **Resid:** Radiation Oncology, NYU Med Ctr 1987

Rotman, Marvin Z MD (RadRO) - **Spec Exp:** Bladder Cancer; Gynecologic Cancer; Eye Tumors/Cancer; Prostate Cancer; **Hospital:** SUNY Downstate Med Ctr (Univ Hosp Brooklyn) (page 441), VA NY Harbor Hlthcr Sys-Brooklyn Campus; **Address:** 450 Clarkson Ave, Box 1211, Brooklyn, NY 11203-2056; **Phone:** 718-270-2181; **Board Cert:** Diagnostic Radiology 1966; **Med School:** Jefferson Med Coll 1958; **Resid:** Internal Medicine, Albert Einstein Med Ctr 1962; Radiation Oncology, Montefiore Hosp Med Ctr 1966; **Fac Appt:** Prof RadRO, SUNY Downstate

Reproductive Endocrinology

Grazi, Richard MD (RE) - **Spec Exp:** Infertility-IVF; Preimplantation Genetic Diagnosis; Fertility Preservation in Cancer; **Hospital:** Maimonides Med Ctr (page 98), Richmond Univ Med Ctr; **Address:** 1355 84th St, Brooklyn, NY 11228-3030; **Phone:** 718-283-8600; **Board Cert:** Obstetrics & Gynecology 2006; Reproductive Endocrinology/Infertility 2006; **Med School:** SUNY Buffalo 1981; **Resid:** Obstetrics & Gynecology, NYU Med Ctr 1985; **Fellow:** Reproductive Endocrinology, UMDNJ Med Ctr 1987; **Fac Appt:** Assoc Clin Prof ObG, Mount Sinai Sch Med

Kofinas, George D MD (RE) - **Spec Exp:** Infertility-IVF; Fertility Preservation; Robotic Assisted Laparoscopic Surgery; Hysteroscopic Surgery; **Hospital:** New York Methodist Hosp (page 440); **Address:** The Fertility Institute, 506 6th St, WKP Bldg Fl 6, Brooklyn, NY 11215-3609; **Phone:** 718-780-5065; **Board Cert:** Obstetrics & Gynecology 2012; Reproductive Endocrinology 2012; **Med School:** Greece 1975; **Resid:** Obstetrics & Gynecology, NY Methodist Hosp 1982; Obstetrics & Gynecology, Brooklyn Caledonian Hosp 1984; **Fellow:** Reproductive Endocrinology, Univ Hosp 1986

Seifer, David B MD (RE) - **Spec Exp:** Infertility-IVF; Infertility-Advanced Maternal Age; Fertility Preservation in Cancer; **Hospital:** Maimonides Med Ctr (page 98); **Address:** Genesis Fertility & Reproductive Med, 1355 84th St, Brooklyn, NY 11228; **Phone:** 718-283-8600; **Board Cert:** Obstetrics & Gynecology 2012; Reproductive Endocrinology/Infertility 2012; **Med School:** Univ IL Coll Med 1981; **Resid:** Obstetrics & Gynecology, Stanford Univ Hosp & Clins 1985; **Fellow:** Reproductive Endocrinology, Yale-New Haven Hosp 1991; **Fac Appt:** Prof ObG, Mount Sinai Sch Med

Rheumatology

Garner, Bruce F MD (Rhu) - **Spec Exp:** Rheumatoid Arthritis; Osteoporosis; Osteoarthritis; Lupus/SLE; **Hospital:** Lutheran Med Ctr - Brooklyn; **Address:** 7901 4th Ave, Ste A5, Brooklyn, NY 11209-3915; **Phone:** 718-921-5239; **Board Cert:** Internal Medicine 1987; Rheumatology 1988; **Med School:** Mexico 1981; **Resid:** Internal Medicine, Lutheran Med Ctr 1985; **Fellow:** Rheumatology, Washington Hosp Ctr 1987; **Fac Appt:** Asst Clin Prof Med, SUNY Downstate

Green, Stuart A MD (Rhu) - **Spec Exp:** Rheumatoid Arthritis; Osteoporosis; Lupus/SLE; **Hospital:** Brooklyn Hosp Ctr; **Address:** 121 DeKalb Ave Fl 7, Brooklyn, NY 11201-5425; **Phone:** 718-250-6921; **Board Cert:** Internal Medicine 1982; Rheumatology 1986; **Med School:** Georgetown Univ 1979; **Resid:** Internal Medicine, St Lukes-Roosevelt Hosp 1982; **Fellow:** Rheumatology, SUNY Downstate Med Ctr 1985; **Fac Appt:** Asst Clin Prof Med, NYU Sch Med

Lesser, Robert S MD (Rhu) - **Spec Exp:** Polymyalgia Rheumatica; Rheumatoid Arthritis; Lupus/SLE; **Hospital:** Beth Israel Med Ctr- Kings Hwy Div (page 94); **Address:** 4015 Avenue U, Brooklyn, NY 11234-5117; **Phone:** 718-252-5151; **Board Cert:** Internal Medicine 1985; Rheumatology 1988; **Med School:** Univ Hlth Scis, Chicago Med Sch 1982; **Resid:** Internal Medicine, Hahnemann Univ Hosp 1985; **Fellow:** Rheumatology, Hahnemann Univ Hosp 1987; **Fac Appt:** Assoc Clin Prof Med, SUNY Downstate

Patel, Jitendra K MD (Rhu) - **Spec Exp:** Arthritis; Fibromyalgia; Pain-Back; **Hospital:** Kingsbrook Jewish Med Ctr, Beth Israel Med Ctr- Kings Hwy Div (page 94); **Address:** 3420 Ave N, Brooklyn, NY 11234-2607; **Phone:** 718-258-7019; **Board Cert:** Internal Medicine 1979; Rheumatology 1982; **Med School:** India 1975; **Resid:** Internal Medicine, Mem Univ Newfoundland Affil Hosp 1979; **Fellow:** Rheumatology, Georgetown Univ Hosp 1982

Schiff, Carl F MD (Rhu) - **Spec Exp:** Rheumatoid Arthritis; Osteoporosis; **Hospital:** Maimonides Med Ctr (page 98); **Address:** 4915 49th St, Brooklyn, NY 11219; **Phone:** 718-283-8519; **Board Cert:** Internal Medicine 1983; Rheumatology 1986; **Med School:** Yale Univ 1980; **Resid:** Internal Medicine, Mt Sinai Hosp 1983; **Fellow:** Rheumatology, Columbia-Presby Med Ctr 1986; **Fac Appt:** Asst Clin Prof Med, SUNY Hlth Sci Ctr

Surgery

Adler, Harry L MD (S) - **Spec Exp:** Biliary Surgery; Laparoscopic Surgery; Hernia; Colon Surgery; **Hospital:** Maimonides Med Ctr (page 98); **Address:** 948 48th St Fl 3, Brooklyn, NY 11219; **Phone:** 718-283-7952; **Board Cert:** Surgery 2005; Surgical Critical Care 2008; **Med School:** NYU Sch Med 1980; **Resid:** Surgery, Bellevue Hosp/NYU Langone Med Ctr 1985; **Fellow:** Surgical Critical Care, Maimonides Med Ctr 1986; **Fac Appt:** Asst Clin Prof S, SUNY Downstate

Alfonso II, Antonio E MD (S) - **Spec Exp:** Thyroid Cancer; Head & Neck Surgery; Breast Cancer; **Hospital:** SUNY Downstate Med Ctr (Univ Hosp Brooklyn) (page 441); **Address:** 100 Amity St, Brooklyn, NY 11201; **Phone:** 718-875-3244; **Board Cert:** Surgery 1973; **Med School:** Philippines 1968; **Resid:** Surgery, Temple Univ Hosp 1972; **Fellow:** Surgical Oncology, Meml Sloan Kettering Cancer Ctr 1974; **Fac Appt:** Prof Emeritus S, SUNY Downstate

Bernstein, Michael O MD (S) - **Spec Exp:** Breast Cancer; Hernia; Gastrointestinal Surgery; **Hospital:** Richmond Univ Med Ctr; **Address:** 11 Ralph Pl, Ste 204, Staten Island, NY 10301; **Phone:** 718-273-5954; **Board Cert:** Surgery 2007; **Med School:** Penn State Coll Med 1983; **Resid:** Surgery, SUNY-Kings Co Hosp 1988; **Fac Appt:** Assoc Clin Prof S, SUNY Downstate

Borgen, Patrick I MD (S) - **Spec Exp:** Breast Cancer; Breast Cancer & Surgery; **Hospital:** Maimonides Med Ctr (page 98); **Address:** Maimonides Breast Ctr, 745 64th St, Brooklyn, NY 11220; **Phone:** 718-765-2570; **Board Cert:** Surgery 2002; **Med School:** Louisiana State U, New Orleans 1984; **Resid:** Surgery, Ochsner Fdn Hosp 1989; **Fellow:** Surgical Oncology, Meml Sloan Kettering Canc Ctr 1990; **Fac Appt:** Prof S, Cornell Univ-Weill Med Coll

Borriello, Raffaele MD (S) - **Spec Exp:** Laparoscopic Surgery; Hernia; Gastrointestinal Surgery; **Hospital:** New York Methodist Hosp (page 440); **Address:** 100 Clinton St, Ste 2, Brooklyn, NY 11201; **Phone:** 718-625-0767; **Board Cert:** Surgery 2005; **Med School:** SUNY Downstate 1981; **Resid:** Surgery, Kings County Hosp Ctr 1986; **Fac Appt:** Assoc Prof S, SUNY Downstate

Chiariello, Mario MD (S) - **Spec Exp:** Cancer Surgery; **Hospital:** New York Methodist Hosp (page 440); **Address:** 1479 73rd St, Brooklyn, NY 11228-2111; **Phone:** 718-331-4938; **Board Cert:** Surgery 2010; **Med School:** Italy 1977; **Resid:** Surgery, Brooklyn Cumberland Hosp 1984

Dresner, Lisa S MD (S) - **Spec Exp:** Breast Surgery; Critical Care; **Hospital:** SUNY Downstate Med Ctr (Univ Hosp Brooklyn) (page 441); **Address:** SUNY HSC, Dept Surg, 450 Clarkson Ave, MS 40, Brooklyn, NY 11203-2056; **Phone:** 718-270-1973; **Board Cert:** Surgery 2011; Surgical Critical Care 2003; **Med School:** SUNY Downstate 1985; **Resid:** Surgery, SUNY Downstate Med Ctr 1992; **Fellow:** Surgical Critical Care, Jackson Meml Hosp 1993; **Fac Appt:** Assoc Prof S, SUNY Downstate

Fahoum, Bashar H MD (S) - **Spec Exp:** Laparoscopic Surgery; Critical Care; Trauma; **Hospital:** New York Methodist Hosp (page 440); **Address:** 506 6th St, Brooklyn, NY 11215-3609; **Phone:** 718-780-3288; **Board Cert:** Surgery 2003; Surgical Critical Care 2012; **Med School:** Syria 1987; **Resid:** Surgery, NY Methodist Hosp 1993; **Fac Appt:** Asst Prof S, Cornell Univ-Weill Med Coll

Fogler, Richard MD (S) - **Spec Exp:** Breast Surgery; Colon & Rectal Surgery; Gastrointestinal Surgery; **Hospital:** Brookdale Univ Hosp Med Ctr; **Address:** 1 Brookdale Plaza, rm 122, Brooklyn, NY 11212-3139; **Phone:** 718-240-5437; **Board Cert:** Surgery 1975; **Med School:** NY Med Coll 1968; **Resid:** Surgery, Brookdale Hosp 1973; **Fac Appt:** Clin Prof S, SUNY Hlth Sci Ctr

Genato, Romulo L MD (S) - **Spec Exp:** Breast Surgery; Laparoscopic Surgery; Hernia; **Hospital:** Brooklyn Hosp Ctr; **Address:** 240 Willoughby St, Ste 8E, Brooklyn, NY 11201; **Phone:** 718-250-8970; **Board Cert:** Surgery 2010; **Med School:** Philippines 1972; **Resid:** Surgery, Brooklyn Hosp 1979

Gorecki, Piotr J MD (S) - **Hospital:** New York Methodist Hosp (page 440); **Address:** 263 7th Ave, Ste 5A, Brooklyn, NY 11215; **Phone:** 718-246-8600; **Board Cert:** Surgery 2009; **Med School:** Poland 1991; **Resid:** Surgery, NY Methodist Hosp 1998; **Fellow:** Laparoscopic Surgery, Mayo Clin 1999; **Fac Appt:** Asst Prof S, Cornell Univ-Weill Med Coll

Kaleya, Ronald N MD (S) - **Spec Exp:** Pancreatic Cancer; Breast Cancer; Colon & Rectal Cancer; **Hospital:** Maimonides Med Ctr (page 98); **Address:** 948 48th St Fl 3, Brooklyn, NY 11219; **Phone:** 718-283-7952; **Board Cert:** Surgery 2008; **Med School:** Cornell Univ-Weill Med Coll 1980; **Resid:** Surgery, Montefiore Med Ctr-Einstein Campus 1985; **Fellow:** Surgical Oncology, Meml Sloan Kettering Canc Ctr 1987

Lewis, Theophilus MD (S) - **Spec Exp:** Breast Cancer & Surgery; **Hospital:** SUNY Downstate Med Ctr (Univ Hosp Brooklyn) (page 441); **Address:** SUNY Downstate Med Ctr - Dept Surgery, 451 Clarkson Ave, rm 4121, Brooklyn, NY 11203-0040; **Phone:** 718-270-2155; **Board Cert:** Surgery 2003; **Med School:** SUNY Downstate 1978; **Resid:** Surgery, Kings Co Hosp Ctr 1983

Lois, William A MD (S) - **Spec Exp:** Dialysis Access Surgery; Vascular Surgery; Wound Healing/Care; **Hospital:** Kingsbrook Jewish Med Ctr; **Address:** 5723 Avenue N, Brooklyn, NY 11234; **Phone:** 718-251-1111; **Board Cert:** Surgery 2010; **Med School:** Spain 1982; **Resid:** Surgery, Interfaith Med Ctr 1987

Manasseh, Donna-Marie MD (S) - **Spec Exp:** Breast Surgery; **Hospital:** Maimonides Med Ctr (page 98); **Address:** 745 64th St, Brooklyn, NY 11220; **Phone:** 718-765-2570; **Board Cert:** Surgery 2005; **Med School:** Harvard Med Sch 1996; **Resid:** Surgery, NY Presby Hosp 2002; **Fellow:** Surgical Breast Oncology, Meml Sloan Kettering Canc Ctr 2005; **Fac Appt:** Asst Clin Prof S, Columbia P&S

Rajpal, Sanjeev MD (S) - **Spec Exp:** Laparoscopic Surgery; Obesity/Bariatric Surgery; Cancer Surgery; **Hospital:** Brookdale Univ Hosp Med Ctr; **Address:** 9413 Flatlands Ave, Ste 203E, Brooklyn, NY 11236-5233; **Phone:** 718-251-1212; **Board Cert:** Surgery 2002; **Med School:** India 1975; **Resid:** Surgery, Brookdale Hosp Med Ctr 1980; **Fellow:** Surgical Oncology, Roswell Park Meml Inst 1982; Laparoscopic Surgery, Yale Univ 2001; **Fac Appt:** Asst Prof S, SUNY Downstate

Schwartzman, Alexander MD (S) - **Spec Exp:** Breast Cancer; Colon Surgery; Laparoscopic Surgery; Gallbladder Surgery; **Hospital:** SUNY Downstate Med Ctr (Univ Hosp Brooklyn) (page 441); **Address:** SUNY Downstate Med Ctr - Dept Surgery, 450 Clarkson Ave, MS 40, Brooklyn, NY 11203; **Phone:** 718-270-1791; **Board Cert:** Surgery 2010; **Med School:** Dominican Republic 1983; **Resid:** Surgery, Brooklyn Hosp Ctr 1988

Thoracic & Cardiac Surgery

Abrol, Sunil MD (T&CS) - **Spec Exp:** Cardiac Surgery; Aneurysm-Thoracic Aortic; Heart Valve Surgery; Aortic Surgery; **Hospital:** Maimonides Med Ctr (page 98), Jamaica Hosp Med Ctr; **Address:** Maimonides Med Ctr - Cardiothoracic Surg, 4802 10th Ave Fl 4 - rm D, Brooklyn, NY 11219; **Phone:** 718-283-7686; **Board Cert:** Surgery 2009; Thoracic Surgery 2011; **Med School:** India 1986; **Resid:** Surgery, Maimonides Med Ctr 1998; **Fellow:** Thoracic Surgery, SUNY Hlth Sci Ctr 2001; **Fac Appt:** Asst Prof S, Mount Sinai Sch Med

Harris, Loren MD (T&CS) - **Spec Exp:** Thoracic Cancers; Esophageal Cancer; **Hospital:** Maimonides Med Ctr (page 98); **Address:** Maimonedes Med Ctr - Dept Surgery, 4802 Tenth Ave Fl 4 - rm D, Brooklyn, NY 11219; **Phone:** 718-283-7686; **Board Cert:** Thoracic Surgery 2006; **Med School:** NYU Sch Med 1987; **Resid:** Surgery, NYU Langone Med Ctr 1994; **Fellow:** Cardiovascular Surgery, NYU Langone Med Ctr 1996; **Fac Appt:** Asst Prof S, Albert Einstein Coll Med

Ribakove, Greg MD (T&CS) - **Spec Exp:** Minimally Invasive Cardiac Surgery; Heart Valve Surgery; Coronary Artery Surgery; **Hospital:** Maimonides Med Ctr (page 98); **Address:** Maimonides, Cardiothoracic Surgery, 4802 10 Ave Fl 4, Brooklyn, NY 11219; **Phone:** 718-283-7686; **Board Cert:** Thoracic Surgery 2010; **Med School:** Univ Chicago-Pritzker Sch Med 1980; **Resid:** Surgery, NYU Med Ctr 1982; **Fellow:** Cardiovascular Surgery, Natl Inst Hlth-Clin Ctr 1984; Thoracic Surgery, Stanford Univ Hosp & Clins 1994; **Fac Appt:** Assoc Prof T&CS, NYU Sch Med

Tortolani, Anthony J MD (T&CS) - **Spec Exp:** Transfusion Free Surgery; Heart Valve Surgery; Coronary Artery Surgery; **Hospital:** New York Methodist Hosp (page 440), NY-Presby/Weill Cornell Med Ctr, NY (page 104); **Address:** New York Methodist Hosp - Dept Surgery, 506 6th St Fl 6, Brooklyn, NY 11215; **Phone:** 718-780-5990; **Board Cert:** Surgery 1975; Thoracic Surgery 2009; **Med School:** Geo Wash Univ 1969; **Resid:** Surgery, N Shore Univ Hosp 1974; **Fellow:** Cardiothoracic Surgery, NYU Langone Med Ctr 1978; **Fac Appt:** Assoc Prof S, Cornell Univ-Weill Med Coll

Urology

Grunberger, Ivan MD (U) - **Spec Exp:** Prostate Cancer; Impotence; Minimally Invasive Surgery; Kidney Stones; **Hospital:** New York Methodist Hosp (page 440); **Address:** One Prospect Park West, Ste C, Brooklyn, NY 11215; **Phone:** 718-230-7788; **Board Cert:** Urology 2007; **Med School:** NYU Sch Med 1980; **Resid:** Surgery, N Shore Univ Hosp 1982; Urology, NYU Langone Med Ctr 1988; **Fac Appt:** Clin Prof U, Cornell Univ-Weill Med Coll

Meisenberg, Gene MD (U) - **Spec Exp:** Prostate Disease; Kidney Stones; Impotence; **Hospital:** NY-Presby/Weill Cornell Med Ctr, NY (page 104); **Address:** 1523 Voorhies Ave, Fl 5th, MS 11235, Brooklyn, NY 11235; **Phone:** 718-743-2200; **Board Cert:** Urology 2011; **Med School:** Russia 1981; **Resid:** Surgery, Beth Israel Med Ctr - Petrie Div 1993; Urology, UNDNJ - RW Johnson Med Sch Affil Hosps 1998

Rosenthal, Sheldon MD (U) - **Spec Exp:** Kidney Stones; Prostate Disease; **Hospital:** Wyckoff Heights Med Ctr; **Address:** 359 Stockholm St Fl 1, Brooklyn, NY 11237; **Phone:** 718-821-3200; **Board Cert:** Urology 1977; **Med School:** Ros Franklin Univ/Chicago Med Sch 1967; **Resid:** Surgery, Albert Einstein Coll Med Affil Hosps 1970; Urology, NY Med Coll Affil Hosps 1975

Saada, Simon MD (U) - **Spec Exp:** Kidney Stones; Prostate Cancer; Kidney Cancer; **Hospital:** Maimonides Med Ctr (page 98), Richmond Univ Med Ctr; **Address:** 705 86th St, Ste M2, Brooklyn, NY 11228-3219; **Phone:** 718-238-1075; **Board Cert:** Urology 1981; **Med School:** Egypt 1970; **Resid:** Surgery, LI Coll Med Ctr 1974; Urology, Charleston Area Med Ctr 1981

Shabsigh, Ridwan MD (U) - **Spec Exp:** Erectile Dysfunction; Hypogonadism; Clinical Trials; Incontinence; **Hospital:** Maimonides Med Ctr (page 98); **Address:** 6300 8th Ave, Brooklyn, NY 11220; **Phone:** 718-283-7746; **Board Cert:** Urology 2011; **Med School:** Syria 1976; **Resid:** Urology, Seepark Hosp 1983; Urology, Baylor Med Ctr 1990; **Fellow:** Urology, Baylor Med Ctr 1987; **Fac Appt:** Clin Prof U, Columbia P&S

Sharaby, Jacob S MD (U) - **Hospital:** Maimonides Med Ctr (page 98), Beth Israel Med Ctr-Kings Hwy Div (page 94); **Address:** 770 Ocean Pkwy, Brooklyn, NY 11217; **Phone:** 718-941-2002; **Board Cert:** Urology 2011; **Med School:** Israel 1992; **Resid:** Surgery, Beth Israel Med Ctr 1994; Urology, Maimonides Med Ctr 1999

Silver, David A MD (U) - **Spec Exp:** Laparoscopic Surgery; Urologic Cancer; Robotic Surgery; Continent Urinary Diversions; **Hospital:** Maimonides Med Ctr (page 98), Lutheran Med Ctr - Brooklyn; **Address:** 6323 7th Ave, Brooklyn, NY 11220; **Phone:** 718-283-7153; **Board Cert:** Urology 2007; **Med School:** Albert Einstein Coll Med 1989; **Resid:** Urology, Maimonides Med Ctr 1995; **Fellow:** Urologic Oncology, Meml Sloan-Kettering Canc Ctr 1997

Wainstein, Sasha MD (U) - **Spec Exp:** Impotence; Voiding Dysfunction; Endourology; **Hospital:** Maimonides Med Ctr (page 98), Forest Hills Hosp (page 106); **Address:** 4720 Fort Hamilton Pkwy, Brooklyn, NY 11219-2500; **Phone:** 718-436-3900; **Board Cert:** Urology 1977; **Med School:** Colombia 1969; **Resid:** Urology, Maimonides Med Ctr 1975

Vascular & Interventional Radiology

Sclafani, Salvatore JA MD (VIR) - **Spec Exp:** Uterine Fibroid Embolization; Varicocele Embolization; Trauma; Pelvic Congestion Syndrome; **Hospital:** SUNY Downstate Med Ctr (Univ Hosp Brooklyn) (page 441); **Address:** American Access Care Physicians, 577 Prospect Ave, Brooklyn, NY 11215; **Phone:** 718-369-1444; **Board Cert:** Diagnostic Radiology 1976; Vascular & Interventional Radiology 2009; **Med School:** SUNY Upstate Med Univ 1972; **Resid:** Diagnostic Radiology, Univ Hosp-SUNY 1976; **Fac Appt:** Prof Emeritus Rad, SUNY Downstate

Vascular Surgery

Ascher, Enrico MD (VascS) - **Spec Exp:** Endovascular Surgery; Carotid Artery Surgery; Limb Sparing Surgery; Aneurysm; **Hospital:** Lutheran Med Ctr - Brooklyn; **Address:** Vascular Inst, 960 50th St, Brooklyn, NY 11219; **Phone:** 718-438-3800; **Board Cert:** Vascular Surgery 2004; **Med School:** Brazil 1974; **Resid:** Surgery, NY Med Coll 1981; **Fellow:** Vascular Surgery, Montefiore Med Ctr 1982; **Fac Appt:** Prof S, SUNY Downstate

D'Ayala, Marcus D MD (VascS) - **Spec Exp:** Endovascular Surgery; Aneurysm-Abdominal Aortic; Carotid Artery Surgery; Peripheral Vascular Disease; **Hospital:** New York Methodist Hosp (page 440); **Address:** NY Methodist Hospital, Vascular Surgery, 506 Sixth St, Brooklyn, NY 11215; **Phone:** 718-780-3288; **Board Cert:** Surgery 2008; Vascular Surgery 2009; **Med School:** Univ Wisc 1992; **Resid:** Surgery, Montefiore Med Ctr 1997; **Fellow:** Vascular Surgery, Mt Sinai Med Ctr 1998; **Fac Appt:** Assoc Clin Prof S, Cornell Univ-Weill Med Coll

Menezes, Nelson MD (VascS) - **Spec Exp:** Varicose Veins; Peripheral Vascular Disease; Carotid Artery Surgery; **Hospital:** Brooklyn Hosp Ctr, New York Methodist Hosp (page 440); **Address:** 186 Joralemon St, Ste 1002, Brooklyn, NY 11201; **Phone:** 718-625-4100; **Board Cert:** Surgery 2006; Vascular Surgery 2007; **Med School:** India 1984; **Resid:** Surgery, Brooklyn Hosp Ctr 1995; **Fellow:** Vascular Surgery, Baptist Memorial Hosp 1996; Vascular Surgery, Stony Brook Univ Med Ctr 1997; **Fac Appt:** Asst Clin Prof VascS, Cornell Univ-Weill Med Coll

Weiser, Robert MD (VascS) - **Spec Exp:** Lower Limb Arterial Disease; Carotid Artery Surgery; Lower Limb Ulcers; **Hospital:** New York Methodist Hosp (page 440); **Address:** 186 Joralemon St Fl 7, Brooklyn, NY 11201-4326; **Phone:** 718-797-1101; **Board Cert:** Surgery 2005; **Med School:** Albert Einstein Coll Med 1977; **Resid:** Surgery, Montefiore Med Ctr 1982; **Fellow:** Vascular Surgery, Montefiore Med Ctr 1983

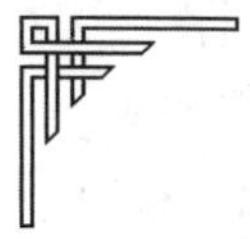

The Best in American Medicine
www.CastleConnolly.com

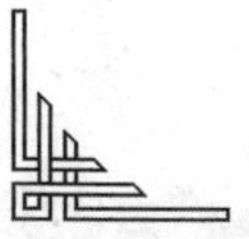
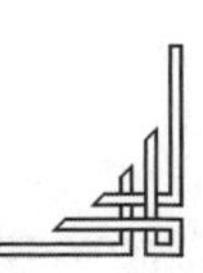

Queens

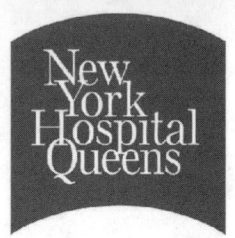

56-45 Main Street, Flushing, NY 11355
(718) 670-2000
www.nyhq.org

There is a place in Queens where medical expertise, the latest technology, and a strong dose of personal service help people feel better and return to daily living faster. A place where you can find remarkable medicine and remarkable results – results that show our care is among the very best you can find.

A place where we use sophisticated diagnostic and surgical procedures every day. Here, we treat everything from heart conditions and childhood obesity to diabetes and dental disease to tough cancers, high -risk pregnancies and serious emergencies. Even your aching knees can find relief here.

And, when you are *our* patient, we treat you like a member of our own family.
This is New York Hospital Queens. Right here, its New York Hospital Queens.

Designations, Affiliations & Accomplishments

- 535-bed tertiary care facility and community teaching hospital, accredited by the Joint Commission
- Member of the New York-Presbyterian Healthcare System, affiliated with the Joan & Sanford I. Weill Medical College of Cornell University
- West Building opened in 2010, adding 80 certified beds, a state-of-the-art ambulatory surgery center and interventional procedure area with a hybrid operating room
- One of the largest employers in Queens County with approximately 3,500+ employees and 1,700 voluntary attending physicians
- Recognized by Thomson Reuters as one of the Thomson Top 100 performance improvement leader among major teaching hospitals in the U.S. in 2007 and 2008
- Designated New York State Level 1 Regional Trauma Center and Emergency Heart Care Station
- Designated New York State Stroke Center
- Designated Level 3 Neonatal Intensive Care Unit
- Cancer Center accredited by the American College of Surgeon's Commission on Cancer
- Theresa and Eugene M. Lang Center for Research and Education with 200+ ongoing clinical trials

Expertise You Can Trust

13 Clinical Departments:

- Surgery
- Cardiothoracic Surgery
- Orthopaedics & Rehabilitation
- Anesthesiology
- Medicine
- Emergency Medicine
- Obstetrics & Gynecology
- Pediatrics
- Community Health
- Dental & Oral Medicine
- Pathology & Clinical Laboratories
- Radiation Oncology
- Radiology

Plus numerous sub specialties...

And, 23 community health centers throughout Queens

New in 2013

- Expanded Orthopaedic and Rehabilitation facility
- Community based primary care and multi specialty practices in Maspeth, Whitestone, Astoria, Fresh Meadows and Bayside

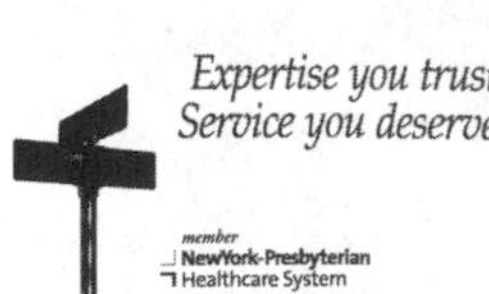

Expertise you trust.
Service you deserve.
member
NewYork-Presbyterian
Healthcare System

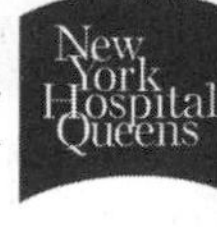

To find a doctor affiliated with New York Hospital Queens call: (800) 282-6684 or go to www.nyhq.org

Allergy & Immunology

Menchell, David L MD (A&I) - **Spec Exp:** Asthma; Nasal Allergy; Sinus Disorders; **Hospital:** NY Hosp Queens (page 488); **Address:** 73-03 198th St, Fresh Meadows, NY 11366; **Phone:** 718-465-4100; **Board Cert:** Internal Medicine 1980; Allergy & Immunology 1983; **Med School:** NYU Sch Med 1977; **Resid:** Internal Medicine, NY Hosp Queens 1980; **Fellow:** Allergy & Immunology, NY Hosp Queens 1983

Cardiovascular Disease

Akinboboye, Olakunle MD (Cv) - **Spec Exp:** Diabetes & Heart Disease; Nuclear Stress Testing; Hypertension; Coronary Artery Disease; **Hospital:** NY Hosp Queens (page 488), St. Francis Hosp - The Heart Ctr (page 116); **Address:** Laurelton Heart Specialists, 234-36 Merrick Blvd Fl 2, Rosedale, NY 11422; **Phone:** 718-949-9400; **Board Cert:** Internal Medicine 2005; Cardiovascular Disease 2005; Nuclear Cardiology 1996; **Med School:** Nigeria 1984; **Resid:** Internal Medicine, Nassau County Med Ctr 1991; **Fellow:** Cardiovascular Disease, NY-Presby/Columbia Univ Med Ctr 1995; Nuclear Cardiology, NY-Presby/Columbia Univ Med Ctr 1994; **Fac Appt:** Asst Clin Prof Med, NYU Sch Med

Hsueh, John Tzu-Lang MD (Cv) - **Spec Exp:** Coronary Artery Disease; Heart Valve Disease; **Hospital:** NY Hosp Queens (page 488), Flushing Hosp Med Ctr; **Address:** 136-17 39th Ave, Ste 4CFE, Flushing, NY 11354; **Phone:** 718-559-3600; **Board Cert:** Internal Medicine 1987; Cardiovascular Disease 1979; **Med School:** Taiwan 1970; **Resid:** Internal Medicine, Flushing Hosp Med Ctr 1976; **Fellow:** Cardiovascular Disease, Wayne State Univ 1978

Kirtane, Sanjay S MD (Cv) - **Spec Exp:** Coronary Artery Disease; Nuclear Cardiology; Heart Failure; Nuclear Cardiology; **Hospital:** St. John's Episcopal Hosp - Queens, South Nassau Comm Hosp; **Address:** 114-12 Beach Channel Drive, Ste 7, Rockaway Park, NY 11694; **Phone:** 718-318-1029; **Board Cert:** Internal Medicine 1980; Cardiovascular Disease 1983; Nuclear Cardiology 2009; **Med School:** India 1974; **Resid:** Internal Medicine, St John's Episcopal Hosp 1980; **Fellow:** Cardiovascular Disease, LI Jewish Med Ctr/St John's Episcopal Hosp 1982

Robbins, Michael J MD (Cv) - **Spec Exp:** Echocardiography; Non-Invasive Cardiology; **Hospital:** Mt Sinai Med Ctr (page 102); **Address:** 94-36 58th Ave, Ste G4, Elmhurst, NY 11373; **Phone:** 718-760-0011; **Board Cert:** Internal Medicine 1984; Cardiovascular Disease 1987; **Med School:** Cornell Univ 1981; **Resid:** Internal Medicine, Albert Einstein Coll Med Affil Hosp 1985; **Fellow:** Cardiovascular Disease, Mount Sinai Med Ctr 1987; **Fac Appt:** Assoc Prof Med, Mount Sinai Sch Med

Rydzinski, Mayer MD (Cv) - **Spec Exp:** Echocardiography; **Hospital:** NY Hosp Queens (page 488), Forest Hills Hosp (page 106); **Address:** 80-02 Kew Gardens Road, Ste 323, Kew Gardens, NY 11415; **Phone:** 718-268-7633; **Board Cert:** Internal Medicine 1979; Cardiovascular Disease 1981; Echocardiography 2008; **Med School:** Albert Einstein Coll Med 1976; **Resid:** Internal Medicine, Metropolitan Hosp Ctr 1977; Internal Medicine, Montefiore Hosp Med Ctr 1979; **Fellow:** Cardiovascular Disease, LI Jewish Hosp 1981

Siskind, Steven J MD (Cv) - **Spec Exp:** Angina; Heart Failure; Arrhythmias; Non-Invasive Cardiology; **Hospital:** NYU Langone Med Ctr (page 108), NY Hosp Queens (page 488); **Address:** NYU Cardiovascular Assocs, 142-42 Booth Memorial Ave, Flushing, NY 11355; **Phone:** 718-353-4004; **Board Cert:** Internal Medicine 1979; Cardiovascular Disease 1981; **Med School:** Albert Einstein Coll Med 1976; **Resid:** Internal Medicine, Jacobi Med Ctr 1979; **Fellow:** Cardiovascular Disease, Albert Einstein Med Coll Affil Hosp 1981; **Fac Appt:** Asst Prof, Cornell Univ-Weill Med Coll

Child & Adolescent Psychiatry

Fornari, Victor M MD (ChAP) - **Spec Exp:** Eating Disorders; Trauma Psychiatry; Post Traumatic Stress Disorder; **Hospital:** Zucker Hillside Hosp (page 106); **Address:** Zucker Hillside Hosp, Ambulatory Care Pav Lower Level, 75-59 263rd St, Glen Oaks, NY 11004; **Phone:** 718-470-3510; **Board Cert:** Psychiatry 1984; Child & Adolescent Psychiatry 1985; **Med School:** SUNY Downstate 1979; **Resid:** Psychiatry, Hosp Univ Penn - UPHS 1982; **Fellow:** Child & Adolescent Psychiatry, NS-LIJ Hlth Sys 1984; **Fac Appt:** Prof Psyc, NYU Sch Med

Kafantaris, Vivian P MD (ChAP) - **Spec Exp:** Bipolar/Mood Disorders; ADD/ADHD; Aggression Disorders; Clinical Trials; **Hospital:** Zucker Hillside Hosp (page 106); **Address:** The Zucker Hillside Hospital, Psychiatry Rsch, 75-59 263rd St, Glen Oaks, NY 11004; **Phone:** 718-470-8556; **Board Cert:** Psychiatry 1989; Child & Adolescent Psychiatry 1990; Addiction Psychiatry 2007; **Med School:** Albert Einstein Coll Med 1983; **Resid:** Psychiatry, Albert Einstein Coll Med 1987; **Fellow:** Child & Adolescent Psychiatry, NYU/Bellevue Hosp Ctr 1989; Research, NYU/Bellevue Hosp Ctr 1991

Colon & Rectal Surgery

Tiszenkel, Howard I MD (CRS) - **Spec Exp:** Colon & Rectal Cancer; Laparoscopic Surgery; **Hospital:** NY Hosp Queens (page 488); **Address:** 56-45 Main St, rm WLL300, Flushing, NY 11355-5000; **Phone:** 718-445-0220; **Board Cert:** Surgery 2006; Colon & Rectal Surgery 1988; **Med School:** NY Med Coll 1981; **Resid:** Surgery, St Luke's Hosp 1986; Colon & Rectal Surgery, Carle Clinic 1987

Critical Care Medicine

Nierman, David M MD (CCM) - **Spec Exp:** Critical Illness-Prolonged; Respiratory Failure; Sepsis; **Hospital:** Mount Sinai Hosp of Queens (page 102), Mt Sinai Med Ctr (page 102); **Address:** 27-53 Crescent St, Astoria, NY 11102; **Phone:** 718-267-4293; **Board Cert:** Internal Medicine 1984; Pulmonary Disease 1988; Critical Care Medicine 2012; **Med School:** Israel 1981; **Resid:** Internal Medicine, LIJ-Hillside Med Ctr 1984; Emergency Medicine, LIJ-Hillside Med Ctr 1984; **Fellow:** Pulmonary Disease, St Lukes-Roosevelt Hosp 1988; **Fac Appt:** Assoc Prof CCM, Mount Sinai Sch Med

Dermatology

Beyda, Bernadette A MD (D) - **Hospital:** NY Hosp Queens (page 488); **Address:** 141-23 59th Ave, Flushing, NY 11355-5304; **Phone:** 718-445-0566; **Board Cert:** Dermatology 1982; **Med School:** France 1976; **Resid:** Pathology, Booth Meml Med Ctr 1979; Dermatology, NY Hosp 1982

Fox, Joshua MD (D) - **Spec Exp:** Skin Cancer; Cosmetic Dermatology; **Hospital:** Long Is Jewish Med Ctr (page 106); **Address:** Advanced Dermatology, 58-47 188th St, Fresh Meadows, NY 11365; **Phone:** 718-357-8200; **Board Cert:** Dermatology ; **Med School:** Mount Sinai Sch Med 1982; **Resid:** Dermatology, NYU Med Ctr 1986

Gladstein, Michael J MD (D) - ; **Address:** 3062 36th Street, Astoria, NY 11103-4798; **Phone:** 718-728-8979; **Board Cert:** Dermatology 1987; **Med School:** NYU Sch Med 1979; **Resid:** Dermatology, NYU Med Ctr 1983

Pereira, Frederick A MD (D) - **Spec Exp:** Skin Cancer; Geriatric Dermatology; **Hospital:** NY Hosp Queens (page 488), Mt Sinai Med Ctr (page 102); **Address:** 51-14 Kissena Blvd, Flushing, NY 11355-4163; **Phone:** 718-359-4425; **Board Cert:** Dermatology 2009; **Med School:** UMDNJ-NJ Med Sch, Newark 1968; **Resid:** Dermatology, Mt Sinai Hosp 1974; Dermatology, Metro Hosp 1975

Diagnostic Radiology

Mollin, Joel MD (DR) - **Spec Exp:** Ultrasound; CT Scan; **Hospital:** Elmhurst Hosp Ctr; **Address:** 79-01 Broadway, E1-18, Radiology, Elmhurst, NY 11373; **Phone:** 718-334-2061; **Board Cert:** Psychiatry 1976; Diagnostic Radiology 1985; **Med School:** SUNY Downstate 1969; **Resid:** Diagnostic Radiology, USPHS Hosp-Staten Island 1981; Diagnostic Radiology, Mt Sinai Hosp 1983; **Fac Appt:** Asst Prof, Mount Sinai Sch Med

Tartell, Jay D MD (DR) - **Hospital:** Mount Sinai Hosp of Queens (page 102); **Address:** Advanced Radiological Imaging, 89-40 56th Ave, Elmhurst, NY 11373-4943; **Phone:** 718-335-5532; **Board Cert:** Diagnostic Radiology 1987; **Med School:** NY Med Coll 1982; **Resid:** Diagnostic Radiology, Bronx Muni Hosp 1986; **Fellow:** Ultrasound/CT/MRI, North Shore Univ Hosp 1987

Youner, Craig J MD (DR) - **Hospital:** Mount Sinai Hosp of Queens (page 102); **Address:** Advanced Radiological Imaging, 29-16 Astoria Blvd, Astoria, NY 11102-1742; **Phone:** 718-204-5800; **Board Cert:** Diagnostic Radiology 1978; **Med School:** Albany Med Coll 1973; **Resid:** Internal Medicine, N Shore Univ Hosp 1975; Diagnostic Radiology, N Shore Univ Hosp 1978; **Fac Appt:** Asst Clin Prof Rad, Mount Sinai Sch Med

Endocrinology, Diabetes & Metabolism

Lorber, Daniel L MD (EDM) - **Spec Exp:** Diabetes; **Hospital:** NY Hosp Queens (page 488); **Address:** Queens Diabetes & Endocrinology, 59-45 161st St, Fresh Meadows, NY 11365-1414; **Phone:** 718-762-3111; **Board Cert:** Internal Medicine 1987; Endocrinology, Diabetes & Metabolism 1977; **Med School:** Albert Einstein Coll Med 1972; **Resid:** Internal Medicine, Jacobi Med Ctr 1975; **Fellow:** Endocrinology, Diabetes & Metabolism, Vanderbilt Univ Hosp 1977; **Fac Appt:** Assoc Clin Prof Med, Cornell Univ-Weill Med Coll

Rosman, Lawrence D MD (EDM) - **Spec Exp:** Thyroid Disorders; Osteoporosis; Diabetes; Pituitary Disorders; **Hospital:** NY Hosp Queens (page 488), NYU Langone Med Ctr (page 108); **Address:** 112-03 Queens Blvd, Ste 207, Forest Hills, NY 11375-5550; **Phone:** 718-263-3718; **Board Cert:** Internal Medicine 1978; Endocrinology 1983; **Med School:** NYU Sch Med 1975; **Resid:** Internal Medicine, NYU Langone Med Ctr 1978; **Fellow:** Endocrinology, Diabetes & Metabolism, NYU Langone Med Ctr 1980; **Fac Appt:** Asst Clin Prof Med, NYU Sch Med

Tibaldi, Joseph M MD (EDM) - **Spec Exp:** Diabetes; Thyroid Disorders; Geriatric Endocrinology; **Hospital:** NY Hosp Queens (page 488); **Address:** 59-45 161st St, Fresh Meadows, NY 11365-1414; **Phone:** 718-762-3111; **Board Cert:** Internal Medicine 1982; Endocrinology, Diabetes & Metabolism 1985; **Med School:** Mount Sinai Sch Med 1979; **Resid:** Internal Medicine, Mount Sinai Med Ctr 1982; **Fellow:** Endocrinology, Montefiore Med Ctr 1984; **Fac Appt:** Asst Clin Prof Med, Cornell Univ-Weill Med Coll

Family Medicine

Fisher, George C MD (FMed) *PCP* - **Spec Exp:** Preventive Medicine; Hypertension; Cholesterol/Lipid Disorders; Diabetes; **Hospital:** Mount Sinai Hosp of Queens (page 102), Mt Sinai Med Ctr (page 102); **Address:** 22-33 33rd St, Astoria, NY 11105; **Phone:** 718-726-1000; **Board Cert:** Family Medicine 2008; **Med School:** England, UK 1979; **Resid:** Family Medicine, St Joseph Med Ctr 1993

Istrico, Richard A DO (FMed) *PCP* - **Spec Exp:** Sports Injuries; Nutrition; Preventive Medicine; **Hospital:** Long Is Jewish Med Ctr (page 106); **Address:** 158-01 Crossbay Blvd, Jamaica, NY 11414-3137; **Phone:** 718-738-9115; **Board Cert:** Family Medicine 1981; **Med School:** Philadelphia Coll Osteo Med 1978; **Resid:** Family Medicine, Interboro Hosp 1979; Sports Medicine, Baptist Med Ctr 1980

Molnar, Thomas G MD (FMed) *PCP* - **Spec Exp:** Hypertension; Diabetes; **Hospital:** NY Hosp Queens (page 488), Flushing Hosp Med Ctr; **Address:** 83-39 Daniels St, Jamaica, NY 11435-1208; **Phone:** 718-291-5151; **Board Cert:** Family Medicine 2007; **Med School:** Hungary 1982; **Resid:** Surgery, Flushing Hosp 1985; Family Medicine, Downstate Med Ctr 1988

Muraca, Glenn J DO (FMed) *PCP* - **Spec Exp:** Sports Medicine; Nutrition; **Hospital:** Flushing Hosp Med Ctr; **Address:** 104-01 Corona Ave, Corona, NY 11368; **Phone:** 718-271-2020; **Board Cert:** Family Medicine 1994; **Med School:** NY Coll Osteo Med 1990; **Resid:** Family Medicine, Peninsula Hosp 1994

Reddy, Mallikarjuna D MD (FMed) *PCP* - **Spec Exp:** Geriatric Care; **Hospital:** NY Hosp Queens (page 488); **Address:** 72-18 164th St, Flushing, NY 11365-4222; **Phone:** 718-969-6640; **Board Cert:** Family Medicine 2009; **Med School:** India 1981; **Resid:** Family Medicine, Catholic Med Ctr 1990

Roth, Alan R DO (FMed) *PCP* - **Spec Exp:** Palliative Care; Diabetes; Hypertension; **Hospital:** Jamaica Hosp Med Ctr, Flushing Hosp Med Ctr; **Address:** 11940 Metropolitan Ave, Kew Gardens, NY 11415; **Phone:** 718-849-0624; **Board Cert:** Family Medicine 2009; Hospice & Palliative Medicine 2008; **Med School:** NY Coll Osteo Med 1986; **Resid:** Family Medicine, Jamaica Hosp Med Ctr 1989; **Fac Appt:** Asst Clin Prof FMed, Albert Einstein Coll Med

Gastroenterology

Esposito, Stephen P MD (Ge) - **Hospital:** NY Hosp Queens (page 488), NY-Presby/Columbia Univ Med Ctr, NY (page 104); **Address:** 26-19 Francis Lewis Blvd, Bayside, NY 11358; **Phone:** 718-224-7186; **Board Cert:** Internal Medicine 1989; Gastroenterology 2002; **Med School:** SUNY Upstate Med Univ 1986; **Resid:** Internal Medicine, LI Jewish Hosp 1989; **Fellow:** Gastroenterology, Booth Meml Hosp 1991

Harooni, Robert B MD (Ge) - **Spec Exp:** Colonoscopy; Peptic Ulcer Disease; Capsule Endoscopy; **Hospital:** NY Hosp Queens (page 488); **Address:** 55-16 Main St, Lower Level, Flushing, NY 11355; **Phone:** 718-461-6161; **Board Cert:** Internal Medicine 1981; Gastroenterology 1985; **Med School:** Iran 1973; **Resid:** Internal Medicine, Booth Meml Hosp 1982; **Fellow:** Gastroenterology, Booth Meml Hosp 1984; **Fac Appt:** Asst Prof Med, Cornell Univ-Weill Med Coll

Nussbaum, Michel E MD (Ge) - **Spec Exp:** Endoscopy & Colonoscopy; Colon Cancer Screening; Inflammatory Bowel Disease; Peptic Ulcer Disease; **Hospital:** NY Hosp Queens (page 488); **Address:** 142-43 Booth Memorial Ave, Flushing, NY 11355-5343; **Phone:** 718-886-1919; **Board Cert:** Internal Medicine 1981; Gastroenterology 1983; **Med School:** Belgium 1977; **Resid:** Internal Medicine, NY Hosp Queens 1980; **Fellow:** Gastroenterology, NY Hosp Queens 1982; **Fac Appt:** Assoc Clin Prof

Ramgopal, Mekala MD (Ge) - **Spec Exp:** Peptic Acid Disorders; Inflammatory Bowel Disease; Colon & Rectal Cancer Detection; **Hospital:** St. John's Episcopal Hosp - Queens, Mercy Med Ctr - Rockville Centre; **Address:** 21-24 Camp Rd, Far Rockaway, NY 11691; **Phone:** 718-327-0207; **Board Cert:** Internal Medicine 1978; Gastroenterology 1979; **Med School:** India 1974; **Resid:** Internal Medicine, Jersey City Med Ctr 1976; Internal Medicine, VA Med Ctr 1977; **Fellow:** Gastroenterology, Univ Hosp 1979

Rand, James A MD (Ge) - **Spec Exp:** Colonoscopy; Endoscopy; **Hospital:** NY Hosp Queens (page 488); **Address:** 200-12 44th Ave, Bayside, NY 11361; **Phone:** 718-224-7454; **Board Cert:** Internal Medicine 1978; Gastroenterology 1981; **Med School:** Albert Einstein Coll Med 1975; **Resid:** Internal Medicine, Strong Meml Hosp 1977; Internal Medicine, Columbia-Presby Med Ctr 1978; **Fellow:** Gastroenterology, Montefiore Hosp Med Ctr 1980

Vogelman, Arthur MD (Ge) - **Spec Exp:** Colon Cancer; Peptic Ulcer Disease; Gastroesophageal Reflux Disease (GERD); **Hospital:** Forest Hills Hosp (page 106), NY Hosp Queens (page 488); **Address:** 7146 110th St, Forest Hills, NY 11375-4842; **Phone:** 718-261-2500; **Board Cert:** Internal Medicine 1979; Gastroenterology 1981; **Med School:** Univ Pittsburgh 1975; **Resid:** Internal Medicine, Mt Sinai Hosp 1978; **Fellow:** Gastroenterology, Mt Sinai Hosp 1980

Weg, Arnold L MD (Ge) - **Spec Exp:** Endoscopy; Inflammatory Bowel Disease/Crohn's; **Hospital:** NY-Presby/Weill Cornell Med Ctr, NY (page 104); **Address:** 71-36 110th St, Ste 1G, Forest Hills, NY 11375-4836; **Phone:** 718-520-2210; **Board Cert:** Internal Medicine 1985; Gastroenterology 1987; **Med School:** NYU Sch Med 1982; **Resid:** Internal Medicine, Columbia-Presby 1985; **Fellow:** Gastroenterology, NY Hosp 1987

Geriatric Medicine

Brody, Samuel A MD (Ger) - **Spec Exp:** Frail Elderly; Geriatric Care; Preventive Medicine; **Hospital:** Forest Hills Hosp (page 106), NY Hosp Queens (page 488); **Address:** 69-15 Yellowstone Blvd, Forest Hills, NY 11375; **Phone:** 718-268-4500; **Board Cert:** Internal Medicine 1980; Gastroenterology 1983; Geriatric Medicine 2008; **Med School:** Vanderbilt Univ 1977; **Resid:** Internal Medicine, Vanderbilt Med Ctr 1980; **Fellow:** Gastroenterology, Temple Univ Hosp 1983

Geriatric Psychiatry

Greenwald, Blaine MD (GerPsy) - **Spec Exp:** Depression; Dementia; **Hospital:** Zucker Hillside Hosp (page 106), N Shore Univ Hosp (page 106); **Address:** Zucker Hillside Hosp - ACP 2102, N Shore-Long Is Jewish Hlth Sys, 75-59 263rd St, Glen Oaks, NY 11004; **Phone:** 718-470-8159; **Board Cert:** Psychiatry 1983; Geriatric Psychiatry 2011; **Med School:** NY Med Coll 1978; **Resid:** Psychiatry, Mt Sinai Med Ctr 1982; **Fellow:** Geriatric Psychiatry, Mt Sinai Med Ctr/Bronx VA Hosp 1983; **Fac Appt:** Assoc Prof Psyc, Hofstra N Shore-LIJ Sch Med

Gynecologic Oncology

Hagopian, George MD (GO) - **Spec Exp:** Gynecologic Cancer; Minimally Invasive Surgery; **Hospital:** Elmhurst Hosp Ctr, Queens Hosp Ctr - Jamaica; **Address:** Elmhurst Hosp, dept Ob/Gyn, 79-01 Broadway, Elmhurst, NY 11373; **Phone:** 718-334-5366; **Board Cert:** Obstetrics & Gynecology 2012; Gynecologic Oncology 2012; **Med School:** Wayne State Univ 1998; **Resid:** Obstetrics & Gynecology, Northwestern Univ Med Ctr 2002; **Fellow:** Gynecologic Oncology, Mount Sinai Hosp 2004; Gynecologic Oncology, UT MD Anderson Cancer Ctr 2005

Welshinger, Marie MD (GO) - **Spec Exp:** Gynecologic Cancer; **Hospital:** NY Hosp Queens (page 488); **Address:** 56-45 Main St, West Wing, lower level, rm 100, Flushing, NY 11355; **Phone:** 718-670-1170; **Board Cert:** Obstetrics & Gynecology 2012; Gynecologic Oncology 2012; **Med School:** Univ Minn 1988; **Resid:** Obstetrics & Gynecology, SUNY Stony Brook Hosp 1992; **Fellow:** Gynecologic Oncology, Meml Sloan Kett Cancer Ctr 1996

Hand Surgery

Caligiuri, Daniel A MD (HS) - **Spec Exp:** Hand & Wrist Surgery; Nerve & Tendon Reconstruction; **Hospital:** Kings Co Hosp Ctr; **Address:** 23-18 31st St, Ste 210, Astoria, NY 11105; **Phone:** 718-777-1885; **Board Cert:** Orthopaedic Surgery 2005; Hand Surgery 2005; **Med School:** SUNY Downstate 1986; **Resid:** Orthopaedic Surgery, SUNY Downstate Med Ctr 1991; **Fellow:** Hand Surgery, Thomas Jefferson Univ Hosp 1992; **Fac Appt:** Asst Prof OrS, SUNY Downstate

Kamler, Kenneth M MD (HS) - **Spec Exp:** Carpal Tunnel Syndrome; Arthritis; Fractures; **Hospital:** Long Is Jewish Med Ctr (page 106); **Address:** 66-55 Fresh Pond Rd, Ridgewood, NY 11385; **Phone:** 516-326-2266; **Med School:** France 1975; **Resid:** Orthopaedic Surgery, LI Jewish Med Ctr 1979; **Fellow:** Hand Surgery, Columbia-Presby Med Ctr 1981

Hospice & Palliative Medicine

Pan, Cynthia MD (H & PM) - **Spec Exp:** Palliative Care; Pain Management; Geriatric Care; **Hospital:** NY Hosp Queens (page 488); **Address:** NY Hosp Queens-Dept of Medicine, 56-45 Main St, Flushing, NY 11355; **Phone:** 718-670-2413; **Board Cert:** Internal Medicine 2005; Geriatric Medicine 2008; Hospice & Palliative Medicine ; **Med School:** SUNY Stony Brook 1988; **Resid:** Internal Medicine, Univ Rochester Med Ctr 1995; **Fellow:** Geriatric Medicine, Harvard Univ Affil Hosp 1996; **Fac Appt:** Assoc Clin Prof Med, Cornell Univ-Weill Med Coll

Infectious Disease

Asnis, Deborah S MD (Inf) - **Spec Exp:** West Nile Virus; AIDS/HIV; Meningitis; **Hospital:** Flushing Hosp Med Ctr; **Address:** Flushing Hosp Med Ctr-Dept Medicine, 4500 Parsons Blvd, Ste 11B, Flushing, NY 11355; **Phone:** 718-670-3012; **Board Cert:** Internal Medicine 1985; Infectious Disease 1988; **Med School:** Northwestern Univ 1981; **Resid:** Ophthalmology, LI Jewish Hosp 1983; Internal Medicine, LI Jewish Hosp 1985; **Fellow:** Infectious Disease, LI Jewish Hosp 1987; **Fac Appt:** Asst Clin Prof Med, Cornell Univ-Weill Med Coll

Masci, Joseph R MD (Inf) - **Spec Exp:** AIDS/HIV; Tropical Diseases; Disaster Preparedness; **Hospital:** Elmhurst Hosp Ctr, Mt Sinai Med Ctr (page 102); **Address:** Elmhurst Hosp, Dept Med, 79-01 Broadway, rm C 6-10, Elmhurst, NY 11373; **Phone:** 718-334-3446; **Board Cert:** Internal Medicine 1979; Infectious Disease 1982; **Med School:** NYU Sch Med 1976; **Resid:** Internal Medicine, Boston City Hosp 1979; **Fellow:** Infectious Disease, Mt Sinai Hosp 1982; **Fac Appt:** Prof Med, Mount Sinai Sch Med

Segal-Maurer, Sorana MD (Inf) - **Spec Exp:** AIDS/HIV; Viral Infections; Tuberculosis; **Hospital:** NY Hosp Queens (page 488); **Address:** NY Hosp Queens, Div Infectious Dis, 56-45 Main St, Flushing, NY 11355-5000; **Phone:** 718-670-1525; **Board Cert:** Infectious Disease 2000; **Med School:** Mount Sinai Sch Med 1988; **Resid:** Internal Medicine, Jacobi Med Ctr 1991; **Fellow:** Infectious Disease, Montefiore Med Ctr 1993

Internal Medicine

Amin, Mahendra MD (IM) *PCP* - **Hospital:** Long Is Jewish Med Ctr (page 106); **Address:** 89-02 Springfield Blvd, Queens Village, NY 11427-2514; **Phone:** 718-776-4444; **Board Cert:** Internal Medicine 1984; **Med School:** India 1978; **Resid:** Internal Medicine, Metro Hosp Ctr 1982; **Fellow:** Internal Medicine, Metro Hosp Ctr 1985

Beyda, Allan E MD (IM) *PCP* - **Spec Exp:** Preventive Medicine; Cholesterol/Lipid Disorders; **Hospital:** NY Hosp Queens (page 488), N Shore Univ Hosp (page 106); **Address:** 141-23 59th Ave, Flushing, NY 11355-5304; **Phone:** 718-359-7406; **Board Cert:** Internal Medicine 1979; **Med School:** France 1976; **Resid:** Internal Medicine, New York Hosp Med Ctr 1979

Blum, Daniel N MD (IM) *PCP* - **Spec Exp:** Geriatric Care; Hypertension; Diabetes; Complex Diagnosis; **Hospital:** NY Hosp Queens (page 488); **Address:** 13806 Jewel Ave, Flushing, NY 11367-1933; **Phone:** 718-520-0248; **Board Cert:** Internal Medicine 1984; **Med School:** Albert Einstein Coll Med 1980; **Resid:** Internal Medicine, NY Hosp of Queens 1984

Brewer, Marlon E MD (IM) *PCP* - **Spec Exp:** Diabetes; Hypertension; Preventive Medicine; **Hospital:** Elmhurst Hosp Ctr; **Address:** 79-01 Broadway, rm A1-16, Elmhurst, NY 11373; **Phone:** 718-334-2490; **Board Cert:** Internal Medicine 2004; **Med School:** Spain 1986; **Resid:** Internal Medicine, Elmhurst Hosp 1992; **Fac Appt:** Asst Prof Med, Mount Sinai Sch Med

Fukilman, Oscar J MD (IM) *PCP* - **Spec Exp:** Preventive Medicine; **Hospital:** Mount Sinai Hosp of Queens (page 102); **Address:** 25-31 30th Road, Ste 1A, Astoria, NY 11102; **Phone:** 718-267-1102; **Board Cert:** Internal Medicine 1979; **Med School:** Argentina 1968; **Resid:** Internal Medicine, Elmhurst Hosp/Mt Sinai Hosp Svc 1972

Joseph, John L MD (IM) - **Spec Exp:** Rheumatology; Osteoporosis; Arthritis; **Hospital:** NY Hosp Queens (page 488); **Address:** 66-20 108th St, Forest Hills, NY 11375; **Phone:** 718-896-8920; **Board Cert:** Internal Medicine 1983; **Med School:** Mexico 1977; **Resid:** Internal Medicine, Coney Island Hosp 1982; **Fellow:** Rheumatology, Long Island Coll Hosp 1984

Messana, Ida MD (IM) *PCP* - **Spec Exp:** Geriatric Medicine; Preventive Medicine; **Hospital:** Long Is Jewish Med Ctr (page 106), N Shore Univ Hosp (page 106); **Address:** 109-33 71st Rd, Ste 2E, Forest Hills, NY 11375; **Phone:** 718-263-4345; **Board Cert:** Internal Medicine 1988; **Med School:** SUNY Stony Brook 1984; **Resid:** Internal Medicine, Montefiore Med Ctr 1987; **Fellow:** Geriatric Medicine, Montefiore Med Ctr 1989

Pasquale, Jack MD (IM) - **Spec Exp:** Nutrition; Nutrition & Cancer Prevention/Control; Nutrition in Cancer Therapy; **Hospital:** NY Hosp Queens (page 488); **Address:** Clinical Nutrition Service, 73-03 198th St, Fresh Meadows, NY 11366-1818; **Phone:** 718-465-0041; **Board Cert:** Internal Medicine 1987; **Med School:** Grenada 1981; **Resid:** Internal Medicine, Millard Fillmore Hosp 1984; **Fellow:** Nutrition, Hosp Univ Penn 1985

Somogyi, Anthony MD (IM) *PCP* - **Hospital:** NY Hosp Queens (page 488); **Address:** 42-23 Francis Lewis Blvd, Ste 201, Bayside, NY 11361; **Phone:** 718-224-5687; **Board Cert:** Internal Medicine 1979; **Med School:** Belgium 1976; **Resid:** Internal Medicine, NY Hosp Queens 1980

Interventional Cardiology

Papadakos, Stylianos P MD (IC) - **Spec Exp:** Cardiac Catheterization; Percutaneous Myocardial Revasc (PMR); Angioplasty & Stent Placement; **Hospital:** NYU Langone Med Ctr (page 108), NS-LIJ Hlth Sys (page 106); **Address:** Cardiovascular Assocs of New York, 44-01 Francis Lewis Blvd, Level 3, Bayside, NY 11361; **Phone:** 718-423-3355; **Board Cert:** Cardiovascular Disease 2004; Interventional Cardiology 2010; **Med School:** Greece 1985; **Resid:** Internal Medicine, Booth Meml Med Ctr 1989; Internal Medicine, Mt Sinai Hosp 1990; **Fellow:** Cardiovascular Disease, Univ Conn Hosp 1994; **Fac Appt:** Asst Clin Prof Med, Cornell Univ-Weill Med Coll

Maternal & Fetal Medicine

Eglinton, Gary Scott MD (MF) - **Spec Exp:** Obstetric Ultrasound; Fetal Diagnosis & Therapy; Pregnancy-High Risk; **Hospital:** NY Hosp Queens (page 488); **Address:** NY Hosp Queens, Ob/Gyn Dept, 56-45 Main St, rm M36, Flushing, NY 11355; **Phone:** 718-670-1534; **Board Cert:** Obstetrics & Gynecology 2012; Maternal & Fetal Medicine 2012; **Med School:** Univ Ariz Coll Med 1976; **Resid:** Obstetrics & Gynecology, David Grant USAF Med Ctr 1980; **Fellow:** Maternal & Fetal Medicine, LAC-USC Med Ctr 1982; **Fac Appt:** Assoc Prof ObG, Cornell Univ-Weill Med Coll

Inglis, Steven R MD (MF) - **Spec Exp:** Pregnancy-High Risk; Obstetric Ultrasound; Prenatal Diagnosis; **Hospital:** Jamaica Hosp Med Ctr; **Address:** Jamaica Hosp, Dept Ob/Gyn, 89-06 135th St, Ste 6A, Jamaica, NY 11418; **Phone:** 718-206-7642; **Board Cert:** Obstetrics & Gynecology 2012; Maternal & Fetal Medicine 2012; **Med School:** NY Med Coll 1986; **Resid:** Obstetrics & Gynecology, Albany Med Ctr 1990; **Fellow:** Maternal & Fetal Medicine, NY-Presby/Weill Cornell Med Ctr 1992; **Fac Appt:** Assoc Prof ObG, Cornell Univ-Weill Med Coll

Skupski, Daniel MD (MF) - **Spec Exp:** Fetal Diagnosis & Therapy; Multiple Gestation; **Hospital:** NY Hosp Queens (page 488), NY-Presby/Weill Cornell Med Ctr, NY (page 104); **Address:** 56-45 Main St, Flushing, NY 11355-5060; **Phone:** 718-670-1534; **Board Cert:** Obstetrics & Gynecology 2012; Maternal & Fetal Medicine 2012; **Med School:** Univ Mich Med Sch 1985; **Resid:** Obstetrics & Gynecology, Hurley Med Ctr 1989; **Fellow:** Maternal & Fetal Medicine, NY-Presby/Weill Cornell Med Ctr 1994; **Fac Appt:** Prof ObG, Cornell Univ-Weill Med Coll

Medical Oncology

Abramowitz, Avram L MD (Onc) - **Spec Exp:** Breast Cancer; Colon & Rectal Cancer; Lung Cancer; Leukemia & Lymphoma; **Hospital:** Mt Sinai Med Ctr (page 102), Forest Hills Hosp (page 106); **Address:** 176-60 Union Tpke, Ste 360, Fresh Meadows, NY 11366; **Phone:** 718-460-2300; **Board Cert:** Internal Medicine 1987; Hematology 2004; Medical Oncology 2004; **Med School:** NY Med Coll 1984; **Resid:** Internal Medicine, Roosevelt Hosp 1987; **Fellow:** Hematology & Oncology, Roosevelt Hosp 1989; Bone Marrow Transplant, Mt Sinai Med Ctr 1993

Benisovich, Vladimir I MD (Onc) - **Spec Exp:** Breast Cancer; Lung Cancer; Colon Cancer; **Hospital:** Elmhurst Hosp Ctr, Mt Sinai Med Ctr (page 102); **Address:** 79-01 Broadway, Ste H2-04, Elmhurst, NY 11373-1329; **Phone:** 718-334-3723; **Board Cert:** Internal Medicine 1982; Hematology 1984; Medical Oncology 1985; **Med School:** Russia 1966; **Resid:** Internal Medicine, Bronx Lebanon Hosp 1980; **Fellow:** Hematology, NYU Med Ctr 1982; Medical Oncology, Mt Sinai Med Ctr 1983

Cortes, Engracio P MD (Onc) - **Spec Exp:** Breast Cancer; Gastrointestinal Cancer; Lung Cancer; Lymphoma; **Hospital:** NY Hosp Queens (page 488), Long Is Jewish Med Ctr (page 106); **Address:** 200-20 44th Ave, Bayside, NY 11361; **Phone:** 718-279-9101; **Board Cert:** Internal Medicine 1976; Medical Oncology 1977; **Med School:** Philippines 1964; **Resid:** Internal Medicine, Lemuel Shattuck Hosp 1968; **Fellow:** Medical Oncology, Roswell Park Cancer Inst 1971; **Fac Appt:** Assoc Clin Prof Med, Cornell Univ-Weill Med Coll

Daly, Jane E MD (Onc) - **Hospital:** NY Hosp Queens (page 488); **Address:** 87-23 Myrtle Ave, Glendale, NY 11385-7431; **Phone:** 718-441-5581; **Board Cert:** Internal Medicine 1978; Hematology 1980; Medical Oncology 1981; **Med School:** NY Med Coll 1975; **Resid:** Internal Medicine, Kings County Hosp 1978; **Fellow:** Hematology, LI Jewish Med Ctr 1980; Medical Oncology, Albert Einstein Coll Med Affil Hosp 1981

Greenberg, Howard J MD (Onc) - **Spec Exp:** Breast Cancer; Colon Cancer; Lymphoma; Coagulation/Bleeding Disorders; **Hospital:** Mount Sinai Hosp of Queens (page 102), Mt Sinai Med Ctr (page 102); **Address:** 2715 30th Ave, Astoria, NY 11102; **Phone:** 718-278-3569; **Board Cert:** Internal Medicine 1976; Hematology 1978; Medical Oncology 1979; **Med School:** SUNY Downstate 1973; **Resid:** Internal Medicine, Mt Sinai Hosp 1976; **Fellow:** Hematology, Mt Sinai Hosp 1978; Medical Oncology, Meml Sloan-Kettering Cancer Ctr 1979; **Fac Appt:** Asst Clin Prof Med, Mount Sinai Sch Med

Shum, Kee Y MD (Onc) - **Spec Exp:** Breast Cancer; Lung Cancer; Colon Cancer; **Hospital:** NY Hosp Queens (page 488), Flushing Hosp Med Ctr; **Address:** 136-25 Maple Ave, Ste 205, Flushing, NY 11355-3891; **Phone:** 718-463-2245; **Board Cert:** Internal Medicine 1984; Medical Oncology 1987; **Med School:** Cornell Univ-Weill Med Coll 1981; **Resid:** Internal Medicine, Kings County Hosp 1985; **Fellow:** Medical Oncology, Meml Sloan-Kettering Cancer Ctr 1987

Neonatal-Perinatal Medicine

Hand, Ivan L MD (NP) - **Spec Exp:** Respiratory Distress Syndrome; Prematurity/Low Birth Weight Infants; Nutrition; Breast Feeding Problems; **Hospital:** Kings Co Hosp Ctr, Queens Hosp Ctr - Jamaica; **Address:** Director, Division of Neonatology, 451 Clarkson Ave, Brooklyn, NY 11203; **Phone:** 718-245-4753; **Board Cert:** Pediatrics 1986; Neonatal-Perinatal Medicine 2004; **Med School:** Albert Einstein Coll Med 1982; **Resid:** Pediatrics, Montefiore Med Ctr 1985; Pediatrics, Bronx Lebanon Hosp 1986; **Fellow:** Neonatal-Perinatal Medicine, NY Hosp-Cornell Med Ctr 1988; **Fac Appt:** Assoc Prof Ped, SUNY Downstate

Nephrology

Galler, Marilyn MD (Nep) - **Spec Exp:** Hypertension; Kidney Disease; **Hospital:** NY Hosp Queens (page 488); **Address:** 56-45 Main St, rm M201, Flushing, NY 11355-5045; **Phone:** 718-670-1151; **Board Cert:** Internal Medicine 1979; Nephrology 1984; **Med School:** NYU Sch Med 1975; **Resid:** Internal Medicine, Bronx Muni Hosp 1979; **Fellow:** Nephrology, Montefiore Med Ctr 1981; **Fac Appt:** Asst Clin Prof Med, Cornell Univ-Weill Med Coll

Mattoo, Nirmal K MD (Nep) - **Spec Exp:** Kidney Failure; Hypertension; Dialysis Care; **Hospital:** Wyckoff Heights Med Ctr, Forest Hills Hosp (page 106); **Address:** 385 Seneca Ave, Ridgewood, NY 11385; **Phone:** 347-312-3041; **Board Cert:** Internal Medicine 1974; Nephrology 1978; **Med School:** India 1967; **Resid:** Internal Medicine, Queens Hosp Ctr 1971; Internal Medicine, Catholic Med Ctr 1972; **Fellow:** Nephrology, Elmhurst Hosp Ctr 1975

Scott III, David MD (Nep) - **Spec Exp:** Hypertension; Kidney Disease; Diabetes; **Hospital:** NY Hosp Queens (page 488), NY-Presby/Weill Cornell Med Ctr, NY (page 104); **Address:** 1 Cross Island Plaza, Rosedale, NY 11422; **Phone:** 718-276-4750; **Board Cert:** Internal Medicine 2003; Nephrology 2005; **Med School:** Tufts Univ 1985; **Resid:** Internal Medicine, Harlem Hosp 1988; **Fellow:** Nephrology, Harlem Hosp 1990

Spinowitz, Bruce S MD (Nep) - **Spec Exp:** Diabetic Kidney Disease; Hypertension; Kidney Stones; **Hospital:** NY Hosp Queens (page 488), Montefiore Med Ctr-Einstein Campus (page 100); **Address:** 56-45 Main St, rm M201, Flushing, NY 11355-5045; **Phone:** 718-670-1151; **Board Cert:** Internal Medicine 1976; Nephrology 1978; **Med School:** NYU Sch Med 1973; **Resid:** Internal Medicine, Bellevue Hosp 1976; **Fellow:** Nephrology, Bellevue Hosp 1978; **Fac Appt:** Assoc Clin Prof Med, Cornell Univ-Weill Med Coll

Neurology

Appelbaum, Jeffrey C DO (N) - **Spec Exp:** Multiple Sclerosis; Peripheral Neuropathy; **Hospital:** NY Hosp Queens (page 488), Long Is Jewish Med Ctr (page 106); **Address:** 59-07 175 Pl, Flushing, NY 11365; **Phone:** 718-939-0800; **Board Cert:** Neurology 1982; **Med School:** Philadelphia Coll Osteo Med 1977; **Resid:** Neurology, Downstate Med Ctr 1981; **Fac Appt:** Assoc Prof N, NY Coll Osteo Med

Casson, Ira R MD (N) - **Spec Exp:** Sports Neurology; Headache; Head Injury; Concussion; **Hospital:** Long Is Jewish Med Ctr (page 106); **Address:** 112-03 Queens Blvd, Ste 201, Forest Hills, NY 11375-5550; **Phone:** 718-544-6633; **Board Cert:** Neurology ; **Med School:** NYU Sch Med 1975; **Resid:** Neurology, NYU Med Ctr 1979; **Fac Appt:** Asst Prof N, Albert Einstein Coll Med

Oribe, Emilio M MD (N) - **Spec Exp:** Movement Disorders; Stroke; **Hospital:** NY Hosp Queens (page 488), NY-Presby/Weill Cornell Med Ctr, NY (page 104); **Address:** 27-47 Crescent St, Astoria, NY 11102; **Phone:** 718-606-9193; **Board Cert:** Therapeutic Radiology 1986; Neurology 1991; **Med School:** Uruguay 1981; **Resid:** Internal Medicine, NYU Downtown Hosp 1986; Neurology, Mt Sinai Med Ctr 1989; **Fellow:** Movement Disorders, Mt Sinai Med Ctr 1991

Obstetrics & Gynecology

Benedicto, Milagros A MD (ObG) - **Hospital:** Wyckoff Heights Med Ctr; **Address:** 68-52 Fresh Pond Rd, Ridgewood, NY 11385; **Phone:** 718-381-7016; **Board Cert:** Obstetrics & Gynecology 2012; **Med School:** Philippines 1964; **Resid:** Obstetrics & Gynecology, Wyckoff Heights Hosp 1969; **Fellow:** Wyckoff Heights Hosp 1971

Ophthalmology

Aharon, Raphael MD (Oph) - **Spec Exp:** Diagnostic Problems; Eye Infections; **Hospital:** Montefiore Med Ctr-Moses Campus (page 100), NY Hosp Queens (page 488); **Address:** 108-37 71st Ave, Forest Hills, NY 11375-4566; **Phone:** 718-268-6120; **Board Cert:** Ophthalmology 1987; **Med School:** Albert Einstein Coll Med 1980; **Resid:** Internal Medicine, Brookdale Hosp 1981; Ophthalmology, Albert Einstein Coll Med Affil Hosp 1984; **Fac Appt:** Asst Clin Prof Oph, Albert Einstein Coll Med

Fishman, Allen J MD (Oph) - **Spec Exp:** Cataract Surgery-Lens Implant; LASIK-Refractive Surgery; **Hospital:** Flushing Hosp Med Ctr; **Address:** 92-29 Queens Blvd, Ste 2I, Rego Park, NY 11374; **Phone:** 718-261-7007; **Board Cert:** Ophthalmology 1981; **Med School:** Ros Franklin Univ/Chicago Med Sch 1976; **Resid:** Surgery, Beth Israel Med Ctr 1977; Ophthalmology, Brookdale Hosp 1980

Grasso, Cono M MD (Oph) - **Spec Exp:** Cataract Surgery; Glaucoma; Oculoplastic Surgery; **Hospital:** Jamaica Hosp Med Ctr, Flushing Hosp Med Ctr; **Address:** Comprehensive Ophthalmology, 83-05 Grand Ave, Elmhurst, NY 11373-4104; **Phone:** 718-429-0300; **Board Cert:** Ophthalmology 1979; **Med School:** NY Med Coll 1974; **Resid:** Internal Medicine, Metropolitan Hosp Ctr 1975; Ophthalmology, Wills Eye 1978; **Fac Appt:** Assoc Prof Oph, NY Med Coll

Mackool, Richard J MD (Oph) - **Spec Exp:** Cataract Surgery; LASIK-Refractive Surgery; Lens Implants-Multifocal; Corneal Disease & Surgery; **Hospital:** New York Eye & Ear Infirm (page 115), NYU Langone Med Ctr (page 108); **Address:** Mackool Eye Institute, 31-27 41st St, Astoria, NY 11103; **Phone:** 718-728-3400; **Board Cert:** Ophthalmology 1976; **Med School:** Boston Univ 1968; **Resid:** Ophthalmology, New York EE Infirm 1973; **Fac Appt:** Clin Prof Oph, NYU Sch Med

Winterkorn, Jacqueline S MD/PhD (Oph) - **Spec Exp:** Neuro-Ophthalmology; Brain Tumors; Eye Muscle Disorders; **Hospital:** NY-Presby/Weill Cornell Med Ctr, NY (page 104); **Address:** 161-10 Union Tpke, Flushing, NY 11366; **Phone:** 718-380-5346; **Board Cert:** Ophthalmology 1989; **Med School:** Cornell Univ-Weill Med Coll 1983; **Resid:** Ophthalmology, Mount Sinai Med Ctr 1987; **Fellow:** Neuro-Ophthalmology, Columbia Presby Med Ctr 1988; **Fac Appt:** Clin Prof Oph, Cornell Univ-Weill Med Coll

Orthopaedic Surgery

Besser Sr, Walter A MD (OrS) - **Spec Exp:** Joint Replacement; Fractures; Trauma; **Hospital:** Mount Sinai Hosp of Queens (page 102), NY Hosp Queens (page 488); **Address:** 30-71 29th St, Astoria, NY 11102; **Phone:** 718-204-7752; **Board Cert:** Orthopaedic Surgery 1977; **Med School:** Spain 1968; **Resid:** Orthopaedic Surgery, LI Jewish Hosp 1971; Orthopaedic Surgery, Brooklyn Jewish Hosp 1974; **Fellow:** Orthopaedic Surgery, Hosp Special Surg 1977; **Fac Appt:** Asst Clin Prof OrS, NYU Sch Med

Schwartz, Evan G MD (OrS) - **Spec Exp:** Sports Medicine; Shoulder Surgery; Knee Surgery; Joint Replacement; **Hospital:** Lenox Hill Hosp (page 106); **Address:** Hellenic Medical Ctr, 30-16 30th Drive, Ste 1B, Astoria, NY 11102; **Phone:** 718-558-1975; **Board Cert:** Orthopaedic Surgery 2010; **Med School:** SUNY Buffalo 1981; **Resid:** Orthopaedic Surgery, Montefiore Med Ctr 1986; **Fellow:** Sports Medicine, Hosp Special Surg 1987; Shoulder Surgery, Hosp Special Surg 1987; **Fac Appt:** Asst Prof OrS, NY Med Coll

Touliopoulos, Steven J MD (OrS) - **Spec Exp:** Sports Medicine; Fractures; Hip Replacement; Knee Replacement; **Hospital:** Mount Sinai Hosp of Queens (page 102), NY-Presby/Lower Manhattan Hosp (page 104); **Address:** Univ Orthopedics of NY, 23-18 31st St, Ste 210, Astoria, NY 11105; **Phone:** 718-777-1885; **Board Cert:** Orthopaedic Surgery 2010; Orthopaedic Sports Medicine 2007; **Med School:** SUNY Downstate 1991; **Resid:** Orthopaedic Surgery, SUNY Hlth Sci Ctr 1996; **Fellow:** Orthopaedic Sports Medicine, Lenox Hill Hosp 1997

Otolaryngology

Huo, Jerry MD (Oto) - **Spec Exp:** Endoscopic Sinus Surgery; Thyroid Surgery; Parotid Gland Surgery; Vocal Cord Disorders; **Hospital:** NY Hosp Queens (page 488); **Address:** 136-20 38th Ave, Ste 7J, Flushing, NY 11354; **Phone:** 718-670-0006; **Board Cert:** Otolaryngology 1998; **Med School:** Mount Sinai Sch Med 1991; **Resid:** Surgery, Lenox Hill Hosp 1993; Otolaryngology, Manhattan EE&T Hosp 1997; **Fac Appt:** Asst Clin Prof Oto, Cornell Univ-Weill Med Coll

La Marca, Charles A MD (Oto) - **Hospital:** Glen Cove Hosp (page 106); **Address:** 75-06 Eliot Ave, Middle Village, NY 11379-1207; **Phone:** 718-335-2224; **Board Cert:** Otolaryngology 1984; **Med School:** Mexico 1977; **Resid:** Otolaryngology, Downstate Med Ctr 1982

Snyder, Gary M MD (Oto) - **Spec Exp:** Cosmetic Surgery-Face; Endoscopic Sinus Surgery; Voice Disorders; Sinus Surgery; **Hospital:** Flushing Hosp Med Ctr, N Shore Univ Hosp (page 106); **Address:** 26-01 Corporal Kennedy St, FL 1 Bldg, Bayside, NY 11360-2452; **Phone:** 718-423-4091; **Board Cert:** Otolaryngology 1983; **Med School:** NY Med Coll 1979; **Resid:** Surgery, North Shore Univ Hosp 1980; Otolaryngology, Manhattan EET Hosp 1983

Pediatric Cardiology

Rutkovsky, Lisa E MD (PCd) - **Spec Exp:** Congenital Heart Disease; Arrhythmias; **Hospital:** NY Hosp Queens (page 488); **Address:** 14223 Booth Memorial Ave, Flushing, NY 11355; **Phone:** 718-460-9776; **Board Cert:** Pediatrics 2007; Pediatric Cardiology 2007; **Med School:** NYU Sch Med 1986; **Resid:** Pediatrics, N Shore Univ Hosp 1989; **Fellow:** Pediatric Cardiology, NYU-Bellevue Hosp 1992; **Fac Appt:** Asst Prof Ped, NYU Sch Med

Pediatrics

Abularrage, Joseph J MD (Ped) *PCP* - **Hospital:** NY Hosp Queens (page 488); **Address:** NY Hosp Queens, Dept Pediatrics, 56-45 Main St, Flushing, NY 11355-5045; **Phone:** 718-670-1033; **Board Cert:** Pediatrics 1981; **Med School:** NYU Sch Med 1975; **Resid:** Pediatrics, NYU-Bellevue Hosp 1979; **Fellow:** Public Health & Genl Preventive Med, NY-Presby/Columbia Univ Med Ctr 1981

Goldstein, Steven J MD (Ped) *PCP* - **Spec Exp:** Nutrition; Asthma; Vaccines; **Hospital:** Long Is Jewish Med Ctr (page 106), NY Hosp Queens (page 488); **Address:** Kew Garden Hills Pediatrics, 141-49 70th Rd, Flushing, NY 11367; **Phone:** 718-268-5282; **Board Cert:** Pediatrics ; **Med School:** SUNY Downstate 1978; **Resid:** Pediatrics, LI Jewish Med Ctr 1981

Yadoo, Moshe MD (Ped) *PCP* - **Hospital:** St. Mary's Hosp for Chldn, Long Is Jewish Med Ctr (page 106); **Address:** St Mary's Hosp for Children, 29-01 216 St, Bayside, NY 11360; **Phone:** 718-281-8525; **Board Cert:** Pediatrics 1987; **Med School:** SUNY Hlth Sci Ctr 1983; **Resid:** Pediatrics, Brookdale Hosp 1986; **Fellow:** Neonatal-Perinatal Medicine, Schneider Chldns Hosp 1988

Physical Medicine & Rehabilitation

Vallarino, Ramon MD (PMR) - **Spec Exp:** Functional Ability Loss; Electromyography; Musculoskeletal Disorders; **Hospital:** New York Methodist Hosp (page 440); **Address:** 37-04 91st St, Jackson Heights, NY 11372; **Phone:** 516-418-0675; **Board Cert:** Physical Medicine & Rehabilitation 1977; **Med School:** Peru 1966; **Resid:** Physical Medicine & Rehabilitation, Mt Sinai Hosp 1968; **Fellow:** Rheumatology, Mt Sinai Hosp 1968; **Fac Appt:** Asst Clin Prof PMR, SUNY Hlth Sci Ctr

Psychiatry

Kalash, Glenn DO (Psyc) - **Spec Exp:** Psychiatry in Physical Illness; Psychosomatic Disorders; Forensic Psychiatry; Liaison Psychiatry; **Hospital:** Jamaica Hosp Med Ctr, St. Francis Hosp - The Heart Ctr (page 116); **Address:** Jamaica Hosp, Dept Psychiatry, 8900 Van Wyck Expressway, Jamaica, NY 11418; **Phone:** 718-206-7167; **Board Cert:** Psychiatry 2008; Forensic Psychiatry 2009; Psychosomatic Medicine 2005; **Med School:** NY Coll Osteo Med 1992; **Resid:** Psychiatry, NS-LIJ Hlth Sys 1996; **Fellow:** Liaison Psychiatry, Meml Sloan-Kettering Cancer Ctr 1997

Mendelowitz, Alan MD (Psyc) - **Spec Exp:** Schizophrenia; Psychopharmacology; **Hospital:** Zucker Hillside Hosp (page 106); **Address:** 75-59 263rd St, rm 208, Glen Oaks, NY 11004; **Phone:** 718-470-8397; **Board Cert:** Psychiatry 1992; **Med School:** UMDNJ-Rutgers Med Sch 1987; **Resid:** Psychiatry, Hillside Hosp 1991

Selzer, Jeffrey A MD (Psyc) - **Spec Exp:** Mood Disorders; Depression; Addiction/Substance Abuse; **Hospital:** Zucker Hillside Hosp (page 106), N Shore Univ Hosp (page 106); **Address:** 75-59 263rd St, Glen Oaks, NY 11004-1150; **Phone:** 718-470-8023; **Board Cert:** Psychiatry 1985; Addiction Psychiatry 2003; **Med School:** Univ Mich Med Sch 1979; **Resid:** Psychiatry, UCLA Med Ctr 1983; **Fac Appt:** Assoc Prof Psyc, Albert Einstein Coll Med

Vivek, Seeth MD (Psyc) - **Spec Exp:** Depression; Panic Disorder; Obsessive-Compulsive Disorder; Liaison Psychiatry; **Hospital:** Jamaica Hosp Med Ctr, Flushing Hosp Med Ctr; **Address:** 75-58 113th St, Ste 1A, Forest Hills, NY 11375-7429; **Phone:** 718-268-9595; **Board Cert:** Psychiatry 1980; Addiction Psychiatry 2011; Geriatric Psychiatry 2011; Psychosomatic Medicine 2005; **Med School:** India 1972; **Resid:** Psychiatry, Natl Inst Mental Hlth 1976; Psychiatry, Mt Sinai Hosp 1979; **Fellow:** Liaison Psychiatry, Montefiore Hosp 1981; **Fac Appt:** Prof Psyc, NY Coll Osteo Med

Pulmonary Disease

Chadha, Jang B S MD (Pul) - **Spec Exp:** Sleep Disorders; Asthma; Emphysema; Critical Care Medicine; **Hospital:** Flushing Hosp Med Ctr, Forest Hills Hosp (page 106); **Address:** 11203 Queens Blvd, Ste 201, Forest Hills, NY 11375; **Phone:** 718-544-6660; **Board Cert:** Internal Medicine 1982; Pulmonary Disease 1984; Critical Care Medicine 2008; Sleep Medicine 2007; **Med School:** India 1976; **Resid:** Internal Medicine, Lincoln Hosp 1982; **Fellow:** Pulmonary Disease, NY Med Coll 1984

Fleischman, Jean K MD (Pul) - **Hospital:** Queens Hosp Ctr - Jamaica; **Address:** Queens Hosp Ctr, Dept Medicine, 82-68 164th St, N Bldg Fl 7, Jamaica, NY 11432-1140; **Phone:** 718-883-4050; **Board Cert:** Internal Medicine 1985; Pulmonary Disease 1988; **Med School:** NYU Sch Med 1982; **Resid:** Internal Medicine, Manhattan VA/NYU Med Ctr 1985; **Fellow:** Pulmonary Disease, NYU Med Ctr 1987; **Fac Appt:** Assoc Clin Prof Med, Mount Sinai Sch Med

Kassapidis, Sotirios MD (Pul) - **Hospital:** Mount Sinai Hosp of Queens (page 102), N Shore Univ Hosp (page 106); **Address:** 22-31 33rd Street, Astoria, NY 11105; **Phone:** 718-278-6595; **Board Cert:** Critical Care Medicine 2010; **Med School:** Grenada 1987; **Resid:** Internal Medicine, SUNY Hlth Sci Ctr 1993; **Fellow:** Pulmonary Disease, SUNY Hlth Sci Ctr 1995; Critical Care Medicine, SUNY Hlth Sci Ctr 1996; **Fac Appt:** Asst Clin Prof Med, NYU Sch Med

Nath, Sunil MD (Pul) - **Spec Exp:** Asthma; Emphysema; Lung Cancer; **Hospital:** NY Hosp Queens (page 488); **Address:** 55-14 Main St, Flushing, NY 11355-5044; **Phone:** 718-359-3131; **Board Cert:** Internal Medicine 1980; Pulmonary Disease 1982; **Med School:** India 1976; **Resid:** Internal Medicine, NY Hosp Med Ctr 1980; **Fellow:** Pulmonary Disease, NY Hosp Med Ctr 1982

Silverman, Joel R MD (Pul) - **Spec Exp:** Emphysema; Asthma; Pulmonary Rehabilitation; Sarcoidosis; **Hospital:** Flushing Hosp Med Ctr, N Shore Univ Hosp (page 106); **Address:** 111-20 Queens Blvd, Forest Hills, NY 11375-6341; **Phone:** 718-544-4224; **Board Cert:** Internal Medicine 1977; Pulmonary Disease 1980; Critical Care Medicine 2005; **Med School:** Univ Okla Coll Med 1974; **Resid:** Internal Medicine, N Shore Univ Hosp 1977; **Fellow:** Pulmonary Disease, Bellevue Hosp 1979

Thurm, Craig A MD (Pul) - **Spec Exp:** Asthma; Chronic Obstructive Lung Disease (COPD); Interstitial Lung Disease; Pulmonary Fibrosis; **Hospital:** Jamaica Hosp Med Ctr; **Address:** Jamaica Hospital, Div Pulmonology, 134-20 Jamaica Ave, Fl 1, Jamaica, NY 11418; **Phone:** 718-206-8776; **Board Cert:** Pulmonary Disease 2012; Critical Care Medicine 2000; **Med School:** Albert Einstein Coll Med 1987; **Resid:** Internal Medicine, Francis Scott Key Med Ctr 1990; **Fellow:** Pulmonary Critical Care Medicine, Univ Maryland 1993; **Fac Appt:** Assoc Clin Prof Med, NY Coll Osteo Med

Radiation Oncology

Dalton, Jack F MD (RadRO) - **Spec Exp:** Brain Tumors; Head & Neck Cancer; Breast Cancer; **Hospital:** Mt Sinai Med Ctr (page 102), Lenox Hill Hosp (page 106); **Address:** 106-14 70th Ave, Forest Hills, NY 11375-4253; **Phone:** 718-520-6620; **Board Cert:** Internal Medicine 1974; Hematology 1976; Medical Oncology 1981; Therapeutic Radiology 1983; **Med School:** Univ Pittsburgh 1970; **Resid:** Internal Medicine, G Washington Univ Hosp 1972; Therapeutic Radiology, Mt Sinai Hosp 1981; **Fellow:** Hematology, Mt Sinai Hosp 1975; **Fac Appt:** Asst Clin Prof RadRO, Mount Sinai Sch Med

Katz, Alan J MD (RadRO) - **Spec Exp:** Stereotactic Body Radiotherapy; Prostate Cancer; Intensity Modulated Radiotherapy (IMRT); **Address:** 40-20 Main St, Queens, NY 11354; **Phone:** 888-880-6646; **Board Cert:** Therapeutic Radiology 1981; **Med School:** NYU Sch Med 1977; **Resid:** Therapeutic Radiology, NYU Med Ctr 1981

Lipsztein, Roberto MD (RadRO) - **Hospital:** Lenox Hill Hosp (page 106), Mt Sinai Med Ctr (page 102); **Address:** 106-14 70th Ave, Forest Hills, NY 11375-4253; **Phone:** 718-520-6620; **Board Cert:** Therapeutic Radiology 1982; **Med School:** Brazil 1974; **Resid:** Radiation Oncology, Mount Sinai Hosp 1981; **Fellow:** Radiation Oncology, Mount Sinai Hosp 1981; **Fac Appt:** Asst Clin Prof RadRO, Mount Sinai Sch Med

Varsos, George MD (RadRO) - **Spec Exp:** Gynecologic Cancer; Urologic Cancer; **Hospital:** Mount Sinai Hosp of Queens (page 102), Mt Sinai Med Ctr (page 102); **Address:** 23-22 30th Ave, Astoria, NY 11102; **Phone:** 718-267-2763; **Board Cert:** Radiation Oncology 1992; **Med School:** Mount Sinai Sch Med 1985; **Resid:** Surgery, Univ Hosp 1987; Radiation Oncology, Univ Hosp 1990; **Fellow:** Radiation Oncology, Meml Sloan-Kettering Cancer Ctr 1992; **Fac Appt:** Asst Clin Prof RadRO, Mount Sinai Sch Med

Rheumatology

Sharon, Ezra MD (Rhu) - **Spec Exp:** Rheumatoid Arthritis; Lupus/SLE; Fibromyalgia; Gout; **Hospital:** Mount Sinai Hosp of Queens (page 102); **Address:** 70-31 108 St, Forest Hills, NY 11375; **Phone:** 718-793-6832; **Board Cert:** Internal Medicine 1973; Rheumatology 1974; **Med School:** Israel 1967; **Resid:** Internal Medicine, Mt Sinai Med Ctr 1971; Rheumatology, SUNY Downstate Med Ctr 1973

Sonpal, Girish M MD (Rhu) - **Spec Exp:** Osteoporosis; Rheumatoid Arthritis; Lupus/SLE; Autoimmune Disease; **Hospital:** NY Hosp Queens (page 488), Flushing Hosp Med Ctr; **Address:** 149-65 24th Ave, Flushing, NY 11357-3646; **Phone:** 718-445-0500; **Board Cert:** Internal Medicine 1974; Rheumatology 1976; **Med School:** India 1969; **Resid:** Internal Medicine, Catholic Med Ctr 1974; **Fellow:** Rheumatology, Worcester City Hosp 1975; Rheumatology, Queens Hosp Ctr 1976; **Fac Appt:** Asst Prof Med, Cornell Univ-Weill Med Coll

Sports Medicine

Rosen, Jeffrey E MD (SM) - **Spec Exp:** Pediatric Sports Medicine; **Hospital:** NY Hosp Queens (page 488), NYU Hosp For Joint Dis (page 108); **Address:** NYHQ Ctr Orthopaedic & Rehab Medicine, 163-03 Horace Harding Expressway, Fl 2, Fresh Meadows, NY 11365; **Phone:** 866-670-6824; **Board Cert:** Orthopaedic Surgery 2012; **Med School:** Columbia P&S 1993; **Resid:** Orthopaedic Surgery, Hosp for Joint Diseases 1998; **Fellow:** Sports Medicine & Arthroscopic Surgery, Kerlan-Jobe Orthopaedic Clinic 1999; **Fac Appt:** Asst Prof OrS, NYU Sch Med

Surgery

Biviano, Bernard J MD (S) - **Spec Exp:** Critical Care; **Hospital:** Mount Sinai Hosp of Queens (page 102); **Address:** 25-10 30th Ave, Astoria, NY 11102; **Phone:** 718-267-4363; **Board Cert:** Surgery 2006; Surgical Critical Care 2007; **Med School:** UMDNJ-RW Johnson Med Sch 1990; **Resid:** Surgery, Cabrini Med Ctr 1995; **Fellow:** Surgical Critical Care, Metropolitan Hosp Ctr 1996; **Fac Appt:** S, Mount Sinai Sch Med

Kemeny, M Margaret MD (S) - **Spec Exp:** Liver Cancer; Pancreatic Cancer; Colon & Rectal Cancer; Cancer Surgery; **Hospital:** Queens Hosp Ctr - Jamaica, N Shore Univ Hosp (page 106); **Address:** Queens Cancer Ctr at Queens Hosp, 82-68 164th St, Jamaica, NY 11432-1140; **Phone:** 718-883-4031; **Board Cert:** Surgery 2003; **Med School:** Columbia P&S 1972; **Resid:** Surgery, Columbia-Presby Hosp 1974; Surgery, Univ Colorado Med Ctr 1976; **Fellow:** Surgery, Meml Sloan Kettering Cancer Ctr 1977; Surgical Oncology, National Cancer Inst 1981; **Fac Appt:** Prof S, Mount Sinai Sch Med

Manolas, Panagiotis A MD (S) - **Spec Exp:** Breast Cancer; Laparoscopic Surgery; **Hospital:** Mount Sinai Hosp of Queens (page 102), Mt Sinai Med Ctr (page 102); **Address:** 30-16 30th Drive, Astoria, NY 11102-1874; **Phone:** 718-626-0707; **Board Cert:** Surgery 1999; **Med School:** Greece 1982; **Resid:** Surgery, NY Methodist Hosp 1989; **Fac Appt:** Asst Clin Prof S, Mount Sinai Sch Med

Mendoza, Ernesto A MD (S) - **Spec Exp:** Parathyroid Surgery; Throat Disorders; Head & Neck Surgery; **Hospital:** New York Methodist Hosp (page 440); **Address:** 40-45 78th St, Elmhurst, NY 11373-1152; **Phone:** 718-397-9058; **Board Cert:** Surgery 2009; **Med School:** Peru 1974; **Resid:** Surgery, Kingsbrook Jewish Med Ctr 1983; **Fellow:** Head and Neck Surgery, Tulane Med Ctr 1985; Surgical Oncology, Roswell Park Canc Inst 1986

Pace, Benjamin W MD (S) - **Spec Exp:** Breast Surgery; Breast Cancer; **Hospital:** Queens Hosp Ctr - Jamaica; **Address:** Queens Hosp Ctr - Dept Surgery, 82-68 164th St, rm A-365, Jamaica, NY 11432-1140; **Phone:** 718-883-4640; **Board Cert:** Surgery 2004; **Med School:** Mexico 1977; **Resid:** Surgery, Long Is Jewish Med Ctr 1983; **Fac Appt:** Assoc Prof S, Mount Sinai Sch Med

Siegel, Beth M MD (S) - **Spec Exp:** Breast Cancer; Breast Disease; **Hospital:** NY Hosp Queens (page 488); **Address:** NY Hosp Queen - Breast Ctr, 56-26 Main St, Flushing, NY 11355; **Phone:** 718-670-1185; **Board Cert:** Surgery 2011; **Med School:** Dominica 1982; **Resid:** Surgery, NY Hosp Queens 1988

Sung, Kap-Jae MD (S) - **Spec Exp:** Breast Cancer; Ultrasound; **Hospital:** NY Hosp Queens (page 488), Forest Hills Hosp (page 106); **Address:** 66-83 70 St, Middle Village, NY 11379-1130; **Phone:** 718-651-2929; **Board Cert:** Surgery 2005; **Med School:** South Korea 1973; **Resid:** Surgery, Wyckoff Heights Hosp 1986; **Fac Appt:** Asst Prof S, NY Med Coll

Zeitlin, Alan P MD (S) - **Spec Exp:** Vascular Surgery; Breast Cancer; Laparoscopic Abdominal Surgery; Gastrointestinal Surgery; **Hospital:** Flushing Hosp Med Ctr; **Address:** 69-60 108th St, Forest Hills, NY 11375-4323; **Phone:** 718-544-0442; **Board Cert:** Surgery 2012; **Med School:** Univ Miami Sch Med 1974; **Resid:** Surgery, Montefiore Med Ctr 1979

Thoracic & Cardiac Surgery

Graver, L. Michael MD (T&CS) - **Spec Exp:** Minimally Invasive Cardiac Surgery; Coronary Artery Surgery; Aortic Surgery; Heart Valve Surgery; **Hospital:** Long Is Jewish Med Ctr (page 106); **Address:** LIJ Med Ctr, Cardiothoracic Surgery, 270-05 76th Ave, Ste O-4000, New Hyde Park, NY 11040; **Phone:** 718-470-7460; **Board Cert:** Surgery 2003; Thoracic Surgery 2004; **Med School:** Albany Med Coll 1977; **Resid:** Surgery, St Lukes-Roosevelt Hosp Ctr 1982; Cardiovascular Surgery, Beth Israel Deaconess Hosp 1983; **Fellow:** Cardiovascular Pathology, NY-Presby/Weill Cornell Med Ctr 1985; **Fac Appt:** Prof TS, Hofstra N Shore-LIJ Sch Med

Lang, Samuel J MD (T&CS) - **Spec Exp:** Minimally Invasive Cardiac Surgery; Heart Valve Surgery; Cardiothoracic Surgery; **Hospital:** NY Hosp Queens (page 488), NY-Presby/Weill Cornell Med Ctr, NY (page 104); **Address:** NY Hosp, Cardiothoracic Surgery Dept, 56-45 Main St, rm 387, Flushing, NY 11355; **Phone:** 718-670-1137; **Board Cert:** Thoracic & Cardiac Surgery 2006; **Med School:** UAB Sch Med 1978; **Resid:** Surgery, UCLA Med Ctr 1982; Thoracic Surgery, NYU Med Ctr 1983; **Fellow:** Cardiothoracic Surgery, UCLA Med Ctr 1985; Pediatric Cardiac Surgery, Hosp Sick Chldn 1986; **Fac Appt:** Prof S, Cornell Univ-Weill Med Coll

Lee, Paul C MD (T&CS) - **Spec Exp:** Lung Cancer; Esophageal Cancer; Gastroesophageal Reflux Disease (GERD); Minimally Invasive Thoracic Surgery; **Hospital:** NY Hosp Queens (page 488), NY-Presby/Weill Cornell Med Ctr, NY (page 104); **Address:** 56-45 Main St, Ste WA-100, Flushing, NY 11355; **Phone:** 718-670-2707; **Board Cert:** Surgery 2010; Thoracic Surgery 2013; **Med School:** Johns Hopkins Univ 1995; **Resid:** Cardiothoracic Surgery, NY Presby Hosp-Cornell 2003; Thoracic Surgery, Meml Sloan Kettering Cancer Ctr 2003; **Fellow:** Minimally Invasive Surgery, Univ Pittsburgh Med Ctr 2003; **Fac Appt:** Prof T&CS, Cornell Univ-Weill Med Coll

Urology

Farrell, Robert M MD (U) - **Spec Exp:** Endourology; Urologic Cancer; **Hospital:** NY Hosp Queens (page 488), Flushing Hosp Med Ctr; **Address:** NY Hosp Queens - Dept Urology, 58-42 Main St, Flushing, NY 11355; **Phone:** 718-353-3710; **Board Cert:** Urology 1976; **Med School:** Cornell Univ-Weill Med Coll 1966; **Resid:** Surgery, NY-Presby/Weill Cornell Med Ctr 1968; Urology, NY-Presby/Weill Cornell Med Ctr 1975

Sandhaus, Jeffrey J MD (U) - **Spec Exp:** Prostate Cancer; Minimally Invasive Surgery; Vasectomy-Scalpelless; **Hospital:** Mount Sinai Hosp of Queens (page 102), NY-Presby/Weill Cornell Med Ctr, NY (page 104); **Address:** 36-01 31st Ave Fl 1, Astoria, NY 11106-1051; **Phone:** 718-932-3535; **Board Cert:** Urology 1976; **Med School:** NY Med Coll 1966; **Resid:** Urology, Kings Co Hosp Ctr 1973; **Fac Appt:** Asst Clin Prof U, Mount Sinai Sch Med

Tarasuk, Albert P MD (U) - **Spec Exp:** Prostate Disease; Bladder Surgery; Kidney Stones; **Hospital:** NY Hosp Queens (page 488), Flushing Hosp Med Ctr; **Address:** NY Hosp Queens - Dept Urology, 58-42 Main St, Flushing, NY 11355-5336; **Phone:** 718-353-3710; **Board Cert:** Urology 1972; **Med School:** Geo Wash Univ 1964; **Resid:** Urology, Beth Israel Med Ctr - Petrie Div 1971

Tillem, Steven M MD (U) - **Hospital:** Mount Sinai Hosp of Queens (page 102), NY Hosp Queens (page 488); **Address:** 31-19 Newton Ave, Ste 801, Astoria, NY 11102; **Phone:** 718-777-2111; **Board Cert:** Urology 2009; **Med School:** UMDNJ-NJ Med Sch, Newark 1992; **Resid:** Surgery, Long Is Jewish Med Ctr 1994; Urology, Long Is Jewish Med Ctr 1998

Vascular & Interventional Radiology

Rogers, David M MD (VIR) - **Hospital:** NY Hosp Queens (page 488), Wyckoff Heights Med Ctr; **Address:** NY Hosp Queens - Dept Radiology, 56-45 Main St, Flushing, NY 11355; **Phone:** 718-670-1496; **Board Cert:** Diagnostic Radiology 1987; **Med School:** Columbia P&S 1981; **Resid:** Diagnostic Radiology, Mt Sinai Med Ctr 1987; **Fellow:** Vascular & Interventional Radiology, NYU Langone Med Ctr 1988

Richmond (Staten Island)

Richmond (Staten Island)

Adolescent Medicine

Lee, April C MD (AM) - **Hospital:** Staten Island Univ Hosp - North (page 106), NS-LIJ Hlth Sys (page 106); **Address:** Staten Island Univ Hosp, Adolescent Med, 242 Mason Ave, Staten Island, NY 10305; **Phone:** 718-226-6294; **Board Cert:** Pediatrics 1986; Adolescent Medicine 2009; **Med School:** NYU Sch Med 1980; **Resid:** Pediatrics, NYU Med Ctr 1983; **Fellow:** Adolescent Medicine, Brookdale Hosp 1986; **Fac Appt:** Asst Clin Prof Ped, SUNY Hlth Sci Ctr

Allergy & Immunology

Rao, Yalamanchili A.K. MD (A&I) - **Spec Exp:** Pediatric Allergy & Immunology; **Hospital:** Staten Island Univ Hosp - North (page 106), Richmond Univ Med Ctr; **Address:** 896 Targee St, Staten Island, NY 10304; **Phone:** 718-816-8200; **Board Cert:** Internal Medicine 1977; Allergy & Immunology 1977; **Med School:** India 1968; **Resid:** Allergy & Immunology, LI Coll Hosp 1975; Internal Medicine, LI Coll Hosp 1977

Cardiovascular Disease

Besser, Louis M MD (Cv) - **Spec Exp:** Coronary Artery Disease; Arrhythmias; **Hospital:** Richmond Univ Med Ctr, Staten Island Univ Hosp - North (page 106); **Address:** 11 Ralph Pl, Ste 310, Staten Island, NY 10304-4419; **Phone:** 718-442-1777; **Board Cert:** Internal Medicine 1988; Cardiovascular Disease 1989; **Med School:** Mexico 1981; **Resid:** Internal Medicine, St Vincents Med Ctr 1986; **Fellow:** Cardiovascular Disease, St Vincents Med Ctr 1988; **Fac Appt:** Asst Clin Prof Med, NY Med Coll

Bogin, Marc MD (Cv) - **Spec Exp:** Echocardiography; Cardiac Catheterization; **Hospital:** Staten Island Univ Hosp - North (page 106), Richmond Univ Med Ctr; **Address:** Heart, Lung & Surgery Ctr, 501 Seaview Ave, Ste 200, Staten Island, NY 10305; **Phone:** 718-663-6400; **Board Cert:** Internal Medicine 1989; Cardiovascular Disease 2003; **Med School:** Mexico 1985; **Resid:** Internal Medicine, Booth Meml Hosp 1990; **Fellow:** Cardiovascular Disease, St Vincent's Hosp & Med Ctr 1993; **Fac Appt:** Asst Clin Prof Med, NY Med Coll

Grodman, Richard S MD (Cv) - **Spec Exp:** Echocardiography; Cardiac Catheterization; **Hospital:** Richmond Univ Med Ctr; **Address:** Richmond University Medical Center, 355 Bard Ave, Staten Island, NY 10310-1664; **Phone:** 718-818-4642; **Board Cert:** Internal Medicine 1976; Cardiovascular Disease 1979; **Med School:** SUNY Downstate 1973; **Resid:** Internal Medicine, SUNY Downstate 1976; Critical Care Medicine, SUNY Downstate 1977; **Fellow:** Cardiovascular Disease, Rhode Island Hosp-Brown 1979; **Fac Appt:** Assoc Clin Prof Med, NY Med Coll

Lafferty, James C MD (Cv) - **Spec Exp:** Electrophysiologic Testing; **Hospital:** Staten Island Univ Hosp - North (page 106); **Address:** Staten Island Heart, 501 Seaview Ave, Ste 300, Staten Island, NY 10305; **Phone:** 718-663-7000 x6; **Board Cert:** Internal Medicine 1985; Cardiovascular Disease 1987; Cardiac Electrophysiology 2006; **Med School:** SUNY Hlth Sci Ctr 1982; **Resid:** Internal Medicine, Staten Island Hosp 1985; **Fellow:** Cardiovascular Disease, Downstate Med Ctr 1987; **Fac Appt:** Assoc Prof Med, SUNY Downstate

Schwartz, Charles A MD (Cv) - **Spec Exp:** Echocardiography; Cardiac Catheterization; Transesophageal Echocardiogram (TEE); **Hospital:** Staten Island Univ Hosp - North (page 106); **Address:** 501 Seaview Ave, Ste 300, Staten Island, NY 10305; **Phone:** 718-663-7000; **Board Cert:** Internal Medicine 1983; Cardiovascular Disease 1985; Echocardiography 2011; **Med School:** SUNY Downstate 1980; **Resid:** Internal Medicine, Staten Island Hosp 1983; **Fellow:** Cardiovascular Disease, St Vincent's Hosp & Med Ctr 1985; **Fac Appt:** Asst Clin Prof Med, SUNY Downstate

Vazzana, Thomas MD (Cv) - **Spec Exp:** Invasive Cardiology; Non-Invasive Cardiology; Interventional Cardiology; **Hospital:** Staten Island Univ Hosp - North (page 106), Richmond Univ Med Ctr; **Address:** Heart, Lung & Surgery Ctr, 501 Seaview Ave, Ste 200, Staten Island, NY 10305; **Phone:** 718-663-6400; **Board Cert:** Internal Medicine 1989; Cardiovascular Disease 2011; **Med School:** Grenada 1985; **Resid:** Internal Medicine, St Joseph's Hosp & Med Ctr 1989; **Fellow:** Cardiovascular Disease, St Vincent's Hosp & Med Ctr 1991; **Fac Appt:** Asst Prof Med, NY Med Coll

Winter, Steven MD (Cv) - **Spec Exp:** Cholesterol/Lipid Disorders; Preventive Cardiology; Non-Invasive Cardiology; **Hospital:** Staten Island Univ Hosp - North (page 106), Richmond Univ Med Ctr; **Address:** 2627 Hylan Blvd, Bldg B, Staten Island, NY 10306-4339; **Phone:** 718-351-5600; **Board Cert:** Internal Medicine 1979; Cardiovascular Disease 1981; **Med School:** UMDNJ-NJ Med Sch, Newark 1976; **Resid:** Internal Medicine, N Shore Univ Hosp 1979; **Fellow:** Cardiovascular Disease, Rhode Island Hosp 1981; **Fac Appt:** Asst Clin Prof Med, SUNY Hlth Sci Ctr

Child Neurology

De Carlo, Regina MD (ChiN) - **Spec Exp:** Autism & Developmental Disorders; Headache; Learning Disorders; ADD/ADHD; **Hospital:** Richmond Univ Med Ctr, NYU Langone Med Ctr (page 108); **Address:** 2550 Victory Blvd, Staten Island, NY 10314-6635; **Phone:** 718-983-0923; **Board Cert:** Pediatrics 1984; Child Neurology 1984; **Med School:** UMDNJ-NJ Med Sch, Newark 1977; **Resid:** Pediatrics, NYU Med Ctr 1979; Neurology, NYU Med Ctr 1981; **Fellow:** Child Neurology, NYU Med Ctr 1982; **Fac Appt:** Asst Clin Prof N, NYU Sch Med

Colon & Rectal Surgery

Lacqua, Frank MD (CRS) - **Spec Exp:** Colonoscopy; Colon Cancer; Anal Disorders & Reconstruction; **Hospital:** Richmond Univ Med Ctr, Lutheran Med Ctr - Brooklyn; **Address:** 2372 Victory Blvd, Staten Island, NY 10314; **Phone:** 718-761-3700; **Board Cert:** Colon & Rectal Surgery 2011; Surgery 2009; **Med School:** SUNY Buffalo 1985; **Resid:** Surgery, St Luke's-Roosevelt Hosp 1990; **Fellow:** Colon & Rectal Surgery, Univ Tex Hlth Sci Ctr 1991

Dermatology

Bernstein, Charles MD (D) - **Hospital:** Staten Island Univ Hosp - North (page 106); **Address:** 244 Buel Ave Fl 2, Staten Island, NY 10305; **Phone:** 718-980-5767; **Board Cert:** Internal Medicine 1983; Dermatology 1987; **Med School:** SUNY Downstate 1980; **Resid:** Internal Medicine, Staten Island Hosp 1984; Dermatology, Downstate Med Ctr 1987; **Fac Appt:** Assoc Clin Prof D, SUNY Hlth Sci Ctr

Lederman, Josiane MD (D) - **Spec Exp:** Cosmetic Dermatology; Skin Cancer; Laser Surgery; **Address:** 116 Lamberts Ln, Staten Island, NY 10314-7210; **Phone:** 718-370-0422; **Board Cert:** Dermatology 1986; **Med School:** France 1981; **Resid:** Dermatology, Saint Louis Hosp 1983; **Fellow:** Dermatology, Mass Genl Hosp/Harvard 1986

McCormack, Patricia C MD (D) - **Spec Exp:** Psoriasis; Skin Cancer; Skin Laser Surgery; Cosmetic Dermatology; **Hospital:** Richmond Univ Med Ctr; **Address:** 1550 Richmond Ave, Ste 207, Staten Island, NY 10314; **Phone:** 718-698-1616; **Board Cert:** Dermatology 1985; **Med School:** UMDNJ-Rutgers Med Sch 1981; **Resid:** Dermatology, Westchester Med Ctr/NY Med Coll 1985

Diagnostic Radiology

Raia, Carolyn MD (DR) - **Spec Exp:** Breast Imaging; Breast Cancer; Mammography; **Hospital:** Staten Island Univ Hosp - North (page 106); **Address:** SIUH Breast Imaging Ctr, 256 B Mason Ave, Staten Island, NY 10305; **Phone:** 718-226-7700; **Board Cert:** Diagnostic Radiology ; **Med School:** SUNY Downstate 1989; **Resid:** Diagnostic Radiology, St Lukes-Roosevelt Hosp 1994; **Fellow:** Breast Surgery, Columbia-Presby Med Ctr 1995

Endocrinology, Diabetes & Metabolism

Cohen, Neil D MD (EDM) - **Spec Exp:** Diabetes; Thyroid Disorders; Osteoporosis; **Hospital:** Staten Island Univ Hosp - North (page 106), Staten Island Univ Hosp - South (page 106); **Address:** 1460 Victory Blvd, Staten Island, NY 10301-3914; **Phone:** 718-442-0300; **Board Cert:** Internal Medicine 2003; Endocrinology, Diabetes & Metabolism 2005; **Med School:** Med Coll PA Hahnemann 1990; **Resid:** Internal Medicine, N Shore Univ Hosp 1993; **Fellow:** Endocrinology, Diabetes & Metabolism, Montefiore Med Ctr 1995

Das, Seshadri MD (EDM) - **Spec Exp:** Diabetes; Thyroid Disorders; **Hospital:** Richmond Univ Med Ctr, Staten Island Univ Hosp - South (page 106); **Address:** 45 Little Clove Rd, Staten Island, NY 10301; **Phone:** 718-273-5522; **Board Cert:** Internal Medicine 1983; Endocrinology, Diabetes & Metabolism 2008; **Med School:** India 1968; **Resid:** Internal Medicine, North Middlesex Hosp 1975; Internal Medicine, Whittington Hosp/Royal Free Hosp 1977; **Fellow:** Endocrinology, Diabetes & Metabolism, SUNY Downstate 1980

Hoffman, Richard S MD (EDM) - **Spec Exp:** Diabetes; Thyroid Disorders; Parathyroid Disorders; Adrenal Disorders; **Hospital:** Staten Island Univ Hosp - North (page 106); **Address:** 1460 Victory Blvd, Staten Island, NY 10301; **Phone:** 718-442-0300; **Board Cert:** Internal Medicine 1971; Endocrinology, Diabetes & Metabolism 1975; **Med School:** SUNY Hlth Sci Ctr 1965; **Resid:** Internal Medicine, Long Island Coll Hosp 1967; Internal Medicine, Boston City Hosp 1968; **Fellow:** Endocrinology, Boston City Hosp 1970

Rothman, Jeffrey G MD (EDM) - **Spec Exp:** Diabetes; Osteoporosis; Thyroid Disorders; **Hospital:** Staten Island Univ Hosp - North (page 106), Staten Island Univ Hosp - South (page 106); **Address:** 1460 Victory Blvd, Staten Island, NY 10301-3914; **Phone:** 718-442-0300; **Board Cert:** Internal Medicine 1973; Endocrinology, Diabetes & Metabolism 1977; **Med School:** SUNY Buffalo 1970; **Resid:** Internal Medicine, Hosp Univ Penn 1973; **Fellow:** Endocrinology, Diabetes & Metabolism, Hosp Univ Penn 1977

Family Medicine

Nepola, Neil MD (FMed) *PCP* - **Hospital:** Staten Island Univ Hosp - South (page 106); **Address:** 217 Rose Ave, Staten Island, NY 10306-2918; **Phone:** 718-667-6767; **Board Cert:** Family Medicine 2004; **Med School:** Philippines 1979; **Resid:** Family Medicine, UMDNJ-St Peter's Hosp 1983

Gastroenterology

Bruckstein, Alex H MD (Ge) - **Spec Exp:** Colonoscopy; Gastroscopy; Gastroesophageal Reflux Disease (GERD); Hepatitis; **Hospital:** Staten Island Univ Hosp - North (page 106), Staten Island Univ Hosp - South (page 106); **Address:** 2627 Hylan Blvd, Staten Island, NY 10306-4339; **Phone:** 718-667-3200; **Board Cert:** Internal Medicine 1979; Gastroenterology 1983; **Med School:** Albert Einstein Coll Med 1975; **Resid:** Internal Medicine, Roosevelt Hosp 1977; Internal Medicine, St Luke's Hosp 1978; **Fellow:** Gastroenterology, NY VA Med Ctr 1980; **Fac Appt:** Asst Clin Prof Med, SUNY Downstate

Fazio, Richard A MD (Ge) - **Spec Exp:** Colonoscopy; Gastroesophageal Reflux Disease (GERD); **Hospital:** Richmond Univ Med Ctr; **Address:** 78 Todt Hill Rd, Ste 203, Staten Island, NY 10314-4528; **Phone:** 718-448-1122; **Board Cert:** Internal Medicine 1982; Gastroenterology 1983; **Med School:** Italy 1978; **Resid:** Internal Medicine, Maimonides Med Ctr 1981; **Fellow:** Gastroenterology, St Vincent's Med Ctr 1983

Wickremesinghe, Prasanna C MD (Ge) - **Spec Exp:** Inflammatory Bowel Disease/Crohn's; Hepatitis; Endoscopy; **Hospital:** Richmond Univ Med Ctr; **Address:** 481 Bard Ave, Staten Island, NY 10310; **Phone:** 718-448-0865; **Board Cert:** Internal Medicine 1980; Gastroenterology 1975; **Med School:** Sri Lanka 1968; **Resid:** Internal Medicine, Coney Island Hosp 1972; **Fellow:** Gastroenterology, Maimonides Medical Ctr 1975

Geriatric Medicine

Seminara, Donna P MD (Ger) - **Spec Exp:** Geriatric Care; Frail Elderly; Preventive Medicine; **Hospital:** Staten Island Univ Hosp - North (page 106); **Address:** Island Internists, 420 Lyndale Ave, Staten Island, NY 10312-6131; **Phone:** 718-967-5630; **Board Cert:** Internal Medicine 2010; Geriatric Medicine 2000; **Med School:** Mexico 1986; **Resid:** Internal Medicine, Staten Island Univ Hosp 1990

Gynecologic Oncology

Maiman, Mitchell MD (GO) - **Spec Exp:** Cervical Cancer; Ovarian Cancer; Uterine Cancer; **Hospital:** Staten Island Univ Hosp - North (page 106); **Address:** 256 Mason Ave Fl C, Staten Island, NY 10305-3408; **Phone:** 718-226-9269; **Board Cert:** Obstetrics & Gynecology 2012; Gynecologic Oncology 2012; **Med School:** SUNY Hlth Sci Ctr 1981; **Resid:** Obstetrics & Gynecology, Montefiore Med Ctr 1985; **Fellow:** Gynecologic Oncology, SUNY Downstate Med Ctr 1987; **Fac Appt:** Prof ObG, SUNY Downstate

Infectious Disease

Glaser, Jordan B MD (Inf) - **Spec Exp:** AIDS/HIV; **Hospital:** Staten Island Univ Hosp - North (page 106), Staten Island Univ Hosp - South (page 106); **Address:** 1408 Richmond Rd, Staten Island, NY 10304; **Phone:** 718-816-3362; **Board Cert:** Internal Medicine 1982; Infectious Disease 1984; **Med School:** SUNY Downstate 1979; **Resid:** Internal Medicine, Staten Island Hosp 1982; **Fellow:** Infectious Disease, SUNY Downstate Med Ctr 1984; **Fac Appt:** Assoc Clin Prof Med, SUNY Hlth Sci Ctr

Internal Medicine

Fulop, Robert MD (IM) *PCP* - **Spec Exp:** Diagnostic Problems; Geriatric Medicine; **Hospital:** Richmond Univ Med Ctr, Staten Island Univ Hosp - North (page 106); **Address:** 476 Klondike Ave, Staten Island, NY 10314-6216; **Phone:** 718-761-1156; **Board Cert:** Internal Medicine 1982; Geriatric Medicine 2005; **Med School:** SUNY Upstate Med Univ 1978; **Resid:** Internal Medicine, Brookdale Hosp 1981

Gazzara, Paul MD (IM) *PCP* - **Spec Exp:** Complementary Medicine; Acupuncture; Addiction/Substance Abuse; **Hospital:** Staten Island Univ Hosp - North (page 106); **Address:** 3589 Hylan Blvd, Staten Island, NY 10308-3513; **Phone:** 718-966-3700; **Board Cert:** Internal Medicine 1986; **Med School:** SUNY Downstate 1983; **Resid:** Internal Medicine, Staten Island Hosp 1986; **Fac Appt:** Asst Clin Prof Med, SUNY Hlth Sci Ctr

Malach, Barbara S MD (IM) *PCP* - **Spec Exp:** Geriatric Medicine; **Hospital:** Staten Island Univ Hosp - North (page 106); **Address:** 2627B Hylan Blvd, Staten Island, NY 10306-4339; **Phone:** 718-987-6000; **Board Cert:** Internal Medicine 1983; Geriatric Medicine 2008; **Med School:** SUNY Downstate 1979; **Resid:** Internal Medicine, Staten Island Hosp 1982

Strange, Theodore MD (IM) *PCP* - **Spec Exp:** Geriatric Medicine; **Hospital:** Staten Island Univ Hosp - South (page 106), Staten Island Univ Hosp - North (page 106); **Address:** 68 Seguine Ave, Staten Island, NY 10309-3723; **Phone:** 718-356-6500; **Board Cert:** Internal Medicine 2001; Geriatric Medicine 2012; **Med School:** SUNY Hlth Sci Ctr 1985; **Resid:** Internal Medicine, Staten Island Univ Hosp 1988; **Fac Appt:** Assoc Clin Prof Med, SUNY Downstate

Interventional Cardiology

Malpeso, James V MD (IC) - **Spec Exp:** Cardiac Catheterization; Angioplasty & Stent Placement; Cardiac CT Angiography; **Hospital:** Staten Island Univ Hosp - North (page 106); **Address:** 501 Seaview Ave, HLS Bldg Fl 2 - Ste 200, Staten Island, NY 10305; **Phone:** 718-226-9600; **Board Cert:** Internal Medicine 1979; Cardiovascular Disease 1981; Cardiovascular Computed Tomography 2008; **Med School:** Albert Einstein Coll Med 1975; **Resid:** Internal Medicine, Kings County Hosp 1978; **Fellow:** Cardiovascular Disease, St Vincent Hosp Med Ctr 1980; **Fac Appt:** Asst Prof Med, SUNY Downstate

Medical Oncology

Forlenza, Thomas J MD (Onc) - **Spec Exp:** Palliative Care; Bleeding/Coagulation Disorders; Breast Cancer; Lung Cancer; **Hospital:** Richmond Univ Med Ctr; **Address:** 1366 Victory Blvd, Ste A, Staten Island, NY 10301; **Phone:** 718-816-4949; **Board Cert:** Internal Medicine 1981; Hematology 1984; Blood Banking 1984; Medical Oncology 1985; **Med School:** Boston Univ 1977; **Resid:** Internal Medicine, Univ Kentucky Med Ctr 1980; **Fellow:** Hematology, NYU Med Ctr 1982; Medical Oncology, Kings County Hosp 1983; **Fac Appt:** Asst Prof Med, NYU Sch Med

Friscia, Philip MD (Onc) - **Spec Exp:** Lung Cancer; Colon Cancer; Hematology; **Hospital:** Staten Island Univ Hosp - North (page 106), Staten Island Univ Hosp - South (page 106); **Address:** Nalitt Cancer Inst, 256 Mason Ave C Bldg Fl 1, Staten Island, NY 10305-3408; **Phone:** 718-226-6400; **Board Cert:** Internal Medicine 1978; Medical Oncology 1981; **Med School:** Italy 1972; **Resid:** Internal Medicine, Long Island Coll Hosp 1976; **Fellow:** Hematology & Oncology, Long Island Coll Hosp 1979; **Fac Appt:** Asst Clin Prof Med, SUNY Downstate

Odaimi, Marcel MD (Onc) - **Spec Exp:** Brain Tumors; **Hospital:** Staten Island Univ Hosp - South (page 106), Staten Island Univ Hosp - North (page 106); **Address:** Nalitt Inst, 256 Mason Ave C Bldg, Staten Island, NY 10305-3408; **Phone:** 718-226-6400; **Board Cert:** Internal Medicine 1987; Medical Oncology 1989; **Med School:** Amer Univ Beirut 1981; **Resid:** Internal Medicine, American Univ 1983; Internal Medicine, Staten Island Hosp 1987; **Fellow:** Medical Oncology, Univ Tex-MD Anderson Cancer Ctr 1985

Terjanian, Terenig O MD (Onc) - **Hospital:** Staten Island Univ Hosp - North (page 106); **Address:** Nalitt Cancer Inst, 256 Mason Ave C Bldg Fl 1, Staten Island, NY 10305-3408; **Phone:** 718-226-6400; **Board Cert:** Internal Medicine 1984; Medical Oncology 1987; Hematology 1988; **Med School:** France 1978; **Resid:** Anatomic Pathology, Amer Univ Beirut 1981; Internal Medicine, Staten Island Univ Hosp 1984; **Fellow:** Medical Oncology, Univ Tex-MD Anderson Cancer Ctr 1986; Hematology, NYU Med Ctr 1988

Neonatal-Perinatal Medicine

Roth, Philip MD/PhD (NP) - **Spec Exp:** Neonatal Care; Breast Feeding Problems; Neonatal Infections/Immunity; **Hospital:** Staten Island Univ Hosp - North (page 106); **Address:** 475 Seaview Ave Fl 4 East, Staten Island, NY 10305-3436; **Phone:** 718-226-9796; **Board Cert:** Pediatrics 1987; Neonatal-Perinatal Medicine 2011; **Med School:** Columbia P&S 1982; **Resid:** Pediatrics, Chldns Hosp 1986; **Fellow:** Neonatal-Perinatal Medicine, Hosp Univ Penn 1988; **Fac Appt:** Assoc Prof Ped, SUNY Downstate

Nephrology

Grossman, Susan D MD (Nep) - **Hospital:** Richmond Univ Med Ctr; **Address:** 1366 Victory Blvd, Staten Island, NY 10310; **Phone:** 718-273-3400; **Board Cert:** Internal Medicine 1980; Nephrology 1982; **Med School:** UMDNJ-NJ Med Sch, Newark 1977; **Resid:** Internal Medicine, Univ Hosp 1980; **Fellow:** Nephrology, New England Med Ctr 1982

Kleiner, Morton MD (Nep) - **Spec Exp:** Hypertension; Kidney Disease; **Hospital:** Staten Island Univ Hosp - North (page 106); **Address:** 470 Seaview Ave, Staten Island, NY 10305-3034; **Phone:** 718-987-5942; **Board Cert:** Internal Medicine 1977; Nephrology 1982; **Med School:** NY Med Coll 1974; **Resid:** Internal Medicine, N Shore Univ Hosp 1977; **Fellow:** Nephrology, NY Hosp-Cornell Med Ctr 1979; **Fac Appt:** Asst Clin Prof Med, SUNY Downstate

Pepe, John M MD (Nep) - **Spec Exp:** Transplant Medicine-Kidney; **Hospital:** Richmond Univ Med Ctr, Staten Island Univ Hosp - South (page 106); **Address:** 1550 Richmond Ave, Ste 205, Staten Island, NY 10314-1519; **Phone:** 718-982-7800; **Board Cert:** Internal Medicine 1978; Nephrology 1980; **Med School:** Med Coll PA Hahnemann 1975; **Resid:** Internal Medicine, Univ Hosp 1978; **Fellow:** Nephrology, Bronx Muni Hosp/ Einstein 1980; **Fac Appt:** Asst Prof Med, NY Med Coll

Neurology

Jutkowitz, Robert S MD (N) - **Spec Exp:** Headache; Seizure Disorders; **Hospital:** Richmond Univ Med Ctr; **Address:** 78 Todt Hill Rd, Ste 205, Staten Island, NY 10314-4528; **Phone:** 718-442-7133; **Board Cert:** Neurology 1976; **Med School:** Univ Louisville Sch Med 1968; **Resid:** Internal Medicine, St Viincents Hosp 1970; Neurology, Mt Sinai Hosp 1974

Najjar, Souhel MD (N) - **Spec Exp:** Epilepsy; Seizure Disorders; **Hospital:** Staten Island Univ Hosp - North (page 106), NYU Langone Med Ctr (page 108); **Address:** 501 Seaview Ave, Ste 104, Staten Island, NY 10305; **Phone:** 718-683-3766; **Board Cert:** Neurology 1993; **Med School:** Syria 1983; **Resid:** Pathology, Albany Med Ctr 1988; Neurology, Albany Med Ctr 1992; **Fellow:** Neurological Pathology, NYU Med Ctr 1994; **Fac Appt:** Assoc Prof N, NYU Sch Med

Neuroradiology

Raden, Mark J MD (NRad) - **Spec Exp:** Invertentional Radiology; Vascular Malformations; **Hospital:** Staten Island Univ Hosp - North (page 106); **Address:** Staten Island Univ Hosp, 475 Seaview Ave, Staten Island, NY 10305; **Phone:** 718-226-1784; **Board Cert:** Diagnostic Radiology ; Neuroradiology 2010; **Med School:** Albert Einstein Coll Med 1989; **Resid:** Diagnostic Radiology, UMDNJ Affil Hosp 1994; **Fellow:** Neurological Radiology, Montefiore Med Ctr 1995

Obstetrics & Gynecology

Ponterio, Jane M MD (ObG) *PCP* - **Spec Exp:** Menopause Problems; Hysterectomy Alternatives; Adolescent Gynecology; HPV-Human Papilloma Virus; **Hospital:** Richmond Univ Med Ctr, Staten Island Univ Hosp North (page 106), **Address:** 1583 Richmond Ave, Staten Island, NY 10314; **Phone:** 718-983-0204; **Board Cert:** Obstetrics & Gynecology 2013; **Med School:** NY Med Coll 1981; **Resid:** Obstetrics & Gynecology, St Luke's Hosp Ctr 1985; **Fac Appt:** Asst Prof ObG, NY Med Coll

Reilly, James G DO (ObG) - **Spec Exp:** Colposcopy; Laparoscopic Surgery; Hysterectomy Alternatives; **Hospital:** Richmond Univ Med Ctr, Staten Island Univ Hosp - North (page 106); **Address:** 668 Castleton Ave, Staten Island, NY 10301-2044; **Phone:** 718-448-4300; **Board Cert:** Obstetrics & Gynecology 2012; **Med School:** NY Coll Osteo Med 1991; **Resid:** Obstetrics & Gynecology, St Vincent Cath Med Ctr 1996; **Fac Appt:** Asst Clin Prof ObG, NY Coll Osteo Med

Ophthalmology

Derespinis Sr, Patrick A MD (Oph) - **Spec Exp:** Eye Muscle Disorders; Pediatric Ophthalmology; Eye Disorders-Congenital; **Hospital:** Staten Island Univ Hosp - South (page 106), Univ Hosp (Newark); **Address:** Pediatric Eye Care, 2504 Richmond Rd, Staten Island, NY 10306; **Phone:** 718-667-1010; **Board Cert:** Ophthalmology 1989; **Med School:** Mexico 1981; **Resid:** Internal Medicine, NY Hosp Med Ctr 1983; Ophthalmology, UMDNJ 1987; **Fellow:** Pediatric Ophthalmology, Manhattan EE&T Hosp 1988; **Fac Appt:** Assoc Clin Prof Oph, UMDNJ-NJ Med Sch, Newark

Kramer, Philip W MD (Oph) - **Spec Exp:** Diabetic Eye Disease/Retinopathy; Cataract Surgery; Glaucoma; **Hospital:** Staten Island Univ Hosp - South (page 106), New York Eye & Ear Infirm (page 115); **Address:** Ophthalmology Assocs of Staten Island, 1460 Victory Blvd, Staten Island, NY 10301-3914; **Phone:** 718-447-0022; **Board Cert:** Ophthalmology 1985; **Med School:** Temple Univ 1980; **Resid:** Ophthalmology, NY Eye & Ear Infirmary 1984

Zerykier, Abraham L MD (Oph) - **Spec Exp:** Cataract Surgery; Diabetic Eye Disease/Retinopathy; Glaucoma; **Hospital:** Staten Island Univ Hosp - South (page 106), Beth Israel Med Ctr- Kings Hwy Div (page 94); **Address:** 16 Ross Ave, Staten Island, NY 10306-2216; **Phone:** 718-667-4444; **Board Cert:** Ophthalmology 1980; **Med School:** Hahnemann Univ 1975; **Resid:** Internal Medicine, Brookdale Hosp 1976; Ophthalmology, Jewish Hosp 1979; **Fac Appt:** Asst Clin Prof Oph, SUNY Downstate

Orthopaedic Surgery

Drucker, David A MD (OrS) - **Spec Exp:** Hip & Knee Replacement; Joint Replacement; Arthritis; **Hospital:** Beth Israel Med Ctr - Petrie Div (page 94), Staten Island Univ Hosp - North (page 106); **Address:** New York Hip & Knee, 11 Ralph Pl, Ste 103A, Staten Island, NY 10304; **Phone:** 718-727-6945; **Board Cert:** Orthopaedic Surgery 2004; **Med School:** Univ Chicago-Pritzker Sch Med 1983; **Resid:** Orthopaedic Surgery, UNDMJ Univ Hosp 1989; **Fellow:** Reconstructive Surgery, Indiana Univ Affil Hosp 1990; Joint Replacement Surgery, Mass Genl Hosp 1991; **Fac Appt:** Asst Clin Prof OrS, UMDNJ-NJ Med Sch, Newark

Flynn, Maryirene MD (OrS) - **Spec Exp:** Arthroscopic Surgery; Sports Medicine; **Hospital:** Richmond Univ Med Ctr, Staten Island Univ Hosp - North (page 106); **Address:** Staten Island Orthopedics, 2052 Richmond Rd, Staten Island, NY 10306; **Phone:** 718-351-6500 x101; **Board Cert:** Orthopaedic Surgery 2005; **Med School:** Albert Einstein Coll Med 1986; **Resid:** Orthopaedic Surgery, Montefiore Hosp Med Ctr 1991; **Fellow:** Sports Medicine, Staten Island Hosp 1992

Jayaram, Nadubeethi MD (OrS) - **Spec Exp:** Hand Surgery; **Hospital:** Richmond Univ Med Ctr; **Address:** Richmond Orthopaedic Assocs, 11 Ralph Pl, Ste 102, Staten Island, NY 10304; **Phone:** 718-447-6545; **Board Cert:** Orthopaedic Surgery 2003; **Med School:** India 1973; **Resid:** Surgery, Univ Hosp 1981; Orthopaedic Surgery, Univ Hosp 1985; **Fellow:** Vascular Surgery, Lutheran Med Ctr 1982; Hand Surgery, Univ Alabama Hosp 1988

Reilly, John P MD (OrS) - **Spec Exp:** Sports Medicine; Trauma; **Hospital:** Staten Island Univ Hosp - North (page 106); **Address:** Ortho Assocs of NY, 3333 Hylan Blvd, Staten Island, NY 10306; **Phone:** 718-667-7500; **Board Cert:** Orthopaedic Surgery 2010; **Med School:** SUNY Downstate 1981; **Resid:** Orthopaedic Surgery, Lenox Hill Hosp 1986; **Fellow:** Trauma, Univ MD Hosp 1987

Otolaryngology

Castellano, Bartolomeo V MD (Oto) - **Hospital:** Mt Sinai Med Ctr (page 102); **Address:** 78 Todt Hill Rd, Ste 204, Staten Island, NY 10314-4528; **Phone:** 718-273-2626; **Board Cert:** Otolaryngology 1985; **Med School:** Mexico 1979; **Resid:** Otolaryngology, NYU Med Ctr 1984; **Fellow:** Facial Plastic Surgery, Mt Sinai Med Ctr 1985; **Fac Appt:** Asst Clin Prof Oto, NYU Sch Med

Sinnreich, Abraham MD (Oto) - **Spec Exp:** Sinus Disorders; Sleep Disorders/Apnea; **Hospital:** Richmond Univ Med Ctr, Mt Sinai Med Ctr (page 102); **Address:** 1887 Richmond Ave, Ste 5, Staten Island, NY 10314; **Phone:** 718-370-0072; **Board Cert:** Otolaryngology 1984; **Med School:** Albert Einstein Coll Med 1979; **Resid:** Otolaryngology, Mount Sinai Hosp 1983; **Fac Appt:** Asst Clin Prof Oto, SUNY Downstate

Pain Medicine

Stilwell, Anne Marie MD (PM) - **Spec Exp:** Pain-Spine; Pain-after Spinal Intervention; **Hospital:** Richmond Univ Med Ctr; **Address:** 45 McLean Ave, Staten Island, NY 10305; **Phone:** 718-448-6373; **Board Cert:** Anesthesiology 2009; Pain Medicine 2007; **Med School:** Univ Rochester 1990; **Resid:** Anesthesiology, NY Hosp-Cornell Med Ctr 1994; **Fellow:** Pain Management, NY Hosp-Cornell Med Ctr 1996

Pediatric Endocrinology

Torrado-Jule, Carmen MD (PEn) - **Spec Exp:** Diabetes; Thyroid Disorders; Growth Disorders; Obesity; **Hospital:** Staten Island Univ Hosp - North (page 106), N Shore Univ Hosp (page 106); **Address:** 584 Forest Ave, Staten Island, NY 10310-2512; **Phone:** 718-226-5619; **Board Cert:** Pediatrics 2008; Pediatric Endocrinology 2012; **Med School:** Dominican Republic 1983; **Resid:** Pediatrics, Kings County Hosp 1987; **Fellow:** Pediatric Endocrinology, Kings County Hosp 1990; **Fac Appt:** Asst Prof Ped, SUNY Hlth Sci Ctr

Pediatric Pulmonology

Chan, Siu-Pun MD (PPul) - **Spec Exp:** Asthma; Critical Care; Sleep Medicine; **Hospital:** Staten Island Univ Hosp - North (page 106); **Address:** Chldns Subspecialty Ctr, 584 Forest Ave Ste 4, Staten Island, NY 10308; **Phone:** 718-226-5619; **Board Cert:** Pediatrics 2012; Pediatric Pulmonology 2009; Sleep Medicine 2007; **Med School:** Hong Kong 1980; **Resid:** Pediatrics, SUNY Downstate Med Ctr 1990; **Fellow:** Pediatric Pulmonology, SUNY Downstate Med Ctr 1994

Pediatric Urology

Horowitz, Mark MD (Ped Uro) - **Hospital:** Staten Island Univ Hosp - North (page 106), SUNY Downstate Med Ctr (Univ Hosp Brooklyn) (page 441); **Address:** 256 Mason Ave C Bldg Fl 3, Staten Island, NY 10305; **Phone:** 718-226-1271; **Board Cert:** Urology 2006; **Med School:** NY Med Coll 1986; **Resid:** Urology, SUNY Downstate Med Ctr 1992; **Fellow:** Pediatric Urology, Chldns Hosp 1994; **Fac Appt:** Assoc Prof U, SUNY Downstate

Pediatrics

Bastawros, Mary N MD (Ped) *PCP* - **Hospital:** Richmond Univ Med Ctr, Staten Island Univ Hosp - North (page 106); **Address:** 314 Seaview Ave, Staten Island, NY 10305; **Phone:** 718-668-3417; **Board Cert:** Pediatrics 1985; **Med School:** Egypt 1966; **Resid:** Pediatrics, NY Methodist Hosp 1975; Pediatrics, Kingsbrook Jewish Med Ctr 1976

Duchnowska, Alicja B MD (Ped) *PCP* - **Hospital:** Staten Island Univ Hosp - North (page 106); **Address:** 934 Ionia Ave, Staten Island, NY 10309-2308; **Phone:** 718-984-5255; **Board Cert:** Pediatrics 1985; **Med School:** Poland 1965; **Resid:** Pediatrics, Natl Inst of Mother & Child 1970; Pediatrics, Staten Island Hosp 1982; **Fellow:** Pediatrics, Staten Island Hosp 1984

Visconti, Ernest B MD (Ped) *PCP* - **Spec Exp:** Infectious Disease; **Hospital:** Lutheran Med Ctr - Brooklyn, Richmond Univ Med Ctr; **Address:** 314 Seaview Ave, Staten Island, NY 10305-2246; **Phone:** 718-668-3417; **Board Cert:** Pediatrics 1992; Pediatric Infectious Disease 2009; **Med School:** SUNY Upstate Med Univ 1971; **Resid:** Pediatrics, NY Hosp 1974; **Fellow:** Infectious Disease, Rhode Island Hosp 1978

Physical Medicine & Rehabilitation

Weinberg, Jeffrey B MD (PMR) - **Spec Exp:** Geriatric Rehabilitation; Musculoskeletal Injuries; **Hospital:** Staten Island Univ Hosp - North (page 106); **Address:** Staten Island Univ Hosp, Dept Rehab Med, 475 Seaview Ave, Staten Island, NY 10305; **Phone:** 718-226-6362; **Board Cert:** Physical Medicine & Rehabilitation 1985; **Med School:** NY Med Coll 1980; **Resid:** Physical Medicine & Rehabilitation, NYU Med Ctr 1983; **Fellow:** Geriatric Medicine, NYU Med Ctr 1986; **Fac Appt:** Asst Clin Prof PMR, SUNY Downstate

Weiner, Kevin H MD (PMR) - **Hospital:** Morristown Med Ctr (page 92), NS-LIJ Hlth Sys (page 106); **Address:** 262 Nelson Ave, Staten Island, NY 10308; **Phone:** 718-442-4422; **Board Cert:** Physical Medicine & Rehabilitation 2009; **Med School:** Univ Hlth Scis, Chicago Med Sch 1994; **Resid:** Physical Medicine & Rehabilitation, NYU Med Ctr 1998

Plastic Surgery

Cherofsky, Alan MD (PlS) - **Spec Exp:** Breast Surgery; Pediatric Plastic Surgery; Cosmetic Surgery-Body; **Hospital:** Staten Island Univ Hosp - South (page 106), Richmond Univ Med Ctr; **Address:** 4546 Hylan Blvd, Staten Island, NY 10312-6400; **Phone:** 718-967-3300; **Board Cert:** Plastic Surgery 1993; **Med School:** SUNY Downstate 1982; **Resid:** Surgery, Staten Island Univ Hosp 1987; Plastic Surgery, Univ Missouri Hosp 1989

Cutolo Jr, Louis C MD (PlS) - **Spec Exp:** Breast Augmentation; Liposuction; Eyelid Surgery; Cosmetic Surgery-Face & Neck; **Hospital:** Staten Island Univ Hosp - North (page 106), Richmond Univ Med Ctr; **Address:** 1557 Victory Blvd, Staten Island, NY 10314; **Phone:** 718-720-9400; **Board Cert:** Plastic Surgery 2003; **Med School:** SUNY Downstate 1985; **Resid:** Surgery, Staten Island Hosp 1990; **Fellow:** Plastic Surgery, Univ Florida/Shands Hosp 1992

Psychiatry

Di Buono, Mark MD (Psyc) - **Spec Exp:** Geriatric Psychiatry; Depression; Autism; **Hospital:** Staten Island Univ Hosp - South (page 106); **Address:** Richmond Behavioral Assocs, 4349 Hylan Blvd, Staten Island, NY 10312; **Phone:** 718-227-1897; **Board Cert:** Psychiatry 1990; Geriatric Psychiatry 2008; **Med School:** Mexico 1981; **Resid:** Psychiatry, Stony Brook Univ Med Ctr 1987; **Fac Appt:** Asst Clin Prof Psyc, SUNY Downstate

Pulmonary Disease

Castellano, Michael A MD (Pul) - **Spec Exp:** Asthma; Emphysema; **Hospital:** Staten Island Univ Hosp - North (page 106); **Address:** 501 Seaview Ave, Ste 102, Staten Island, NY 10305; **Phone:** 718-980-5700; **Board Cert:** Internal Medicine 1974; Pulmonary Disease 1978; Critical Care Medicine 2007; Geriatric Medicine 2004; **Med School:** Italy 1968; **Resid:** Internal Medicine, Staten Island Hosp 1972; **Fellow:** Pulmonary Disease, NYU-Bellvue Hosp 1974; **Fac Appt:** Asst Prof Med, SUNY Downstate

Maniatis, Theodore MD (Pul) - **Spec Exp:** Asthma; Lung Cancer; Chronic Obstructive Lung Disease (COPD); Interstitial Lung Disease; **Hospital:** Staten Island Univ Hosp - North (page 106), Staten Island Univ Hosp - South (page 106); **Address:** 501 Seaview Ave, Ste 102, Staten Island, NY 10305; **Phone:** 718-980-5700; **Board Cert:** Internal Medicine 1983; Pulmonary Disease 1986; Critical Care Medicine 2007; **Med School:** SUNY Hlth Sci Ctr 1980; **Resid:** Internal Medicine, Staten Island Univ Hosp 1983; **Fellow:** Pulmonary Disease, UMDNJ Med Ctr 1985; **Fac Appt:** Asst Clin Prof Med, SUNY Downstate

Martins, Publius MD (Pul) - **Spec Exp:** Asthma; Emphysema; **Hospital:** Richmond Univ Med Ctr; **Address:** 283 Bard Ave, Staten Island, NY 10310-1664; **Phone:** 718-816-8068; **Board Cert:** Internal Medicine 1984; **Med School:** Portugal 1975; **Resid:** Internal Medicine, St Vincent's Hosp 1981; **Fellow:** Pulmonary Disease, Meml Hosp 1983; **Fac Appt:** Assoc Clin Prof Med, NY Med Coll

Sasso, Louis MD (Pul) - **Spec Exp:** Asthma; Chronic Obstructive Lung Disease (COPD); Interstitial Lung Disease; **Hospital:** Staten Island Univ Hosp - North (page 106); **Address:** 501 Seaview Ave, Ste 102, Staten Island, NY 10305-3400; **Phone:** 718-980-5700; **Board Cert:** Internal Medicine 1976; Pulmonary Disease 1978; Critical Care Medicine 2005; Geriatric Medicine 2009; **Med School:** UMDNJ-NJ Med Sch, Newark 1972; **Resid:** Internal Medicine, St Vincent's Hosp & Med Ctr 1974; Internal Medicine, CMDNJ-Martland Hosp 1975; **Fellow:** Pulmonary Disease, Bellevue Hosp/NYU Med Ctr 1977; **Fac Appt:** Asst Clin Prof Med, SUNY Downstate

Radiation Oncology

Adams, Marc T MD (RadRO) - **Spec Exp:** Prostate Cancer; Breast Cancer; Lung Cancer; Brain Tumors; **Hospital:** Richmond Univ Med Ctr; **Address:** Regional Radiology, 360 Bard Ave, Staten Island, NY 10310; **Phone:** 718-876-2023; **Board Cert:** Radiation Oncology 1990; **Med School:** UAB Sch Med 1985; **Resid:** Radiation Oncology, St Barnabas Hosp 1989; **Fac Appt:** Asst Prof Rad, NY Med Coll

Schwartz, David Lawrence MD (RadRO) - **Spec Exp:** Prostate Cancer; Brachytherapy; Breast Cancer; **Hospital:** SUNY Downstate Med Ctr (Univ Hosp Brooklyn) (page 441), VA NY Harbor Hlthcr Sys-Brooklyn Campus; **Address:** Staten Island Radiation Oncology, 1781 Hyland Blvd, Staten Island, NY 10305; **Phone:** 718-351-9750; **Board Cert:** Radiation Oncology 1993; **Med School:** SUNY Downstate 1988; **Resid:** Radiation Oncology, SUNY Downstate Med Ctr 1992

Rheumatology

Goldstein, Mark A MD (Rhu) - **Spec Exp:** Rheumatoid Arthritis; Osteoporosis; Lupus/SLE; **Hospital:** Staten Island Univ Hosp - South (page 106), Staten Island Univ Hosp - North (page 106); **Address:** 1534 Victory Blvd, Staten Island, NY 10314; **Phone:** 718-447-0055; **Board Cert:** Internal Medicine 1982; Rheumatology 1988; **Med School:** NY Med Coll 1979; **Resid:** Internal Medicine, Montefiore Med Ctr 1982; **Fellow:** Rheumatology, Montefiore Med Ctr 1987

Surgery

D'Anna Jr, John A MD (S) - **Spec Exp:** Vascular Surgery; **Hospital:** Staten Island Univ Hosp - North (page 106), Staten Island Univ Hosp - South (page 106); **Address:** 375 Seguine Ave, Staten Island, NY 10309; **Phone:** 718-226-2950; **Board Cert:** Surgery 2011; **Med School:** Georgetown Univ 1977; **Resid:** Surgery, St Vincent's Hosp Med Ctr 1982; **Fellow:** Vascular Surgery, St Vincent's Hosp Med Ctr 1983; **Fac Appt:** Assoc Clin Prof S, SUNY Downstate

Hornyak, Stephen W MD (S) - **Spec Exp:** Breast Surgery; Laparoscopic Surgery; Gastrointestinal Surgery; **Hospital:** Staten Island Univ Hosp - North (page 106), Richmond Univ Med Ctr; **Address:** 1130 Victory Blvd, Staten Island, NY 10301; **Phone:** 718-442-3400; **Board Cert:** Surgery 2010; **Med School:** SUNY Hlth Sci Ctr 1974; **Resid:** Surgery, Kings County Hosp 1979; **Fellow:** Research, Meml Sloan Kettering Cancer Ctr 1980; **Fac Appt:** Asst Clin Prof S, SUNY Downstate

Lutchman, Gordon MD (S) - **Spec Exp:** Wound Healing/Care; Vein Disorders; Laser Surgery; **Hospital:** Maimonides Med Ctr (page 98); **Address:** Laser & Varicose Vein Treatment Ctr, 500 Seaview Ave, Ste 240, Staten Island, NY 10305; **Phone:** 718-667-1777; **Board Cert:** Surgery 2007; **Med School:** Jamaica 1976; **Resid:** Surgery, Royal United Hosp 1982; Surgery, Maimonides Med Ctr 1987; **Fellow:** Vascular Surgery, Maimonides Med Ctr 1988

Pahuja, Murlidhar MD (S) - **Spec Exp:** Breast Cancer; Laparoscopic Surgery; Wound Healing/Care; **Hospital:** Staten Island Univ Hosp - North (page 106), Staten Island Univ Hosp - South (page 106); **Address:** 4287 Richmond Ave, Staten Island, NY 10312; **Phone:** 718-967-6230; **Board Cert:** Surgery 2004; **Med School:** Pakistan 1971; **Resid:** Surgery, Stamford Hosp 1978; Surgery, Staten Island Hosp 1982; **Fellow:** Burn Surgery, NY Hosp 1980

Thoracic & Cardiac Surgery

McGinn Jr, Joseph T MD (T&CS) - **Spec Exp:** Minimally Invasive Cardiac Surgery; Heart Valve Surgery; **Hospital:** Staten Island Univ Hosp - North (page 106); **Address:** 501 Seaview Ave, Ste 202, Staten Island, NY 10305; **Phone:** 718-226-1612; **Board Cert:** Surgery 2009; Thoracic Surgery 2009; Surgical Critical Care 2003; **Med School:** SUNY Downstate 1981; **Resid:** Surgery, SUNY Downstate Med Ctr 1985; Thoracic Surgery, Long Is Jewish Med Ctr 1987; **Fellow:** Cardiothoracic Surgery, Long Is Jewish Med Ctr 1988; **Fac Appt:** Asst Clin Prof S, SUNY Downstate

Rosell, Frank M MD (T&CS) - **Hospital:** Staten Island Univ Hosp - North (page 106); **Address:** 501 Seaview Ave, Ste 202, Staten Island, NY 10305; **Phone:** 718-226-1612; **Board Cert:** Surgery 2006; Thoracic Surgery 2010; **Med School:** NYU Sch Med 1992; **Resid:** Surgery, NY Med Coll Affil Hosp 1997; **Fellow:** Thoracic Surgery, Long Is Jewish Med Ctr 2000

Urology

Lessing, Jeffrey A MD (U) - **Spec Exp:** Prostate Disease; Impotence; Kidney Stones; Infertility-Male; **Hospital:** Staten Island Univ Hosp - North (page 106), Staten Island Univ Hosp - South (page 106); **Address:** 78 Todt Hill Rd, Ste 112, Staten Island, NY 10314; **Phone:** 718-448-3880; **Board Cert:** Urology 1982; **Med School:** NYU Sch Med 1975; **Resid:** Surgery, Mt Sinai Med Ctr 1977; Urology, Mt Sinai Med Ctr 1982

Raboy, Adley MD (U) - **Spec Exp:** Prostate Disease; Kidney Stones; Minimally Invasive Surgery; **Hospital:** Staten Island Univ Hosp - North (page 106), Staten Island Univ Hosp - South (page 106); **Address:** Staten Is Urological Assocs, 1460 Victory Blvd, Staten Island, NY 10301-3914; **Phone:** 718-273-8100; **Board Cert:** Urology 2012; **Med School:** SUNY Downstate 1984; **Resid:** Surgery, Staten Is Hosp 1986; **Fellow:** Urology, SUNY Downstate Med Ctr 1991; **Fac Appt:** Asst Clin Prof U, SUNY Downstate

Savino, Michael A MD (U) - **Spec Exp:** Robotic Surgery; Prostate Cancer; Kidney Stones; Laparoscopic Surgery; **Hospital:** Staten Island Univ Hosp - South (page 106), Maimonides Med Ctr (page 98); **Address:** 375 Seguine Ave Fl 1, Staten Island, NY 10309; **Phone:** 718-226-2950; **Board Cert:** Urology 2007; **Med School:** Mexico 1979; **Resid:** Surgery, Maimonides Med Ctr 1982; Urology, Maimonides Med Ctr 1986

Vascular & Interventional Radiology

Scheiner, Jonathan E MD (VIR) - **Spec Exp:** Endovascular Surgery; Carotid Artery Stent Placement; Varicocele Embolization; **Hospital:** Staten Island Univ Hosp - North (page 106); **Address:** Staten Island Univ Hosp-North, 475 Seaview Ave, Staten Island, NY 10305; **Phone:** 718-226-7700; **Board Cert:** Diagnostic Radiology ; **Med School:** Albert Einstein Coll Med 1994; **Resid:** Diagnostic Radiology, Montefiore Med Ctr 1999; **Fellow:** Vascular & Interventional Radiology, NY Presby Hosp/Sloan-Kettering Cancer Ctr 2000

Vascular Surgery

Deitch, Jonathan MD (VascS) - **Spec Exp:** Aneurysm-Aortic; Carotid Artery Surgery; Endovascular Surgery; **Hospital:** Staten Island Univ Hosp - North (page 106); **Address:** 501 Seaview Ave, Ste 302, Staten Island, NY 10305; **Phone:** 718-226-6800; **Board Cert:** Vascular Surgery 2009; **Med School:** NY Med Coll 1991; **Resid:** Surgery, Montefiore Med Ctr 1996; **Fellow:** Vascular Surgery, Wake Forest Baptist Med Ctr 1998; Endovascular Surgery, UMDNJ Med Ctr 1998

Rodino, William MD (VascS) - **Spec Exp:** Aneurysm-Aortic; Peripheral Vascular Disease; Dialysis Access; Varicose Veins; **Hospital:** New York Methodist Hosp (page 440), Richmond Univ Med Ctr; **Address:** ACC, Verrazano Vascular Assocs, 2025 Richmond Ave, Ste 1LL, Staten Island, NY 10314; **Phone:** 718-259-3436; **Board Cert:** Surgery 2006; Vascular Surgery 2007; **Med School:** SUNY Downstate 1990; **Resid:** Surgery, SUNY Downstate Med Ctr 1995; **Fellow:** Vascular Surgery, SUNY Downstate Med Ctr 1997

The Best in American Medicine
www.CastleConnolly.com

Nassau

259 First Street, Mineola, NY 11501
Tel: 1-866-WINTHROP
www.winthrop.org

WINTHROP University Hospital
Your Health Means Everything.®

Sponsorship: Voluntary, Not-for-Profit
Beds: 591
Accreditation: The Joint Commission

General Overview

Founded in 1896 by a group of local physicians and concerned citizens, Winthrop-University Hospital is Long Island's first voluntary hospital. The university-affiliated medical center and New York State-designated Regional Trauma Center offers sophisticated diagnostic and therapeutic care in virtually every specialty and subspecialty of medicine and surgery.

Winthrop has earned many prestigious accreditations, including designations as a New York State (NYS) Stroke Center and NYS Regional Perinatal Center, and is known across the State for its excellent outcomes in interventional cardiology and cardiac surgery. In addition to Orthopaedics, Winthrop boasts several specialized Centers that are dedicated to Cancer Care, Digestive Disorders, Women's and Children's Health Services, Lung Care and Neurosciences. Winthrop was also recently accredited by the Joint Commission for Inpatient Diabetes Care, the first major teaching hospital in New York State to hold this accreditation.

Patient care, academics and research are the three components of Winthrop's mission. Winthrop has initiated the construction of a new four-floor, 95,000-square-foot Research and Academic Center which will house basic science research, clinical/translational research, outcomes research, medical education classrooms.

***Staff* -** The Hospital employs over 6,900 dedicated and caring individuals, including nearly 1,500 nurses and more than 1,800 full-time and voluntary attending physicians.

***Academic and Clinical Affiliations* -** Winthrop is the Clinical Campus of Stony Brook University School of Medicine and an affiliated member of the New York-Presbyterian Healthcare System.

Special Programs and Services

Advances in Neuroscience: Within Winthrop's Department of Neuroscience, an interdisciplinary team of healthcare professionals are pioneering the use of advanced approaches for diagnosis and treatment, including computerized imaging systems, state-of-the-art surgical interventions, such as deep brain stimulation, and the latest generation of medication therapies. In addition to a 14-bed Neurosciences Special Care Unit, the Department offers special programs for conditions including Multiple Sclerosis, Movement Disorders, and Epilepsy.

Innovative Prostate Cancer Treatment: At Winthrop, prostate cancer patients are offered a full array of treatment options. Minimally invasive robotic surgery is available, as well as cryotherapy, and more. In addition, Winthrop pioneered the use of CyberKnife for prostate cancer. Winthrop is the second largest site in the world for treating prostate cancer with CyberKnife and is a designated CyberKnife training site.

Excellence in Women's Healthcare: Winthrop is a nationally recognized, regional leader in women's health services. The experts at the Winthrop Breast Health Center – the first center in Nassau County to earn accreditation by the National Accreditation Program for Breast Centers (NAPBC) – provide comprehensive risk assessment, diagnosis, treatment and follow-up care to patients. Winthrop is also the only site in the tri-state area to earn accreditation by the American Institute of Ultrasound in Medicine (AIUM) for fetal echocardiograms. Winthrop has been ranked by HealthGrades® among the top 10% in the nation for Women's Health four years in a row.

No Place Like Home: *Winthrop's award-winning certified home healthcare agency offers nursing, as well as physical, speech and occupational therapies in conjunction with medical social work and home health aide services to Nassau, Suffolk and Queens County residents.*

Select National Performance Recognitions

2013-14 Best Regional Hospitals in the New York Metro Area - ***U.S. News & World Report*** with 12 high-performing specialties

2013-14 Best Children's Hospitals - ***U.S. News & World Report*** **for excellence in pediatric diabetes & endocrinology, urology and pulmonology**

Healthgrades® Top 5% in the Nation for Cardiac Care, Cardiology Services, Cardiac Surgery and Angioplasty/Stent Procedures, 2013

"100 Hospitals with Great Women's Health Programs" - *Becker's Hospital Review*

"100 Hospitals and Health Systems with Great Oncology Programs" - *Becker's Hospital Review*

"Most Wired" Hospital by ***Hospitals & Health Networks*** Magazine, 2012 and 2013

NAEC Level 4 Epilepsy Center

HCM Center of Excellence by The National Hypertrophic Cardiomyopathy Association

NAPBC National Breast Center

New York State Designated Regional Trauma Center

New York State Regional Perinatal Center

New York State Stroke Center

The Joint Commission: *Accreditation – Hospital, Certified Home Health Agency*

The Joint Commission*:* *Gold Seal of Approval™ for Advanced Certification* – Inpatient Diabetes

Adolescent Medicine

Arden, Martha MD (AM) - **Spec Exp:** Adolescent Gynecology; Nutrition; Eating Disorders; **Hospital:** Steven & Alexandra Cohen Chldn's Med Ctr of NY (page 106), N Shore Univ Hosp (page 106); **Address:** 2001 Marcus Ave, Ste N204, New Hyde Park, NY 11040; **Phone:** 347-882-1321; **Board Cert:** Adolescent Medicine 2009; **Med School:** Yale Univ 1984; **Resid:** Pediatrics, NY-Presby/Columbia Univ Med Ctr 1987; **Fellow:** Adolescent Medicine, Schneider Chldns Hosp 1990; **Fac Appt:** Assoc Clin Prof Ped, Albert Einstein Coll Med

Carmine, Linda MD (AM) - **Spec Exp:** Eating Disorders; **Hospital:** Steven & Alexandra Cohen Chldn's Med Ctr of NY (page 106); **Address:** Division of Adolescent Medicine, 410 Lakeville Rd, Ste 108, New Hyde Park, NY 11042; **Phone:** 516-465-3270; **Board Cert:** Pediatrics 1987; Adolescent Medicine 2009; **Med School:** NYU Sch Med 1982; **Resid:** Pediatrics, Montefiore Med Ctr 1985; **Fellow:** Adolescent Medicine, Montefiore Med Ctr 1986; **Fac Appt:** Assoc Prof Ped, Mount Sinai Sch Med

Feinstein, Ronald A MD (AM) - **Spec Exp:** Weight Management; Obesity; Eating Disorders; **Hospital:** Steven & Alexandra Cohen Chldn's Med Ctr of NY (page 106); **Address:** 410 Lakeville Rd, Ste 108, New Hyde Park, NY 11042; **Phone:** 516-465-3270; **Board Cert:** Pediatrics ; Adolescent Medicine 2009; **Med School:** NY Med Coll 1976; **Resid:** Pediatrics, LI Jewish Med Ctr 1979; **Fellow:** Adolescent Medicine, UAB Hosp 1981; **Fac Appt:** Prof Ped, Hofstra N Shore-LIJ Sch Med

Fisher, Martin M MD (AM) - **Spec Exp:** Eating Disorders; Chronic Fatigue Syndrome; **Hospital:** Steven & Alexandra Cohen Chldn's Med Ctr of NY (page 106), N Shore Univ Hosp (page 106); **Address:** Cohen Chldns Med Ctr, Adolescent Med, 410 Lakeville Rd, Ste 108, New Hyde Park, NY 11042; **Phone:** 516-465-3270; **Board Cert:** Pediatrics 1979; Adolescent Medicine 2009; **Med School:** Albert Einstein Coll Med 1975; **Resid:** Pediatrics, LI Jewish Med Ctr 1978; **Fellow:** Adolescent Medicine, LI Jewish Med Ctr 1980

Jacobson, Marc S MD (AM) - **Spec Exp:** Cholesterol/Lipid Disorders; Obesity; Preventive Cardiology; **Hospital:** NS-LIJ Hlth Sys (page 106); **Address:** ProHealth Care Assocs, 2 Prohealth Plaza, Ste 200, Lake Success, NY 11042; **Phone:** 516-304-3950; **Board Cert:** Pediatrics ; Adolescent Medicine 2009; **Med School:** Univ Kansas 1973; **Resid:** Pediatrics, Univ Kansas Hosp 1976; **Fellow:** Adolescent Medicine, Univ MD Med Ctr 1979; **Fac Appt:** Prof Ped, Albert Einstein Coll Med

Swedler, Jane MD (AM) - **Spec Exp:** Adolescent Gynecology; **Hospital:** Winthrop Univ Hosp (page 524); **Address:** Winthrop Pediatric Assocs, 222 Station Plaza N, Ste 611, Mineola, NY 11501; **Phone:** 516-663-2532; **Board Cert:** Family Medicine 2009; Adolescent Medicine 2011; **Med School:** McGill Univ 1987; **Resid:** Family Medicine, Queen Elizabeth Hosp 1989; Family Medicine, Stony Brook Univ Med Ctr 1990; **Fellow:** Adolescent Medicine, Montefiore Med Ctr 1992; **Fac Appt:** Asst Prof Med, Mount Sinai Sch Med

Allergy & Immunology

Boxer, Mitchell MD (A&I) - **Spec Exp:** Asthma; Drug Sensitivity; Churg-Strauss Vasculitis; Sinusitis; **Hospital:** Long Is Jewish Med Ctr (page 106); **Address:** 2001 Marcus Ave, Ste N220, Lake Success, NY 11042; **Phone:** 516-482-0910; **Board Cert:** Internal Medicine 1984; Allergy & Immunology 1987; **Med School:** NY Med Coll 1981; **Resid:** Internal Medicine, LI Jewish Med Ctr 1984; **Fellow:** Allergy & Immunology, Northwestern Meml Hosp 1987; **Fac Appt:** Asst Clin Prof Med, Albert Einstein Coll Med

Corriel, Robert N MD (A&I) - **Spec Exp:** Asthma & Allergy; Sinus Disorders; Rhinitis; Food Allergy; **Hospital:** N Shore Univ Hosp (page 106), Long Is Jewish Med Ctr (page 106); **Address:** Manhasset Allergy & Asthma Assocs, 1129 Northern Blvd, Ste 300, Manhasset, NY 11030; **Phone:** 516-365-6077; **Board Cert:** Pediatrics 1983; Allergy & Immunology 1985; **Med School:** Wake Forest Univ 1976; **Resid:** Pediatrics, N Shore Univ Hosp 1979; **Fellow:** Allergy & Immunology, Univ Hosp 1981; **Fac Appt:** Asst Clin Prof Ped, Hofstra N Shore-LIJ Sch Med

Edwards, Bruce L MD (A&I) - **Spec Exp:** Asthma; Sinus Disorders; Food Allergy; **Hospital:** Long Is Jewish Med Ctr (page 106), Plainview Hosp (page 106); **Address:** 700 Old Country Rd, Ste 105, Plainview, NY 11803-4932; **Phone:** 516-933-1125; **Board Cert:** Allergy & Immunology 2009; **Med School:** Case West Res Univ 1984; **Resid:** Pediatrics, Babies Hosp/Columbia Presby 1987; **Fellow:** Allergy & Immunology, Schneider Chldns Hosp-LIJ 1989

Fonacier, Luz MD (A&I) - **Spec Exp:** Skin Allergies; Drug Sensitivity; Asthma & Allergy; **Hospital:** Winthrop Univ Hosp (page 524); **Address:** 120 Mineola Blvd, Ste 410, Mineola, NY 11501; **Phone:** 516-663-2097; **Board Cert:** Internal Medicine 1989; Allergy & Immunology 2011; **Med School:** Philippines 1978; **Resid:** Dermatology, Univ Philippines 1983; Internal Medicine, Lutheran Med Ctr 1989; **Fellow:** Dermatology, NYU Med Ctr 1986; Allergy & Immunology, NY Hosp-Cornell Med Ctr 1991; **Fac Appt:** Clin Prof A&I, SUNY Stony Brook

Frieri, Marianne MD/PhD (A&I) - **Spec Exp:** Asthma; Food Allergy; Immune Deficiency; Rhinitis; **Hospital:** N Shore Univ Hosp (page 106), Nassau Univ Med Ctr; **Address:** 566 Broadway, Massapequa, NY 11758; **Phone:** 516-541-6262; **Board Cert:** Internal Medicine 1984; Allergy & Immunology 1985; Diagnostic Lab Immunology 1990; **Med School:** Loyola Univ-Stritch Sch Med 1978; **Resid:** Internal Medicine, St Josephs Hosp 1980; **Fellow:** Allergy & Immunology, NIH/NIAID 1983; **Fac Appt:** Prof Med, SUNY Stony Brook

Goldstein, Stanley MD (A&I) - **Spec Exp:** Asthma; Pulmonary Disease; **Hospital:** Long Is Jewish Med Ctr (page 106), Mercy Med Ctr - Rockville Centre; **Address:** Allergy & Asthma Care, 242 Merrick Rd, Ste 401, Rockville Centre, NY 11570; **Phone:** 516-536-7336; **Board Cert:** Pediatrics 1979; Allergy & Immunology 1981; Pediatric Pulmonology 2011; **Med School:** NY Med Coll 1975; **Resid:** Pediatrics, LI Jewish Med Ctr 1978; **Fellow:** Allergy & Immunology, Chldns Hosp 1982

Lang, Paul MD (A&I) - **Spec Exp:** Asthma; Food Allergy; Insect Allergies; **Hospital:** N Shore Univ Hosp (page 106), Winthrop Univ Hosp (page 524); **Address:** N Shore Allergy Asthma Inst, 1 Hollow Ln, Ste 110, New Hyde Park, NY 11042; **Phone:** 516-365-6666; **Board Cert:** Pediatrics 1978; Allergy & Immunology 1979; **Med School:** Cornell Univ-Weill Med Coll 1973; **Resid:** Pediatrics, LAC & USC Med Ctr 1975; Allergy & Immunology, St Lukes-Roosevelt Hosp 1977; **Fac Appt:** Assoc Clin Prof Ped, NYU Sch Med

Markovics, Sharon B MD (A&I) - **Spec Exp:** Allergy; Asthma; Rhinitis; Sinus Disorders; **Hospital:** N Shore Univ Hosp (page 106), Long Is Jewish Med Ctr (page 106); **Address:** 1129 Northern Blvd, Ste 300, Manhasset, NY 11030-3527; **Phone:** 516-365-6077; **Board Cert:** Pediatrics 1979; Allergy & Immunology 1981; **Med School:** Albert Einstein Coll Med 1975; **Resid:** Pediatrics, Bellevue Hosp 1977; **Fellow:** Allergy & Immunology, Montreal Chldns Hosp 1979; **Fac Appt:** Asst Clin Prof Ped, NYU Sch Med

Novick, Brian MD (A&I) - **Spec Exp:** Asthma; Sinus Disorders; Food Allergy; Hives; **Hospital:** Nassau Univ Med Ctr, Lenox Hill Hosp (page 106); **Address:** ProHlth, Allergy Testing, 30 Newbridge Rd, Ste 100, East Meadow, NY 11554; **Phone:** 516-731-5740; **Board Cert:** Pediatrics 1984; Allergy & Immunology 2012; **Med School:** Mexico 1978; **Resid:** Pediatrics, Albert Einstein Coll Med Affil Hosp 1982; **Fellow:** Allergy & Immunology, Albert Einstein Coll Med Affil Hosp 1984; **Fac Appt:** Asst Clin Prof A&I, Albert Einstein Coll Med

Sicklick, Marc MD (A&I) - **Spec Exp:** Asthma; Immune Deficiency; Insect Allergies; **Hospital:** N Shore Univ Hosp (page 106), Long Is Jewish Med Ctr (page 106); **Address:** 123 Grove Ave, Ste 110, Cedarhurst, NY 11516; **Phone:** 516-569-5550; **Board Cert:** Pediatrics 1979; Allergy & Immunology 1987; **Med School:** Albert Einstein Coll Med 1974; **Resid:** Pediatrics, Bronx Muni Hosp Ctr 1977; **Fellow:** Allergy & Immunology, Montefiore Med Ctr 1979; **Fac Appt:** Assoc Clin Prof Ped, Albert Einstein Coll Med

Weinstock, Gary A MD (A&I) - **Spec Exp:** Asthma; Allergy; Hives; **Hospital:** N Shore Univ Hosp (page 106), Glen Cove Hosp (page 106); **Address:** 310 E Shore Rd, Ste 207, Great Neck, NY 11023; **Phone:** 516-487-1073; **Board Cert:** Internal Medicine 1982; Pulmonary Disease 1984; Allergy & Immunology 1985; **Med School:** Albany Med Coll 1979; **Resid:** Internal Medicine, N Shore Univ Hosp 1982; **Fellow:** Pulmonary Disease, Stony Brook Univ Med Ctr 1983; Allergy & Immunology, Stony Brook Univ Med Ctr 1986; **Fac Appt:** Asst Clin Prof Med, NYU Sch Med

Wertheim, David MD (A&I) - **Spec Exp:** Pediatric Allergy & Immunology; **Hospital:** Long Is Jewish Med Ctr (page 106), St. Francis Hosp - The Heart Ctr (page 116); **Address:** ProHlth, Allergy & Immunology, 2800 Marcus Ave, Ste 202, Lake Success, NY 11042; **Phone:** 516-608-2898; **Board Cert:** Allergy & Immunology 2006; **Med School:** Med Coll PA 1988; **Resid:** Pediatrics, Schneider Chldns Hosp 1992; **Fellow:** Allergy & Immunology, LI Jewish Med Ctr 1994; **Fac Appt:** Asst Clin Prof Ped, Albert Einstein Coll Med

Cardiac Electrophysiology

Evans, Steven J MD (CE) - **Spec Exp:** Arrhythmias; Defibrillators; Pacemakers; **Hospital:** Beth Israel Med Ctr - Petrie Div (page 94); **Address:** BIMC, Cardiac Electrophysiology, 300 Union Tpke, Ste 305A, New Hyde Park, NY 11040; **Phone:** 516-616-5902; **Board Cert:** Internal Medicine 1987; Cardiovascular Disease 1989; **Med School:** NYU Sch Med 1984; **Resid:** Internal Medicine, VA Med Ctr 1987; **Fellow:** Cardiovascular Disease, Cedars-Sinai Med Ctr 1990; Cardiac Electrophysiology, Cedars-Sinai Med Ctr 1990; **Fac Appt:** Asst Prof Med, Albert Einstein Coll Med

Jadonath, Ram L MD (CE) - **Spec Exp:** Arrhythmias; Atrial Fibrillation; Pacemakers/Defibrillators; Syncope; **Hospital:** N Shore Univ Hosp (page 106); **Address:** N Shore Univ Hosp, Cardiology Dept, 300 Community Drive, Manhasset, NY 11030; **Phone:** 516-562-2300; **Board Cert:** Internal Medicine 1989; Cardiovascular Disease 2006; Cardiac Electrophysiology 2006; **Med School:** Columbia P&S 1986; **Resid:** Internal Medicine, St Lukes-Roosevelt Hosp 1989; **Fellow:** Cardiovascular Disease, St Lukes-Roosevelt Hosp 1992; Cardiac Electrophysiology, Philadelphia Heart Inst 1993; **Fac Appt:** Assoc Prof Med, Albert Einstein Coll Med

Levine, Joseph H MD (CE) - **Spec Exp:** Arrhythmias; Sudden Death Prevention; Atrial Fibrillation; Pacemakers; **Hospital:** St. Francis Hosp - The Heart Ctr (page 116); **Address:** 100 Port Washington Blvd, Roslyn, NY 11576; **Phone:** 516-622-1011; **Board Cert:** Internal Medicine 1983; Cardiovascular Disease 1987; Cardiac Electrophysiology 2003; **Med School:** Univ Rochester 1980; **Resid:** Internal Medicine, Yale-New Haven Hosp 1983; **Fellow:** Cardiovascular Disease, Johns Hopkins Hosp 1986; Cardiac Electrophysiology, Hosp U Penn 1987

Cardiovascular Disease

Anto, Maliakal Joseph MD (Cv) - **Spec Exp:** Hypertension; Coronary Artery Disease; Non-Invasive Cardiology; Congestive Heart Failure; **Hospital:** Syosset Hosp (page 106), Plainview Hosp (page 106); **Address:** 8 Greenfield Rd, Syosset, NY 11791; **Phone:** 516-496-7900; **Board Cert:** Internal Medicine 1980; Cardiovascular Disease 1989; **Med School:** India 1974; **Resid:** Internal Medicine, Our Lady of Mercy Med Ctr 1979; **Fellow:** Cardiovascular Disease, Nassau County Med Ctr 1981

Bhansali, Rohan D MD (Cv) - **Spec Exp:** Echocardiography; Nuclear Cardiology; Nuclear Stress Testing; **Hospital:** Long Is Jewish Med Ctr (page 106), N Shore Univ Hosp (page 106); **Address:** LIJ Med Ctr, Cardiology Dept, 270-05 76th Ave Fl 4, New Hyde Park, NY 11040; **Phone:** 718-470-7330; **Board Cert:** Cardiovascular Disease 2004; **Med School:** SUNY Upstate Med Univ 1998; **Resid:** Internal Medicine, LIJ Med Ctr 2001; **Fellow:** Cardiovascular Disease, LIJ Med Ctr 2004

Breen, William John MD (Cv) - **Spec Exp:** Echocardiography; **Hospital:** Plainview Hosp (page 106); **Address:** 43 Crossways Park Drive, Woodbury, NY 11797; **Phone:** 516-938-3000; **Board Cert:** Internal Medicine 1980; Cardiovascular Disease 1983; **Med School:** NY Med Coll 1977; **Resid:** Internal Medicine, North Shore Univ Hosp 1980; **Fellow:** Cardiovascular Disease, North Shore Univ Hosp 1982; **Fac Appt:** Assoc Prof Med, NYU Sch Med

Chadda, Kul MD (Cv) - **Hospital:** South Nassau Comm Hosp, Wyckoff Heights Med Ctr; **Address:** South Nassau Comm Hosp, Electrophysiology Svcs, 1 Healthy Way, Oceanside, NY 11572; **Phone:** 516-632-3418; **Board Cert:** Internal Medicine 1974; Cardiovascular Disease 1977; **Med School:** India 1966; **Resid:** Internal Medicine, Elmhurst City Hosp 1972; **Fellow:** Cardiovascular Disease, Univ Penn Hosp 1973; **Fac Appt:** Clin Prof Med, SUNY Stony Brook

Chen, Timothy T MD (Cv) - **Spec Exp:** Congestive Heart Failure; Cardiovascular Disease/Young Adult; Pacemakers; **Hospital:** Winthrop Univ Hosp (page 524), South Nassau Comm Hosp; **Address:** South Shore Heart Assocs, 242 Merrick Rd, Ste 402, Rockville Center, NY 11570; **Phone:** 516-763-2800; **Board Cert:** Cardiovascular Disease 2004; Echocardiography 2004; Nuclear Cardiology 2004; **Med School:** Columbia P&S 1998; **Resid:** Internal Medicine, Montefiore Med Ctr 2001; **Fellow:** Cardiovascular Disease, Montefiore Med Ctr 2004

Chesner, Michael D MD (Cv) - **Spec Exp:** Preventive Cardiology; Cholesterol/Lipid Disorders; Cardiac Stress Testing; **Hospital:** Long Beach Med Ctr; **Address:** 325 W Park Ave, Long Beach, NY 11561; **Phone:** 516-432-2004; **Board Cert:** Internal Medicine 2004; Cardiovascular Disease 2007; **Med School:** Albert Einstein Coll Med 1987; **Resid:** Internal Medicine, Bronx Municipal Hosp 1990; **Fellow:** Cardiovascular Disease, LI Jewish Hosp 1993; **Fac Appt:** Assoc Prof Med, NY Coll Osteo Med

Cramer, Marvin MD (Cv) - **Spec Exp:** Coronary Artery Disease; Echocardiography; Stress Echocardiography; **Hospital:** N Shore Univ Hosp (page 106), St. Francis Hosp - The Heart Ctr (page 116); **Address:** 225 Community Drive, Ste 130, Great Neck, NY 11021; **Phone:** 516-504-0474; **Board Cert:** Internal Medicine 1974; Cardiovascular Disease 1977; Nuclear Cardiology 2005; Echocardiography 2007; **Med School:** Jefferson Med Coll 1969; **Resid:** Internal Medicine, St Lukes Med Ctr 1973; **Fellow:** Cardiovascular Disease, Columbia-Presby Med Ctr 1976; **Fac Appt:** Assoc Clin Prof Med, NYU Sch Med

D'Agostino, Ronald DO (Cv) - **Spec Exp:** Hypertension; Cholesterol/Lipid Disorders; Mitral Valve Disease; **Hospital:** Long Is Jewish Med Ctr (page 106), N Shore Univ Hosp (page 106); **Address:** 1129 Northern Blvd, Ste 408, Manhasset, NY 11030; **Phone:** 516-627-2121; **Board Cert:** Internal Medicine 2000; Cardiovascular Disease 2011; **Med School:** NY Coll Osteo Med 1985; **Resid:** Internal Medicine, LI Jewish Med Ctr 1989; Internal Medicine, LI Jewish Med Ctr 1993; **Fellow:** Cardiovascular Disease, LI Jewish Med Ctr 1992; **Fac Appt:** Asst Prof Med, NY Coll Osteo Med

Dresdale, Robert J MD (Cv) - **Spec Exp:** Heart Disease in Women; Pulmonary Hypertension; **Hospital:** N Shore Univ Hosp (page 106), St. Francis Hosp - The Heart Ctr (page 116); **Address:** 225 Community Drive, Ste 130, Great Neck, NY 11021-5506; **Phone:** 516-504-0474; **Board Cert:** Internal Medicine 1975; Cardiovascular Disease 1977; **Med School:** Columbia P&S 1972; **Resid:** Internal Medicine, Columbia-Presby Med Ctr 1974; **Fellow:** Cardiovascular Disease, Columbia-Presby Med Ctr 1976; **Fac Appt:** Assoc Clin Prof Med, NYU Sch Med

Ezratty, Ari M MD (Cv) - **Spec Exp:** Interventional Cardiology; **Hospital:** St. Francis Hosp - The Heart Ctr (page 116); **Address:** 100 Port Washington Blvd, Roslyn, NY 11576; **Phone:** 516-570-6907; **Board Cert:** Internal Medicine 1988; **Med School:** Mount Sinai Sch Med 1985; **Resid:** Internal Medicine, Mt Sinai Hosp 1989; **Fellow:** Cardiovascular Disease, Brigham & Womens Hosp 1992; Interventional Cardiology, Mt Sinai Hosp 1994

Fein, Frederick S MD (Cv) - **Spec Exp:** Heart Disease; **Hospital:** Winthrop Univ Hosp (page 524); **Address:** 120 Mineola Blvd, Ste 500, Mineola, NY 11501; **Phone:** 516-663-4480; **Board Cert:** Internal Medicine 1975; Cardiovascular Disease 1977; **Med School:** NYU Sch Med 1972; **Resid:** Internal Medicine, Montefiore Hosp Med Ctr 1975; **Fellow:** Cardiovascular Disease, Montefiore Hosp Med Ctr 1977; **Fac Appt:** Assoc Prof Med, Albert Einstein Coll Med

Gindea, Aaron J MD (Cv) - **Spec Exp:** Heart Valve Disease; Congestive Heart Failure; Congenital Heart Disease; **Hospital:** N Shore Univ Hosp (page 106), St. Francis Hosp - The Heart Ctr (page 116); **Address:** 800 Community Drive, Manhasset, NY 11030-3803; **Phone:** 516-627-6622; **Board Cert:** Internal Medicine 1985; Cardiovascular Disease 1989; **Med School:** NYU Sch Med 1982; **Resid:** Internal Medicine, Bellevue Hosp 1985; **Fellow:** Cardiovascular Disease, Bellevue Hosp 1987; **Fac Appt:** Assoc Prof Med, Hofstra N Shore-LIJ Sch Med

Gleckel, Louis W MD (Cv) - **Spec Exp:** Preventive Cardiology; Cardiac Stress Testing; Cholesterol/Lipid Disorders; Hypertension; **Hospital:** Long Is Jewish Med Ctr (page 106); **Address:** 2 Ohio Drive, Fl 2, Lake Success, NY 11042-1052; **Phone:** 516-622-6060; **Board Cert:** Internal Medicine 1986; **Med School:** SUNY Hlth Sci Ctr 1983; **Resid:** Internal Medicine, LI Jewish Hosp 1986; **Fellow:** Cardiovascular Disease, LI Jewish Hosp 1989; **Fac Appt:** Asst Clin Prof Med, SUNY Downstate

Goldberg, Steven Mark MD (Cv) - **Spec Exp:** Cholesterol/Lipid Disorders; Preventive Cardiology; **Hospital:** N Shore Univ Hosp (page 106); **Address:** 1010 Northern Blvd, Ste 110, Great Neck, NY 11021-5306; **Phone:** 516-390-2430; **Board Cert:** Internal Medicine 1982; Cardiovascular Disease 1985; **Med School:** Univ Pennsylvania 1979; **Resid:** Internal Medicine, N Shore Univ Hosp 1982; **Fellow:** Cardiovascular Disease, N Shore Univ Hosp 1984

Gomez, Henry Esteban MD (Cv) - **Spec Exp:** Echocardiography; Non-Invasive Cardiology; **Hospital:** N Shore Univ Hosp (page 106); **Address:** Long Island Cardiovascular, 1129 Northen Blvd, Ste 408, Manhasset, NY 11030; **Phone:** 516-627-2121; **Board Cert:** Internal Medicine 2004; Cardiovascular Disease 2008; **Med School:** Mount Sinai Sch Med 1990; **Resid:** Internal Medicine, Montefiore Med Ctr 1993; **Fellow:** Cardiovascular Disease, Long Island Jewish Med Ctr 1996

Goodman, Mark A MD (Cv) - **Spec Exp:** Cholesterol/Lipid Disorders; Pacemakers/Defibrillators; Coronary Artery Disease; Congestive Heart Failure; **Hospital:** Winthrop Univ Hosp (page 524), N Shore Univ Hosp (page 106); **Address:** 975 Stewart Ave, Garden City, NY 11530-4816; **Phone:** 516-222-8610; **Board Cert:** Internal Medicine 1972; Cardiovascular Disease 1973; **Med School:** SUNY Upstate Med Univ 1967; **Resid:** Internal Medicine, Montefiore Med Ctr 1969; Internal Medicine, Mt Sinai Hosp 1970; **Fellow:** Cardiovascular Disease, Montefiore Med Ctr 1972; **Fac Appt:** Assoc Clin Prof Med, SUNY Stony Brook

Green, Stephen J MD (Cv) - **Spec Exp:** Heart Attack; Angioplasty; Cholesterol/Lipid Disorders; Interventional Cardiology; **Hospital:** Winthrop Univ Hosp (page 524); **Address:** Winthrop Cardiology Associates, Division of Cardiology, 120 Mineola Blvd, Ste 500, Mineola, NY 11501; **Phone:** 516-663-4480; **Board Cert:** Internal Medicine 1983; Cardiovascular Disease 1985; Interventional Cardiology 2009; **Med School:** Tufts Univ 1980; **Resid:** Internal Medicine, N Shore Univ Hosp 1983; **Fellow:** Cardiovascular Disease, N Shore Univ Hosp 1985

Hershman, Ronnie MD (Cv) - **Spec Exp:** Invasive Cardiology; **Hospital:** St. Francis Hosp - The Heart Ctr (page 116); **Address:** 1 Hollow Ln, Ste 103, Lake Success, NY 11042; **Phone:** 516-869-5400; **Board Cert:** Internal Medicine 1985; Cardiovascular Disease 1987; **Med School:** Mount Sinai Sch Med 1982; **Resid:** Internal Medicine, Mt Sinai Med Ctr 1985; **Fellow:** Cardiovascular Disease, Mt Sinai Med Ctr 1989

Jauhar, Rajiv MD (Cv) - **Spec Exp:** Angioplasty & Stent Placement; Cardiac Catheterization; Cardiac Imaging; Interventional Cardiology; **Hospital:** Long Is Jewish Med Ctr (page 106); **Address:** LIJ Med Ctr, Cardiology Dept, 270-05 76 Ave Fl 4, New Hyde Park, NY 11040; **Phone:** 718-470-7330; **Board Cert:** Internal Medicine 1994; Cardiovascular Disease 2009; Interventional Cardiology 2010; **Med School:** Univ Chicago-Pritzker Sch Med 1991; **Resid:** Internal Medicine, UCSD Med Ctr 1994; **Fellow:** Cardiovascular Disease, NY-Presby/Weill Cornell Med Ctr 1999

Jelveh, Mansoor MD (Cv) - **Hospital:** N Shore Univ Hosp (page 106), St. Joseph's Hosp-Nassau; **Address:** 875 Old Country Rd, Ste 102, Plainview, NY 11803; **Phone:** 516-935-8877; **Board Cert:** Internal Medicine 1975; Cardiovascular Disease 1977; **Med School:** Iran 1968; **Resid:** Internal Medicine, Winthrop-Univ Hosp 1975; **Fellow:** Cardiovascular Disease, Beth Israel Med Ctr 1977

Kaplan, Barry M MD (Cv) - **Spec Exp:** Interventional Cardiology; **Hospital:** Long Is Jewish Med Ctr (page 106); **Address:** LIJ Med Ctr, Cardiology Dept, 270-05 76 Ave Fl 4, New Hyde Park, NY 11040; **Phone:** 718-470-7330; **Board Cert:** Cardiovascular Disease 2005; Interventional Cardiology 1999; **Med School:** Israel 1987; **Resid:** Internal Medicine, NYU/VA Med Ctr 1991; **Fellow:** Cardiovascular Disease, Montefiore Med Ctr 1994; Interventional Cardiology, William Beaumont Hosp 1995; **Fac Appt:** Asst Prof Med, NYU Sch Med

Kobren, Steven M MD (Cv) - **Spec Exp:** Heart Failure; Mitral Valve Prolapse; Nuclear Stress Testing; **Hospital:** NYU Langone Med Ctr (page 108), Long Is Jewish Med Ctr (page 106); **Address:** NYU Langone, Cardiology Dept, 488 Great Neck Rd, Great Neck, NY 11021; **Phone:** 516-482-6747; **Board Cert:** Internal Medicine 1986; Cardiovascular Disease 1989; Critical Care Medicine 2011; Echocardiography 2007; **Med School:** SUNY Downstate 1983; **Resid:** Internal Medicine, LIJ Med Ctr 1986; **Fellow:** Cardiovascular Disease, LIJ Med Ctr 1988

Koss, Jerome MD (Cv) - **Spec Exp:** Interventional Cardiology; Heart Valve Disease; Nuclear Cardiology; Atrial Fibrillation; **Hospital:** Long Is Jewish Med Ctr (page 106), St. Francis Hosp - The Heart Ctr (page 116); **Address:** 3003 New Hyde Park Rd, Ste 406, New Hyde Park, NY 11042; **Phone:** 516-358-5401; **Board Cert:** Internal Medicine 1977; Cardiovascular Disease 1981; Interventional Cardiology 2010; **Med School:** Albert Einstein Coll Med 1974; **Resid:** Internal Medicine, Jacobi Med Ctr 1978; **Fellow:** Cardiovascular Disease, Montefiore Med Ctr 1980; **Fac Appt:** Asst Prof Med, Albert Einstein Coll Med

Lituchy, Andrew MD (Cv) - **Spec Exp:** Coronary Artery Disease; Peripheral Vascular Disease; Interventional Cardiology; **Hospital:** St. Francis Hosp - The Heart Ctr (page 116), South Nassau Comm Hosp; **Address:** 100 Port Washington Blvd, Ste G-05, Roslyn, NY 11576-1353; **Phone:** 516-365-4888; **Board Cert:** Cardiovascular Disease 2005; **Med School:** Hahnemann Univ 1988; **Resid:** Internal Medicine, Bronx Muni/Albert Einstein Med Ctr 1991; **Fellow:** Cardiovascular Disease, NY-Cornell Med Ctr 1994; Interventional Cardiology, NY-Cornell Med Ctr 1995

Mintz, Guy L MD (Cv) - **Spec Exp:** Preventive Cardiology; Cholesterol/Lipid Disorders; Coronary Artery Disease; Hypertension; **Hospital:** N Shore Univ Hosp (page 106), St. Francis Hosp - The Heart Ctr (page 116); **Address:** 287 Northern Blvd, Ste 211, Great Neck, NY 11021; **Phone:** 516-482-3401; **Board Cert:** Internal Medicine 1987; Cardiovascular Disease 2003; **Med School:** Boston Univ 1984; **Resid:** Internal Medicine, N Shore Univ Hosp 1987; **Fellow:** Cardiovascular Disease, N Shore Univ Hosp 1989; **Fac Appt:** Assoc Prof Med, NYU Sch Med

Nicosia, Thomas A MD (Cv) - **Spec Exp:** Coronary Artery Disease; Congestive Heart Failure; **Hospital:** St. Francis Hosp - The Heart Ctr (page 116), N Shore Univ Hosp (page 106); **Address:** 1615 Northern Blvd, Ste 301, Manhasset, NY 11030; **Phone:** 516-627-9355; **Board Cert:** Internal Medicine 1979; Cardiovascular Disease 1981; **Med School:** Univ Cincinnati 1974; **Resid:** Internal Medicine, University Hosp 1978; **Fellow:** Cardiovascular Disease, Bellevue Hosp 1980

Pappas, Thomas W MD (Cv) - **Spec Exp:** Interventional Cardiology; Coronary Angioplasty/Stents; Angiography-Coronary; Cardiac Imaging; **Hospital:** St. Francis Hosp - The Heart Ctr (page 116); **Address:** 1155 Northern Blvd, Ste 330, Manhasset, NY 11030; **Phone:** 516-726-7575; **Board Cert:** Internal Medicine 1986; Cardiovascular Disease 1989; Interventional Cardiology 2010; **Med School:** Cornell Univ-Weill Med Coll 1983; **Resid:** Internal Medicine, New York Hosp 1986; **Fellow:** Cardiovascular Disease, New York Hosp-Cornell 1988; Interventional Cardiology, NYU Med Ctr 1990

Ragno, Philip D MD (Cv) - **Spec Exp:** Cholesterol/Lipid Disorders; Congestive Heart Failure; **Hospital:** Winthrop Univ Hosp (page 524), N Shore Univ Hosp (page 106); **Address:** 1401 Franklin Ave, Garden City, NY 11501; **Phone:** 516-877-2626; **Board Cert:** Internal Medicine 1987; Cardiovascular Disease 1989; **Med School:** SUNY Stony Brook 1984; **Resid:** Internal Medicine, Winthrop Univ Hosp 1987; **Fellow:** Cardiovascular Disease, Winthrop Univ Hosp 1989

Rutkovsky, Edward V MD (Cv) - **Spec Exp:** Nuclear Stress Testing; Echocardiography; **Hospital:** N Shore Univ Hosp (page 106), St. Francis Hosp - The Heart Ctr (page 116); **Address:** 2035 Lakeville Rd, Ste 101, New Hyde Park, NY 11040-1661; **Phone:** 516-328-9797; **Board Cert:** Internal Medicine 1987; Cardiovascular Disease 1989; **Med School:** NYU Sch Med 1984; **Resid:** Internal Medicine, NYU Med Ctr 1987; **Fellow:** Cardiovascular Disease, N Shore Univ Hosp 1989; **Fac Appt:** Asst Clin Prof Med, NYU Sch Med

Schreiber, Carl MD (Cv) - **Spec Exp:** Coronary Artery Disease; Nuclear Cardiology; Non-Invasive Cardiology; **Hospital:** Glen Cove Hosp (page 106), N Shore Univ Hosp (page 106); **Address:** 70 Glen St, Glen Cove, NY 11542-2853; **Phone:** 516-484-7893; **Board Cert:** Internal Medicine 1982; Cardiovascular Disease 1985; **Med School:** Med Coll GA 1979; **Resid:** Internal Medicine, Columbia-Presby Med Ctr 1982; **Fellow:** Cardiovascular Disease, Westchester Med Ctr 1984

Shayani, Steven S MD (Cv) - **Spec Exp:** Coronary Artery Disease; Congestive Heart Failure; Nuclear Cardiology; Cholesterol/Lipid Disorders; **Hospital:** Mt Sinai Med Ctr (page 102), St. Francis Hosp - The Heart Ctr (page 116); **Address:** 200 Old Country Rd, Ste 278, Mineola, NY 11501; **Phone:** 516-877-0977; **Board Cert:** Cardiovascular Disease 2005; **Med School:** SUNY Upstate Med Univ 1988; **Resid:** Internal Medicine, Winthrop Univ Hosp 1991; **Fellow:** Cardiovascular Disease, Winthrop Univ Hosp 1994; **Fac Appt:** Asst Clin Prof Med, Mount Sinai Sch Med

Shlofmitz, Richard A MD (Cv) - **Spec Exp:** Interventional Cardiology; Cardiac Catheterization; **Hospital:** St. Francis Hosp - The Heart Ctr (page 116); **Address:** 100 Port Washington Blvd, Ste 105, Vizza Pavilion, Roslyn, NY 11576; **Phone:** 516-390-9640; **Board Cert:** Internal Medicine 1984; Cardiovascular Disease 1987; **Med School:** NYU Sch Med 1980; **Resid:** Internal Medicine, N Shore Univ Hosp 1984; **Fellow:** Cardiovascular Disease, Presby/Columbia Univ Med Ctr 1987

Sokol, Sergio MD (Cv) - **Spec Exp:** Echocardiography; **Hospital:** St. John's Episcopal Hosp - Queens; **Address:** Five Towns Heart Imaging, 650 Central Ave, Ste K, Cedarhurst, NY 11516; **Phone:** 516-804-8590; **Board Cert:** Cardiovascular Disease 2004; **Med School:** Israel 1994; **Resid:** Internal Medicine, Montefiore Med Ctr 1998; **Fellow:** Cardiovascular Disease, N Shore Univ Hosp 2001

Spadaro, Louise A MD (Cv) - **Spec Exp:** Preventive Cardiology; Heart Disease in Women; **Hospital:** St. Francis Hosp - The Heart Ctr (page 116); **Address:** 100 Port Washington Blvd, Vizza Bldg Fl 1 - Ste 101, Roslyn, NY 11576; **Phone:** 516-562-6653; **Board Cert:** Internal Medicine 1987; Cardiovascular Disease 1989; **Med School:** NYU Sch Med 1984; **Resid:** Internal Medicine, Bellevue Hosp 1987; **Fellow:** Cardiovascular Disease, Bellevue Hosp/NYU Med Ctr 1989

Tenet, William MD (Cv) - **Spec Exp:** Congestive Heart Failure; Coronary Artery Disease; **Hospital:** N Shore Univ Hosp (page 106), Lenox Hill Hosp (page 106); **Address:** 1155 Northern Blvd, Ste 330, Manhasset, NY 11030; **Phone:** 516-627-4330; **Board Cert:** Internal Medicine 1983; Cardiovascular Disease 1987; **Med School:** Italy 1980; **Resid:** Internal Medicine, Booth Meml Med Ctr 1984; **Fellow:** Cardiovascular Disease, Univ Conn Hlth Ctr 1986; **Fac Appt:** Asst Clin Prof Med, Cornell Univ-Weill Med Coll

Weg, Ira L MD (Cv) - **Spec Exp:** Congestive Heart Failure; Coronary Artery Disease; **Hospital:** South Nassau Comm Hosp; **Address:** 158 Hempstead Ave, Lynbrook, NY 11563; **Phone:** 516-593-3541; **Board Cert:** Internal Medicine 1979; Cardiovascular Disease 1981; **Med School:** SUNY Hlth Sci Ctr 1976; **Resid:** Internal Medicine, Kings County Hosp 1979; **Fellow:** Cardiovascular Disease, Montefiore Med Ctr 1981; **Fac Appt:** Asst Clin Prof Med, Albert Einstein Coll Med

Zeldis, Steven M MD (Cv) - **Spec Exp:** Echocardiography; Cardiac Stress Testing; Cardiac Imaging; **Hospital:** Winthrop Univ Hosp (page 524); **Address:** 200 Old Country Rd, Ste 278, Mineola, NY 11501-4298; **Phone:** 516-877-0977; **Board Cert:** Internal Medicine 1975; Cardiovascular Disease 1977; **Med School:** Yale Univ 1972; **Resid:** Internal Medicine, Yale Med Ctr 1975; **Fellow:** Cardiovascular Disease, Hosp Univ Penn 1977; **Fac Appt:** Assoc Prof Med, SUNY Stony Brook

Child & Adolescent Psychiatry

Foley, Carmel A MD (ChAP) - **Spec Exp:** Mood Disorders; **Hospital:** Steven & Alexandra Cohen Chldn's Med Ctr of NY (page 106); **Address:** 420 Lakeville Rd, 1st Floor, Ste 110, New Hyde Park, NY 11040; **Phone:** 718-470-3550; **Board Cert:** Psychiatry 1979; Child & Adolescent Psychiatry 1981; Psychosomatic Medicine 2009; **Med School:** Ireland 1972; **Resid:** Psychiatry, St Patricks Hosp 1976; Psychiatry, Lafayette Clin 1977; **Fellow:** Child & Adolescent Psychiatry, Lafayette Clin 1979

Williams, Daniel T MD (ChAP) - **Spec Exp:** Neuro-Psychiatry; Psychopharmacology; Psychosomatic Disorders; **Hospital:** NY-Presby/Columbia Univ Med Ctr, NY (page 104), NS-LIJ Hlth Sys (page 106); **Address:** 2001 Marcus Ave, Ste N-218, New Hyde Park, NY 11042; **Phone:** 516-488-3636; **Board Cert:** Psychiatry 1975; Child & Adolescent Psychiatry 1976; **Med School:** Cornell Univ-Weill Med Coll 1969; **Resid:** Psychiatry, Mount Sinai Hosp 1972; **Fellow:** Child & Adolescent Psychiatry, Columbia-Presby Hosp 1974

Child Neurology

Atluru, Vijaya MD (ChiN) - **Spec Exp:** Epilepsy; Migraine; Developmental Disorders; Autism; **Hospital:** Winthrop Univ Hosp (page 524); **Address:** Winthrop Child Neurology Assocs, 120 Mineola Blvd, Ste 430, Mineola, NY 11501; **Phone:** 516-663-9494; **Board Cert:** Pediatrics 1979; Child Neurology 1983; **Med School:** India 1973; **Resid:** Pediatrics, Nassau Co Med Ctr 1977; **Fellow:** Child Neurology, Stony Brook Univ Med Ctr 1980; **Fac Appt:** Assoc Prof N, SUNY Stony Brook

Bergtraum, Marcia MD (ChiN) - **Hospital:** Long Is Jewish Med Ctr (page 106); **Address:** 2001 Marcus Ave, Ste N-218, New Hyde Park, NY 11042-1214; **Phone:** 516-488-2323; **Board Cert:** Pediatrics 1981; Child Neurology 1988; **Med School:** Georgetown Univ 1974; **Resid:** Pediatrics, LI Jewish Hosp 1977; **Fellow:** Pediatric Hematology-Oncology, LI Jewish Hosp 1978; Pediatric Neurology, LI Jewish Hosp 1982

LaJoie, Josiane M MD (ChiN) - **Spec Exp:** Epilepsy/Seizure Disorders; Neurophysiology; **Hospital:** Steven & Alexandra Cohen Chldn's Med Ctr of NY (page 106); **Address:** Steven & Alexandra Cohen Chldns Med Ctr, Div of Pediatric Neurology, 410 Lakeville Rd, Ste 105, Lake Success, NY 11042; **Phone:** 516-465-5255; **Board Cert:** Pediatrics 2013; Child Neurology 2012; Clinical Neurophysiology 2005; **Med School:** Univ Pennsylvania 1996; **Resid:** Pediatrics, Montefiore Med Ctr 1998; **Fellow:** Child Neurology, Montefiore Med Ctr 2001; Clinical Neurophysiology, Montefiore Med Ctr 2002; **Fac Appt:** Asst Prof N, NYU Sch Med

Maytal, Joseph MD (ChiN) - **Spec Exp:** Epilepsy/Seizure Disorders; Migraine; **Hospital:** Steven & Alexandra Cohen Chldn's Med Ctr of NY (page 106); **Address:** Div Pediatric Neurology, 410 Lakeville Rd, Ste 105, Lake Success, NY 11042; **Phone:** 516-465-5255; **Board Cert:** Pediatrics 1986; Child Neurology 1988; **Med School:** Israel 1979; **Resid:** Pediatrics, Brookdale Univ Hosp Med Ctr 1983; Child Neurology, Montefiore Med Ctr-Einstein Campus 1986; **Fellow:** Neurophysiology, Montefiore Med Ctr-Einstein Campus 1987; **Fac Appt:** Clin Prof N, Albert Einstein Coll Med

Smith, Robin E MD (ChiN) - **Spec Exp:** Cerebral Palsy; Neuromuscular Disorders; Headache; Epilepsy/Seizure Disorders; **Hospital:** Steven & Alexandra Cohen Chldn's Med Ctr of NY (page 106); **Address:** NRAD Medical Assocs, 105 Froehlich Farm Blvd, Woodbury, NY 11797; **Phone:** 516-222-2022 x7776; **Board Cert:** Pediatrics 2013; Child Neurology 2008; **Med School:** South Africa 1985; **Resid:** Pediatrics, Johannesburg Hosp 1993; Pediatrics, Schneider Childrens Hosp 1998; **Fellow:** Child Neurology, Schneider Childrens Hosp 1997; **Fac Appt:** Asst Prof N, Hofstra N Shore-LIJ Sch Med

Clinical Genetics

Bialer, Martin G MD/PhD (CG) - **Spec Exp:** Marfan's Syndrome; Neurofibromatosis; Metabolic Genetic Disorders; Cancer Genetics; **Hospital:** Steven & Alexandra Cohen Chldn's Med Ctr of NY (page 106), NS-LIJ Hlth Sys (page 106); **Address:** 1554 Northern Blvd, Ste 204, Manhasset, NY 11030; **Phone:** 516-365-3996; **Board Cert:** Pediatrics 1987; Clinical Biochemical Genetics 1990; Clinical Genetics 1990; **Med School:** Med Univ SC 1983; **Resid:** Pediatrics, N Shore Univ Hosp 1986; **Fellow:** Clinical Genetics, Univ of VA Hlth Sys 1989; **Fac Appt:** Clin Prof Ped, NYU Sch Med

Fox, Joyce MD (CG) - **Hospital:** Steven & Alexandra Cohen Chldn's Med Ctr of NY (page 106), Long Is Jewish Med Ctr (page 106); **Address:** 1554 Northern Blvd, Ste 204, Manhasset, NY 11030; **Phone:** 516-365-3996; **Board Cert:** Pediatrics 1986; Clinical Genetics 1987; **Med School:** Columbia P&S 1980; **Resid:** Pediatrics, Case Western Univ Hosp 1983; **Fellow:** Clinical Genetics, Yale-New Haven Hosp 1986; **Fac Appt:** , Albert Einstein Coll Med

Colon & Rectal Surgery

Greenwald, Marc MD (CRS) - **Spec Exp:** Laparoscopic Surgery; Colonoscopy; Anorectal Disorders; Colon & Rectal Cancer; **Hospital:** N Shore Univ Hosp (page 106), St. Francis Hosp - The Heart Ctr (page 116); **Address:** North Shore Surgical Specialists, 310 E Shore Rd, Ste 203, Great Neck, NY 11023-2432; **Phone:** 516-482-8657; **Board Cert:** Surgery 2009; Colon & Rectal Surgery 2011; **Med School:** Albert Einstein Coll Med 1985; **Resid:** Surgery, Montefiore Hosp Med Ctr 1990; **Fellow:** Colon & Rectal Surgery, St Francis Hosp 1991

Moseson, Michael J MD (CRS) - **Spec Exp:** Anorectal Disorders; Colonoscopy/Polypectomy; **Hospital:** St. Francis Hosp - The Heart Ctr (page 116), N Shore Univ Hosp (page 106); **Address:** 3 Vermont Drive, Lake Success, NY 11042; **Phone:** 516-608-6848; **Board Cert:** Colon & Rectal Surgery 1982; **Med School:** Spain 1975; **Resid:** Surgery, North Shore Univ Hosp 1980; Colon & Rectal Surgery, UMDNJ-RWJohnson Med Ctr 1981

Procaccino Jr, John A MD (CRS) - **Spec Exp:** Inflammatory Bowel Disease/Crohn's; Colon & Rectal Cancer; Anorectal Disorders; Colon & Rectal Cancer-Familial Polyposis; **Hospital:** N Shore Univ Hosp (page 106), Long Is Jewish Med Ctr (page 106); **Address:** Chief, Div of Colon & Rectal Surg, 900 Northern Blvd, Ste 100, Great Neck, NY 11021; **Phone:** 516-730-2100; **Board Cert:** Surgery 2009; Colon & Rectal Surgery 2011; **Med School:** NYU Sch Med 1984; **Resid:** Surgery, N Shore Univ Hosp 1989; **Fellow:** Colon & Rectal Surgery, Cleveland Clin 1990; **Fac Appt:** Asst Clin Prof S, Cornell Univ-Weill Med Coll

Sullivan III, James D MD (CRS) - **Spec Exp:** Cancer Surgery; Colon & Rectal Cancer & Surgery; **Hospital:** N Shore Univ Hosp (page 106), St. Francis Hosp - The Heart Ctr (page 116); **Address:** North Shore Oncology Associates, 600 Northern Blvd, Ste 111, Great Neck, NY 11021; **Phone:** 516-941-1213; **Board Cert:** Surgery 2004; Colon & Rectal Surgery 2005; **Med School:** NY Med Coll 1987; **Resid:** Surgery, N Shore Univ Hosp 1992; **Fellow:** Colon & Rectal Surgery, Cleveland Clinic 1993

Dermatology

Aprile, Georgette MD (D) - **Spec Exp:** Acne; Atopic Dermatitis; Laser Surgery; Laser Hair Removal; **Hospital:** Glen Cove Hosp (page 106); **Address:** 8 Med Plaza, Lower Level, Ste 103, Glen Cove, NY 11542; **Phone:** 516-759-9200; **Board Cert:** Dermatology 1978; **Med School:** NY Med Coll 1974; **Resid:** Dermatology, New York Hosp 1978

Bruckstein, Robert MD (D) - **Spec Exp:** Acne; Skin Cancer; Cosmetic Dermatology; Skin Laser Surgery; **Hospital:** St. John's Episcopal Hosp - Queens; **Address:** 290 Central Ave, Ste 206, Lawrence, NY 11559-8507; **Phone:** 516-239-2332; **Board Cert:** Dermatology 1977; **Med School:** NYU Sch Med 1972; **Resid:** Dermatology, Bellevue Hosp Ctr 1975; **Fac Appt:** Asst Clin Prof D, NYU Sch Med

De Pietro, William MD (D) - **Spec Exp:** Skin Laser Surgery; Dermatologic Surgery; **Hospital:** Glen Cove Hosp (page 106); **Address:** 10 Medical Plaza, Ste 102, Glen Cove, NY 11542; **Phone:** 516-671-1780; **Board Cert:** Dermatology 1980; **Med School:** Georgetown Univ 1976; **Resid:** Dermatology, St Luke's Hosp 1980

Demento, Frank MD (D) - **Spec Exp:** Dermatologic Surgery; Skin Cancer; **Hospital:** Winthrop Univ Hosp (page 524), NY-Presby/Columbia Univ Med Ctr, NY (page 104); **Address:** 520 Franklin Ave, Ste 229, Garden City, NY 11530; **Phone:** 516-746-1227; **Board Cert:** Dermatology 1969; **Med School:** UMDNJ-NJ Med Sch, Newark 1964; **Resid:** Dermatology, USPHS Hosp 1966; **Fellow:** Dermatology, Columbia-Presby Hosp 1968

Dolitsky, Charisse MD (D) - **Spec Exp:** Acne; Skin Cancer; Botox Therapy; Facial Rejuvenation; **Hospital:** Long Beach Med Ctr; **Address:** 604 E Park Ave, Long Beach, NY 11561; **Phone:** 516-432-0011; **Board Cert:** Dermatology 1989; **Med School:** SUNY Downstate 1985; **Resid:** Dermatology, SUNY Downstate Med Ctr 1989

Falcon, Ronald MD (D) - **Spec Exp:** Skin Cancer; Acne; Psoriasis; **Hospital:** Long Beach Med Ctr; **Address:** 604 E Park Ave, Long Beach, NY 11561; **Phone:** 516-432-0011; **Board Cert:** Dermatology 1989; **Med School:** SUNY Downstate 1985; **Resid:** Dermatology, SUNY Downstate Med Ctr 1989

Franck, Jeanne M MD (D) - **Spec Exp:** Mohs' Surgery; **Hospital:** NY-Presby/Columbia Univ Med Ctr, NY (page 104); **Address:** 520 Franklin Ave, Ste 207, Garden City, NY 11530; **Phone:** 516-741-1055; **Board Cert:** Dermatology 2013; **Med School:** Columbia P&S 1991; **Resid:** Dermatology, Columbia Presby Med Ctr 1995; **Fellow:** Mohs Surgery, Univ Minn Med Ctr 1996

Hefter, Harold MD (D) - **Spec Exp:** Cosmetic Dermatology; Dermatologic Surgery; Acne; **Hospital:** Franklin Hosp (page 106), Jacobi Med Ctr; **Address:** 135 Rockaway Tpke, Ste 100, Lawrence, NY 11559-1033; **Phone:** 516-371-1600; **Board Cert:** Dermatology 1985; **Med School:** Albert Einstein Coll Med 1981; **Resid:** Dermatology, Albert Einstein Affil Hosp 1985; **Fac Appt:** Asst Prof D, Albert Einstein Coll Med

Hisler, Barbara M MD (D) - **Spec Exp:** Skin Cancer; Acne; Psoriasis; **Hospital:** Long Is Jewish Med Ctr (page 106); **Address:** 1300 Union Tpke, Ste 303, New Hyde Park, NY 11040-1759; **Phone:** 516-326-0333; **Board Cert:** Internal Medicine 1986; Dermatology 1989; **Med School:** NY Med Coll 1983; **Resid:** Internal Medicine, LI Jewish Med Ctr 1985; Dermatology, Detroit Med Ctr 1988; **Fac Appt:** Asst Prof Med, Albert Einstein Coll Med

Levine, Laurie J MD (D) - **Spec Exp:** Skin Laser Surgery; Botox Therapy; Cosmetic Dermatology; **Hospital:** Winthrop Univ Hosp (page 524); **Address:** 200 Old Country Rd, Ste 140, Mineola, NY 11501-4237; **Phone:** 516-742-6136; **Board Cert:** Dermatology 1988; **Med School:** SUNY Stony Brook 1984; **Resid:** Dermatology, T Jefferson Univ Hosp 1988; **Fellow:** Dermatologic Surgery, T Jefferson Univ Hosp 1989; **Fac Appt:** Asst Clin Prof D, SUNY Stony Brook

Paltzik, Robert L MD (D) - **Spec Exp:** Pediatric Dermatology; Dermatologic Surgery; Facial Rejuvenation; **Hospital:** N Shore Univ Hosp (page 106), Winthrop Univ Hosp (page 524); **Address:** 2 Hillside Ave, Ste G, Williston Park, NY 11596; **Phone:** 516-747-2230; **Board Cert:** Dermatology 1977; Pediatrics 1976; **Med School:** NYU Sch Med 1971; **Resid:** Pediatrics, Yale-New Haven Hosp 1973; Dermatology, SUNY Downstate Med Ctr 1977; **Fac Appt:** Asst Prof D, NYU Sch Med

Sarnoff, Deborah S MD (D) - **Spec Exp:** Mohs' Surgery; Skin Cancer; Dermatologic Surgery; Skin Laser Surgery; **Hospital:** NYU Langone Med Ctr (page 108); **Address:** 31 Northern Blvd, 625 Park Ave, Greenvale, NY 11548; **Phone:** 516-484-9000; **Board Cert:** Dermatology 2009; **Med School:** Geo Wash Univ 1980; **Resid:** Dermatology, NYU Med Ctr 1984; **Fellow:** Dermatologic Surgery, NYU Med Ctr 1986; **Fac Appt:** Clin Prof D, NYU Sch Med

Silverman, Mark K MD (D) - **Spec Exp:** Melanoma; Skin Cancer; Skin Laser Surgery; **Hospital:** South Nassau Comm Hosp; **Address:** 258 Merrick Rd, Oceanside, NY 11572; **Phone:** 516-766-0345; **Board Cert:** Internal Medicine 1989; Dermatology 2001; **Med School:** Tufts Univ 1986; **Resid:** Internal Medicine, Montefiore Med Ctr 1989; Dermatology, Montefiore Med Ctr 1994; **Fellow:** Research, NYU 1991

Sklar, Jeffrey Alan MD (D) - **Spec Exp:** Facial Rejuvenation; Cosmetic Dermatology; Botox Therapy; **Hospital:** NY-Presby/Columbia Univ Med Ctr, NY (page 104), Syosset Hosp (page 106); **Address:** 800 Woodbury Rd, Ste A, Woodbury, NY 11797-2503; **Phone:** 516-496-9400; **Board Cert:** Dermatology 1986; **Med School:** Columbia P&S 1982; **Resid:** Dermatology, Columbia Presby Hosp 1986; **Fac Appt:** Asst Clin Prof D, Columbia P&S

Spinowitz, Alan MD (D) - **Spec Exp:** Skin Cancer; Mohs' Surgery; **Hospital:** Franklin Hosp (page 106); **Address:** 877 Stewart Ave, Ste 27, Garden City, NY 11530-4803; **Phone:** 516-745-0606; **Board Cert:** Dermatology 1985; **Med School:** SUNY Hlth Sci Ctr 1981; **Resid:** Dermatology, Univ IL Med Ctr 1985; **Fellow:** Dermatologic Surgery, Univ IL Med Ctr 1987

Walczyk, John MD (D) - **Spec Exp:** Cosmetic Dermatology; **Hospital:** NY-Presby/Columbia Univ Med Ctr, NY (page 104), Plainview Hosp (page 106); **Address:** 1165 Northern Blvd, Ste 405, Manhasset, NY 11030; **Phone:** 516-365-8030; **Board Cert:** Dermatology 2013; **Med School:** Columbia P&S 1990; **Resid:** Dermatology, Columbia Presby Hosp 1994

Diagnostic Radiology

Goodman, Kenneth J MD (DR) - **Spec Exp:** Urologic Imaging; Ultrasound; CT Scan; **Hospital:** St. Francis Hosp - The Heart Ctr (page 116); **Address:** St Francis Hosp-The Heart Ctr, Dept Radiology, 100 Port Washington Blvd, Roslyn, NY 11576-1353; **Phone:** 516-562-6500; **Board Cert:** Diagnostic Radiology 1977; **Med School:** Univ Tex, San Antonio 1972; **Resid:** Diagnostic Radiology, Cornell Med Ctr 1977; **Fellow:** Brain Imaging, Cornell Med Ctr 1978

Hammel, Jay D MD (DR) - **Spec Exp:** MRI; **Hospital:** N Shore Univ Hosp (page 106), Syosset Hosp (page 106); **Address:** 4277 Hempstead Tpke, Ste 200, Bethpage, NY 11714; **Phone:** 516-796-4340; **Board Cert:** Diagnostic Radiology 1989; **Med School:** SUNY Upstate Med Univ 1984; **Resid:** Diagnostic Radiology, St Vincent's Med Ctr 1989

Hoffman, Janet C MD (DR) - **Hospital:** Long Is Jewish Med Ctr (page 106); **Address:** 270-05 76th Ave, rm C-204, New Hyde Park, NY 11040; **Phone:** 718-470-3456; **Board Cert:** Diagnostic Radiology 1978; **Med School:** SUNY Downstate 1974; **Resid:** Diagnostic Radiology, Colum Presby Hosp 1978; **Fellow:** Ultrasound, NY Hosp-Cornell Med Ctr 1979

Khan, Arfa MD (DR) - **Spec Exp:** Thoracic Radiology; **Hospital:** Long Is Jewish Med Ctr (page 106), Syosset Hosp (page 106); **Address:** 270-05 76th Ave, rm C204, New Hyde Park, NY 11040; **Phone:** 718-470-7164; **Board Cert:** Diagnostic Radiology 1971; **Med School:** India 1964; **Resid:** Diagnostic Radiology, Queens Hosp 1970; **Fellow:** Diagnostic Radiology, LI Jewish Med Ctr 1971; **Fac Appt:** Prof Rad, Albert Einstein Coll Med

Luchs, Jonathan S MD (DR) - ; **Address:** 224 Seventh St, Garden City, NY 11530; **Phone:** 516-747-0161; **Board Cert:** Diagnostic Radiology 2003; **Med School:** Israel 1996; **Resid:** Surgery, Maimonides Med Ctr 1999; **Fellow:** Diagnostic Radiology, Winthrop Univ Hosp 2003; Musculoskeletal Imaging, Hosp for Special Surgery 2004

Port, Abraham MD (DR) - **Spec Exp:** Breast Cancer; Mammogrpahy; **Hospital:** South Nassau Comm Hosp; **Address:** Complete Women's Imaging, 990 Stewart Ave, Ste 100, Garden City, NY 11530; **Phone:** 516-222-4294; **Board Cert:** Diagnostic Radiology 1985; **Med School:** Albert Einstein Coll Med 1981; **Resid:** Diagnostic Radiology, Montefiore Med Ctr 1985; **Fellow:** Body Imaging, NY Hosp-Cornell Med Ctr 1986

Rifkin, Matthew D MD (DR) - **Spec Exp:** CT Scan; MRI; Ultrasound; **Hospital:** South Nassau Comm Hosp; **Address:** S Nassau Comm Hosp, Radiology Dept, 1 Healthy Way, Oceanside, NY 11572; **Phone:** 516-632-3921; **Board Cert:** Diagnostic Radiology 1978; **Med School:** Albert Einstein Coll Med 1974; **Resid:** Diagnostic Radiology, Montefiore Hosp 1978; **Fellow:** Ultrasound/CT, Johns Hopkins Hosp 1979

Rossi, Dennis R MD (DR) - **Spec Exp:** MRI; **Hospital:** Long Beach Med Ctr; **Address:** Elmont Open MRI, 545 Elmont Rd, Elmont, NY 11003; **Phone:** 516-328-7200; **Board Cert:** Diagnostic Radiology 1973; **Med School:** SUNY Downstate 1968; **Resid:** Diagnostic Radiology, Montefiore Hosp Med Ctr 1972; **Fac Appt:** Asst Prof Rad, SUNY Stony Brook

Sherman, Scott J MD (DR) - **Spec Exp:** CT Scan; PET Imaging; **Hospital:** St. Francis Hosp - The Heart Ctr (page 116), St. Joseph's Hosp-Nassau; **Address:** 100 Port Washington Blvd, Roslyn, NY 11576; **Phone:** 516-562-6500; **Board Cert:** Diagnostic Radiology 1983; Nuclear Medicine 1984; **Med School:** Northwestern Univ 1979; **Resid:** Diagnostic Radiology, NY Hosp 1983; Nuclear Medicine, NY Hosp 1984; **Fellow:** Ultrasound, NY Hosp 1985

Weck, Steven D MD (DR) - **Spec Exp:** Interventional Radiology; **Hospital:** Glen Cove Hosp (page 106); **Address:** 101 St. Andrews Ln, Fl 1st, Glen Cove, NY 11542; **Phone:** 516-674-7540; **Board Cert:** Diagnostic Radiology 1977; **Med School:** NYU Sch Med 1973; **Resid:** Diagnostic Radiology, NYU Med Ctr 1977

Yoon, Sydney S MD (DR) - **Spec Exp:** MRI; CT Scan; Neuroradiology; Interventional Radiology; **Hospital:** South Nassau Comm Hosp; **Address:** South Nassau Comm Hosp, Dept Radiology, 1 Healthy Way, Oceanside, NY 11572; **Phone:** 516-632-4660; **Board Cert:** Internal Medicine 1989; Diagnostic Radiology 1993; Vascular & Interventional Radiology 2011; Neuroradiology 2006; **Med School:** Univ Chicago-Pritzker Sch Med 1986; **Resid:** Internal Medicine, Johns Hopkins Hosp 1989; Diagnostic Radiology, UCLA Ronald Reagan Med Ctr 1993; **Fellow:** Neuroradiology, NY-Presby/Columbia Univ Med Ctr 1995; Vascular & Interventional Radiology, UCLA Ronald Reagan Med Ctr 1997

Endocrinology, Diabetes & Metabolism

Bhatt, Anjani A MD (EDM) - **Spec Exp:** Thyroid Disorders; Diabetes; **Address:** 871 E Park Ave, Long Beach, NY 11561; **Phone:** 516-889-8853; **Board Cert:** Internal Medicine 1983; Endocrinology, Diabetes & Metabolism 1985; **Med School:** India 1976; **Resid:** Internal Medicine, Brooklyn Hosp 1981; **Fellow:** Endocrinology, Brooklyn Hosp 1984

Bitton, Rachelle N MD (EDM) - **Spec Exp:** Osteoporosis; Thyroid Disorders; Diabetes; Pituitary Disorders; **Hospital:** Long Is Jewish Med Ctr (page 106), N Shore Univ Hosp (page 106); **Address:** ProHealth Care Assocs, 2 ProHealth Plaza, Ste 201, Lake Success, NY 11042; **Phone:** 516-390-5760; **Board Cert:** Internal Medicine 1981; Endocrinology, Diabetes & Metabolism 1985; **Med School:** SUNY Downstate 1978; **Resid:** Internal Medicine, Brookdale Hosp 1981; **Fellow:** Endocrinology, Diabetes & Metabolism, Univ Hosp 1984

Friedman, Seth G MD (EDM) - **Spec Exp:** Thyroid Disorders; Pituitary Disorders; Diabetes; Osteoporosis; **Hospital:** N Shore Univ Hosp (page 106), Long Is Jewish Med Ctr (page 106); **Address:** 560 Northern Blvd, Ste 207, Great Neck, NY 11021; **Phone:** 516-466-6165; **Board Cert:** Internal Medicine 2002; Endocrinology, Diabetes & Metabolism 2003; **Med School:** Mount Sinai Sch Med 1988; **Resid:** Internal Medicine, LI Jewish Med Ctr 1991; **Fellow:** Endocrinology, Diabetes & Metabolism, Albert Einstein 1993

Gordon, Jeffrey H MD (EDM) - **Spec Exp:** Diabetes; Thyroid Disorders; Pituitary Disorders; **Hospital:** St. Francis Hosp - The Heart Ctr (page 116), N Shore Univ Hosp (page 106); **Address:** 3 School St, Ste 306, Glen Cove, NY 11542-2548; **Phone:** 516-759-2420; **Board Cert:** Internal Medicine 1972; Endocrinology, Diabetes & Metabolism 1973; **Med School:** Cornell Univ-Weill Med Coll 1965; **Resid:** Internal Medicine, Bellevue Hosp 1967; **Fellow:** Endocrinology, Duke Univ Med Ctr 1970; Endocrinology, VA Hosp 1972; **Fac Appt:** Asst Clin Prof Med, NYU Sch Med

Greenfield, Martin MD (EDM) - **Spec Exp:** Diabetes; Thyroid Disorders; Osteoporosis; Adrenal Disorders; **Hospital:** Long Is Jewish Med Ctr (page 106), N Shore Univ Hosp (page 106); **Address:** ProHealth Care Assocs, 2 ProHealth Plaza, Ste 201, Lake Success, NY 11042; **Phone:** 516-608-6823; **Board Cert:** Internal Medicine 1987; Endocrinology, Diabetes & Metabolism 1979; **Med School:** SUNY Downstate 1968; **Resid:** Internal Medicine, LI Jewish Med Ctr 1971; **Fellow:** Endocrinology, Diabetes & Metabolism, Brigham & Womens Hosp 1975

Hupart, Kenneth H MD (EDM) - **Spec Exp:** Thyroid Disorders; Osteoporosis; Diabetes; Cholesterol/Lipid Disorders; **Hospital:** Nassau Univ Med Ctr; **Address:** Nassau Univ Med Ctr, Div Endocrinology, 2201 Heampstead Tpke, East Meadow, NY 11554; **Phone:** 516-572-4848; **Board Cert:** Internal Medicine 1985; Endocrinology 1989; **Med School:** SUNY Stony Brook 1982; **Resid:** Internal Medicine, Montefiore Hosp Med Ctr 1986; **Fellow:** Endocrinology, Diabetes & Metabolism, Montefiore Hosp Med Ctr 1988; **Fac Appt:** Assoc Clin Prof Med, Albert Einstein Coll Med

Kaplan, Jonathan MD (EDM) - **Spec Exp:** Diabetes; **Hospital:** N Shore Univ Hosp (page 106); **Address:** 1000 Northern Blvd, Ste 240, Great Neck, NY 11021; **Phone:** 516-829-0802; **Board Cert:** Internal Medicine 2006; Endocrinology, Diabetes & Metabolism 2008; **Med School:** Israel 1990; **Resid:** Internal Medicine, Rambam Med Ctr 1994; Internal Medicine, N Shore Univ Hosp 1996; **Fellow:** Endocrinology, Diabetes & Metabolism, Albert Einstein 1998

Lomasky, Steven MD (EDM) - **Spec Exp:** Diabetes; Cholesterol/Lipid Disorders; Thyroid Disorders; **Hospital:** South Nassau Comm Hosp; **Address:** 242 Merrick Rd, rm 403, Rockville Ctr, NY 11570; **Phone:** 516-536-3700; **Board Cert:** Endocrinology, Diabetes & Metabolism 1989; Internal Medicine 1985; **Med School:** Israel 1982; **Resid:** Internal Medicine, Montefiore Med Ctr 1986; **Fellow:** Endocrinology, Diabetes & Metabolism, Montefiore Med Ctr 1987; **Fac Appt:** Asst Clin Prof Med, Albert Einstein Coll Med

Margulies, Paul MD (EDM) - **Spec Exp:** Thyroid Disorders; Adrenal Disorders; Pituitary Disorders; Addison's Disease; **Hospital:** N Shore Univ Hosp (page 106); **Address:** 444 Community, Ste 312, Manhasset, NY 11030-3820; **Phone:** 516-627-1366; **Board Cert:** Internal Medicine 1975; Endocrinology, Diabetes & Metabolism 1977; **Med School:** Univ Chicago-Pritzker Sch Med 1970; **Resid:** Internal Medicine, NY Hosp/Cornell 1974; Endocrinology, Diabetes & Metabolism, NY Hosp/Cornell 1975; **Fellow:** Endocrinology, Diabetes & Metabolism, NY Hosp/Cornell 1976; **Fac Appt:** Assoc Prof Med, NYU Sch Med

Rosenthal, David S MD (EDM) - **Spec Exp:** Thyroid Disorders; Pituitary Disorders; Adrenal Disorders; Osteoporosis; **Hospital:** Nassau Univ Med Ctr; **Address:** Nassau Univ Med Ctr, Div Endocrinology, 2201 Hempstead Tpke, Box 49, East Meadow, NY 11554; **Phone:** 516-572-4848; **Board Cert:** Internal Medicine 1969; Endocrinology, Diabetes & Metabolism 1972; **Med School:** NYU Sch Med 1963; **Resid:** Internal Medicine, Wilford Hall USAF Med Ctr 1967; **Fellow:** Endocrinology, Diabetes & Metabolism, Boston Univ Med Ctr 1972; Nuclear Medicine, Boston Univ Med Ctr 1972; **Fac Appt:** Asst Prof Med, SUNY Stony Brook

Shapiro, Lawrence E MD (EDM) - **Spec Exp:** Thyroid Disorders; Diabetes; **Hospital:** Winthrop Univ Hosp (page 524); **Address:** 1300 Franklin Ave, Ste ML6, Garden City, NY 11530; **Phone:** 516-663-3511; **Board Cert:** Internal Medicine 1975; Endocrinology 1977; **Med School:** SUNY Downstate 1971; **Resid:** Internal Medicine, Bellevue Hosp 1974; **Fellow:** Endocrinology, Diabetes & Metabolism, NYU Med Ctr 1975; **Fac Appt:** Prof Med, SUNY Stony Brook

Family Medicine

Arcati, Anthony T MD (FMed) *PCP* - **Hospital:** Winthrop Univ Hosp (page 524); **Address:** 530 Hicksville Rd, Bethpage, NY 11714; **Phone:** 516-937-5000; **Board Cert:** Family Medicine 2003; **Med School:** Mexico 1975; **Resid:** Family Medicine, Nassau Co Med Ctr 1979

Arcati, Robert J MD (FMed) *PCP* - **Hospital:** Winthrop Univ Hosp (page 524); **Address:** 530 Hicksville Rd, Bethpage, NY 11714; **Phone:** 516-937-5000; **Board Cert:** Family Medicine 2008; **Med School:** Mount Sinai Sch Med 1986; **Resid:** Family Medicine, Somerset Med Ctr 1989

Capobianco, Luigi MD (FMed) *PCP* - **Spec Exp:** Geriatric Care; **Hospital:** Glen Cove Hosp (page 106); **Address:** One School St, Ste 203, Glen Cove, NY 11542; **Phone:** 516-671-9800; **Board Cert:** Family Medicine 2007; Geriatric Medicine 2008; **Med School:** Italy 1984; **Resid:** Family Medicine, N Shore Univ Hosp 1988

Edelstein, Martin P MD (FMed) *PCP* - **Spec Exp:** Preventive Medicine; **Hospital:** N Shore Univ Hosp (page 106); **Address:** 11 Beverly Rd, Great Neck, NY 11021-1320; **Phone:** 516-487-1614; **Board Cert:** Family Medicine 2008; **Med School:** McGill Univ 1971; **Resid:** Family Medicine, Jewish Genl Hosp 1973; **Fac Appt:** Asst Clin Prof FMed, Albert Einstein Coll Med

Moynihan, Brian T DO (FMed) *PCP* - **Spec Exp:** Hypertension; Diabetes; Skin Diseases; **Hospital:** St. Joseph's Hosp-Nassau, N Shore Univ Hosp (page 106); **Address:** 2840 Jerusalem Ave, Wantagh, NY 11793-2017; **Phone:** 516-781-1141; **Med School:** NY Coll Osteo Med 1983; **Resid:** Family Medicine, Massapequa Genl Hosp 1984; Family Medicine, Kennedy Meml Hosp 1985; **Fac Appt:** Asst Prof FMed, NY Coll Osteo Med

Rechter, Lesley MD (FMed) *PCP* - **Spec Exp:** Women's Health; **Hospital:** Stony Brook Univ Med Ctr; **Address:** 54 Birchwood Park Drive, Jericho, NY 11753-2202; **Phone:** 516-933-6850; **Board Cert:** Family Medicine 2003; **Med School:** NY Med Coll 1976; **Resid:** Family Medicine, Nassau County Med Ctr 1979; **Fac Appt:** Assoc Clin Prof FMed, SUNY Stony Brook

Soskel, Neil DO (FMed) *PCP* - **Spec Exp:** Sports Medicine; **Hospital:** South Nassau Comm Hosp; **Address:** 185 Merrick Rd, Ste 1B, Lynbrook, NY 11563; **Phone:** 516-887-0077; **Board Cert:** Family Medicine 2008; **Med School:** NY Coll Osteo Med 1986; **Resid:** Family Medicine, S Nassau Comm Hosp 1989; **Fac Appt:** Assoc Prof FMed, NY Coll Osteo Med

Gastroenterology

Bartolomeo, Robert S MD (Ge) - **Spec Exp:** Colonoscopy; Inflammatory Bowel Disease; Gastroesophageal Reflux Disease (GERD); Colon Cancer Screening; **Hospital:** Winthrop Univ Hosp (page 524); **Address:** Gastroenterology Assocs, 1103 Stewart Ave, Ste 300, Garden City, NY 11530; **Phone:** 516-248-3737; **Board Cert:** Internal Medicine 1974; Gastroenterology 1977; **Med School:** NY Med Coll 1971; **Resid:** Internal Medicine, Metropolitan Hosp Ctr 1973; Internal Medicine, Beth Israel Hosp 1974; **Fellow:** Gastroenterology, Bridgeport Hosp 1977

Bernstein, David E MD (Ge) - **Spec Exp:** Liver Disease; Hepatitis; **Hospital:** N Shore Univ Hosp (page 106); **Address:** North Shore Univ Hosp, Div Gastroenterology, 300 Community Drive, Manhasset, NY 11030-3816; **Phone:** 516-562-4281; **Board Cert:** Internal Medicine 2011; Gastroenterology 2013; **Med School:** SUNY Stony Brook 1988; **Resid:** Internal Medicine, Montefiore Med Ctr 1991; **Fellow:** Gastroenterology, Jackson Meml Hosp 1993

Blumstein, Meyer MD (Ge) - **Spec Exp:** Endoscopy; Gastroesophageal Reflux Disease (GERD); Inflammatory Bowel Disease; **Hospital:** Long Is Jewish Med Ctr (page 106), South Nassau Comm Hosp; **Address:** 158 Hempstead Ave, Lynbrook, NY 11563-1605; **Phone:** 516-593-3541; **Board Cert:** Internal Medicine 1989; **Med School:** SUNY Hlth Sci Ctr 1986; **Resid:** Internal Medicine, LI Jewish Med Ctr 1989; **Fellow:** Gastroenterology, LI Jewish Med Ctr 1991; **Fac Appt:** Asst Prof Med, Albert Einstein Coll Med

Caccese, William MD (Ge) - **Spec Exp:** Endoscopy; Colon Cancer; **Hospital:** Plainview Hosp (page 106); **Address:** 700 Old Country Rd, Ste 206, Plainview, NY 11803-4932; **Phone:** 516-681-1200; **Board Cert:** Internal Medicine 1981; Gastroenterology 1983; **Med School:** SUNY Hlth Sci Ctr 1978; **Resid:** Internal Medicine, N Shore Univ Hosp 1981; **Fellow:** Gastroenterology, N Shore Univ Hosp 1983

Cerulli, Maurice A MD (Ge) - **Spec Exp:** Inflammatory Bowel Disease; Gastroesophageal Reflux Disease (GERD); Colon Cancer Screening; Hepatitis B & C; **Hospital:** Long Is Jewish Med Ctr (page 106), N Shore Univ Hosp (page 106); **Address:** 270-05 76th Ave, rm B202, 410 Lakeville Rd, Ste 107, New Hyde Park, NY 11040; **Phone:** 718-470-7281; **Board Cert:** Internal Medicine 1975; Gastroenterology 1977; **Med School:** SUNY Hlth Sci Ctr 1972; **Resid:** Internal Medicine, Kings County Hosp 1975; **Fellow:** Gastroenterology, Johns Hopkins Hosp 1977; **Fac Appt:** Assoc Prof Med, Hofstra N Shore-LIJ Sch Med

DeVito, Bethany S MD (Ge) - **Spec Exp:** Women's Health; Capsule Endoscopy; **Hospital:** N Shore Univ Hosp (page 106), Long Is Jewish Med Ctr (page 106); **Address:** N Shore Univ Hospital, 4 Levitt Pavilion, 300 Community Drive, Manhasset, NY 11030; **Phone:** 516-562-4281; **Board Cert:** Gastroenterology 2007; **Med School:** SUNY Upstate Med Univ 1992; **Resid:** Internal Medicine, St Vincents Hosp 1995; **Fellow:** Gastroenterology, NY Hosp 1997

Eskreis, David MD (Ge) - **Spec Exp:** Ulcerative Colitis/Crohn's; **Hospital:** N Shore Univ Hosp (page 106), Long Is Jewish Med Ctr (page 106); **Address:** 2001 Marcus Ave, Ste W85, Lake Success, NY 11042; **Phone:** 516-326-2700; **Board Cert:** Internal Medicine 1986; Gastroenterology 1987; **Med School:** Geo Wash Univ 1982; **Resid:** Internal Medicine, Bronx Muni Hosp Ctr 1985; **Fellow:** Gastroenterology, Bronx Muni Hosp Ctr 1987

Farber, Charles MD (Ge) - **Spec Exp:** Colon Cancer; Gastroesophageal Reflux Disease (GERD); **Hospital:** Plainview Hosp (page 106); **Address:** 146A Manetto Hill Rd, Ste 205, Plainview, NY 11803; **Phone:** 516-822-4404; **Board Cert:** Internal Medicine 1981; Gastroenterology 1983; **Med School:** SUNY Hlth Sci Ctr 1978; **Resid:** Internal Medicine, N Shore Univ Hosp 1981; **Fellow:** Gastroenterology, Albert Einstein 1983

Goldblum, Lester DO (Ge) - **Spec Exp:** Endoscopy; Colon Cancer; Capsule Endoscopy; **Hospital:** St. Joseph's Hosp-Nassau, Plainview Hosp (page 106); **Address:** Massapequa Gastroenterology, 850 Hicksville Rd, Ste 100, Seaford, NY 11783; **Phone:** 516-796-9000; **Board Cert:** Internal Medicine 1983; **Med School:** Univ Osteo Med & Hlth Sci, Des Moines 1979; **Resid:** Internal Medicine, Nassau County Med Ctr 1983; **Fellow:** Gastroenterology, Nassau County Med Ctr 1985; **Fac Appt:** Asst Clin Prof Med, NY Coll Osteo Med

Gould, Perry C MD (Ge) - **Spec Exp:** Ulcerative Colitis; Colon & Rectal Cancer; Gastroesophageal Reflux Disease (GERD); Capsule Endoscopy; **Hospital:** Winthrop Univ Hosp (page 524); **Address:** Gastroenterology Assocs, 1103 Stewart Ave, Ste 300, Garden City, NY 11530; **Phone:** 516-248-3737; **Board Cert:** Internal Medicine 1980; Gastroenterology 1983; **Med School:** NY Med Coll 1977; **Resid:** Internal Medicine, LI Jewish Hosp 1980; **Fellow:** Gastroenterology, NY Med Coll 1983; **Fac Appt:** Asst Clin Prof Med, SUNY Stony Brook

Greenberg, Ronald MD (Ge) - **Spec Exp:** Inflammatory Bowel Disease; Peptic Acid Disorders; **Hospital:** Long Is Jewish Med Ctr (page 106); **Address:** 410 Lakeville Rd, New Hyde Park, NY 11042; **Phone:** 718-470-7281; **Board Cert:** Internal Medicine 1982; Gastroenterology 1985; **Med School:** Hahnemann Univ 1979; **Resid:** Internal Medicine, Albany Med Ctr 1982; **Fellow:** Gastroenterology, St Luke's Hosp 1985

Grendell, James H MD (Ge) - **Spec Exp:** Pancreatic Disease; Nutrition; Liver Disease; Vomiting-Cyclic; **Hospital:** Winthrop Univ Hosp (page 524); **Address:** 222 Station Plaza N, Ste 428, Mineola, NY 11501-3819; **Phone:** 516-663-2066; **Board Cert:** Internal Medicine 1978; Gastroenterology 1981; **Med School:** Ohio State Univ 1975; **Resid:** Internal Medicine, Beth Israel Hosp 1978; **Fellow:** Gastroenterology, UCSF Med Ctr 1981; **Fac Appt:** Prof Med, SUNY Stony Brook

Katz, Seymour MD (Ge) - **Spec Exp:** Inflammatory Bowel Disease; Colonoscopy; Endoscopy; **Hospital:** N Shore Univ Hosp (page 106), Long Is Jewish Med Ctr (page 106); **Address:** 1000 Northern Blvd, Ste 140, Great Neck, NY 11021; **Phone:** 516-466-2340; **Board Cert:** Internal Medicine 1971; Gastroenterology 1972; **Med School:** NYU Sch Med 1964; **Resid:** Internal Medicine, Albert Einstein Sch Med 1966; Internal Medicine, Jacobi Med Ctr 1969; **Fellow:** Gastroenterology, NY Hosp 1971; **Fac Appt:** Clin Prof Med, NYU Sch Med

McKinley, Matthew John MD (Ge) - **Spec Exp:** Gastroesophageal Reflux Disease (GERD); Barrett's Esophagus; Biliary Disease; **Hospital:** N Shore Univ Hosp (page 106); **Address:** 2800 Marcus Ave, Ste 201, Lake Success, NY 11042; **Phone:** 516-622-6076; **Board Cert:** Internal Medicine 1978; Gastroenterology 1981; **Med School:** Creighton Univ 1975; **Resid:** Internal Medicine, N Shore Univ Hosp 1978; Internal Medicine, Meml Sloan Kettering Cancer Ctr 1978; **Fellow:** Gastroenterology, Yale-New Haven Hosp 1980; **Fac Appt:** Assoc Prof Med, NYU Sch Med

Miller, Seth L MD (Ge) - **Hospital:** Long Beach Med Ctr; **Address:** 206 West Park Ave, Long Beach, NY 11561; **Phone:** 516-432-8021; **Board Cert:** Internal Medicine 1983; Gastroenterology 1987; **Med School:** Mount Sinai Sch Med 1980; **Resid:** Internal Medicine, Beth Israel Med Ctr 1983; **Fellow:** Gastroenterology, Beth Israel Med Ctr 1985

Milman, Perry J MD (Ge) - **Spec Exp:** Gastroesophageal Reflux Disease (GERD); Colon Cancer; Inflammatory Bowel Disease; Endoscopy; **Hospital:** Long Is Jewish Med Ctr (page 106), N Shore Univ Hosp (page 106); **Address:** 2001 Marcus Ave, Ste N18, Lake Success, NY 11042-1011; **Phone:** 516-775-7770; **Board Cert:** Internal Medicine 1976; Gastroenterology 1979; **Med School:** SUNY Downstate 1973; **Resid:** Internal Medicine, LI Jewish Med Ctr 1976; **Fellow:** Gastroenterology, VA Hosp/NYU 1978; **Fac Appt:** Asst Clin Prof Med, Albert Einstein Coll Med

Schwartz, Gary J MD (Ge) - **Spec Exp:** Colon Cancer Screening; Gastroesophageal Reflux Disease (GERD); **Hospital:** Winthrop Univ Hosp (page 524); **Address:** Gastroenterology Assocs, 1103 Stewart Ave, Ste 300, Garden City, NY 11530; **Phone:** 516-248-3737; **Board Cert:** Internal Medicine 1985; Gastroenterology 1987; **Med School:** Mexico 1979; **Resid:** Internal Medicine, Winthrop Univ Hosp 1983; **Fellow:** Gastroenterology, Univ Hosp/SUNY Hlth Sci Ctr 1986

Talansky, Arthur L MD (Ge) - **Spec Exp:** Crohn's Disease; Ulcerative Colitis; Colonoscopy; **Hospital:** N Shore Univ Hosp (page 106), St. Francis Hosp - The Heart Ctr (page 116); **Address:** 233 E Shore Rd, Ste 101, Great Neck, NY 11023-2433; **Phone:** 516-487-2444; **Board Cert:** Internal Medicine 1980; Gastroenterology 1983; **Med School:** Mount Sinai Sch Med 1977; **Resid:** Internal Medicine, Meml Sloan Kettering Cancer Ctr 1980; **Fellow:** Gastroenterology, Mount Sinai Hosp 1982; **Fac Appt:** Assoc Clin Prof Med, Hofstra N Shore-LIJ Sch Med

Weissman, Gary S MD (Ge) - **Spec Exp:** Gastrointestinal Cancer; Inflammatory Bowel Disease; Esophageal Disorders; **Hospital:** N Shore Univ Hosp (page 106), Long Is Jewish Med Ctr (page 106); **Address:** 2800 Marcus Ave, Ste 201, Lake Success, NY 11042; **Phone:** 516-622-6076; **Board Cert:** Internal Medicine 1980; Gastroenterology 1983; **Med School:** NY Med Coll 1976; **Resid:** Internal Medicine, North Shore Univ Hosp 1980; **Fellow:** Gastroenterology, Meml Sloan Kettering Cancer Ctr 1982

Geriatric Medicine

Gomolin, Irving H MD (Ger) - **Spec Exp:** Medications in the Elderly; Dementia; Polypharmacology (Excess Medications); **Hospital:** Winthrop Univ Hosp (page 524); **Address:** Winthrop Geriatric Medicine Assocs, 222 Station Plaza N Fl 5th - Ste 518, Mineola, NY 11501; **Phone:** 516-663-2588; **Board Cert:** Internal Medicine 1979; Geriatric Medicine 2008; **Med School:** McGill Univ 1976; **Resid:** Internal Medicine, Jewish Genl Hosp 1978; Internal Medicine, Beth Israel Hosp 1981; **Fellow:** Clinical Pharmacology, Harvard Med Sch 1980; **Fac Appt:** Clin Prof Med, SUNY Stony Brook

Guzik, Howard J MD (Ger) *PCP* - **Spec Exp:** Palliative Care; Geriatric Care; Preventive Medicine; **Hospital:** N Shore Univ Hosp (page 106), Long Is Jewish Med Ctr (page 106); **Address:** 865 Northern Blvd, Ste 201, Great Neck, NY 11021; **Phone:** 516-708-2520; **Board Cert:** Internal Medicine 1984; Geriatric Medicine 2008; Hospice & Palliative Medicine 2010; **Med School:** Albert Einstein Coll Med 1981; **Resid:** Internal Medicine, Montefiore Med Ctr 1984; **Fellow:** Geriatric Medicine, Montefiore Med Ctr 1986

Lanman, Geraldine M MD (Ger) *PCP* - **Spec Exp:** Geriatric Care; Preventive Medicine; **Hospital:** Long Is Jewish Med Ctr (page 106); **Address:** 1 Delaware Drive, Ste 48, New Hyde Park, NY 11042; **Phone:** 516-326-5320; **Board Cert:** Internal Medicine 1983; **Med School:** Univ Calgary 1980; **Resid:** Internal Medicine, LIJ Med Ctr 1983; **Fellow:** Geriatric Medicine, Parker Jewish Inst for Hlthcare & Rehab 1985; **Fac Appt:** Asst Clin Prof Med, Albert Einstein Coll Med

Macina, Lucy O MD (Ger) *PCP* - **Spec Exp:** Frail Elderly; Dementia; Geriatric Care; **Hospital:** Winthrop Univ Hosp (page 524); **Address:** Winthrop Geriatric Medicine Assocs, 222 Station Plaza N, Ste 518, Mineola, NY 11501-3893; **Phone:** 516-663-2588; **Board Cert:** Internal Medicine 1982; Geriatric Medicine 2012; **Med School:** Loyola Univ-Stritch Sch Med 1978; **Resid:** Internal Medicine, VA Hosp 1980; Internal Medicine, Loyola Univ Med Ctr 1982; **Fellow:** Geriatric Medicine, Roger Williams Hosp 1985; **Fac Appt:** Asst Clin Prof Med, SUNY Stony Brook

Wolf-Klein, Gisele P MD (Ger) *PCP* - **Spec Exp:** Dementia; Falls in the Elderly; Alzheimer's Disease; **Hospital:** Long Is Jewish Med Ctr (page 106); **Address:** 865 Northern Blvd, Ste 201, Great Neck, NY 11021; **Phone:** 516-708-2520; **Board Cert:** Internal Medicine 1984; Geriatric Medicine 2012; **Med School:** Switzerland 1975; **Resid:** Internal Medicine, LIJ Med Ctr 1978; **Fellow:** Geriatric Medicine, Parker Jewish Inst 1979; **Fac Appt:** Clin Prof Med, Albert Einstein Coll Med

Gynecologic Oncology

Chalas, Eva MD (GO) - **Spec Exp:** Gynecologic Cancer; Minimally Invasive Surgery; **Hospital:** Winthrop Univ Hosp (page 524); **Address:** 200 Old Country Rd, Ste 365, Mineola, NY 11501; **Phone:** 516-294-5440; **Board Cert:** Obstetrics & Gynecology 2012; Gynecologic Oncology 2012; **Med School:** SUNY Stony Brook 1981; **Resid:** Obstetrics & Gynecology, Univ Hosp 1985; **Fellow:** Gynecologic Oncology, Meml Sloan Kettering Cancer Ctr 1987; **Fac Appt:** Prof ObG, SUNY Stony Brook

Lovecchio, John L MD (GO) - **Spec Exp:** Ovarian Cancer; Uterine Cancer; Cervical Cancer; Vulvar Disease/Cancer; **Hospital:** N Shore Univ Hosp (page 106), Long Is Jewish Med Ctr (page 106); **Address:** North Shore Hospital, 10th Fl Monti, 300 Community Drive, Manhasset, NY 11030-3816; **Phone:** 516-562-4438; **Board Cert:** Obstetrics & Gynecology 2005; Gynecologic Oncology 2005; **Med School:** SUNY Buffalo 1975; **Resid:** Obstetrics & Gynecology, Univ Hosp Case West Res 1979; **Fellow:** Gynecologic Oncology, Jackson Meml Hosp 1982; **Fac Appt:** Prof ObG, NYU Sch Med

Menzin, Andrew William MD (GO) - **Spec Exp:** Uterine Cancer; Ovarian Cancer; Cervical Cancer; Robotic Surgery; **Hospital:** N Shore Univ Hosp (page 106), Long Is Jewish Med Ctr (page 106); **Address:** N Shore Univ Hosp-OB/GYN Dept, 300 Community Drive, 10 Monti, Manhasset, NY 11030-3816; **Phone:** 516-562-4438; **Board Cert:** Obstetrics & Gynecology 2012; Gynecologic Oncology 2012; **Med School:** NYU Sch Med 1989; **Resid:** Obstetrics & Gynecology, Hosp Univ Penn 1993; **Fellow:** Gynecologic Oncology, Hosp Univ Penn 1995; **Fac Appt:** Prof ObG, Hofstra N Shore-LIJ Sch Med

Hand Surgery

Gluck, Robert I MD (HS) - **Spec Exp:** Microvascular Surgery; Dupuytren's Contracture; Carpal Tunnel Syndrome; Elbow Surgery; **Hospital:** Long Is Jewish Med Ctr (page 106); **Address:** The Healthy Hands Ctr-Long Island NY, 410 Lakeville Rd, Ste 310, New Hyde Park, NY 11042; **Phone:** 516-280-5844; **Board Cert:** Hand Surgery 2012; **Med School:** Albert Einstein Coll Med 1982; **Resid:** Surgery, Long Island Jewish Hosp 1987; **Fellow:** Hand & Microvascular Surgery, Stony Brook Univ Med Ctr 1989; **Fac Appt:** Asst Clin Prof S, Albert Einstein Coll Med

Lane, Lewis B MD (HS) - **Spec Exp:** Carpal Tunnel Syndrome; Arthritis; Sports Injuries; Hand Reconstruction; **Hospital:** N Shore Univ Hosp (page 106); **Address:** University Orthopaedics, 611 Northern Blvd, Ste 200, Great Neck, NY 11021; **Phone:** 516-723-2663; **Board Cert:** Orthopaedic Surgery 1981; Hand Surgery 2010; **Med School:** Columbia P&S 1974; **Resid:** Surgery, NY Hosp 1975; Orthopaedic Surgery, Hosp Special Surgery 1979; **Fellow:** Research, Hosp Special Surgery 1976; Hand Surgery, St Lukes-Roosevelt Hosp Ctr 1980; **Fac Appt:** Prof OrS, Hofstra N Shore-LIJ Sch Med

Teplitz, Glenn A MD (HS) - **Spec Exp:** Carpal Tunnel Syndrome; Fractures; Sports Injuries; Wrist/Hand Injuries; **Hospital:** Winthrop Univ Hosp (page 524); **Address:** Winthrop Orthopaedic Assocs, 1300 Franklin Ave, Ste UL-3A, Garden City, NY 11530; **Phone:** 516-747-8900; **Board Cert:** Orthopaedic Surgery 2007; **Med School:** Tulane Univ 1987; **Resid:** Orthopaedic Surgery, UMDNJ Med Ctr 1993; **Fellow:** Hand Surgery, Hosp for Special Surgery 1994; **Fac Appt:** Asst Clin Prof OrS, SUNY Stony Brook

Tuckman, David V MD (HS) - **Spec Exp:** Carpal Tunnel Syndrome; **Hospital:** Long Is Jewish Med Ctr (page 106), St. Francis Hosp - The Heart Ctr (page 116); **Address:** Orthopedic Assocs Manhasset, 600 Northern Blvd, Ste 300, Great Neck, NY 11021; **Phone:** 516-627-8717; **Board Cert:** Orthopaedic Surgery 2007; Hand Surgery 2009; **Med School:** Albert Einstein Coll Med 1998; **Resid:** Orthopaedic Surgery, Long Island Jewish Med Ctr 2003; **Fellow:** Sports Medicine & Shoulder Surgery, Hosp for Joint Diseases 2004; Hand Surgery, Hosp for Joint Diseases 2005

Hematology

Allen, Steven Lee MD (Hem) - **Spec Exp:** Bleeding/Coagulation Disorders; Leukemia & Lymphoma; Multiple Myeloma; Gaucher Disease; **Hospital:** N Shore Univ Hosp (page 106), Long Is Jewish Med Ctr (page 106); **Address:** Monter Cancer Ctr, 450 Lakeville Rd, Lake Success, NY 11042; **Phone:** 516-734-8959; **Board Cert:** Internal Medicine 1980; Hematology 1982; Medical Oncology 1983; **Med School:** Johns Hopkins Univ 1977; **Resid:** Internal Medicine, NY Hosp-Cornell 1980; **Fellow:** Hematology & Oncology, NY Hosp-Cornell 1983; **Fac Appt:** Prof Hem & Onc, Hofstra N Shore-LIJ Sch Med

Kolitz, Jonathan E MD (Hem) - **Spec Exp:** Leukemia & Lymphoma; Hodgkin's Lymphoma; Multiple Myeloma; Myelodysplastic Syndromes; **Hospital:** N Shore Univ Hosp (page 106), Long Is Jewish Med Ctr (page 106); **Address:** 450 Lakeville Rd, Lake Success, NY 11042; **Phone:** 516-734-8970; **Board Cert:** Internal Medicine 1982; Medical Oncology 1985; Hematology 1988; **Med School:** Yale Univ 1979; **Resid:** Internal Medicine, N Shore Univ Hosp 1982; **Fellow:** Hematology & Oncology, Meml Sloan Kettering Cancer Ctr 1985; **Fac Appt:** Prof Hem, Hofstra N Shore-LIJ Sch Med

Rai, Kanti R MD (Hem) - **Spec Exp:** Leukemia; Lymphoma; **Hospital:** Long Is Jewish Med Ctr (page 106); **Address:** Long Island Jewish Med Ctr, Div Hem-Onc, CLL Research & Treatment Program, 410 Lakeville Rd, Ste 212, New Hyde Park, NY 10042; **Phone:** 718-470-4050; **Board Cert:** Pediatrics 1959; **Med School:** India 1955; **Resid:** Pediatrics, Lincoln Hosp 1958; Pediatrics, North Shore Univ Hosp 1959; **Fellow:** Hematology, LI Jewish Med Ctr 1960; **Fac Appt:** Prof Onc, Hofstra N Shore-LIJ Sch Med

Staszewski, Harry MD (Hem) - **Spec Exp:** Hematologic Malignancies; Clinical Trials; **Hospital:** Winthrop Univ Hosp (page 524); **Address:** Winthrop Hematology Oncology Assocs, 200 Old Country Rd, Ste 450, Mineola, NY 11501; **Phone:** 516-663-9500; **Board Cert:** Internal Medicine 1981; Medical Oncology 1983; Hematology 1984; **Med School:** Yale Univ 1978; **Resid:** Internal Medicine, N Shore Univ Hosp 1981; **Fellow:** Medical Oncology, Meml Sloan Kettering Cancer Ctr 1983; Hematology, LI Jewish Hosp 1984; **Fac Appt:** Asst Prof Med, SUNY Stony Brook

Hospice & Palliative Medicine

Berger, Jeffrey MD (H & PM) - **Spec Exp:** Ethics; Palliative Care; Geriatric Care; **Hospital:** Winthrop Univ Hosp (page 524); **Address:** 222 Station Plaza North, Ste 518, Mineola, NY 11501-3893; **Phone:** 516-663-2588; **Board Cert:** Internal Medicine 2011; Hospice & Palliative Medicine 2008; **Med School:** SUNY Stony Brook 1988; **Resid:** Internal Medicine, Winthrop Univ Hosp 1991; **Fac Appt:** Prof Med, SUNY Stony Brook

Infectious Disease

Cervia, Joseph S MD (Inf) - **Spec Exp:** AIDS/HIV; Travel Medicine; Pediatric Infections; Immune Deficiency; **Hospital:** N Shore Univ Hosp (page 106), Steven & Alexandra Cohen Chldn's Med Ctr of NY (page 106); **Address:** North Shore Div Infectious Diseases, 400 Community Drive, Manhasset, NY 11030; **Phone:** 516-562-4280; **Board Cert:** Internal Medicine 1989; Pediatrics 2010; Infectious Disease 2010; Pediatric Infectious Disease 2009; **Med School:** NY Med Coll 1984; **Resid:** Internal Medicine & Pediatrics, Brookdale Hosp 1988; **Fellow:** Infectious Disease, New York Hosp/Cornell 1990; **Fac Appt:** Clin Prof Med, Hofstra N Shore-LIJ Sch Med

Cunha, Burke A MD (Inf) - **Spec Exp:** Infections in Immunocompromised Patients; Fevers of Unknown Origin; Pneumonia; Chronic Fatigue Syndrome; **Hospital:** Winthrop Univ Hosp (page 524); **Address:** 222 Station Plz N, Ste 432, Mineola, NY 11501; **Phone:** 516-663-2507; **Board Cert:** Internal Medicine 1977; Infectious Disease 1978; **Med School:** Penn State Coll Med 1972; **Resid:** Internal Medicine, Hartford Hosp 1975; **Fellow:** Infectious Disease, Hartford Hosp 1977; **Fac Appt:** Prof Med, SUNY Stony Brook

Epstein, Marcia E MD (Inf) - **Spec Exp:** Infections in Immunocompromised Patients; Antibiotic Resistance; **Hospital:** N Shore Univ Hosp (page 106); **Address:** N Shore Univ Hosp, Infectious Disease, 400 Community Drive, Manhasset, NY 11030; **Phone:** 516-562-4280; **Board Cert:** Internal Medicine 1987; Infectious Disease 2012; **Med School:** Harvard Med Sch 1983; **Resid:** Internal Medicine, Montefiore Med Ctr 1986; **Fellow:** Infectious Disease, Montefiore Med Ctr 1990

Farber, Bruce F MD (Inf) - **Spec Exp:** AIDS/HIV; **Hospital:** NS-LIJ Hlth Sys (page 106); **Address:** N Shore LIJ Hlth Sys, Div Infectious Dis, 400 Community Drive, Manhasset, NY 11030; **Phone:** 516-562-4280; **Board Cert:** Internal Medicine 1979; Infectious Disease 1984; **Med School:** Northwestern Univ 1976; **Resid:** Internal Medicine, Univ Va Hosp 1979; **Fellow:** Infectious Disease, Mass Genl Hosp 1982; **Fac Appt:** Assoc Prof Med, NYU Sch Med

Hirsch, Bruce E MD (Inf) - **Spec Exp:** Infectious Disease in Elderly; **Hospital:** N Shore Univ Hosp (page 106), Long Is Jewish Med Ctr (page 106); **Address:** N Shore Univ Hosp, Infectious Disease, 400 Community Drive, Manhasset, NY 11030; **Phone:** 516-562-4280; **Board Cert:** Internal Medicine 1986; Geriatric Medicine 2007; Infectious Disease 2004; **Med School:** Cornell Univ-Weill Med Coll 1982; **Resid:** Internal Medicine, N Shore Univ Hosp 1986; Geriatric Medicine, NY-Presby/Weill Cornell Med Ctr 1988; **Fellow:** Infectious Disease, Jacobi Med Ctr 1989; Infectious Disease, N Shore Univ Hosp 1994

Johnson, Diane H MD (Inf) - **Spec Exp:** AIDS/HIV; Sexually Transmitted Diseases; Travel Medicine; **Hospital:** Winthrop Univ Hosp (page 524); **Address:** Winthrop Infectious Disease Assocs, 222 Station Plaza N, Ste 432, Mineola, NY 11501; **Phone:** 516-663-2507; **Board Cert:** Internal Medicine 2004; Infectious Disease 2004; **Med School:** Univ VT Coll Med 1989; **Resid:** Internal Medicine, Winthrop Univ Hosp 1992; **Fellow:** Infectious Disease, Winthrop Univ Hosp 1994; **Fac Appt:** Asst Prof Med, SUNY Stony Brook

Klein, Natalie C MD (Inf) - **Spec Exp:** HIV; Lyme Disease; Tuberculosis; **Hospital:** Winthrop Univ Hosp (page 524); **Address:** Winthrop Infectious Disease Assocs, 222 Station Plaza N, Ste 432, Mineola, NY 11501-3957; **Phone:** 516-663-2507; **Board Cert:** Internal Medicine 1982; Infectious Disease 1984; **Med School:** Jefferson Med Coll 1979; **Resid:** Internal Medicine, Mount Sinai Hosp 1982; **Fellow:** Infectious Disease, Mount Sinai Hosp 1984; **Fac Appt:** Assoc Clin Prof Med, SUNY Stony Brook

McGowan, Joseph MD (Inf) - **Spec Exp:** AIDS/HIV; HIV in Pregnancy; HIV & Hepatitis co-infection; AIDS/HIV in Elderly; **Hospital:** N Shore Univ Hosp (page 106); **Address:** N Shore Univ Hosp-Div Infectious Dis, 400 Community Drive, Manhasset, NY 11030; **Phone:** 516-562-4280; **Board Cert:** Internal Medicine 2002; Infectious Disease 2002; **Med School:** Mount Sinai Sch Med 1987; **Resid:** Internal Medicine, Montefiore Med Ctr 1990; **Fellow:** Infectious Disease, Montefiore Med Ctr 1993

Scheer, Max S MD (Inf) - **Spec Exp:** Skin/Soft Tissue Infections; Infections-Respiratory; Sexually Transmitted Diseases; **Hospital:** N Shore Univ Hosp (page 106); **Address:** Woodmere Medical Assocs, 15 Irving Pl, Woodmere, NY 11598-1229; **Phone:** 516-374-6750; **Board Cert:** Internal Medicine 1979; Infectious Disease 1982; **Med School:** SUNY Downstate 1975; **Resid:** Family Medicine, Kings Co Hosp-SUNY 1978; Internal Medicine, Morristown Meml Hosp 1979; **Fellow:** Infectious Disease, Mt Sinai Hosp 1981; **Fac Appt:** Asst Clin Prof Med, NYU Sch Med

Internal Medicine

Berbari, Nicholas E MD (IM) *PCP* - **Hospital:** Winthrop Univ Hosp (page 524); **Address:** 222 Station Plaza N, Ste 310, Mineola, NY 11501; **Phone:** 516-663-2051; **Board Cert:** Internal Medicine 2006; **Med School:** SUNY Stony Brook 1993; **Resid:** Internal Medicine, Winthrop Univ Hosp 1997; **Fac Appt:** Asst Prof Med, SUNY Stony Brook

Corapi, Mark MD (IM) *PCP* - **Hospital:** Winthrop Univ Hosp (page 524); **Address:** 222 Station Plaza N, Ste 310, Mineola, NY 11501; **Phone:** 516-663-2051; **Board Cert:** Internal Medicine 1985; **Med School:** SUNY Downstate 1982; **Resid:** Internal Medicine, LI Jewish Med Ctr 1985; **Fellow:** Internal Medicine, LI Jewish Med Ctr 1986; **Fac Appt:** Assoc Prof Med, SUNY Stony Brook

Cusumano, Stephen P MD (IM) *PCP* - **Spec Exp:** Hypertension; Asthma; **Hospital:** St. Joseph's Hosp-Nassau, Winthrop Univ Hosp (page 524); **Address:** 850 Hicksville Rd, Ste 104, Seaford, NY 11783; **Phone:** 516-735-5454; **Board Cert:** Internal Medicine 1988; **Med School:** Univ Hlth Scis, Chicago Med Sch 1985; **Resid:** Internal Medicine, Winthrop Univ Hosp 1988

Edelson, David G MD (IM) *PCP* - **Spec Exp:** Concierge Medicine; **Hospital:** NS-LIJ Hlth Sys (page 106); **Address:** Healthbridge, 1000 Northern Blvd, Ste 230, Great Neck, NY 11021; **Phone:** 516-627-4433; **Board Cert:** Internal Medicine 1985; **Med School:** Northwestern Univ 1982; **Resid:** Internal Medicine, LI Jewish Med Ctr 1987; **Fac Appt:** Asst Clin Prof Med, Hofstra N Shore-LIJ Sch Med

Federbush, Richard MD (IM) *PCP* - **Spec Exp:** Hypertension; Cholesterol/Lipid Disorders; Diabetes; **Hospital:** Plainview Hosp (page 106), Syosset Hosp (page 106); **Address:** 175 Jericho Tpke, Ste 216, Syosset, NY 11791; **Phone:** 516-364-9800; **Board Cert:** Internal Medicine 2012; **Med School:** Mexico 1985; **Resid:** Internal Medicine, Univ Hosp-SUNY 1989; **Fac Appt:** Asst Clin Prof Med, Hofstra N Shore-LIJ Sch Med

Gelberg, Burt W MD (IM) *PCP* - **Spec Exp:** Preventive Medicine; Colonoscopy; Gastroscopy; **Hospital:** Franklin Hosp (page 106); **Address:** 401 Franklin Ave, Franklin Square, NY 11010-1227; **Phone:** 516-326-2255; **Board Cert:** Internal Medicine 1975; **Med School:** SUNY Downstate 1972; **Resid:** Internal Medicine, Montefiore Hosp 1973; Internal Medicine, Lenox Hill Hosp 1975; **Fellow:** Gastroenterology, Lenox Hill Hosp 1977

Goodman, Michael MD (IM) - **Hospital:** South Nassau Comm Hosp; **Address:** 2495 Newbridge Rd, Bellmore, NY 11710; **Phone:** 516-826-1200; **Board Cert:** Internal Medicine 1980; **Med School:** Italy 1975; **Resid:** Internal Medicine, Nassau Co Med Ctr 1978

Gorski, Lydia E MD (IM) *PCP* - **Spec Exp:** Women's Health; Geriatric Medicine; Preventive Medicine; **Hospital:** Winthrop Univ Hosp (page 524), N Shore Univ Hosp (page 106); **Address:** 820 Jericho Tpke, New Hyde Park, NY 11040-4514; **Phone:** 516-352-0430; **Board Cert:** Internal Medicine 1988; **Med School:** Poland 1982; **Resid:** Internal Medicine, St Vincent Hosp Med Ctr 1987

Gottridge, Joanne MD (IM) *PCP* - **Hospital:** N Shore Univ Hosp (page 106), Long Is Jewish Med Ctr (page 106); **Address:** 865 Northern Blvd, Ste 102, Great Neck, NY 11021; **Phone:** 516-622-5000; **Board Cert:** Internal Medicine 1983; **Med School:** Case West Res Univ 1980; **Resid:** Internal Medicine, N Shore Univ Hosp 1983; **Fac Appt:** Assoc Prof Med, NYU Sch Med

Hotchkiss, Edward MD (IM) *PCP* - **Hospital:** South Nassau Comm Hosp; **Address:** 158 Hempstead Ave, Lynbrook, NY 11563; **Phone:** 516-593-3541; **Board Cert:** Internal Medicine 1972; **Med School:** SUNY Downstate 1965; **Resid:** Internal Medicine, LI Jewish Med Ctr 1970; **Fellow:** Psychiatry, SUNY Downstate Med Ctr 1971; **Fac Appt:** Assoc Prof Med, Albert Einstein Coll Med

Leong, Pauline MD (IM) *PCP* - **Hospital:** N Shore Univ Hosp (page 106), Long Is Jewish Med Ctr (page 106); **Address:** 865 Northern Blvd, Ste 102, Great Neck, NY 11021; **Phone:** 516-622-5000; **Board Cert:** Internal Medicine 1988; **Med School:** NYU Sch Med 1983; **Resid:** Internal Medicine, New York Hosp Queens 1988

Pollak, Harvey MD (IM) *PCP* - **Spec Exp:** Hypertension; Heart Disease; Cholesterol/Lipid Disorders; **Hospital:** N Shore Univ Hosp (page 106); **Address:** 2 ProHealth Plaza, Ste 101, Lake Success, NY 11042; **Phone:** 516-622-6020; **Board Cert:** Internal Medicine 1974; **Med School:** Ros Franklin Univ/Chicago Med Sch 1971; **Resid:** Internal Medicine, Meml Sloan-Kettering Cancer Ctr 1973; Internal Medicine, N Shore Univ Hosp 1975; **Fac Appt:** Clin Prof Med, NYU Sch Med

Rubenstein, Jack MD (IM) *PCP* - **Spec Exp:** Complex Diagnosis; Kidney Failure-Chronic; Geriatric Care; Hypertension; **Hospital:** Franklin Hosp (page 106), N Shore Univ Hosp (page 106); **Address:** 70 Glen Cove Rd, Ste 301, Roslyn Heights, NY 11577-1731; **Phone:** 516-621-1502; **Board Cert:** Internal Medicine 2008; Nephrology 2009; Geriatric Medicine 2008; **Med School:** NY Med Coll 1976; **Resid:** Internal Medicine, North Shore Univ Hosp 1979; Nephrology, North Shore Univ Hosp 1980; **Fellow:** Nephrology, NYU Med Ctr 1982; **Fac Appt:** Assoc Clin Prof Med, Hofstra N Shore-LIJ Sch Med

Rucker, Steve MD (IM) *PCP* - **Spec Exp:** Hypertension; Kidney Disease; Kidney Stones; **Hospital:** St. Francis Hosp - The Heart Ctr (page 116), NS-LIJ Hlth Sys (page 106); **Address:** 1999 Marcus Ave, Ste 216, Lake Success, NY 11042; **Phone:** 516-775-4545; **Board Cert:** Internal Medicine 1986; Nephrology 1988; **Med School:** Univ Pittsburgh 1983; **Resid:** Internal Medicine, LI Jewish Med Ctr 1986; **Fellow:** Nephrology, Mount Sinai Med Ctr 1988

Taubman, Lowell B MD (IM) *PCP* - **Spec Exp:** Dementia; Alzheimer's Disease; Preventive Medicine; Geriatric Care; **Hospital:** Long Beach Med Ctr; **Address:** 206 Riverside Blvd, Long Beach, NY 11561; **Phone:** 516-432-5670; **Board Cert:** Internal Medicine 1988; **Med School:** Mexico 1980; **Resid:** Internal Medicine, Montefiore Hosp 1983; Internal Medicine, St Clares Hosp 1984; **Fellow:** Geriatric Medicine, Jewish Inst Geriatric Care 1986

Timpone, Leonard MD (IM) *PCP* - **Spec Exp:** Geriatric Medicine; Headache; Preventive Medicine; **Hospital:** Franklin Hosp (page 106), Mercy Med Ctr - Rockville Centre; **Address:** 1051 Adams Ave, Franklin Square, NY 11010-2251; **Phone:** 516-354-4858; **Board Cert:** Internal Medicine 2004; **Med School:** France 1984; **Resid:** Internal Medicine, NY Downtown Hosp 1988

Weinstein, Mark J MD (IM) *PCP* - **Spec Exp:** Hypertension; Diabetes; Cholesterol/Lipid Disorders; **Hospital:** Plainview Hosp (page 106); **Address:** 4045 Hempstead Tpke, Fl 3, Bethpage, NY 11714-5706; **Phone:** 516-731-7770; **Board Cert:** Internal Medicine 1978; Infectious Disease 1980; **Med School:** Harvard Med Sch 1975; **Resid:** Internal Medicine, Univ Hosp 1978; **Fellow:** Infectious Disease, Univ Hosp 1980

Wolff, Edward MD (IM) *PCP* - **Spec Exp:** Asthma; Heart Disease; **Hospital:** St. Francis Hosp - The Heart Ctr (page 116), N Shore Univ Hosp (page 106); **Address:** 107 Northern Blvd, Ste 404, Great Neck, NY 11021; **Phone:** 516-498-1818; **Board Cert:** Internal Medicine 1987; **Med School:** Georgetown Univ 1966; **Resid:** Internal Medicine, Metropolitan Hosp Ctr 1970; **Fellow:** Pulmonary Disease, Metropolitan Hosp Ctr 1971; **Fac Appt:** Med, Cornell Univ-Weill Med Coll

Interventional Cardiology

Abittan, Meyer H MD (IC) - **Spec Exp:** Angiography-Coronary; Preventive Cardiology; **Hospital:** St. Francis Hosp - The Heart Ctr (page 116); **Address:** St Francis Hosp, The Heart Ctr, 100 Port Washington Blvd, Ste G-03, Roslyn, NY 11576; **Phone:** 516-627-1155; **Board Cert:** Internal Medicine 1989; **Med School:** Mount Sinai Sch Med 1986; **Resid:** Internal Medicine, Brookdale Univ Hosp Med Ctr 1989; **Fellow:** Cardiovascular Disease, Mt Sinai Med Ctr 1990; Interventional Cardiology, Maimonides Med Ctr

Berke, Andrew D MD (IC) - **Hospital:** St. Francis Hosp - The Heart Ctr (page 116), South Nassau Comm Hosp; **Address:** 100 Port Washington Blvd, Roslyn, NY 11576; **Phone:** 516-365-2211; **Board Cert:** Internal Medicine 1982; Cardiovascular Disease 1985; Interventional Cardiology 2009; **Med School:** Brown Univ 1979; **Resid:** Internal Medicine, NY-Presby/Columbia Univ Med Ctr 1982; **Fellow:** Cardiovascular Disease, NY-Presby/Columbia Univ Med Ctr 1985; **Fac Appt:** Asst Clin Prof Med, Columbia P&S

Petrossian, George A MD (IC) - **Spec Exp:** Carotid Artery Stent Placement; Peripheral Vascular Disease; Coronary Angioplasty/Stents; Renovascular Disease; **Hospital:** St. Francis Hosp - The Heart Ctr (page 116), South Nassau Comm Hosp; **Address:** 1405 Old Northern Blvd, 1st Floor, Roslyn, NY 11576-1353; **Phone:** 516-484-6777; **Board Cert:** Internal Medicine 1986; Cardiovascular Disease 1989; Interventional Cardiology 2010; **Med School:** Mount Sinai Sch Med 1983; **Resid:** Internal Medicine, Columbia-Presby Med Ctr 1987; **Fellow:** Cardiovascular Disease, Columbia -Presby Med Ctr 1989; Interventional Cardiology, Mass Genl Hosp 1990

Zisfein, Jerome B MD (IC) - **Spec Exp:** Coronary Angioplasty/Stents; Pacemakers; Cardiac Catheterization; **Hospital:** Winthrop Univ Hosp (page 524), South Nassau Comm Hosp; **Address:** South Shore Heart Assocs, 242 Merrick Rd, Ste 402, Rockville Centre, NY 11570; **Phone:** 516-763-2800; **Board Cert:** Internal Medicine 1984; Cardiovascular Disease 1987; Interventional Cardiology 2010; **Med School:** NY Med Coll 1981; **Resid:** Internal Medicine, Rhode Island Hosp 1984; **Fellow:** Cardiovascular Disease, Mass Genl Hosp 1989

Maternal & Fetal Medicine

Fleischer, Adiel MD (MF) - **Spec Exp:** Pregnancy-High Risk; **Hospital:** Long Is Jewish Med Ctr (page 106), N Shore Univ Hosp (page 106); **Address:** LIJ Med Ctr, Dept Ob/Gyn, 270-05 76th Ave, Ste I-457A - rm 464, New Hyde Park, NY 11040-1433; **Phone:** 718-470-5466; **Board Cert:** Obstetrics & Gynecology 1999; Maternal & Fetal Medicine 1999; **Med School:** Romania 1972; **Resid:** Obstetrics & Gynecology, Maimonides Med Ctr 1979; **Fellow:** Maternal & Fetal Medicine, Montefiore Med Ctr 1982; **Fac Appt:** Assoc Prof ObG, Hofstra N Shore-LIJ Sch Med

Kinzler, Wendy MD (MF) - **Spec Exp:** Pregnancy-High Risk; Miscarriage-Recurrent; Prematurity Prevention; **Hospital:** Winthrop Univ Hosp (page 524); **Address:** Perinatal Associates, 120 Mineola Blvd, Ste 110, Mineola, NY 11501; **Phone:** 516-663-3061; **Board Cert:** Obstetrics & Gynecology 2012; Maternal & Fetal Medicine 2012; **Med School:** Boston Univ 1994; **Resid:** Obstetrics & Gynecology, Albert Einstein Med Ctr 1998; **Fellow:** Maternal & Fetal Medicine, UMDNJ RWJ Hosp 2001; **Fac Appt:** , Afghanistan

Klein, Victor R MD (MF) - **Spec Exp:** Multiple Gestation; Pregnancy-High Risk; Genetic Disorders; **Hospital:** N Shore Univ Hosp (page 106), Long Is Jewish Med Ctr (page 106); **Address:** 600 Northern Blvd, Ste 212, Great Neck, NY 11021; **Phone:** 516-472-5700; **Board Cert:** Obstetrics & Gynecology 2012; Maternal & Fetal Medicine 2012; Clinical Genetics 1987; **Med School:** SUNY Downstate 1980; **Resid:** Internal Medicine, Kings Co Hosp Ctr 1981; Obstetrics & Gynecology, Johns Hopkins Hosp 1985; **Fellow:** Clinical Genetics, Univ Texas SW Med Ctr 1987; Maternal & Fetal Medicine, Univ Texas SW Med Ctr 1987; **Fac Appt:** Assoc Clin Prof ObG, Hofstra N Shore-LIJ Sch Med

Meirowitz, Natalie MD (MF) - **Spec Exp:** Prenatal Diagnosis; Pregnancy Loss; Pregnancy-High Risk; **Hospital:** Long Is Jewish Med Ctr (page 106); **Address:** NS-LIJ Med Ctr, Dept Ob/Gyn, 270-05 76th Ave, Ste T-457A, New Hyde Park, NY 11040; **Phone:** 516-470-7636; **Board Cert:** Obstetrics & Gynecology 2012; Maternal & Fetal Medicine 2012; **Med School:** Harvard Med Sch 1993; **Resid:** Obstetrics & Gynecology, North Shore Univ Med Ctr 1997; **Fellow:** Maternal & Fetal Medicine, Univ Hosp-UMDNJ 2000; **Fac Appt:** Asst Prof ObG, Albert Einstein Coll Med

Rochelson, Burton L MD (MF) - **Spec Exp:** Pregnancy-High Risk; Ultrasound; Prenatal Diagnosis; **Hospital:** N Shore Univ Hosp (page 106); **Address:** 300 Community Drive, Levitt Bldg Fl 3, Manhasset, NY 11030-3876; **Phone:** 516-562-2892; **Board Cert:** Obstetrics & Gynecology 2012; Maternal & Fetal Medicine 2012; **Med School:** Univ Mich Med Sch 1978; **Resid:** Obstetrics & Gynecology, LI Jewish Med Ctr 1982; **Fellow:** Maternal & Fetal Medicine, Univ Hosp 1986; **Fac Appt:** Prof ObG, Hofstra N Shore-LIJ Sch Med

Vintzileos, Anthony M MD (MF) - **Spec Exp:** Ultrasound; Fetal Therapy; **Hospital:** Winthrop Univ Hosp (page 524); **Address:** Women's Contemporary Care Assocs, 120 Mineola Blvd Ste 100, Mineola, NY 11501; **Phone:** 516-663-3010; **Board Cert:** Obstetrics & Gynecology 1999; Maternal & Fetal Medicine 1999; **Med School:** Greece 1975; **Resid:** Obstetrics & Gynecology, St Joseph's Hosp Med Ctr 1981; **Fellow:** Maternal & Fetal Medicine, Univ Conn Hlth Ctr 1983; **Fac Appt:** Prof ObG, SUNY Stony Brook

Medical Oncology

Arena, Francis P MD (Onc) - **Spec Exp:** Breast Cancer; **Hospital:** N Shore Univ Hosp (page 106), NYU Langone Med Ctr (page 108); **Address:** NYU Langone Arena Onc Assocs, 1999 Marcus Ave, Ste 120, Lake Success, NY 11042; **Phone:** 516-466-6611; **Board Cert:** Internal Medicine 1978; Medical Oncology 2006; **Med School:** Cornell Univ-Weill Med Coll 1975; **Resid:** Internal Medicine, NY Hosp-Cornell Med Ctr 1978; Internal Medicine, Meml Sloan-Kettering Cancer Ctr 1979; **Fellow:** Hematology & Oncology, Meml Sloan-Kettering Cancer Ctr 1980; **Fac Appt:** Assoc Clin Prof Med, NYU Sch Med

Bradley, Thomas P MD (Onc) - **Spec Exp:** Bladder Cancer; Prostate Cancer; Kidney Cancer; **Hospital:** N Shore Univ Hosp (page 106); **Address:** Monter Cancer Ctr, 450 Lakeville Rd, Lake Success, NY 11042; **Phone:** 516-734-8963; **Board Cert:** Internal Medicine 1987; Medical Oncology 2011; Hematology 2012; **Med School:** Mexico 1982; **Resid:** Internal Medicine, SUNY Downstate Med Ctr 1988; **Fellow:** Hematology & Oncology, SUNY Downstate Med Ctr 1991; **Fac Appt:** Assoc Prof Med, Albert Einstein Coll Med

Budman, Daniel MD (Onc) - **Spec Exp:** Breast Cancer; Lymphoma; Drug Discovery & Development; Psychopharmacology; **Hospital:** N Shore Univ Hosp (page 106), Long Is Jewish Med Ctr (page 106); **Address:** 450 Lakeville Rd, Monter Cancer Ctr A Bldg, Lake Success, NY 11042; **Phone:** 516-734-8900; **Board Cert:** Internal Medicine 1975; Hematology 1978; Medical Oncology 1979; **Med School:** Albert Einstein Coll Med 1972; **Resid:** Internal Medicine, Hosp Univ Penn 1974; Hematology, Natl Inst Hlth 1976; **Fellow:** Medical Oncology, Sloan Kettering Cancer Ctr 1977; Hematology, NYU Med Ctr 1978; **Fac Appt:** Prof Med, Hofstra N Shore-LIJ Sch Med

Citron, Marc L MD (Onc) - **Spec Exp:** Breast Cancer; Lung Cancer; **Hospital:** Long Is Jewish Med Ctr (page 106); **Address:** ProHealth Care Assocs, Div Oncology, 2800 Marcus Ave, Ste 205, Lake Success, NY 11042-1008; **Phone:** 516-622-6150; **Board Cert:** Internal Medicine 1977; Medical Oncology 1979; **Med School:** Wayne State Univ 1974; **Resid:** Internal Medicine, Georgetown Univ Hosp 1977; **Fellow:** Medical Oncology, Georgetown Univ Hosp 1979; **Fac Appt:** Clin Prof Med, Albert Einstein Coll Med

Hindenburg, Alexander A MD (Onc) - **Spec Exp:** Pancreatic Cancer; Breast Cancer; Gynecologic Cancer; Myelodysplastic Syndromes; **Hospital:** Winthrop Univ Hosp (page 524); **Address:** Winthrop Oncology/Hematology Assocs, 200 Old Country Rd, Ste 450, Mineola, NY 11501; **Phone:** 516-663-9500; **Board Cert:** Internal Medicine 1981; Medical Oncology 1983; Hematology 1988; **Med School:** UMDNJ-RW Johnson Med Sch 1978; **Resid:** Internal Medicine, Mt Sinai Hosp 1981; **Fellow:** Hematology & Oncology, NY-Presby/Columbia Univ Med Ctr 1984; **Fac Appt:** Asst Prof Med, SUNY Stony Brook

Kappel, Bruce I MD (Onc) - **Spec Exp:** Breast Cancer; Colon Cancer; **Hospital:** Plainview Hosp (page 106), St. Joseph's Hosp-Nassau; **Address:** 40 Crossways Park Drive, Ste 103, Woodbury, NY 11797; **Phone:** 516-921-5533; **Board Cert:** Internal Medicine 1985; Medical Oncology 1987; Hematology 1988; **Med School:** Emory Univ 1982; **Resid:** Internal Medicine, Emory Univ Hosp 1985; **Fellow:** Medical Oncology, NY-Presby/Columbia Univ Med Ctr 1988

Kessler, Leonard MD (Onc) - **Hospital:** South Nassau Comm Hosp, Mercy Med Ctr - Rockville Centre; **Address:** 242 Merrick Rd, Ste 301, Rockville Centre, NY 11570; **Phone:** 516-536-1455; **Board Cert:** Internal Medicine 1979; Medical Oncology 1981; Hematology 1982; **Med School:** Albert Einstein Coll Med 1975; **Resid:** Internal Medicine, Montefiore Med Ctr 1977; **Fellow:** Hematology, Montefiore Med Ctr 1981; Medical Oncology, Meml Sloan-Kettering Cancer Ctr 1980

Marino, John S MD (Onc) - **Spec Exp:** Breast Cancer; Colon Cancer; Lung Cancer; **Hospital:** N Shore Univ Hosp (page 106), St. Francis Hosp - The Heart Ctr (page 116); **Address:** 2001 Marcus Ave, Ste S265, Lake Success, NY 11042; **Phone:** 516-883-0122; **Board Cert:** Internal Medicine 1982; Medical Oncology 1985; **Med School:** NY Med Coll 1979; **Resid:** Internal Medicine, N Shore Univ Hosp 1982; **Fellow:** Medical Oncology, Jacobi Med Ctr 1983; Medical Oncology, N Shore Univ Hosp 1984; **Fac Appt:** Asst Clin Prof Med, NYU Sch Med

Mehrotra, Bhoomi MD (Onc) - **Spec Exp:** Lung Cancer; Head & Neck Cancer; Gastrointestinal Cancer; **Hospital:** St. Francis Hosp - The Heart Ctr (page 116); **Address:** 100 Port Washington Blvd, Roslyn, NY 11576; **Phone:** 516-325-7500; **Board Cert:** Hematology 2004; Medical Oncology 2003; **Med School:** India 1986; **Resid:** Internal Medicine, LI Jewish Med Ctr 1990; **Fellow:** Hematology & Oncology, UCSF Med Ctr 1993; **Fac Appt:** Assoc Prof Med, Hofstra N Shore-LIJ Sch Med

Raptis, George MD (Onc) - **Spec Exp:** Breast Cancer; **Hospital:** N Shore Univ Hosp (page 106), Long Is Jewish Med Ctr (page 106); **Address:** 450 Lakeville Rd, Monter Cancer Ctr A Bldg, Lake Success, NY 11042; **Phone:** 516-734-8900; **Board Cert:** Medical Oncology 2003; **Med School:** Mount Sinai Sch Med 1987; **Resid:** Internal Medicine, Mt Sinai Med Ctr 1990; **Fellow:** Hematology & Oncology, Meml Sloan-Kettering Canc Ctr 1993; **Fac Appt:** Assoc Prof Med, Hofstra N Shore-LIJ Sch Med

Schwartz, Paula R MD (Onc) - **Spec Exp:** Breast Cancer; Colon Cancer; **Hospital:** N Shore Univ Hosp (page 106), Long Is Jewish Med Ctr (page 106); **Address:** 3003 New Hyde Park Rd Bldg 401, New Hyde Park, NY 11042; **Phone:** 516-354-5700; **Board Cert:** Internal Medicine 1986; Hematology 1988; **Med School:** SUNY Downstate 1980; **Resid:** Internal Medicine, LI Jewish Med Ctr 1983; **Fellow:** Hematology, Mt Sinai Hosp 1985; Hematology, N Shore Univ Hosp 1989

Shapira, Iuliana T MD (Onc) - **Spec Exp:** Breast Cancer; **Hospital:** N Shore Univ Hosp (page 106), Long Is Jewish Med Ctr (page 106); **Address:** N Shore Univ Hosp, Cancer Ctr, 450 Lakeville Rd, Lake Success, NY 11042; **Phone:** 516-734-8866; **Board Cert:** Internal Medicine 2008; Hematology 2005; Medical Oncology 2005; **Med School:** Romania 1990; **Resid:** Internal Medicine, St Barnabas Med Ctr 1998; **Fellow:** Medical Oncology, SUNY Hlth Sci Ctr 2005; **Fac Appt:** Asst Prof Onc, Hofstra N Shore-LIJ Sch Med

Tomao, Frank A MD (Onc) - **Spec Exp:** Lung Cancer; Breast Cancer; **Hospital:** Long Is Jewish Med Ctr (page 106), St. Francis Hosp - The Heart Ctr (page 116); **Address:** 2001 Marcus Ave, Ste S265, Lake Success, NY 11042; **Phone:** 516-883-0122; **Board Cert:** Internal Medicine 1974; Medical Oncology 1975; **Med School:** Cornell Univ-Weill Med Coll 1965; **Resid:** Internal Medicine, Meml Sloan-Kettering Cancer Ctr 1967; Internal Medicine, Bellevue Hosp 1968; **Fellow:** Medical Oncology, Meml Sloan-Kettering Cancer Ctr 1969

Vinciguerra, Vincent P MD (Onc) - **Spec Exp:** Breast Cancer; Gastrointestinal Cancer; Lung Cancer; Cancer Prevention; **Hospital:** N Shore Univ Hosp (page 106), Glen Cove Hosp (page 106); **Address:** Monter Cancer Ctr, 450 Lakeville Rd, Lake Success, NY 11042; **Phone:** 516-734-8954; **Board Cert:** Internal Medicine 1971; Hematology 1974; Medical Oncology 1975; **Med School:** Georgetown Univ 1966; **Resid:** Internal Medicine, NY Hosp-Cornell 1969; Internal Medicine, N Shore Univ Hosp 1971; **Fellow:** Hematology & Oncology, NY Hosp-Cornell 1973; Hematology & Oncology, N Shore Univ Hosp 1974; **Fac Appt:** Prof Med, NYU Sch Med

Weiselberg, Lora MD (Onc) - **Spec Exp:** Breast Cancer; Cancer Prevention; **Hospital:** N Shore Univ Hosp (page 106), Long Is Jewish Med Ctr (page 106); **Address:** Monter Cancer Ctr, 450 Lakeville Rd, Lake Success, NY 11042; **Phone:** 516-734-8963; **Board Cert:** Internal Medicine 1978; Medical Oncology 1981; Hematology 1982; **Med School:** NY Med Coll 1975; **Resid:** Internal Medicine, Stamford Hosp 1978; **Fellow:** Medical Oncology, N Shore Univ Hosp 1980; Hematology, N Shore Univ Hosp 1981; **Fac Appt:** Assoc Prof Med, Hofstra N Shore-LIJ Sch Med

Weiss, Rita MD/PhD (Onc) - **Hospital:** St. Francis Hosp - The Heart Ctr (page 116), N Shore Univ Hosp (page 106); **Address:** 107 Northern Blvd, Ste 306, Great Neck, NY 11021-4309; **Phone:** 516-482-0080; **Board Cert:** Internal Medicine 1984; Medical Oncology 1989; **Med School:** Mexico 1977; **Resid:** Internal Medicine, Winthrop Univ Hosp 1980; **Fellow:** Medical Oncology, Mount Sinai 1982; **Fac Appt:** Asst Clin Prof Onc, NYU Sch Med

Neonatal-Perinatal Medicine

Boxer, Harriet S MD (NP) - **Spec Exp:** Prematurity/Low Birth Weight Infants; Chronic Obstructive Lung Disease (COPD); **Hospital:** Nassau Univ Med Ctr; **Address:** Nassau Univ Med Ctr, Div Neonatology, 2201 Hempstead Tpke, Box 30, East Meadow, NY 11554; **Phone:** 516-572-3318; **Board Cert:** Pediatrics 1977; Neonatal-Perinatal Medicine 1977; **Med School:** SUNY Downstate 1972; **Resid:** Pediatrics, Babies Hosp 1974; Pediatrics, Children's Hosp 1975; **Fellow:** Neonatal-Perinatal Medicine, LI Jewish-Hillside Med Ctr 1977; **Fac Appt:** Asst Prof Ped, SUNY Stony Brook

Schanler, Richard J MD (NP) - **Spec Exp:** Neonatal Care; **Hospital:** Steven & Alexandra Cohen Chldn's Med Ctr of NY (page 106), N Shore Univ Hosp (page 106); **Address:** 269-01 76th Ave, rm CH 344, New Hyde Park, NY 11040; **Phone:** 718-470-3440; **Board Cert:** Pediatrics 1979; Neonatal-Perinatal Medicine 2009; **Med School:** UMDNJ-NJ Med Sch, Newark 1974; **Resid:** Pediatrics, Univ Colorado Hosp 1977; **Fellow:** Neonatology, Women & Infants Hosp 1980; **Fac Appt:** Prof Ped, Albert Einstein Coll Med

Steele, Andrew M MD (NP) - **Spec Exp:** Lung Disease in Newborns; Sudden Infant Death Syndrome (SIDS); Breathing Disorders; **Hospital:** Steven & Alexandra Cohen Chldn's Med Ctr of NY (page 106), N Shore Univ Hosp (page 106); **Address:** Steven & Alexandra Cohen Chldn's Med Ctr, 269-01 76th Ave, New Hyde Park, NY 11040-1433; **Phone:** 718-470-3013; **Board Cert:** Pediatrics 1981; Neonatal-Perinatal Medicine 2009; **Med School:** SUNY Hlth Sci Ctr 1976; **Resid:** Pediatrics, LI Jewish Med Ctr 1978; **Fellow:** Neonatal-Perinatal Medicine, LI Jewish Med Ctr 1980; **Fac Appt:** Assoc Prof Ped, Hofstra N Shore-LIJ Sch Med

Nephrology

Bellucci, Alessandro G MD (Nep) - **Spec Exp:** Hypertension; Kidney Stones; Kidney Disease; Kidney Failure; **Hospital:** N Shore Univ Hosp (page 106); **Address:** North Shore Univ Hosp, Dept Nephrology, 100 Community Drive, Great Neck, NY 11021; **Phone:** 516-562-4312; **Board Cert:** Internal Medicine 1979; Nephrology 1982; **Med School:** Italy 1975; **Resid:** Internal Medicine, Cabrini Med Ctr 1979; **Fellow:** Nephrology, N Shore Univ Hosp 1982; **Fac Appt:** Assoc Prof Med, NYU Sch Med

Bourla, Steven L MD (Nep) - **Spec Exp:** Kidney Disease; **Hospital:** Plainview Hosp (page 106), St. Joseph's Hosp-Nassau; **Address:** Island Medical Group, 789 Old Country Rd, Plainview, NY 11803; **Phone:** 516-433-3600; **Board Cert:** Internal Medicine 1979; Nephrology 1982; **Med School:** NY Med Coll 1975; **Resid:** Internal Medicine, LI Jewish Med Ctr 1979; **Fellow:** Nephrology, NYU Med Ctr 1981

Mailloux, Lionel U MD (Nep) - **Spec Exp:** Hypertension; Dialysis Care; **Hospital:** N Shore Univ Hosp (page 106), Glen Cove Hosp (page 106); **Address:** 50 Seaview Blvd, Port Washington, NY 11050; **Phone:** 516-484-6093; **Board Cert:** Internal Medicine 1977; Nephrology 1972; **Med School:** Hahnemann Univ 1962; **Resid:** Internal Medicine, Hartford Hosp 1965; **Fellow:** Nephrology, Hahnemann Hosp 1966; **Fac Appt:** Assoc Prof Med, NYU Sch Med

Masani, Naveed N MD (Nep) - **Spec Exp:** Dialysis Care; **Hospital:** Winthrop Univ Hosp (page 524); **Address:** Winthrop Nephrology Assocs, 200 Old Country Rd, Ste 135, Mineola, NY 11501; **Phone:** 516-663-2169; **Board Cert:** Nephrology 2004; **Med School:** SUNY Stony Brook 1999; **Resid:** Internal Medicine, Winthrop Univ Hosp 2002; **Fellow:** Nephrology, Winthrop Univ Hosp 2004

Mattana, Joseph MD (Nep) - **Spec Exp:** Diabetic Kidney Disease; Hypertension; Glomerulonephritis; **Hospital:** Winthrop Univ Hosp (page 524); **Address:** Winthrop Nephrology Assocs, 200 Old Country Rd, Ste 135, Mineola, NY 11501; **Phone:** 516-663-2169; **Board Cert:** Nephrology 2004; **Med School:** SUNY Hlth Sci Ctr 1987; **Resid:** Internal Medicine, LI Jewish Hosp 1990; **Fellow:** Nephrology, LI Jewish Hosp 1993

Singhal, Pravin C MD (Nep) - **Spec Exp:** Hypertension; Diabetic Kidney Disease; HIV Related Kidney Disease; **Hospital:** Long Is Jewish Med Ctr (page 106), N Shore Univ Hosp (page 106); **Address:** 100 Community Drive, Fl 2, Great Neck, NY 11021; **Phone:** 516-465-3010; **Board Cert:** Internal Medicine 1983; Nephrology 1986; **Med School:** India 1970; **Resid:** Internal Medicine, Postgrad Inst Med Ed. 1972; Internal Medicine, Brigham Womens Hosp 1983; **Fellow:** Nephrology, Montefiore Med Ctr 1985; **Fac Appt:** Prof Med, Albert Einstein Coll Med

Wagner, John D MD (Nep) - **Spec Exp:** Hypertension; Dialysis Care; Kidney Failure-Chronic; **Hospital:** Long Is Jewish Med Ctr (page 106), N Shore Univ Hosp (page 106); **Address:** 100 Community Drive Fl 2, Great Neck, NY 11021; **Phone:** 516-465-3010; **Board Cert:** Internal Medicine 1981; Nephrology 1984; **Med School:** Yale Univ 1978; **Resid:** Internal Medicine, Bellevue Hosp Ctr 1982; **Fellow:** Nephrology, NYU-Bellevue Hosp-VA Med Ctr 1984; **Fac Appt:** Assoc Clin Prof Med, Albert Einstein Coll Med

Neurological Surgery

Brisman, Jonathan L MD (NS) - **Spec Exp:** Aneurysm-Cerebral; Arteriovenous Malformations; Carotid Stenosis; Endovascular Neurosurgery; **Hospital:** Winthrop Univ Hosp (page 524), St. Francis Hosp - The Heart Ctr (page 116); **Address:** Neurological Surgery, 1991 Marcus Ave, Ste 108, Lake Success, NY 11042; **Phone:** 516-442-2250; **Board Cert:** Neurological Surgery 2008; **Med School:** Columbia P&S 1995; **Resid:** Surgery, Mass Genl Hosp 1996; Neurological Surgery, Mass Genl Hosp 2002; **Fellow:** Interventional Neuroradiology, Roosevelt Hosp 2003; Cerebrovascular Neurosurgery, Swedish Med Ctr 2005

Brown, Jeffrey A MD (NS) - **Spec Exp:** Trigeminal Neuralgia; Pain-Chronic; **Hospital:** Winthrop Univ Hosp (page 524), N Shore Univ Hosp (page 106); **Address:** 600 Northern Blvd, Ste 118, Great Neck, NY 11021-5200; **Phone:** 516-478-0008; **Board Cert:** Neurological Surgery 1986; **Med School:** Univ Chicago-Pritzker Sch Med 1976; **Resid:** Surgery, Univ Chicago Hosps 1977; Neurological Surgery, Univ Chicago Hosps 1982

Eisenberg, Mark B MD (NS) - **Spec Exp:** Skull Base Surgery; Spinal Surgery-Minimally Invasive; Pituitary Tumors; Brain Tumors; **Hospital:** Long Is Jewish Med Ctr (page 106); **Address:** 900 Northern Blvd, Ste 260, Great Neck, NY 11021; **Phone:** 516-773-7737; **Board Cert:** Neurological Surgery 2010; **Med School:** Univ Miami Sch Med 1988; **Resid:** Neurological Surgery, Mount Sinai Med Ctr 1994; **Fellow:** Skull Base Surgery, Univ Arkansas Med Ctr 1995; **Fac Appt:** Asst Clin Prof NS, NYU Sch Med

Epstein, Nancy E MD (NS) - **Spec Exp:** Spinal Surgery; Spinal Surgery-Neck; Transfusion Free Surgery; **Hospital:** Winthrop Univ Hosp (page 524); **Address:** 410 Lakeville Rd, Ste 204, New Hyde Park, NY 11042-1199; **Phone:** 516-354-3401; **Board Cert:** Neurological Surgery 1984; **Med School:** Columbia P&S 1976; **Resid:** Neurological Surgery, Bellevue Hosp Ctr-NYU 1981; **Fac Appt:** Clin Prof NS, Albert Einstein Coll Med

Grant, John A MD (NS) - **Spec Exp:** Pediatric Neurosurgery; Epilepsy; **Hospital:** Winthrop Univ Hosp (page 524), Good Samaritan Hosp Med Ctr - West Islip; **Address:** Neurological Surgery, PC, 100 Merrick Rd, Ste 200, Rockville Centre, NY 11570; **Phone:** 516-255-9031; **Board Cert:** Neurological Surgery 1998; **Med School:** Ireland 1985; **Resid:** Surgery, Johns Hopkins Univ Hosp 1987; Neurological Surgery, Columbia Univ Med Ctr 1992; **Fellow:** Pediatric Neurological Surgery, Chldn's Meml Hosp 1993

Holtzman, Robert N MD (NS) - **Spec Exp:** Brain & Spinal Cord Tumors; Spinal Surgery; Aneurysm-Cerebral; Chiari's Deformity; **Hospital:** Winthrop Univ Hosp (page 524); **Address:** 1991 Marcus Ave, Ste 108, Lake Success, NY 11042; **Phone:** 516-442-2250; **Board Cert:** Neurology 1978; Neurological Surgery 1980; **Med School:** Columbia P&S 1969; **Resid:** Surgery, Harbor Genl Hosp 1973; Neurological Surgery, Neurological Inst 1977; **Fac Appt:** Assoc Clin Prof NS, Columbia P&S

Levine, Mitchell E MD (NS) - **Spec Exp:** Brain Tumors; Minimally Invasive Spinal Surgery; Cerebrovascular Surgery; **Hospital:** N Shore Univ Hosp (page 106); **Address:** 900 Northern Blvd, Ste 260, Great Neck, NY 11021; **Phone:** 516-773-7737; **Board Cert:** Neurological Surgery 1987; **Med School:** Mount Sinai Sch Med 1977; **Resid:** Surgery, Mt Sinai Hosp 1978; Neurological Surgery, Mt Sinai Hosp 1983; **Fac Appt:** Asst Prof NS, Mount Sinai Sch Med

Mittler, Mark A MD (NS) - **Spec Exp:** Pediatric Neurosurgery; Brain & Spinal Tumors; Vascular Malformations; Hydrocephalus; **Hospital:** Steven & Alexandra Cohen Chldn's Med Ctr of NY (page 106), N Shore Univ Hosp (page 106); **Address:** LI Neurosurgical Assocs, 410 Lakeville Rd, Ste 204, New Hyde Park, NY 11042; **Phone:** 516-354-3401; **Board Cert:** Neurological Surgery 2012; Pediatric Neurological Surgery 2003; **Med School:** Univ Rochester 1991; **Resid:** Neurological Surgery, Rhode Island Hosp 1998; **Fellow:** Pediatric Neurological Surgery, Chldns Hosp 1999; **Fac Appt:** Asst Prof NS, Hofstra N Shore-LIJ Sch Med

Onesti, Stephen T MD (NS) - **Spec Exp:** Spinal Surgery; Minimally Invasive Spinal Surgery; Spinal Disorders-Degenerative; Pain-Chronic; **Hospital:** South Nassau Comm Hosp; **Address:** 100 Merrick Rd, Rockville Centre, NY 11570; **Phone:** 516-632-7050; **Board Cert:** Neurological Surgery 1995; **Med School:** Harvard Med Sch 1986; **Resid:** Neurological Surgery, Columbia-Presby Med Ctr 1993; **Fellow:** Neurological Science, Columbia-Presby Med Ctr 1988; **Fac Appt:** Prof NS, SUNY Downstate

Rekate, Harold L MD (NS) - **Spec Exp:** Chiari's Deformity; Hydrocephalus; Pediatric Neurosurgery; Brain Tumors; **Hospital:** N Shore Univ Hosp (page 106), Long Is Jewish Med Ctr (page 106); **Address:** The Chiari Institute, 611 Northern Blvd, Ste 150, Great Neck, NY 11021; **Phone:** 516-570-4400; **Board Cert:** Neurological Surgery 1980; **Med School:** Med Coll VA 1970; **Resid:** Neurological Surgery, Univ Hosps-Case West Res 1978; **Fac Appt:** Prof NS, Hofstra N Shore-LIJ Sch Med

Schulder, Michael MD (NS) - **Spec Exp:** Brain Tumors; Movement Disorders; Skull Base Surgery; **Hospital:** N Shore Univ Hosp (page 106), Long Is Jewish Med Ctr (page 106); **Address:** North Shore University Hospital, 300 Community Drive, Tower 9, Manhasset, NY 11030; **Phone:** 516-562-3062; **Board Cert:** Neurological Surgery 1991; **Med School:** Columbia P&S 1982; **Resid:** Neurological Surgery, Montefiore Hosp Med Ctr/Albert Einstein 1988; **Fac Appt:** Assoc Prof NS, UMDNJ-NJ Med Sch, Newark

Neurology

Blanck, Richard H MD (N) - **Spec Exp:** Multiple Sclerosis; Pain-Back; **Hospital:** N Shore Univ Hosp (page 106), St. Francis Hosp - The Heart Ctr (page 116); **Address:** 1991 Marcus Ave, Ste 110, Lake Success, NY 11042; **Phone:** 516-466-4700; **Board Cert:** Internal Medicine 1976; Neurology 1980; **Med School:** UMDNJ-NJ Med Sch, Newark 1973; **Resid:** Internal Medicine, N Shore Univ Hosp 1975; Neurology, N Shore Univ Hosp 1978; **Fac Appt:** Assoc Clin Prof N, NYU Sch Med

Ettinger, Alan MD (N) - **Spec Exp:** Epilepsy; Seizure Disorders; **Hospital:** Winthrop Univ Hosp (page 524), Huntington Hosp (page 106); **Address:** Neurological Surgery, PC, 1991 Marcus Ave, Ste 108, Lake Success, NY 11042; **Phone:** 516-442-2250; **Board Cert:** Neurology 1989; **Med School:** Boston Univ 1983; **Resid:** Internal Medicine, Hartford Hosp 1985; Neurology, Montefiore Med Ctr 1988; **Fellow:** Epilepsy, Montefiore Med Ctr 1989; **Fac Appt:** Prof N, Albert Einstein Coll Med

Gordon, Marc L MD (N) - **Spec Exp:** Dementia; Headache; Multiple Sclerosis; Alzheimer's Disease; **Hospital:** Long Is Jewish Med Ctr (page 106), NS-LIJ Hlth Sys (page 106); **Address:** 611 Northern Blvd, Ste 150, Great Neck, NY 11021-5207; **Phone:** 516-325-7000; **Board Cert:** Neurology 1990; **Med School:** Columbia P&S 1985; **Resid:** Neurology, Jacobi Med Ctr 1989; **Fellow:** Neuropsychopharmacology, Albert Einstein Coll Med 1990; **Fac Appt:** Assoc Prof N, Hofstra N Shore-LIJ Sch Med

Gottesman, Malcolm MD (N) - **Spec Exp:** Multiple Sclerosis; Stroke; **Hospital:** Winthrop Univ Hosp (page 524); **Address:** Winthrop Neuroscience, 200 Old Country Rd, Ste 370, Mineola, NY 11501; **Phone:** 516-663-4525; **Board Cert:** Neurology 1989; Psychiatry 1983; **Med School:** Albany Med Coll 1978; **Resid:** Psychiatry, Boston Med Ctr 1982; Neurology; **Fellow:** Behavioral Medicine, Boston Med Ctr 1983LIJ Med Ctr 1988; **Fac Appt:** Assoc Prof N, SUNY Stony Brook

Haimovic, Itzhak C MD (N) - **Spec Exp:** Spinal Disorders; Epilepsy; Headache; **Hospital:** N Shore Univ Hosp (page 106), Long Is Jewish Med Ctr (page 106); **Address:** 170 Great Neck Rd, Great Neck, NY 11021; **Phone:** 516-487-4464; **Board Cert:** Neurology 1981; Clinical Neurophysiology 2010; **Med School:** NY Med Coll 1975; **Resid:** Internal Medicine, N Shore Univ Hosp 1977; Neurology, NY Hosp-Cornell Univ 1980; **Fac Appt:** Assoc Clin Prof N, NYU Sch Med

Harden, Cynthia L MD (N) - **Spec Exp:** Epilepsy/Seizure Disorders; **Hospital:** Long Is Jewish Med Ctr (page 106), N Shore Univ Hosp (page 106); **Address:** LIJ Cushing Neuroscience Inst, 611 Northern Blvd, Ste 150, Great Neck, NY 11021; **Phone:** 516-325-7060; **Board Cert:** Neurology 1989; **Med School:** Univ Wisc 1983; **Resid:** Internal Medicine, St Luke's Roosevelt Hosp 1985; Neurology, Mt Sinai Hosp 1988; **Fellow:** Clinical Neurophysiology, Albert Einstein Med Coll 1989

Kanner, Ronald M MD (N) - **Spec Exp:** Headache; Pain-Chronic; Migraine; **Hospital:** Long Is Jewish Med Ctr (page 106); **Address:** 611 Northern Blvd, Ste 150, Great Neck, NY 11021; **Phone:** 516-325-7000; **Board Cert:** Neurology 1980; **Med School:** Spain 1975; **Resid:** Internal Medicine, Philadelphia Genl Hosp 1976; Neurology, Montefiore Med Ctr 1979; **Fellow:** Neurology, Meml Sloan-Kettering Cancer Ctr 1981; **Fac Appt:** Prof N, Albert Einstein Coll Med

Kelemen, John MD (N) - **Spec Exp:** Electromyography; Neuromuscular Disorders; Botox for Muscle Overactivity; Dystonia; **Hospital:** Plainview Hosp (page 106); **Address:** Island Neurological Assocs, 824 Old Country Rd, Plainview, NY 11803-4935; **Phone:** 516-822-2230; **Board Cert:** Neurology 1979; **Med School:** Georgetown Univ 1974; **Resid:** Internal Medicine, Nassau County Med Ctr 1978; **Fellow:** Neuromuscular Medicine, New England Med Ctr 1980

Kessler, Jeffrey T MD (N) - **Spec Exp:** Parkinson's Disease; Dementia; Pain-Facial; **Hospital:** N Shore Univ Hosp (page 106), St. Francis Hosp - The Heart Ctr (page 116); **Address:** 1991 Marcus Ave, Ste 110, Lake Success, NY 11042; **Phone:** 516-466-4700; **Board Cert:** Internal Medicine 1974; Neurology 1976; **Med School:** Cornell Univ-Weill Med Coll 1969; **Resid:** Internal Medicine, NY Hosp-Cornell Med Ctr 1971; **Fellow:** Neurology, NY Hosp-Cornell Med Ctr 1974; **Fac Appt:** Assoc Clin Prof N, NYU Sch Med

Kula, Roger W MD (N) - **Spec Exp:** Neuromuscular Disorders; Chiari's Deformity; Syringomyelia & Spinal Cord Diseases; Myasthenia Gravis; **Hospital:** N Shore Univ Hosp (page 106), Steven & Alexandra Cohen Chldn's Med Ctr of NY (page 106); **Address:** 611 Northern Blvd, Ste 150, Great Neck, NY 11021; **Phone:** 516-570-4400 x4; **Board Cert:** Internal Medicine 1975; Neurology 1977; Neuromuscular Medicine 2008; **Med School:** Johns Hopkins Univ 1970; **Resid:** Internal Medicine, New York Hosp 1972; Neurology, UCSF Med Ctr 1974; **Fellow:** Neuromuscular Medicine, Natl Inst Hlth 1977; **Fac Appt:** Assoc Prof N, Hofstra N Shore-LIJ Sch Med

Levy, Lewis A MD (N) - **Spec Exp:** Tourette's Syndrome; Parkinson's Disease; **Hospital:** South Nassau Comm Hosp; **Address:** Long Island Neurology Consultants, 777 Sunrise Hwy, Ste 200, Lynbrook, NY 11563; **Phone:** 516-887-3516; **Board Cert:** Neurology 1979; **Med School:** SUNY Downstate 1973; **Resid:** Neurology, Albert Einstein 1977; **Fac Appt:** Asst Clin Prof N, Albert Einstein Coll Med

Libman, Richard MD (N) - **Spec Exp:** Stroke; **Hospital:** Long Is Jewish Med Ctr (page 106); **Address:** 270-05 76th Ave, Ste M2006, New Hyde Park, NY 11040-1433; **Phone:** 718-470-7311; **Board Cert:** Neurology 1991; Vascular Neurology 2005; **Med School:** McGill Univ 1986; **Resid:** Neurology, Montefiore Med Ctr 1990; **Fellow:** Stroke, Columbia-Presby Med Ctr 1993; **Fac Appt:** Assoc Prof N, Albert Einstein Coll Med

Newman, Stephen M MD (N) - **Spec Exp:** Multiple Sclerosis; Migraine; **Hospital:** Plainview Hosp (page 106); **Address:** Island Neurological Assocs, 824 Old Country Rd, Plainview, NY 11803; **Phone:** 516-822-2230; **Board Cert:** Neurology 1978; **Med School:** SUNY Buffalo 1972; **Resid:** Neurology, Nassau County Med Ctr 1976

Ragone, Philip S MD (N) - **Spec Exp:** Electromyography; **Hospital:** St. Francis Hosp - The Heart Ctr (page 116), N Shore Univ Hosp (page 106); **Address:** 1010 Northern Blvd, Ste 136, Great Neck, NY 11021; **Phone:** 516-482-4100; **Board Cert:** Internal Medicine 1985; Neurology 1989; Electrodiagnostic Medicine 1990; **Med School:** NY Med Coll 1982; **Resid:** Internal Medicine, Lenox Hill Hosp 1985; Neurology, Albert Einstein 1988; **Fellow:** Electromyography, Albert Einstein 1989

Schaul, Neil S MD (N) - **Spec Exp:** Epilepsy/Seizure Disorders; Electrodiagnosis; **Hospital:** NY Hosp Queens (page 488); **Address:** 1575 Hillside Ave, Ste 100, New Hyde Park, NY 11040; **Phone:** 516-616-6286; **Board Cert:** Neurology 1976; **Med School:** SUNY Hlth Sci Ctr 1966; **Resid:** Internal Medicine, DC General Hosp 1968; Neurology, Montreal Neur Inst 1974; **Fellow:** Neurophysiology, Montreal Neur Inst 1977; **Fac Appt:** Assoc Prof Med, Cornell Univ-Weill Med Coll

Turner, Ira MD (N) - **Spec Exp:** Headache; **Hospital:** Plainview Hosp (page 106); **Address:** Island Neurological Assocs, 824 Old Country Rd, Plainview, NY 11803; **Phone:** 516-822-2230; **Board Cert:** Neurology 1978; Headache Medicine 2007; **Med School:** SUNY Downstate 1972; **Resid:** Neurology, Nassau Co Med Ctr 1976

Neuroradiology

Johnson, Alan A MD (NRad) - **Hospital:** Long Is Jewish Med Ctr (page 106); **Address:** 270-05 76th Ave, New Hyde Park, NY 11040; **Phone:** 718-470-7175; **Board Cert:** Neuroradiology 2007; Diagnostic Radiology 2001; **Med School:** SUNY Upstate Med Univ 1996; **Resid:** Diagnostic Radiology, NY Presby Med Ctr 2001; **Fellow:** Neuroradiology, NY Presby Med Ctr 2003

Ortiz, Orlando MD (NRad) - **Spec Exp:** Interventional Neuroradiology; Spine Imaging & Intervention; **Hospital:** Winthrop Univ Hosp (page 524); **Address:** 259 First St, Mineola, NY 11501; **Phone:** 516-663-2123; **Board Cert:** Diagnostic Radiology 1990; Neuroradiology 2006; **Med School:** Harvard Med Sch 1985; **Resid:** Diagnostic Radiology, LIJ Med Ctr 1990; **Fellow:** Neurological Radiology, NY Presby-Columbia Med Ctr 1992; **Fac Appt:** Clin Prof Rad, SUNY Stony Brook

Pile-Spellman, John M MD (NRad) - **Spec Exp:** Interventional Neuroradiology; Cerebrovascular Disease; Aneurysm; Arteriovenous Malformations; **Hospital:** Winthrop Univ Hosp (page 524); **Address:** Neurological Surgery, 1991 Marcus Ave, Ste 108, Lake Success, NY 11042; **Phone:** 516-442-2250; **Board Cert:** Diagnostic Radiology 1984; **Med School:** Tufts Univ 1978; **Resid:** Neurological Surgery, New England Med Ctr 1981; Neurological Radiology, Mass Genl Hosp 1984; **Fellow:** Interventional Neuroradiology, NYU Med Ctr 1986; **Fac Appt:** Prof Rad, Columbia P&S

Setton, Avi MD (NRad) - **Spec Exp:** Cerebrovascular Disease; Stroke; **Hospital:** N Shore Univ Hosp (page 106); **Address:** N Shore Univ Hospital, 300 Community Drive, 9 Tower, Manhasset, NY 11030; **Phone:** 516-562-3021; **Med School:** Israel 1978; **Resid:** Diagnostic Radiology, Bellevue Med Ctr 1991; **Fellow:** Neurological Radiology, NYU Med Ctr 1992

Nuclear Medicine

Palestro, Christopher J MD (NuM) - **Hospital:** Long Is Jewish Med Ctr (page 106), N Shore Univ Hosp (page 106); **Address:** Nuclear Medicine, 270-05 76th Ave, Fl 4, New Hyde Park, NY 11040-1402; **Phone:** 718-470-7080; **Board Cert:** Nuclear Medicine 1982; **Med School:** Mexico 1975; **Resid:** Diagnostic Radiology, Roosevelt Hosp 1980; **Fellow:** Nuclear Medicine, Meml Sloan Kettering Cancer Ctr 1982; **Fac Appt:** Prof Rad, Hofstra N Shore-LIJ Sch Med

Yung, Elizabeth Ying-Kou MD (NuM) - **Spec Exp:** PET Imaging; **Hospital:** Winthrop Univ Hosp (page 524); **Address:** 259 First St, Mineola, NY 11501; **Phone:** 516-663-2778; **Board Cert:** Diagnostic Radiology 1984; Nuclear Radiology 1991; **Med School:** Tufts Univ 1980; **Resid:** Diagnostic Radiology, St Vincent's Hosp & Med Ctr 1984; **Fellow:** Nuclear Medicine, Yale-New Haven Hosp 1991

Obstetrics & Gynecology

Benedict, Leonard A MD (ObG) - **Spec Exp:** Pregnancy-High Risk; Gynecologic Surgery; **Hospital:** N Shore Univ Hosp (page 106); **Address:** 433 Uniondale Ave, Uniondale, NY 11553; **Phone:** 516-483-8798; **Board Cert:** Obstetrics & Gynecology 1981; **Med School:** Scotland, UK 1972; **Resid:** Obstetrics & Gynecology, Brooklyn Jewish Hosp 1978; **Fac Appt:** Asst Clin Prof ObG, NYU Sch Med

Haselkorn, Joan MD (ObG) *PCP* - **Spec Exp:** Laparoscopic Surgery; Hysteroscopic Surgery; Uterine Fibroids; Gynecology Only; **Hospital:** South Nassau Comm Hosp; **Address:** 556 Merrick Rd, Ste 200, Rockville Centre, NY 11570; **Phone:** 516-255-2044; **Board Cert:** Obstetrics & Gynecology 2012; **Med School:** Israel 1982; **Resid:** Obstetrics & Gynecology, NYU Med Ctr 1986

Jacob, Jessica MD (ObG) *PCP* - **Hospital:** N Shore Univ Hosp (page 106); **Address:** 3003 New Hyde Park Rd, Ste 407, New Hyde Park, NY 11042-1214; **Phone:** 516-488-8145; **Board Cert:** Obstetrics & Gynecology 2012; **Med School:** NYU Sch Med 1983; **Resid:** Obstetrics & Gynecology, N Shore Univ Hosp 1987; **Fac Appt:** Asst Clin Prof ObG, NYU Sch Med

Krim, Eileen Y MD (ObG) - **Spec Exp:** Menopause Problems; Adolescent Gynecology; Osteoporosis; Laparoscopic Surgery; **Hospital:** N Shore Univ Hosp (page 106); **Address:** 3111 New Hyde Park Rd, North Hills, NY 11040-3500; **Phone:** 516-365-6100; **Board Cert:** Obstetrics & Gynecology 1982; **Med School:** NY Med Coll 1975; **Resid:** Obstetrics & Gynecology, Beth Israel 1979; **Fellow:** Maternal & Fetal Medicine, N Shore Univ Hosp 1981; **Fac Appt:** Assoc Clin Prof ObG, NYU Sch Med

Leong, Mary MD (ObG) - **Spec Exp:** Pelvic Reconstruction; Menopause Problems; Uterine Fibroids; **Hospital:** Long Is Jewish Med Ctr (page 106); **Address:** Womens Comprehensive Hlth Ctr, 1554 Northern Blvd Fl 5th, Manhasset, NY 11030; **Phone:** 516-390-9242; **Board Cert:** Obstetrics & Gynecology 2012; **Med School:** NYU Sch Med 1978; **Resid:** Obstetrics & Gynecology, Bellevue Hosp Ctr 1982; **Fac Appt:** Asst Prof ObG, Albert Einstein Coll Med

Lind, Lawrence R MD (ObG) - **Spec Exp:** Uro-Gynecology; Pelvic Reconstruction; **Hospital:** N Shore Univ Hosp (page 106), Long Is Jewish Med Ctr (page 106); **Address:** 865 Northern Blvd, Ste 202, Great Neck, NY 11021; **Phone:** 516-622-5114; **Board Cert:** Obstetrics & Gynecology 2012; **Med School:** Cornell Univ-Weill Med Coll 1990; **Resid:** Obstetrics & Gynecology, N Shore Univ Hosp 1994; **Fellow:** Gynecologic Urology, UCLA Med Ctr 1996

Mack, Laurence F MD (ObG) *PCP* - **Spec Exp:** Infertility; Pregnancy-High Risk; Autoimmune Disease in Pregnancy; Pap Smear Abnormalities; **Hospital:** Plainview Hosp (page 106), Mercy Med Ctr - Rockville Centre; **Address:** 1130 N Broadway, North Massapequa, NY 11758-0910; **Phone:** 516-799-3462; **Board Cert:** Obstetrics & Gynecology 2012; **Med School:** Univ Hlth Scis, Chicago Med Sch 1985; **Resid:** Obstetrics & Gynecology, Brookdale Hosp 1989

Nimaroff, Michael L MD (ObG) *PCP* - **Spec Exp:** Laparoscopic Surgery; Hysterectomy Alternatives; Hysteroscopic Surgery; **Hospital:** N Shore Univ Hosp (page 106), Long Is Jewish Med Ctr (page 106); **Address:** 600 Northern Blvd, Ste 212, Great Neck, NY 11021; **Phone:** 516-472-5700; **Board Cert:** Obstetrics & Gynecology 2012; **Med School:** UMDNJ-NJ Med Sch, Newark 1987; **Resid:** Obstetrics & Gynecology, N Shore Univ Hosp 1991; **Fac Appt:** Asst Clin Prof ObG, NYU Sch Med

Salzman, Ronnie M MD (ObG) - **Spec Exp:** Gynecology Only; **Hospital:** Long Is Jewish Med Ctr (page 106); **Address:** Long Island Womens Healthcare Assocs, 2428 Merrick Rd Unit A, Bellmore, NY 11710; **Phone:** 516-379-2689; **Board Cert:** Obstetrics & Gynecology 2012; **Med School:** SUNY Stony Brook 1980; **Resid:** Obstetrics & Gynecology, Mass Genl Hosp 1984

Toles, Allen W MD (ObG) - **Spec Exp:** Pregnancy-High Risk; **Hospital:** Long Is Jewish Med Ctr (page 106); **Address:** 1554 Northern Blvd Fl 5, Manhasset, NY 11030; **Phone:** 516-390-9242; **Board Cert:** Obstetrics & Gynecology 2012; **Med School:** Meharry Med Coll 1986; **Resid:** Obstetrics & Gynecology, Howard Univ Hosp 1990; **Fac Appt:** Asst Prof ObG, Albert Einstein Coll Med

Vasudeva, Kusum MD (ObG) - **Spec Exp:** Pregnancy-High Risk; Menopause Problems; **Hospital:** N Shore Univ Hosp (page 106); **Address:** 2 Ohio Drive, Ste 200, Pro Health Plaza, Lake Success, NY 11042; **Phone:** 516-608-6800; **Board Cert:** Obstetrics & Gynecology 1975; **Med School:** India 1967; **Resid:** Obstetrics & Gynecology, N Shore Univ Hosp 1974; **Fellow:** Maternal & Fetal Medicine, N Shore Univ Hosp 1976

Occupational Medicine

Mendelsohn, Sara L MD (OM) - **Spec Exp:** Travel Medicine; Occupational Disease & Injury; Preventive Medicine; **Address:** 800 Woodbury Rd, Ste K, Woodbury, NY 11797; **Phone:** 516-682-9142; **Board Cert:** Occupational Medicine 1993; **Med School:** Boston Univ 1988; **Resid:** Occupational Medicine, Univ of Illinois Med Ctr 1991; **Fac Appt:** Asst Clin Prof Med, SUNY Stony Brook

Wilkenfeld, Marc MD (OM) - **Spec Exp:** Environmental Medicine; **Hospital:** Winthrop Univ Hosp (page 524); **Address:** 1300 Franklin Ave, Ste UL4A, Garden City, NY 11530; **Phone:** 516-663-8890; **Board Cert:** Occupational Medicine 1991; **Med School:** Univ VT Coll Med 1985; **Resid:** Occupational Medicine, Mt Sinai Med Ctr 1989; **Fac Appt:** Asst Clin Prof OM, Columbia P&S

Ophthalmology

Berke, Stanley J MD (Oph) - **Spec Exp:** Glaucoma; Cataract Surgery-Lens Implant; Laser Surgery; **Hospital:** Long Is Jewish Med Ctr (page 106), Nassau Univ Med Ctr; **Address:** Berke Eye Care, 1600 Stewart Ave, Ste 306, Westbury, NY 11590; **Phone:** 516-794-2020; **Board Cert:** Ophthalmology 1987; **Med School:** SUNY Buffalo 1981; **Resid:** Internal Medicine, Lenox Hill Hosp 1982; Ophthalmology, Nassau Univ Med Ctr 1985; **Fellow:** Glaucoma, Mass Eye & Ear Infirm 1986; Cataract/Lens Implant Surgery, Mass Eye & Ear Infirm 1986; **Fac Appt:** Assoc Clin Prof Oph, Albert Einstein Coll Med

Boniuk, Vivien MD (Oph) - **Spec Exp:** Diagnostic Problems; **Hospital:** Queens Hosp Ctr - Jamaica, Long Is Jewish Med Ctr (page 106); **Address:** 600 Northern Blvd, Ste 214, Great Neck, NY 11021; **Phone:** 516-470-2020; **Board Cert:** Ophthalmology 1969; **Med School:** Dalhousie Univ 1964; **Resid:** Ophthalmology, Barnes Hosp-Washington Univ 1967; **Fellow:** Ophthalmological Pathology, Baylor Coll Affil Hosp 1968; **Fac Appt:** Assoc Prof Oph, Hofstra N Shore-LIJ Sch Med

D'Aversa, Gerard MD (Oph) - **Spec Exp:** Cataract Surgery; Refractive Surgery; Corneal Disease; **Hospital:** Long Is Jewish Med Ctr (page 106); **Address:** Ophthalmic Consultants of LI, 65 Roosevelt Ave, rm 204, Valley Stream, NY 11580-1106; **Phone:** 516-374-4199; **Board Cert:** Ophthalmology 2006; **Med School:** Albert Einstein Coll Med 1989; **Resid:** Internal Medicine, Winthrop Univ Hosp 1990; Ophthalmology, LI Jewish Med Ctr 1993; **Fellow:** Cornea & Ext Eye Disease, Shands Hosp 1994; **Fac Appt:** Asst Prof Oph, Albert Einstein Coll Med

Fastenberg, David M MD (Oph) - **Spec Exp:** Retina/Vitreous Surgery; Macular Degeneration; Diabetic Eye Disease/Retinopathy; **Hospital:** Syosset Hosp (page 106), Long Is Jewish Med Ctr (page 106); **Address:** LI Vitreoretinal Consultants, 600 Northern Blvd, rm 216, Great Neck, NY 11021; **Phone:** 516-466-0390; **Board Cert:** Ophthalmology 1981; **Med School:** NY Med Coll 1976; **Resid:** Ophthalmology, Northwestern Meml Hosp 1980; **Fellow:** Retina, USC-Doheny Eye Inst 1982; **Fac Appt:** Assoc Clin Prof Oph, Albert Einstein Coll Med

Ferrone, Philip J MD (Oph) - **Spec Exp:** Retinal Disorders; Retina/Vitreous Surgery; Retinal Disorders-Pediatric; **Hospital:** Syosset Hosp (page 106), Long Is Jewish Med Ctr (page 106); **Address:** Long Island Vitreoretinal Consultants, 600 Northern Blvd, Ste 216, Great Neck, NY 11021; **Phone:** 516-466-0390; **Board Cert:** Ophthalmology 2006; **Med School:** Harvard Med Sch 1989; **Resid:** Ophthalmology, Duke Univ Eye Ctr 1993; **Fellow:** Vitreoretinal Surgery, Associated Retinal Consultants 1995

Girardi, Anthony MD (Oph) - **Spec Exp:** Cataract Surgery; Glaucoma; **Hospital:** Glen Cove Hosp (page 106); **Address:** 8 Medical Plaza, Ste 201, Glen Cove, NY 11542; **Phone:** 516-676-4596; **Board Cert:** Ophthalmology 1985; **Med School:** SUNY Stony Brook 1980; **Resid:** Ophthalmology, Kings Co Hosp 1984; **Fac Appt:** Asst Clin Prof Oph, SUNY Downstate

Goldberg, Leslie P MD (Oph) - **Spec Exp:** Cataract Surgery; LASIK-Refractive Surgery; Eyelid Cosmetic Surgery; **Hospital:** St. Francis Hosp - The Heart Ctr (page 116), N Shore Univ Hosp (page 106); **Address:** Long Island Eye Surgeons, 1981 Marcus Ave, Ste E115, Lake Success, NY 11042; **Phone:** 516-627-5113; **Board Cert:** Ophthalmology 1977; **Med School:** Ros Franklin Univ/Chicago Med Sch 1970; **Resid:** Ophthalmology, NYU Med Ctr 1976; **Fac Appt:** Asst Clin Prof Oph, NYU Sch Med

Hatsis, Alexander MD (Oph) - **Spec Exp:** LASIK-Refractive Surgery; Cataract Surgery; Corneal Disease & Surgery; Keratoconus; **Hospital:** South Nassau Comm Hosp, Nassau Univ Med Ctr; **Address:** 2 Lincoln Ave, Ste 401, Rockville Centre, NY 11570; **Phone:** 516-763-4106; **Board Cert:** Ophthalmology 2013; **Med School:** Italy 1978; **Resid:** Surgery, Nassau County Med Ctr 1980; Ophthalmology, Nassau County Med Ctr 1981; **Fellow:** Ophthalmology, Nassau County Med Ctr 1983; **Fac Appt:** Asst Clin Prof Oph, SUNY Stony Brook

Kasper, William S MD (Oph) - **Spec Exp:** Cataract Surgery; Glaucoma; Cornea & External Eye Disease; **Hospital:** Winthrop Univ Hosp (page 524), Nassau Univ Med Ctr; **Address:** 520 Franklin Ave, Ste L9, Garden City, NY 11530; **Phone:** 516-742-3937; **Board Cert:** Ophthalmology 1974; **Med School:** Belgium 1967; **Resid:** Ophthalmology, Nassau Univ Med Ctr 1971; **Fac Appt:** Assoc Clin Prof Oph, Belgium

Kodsi, Sylvia R MD (Oph) - **Spec Exp:** Pediatric Ophthalmology; **Hospital:** Long Is Jewish Med Ctr (page 106); **Address:** 600 Northern Blvd, Ste 220, Great Neck, NY 11021; **Phone:** 516-470-2020; **Board Cert:** Ophthalmology 2013; **Med School:** NYU Sch Med 1987; **Resid:** Ophthalmology, St Vincent's Hosp & Med Ctr 1991; **Fellow:** Neuro-Ophthalmology, Mayo Clinic 1992; Pediatric Ophthalmology, U Minn Med Ctr 1993

Malik, Sajid MD (Oph) - **Spec Exp:** Cataract Surgery; Lens Implants-Multifocal; **Hospital:** Winthrop Univ Hosp (page 524); **Address:** Woodbury Optical, 185 Woodbury Rd, Hicksville, NY 11801; **Phone:** 516-681-3937; **Board Cert:** Ophthalmology 2010; **Med School:** SUNY Stony Brook 1989; **Resid:** Ophthalmology, Harlem Hosp 1994

Marks, Alan B MD (Oph) - **Spec Exp:** Cataract Surgery; Laser-Refractive Surgery; Eyelid Cosmetic Surgery; **Hospital:** St. Francis Hosp - The Heart Ctr (page 116), Syosset Hosp (page 106); **Address:** Long Island Eye Surgeons, 1981 Marcus Ave, Ste E115, Lake Success, NY 11042; **Phone:** 516-627-5113; **Board Cert:** Ophthalmology 1983; **Med School:** NY Med Coll 1978; **Resid:** Ophthalmology, N Shore Univ Hosp 1982

Nauheim, Richard MD (Oph) - **Spec Exp:** Corneal Disease; Cataract Surgery; **Hospital:** South Nassau Comm Hosp, NS-LIJ Hlth Sys (page 106); **Address:** 2025 Merrick Ave, Merrick, NY 11566; **Phone:** 516-868-7110; **Board Cert:** Ophthalmology 1989; **Med School:** SUNY Buffalo 1984; **Resid:** Ophthalmology, Nassau Univ Med Ctr 1988; **Fellow:** Cornea & Ext Eye Disease, Eye & Ear Inst - UPMC 1989; **Fac Appt:** Asst Prof Oph, SUNY Stony Brook

Nelson, David B MD (Oph) - **Spec Exp:** Cataract Surgery; **Hospital:** Mercy Med Ctr - Rockville Centre; **Address:** Ophthalmic Consultants of LI, 2000 N Village Ave, Ste 402, Ryan Medical Arts Bldg, Rockville Center, NY 11570-1001; **Phone:** 516-766-2519; **Board Cert:** Ophthalmology 1977; **Med School:** SUNY Hlth Sci Ctr 1972; **Resid:** Internal Medicine, Nassau Co Med Ctr 1973; Ophthalmology, NY Eye & Ear Infirm 1976; **Fac Appt:** Asst Prof Oph, SUNY Stony Brook

Packer, Samuel MD (Oph) - **Spec Exp:** Glaucoma; **Hospital:** N Shore Univ Hosp (page 106), Long Is Jewish Med Ctr (page 106); **Address:** 600 Northern Blvd, Ste 100, Great Neck, NY 11021; **Phone:** 516-465-8400; **Board Cert:** Ophthalmology 1973; **Med School:** SUNY Hlth Sci Ctr 1966; **Resid:** Ophthalmology, Yale-New Haven Hosp 1971; **Fac Appt:** Clin Prof Oph, NYU Sch Med

Perry, Henry D MD (Oph) - **Spec Exp:** Laser-Refractive Surgery; Cornea Transplant; Cataract Surgery; Eyelid/Tear Duct Disorders; **Hospital:** Mercy Med Ctr - Rockville Centre, N Shore Univ Hosp (page 106); **Address:** Ophthalmic Consultants of LI, 2000 N Village Ave, Ste 402, Ryan Medical Arts Bldg, Rockville Centre, NY 11570-1001; **Phone:** 516-766-2519; **Board Cert:** Ophthalmology 1976; **Med School:** Univ Cincinnati 1971; **Resid:** Ophthalmology, Nassau Univ Med Ctr 1975; Ophthalmology, Hosp Univ Penn 1974; **Fellow:** Cornea, Mass Eye & Ear Infirmary 1977; Ophthalmic Pathology, Armed Forces Inst of Pathology 1976; **Fac Appt:** Assoc Clin Prof Oph, Cornell Univ-Weill Med Coll

Prywes, Arnold S MD (Oph) - **Spec Exp:** Glaucoma; Cataract Surgery; **Hospital:** N Shore Univ Hosp (page 106); **Address:** Eye Care Assocs & Glaucoma Consultants of LI, 4212 Hempstead Tpke, Bethpage, NY 11714-5709; **Phone:** 516-731-4800; **Board Cert:** Ophthalmology 1978; **Med School:** Mount Sinai Sch Med 1972; **Resid:** Ophthalmology, Mount Sinai Hosp 1977; **Fellow:** Ophthalmology, Mount Sinai Hosp 1978; **Fac Appt:** Assoc Clin Prof Oph, Albert Einstein Coll Med

Rosenthal, Kenneth J MD (Oph) - **Spec Exp:** Intraocular Lenses; Cataract Surgery; Laser Surgery; Cosmetic Surgery-Face; **Hospital:** New York Eye & Ear Infirm (page 115), St. Francis Hosp - The Heart Ctr (page 116); **Address:** Rosenthal Eye Surgery, 310 E Shore Rd, rm 102, Great Neck, NY 11023; **Phone:** 516-466-8989; **Board Cert:** Ophthalmology 1986; **Med School:** Albany Med Coll 1978; **Resid:** Ophthalmology, N Shore Univ Hosp 1983

Rubin, Laurence MD (Oph) - **Spec Exp:** Cataract Surgery; Intraocular Lenses; Glaucoma; **Hospital:** St. Joseph's Hosp-Nassau, N Shore Univ Hosp (page 106); **Address:** Mid-Island Eye Phys & Surgeons, 4277 Hempstead Tpke, Ste 109, Bethpage, NY 11714-5706; **Phone:** 516-796-4030; **Board Cert:** Ophthalmology 1987; **Med School:** NY Med Coll 1980; **Resid:** Ophthalmology, New York Eye & Ear Infirm 1984

Rubin, Steven E MD (Oph) - **Spec Exp:** Strabismus; Pediatric Ophthalmology; Amblyopia; **Hospital:** N Shore Univ Hosp (page 106), Long Is Jewish Med Ctr (page 106); **Address:** 600 Northern Blvd, Ste 220, Great Neck, NY 11021-5200; **Phone:** 516-465-8444; **Board Cert:** Ophthalmology 1983; **Med School:** SUNY Downstate 1978; **Resid:** Ophthalmology, Univ Penn-Scheie Eye Inst 1982; **Fellow:** Pediatric Ophthalmology, Wills Eye Hosp 1983; **Fac Appt:** Prof Oph, NYU Sch Med

Schlessinger, David A MD (Oph) - **Spec Exp:** Eyelid Cosmetic & Reconstructive Surgery; Oculoplastic Surgery; Neuro-Ophthalmology; **Hospital:** Syosset Hosp (page 106), Winthrop Univ Hosp (page 524); **Address:** 75 Froehlich Farm Blvd, Woodbury, NY 11797; **Phone:** 516-496-2122; **Board Cert:** Ophthalmology 2005; **Med School:** Univ Pittsburgh 1988; **Resid:** Ophthalmology, Interfaith Med Ctr 1992; **Fellow:** Ophthalmic Plastic & Reconstructive Surgery, Univ Minnesota Hosp 1993; Neuro-Ophthalmology, Univ Minnesota Hosp 1993

Sturm, Richard T MD (Oph) - **Spec Exp:** Glaucoma; Cataract Surgery; **Address:** 360 Merrick Rd Fl 3, Lynbrook, NY 11563; **Phone:** 516-593-7709; **Board Cert:** Ophthalmology 1989; **Med School:** NY Med Coll 1983; **Resid:** Ophthalmology, St Luke's-Roosevelt Hosp Ctr 1987; **Fellow:** Glaucoma, Mass Eye & Ear Infirm 1988; **Fac Appt:** Asst Clin Prof Oph, Albert Einstein Coll Med

Svitra, Paul P MD (Oph) - **Spec Exp:** Diabetic Eye Disease/Retinopathy; Macular Degeneration; Retinal Detachment; Retinal Disorders; **Hospital:** N Shore Univ Hosp (page 106), Long Is Jewish Med Ctr (page 106); **Address:** 3003 New Hyde Park Rd, Ste 203, New Hyde Park, NY 11042; **Phone:** 516-327-0505; **Board Cert:** Ophthalmology 1990; **Med School:** Cornell Univ-Weill Med Coll 1984; **Resid:** Ophthalmology, Mass Eye & Ear Infirmary 1989; **Fellow:** Retina/Vitreous Surgery, Duke Eye Ctr 1990; **Fac Appt:** Asst Prof Oph, Cornell Univ-Weill Med Coll

Udell, Ira J MD (Oph) - **Spec Exp:** Cornea Transplant; Corneal Disease; Keratoconus; PROSE Contact Lens; **Hospital:** Long Is Jewish Med Ctr (page 106), N Shore Univ Hosp (page 106); **Address:** LI Jewish Med Ctr, Dept Ophthalmology, 600 Northern Blvd, Ste 214, Great Neck, NY 11021-5200; **Phone:** 516-470-2020; **Board Cert:** Ophthalmology 1980; **Med School:** Tulane Univ 1974; **Resid:** Ophthalmology, LI Jewish Med Ctr 1979; **Fellow:** Cornea, Mass Eye & Ear Infirm 1981; **Fac Appt:** Prof Oph, Hofstra N Shore-LIJ Sch Med

Weinstein, Joseph MD (Oph) - **Spec Exp:** Cataract Surgery; Refractive Surgery; Contact Lenses; Botox Therapy; **Hospital:** N Shore Univ Hosp (page 106), Syosset Hosp (page 106); **Address:** Eye Care Assocs & Glaucoma Consultants of LI, 4212 Hempstead Tpke, Bethpage, NY 11714-5712; **Phone:** 516-731-4800; **Board Cert:** Ophthalmology 1982; **Med School:** Albert Einstein Coll Med 1977; **Resid:** Ophthalmology, Long Island Jewish Med Ctr 1981

Orthopaedic Surgery

Asnis, Stanley E MD (OrS) - **Spec Exp:** Hip Replacement; Knee Replacement; Joint Replacement; **Hospital:** N Shore Univ Hosp (page 106); **Address:** Univ Ortho Assocs, 611 Northern Blvd, Ste 200, Great Neck, NY 11021; **Phone:** 516-723-2663; **Board Cert:** Orthopaedic Surgery 1976; **Med School:** Washington Univ, St Louis 1968; **Resid:** Surgery, NY Hosp 1971; Orthopaedic Surgery, Hosp for Special Surg 1975; **Fellow:** Research, Hosp for Special Surg 1972; **Fac Appt:** Assoc Prof OrS, Albert Einstein Coll Med

Capozzi, James D MD (OrS) - **Spec Exp:** Joint Replacement; Fractures in the Elderly; Arthroscopic Surgery; **Hospital:** Winthrop Univ Hosp (page 524); **Address:** Winthrop Ortho Assocs of Long Island, 1300 Franklin Ave, Ste UL3A/B, Garden City, NY 11530; **Phone:** 516-747-8900; **Board Cert:** Orthopaedic Surgery 2010; **Med School:** Mount Sinai Sch Med 1981; **Resid:** Orthopaedic Surgery, Mount Sinai Hosp 1986; **Fellow:** Joint Replacement Surgery, New England Baptist Hosp 1987; **Fac Appt:** Asst Clin Prof OrS, Mount Sinai Sch Med

D'Agostino, Richard J MD (OrS) - **Spec Exp:** Sports Medicine; Knee Surgery; Shoulder Surgery; Arthroscopic Surgery; **Hospital:** St. Francis Hosp - The Heart Ctr (page 116), N Shore Univ Hosp (page 106); **Address:** Orthopaedic Assocs of Manhasset, 600 Northern Blvd, Ste 300, Great Neck, NY 11021; **Phone:** 516-627-8717; **Board Cert:** Orthopaedic Surgery 2011; **Med School:** Mount Sinai Sch Med 1982; **Resid:** Orthopaedic Surgery, Mt Sinai Med Ctr 1987; **Fellow:** Sports Medicine, New Eng Baptist Hosp 1988; **Fac Appt:** Asst Clin Prof OrS, Albert Einstein Coll Med

Dines, David M MD (OrS) - **Spec Exp:** Shoulder Arthroscopic Surgery; Shoulder Surgery; Shoulder Replacement; Sports Medicine; **Hospital:** Long Is Jewish Med Ctr (page 106), Hosp For Special Surgery (page 113); **Address:** 333 Earl Ovington Blvd, Ste 106, Uniondale, NY 11553; **Phone:** 516-482-1037; **Board Cert:** Orthopaedic Surgery 1980; **Med School:** UMDNJ-NJ Med Sch, Newark 1974; **Resid:** Surgery, NY Hosp-Cornell Med Ctr 1976; Orthopaedic Surgery, Hosp Special Surg 1979; **Fac Appt:** Clin Prof OrS, Albert Einstein Coll Med

Kenan, Samuel MD (OrS) - **Spec Exp:** Bone Tumors; Limb Sparing Surgery; Pediatric Orthopaedic Surgery; Reconstructive Surgery-Complex; **Hospital:** Lenox Hill Hosp (page 106), N Shore Univ Hosp (page 106); **Address:** 1001 Franklin Ave, Ste 110, Garden City, NY 11530; **Phone:** 212-684-5511; **Med School:** Israel 1976; **Resid:** Orthopaedic Surgery, Hadassah Univ Hosp 1984; **Fellow:** Orthopaedic Pathology, Hosp for Joint Diseases 1987; **Fac Appt:** Prof OrS, NYU Sch Med

Kipnis, James MD (OrS) - **Spec Exp:** Knee Surgery; Hip Surgery; Shoulder Surgery; Sports Surgery; **Hospital:** N Shore Univ Hosp (page 106), Long Is Jewish Med Ctr (page 106); **Address:** Orthopaedic Care of Long Island, 1000 Northern Blvd, Ste 110, Great Neck, NY 11021; **Phone:** 516-482-0302; **Board Cert:** Orthopaedic Surgery 2016; **Med School:** UCSF 1986; **Resid:** Surgery, Jacobi Med Ctr 1987; Orthopaedic Surgery, Montefiore Med Ctr 1991

Levitz, Craig L MD (OrS) - **Spec Exp:** Sports Medicine; Shoulder Surgery; Knee Injuries/ACL; Cartilage Damage & Transplant; **Hospital:** South Nassau Comm Hosp; **Address:** Orlin & Cohen Ortho Assocs, 36 Lincoln Ave Fl 3rd, Rockville Centre, NY 11570; **Phone:** 516-536-2800; **Board Cert:** Orthopaedic Surgery 2011; Orthopaedic Sports Medicine 2007; **Med School:** Univ Pennsylvania 1992; **Resid:** Orthopaedic Surgery, Hosp Univ Penn 1997; **Fellow:** Sports Medicine, Amer Sports Med Inst 1998

Mauri, Thomas M MD (OrS) - **Spec Exp:** Spinal Surgery; Scoliosis; Spinal Disc Replacement; **Hospital:** N Shore Univ Hosp (page 106), Long Is Jewish Med Ctr (page 106); **Address:** Univ Ortho Assocs, 611 Northern Blvd, Ste 200, Great Neck, NY 11021; **Phone:** 516-723-2663; **Board Cert:** Orthopaedic Surgery 2009; **Med School:** Albany Med Coll 1980; **Resid:** Neurological Surgery, North Shore Univ Hosp 1982; Orthopaedic Surgery, Hosp for Special Surgery 1985; **Fellow:** Spine Surgery, Rancho Los Amigos Natl Rehab Ctr 1986

Montero, Carlos F MD (OrS) - **Spec Exp:** Hand Surgery; **Hospital:** St. Joseph's Hosp-Nassau, Plainview Hosp (page 106); **Address:** ProHEALTH Care Assocs, 2920 Hempstead Tpke, Ste 7, Levittown, NY 11756; **Phone:** 516-735-4048; **Board Cert:** Orthopaedic Surgery 1974; **Med School:** Argentina 1968; **Resid:** Surgery, Bronx VA Hosp 1970; Orthopaedic Surgery, Nassau County Med Ctr 1974; **Fellow:** Hand Surgery, Nassau County Med Ctr 1975; **Fac Appt:** Asst Clin Prof OrS, SUNY Stony Brook

Rich, Daniel Stephen MD (OrS) - **Spec Exp:** Knee Replacement; Hip Replacement; **Hospital:** Hosp For Special Surgery (page 113), St. Francis Hosp - The Heart Ctr (page 116); **Address:** 585 Plandome Rd, Ste 103, Manhasset, NY 11030-1971; **Phone:** 516-627-1525; **Board Cert:** Orthopaedic Surgery 1984; **Med School:** Harvard Med Sch 1977; **Resid:** Surgery, St Luke's-Roosevelt Hosp Ctr 1979; Orthopaedic Surgery, Hosp for Special Surgery 1982; **Fac Appt:** Asst Clin Prof OrS, Cornell Univ-Weill Med Coll

Seideman, Bruce MD (OrS) - **Spec Exp:** Hip Replacement; Knee Replacement; Arthritis; **Hospital:** St. Francis Hosp - The Heart Ctr (page 116), N Shore Univ Hosp (page 106); **Address:** Orthopaedic Assocs of Manhasset, 600 Northern Blvd, Ste 300, Great Neck, NY 11021; **Phone:** 516-627-8717; **Board Cert:** Orthopaedic Surgery 2010; **Med School:** Albany Med Coll 1981; **Resid:** Orthopaedic Surgery, NY Presby/Columbia Med Ctr 1986; **Fellow:** Joint Replacement Surgery, Mayo Clinic 1987

Sgaglione, Nicholas A MD (OrS) - **Spec Exp:** Sports Medicine; Shoulder Surgery; Elbow Surgery; Arthroscopic Surgery; **Hospital:** N Shore Univ Hosp (page 106), Long Is Jewish Med Ctr (page 106); **Address:** Univ Orthopaedic Assocs, 611 Northern Blvd, Ste 200, Great Neck, NY 11021; **Phone:** 516-723-2663; **Board Cert:** Orthopaedic Surgery 2012; **Med School:** Mount Sinai Sch Med 1983; **Resid:** Surgery, Mt Sinai Med Ctr 1984; Orthopaedic Surgery, Hosp Special Surg 1988; **Fellow:** Sports Medicine, Southern CA Ortho Inst 1989; **Fac Appt:** Prof OrS, Hofstra N Shore-LIJ Sch Med

Shapiro, Jeffrey F MD (OrS) - **Spec Exp:** Knee Surgery; Knee Replacement; **Hospital:** N Shore Univ Hosp (page 106), Long Is Jewish Med Ctr (page 106); **Address:** Orthopaedic Care of Long Island, 1000 Northern Blvd, Ste 110, Great Neck, NY 11021; **Phone:** 516-482-0302; **Board Cert:** Neurology 2009; **Med School:** NY Med Coll 1977; **Resid:** Surgery, Mount Sinai Med Ctr 1978; Orthopaedic Surgery, LIJ Med Ctr 1983

Shebairo, Raymond A MD (OrS) - **Spec Exp:** Arthroscopic Surgery; Shoulder & Knee Surgery; Joint Replacement; Sports Medicine; **Hospital:** Long Is Jewish Med Ctr (page 106); **Address:** 1575 Hillside Ave, Ste 303, New Hyde Park, NY 11040; **Phone:** 516-437-5500; **Board Cert:** Orthopaedic Surgery 1982; **Med School:** Med Coll Wisc 1973; **Resid:** Orthopaedic Surgery, LIJ Med Ctr 1977

Simonson, Barry G MD (OrS) - **Spec Exp:** Sports Medicine; Arthroscopic Surgery; Hip & Knee Reconstruction; Hip & Knee Replacement; **Hospital:** Glen Cove Hosp (page 106), NS-LIJ Hlth Sys (page 106); **Address:** Orthopaedic Assocs of Great Neck, 825 Northern Blvd, Ste 201, Great Neck, NY 11021-5323; **Phone:** 516-773-7500; **Board Cert:** Orthopaedic Surgery 2004; **Med School:** Mount Sinai Sch Med 1984; **Resid:** Surgery, LI Jewish Med Ctr 1986; Orthopaedic Surgery, LI Jewish Med Ctr 1990; **Fellow:** Sports Medicine, New York Univ Med Ctr 1991

Ticker, Jonathan B MD (OrS) - **Spec Exp:** Shoulder Surgery; Shoulder Arthroscopic Surgery; Rotator Cuff Surgery; Sports Medicine; **Hospital:** South Nassau Comm Hosp, Long Is Jewish Med Ctr (page 106); **Address:** Orlin & Cohen Orthopaedic Group, 1728 Sunrise Hwy, Merrick, NY 11566; **Phone:** 516-992-4700; **Board Cert:** Orthopaedic Surgery 2008; **Med School:** UMDNJ-NJ Med Sch, Newark 1988; **Resid:** Orthopaedic Surgery, NY Presby-Columbia Med Ctr 1994; **Fellow:** Shoulder Surgery, NY Presby-Columbia Med Ctr 1991; Sports Medicine & Shoulder Surgery, Univ Pittsburgh 1995; **Fac Appt:** Asst Prof OrS, Columbia P&S

Otolaryngology

Draizin, Dennis L MD (Oto) - **Spec Exp:** Hearing Disorders; Nasal & Sinus Disorders; Voice Disorders; **Hospital:** South Nassau Comm Hosp, Winthrop Univ Hosp (page 524); **Address:** 195 N Village Ave, Ste 1, Rockville Centre, NY 11570-3814; **Phone:** 516-536-7777; **Board Cert:** Otolaryngology 1980; **Med School:** Univ VA Sch Med 1975; **Resid:** Surgery, Northshore Univ Hosp 1977; Otolaryngology, Mt Sinai Sch Med 1980

Durante, Anthony J MD (Oto) - **Hospital:** Winthrop Univ Hosp (page 524); **Address:** 134 Mineola Blvd, Ste 201, Mineola, NY 11501; **Phone:** 516-294-9363; **Board Cert:** Otolaryngology 1975; **Med School:** Italy 1967; **Resid:** Surgery, Nassau Hosp 1970; Otolaryngology, Albert Einstein Coll Med 1975; **Fac Appt:** Asst Clin Prof S, SUNY Stony Brook

Frank, Douglas K MD (Oto) - **Spec Exp:** Head & Neck Cancer & Surgery; Thyroid & Parathyroid Surgery; Salivary Gland Tumors & Surgery; Skull Base Surgery; **Hospital:** Long Is Jewish Med Ctr (page 106), N Shore Univ Hosp (page 106); **Address:** 430 Lakeville Rd, New Hyde Park, NY 11042; **Phone:** 718-470-7552; **Board Cert:** Otolaryngology 1997; **Med School:** Univ Pennsylvania 1990; **Resid:** Surgery, St Vincent Hosp 1992; Otolaryngology, NY Ear & Ear Infirm 1996; **Fellow:** Head and Neck Surgery, UT MD Anderson Cancer Ctr 1997; **Fac Appt:** Assoc Prof Oto, Albert Einstein Coll Med

Gordon, Michael A MD (Oto) - **Spec Exp:** Balance Disorders; Hearing Disorders; Otosclerosis; Ear Surgery; **Hospital:** Long Is Jewish Med Ctr (page 106); **Address:** ENT & Allergy Assocs, 990 Stewart Ave, Ste 610, Garden City, NY 11530; **Phone:** 516-222-1881; **Board Cert:** Otolaryngology 1993; **Med School:** Albert Einstein Coll Med 1986; **Resid:** Surgery, Montefiore Hosp Med Ctr 1988; Otolaryngology, Montefiore Hosp Med Ctr 1992; **Fellow:** Otology & Neurotology, Ear Research Foundation 1993; **Fac Appt:** Asst Prof Oto, Albert Einstein Coll Med

Grosso, John J MD (Oto) - **Spec Exp:** Pediatric Otolaryngology; Otology; **Hospital:** Plainview Hosp (page 106), Syosset Hosp (page 106); **Address:** Long Island ENT Assocs, 875 Old Country Rd, Ste 200, Plainview, NY 11803-4934; **Phone:** 516-931-5552; **Board Cert:** Otolaryngology 1993; **Med School:** SUNY Upstate Med Univ 1986; **Resid:** Otolaryngology, Univ Hosp 1992

Jacono, Andrew A MD (Oto) - **Spec Exp:** Cosmetic Surgery-Face; Rhinoplasty; **Hospital:** Lenox Hill Hosp (page 106), New York Eye & Ear Infirm (page 115); **Address:** 990 5th Ave, New York, NY 10075; **Phone:** 212-570-2500; **Board Cert:** Otolaryngology 2002; Facial Plastic & Reconstr Surgery 2004; **Med School:** Albert Einstein Coll Med 1996; **Resid:** Otolaryngology, New York Eye & Ear Infirmary 2001; **Fellow:** Facial Plastic Surgery, Univ of Rochester 2002; **Fac Appt:** Asst Prof Oto, NY Med Coll

Mattucci, Kenneth MD (Oto) - **Spec Exp:** Otology; Neuro-Otology; Nasal & Sinus Disorders; **Hospital:** St. Francis Hosp - The Heart Ctr (page 116), N Shore Univ Hosp (page 106); **Address:** 29 Barstow Rd, Ste 203, Great Neck, NY 11021; **Phone:** 516-482-7960; **Board Cert:** Otolaryngology 1970; **Med School:** Wake Forest Univ 1964; **Resid:** Surgery, New York Hosp 1966; Otolaryngology, NY Eye & Ear Infirm 1969; **Fellow:** Otolaryngology, New York Hosp 1970; **Fac Appt:** Clin Prof Oto, NY Med Coll

Moisa, Idel I MD (Oto) - **Spec Exp:** Thyroid Surgery; Sinus Disorders; Snoring/Sleep Apnea; Endoscopic Sinus Surgery; **Hospital:** Glen Cove Hosp (page 106); **Address:** Prohealth Care Assocs-Glen Cove ENT, 3 School St, Ste 304, Glen Cove, NY 11542-2548; **Phone:** 516-671-0085; **Board Cert:** Otolaryngology 1988; **Med School:** Albert Einstein Coll Med 1983; **Resid:** Otolaryngology, Montefiore Med Ctr 1988; **Fellow:** Head and Neck Surgery, Montefiore Med Ctr 1989; **Fac Appt:** Asst Clin Prof Oto, NYU Sch Med

Perlman, Philip W MD (Oto) - **Spec Exp:** Pediatric & Adult Otolaryngology; Endoscopic Sinus Surgery; Head & Neck Surgery; Snoring/Sleep Apnea; **Hospital:** St. Francis Hosp - The Heart Ctr (page 116), N Shore Univ Hosp (page 106); **Address:** Progressive Ear, Nose & Throat Assocs, 333 E Shore Rd, Ste 102, Manhasset, NY 11030-2911; **Phone:** 516-466-5100; **Board Cert:** Otolaryngology 1988; Facial Plastic & Reconstr Surgery 1994; **Med School:** SUNY Downstate 1983; **Resid:** Surgery, Staten Island Hosp 1985; Otolaryngology, Albany Meml Hosp 1988; **Fellow:** Facial Plastic & Reconstr Surgery, AAFPRS 1989

Rosner, Louis M MD (Oto) - **Spec Exp:** Rhinoplasty; Endoscopic Sinus Surgery; Head & Neck Cancer; **Hospital:** South Nassau Comm Hosp, Mercy Med Ctr - Rockville Centre; **Address:** 176 N Village Ave, Ste 1A, Rockville Centre, NY 11570-3800; **Phone:** 516-678-0303; **Board Cert:** Otolaryngology 1982; **Med School:** Ros Franklin Univ/Chicago Med Sch 1978; **Resid:** Otolaryngology, NY Eye & Ear Infirm 1982

Setzen, Michael MD (Oto) - **Spec Exp:** Nasal & Sinus Surgery; Rhinoplasty; Sleep Disorders/Apnea; Snoring/Sleep Apnea; **Hospital:** N Shore Univ Hosp (page 106), St. Francis Hosp - The Heart Ctr (page 116); **Address:** 600 Northern Blvd, Ste 312, Great Neck, NY 11021-5200; **Phone:** 516-829-0045; **Board Cert:** Otolaryngology 1982; **Med School:** South Africa 1974; **Resid:** Surgery, Cleveland Clinic Fdn 1978; Otolaryngology, Barnes Jewish Hosp 1982; **Fac Appt:** Assoc Clin Prof Oto, NYU Sch Med

Shikowitz, Mark J MD (Oto) - **Spec Exp:** Pituitary Tumors; Rhinoplasty; Head & Neck Surgery; Facial Plastic Surgery; **Hospital:** Long Is Jewish Med Ctr (page 106), N Shore Univ Hosp (page 106); **Address:** 430 Lakeville Rd, Hearing & Speech Bldg, New Hyde Park, NY 11042; **Phone:** 718-470-7552; **Board Cert:** Otolaryngology 1987; **Med School:** Dominica 1981; **Resid:** Surgery, Maimonides Med Ctr 1982; Otolaryngology, LI Jewish Med Ctr 1986; **Fac Appt:** Prof Oto, Albert Einstein Coll Med

Soletic, Raymond MD (Oto) - **Spec Exp:** Endoscopic Sinus Surgery; Cosmetic Surgery-Face; **Hospital:** St. Francis Hosp - The Heart Ctr (page 116); **Address:** 1615 Northern Blvd, Ste 201, Manhasset, NY 11030; **Phone:** 516-365-7952; **Board Cert:** Otolaryngology 1990; **Med School:** Mexico 1982; **Resid:** Surgery, Baystate/Tufts 1985; Otolaryngology, Manhattan EE&T Hosp 1989

Tawfik, Bernard MD (Oto) - **Spec Exp:** Thyroid Disorders; Sinus Disorders; Snoring/Sleep Apnea; Sleep Disorders/Apnea; **Hospital:** Glen Cove Hosp (page 106); **Address:** Prohealth Care Assocs-Glen Cove ENT, 3 School St, Ste 304, Glen Cove, NY 11542; **Phone:** 516-671-0085; **Board Cert:** Otolaryngology 1977; **Med School:** Johns Hopkins Univ 1971; **Resid:** Surgery, USPHS Hosp 1974; Otolaryngology, Manhattan Eye & Ear 1977

Turk, Jon B MD (Oto) - **Spec Exp:** Facial Plastic & Reconstructive Surgery; Cosmetic Surgery-Face; **Hospital:** N Shore Univ Hosp (page 106); **Address:** 173 Froehlich Farm Blvd, Woodbury, NY 11797; **Phone:** 516-921-8989; **Board Cert:** Otolaryngology ; Facial Plastic & Reconstr Surgery ; **Med School:** SUNY Downstate 1988; **Resid:** Surgery, Mt Sinai Hosp 1990; Otolaryngology, Mt Sinai Hosp 1993; **Fellow:** Facial Plastic Surgery, University Hosp of Bern 1994

Vambutas, Andrea MD (Oto) - **Spec Exp:** Hearing & Balance Disorders; Pediatric Otolaryngology; Cochlear Implants; **Hospital:** Long Is Jewish Med Ctr (page 106), N Shore Univ Hosp (page 106); **Address:** LIJ Med Ctr-Apelian Cochlear Implant Ctr, 430 Lakeville Rd, Hearing & Speech Bldg, New Hyde Park, NY 11042; **Phone:** 718-470-7552; **Board Cert:** Otolaryngology 1998; **Med School:** Albert Einstein Coll Med 1992; **Resid:** Otolaryngology, LIJ Med Ctr 1997; **Fellow:** Otology, Minnesota Ear Head & Neck Clin 1998; **Fac Appt:** Prof Oto, Albert Einstein Coll Med

Youngerman, Jay S MD (Oto) - **Spec Exp:** Pediatric Otolaryngology; Head & Neck Surgery; Sleep & Snoring Disorders; Ear Disorders/Surgery; **Hospital:** Plainview Hosp (page 106), Syosset Hosp (page 106); **Address:** Long Island ENT Assocs, 875 Old Country Rd, Ste 200, Plainview, NY 11803-4934; **Phone:** 516-931-5552; **Board Cert:** Otolaryngology 1984; **Med School:** Med Coll VA 1979; **Resid:** Otolaryngology, LI Jewish Med Ctr 1983

Zahtz, Gerald D MD (Oto) - **Spec Exp:** Sinus Disorders/Surgery; Pediatric Otolaryngology; **Hospital:** Long Is Jewish Med Ctr (page 106), N Shore Univ Hosp (page 106); **Address:** L I Jewish Med Ctr, 270-05 76th Ave, New Hyde Park, NY 11040; **Phone:** 718-470-7552; **Board Cert:** Otolaryngology 1981; **Med School:** St Louis Univ 1977; **Resid:** Surgery, LIJ-Hillside Med Ctr 1978; Otolaryngology, LIJ-Hillside Med Ctr 1981; **Fac Appt:** Assoc Clin Prof Oto, Albert Einstein Coll Med

Zelman, Warren H MD (Oto) - **Spec Exp:** Head & Neck Surgery; Sinus Disorders/Surgery; Pediatric & Adult Otolaryngology; **Hospital:** Winthrop Univ Hosp (page 524); **Address:** 990 Stewart Ave, Ste 610, Garden City, NY 11530; **Phone:** 516-739-3999; **Board Cert:** Otolaryngology 1987; **Med School:** Ros Franklin Univ/Chicago Med Sch 1982; **Resid:** Surgery, Univ Hosp-SUNY 1984; Otolaryngology, Manhattan EE&T Hosp 1987

Pain Medicine

Agin, Carole A MD (PM) - **Spec Exp:** Acupuncture; Complex Regional Pain Syndromes; Pain-Neuropathic; Pain-Back; **Address:** 3 Delaware Drive, Lake Success, NY 11042; **Phone:** 516-622-6105; **Board Cert:** Anesthesiology 1992; Pain Medicine 2004; **Med School:** Ros Franklin Univ/Chicago Med Sch 1986; **Resid:** Anesthesiology, Beth Israel Med Ctr 1990; **Fellow:** Pain Medicine, Meml Sloan Kettering Cancer Ctr 1991

Pinsky, Steven H MD (PM) - **Hospital:** Mercy Med Ctr - Rockville Centre; **Address:** 55 Maple Ave, Ste 106, Rockville Centre, NY 11570; **Phone:** 516-764-4875; **Board Cert:** Anesthesiology 1994; Pain Medicine 2007; **Med School:** Albert Einstein Coll Med 1989; **Resid:** Anesthesiology, SUNY Downstate 1993; **Fellow:** Pain Medicine, St Lukes Roosevelt Med Ctr 1994

Pathology

Crawford, James M MD/PhD (Path) - **Spec Exp:** Liver Pathology; Gastrointestinal Pathology; Gastrointestinal Cancer; **Hospital:** N Shore Univ Hosp (page 106), Long Is Jewish Med Ctr (page 106); **Address:** N Shore-LIJHS Laboratories, 10 Nevada Drive, Lake Success, NY 11042-1114; **Phone:** 516-719-1061; **Board Cert:** Anatomic Pathology 1987; **Med School:** Duke Univ 1982; **Resid:** Pathology, Duke Univ Med Ctr 1983; Pathology, Brigham & Women's Hosp 1987; **Fellow:** Gastrointestinal Pathology, Brigham & Women's Hosp 1987; Research, Royal Free hosp 1989; **Fac Appt:** Prof Path, Hofstra N Shore-LIJ Sch Med

Esposito, Michael John MD (Path) - **Hospital:** N Shore Univ Hosp (page 106); **Address:** 6 Ohio Drive, Ste 202, Lake Success, NY 11042; **Phone:** 516-304-7271; **Board Cert:** Anatomic & Clinical Pathology 1995; **Med School:** NE Ohio Univ 1989; **Resid:** Anatomic & Clinical Pathology, LI Jewish Med Ctr 1994

Kahn, Leonard B MD (Path) - **Spec Exp:** Bone Pathology; Head & Neck Pathology; Soft Tissue Tumors; Jaw Tumors; **Hospital:** Long Is Jewish Med Ctr (page 106), N Shore Univ Hosp (page 106); **Address:** 6 Ohio Drive, Ste 202 - rm 21, Lake Success, NY 10042; **Phone:** 516-304-7264; **Board Cert:** Anatomic Pathology 1980; **Med School:** South Africa 1960; **Resid:** Pathology, Univ Cape Town Affil Hosp 1966; **Fellow:** Surgical Pathology, Washington Univ Affil Hosp 1969; **Fac Appt:** Prof Path, Albert Einstein Coll Med

Pediatric Allergy & Immunology

Bonagura, Vincent R MD (PA&I) - **Hospital:** Long Is Jewish Med Ctr (page 106), NS-LIJ Hlth Sys (page 106); **Address:** 865 Northern Blvd, Ste 101, Great Neck, NY 11021; **Phone:** 516-622-5070; **Board Cert:** Pediatrics 1979; Allergy & Immunology 1981; Clinical & Laboratory Immunology 1986; **Med School:** Columbia P&S 1975; **Resid:** Pediatrics, Columbia Presby Hosp 1978; **Fellow:** Allergy & Immunology, Columbia Presby Hosp 1981; **Fac Appt:** Prof Ped, Hofstra N Shore-LIJ Sch Med

Fagin, James C MD (PA&I) - **Spec Exp:** Asthma; Allergy; Immunodeficiency Disorders; Rhinitis; **Hospital:** N Shore Univ Hosp (page 106); **Address:** Manhasset Allergy & Asthma, 1129 Northern Blvd, Ste 300, Manhasset, NY 11030; **Phone:** 516-365-6077; **Board Cert:** Pediatrics 1980; Allergy & Immunology 1983; **Med School:** Belgium 1976; **Resid:** Pediatrics, N Shore Univ Hosp 1979; **Fellow:** Allergy & Immunology, Chldns Hosp Pittsburgh 1981

Pediatric Cardiology

Better, Donna J MD (PCd) - **Spec Exp:** Echocardiography; Fetal Echocardiography; Congenital Heart Disease; **Hospital:** Winthrop Univ Hosp (page 524), Morgan Stanley Children's Hosp of NY-Presby, NY (page 104); **Address:** 120 Mineola Blvd, Ste 210, Mineola, NY 11501; **Phone:** 516-663-4600; **Board Cert:** Pediatric Cardiology 2011; **Med School:** Albert Einstein Coll Med 1989; **Resid:** Pediatrics, Mt Sinai Hosp 1992; **Fellow:** Pediatric Cardiology, Columbia-Presby Med Ctr 1995

Blaufox, Andrew D MD (PCd) - **Hospital:** Steven & Alexandra Cohen Chldn's Med Ctr of NY (page 106), NS-LIJ Hlth Sys (page 106); **Address:** Steven & Alexandra Cohen Children's Med Ctr, 269-01 76th Ave, New Hyde Park, NY 11040; **Phone:** 718-470-7350; **Board Cert:** Pediatric Cardiology 2008; **Med School:** Albert Einstein Coll Med 1993; **Resid:** Pediatrics, Mt Sinai Med Ctr 1996; **Fellow:** Pediatric Cardiology, Mt Sinai Med Ctr 1999; **Fac Appt:** Clin Prof Ped, Albert Einstein Coll Med

Cooper, Rubin MD (PCd) - **Spec Exp:** Congenital Heart Disease; Rheumatic Heart Disease; Kawasaki Disease; **Hospital:** Steven & Alexandra Cohen Chldn's Med Ctr of NY (page 106), Long Is Jewish Med Ctr (page 106); **Address:** Steven & Alexandra Cohen Chldns Med Ctr, 269-01 76th Ave, Ste 139, New Hyde Park, NY 11040; **Phone:** 718-470-3661; **Board Cert:** Pediatrics 1976; Pediatric Cardiology 1979; **Med School:** NY Med Coll 1971; **Resid:** Pediatrics, Strong Meml Hosp 1976; **Fellow:** Pediatric Cardiology, Strong Meml Hosp 1979; **Fac Appt:** Prof Ped, Cornell Univ-Weill Med Coll

Levchuck, Sean G MD (PCd) - **Spec Exp:** Interventional Cardiology; Congenital Heart Disease; Atrial Septal Defect; **Hospital:** St. Francis Hosp - The Heart Ctr (page 116), Steven & Alexandra Cohen Chldn's Med Ctr of NY (page 106); **Address:** 100 Port Washington Blvd, Ste 108, Roslyn, NY 11576-1353; **Phone:** 516-365-3340; **Board Cert:** Pediatrics 2008; Pediatric Cardiology 2011; **Med School:** Grenada 1989; **Resid:** Pediatrics, Winthrop Univ Hosp 1992; **Fellow:** Pediatric Cardiology, St Christophers Hosp 1995

Luxenberg, Douglas M DO (PCd) - **Spec Exp:** Echocardiography; Congenital Heart Disease; **Hospital:** St. Francis Hosp - The Heart Ctr (page 116); **Address:** St Francis Hosp, Ped Cardiology, 100 Port Washington Blvd, Ste 108, Roslyn, NY 11576; **Phone:** 516-365-3340; **Board Cert:** Pediatrics 2012; Pediatric Cardiology 2006; **Med School:** Philadelphia Coll Osteo Med 1999; **Resid:** Pediatrics, Winthrop Univ Hosp 2003; **Fellow:** Pediatric Cardiology, St Christophers Hosp Chldn 2004; Pediatric Cardiology, Univ Chicago Med Ctr 2006

Montoya-Iraheta, Carlos MD (PCd) - **Spec Exp:** Congenital Heart Disease; **Hospital:** Winthrop Univ Hosp (page 524); **Address:** Winthrop Pediatric Assocs, 120 Mineola Blvd, Ste 210, Mineola, NY 11501; **Phone:** 516-663-4600; **Board Cert:** Pediatrics 1999; Pediatric Cardiology 2008; **Med School:** Guatemala 1982; **Resid:** Pediatrics, SUNY Downstate Med Ctr 1987; **Fellow:** Pediatric Cardiology, NY-Presby-Cornell Med Ctr 1992; **Fac Appt:** Asst Prof Ped, Columbia P&S

Romano, Angela MD (PCd) - **Spec Exp:** Echocardiography; Marfan's Syndrome; Kawasaki Disease; **Hospital:** Steven & Alexandra Cohen Chldn's Med Ctr of NY (page 106); **Address:** Dept Pediatric Cardiology, 269-01 76th Ave, New Hyde Park, NY 11040; **Phone:** 718-470-7350; **Board Cert:** Pediatrics 1984; Pediatric Cardiology 2010; **Med School:** Columbia P&S 1980; **Resid:** Pediatrics, Babies Hosp/Columbia Univ Med Ctr 1984; **Fellow:** Pediatric Cardiology, Children's Hosp 1987; **Fac Appt:** Asst Prof Ped, Albert Einstein Coll Med

Schiff, Russell J MD (PCd) - **Spec Exp:** Echocardiography; Fetal Echocardiography; Cardiomyopathy; Congenital Heart Disease; **Hospital:** Huntington Hosp (page 106), Steven & Alexandra Cohen Chldn's Med Ctr of NY (page 106); **Address:** 43 Crossways Park Drive W, Woodbury, NY 11797; **Phone:** 516-992-5205; **Board Cert:** Pediatrics 1986; Pediatric Cardiology 2010; **Med School:** SUNY Stony Brook 1981; **Resid:** Pediatrics, Long Island Jewish Med Ctr 1984; **Fellow:** Pediatric Cardiology, Long Island Jewish Med Ctr 1986

Shapir, Yehuda MD (PCd) - **Spec Exp:** Congenital Heart Disease & Acquired; Echocardiography; Fetal Echocardiography; **Hospital:** Steven & Alexandra Cohen Chldn's Med Ctr of NY (page 106); **Address:** Steven & Alexandra Cohen Chldn's Med Ctr, 269-01 76th Ave, New Hyde Park, NY 11040-1433; **Phone:** 718-470-7350; **Board Cert:** Pediatric Cardiology 2013; **Med School:** Israel 1977; **Resid:** Pediatrics, Rambam Med Ctr 1981; **Fellow:** Pediatric Cardiology, UCLA Med Ctr 1985

Vallone, Ambrose M MD (PCd) - **Spec Exp:** Cardiac Catheterization; Syncope; Fetal Echocardiography; **Hospital:** St. Francis Hosp - The Heart Ctr (page 116), NS-LIJ Hlth Sys (page 106); **Address:** 100 Port Washington Blvd, Ste 108, Roslyn, NY 11576-1353; **Phone:** 516-365-3340; **Board Cert:** Pediatrics 1983; Pediatric Cardiology 2010; **Med School:** Johns Hopkins Univ 1977; **Resid:** Pediatrics, Johns Hopkins Hosp 1980; **Fellow:** Pediatric Cardiology, Yale-New Haven Hosp 1983; Pediatric Critical Care Medicine, Yale-New Haven Hosp 1983

Pediatric Endocrinology

Accacha, Siham D MD (PEn) - **Spec Exp:** Diabetes; Growth Disorders; Metabolic Syndrome; **Hospital:** Winthrop Univ Hosp (page 524); **Address:** 120 Mineola Blvd, Ste 210, Mineola, NY 11501; **Phone:** 516-663-4600; **Board Cert:** Pediatric Endocrinology 2013; **Med School:** France 1993; **Resid:** Pediatrics, Westchester Med Ctr 2001; **Fellow:** Pediatric Endocrinology, Winthrop Univ Hosp 2005

Carey, Dennis E MD (PEn) - **Spec Exp:** Diabetes; Calcium Disorders; Growth Disorders; Thyroid Disorders; **Hospital:** Steven & Alexandra Cohen Chldn's Med Ctr of NY (page 106); **Address:** 1991 Marcus Ave, Ste M100, Lake Success, NY 11042-2057; **Phone:** 516-472-3750; **Board Cert:** Pediatrics 1979; Pediatric Endocrinology 1983; **Med School:** SUNY Downstate 1973; **Resid:** Pediatric Surgery, LI Jewish Med Ctr 1976; **Fellow:** Pediatric Endocrinology, UCSD Med Ctr 1979

Castro-Magana, Mariano MD (PEn) - **Spec Exp:** Growth/Development Disorders; Adrenal Disorders; Sexual Development Problems; **Hospital:** Winthrop Univ Hosp (page 524); **Address:** Winthrop Univ Hosp, Div Ped Endo, 120 Mineola Blvd, Ste 210, Mineola, NY 11501; **Phone:** 516-663-4600 x2; **Board Cert:** Pediatrics 1983; Pediatric Endocrinology 1983; **Med School:** El Salvador 1974; **Resid:** Pediatrics, Nassau County Med Ctr 1980; **Fellow:** Pediatric Endocrinology, Nassau County Med Ctr 1982; **Fac Appt:** Clin Prof Ped, SUNY Stony Brook

Frank, Graeme R MD (PEn) - **Spec Exp:** Pubertal Disorders; Growth/Development Disorders; Diabetes; Thyroid Disorders; **Hospital:** Steven & Alexandra Cohen Chldn's Med Ctr of NY (page 106); **Address:** 1991 Marcus Ave, Ste M100, Lake Success, NY 11042-2057; **Phone:** 516-472-3750; **Board Cert:** Pediatrics 2005; Pediatric Endocrinology 2010; **Med School:** South Africa 1982; **Resid:** Pediatrics, LIJ-Schneider Chldns Hosp 1991; **Fellow:** Pediatric Endocrinology, Children's Hosp 1994

Kreitzer, Paula MD (PEn) - **Spec Exp:** Diabetes; Growth/Development Disorders; **Hospital:** Steven & Alexandra Cohen Chldn's Med Ctr of NY (page 106), Long Is Jewish Med Ctr (page 106); **Address:** 1991 Marcus Ave, Ste M100, Lake Success, NY 11042-2057; **Phone:** 516-472-3750; **Board Cert:** Pediatrics 1987; Pediatric Endocrinology 2011; **Med School:** Univ NC Sch Med 1982; **Resid:** Pediatrics, LIJ-Schneider Chldns Hosp 1987; **Fellow:** Pediatric Endocrinology, LIJ-Schneider Chldns Hosp 1989

Speiser, Phyllis W MD (PEn) - **Spec Exp:** Pubertal Disorders; Growth/Development Disorders; Adrenal Disorders; Thyroid Disorders; **Hospital:** Steven & Alexandra Cohen Chldn's Med Ctr of NY (page 106), N Shore Univ Hosp (page 106); **Address:** 1991 Marcus Ave, Ste M100, Div Ped Endocrinology, Lake Success, NY 11042-2057; **Phone:** 516-472-3750; **Board Cert:** Pediatrics 1984; Pediatric Endocrinology 1986; **Med School:** Columbia P&S 1979; **Resid:** Pediatrics, Jacobi Med Ctr 1982; **Fellow:** Pediatric Endocrinology, New York Hosp-Cornell 1984; **Fac Appt:** Prof Ped, Hofstra N Shore-LIJ Sch Med

Pediatric Gastroenterology

Daum, Fredric MD (PGe) - **Spec Exp:** Inflammatory Bowel Disease; Liver Disease; Incontinence-Fecal; **Hospital:** Winthrop Univ Hosp (page 524); **Address:** 120 Mineola Blvd, Ste 210, Mineola, NY 11501; **Phone:** 516-663-4600; **Board Cert:** Pediatrics 1972; Pediatric Gastroenterology 2012; **Med School:** Tufts Univ 1967; **Resid:** Pediatrics, Jacobi Med Ctr 1969; **Fellow:** Adolescent Medicine, Montefiore Med Ctr 1972

Markowitz, James MD (PGe) - **Spec Exp:** Inflammatory Bowel Disease/Crohn's; Gastroesophageal Reflux Disease (GERD); **Hospital:** Steven & Alexandra Cohen Chldn's Med Ctr of NY (page 106); **Address:** Pediatric Gastroenterology, 1991 Marcus Ave, Ste M100, Lake Success, NY 11042; **Phone:** 516-472-3650; **Board Cert:** Pediatrics 1981; Pediatric Gastroenterology 2005; **Med School:** Cornell Univ-Weill Med Coll 1977; **Resid:** Pediatrics, NY Hosp 1980; **Fellow:** Pediatric Gastroenterology, N Shore Univ Hosp 1983

Pettei, Michael J MD/PhD (PGe) - **Spec Exp:** Cholesterol/Lipid Disorders; Nutrition; Celiac Disease; **Hospital:** Steven & Alexandra Cohen Chldn's Med Ctr of NY (page 106); **Address:** Pediatric Gastroenterology, 1991 Marcus Ave, Ste M100, Lake Success, NY 11042; **Phone:** 516-472-3650; **Board Cert:** Pediatrics 1986; Pediatric Gastroenterology 2012; **Med School:** Univ Miami Sch Med 1980; **Resid:** Pediatrics, Mt Sinai Med Ctr 1982; **Fellow:** Pediatric Gastroenterology, Columbia-Presby Med Ctr 1984

Weinstein, Toba MD (PGe) - **Spec Exp:** Inflammatory Bowel Disease/Crohn's; Gastroesophageal Reflux Disease (GERD); Irritable Bowel Syndrome; Constipation; **Hospital:** Steven & Alexandra Cohen Chldn's Med Ctr of NY (page 106); **Address:** 1991 Marcus Ave, Ste M100, Lake Success, NY 11042; **Phone:** 516-472-3650; **Board Cert:** Pediatrics 2007; Pediatric Gastroenterology 2007; **Med School:** Columbia P&S 1986; **Resid:** Pediatrics, Chldn's Hosp Natl Med Ctr 1989; **Fellow:** Pediatric Gastroenterology, Schneider Children's Hosp-LIJ 1991; **Fac Appt:** Assoc Prof Ped, Hofstra N Shore-LIJ Sch Med

Pediatric Hematology-Oncology

Atlas, Mark MD (PHO) - **Spec Exp:** Hematologic Malignancies; Bone Marrow Transplant; Thalassemia; Brain Tumors; **Hospital:** Steven & Alexandra Cohen Chldn's Med Ctr of NY (page 106); **Address:** CCMC, Ped Hem/Onc Dept, 269-01 76 Ave, rm 253, New Hyde Park, NY 11040; **Phone:** 718-470-3460; **Board Cert:** Pediatric Hematology-Oncology 2013; Pediatrics 2007; **Med School:** Albert Einstein Coll Med 1989; **Resid:** Pediatrics, Chldns Hosp 1992; **Fellow:** Pediatric Hematology-Oncology, Northwestern Meml Hosp 1996

Lipton, Jeffrey M MD/PhD (PHO) - **Spec Exp:** Bone Marrow Failure Disorders; Stem Cell Transplant; Bone Marrow Transplant; **Hospital:** Steven & Alexandra Cohen Chldn's Med Ctr of NY (page 106), N Shore Univ Hosp (page 106); **Address:** Steven & Alexandra Chldns Med Ctr NY, Pediatric Hema/Onc Dept, 269-01 76th Ave, New Hyde Park, NY 11040-1433; **Phone:** 718-470-3460; **Board Cert:** Pediatrics 1981; **Med School:** St Louis Univ 1975; **Resid:** Pediatrics, Boston Chldns Hosp 1978; **Fellow:** Pediatric Hematology-Oncology, Boston Chldns Hosp/Dana Farber Cancer Inst 1981; **Fac Appt:** Prof Ped, Hofstra N Shore-LIJ Sch Med

Redner, Arlene S MD (PHO) - **Spec Exp:** Leukemia; Brain Tumors; Solid Tumors; Neuro-Oncology; **Hospital:** Steven & Alexandra Cohen Chldn's Med Ctr of NY (page 106); **Address:** 269-01 76th Ave, rm 255, New Hyde Park, NY 11040-1434; **Phone:** 718-470-3460; **Board Cert:** Pediatrics 1982; Pediatric Hematology-Oncology 1984; **Med School:** Univ Pennsylvania 1977; **Resid:** Pediatrics, Boston Floating Hosp 1980; **Fellow:** Pediatric Hematology-Oncology, Meml Sloan Kettering Hosp 1985; **Fac Appt:** Prof Ped, Hofstra N Shore-LIJ Sch Med

Sabatino, Dominick P MD (PHO) - **Spec Exp:** Cooley's Anemia; Thalassemia; Sickle Cell Disease; **Hospital:** Nassau Univ Med Ctr; **Address:** Nassau Univ Med Ctr, Dept Peds, 2201 Hempstead Tpke, East Meadow, NY 11554; **Phone:** 516-572-6177; **Board Cert:** Pediatrics 1975; Pediatric Hematology-Oncology 1982; **Med School:** Italy 1968; **Resid:** Pediatrics, LI College Hosp 1973; **Fellow:** Pediatric Hematology-Oncology, LI College Hosp 1975

Weinblatt, Mark E MD (PHO) - **Spec Exp:** Leukemia & Lymphoma; Sickle Cell Disease; Bleeding/Coagulation Disorders; Thalassemia; **Hospital:** Winthrop Univ Hosp (page 524); **Address:** 120 Mineola Blvd, Ste 460, Mineola, NY 11501; **Phone:** 516-663-9400; **Board Cert:** Pediatrics 1980; Pediatric Hematology-Oncology 1982; **Med School:** Albert Einstein Coll Med 1976; **Resid:** Pediatrics, Jacobi Med Ctr 1979; **Fellow:** Pediatric Hematology-Oncology, Children's Hosp 1981; **Fac Appt:** Prof Ped, SUNY Stony Brook

Wolfe, Lawrence C MD (PHO) - **Spec Exp:** Palliative Care; Neuroblastoma; Adrenal Cancer; Congenital Hemolytic Anemia; **Hospital:** Steven & Alexandra Cohen Chldn's Med Ctr of NY (page 106); **Address:** Steven & Alexandra Cohen Chldn's Med Ctr, Div Pediatric Hematology/Oncology, 269-01 76th Ave, New Hyde Park, NY 11040; **Phone:** 718-470-3460; **Board Cert:** Pediatrics 1981; Pediatric Hematology-Oncology 1987; Hospice & Palliative Medicine 2010; **Med School:** Harvard Med Sch 1976; **Resid:** Pediatrics, Chldns Hosp 1978; **Fellow:** Pediatric Hematology-Oncology, Chldns Hosp 1991; **Fac Appt:** Prof Ped

Pediatric Infectious Disease

Krilov, Leonard R MD (PInf) - **Spec Exp:** Infections-Respiratory; Infections in Int'l Adopted Children; Chronic Fatigue Syndrome; Lyme Disease; **Hospital:** Winthrop Univ Hosp (page 524), Good Samaritan Hosp Med Ctr - West Islip; **Address:** 120 Mineola Blvd, Ste 210, Mineola, NY 11501; **Phone:** 516-663-9414; **Board Cert:** Pediatrics 1983; Pediatric Infectious Disease 2009; **Med School:** Columbia P&S 1978; **Resid:** Pediatrics, Johns Hopkins Hosp 1981; **Fellow:** Pediatric Infectious Disease, Children's Hosp 1984; **Fac Appt:** Prof Ped, SUNY Stony Brook

Rubin, Lorry G MD (PInf) - **Spec Exp:** Kawasaki Disease; Tuberculosis; Fevers of Unknown Origin; **Hospital:** Steven & Alexandra Cohen Chldn's Med Ctr of NY (page 106), N Shore Univ Hosp (page 106); **Address:** 269-01 76th Ave, Div Infectious Disease, New Hyde Park, NY 11040-1433; **Phone:** 718-470-3480; **Board Cert:** Pediatrics 1983; Pediatric Infectious Disease 2009; **Med School:** Rush Med Coll 1978; **Resid:** Pediatrics, Children's Hosp 1980; **Fellow:** Pediatric Infectious Disease, Johns Hopkins Hosp 1982

Sood, Sunil K MD (PInf) - **Spec Exp:** Fevers of Unknown Origin; Tuberculosis; Lyme Disease; **Hospital:** Steven & Alexandra Cohen Chldn's Med Ctr of NY (page 106); **Address:** 269-01 76th Ave, New Hyde Park, NY 11040-1433; **Phone:** 718-470-3480; **Board Cert:** Pediatrics 1987; Pediatric Infectious Disease 2009; **Med School:** India 1976; **Resid:** Pediatrics, Mercy Med Ctr 1983; Pediatrics, Georgetown Univ Hosp 1985; **Fellow:** Infectious Disease, Tulane Univ 1988; **Fac Appt:** , Albert Einstein Coll Med

Pediatric Otolaryngology

Mendelsohn, Michael G MD (PO) - **Hospital:** Long Is Jewish Med Ctr (page 106); **Address:** 990 Stewart Ave, Ste 610, Garden City, NY 11530; **Phone:** 516-222-1881; **Board Cert:** Otolaryngology 1999; **Med School:** Boston Univ 1990; **Resid:** Otolaryngology, LI Jewish Med Ctr 1995; **Fellow:** Pediatric Otolaryngology, Univ Virginia Med Ctr 1996; **Fac Appt:** Asst Prof Oto, SUNY Downstate

Smith, Lee P MD (PO) - **Spec Exp:** Airway Disorders; Head & Neck Tumors; Tonsil/Adenoid Disorders; Ear Infections; **Hospital:** Steven & Alexandra Cohen Chldn's Med Ctr of NY (page 106), Long Is Jewish Med Ctr (page 106); **Address:** Steven and Alexandra Cohen Childrens Medical Center, Pediatric Otolaryngology, 430 Lakeville Rd, New Hyde Park, NY 11042; **Phone:** 718-470-7550; **Board Cert:** Otolaryngology 2008; **Med School:** NYU Sch Med 2002; **Resid:** Otolaryngology, Jackson Memorial Hosp 2007; **Fellow:** Pediatric Otolaryngology, Chldns Hosp 2009; **Fac Appt:** Asst Prof Oto, Hofstra N Shore-LIJ Sch Med

Pediatric Pulmonology

Pirzada, Melodi MD (PPul) - **Spec Exp:** Asthma; Cystic Fibrosis; Breathing Disorders; **Hospital:** Winthrop Univ Hosp (page 524); **Address:** Winthrop Pediatric Assocs, 120 Mineola Blvd, Ste 210, Mineola, NY 11501; **Phone:** 516-663-4600; **Board Cert:** Pediatrics 2007; Pediatric Pulmonology 2009; **Med School:** Turkey 1986; **Resid:** Pediatrics, Winthrop Univ Hosp 1991; **Fellow:** Pediatric Pulmonology, NY-Presby-Weill Cornell Med Ctr 1994

Schaeffer, Janis I MD (PPul) - **Spec Exp:** Asthma; Cough-Chronic; Lung Disorders-Congenital; **Hospital:** Steven & Alexandra Cohen Chldn's Med Ctr of NY (page 106), N Shore Univ Hosp (page 106); **Address:** 3003 New Hyde Park Rd, Ste 204, New Hyde Park, NY 11042-1214; **Phone:** 516-488-7575; **Board Cert:** Pediatrics 1984; Pediatric Pulmonology 2011; **Med School:** SUNY Downstate 1979; **Resid:** Pediatrics, LI Jewish Med Ctr 1982; **Fellow:** Pediatric Pulmonology, Columbia-Presby Med Ctr 1985; **Fac Appt:** Asst Prof Ped, Albert Einstein Coll Med

Pediatric Rheumatology

Gottlieb, Beth S MD (PRhu) - **Spec Exp:** Juvenile Arthritis; Lupus/SLE; Osteoarthritis; Dermatomyositis; **Hospital:** Steven & Alexandra Cohen Chldn's Med Ctr of NY (page 106), NS-LIJ Hlth Sys (page 106); **Address:** 1991 Marcus Ave, Ste M100, Lake Success, NY 11042; **Phone:** 516-472-3700; **Board Cert:** Pediatrics 2010; Pediatric Rheumatology 2013; **Med School:** Israel 1992; **Resid:** Pediatrics, Long Island Jewish Med Ctr 1995; **Fellow:** Pediatric Rheumatology, Long Island Jewish Med Ctr 1998

Pediatric Surgery

Coren, Charles V MD (PS) - **Hospital:** Winthrop Univ Hosp (page 524), NY Hosp Queens (page 488); **Address:** 320 Post Ave, Ste 101, Westbury, NY 11590; **Phone:** 516-997-1199; **Board Cert:** Pediatric Surgery 2005; **Med School:** Univ Cincinnati 1978; **Resid:** Surgery, NYU Med Ctr 1983; **Fellow:** Pediatric Surgery, Univ Hosp 1985; **Fac Appt:** Asst Clin Prof S, SUNY Hlth Sci Ctr

Dolgin, Stephen E MD (PS) - **Spec Exp:** Neonatal Surgery; Ulcerative Colitis; Inflammatory Bowel Disease/Crohn's; Ovarian Masses in Children/Adolescents; **Hospital:** Steven & Alexandra Cohen Chldn's Med Ctr of NY (page 106), N Shore Univ Hosp (page 106); **Address:** Cohen Chldn's Med Ctr, Dept Ped Surg, 269-01 76th Ave, Ste 171, New Hyde Park, NY 11040; **Phone:** 718-470-3636; **Board Cert:** Surgery 2011; Pediatric Surgery 2003; **Med School:** NYU Sch Med 1977; **Resid:** Surgery, Peter Bent Brigham Hosp/Harvard Univ 1982; **Fellow:** Pediatric Surgery, Chldns Meml Hosp/Northwestern Univ 1984; **Fac Appt:** Prof S, Hofstra N Shore-LIJ Sch Med

Hong, Andrew MD (PS) - **Spec Exp:** Neonatal Surgery; Minimally Invasive Surgery; Chest Wall Deformities; **Hospital:** Steven & Alexandra Cohen Chldn's Med Ctr of NY (page 106), N Shore Univ Hosp (page 106); **Address:** Cohen Chldns Med Ctr, 269-01 76th Ave, Ste CH158, New Hyde Park, NY 11040; **Phone:** 718-470-3636; **Board Cert:** Surgery 2012; Pediatric Surgery 2011; **Med School:** Univ Wisc 1985; **Resid:** Surgery, Med Ctr Hosp 1990; **Fellow:** Pediatric Surgery, Montreal Chldns Hosp 1992; **Fac Appt:** Asst Prof S, Hofstra N Shore-LIJ Sch Med

Parnell, Vincent MD (PS) - **Spec Exp:** Pediatric Cardiothoracic Surgery; Congenital Heart Disease; **Hospital:** Steven & Alexandra Cohen Chldn's Med Ctr of NY (page 106), N Shore Univ Hosp (page 106); **Address:** Steven & Alexandra Cohen Chldn's Med Ctr, Ped Cardiothoracic Surgery, 269-01 76th Ave, New Hyde Park, NY 11040; **Phone:** 718-470-3580; **Board Cert:** Surgery 2000; Thoracic & Cardiac Surgery 2002; Congenital Cardiac Surgery 2011; **Med School:** SUNY Downstate 1976; **Resid:** Surgery, N Shore Univ Hosp 1981; Thoracic Surgery, Harper Hosp 1983; **Fellow:** Pediatric Cardiac Surgery, Chldns Hosp 1984

Pediatric Urology

Gitlin, Jordan MD (Ped Uro) - **Spec Exp:** Reconstructive Surgery; **Hospital:** Steven & Alexandra Cohen Chldn's Med Ctr of NY (page 106); **Address:** Pediatric Urology Associates, 1999 Marcus Ave, M18, Lake Success, NY 11042; **Phone:** 516-466-6953; **Board Cert:** Urology 2008; Pediatric Urology ; **Med School:** SUNY Upstate Med Univ 1994; **Resid:** Urology, NYU Med Ctr 2001; **Fellow:** Pediatric Urology, Riley Chldn's Hosp 2002

Pediatrics

Adesman, Andrew MD (Ped) - **Spec Exp:** Autism; Asperger's Syndrome; Developmental Disorders; Tourette's Syndrome; **Hospital:** Steven & Alexandra Cohen Chldn's Med Ctr of NY (page 106); **Address:** 1983 Marcus Ave Fl 1 - Ste 130, Lake Success, NY 11042; **Phone:** 516-802-6100; **Board Cert:** Pediatrics 1987; Neurodevelopmental Disabilities 2012; Developmental-Behavioral Pediatrics 2010; **Med School:** Univ Pennsylvania 1981; **Resid:** Pediatrics, Chldn's Hosp Natl Med Ctr 1984; **Fellow:** Developmental-Behavioral Pediatrics, Chldn's Hosp 1986; **Fac Appt:** Assoc Prof Ped, Albert Einstein Coll Med

Amer, Jeffrey A MD (Ped) *PCP* - **Hospital:** Winthrop Univ Hosp (page 524), Long Is Jewish Med Ctr (page 106); **Address:** 38 S Oyster Bay Rd, Syosset, NY 11791; **Phone:** 516-682-0555; **Board Cert:** Pediatrics 2009; **Med School:** Jefferson Med Coll 1981; **Resid:** Pediatrics, Bronx Municipal Hosp 1984

Chianese, Maurice J MD (Ped) *PCP* - **Spec Exp:** Pediatric Sports Medicine; Asthma; Developmental & Behavioral Disorders; **Hospital:** Steven & Alexandra Cohen Chldn's Med Ctr of NY (page 106), N Shore Univ Hosp (page 106); **Address:** ProHealthCare Assocs, 7 Vermont Drive, Div Pediatrics, Lake Success, NY 11042; **Phone:** 516-622-7337; **Board Cert:** Pediatrics 2011; **Med School:** NY Med Coll 1986; **Resid:** Pediatrics, N Shore Univ Hosp 1990; **Fac Appt:** Assoc Clin Prof Ped, NYU Sch Med

Cooper, Seymour M MD (Ped) *PCP* - **Hospital:** Winthrop Univ Hosp (page 524), Steven & Alexandra Cohen Chldn's Med Ctr of NY (page 106); **Address:** 1101 Stewart Ave, Ste 306, Garden City, NY 11530; **Phone:** 516-746-2299; **Board Cert:** Pediatrics 1977; **Med School:** NY Med Coll 1972; **Resid:** Pediatrics, Montefiore Hosp Med Ctr 1975

Friedman, Eugene B MD (Ped) *PCP* - **Hospital:** Steven & Alexandra Cohen Chldn's Med Ctr of NY (page 106), Winthrop Univ Hosp (page 524); **Address:** 271 Jericho Tpke, Floral Park, NY 11002; **Phone:** 516-354-7575; **Board Cert:** Pediatrics 1973; **Med School:** NY Med Coll 1968; **Resid:** Pediatrics, Metropolitan Hosp Ctr 1971; **Fac Appt:** Asst Clin Prof Ped, Albert Einstein Coll Med

Galinkin, Lawrence MD (Ped) *PCP* - **Hospital:** N Shore Univ Hosp (page 106), Long Is Jewish Med Ctr (page 106); **Address:** 700 Old Bethpage Rd, Old Bethpage, NY 11804; **Phone:** 516-293-0666; **Board Cert:** Pediatrics 1976; **Med School:** Tulane Univ 1971; **Resid:** Pediatrics, Bronx Muni Hosp 1974

Gerberg, Lynda Frances MD (Ped) *PCP* - **Spec Exp:** Sports Medicine; **Hospital:** N Shore Univ Hosp (page 106), NS-LIJ Hlth Sys (page 106); **Address:** 200 Middle Neck Rd, Great Neck, NY 11021; **Phone:** 516-466-3311; **Board Cert:** Pediatrics 2009; **Med School:** Mexico 1987; **Resid:** Pediatrics, Schneider Chldns Hosp 1993; **Fellow:** Pediatrics, Chldns Hosp 1994; **Fac Appt:** Asst Prof Ped, Albert Einstein Coll Med

Gould, Eric MD (Ped) *PCP* - **Spec Exp:** Developmental Disorders; **Hospital:** Long Is Jewish Med Ctr (page 106), N Shore Univ Hosp (page 106); **Address:** 225 Community Drive, Ste 105, Great Neck, NY 11021-2229; **Phone:** 516-829-9409; **Board Cert:** Pediatrics 1976; **Med School:** NY Med Coll 1970; **Resid:** Pediatrics, Bellevue Hosp Ctr/NYU 1974; **Fellow:** Child Development, Montefiore Med Ctr 1976

Green, Abraham I MD (Ped) *PCP* - **Spec Exp:** Asthma; Nutrition; ADD/ADHD; **Hospital:** Long Is Jewish Med Ctr (page 106), Winthrop Univ Hosp (page 524); **Address:** 115 Franklin Pl, Woodmere, NY 11598; **Phone:** 516-295-1200; **Board Cert:** Pediatrics 2009; **Med School:** Albert Einstein Coll Med 1979; **Resid:** Pediatrics, Jacobi Med Ctr 1983

Grijnsztein, Jacob MD (Ped) *PCP* - **Hospital:** Long Is Jewish Med Ctr (page 106), N Shore Univ Hosp (page 106); **Address:** 107 Northern Blvd, Ste 201, Great Neck, NY 11021; **Phone:** 516-487-6565; **Board Cert:** Pediatrics 1979; **Med School:** NYU Sch Med 1973; **Resid:** Pediatrics, Bellevue Hosp 1976

Hankin, Dorie E MD (Ped) - **Spec Exp:** Developmental Disorders; Behavioral Disorders; **Hospital:** Winthrop Univ Hosp (page 524), Steven & Alexandra Cohen Chldn's Med Ctr of NY (page 106); **Address:** 173 Mineola Blvd, Ste 301B, Mineola, NY 11501; **Phone:** 516-739-1936; **Board Cert:** Pediatrics 1980; Neurodevelopmental Disabilities 2012; Developmental-Behavioral Pediatrics 2010; **Med School:** Albert Einstein Coll Med 1974; **Resid:** Pediatrics, Montefiore Med Ctr 1978; **Fellow:** Child Development, Montefiore Med Ctr 1980

Leavens-Maurer, Jill MD (Ped) *PCP* - **Hospital:** Winthrop Univ Hosp (page 524); **Address:** Winthrop Pediatric Assocs, 222 Station Plaza N, Ste 611, Mineola, NY 11501-3893; **Phone:** 516-663-2532; **Board Cert:** Pediatrics 2011; **Med School:** SUNY Upstate Med Univ 1984; **Resid:** Pediatrics, NY-Presby/Weill Cornell Med Ctr 1987

Levy, Morton G MD (Ped) *PCP* - **Hospital:** N Shore Univ Hosp (page 106), Steven & Alexandra Cohen Chldn's Med Ctr of NY (page 106); **Address:** 133 Andover Rd, Roslyn Heights, NY 11577-1009; **Phone:** 516-621-9360; **Board Cert:** Pediatrics ; **Med School:** SUNY Downstate 1961; **Resid:** Pediatrics, Mt Sinai Hosp 1964; **Fac Appt:** Asst Clin Prof Ped, NYU Sch Med

Marino, Ronald V DO (Ped) *PCP* - **Spec Exp:** Developmental & Behavioral Disorders; **Hospital:** Winthrop Univ Hosp (page 524), Good Samaritan Hosp Med Ctr - West Islip; **Address:** Winthrop Pediatric Assocs, 222 Station Plaza N, Ste 611, Mineola, NY 11501-3808; **Phone:** 516-663-2532; **Board Cert:** Pediatrics 1985; **Med School:** Mich State Univ 1978; **Resid:** Pediatrics, Doctors Hosp 1981; **Fellow:** Behavioral Pediatrics, Univ Maryland Med Ctr 1985; **Fac Appt:** Clin Prof Ped, SUNY Stony Brook

Milanaik, Ruth DO (Ped) - **Spec Exp:** Developmental & Behavioral Disorders; ADD/ADHD; **Hospital:** Steven & Alexandra Cohen Chldn's Med Ctr of NY (page 106), NS-LIJ Hlth Sys (page 106); **Address:** 1983 Marcus Ave, Bldg 1 - Ste 130, Lake Success, NY 11042; **Phone:** 516-802-6100; **Board Cert:** Pediatrics 2009; Developmental-Behavioral Pediatrics 2012; **Med School:** NY Coll Osteo Med 1997; **Resid:** Pediatrics, Winthrop Univ Hosp 2001; **Fellow:** Developmental-Behavioral Pediatrics, NS-LIJ Hlth Sys 2004

Nerwen, Clifford MD (Ped) *PCP* - **Hospital:** Steven & Alexandra Cohen Chldn's Med Ctr of NY (page 106), N Shore Univ Hosp (page 106); **Address:** Steven & Alexandra Cohen Chldn's Med Ctr, 410 Lakeville Rd, Ste 108, Dept Pediatrics, New Hyde Park, NY 11040; **Phone:** 516-465-4377; **Board Cert:** Pediatrics 2010; **Med School:** Univ Conn 1991; **Resid:** Pediatrics, Schneider Chldns Hosp 1994

Rabinowicz, Morris MD (Ped) *PCP* - **Hospital:** Plainview Hosp (page 106), Steven & Alexandra Cohen Chldn's Med Ctr of NY (page 106); **Address:** 995 Old Country Rd, Plainview, NY 11803; **Phone:** 516-935-7333; **Board Cert:** Pediatrics 1985; **Med School:** SUNY Downstate 1978; **Resid:** Surgery, LIJ Med Ctr 1982; Pediatrics, Brookdale Hosp 1983; **Fac Appt:** Asst Prof Ped, Hofstra N Shore-LIJ Sch Med

Resmovits, Marvin MD (Ped) *PCP* - **Hospital:** Steven & Alexandra Cohen Chldn's Med Ctr of NY (page 106), N Shore Univ Hosp (page 106); **Address:** 107 NE Northern Blvd, Fl s, Ste 201, Great Neck, NY 11021-4309; **Phone:** 516-487-6565; **Board Cert:** Pediatrics 1984; **Med School:** SUNY Buffalo 1979; **Resid:** Pediatrics, LI Jewish Hosp 1982

Physical Medicine & Rehabilitation

Beer, Jeffry R MD (PMR) - **Spec Exp:** Spinal Rehabilitation; Pain Medicine; Pain-Interventional Techniques; Pain-Musculoskeletal; **Hospital:** N Shore Univ Hosp (page 106), NS-LIJ Hlth Sys (page 106); **Address:** Long Island Spine Rehabilitation Med, 801 Merrick Ave, East Meadow, NY 11554; **Phone:** 516-393-8941; **Board Cert:** Physical Medicine & Rehabilitation 2005; Pain Medicine 2005; **Med School:** SUNY Downstate 2000; **Resid:** Physical Medicine & Rehabilitation, Long Island Jewish Med Ctr 2004; **Fellow:** Interventional Spine Medicine, Beth Israel Med Ctr - Petrie Division 2005

Lipetz, Jason S MD (PMR) - **Spec Exp:** Spinal Rehabilitation; Pain-Spine; **Hospital:** NS-LIJ Hlth Sys (page 106), N Shore Univ Hosp (page 106); **Address:** LI Spine Rehab Medicine, 801 Merrick Ave, East Meadow, NY 11554; **Phone:** 516-393-8941; **Board Cert:** Physical Medicine & Rehabilitation 2009; Pain Medicine 2012; **Med School:** Columbia P&S 1994; **Resid:** Physical Medicine & Rehabilitation, Kessler Inst-UMDNJ 1998; **Fellow:** Interventional Spine Medicine, Univ Penn Affil Hosp 1999; **Fac Appt:** Asst Prof PMR, Albert Einstein Coll Med

Root, Barry C MD (PMR) - **Spec Exp:** Spinal Cord Injury; Electromyography; Spinal Rehabilitation; **Hospital:** N Shore Univ Hosp (page 106), St. Francis Hosp - The Heart Ctr (page 116); **Address:** N Shore Univ Hosp, Dept Physical Med & Rehab, 101 St Andrew's Ln Fl 1-North, Glen Cove, NY 11542-2254; **Phone:** 516-674-7501; **Board Cert:** Physical Medicine & Rehabilitation 1988; Spinal Cord Injury Medicine 2003; **Med School:** Ohio State Univ 1984; **Resid:** Physical Medicine & Rehabilitation, Nassau County Med Ctr 1987

Stein, Adam B MD (PMR) - **Spec Exp:** Spinal Cord Injury; Multiple Sclerosis; Stroke Rehabilitation; **Hospital:** Glen Cove Hosp (page 106), Long Is Jewish Med Ctr (page 106); **Address:** 825 Northern Blvd Fl 1 - Ste 105, Great Neck, NY 11021; **Phone:** 516-465-8609; **Board Cert:** Physical Medicine & Rehabilitation 1992; Spinal Cord Injury Medicine 2003; **Med School:** NYU Sch Med 1987; **Resid:** Physical Medicine & Rehabilitation, Rusk Inst-NYU Med Ctr 1991

Weiss, Lyn D MD (PMR) - **Spec Exp:** Stroke Rehabilitation; Electrodiagnosis; **Hospital:** Nassau Univ Med Ctr; **Address:** Nassau Univ Med Ctr, Phys Med & Rehab, 2201 Hempstead Tpke, East Meadow, NY 11554; **Phone:** 516-572-6525; **Board Cert:** Physical Medicine & Rehabilitation 1990; **Med School:** SUNY Downstate 1985; **Resid:** Physical Medicine & Rehabilitation, Nassau Univ Med Ctr 1989; **Fac Appt:** Prof PMR, SUNY Stony Brook

Plastic Surgery

Alizadeh, Kaveh MD (PlS) - **Spec Exp:** Breast Cosmetic & Reconstructive Surgery; Facial Plastic & Reconstructive Surgery; Liposuction & Body Contouring; Migraine; **Hospital:** South Nassau Comm Hosp, Lenox Hill Hosp (page 106); **Address:** Long Island Plastic Surgical Group, 999 Franklin Ave, Garden City, NY 11530; **Phone:** 516-742-3404; **Board Cert:** Plastic Surgery 2011; **Med School:** Cornell Univ 1993; **Resid:** Plastic Surgery, Univ Chicago Hosps 1999; **Fellow:** Microsurgery, Meml Sloan-Kettering Cancer Ctr 2000; Cosmetic Plastic Surgery, Manhattan Eye, Ear & Throat Hosp 2000

Breitbart, Arnold MD (PlS) - **Spec Exp:** Cosmetic Surgery-Face & Body; Liposuction; Breast Reconstruction; Cosmetic Surgery-Breast; **Hospital:** N Shore Univ Hosp (page 106), NY-Presby/Weill Cornell Med Ctr, NY (page 104); **Address:** 1155 Northern Blvd, Ste 110, Manhasset, NY 11030; **Phone:** 516-365-3511; **Board Cert:** Surgery 2003; Plastic Surgery 2004; **Med School:** NYU Sch Med 1985; **Resid:** Surgery, NYU Med Ctr 1991; Plastic Surgery, NYU Med Ctr 1993; **Fellow:** Craniofacial Surgery, NYU Med Ctr 1994; Microsurgery, Meml Sloan-Kettering Cancer Ctr 1995; **Fac Appt:** Asst Prof S, Cornell Univ-Weill Med Coll

DeVita, Gregory A MD (PlS) - **Spec Exp:** Rhinoplasty; Rhinoplasty Revision; Cosmetic Surgery-Face; Cosmetic Surgery-Breast; **Hospital:** St. Francis Hosp - The Heart Ctr (page 116), N Shore Univ Hosp (page 106); **Address:** 650 Northern Blvd, Great Neck, NY 11021-5204; **Phone:** 516-466-7000; **Board Cert:** Plastic Surgery 1989; **Med School:** SUNY Downstate 1980; **Resid:** Surgery, St Luke's Hosp 1982; Surgery, Jersey City Med Ctr 1983; **Fellow:** Plastic Surgery, New York Methodist Hosp 1984; Plastic Surgery, SUNY Downstate Med Ctr 1986

DiGregorio, Vincent R MD (PlS) - **Spec Exp:** Rhinoplasty Revision; Cosmetic Surgery-Face; Breast Reconstruction & Augmentation; Eyelid Surgery; **Hospital:** Winthrop Univ Hosp (page 524), Mercy Med Ctr - Rockville Centre; **Address:** 999 Franklin Ave, Garden City, NY 11530; **Phone:** 516-742-3404; **Board Cert:** Plastic Surgery 1978; **Med School:** Albany Med Coll 1968; **Resid:** Surgery, Thomas Jefferson Univ Hosp 1974; Plastic Surgery, Nassau Co Med Ctr 1976; **Fac Appt:** Assoc Prof PlS, SUNY Stony Brook

Doctor, Naishad M MD (PlS) - **Spec Exp:** Cosmetic & Reconstructive Surgery; **Hospital:** Mercy Med Ctr - Rockville Centre, Winthrop Univ Hosp (page 524); **Address:** 2000 N Village Ave, Ste 103, Rockville Centre, NY 11570-1001; **Phone:** 516-678-2517; **Board Cert:** Plastic Surgery ; **Med School:** India 1974; **Resid:** Surgery, Univ Hosp 1987; Plastic Surgery, Univ Utah Hosp 1990; **Fellow:** Burn Surgery, Univ Hosp 1988

Dubner, Sanford MD (PlS) - **Spec Exp:** Head & Neck Tumors; Melanoma; Reconstructive Plastic Surgery; **Hospital:** Long Is Jewish Med Ctr (page 106), N Shore Univ Hosp (page 106); **Address:** 410 Lakeville Rd, Ste 310, Lake Success, NY 11042; **Phone:** 516-437-1111; **Board Cert:** Surgery 2006; Plastic Surgery 1992; **Med School:** SUNY Stony Brook 1982; **Resid:** Surgery, Booth Meml Med Ctr 1987; Plastic Surgery, Montefiore Med Ctr 1989; **Fellow:** Head and Neck Surgery, Meml Sloan-Kettering Cancer Ctr 1990; **Fac Appt:** Clin Prof S, Hofstra N Shore-LIJ Sch Med

Elkowitz, Marc J MD (PlS) - **Spec Exp:** Cosmetic Surgery; Reconstructive Surgery; **Hospital:** Long Is Jewish Med Ctr (page 106), N Shore Univ Hosp (page 106); **Address:** 107 Northern Blvd, Ste 203, Great Neck, NY 11021; **Phone:** 516-773-9200; **Board Cert:** Surgery 2007; Plastic Surgery 2012; **Med School:** Albany Med Coll 1993; **Resid:** Surgery, NY Med Coll 1998; **Fellow:** Plastic Surgery, Montefiore Med Ctr 2000; **Fac Appt:** Asst Clin Prof PlS, Albert Einstein Coll Med

Feinberg, Joseph MD (PlS) - **Spec Exp:** Cosmetic Surgery-Face & Eyes; Breast Augmentation; Abdominoplasty; **Hospital:** St. Francis Hosp - The Heart Ctr (page 116), N Shore Univ Hosp (page 106); **Address:** 1201 Northern Blvd, Ste 202, Manhasset, NY 11030; **Phone:** 516-869-6200; **Board Cert:** Plastic Surgery 1980; **Med School:** Cornell Univ-Weill Med Coll 1973; **Resid:** Surgery, NY Hosp 1976; Plastic Surgery, NY Hosp 1978; **Fellow:** Plastic/Reconstructive Surgery, Meml Sloan Kettering Cancer Ctr 1978; **Fac Appt:** Asst Clin Prof S, Cornell Univ-Weill Med Coll

Funt, David K MD (PlS) - **Spec Exp:** Cosmetic Surgery-Face & Body; Liposuction; Botox Therapy; Facial Rejuvenation; **Hospital:** South Nassau Comm Hosp, N Shore Univ Hosp (page 106); **Address:** 19 Irving Pl, Woodmere, NY 11598; **Phone:** 516-295-0404; **Board Cert:** Plastic Surgery 1987; **Med School:** Geo Wash Univ 1979; **Resid:** Surgery, Montefiore Med Ctr 1983; Plastic Surgery, Montefiore Med Ctr 1985; **Fac Appt:** Asst Clin Prof PlS, Albert Einstein Coll Med

Gallagher, Pamela M MD (PlS) - **Spec Exp:** Abdominoplasty; Body Contouring; Facial Rejuvenation; Breast Augmentation; **Hospital:** Good Samaritan Hosp Med Ctr - West Islip, N Shore Univ Hosp (page 106); **Address:** 190 E Jericho Tpke, Mineola, NY 11501; **Phone:** 516-977-9922; **Board Cert:** Plastic Surgery 1980; **Med School:** Univ Chicago-Pritzker Sch Med 1974; **Resid:** Surgery, NY-Presby/Weill Cornell Med Ctr 1977; Plastic Surgery, NY-Presby/Weill Cornell Med Ctr 1979

Gold, Alan H MD (PlS) - **Spec Exp:** Cosmetic Surgery-Face & Eyes; Cosmetic Surgery-Breast; Cosmetic Surgery-Body; Nasal Surgery; **Hospital:** N Shore Univ Hosp (page 106), Long Is Jewish Med Ctr (page 106); **Address:** 833 Northern Blvd, Ste 240, Great Neck, NY 11021-5322; **Phone:** 516-498-2800; **Board Cert:** Plastic Surgery 1979; **Med School:** SUNY Downstate 1971; **Resid:** Surgery, N Shore Univ Hosp 1975; Plastic Surgery, Kings County-Suny Med Ctr 1978; **Fellow:** Hand Surgery, Nassau County Med Ctr 1976

Gotkin, Robert MD (PlS) - **Spec Exp:** Cosmetic Surgery-Face & Breast; Liposuction; Skin Laser Surgery; **Hospital:** Long Is Jewish Med Ctr (page 106), NS-LIJ Hlth Sys (page 106); **Address:** 31 Northern Blvd, Greenvale, NY 11548; **Phone:** 516-484-9000; **Board Cert:** Plastic Surgery 1990; **Med School:** Howard Univ 1980; **Resid:** Surgery, SUNY Stony Brook 1985; Plastic Surgery, Georgetown Univ 1988; **Fellow:** Surgical Critical Care, SUNY Stony Brook 1986

Groeger, William E MD (PlS) - **Spec Exp:** Skin Cancer; **Hospital:** South Nassau Comm Hosp, Mercy Med Ctr - Rockville Centre; **Address:** 1490 Broadway Fl 2, Hewlett, NY 11557-1645; **Phone:** 516-887-5502; **Board Cert:** Plastic Surgery 1982; **Med School:** SUNY Downstate 1972; **Resid:** Surgery, Beth Israel Hosp 1977; Plastic Surgery, Univ Hosp 1979

Israeli, Ron MD (PlS) - **Spec Exp:** Plastic & Reconstructive Surgery; Breast Reconstruction; Microsurgery; **Hospital:** N Shore Univ Hosp (page 106), St. Francis Hosp - The Heart Ctr (page 116); **Address:** 833 Northern Blvd, Ste 160, Great Neck, NY 11021; **Phone:** 516-498-8400; **Board Cert:** Plastic Surgery 2009; **Med School:** Boston Univ 1990; **Resid:** Surgery, Mt Sinai Hosp 1995; Plastic Surgery, Mass Genl Hosp 1997; **Fellow:** Microsurgery, Mt Sinai Hosp 1992

Kasabian, Armen K MD (PlS) - **Spec Exp:** Hand Reconstruction; Plastic & Reconstructive Surgery; Microsurgery; **Hospital:** Long Is Jewish Med Ctr (page 106), NS-LIJ Hlth Sys (page 106); **Address:** Dept Plastic Surgery, 1991 Marcus Ave, Ste 102, Lake Success, NY 11042; **Phone:** 516-497-7900; **Board Cert:** Plastic Surgery 1992; Hand Surgery 2004; **Med School:** Cornell Univ-Weill Med Coll 1982; **Resid:** Surgery, NYU Med Ctr 1987; Plastic Surgery, NYU Med Ctr 1989; **Fellow:** Microsurgery, NYU Med Ctr 1990; **Fac Appt:** Asst Prof PlS, NYU Sch Med

Kessler, Martin E MD (PlS) - **Spec Exp:** Cosmetic Surgery-Face & Body; Reconstructive Surgery-Face; Breast Reconstruction; Hand Surgery; **Hospital:** South Nassau Comm Hosp, N Shore Univ Hosp (page 106); **Address:** 242 Merrick Rd, Ste 302, Rockville Centre, NY 11570-5254; **Phone:** 516-536-5858; **Board Cert:** Plastic Surgery 1987; **Med School:** Cornell Univ-Weill Med Coll 1980; **Resid:** Surgery, NY Hosp 1983; Plastic Surgery, NY Hosp 1985; **Fellow:** Hand Surgery, Cleveland Clin 1986; Microsurgery, Univ Louisville Hosp 1986; **Fac Appt:** Assoc Clin Prof PlS, Cornell Univ-Weill Med Coll

Leipziger, Lyle S MD (PlS) - **Spec Exp:** Cosmetic Surgery-Face & Eyes; Cosmetic Surgery-Breast; Breast Reconstruction; Liposuction & Body Contouring; **Hospital:** N Shore Univ Hosp (page 106), Long Is Jewish Med Ctr (page 106); **Address:** 825 Northern Blvd Fl 3, Great Neck, NY 11021; **Phone:** 516-465-8787; **Board Cert:** Plastic Surgery 1994; **Med School:** Cornell Univ-Weill Med Coll 1985; **Resid:** Plastic Surgery, NY Hosp 1990; **Fellow:** Craniofacial Surgery, Johns Hopkins Hosp 1991

Lukash, Frederick N MD (PlS) - **Spec Exp:** Pediatric Plastic Surgery; Cosmetic Surgery-Face; Breast Cosmetic & Reconstructive Surgery; Rhinoplasty; **Hospital:** Long Is Jewish Med Ctr (page 106), Steven & Alexandra Cohen Chldn's Med Ctr of NY (page 106); **Address:** 2110 Northern Blvd, Ste 210, Manhasset, NY 11030-3022; **Phone:** 516-365-1040; **Board Cert:** Plastic Surgery 1982; **Med School:** Tulane Univ 1973; **Resid:** Surgery, Emory Univ Hosp 1975; Surgery, Univ Hosp 1980; **Fellow:** Plastic Surgery, Mass Genl Hosp 1981; **Fac Appt:** Asst Prof S, Albert Einstein Coll Med

Silberman, Mark Illan MD (PlS) - **Spec Exp:** Cosmetic Surgery-Face; Breast Cosmetic & Reconstructive Surgery; Facial Rejuvenation; Body Contouring; **Hospital:** N Shore Univ Hosp (page 106), St. Francis Hosp - The Heart Ctr (page 116); **Address:** 650 Northern Blvd, Great Neck, NY 11021-5204; **Phone:** 516-466-7000; **Board Cert:** Plastic Surgery 1988; **Med School:** SUNY Downstate 1980; **Resid:** Surgery, Beth Israel Med Ctr 1983; Plastic Surgery, SUNY Downstate Med Ctr 1985

Simpson, Roger MD (PlS) - **Spec Exp:** Eyelid Surgery; Liposuction & Body Contouring; Cosmetic Surgery-Face & Breast; Burn Care; **Hospital:** Winthrop Univ Hosp (page 524), NS-LIJ Hlth Sys (page 106); **Address:** 999 Franklin Ave, Garden City, NY 11530; **Phone:** 516-742-3404; **Board Cert:** Plastic Surgery 1981; **Med School:** Belgium 1974; **Resid:** Surgery, Nassau Co Med Ctr 1978; Plastic Surgery, Nassau Co Med Ctr 1980; **Fellow:** Hand Surgery, St Luke's-Roosevelt Hosp Ctr 1981; **Fac Appt:** Asst Clin Prof S, SUNY Stony Brook

Psychiatry

Bailine, Samuel MD (Psyc) - **Spec Exp:** Depression; Psychopharmacology; Electroconvulsive Therapy (ECT); **Hospital:** Zucker Hillside Hosp (page 106); **Address:** 5 Ridgeway Rd, Port Washington, NY 11050; **Phone:** 516-883-3304; **Board Cert:** Psychiatry ; **Med School:** NYU Sch Med 1964; **Resid:** Psychiatry, Tulane Med Ctr 1968; **Fac Appt:** Assoc Prof Psyc, Hofstra N Shore-LIJ Sch Med

Behr, Raymond MD (Psyc) - **Spec Exp:** Depression; Bipolar/Mood Disorders; Addiction/Substance Abuse; **Hospital:** Long Is Jewish Med Ctr (page 106); **Address:** 81-A Arleigh Rd, Great Neck, NY 11021-1442; **Phone:** 516-482-1980; **Board Cert:** Psychiatry 1981; Child & Adolescent Psychiatry 1982; **Med School:** South Africa 1973; **Resid:** Psychiatry, LI Jewish Med Ctr 1978; **Fellow:** Child & Adolescent Psychiatry, LI Jewish Med Ctr 1980; **Fac Appt:** Asst Clin Prof Psyc, Albert Einstein Coll Med

Benjamin, John MD (Psyc) - **Spec Exp:** Depression; Anxiety Disorders; Schizophrenia; **Hospital:** N Shore Univ Hosp (page 106); **Address:** 1983 Marcus Ave, Ste E132, Lake Success, NY 11042; **Phone:** 516-216-1780; **Board Cert:** Psychiatry 1983; **Med School:** India 1969; **Resid:** Psychiatry, N Shore Univ Hosp 1981; **Fac Appt:** Asst Clin Prof Psyc, NYU Sch Med

Berman, Sheldon S MD (Psyc) - **Spec Exp:** Psychodynamic Psychotherapy; Psychopharmacology; Palliative Care; **Address:** 8 Payne Circle, Hewlett Harbor, NY 11557-2735; **Phone:** 516-374-4417; **Board Cert:** Psychiatry 1979; **Med School:** Ros Franklin Univ/Chicago Med Sch 1969; **Resid:** Psychiatry, Brookdale Hosp 1973; **Fac Appt:** Asst Clin Prof Psyc, SUNY Downstate

Bhatt, Ashok MD (Psyc) - **Spec Exp:** Depression; Psychopharmacology; **Hospital:** Long Beach Med Ctr; **Address:** 871 E Park Ave, Long Beach, NY 11561; **Phone:** 516-889-8844; **Board Cert:** Psychiatry 1985; **Med School:** India 1976; **Resid:** Psychiatry, LI Jewish Med Ctr 1981; **Fellow:** Psychiatry, LI Jewish Med Ctr 1983

Budman, Cathy L MD (Psyc) - **Spec Exp:** Tourette's Syndrome; ADD/ADHD; Obsessive-Compulsive Disorder; Neuro-Psychiatry; **Hospital:** N Shore Univ Hosp (page 106), Long Is Jewish Med Ctr (page 106); **Address:** 400 Community Drive, Dept Psychiatry North Shore-LIJHS, Manhasset, NY 11030; **Phone:** 516-562-3223; **Board Cert:** Psychiatry 1991; **Med School:** SUNY Buffalo 1984; **Resid:** Psychiatry, Langley Porter Psych Inst/UCSF 1986; Psychiatry, N Shore Univ Hosp 1990; **Fellow:** Family Medicine, Sydney Univ-Royal Price Albert Hosp 1988; Neuropsychiatry, N Shore Univ Hosp 1991; **Fac Appt:** Prof Psyc, Hofstra N Shore-LIJ Sch Med

Crasta, Jovita M MD (Psyc) - **Spec Exp:** Anxiety Disorders; Depression; Bipolar/Mood Disorders; Women's Health-Mental Health; **Hospital:** South Nassau Comm Hosp; **Address:** 2277 Grand Ave, Baldwin, NY 11510-3148; **Phone:** 516-377-5400; **Board Cert:** Psychiatry 1991; **Med School:** India 1981; **Resid:** Psychiatry, Nassau County Med Ctr 1987

Gupta, Adarsh MD/PhD (Psyc) - **Spec Exp:** Psychosomatic Disorders; Psychiatry in Physical Illness; Neuro-Psychiatry; Sleep Medicine; **Hospital:** Long Is Jewish Med Ctr (page 106); **Address:** Great Neck Psychiatry, 1010 Northern Blvd, Ste 208, Great Neck, NY 11021; **Phone:** 516-336-2544; **Board Cert:** Surgery 2007; Psychosomatic Medicine 2005; Sleep Medicine 2011; **Med School:** India 1978; **Resid:** Internal Medicine, St Vincent Hosp Med Ctr 1992; Psychiatry, NYU Med Ctr 1995

Gurevich, Michael I MD (Psyc) - **Spec Exp:** Psychotherapy & Psychopharmacology; Complementary Medicine; Addiction/Substance Abuse; Psychiatry in Physical Illness; **Address:** 997 Glen Cove Avenue, Glen Head, NY 11545-1584; **Phone:** 516-674-9489; **Board Cert:** Psychiatry 1989; **Med School:** Lithuania 1974; **Resid:** Psychiatry, Elmhurst Hosp Ctr 1987; **Fellow:** Child Psychiatry, Elmhurst Hosp Ctr 1989

Katus, Eli Margrethe MD (Psyc) - **Spec Exp:** Psychopharmacology; Psychotherapy; Child & Adolescent Psychiatry; **Hospital:** N Shore Univ Hosp (page 106), Winthrop Univ Hosp (page 524); **Address:** 1035 Route 106, East Norwich, NY 11732-1005; **Phone:** 516-922-5607; **Board Cert:** Psychiatry 1990; Child & Adolescent Psychiatry 1991; **Med School:** Germany 1982; **Resid:** Psychiatry, N Shore Univ Hosp 1986; **Fellow:** Child & Adolescent Psychiatry, N Shore Univ Hosp 1988

Katz, Jack L MD (Psyc) - **Spec Exp:** Eating Disorders; Mood Disorders; Anxiety Disorders; **Hospital:** N Shore Univ Hosp (page 106), Long Is Jewish Med Ctr (page 106); **Address:** 1010 Northern Blvd, Ste 208, Great Neck, NY 11021; **Phone:** 516-336-2565; **Board Cert:** Psychiatry 1968; **Med School:** Albert Einstein Coll Med 1960; **Resid:** Psychiatry, Montefiore Med Ctr 1966; Internal Medicine, Jackson Meml Hosp 1961; **Fellow:** Psychiatry, Montefiore Med Ctr-Einstein 1968; **Fac Appt:** Prof Psyc, Hofstra N Shore-LIJ Sch Med

Liang, Vera T MD (Psyc) - **Spec Exp:** Women's Health-Mental Health; Depression; Anxiety Disorders; **Hospital:** Long Is Jewish Med Ctr (page 106); **Address:** 1 Expressway Plaza, Ste 201, Roslyn Heights, NY 11577; **Phone:** 516-484-5869; **Board Cert:** Psychiatry 1977; Child & Adolescent Psychiatry 1981; **Med School:** Hong Kong 1969; **Resid:** Psychiatry, LI Jewish Med Ctr 1973; **Fellow:** Child & Adolescent Psychiatry, Jacobi Med Ctr 1975

Sami, Sherif F MD (Psyc) - **Spec Exp:** Depression; Anxiety & Mood Disorders; Geriatric Psychiatry; **Hospital:** Winthrop Univ Hosp (page 524), N Shore Univ Hosp (page 106); **Address:** 7 Bond St, Great Neck, NY 11021; **Phone:** 516-487-9191; **Board Cert:** Psychiatry 1973; **Med School:** Egypt 1961; **Resid:** Psychiatry, Cairo Univ Hosp 1966; Psychiatry, Elmhurst Hosp 1969; **Fellow:** Community Psychiatry, Albert Einstein 1970

Pulmonary Disease

Altus, Jonathan D MD (Pul) - **Spec Exp:** Breathing Disorders; Asthma; Chronic Obstructive Lung Disease (COPD); Cough; **Hospital:** South Nassau Comm Hosp, Franklin Hosp (page 106); **Address:** South Shore Pulmonary Medicine, 920 Atlantic Ave, Baldwin Harbor, NY 11510; **Phone:** 516-623-8700; **Board Cert:** Internal Medicine 1988; Pulmonary Disease 2012; **Med School:** SUNY Downstate 1984; **Resid:** Internal Medicine, Beth Israel Med Ctr 1987; **Fellow:** Pulmonary Disease, New York Univ Med Ctr 1989

Blum, Alan I MD (Pul) - **Spec Exp:** Cough-Chronic; Asthma; Sleep Disorders; **Hospital:** South Nassau Comm Hosp, Franklin Hosp (page 106); **Address:** 444 Merrick Rd Fl Lower Level 1, Lynbrook, NY 11563-2400; **Phone:** 516-593-9500; **Board Cert:** Internal Medicine 1981; Pulmonary Disease 1984; **Med School:** Mexico 1977; **Resid:** Internal Medicine, Mt Sinai Hosp Ctr 1981; **Fellow:** Pulmonary Disease, Mt Sinai Hosp Ctr 1983

Breidbart, David M MD (Pul) - **Spec Exp:** Asthma; Chronic Obstructive Lung Disease (COPD); Sarcoidosis; **Hospital:** N Shore Univ Hosp (page 106), St. Francis Hosp - The Heart Ctr (page 116); **Address:** 6 Ohio Drive, Ste 201, Lake Success, NY 11042-1129; **Phone:** 516-328-8700; **Board Cert:** Internal Medicine 1982; Pulmonary Disease 1984; **Med School:** SUNY Downstate 1979; **Resid:** Internal Medicine, North Shore Univ Hosp 1982; **Fellow:** Pulmonary Disease, Meml Sloan-Kettering Hosp 1983; Pulmonary Disease, Montefiore-Albert Einstein Med Ctr 1985; **Fac Appt:** Asst Clin Prof Med, NYU Sch Med

Cohen, Michael L MD (Pul) - **Spec Exp:** Asthma; Bronchitis; Emphysema; **Hospital:** N Shore Univ Hosp (page 106); **Address:** N Shore Internal Med Assocs, 560 Northern Blvd, Ste 203, Great Neck, NY 11021-5100; **Phone:** 516-482-0600; **Board Cert:** Internal Medicine 1972; Pulmonary Disease 1974; **Med School:** SUNY Upstate Med Univ 1967; **Resid:** Internal Medicine, Montefiore Hosp Med Ctr 1970; **Fellow:** Pulmonary Disease, Montefiore Hosp Med Ctr 1971; Pulmonary Disease, LI Jewish Med Ctr 1974; **Fac Appt:** Asst Clin Prof Med, NYU Sch Med

Donath, Joseph MD (Pul) - **Spec Exp:** Asthma; Lung Cancer; Critical Care; **Hospital:** NY Hosp Queens (page 488), Flushing Hosp Med Ctr; **Address:** 360 Central Ave, Lawrence, NY 11559; **Phone:** 516-569-6966; **Board Cert:** Internal Medicine 1980; Pulmonary Disease 1982; Critical Care Medicine 2009; **Med School:** Hungary 1972; **Resid:** Internal Medicine, VA Med Ctr 1980; **Fellow:** Pulmonary Disease, Mt Sinai Hosp 1982; **Fac Appt:** Asst Clin Prof Med, NY Med Coll

Fein, Alan MD (Pul) - **Spec Exp:** Chronic Obstructive Lung Disease (COPD); Asthma; Pneumonia; **Hospital:** N Shore Univ Hosp (page 106), Long Is Jewish Med Ctr (page 106); **Address:** 2800 Marcus Ave, Ste 202, Lake Success, NY 11042; **Phone:** 516-608-2890; **Board Cert:** Internal Medicine 1976; Pulmonary Disease 1978; Critical Care Medicine 2008; **Med School:** SUNY Downstate 1973; **Resid:** Internal Medicine, Albert Einstein Affil Hosp 1976; **Fellow:** Pulmonary Disease, UC San Francisco Med Ctr 1978

Gordon, Richard Eric MD (Pul) - **Spec Exp:** Emphysema; Sleep Disorders; Asthma; **Hospital:** St. Joseph's Hosp-Nassau, Plainview Hosp (page 106); **Address:** Island Pulmonary Associates, 4271 Hempstead Tpke, Ste 1, Bethpage, NY 11714-5718; **Phone:** 516-796-3700; **Board Cert:** Internal Medicine 1984; Pulmonary Disease 1986; **Med School:** Mount Sinai Sch Med 1980; **Resid:** Internal Medicine, Beth Israel Med Ctr 1983; **Fellow:** Pulmonary Disease, Queens Hosp Ctr 1985

Greenberg, Harly MD (Pul) - **Spec Exp:** Sleep Disorders/Apnea; Lung Disease; Critical Care; **Hospital:** Long Is Jewish Med Ctr (page 106), N Shore Univ Hosp (page 106); **Address:** N Shore-LIJ Sleep Disorders Ctr, 410 Lakeville Rd, Ste 107, New Hyde Park, NY 11042; **Phone:** 516-465-3899; **Board Cert:** Internal Medicine 1985; Pulmonary Disease 1988; Sleep Medicine 2011; **Med School:** NYU Sch Med 1982; **Resid:** Internal Medicine, North Shore Univ Hosp 1985; **Fellow:** Pulmonary Disease, Bellevue Hosp Ctr 1987; **Fac Appt:** Prof Med, Hofstra N Shore-LIJ Sch Med

Leeman, Benjamin J MD (Pul) - **Spec Exp:** Asthma; Pneumonia; Chronic Obstructive Lung Disease (COPD); **Hospital:** Franklin Hosp (page 106), South Nassau Comm Hosp; **Address:** 20 W Lincoln Ave, Ste 306, Valley Stream, NY 11580; **Phone:** 516-599-8787; **Board Cert:** Internal Medicine 2006; Pulmonary Disease 2007; **Med School:** SUNY Stony Brook 1988; **Resid:** Internal Medicine, Montefiore Med Ctr-Weiler Div 1991; **Fellow:** Pulmonary Disease, NY Presby-Columbia Med Ctr 1993

Mermelstein, Steve A MD (Pul) - **Spec Exp:** Asthma; Chronic Obstructive Lung Disease (COPD); Cough-Chronic; **Hospital:** South Nassau Comm Hosp, Franklin Hosp (page 106); **Address:** 444 Merrick Rd, Lower Level 1, Lynbrook, NY 11563-2456; **Phone:** 516-593-9500; **Board Cert:** Internal Medicine 1980; Pulmonary Disease 1982; **Med School:** Albert Einstein Coll Med 1977; **Resid:** Internal Medicine, Metropolitan Hosp Ctr 1980; **Fellow:** Pulmonary Disease, St Luke's-Roosevelt Hosp Ctr 1982

Multz, Alan S MD (Pul) - **Spec Exp:** Respiratory Distress Syndrome; Chronic Obstructive Lung Disease (COPD); **Hospital:** Nassau Univ Med Ctr, N Shore Univ Hosp (page 106); **Address:** Nassau Univ Med Ctr, Div Pulmonology, 2201 Hempstead Tpke Fl 6, East Meadow, NY 11554; **Phone:** 516-572-6501; **Board Cert:** Internal Medicine 1988; Pulmonary Disease 2010; Critical Care Medicine 2011; **Med School:** Boston Univ 1985; **Resid:** Internal Medicine, Montefiore Med Ctr 1988; **Fellow:** Pulmonary Disease, Montefiore Med Ctr 1990; Critical Care Medicine, Montefiore Med Ctr 1991; **Fac Appt:** Assoc Prof Med, Albert Einstein Coll Med

Newmark, Ian H MD (Pul) - **Spec Exp:** Critical Care; Asthma; Lung Cancer; **Hospital:** Plainview Hosp (page 106), Syosset Hosp (page 106); **Address:** 8 Greenfield Rd, Syosset, NY 11791-4831; **Phone:** 516-496-3001; **Board Cert:** Internal Medicine 1982; Pulmonary Disease 1986; Critical Care Medicine 2010; **Med School:** SUNY Hlth Sci Ctr 1979; **Resid:** Internal Medicine, Nassau Co Med Ctr 1982; **Fellow:** Pulmonary Intensive Care, Nassau Co Med Ctr 1984; **Fac Appt:** Asst Clin Prof Med, Hofstra N Shore-LIJ Sch Med

Niederman, Michael S MD (Pul) - **Spec Exp:** Infections-Respiratory; Emphysema; Respiratory Failure; Pneumonia; **Hospital:** Winthrop Univ Hosp (page 524); **Address:** 222 Station Plaza N, Ste 400, Mineola, NY 11501-3893; **Phone:** 516-663-2834; **Board Cert:** Internal Medicine 1980; Pulmonary Disease 1982; Critical Care Medicine 2007; **Med School:** Boston Univ 1977; **Resid:** Internal Medicine, Northwestern Univ Med Ctr 1980; **Fellow:** Pulmonary Disease, Yale-New Haven Hosp 1983; **Fac Appt:** Prof Med, SUNY Stony Brook

Schulster, Rita B MD (Pul) - **Spec Exp:** Asthma; Bronchitis; **Hospital:** Long Beach Med Ctr, South Nassau Comm Hosp; **Address:** 442 E Waukena Ave, Oceanside, NY 11572; **Phone:** 516-599-8234; **Board Cert:** Internal Medicine 1977; Pulmonary Disease 1978; **Med School:** Albert Einstein Coll Med 1970; **Resid:** Internal Medicine, Beth Israel Med Ctr 1973; Internal Medicine, Beth Israel Med Ctr 1974; **Fellow:** Pulmonary Disease, LI Jewish Med Ctr 1975; Pulmonary Disease, Beth Israel Med Ctr 1976

Steinberg, Harry MD (Pul) - **Spec Exp:** Asthma; Emphysema; Lung Cancer; Pulmonary Hypertension; **Hospital:** Long Is Jewish Med Ctr (page 106), N Shore Univ Hosp (page 106); **Address:** 410 Lakeville Rd, Ste 107, New Hyde Park, NY 11042; **Phone:** 516-465-5400; **Med School:** Temple Univ 1966; **Resid:** Internal Medicine, LI Jewish Med Ctr 1969; Pulmonary Critical Care Medicine, LI Jewish Med Ctr 1970; **Fellow:** Pulmonary Disease, Hosp Univ Penn 1974; **Fac Appt:** Prof Med, Hofstra N Shore-LIJ Sch Med

Wyner, Perry A MD (Pul) - **Spec Exp:** Asthma; Cough-Chronic; Emphysema; Preventive Medicine; **Hospital:** Mercy Med Ctr - Rockville Centre; **Address:** 2 Lincoln Ave, Ste 201, Rockville Centre, NY 11570; **Phone:** 516-536-4960; **Board Cert:** Internal Medicine 1980; Pulmonary Disease 1982; **Med School:** Cornell Univ-Weill Med Coll 1977; **Resid:** Internal Medicine, Med Coll Virginia Hosps 1980; **Fellow:** Pulmonary Disease, Bellevue Hosp 1982

Zupnick, Henry Michael MD (Pul) - **Spec Exp:** Asthma; Bronchitis; Cough; **Hospital:** South Nassau Comm Hosp; **Address:** 158 Hempstead Ave, Lynbrook, NY 11563; **Phone:** 516-593-3541; **Board Cert:** Internal Medicine 1983; Pulmonary Disease 1988; **Med School:** Albert Einstein Coll Med 1980; **Resid:** Internal Medicine, Brookdale Hosp Med Ctr 1983; **Fellow:** Pulmonary Disease, Columbia-Presby Med Ctr 1985; Critical Care Medicine, Mount Sinai Hosp 1987; **Fac Appt:** Asst Clin Prof Med, SUNY Downstate

Radiation Oncology

Bosworth, Jay L MD (RadRO) - **Spec Exp:** Breast Cancer; Prostate Cancer; **Hospital:** St. Francis Hosp - The Heart Ctr (page 116), N Shore Univ Hosp (page 106); **Address:** NRAD Medical Associates, 6 Ohio Drive, Ste 103, Lake Success, NY 11042; **Phone:** 516-222-2022; **Board Cert:** Therapeutic Radiology 1974; **Med School:** Albert Einstein Coll Med 1970; **Resid:** Radiation Oncology, Bronx Muni Hosp Ctr 1974

Diamond, Ezriel MD (RadRO) - **Spec Exp:** Breast Cancer; Lung Cancer; Prostate Cancer; **Hospital:** Plainview Hosp (page 106); **Address:** Advanced Radiation Centers of New York, 688 Old Country Rd, Plainview, NY 11803; **Phone:** 516-932-6007; **Board Cert:** Therapeutic Radiology 1982; **Med School:** NYU Sch Med 1978; **Resid:** Radiation Oncology, NYU Med Ctr 1981; **Fellow:** Radiation Oncology, NY Methodist Hosp 1982

Gewanter, Richard M MD (RadRO) - **Spec Exp:** Prostate Cancer; Lung Cancer; **Hospital:** Meml Sloan-Kettering Canc Ctr (page 114); **Address:** MSKCC Rockville Centre, 1000 N Village Ave, Rockville Centre, NY 11570; **Phone:** 516-256-3600; **Board Cert:** Radiation Oncology 2012; **Med School:** Albert Einstein Coll Med 1995; **Resid:** Radiation Oncology, Columbia Presby Med Ctr 2002

Ghaly, Maged M MD (RadRO) - **Spec Exp:** Brachytherapy; Stereotactic Body Radiotherapy; Radiation Therapy-Intraoperative; **Hospital:** Long Is Jewish Med Ctr (page 106); **Address:** LIJ Dept Radiation Medicine, 270-05 76th Ave, New Hyde Park, NY 11040; **Phone:** 516-470-7190; **Board Cert:** Radiation Oncology 2013; **Med School:** Egypt 1992; **Resid:** Radiation Oncology, New York Methodist Hosp 2002; **Fellow:** Radiation Oncology, New York Methodist Hsop 2003

Haas, Jonathan A MD (RadRO) - **Spec Exp:** Brachytherapy; Prostate Cancer; Gynecologic Cancer; Intensity Modulated Radiotherapy (IMRT); **Hospital:** Winthrop Univ Hosp (page 524); **Address:** Winthrop Univ Hosp, Dept Radiation Oncology, 264 Old Country Rd, Mineola, NY 11501; **Phone:** 516-663-2501; **Board Cert:** Radiation Oncology 2009; **Med School:** Washington Univ, St Louis 1993; **Resid:** Radiation Oncology, Hosp Univ Penn 1997; **Fac Appt:** Asst Clin Prof RadRO, SUNY Stony Brook

Knisely, Jonathan P S MD (RadRO) - **Spec Exp:** Brain Tumors; Stereotactic Radiosurgery; Skull Base Tumors; **Hospital:** N Shore Univ Hosp (page 106), Glen Cove Hosp (page 106); **Address:** North Shore University Hospital, 300 Community Drive, Manhasset, NY 11030; **Phone:** 516-470-7190; **Board Cert:** Internal Medicine 1989; Radiation Oncology 1993; **Med School:** Univ Pennsylvania 1986; **Resid:** Internal Medicine, Michael Reese Hosp 1989; Radiation Oncology, Univ Toronto Med Ctr 1992; **Fac Appt:** Assoc Prof RadRO, Hofstra N Shore-LIJ Sch Med

Lee, Lucille MD (RadRO) - **Spec Exp:** Breast Cancer; Prostate Cancer; Gastrointestinal Cancer; **Hospital:** Long Is Jewish Med Ctr (page 106); **Address:** LIJ Dept Radiation Medicine, 270-05 76th Ave, New Hyde Park, NY 11040; **Phone:** 516-470-7190; **Board Cert:** Radiation Oncology 2011; **Med School:** UMDNJ-RW Johnson Med Sch 1996; **Resid:** Radiation Oncology, Mount Sinai Med Ctr 2001

Marienberg, Evelyn MD (RadRO) - **Spec Exp:** Breast Cancer; Head & Neck Cancer; Vulvar & Vaginal Cancer; **Hospital:** Glen Cove Hosp (page 106); **Address:** 101 St Andrews Ln, Glen Cove, NY 11542; **Phone:** 516-470-7190; **Board Cert:** Radiation Oncology 1996; **Med School:** SUNY Stony Brook 1988; **Resid:** Radiation Oncology, Univ of Miami Hosp & Clins/Sylvester Comp Canc Ctr 1992; **Fac Appt:** Asst Prof RadRO, SUNY Downstate

Mullen, Edward E MD (RadRO) - **Spec Exp:** Brain Tumors; Breast Cancer; Stereotactic Radiosurgery; **Hospital:** South Nassau Comm Hosp; **Address:** South Nassau Comm Hosp, Dept Radiation Oncology, One Healthy Way, Oceanside, NY 11572; **Phone:** 516-632-3370; **Board Cert:** Radiation Oncology 1991; **Med School:** Univ VA Sch Med 1986; **Resid:** Radiation Oncology, Columbia-Presby Med Ctr 1990

Potters, Louis MD (RadRO) - **Spec Exp:** Prostate Cancer; Intensity Modulated Radiotherapy (IMRT); Brachytherapy; **Hospital:** Long Is Jewish Med Ctr (page 106), N Shore Univ Hosp (page 106); **Address:** LIJ Medical Ctr, 270-05 76th Ave, New Hyde Park, NY 11040; **Phone:** 718-470-7190; **Board Cert:** Internal Medicine 1988; Radiation Oncology 1999; **Med School:** UMDNJ-NJ Med Sch, Newark 1985; **Resid:** Internal Medicine, Beth Israel Med Ctr 1988; Radiation Oncology, SUNY Downstate Med Ctr 1991; **Fac Appt:** Prof RadRO, Hofstra N Shore-LIJ Sch Med

Reproductive Endocrinology

Brenner, Steven H MD (RE) - **Spec Exp:** Infertility-IVF; Polycystic Ovarian Syndrome; **Hospital:** Long Is Jewish Med Ctr (page 106); **Address:** 2001 Marcus Ave, Ste N213, Lake Success, NY 11042; **Phone:** 516-358-6363; **Board Cert:** Obstetrics & Gynecology 1985; Reproductive Endocrinology 1987; **Med School:** SUNY Downstate 1978; **Resid:** Obstetrics & Gynecology, Beth Israel Med Ctr 1982; **Fellow:** Reproductive Endocrinology, NYU Med Ctr 1984; **Fac Appt:** Assoc Clin Prof ObG, Hofstra N Shore-LIJ Sch Med

Hershlag, Avner MD (RE) - **Spec Exp:** Fertility Preservation; Preimplantation Genetic Diagnosis; **Hospital:** N Shore Univ Hosp (page 106); **Address:** Center for Human Reproduction, 300 Community Drive, Manhasset, NY 11030; **Phone:** 516-562-2229; **Board Cert:** Obstetrics & Gynecology 2012; Reproductive Endocrinology 2012; **Med School:** Israel 1977; **Resid:** Surgery, Hadassah Affil Hosp 1984; Obstetrics & Gynecology, George Washington Univ Med Ctr 1988; **Fellow:** Reproductive Endocrinology, Yale-New Haven Hosp 1990; **Fac Appt:** Prof ObG, Hofstra N Shore-LIJ Sch Med

Rheumatology

Belilos, Elise MD (Rhu) - **Spec Exp:** Polymyalgia Rheumatica; Giant Cell Arteritis; Rheumatoid Arthritis; **Hospital:** Winthrop Univ Hosp (page 524); **Address:** Winthrop Univ Hosp, Div Rheum, 120 Mineola Blvd, Ste 410, Mineola, NY 11501; **Phone:** 516-663-2097; **Board Cert:** Internal Medicine 1989; Rheumatology 2004; **Med School:** SUNY Stony Brook 1986; **Resid:** Internal Medicine, Winthrop Univ Hosp 1990; **Fellow:** Rheumatology, Winthrop UnivHosp 1993; **Fac Appt:** Asst Clin Prof Med, SUNY Stony Brook

Blau, Sheldon P MD (Rhu) - **Spec Exp:** Lupus/SLE; Scleroderma; Rheumatoid Arthritis; Osteoporosis; **Hospital:** Winthrop Univ Hosp (page 524); **Address:** 566 Broadway, Massapequa, NY 11758-5017; **Phone:** 516-541-6262; **Board Cert:** Internal Medicine 1969; Rheumatology 1972; **Med School:** Albert Einstein Coll Med 1961; **Resid:** Internal Medicine, Montefiore Med Ctr 1964; **Fellow:** Rheumatology, Albert Einstein Coll Med 1965; **Fac Appt:** Clin Prof Med, SUNY Stony Brook

Carsons, Steven E MD (Rhu) - **Spec Exp:** Rheumatoid Arthritis; Sjogren's Syndrome; Vasculitis; **Hospital:** Winthrop Univ Hosp (page 524); **Address:** Winthrop Univ Hosp, Div Rhematology, 120 Mineola Blvd, Ste 410, Mineola, NY 11501; **Phone:** 516-663-2097; **Board Cert:** Internal Medicine 1978; Rheumatology 1980; Clinical & Laboratory Immunology 1988; **Med School:** NY Med Coll 1975; **Resid:** Internal Medicine, Maimonides Med Ctr 1978; **Fellow:** Rheumatology, SUNY Brooklyn Med Ctr 1980; **Fac Appt:** Prof Med, SUNY Hlth Sci Ctr

Cohen, Daniel Henry MD (Rhu) - **Spec Exp:** Osteoporosis; Amyloidosis; **Hospital:** South Nassau Comm Hosp, Franklin Hosp (page 106); **Address:** 1157 Broadway, Hewlett, NY 11557; **Phone:** 516-295-4481; **Board Cert:** Internal Medicine 1981; Rheumatology 1984; **Med School:** NYU Sch Med 1978; **Resid:** Internal Medicine, Columbia-Presby Med Ctr 1981; **Fellow:** Rheumatology, NYU Med Ctr 1983

Furie, Richard A MD (Rhu) - **Spec Exp:** Lupus/SLE; Antiphospholipid Syndrome (APS); Rheumatoid Arthritis; **Hospital:** N Shore Univ Hosp (page 106), Long Is Jewish Med Ctr (page 106); **Address:** 865 Northern Blvd, Ste 302, Great Neck, NY 11021; **Phone:** 516-708-2550; **Board Cert:** Internal Medicine 1982; Rheumatology 1984; **Med School:** Cornell Univ-Weill Med Coll 1979; **Resid:** Internal Medicine, NY Hosp 1982; **Fellow:** Rheumatology, Hosp Spec Surg 1984; **Fac Appt:** Prof Med, Albert Einstein Coll Med

Greenwald, Robert A MD (Rhu) - **Spec Exp:** Rheumatoid Arthritis; Psoriatic Arthritis; Osteoarthritis; Gout; **Hospital:** Long Is Jewish Med Ctr (page 106); **Address:** ProHealth Care Assocs, 2 ProHealth Plaza, Ste 103, Lake Success, NY 11042; **Phone:** 516-622-6090; **Board Cert:** Internal Medicine 1973; Rheumatology 1974; **Med School:** Johns Hopkins Univ 1967; **Resid:** Internal Medicine, LI Jewish-Hillside Med Ctr 1970; **Fellow:** Rheumatology, SUNY Brooklyn Med Ctr 1972; **Fac Appt:** Prof Med, Albert Einstein Coll Med

Hoffman, Michael L MD (Rhu) - **Spec Exp:** Lupus/SLE; Rheumatoid Arthritis; Osteoarthritis; Osteoporosis; **Hospital:** Long Is Jewish Med Ctr (page 106), N Shore Univ Hosp (page 106); **Address:** 560 Northern Blvd, Ste 107, Great Neck, NY 11021; **Phone:** 516-498-3500; **Board Cert:** Internal Medicine 1971; **Med School:** SUNY Downstate 1965; **Resid:** Internal Medicine, Maimonides Med Ctr 1967; Internal Medicine, Jacobi Med Ctr 1968; **Fellow:** Rheumatology, Hosp for Special Surg 1970; **Fac Appt:** Assoc Clin Prof Med, Albert Einstein Coll Med

Jarrett, Mark MD (Rhu) - **Spec Exp:** Lupus/SLE; Osteoporosis; Rheumatoid Arthritis; **Hospital:** Staten Island Univ Hosp - North (page 106), NS-LIJ Hlth Sys (page 106); **Address:** 145 Community Drive, Great Neck, NY 11021; **Phone:** 516-465-3214; **Board Cert:** Internal Medicine 1978; Rheumatology 1980; Geriatric Medicine 2008; **Med School:** NYU Sch Med 1975; **Resid:** Internal Medicine, Montefiore Med Ctr 1978; **Fellow:** Rheumatology, Montefiore Med Ctr 1980; **Fac Appt:** Prof D, Hofstra N Shore-LIJ Sch Med

Lipstein-Kresch, Esther MD (Rhu) - **Spec Exp:** Rheumatoid Arthritis; Osteoarthritis; Osteoporosis; Fibromyalgia; **Hospital:** Long Is Jewish Med Ctr (page 106), N Shore Univ Hosp (page 106); **Address:** ProHealth Care Assocs, 2 ProHealth Plaza, Ste 103, Lake Success, NY 11042-1111; **Phone:** 516-622-6090; **Board Cert:** Internal Medicine 1982; Rheumatology 1984; **Med School:** SUNY Hlth Sci Ctr 1979; **Resid:** Internal Medicine, LI Jewish Med Ctr 1982; **Fellow:** Rheumatology, LI Jewish Med Ctr 1984

Meredith, Gary S MD (Rhu) - **Spec Exp:** Gout; Lupus/SLE; Rheumatoid Arthritis; **Hospital:** St. Francis Hosp - The Heart Ctr (page 116); **Address:** 2 ProHEALTH Plaza, Ste 200, Lake Success, NY 11042; **Phone:** 516-622-6125; **Board Cert:** Internal Medicine 1984; Rheumatology 1986; **Med School:** NYU Sch Med 1981; **Resid:** Internal Medicine, Bellevue Hosp 1984; **Fellow:** Rheumatology, NYU Med Ctr 1986; **Fac Appt:** Asst Clin Prof Med, NYU Sch Med

Porges, Andrew J MD (Rhu) - **Spec Exp:** Osteoporosis; Rheumatoid Arthritis; Vasculitis; Lupus/SLE; **Hospital:** N Shore Univ Hosp (page 106), Glen Cove Hosp (page 106); **Address:** 1044 Northern Blvd, Ste 104, Roslyn, NY 11576; **Phone:** 516-484-6880; **Board Cert:** Internal Medicine 1989; Rheumatology 2012; **Med School:** Cornell Univ 1986; **Resid:** Internal Medicine, New York Hosp 1989; **Fellow:** Rheumatology, Hosp Special Surg 1992

Sullivan, James M MD (Rhu) - **Spec Exp:** Rheumatoid Arthritis; Lupus/SLE; Osteoarthritis; **Hospital:** Winthrop Univ Hosp (page 524); **Address:** 711 Stewart Ave, Ste 100, Garden City, NY 11530; **Phone:** 516-222-8654; **Board Cert:** Internal Medicine 1977; Rheumatology 1980; **Med School:** SUNY Upstate Med Univ 1974; **Resid:** Internal Medicine, Univ Michigan Med Ctr 1977; **Fellow:** Rheumatology, Univ Michigan Med Ctr 1979

Tiger, Louis MD (Rhu) - **Spec Exp:** Rheumatoid Arthritis; Lupus/SLE; Osteoarthritis; **Hospital:** Winthrop Univ Hosp (page 524); **Address:** 566 Broadway, Massapequa, NY 11758-5017; **Phone:** 516-541-6262; **Board Cert:** Internal Medicine 1975; Rheumatology 1976; **Med School:** Univ Louisville Sch Med 1967; **Resid:** Internal Medicine, Maimonides Medical Ctr 1970; **Fellow:** Rheumatology, Albert Einstein Med Ctr 1974; **Fac Appt:** Asst Clin Prof Med, SUNY Stony Brook

Sports Medicine

Briner Jr, William W MD (SM) - **Spec Exp:** Primary Care Sports Medicine; **Hospital:** Hosp For Special Surgery (page 113); **Address:** 333 Earle Ovington Blvd, Omni Bldg - Ste 106, Uniondale, NY 11553; **Phone:** 516-222-6803; **Board Cert:** Family Medicine 2007; Sports Medicine 2013; **Med School:** Ohio State Univ 1985; **Resid:** Family Medicine, Macneal Meml Hosp 1988; **Fellow:** Sports Medicine, Marshall Univ 1990; **Fac Appt:** Asst Clin Prof FMed, Univ IL Coll Med

Surgery

Auguste, Louis J MD (S) - **Spec Exp:** Breast Disease; Melanoma; Thyroid & Parathyroid Surgery; Hernia; **Hospital:** Long Is Jewish Med Ctr (page 106), N Shore Univ Hosp (page 106); **Address:** 2035 Lakeville Rd, Ste 206, New Hyde Park, NY 11042-1102; **Phone:** 516-775-2070; **Board Cert:** Surgery 2011; **Med School:** Haiti 1973; **Resid:** Surgery, Long Is Jewish Med Ctr 1980; **Fellow:** Surgical Oncology, Roswell Park Canc Inst 1982; **Fac Appt:** Assoc Clin Prof S, Albert Einstein Coll Med

Bank, Matthew A MD (S) - **Spec Exp:** Trauma; **Hospital:** N Shore Univ Hosp (page 106), NS-LIJ Hlth Sys (page 106); **Address:** 1999 Marcus Ave, Ste 106C, Lake Success, NY 11030; **Phone:** 516-233-3610; **Board Cert:** Surgery 2011; Surgical Critical Care 2003; **Med School:** NY Med Coll 1995; **Resid:** Surgery, Long Is Jewish Med Ctr 2000; **Fellow:** Surgical Critical Care, Yale-New Haven Hosp 2001

Benowitz, Joel MD (S) - **Spec Exp:** Breast Cancer; Breast Disease; Minimally Invasive Surgery; Breast Reconstruction; **Hospital:** Mercy Med Ctr - Rockville Centre; **Address:** 1000 North Village Ave, Rockville Centre, NY 11570; **Phone:** 516-889-9100; **Board Cert:** Surgery 2012; **Med School:** Mexico 1975; **Resid:** Surgery, Brookdale Hosp Med Ctr 1981

Brathwaite, Collin MD (S) - **Spec Exp:** Obesity/Bariatric Surgery; Trauma; Minimally Invasive Surgery; Gastrointestinal Surgery; **Hospital:** Winthrop Univ Hosp (page 524); **Address:** Winthrop Surgical Weight Loss, 120 Mineola Blvd, Ste 320, Mineola, NY 11501; **Phone:** 855-678-7436; **Board Cert:** Surgery 2011; **Med School:** Howard Univ 1983; **Resid:** Surgery, St Vincents Hosp & Med Ctr 1998; **Fellow:** Surgical Critical Care, Univ Maryland Med Ctr 1998; **Fac Appt:** Assoc Prof S, SUNY Stony Brook

Conte, Charles C MD (S) - **Spec Exp:** Cancer Surgery; Breast Cancer; Pancreatic Cancer; **Hospital:** N Shore Univ Hosp (page 106), Forest Hills Hosp (page 106); **Address:** 600 Northern Blvd, Ste 111, Great Neck, NY 11021; **Phone:** 516-487-9454; **Board Cert:** Surgery 2005; **Med School:** Dartmouth Med Sch 1981; **Resid:** Surgery, Hartford Hosp 1986; **Fellow:** Surgical Oncology, Roswell Pk Canc Inst 1988

Coppa, Gene F MD (S) - **Spec Exp:** Minimally Invasive Surgery; Hepatobiliary Surgery; Gastrointestinal Surgery; Pancreatic Surgery; **Hospital:** N Shore Univ Hosp (page 106); **Address:** N Shore Univ Hosp, 300 Community Drive, Manhasset, NY 11030; **Phone:** 516-562-2870; **Board Cert:** Surgery 2010; **Med School:** NYU Sch Med 1974; **Resid:** Surgery, NYU/Bellevue Med Ctr 1979; **Fac Appt:** Prof S, Hofstra N Shore-LIJ Sch Med

Datta, Rajiv V MD (S) - **Spec Exp:** Breast Cancer; Colon & Rectal Cancer; Gastrointestinal Cancer; Head & Neck Cancer; **Hospital:** South Nassau Comm Hosp; **Address:** South Nassau Comm Hosp Canc Ctr, 1 S Central Ave, Valley Stream, NY 11580; **Phone:** 516-632-3350; **Board Cert:** Surgery 2009; **Med School:** India 1984; **Resid:** Surgery, Maimonides Med Ctr 1998; **Fellow:** Surgical Oncology, Roswell Park Canc Inst 1999; Head and Neck Surgery, Roswell Park Canc Inst 2000; **Fac Appt:** Assoc Clin Prof S, NY Coll Osteo Med

Denoto, George MD (S) - **Spec Exp:** Laparoscopic Surgery; Hernia; **Hospital:** St. Francis Hosp - The Heart Ctr (page 116); **Address:** 139 Plandome Rd, Manhasset, NY 11030; **Phone:** 516-627-5262; **Board Cert:** Surgery 2006; **Med School:** SUNY Stony Brook 1988; **Resid:** Surgery, Mt Sinai Med Ctr 1994

Gecelter, Gary MD (S) - **Spec Exp:** Pancreatic Cancer; Esophageal Surgery; Laparoscopic Surgery; Biliary Surgery; **Hospital:** St. Francis Hosp - The Heart Ctr (page 116); **Address:** 139 Plandome Rd, Manhasset, NY 11030; **Phone:** 516-627-5262; **Med School:** South Africa 1981; **Resid:** Surgery, Johannesburg Hosp 1990; **Fellow:** Gastroenterology, Johannesburg Hosp 1992

Grieco, Michael B MD (S) - **Spec Exp:** Breast Surgery; Laparoscopic Abdominal Surgery; Hernia; Laparoscopic Cholecystectomy; **Hospital:** Glen Cove Hosp (page 106), St. Francis Hosp - The Heart Ctr (page 116); **Address:** 10 Medical Plaza, Ste 105, Glen Cove, NY 11542; **Phone:** 516-676-1060; **Board Cert:** Surgery 2010; Colon & Rectal Surgery 1982; **Med School:** Albany Med Coll 1974; **Resid:** Surgery, N Shore Univ Hosp 1979; **Fellow:** Surgery, Lahey Clinic 1980; Colon & Rectal Surgery, Greater Baltimore Med Ctr 1981

Khalife, Michael E MD (S) - **Spec Exp:** Laparoscopic Surgery; Breast Surgery; **Hospital:** Winthrop Univ Hosp (page 524), N Shore Univ Hosp (page 106); **Address:** Nassau Surgical Assocs, 300 Old Country Rd, Ste 101, Mineola, NY 11501; **Phone:** 516-741-4138; **Board Cert:** Surgery 2003; **Med School:** France 1978; **Resid:** Surgery, Stony Brook Univ Med Ctr 1984; **Fac Appt:** Asst Clin Prof S, SUNY Stony Brook

Kurtz, Lewis M MD (S) - **Spec Exp:** Breast Surgery; Gallbladder Surgery; Hernia; **Hospital:** St. Francis Hosp - The Heart Ctr (page 116), Long Is Jewish Med Ctr (page 106); **Address:** 310 E Shore Rd, Ste 203, Great Neck, NY 11023; **Phone:** 516-482-8657; **Board Cert:** Surgery 2010; **Med School:** Italy 1972; **Resid:** Surgery, Long Is Jewish Med Ctr 1977; **Fellow:** Research, Long Is Jewish Med Ctr 1978

Mansouri, Hormoz MD (S) - **Spec Exp:** Varicose Veins; **Hospital:** N Shore Univ Hosp (page 106); **Address:** 175 Jericho Tpke, Ste 201, Syosset, NY 11791; **Phone:** 516-682-4800; **Board Cert:** Surgery 1980; **Med School:** Iran 1964; **Resid:** Surgery, Henry Ford Hosp 1969; Surgery, Nassau Univ Med Ctr 1971; **Fac Appt:** Asst Prof S, SUNY Stony Brook

Molmenti, Ernesto P MD/PhD (S) - **Spec Exp:** Transplant-Kidney; **Hospital:** Long Is Jewish Med Ctr (page 106), NS-LIJ Hlth Sys (page 106); **Address:** 1554 Northern Blvd, Manhasset, NY 11030; **Phone:** 516-472-5800; **Board Cert:** Surgery 2006; **Med School:** Boston Univ 1989; **Resid:** Surgery, Barnes Jewish Med Ctr 1996; **Fellow:** Research, Wash Univ Affil Hosp 1994; Research, Thomas E. Starzl Transplantation Inst 1998; **Fac Appt:** Prof S, Boston Univ

Reiner, Dan S MD (S) - **Spec Exp:** Laparoscopic Surgery; Hernia; Gastrointestinal Surgery; **Hospital:** N Shore Univ Hosp (page 106), Syosset Hosp (page 106); **Address:** 2800 Marcus Ave, Ste 204, Lake Success, NY 11042-1008; **Phone:** 516-622-6120; **Board Cert:** Surgery 2005; Surgical Critical Care 2007; **Med School:** St Louis Univ 1980; **Resid:** Surgery, St Louis Univ Hosp 1985; **Fellow:** Surgical Critical Care, UMDNJ-NJ Med Sch Affil Hosp 1986; **Fac Appt:** Assoc Clin Prof S, NYU Sch Med

Romero, Carlos A MD (S) - **Spec Exp:** Laparoscopic Surgery; Head & Neck Surgery; Breast Surgery; **Hospital:** Winthrop Univ Hosp (page 524); **Address:** 173 Mineola Blvd, Ste 401, Mineola, NY 11501-2555; **Phone:** 516-741-6464; **Board Cert:** Surgery 2007; **Med School:** Argentina 1969; **Resid:** Surgery, Winthrop Univ Hosp 1975; **Fellow:** Surgical Oncology, Med Coll VA Affil Hosp 1977; **Fac Appt:** Assoc Prof S, SUNY Stony Brook

Vitale, Gerard F MD (S) - **Spec Exp:** Aneurysm; Carotid Artery Surgery; Varicose Veins; Arterial Bypass Surgery; **Hospital:** Glen Cove Hosp (page 106); **Address:** 10 Medical Plaza, Ste 305, Glen Cove, NY 11542; **Phone:** 516-759-5559; **Board Cert:** Surgery 2010; **Med School:** SUNY Buffalo 1982; **Resid:** Surgery, N Shore Univ Hosp 1987; **Fellow:** Vascular Surgery, St Vincents Hosp 1988

Thoracic & Cardiac Surgery

Andaz, Shahriyour J MD (T&CS) - **Spec Exp:** Thoracic Cancers; Lung Cancer; **Hospital:** South Nassau Comm Hosp, Franklin Hosp (page 106); **Address:** 444 Merrick Rd, Ste 380, Lynbrook, NY 11563; **Phone:** 516-255-5010; **Board Cert:** Surgery 2009; Thoracic & Cardiac Surgery 2010; **Med School:** India 1983; **Resid:** Surgery, Bronx Lebanon Hosp Ctr 1998; **Fellow:** Thoracic Surgery, SUNY Hlth Sci Ctr 2001

Barrett, Leonard O MD (T&CS) - **Spec Exp:** Chest Trauma; Esophageal Tumors; Critical Care; **Hospital:** Nassau Univ Med Ctr; **Address:** Nassau Univ Med Ctr, 2201 Hempstead Tpke, Fl 8, East Meadow, NY 11554; **Phone:** 516-572-6703; **Board Cert:** Surgery 2009; Surgical Critical Care 2010; Thoracic Surgery 2005; **Med School:** SUNY Downstate 1983; **Resid:** Surgery, SUNY Stony Brook Med Ctr 1989; Cardiothoracic Surgery, Beth Israel Med Ctr 1993; **Fellow:** Surgical Critical Care, Winthrop Univ Med Ctr 1990

Esposito, Rick A MD (T&CS) - **Spec Exp:** Cardiac Surgery; Coronary Artery Surgery; Mitral Valve Minimally Invasive Surgery; **Hospital:** N Shore Univ Hosp (page 106); **Address:** N Shore Univ Hosp, Dept Cardiothoracic Surgery, 300 Community Drive, Manhasset, NY 11030; **Phone:** 516-562-4970; **Board Cert:** Thoracic Surgery 2006; **Med School:** Univ Chicago-Pritzker Sch Med 1979; **Resid:** Surgery, NYU Langone Med Ctr 1984; **Fellow:** Thoracic Surgery, NYU Langone Med Ctr 1986; **Fac Appt:** Assoc Clin Prof S, NYU Sch Med

Fernandez, Harold A MD (T&CS) - **Spec Exp:** Cardiac Surgery-High Risk; Minimally Invasive Heart Valve Surgery; Ventricular Assist Device (LVAD); Atrial Fibrillation; **Hospital:** Stony Brook Univ Med Ctr; **Address:** Stony Brook Surgical Assocs, 101 Nicolls Rd, HSC T19-080, Stony Brook, NY 11794-8191; **Phone:** 631-444-1820; **Board Cert:** Surgery 2012; Thoracic Surgery 2005; **Med School:** Harvard Med Sch 1993; **Resid:** Surgery, NYU Med Ctr 1999; **Fellow:** Cardiothoracic Surgery, NYU Med Ctr 2001; **Fac Appt:** Clin Prof T&CS, SUNY Stony Brook

Glassman, Lawrence R MD (T&CS) - **Spec Exp:** Lung Cancer; Esophageal Cancer; Emphysema; Tracheal Surgery; **Hospital:** N Shore Univ Hosp (page 106); **Address:** 225 Community Drive, Ste 110, Great Neck, NY 11021; **Phone:** 516-918-4388; **Board Cert:** Thoracic Surgery 2013; **Med School:** NYU Sch Med 1981; **Resid:** Surgery, Univ Minn Affil Hosps 1983; Surgery, NYU Langone Med Ctr 1987; **Fellow:** Thoracic Surgery, Meml Sloan-Kettering Canc Ctr 1988; Thoracic Surgery, NYU Langone Med Ctr 1990

Hyman, Kevin M MD (T&CS) - **Spec Exp:** Lung Cancer; Esophageal Cancer; Emphysema; Minimally Invasive Thoracic Surgery; **Hospital:** N Shore Univ Hosp (page 106); **Address:** NS-LIJ Med Grp, Div Thoracic Surg, 225 Community Drive, Ste 110, Great Neck, NY 11021; **Phone:** 516-918-4388; **Board Cert:** Surgery 2006; Thoracic & Cardiac Surgery 2007; **Med School:** Cornell Univ-Weill Med Coll 1997; **Resid:** Surgery, NYU Med Ctr 2004; **Fellow:** Cardiothoracic Surgery, NYU Med Ctr 2006; Thoracic Surgery, Mount Sinai Med Ctr 2007; **Fac Appt:** Asst Prof S, Hofstra N Shore-LIJ Sch Med

Kline, Gary M MD (T&CS) - **Spec Exp:** Lung Cancer; Emphysema; Mediastinal Tumors; **Hospital:** Holy Name Med Ctr (page 720); **Address:** Summit Surgical Inst, 332 Summit Ave, Hackensack, NJ 07601; **Phone:** 201-488-6445; **Board Cert:** Surgery 2004; Thoracic & Cardiac Surgery 2005; **Med School:** Wayne State Univ 1986; **Resid:** Surgery, Detroit Med Ctr 1991; **Fellow:** Thoracic Surgery, Hosp Univ Penn 1994

Meyer, David B MD (T&CS) - **Spec Exp:** Pediatric Cardiac Surgery; Congenital Heart Disease-Adult & Child; **Hospital:** Steven & Alexandra Cohen Chldn's Med Ctr of NY (page 106); **Address:** Steven & Alexandra Cohen Children's Med Ctr, 269-01 76th Ave, Ste 139, New Hyde Park, NY 11040; **Phone:** 718-470-3580; **Board Cert:** Surgery 2003; Thoracic Surgery 2005; Congenital Cardiac Surgery 2010; **Med School:** Yale Univ 1997; **Resid:** Surgery, NYU Med Ctr 2002; **Fellow:** Cardiothoracic Surgery, NYU Med Ctr 2004

Pogo, Gustave MD (T&CS) - **Spec Exp:** Aneurysm-Aortic; **Hospital:** N Shore Univ Hosp (page 106); **Address:** N Shore, Thoracic & Cardiac Surgery, 300 Community Drive, Manhasset, NY 11030; **Phone:** 516-562-4970; **Board Cert:** Thoracic & Cardiac Surgery 2011; **Med School:** NYU Sch Med 1983; **Resid:** Surgery, N Shore Univ Hosp 1988; Cardiothoracic Surgery, Mount Sinai Med Ctr 1991

Robinson, Newell B MD (T&CS) - **Spec Exp:** Minimally Invasive Cardiac Surgery; Maze Procedure for Atrial Fibrillation; **Hospital:** St. Francis Hosp - The Heart Ctr (page 116); **Address:** St Francis Hosp-The Heart Ctr, 100 Port Washington Blvd, Ste G01, Roslyn, NY 11576; **Phone:** 516-627-2173; **Board Cert:** Surgery 2005; Thoracic Surgery 2006; **Med School:** Univ Miss 1973; **Resid:** Surgery, NY-Presby/Weill Cornell Med Ctrr 1984; Surgery, Meml Sloan Kettering Canc Ctr 1984; **Fellow:** Trauma, Univ Washington Med Ctr 1981; Cardiothoracic Surgery, NY-Presby/Weill Cornell Med Ctr 1986

Schubach, Scott L MD (T&CS) - **Spec Exp:** Cardiac Surgery; Coronary Artery Surgery; Heart Valve Surgery; Minimally Invasive Surgery; **Hospital:** Winthrop Univ Hosp (page 524); **Address:** 120 Mineola Blvd, Ste 300, Mineola, NY 11501; **Phone:** 516-663-4400; **Board Cert:** Surgery 2007; Thoracic Surgery 2010; Surgical Critical Care 2010; **Med School:** Baylor Coll Med 1983; **Resid:** Surgery, Dartmouth Hitchcock Med Ctr Ctr. 1988; Cardiothoracic Surgery, Univ of Pittsburgh Med Ctr 1991

Zeltsman, Vadim MD (T&CS) - **Spec Exp:** Thoracic Cancers; Video Assisted Thoracic Surgery (VATS); **Hospital:** Long Is Jewish Med Ctr (page 106), N Shore Univ Hosp (page 106); **Address:** 225 Community Drive, Ste 110, Great Neck, NY 11021; **Phone:** 516-918-4388; **Board Cert:** Surgery 2011; Thoracic Surgery 2013; **Med School:** Russia 1986; **Resid:** Surgery, Mercy Catholic Med Ctr 1997; **Fellow:** Cardiothoracic Surgery, UMDNJ Affil Hosp 2000

Urology

Ashley, Richard N MD (U) - **Hospital:** N Shore Univ Hosp (page 106); **Address:** 233 7th St, Ste 203, Garden City, NY 11530; **Phone:** 516-294-7666; **Board Cert:** Urology 1980; **Med School:** NY Med Coll 1972; **Resid:** Surgery, St Vincents Hosp 1975; Urology, SUNY Downstate Med Ctr 1980; **Fac Appt:** Asst Clin Prof U, SUNY Stony Brook

Bruno, Anthony M MD (U) - **Spec Exp:** Prostate Cancer; Kidney Stones; Voiding Dysfunction; **Hospital:** Winthrop Univ Hosp (page 524); **Address:** 1305 Franklin Ave, Ste 100, Garden City, NY 11530; **Phone:** 516-746-5550; **Board Cert:** Urology 1977; **Med School:** Italy 1968; **Resid:** Surgery, Winthrop Univ Hosp 1972; Urology, Bellevue Hosp Ctr 1975; **Fac Appt:** Asst Prof U, SUNY Stony Brook

D'Esposito, Robert F MD (U) - **Hospital:** Winthrop Univ Hosp (page 524); **Address:** 601 Franklin Ave, Ste 300, Garden City, NY 11530-5759; **Phone:** 516-742-3200; **Board Cert:** Urology 1981; **Med School:** Italy 1971; **Resid:** Surgery, Winthrop Univ Hosp 1972; Urology, Winthrop Univ Hosp 1978; **Fac Appt:** Assoc Clin Prof U, SUNY Stony Brook

Edelman, Robert A MD (U) - **Hospital:** Winthrop Univ Hosp (page 524); **Address:** 601 Franklin Ave, Ste 300, Garden City, NY 11530-5729; **Phone:** 516-742-3200; **Board Cert:** Urology 1981; **Med School:** SUNY Upstate Med Univ 1974; **Resid:** Surgery, Montefiore Med Ctr 1976; Urology, Montefiore Med Ctr 1981; **Fac Appt:** Assoc Clin Prof U, SUNY Stony Brook

Gershbaum, Meyer D MD (U) - **Spec Exp:** Robotic Surgery; Laparoscopic Surgery; **Hospital:** Winthrop Univ Hosp (page 524), NS-LIJ Hlth Sys (page 106); **Address:** 601 Franklin Ave, Ste 300, Garden City, NY 11530; **Phone:** 516-742-3200; **Board Cert:** Urology 2013; **Med School:** Albert Einstein Coll Med 1996; **Resid:** Surgery, LI Jewish Med Ctr 1998; Urology, LI Jewish Med Ctr 2002; **Fellow:** Laparoscopic Surgery, VA Med Ctr 2003

Girardi, Sarah K MD (U) - **Spec Exp:** Urology-Female; Infertility-Male; **Hospital:** N Shore Univ Hosp (page 106), St. Francis Hosp - The Heart Ctr (page 116); **Address:** 535 Plandome Rd, Ste 3, Manhasset, NY 11030; **Phone:** 516-627-6188; **Board Cert:** Urology 2006; **Med School:** Univ NC Sch Med 1989; **Resid:** Urology, NY-Presby/Weill Cornell Med Ctr 1995; **Fellow:** Urology, Yale-New Haven Hosp 1996; **Fac Appt:** Assoc Prof U, Cornell Univ

Hanna, Moneer K MD (U) - **Spec Exp:** Pediatric Urology; Reconstructive Surgery; Hypospadias; Bladder Surgery; **Hospital:** Steven & Alexandra Cohen Chldn's Med Ctr of NY (page 106), NY-Presby/Weill Cornell Med Ctr, NY (page 104); **Address:** 935 Northern Blvd, Ste 303, Great Neck, NY 11021; **Phone:** 516-466-6950; **Board Cert:** Urology 1978; **Med School:** Egypt 1963; **Resid:** Urology, London Univ Affil Hosp 1972; Urology, Univ West Ont Affil Hosps 1976; **Fellow:** Pediatric Urology, Hosp For Sick Chldn 1975; **Fac Appt:** Clin Prof U, Cornell Univ-Weill Med Coll

Harris, Steven M MD (U) - **Spec Exp:** Impotence; Prostate Disease; Kidney Stones; **Hospital:** Long Beach Med Ctr, South Nassau Comm Hosp; **Address:** 711 Lincoln Blvd, Long Beach, NY 11561-3241; **Phone:** 516-431-9800; **Board Cert:** Urology 1984; **Med School:** Albert Einstein Coll Med 1976; **Resid:** Urology, Mt Sinai Med Ctr 1982; **Fac Appt:** Asst Prof U, NY Coll Osteo Med

Katz, Aaron E MD (U) - **Spec Exp:** Prostate Cancer-Cryosurgery; Kidney Cancer-Cryosurgery; Complementary Medicine; Nutrition & Cancer Prevention; **Hospital:** Winthrop Univ Hosp (page 524); **Address:** Winthrop Urology, 1401 Franklin Ave, Garden City, NY 11530; **Phone:** 516-535-1900; **Board Cert:** Urology 2006; **Med School:** NY Med Coll 1986; **Resid:** Urology, Maimonides Med Ctr 1992; **Fellow:** Urologic Oncology, Columbia Presby Med Ctr 1993; **Fac Appt:** Assoc Clin Prof U, Columbia P&S

Kavoussi, Louis R MD (U) - **Spec Exp:** Robotic Surgery; Urologic Cancer; Prostate Cancer; Kidney Cancer; **Hospital:** Long Is Jewish Med Ctr (page 106), N Shore Univ Hosp (page 106); **Address:** Arthur Smith Institute for Urology, 450 Lakeville Rd, Ste M-41, New Hyde Park, NY 11042; **Phone:** 516-734-8558; **Board Cert:** Urology 2009; **Med School:** SUNY Buffalo 1983; **Resid:** Surgery, Barnes Jewish Hosp 1985; Urology, Barnes Jewish Hosp 1989; **Fac Appt:** Prof U, Hofstra N Shore-LIJ Sch Med

Layne, Jeffrey MD (U) - **Spec Exp:** Kidney Stones; Incontinence; Impotence; **Hospital:** St. Joseph's Hosp-Nassau, N Shore Univ Hosp (page 106); **Address:** Advn Urology Ctrs NY, 1181 Old Country Rd, Ste 1, Plainview, NY 11803-5018; **Phone:** 516-933-6060; **Board Cert:** Urology 2007; **Med School:** SUNY Stony Brook 1989; **Resid:** Surgery, Tufts-New England Med Ctr 1991; Urology, Tufts-New England Med CtrTufts-New England Med Ctr 1996

Levine, Michael MD (U) - **Spec Exp:** Urologic Cancer; Kidney Stones; Erectile Dysfunction; Incontinence; **Hospital:** Long Is Jewish Med Ctr (page 106), N Shore Univ Hosp (page 106); **Address:** Lake Success Urological Assocs, 2001 Marcus Ave, Ste N214, Lake Success, NY 11042; **Phone:** 516-437-4228; **Board Cert:** Urology 2008; **Med School:** SUNY Downstate 1992; **Resid:** Urology, NYU Med Ctr 1998; **Fac Appt:** Asst Clin Prof U, SUNY Upstate Med Univ

Lieberman, Elliott MD (U) - **Hospital:** Plainview Hosp (page 106); **Address:** Advanced Urology Ctrs NY, 875 Old Country Rd, Ste 301, Plainview, NY 11803-4934; **Phone:** 516-931-1710; **Board Cert:** Urology 1983; **Med School:** SUNY Downstate 1976; **Resid:** Surgery, Mt Sinai Med Ctr 1978; Urology, SUNY Downstate Med Ctr 1983

Mellinger, Brett C MD (U) - **Spec Exp:** Infertility-Male; Impotence; **Hospital:** Winthrop Univ Hosp (page 524), N Shore Univ Hosp (page 106); **Address:** Advanced Urology Ctrs of NY, Garden City East Div, 100 Garden City Plaza, Ste 101, Garden City, NY 11530; **Phone:** 516-873-5353; **Board Cert:** Urology 2010; **Med School:** Indiana Univ 1981; **Resid:** Urology, SUNY Downstate Med Ctr 1985; Urology, NY-Presby/Weill Cornell Med Ctr 1986; **Fellow:** Male Infertility, NY-Presby/Weill Cornell Med Ctr 1988; **Fac Appt:** Assoc Clin Prof U, SUNY Stony Brook

Moldwin, Robert MD (U) - **Spec Exp:** Urinary Tract Infections; **Hospital:** Long Is Jewish Med Ctr (page 106), NS-LIJ Hlth Sys (page 106); **Address:** 450 Lakeville Rd B Bldg - Ste M41, New Hyde Park, NY 11040-1433; **Phone:** 516-734-8500; **Board Cert:** Urology 2012; **Med School:** Univ Chicago-Pritzker Sch Med 1984; **Resid:** Surgery, LI Jewish Med Ctr 1986; Urology, Thomas Jefferson Univ Hosp 1992; **Fac Appt:** Assoc Clin Prof U, Albert Einstein Coll Med

Paul, Elliot M MD (U) - **Spec Exp:** Prostate Cancer; Kidney Stones; Laparoscopic Surgery; **Hospital:** Long Is Jewish Med Ctr (page 106), St. Francis Hosp - The Heart Ctr (page 116); **Address:** Advanced Urology Centers of NY, Integrated Medical Professionals, 2001 Marcus Ave, Ste N214, Lake Success, NY 11042; **Phone:** 516-437-4228; **Board Cert:** Urology 2007; **Med School:** Albert Einstein Coll Med 2000; **Resid:** Urology, Long Island Jewish Med Ctr 2005

Richstone, Lee MD (U) - **Hospital:** Long Is Jewish Med Ctr (page 106), NS-LIJ Hlth Sys (page 106); **Address:** Arthur Smith Inst, 450 Lakeville Rd, Ste M41, New Hyde Park, NY 11042; **Phone:** 516-734-8500; **Board Cert:** Urology 2009; **Med School:** Cornell Univ-Weill Med Coll 2000; **Resid:** Urology, NY-Presby/Weill Cornell Med Ctr 2006

Shepard, Barry R MD (U) - **Spec Exp:** Kidney Stones; Urologic Cancer; **Hospital:** Winthrop Univ Hosp (page 524), N Shore Univ Hosp (page 106); **Address:** 601 Franklin Ave, Ste 300, Garden City, NY 11530; **Phone:** 516-742-3200; **Board Cert:** Urology 2006; **Med School:** SUNY Downstate 1979; **Resid:** Surgery, Long Is Jewish Med Ctr 1981; Urology, NY-Presby/Columbia Univ Med Ctr 1984

Sunshine, Robert D MD (U) - **Spec Exp:** Vasectomy-Scalpelless; Prostate Disease; **Hospital:** St. Joseph's Hosp-Nassau, Plainview Hosp (page 106); **Address:** Advanced Urology Ctrs of NY, 480 Hicksville Rd, Bethpage, NY 11714-5700; **Phone:** 516-796-2222; **Board Cert:** Urology 2005; **Med School:** Mexico 1977; **Resid:** Surgery, Long Island Jewish Hosp 1981; Urology, Mount Sinai Med Ctr 1985

Ziegelbaum, Michael M MD (U) - **Spec Exp:** Incontinence-Male & Female; Prostate Disease; Laparoscopic Surgery; Kidney Stones; **Hospital:** Long Is Jewish Med Ctr (page 106), St. Francis Hosp - The Heart Ctr (page 116); **Address:** 2001 Marcus Ave, Ste N214, Lake Success, NY 11042; **Phone:** 516-437-4228; **Board Cert:** Urology 2010; **Med School:** Cornell Univ-Weill Med Coll 1982; **Resid:** Urology, Cleveland Clin 1988; **Fellow:** Stone Disease, Stony Brook Univ Med Ctr 1989; **Fac Appt:** Asst Clin Prof S, Albert Einstein Coll Med

Vascular & Interventional Radiology

Cooper, Stanley G MD (VIR) - **Spec Exp:** Interventional Radiology; Dialysis Access; **Address:** ProHEALTH Care Associates, 2800 Marcus Ave, Lake Success, NY 11042; **Phone:** 516-622-7485; **Board Cert:** Diagnostic Radiology ; Vascular & Interventional Radiology 2006; **Med School:** Albert Einstein Coll Med 1984; **Resid:** Diagnostic Radiology, Norwalk Hosp 1989; **Fellow:** Vascular & Interventional Radiology, Yale-New Haven Hosp 1990

Crystal, Kenneth S MD (VIR) - **Spec Exp:** Interventional Radiology; Uterine Fibroid Embolization; Angioplasty; **Hospital:** St. Francis Hosp - The Heart Ctr (page 116); **Address:** 100 Port Washington Blvd, Roslyn, NY 11576; **Phone:** 516-562-6509; **Board Cert:** Diagnostic Radiology 1986; **Med School:** Univ Rochester 1981; **Resid:** Internal Medicine, Beth Israel Med Ctr - Petrie Div 1982; Diagnostic Radiology, NYU Langone Med Ctr 1986; **Fellow:** Vascular & Interventional Radiology, NYU Langone Med Ctr 1986; **Fac Appt:** Asst Prof Rad, NYU Sch Med

Hon, Man MD (VIR) - **Hospital:** Winthrop Univ Hosp (page 524); **Address:** Winthrop Univ Hosp, 259 1st St, Mineola, NY 11501; **Phone:** 516-663-2452; **Board Cert:** Diagnostic Radiology 1990; Vascular & Interventional Radiology 2009; **Med School:** Albert Einstein Coll Med 1985; **Resid:** Diagnostic Radiology, Montefiore Med Ctr 1990; **Fellow:** Vascular & Interventional Radiology, NY-Presby/Weill Cornell Med Ctr 1991; **Fac Appt:** Asst Prof Rad, SUNY Stony Brook

Naidich, Jason MD (VIR) - **Hospital:** N Shore Univ Hosp (page 106); **Address:** North Shore Dept Radiology, 300 Community Drive, Manhasset, NY 11030; **Phone:** 516-562-4797; **Board Cert:** Diagnostic Radiology 2000; Vascular & Interventional Radiology 2002; **Med School:** Cornell Univ 1995; **Resid:** Diagnostic Radiology, NYU Med Ctr 2000; **Fellow:** Vascular & Interventional Radiology, NYU Med Ctr 2001; Magnetic Resonance Imaging, Beth Israel Deaconess Med Ctr 2002; **Fac Appt:** Clin Prof Rad

Siegel, David N MD (VIR) - **Spec Exp:** Uterine Fibroid Embolization; **Hospital:** Long Is Jewish Med Ctr (page 106); **Address:** LIJ Interventional Radiology, 270-05 76th Ave, New Hyde Park, NY 11040; **Phone:** 718-470-7134; **Board Cert:** Diagnostic Radiology 1991; Vascular & Interventional Radiology 2006; **Med School:** UMDNJ-NJ Med Sch, Newark 1986; **Resid:** Diagnostic Radiology, Hackensack Univ Med Ctr 1991; **Fellow:** Vascular & Interventional Radiology, LIJ Med Ctr 1996; **Fac Appt:** Asst Prof Rad, Albert Einstein Coll Med

Vascular Surgery

Chaudhry, Saqib S MD (VascS) - **Spec Exp:** Aneurysm-Aortic; Carotid Artery Surgery; Dialysis Access Surgery; Limb Sparing Surgery; **Hospital:** Forest Hills Hosp (page 106), Flushing Hosp Med Ctr; **Address:** 1044 Northern Blvd, Ste 302, Roslyn, NY 11576; **Phone:** 516-621-1313; **Board Cert:** Vascular Surgery 2009; Thoracic & Cardiac Surgery 2011; **Med School:** Iraq 1972; **Resid:** Surgery, Flushing Hosp Med Ctr 1978; Thoracic Surgery, Wayne State Univ Affil Hosps 1980

Faust, Glenn R MD (VascS) - **Spec Exp:** Carotid Artery Surgery; Diabetic Leg/Foot; Aneurysm-Abdominal Aortic; Vein Disorders; **Hospital:** Nassau Univ Med Ctr; **Address:** 2201 Hempstead Tpke, East Meadow, NY 11554; **Phone:** 516-572-4848; **Board Cert:** Vascular Surgery 2004; **Med School:** Yale Univ 1986; **Resid:** Surgery, LI Jewish Med Ctr 1991; **Fellow:** Vascular Surgery, LI Jewish Med Ctr 1992; **Fac Appt:** Asst Prof S, Albert Einstein Coll Med

Landis, Gregg S MD (VascS) - **Spec Exp:** Endovascular Surgery; Carotid Artery Surgery; Aortic Surgery; **Hospital:** Long Is Jewish Med Ctr (page 106); **Address:** 1999 Marcus Ave Fl 1 - Ste 106B, New Hyde Park, NY 11042; **Phone:** 516-470-4505; **Board Cert:** Surgery 2009; Vascular Surgery 2011; **Med School:** UMDNJ-NJ Med Sch, Newark 1995; **Resid:** Surgery, Montefiore Med Ctr 2000; **Fellow:** Vascular Surgery, SUNY Downstate Med Ctr 2002; **Fac Appt:** Assoc Clin Prof VascS, Cornell Univ-Weill Med Coll

Purtill, William A MD (VascS) - **Spec Exp:** Carotid Artery Surgery; Endovascular Surgery; Lower Limb Arterial Disease; Aneurysm-Aortic; **Hospital:** N Shore Univ Hosp (page 106), St. Francis Hosp - The Heart Ctr (page 116); **Address:** 990 Stewart Ave, Ste L32, Garden City, NY 11530; **Phone:** 516-466-0485; **Board Cert:** Surgery 2007; Vascular Surgery 2007; **Med School:** Ireland 1989; **Resid:** Surgery, Johns Hopkins Hosp 1993; Surgery, Stony Brook Univ Med Ctr 1996; **Fellow:** Vascular Surgery, Univ MD Med Ctr 1997; **Fac Appt:** Asst Prof S, SUNY Stony Brook

Rockland

Rockland

Allergy & Immunology

Bosso, John MD (A&I) - **Spec Exp:** Asthma; Food Allergy; Drug Sensitivity; **Hospital:** Nyack Hosp, Valley Hosp (page 721); **Address:** Allergy & Asthma Consultants, 2 Crosfield Ave, Ste 406, West Nyack, NY 10994; **Phone:** 845-353-9600; **Board Cert:** Internal Medicine 1988; Allergy & Immunology 2011; **Med School:** SUNY Buffalo 1985; **Resid:** Internal Medicine, Staten Island Univ Hosp 1988; **Fellow:** Allergy & Immunology, Scripps Green Hosp 1990

LoGalbo, Peter MD (A&I) - **Spec Exp:** Asthma; Food Allergy; **Hospital:** Good Samaritan Regional Med Ctr, Nyack Hosp; **Address:** ENT & Allergy Assocs, 1 Crosfield Ave, Ste 201, West Nyack, NY 10994; **Phone:** 845-727-1370; **Board Cert:** Pediatrics 1983; Allergy & Immunology 1983; **Med School:** SUNY Stony Brook 1978; **Resid:** Pediatrics, Mount Sinai Med Ctr 1980; **Fellow:** Pediatric Allergy & Immunology, Duke Univ Hosp 1982; **Fac Appt:** Asst Clin Prof Ped, Albert Einstein Coll Med

Cardiovascular Disease

Beniaminovitz, Ainat MD (Cv) - **Spec Exp:** Heart Failure; Transplant Medicine-Heart; **Hospital:** Good Samaritan Regional Med Ctr; **Address:** Columbia Doctors Hudson Vly, 222 Route 59, Ste 302, Suffern, NY 10901; **Phone:** 845-368-0100; **Board Cert:** Internal Medicine 2003; Cardiovascular Disease 2007; **Med School:** Columbia P&S 1990; **Resid:** Internal Medicine, NY-Presby/Columbia Univ Med Ctr 1994; **Fellow:** Cardiovascular Disease, NY-Presby/Columbia Univ Med Ctr 1997; **Fac Appt:** Asst Prof Med, Columbia P&S

Roth, Richard L MD (Cv) - **Spec Exp:** Cholesterol/Lipid Disorders; Non-Invasive Cardiology; **Hospital:** Good Samaritan Regional Med Ctr, Nyack Hosp; **Address:** 222 Route 59, Ste 302, Suffern, NY 10901; **Phone:** 845-368-0100; **Board Cert:** Internal Medicine 1978; Cardiovascular Disease 1981; **Med School:** Yale Univ 1975; **Resid:** Internal Medicine, Boston Med Ctr 1978; **Fellow:** Cardiovascular Disease, Boston Med Ctr 1980; **Fac Appt:** Asst Clin Prof Med, Columbia P&S

Southren, David MD (Cv) - **Spec Exp:** Cholesterol/Lipid Disorders; Non-Invasive Cardiology; Preventive Cardiology; **Hospital:** Nyack Hosp, Good Samaritan Regional Med Ctr; **Address:** Advanced Cardiovascular Care, 206 Route 303, Valley Cottage, NY 10989; **Phone:** 845-268-0880; **Board Cert:** Internal Medicine 1984; Cardiovascular Disease 1987; Critical Care Medicine 2011; **Med School:** NY Med Coll 1981; **Resid:** Internal Medicine, Barnes-Jewish Hosp 1984; **Fellow:** Cardiovascular Disease, Emory Univ Hosp 1985; Cardiovascular Disease, Westchester Med Ctr 1986

Child & Adolescent Psychiatry

Leventhal, Bennett L MD (ChAP) - **Spec Exp:** Autism; ADD/ADHD; Psychopharmacology; **Hospital:** NYU Langone Med Ctr (page 108); **Address:** 140 Old Orangeburg Rd, Bldg 35, Orangeburg, NY 10962; **Phone:** 845-398-5502; **Board Cert:** Psychiatry 1979; Child & Adolescent Psychiatry 1980; **Med School:** Louisiana State U, New Orleans 1974; **Resid:** Psychiatry, Duke Univ Med Ctr 1978; **Fellow:** Child & Adolescent Psychiatry, Duke Univ Med Ctr 1977; **Fac Appt:** Prof Psyc, NYU Sch Med

Dermatology

Waldorf, Donald MD (D) - **Spec Exp:** Skin Cancer; Acne; Psoriasis; Cosmetic Dermatology; **Hospital:** Rockland Psych Ctr; **Address:** 57 N Middletown Rd, Nanuet, NY 10954-2312; **Phone:** 845-623-7077; **Board Cert:** Dermatology 1967; **Med School:** Univ Pennsylvania 1962; **Resid:** Dermatology, Hosp Univ Penn 1964; Dermatology, NYU Medical Center 1967; **Fellow:** Dermatology, Natl Cancer Inst 1966

Waldorf, Heidi A MD (D) - **Spec Exp:** Cosmetic Dermatology; Skin Laser Surgery; Mohs' Surgery; **Hospital:** Mt Sinai Med Ctr (page 102); **Address:** 57 N Middletown Rd, Nanuet, NY 10954; **Phone:** 845-623-7077; **Board Cert:** Dermatology 2013; **Med School:** Univ Pennsylvania 1990; **Resid:** Dermatology, Mass Genl Hosp 1994; **Fellow:** Mohs Surgery, Laser & Skin Surg Ctr 1995; **Fac Appt:** Assoc Clin Prof D, Mount Sinai Sch Med

Diagnostic Radiology

Bobroff, Lewis M MD (DR) - **Spec Exp:** Mammography; Nuclear Medicine; PET Imaging; **Hospital:** Good Samaritan Regional Med Ctr; **Address:** Ramapo Radiology Assocs, 255 Lafayette Ave, Suffern, NY 10901-5103; **Phone:** 845-368-5196; **Board Cert:** Diagnostic Radiology 1974; **Med School:** Harvard Med Sch 1969; **Resid:** Diagnostic Radiology, Montefiore Med Ctr 1973; **Fellow:** Interventional Radiology, Montefiore Med Ctr 1973

Geller, Mark E MD (DR) - **Spec Exp:** MRI; CT Scan; Nuclear Radiology; **Hospital:** Nyack Hosp; **Address:** Hudson Vly Radiology Assocs, 18 Squadron Blvd, New City, NY 10956; **Phone:** 845-634-9729; **Board Cert:** Diagnostic Radiology 1989; **Med School:** SUNY Downstate 1985; **Resid:** Diagnostic Radiology, Westchester Med Ctr 1989

Endocrinology, Diabetes & Metabolism

Cosman, Felicia MD (EDM) - **Spec Exp:** Osteoporosis; **Hospital:** Helen Hayes Hosp; **Address:** Helen Hayes Hosp, Regl Bone Ctr, Route 9W, West Haverstraw, NY 10993-1195; **Phone:** 845-786-4489; **Board Cert:** Internal Medicine 1986; Endocrinology, Diabetes & Metabolism 1989; **Med School:** SUNY Stony Brook 1983; **Resid:** Internal Medicine, NY-Presby/Columbia Univ Med Ctr 1986; **Fellow:** Endocrinology, NY-Presby/Columbia Univ Med Ctr 1988

Family Medicine

Ibelli, Vincent MD (FMed) *PCP* - **Spec Exp:** Asthma; Hypertension; Osteoporosis; Gastroesophageal Reflux Disease (GERD); **Hospital:** Nyack Hosp; **Address:** Orangetown Family Practice, 97 Route 303, Tappan, NY 10983-2514; **Phone:** 845-359-5005; **Board Cert:** Family Medicine 2007; **Med School:** Italy 1983; **Resid:** Family Medicine, JFK Med Ctr 1986

Ingrassia, Joseph T MD (FMed) *PCP* - **Hospital:** Good Samaritan Regional Med Ctr, Nyack Hosp; **Address:** 36 College Ave, Nanuet, NY 10954; **Phone:** 845-623-2456; **Board Cert:** Family Medicine 2003; **Med School:** Mexico 1974; **Resid:** Family Medicine, Nassau Univ Med Ctr 1978

Gastroenterology

May, Louis D MD (Ge) - **Spec Exp:** Hepatitis; Endoscopy; Pancreatic/Biliary Endoscopy (ERCP); **Hospital:** Good Samaritan Regional Med Ctr, Nyack Hosp; **Address:** Gastrointestinal Assocs of Rockland, 500 New Henpstead Rd, New City, NY 10956; **Phone:** 845-362-3200; **Board Cert:** Internal Medicine 1981; Gastroenterology 1983; **Med School:** Univ Miami Sch Med 1978; **Resid:** Internal Medicine, Univ Utah Med Ctr 1981; **Fellow:** Gastroenterology, Univ Utah Med Ctr 1983

Internal Medicine

Glassman, Charles F MD (IM) *PCP* - **Spec Exp:** Concierge Medicine; Preventive Medicine; Complementary Medicine; **Hospital:** Good Samaritan Regional Med Ctr, Nyack Hosp; **Address:** 7C Medical Park Drive, Pomona, NY 10970; **Phone:** 845-362-1110; **Board Cert:** Internal Medicine 1989; **Med School:** NY Med Coll 1985; **Resid:** Internal Medicine, Westchester Co Med Ctr 1988; **Fac Appt:** Asst Clin Prof Med, NY Med Coll

Handelsman, Richard E DO (IM) *PCP* - **Spec Exp:** Concierge Medicine; Preventive Medicine; **Hospital:** Nyack Hosp, Good Samaritan Regional Med Ctr; **Address:** 7 Medical Park Drive, Ste C, Pomona, NY 10970-3562; **Phone:** 845-362-1169; **Board Cert:** Internal Medicine 1981; **Med School:** Univ Osteo Med & Hlth Sci, Des Moines 1976; **Resid:** Internal Medicine, UMDNJ Med Ctr 1978; Internal Medicine, Norwalk Hosp 1980; **Fac Appt:** Asst Clin Prof Med, NY Med Coll

Interventional Cardiology

Brogno, David MD (IC) - **Spec Exp:** Cardiac Catheterization; Angioplasty; Coronary Angioplasty/Stents; **Hospital:** NY-Presby/Columbia Univ Med Ctr, NY (page 104), Good Samaritan Regional Med Ctr; **Address:** Columbia Doctors-Hudson Valley, 222 Route 59, Ste 302, Suffern, NY 10901; **Phone:** 845-368-0100; **Board Cert:** Internal Medicine 1986; Cardiovascular Disease 1989; Interventional Cardiology 2009; **Med School:** Univ Mich Med Sch 1983; **Resid:** Internal Medicine, St Lukes-Roosevelt Hosp Ctr 1987; **Fellow:** Cardiovascular Disease, St Lukes-Roosevelt Hosp Ctr 1989; Interventional Cardiology, St Lukes-Roosevelt Hosp Ctr 1991; **Fac Appt:** Asst Clin Prof Med, Columbia P&S

Innerfield, Michael MD (IC) - **Spec Exp:** Coronary Artery Disease; Preventive Cardiology; Peripheral Vascular Disease; **Hospital:** Good Samaritan Regional Med Ctr, Nyack Hosp; **Address:** Good Samaritan Hosp, Cardiology, 257 Lafayette Ave, Ste 330, Suffern, NY 10901; **Phone:** 845-368-0048; **Board Cert:** Internal Medicine 1984; Cardiovascular Disease 1987; Interventional Cardiology 2009; **Med School:** NY Med Coll 1981; **Resid:** Internal Medicine, Albert Einstein/Jacobi Med Ctr 1984; **Fellow:** Cardiovascular Disease, Montefiore Med Ctr 1986; Cardiovascular Disease, Cooper Univ Hosp 1987; **Fac Appt:** Asst Prof S, Mount Sinai Sch Med

Medical Oncology

Goldberg, Robert MD (Onc) - **Spec Exp:** Brain Tumors; Bone Tumors; **Hospital:** Good Samaritan Regional Med Ctr, Nyack Hosp; **Address:** 10 Esquire Rd, Ste 6, New City, NY 10956; **Phone:** 845-634-2727; **Board Cert:** Internal Medicine 1982; Medical Oncology 1985; Hematology 1984; **Med School:** Mount Sinai Sch Med 1979; **Resid:** Internal Medicine, Beth Israel Med Ctr 1982; **Fellow:** Hematology & Oncology, Univ Minnesota Hosp 1985

Lonberg, Mathew MD (Onc) - **Spec Exp:** Lung Cancer; Breast Cancer; Lymphoma; Melanoma; **Hospital:** Nyack Hosp, NY-Presby/Columbia Univ Med Ctr, NY (page 104); **Address:** 255 5th Ave, Nyack, NY 10960; **Phone:** 845-362-1750; **Board Cert:** Internal Medicine 1984; Medical Oncology 1987; Hematology 1988; **Med School:** Univ VA Sch Med 1981; **Resid:** Internal Medicine, Bellevue Hosp Ctr 1984; **Fellow:** Hematology & Oncology, Meml Sloan-Kettering Cancer Ctr 1985; **Fac Appt:** Asst Clin Prof Med, Columbia P&S

Zimmerman, Marc MD (Onc) - **Hospital:** Nyack Hosp, Good Samaritan Regional Med Ctr; **Address:** Pomona Professional Plaza, 974 Rte 45, Ste 1200, Pomona, NY 10970; **Phone:** 845-362-3970; **Board Cert:** Internal Medicine 1980; Medical Oncology 1981; Hematology 1984; **Med School:** Albany Med Coll 1977; **Resid:** Internal Medicine, Albany Med Ctr 1979; **Fellow:** Medical Oncology, Albany Med Ctr 1982

Neonatal-Perinatal Medicine

Mendoza, Glenn MD (NP) - **Hospital:** Good Samaritan Regional Med Ctr, Children's & Women's Phys.of Westchester (page 638); **Address:** Good Samaritan Hosp, Dept Neonatology, 255 Lafayette Ave, Suffern, NY 10901-4817; **Phone:** 845-368-5104; **Board Cert:** Pediatrics 1985; **Med School:** Philippines 1976; **Resid:** Family Medicine, Elyria Meml Hosp 1980; Pediatrics, Brooklyn Jewish Med Ctr 1983; **Fellow:** Neonatal-Perinatal Medicine, Mt Sinai Hosp 1985; **Fac Appt:** Asst Prof Ped, Columbia P&S

Nephrology

Kozin, Arthur M MD (Nep) - **Spec Exp:** Hypertension; Kidney Failure-Chronic; Diabetic Kidney Disease; **Hospital:** Nyack Hosp, Good Samaritan Regional Med Ctr; **Address:** 2 Crosfield Ave, Ste 312, West Nyack, NY 10994-2212; **Phone:** 845-358-2400; **Board Cert:** Internal Medicine 1985; Nephrology 1988; Critical Care Medicine 2002; **Med School:** Albert Einstein Coll Med 1982; **Resid:** Internal Medicine, Montefiore Hosp Med Ctr 1985; **Fellow:** Nephrology, Bellevue Hosp 1987

Shapiro, Kenneth S MD (Nep) - **Spec Exp:** Hypertension; Diabetic Kidney Disease; Transplant Medicine-Kidney; **Hospital:** Nyack Hosp, Good Samaritan Regional Med Ctr; **Address:** Rockland Renal Assocs, 2 Crosfield Ave, Ste 312, West Nyack, NY 10994; **Phone:** 845-358-2400; **Board Cert:** Internal Medicine 1978; Nephrology 1980; **Med School:** Rush Med Coll 1975; **Resid:** Internal Medicine, Albany Meml Hosp 1978; **Fellow:** Nephrology, Tufts Med Ctr 1980; **Fac Appt:** Asst Clin Prof Med, NY Med Coll

Yablon, Steven MD (Nep) - **Spec Exp:** Hypertension; Kidney Failure; Dialysis Care; **Hospital:** Nyack Hosp, Good Samaritan Regional Med Ctr; **Address:** Rockland Renal Assocs, 2 Crosfield Ave, Ste 312, West Nyack, NY 10994-2220; **Phone:** 845-358-2400; **Board Cert:** Internal Medicine 1976; Nephrology 1978; **Med School:** UMDNJ-NJ Med Sch, Newark 1973; **Resid:** Internal Medicine, Tufts Med Ctr 1975; **Fellow:** Renal Disease, Hosp Univ Penn-UPHS 1977

Neurological Surgery

Degen, Jeffrey W MD (NS) - **Spec Exp:** Neuro-Endoscopy; Minimally Invasive Spinal Surgery; Brain & Spinal Tumors; **Hospital:** St. Luke's Newburgh, Orange Regl Med Ctr-Horton Campus; **Address:** Hudson Vly Brain & Spine Surg, 222 Route 59, Ste 205, Suffern, NY 10901; **Phone:** 845-368-0286; **Board Cert:** Neurological Surgery 2007; **Med School:** Cornell Univ-Weill Med Coll 1998; **Resid:** Neurological Surgery, Georgetown Univ Hosp 2005; **Fac Appt:** Asst Clin Prof NS, NY Med Coll

Oppenheim, Jeffrey S MD (NS) - **Spec Exp:** Spinal Disorders-Degenerative; Brain Tumors; Spinal Surgery; Microsurgery; **Hospital:** Nyack Hosp, Good Samaritan Regional Med Ctr; **Address:** Hudson Vly Brain & Spine Surgery, 222 Route 59, Ste 205, Suffern, NY 10901; **Phone:** 845-368-0286; **Board Cert:** Neurological Surgery 1996; **Med School:** Cornell Univ-Weill Med Coll 1988; **Resid:** Neurological Surgery, Mount Sinai Med Ctr 1994

Spitzer, Daniel MD (NS) - **Spec Exp:** Brain Tumors; Spinal Surgery; Stereotactic Radiosurgery; **Hospital:** Nyack Hosp, Good Samaritan Regional Med Ctr; **Address:** Hudson Vly Brain & Spine Surgery, 222 Route 59, Ste 205, Suffern, NY 10901-5206; **Phone:** 845-368-0286; **Board Cert:** Neurological Surgery 1992; **Med School:** NYU Sch Med 1983; **Resid:** Neurological Surgery, Montefiore Med Ctr 1989; **Fac Appt:** Asst Clin Prof NS, Columbia P&S

Neurology

Ober, David T MD (N) - **Spec Exp:** Neuromuscular Disorders; Botox Therapy; Electrodiagnosis; **Hospital:** Nyack Hosp; **Address:** Rockland Neurological Assocs, 2 Crosfield Ave, Ste 202, West Nyack, NY 10994; **Phone:** 845-353-4344; **Board Cert:** Neurology 2009; **Med School:** Albany Med Coll 1994; **Resid:** Neurology, Mount Sinai Med Ctr 1998; **Fellow:** Neuroelectrophysiology, St Elizabeths Med Ctr 1999

Seliger, Glenn M MD (N) - **Spec Exp:** Head Injury; **Hospital:** Helen Hayes Hosp; **Address:** Helen Hayes Hosp, Dept Neurology, Route 9W, West Haverstraw, NY 10993; **Phone:** 845-786-4459; **Board Cert:** Neurology 1988; **Med School:** SUNY Downstate 1983; **Resid:** Neurology, Neurological Inst 1987; **Fellow:** Neurological Rehabilitation, Braintree Rehab Hosp 1988; **Fac Appt:** Assoc Clin Prof N, Columbia P&S

Neuroradiology

Schwartz, Joel M MD (NRad) - **Spec Exp:** Head & Neck Imaging; **Hospital:** Nyack Hosp; **Address:** Hudson Vly Radiology Assocs, 18 Squadron Blvd, New City, NY 10956; **Phone:** 845-634-9729; **Board Cert:** Diagnostic Radiology 1990; Neuroradiology 2006; **Med School:** SUNY Upstate Med Univ 1985; **Resid:** Diagnostic Radiology, NYU Med Ctr 1990; **Fellow:** Neuroradiology, NYU Med Ctr 1993

Obstetrics & Gynecology

Hostin, Helen MD (ObG) - **Hospital:** Nyack Hosp; **Address:** Comprehensive Ob/Gyn, 26 Firemans Memorial Drive, Ste 120, Pomona, NY 10970; **Phone:** 845-362-5900; **Board Cert:** Obstetrics & Gynecology 2012; **Med School:** NYU Sch Med 1997; **Resid:** Obstetrics & Gynecology, Westchester Med Ctr 2001

Ophthalmology

Weingarten, Phyllis E MD (Oph) - **Spec Exp:** Pediatric Ophthalmology; Strabismus; **Hospital:** Good Samaritan Regional Med Ctr, Beth Israel Med Ctr - Petrie Div (page 94); **Address:** Pomona Eye Assocs, 4A Medical Park Drive, Pomona, NY 10970; **Phone:** 718-369-4851; **Board Cert:** Ophthalmology 1991; **Med School:** NY Med Coll 1986; **Resid:** Internal Medicine, Lenox Hill Hosp 1987; Ophthalmology, Brookdale Univ Hosp Med Ctr 1990; **Fellow:** Strabismus, SUNY Downstate Med Ctr 1991; Pediatric Ophthalmology, Johns Hopkins Hosp 1992

Orthopaedic Surgery

Austin, Kenneth S MD (OrS) - **Spec Exp:** Hip Replacement; Knee Replacement; Sports Medicine; Trauma; **Hospital:** Good Samaritan Regional Med Ctr; **Address:** Rockland Orthopedics & Sports Med, 327 Route 59, Colonial Square, Airmont, NY 10952; **Phone:** 845-356-2900; **Board Cert:** Orthopaedic Surgery 2007; **Med School:** NYU Sch Med 1988; **Resid:** Surgery, Bellevue Hosp-NYU Sch Med 1989; Orthopaedic Surgery, Bellevue Hosp-NYU Sch Med 1993; **Fellow:** Sports Medicine, Mass Genl Hosp 1994

Medici, Mark D MD (OrS) - **Spec Exp:** Sports Medicine; Joint Replacement; Trauma; **Hospital:** Nyack Hosp, Good Samaritan Regional Med Ctr; **Address:** Clarkstown Orthopedics, 2 Crosfield Ave, Ste 422, West Nyack, NY 10994; **Phone:** 845-358-1000; **Board Cert:** Orthopaedic Surgery 2012; **Med School:** NY Med Coll 1993; **Resid:** Orthopaedic Surgery, Westchester Med Ctr 1994; Orthopaedic Surgery, Montefiore Med Ctr 1998; **Fellow:** Sports Medicine, Staten Island Orthopedics & Sports Med 1999

Rubin, Cheryl J MD (OrS) - **Spec Exp:** Shoulder Arthroscopic Surgery; Knee Surgery; **Hospital:** Good Samaritan Regional Med Ctr; **Address:** Rockland Ortho & Sports Med, 327 Route 59, Colonial Square, Airmont, NY 10952; **Phone:** 845-356-2900; **Board Cert:** Orthopaedic Surgery 2013; **Med School:** Mount Sinai Sch Med 1983; **Resid:** Orthopaedic Surgery, Montefiore Hosp Med Ctr 1988; **Fellow:** Arthroscopic Surgery, Ortho Research Of Virginia 1989

Pain Medicine

Burns, Paul MD (PM) - **Spec Exp:** Pain-Cancer; Pain-Chronic; **Hospital:** Good Samaritan Regional Med Ctr; **Address:** Ramapo Med Assocs, 100 Route 59, Ste 105, Suffern, NY 10901; **Phone:** 845-357-5745; **Board Cert:** Anesthesiology 1984; Pain Medicine 2007; **Med School:** SUNY Buffalo 1978; **Resid:** Anesthesiology, NY-Presby/Weill Cornell Med Ctr 1981

Pediatric Infectious Disease

Arlievsky, Nina Z MD (PInf) - **Spec Exp:** Lyme Disease; **Hospital:** Westchester Med Ctr; **Address:** 19 Bradhurst Ave Fl 1 - rm 1400, Hawthorne, NY 10532; **Phone:** 914-493-8333; **Board Cert:** Pediatric Infectious Disease 2012; **Med School:** Mount Sinai Sch Med 1989; **Resid:** Pediatrics, Northshore Univ Hosp 1992; **Fellow:** Pediatric Infectious Disease, NYU/Bellevue Hosp 1994; **Fac Appt:** Asst Prof Ped, NY Med Coll

Pediatrics

Bernstein, William H MD (Ped) *PCP* - **Hospital:** Nyack Hosp; **Address:** 67 N Main St Fl 2, New City, NY 10956; **Phone:** 845-634-8911; **Board Cert:** Pediatrics 1966; **Med School:** Vanderbilt Univ 1960; **Resid:** Pediatrics, Bellevue Hosp 1962; Pediatrics, Mt Sinai Hosp 1965; **Fellow:** Neonatology, Mt Sinai Hosp 1966

Diamant, Esther MD (Ped) *PCP* - **Spec Exp:** Infectious Disease; **Address:** Refuah Hlth Ctr, Pediatrics, 728 N Main St Fl 4, Spring Valley, NY 10977; **Phone:** 845-354-9300; **Board Cert:** Pediatrics 2010; **Med School:** Mount Sinai Sch Med 1987; **Resid:** Pediatrics, Mount Sinai Med Ctr 1991; **Fellow:** Pediatric Infectious Disease, Mount Sinai Med Ctr 1993

Katzenstein, Martin S MD (Ped) - **Spec Exp:** Neonatal Nutrition; Ethics; Neonatal Respiratory Care; **Hospital:** Good Samaritan Regional Med Ctr, Westchester Med Ctr; **Address:** Good Samaritan Hosp, Div Neonatal Med, 255 Lafayette Ave, Suffern, NY 10901; **Phone:** 845-368-5705; **Board Cert:** Pediatrics 2011; **Med School:** NY Med Coll 1978; **Resid:** Pediatrics, NY Hosp-Cornell 1981; **Fellow:** Neonatal-Perinatal Medicine, NY Hosp-Cornell 1982; Neonatal-Perinatal Medicine, Westchester Co Med Ctr 1984; **Fac Appt:** Assoc Clin Prof Ped, NY Med Coll

Puder, Douglas R MD (Ped) *PCP* - **Spec Exp:** Asthma; Developmental Disorders; **Hospital:** Nyack Hosp; **Address:** 35 Smith St, Nanuet, NY 10954; **Phone:** 845-623-7100; **Board Cert:** Pediatrics 1987; **Med School:** NYU Sch Med 1982; **Resid:** Pediatrics, NYU/Bellevue Hosp 1985; **Fellow:** Ambulatory Pediatrics, NYU Med Ctr 1987; **Fac Appt:** Assoc Clin Prof Ped, Columbia P&S

Siegal, Elliot MD (Ped) *PCP* - **Spec Exp:** Thyroid Disorders; Growth Disorders; Diabetes; **Hospital:** Nyack Hosp; **Address:** Clarkstown Pediatrics, 200 E Eckerson Rd, New City, NY 10956-7169; **Phone:** 845-352-5511; **Board Cert:** Pediatrics 1973; Pediatric Endocrinology 1978; **Med School:** Univ Pennsylvania 1968; **Resid:** Pediatrics, NY Hosp 1971; **Fellow:** Pediatric Endocrinology, NY Hosp 1972

Physical Medicine & Rehabilitation

Brief, Rochelle MD (PMR) - **Spec Exp:** Electrodiagnosis; **Hospital:** Nyack Hosp; **Address:** 365 Route 304, Bardonia, NY 10954-2042; **Phone:** 845-623-7949; **Board Cert:** Physical Medicine & Rehabilitation 2013; **Med School:** Albert Einstein Coll Med 1987; **Resid:** Physical Medicine & Rehabilitation, Montefiore Med Ctr 1992

Guarracini, Mary MD (PMR) - **Spec Exp:** Amputee Rehabilitation; **Hospital:** Helen Hayes Hosp; **Address:** Helen Hayes Hosp, Dept Rehabilitation, Route 9W, West Haverstraw, NY 10993; **Phone:** 845-786-4967; **Board Cert:** Physical Medicine & Rehabilitation 1986; **Med School:** St Louis Univ 1982; **Resid:** Physical Medicine & Rehabilitation, Northwestern Meml Hosp 1985

Robinson, Michael MD (PMR) - **Spec Exp:** Pain-Neuropathic; Pain-Back & Neck; Musculoskeletal Disorders; **Hospital:** Good Samaritan Regional Med Ctr; **Address:** Rockland Orthopedic & Sports Med, 327 Rte 59, Colonial Square, Airmont, NY 10952; **Phone:** 845-356-2900; **Board Cert:** Physical Medicine & Rehabilitation 2013; Pain Medicine 2011; Electrodiagnostic Medicine 2000; **Med School:** Tufts Univ 1988; **Resid:** Rehabilitation, Walter Reed Army Med Ctr 1992

Psychiatry

Levy, Michael I MD (Psyc) - **Spec Exp:** Psychopharmacology; Geriatric Psychiatry; Anxiety & Depression; **Hospital:** Nyack Hosp; **Address:** 160 N Midland Ave, Nyack, NY 10960; **Phone:** 845-348-2116; **Board Cert:** Psychiatry 1982; **Med School:** Albert Einstein Coll Med 1977; **Resid:** Psychiatry, Mt Sinai Med Ctr 1981

Schroeder, Karl J MD (Psyc) - **Spec Exp:** Addiction/Substance Abuse; Psychiatry in Physical Illness; Post Traumatic Stress Disorder; **Address:** 104 Montebello Rd, Suffern, NY 10901; **Phone:** 845-357-9367; **Board Cert:** Psychiatry 1980; **Med School:** Columbia P&S 1974; **Resid:** Psychiatry, NY State Psychiatric Inst 1977; **Fac Appt:** Asst Clin Prof Med, Columbia P&S

Pulmonary Disease

Chang, Benjamin G MD (Pul) - **Spec Exp:** Sleep Disorders/Apnea; **Hospital:** Nyack Hosp; **Address:** Rockland Pulmonary & Med Assocs, 2 Crosfield Ave, Ste 318, West Nyack, NY 10994; **Phone:** 845-353-5600; **Board Cert:** Internal Medicine 2011; Pulmonary Disease 2003; Critical Care Medicine 2004; Sleep Medicine 2007; **Med School:** Columbia P&S 1998; **Resid:** Internal Medicine, Georgetown Univ Hosp 2001; **Fellow:** Pulmonary Disease, NYU Med Ctr 2004

Harris, Leon MD (Pul) - **Hospital:** Good Samaritan Regional Med Ctr; **Address:** 2 Crossfield Ave, Ste 318, West Nyack, NY 10994-2212; **Phone:** 845-353-5600; **Board Cert:** Internal Medicine 1979; Pulmonary Disease 1982; Critical Care Medicine 2004; **Med School:** Mount Sinai Sch Med 1976; **Resid:** Internal Medicine, Mt Sinai Hosp 1979; **Fellow:** Pulmonary Disease, Mass Genl Hosp 1981

Hodes, David L MD (Pul) - **Hospital:** Nyack Hosp, Good Samaritan Regional Med Ctr; **Address:** 2 Medical Park Drive, Ste 3, West Nyack, NY 10994; **Phone:** 845-727-7733; **Board Cert:** Internal Medicine 1976; Pulmonary Disease 1978; **Med School:** NYU Sch Med 1973; **Resid:** Internal Medicine, St Luke's Hosp 1976; **Fellow:** Pulmonary Disease, Bellevue Hosp/NYU 1978

Menitove, Stephen MD (Pul) - **Hospital:** Nyack Hosp, Good Samaritan Regional Med Ctr; **Address:** Rockland Pulmonary & Medical Assocs, 2 Crosfield Ave, Ste 318, West Nyack, NY 10994-2212; **Phone:** 845-353-5600; **Board Cert:** Internal Medicine 1980; Pulmonary Disease 1982; **Med School:** Mount Sinai Sch Med 1977; **Resid:** Internal Medicine, Mount Sinai Hospital 1983; **Fellow:** Pulmonary Disease, Bellevue/NYU Med Ctr 1982; **Fac Appt:** Med, Mount Sinai Sch Med

Pellicone, John MD (Pul) - **Hospital:** Helen Hayes Hosp, Nyack Hosp; **Address:** Helen Hayes Hosp, Pulmonary Dept, 51-55 Route 9W, West Haverstraw, NY 10993; **Phone:** 845-786-4060; **Board Cert:** Internal Medicine 1984; Pulmonary Disease 2010; Critical Care Medicine 2012; **Med School:** Columbia P&S 1981; **Resid:** Internal Medicine, Montefiore Med Ctr 1984; **Fellow:** Pulmonary Disease, Bellevue Hosp 1986

Rheumatology

Becker, Alfred MD (Rhu) - **Spec Exp:** Arthritis; **Hospital:** Good Samaritan Regional Med Ctr, Nyack Hosp; **Address:** 222 Rte 59, Ste 204, Suffern, NY 10901; **Phone:** 845-357-6464; **Board Cert:** Internal Medicine 1969; Rheumatology 1972; **Med School:** Albert Einstein Coll Med 1962; **Resid:** Internal Medicine, Univ Pittsburgh Med Ctr 1967; **Fellow:** Rheumatology, Montefiore Med Ctr 1968

Kurucz, Oliver MD (Rhu) - **Spec Exp:** Rheumatoid Arthritis; Immunodeficiency Disorders; **Hospital:** Nyack Hosp; **Address:** 300 N Middletown Rd, Ste 11, Pearl River, NY 10965; **Phone:** 845-735-4114; **Board Cert:** Rheumatology ; **Med School:** SUNY Downstate 1999; **Resid:** Internal Medicine, St Vincents Hosp 2002; **Fellow:** Rheumatology, NYU Med Ctr 2004

Sports Medicine

Berezin, Marc A MD (SM) - **Spec Exp:** Arthroscopic Surgery; Knee Surgery; **Hospital:** Nyack Hosp, Good Samaritan Regional Med Ctr; **Address:** Orangetown Orthopaedic Assocs, 99 Dutch Hill Rd, Orangeburg, NY 10962-2106; **Phone:** 845-359-1877; **Board Cert:** Orthopaedic Surgery 2013; **Med School:** NY Med Coll 1985; **Resid:** Orthopaedic Surgery, NY Med Coll Affil Hosps 1990; **Fellow:** Sports Medicine, Orthopaedic Assocs 1991

Kraushaar, Barry S MD (SM) - **Spec Exp:** Shoulder Arthroscopic Surgery; Rotator Cuff Surgery; Knee Injuries; Sports Injuries; **Hospital:** Nyack Hosp, Good Samaritan Regional Med Ctr; **Address:** Advanced Orthopedics & Sports Med, 408 Airport Executive Park, Nanuet, NY 10954; **Phone:** 845-425-0555; **Board Cert:** Orthopaedic Surgery 2009; Orthopaedic Sports Medicine 2007; **Med School:** Albert Einstein Coll Med 1990; **Resid:** Orthopaedic Surgery, Bronx Lebanon Hosp Ctr 1995; **Fellow:** Sports Medicine, Virginia Sports Med Inst 1996

Surgery

Fleischer, Lee S MD (S) - **Spec Exp:** Breast Disease; Laparoscopic Surgery; Gastrointestinal Surgery; Hernia; **Hospital:** Nyack Hosp; **Address:** Highland Surgical Assocs, 1 Crosfield Ave, Ste 105, West Nyack, NY 10994; **Phone:** 845-535-3362; **Board Cert:** Surgery 2012; **Med School:** McGill Univ 1987; **Resid:** Surgery, Beth Israel Med Ctr 1992

Joseph, Patricia K MD (S) - **Spec Exp:** Breast Cancer; **Hospital:** Nyack Hosp; **Address:** Nyack Breast & Women's Hlth Ctr, 160 N Midland Ave, Nyack, NY 10960; **Phone:** 845-348-8507; **Board Cert:** Surgery 2005; **Med School:** Univ Fla Coll Med 1979; **Resid:** Surgery, Montefiore Med Ctr-Einstein Campus 1985

Urology

Giella, John G MD (U) - **Spec Exp:** Kidney Stones; Prostate Cancer; Prostate Disease; **Hospital:** Nyack Hosp, Good Samaritan Regional Med Ctr; **Address:** AUCNY, Rockland Co, 2 Medical Park Drive, Ste 10, West Nyack, NY 10994; **Phone:** 845-354-5000; **Board Cert:** Urology 2012; **Med School:** Harvard Med Sch 1986; **Resid:** Surgery, St Vincents Hosp 1988; Urology, NY-Presby/Columbia Univ Med Ctr 1992

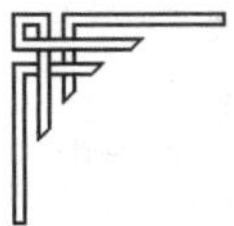

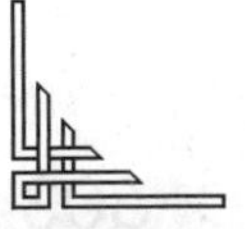
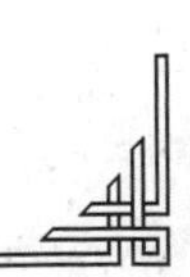

Suffolk

Suffolk

Allergy & Immunology

Cancellieri, Russell P MD (A&I) - **Spec Exp:** Asthma; **Hospital:** Southampton Hosp; **Address:** 596 Hampton Rd, Southampton, NY 11968; **Phone:** 631-283-3300; **Board Cert:** Pediatrics 1979; Allergy & Immunology 1981; **Med School:** Georgetown Univ 1974; **Resid:** Pediatrics, Georgetown Univ Hosp 1977; Allergy & Immunology, St Lukes-Roosevelt Hosp 1979

Guida Jr, Louis E MD (A&I) - **Spec Exp:** Allergy; Urticaria; Asthma; Cystic Fibrosis; **Hospital:** Good Samaritan Hosp Med Ctr - West Islip, St. Charles Hosp; **Address:** Bay Shore Allergy & Asthma Specialists, 649 Montauk Hwy, West Bay Shore, NY 11706; **Phone:** 631-665-2700; **Board Cert:** Pediatrics 2011; **Med School:** Grenada 1984; **Resid:** Pediatrics, Monmouth Med Ctr 1987; Allergy & Immunology, Nassau Co Med Ctr 1993; **Fellow:** Pediatric Pulmonology, Hahnemann Univ Hosp 1990

Lusman, Paul A MD (A&I) - **Spec Exp:** Asthma; Sinus Disorders; Hives; **Hospital:** John T Mather Meml Hosp, St. Charles Hosp; **Address:** 120 N Country Rd, Port Jefferson, NY 11777; **Phone:** 631-928-4990; **Board Cert:** Pediatrics 1971; Allergy & Immunology 1974; **Med School:** Albert Einstein Coll Med 1965; **Resid:** Pediatrics, Bellevue Hosp 1968; **Fellow:** Allergy & Immunology, Duke Univ Hosp 1972; **Fac Appt:** Asst Clin Prof Med, SUNY Stony Brook

Mayer, Daniel L MD (A&I) - **Spec Exp:** Asthma; Allergic Rhinitis; Food Allergy; Sinusitis; **Hospital:** Stony Brook Univ Med Ctr, St. Catherine's of Siena Med Ctr; **Address:** 263 E Main St, Smithtown, NY 11787; **Phone:** 631-366-5252; **Board Cert:** Pediatrics 1983; **Med School:** Italy 1978; **Resid:** Pediatrics, Albany Med Ctr 1985; **Fellow:** Allergy & Immunology, LI Coll Hosp 1987; **Fac Appt:** Asst Prof A&I, SUNY Stony Brook

Richheimer, Michael Steven MD (A&I) - **Spec Exp:** Asthma; Skin Allergies; Sinus Disorders; Immunodeficiency Disorders; **Hospital:** Stony Brook Univ Med Ctr, Maimonides Med Ctr (page 98); **Address:** 1855 Union Blvd, Bayshore, NY 11706; **Phone:** 631-665-6363; **Board Cert:** Allergy & Immunology 2006; **Med School:** Grenada 1985; **Resid:** Internal Medicine, St Joseph's Hosp-Seton Hall Univ 1988; **Fellow:** Allergy & Immunology, SUNY Stony Brook Med Ctr 1990; **Fac Appt:** Assoc Clin Prof A&I, SUNY Stony Brook

Satnick, Steven MD (A&I) - **Spec Exp:** Asthma; Urticaria; **Hospital:** Stony Brook Univ Med Ctr; **Address:** 900 Main St, Ste 102, Holbrook, NY 11741-1813; **Phone:** 631-588-4486; **Board Cert:** Internal Medicine 1983; Allergy & Immunology 1987; **Med School:** SUNY Downstate 1980; **Resid:** Internal Medicine, SUNY Downstate Med Ctr 1984; **Fellow:** Allergy & Immunology, SUNY Downstate Med Ctr 1987

Cardiac Electrophysiology

Rashba, Eric J MD (CE) - **Spec Exp:** Arrhythmias; Pacemakers; Syncope; Atrial Fibrillation; **Hospital:** Stony Brook Univ Med Ctr; **Address:** Stony Brook Univ Med Ctr, 101 Nicolls Rd, Stony Brook, NY 11794-8167; **Phone:** 631-444-3575; **Board Cert:** Internal Medicine 2006; Cardiovascular Disease 2008; Cardiac Electrophysiology 2009; **Med School:** Yale Univ 1992; **Resid:** Internal Medicine, Strong Meml Hosp 1995; **Fellow:** Cardiovascular Disease, New England Med Ctr 1999; Cardiac Electrophysiology, New England Med Ctr 1999; **Fac Appt:** Prof Med, SUNY Stony Brook

Cardiovascular Disease

Altschul, Larry MD (Cv) - **Spec Exp:** Non-Invasive Cardiology; Echocardiography; Nuclear Cardiology; **Hospital:** St. Francis Hosp - The Heart Ctr (page 116), Good Samaritan Hosp Med Ctr - West Islip; **Address:** St Francis, South Bay Cardiovascular, 540 Union Blvd, West Islip, NY 11795; **Phone:** 631-669-2555; **Board Cert:** Internal Medicine 1980; Cardiovascular Disease 1983; **Med School:** SUNY Buffalo 1977; **Resid:** Internal Medicine, Nassau Univ Med Ctr 1980; **Fellow:** Cardiovascular Disease, Nassau Univ Med Ctr 1982

Borek, Mark G MD (Cv) - **Spec Exp:** Nuclear Cardiology; Echocardiography; Cardiac Catheterization; **Hospital:** Stony Brook Univ Med Ctr; **Address:** Island Cardiovascular Assocs, 496 Smithtown ByPass, Ste 101, Smithtown, NY 11787; **Phone:** 631-979-8880; **Board Cert:** Internal Medicine 1985; Cardiovascular Disease 1987; **Med School:** SUNY Downstate 1981; **Resid:** Internal Medicine, Nassau Univ Med Ctr 1984; **Fellow:** Cardiovascular Disease, Long Island Coll Hosp 1987; **Fac Appt:** Asst Prof Med, SUNY Stony Brook

Brown, David Lloyd MD (Cv) - **Spec Exp:** Heart Valve Disease; Critical Care Medicine; Preventive Cardiology; Coronary Artery Disease; **Hospital:** Stony Brook Univ Med Ctr; **Address:** Stony Brook Univ Med Ctr, Div Cardiology, 26 Research Way, Stony Brook, NY 11733; **Phone:** 631-444-9885; **Board Cert:** Internal Medicine 1986; Cardiovascular Disease 2005; **Med School:** Baylor Coll Med 1982; **Resid:** Internal Medicine, Baylor Coll Med 1986; Cardiovascular Disease, UCSF Med Ctr 1990; **Fellow:** Interventional Cardiology, Cleveland Clinic 1993; Hematology, USCF Med Ctr 1988; **Fac Appt:** Prof Med, SUNY Stony Brook

Chengot, Mathew T MD (Cv) - **Spec Exp:** Nuclear Cardiology; Interventional Cardiology; Heart Failure; Echocardiography; **Hospital:** Good Samaritan Hosp Med Ctr - West Islip, St. Joseph's Hosp-Nassau; **Address:** Amityville Heart Ctr, 129 Broadway, Amityville, NY 11701; **Phone:** 631-598-3434; **Board Cert:** Internal Medicine 1980; Cardiovascular Disease 1983; **Med School:** India 1976; **Resid:** Internal Medicine, Lincoln Med Ctr 1982; **Fellow:** Cardiovascular Disease, Mount Sinai Med Ctr 1984

Dervan, John MD (Cv) - **Spec Exp:** Interventional Cardiology; Cholesterol/Lipid Disorders; Heart Failure; **Hospital:** Stony Brook Univ Med Ctr, St. Charles Hosp; **Address:** Heart Associates of Long Island, 220 Belle Mead Rd, Ste A, East Setauket, NY 11733; **Phone:** 631-941-2273; **Board Cert:** Internal Medicine 1979; Cardiovascular Disease 1985; Interventional Cardiology 2009; **Med School:** St Louis Univ 1976; **Resid:** Internal Medicine, Faulkner Hosp 1980; **Fellow:** Cardiovascular Disease, Beth Israel Deaconess Med Ctr 1983; **Fac Appt:** Assoc Clin Prof Med, SUNY Stony Brook

Falco, Thomas MD (Cv) - **Hospital:** Peconic Bay Med Ctr, Eastern Long Island Hosp; **Address:** 1279 E Main St, Riverhead, NY 11901; **Phone:** 631-727-2100; **Board Cert:** Internal Medicine 1985; Cardiovascular Disease 1987; **Med School:** Mexico 1980; **Resid:** Internal Medicine, Winthrop Univ Hosp 1985; **Fellow:** Cardiovascular Disease, Albany Med Ctr 1987

Jeremias, Allen MD (Cv) - **Spec Exp:** Interventional Cardiology; Peripheral Vascular Disease; Percutaneous Vascular Interventions; Vascular Disease; **Hospital:** Stony Brook Univ Med Ctr; **Address:** Stony Brook Univ Med Ctr, Div Cardiology, 26 Research Way, Stony Brook, NY 11733; **Phone:** 631-444-9970; **Board Cert:** Cardiovascular Disease 2005; Interventional Cardiology 2006; **Med School:** Germany 1995; **Resid:** Internal Medicine, Cleveland Clinic Hosp 2002; **Fellow:** Cardiovascular Disease, Beth Israel-Deaconess Med Ctr 2004; Interventional Cardiology, Beth Israel-Deaconess Med Ctr 2005; **Fac Appt:** Assoc Prof Med, SUNY Stony Brook

Lense, Lloyd D MD (Cv) - **Spec Exp:** Cholesterol/Lipid Disorders; Hypertension; Coronary Artery Disease; Congestive Heart Failure; **Hospital:** Stony Brook Univ Med Ctr; **Address:** Stony Brook Univ Med Ctr, Div Cardiology, 26 Research Way, East Setauket, NY 11733; **Phone:** 631-444-9970; **Board Cert:** Internal Medicine 1980; Cardiovascular Disease 1983; **Med School:** NYU Sch Med 1977; **Resid:** Internal Medicine, Mt Sinai Hosp 1980; **Fellow:** Cardiovascular Disease, Montefiore Med Ctr 1983; **Fac Appt:** Assoc Clin Prof Med, SUNY Stony Brook

Masciello, Michael A MD (Cv) - **Spec Exp:** Coronary Artery Disease; Congestive Heart Failure; **Hospital:** Southside Hosp (page 106), Good Samaritan Hosp Med Ctr - West Islip; **Address:** 540 Union Blvd, West Islip, NY 11795; **Phone:** 631-669-2555; **Board Cert:** Internal Medicine 1983; Cardiovascular Disease 1985; Critical Care Medicine 2003; **Med School:** Univ Miami Sch Med 1980; **Resid:** Internal Medicine, Nassau County Med Ctr 1983; **Fellow:** Cardiovascular Disease, Nassau County Med Ctr 1985

Matilsky, Michael A MD (Cv) - **Spec Exp:** Cholesterol/Lipid Disorders; Hypertension; Coronary Artery Disease; Atrial Fibrillation; **Hospital:** St. Charles Hosp, John T Mather Meml Hosp; **Address:** Three Village Cardiology, 210 Belle Mead Rd, East Setauket, NY 11733-3327; **Phone:** 631-689-1400; **Board Cert:** Internal Medicine 1985; Cardiovascular Disease 1987; **Med School:** SUNY Stony Brook 1982; **Resid:** Internal Medicine, Mt Sinai Hosp 1985; **Fellow:** Cardiovascular Disease, New York Hosp-Cornell 1988

Skopicki, Hal A MD/PhD (Cv) - **Spec Exp:** Heart Failure; Cardiomyopathy; **Hospital:** Stony Brook Univ Med Ctr; **Address:** 200 Motor Pkwy, Ste C-16, Hauppauge, NY 11788; **Phone:** 631-444-9600; **Board Cert:** Internal Medicine 2003; Cardiovascular Disease 2007; Advanced Heart Failure & Transplant Cardiology 2012; **Med School:** Ros Franklin Univ/Chicago Med Sch 1990; **Resid:** Internal Medicine, Yale-New Haven Hosp 1993; **Fellow:** Cardiovascular Disease, Mass Genl Hosp 1994; **Fac Appt:** Asst Prof Med, SUNY Stony Brook

Weinberg, Marc MD (Cv) - **Hospital:** Huntington Hosp (page 106); **Address:** West Carver Med Assocs, 200 W Carver St, Ste 8, Huntington, NY 11743-3303; **Phone:** 631-421-0020; **Board Cert:** Internal Medicine 1976; Cardiovascular Disease 1979; Critical Care Medicine 2007; **Med School:** Yale Univ 1973; **Resid:** Internal Medicine, New Haven Hosp 1977; **Fellow:** Cardiovascular Disease, New Haven Hosp 1979

Child & Adolescent Psychiatry

Carlson, Gabrielle A MD (ChAP) - **Spec Exp:** Child Psychiatry; Bipolar/Mood Disorders; ADD/ADHD; **Hospital:** Stony Brook Univ Med Ctr; **Address:** Stony Brook Univ Med Ctr, Div Child & Adolescent Psych, Putnam Hall, rm 103, Stony Brook, NY 11794-8790; **Phone:** 631-632-8840; **Board Cert:** Psychiatry 1975; Child & Adolescent Psychiatry 1978; **Med School:** Cornell Univ-Weill Med Coll 1968; **Resid:** Psychiatry, Barnes Hosp-Washington Univ 1970; Psychiatry, Nat Inst Mental Hlth 1972; **Fellow:** Child & Adolescent Psychiatry, UCLA Med Ctr 1978; **Fac Appt:** Prof Psyc, SUNY Stony Brook

Gandhi, Lajpat R MD (ChAP) - **Spec Exp:** Anxiety & Mood Disorders; ADD/ADHD; **Hospital:** Huntington Hosp (page 106); **Address:** 110 E Main St, Ste 5, Huntington, NY 11743; **Phone:** 631-427-6411; **Board Cert:** Psychiatry 1981; Child & Adolescent Psychiatry 1985; **Med School:** India 1975; **Resid:** Psychiatry, Metropolitan Hosp 1979; **Fellow:** Psychiatry, Elmhurst Hosp-Mt Sinai 1980; Child & Adolescent Psychiatry, LI Jewish-Hillside Med Ctr 1981

Pomeroy, John C MD (ChAP) - **Spec Exp:** Autism; Mental Retardation; Developmental Disorders; **Hospital:** Stony Brook Univ Med Ctr; **Address:** The Cody Center for Autism, 37 Research Way, East Setauket, NY 11733; **Phone:** 631-444-3070; **Board Cert:** Psychiatry 1984; Child & Adolescent Psychiatry 1988; **Med School:** England, UK 1973; **Resid:** Psychiatry, St Mary's Hosp 1979; **Fellow:** Child & Adolescent Psychiatry, Univ Iowa Hosps 1981; **Fac Appt:** Assoc Prof Psyc, SUNY Stony Brook

Weisbrot, Deborah M MD (ChAP) - **Spec Exp:** Anxiety & Mood Disorders; Neuro-Psychiatry; **Hospital:** Stony Brook Univ Med Ctr; **Address:** SUNY Stony Brook, Div Child & Adolescent Psych, Putnam Hall-South Campus, room 169, Stony Brook, NY 11794-8790; **Phone:** 631-632-8840; **Board Cert:** Psychiatry 1985; Child & Adolescent Psychiatry 1991; **Med School:** SUNY Buffalo 1979; **Resid:** Psychiatry, Yale-New Haven Hosp 1983; **Fellow:** Child Psychiatry, NY Hosp-Payne Whitney Clin 1986; **Fac Appt:** Assoc Prof Psyc, SUNY Stony Brook

Child Neurology

Andriola, Mary R MD (ChiN) - **Spec Exp:** Epilepsy; ADD/ADHD; Headache; Developmental Disorders; **Hospital:** Stony Brook Univ Med Ctr; **Address:** Neurology Associates of Stony Brook, 179 N Belle Mead Rd, East Setauket, NY 11733; **Phone:** 631-444-2599; **Board Cert:** Pediatrics 1970; Child Neurology 1972; Clinical Neurophysiology 2012; Neurodevelopmental Disabilities 2005; **Med School:** Duke Univ 1965; **Resid:** Pediatrics, Univ Fla Shands Hosp 1967; **Fellow:** Neurology, Univ Fla Shands Hosp 1970; **Fac Appt:** Prof N, SUNY Stony Brook

Clinical Genetics

Hyman, David B MD (CG) - **Spec Exp:** Prenatal Diagnosis; Genetic Disorders; Cancer Risk Assessment; **Hospital:** Stony Brook Univ Med Ctr, St. Catherine's of Siena Med Ctr; **Address:** The Genetics Center, 48 Route 25A, Ste 205, Smithtown, NY 11787-1448; **Phone:** 631-862-3620; **Board Cert:** Pediatrics 1983; Clinical Genetics 1984; Clinical Biochemical Genetics 1990; Clinical Molecular Genetics 1990; **Med School:** Univ IL Coll Med 1978; **Resid:** Pediatrics, Yale Univ Sch Med 1980; **Fellow:** Clinical Genetics, Yale Univ Sch Med 1983

McGovern, Margaret MD/PhD (CG) - **Hospital:** Stony Brook Univ Med Ctr; **Address:** Stony Brook Childrens Services, 37 Research Way, East Setauket, NY 11733; **Phone:** 631-444-5437; **Board Cert:** Pediatrics 2012; Clinical Genetics 1990; **Med School:** Mount Sinai Sch Med 1986; **Resid:** Pediatrics, Mt Sinai Hosp 1988; **Fellow:** Genetics, Mt Sinai Hosp 1990; **Fac Appt:** Prof Ped, SUNY Stony Brook

Colon & Rectal Surgery

Leiboff, Arnold R MD (CRS) - **Hospital:** John T Mather Meml Hosp, St. Charles Hosp; **Address:** 3400 Nesconset Hwy, Ste 100, East Setauket, NY 11733; **Phone:** 631-689-2600; **Board Cert:** Surgery 2007; Colon & Rectal Surgery 2010; **Med School:** NY Med Coll 1978; **Resid:** Surgery, SUNY at Stony Brook 1987; **Fellow:** Colon & Rectal Surgery, Carle Foundation Hosp-Univ Ill 1989

Rivadeneira, David E MD (CRS) - **Spec Exp:** Colon & Rectal Cancer & Surgery; Inflammatory Bowel Disease; Gastrointestinal Surgery; Incontinence/Pelvic Floor Disorders; **Hospital:** Huntington Hosp (page 106), Southside Hosp (page 106); **Address:** 755 New York Ave, Ste 108, Huntington, NY 11743; **Phone:** 631-470-1450; **Board Cert:** Colon & Rectal Surgery ; Surgery ; **Med School:** Howard Univ 1995; **Resid:** Surgery, NY-Presby/Weill Cornell Med Ctr 2002; **Fellow:** Colon & Rectal Surgery, Lahey Clinic 2003

Savoca, Paul MD (CRS) - **Spec Exp:** Anal Sphincter Repair; Constipation; Hemorrhoids; **Hospital:** St. Catherine's of Siena Med Ctr; **Address:** St Catherine of Siena Med Ctr, 48 Route 25A, Ste 301, Smithtown, NY 11787; **Phone:** 631-862-3600; **Board Cert:** Colon & Rectal Surgery 2012; Surgery 2012; **Med School:** SUNY Downstate 1985; **Resid:** Surgery, Yale-New Haven Hosp 1991; **Fellow:** Colon & Rectal Surgery, Univ Minn Med Ctr 1992

Smithy, William B MD (CRS) - **Spec Exp:** Colon & Rectal Cancer; Anorectal Disorders; Colonoscopy; **Hospital:** Stony Brook Univ Med Ctr, St. Catherine's of Siena Med Ctr; **Address:** 222 Middle Country Rd, Ste 209, Smithtown, NY 11787; **Phone:** 631-638-2800; **Board Cert:** Surgery 2009; Colon & Rectal Surgery 1989; **Med School:** Columbia P&S 1981; **Resid:** Surgery, Roosevelt Hosp 1987; **Fellow:** Colon & Rectal Surgery, RWJ Univ Hosp 1988; **Fac Appt:** Asst Clin Prof S, SUNY Stony Brook

Dermatology

Basuk, Pamela MD (D) - **Spec Exp:** Cosmetic Dermatology; Melanoma; Skin Laser Surgery; Skin Cancer; **Hospital:** Southside Hosp (page 106); **Address:** 2011 Union Blvd, Ste 1, Bayshore, NY 11706; **Phone:** 631-666-2900; **Board Cert:** Dermatology 1988; **Med School:** NYU Sch Med 1984; **Resid:** Dermatology, Brown Univ Hosp 1988

Berger, Bernard W MD (D) - ; **Address:** 319 Hampton Rd, Southampton, NY 11968-5029; **Phone:** 631-283-7722; **Board Cert:** Dermatology 1975; **Med School:** UC Irvine 1963; **Resid:** Dermatology, Mount Sinai Hosp 1971

Clark, Richard A MD (D) - **Spec Exp:** Eczema; Contact Dermatitis; Skin Cancer; **Hospital:** Stony Brook Univ Med Ctr; **Address:** 181 N Belle Mead Rd, Ste 5, East Setauket, NY 11733; **Phone:** 631-444-4200; **Board Cert:** Internal Medicine 1974; Allergy & Immunology 1977; Dermatology 1980; **Med School:** Univ Rochester 1971; **Resid:** Internal Medicine, Strong Meml Hosp 1973; **Fellow:** Allergy & Immunology, Nat Inst Health 1976; Dermatology, Mass Genl Hosp 1980; **Fac Appt:** Prof D, SUNY Stony Brook

Huh, Julie MD (D) - **Spec Exp:** Acne; Skin Cancer; Eczema; **Hospital:** Good Samaritan Hosp Med Ctr - West Islip, Southside Hosp (page 106); **Address:** 332 E Main St, Bayshore, NY 11706-8404; **Phone:** 631-666-0500; **Board Cert:** Dermatology 2013; **Med School:** Columbia P&S 1991; **Resid:** Dermatology, Columbia-Presby Med Ctr 1995

Kristal, Leonard MD (D) - **Spec Exp:** Pediatric Dermatology; **Hospital:** Stony Brook Univ Med Ctr, Steven & Alexandra Cohen Chldn's Med Ctr of NY (page 106); **Address:** Stony Brook Dermatology Associates, 181 N Belle Mead Rd, Ste 5, East Setauket, NY 11733; **Phone:** 631-444-4200; **Board Cert:** Pediatrics 2011; Dermatology 2013; Pediatric Dermatology 2004; **Med School:** Univ Hlth Scis, Chicago Med Sch 1986; **Resid:** Pediatrics, Childrens Hosp 1989; Dermatology, Univ Hosp-SUNY 1993; **Fellow:** Pediatric Dermatology, Childrens Hosp 1994; **Fac Appt:** Asst Clin Prof Ped, SUNY Stony Brook

Marghoob, Ashfaq A MD (D) - **Spec Exp:** Skin Cancer; Melanoma; **Hospital:** Meml Sloan-Kettering Canc Ctr (page 114); **Address:** Meml Sloan Kettering Cancer Ctr, 800 Veterans Memorial Hwy, Fl 2, Hauppage, NY 11788; **Phone:** 631-863-5150; **Board Cert:** Dermatology 2005; **Med School:** SUNY Stony Brook 1987; **Resid:** Family Medicine, SUNY Stony Brook Med Ctr 1990; **Fellow:** Dermatology, SUNY Stony Brook Med Ctr 1995

Moynihan, Gavan D MD (D) - **Spec Exp:** Melanoma; Skin Cancer; **Hospital:** Good Samaritan Hosp Med Ctr - West Islip, Southside Hosp (page 106); **Address:** 332 E Main St, Bay Shore, NY 11706-8404; **Phone:** 631-666-0500; **Board Cert:** Dermatology 2009; **Med School:** Howard Univ 1973; **Resid:** Dermatology, USPHS Hosp 1976; **Fellow:** Dermatology, Columbia-Presby Med Ctr 1977; **Fac Appt:** Asst Prof D, SUNY Stony Brook

Notaro, Antoinette MD (D) - **Spec Exp:** Skin Cancer; Botox Therapy; Psoriasis; Acne; **Hospital:** Eastern Long Island Hosp, Peconic Bay Med Ctr; **Address:** 13405 Main Rd, Box 93, Mattituck, NY 11952-0093; **Phone:** 631-298-1122; **Board Cert:** Dermatology 1982; **Med School:** SUNY Downstate 1978; **Resid:** Dermatology, Montefiore Med Ctr 1982; **Fac Appt:** Asst Clin Prof D, SUNY Stony Brook

Siegel, Daniel M MD (D) - **Spec Exp:** Mohs' Surgery; Dermatologic Surgery; Skin Cancer; **Hospital:** SUNY Downstate Med Ctr (Univ Hosp Brooklyn) (page 441), VA NY Harbor Hlthcr Sys-Brooklyn Campus; **Address:** 994 W Jericho Tpke, Ste 103, Smithtown, NY 11787; **Phone:** 631-864-6647; **Board Cert:** Dermatology 2009; **Med School:** Albany Med Coll 1981; **Resid:** Dermatology, Parkland Univ Texas SW Med Ctr 1985; **Fellow:** Mohs Surgery, Baylor Coll Med 1986; **Fac Appt:** Clin Prof D, SUNY Downstate

Skrokov, Robert MD (D) - **Spec Exp:** Vascular Malformations/Birthmarks; Psoriasis; Skin Cancer; **Hospital:** Good Samaritan Hosp Med Ctr - West Islip, Southside Hosp (page 106); **Address:** 332 E Main St, Bay Shore, NY 11706-8404; **Phone:** 631-666-0500; **Board Cert:** Dermatology 2009; **Med School:** SUNY Downstate 1982; **Resid:** Dermatology, SUNY-Downstate Med Ctr 1986; **Fac Appt:** Asst Clin Prof D, SUNY Stony Brook

Tom, Jack MD (D) - **Spec Exp:** Acne; Geriatric Dermatology; **Hospital:** Mt Sinai Med Ctr (page 102); **Address:** 207 Hallock Rd, Ste 210, Stony Brook, NY 11790-3076; **Phone:** 631-444-0004; **Board Cert:** Dermatology 1986; **Med School:** NYU Sch Med 1982; **Resid:** Internal Medicine, NYU Med Ctr 1983; Dermatology, Mount Sinai Med Ctr 1986; **Fac Appt:** Asst Clin Prof D, Mount Sinai Sch Med

Wong, Anthony L MD (D) - **Spec Exp:** Mohs' Surgery; Skin Cancer; **Address:** Skin Cancer & Dermatologic Surgery, 994 W Jericho Tpke, Ste 103, Smithtown, NY 11787; **Phone:** 631-864-6647; **Board Cert:** Dermatology 2004; **Med School:** SUNY Downstate 2000; **Resid:** Dermatology, SUNY Hlth Sci Ctr 2004; **Fellow:** Mohs Surgery, SUNY Hlth Sci Ctr 2005

Diagnostic Radiology

Brancaccio, William R MD (DR) - **Spec Exp:** Abdominal Imaging; Mammography; **Hospital:** Southampton Hosp, Eastern Long Island Hosp; **Address:** 240 Meeting House Ln, Radiology Dept, Southampton, NY 11968; **Phone:** 631-726-8411; **Board Cert:** Diagnostic Radiology 1981; **Med School:** Geo Wash Univ 1976; **Resid:** Diagnostic Radiology, Univ Hosp 1979; **Fellow:** Diagnostic Radiology, NYU Med Ctr 1980

Gould, Elaine S MD (DR) - **Spec Exp:** Musculoskeletal Imaging; Bone Imaging; **Hospital:** Stony Brook Univ Med Ctr; **Address:** Stony Brook Univ Med Ctr-Radiology, Level 4, Room 120, Nicolls Rd, Stony Brook, NY 11794-8460; **Phone:** 516-482-6700; **Board Cert:** Diagnostic Radiology ; **Med School:** SUNY Downstate 1980; **Resid:** Diagnostic Radiology, Winthrop Univ Hosp 1982; Diagnostic Radiology, SUNY Stony Brook Univ Hosp 1985; **Fellow:** Skeletal Radiology, Hosp for Joint Diseases 1986; **Fac Appt:** Assoc Prof Rad, SUNY Stony Brook

Kirshy, David MD (DR) - **Spec Exp:** CT Scan; MRI; PET Imaging; **Hospital:** Southampton Hosp; **Address:** 1333 Roanoke Ave, Riverhead, NY 11901; **Phone:** 631-727-2755; **Board Cert:** Diagnostic Radiology 1993; **Med School:** SUNY Downstate 1988; **Resid:** Diagnostic Radiology, SUNY Hlth Sci Ctr 1993

Mankes, Seth O MD (DR) - **Hospital:** Stony Brook Univ Med Ctr; **Address:** Stony Brook Univ Med Ctr, Radiology Dept, HSC Level 4, rm 120, Stony Brook, NY 11794-8460; **Phone:** 631-444-7901; **Board Cert:** Diagnostic Radiology 1981; **Med School:** NYU Sch Med 1976; **Resid:** Diagnostic Radiology, NYU Med Ctr 1981; **Fellow:** Ultrasound, NYU Med Ctr 1982; **Fac Appt:** Assoc Clin Prof Rad, SUNY Stony Brook

Schweitzer, Mark MD (DR) - **Spec Exp:** Musculoskeletal Imaging; Bone Imaging; **Hospital:** Stony Brook Univ Med Ctr; **Address:** Stony Brook Univ Med Ctr-Radiology, Level 4, Room 120, Nicolls Rd, Stony Brook, NY 11794-8460; **Phone:** 631-638-2121; **Board Cert:** Diagnostic Radiology ; **Med School:** SUNY Buffalo 1986; **Resid:** Diagnostic Radiology, Stony Brook Univ Hosp/Nassau Co Med Ctr 1990; **Fellow:** Musculoskeletal Imaging, UCSF Med Ctr 1991; **Fac Appt:** Prof Rad, SUNY Stony Brook

Endocrinology, Diabetes & Metabolism

Balkin, Michael S MD (EDM) - **Spec Exp:** Diabetes; Thyroid Disorders; Hirsutism (Excessive Body Hair); Osteoporosis; **Hospital:** Huntington Hosp (page 106), Nassau Univ Med Ctr; **Address:** 191 E Main St, Huntington, NY 11743-2921; **Phone:** 631-549-2525; **Board Cert:** Internal Medicine 1976; Endocrinology 1977; **Med School:** Mount Sinai Sch Med 1972; **Resid:** Internal Medicine, Kings County Med Ctr 1975; **Fellow:** Endocrinology, Diabetes & Metabolism, Mt Sinai Med Ctr 1977; Endocrinology, Diabetes & Metabolism, Meml Sloan Kettering Cancer Ctr 1980

Brand, Howard A MD (EDM) - **Spec Exp:** Thyroid Disorders; Pituitary Disorders; Diabetes; Cholesterol/Lipid Disorders; **Hospital:** St. Charles Hosp, John T Mather Meml Hosp; **Address:** 2500 Nesconset Hwy, Bldg 3C, Stony Brook, NY 11790; **Phone:** 631-751-2400; **Board Cert:** Internal Medicine 1987; Endocrinology, Diabetes & Metabolism 2011; **Med School:** UMDNJ-Rutgers Med Sch 1984; **Resid:** Internal Medicine, Mt Sinai Hosp 1987; Internal Medicine, Bronx VA Med Ctr 1988; **Fellow:** Endocrinology, Diabetes & Metabolism, NYU Med Ctr 1990

Carlson, Harold E MD (EDM) - **Spec Exp:** Thyroid Disorders; Pituitary Disorders; Gynecomastia; **Hospital:** Stony Brook Univ Med Ctr; **Address:** Stony Brook Univ Med Ctr, Div Endocrinology & Metabolism, 24 Research Way, East Setauket, NY 11733-3453; **Phone:** 631-444-0580; **Board Cert:** Internal Medicine 1974; Endocrinology, Diabetes & Metabolism 1975; **Med School:** Cornell Univ-Weill Med Coll 1968; **Resid:** Internal Medicine, Barnes-Jewish Hosp 1970; Internal Medicine, Natl Inst Hlth 1972; **Fellow:** Endocrinology, Washington Univ 1974; **Fac Appt:** Prof Med, SUNY Stony Brook

Gelato, Marie MD (EDM) - **Spec Exp:** Thyroid Disorders; Pituitary Disorders; Adrenal Disorders; Polycystic Ovarian Syndrome; **Hospital:** Stony Brook Univ Med Ctr; **Address:** Stony Brook Internist, Specialty Care, 26 Research Way, East Setauket, NY 11733; **Phone:** 631-444-0580; **Board Cert:** Internal Medicine 1982; Endocrinology 1985; **Med School:** Mich State Univ 1979; **Resid:** Internal Medicine, Dartmouth Med Ctr 1982; **Fellow:** Endocrinology, Natl Inst Hlth 1985; **Fac Appt:** Prof Med, SUNY Stony Brook

Gioia, Leonard V MD (EDM) - **Spec Exp:** Diabetes; Thyroid Disorders; **Hospital:** Southside Hosp (page 106), Good Samaritan Hosp Med Ctr - West Islip; **Address:** 53 Brentwood Rd, Ste E, Bay Shore, NY 11706; **Phone:** 631-666-6275; **Board Cert:** Internal Medicine 1979; Endocrinology, Diabetes & Metabolism 1981; **Med School:** SUNY Downstate 1976; **Resid:** Internal Medicine, St Vincent's Hosp & Med Ctr 1979; **Fellow:** Endocrinology, Diabetes & Metabolism, Boston Univ Med Ctr 1981

Goldenberg, Alan MD (EDM) - **Spec Exp:** Diabetes; Thyroid Disorders; Hormonal Disorders; Addison's Disease; **Hospital:** Southampton Hosp, Peconic Bay Med Ctr; **Address:** East End Endocrine Assocs, 189 Main Rd, Riverhead, NY 11901; **Phone:** 631-288-7120; **Board Cert:** Internal Medicine 2008; Endocrinology, Diabetes & Metabolism 2008; **Med School:** SUNY Stony Brook 1993; **Resid:** Internal Medicine, Winthrop Univ Hosp 1996; **Fellow:** Endocrinology, Diabetes & Metabolism, Winthrop Univ Hosp 1998

Weitzman, Steven P MD (EDM) - **Spec Exp:** Hashimoto's Disease; Adrenal Disorders; Thyroid Disorders; **Hospital:** Stony Brook Univ Med Ctr; **Address:** Stony Brook Univ Med Ctr, Internal Med, 26 Research Way, East Setauket, NY 11733; **Phone:** 631-444-0538; **Board Cert:** Internal Medicine 2005; Endocrinology, Diabetes & Metabolism 2008; **Med School:** SUNY Buffalo 2002; **Resid:** Internal Medicine, Long Island Jewish Med Ctr 2005; **Fellow:** Endocrinology, Diabetes & Metabolism, Stony Brook Univ Med Ctr 2008; **Fac Appt:** Asst Prof Med, SUNY Stony Brook

Wexler, Craig B MD (EDM) - **Spec Exp:** Diabetes; Thyroid Disorders; Hormonal Disorders; Cholesterol/Lipid Disorders; **Hospital:** Brookhaven Meml Hosp & Med Ctr; **Address:** 1723A North Ocean Ave, Medford, NY 11763; **Phone:** 631-758-5858; **Board Cert:** Internal Medicine 1981; Endocrinology, Diabetes & Metabolism 1989; **Med School:** Ros Franklin Univ/Chicago Med Sch 1978; **Resid:** Internal Medicine, LIJ-Hillside Med Ctr 1981; **Fellow:** Endocrinology, Diabetes & Metabolism, LIJ-Hillside Med Ctr 1989

Family Medicine

Aponte, Alex M MD (FMed) *PCP* - **Spec Exp:** Preventive Medicine; **Hospital:** Southampton Hosp; **Address:** Westhampton Primary Care, 80 Old Riverhead Rd, Westhampton Beach, NY 11978; **Phone:** 631-288-7746; **Board Cert:** Family Medicine 2009; **Med School:** SUNY Buffalo 1992; **Resid:** Family Medicine, Overlook Hosp 1995

Ebarb, Raymond MD (FMed) *PCP* - **Spec Exp:** Cholesterol/Lipid Disorders; **Hospital:** Southside Hosp (page 106), Good Samaritan Hosp Med Ctr - West Islip; **Address:** 213 Montauk Hwy, West Sayville, NY 11796; **Phone:** 631-563-6205; **Board Cert:** Family Medicine 2005; **Med School:** Mexico 1982; **Resid:** Family Medicine, Southside Hosp 1987; **Fac Appt:** Asst Clin Prof FMed, SUNY Stony Brook

Fishkin, Michael DO (FMed) *PCP* - **Hospital:** John T Mather Meml Hosp, St. Charles Hosp; **Address:** 2500 Nesconset Hwy, Building 7D, Stony Brook, NY 11790-2566; **Phone:** 631-751-3322; **Board Cert:** Family Medicine 2006; **Med School:** Univ Osteo Med & Hlth Sci, Des Moines 1973; **Resid:** Family Medicine, Nassau County Med Ctr 1976

Giugliano, James E DO (FMed) *PCP* - **Spec Exp:** Lyme Disease; **Hospital:** Southampton Hosp; **Address:** 290 N Sea Rd, Southampton, NY 11968; **Phone:** 631-283-5900; **Board Cert:** Family Medicine 2012; **Med School:** NY Coll Osteo Med 1988; **Resid:** Family Medicine, Southside Hosp 1991; **Fac Appt:** Clin Prof FMed, NY Coll Osteo Med

Greenblatt, Louis L DO (FMed) *PCP* - **Spec Exp:** Preventive Medicine; Geriatric Medicine; **Hospital:** St. Catherine's of Siena Med Ctr, Stony Brook Univ Med Ctr; **Address:** 533 Rte 111, Hauppauge, NY 11788; **Phone:** 631-366-1788; **Board Cert:** Family Medicine 2007; Geriatric Medicine 2006; **Med School:** NY Coll Osteo Med 1983; **Resid:** Family Medicine, Stony Brook Med Ctr 1986; **Fac Appt:** Asst Clin Prof FMed, SUNY Stony Brook

Johnson, Sabrina MD (FMed) *PCP* - ; **Address:** Shirley Health Ctr, 550 Montauk Hwy, Shirley, NY 11967; **Phone:** 631-852-1022; **Board Cert:** Family Medicine 2003; **Med School:** SUNY Downstate 1987; **Resid:** Family Medicine, Stony Brook Univ Hosp 1991

Schwinn, Hans D MD (FMed) *PCP* - **Hospital:** Southampton Hosp; **Address:** Westhampton Primary Care Center, 80 Old Riverhead Rd, Westhampton Beach, NY 11978-1401; **Phone:** 631-288-7746; **Board Cert:** Family Medicine 2007; **Med School:** Germany 1978; **Resid:** Family Medicine, Community Hosp 1981

Gastroenterology

Buscaglia, Jonathan M MD (Ge) - **Spec Exp:** Endoscopy; Pancreatic/Biliary Endoscopy (ERCP); **Hospital:** Stony Brook Univ Med Ctr; **Address:** Univ Gastroenterology & Hepatology, 3 Technology Drive, Ste 300, East Setauket, NY 11733-4073; **Phone:** 631-444-5220; **Board Cert:** Internal Medicine 2004; Gastroenterology 2007; **Med School:** SUNY Buffalo 2001; **Resid:** Internal Medicine, Montefiore Med Ctr 2004; **Fellow:** Gastroenterology, Johns Hopkins Hosp 2007; Advanced Endoscopy, Johns Hopkins Hosp 2008; **Fac Appt:** Asst Prof Med, SUNY Stony Brook

Cohn, William J MD (Ge) - **Spec Exp:** Liver Disease; **Hospital:** John T Mather Meml Hosp, St. Charles Hosp; **Address:** LI Digestive Disease Consultants, 8 Technology Drive, Ste 101, East Setauket, NY 11733-3327; **Phone:** 631-751-8700; **Board Cert:** Internal Medicine 1975; Gastroenterology 1979; **Med School:** Med Coll VA 1972; **Resid:** Internal Medicine, Med Coll Virginia Affil Hosp 1975; **Fellow:** Gastroenterology, Albert Einstein Med Ctr 1978; **Fac Appt:** Asst Clin Prof Med, SUNY Stony Brook

Duva, Joseph M MD (Ge) - **Spec Exp:** Endoscopy & Colonoscopy; Gastroesophageal Reflux Disease (GERD); Irritable Bowel Syndrome; Colonoscopy/Polypectomy; **Hospital:** Peconic Bay Med Ctr; **Address:** 887 Old Country Rd, Ste A, Riverhead, NY 11901-2115; **Phone:** 631-727-6122; **Board Cert:** Internal Medicine 1981; Gastroenterology 2007; **Med School:** Mount Sinai Sch Med 1978; **Resid:** Internal Medicine, Nassau County Med Ctr 1981; **Fellow:** Gastroenterology, Nassau County Med Ctr 1983

Glanzman, Barry MD (Ge) - **Spec Exp:** Colonoscopy; Gastroesophageal Reflux Disease (GERD); Liver Disease; **Hospital:** Huntington Hosp (page 106); **Address:** 152 E Main St, Ste C, Huntington, NY 11743; **Phone:** 631-421-2185; **Board Cert:** Gastroenterology 1989; Internal Medicine 1984; **Med School:** SUNY Downstate 1980; **Resid:** Internal Medicine, LI Jewish hosp 1983; **Fellow:** Gastroenterology, Med Coll of VA 1986

Harrison, Aaron R MD (Ge) - **Spec Exp:** Gastroesophageal Reflux Disease (GERD); Colon Cancer; Crohn's Disease; **Hospital:** Southside Hosp (page 106); **Address:** North Shore LIJ Western Suffolk Gastro Assocs, 375 E Main St, Ste 21, Bay Shore, NY 11706; **Phone:** 631-968-8288; **Board Cert:** Internal Medicine 1977; Gastroenterology 1979; **Med School:** Albert Einstein Coll Med 1974; **Resid:** Internal Medicine, Jacobi Med Ctr 1977; **Fellow:** Gastroenterology, UCLA Med Ctr 1979; **Fac Appt:** Asst Clin Prof Med, SUNY Stony Brook

Khokhar, Asim MD (Ge) - **Spec Exp:** Liver Disease; Hepatitis B & C; **Hospital:** Stony Brook Univ Med Ctr; **Address:** Univ Gastroenterology & Hepatology, 3 Technology Drive, Ste 300, East Setauket, NY 11733-4073; **Phone:** 631-444-5220; **Board Cert:** Internal Medicine 2003; Gastroenterology 2008; **Med School:** Pakistan 1998; **Resid:** Internal Medicine, Parkridge Hosp 2003; **Fellow:** Gastroenterology, Beth Israel Deaconess Med Ctr 2004; Hepatology, Beth Isreal Deaconess Med Ctr 2005; **Fac Appt:** Asst Prof Med, SUNY Stony Brook

Lazar, Robert M MD (Ge) - **Spec Exp:** Endoscopy; Colonoscopy; **Hospital:** St. Catherine's of Siena Med Ctr; **Address:** 48 Route 25A, Ste 107, Smithtown, NY 11787-1431; **Phone:** 631-862-3680; **Board Cert:** Internal Medicine 1986; Gastroenterology 2011; **Med School:** Mexico 1981; **Resid:** Internal Medicine, Univ Hosp/SUNY Hlth Sci Ctr 1986

Spielberg, Alan L MD (Ge) - **Spec Exp:** Inflammatory Bowel Disease, Colitis; **Hospital:** St. Catherine's of Siena Med Ctr; **Address:** 48 Route 25A, Ste 203, Smithtown, NY 11787-1448; **Phone:** 631-724-1178; **Board Cert:** Internal Medicine 1977; Gastroenterology 1979; **Med School:** Belgium 1974; **Resid:** Internal Medicine, Albany Med Ctr 1977; **Fellow:** Gastroenterology, Albany Med Ctr 1979; **Fac Appt:** Asst Clin Prof Med, SUNY Stony Brook

Zinkin, Noah T MD (Ge) - **Spec Exp:** Celiac Disease; Crohn's Disease; Hepatitis; **Hospital:** Huntington Hosp (page 106); **Address:** 775 Park Ave, Ste 225, Huntington, NY 11743; **Phone:** 631-923-1420; **Board Cert:** Internal Medicine 2003; Gastroenterology 2006; **Med School:** Univ Rochester 2000; **Resid:** Internal Medicine, Brigham & Women's Hosp 2003; **Fellow:** Gastroenterology, Beth Israel Deaconess Med Ctr 2006

Geriatric Medicine

Fields, Suzanne D MD (Ger) *PCP* - **Spec Exp:** Geriatric Care; Preventive Medicine; **Hospital:** Stony Brook Univ Med Ctr; **Address:** 205 N Belle Mead Rd, East Setauket, NY 11733; **Phone:** 631-444-4630; **Board Cert:** Internal Medicine 1982; Geriatric Medicine 2008; Hospice & Palliative Medicine 2012; **Med School:** Univ Conn 1979; **Resid:** Internal Medicine, Waterbury Hosp 1983; **Fellow:** Geriatric Medicine, New York Hosp-Cornell 1985; **Fac Appt:** Prof Med, SUNY Stony Brook

Gynecologic Oncology

Pearl, Michael L MD (GO) - **Spec Exp:** Gynecologic Cancer; Gynecologic Surgery-Complex; **Hospital:** Stony Brook Univ Med Ctr; **Address:** Stony Brook, Gynecolgoic Oncology, 3 Edmund D Pellegrino Rd, Stony Brook, NY 11794-9456; **Phone:** 631-444-2989; **Board Cert:** Obstetrics & Gynecology 2012; Gynecologic Oncology 2012; Hospice & Palliative Medicine 2010; **Med School:** UCSF 1986; **Resid:** Obstetrics & Gynecology, UCSF Med Ctr 1990; **Fellow:** Gynecologic Oncology, Univ Michigan 1994; **Fac Appt:** Prof ObG, SUNY Stony Brook

Hand Surgery

Hurst, Lawrence C MD (HS) - **Spec Exp:** Microvascular Surgery; Nerve Disorders/Surgery; Dupuytren's Contracture; **Hospital:** Stony Brook Univ Med Ctr; **Address:** Stony Brook Orthopaedic Associates, 14 Technology Drive, Ste 11, East Setauket, NY 11733-3464; **Phone:** 631-444-3145; **Board Cert:** Orthopaedic Surgery 1980; Hand Surgery 2010; **Med School:** Univ VT Coll Med 1973; **Resid:** Orthopaedic Surgery, N Carolina Meml Hosp 1978; **Fellow:** Hand Surgery, Columbia-Presby Med Ctr 1979; **Fac Appt:** Prof OrS, SUNY Stony Brook

Wang, Edward D MD (HS) - **Spec Exp:** Hand & Upper Extremity Surgery; Arthritis; Wrist Surgery; Shoulder Surgery; **Hospital:** Stony Brook Univ Med Ctr; **Address:** 14 Technology Drive, Ste 11, East Setauket, NY 11733-3464; **Phone:** 631-444-4233; **Board Cert:** Orthopaedic Surgery 2009; Headache Medicine 2009; **Med School:** Yale Univ 1990; **Resid:** Orthopaedic Surgery, Hosp Univ Penn 1995; **Fellow:** Hand Surgery, Mass Genl Hosp 1996; **Fac Appt:** Assoc Clin Prof OrS, SUNY Stony Brook

Hematology

Avvento, Louis J MD (Hem) - **Spec Exp:** Breast Cancer; Lymphoma; **Hospital:** Peconic Bay Med Ctr, Southampton Hosp; **Address:** 1333 E Main St, Riverhead, NY 11901; **Phone:** 631-727-8500; **Board Cert:** Internal Medicine 1985; Medical Oncology 1987; Hematology 2004; Hospice & Palliative Medicine 2012; **Med School:** Italy 1981; **Resid:** Internal Medicine, Jamaica Med Ctr 1985; **Fellow:** Hematology, Univ Hosp-SUNY 1988

Schuster, Michael W MD (Hem) - **Spec Exp:** Bone Marrow Transplant; Hematologic Malignancies; Myelodysplastic Syndromes; Anemia-Aplastic; **Hospital:** Stony Brook Univ Med Ctr; **Address:** Stony Brook Univ Cancer Ctr, 3 Edmund D Pellegrino Rd, Stony Brook, NY 11794; **Phone:** 631-444-3577; **Board Cert:** Internal Medicine 1984; Hematology 1986; **Med School:** Dartmouth Med Sch 1980; **Resid:** Internal Medicine, Beth Israel Deaconess Med Ctr 1983; **Fellow:** Hematology & Oncology, Beth Israel Deaconess Med Ctr 1987; **Fac Appt:** Prof Hem & Onc, SUNY Stony Brook

Hospice & Palliative Medicine

Hallarman, Lynn E MD (H & PM) - **Spec Exp:** Palliative Care; Pain-Cancer; Ethics; **Hospital:** Stony Brook Univ Med Ctr; **Address:** Stony Brook Univ Med Ctr-Palliative Care, 101 Nicolls Road, Stony Brook, NY 11794-8160; **Phone:** 631-638-2801; **Board Cert:** Internal Medicine 2006; Hospice & Palliative Medicine ; **Med School:** Yale Univ 1993; **Resid:** Internal Medicine, Strong Meml Hosp 1996; **Fellow:** Hospice & Palliative Medicine, Harvard Med School; **Fac Appt:** Asst Prof Med, SUNY Stony Brook

Infectious Disease

Nash, Bernard J MD (Inf) - **Spec Exp:** Hospital Acquired Infections; Viral Infections; **Hospital:** Good Samaritan Hosp Med Ctr - West Islip, Southside Hosp (page 106); **Address:** Suffolk Internal Med Assocs, 500 Montauk Hwy, Ste S, West Islip, NY 11795; **Phone:** 631-587-7733; **Board Cert:** Internal Medicine 1978; Infectious Disease 1982; **Med School:** Georgetown Univ 1975; **Resid:** Internal Medicine, St Elizabeth Hosp 1978; **Fellow:** Infectious Disease, Boston Univ Med Ctr 1981

Sacks-Berg, Anne C MD (Inf) - **Spec Exp:** Travel Medicine; **Hospital:** Huntington Hosp (page 106); **Address:** Long Island Infectious Disease Assocs, 120 New York Ave, Ste 5W, Huntington, NY 11743-2743; **Phone:** 631-423-9809; **Board Cert:** Internal Medicine 1986; Infectious Disease 1988; Hospice & Palliative Medicine 2012; **Med School:** SUNY Stony Brook 1983; **Resid:** Internal Medicine, Winthrop Univ Hosp 1986; **Fellow:** Infectious Disease, Winthrop Univ Hosp 1988

Samuels, Steven MD (Inf) - **Spec Exp:** Lyme Disease; AIDS/HIV; **Hospital:** Good Samaritan Hosp Med Ctr - West Islip, Southside Hosp (page 106); **Address:** Suffolk Internal Med Assocs, 500 Montauk Hwy, Ste S, West Islip, NY 11795; **Phone:** 631-587-7733; **Board Cert:** Internal Medicine 1977; Infectious Disease 1982; **Med School:** NY Med Coll 1974; **Resid:** Internal Medicine, Nassau County Med Ctr 1977; **Fellow:** Infectious Disease, UC Irvine Med Ctr 1979; **Fac Appt:** Asst Prof Med, SUNY Stony Brook

Internal Medicine

Balot, Barry H DO (IM) *PCP* - **Spec Exp:** Geriatric Medicine; Preventive Medicine; **Hospital:** Good Samaritan Hosp Med Ctr - West Islip, Southside Hosp (page 106); **Address:** 150 E Sunrise Hwy, Ste 101, Lindenhurst, NY 11757; **Phone:** 631-225-6200; **Board Cert:** Internal Medicine 1989; **Med School:** NY Coll Osteo Med 1985; **Resid:** Internal Medicine, Univ Hosp 1987; Internal Medicine, Overlook Hosp 1989

Covey, Alexander J MD (IM) - **Spec Exp:** Aging Skin; **Address:** 445 Main St, Center Moriches, NY 11934; **Phone:** 631-878-9200; **Board Cert:** Internal Medicine 1988; **Med School:** Ros Franklin Univ/Chicago Med Sch 1985; **Resid:** Internal Medicine, Winthrop Univ Hosp 1988

Friedling, Steven MD (IM) *PCP* - **Spec Exp:** Preventive Medicine; Chronic Illness; **Hospital:** St. Catherine's of Siena Med Ctr, Stony Brook Univ Med Ctr; **Address:** 267 E Main St A Bldg, Smithtown, NY 11787-2580; **Phone:** 631-724-8348; **Board Cert:** Internal Medicine 1973; Infectious Disease 1980; **Med School:** SUNY Downstate 1968; **Resid:** Medical Oncology, Natl Cancer Inst 1971; Internal Medicine, Barnes Hosp 1973; **Fellow:** Infectious Disease, Barnes Hosp 1974; **Fac Appt:** Asst Prof Med, SUNY Stony Brook

German, Harold J MD (IM) *PCP* - **Spec Exp:** Hematology; Preventive Medicine; **Hospital:** Huntington Hosp (page 106); **Address:** 150 Main St, Huntington, NY 11743-6908; **Phone:** 631-271-8700; **Board Cert:** Internal Medicine 1973; Hematology 1978; **Med School:** Columbia P&S 1967; **Resid:** Internal Medicine, Harlem Hosp Med Ctr 1971; Internal Medicine, Columbia Presby Hosp 1972; **Fellow:** Hematology, Columbia Presby Hosp 1973

Hallal Jr, Edward J MD (IM) *PCP* - **Hospital:** Southside Hosp (page 106); **Address:** 180 E Main St, Bay Shore, NY 11706; **Phone:** 631-665-0027; **Board Cert:** Internal Medicine 1987; **Med School:** Grenada 1984; **Resid:** Internal Medicine, NY Methodist Hosp 1987

Lalli, Corradino Michael MD (IM) *PCP* - **Spec Exp:** Geriatric Medicine; **Hospital:** St. Catherine's of Siena Med Ctr; **Address:** 59 Southern Blvd, Nesconset, NY 11767; **Phone:** 631-659-1700; **Board Cert:** Internal Medicine 1979; Geriatric Medicine 2008; **Med School:** Albert Einstein Coll Med 1976; **Resid:** Internal Medicine, Nassau County Med Ctr 1979; **Fellow:** Pulmonary Disease, Nassau County Med Ctr 1980; **Fac Appt:** Asst Clin Prof Med, SUNY Stony Brook

Oppenheimer, John MD (IM) *PCP* - **Spec Exp:** Geriatric Medicine; AIDS/HIV; **Hospital:** Southampton Hosp; **Address:** 60 Bay St, Sag Harbor, NY 11963; **Phone:** 631-725-4600; **Board Cert:** Internal Medicine 1984; Geriatric Medicine 2009; **Med School:** Tulane Univ 1981; **Resid:** Internal Medicine, Tulane Univ Hosp 1982; Internal Medicine, Harlem Hosp 1983

Romano, Rosario MD (IM) *PCP* - **Spec Exp:** Geriatric Care; Cholesterol/Lipid Disorders; **Hospital:** John T Mather Meml Hosp, St. Charles Hosp; **Address:** 5225-15 Rte 347, Port Jefferson Station, NY 11776-2054; **Phone:** 631-331-1000; **Board Cert:** Internal Medicine 1977; **Med School:** NY Med Coll 1973; **Resid:** Internal Medicine, Lenox Hill Hosp 1977; **Fac Appt:** Asst Clin Prof Med, SUNY Stony Brook

Simon, Lloyd D MD (IM) *PCP* - **Spec Exp:** Addiction/Substance Abuse; **Hospital:** Eastern Long Island Hosp; **Address:** East End Physicians Services, 44210 County Road 48, P O Box 1341, Southold, NY 11971; **Phone:** 631-765-4150; **Board Cert:** Internal Medicine 1983; **Med School:** SUNY Buffalo 1980; **Resid:** Internal Medicine, Univ Mass Med Ctr 1983

Singer, Mark DO (IM) *PCP* - **Hospital:** Huntington Hosp (page 106); **Address:** Mt Sinai/North Shore Medical Group, 325 Park Ave, Huntington, NY 11743; **Phone:** 631-351-8487; **Board Cert:** Internal Medicine 2009; **Med School:** NY Coll Osteo Med 1995; **Resid:** Internal Medicine, North Shore Univ Hosp 1999

Stallone, James A DO (IM) *PCP* - **Spec Exp:** Preventive Medicine; **Hospital:** Good Samaritan Hosp Med Ctr - West Islip; **Address:** 400 W Main St, Ste 234, Babylon, NY 11702; **Phone:** 631-321-4200; **Board Cert:** Internal Medicine 1989; **Med School:** NY Coll Osteo Med 1986; **Resid:** Internal Medicine, Booth Meml Med Ctr/Einstein 1989; **Fac Appt:** Asst Clin Prof Med, NY Coll Osteo Med

weiss, Deborah MD (IM) *PCP* - **Hospital:** Huntington Hosp (page 106); **Address:** Mt Sinai/North Shore Medical Group, 325 Park Ave, Huntington, NY 11743; **Phone:** 631-367-5024; **Board Cert:** Internal Medicine 2010; **Med School:** Cornell Univ-Weill Med Coll 1997; **Resid:** Internal Medicine, North Shore Univ Hosp 2000

Wertheim, William A MD (IM) *PCP* - **Spec Exp:** Geriatric Care; **Hospital:** Stony Brook Univ Med Ctr; **Address:** Stony Brook Internists, Primary Care, 205 N Belle Mead Rd, East Setauket, NY 11733; **Phone:** 631-444-4630; **Board Cert:** Internal Medicine 2003; **Med School:** NYU Sch Med 1989; **Resid:** Internal Medicine, Univ Michigan Med Ctr 1992; **Fac Appt:** Clin Prof Med, SUNY Stony Brook

Interventional Cardiology

Lawson, William E MD (IC) - **Spec Exp:** Angioplasty & Stent Placement; Preventive Cardiology; Non-Invasive Cardiology; Heart Failure; **Hospital:** Stony Brook Univ Med Ctr; **Address:** Stony Brook Heart Ctr, 101 Nicholls Rd, Stony Brook, NY 11794; **Phone:** 631-444-1066; **Board Cert:** Internal Medicine 1980; Cardiovascular Disease 1983; Interventional Cardiology 2009; Advanced Heart Failure & Transplant Cardiology 2010; **Med School:** UMDNJ-Rutgers Med Sch 1977; **Resid:** Internal Medicine, Nassau Univ Med Ctr 1980; **Fellow:** Cardiovascular Disease, Stony Brook Univ Med Ctr 1982; **Fac Appt:** Prof Med, SUNY Stony Brook

Ong, Lawrence MD (IC) - **Spec Exp:** Angioplasty & Stent Placement; **Hospital:** Huntington Hosp (page 106), N Shore Univ Hosp (page 106); **Address:** 270 Park Ave, Huntington, NY 11743; **Phone:** 631-351-7948; **Board Cert:** Internal Medicine 1979; Cardiovascular Disease 1981; Interventional Cardiology 2009; **Med School:** UCSF 1976; **Resid:** Internal Medicine, N Shore Univ Hosp 1979; **Fellow:** Cardiovascular Disease, N Shore Univ Hosp 1981; **Fac Appt:** Assoc Prof Med, NYU Sch Med

Maternal & Fetal Medicine

Bernasko, James MD (MF) - **Spec Exp:** Pregnancy-High Risk; Diabetes in Pregnancy; Prenatal Diagnosis; **Hospital:** Stony Brook Univ Med Ctr; **Address:** Stony Brook OB/GYN, 4875 Sunrise Hwy, Bohemia, NY 11716; **Phone:** 631-444-4686; **Board Cert:** Obstetrics & Gynecology 2012; Maternal & Fetal Medicine 2012; **Med School:** Ghana 1987; **Resid:** Obstetrics & Gynecology, Columbia/Harlem Hosp Ctr 1994; **Fellow:** Maternal & Fetal Medicine, Mt Sinai Med Ctr 1996; **Fac Appt:** Assoc Prof ObG, SUNY Stony Brook

Medical Oncology

Akhund, Birjis G MD (Onc) - **Spec Exp:** Breast Cancer; Lymphoma; Lung Cancer; **Hospital:** Huntington Hosp (page 106); **Address:** 180 E Pulaski Rd, Huntington Station, NY 11746; **Phone:** 631-425-2280; **Board Cert:** Internal Medicine 1989; Medical Oncology 2003; Hematology 2004; **Med School:** Lebanon 1986; **Resid:** Internal Medicine, Beth Israel Med Ctr 1990; **Fellow:** Hematology & Oncology, NYU Med Ctr 1992; Hematology Research, NYU Med Ctr 1993

Caruso, Rocco MD (Onc) - **Spec Exp:** Lymphoma; **Hospital:** St. Catherine's of Siena Med Ctr, St. Charles Hosp; **Address:** North Island Hematology Oncology, 2500 Nesconset Hwy, Bldg 26-B, Stony Brook, NY 11790; **Phone:** 631-751-8305; **Board Cert:** Internal Medicine 1982; Hematology 1984; Medical Oncology 2005; **Med School:** Univ Pennsylvania 1979; **Resid:** Internal Medicine, St Luke's-Roosevelt Hosp Ctr 1982; **Fellow:** Hematology, NYU Med Ctr 1985; Medical Oncology, LI Jewish Med Ctr 1994; **Fac Appt:** Asst Prof Med, SUNY Stony Brook

DaCosta, Noshir Anthony MD (Onc) - **Spec Exp:** Breast Cancer; Hematologic Malignancies; **Hospital:** Stony Brook Univ Med Ctr, John T Mather Meml Hosp; **Address:** North Shore Hematology Oncology Assocs, 235 N Belle Mead Rd, East Setauket, NY 11733; **Phone:** 631-751-3000; **Board Cert:** Internal Medicine 1989; Hematology 2012; Medical Oncology 2012; **Med School:** India 1985; **Resid:** Internal Medicine, LaGuardia Hosp 1989; **Fellow:** Hematology & Oncology, SUNY Stony Brook Hosp 1992; **Fac Appt:** Asst Clin Prof Onc, SUNY Stony Brook

Fiore, John J MD (Onc) - **Spec Exp:** Lung Cancer; **Hospital:** St. Catherine's of Siena Med Ctr; **Address:** Meml Sloan-Kettering Ctr, 650 Commack Rd, Commack, NY 11725; **Phone:** 631-623-4100; **Board Cert:** Internal Medicine 1978; Hematology 1982; Medical Oncology 1983; **Med School:** Tufts Univ 1975; **Resid:** Internal Medicine, VA Med Ctr 1979; **Fellow:** Hematology, VA Med Ctr 1981; Medical Oncology, Meml Sloan-Kettering Cancer Ctr 1984

Kudelka, Andrzej P MD (Onc) - **Spec Exp:** Head & Neck Cancer; Breast Cancer; Pancreatic Cancer; **Hospital:** Stony Brook Univ Med Ctr; **Address:** Stony Brook Cancer Ctr, Hematology/Onc, 3 Edmund D Pellegrino Rd, Stony Brook, NY 11794; **Phone:** 631-638-1000; **Board Cert:** Internal Medicine 1987; Medical Oncology 1989; Hospice & Palliative Medicine 2010; **Med School:** Poland 1982; **Resid:** Internal Medicine, Coney Island Hosp 1987; **Fellow:** Hematology & Oncology, Stony Brook Univ Hosp 1990

Ostrow, Stanley MD (Onc) - **Spec Exp:** Lymphoma; Breast Cancer; Leukemia; Carcinoid Tumors; **Hospital:** John T Mather Meml Hosp, Brookhaven Meml Hosp & Med Ctr; **Address:** 235 N Belle Mead Rd, East Setauket, NY 11733; **Phone:** 631-751-5151; **Board Cert:** Internal Medicine 1978; Medical Oncology 1979; Hematology 1982; **Med School:** SUNY Downstate 1974; **Resid:** Internal Medicine, Jewish Meml Hosp 1976; **Fellow:** Hematology & Oncology, Natl Cancer Inst 1980; **Fac Appt:** Asst Prof Med, SUNY Stony Brook

Rizvi, Hasan A MD (Onc) - **Hospital:** Good Samaritan Hosp Med Ctr - West Islip, Southside Hosp (page 106); **Address:** 180 E Main St, Bay Shore, NY 11706-8427; **Phone:** 631-666-0262; **Board Cert:** Hematology 2002; **Med School:** Pakistan 1975; **Resid:** Clinical Pathology, Ellis Hosp 1978; Internal Medicine, Mt Sinai Med Ctr 1981; **Fellow:** Hematology & Oncology, Winthrop Univ Hosp 1983; Hematology & Oncology, St Elizabeth Hosp 1984

Strauss, Barry MD (Onc) - **Spec Exp:** Lung Cancer; Breast Cancer; Colon Cancer; Ovarian Cancer; **Hospital:** Southampton Hosp; **Address:** 353 Meeting House Ln, Southampton, NY 11968-5051; **Phone:** 631-283-6611; **Board Cert:** Internal Medicine 1975; Medical Oncology 1975; **Med School:** Geo Wash Univ 1971; **Resid:** Internal Medicine, Beth Israel Hosp 1973; **Fellow:** Medical Oncology, Natl Cancer Inst 1975

Neonatal-Perinatal Medicine

Davidson, Dennis MD (NP) - **Spec Exp:** Lung Disease in Newborns; **Hospital:** Stony Brook Univ Med Ctr; **Address:** Stony Brook Univ Med Ct, Dept Pediatrics, 101 Nicholls Rd, HSC T11-060, Stony Brook, NY 11794-8111; **Phone:** 631-444-7653; **Board Cert:** Pediatrics 1980; Neonatal-Perinatal Medicine 2009; **Med School:** Loyola Univ-Stritch Sch Med 1974; **Resid:** Pediatrics, Babies Hosp-Columbia Univ 1978; **Fellow:** Neonatal-Perinatal Medicine, Babies Hosp-Columbia Univ 1981; **Fac Appt:** Clin Prof Ped, Albert Einstein Coll Med

Parekh, Aruna J MD (NP) - **Hospital:** Stony Brook Univ Med Ctr; **Address:** Stony Brook Dept Pediatrics, 37 Research Way, East Setauket, NY 11733; **Phone:** 631-444-4660; **Board Cert:** Pediatrics 1976; Neonatal-Perinatal Medicine 1985; **Med School:** India 1970; **Resid:** Pediatrics, LI Coll Hosp 1975; **Fellow:** Neonatal-Perinatal Medicine, N Shore Univ Hosp 1977

Neurological Surgery

Davis, Raphael P MD (NS) - **Spec Exp:** Acoustic Neuroma; Skull Base Surgery; Spinal Disc Replacement; Brain & Spinal Surgery; **Hospital:** Stony Brook Univ Med Ctr, St. Charles Hosp; **Address:** New York Spine & Brain Surgery, 24 Research Way, Ste 200, East Setauket, NY 11733; **Phone:** 631-444-1213; **Board Cert:** Neurological Surgery 1990; **Med School:** Mount Sinai Sch Med 1981; **Resid:** Neurological Surgery, Mt Sinai Med Ctr 1987; **Fac Appt:** Prof NS, SUNY Stony Brook

Leon, Steven P MD (NS) - **Spec Exp:** Minimally Invasive Spinal Surgery; Spinal Disorders-Degenerative; Spinal Disc Replacement; Spinal Tumors; **Hospital:** St. Charles Hosp, Brookhaven Meml Hosp & Med Ctr; **Address:** Long Island Neuroscience Specialists, 100 Hospital Rd, Ste 216, East Patchogue, NY 11772; **Phone:** 631-475-5511; **Board Cert:** Neurological Surgery 2004; **Med School:** Harvard Med Sch 1994; **Resid:** Neurological Surgery, Brigham & Women's Hosp 2000; **Fellow:** Spine Surgery, Cleveland Clin 2001; **Fac Appt:** Asst Clin Prof NS, Cornell Univ-Weill Med Coll

Woo, Henry H MD (NS) - **Spec Exp:** Brain Tumors; Aneurysm-Cerebral; Cerebrovascular Surgery; Stroke; **Hospital:** Stony Brook Univ Med Ctr; **Address:** New York Spine & Brain Surgery, 24 Research Way, Ste 200, East Setauket, NY 11733; **Phone:** 631-444-1213; **Board Cert:** Neurological Surgery 2008; **Med School:** NYU Sch Med 1995; **Resid:** Neurological Surgery, NYU Med Ctr 2002; **Fellow:** Interventional Neuroradiology, NYU Med Ctr 2003; **Fac Appt:** Prof NS, SUNY Stony Brook

Neurology

Cohen, Daniel H MD/PhD (N) - **Spec Exp:** Stroke; Neuromuscular Disorders; Multiple Sclerosis; Dementia; **Hospital:** Good Samaritan Hosp Med Ctr - West Islip, Southside Hosp (page 106); **Address:** 370 E Main St, Ste 1, Bay Shore, NY 11706; **Phone:** 631-666-4767; **Board Cert:** Neurology 1986; **Med School:** Univ Miami Sch Med 1980; **Resid:** Neurology, Jackson Meml Hosp 1984

Coyle, Patricia K MD (N) - **Spec Exp:** Multiple Sclerosis; Neuro-Immunology; Lyme Disease; Infections-Neurologic; **Hospital:** Stony Brook Univ Med Ctr; **Address:** Stony Brook Univ Med Ctr, 179 Belle Mead Rd, East Setauket, NY 11733; **Phone:** 631-444-2599; **Board Cert:** Neurology 2004; **Med School:** Johns Hopkins Univ 1974; **Resid:** Neurology, Johns Hopkins Hosp 1978; **Fellow:** Neurological Immunology, Johns Hopkins Hosp 1980; **Fac Appt:** Prof N, SUNY Stony Brook

Gerber, Oded MD (N) - **Spec Exp:** Stroke; Parkinson's Disease; Neuromuscular Disorders; **Hospital:** Stony Brook Univ Med Ctr; **Address:** Neurology Associates of Stony Brook, 179 N Belle Mead Rd, East Setauket, NY 11733; **Phone:** 631-444-2599; **Board Cert:** Neurology 1979; **Med School:** SUNY Downstate 1972; **Resid:** Internal Medicine, Kings County Hosp 1974; Neurology, Mt Sinai Hosp 1977; **Fac Appt:** Asst Clin Prof N, Mount Sinai Sch Med

Moreta, Henry G MD (N) - **Hospital:** Peconic Bay Med Ctr; **Address:** 877 E Main St, Ste 106, South Shore Neurologic Associates, P.C., Riverhead, NY 11901; **Phone:** 631-727-0660; **Board Cert:** Neurology 1987; **Med School:** Harvard Med Sch 1977; **Resid:** Neurology, New York Hosp 1981

Neuroradiology

Fiorella, David J MD (NRad) - **Spec Exp:** Stroke; Endovascular Surgery; Arteriovenous Malformations; Interventional Neuroradiology; **Hospital:** Stony Brook Univ Med Ctr; **Address:** Stony Brook University Medical Center, Dept of Neurological Surgery, HSC T12, rn 080, Stony Brook, NY 11794; **Phone:** 631-444-1213; **Board Cert:** Diagnostic Radiology 2001; Neuroradiology 2004; **Med School:** SUNY Buffalo 1986; **Resid:** Diagnostic Radiology, Duke Univ Med Ctr 2001; **Fellow:** Neurological Radiology, Barrow Neuro Inst 2004; **Fac Appt:** Prof NS, SUNY Stony Brook

Peyster, Robert MD (NRad) - **Hospital:** Stony Brook Univ Med Ctr; **Address:** Stony Brook Univ Med Ctr-Radiology, L4, Room 120, Nicolls Rd, Stony Brook, NY 11794-8460; **Phone:** 631-638-2121; **Board Cert:** Diagnostic Radiology ; Neuroradiology 2007; **Med School:** SUNY Downstate 1973; **Resid:** Diagnostic Radiology, Mass Genl Hosp 1977; **Fellow:** Neurological Radiology, Mass Genl Hosp 1979; **Fac Appt:** Prof Rad, SUNY Stony Brook

Obstetrics & Gynecology

Baker, David A MD (ObG) - **Spec Exp:** Infectious Disease; Premature Labor; Vulvar & Vaginal Disorders; Sexually Transmitted Diseases; **Hospital:** Stony Brook Univ Med Ctr; **Address:** University Assocs in Ob/Gyn, 6 Technology Drive, East Setauket, NY 11733-9254; **Phone:** 631-444-4686; **Board Cert:** Obstetrics & Gynecology 1979; Maternal & Fetal Medicine 1981; **Med School:** SUNY Hlth Sci Ctr 1973; **Resid:** Obstetrics & Gynecology, Hosp Univ Penn 1977; **Fellow:** Maternal & Fetal Medicine, Med Ctr Hosp 1979; **Fac Appt:** Prof ObG, SUNY Stony Brook

Berlin, Scott F MD (ObG) - **Hospital:** Southside Hosp (page 106); **Address:** 2330 Union Blvd, Islip, NY 11751; **Phone:** 631-224-4200; **Board Cert:** Obstetrics & Gynecology 2012; **Med School:** Univ Chicago-Pritzker Sch Med 1990; **Resid:** Obstetrics & Gynecology, Univ of Illinois Hosps 1994

Davenport, Deborah M MD (ObG) - **Spec Exp:** Menopause Problems; **Hospital:** Stony Brook Univ Med Ctr; **Address:** Three Village Women's Health Care, 100-16 S Jersey Ave, East Setauket, NY 11733-2036; **Phone:** 631-689-6400; **Board Cert:** Obstetrics & Gynecology 2009; **Med School:** Univ Pennsylvania 1975; **Resid:** Obstetrics & Gynecology, Univ Hosp 1983; **Fac Appt:** Asst Clin Prof ObG, SUNY Stony Brook

Droesch, James N MD (ObG) - **Spec Exp:** Gynecology Only; Menstrual Disorders; Endometriosis; Uterine Fibroids; **Hospital:** Stony Brook Univ Med Ctr; **Address:** University Assocs in OB/GYN, 6 Technology Drive, Ste 200, East Setauket, NY 11733-9254; **Phone:** 631-444-4686; **Board Cert:** Obstetrics & Gynecology 2012; **Med School:** SUNY Downstate 1982; **Resid:** Obstetrics & Gynecology, Long Island Jewish Med Ctr 1988; **Fac Appt:** Assoc Prof ObG, SUNY Stony Brook

Gentilesco, Michael MD (ObG) *PCP* - **Spec Exp:** Gynecology Only; **Hospital:** St. Catherine's of Siena Med Ctr, Stony Brook Univ Med Ctr; **Address:** 48 Route 25A, Ste 207, Smithtown, NY 11787; **Phone:** 631-862-3800; **Board Cert:** Obstetrics & Gynecology 2012; **Med School:** Albert Einstein Coll Med 1980; **Resid:** Obstetrics & Gynecology, NY Presby/Columbia Med Ctr 1984

Hirt, Paula Sue MD (ObG) - **Hospital:** Good Samaritan Hosp Med Ctr - West Islip; **Address:** 83 W Main St, East Islip, NY 11730; **Phone:** 631-277-5800; **Board Cert:** Obstetrics & Gynecology 1985; **Med School:** NYU Sch Med 1979; **Resid:** Obstetrics & Gynecology, NYU Med Ctr 1983

Kramer, Mitchell MD (ObG) - **Spec Exp:** Gynecologic Surgery-Complex; Menopause Problems; Minimally Invasive Surgery; Cervical Disease; **Hospital:** Huntington Hosp (page 106), N Shore Univ Hosp (page 106); **Address:** 180 E Pulaski Rd, Huntington Station, NY 11746; **Phone:** 631-425-2218; **Board Cert:** Obstetrics & Gynecology 2012; **Med School:** NY Med Coll 1985; **Resid:** Obstetrics & Gynecology, LI Jewish Med Ctr 1989; **Fac Appt:** Asst Clin Prof ObG, Hofstra N Shore-LIJ Sch Med

Lee, Douglas S MD (ObG) *PCP* - **Spec Exp:** Gynecology Only; Menopause Problems; Cervical Disease; **Hospital:** John T Mather Meml Hosp, St. Charles Hosp; **Address:** 118 N Country Road, Port Jefferson, NY 11777; **Phone:** 631-473-7171; **Board Cert:** Obstetrics & Gynecology 1979; **Med School:** NYU Sch Med 1973; **Resid:** Obstetrics & Gynecology, Bronx Municipal Hosp 1977; **Fac Appt:** Asst Clin Prof ObG, SUNY Stony Brook

Ott, Allen Edwin MD (ObG) - **Spec Exp:** Infertility; Colposcopy; Gynecology Only; **Hospital:** Southampton Hosp; **Address:** 595 Hampton Rd, Southampton, NY 11968-3021; **Phone:** 631-283-0918; **Board Cert:** Obstetrics & Gynecology 1979; **Med School:** Boston Univ 1972; **Resid:** Obstetrics & Gynecology, Hosp Univ Penn 1976

San Roman, Gerardo A MD (ObG) - **Spec Exp:** Minimally Invasive Surgery; Robotic Surgery; **Hospital:** St. Charles Hosp, John T Mather Meml Hosp; **Address:** Suffolk OB/GYN, 118 N Country Rd, Port Jefferson, NY 11777; **Phone:** 631-473-7171; **Board Cert:** Obstetrics & Gynecology 2012; **Med School:** Johns Hopkins Univ 1981; **Resid:** Obstetrics & Gynecology, NY Hosp 1985

Segarra, Pedro R MD (ObG) - **Spec Exp:** Pelvic Organ Prolapse Repair; Breast Disease; Gynecologic Surgery; Vaginal Reconstruction; **Hospital:** Southampton Hosp; **Address:** 595 Hampton Rd, Southampton, NY 11968; **Phone:** 631-283-0918; **Board Cert:** Obstetrics & Gynecology 2012; **Med School:** NY Med Coll 1983; **Resid:** Obstetrics & Gynecology, Lenox Hill Hosp 1987

Ophthalmology

Aries, Philip M MD (Oph) - **Spec Exp:** Diabetic Eye Disease; **Hospital:** Southside Hosp (page 106), Good Samaritan Hosp Med Ctr - West Islip; **Address:** Suffolk Ophthalmology Assocs, 375 E Main St, Ste 24, Bay Shore, NY 11706; **Phone:** 631-665-1330; **Board Cert:** Ophthalmology 1975; **Med School:** NY Med Coll 1967; **Resid:** Ophthalmology, Nassau Univ Med Ctr 1973

Cossari Jr, Alfred J MD (Oph) - **Spec Exp:** Pediatric Ophthalmology; Strabismus; **Hospital:** John T Mather Meml Hosp, St. Charles Hosp; **Address:** Village Eye Care, 311 Barnum Ave, Port Jefferson, NY 11777-1682; **Phone:** 631-928-6400; **Board Cert:** Ophthalmology 1976; **Med School:** Italy 1969; **Resid:** Ophthalmology, Nassau County Med Ctr 1974; **Fellow:** Retina, Johns Hopkins Hosp 1974; Pediatric Ophthalmology, Chldns Natl Med Ctr 1975

Di Leo, Frank MD (Oph) - **Spec Exp:** Oculoplastic Surgery; **Hospital:** Southampton Hosp, St. Luke's - Roosevelt Hosp Ctr - Roosevelt Div (page 94); **Address:** 365 County Road 39A, Ste 2, Southampton, NY 11968-5243; **Phone:** 631-283-3677; **Board Cert:** Ophthalmology 1987; **Med School:** Albert Einstein Coll Med 1981; **Resid:** Ophthalmology, St Luke's-Roosevelt Hosp Ctr 1985

El Baba, Fadi Z MD (Oph) - **Spec Exp:** Retina/Vitreous Surgery; Diabetic Eye Disease/Retinopathy; Macular Degeneration; HIV Retinitis; **Hospital:** Stony Brook Univ Med Ctr; **Address:** Stony Brook Ophthalmology, 33 Research Way, Ste 13, East Setauket, NY 11733; **Phone:** 631-444-4090; **Board Cert:** Ophthalmology 2013; **Med School:** Amer Univ Beirut 1982; **Resid:** Ophthalmology, Doheny Eye Inst/USC Med Ctr 1991; **Fellow:** Eye Pathology, Wilmer Eye Inst/Johns Hopkins 1986; Retina, Oregon Lions Sight & Hearing Inst 1987; **Fac Appt:** Assoc Clin Prof Oph, SUNY Stony Brook

Martin, Jeffrey Lawrence MD (Oph) - **Spec Exp:** Cataract Surgery; Laser Vision Surgery; **Hospital:** St. Catherine's of Siena Med Ctr, Stony Brook Univ Med Ctr; **Address:** 260 Middle Country Rd, Ste 201, Smithtown, NY 11787; **Phone:** 631-265-8780; **Board Cert:** Ophthalmology 2010; **Med School:** SUNY Stony Brook 1994; **Resid:** Ophthalmology, Nassau Co Med Ctr 1998; **Fac Appt:** Asst Clin Prof Oph, SUNY Stony Brook

Morris, Robert P MD (Oph) - **Spec Exp:** Cataract Surgery; Glaucoma; **Hospital:** St. Catherine's of Siena Med Ctr; **Address:** Morris & Romanelli, 222 E Main St, Ste 330, Smithtown, NY 11787; **Phone:** 631-724-4488; **Board Cert:** Ophthalmology 1974; **Med School:** SUNY Upstate Med Univ 1966; **Resid:** Ophthalmology, SUNY Downstate Med Ctr 1972

Nattis, Richard J MD (Oph) - **Spec Exp:** Cataract Surgery; Laser Vision Surgery; **Hospital:** Southside Hosp (page 106), Syosset Hosp (page 106); **Address:** Lindenhurst Eye Physicians & Surgeons, 500 W Main St, Ste 210, Babylon, NY 11702; **Phone:** 631-957-3355; **Board Cert:** Ophthalmology 1985; **Med School:** NY Med Coll 1980; **Resid:** Ophthalmology, St Vincent's Hosp 1984; **Fac Appt:** Asst Clin Prof Oph, NY Coll Osteo Med

O'Malley, Grace M MD (Oph) - **Spec Exp:** Cataract Surgery; **Hospital:** Southampton Hosp; **Address:** North Shore Eye Care & Hampton Eye, 186 Old Towne Rd, Southampton, NY 11968; **Phone:** 631-283-3533; **Board Cert:** Ophthalmology 1987; **Med School:** NY Med Coll 1981; **Resid:** Ophthalmology, NY Med Coll 1985

Pizzarello, Louis MD (Oph) - **Spec Exp:** Diabetic Eye Disease/Retinopathy; Oculoplastic Surgery; **Hospital:** Southampton Hosp, Eastern Long Island Hosp; **Address:** 137 Hampton Rd, Southampton, NY 11968; **Phone:** 631-283-5152; **Board Cert:** Ophthalmology 1980; **Med School:** Univ VA Sch Med 1975; **Resid:** Ophthalmology, Columbia-Presby Med Ctr 1979

Romanelli, John F MD (Oph) - **Spec Exp:** Cataract Surgery; Glaucoma; **Hospital:** St. Catherine's of Siena Med Ctr, Stony Brook Univ Med Ctr; **Address:** Morris & Romanelli, 222 E Main St, Ste 330, Smithtown, NY 11787-2814; **Phone:** 631-724-4488; **Board Cert:** Ophthalmology 2013; **Med School:** Harvard Med Sch 1987; **Resid:** Ophthalmology, Manhattan EET Hosp 1991

Rothberg, Charles MD (Oph) - **Spec Exp:** Cataract Surgery; Glaucoma; **Hospital:** Brookhaven Meml Hosp & Med Ctr; **Address:** 331 E Main St, Patchogue, NY 11772-3114; **Phone:** 631-758-5300; **Board Cert:** Ophthalmology 1989; **Med School:** SUNY Downstate 1983; **Resid:** Internal Medicine, Nassau Univ Med Ctr 1984; Ophthalmology, SUNY Downstate Med Ctr 1987

Schneck, Gideon L MD (Oph) - **Spec Exp:** Eyelid Cosmetic Surgery; Thyroid Eye Disease; Orbital Surgery; **Hospital:** Stony Brook Univ Med Ctr, St. Charles Hosp; **Address:** 2500 Nesconset Hwy, 17 B Bldg, Stony Brook, NY 11790; **Phone:** 631-246-9140; **Board Cert:** Ophthalmology 1991; **Med School:** Boston Univ 1986; **Resid:** Ophthalmology, Northwestern Univ Med Sch 1990; **Fellow:** Oculoplastic Surgery, IL Eye & Ear Infirmary 1991; **Fac Appt:** Asst Clin Prof Oph, SUNY Stony Brook

Sibony, Patrick A MD (Oph) - **Spec Exp:** Neuro-Ophthalmology; Orbital Diseases; **Hospital:** Stony Brook Univ Med Ctr; **Address:** Stony Brook Ophthalmology, 33 Research Way, Ste 13, East Setauket, NY 11733; **Phone:** 631-444-4090; **Board Cert:** Ophthalmology 1982; **Med School:** Boston Univ 1977; **Resid:** Ophthalmology, Boston Univ Med Ctr 1981; **Fellow:** Ophthalmology, Eye & Ear Hosp 1982; **Fac Appt:** Prof Oph, SUNY Stony Brook

Weber, Pamela A MD (Oph) - **Spec Exp:** Retinal Disorders; Macular Degeneration; Diabetic Eye Disease/Retinopathy; **Hospital:** Stony Brook Univ Med Ctr; **Address:** Island Retina, 1500 William Floyd Pkwy, Ste 304, Shirley, NY 11967; **Phone:** 631-924-4300; **Board Cert:** Ophthalmology 1989; **Med School:** Columbia P&S 1984; **Resid:** Ophthalmology, New York Eye & Ear Infirm 1988; **Fellow:** Vitreoretinal Surgery, Retina Assoc 1990; **Fac Appt:** Asst Prof Oph, SUNY Stony Brook

Zweibel, Lawrence C MD (Oph) - **Spec Exp:** LASIK-Refractive Surgery; Cataract Surgery; Glaucoma; **Hospital:** St. Catherine's of Siena Med Ctr; **Address:** North Shore Eye Care, 260 Middle Country Rd, Ste 201, Smithtown, NY 11787-2982; **Phone:** 631-265-8780; **Board Cert:** Ophthalmology 1977; **Med School:** Albany Med Coll 1972; **Resid:** Ophthalmology, French-Polyclinic Hosp 1976

Orthopaedic Surgery

Arvan, Glenn D MD (OrS) - **Spec Exp:** Trauma; Pediatric Orthopaedic Surgery; Joint Replacement; Geriatric Orthopaedic Surgery; **Hospital:** Good Samaritan Hosp Med Ctr - West Islip; **Address:** 400 W Main St, Ste 120, Babylon, NY 11702; **Phone:** 631-661-0202; **Board Cert:** Orthopaedic Surgery 1979; **Med School:** Duke Univ 1972; **Resid:** Orthopaedic Surgery, NY Hosp 1974; Orthopaedic Surgery, Case Western Res Med Ctr 1977

Dowling Jr, Thomas J MD (OrS) - **Spec Exp:** Spinal Surgery; Spinal Deformity; **Hospital:** St. Catherine's of Siena Med Ctr, Huntington Hosp (page 106); **Address:** 763 Larkfield Rd, Fl 2, Commack, NY 11725-2900; **Phone:** 631-462-2225; **Board Cert:** Orthopaedic Surgery 2011; **Med School:** Boston Univ 1981; **Resid:** Surgery, North Shore Univ Hosp 1983; Orthopaedic Surgery, SUNY Univ Hosp 1987; **Fellow:** Spine Surgery, North Shore Univ Hosp 1983; Spine Surgery, Univ Toronto 1988; **Fac Appt:** Asst Clin Prof OrS, Hofstra N Shore-LIJ Sch Med

Kottmeier, Stephen A MD (OrS) - **Spec Exp:** Trauma; Sports Injuries; **Hospital:** Stony Brook Univ Med Ctr; **Address:** Stony Brook Orthopaedic Associates, 14 Technology Drive, Ste 11, East Setauket, NY 11733; **Phone:** 631-444-4233; **Board Cert:** Orthopaedic Surgery 2013; **Med School:** SUNY Downstate 1984; **Resid:** Orthopaedic Surgery, SUNY Downstate Med Ctr 1989; **Fellow:** Sports Medicine, Penn State Hershey Med Ctr 1990; Orthopaedic Trauma Surgery, Southern NJ Regl Trauma Ctr 1991; **Fac Appt:** Prof OrS, SUNY Stony Brook

Lewis, Ronald MD (OrS) - **Spec Exp:** Pediatric Orthopaedic Surgery; Arthroscopic Surgery; Sports Medicine; Scoliosis; **Hospital:** Winthrop Univ Hosp (page 524), Huntington Hosp (page 106); **Address:** Pediatric Orthopaedics of LI, 205 E Main St, Ste 2-6, Huntington, NY 11743; **Phone:** 631-923-2370; **Board Cert:** Orthopaedic Surgery 2012; **Med School:** SUNY Stony Brook 1993; **Resid:** Surgery, Univ Hosp-SUNY Stony Brook 1994; Orthopaedic Surgery, Univ Hosp-SUNY Stony Brook 1998; **Fellow:** Pediatric Orthopaedic Surgery, Chldns Hosp Med Ctr 1999

Sampson, Steven MD (OrS) - **Spec Exp:** Hand & Wrist Surgery; Foot & Ankle Surgery; **Hospital:** Stony Brook Univ Med Ctr; **Address:** 14 Technology Drive, Ste 11, East Setauket, NY 11733-3464; **Phone:** 631-444-4233; **Board Cert:** Orthopaedic Surgery 2008; Hand Surgery 2008; **Med School:** UMDNJ-Rutgers Med Sch 1978; **Resid:** Orthopaedic Surgery, Hosp Univ Penn 1983; **Fellow:** Hand Surgery, St Luke's-Roosevelt Hosp 1984; **Fac Appt:** Assoc Prof OrS, SUNY Stony Brook

Tabershaw, Richard J MD (OrS) - **Spec Exp:** Shoulder Surgery; Sports Medicine; Arthroscopic Surgery; **Address:** Suffolk Orthopedic Assocs, 375 E Main St, Ste 1, Bay Shore, NY 11706-8418; **Phone:** 631-665-8790; **Board Cert:** Orthopaedic Surgery 2009; **Med School:** Georgetown Univ 1980; **Resid:** Surgery, St Vincent Med Ctr 1983; Orthopaedic Surgery, Columbia-Presby Hosp 1986

Otolaryngology

Gargano, Robert M MD (Oto) - **Spec Exp:** Ear Disorders/Surgery; Nasal Surgery; **Hospital:** Southside Hosp (page 106), Good Samaritan Hosp Med Ctr - West Islip; **Address:** 375 E Main St, Ste 17, Bay Shore, NY 11706; **Phone:** 631-665-2430; **Board Cert:** Otolaryngology 1989; **Med School:** Tufts Univ 1984; **Resid:** Otolaryngology, New England Med Ctr 1989

Lipinsky, Edward J MD (Oto) - **Spec Exp:** Head & Neck Surgery; **Hospital:** St. Catherine's of Siena Med Ctr; **Address:** 300 E Main St, 2nd Fl, Ste 1, Smithtown, NY 11787-2900; **Phone:** 631-265-3727; **Board Cert:** Otolaryngology 1976; **Med School:** NYU Sch Med 1972; **Resid:** Otolaryngology, Washington Hosp 1976

Litman, Richard S MD (Oto) - **Spec Exp:** Pediatric Otolaryngology; Head & Neck Surgery; Otology; Sinus Surgery; **Hospital:** John T Mather Meml Hosp, St. Charles Hosp; **Address:** ENT & Allergy Assocs, 251 E Oakland Ave, Port Jefferson, NY 11777; **Phone:** 631-928-0188; **Board Cert:** Otolaryngology 1976; **Med School:** Wake Forest Univ 1971; **Resid:** Surgery, LIJ Med Ctr 1973; Otolaryngology, Bronx Muni Hosp 1976; **Fac Appt:** Asst Clin Prof Oto, SUNY Stony Brook

Pain Medicine

Gargiulo, Juan J MD (PM) - **Spec Exp:** Pain-Chronic; Pain-Back; Pain-Cancer; **Hospital:** Southampton Hosp; **Address:** 365 County Rd 39A, Ste 15-16, Southampton, NY 11968; **Phone:** 631-702-2300; **Board Cert:** Anesthesiology 1993; Pain Medicine 2009; **Med School:** Uruguay 1984; **Resid:** Anesthesiology, Westchester Med Ctr 1991; Pain Medicine, Westchester Med Ctr 1991

Litman, Steven J MD (PM) - **Spec Exp:** Pain-Back & Neck; **Hospital:** Good Samaritan Hosp Med Ctr - West Islip, St. Charles Hosp; **Address:** All Island Pain Consultants, 387 E Main St, Ste 102, Bay Shore, NY 11706; **Phone:** 631-665-0075; **Board Cert:** Anesthesiology 2003; Pain Medicine 2007; **Med School:** NY Med Coll 1987; **Resid:** Anesthesiology, Westchester Co Med Ctr 1991

Vaillancourt, Philippe D MD (PM) - **Spec Exp:** Headache; Pain-Chronic; **Hospital:** Southampton Hosp, Peconic Bay Med Ctr; **Address:** 877 E Main St, Ste 106, Riverhead, NY 11901; **Phone:** 631-727-0660; **Board Cert:** Neurology 1986; Pain Medicine 2010; **Med School:** McGill Univ 1978; **Resid:** Neurology, Mount Sinai Med Ctr 1983

Pathology

Tornos, Carmen MD (Path) - **Spec Exp:** Gynecologic Cancer; Breast Cancer; Ovarian Cancer; **Hospital:** Stony Brook Univ Med Ctr; **Address:** Stony Brook Univ Hosp, Dept Pathology, 10 Nicolls Rd, HSC Level 2, rm 766, Stony Brook, NY 11794; **Phone:** 631-444-2222; **Board Cert:** Anatomic & Clinical Pathology 1989; **Med School:** Spain 1977; **Resid:** Hematology, Ciudad Sanitaria Valle de Hebron 1982; Anatomic & Clinical Pathology, Univ Texas HSC 1989; **Fellow:** Surgical Pathology, MD Anderson Cancer Ctr 1990; **Fac Appt:** Prof Path, SUNY Stony Brook

Pediatric Cardiology

Biancaniello, Thomas MD (PCd) - **Spec Exp:** Congenital Heart Disease; Fetal Echocardiography; Interventional Cardiology; Cardiac Catheterization; **Hospital:** Morgan Stanley Children's Hosp of NY-Presby, NY (page 104); **Address:** 57 Southern Blvd, Ste 3, Nesconset, NY 11767; **Phone:** 631-265-3300; **Board Cert:** Pediatrics 1979; Pediatric Cardiology 1981; **Med School:** NY Med Coll 1975; **Resid:** Pediatrics, North Shore Univ Hosp 1977; **Fellow:** Pediatric Cardiology, Cincinnati Chldns Hosp 1980; **Fac Appt:** Prof Ped, Columbia P&S

Pediatric Endocrinology

Wilson, Thomas A MD (PEn) - **Spec Exp:** Growth Disorders; Adrenal Disorders; Sexual Differentiation Disorders; Thyroid Disorders; **Hospital:** Stony Brook Univ Med Ctr; **Address:** Stony Brook Children's Service, 37 Research Way, E Setauket, NY 11733; **Phone:** 631-444-5437; **Board Cert:** Pediatrics 2009; **Med School:** Univ Pennsylvania 1973; **Resid:** Pediatrics, Chldns Hosp 1976; **Fellow:** Pediatric Endocrinology, Univ Virginia Med Ctr 1982; **Fac Appt:** Prof Ped, SUNY Stony Brook

Pediatric Gastroenterology

Chawla, Anupama MD (PGe) - **Spec Exp:** Gastroesophageal Reflux Disease (GERD); Crohn's Disease; Inflammatory Bowel Disease; **Hospital:** Stony Brook Univ Med Ctr; **Address:** Stony Brook Children Services, 4 Technology Drive, Ste 270, East Setauket, NY 11733; **Phone:** 631-444-5437; **Board Cert:** Pediatrics 2008; Pediatric Gastroenterology 2007; **Med School:** India 1980; **Resid:** Pediatrics, Stony Brook Med Ctr 1987; **Fellow:** Pediatric Gastroenterology, N Shore Univ Hosp 1987; **Fac Appt:** Assoc Clin Prof Ped, SUNY Stony Brook

Gold, David MD (PGe) - **Spec Exp:** Gastroesophageal Reflux Disease (GERD); Irritable Bowel Syndrome; Ulcerative Colitis/Crohn's; **Hospital:** Good Samaritan Hosp Med Ctr - West Islip; **Address:** 655 Deer Park Ave, Babylon, NY 11702; **Phone:** 631-321-2190; **Board Cert:** Pediatric Gastroenterology 2010; **Med School:** Albert Einstein Coll Med 1987; **Resid:** Pediatrics, LI Jewish Med Ctr 1990; **Fellow:** Pediatric Gastroenterology, LI Jewish Med Ctr 1993

Kessler, Bradley MD (PGe) - **Spec Exp:** Inflammatory Bowel Disease/Crohn's; Liver Disease; Malabsorption; **Hospital:** Good Samaritan Hosp Med Ctr - West Islip, Mercy Med Ctr - Rockville Centre; **Address:** 655 Deer Park Ave, Babylon, NY 11702; **Phone:** 631-321-2190; **Board Cert:** Pediatrics 1988; Pediatric Gastroenterology 2012; **Med School:** SUNY Downstate 1982; **Resid:** Pediatrics, N Shore Univ Hosp 1985; **Fellow:** Pediatric Gastroenterology, Baylor-Tex Chldns Hosp 1987; **Fac Appt:** Assoc Prof Ped, NY Coll Osteo Med

Pediatric Hematology-Oncology

Laver, Joseph H MD (PHO) - **Spec Exp:** Stem Cell Transplant; Lymphoma, Non-Hodgkin's; **Hospital:** Stony Brook Univ Med Ctr; **Address:** Stony Brook Univ Hosp, Health Sciences Tower, Level 4, Ste 205, Stony Brook, NY 11794-8410; **Phone:** 631-638-1000; **Board Cert:** Pediatrics 1985; Pediatric Hematology-Oncology 1987; **Med School:** Israel 1979; **Resid:** Pediatrics, Assaf Harofeh Med Ctr 1982; **Fellow:** Pediatric Hematology-Oncology, Meml Sloan Kettering Cancer Ctr 1985; **Fac Appt:** Prof Ped, SUNY Stony Brook

Parker, Robert I MD (PHO) - **Spec Exp:** Pediatric Cancers; Bleeding/Coagulation Disorders; Platelet Disorders; Lymphoma; **Hospital:** Stony Brook Univ Med Ctr; **Address:** Stony Brook Univ Med Ctr, Dept Pediatric Hematology-Oncology, 3 Edmund D Pellegrino Rd, Stony Brook, NY 11794-9448; **Phone:** 631-444-7720; **Board Cert:** Pediatrics 1983; Pediatric Hematology-Oncology 1984; **Med School:** Brown Univ 1976; **Resid:** Internal Medicine, Roger Williams Med Ctr 1977; Pediatrics, Rhode Island Hosp 1979; **Fellow:** Pediatric Hematology-Oncology, Natl Cancer Inst 1981; Hematology, Natl Cancer Inst 1984; **Fac Appt:** Prof Ped, SUNY Stony Brook

Pediatric Infectious Disease

Nachman, Sharon MD (PInf) - **Spec Exp:** Lyme Disease; AIDS/HIV; **Hospital:** Stony Brook Univ Med Ctr; **Address:** Stony Brook Children's Services, 37 Research Way, Stony Brook, NY 11794-3465; **Phone:** 631-444-7692; **Board Cert:** Pediatrics 1987; Pediatric Infectious Disease 2009; **Med School:** SUNY Stony Brook 1983; **Resid:** Pediatrics, Schneiders Chldns Hosp 1986; **Fellow:** Pediatric Infectious Disease, NY Med Coll 1987; **Fac Appt:** Prof Ped, SUNY Stony Brook

Pediatric Nephrology

Whyte, Dilys A MD (PNep) - **Spec Exp:** Kidney Disease; **Hospital:** Good Samaritan Hosp Med Ctr - West Islip; **Address:** 655 Deer Park Ave, Babylon, NY 11702; **Phone:** 631-321-2100; **Board Cert:** Pediatrics 2012; **Med School:** SUNY Buffalo 1991; **Resid:** Pediatrics, Kaleida Hlth Chldn Hosp 1994; **Fellow:** Pediatric Nephrology, Yale-New Haven Hosp 1998

Pediatric Pulmonology

Kier, Catherine E MD (PPul) - **Spec Exp:** Cystic Fibrosis; Sleep Medicine; **Hospital:** Stony Brook Univ Med Ctr; **Address:** Stony Brook Childrens Services, 8 Technology Drive, Ste 270, East Setauket, NY 11733; **Phone:** 631-444-5437; **Board Cert:** Pediatric Pulmonology 2008; **Med School:** Philippines 1990; **Resid:** Pediatrics, North Shore Univ Hosp 1995; **Fellow:** Pediatric Pulmonology, Chldns Hosp 2000; **Fac Appt:** Assoc Prof Ped, SUNY Stony Brook

Pediatric Surgery

Lee, Thomas Kang-Ming MD (PS) - **Spec Exp:** Hernia; Pediatric Cancers; Minimally Invasive Surgery; **Hospital:** Stony Brook Univ Med Ctr; **Address:** Stony Brook Univ Med Ctr, Surg Care Ctr, 37 Research Way, East Setauket, NY 11733; **Phone:** 631-444-4545; **Board Cert:** Surgery 2005; Pediatric Surgery 2007; **Med School:** Univ Chicago-Pritzker Sch Med 1988; **Resid:** Surgery, NY Hosp-Cornell Med Ctr 1995; **Fellow:** Surgery, Hosps Univ Pittsburgh 1992; Pediatric Surgery, Cardinal Glennon Chldns Hosp/St Louis Univ 1997; **Fac Appt:** Clin Prof S, SUNY Stony Brook

Scriven, Richard J MD (PS) - **Spec Exp:** Hernia; Minimally Invasive Surgery; Necrotizing Enterocolitis; Tumor Surgery; **Hospital:** Stony Brook Univ Med Ctr; **Address:** Stony Brook Univ Med Ctr, Surg Care Ctr, 37 Research Way, East Setauket, NY 11733; **Phone:** 631-444-4545; **Board Cert:** Surgery 1998; Pediatric Surgery 2000; **Med School:** Albert Einstein Coll Med 1990; **Resid:** Surgery, SUNY Hlth Sci Ctr 1997; **Fellow:** Pediatric Surgery, SUNY Hlth Sci Ctr 1999; **Fac Appt:** Assoc Prof S, SUNY Stony Brook

Pediatric Urology

Wasnick, Robert MD (Ped Uro) - **Spec Exp:** Undescended Testis; Hydronephrosis; Hypospadias; **Hospital:** Stony Brook Univ Med Ctr, St. Charles Hosp; **Address:** Stony Brook Urology, 24 Research Way, Ste 500, East Setauket, NY 11733; **Phone:** 631-444-1910; **Board Cert:** Urology 1982; Pediatric Urology 2008; **Med School:** Jefferson Med Coll 1974; **Resid:** Surgery, St Vincents Hosp Med Ctr 1977; Urology, Downstate Med Ctr 1980; **Fellow:** Pediatric Urology, Alder Hey Chldns Hosp 1981; **Fac Appt:** Clin Prof U, SUNY Stony Brook

Pediatrics

Bernstein, Harvey E MD (Ped) *PCP* - **Hospital:** St. Catherine's of Siena Med Ctr, Stony Brook Univ Med Ctr; **Address:** Smithtown Pediatric Grp, 260 Middle Country Rd, Ste 107, Smithtown, NY 11787; **Phone:** 631-979-7222; **Board Cert:** Pediatrics 2009; **Med School:** Univ Pennsylvania 1973; **Resid:** Pediatrics, Bronx Muni Hosp 1976; **Fac Appt:** Assoc Clin Prof Ped, SUNY Stony Brook

Chernobilsky, Lev MD (Ped) *PCP* - **Spec Exp:** Asthma; **Hospital:** Stony Brook Univ Med Ctr, St. Catherine's of Siena Med Ctr; **Address:** 269-D E Main St, Smithtown, NY 11787; **Phone:** 631-361-2121; **Board Cert:** Pediatrics 1987; **Med School:** Ukraine 1974; **Resid:** Pediatrics, Stony Brook Univ Med Ctr 1985; **Fac Appt:** Assoc Clin Prof Ped, SUNY Stony Brook

Cusumano, Barbara Jane MD (Ped) *PCP* - **Hospital:** Southampton Hosp; **Address:** 5 Squiretown Rd, MS 11946, Hampton Bays, NY 11946; **Phone:** 631-728-5300; **Board Cert:** Pediatrics 2009; **Med School:** Ros Franklin Univ/Chicago Med Sch 1984; **Resid:** Pediatrics, New York Hosp 1987

Festa, Robert S MD (Ped) *PCP* - **Hospital:** Stony Brook Univ Med Ctr, St. Charles Hosp; **Address:** Pediatric & Adolescent Medicine, 270 Union Ave, Holbrook, NY 11741; **Phone:** 631-588-4442 x5; **Board Cert:** Pediatrics 1978; Pediatric Hematology-Oncology 1980; **Med School:** SUNY Downstate 1972; **Resid:** Pediatrics, Montefiore Med Ctr 1975; **Fellow:** Pediatric Hematology-Oncology, Chldns Hosp 1978

Kaplan, Martin P MD (Ped) *PCP* - **Spec Exp:** Asthma; Developmental Disorders; ADD/ADHD; **Hospital:** Stony Brook Univ Med Ctr, St. Charles Hosp; **Address:** Port Jefferson Pediatrics, 12 Medical Drive, Port Jefferson Station, NY 11776-1588; **Phone:** 631-331-1710; **Board Cert:** Pediatrics 1977; **Med School:** NYU Sch Med 1972; **Resid:** Pediatrics, Bellevue Hosp 1974; Pediatrics, Duke Univ Med Ctr 1975; **Fac Appt:** Asst Clin Prof Ped, SUNY Stony Brook

Kolker, Harvey A MD (Ped) *PCP* - **Hospital:** St. Charles Hosp, Stony Brook Univ Med Ctr; **Address:** 111 Sylvan Ave, Miller Place, NY 11764-2420; **Phone:** 631-928-4888; **Board Cert:** Pediatrics 1971; **Med School:** SUNY Downstate 1966; **Resid:** Pediatrics, Madigan Army Med Ctr 1969; **Fac Appt:** Assoc Clin Prof Ped, SUNY Stony Brook

Kurfist, Lee A MD (Ped) *PCP* - **Spec Exp:** Adolescent Medicine; **Hospital:** Huntington Hosp (page 106); **Address:** 205 E Main St, Ste 2-8, Huntington, NY 11743; **Phone:** 631-424-1741; **Board Cert:** Pediatrics 2007; **Med School:** Italy 1985; **Resid:** Pediatrics, Nassau County Med Ctr 1988; **Fellow:** Pediatric Gastroenterology, Mt Sinai Hosp 1990

Manners, Richard E MD (Ped) *PCP* - **Hospital:** St. Charles Hosp, Stony Brook Univ Med Ctr; **Address:** Mid-Suffolk Pediatrics, 1770 Motor Pkwy, Islandia, NY 11749; **Phone:** 631-434-1770; **Board Cert:** Pediatrics 1980; **Med School:** Albert Einstein Coll Med 1975; **Resid:** Pediatrics, Univ Minn Med Ctr 1978

McMahon, Donna-Marie DO (Ped) *PCP* - **Hospital:** Good Samaritan Hosp Med Ctr - West Islip, Southside Hosp (page 106); **Address:** Family Health Care Center, 267 Carelton Ave, Central Islip, NY 11722; **Phone:** 631-348-3254; **Board Cert:** Pediatrics 2013; **Med School:** NY Coll Osteo Med 1987; **Resid:** Pediatrics, Winthrop Hosp 1990Chldn's Hosp 1991; **Fac Appt:** Asst Prof Ped, NY Coll Osteo Med

Parles, James G MD (Ped) *PCP* - **Hospital:** Stony Brook Univ Med Ctr, St. Catherine's of Siena Med Ctr; **Address:** Smithtown Pediatric Grp, 260 Middle Country Rd, Ste 107, Smithtown, NY 11787; **Phone:** 631-979-7222; **Board Cert:** Pediatrics 2009; **Med School:** NYU Sch Med 1985; **Resid:** Pediatrics, Mt Sinai Hosp 1988; **Fac Appt:** Asst Clin Prof Ped, SUNY Upstate Med Univ

Quinn, Joseph B MD (Ped) *PCP* - **Spec Exp:** ADD/ADHD; **Hospital:** Southampton Hosp; **Address:** Southampton Pediatric Assocs, 325 Meetinghouse Ln Bldg 2 - Ste J, Southampton, NY 11968; **Phone:** 631-283-7733; **Board Cert:** Pediatrics 1987; **Med School:** Univ VT Coll Med 1981; **Resid:** Pediatrics, NY Hosp 1984

Quinn, Leslie MD (Ped) *PCP* - **Spec Exp:** Child Abuse; Pneumonia; **Hospital:** Stony Brook Univ Med Ctr; **Address:** Stony Brook, Pediatrics, 4 Technology Drive, Ste 250, East Setauket, NY 11733; **Phone:** 631-444-5437; **Board Cert:** Pediatrics 2011; Child Abuse Pediatrics 2011; **Med School:** SUNY Downstate 1984; **Resid:** Pediatrics, NY-Presby/Weill Cornell Med Ctr 1987; **Fellow:** Child Abuse & Neglect, Bellevue Hosp 2011; **Fac Appt:** Assoc Prof Ped, SUNY Stony Brook

Sosulski, Richard MD (Ped) *PCP* - **Spec Exp:** Lung Disease in Newborns; Neonatal Critical Care; Neonatology; **Hospital:** Stony Brook Univ Med Ctr, St. Catherine's of Siena Med Ctr; **Address:** 269 E Main St, D Bldg, Smithtown, NY 11787-2807; **Phone:** 631-361-2121; **Board Cert:** Pediatrics 1982; Neonatal-Perinatal Medicine 1983; **Med School:** SUNY Downstate 1977; **Resid:** Pediatrics, LI Jewish Med Ctr 1980; **Fellow:** Neonatal-Perinatal Medicine, Chldns Hosp 1982; **Fac Appt:** Assoc Clin Prof Ped, SUNY Stony Brook

Physical Medicine & Rehabilitation

John, Sylvia T MD (PMR) - **Spec Exp:** Trauma Rehabilitation; Brain Injury Rehabilitation; **Hospital:** Southside Hosp (page 106); **Address:** 301 E Main St, Bay Shore, NY 11706; **Phone:** 631-232-0057; **Board Cert:** Pediatric Rehabilitation Medicine 2004; **Med School:** India 1990; **Resid:** Physical Medicine & Rehabilitation, LIJ Med Ctr 2003

Rosenberg, Craig H MD (PMR) - **Spec Exp:** Pain-Back & Neck; Spasticity Management; Electromyography; Acupuncture; **Hospital:** Southside Hosp (page 106), Stony Brook Univ Med Ctr; **Address:** 301 E Main St, Bay Shore, NY 11706; **Phone:** 631-675-4550; **Board Cert:** Physical Medicine & Rehabilitation 1987; **Med School:** Mexico 1981; **Resid:** Physical Medicine & Rehabilitation, NYU Med Ctr/Rusk Inst 1985; **Fac Appt:** Asst Prof PMR, Hofstra N Shore-LIJ Sch Med

Plastic Surgery

Anton, John R MD (PlS) - **Spec Exp:** Cosmetic Surgery-Face; Eyelid Surgery; Liposuction; **Hospital:** Southampton Hosp, Peconic Bay Med Ctr; **Address:** 138 Old Town Rd, Southampton, NY 11968-5011; **Phone:** 631-283-9100; **Board Cert:** Plastic Surgery 1992; **Med School:** Univ VT Coll Med 1981; **Resid:** Surgery, Mass Genl Hosp 1986; Plastic Surgery, Wayne State Univ Affil Hosp 1987; **Fellow:** Surgery, Mass Genl Hosp 1986; Plastic Surgery, Nassau Co Med Ctr 1988

Dagum, Alexander B MD (PlS) - **Spec Exp:** Reconstructive Plastic Surgery; Cleft Palate/Lip; Hand Surgery; Microsurgery; **Hospital:** Stony Brook Univ Med Ctr; **Address:** Plastic & Cosmetic Surgery Center, 24 Research Way, Ste 100, East Setauket, NY 11733; **Phone:** 631-444-4666; **Board Cert:** Plastic Surgery 2013; Hand Surgery 2012; **Med School:** Canada 1987; **Resid:** Surgery, Univ Ottawa Civic Hosp 1988; Plastic Surgery, Univ Toronto Med Ctr 1993; **Fellow:** Microsurgery, Univ Toronto Med Ctr 1984; Hand Surgery, Stony Brook Univ Hosp 1995; **Fac Appt:** Prof S, SUNY Stony Brook

Duboys, Elliot B MD (PlS) - **Spec Exp:** Cosmetic & Reconstructive Surgery; Pediatric Plastic Surgery; Cosmetic Surgery-Breast; Birth Defects; **Hospital:** Plainview Hosp (page 106), Stony Brook Univ Med Ctr; **Address:** Associated Plastic Surgeons/Consultants, 864 W Jericho Tpke, Huntington, NY 11743; **Phone:** 631-423-1000; **Board Cert:** Plastic Surgery 1985; **Med School:** Belgium 1977; **Resid:** Surgery, Stony Brook Univ Med Ctr 1982; Plastic Surgery, Nassau County Med Ctr 1984; **Fac Appt:** Assoc Prof PlS, SUNY Stony Brook

Marotta, James C MD (PlS) - **Spec Exp:** Facial Plastic & Reconstructive Surgery; Cosmetic Surgery-Face; **Hospital:** Stony Brook Univ Med Ctr, St. Catherine's of Siena Med Ctr; **Address:** 267 E Main St, Ste B5, Smithtown, NY 11787; **Phone:** 631-982-2022; **Board Cert:** Otolaryngology 2005; Facial Plastic & Reconstr Surgery 2008; **Med School:** SUNY Stony Brook 1999; **Resid:** Otolaryngology, Yale-New Haven Hosp 2004; **Fellow:** Facial Plastic & Reconstr Surgery, Quatela Ctr for Plastic Surg 2005; **Fac Appt:** Asst Clin Prof Oto, SUNY Stony Brook

Psychiatry

Aronson, Thomas MD (Psyc) - **Spec Exp:** Depression; Bipolar/Mood Disorders; Personality Disorders-Borderline; **Hospital:** St. Catherine's of Siena Med Ctr; **Address:** 2 Brooksite, Ste 220, Smithtown, NY 11787-3400; **Phone:** 631 265 0909; **Board Cert:** Psychiatry 1985, **Med School:** Washington Univ, St Louis 1980; **Resid:** Psychiatry, Hosp Univ Penn 1984; **Fac Appt:** Assoc Clin Prof Psyc, SUNY Stony Brook

Koreen, Amy R MD (Psyc) - ; **Address:** 28 Elm St, Huntington, NY 11743; **Phone:** 631-423-8368; **Board Cert:** Psychiatry 1993; **Med School:** Mount Sinai Sch Med 1988; **Resid:** Psychiatry, Univ Maryland Med Ctr 1991; Psychiatry, LI Jewish Med Ctr 1992; **Fellow:** Neuropsychopharmacology, LI Jewish Med Ctr 1993

Lee, Kwang Soo MD (Psyc) - ; **Address:** 221 Broadway, Ste 303, Amityville, NY 11701-2726; **Phone:** 631-789-7448; **Board Cert:** Psychiatry 1979; **Med School:** South Korea 1965; **Resid:** Internal Medicine, Booth Meml Hosp 1967; Psychiatry, Bellevue Hosp 1969; **Fellow:** Psychiatry, Amer Inst Psychoanalysis 1969

Nass, Jack MD (Psyc) - **Spec Exp:** Geriatric Rehabilitation; Bipolar/Mood Disorders; Depression; Neuro-Psychiatry; **Hospital:** Good Samaritan Hosp Med Ctr - West Islip; **Address:** 2100 Deer Park Ave, Ste 8, Deer Park, NY 11729; **Phone:** 631-321-7697; **Board Cert:** Psychiatry 1980; **Med School:** Belgium 1975; **Resid:** Psychiatry, LI Jewish Med Ctr 1979

Rosen, Bruce I MD (Psyc) - **Spec Exp:** Depression; Anxiety Disorders; Bipolar/Mood Disorders; Psychopharmacology; **Hospital:** St. Catherine's of Siena Med Ctr; **Address:** North Shore Psychiatric Consultants, 222 Middle Country Rd, Ste 210, Smithtown, NY 11787-2814; **Phone:** 631-265-6868; **Board Cert:** Psychiatry 1976; **Med School:** Loyola Univ-Stritch Sch Med 1971; **Resid:** Psychiatry, LI Jewish-Hillside Med Ctr 1974; **Fellow:** Psychiatry, LI Jewish-Hillside Med Ctr 1975; **Fac Appt:** Assoc Clin Prof Psyc, SUNY Stony Brook

Schwartz, Michael MD (Psyc) - **Spec Exp:** Forensic Psychiatry; Psychotherapy & Psychopharmacology; Mood Disorders; Anxiety Disorders; **Hospital:** Stony Brook Univ Med Ctr; **Address:** 150 Broadhollow Rd, Ste 204, Melville, NY 11747; **Phone:** 631-385-3313; **Board Cert:** Psychiatry 1984; **Med School:** Univ Miami Sch Med 1977; **Resid:** Internal Medicine, Mount Sinai Hosp 1978; Psychiatry, Mount Sinai Hosp 1981; **Fellow:** Research, Natl Inst Aging 1983; **Fac Appt:** Assoc Prof Psyc, SUNY Stony Brook

Pulmonary Disease

Baram, Daniel MD (Pul) - **Spec Exp:** Critical Care Medicine; Lung Cancer; **Hospital:** John T Mather Meml Hosp; **Address:** 70 North Country Rd, Ste 101, Port Jefferson, NY 11777; **Phone:** 631-473-0037; **Board Cert:** Internal Medicine 2004; Critical Care Medicine 2007; Pulmonary Disease 2008; **Med School:** Jefferson Med Coll 1990; **Resid:** Internal Medicine, New York Hosp 1993; **Fellow:** Critical Care Medicine, Natl Inst of Health 1996; Pulmonary Disease, NYU/Bellevue Hosps 1998

Bernardini, Dennis L MD (Pul) - **Spec Exp:** Chronic Obstructive Lung Disease (COPD); Asthma; Sarcoidosis; Pulmonary Fibrosis; **Hospital:** Huntington Hosp (page 106); **Address:** 175 E Main St, Huntington, NY 11743-2939; **Phone:** 631-424-3787; **Board Cert:** Internal Medicine 1983; Pulmonary Disease 1986; **Med School:** Johns Hopkins Univ 1980; **Resid:** Internal Medicine, St Luke's Hosp 1983; **Fellow:** Pulmonary Disease, Univ Hospital 1985; Critical Care Medicine, Univ Hospital 1985

Glaser, Morton L MD (Pul) - **Spec Exp:** Emphysema & Asthma; Interstitial Lung Disease; Lung Cancer; Pulmonary Hypertension; **Hospital:** St. Charles Hosp, John T Mather Meml Hosp; **Address:** 60 N Country Rd, Ste 203, Port Jefferson, NY 11777; **Phone:** 631-509-1888; **Board Cert:** Internal Medicine 1980; Pulmonary Disease 1984; Critical Care Medicine 2010; Undersea & Hyperbaric Medicine 2005; **Med School:** Med Coll Wisc 1976; **Resid:** Internal Medicine, Roger Williams Med Ctr 1979; **Fellow:** Pulmonary Disease, Univ Hosp 1981

Sklarek, Howard MD (Pul) - **Spec Exp:** Asthma; Cough; Chronic Obstructive Lung Disease (COPD); Interstitial Lung Disease; **Hospital:** Southampton Hosp; **Address:** Southampton Pulmonary Medicine, 325 Meeting House Ln Bldg 1 - Ste K, Southampton, NY 11968; **Phone:** 631-283-8008; **Board Cert:** Internal Medicine 1984; Pulmonary Disease 1986; Critical Care Medicine 2010; Hospice & Palliative Medicine 2012; **Med School:** SUNY Buffalo 1981; **Resid:** Internal Medicine, Winthrop Univ Hosp 1984; **Fellow:** Pulmonary Critical Care Medicine, Winthrop Univ Hosp 1986

Walser, Lawrence A MD (Pul) - **Hospital:** Peconic Bay Med Ctr; **Address:** 185 Old Country Rd, Ste 3, Riverhead, NY 11901; **Phone:** 631-727-2523; **Board Cert:** Internal Medicine 1982; Pulmonary Disease 2007; Critical Care Medicine 2007; **Med School:** SUNY Downstate 1979; **Resid:** Internal Medicine, Berkshire Med Ctr 1982; **Fellow:** Pulmonary Disease, SUNY/Univ Hosp 1984

Wohlberg, Gary MD (Pul) - **Spec Exp:** Critical Care Medicine; Sleep Disorders/Apnea; **Hospital:** Southside Hosp (page 106), Good Samaritan Hosp Med Ctr - West Islip; **Address:** 370 E Main St, Ste 5 Bldg, Bay Shore, NY 11706-8405; **Phone:** 631-666-5864; **Board Cert:** Internal Medicine 1985; Pulmonary Disease 1986; Critical Care Medicine 2010; Sleep Medicine 2007; **Med School:** SUNY Hlth Sci Ctr 1981; **Resid:** Internal Medicine, Long Island Jewish Hosp 1984; **Fellow:** Pulmonary Disease, Montefiore Hosp Med Ctr 1986

Radiation Oncology

Park, Tae L MD (RadRO) - **Spec Exp:** Prostate Cancer; Breast Cancer; Gynecologic Cancer; **Hospital:** Stony Brook Univ Med Ctr; **Address:** Stony Brook Univ Med Ctr-Rad Oncology, 100 Nicolls Rd, Level 2, rm 643, Stony Brook, NY 11794-7028; **Phone:** 631-444-2210; **Board Cert:** Therapeutic Radiology 1984; **Med School:** South Korea 1976; **Resid:** Radiation Oncology, Kings Co Downstate Med Ctr. 1984; **Fellow:** Radiation Oncology, MD Anderson Cancer Ctr 1985; **Fac Appt:** Assoc Clin Prof RadRO, SUNY Stony Brook

Pollack, Jed MD (RadRO) - **Spec Exp:** Head & Neck Cancer; Prostate Cancer; Brain Tumors; **Hospital:** Southside Hosp (page 106); **Address:** Southside Hosp Radiation Oncology, 301 E Main St, Bayshore, NY 11706; **Phone:** 718-470-7190; **Board Cert:** Therapeutic Radiology 1985; **Med School:** Univ New Mexico 1981; **Resid:** Therapeutic Radiology, Meml Sloan-Kettering Cancer Ctr 1985; **Fac Appt:** Asst Clin Prof

Reproductive Endocrinology

Bronson, Richard A MD (RE) - **Spec Exp:** Infertility-IVF; Pregnancy Loss-Recurrent; Reproductive Immunology; **Hospital:** Stony Brook Univ Med Ctr; **Address:** Reproductive Specialists of New York, 2500 Nesconset Highway, Bldg 23, Stony Brook, NY 11790; **Phone:** 631-246-9100; **Board Cert:** Obstetrics & Gynecology 1976; Reproductive Endocrinology 1980; **Med School:** NYU Sch Med 1966; **Resid:** Surgery, NYU Med Ctr 1971; Obstetrics & Gynecology, Hosp Univ Penn 1974; **Fellow:** Reproductive Endocrinology, Pennsylvania Hosp 1976; **Fac Appt:** Prof ObG, SUNY Stony Brook

Kenigsberg, Daniel J MD (RE) - **Spec Exp:** Infertility-IVF; Uterine Fibroids; Endometriosis; Reproductive Surgery; **Hospital:** John T Mather Meml Hosp, Stony Brook Univ Med Ctr; **Address:** Long Island IVF, 8 Corporate Center Drive, Melville, NY 11747; **Phone:** 631-752-0606; **Board Cert:** Obstetrics & Gynecology 1995; Reproductive Endocrinology 1995; **Med School:** NY Med Coll 1978; **Resid:** Obstetrics & Gynecology, Johns Hopkins Hosp 1982; **Fellow:** Reproductive Endocrinology, Natl Inst Hlth 1984; **Fac Appt:** Assoc Clin Prof ObG, SUNY Stony Brook

Lydic, Michael L MD (RE) - **Spec Exp:** Polycystic Ovarian Syndrome; Pregnancy Loss-Recurrent; Infertility; Infertility-IVF; **Hospital:** Stony Brook Univ Med Ctr; **Address:** Reproductive Specialists of NY, 2500 Nesconset Hwy Bldg 23, Stony Brook, NY 11790; **Phone:** 631-246-9100; **Board Cert:** Obstetrics & Gynecology 2012; Reproductive Endocrinology 2012; **Med School:** Hahnemann Univ 1989; **Resid:** Obstetrics & Gynecology, Hahnemann Univ Hosp 1993; **Fellow:** Reproductive Endocrinology, Univ of Cincinnati 1995; **Fac Appt:** Assoc Clin Prof ObG, SUNY Stony Brook

Rheumatology

Hamburger, Max Ira MD (Rhu) - **Spec Exp:** Rheumatoid Arthritis; Gout; Vasculitis; **Hospital:** St. Charles Hosp, John T Mather Meml Hosp; **Address:** 1895 Walt Whitman Rd, Rheumatology Associates of Long Island, Melville, NY 11747; **Phone:** 631-249-9525; **Board Cert:** Internal Medicine 1977; Rheumatology 1980; **Med School:** Albert Einstein Coll Med 1973; **Resid:** Internal Medicine, Bellevue Hosp 1976; **Fellow:** Allergy & Immunology, Nat Inst Health 1979; **Fac Appt:** Asst Clin Prof Med, SUNY Stony Brook

Repice, Michael MD (Rhu) - **Spec Exp:** Arthritis; Connective Tissue Disorders; **Hospital:** Huntington Hosp (page 106); **Address:** 5 E Main St, Huntington, NY 11743-2812; **Phone:** 631-271-1640; **Board Cert:** Internal Medicine 1976; Rheumatology 1980; **Med School:** Georgetown Univ 1973; **Resid:** Internal Medicine, Worcester City Hosp 1977; **Fellow:** Rheumatology, Northwestern Univ 1979

Sports Medicine

Putterman, Eric A MD (SM) - **Spec Exp:** Arthroscopic Surgery; **Hospital:** Glen Cove Hosp (page 106); **Address:** Premier Ortho Surgery/Sports Medicine, 1800 Walt Whitman Rd, Ste 120, Melville, NY 11747; **Phone:** 631-293-9540; **Board Cert:** Orthopaedic Surgery 2009; **Med School:** Mount Sinai Sch Med 1980; **Resid:** Orthopaedic Surgery, NYU-Bellevue Med Ctr 1985; **Fellow:** Sports Medicine, NYU-Bellevue Med Ctr 1985

Surgery

Busch-Devereaux, Erna MD (S) - **Spec Exp:** Breast Cancer; Breast Surgery; **Hospital:** Huntington Hosp (page 106), N Shore Univ Hosp (page 106); **Address:** 270 Pulaski Rd, Ste A, Greenlawn, NY 11740; **Phone:** 631-423-1414; **Board Cert:** Surgery 2010; **Med School:** UMDNJ-NJ Med Sch, Newark 1985; **Resid:** Surgery, St Vincent Cath Med Ctr 1990; **Fellow:** Surgical Oncology, Roswell Park Canc Inst 1993; **Fac Appt:** Asst Prof S, NYU Sch Med

Cohen, Bradley D MD (S) - **Spec Exp:** Breast Cancer; Laparoscopic Surgery; Sentinel Node Surgery; Melanoma; **Hospital:** Good Samaritan Hosp Med Ctr - West Islip, Southside Hosp (page 106); **Address:** 15 Park Ave, Bay Shore, NY 11706; **Phone:** 631-581-4400; **Board Cert:** Surgery 2009; **Med School:** Mount Sinai Sch Med 1983; **Resid:** Surgery, Lenox Hill Hosp 1988; **Fellow:** Surgical Oncology, Meml Sloan Kettering Cancer Ctr 1989

Cosgrove, John M MD (S) - **Spec Exp:** Laparoscopic Surgery; Endoscopy; Biliary Surgery; Gastrointestinal Surgery; **Hospital:** Eastern Long Island Hosp; **Address:** 201 Manor Place, Greenport, NY 11944; **Phone:** 631-477-5386; **Board Cert:** Surgery 2008; **Med School:** NY Med Coll 1983; **Resid:** Surgery, Beth Israel Med Ctr 1988

Francfort, John MD (S) - **Spec Exp:** Breast Surgery; Gastrointestinal Surgery; Vascular Surgery; Laparoscopic Surgery; **Hospital:** Good Samaritan Hosp Med Ctr - West Islip, Southside Hosp (page 106); **Address:** 580 Union Blvd, West Islip, NY 11795-3105; **Phone:** 631-321-6801; **Board Cert:** Surgery 2005; Vascular Surgery 2006; **Med School:** UMDNJ-NJ Med Sch, Newark 1980; **Resid:** Surgery, Hosp Univ Penn 1986; **Fellow:** Vascular Surgery, Northwesten Univ 1987; **Fac Appt:** Asst Clin Prof S, SUNY Stony Brook

Klausner, Stanley K MD (S) - **Spec Exp:** Breast Surgery; Breast Cancer; **Hospital:** Brookhaven Meml Hosp & Med Ctr; **Address:** 100 Hospital Rd, Ste 106, Patchogue, NY 11772; **Phone:** 631-475-8846; **Board Cert:** Surgery 1975; **Med School:** NYU Sch Med 1967; **Resid:** Surgery, Bronx Muni Hosp 1973

O'Hea, Brian J MD (S) - **Spec Exp:** Breast Cancer; Sentinel Node Surgery; **Hospital:** Stony Brook Univ Med Ctr; **Address:** Stony Brook Univ Med Ctr, Breast Cancer Ctr, 3 Edmund D Pellegrino Rd, Stony Brook, NY 11794; **Phone:** 631-444-1795; **Board Cert:** Surgery 2012; **Med School:** Georgetown Univ 1986; **Resid:** Surgery, St Vincent's Hosp 1991; **Fellow:** Breast Disease, Meml Sloan-Kettering Cancer Ctr 1996; **Fac Appt:** Asst Prof S, SUNY Stony Brook

Pryor, Aurora D MD (S) - **Spec Exp:** Laparoscopic Surgery-Advanced; Obesity/Bariatric Surgery; Gastroesophageal Reflux Disease (GERD); Achalasia; **Hospital:** Stony Brook Univ Med Ctr; **Address:** Stony Brook Univ Med Ctr, Surg Care Ctr, 37 Research Way, East Setauket, NY 11733-3465; **Phone:** 631-444-4545; **Board Cert:** Surgery 2012; **Med School:** Duke Univ 1995; **Resid:** Surgery, Duke Univ Med Ctr 2002; **Fellow:** Laparoscopic Surgery, Duke Univ 2003; **Fac Appt:** Prof S, SUNY Stony Brook

Sclafani, Lisa M MD (S) - **Spec Exp:** Breast Surgery; Breast Cancer; **Hospital:** Meml Sloan-Kettering Canc Ctr (page 114); **Address:** Meml Sloan-Kettering Canc Ctr - Commack, 650 Commack Rd, Commack, NY 11725; **Phone:** 631-623-4050; **Board Cert:** Surgery 2007; **Med School:** NYU Sch Med 1982; **Resid:** Surgery, Montefiore Med Ctr-Moses Campus 1987; **Fellow:** Surgical Oncology, Meml Sloan Kettering Canc Ctr 1988; **Fac Appt:** Assoc Clin Prof S, Cornell Univ-Weill Med Coll

Shapiro, Marc MD (S) - **Spec Exp:** Laparoscopic Surgery; Gastrointestinal Surgery; Burn Care; Trauma; **Hospital:** Stony Brook Univ Med Ctr; **Address:** Stony Brook Univ Med Ctr, Surg Care Ctr, 37 Research Way, East Setauket, NY 11733; **Phone:** 631-444-4545; **Board Cert:** Surgery 2004; Surgical Critical Care 2005; **Med School:** Univ Mich Med Sch 1979; **Resid:** Surgery, Henry Ford Hosp 1984; **Fellow:** Critical Care Medicine, Univ Pittsburgh Hosp 1985; **Fac Appt:** Prof S, SUNY Stony Brook

Watkins, Kevin T MD (S) - **Spec Exp:** Pancreatic Cancer; Minimally Invasive Surgery; Gastrointestinal Cancer; Esophageal Cancer; **Hospital:** Stony Brook Univ Med Ctr; **Address:** Stony Brook, Surgl Onc Dept, 3 Edmund D Pellegrino Rd, Stony Brook, NY 11794; **Phone:** 631-444-8086; **Board Cert:** Surgery 2005; **Med School:** Univ VA Sch Med 1990; **Resid:** Surgery, Shands at Univ FL 1996; **Fellow:** Surgical Oncology, MD Anderson Cancer Ctr 1998; **Fac Appt:** Assoc Prof S, SUNY Stony Brook

Zingale, Robert MD (S) - **Hospital:** Huntington Hosp (page 106); **Address:** 158 E Main St, Ste 7, Huntington, NY 11743-2988; **Phone:** 631-271-1822; **Board Cert:** Surgery 2007; Surgical Critical Care 2010; **Med School:** SUNY Downstate 1983; **Resid:** Surgery, Maimonides Med Ctr 1988; **Fellow:** Trauma, Coney Is Hosp 1989; **Fac Appt:** Assoc Clin Prof S, NY Med Coll

Thoracic & Cardiac Surgery

Bilfinger, Thomas MD (T&CS) - **Spec Exp:** Cardiac Surgery-Adult; Lung Cancer; **Hospital:** Stony Brook Univ Med Ctr; **Address:** Health Science Center T-19 Rm80, 3 Edmund D Pellegrino Rd, Stony Brook, NY 11794; **Phone:** 631-444-1820; **Board Cert:** Surgery 2006; Thoracic & Cardiac Surgery 2008; Surgical Critical Care 2010; **Med School:** Switzerland 1978; **Resid:** Surgery, Univ Chicago 1982; Surgery, Univ TX Med Branch Hosp 1986; **Fellow:** Thoracic Surgery, Univ TX Med Branch Hosp 1988; **Fac Appt:** Prof T&CS, SUNY Stony Brook

Hartman, Alan R MD (T&CS) - **Spec Exp:** Minimally Invasive Heart Valve Surgery; Aneurysm-Thoracic Aortic; **Hospital:** N Shore Univ Hosp (page 106), Southside Hosp (page 106); **Address:** Southside Hosp - Cardiothoracic Surgery, 301 E Main St, 2 North, Bay Shore, NY 11706; **Phone:** 631-968-3525; **Board Cert:** Surgery 2004; Thoracic Surgery 2005; Surgical Critical Care 2010; **Med School:** Mount Sinai Sch Med 1979; **Resid:** Surgery, Bellevue Hosp/NYU Langone Med Ctr 1984; **Fellow:** Cardiothoracic Surgery, Bellevue Hosp/NYU Langone Med Ctr 1986; **Fac Appt:** Assoc Prof S, NYU Sch Med

Palatt, Terry MD (T&CS) - **Spec Exp:** Lung Cancer; Video Assisted Thoracic Surgery (VATS); **Hospital:** Good Samaritan Hosp Med Ctr - West Islip, Southside Hosp (page 106); **Address:** Is Surgical & Vascular Grp, 15 Park Ave, Bay Shore, NY 11706; **Phone:** 631-581-4400; **Board Cert:** Thoracic Surgery 2008; **Med School:** Grenada 1981; **Resid:** Surgery, Maimonides Med Ctr 1987; Thoracic Surgery, SUNY Downstate Med Ctr 1989

Taylor Jr, James R MD (T&CS) - **Spec Exp:** Thoracic Aortic Surgery; Aneurysm-Aortic; **Hospital:** Stony Brook Univ Med Ctr; **Address:** Stony Brook Univ Med Ctr, Dept Cardiothoracic Surgery, 12 Nicolls Rd, 12 N, rm 046, Stony Brook, NY 11794-8191; **Phone:** 631-444-1820; **Board Cert:** Surgery 2008; Thoracic & Cardiac Surgery 2013; **Med School:** Med Univ SC 1984; **Resid:** Surgery, NY Hosp-Cornell Med Ctr 1989; **Fellow:** Cardiothoracic Surgery, NY Hosp-Cornell Med Ctr 1991; **Fac Appt:** Prof T&CS, SUNY Stony Brook

Urology

Beccia, David J MD (U) - **Spec Exp:** Prostate Cancer; Erectile Dysfunction; **Hospital:** Southside Hosp (page 106), Good Samaritan Hosp Med Ctr - West Islip; **Address:** Suffolk Urology, 332 E Main St, Bay Shore, NY 11706-8404; **Phone:** 631-665-3737; **Board Cert:** Urology 1979; **Med School:** NY Med Coll 1970; **Resid:** Surgery, Hartford Hosp 1973; Urology, Boston Med Ctr 1977

Mills II, Carl MD (U) - **Spec Exp:** Urologic Cancer; **Hospital:** Brookhaven Meml Hosp & Med Ctr, St. Charles Hosp; **Address:** 635 Belle Terre Rd, Ste 201, Port Jefferson, NY 11777; **Phone:** 631-509-4802; **Board Cert:** Urology 1984; **Med School:** Geo Wash Univ 1975; **Resid:** Surgery, New York Hosp 1978; Urology, Meml Sloan-Kettering Canc Ctr 1982

Vascular Surgery

Arnold, Thomas E MD (VascS) - **Spec Exp:** Carotid Artery Surgery; Aneurysm-Abdominal Aortic; Varicose Veins; Dialysis Access Surgery; **Hospital:** John T Mather Meml Hosp, St. Charles Hosp; **Address:** 1110 Hallock Ave, Port Jefferson Station, NY 11776; **Phone:** 631-476-9100; **Board Cert:** Surgery 2003; Vascular Surgery 2003; **Med School:** SUNY Downstate 1985; **Resid:** Surgery, Presbyterian Med Ctr/Univ Penn 1987; Surgery, Medical Coll Penn Affil Hosp 1991; **Fellow:** Vascular Surgery, Hahnemann Univ Hosp 1993

Pollina, Robert M MD (VascS) - **Spec Exp:** Varicose Veins; Aneurysm; Carotid Artery Surgery; Dialysis Access Surgery; **Hospital:** John T Mather Meml Hosp, St. Charles Hosp; **Address:** 1110 Hallock Ave, Port Jefferson Station, NY 11776; **Phone:** 631-476-9100; **Board Cert:** Vascular Surgery 2007; **Med School:** SUNY Hlth Sci Ctr 1988; **Resid:** Surgery, Kings Co Hosp Ctr 1993; **Fellow:** Vascular Surgery, Maimonides Med Ctr 1995

Tassiopoulos, Apostolos K MD (VascS) - **Spec Exp:** Vein Disorders; **Hospital:** Stony Brook Univ Med Ctr; **Address:** Stony Brook Univ Med Ctr, Surg Care Ctr, 37 Research Way, East Setauket, NY 11733; **Phone:** 631-444-4545; **Board Cert:** Surgery 2010; Vascular Surgery 2012; **Med School:** Greece 1989; **Resid:** Surgery, SUNY Upstate Med Ctr 1999; Vascular Surgery, Loyola Univ Med Ctr 2001; **Fac Appt:** Assoc Prof S, SUNY Stony Brook

Westchester

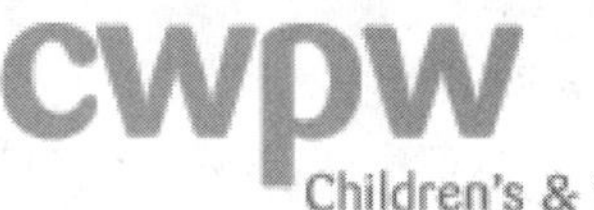

Children's & Women's
Physicians of Westchester, LLP

19 Bradhurst Avenue, Suite 1400, Hawthorne, NY 10532
Tel: 914-593-8838 www.cwpw.org

GENERAL OVERVIEW

Children's & Women's Physicians of Westchester, LLP (CWPW) is one of the largest physician medical and surgical practices in the Tri-State area, providing a wide-reaching system of primary-care and specialty-care services in both the in-patient and out-patient settings. CWPW is committed to providing comprehensive in-patient and out-patient care to infants, children, adolescents and selected adults throughout the greater New York Metropolitan area, extending from New York City, throughout the Hudson Valley, and into parts of Connecticut. CWPW physicians are world leaders in the diagnosis and treatment of complex illnesses and 41 of our doctors were selected as *Top Doctors* by Castle Connolly.

ACADEMIC AND CLINICAL AFFLIATIONS

CWPW consists of more than 275 practicing physicians who are also faculty at New York Medical College in Valhalla, New York. CWPW pediatricians are also teachers and researchers with access to the most advanced diagnostic and therapeutic approaches and the latest technology in the field of pediatric and adult medicine. CWPW attending physicians are core faculty at the following medical centers: Maria Fareri Children's Hospital at Westchester Medical Center and Good Samaritan Hospital. CWPW physicians are also on staff at Vassar Brothers Medical Center, Phelps Memorial Hospital, Hudson Valley Hospital, Northern Westchester Hospital, Orange Regional Medical Center, St. John's Riverside Hospital, St. Vincent's Hospital Westchester, St. Luke's Hospital, Putnam Hospital, Wyckoff Heights Medical Center, Norwalk Hospital, Stamford Hospital and Danbury Hospital. In addition to their academic and clinical affiliations, our physicians also provide an array of primary and specialty-care services in out-patient settings throughout the region.

MEDICAL SPECIALTIES

CWPW physicians are well recognized and renowned in the pediatric medical specialties of: Adolescent and Pediatric Gynecology, Adolescent Medicine, Cardiology, Cardiothoracic Surgery, Critical Care, Developmental Pediatrics, Endocrinology, Gastroenterology, General Pediatrics, Hematology/Oncology/Bone Marrow Transplant, Infectious Disease & Immunology, Medical Genetics, Neonatology, Nephrology, Neurology, Pediatric Surgery, Psychology, Pulmonology, Allergy & Sleep Medicine, Rheumatology and The Medical Home. CWPW physicians are also well recognized in the adult medical specialties of: Gastroenterology, Nephrology and Obstetrics/Gynecology. CWPW doctors are also leading researchers in all of these disciplines.

PIONEERING, COMPREHENSIVE CARE

CWPW's dedicated and skilled physicians care for low and high risk newborns, as well as mildly to seriously ill children, with a broad range of medical conditions. Our pediatricians and health care professionals make parents feel comfortable when asking about their children's medical problems and treatment options.

CWPW pediatric cardiologists are teaming up with interventional cardiologists to perform 'hybrid' procedures in complex cardiac cases in children. The cardiologists treat cardiac disorders less invasively, but still with outstanding results.

CWPW pediatric oncologists are making new discoveries on how the immune system can be strengthened to counteract neuroblastoma. Their work has helped to develop a procedure where antibodies adhere to the surface of cancer cells, enabling the immune system to target the disease, and eliminate it.

CWPW's Children's Environmental Health Center at Children's is one of only eight such centers in New York State, which treats and studies environmental hazards in the home and in the community.

The goal and philosophy of Children's and Women's Physicians of Westchester is to provide the highest quality medical care in a range of specialties for infants, children and adults every day.

Physician Referral -For a physician referral or more information please contact Children's and Women's Physicians of Westchester 914-593- 8838 or visit www.cwpw.org

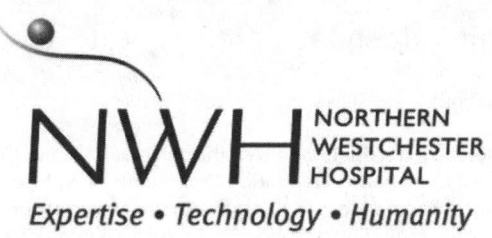

Northern Westchester Hospital (NWH) provides quality, patient centered care that is close to home through the right combination of medical expertise, leading edge technology, and a commitment to humanity. Over 750 highly skilled physicians, state-of-the-art technology and professional staff of caregivers are all in place to ensure that you and your family receive treatment in a caring, respectful and nurturing environment.

NWH has established extensive internal quality measurements that surpass the standards defined by the Centers for Medicare & Medicaid Services (CMS) and the Hospital Quality Alliance (HQA) National Hospital Quality Measures. Our high quality standards help to ensure that the treatment you receive at NWH is among the best in the nation. For a complete list of our services, please visit www.nwhc.net.

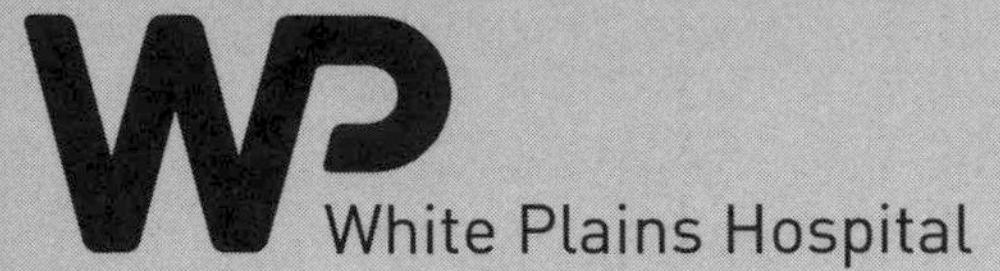

41 East Post Road
White Plains, NY 10601
Tel: (914) 681-0600
www.wphospital.org

Sponsorship: Private, Not-for-Profit
Beds: 292
Accreditation: Joint Commission on Accreditation of Healthcare Organizations, Commission on Cancer of the American College of Surgeons, National Accreditation Program for Breast Centers, College of American Pathologists, American Registry of Radiological Technology, American Society of Radiological Technology, Intersocietal Commission for the Accreditation of Echocardiography Laboratories, American Institute of Ultrasound Medicine, American Academy of Sleep Medicine.

A LEADING COMMUNITY HOSPITAL White Plains Hospital (WPH) is a 292-bed facility that has served Westchester County and the surrounding area since 1893. The Hospital offers much of the technology of large urban specialty teaching hospitals, and combines it with compassionate and personalized care close to home. In addition to a wide range of general acute care services, WPH offers highly sophisticated specialty programs in Oncology, Orthopedics & Joint Replacement, Obstetrics, Neonatal Intensive Care, Radiology, Minimally Invasive & Robotic Surgery, Cardiology, and Stroke Care. An enhanced Emergency Department opened in 2010 and a state-of-the-art Cardiac Catheterization Lab opened in 2008.

The Hospital is an eleven-time winner of the Consumer Choice Award for Westchester County, and the Hospital received Magnet® recognition from the American Nurses Credentialing Center (ANCC) in 2012. WPH is a member of the NewYork-Presbyterian Healthcare System.

CENTERS OF EXCELLENCE

- WILLIAM & SYLVIA SILBERSTEIN NEONATAL & MATERNITY CENTER A Labor & Delivery unit, backed up by a state-of-the-art Level III Neonatal Intensive Care Unit – the highest designation available to a community hospital – is part of the reason why WPH leads Westchester County in number of deliveries, year after year.

- DICKSTEIN CANCER TREATMENT CENTER Part of the Hospital's comprehensive Cancer Program, the Dickstein Center anchors a wide range of services including two linear accelerators for radiation therapy, a state of the art infusion center for chemotherapy and other intravenous treatments, and complementary care programs. Clinical navigation services provide a personal guide for patients at each stage of diagnosis, treatment and follow up care. The Cancer Program has repeatedly received an Outstanding Achievement Award from the American College of Surgeons Commission on Cancer and was recognized by the National Accreditation Program for Breast Centers (NAPBC) in 2012.

- MINIMALLY INVASIVE & ROBOTIC SURGERY White Plains Hospital's surgeons perform more minimally invasive surgeries than any other hospital in Westchester. The Hospital was also the first community hospital in the Westchester-Fairfield region to use the da Vinci® Robotic Surgical System for prostate cancer surgery.

- ORTHOPAEDICS More hip and knee replacement surgeries – many of them using minimally invasive techniques – have been performed at WPH than at any other hospital in Westchester.

- CARDIOLOGY The Hospital's cardiology program includes a new and expansive non-invasive testing center, cardiac catheterization laboratory, and an eight-bed inpatient coronary care unit.

- THE RUTH AND JEROME A. SIEGEL STROKE CENTER The Hospital was the first in Westchester County to receive Stroke Center designation from the New York State Department of Health and the first in the County to receive Gold (Sustained) Award Recognition from the American Stroke Association's Get with the Guidelines[sm] – Stroke program.

PHYSICIAN REFERRAL:
For a physician referral or more information about our services, please call (914) 681-1010 or visit www.wphospital.org

Addiction Psychiatry

Bisaga, Adam MD (AdP) - **Spec Exp:** Opiate Addiction; Alcohol Abuse; Drug Abuse; Dual Diagnosis; **Hospital:** NY-Presby/Columbia Univ Med Ctr, NY (page 104), NY State Psychiatric Inst; **Address:** 547 Saw Mill River Rd, Fl 3, Ste PH, Ardsley, NY 10502; **Phone:** 914-419-8921; **Board Cert:** Psychiatry 2008; Addiction Psychiatry 2011; **Med School:** Poland 1989; **Resid:** Psychiatry, N Shore Univ Hosp 1997; **Fellow:** Addiction Psychiatry, NYSPI-Columbia Univ 1999; **Fac Appt:** Prof Psyc, Columbia P&S

Adolescent Medicine

Browner-Elhanan, Karen MD (AM) - **Hospital:** Westchester Med Ctr, Montefiore Med Ctr-Moses Campus (page 100); **Address:** 222 N Westchester Ave, Ste 201, Bridgespan Medicine, White Plains, NY 10604; **Phone:** 914-698-5544; **Board Cert:** Pediatrics 2011; Adolescent Medicine 2005; **Med School:** Israel 1988; **Resid:** Pediatrics, Maimonides Med Ctr 1996; **Fellow:** Adolescent Medicine, Montefiore Med Ctr 2003; **Fac Appt:** Asst Clin Prof Ped, Cornell Univ-Weill Med Coll

Nackenson, Marcia J MD (AM) - **Spec Exp:** Adolescent Gynecology; Eating Disorders; **Hospital:** Westchester Med Ctr; **Address:** Chldns & Women's Physicians Westchester, 503 Grasslands Rd, Ste 200, Valhalla, NY 10595; **Phone:** 914-304-5288; **Board Cert:** Pediatrics 1987; Adolescent Medicine 2012; **Med School:** Israel 1983; **Resid:** Pediatrics, Brookdale Hosp Med Ctr 1986; **Fellow:** Adolescent Medicine, Brookdale Hosp Med Ctr 1987; **Fac Appt:** Assoc Clin Prof Ped, NY Med Coll

Allergy & Immunology

Geraci-Ciardullo, Kira MD (A&I) - **Spec Exp:** Asthma; Sinus Disorders; Food Allergy; Insect Allergies; **Hospital:** White Plains Hosp (page 640); **Address:** 1600 Harrison Ave, Ste 304, Rockledge Plaza, Mamaroneck, NY 10543-3145; **Phone:** 914-777-1179; **Board Cert:** Pediatrics 1984; Allergy & Immunology 2008; **Med School:** Columbia P&S 1980; **Resid:** Pediatrics, NY-Cornell Hosp 1983; **Fellow:** Allergy & Immunology, NY-Cornell Hosp 1985

Goldman, Neil C MD (A&I) - **Spec Exp:** Asthma; Drug Sensitivity; Sinusitis; Insect Allergies; **Hospital:** Phelps Meml Hosp Ctr; **Address:** Hudson Vly Asthma & Allergy Assocs, 35 S Riverside Ave, Ste 106, Croton On Hudson, NY 10520; **Phone:** 914-271-0001; **Board Cert:** Allergy & Immunology 1977; **Med School:** NY Med Coll 1966; **Resid:** Internal Medicine, Beth Israel Hosp 1968; Internal Medicine, Metropolitan Hosp Ctr 1969; **Fellow:** Allergy & Immunology, Jewish Med Ctr 1970

Maloney, Patrick F MD (A&I) - **Spec Exp:** Food Allergy; **Hospital:** White Plains Hosp (page 640), Westchester Med Ctr; **Address:** Westchester Hlth Assocs, 1600 Harrison Ave, Ste 304, Mamaroneck, NY 10543; **Phone:** 914-777-1179; **Board Cert:** Allergy & Immunology 2005; **Med School:** SUNY Stony Brook 1999; **Resid:** Internal Medicine, Stony Brook Univ Med Ctr 2002; **Fellow:** Allergy & Immunology, Stony Brook Univ Med Ctr 2004

Mechanic, Laura MD (A&I) - **Spec Exp:** Allergic Rhinitis; Eczema; Hives; Immunodeficiency Disorders; **Hospital:** White Plains Hosp (page 640); **Address:** Westchester Medical Group, 210 Westchester Ave, White Plains, NY 10604; **Phone:** 914-831-6850; **Board Cert:** Internal Medicine 2002; Allergy & Immunology 2005; **Med School:** NYU Sch Med 1989; **Resid:** Internal Medicine, Mt Sinai Med Ctr 1992; **Fellow:** Allergy & Immunology, Mt Sinai Med Ctr 1995; Allergy & Immunology, White Plains Hosp 2006

Osleeb, Craig MD (A&I) - **Hospital:** Northern Westchester Hosp (page 639); **Address:** Mount Kisco Medical Grp, 110 S Bedford Rd, Mt Kisco, NY 10549; **Phone:** 914-242-1580; **Board Cert:** Allergy & Immunology 2003; Pediatrics 2006; **Med School:** Univ Wisc 1988; **Resid:** Pediatrics, UConn Med Ctr 1991; **Fellow:** Allergy & Immunology, Chldns Natl Med Ctr 1993

Pollowitz, James Allen MD (A&I) - **Spec Exp:** Asthma; Food Allergy; Hives; Drug Sensitivity; **Hospital:** White Plains Hosp (page 640), Lawrence Hosp Ctr; **Address:** 281 Garth Rd, Ste A, Scarsdale, NY 10583-4034; **Phone:** 914-472-3833; **Board Cert:** Pediatrics 1978; Allergy & Immunology 1979; **Med School:** NYU Sch Med 1973; **Resid:** Pediatrics, Bronx Muni Hosp Ctr 1976; **Fellow:** Allergy & Immunology, St Vincent Med Ctr 1978; **Fac Appt:** Asst Clin Prof Ped, NY Med Coll

Tuerk-Mendelsohn, Lois MD (A&I) - **Spec Exp:** Asthma; Hay Fever; Food Allergy; Eczema; **Hospital:** Northern Westchester Hosp (page 639); **Address:** MKMG, Allergy & Immunology, 103 S Bedford Rd, Ste 208, Mt Kisco, NY 10549; **Phone:** 914-666-7171; **Board Cert:** Internal Medicine 1989; **Med School:** NY Med Coll 1986; **Resid:** Internal Medicine, Lenox Hill Hosp 1989; **Fellow:** Allergy & Immunology, Mount Sinai Med Ctr 1991

Cardiac Electrophysiology

Cohen, Martin B MD (CE) - **Spec Exp:** Arrhythmias; Pacemakers; Defibrillators; Coronary Angioplasty/Stents; **Hospital:** Westchester Med Ctr, White Plains Hosp (page 640); **Address:** Westchester Heart & Vascular, 19 Bradhurst Ave Fl 3 - Ste 3850 South, Hawthorne, NY 10532-2140; **Phone:** 914-909-6900; **Board Cert:** Internal Medicine 1983; Cardiovascular Disease 1985; Cardiac Electrophysiology 2006; Interventional Cardiology 2004; **Med School:** SUNY Downstate 1980; **Resid:** Internal Medicine, Univ Hosp 1983; **Fellow:** Cardiovascular Disease, Univ Hosp 1985; Interventional Cardiology, Westchester Co Med Ctr 1986; **Fac Appt:** Assoc Prof Med, NY Med Coll

Iwai, Sei MD (CE) - **Spec Exp:** Arrhythmias; Atrial Fibrillation; Radiofrequency Ablation; **Hospital:** Westchester Med Ctr; **Address:** Westchester Heart & Vascular, 19 Bradhurst Ave Fl 3 - Ste 3850 South, Valhalla, NY 10595; **Phone:** 914-909-6900; **Board Cert:** Internal Medicine 1997; Cardiovascular Disease 2011; Cardiac Electrophysiology 2001; **Med School:** Columbia P&S 1994; **Resid:** Internal Medicine, NY-Presby/Columbia Univ Med Ctr 1997; **Fellow:** Cardiovascular Disease, NY-Presby/Weill Cornell Med Ctr 2000; Cardiac Electrophysiology, NY-Presby/Weill Cornell Med Ctr 2001; **Fac Appt:** Prof Med, NY Med Coll

Rubin, David A MD (CE) - **Spec Exp:** Arrhythmias; Radiofrequency Ablation; Pacemakers/Defibrillators; **Hospital:** NY-Presby/Columbia Univ Med Ctr, NY (page 104), White Plains Hosp (page 640); **Address:** 222 Westchester Ave, White Plains, NY 10604; **Phone:** 914-428-3888; **Board Cert:** Internal Medicine 1978; Cardiovascular Disease 1981; Cardiac Electrophysiology 2012; **Med School:** Columbia P&S 1975; **Resid:** Internal Medicine, NY-Presby/Columbia Univ Med Ctr 1978; **Fellow:** Cardiovascular Disease, Mount Sinai Med Ctr 1980; **Fac Appt:** Clin Prof Med, Columbia P&S

Sorbera, Carmine A MD (CE) - **Spec Exp:** Arrhythmias; Cardiac Catheterization; **Hospital:** Northern Westchester Hosp (page 639); **Address:** Columbia Med Grp, 19 Bradhurst Ave, Ste 700, Hawthorne, NY 10532; **Phone:** 914-593-7800; **Board Cert:** Internal Medicine 1987; Cardiovascular Disease 1989; Cardiac Electrophysiology 2004; **Med School:** NY Med Coll 1983; **Resid:** Internal Medicine, Westchester Med Ctr 1987; **Fellow:** Cardiovascular Disease, Westchester Med Ctr 1989; Cardiac Electrophysiology, Westchester Med Ctr 1990

Cardiovascular Disease

Cappucci, Roger Vincent MD (Cv) - **Spec Exp:** Echocardiography; Cardiac Stress Testing; **Hospital:** White Plains Hosp (page 640); **Address:** Scarsdale Med Grp, 600 Mamaroneck Ave, Ste 200, Harrison, NY 10528; **Phone:** 914-723-8100; **Board Cert:** Internal Medicine 2003; Cardiovascular Disease 2005; **Med School:** Cornell Univ-Weill Med Coll 1989; **Resid:** Internal Medicine, NY-Presby/Weill Cornell Med Ctr 1992; **Fellow:** Cardiovascular Disease, Montefiore Med Ctr 1995

Catanese, James W MD (Cv) - **Spec Exp:** Coronary Artery Disease; Congestive Heart Failure; Heart Valve Disease; **Hospital:** Northern Westchester Hosp (page 639), Westchester Med Ctr; **Address:** Westchester Health- Cardiology, 105 S Bedford Rd, Ste 320, Mt Kisco, NY 10549; **Phone:** 914-242-9400; **Board Cert:** Cardiovascular Disease 2005; **Med School:** Albany Med Coll 1988; **Resid:** Internal Medicine, Montefiore Med Ctr 1991; **Fellow:** Cardiovascular Disease, Montefiore Med Ctr 1994

Charney, Richard MD (Cv) - **Spec Exp:** Interventional Cardiology; Heart Valve Disease; Coronary Artery Disease; Peripheral Vascular Disease; **Hospital:** Montefiore New Rochelle Hosp, NY-Presby/Weill Cornell Med Ctr, NY (page 104); **Address:** Sound Shore Cardiology Assocs, 175 Memorial Hwy, Ste 1-1, New Rochelle, NY 10801; **Phone:** 914-235-3535; **Board Cert:** Internal Medicine 1989; Cardiovascular Disease 2011; Interventional Cardiology 2010; **Med School:** Mount Sinai Sch Med 1986; **Resid:** Internal Medicine, Mt Sinai Hosp 1989; **Fellow:** Cardiovascular Disease, Montefiore Med Ctr 1992; Interventional Cardiology, Montefiore Med Ctr 1993; **Fac Appt:** Asst Prof Med, Cornell Univ-Weill Med Coll

Cooper, Jerome MD (Cv) - **Spec Exp:** Coronary Artery Disease; Hypertension; Heart Valve Disease; **Hospital:** Montefiore New Rochelle Hosp, NY-Presby/Columbia Univ Med Ctr, NY (page 104); **Address:** Westchester Heart Assocs, 150 Lockwood Ave, Ste 28, New Rochelle, NY 10801; **Phone:** 914-633-7870; **Board Cert:** Internal Medicine 1968; Cardiovascular Disease 1973; **Med School:** SUNY Hlth Sci Ctr 1961; **Resid:** Internal Medicine, Baltimore City Hosps 1963; Internal Medicine, Montefiore Hosp Med Ctr 1965; **Fellow:** Cardiovascular Disease, Johns Hopkins Univ Hosp 1967; **Fac Appt:** Assoc Clin Prof Med, Columbia P&S

Cziner, David MD (Cv) - **Spec Exp:** Coronary Artery Disease; Cholesterol/Lipid Disorders; **Hospital:** White Plains Hosp (page 640), Greenwich Hosp (page 938); **Address:** WestMed Medical Group, 210 Westchester Ave, White Plains, NY 10604; **Phone:** 914-305-2700; **Board Cert:** Internal Medicine 1989; Cardiovascular Disease 2011; Nuclear Cardiology 2003; **Med School:** NYU Sch Med 1986; **Resid:** Internal Medicine, Bellevue/NYU Med Ctr 1989; **Fellow:** Cardiovascular Disease, Bellevue/NYU Med Ctr 1992

DeLuca, Albert J MD (Cv) - **Spec Exp:** Coronary Artery Disease; Cholesterol/Lipid Disorders; **Hospital:** NY-Presby/Columbia Univ Med Ctr, NY (page 104), White Plains Hosp (page 640); **Address:** Columbia Doctors Medical Grp, 15 N Broadway Fl 2, White Plains, NY 10601-2225; **Phone:** 914-428-2600; **Board Cert:** Cardiovascular Disease 2003; Internal Medicine 1989; **Med School:** SUNY Downstate 1986; **Resid:** Internal Medicine, Mount Sinai Med Ctr 1989; **Fellow:** Cardiovascular Disease, Westchester Med Ctr 1991; **Fac Appt:** Asst Prof Med, NY Med Coll

Fass, Arthur MD (Cv) - **Spec Exp:** Preventive Cardiology; Coronary Artery Disease; Hypertension; Cholesterol/Lipid Disorders; **Hospital:** Phelps Meml Hosp Ctr, Westchester Med Ctr; **Address:** 465 N State Rd, Briarcliff Manor, NY 10510; **Phone:** 914-762-5810; **Board Cert:** Internal Medicine 1979; Cardiovascular Disease 1981; **Med School:** NY Med Coll 1976; **Resid:** Internal Medicine, Metropolitan Hosp 1979; **Fellow:** Cardiovascular Disease, Westchester Med Ctr 1981

Feld, Michael MD (Cv) - **Spec Exp:** Pacemakers; Coronary Artery Disease; Congestive Heart Failure; **Hospital:** Phelps Meml Hosp Ctr, St. John's Riverside Hosp-Dobbs Ferry Pavil; **Address:** 150 White Plains Rd, Tarrytown, NY 10591-4500; **Phone:** 914-631-2895; **Board Cert:** Internal Medicine 1980; Cardiovascular Disease 1983; **Med School:** Penn State Coll Med 1977; **Resid:** Internal Medicine, Montefiore Med Ctr 1981; **Fellow:** Cardiovascular Disease, Montefiore Med Ctr 1983; **Fac Appt:** Asst Clin Prof Med, Albert Einstein Coll Med

Fishbach, Mitchell MD (Cv) - **Spec Exp:** Non-Invasive Cardiology; Sports Medicine; Nuclear Cardiology; **Hospital:** Lawrence Hosp Ctr, NY-Presby/Columbia Univ Med Ctr, NY (page 104); **Address:** Westmed Med Grp, Cardiology, 73 Market St, Yonkers, NY 10710; **Phone:** 914-831-6880; **Board Cert:** Internal Medicine 1980; Cardiovascular Disease 1983; **Med School:** Albert Einstein Coll Med 1977; **Resid:** Internal Medicine, Montefiore Med Ctr 1980; **Fellow:** Cardiovascular Disease, Montefiore Med Ctr 1982

Frishman, William MD (Cv) - **Spec Exp:** Coronary Artery Disease; Preventive Cardiology; Hypertension; Heart Failure; **Hospital:** Westchester Med Ctr; **Address:** 19 Bradhurst Ave, Hawthorne, NY 10532; **Phone:** 914-594-4383; **Board Cert:** Internal Medicine 1987; Cardiovascular Disease 1975; **Med School:** Boston Univ 1969; **Resid:** Internal Medicine, Montefiore Med Ctr 1971; Internal Medicine, Bronx Muni Hosp 1972; **Fellow:** Cardiovascular Disease, NY Hosp 1974; **Fac Appt:** Prof Med, NY Med Coll

Gabelman, Gary S MD (Cv) - **Spec Exp:** Non-Invasive Cardiology; Echocardiography; Nuclear Cardiology; Preventive Cardiology; **Hospital:** Lawrence Hosp Ctr, NY-Presby/Columbia Univ Med Ctr, NY (page 104); **Address:** Westmed Med Grp, Cardiology, 73 Market St, Yonkers, NY 10710; **Phone:** 914-831-6880; **Board Cert:** Internal Medicine 1988; Cardiovascular Disease 2011; **Med School:** Mount Sinai Sch Med 1985; **Resid:** Internal Medicine, Montefiore Med Ctr 1989; **Fellow:** Cardiovascular Disease, Montefiore Med Ctr 1991; **Fac Appt:** Assoc Clin Prof Med, Columbia P&S

Gass, Alan MD (Cv) - **Spec Exp:** Heart Failure; Transplant Medicine-Heart; **Hospital:** Westchester Med Ctr; **Address:** 19 Bradhurst Ave, Ste 3850 South, Hawthorne, NY 10532; **Phone:** 914-909-6900; **Board Cert:** Cardiovascular Disease 2002; **Med School:** Italy 1984; **Resid:** Internal Medicine, LIJ Med Ctr 1987; **Fellow:** Cardiovascular Disease, Beth Israel Med Ctr 1988; Transplant Medicine, Stanford Univ Med Ctr 1989; **Fac Appt:** Assoc Prof Med, NY Med Coll

Gitler, Bernard MD (Cv) - **Spec Exp:** Hypertension; Cholesterol/Lipid Disorders; Coronary Artery Disease; Heart Valve Disease; **Hospital:** Montefiore New Rochelle Hosp, Montefiore Med Ctr-Moses Campus (page 100); **Address:** Westchester Heart Specialists, 150 Lockwood Ave, Ste 28, New Rochelle, NY 10801-4913; **Phone:** 914-633-7870; **Board Cert:** Cardiovascular Disease 2009; Advanced Heart Failure & Transplant Cardiology 2012; Critical Care Medicine 2010; Internal Medicine 2009; **Med School:** Cornell Univ-Weill Med Coll 1976; **Resid:** Internal Medicine, Jacobi Med Ctr 1979; **Fellow:** Cardiovascular Disease, Montefiore Med Ctr 1981; **Fac Appt:** Assoc Prof Med, Albert Einstein Coll Med

Greif, Richard H MD (Cv) - **Hospital:** Saint Joseph's Med Ctr - Yonkers; **Address:** 127 S Broadway Fl 4th - Ste 409, Yonkers, NY 10701; **Phone:** 914-378-7583; **Board Cert:** Internal Medicine 1978; Cardiovascular Disease 1981; **Med School:** NY Med Coll 1975; **Resid:** Internal Medicine, Metropolitan Hosp 1978; **Fellow:** Cardiovascular Disease, St Vincents Hosp 1981; **Fac Appt:** Assoc Clin Prof Med, NY Med Coll

Kaplan, Kenneth C MD (Cv) - **Hospital:** Phelps Meml Hosp Ctr; **Address:** 160 N State Rd, Briarcliff Manor, NY 10510; **Phone:** 914-762-3821; **Board Cert:** Internal Medicine 1970; Cardiovascular Disease 1975; Echocardiography 1996; **Med School:** NYU Sch Med 1962; **Resid:** Internal Medicine, Bellevue Hosp 1966; **Fellow:** Cardiovascular Disease, Bellevue Hosp/NYU 1969; **Fac Appt:** Asst Clin Prof Med, NY Med Coll

Kay, Richard H MD (Cv) - **Spec Exp:** Preventive Cardiology; Congestive Heart Failure; Non-Invasive Cardiology; **Hospital:** White Plains Hosp (page 640), NY-Presby/Columbia Univ Med Ctr, NY (page 104); **Address:** Columbia Doctors Medical Group, 19 Bradhurst Ave, Ste 700, Hawthorne, NY 10532-2140; **Phone:** 914-593-7800; **Board Cert:** Internal Medicine 1979; Cardiovascular Disease 1981; **Med School:** Johns Hopkins Univ 1976; **Resid:** Internal Medicine, Columbia-Presby Med Ctr 1979; **Fellow:** Cardiovascular Disease, Mount Sinai Hosp 1981; **Fac Appt:** Assoc Prof Med, NY Med Coll

Keltz, Theodore MD (Cv) - **Spec Exp:** Echocardiography; Nuclear Cardiology; Coronary Artery Disease; Preventive Cardiology; **Hospital:** Montefiore New Rochelle Hosp, NY-Presby/Columbia Univ Med Ctr, NY (page 104); **Address:** Westchester Heart Assocs, 150 Lockwood Ave, Ste 28, New Rochelle, NY 10801-4913; **Phone:** 914-633-7870; **Board Cert:** Internal Medicine 1983; Cardiovascular Disease 1985; Echocardiography 2006; Nuclear Cardiology 1996; **Med School:** Albany Med Coll 1980; **Resid:** Internal Medicine, Mt Sinai Med Ctr 1983; **Fellow:** Cardiovascular Disease, Montefiore Med Ctr 1985; **Fac Appt:** Assoc Clin Prof Med, Albert Einstein Coll Med

Kupersmith, Andrew C MD (Cv) - **Hospital:** Westchester Med Ctr, White Plains Hosp (page 640); **Address:** Columbia Doctors Medical Group, 19 Bradhurst Ave, Ste 700, Hawthorne, NY 10532; **Phone:** 914-593-7800; **Board Cert:** Cardiovascular Disease 2002; **Med School:** Univ MD Sch Med 1995; **Resid:** Internal Medicine, LIJ Med Ctr 1998; **Fellow:** Cardiovascular Disease, Wesctchester Med Ctr 2001; **Fac Appt:** Asst Prof Med, NY Med Coll

Leonard, Daniel MD (Cv) - **Hospital:** Northern Westchester Hosp (page 639), Westchester Med Ctr; **Address:** Mt Kisco Med Grp, 110 S Bedford Rd Bldg 110, Mt Kisco, NY 10549-3433; **Phone:** 914-241-1050; **Board Cert:** Internal Medicine 1984; Cardiovascular Disease 1987; **Med School:** Univ Cincinnati 1981; **Resid:** Internal Medicine, NY-Presby/Weil Cornell Med Ctr 1984; **Fellow:** Cardiovascular Disease, Montefiore Med Ctr 1986; **Fac Appt:** Assoc Clin Prof Med, NY Med Coll

Levine, Evan MD (Cv) - **Spec Exp:** Cardiac Stress Testing; **Hospital:** Montefiore Med Ctr-Moses Campus (page 100), St. John's Riverside Hosp-Andrus Pavil; **Address:** Riverside Cardiology, 955 Yonkers Ave, Ste 200, Yonkers, NY 10704; **Phone:** 914-237-1332; **Board Cert:** Internal Medicine 1988; Cardiovascular Disease 2011; **Med School:** Mount Sinai Sch Med 1985; **Resid:** Internal Medicine, Montefiore Med Ctr 1988; **Fellow:** Cardiovascular Disease, Montefiore Med Ctr 1990; **Fac Appt:** Asst Clin Prof Med, Albert Einstein Coll Med

Lieb, Mark MD (Cv) - **Hospital:** Northern Westchester Hosp (page 639); **Address:** 110 S Bedford Rd, Fl 2, Mount Kisco Medical Group, Mt Kisco, NY 10549-3412; **Phone:** 914-241-1050; **Board Cert:** Cardiovascular Disease 2006; **Med School:** Boston Univ 1988; **Resid:** Internal Medicine, Mt Sinai Med Ctr 1991; **Fellow:** Cardiovascular Disease, Mt Sinai Med Ctr 1995

Matos, Marshall MD (Cv) - **Spec Exp:** Coronary Artery Disease; Preventive Cardiology; Arrhythmias; Cholesterol/Lipid Disorders; **Hospital:** Montefiore New Rochelle Hosp, Lenox Hill Hosp (page 106); **Address:** 140 Lockwood Ave, Ste 310, New Rochelle, NY 10801-4909; **Phone:** 914-576-7171; **Board Cert:** Internal Medicine 1980; Cardiovascular Disease 1985; **Med School:** Albert Einstein Coll Med 1977; **Resid:** Internal Medicine, Bronx Muni Hosp 1981; **Fellow:** Cardiovascular Disease, Albert Einstein Coll Med 1983; **Fac Appt:** Asst Prof Med, NYU Sch Med

McClung, John Arthur MD (Cv) - **Spec Exp:** Echocardiography; **Hospital:** Westchester Med Ctr; **Address:** 19 Bradhurst Ave, Ste 3850 South, Hawthorne, NY 10532; **Phone:** 914-909-6900; **Board Cert:** Internal Medicine 1980; Cardiovascular Disease 1983; **Med School:** NY Med Coll 1975; **Resid:** Internal Medicine, Misericordia Hosp Med Ctr 1976; Internal Medicine, Lincoln Med & Mental Hlth Ctr 1979; **Fellow:** Cardiovascular Disease, Westchester Med Ctr 1982; **Fac Appt:** Prof Med, NY Med Coll

Medina, Emma MD (Cv) - **Spec Exp:** Non-Invasive Cardiology; **Hospital:** Montefiore New Rochelle Hosp, Montefiore Med Ctr-Einstein Campus (page 100); **Address:** 140 Lockwood Ave, Ste 310, New Rochelle, NY 10801-4909; **Phone:** 914-632-1600; **Board Cert:** Internal Medicine 1982; Cardiovascular Disease 1985; **Med School:** NYU Sch Med 1979; **Resid:** Internal Medicine, Jacobi Med Ctr 1982; **Fellow:** Cardiovascular Disease, Jacobi Med Ctr 1984; **Fac Appt:** Asst Clin Prof Med, Albert Einstein Coll Med

Mercando, Anthony MD (Cv) - **Spec Exp:** Cholesterol/Lipid Disorders; Preventive Cardiology; **Hospital:** Lawrence Hosp Ctr, NY-Presby/Columbia Univ Med Ctr, NY (page 104); **Address:** Westmed Med Grp, Cardiology, 73 Market St, Ste 215, Yonkers, NY 10710; **Phone:** 914-831-6880; **Board Cert:** Internal Medicine 1983; Cardiovascular Disease 1987; **Med School:** Harvard Med Sch 1980; **Resid:** Internal Medicine, Montefiore Med Ctr 1984; **Fellow:** Cardiovascular Disease, Montefiore Med Ctr 1986; **Fac Appt:** Clin Prof Med, Albert Einstein Coll Med

Paley, Ari J MD (Cv) - **Spec Exp:** Coronary Artery Disease; **Hospital:** White Plains Hosp (page 640); **Address:** 30 Davis Ave, White Plains, NY 10605; **Phone:** 914-328-2355; **Board Cert:** Integrative Medicine 2006; Cardiovascular Disease 2009; **Med School:** Albert Einstein Coll Med 2002; **Resid:** Internal Medicine, NY Presby-Columbia Med Ctr 2006; **Fellow:** Cardiovascular Disease, NYU Med Ctr 2009

Perry-Bottinger, Lynne V MD (Cv) - **Spec Exp:** Cardiac Catheterization; Coronary Angioplasty/Stents; Heart Disease in Women; Heart Disease in African Americans; **Hospital:** NY-Presby/Columbia Univ Med Ctr, NY (page 104), Montefiore New Rochelle Hosp; **Address:** Clinical & Interventional Cardiology, 140A Lockwood Ave, New Rochelle, NY 10801; **Phone:** 914-576-7577; **Med School:** Yale Univ 1986; **Resid:** Internal Medicine, Yale-New Haven Hosp 1990; **Fellow:** Cardiovascular Disease, Johns Hopkins Hosp 1993; Interventional Cardiology, Johns Hopkins Hosp 1994; **Fac Appt:** Asst Clin Prof Med, Columbia P&S

Pilchik, Robert M MD (Cv) - **Spec Exp:** Cardiac Catheterization; Echocardiography; Nuclear Cardiology; **Hospital:** Northern Westchester Hosp (page 639), White Plains Hosp (page 640); **Address:** Westchester Health Associates, 1888 Commerce St, Yorktown Heights, NY 10598; **Phone:** 914-962-4000; **Board Cert:** Internal Medicine 2013; Cardiovascular Disease 2013; Nuclear Cardiology 2006; **Med School:** Mount Sinai Sch Med 1995; **Resid:** Internal Medicine, St Lukes-Roosevelt Hosp 1998; **Fellow:** Cardiovascular Disease, St Lukes-Roosevelt Hosp 2001

Price Jr, Thomas J MD (Cv) - **Hospital:** Montefiore Mt Vernon Hosp, Montefiore New Rochelle Hosp; **Address:** 105 Stevens Ave, Ste 603, Mt Vernon, NY 10550; **Phone:** 914-664-4052; **Board Cert:** Internal Medicine 1984; Cardiovascular Disease 1987; **Med School:** Univ Cincinnati 1975; **Resid:** Internal Medicine, Harlem Hosp 1979; **Fellow:** Cardiovascular Disease, Harlem Hosp 1983; **Fac Appt:** Asst Clin Prof Med, Columbia P&S

Pucillo, Anthony MD (Cv) - **Spec Exp:** Coronary Angioplasty/Stents; Peripheral Vascular Disease; Cardiac Catheterization; Interventional Cardiology; **Hospital:** Westchester Med Ctr; **Address:** 19 Bradhurst Ave, Ste 700, Hawthorne, NY 10532; **Phone:** 914-593-7800; **Board Cert:** Internal Medicine 1981; Cardiovascular Disease 1983; **Med School:** Mount Sinai Sch Med 1978; **Resid:** Internal Medicine, Columbia-Presby Med Ctr 1981; **Fellow:** Cardiovascular Disease, Columbia-Presby Med Ctr 1984; **Fac Appt:** Assoc Prof Med, NY Med Coll

Sheikh, Shahid H MD (Cv) - **Hospital:** St. John's Riverside Hosp-Andrus Pavil, Montefiore Med Ctr-Wakefield Campus (page 100); **Address:** 970 N Broadway, Ste 210, Yonkers, NY 10701-1311; **Phone:** 914-963-0111; **Board Cert:** Internal Medicine 1977; Cardiovascular Disease 1979; **Med School:** Pakistan 1971; **Resid:** Internal Medicine, Our Lady of Mercy Med Ctr 1977

Silver, Michael M MD (Cv) - **Spec Exp:** Hypertension; Cholesterol/Lipid Disorders; Coronary Artery Disease; **Hospital:** White Plains Hosp (page 640), Greenwich Hosp (page 938); **Address:** WestMed Medical Group, 210 Westchester Ave, White Plains, NY 10604; **Phone:** 914-305-2700 x2; **Board Cert:** Internal Medicine 1980; Cardiovascular Disease 1983; **Med School:** SUNY Downstate 1977; **Resid:** Internal Medicine, Thomas Jefferson Univ Hosp 1980; **Fellow:** Cardiovascular Disease, Presby-Hosp Univ Penn 1982

Tartaglia, Joseph J MD (Cv) - **Spec Exp:** Angina; Congestive Heart Failure; Arrhythmias; **Hospital:** White Plains Hosp (page 640), Greenwich Hosp (page 938); **Address:** 311 North St, Ste 402, White Plains, NY 10605-2232; **Phone:** 914-946-3388; **Board Cert:** Internal Medicine 1988; Cardiovascular Disease 2011; Geriatric Medicine 2004; **Med School:** Italy 1984; **Resid:** Internal Medicine, Our Lady of Mercy Med Ctr 1988; **Fellow:** Cardiovascular Disease, N Shore Univ Hosp 1990; **Fac Appt:** Asst Clin Prof Med, NY Med Coll

Weissman, Ronald MD (Cv) - **Spec Exp:** Coronary Artery Disease; Congestive Heart Failure; Arrhythmias; Hypertrophic Cardiomyopathy; **Hospital:** White Plains Hosp (page 640), Westchester Med Ctr; **Address:** 15 N Broadway Fl 2, White Plains, NY 10601; **Phone:** 914-428-6000; **Board Cert:** Internal Medicine 1980; Cardiovascular Disease 1983; **Med School:** NY Med Coll 1977; **Resid:** Internal Medicine, LI Jewish Hosp 1980; **Fellow:** Cardiovascular Disease, LI Jewish Hosp 1982; **Fac Appt:** Assoc Clin Prof Med, NY Med Coll

Zimmerman, Franklin Harrison MD (Cv) - **Spec Exp:** Preventive Cardiology; Sports Medicine-Cardiology; Cholesterol/Lipid Disorders; Hypertension; **Hospital:** Phelps Meml Hosp Ctr, Westchester Med Ctr; **Address:** 465 N State Rd, Briarcliff Manor, NY 10510-1468; **Phone:** 914-762-5810; **Board Cert:** Internal Medicine 1983; Cardiovascular Disease 1987; Critical Care Medicine 2006; **Med School:** Brown Univ 1980; **Resid:** Internal Medicine, St Lukes-Roosevelt Hosp Ctr 1983; **Fellow:** Cardiovascular Disease, St Lukes-Roosevelt Hosp Ctr 1988; **Fac Appt:** Asst Prof Med, Columbia P&S

Child & Adolescent Psychiatry

Cohen, Lee Steven MD (ChAP) - **Spec Exp:** Anxiety & Mood Disorders; Psychopharmacology; ADD/ADHD; Autism; **Hospital:** Morgan Stanley Children's Hosp of NY-Presby, NY (page 104), NY-Presby/Columbia Univ Med Ctr, NY (page 104); **Address:** 623 Warburton Ave, Hastings On Hudson, NY 10706-1523; **Phone:** 914-478-1330; **Board Cert:** Psychiatry 1987; Child & Adolescent Psychiatry 1988; **Med School:** SUNY Stony Brook 1982; **Resid:** Psychiatry, Mt Sinai Med Ctr 1985; **Fellow:** Child & Adolescent Psychiatry, Columbia-Presby Med Ctr 1987; **Fac Appt:** Asst Clin Prof Psyc, Columbia P&S

Fink, Candida A MD (ChAP) - **Spec Exp:** Anxiety & Mood Disorders; ADD/ADHD; Developmental Disorders; **Address:** 4 Stanton Cir, New Rochelle, NY 10804; **Phone:** 877-534-1090; **Board Cert:** Psychiatry 1994; Child & Adolescent Psychiatry 2006; **Med School:** Boston Univ 1987; **Resid:** Psychiatry, Beth Israel Deaconess Hosp 1990; **Fellow:** Child & Adolescent Psychiatry, Children's Hosp 1992

Greenhill, Laurence L MD (ChAP) - **Spec Exp:** ADD/ADHD; Depression; **Hospital:** NY State Psychiatric Inst, NY-Presby/Columbia Univ Med Ctr, NY (page 104); **Address:** 9 Country Rd, Mamaroneck, NY 10543; **Phone:** 914-381-2436; **Board Cert:** Psychiatry ; Child & Adolescent Psychiatry ; **Med School:** Albert Einstein Coll Med 1967; **Resid:** Psychiatry, Bronx Muni Hosp Ctr 1972; Psychiatry, Bronx Muni Hosp Ctr 1974; **Fellow:** Child & Adolescent Psychiatry, Natl Inst Mental Hlth 1971; **Fac Appt:** Prof Psyc, Columbia P&S

Hyler, Irene MD (ChAP) - **Spec Exp:** Psychotherapy; Psychoanalysis; **Hospital:** NY-Presby/Weill Cornell Med Ctr, NY (page 104); **Address:** 2A Berkeley Rd, Scarsdale, NY 10583-1102; **Phone:** 914-472-8447; **Board Cert:** Psychiatry 1984; Child & Adolescent Psychiatry 1986; **Med School:** Albert Einstein Coll Med 1979; **Resid:** Psychiatry, Bronx Muni Hosp 1982; **Fellow:** Child & Adolescent Psychiatry, Albert Einstein Coll Med 1984; **Fac Appt:** Asst Clin Prof Psyc, Cornell Univ-Weill Med Coll

Kalikow, Kevin T MD (ChAP) - ; **Address:** 83 S Bedford Rd, Mt Kisco, NY 10549; **Phone:** 914-666-3000; **Board Cert:** Psychiatry 1984; Child & Adolescent Psychiatry 1986; **Med School:** Tulane Univ 1979; **Resid:** Psychiatry, NY Hosp-Westchester Div 1983; **Fellow:** Child & Adolescent Psychiatry, NY State Psych Inst 1985; **Fac Appt:** Asst Clin Prof Psyc, NY Med Coll

Lomonaco, Salvatore MD (ChAP) - **Hospital:** Montefiore Med Ctr-Moses Campus (page 100); **Address:** 1815 Palmer Ave, Larchmont, NY 10538; **Phone:** 914-834-0085; **Board Cert:** Psychiatry 1976; **Med School:** SUNY Downstate 1966; **Resid:** Psychiatry, Montefiore Med Ctr 1971; Child Psychiatry, Montefiore Med Ctr 1972

Rabinowitz, Ilene MD (ChAP) - **Spec Exp:** Psychopharmacology; Mood Disorders; Anxiety; **Address:** 50 Main St, Ste 1000, White Plains, NY 10606; **Phone:** 914-682-2047; **Board Cert:** Psychiatry 1993; Child & Adolescent Psychiatry 2008; **Med School:** Mount Sinai Sch Med 1988; **Resid:** Psychiatry, NY-Presby/Westchester Div 1992; **Fellow:** Child & Adolescent Psychiatry, NY-Presby/Columbia Univ Med Ctr 1994

Rubinstein, Boris MD (ChAP) - **Spec Exp:** Psychopharmacology; Neuro-Psychiatry; Anxiety & Mood Disorders; Developmental Disorders; **Hospital:** Morgan Stanley Children's Hosp of NY-Presby, NY (page 104); **Address:** 623 Warburton Ave, Hastings On Hudson, NY 10706; **Phone:** 914-478-1330; **Board Cert:** Pediatrics 1976; Psychiatry 1979; Child & Adolescent Psychiatry 1981; **Med School:** Mexico 1970; **Resid:** Pediatrics, Chldns Hosp 1974; Psychiatry, Jacobi Med Ctr 1976; **Fellow:** Child & Adolescent Psychiatry, Jacobi Med Ctr 1978

Schreiber, Klaus MD (ChAP) - **Spec Exp:** Developmental Disorders; **Address:** 1 Neperan Rd, Tarrytown, NY 10591; **Phone:** 914-332-0270; **Board Cert:** Psychiatry 1976; Child & Adolescent Psychiatry 1986; **Med School:** Germany 1966; **Resid:** Psychiatry, Elmhurst City Hosp Ctr 1971; Psychiatry, Westchester Med Ctr 1972; **Fellow:** Child & Adolescent Psychiatry, Westchester Med Ctr 1973; Child & Adolescent Psychiatry, Albert Einstein Coll Med 1982; **Fac Appt:** Asst Prof Psyc, NY Med Coll

Seaver, Robert MD (ChAP) - **Spec Exp:** Forensic Psychiatry; Art & Creativity; Psychopharmacology; **Address:** 83 S Bedford Rd Fl 2nd, Mt Kisco, NY 10549; **Phone:** 914-241-8979; **Board Cert:** Pediatrics 1978; Psychiatry 1984; Child & Adolescent Psychiatry 1986; **Med School:** Mount Sinai Sch Med 1973; **Resid:** Pediatrics, Mount Sinai Med Ctr 1975; Pediatrics, St Lukes-Roosevelt Hosp 1976; **Fellow:** Psychiatry, NY-Presby/Westchester Div 1984; Child & Adolescent Psychiatry, Jacobi Med Ctr 1985

Silva, Raul R MD (ChAP) - **Spec Exp:** Autism; ADD/ADHD; Depression; Psychopharmacology; **Address:** 2975 Westchester Ave, Ste 308, Purchase, NY 10577; **Phone:** 201-218-1380; **Board Cert:** Psychiatry 1991; Child & Adolescent Psychiatry 1992; **Med School:** Mexico 1983; **Resid:** Psychiatry, St Vincent's Medical Ctr 1988; **Fellow:** Child & Adolescent Psychiatry, St Luke's Hosp 1990; Research, Bellevue Hosp Ctr 1992

Silverman, Amy MD (ChAP) - **Spec Exp:** Anxiety & Depression; ADD/ADHD; **Hospital:** NY-Presby/Westchester Div, NY (page 104); **Address:** 600 Mamaroneck Ave, Ste 400, Harrison, NY 10528; **Phone:** 914-301-9465; **Board Cert:** Psychiatry 2013; Child & Adolescent Psychiatry 2013; **Med School:** Mount Sinai Sch Med 1998; **Resid:** Psychiatry, Brigham and Women's Hosp 2001; **Fellow:** Child Psychiatry, NY Presby/Cornell Med Ctr 2003; **Fac Appt:** Asst Clin Prof ChAP, Cornell Univ

Slater, Jonathan Allen MD (ChAP) - **Spec Exp:** Psychopharmacology; Psychiatry in Physical Illness; **Hospital:** Morgan Stanley Children's Hosp of NY-Presby, NY (page 104); **Address:** 1 Bridge St, Ste 24, Irvington, NY 10533; **Phone:** 914-591-4040; **Board Cert:** Psychiatry 1991; Child & Adolescent Psychiatry 1993; Psychosomatic Medicine 2006; **Med School:** Columbia P&S 1985; **Resid:** Psychiatry, NY State Psych Inst 1990; **Fellow:** Research, Columbia Univ 1986; Child & Adolescent Psychiatry, NY Presby-Columbia Med Ctr 1992; **Fac Appt:** Clin Prof Psyc, Columbia P&S

Walker, Audrey MD (ChAP) - **Spec Exp:** Psychosomatic Disorders; **Hospital:** Montefiore Med Ctr-Moses Campus (page 100); **Address:** 2005 Palmer Ave, Larchmont, NY 10538; **Phone:** 914-834-2214; **Board Cert:** Psychiatry 1992; Child & Adolescent Psychiatry 1994; Psychosomatic Medicine 2005; **Med School:** Albert Einstein Coll Med 1985; **Resid:** Psychiatry, NY Presby-Columbia Med Ctr 1990

Child Neurology

Jacobson, Ronald I MD (ChiN) - **Spec Exp:** Epilepsy; Headache; ADD/ADHD; Autism; **Hospital:** Westchester Med Ctr, Children's & Women's Phys.of Westchester (page 638); **Address:** Pediatric Neurology Associates, 755 N Broadway, Medical Services Bldg, Ste 540, Sleepy Hollow, NY 10591; **Phone:** 914-358-0190; **Board Cert:** Pediatrics 1981; Child Neurology 1984; **Med School:** Albert Einstein Coll Med 1975; **Resid:** Pediatrics, Yale-New Haven Hosp 1978; **Fellow:** Neurological Immunology, Yale Univ School of Med 1979; Pediatric Neurology, Univ Minn Med Ctr 1982; **Fac Appt:** Assoc Clin Prof N, NY Med Coll

Kang, Harriet MD (ChiN) - **Spec Exp:** Epilepsy/Seizure Disorders; **Hospital:** Beth Israel Med Ctr - Petrie Div (page 94); **Address:** 141 S Central Park Ave, Hartsdale, NY 10530; **Phone:** 914-428-0529; **Board Cert:** Pediatrics 1979; Child Neurology 1981; Clinical Neurophysiology 2006; **Med School:** Johns Hopkins Univ 1974; **Resid:** Pediatrics, Johns Hopkins Hosp 1976; Child Neurology, Univ Minn Med Ctr 1979; **Fellow:** Clinical Neurophysiology, Univ Minn Med Ctr 1980; **Fac Appt:** Assoc Prof N, Albert Einstein Coll Med

Kutscher, Martin MD (ChiN) - **Spec Exp:** ADD/ADHD; Asperger's Syndrome; Autism; **Hospital:** Westchester Med Ctr; **Address:** 800 Westchester Ave, Ste N641, Rye Brook, NY 10573; **Phone:** 914-232-1810; **Board Cert:** Pediatrics 1986; Child Neurology 1989; **Med School:** Columbia P&S 1981; **Resid:** Pediatrics, St Christopher's Hosp 1984; **Fellow:** Child Neurology, Montefiore Med Ctr 1987; **Fac Appt:** Asst Clin Prof Ped, NY Med Coll

Roseman, Bruce MD (ChiN) - **Spec Exp:** Asperger's Syndrome; **Hospital:** Westchester Med Ctr; **Address:** 125 S Broadway, White Plains, NY 10605-1405; **Phone:** 914-997-2032; **Board Cert:** Pediatrics 1978; Child Neurology 1982; **Med School:** Georgetown Univ 1973; **Resid:** Pediatrics, Johns Hopkins Hosp 1976; **Fellow:** Child Neurology, NY-Presby/Columbia Univ Med Ctr 1979

Sweeney, Tanya-Marie MD (ChiN) - **Spec Exp:** Neurodevelopmental Disabilities; **Hospital:** Northern Westchester Hosp (page 639); **Address:** 110 S Beford Rd, Mount Kisco, NY 10549-3412; **Phone:** 914-241-1050; **Board Cert:** Pediatrics 2005; Child Neurology 2008; **Med School:** SUNY Stony Brook 2002; **Resid:** Pediatrics, Winthrop Univ Hosp 2005; **Fellow:** Child Neurology, N Shore-LIJ Hlth System 2008

Clinical Genetics

Kronn, David F MD (CG) - **Spec Exp:** Bone Disorders-Metabolic; Bone Disorders-Inherited; **Hospital:** Westchester Med Ctr, Children's & Women's Phys.of Westchester (page 638); **Address:** Regional Medical Genetics, 503 Grasslands Rd, Ste 200, Valhalla, NY 10595; **Phone:** 914-304-5280; **Board Cert:** Clinical Genetics 2010; Clinical Biochemical Genetics 2010; **Med School:** Ireland 1989; **Resid:** Pediatrics, NYU Med Ctr 1996; **Fellow:** Clinical Genetics, NYU Med Ctr 1996; **Fac Appt:** Assoc Prof CG, NY Med Coll

Colon & Rectal Surgery

Krakovitz, Evan K MD (CRS) - **Spec Exp:** Colon & Rectal Cancer & Surgery; Hemorrhoids; Laparoscopic Surgery; Hernia; **Hospital:** Greenwich Hosp (page 938), White Plains Hosp (page 640); **Address:** Westmed Medical Group, 210 Westchester Ave, Ste 106, White Plains, NY 10604; **Phone:** 914-682-6557; **Board Cert:** Surgery 2005; Colon & Rectal Surgery 2007; **Med School:** Hahnemann Univ 1989; **Resid:** Surgery, Graduate Hospital 1994; **Fellow:** Colon & Rectal Surgery, RWJ Univ Hosp 1995; **Fac Appt:** Clin Prof CRS, Cornell Univ-Weill Med Coll

Wishner, Jerald D MD (CRS) - **Spec Exp:** Colon & Rectal Cancer; Laparoscopic Surgery; **Hospital:** Northern Westchester Hosp (page 639); **Address:** Mount Kisco Med Grp, 110 S Bedford Rd, Mount Kisco, NY 10549; **Phone:** 914-241-1050; **Board Cert:** Surgery 2004; Colon & Rectal Surgery 2006; **Med School:** Northwestern Univ 1988; **Resid:** Surgery, St Luke's-Roosevelt Hosp Ctr 1993; Colon & Rectal Surgery, Grtr Baltimore Med Ctr 1994; **Fellow:** Minimally Invasive Surgery, Eastern Va Med Sch 1995; **Fac Appt:** Asst Prof S, Columbia P&S

Dermatology

Bank, David MD (D) - **Spec Exp:** Liposuction; Skin Laser Surgery; Botox Therapy; **Hospital:** Northern Westchester Hosp (page 639), NY-Presby/Columbia Univ Med Ctr, NY (page 104); **Address:** 359 E Main St, Ste 4G, Mt Kisco, NY 10549; **Phone:** 914-241-3003; **Board Cert:** Dermatology 1989; **Med School:** Columbia P&S 1985; **Resid:** Dermatology, Columbia-Presby Med Ctr 1989; **Fac Appt:** Assoc Clin Prof D, Columbia P&S

Berkowitz, Rhonda K MD (D) - **Spec Exp:** Melanoma; Skin Cancer; **Hospital:** NY-Presby/Columbia Univ Med Ctr, NY (page 104); **Address:** 325 S Highland Ave, Briarcliff Manor, NY 10510-2031; **Phone:** 914-941-5769; **Board Cert:** Dermatology 1986; **Med School:** NYU Sch Med 1982; **Resid:** Internal Medicine, N Shore Univ Hosp 1983; Dermatology, Columbia-Presby Med Ctr 1986

Bronin, Andrew MD (D) - **Spec Exp:** Melanoma; Skin Cancer; Complex Diagnosis; **Hospital:** Greenwich Hosp (page 938), Yale-New Haven Hosp; **Address:** 4 Rye Ridge Plaza, Rye Brook, NY 10573-2820; **Phone:** 914-253-8080; **Board Cert:** Dermatology 1981; **Med School:** NY Med Coll 1975; **Resid:** Dermatology, New York Hosp 1979; **Fac Appt:** Assoc Clin Prof D, Yale Univ

Davis, Ira C MD (D) - **Spec Exp:** Mohs' Surgery; Skin Cancer; Laser Surgery; Cosmetic Dermatology; **Hospital:** Westchester Med Ctr; **Address:** 280 N Central Park Ave, Ste 114, Hartsdale, NY 10530; **Phone:** 914-288-0500; **Board Cert:** Dermatology 1990; **Med School:** NYU Sch Med 1986; **Resid:** Dermatology, Duke Univ Med Ctr 1990; **Fellow:** Dermatologic Pharmacology, NYU Med Ctr 1991; Mohs Surgery, Wake Forest Univ Med Ctr 1994; **Fac Appt:** Asst Clin Prof D, NY Med Coll

Evans, Lydia Marion MD (D) - **Spec Exp:** Cosmetic Dermatology; Mohs' Surgery; Facial Rejuvenation; Skin Laser Surgery; **Hospital:** NY-Presby/Columbia Univ Med Ctr, NY (page 104); **Address:** 229 King Street, Chappaqua, NY 10514; **Phone:** 914-238-1500; **Board Cert:** Dermatology 2013; Internal Medicine 1982; **Med School:** Penn State Coll Med 1979; **Resid:** Internal Medicine, Fletcher Allen Hlth Care 1983; Dermatology, NY-Presby/Columbia Univ Med Ctr 1993; **Fellow:** Medical Oncology, Meml Sloan-Kettering Cancer Ctr 1986

Felsenstein, Jerome M MD (D) - **Hospital:** Phelps Meml Hosp Ctr, NYU Langone Med Ctr (page 108); **Address:** 449 N State Rd, Ste 203, Briar Cliff Manor, NY 10510; **Phone:** 914-941-5770; **Board Cert:** Dermatology 1976; **Med School:** NYU Sch Med 1971; **Resid:** Dermatology, Kings County Hosp 1975

Goldberg, Neil S MD (D) - **Spec Exp:** Pediatric Dermatology; Acne; **Hospital:** Lawrence Hosp Ctr; **Address:** 222 Westchester Ave, Ste 203, White Plains, NY 10604-2926; **Phone:** 914-761-8140; **Board Cert:** Dermatology 1986; **Med School:** Northwestern Univ 1982; **Resid:** Dermatology, Northwestern Meml Hosp 1986

Grossman, Marc E MD (D) - **Spec Exp:** Skin Diseases in Transplants/Cancer; Psoriasis; Rare Skin Disorders; Cutaneous Lymphoma; **Hospital:** NY-Presby/Columbia Univ Med Ctr, NY (page 104), White Plains Hosp (page 640); **Address:** 12 Greenridge Ave, White Plains, NY 10605-1238; **Phone:** 914-946-1101; **Board Cert:** Internal Medicine 1977; Dermatology 2009; **Med School:** Univ Pennsylvania 1974; **Resid:** Internal Medicine, Hosp Univ Penn 1976; **Fellow:** Dermatology, Columbia-Presby Med Ctr 1979; **Fac Appt:** Prof D, Columbia P&S

Howanitz, Nancy C MD (D) - **Spec Exp:** Melanoma; Skin Cancer; Rosacea; Cosmetic Dermatology; **Hospital:** Lawrence Hosp Ctr; **Address:** 700 White Plains Rd, Scarsdale, NY 10583-5013; **Phone:** 914-725-5150; **Board Cert:** Dermatology 1980; **Med School:** Baylor Coll Med 1975; **Resid:** Anatomic Pathology, Texas Houston Med Ctr 1977; Dermatology, NYU Med Ctr 1980; **Fac Appt:** Asst Clin Prof D, NYU Sch Med

Hurwitz, Diana S MD (D) - ; **Address:** Westchester Medical Group, 1 Theall Rd, Ste 211, Rye, NY 10580; **Phone:** 914-848-8840; **Board Cert:** Dermatology 2005; **Med School:** Mount Sinai Sch Med 1992; **Resid:** Dermatology, Mt Sinai Med Ctr 1996

Kaplan, Sherri KO MD (D) - **Hospital:** St. John's Riverside Hosp-Dobbs Ferry Pavil; **Address:** 1055 Saw Mill River Rd, Ste 208, Ardsley, NY 10502-1046; **Phone:** 914-693-7191; **Board Cert:** Dermatology 1987; **Med School:** NY Med Coll 1983; **Resid:** Dermatology, Westchester Med Ctr 1987

Kaporis, Athena G MD (D) - **Spec Exp:** Cosmetic Dermatology; Skin Cancer; Laser Surgery; **Hospital:** Northern Westchester Hosp (page 639); **Address:** 185 Kisco Ave, Ste 300, Mt. Kisco, NY 10549; **Phone:** 914-242-2020; **Board Cert:** Dermatology 2006; **Med School:** NYU Sch Med 1994; **Resid:** Dermatology, Downstate Med Ctr 1998

Klar, Tobi MD (D) - **Spec Exp:** Skin Cancer; **Hospital:** Montefiore New Rochelle Hosp; **Address:** 150 Lockwood Ave, Ste 20, New Rochelle, NY 10801; **Phone:** 914-636-2039; **Board Cert:** Dermatology 1989; **Med School:** SUNY Downstate 1981; **Resid:** Dermatology, Downstate Med Ctr 1986

Levy, Ross S MD (D) - **Spec Exp:** Skin Laser Surgery; Dermatologic Surgery; Skin Cancer; **Hospital:** Northern Westchester Hosp (page 639), Montefiore Med Ctr-Moses Campus (page 100); **Address:** Mt Kisco Med Group, 110 S Bedford Rd, Mt Kisco, NY 10549; **Phone:** 914-242-1355; **Board Cert:** Dermatology 1981; **Med School:** Albert Einstein Coll Med 1976; **Resid:** Internal Medicine, Montefiore Med Ctr 1978; **Fellow:** Dermatology, Montefiore Med Ctr 1981; **Fac Appt:** Assoc Clin Prof Med, Albert Einstein Coll Med

Lukash, Barbara MD (D) - **Spec Exp:** Skin Cancer; Acne; Psoriasis; Melanoma; **Hospital:** NY-Presby/Columbia Univ Med Ctr, NY (page 104); **Address:** 14 Lawton St, New Rochelle, NY 10801; **Phone:** 914-712-2800; **Board Cert:** Dermatology 1980; **Med School:** Tulane Univ 1976; **Resid:** Dermatology, Univ Chicago Hosps 1980; **Fac Appt:** Assoc Clin Prof D, Columbia P&S

Mackler, Karen MD (D) - **Spec Exp:** Pediatric Dermatology; Skin Cancer; **Hospital:** Montefiore New Rochelle Hosp, Montefiore Med Ctr-Moses Campus (page 100); **Address:** 150 Lockwood Ave, Ste 34, New Rochelle, NY 10801-4914; **Phone:** 914-576-7070; **Board Cert:** Pediatrics 1978; Dermatology 1983; **Med School:** NYU Sch Med 1973; **Resid:** Pediatrics, NY Hosp 1976; Dermatology, Montefiore Hosp Med Ctr 1983; **Fac Appt:** Asst Prof D, Albert Einstein Coll Med

Mattison, Timothy D MD (D) - **Hospital:** Northern Westchester Hosp (page 639); **Address:** Mt Kisco Medical Group, 90 S Bedford Rd, Mt Kisco, NY 10549-3412; **Phone:** 914-242-1355; **Board Cert:** Dermatology 1980; **Med School:** Dartmouth Med Sch 1976; **Resid:** Dermatology, NYU Med Ctr 1980

Mermelstein, Harold MD (D) - **Spec Exp:** Cosmetic Dermatology; Aging Skin; Sclerotherapy; Laser Surgery; **Hospital:** NYU Langone Med Ctr (page 108), Lawrence Hosp Ctr; **Address:** 559 Gramatan Ave, Ste 205, Mt Vernon, NY 10552; **Phone:** 914-667-2242; **Board Cert:** Dermatology 1979; **Med School:** NY Med Coll 1975; **Resid:** Dermatology, NYU Med Ctr 1979; **Fellow:** Dermatologic Surgery, NYU Med Ctr 1980; **Fac Appt:** Assoc Clin Prof D, NYU Sch Med

Narins, Rhoda S MD (D) - **Spec Exp:** Liposuction; Cosmetic Dermatology; Botox Therapy; Facial Rejuvenation; **Hospital:** NYU Langone Med Ctr (page 108), White Plains Hosp (page 640); **Address:** 222 Westchester Ave, Ste 300, White Plains, NY 10604-2925; **Phone:** 914-684-1000; **Board Cert:** Dermatology 1970; **Med School:** NYU Sch Med 1965; **Resid:** Dermatology, NYU Med Ctr 1969; **Fac Appt:** Clin Prof D, NYU Sch Med

Newburger, Amy E MD (D) - **Spec Exp:** Contact Dermatitis; Cosmetic Dermatology; **Address:** 2 Overhill Rd, Ste 330, Scarsdale, NY 10583; **Phone:** 914-725-1800; **Board Cert:** Dermatology 1979; **Med School:** NYU Sch Med 1974; **Resid:** Dermatology, Univ Miami Hosps 1978

Schachne, Jeffrey P MD (D) - **Spec Exp:** Skin Laser Surgery; **Hospital:** Hudson Valley Hosp Ctr; **Address:** 3630 Hill Blvd, Ste 101, Jefferson Valley, NY 10535; **Phone:** 914-962-6222; **Board Cert:** Dermatology 1988; **Med School:** SUNY Downstate 1984; **Resid:** Dermatology, Einstein Affil Hosp 1988

Schliftman, Alan B MD (D) - **Spec Exp:** Skin Laser Surgery; Skin Cancer; Cosmetic Dermatology; **Hospital:** Westchester Med Ctr; **Address:** 244 Westchester Ave, Ste 211, White Plains, NY 10604-2926; **Phone:** 914-761-1400; **Board Cert:** Dermatology 1981; **Med School:** Geo Wash Univ 1977; **Resid:** Dermatology, Montefiore Med Ctr 1981; **Fac Appt:** Asst Clin Prof D, NY Med Coll

Stillman, Michael MD (D) - **Spec Exp:** Skin Cancer; Acne; Eczema; **Hospital:** Northern Westchester Hosp (page 639); **Address:** Mt Kisco Medical Group, 111 Bedford Rd, Katonah, NY 10536; **Phone:** 914-232-3135; **Board Cert:** Dermatology 1973; **Med School:** SUNY Downstate 1967; **Resid:** Dermatology, NYU Med Ctr 1973; **Fellow:** Dermatology, Letterman Army Inst Rsch 1970

Sturza, Jeffrey MD (D) - **Spec Exp:** Psoriasis; Skin Laser Surgery; Cosmetic Dermatology; **Hospital:** Phelps Meml Hosp Ctr; **Address:** 150 White Plains Rd, Ste 210, Tarrytown, NY 10591; **Phone:** 914-631-4666; **Board Cert:** Dermatology 1988; **Med School:** SUNY Hlth Sci Ctr 1984; **Resid:** Dermatology, Cook Co Hosp 1988

Treiber, Ruth K MD (D) - **Spec Exp:** Botox Therapy; Acne; Facial Rejuvenation; Skin Cancer; **Hospital:** NY-Presby/Columbia Univ Med Ctr, NY (page 104); **Address:** 175 Purchase St, Rye, NY 10580; **Phone:** 914-967-2153; **Board Cert:** Dermatology 1983; **Med School:** Cornell Univ-Weill Med Coll 1978; **Resid:** Internal Medicine, New York Hosp 1980; Dermatology, Columbia-Presby Med Ctr 1983; **Fac Appt:** Assoc Clin Prof D, Columbia P&S

Zeltser, Ross MD (D) - **Spec Exp:** Mohs' Surgery; Skin Cancer; **Hospital:** Northern Westchester Hosp (page 639); **Address:** 185 Kisco Ave, Ste 300, Mt Kisco, NY 10549; **Phone:** 914-242-2020; **Board Cert:** Dermatology ; **Med School:** Univ Rochester 2002; **Resid:** Internal Medicine, Lenox Hill Hosp 2003; Dermatology, Boston Med Ctr/Tufts Med Ctr 2006; **Fellow:** Mohs Surgery, Tufts Med Ctr 2007

Zweibel, Stuart M MD/PhD (D) - **Spec Exp:** Mohs' Surgery; Skin Cancer; Skin Laser Surgery; Cosmetic Dermatology; **Hospital:** Northern Westchester Hosp (page 639); **Address:** 185 Kisco Ave, Ste 300, Mt Kisco, NY 10549; **Phone:** 914-242-2020; **Board Cert:** Dermatology 2009; **Med School:** Mount Sinai Sch Med 1985; **Resid:** Dermatology, Rhode Island Hosp 1989; **Fellow:** Mohs Surgery, Univ Wisconsin 1991

Diagnostic Radiology

Hertz, Marc MD (DR) - **Spec Exp:** CT Scan; MRI; **Address:** Mt Kisco Medical Group, Radiology, 90 S Bedford Rd, Mount Kisco, NY 10549; **Phone:** 914-242-1395; **Board Cert:** Diagnostic Radiology 1985; **Med School:** Howard Univ 1979; **Resid:** Pathology, Lenox Hill Hospital 1981; Diagnostic Radiology, Montefiore Hospital 1984; **Fellow:** Ultrasound/CT, North Shore Univ Hosp 1985

Hibbard, Claire MD (DR) - **Spec Exp:** Women's Imaging; Mammography; **Address:** Mount Kisco Medical Group, Radiology, 110 S Bedford Rd, Mount Kisco, NY 10549-3412; **Phone:** 914-232-3135; **Board Cert:** Diagnostic Radiology 1989; **Med School:** Columbia P&S 1984; **Resid:** Diagnostic Radiology, Hosp U Penn 1989; **Fellow:** Musculoskeletal Imaging, Hosp U Penn 1990; **Fac Appt:** Asst Clin Prof Rad, Albert Einstein Coll Med

Khoury, Paul MD (DR) - **Hospital:** White Plains Hosp (page 640); **Address:** White Plains Hosp Ctr, Dept Radiology, 41 E Post Rd, White Plains, NY 10601; **Phone:** 914-681-1219; **Board Cert:** Diagnostic Radiology 1979; Nuclear Radiology 1980; **Med School:** Lebanon 1973; **Resid:** Diagnostic Radiology, Hotel Dieu de France Hosp 1975; Diagnostic Radiology, St Luke's-Roosevelt Hosp Ctr 1979

Kutcher, Rosalyn MD (DR) - **Spec Exp:** Mammography; Ultrasound; Women's Imaging; **Hospital:** White Plains Hosp (page 640); **Address:** 90 S Ridge St, Women's Imaging Ctr, Rye Brook, NY 10573; **Phone:** 914-935-0011; **Board Cert:** Diagnostic Radiology 1975; **Med School:** SUNY Hlth Sci Ctr 1970; **Resid:** Diagnostic Radiology, Montefiore Med Ctr 1974; **Fac Appt:** Prof Rad, Albert Einstein Coll Med

Lefkovitz, Zvi MD (DR) - **Spec Exp:** Thoracic Radiology; **Hospital:** Westchester Med Ctr; **Address:** WMC Advanced Physician Services, 100 Woods Rd, Valhalla, NY 10595; **Phone:** 914-493-6692; **Board Cert:** Diagnostic Radiology 1986; **Med School:** Ros Franklin Univ/Chicago Med Sch 1982; **Resid:** Diagnostic Radiology, Maimonides Med Ctr 1986; **Fellow:** Interventional Radiology, Univ Hosp 1987; **Fac Appt:** Clin Prof Rad, NY Med Coll

Leslie, Denise MD (DR) - **Spec Exp:** Neuroradiology; **Hospital:** Good Samaritan Regional Med Ctr; **Address:** Hartsdale Imaging, 141 S Central Ave, Hartsdale, NY 10530; **Phone:** 914-345-0376; **Board Cert:** Diagnostic Radiology 1985; **Med School:** SUNY Buffalo 1981; **Resid:** Diagnostic Radiology, Metropolitan Med Ctr 1985; **Fellow:** Neuroradiology, Westchester Co Med Ctr 1987

LoRusso, Diane MD (DR) - **Spec Exp:** Breast Imaging; Women's Health; Ultrasound; Mammography-Digital; **Address:** Rye Radiology Assoc, 30 Rye Ridge Plaza, Rye Brook, NY 10573-2830; **Phone:** 914-253-9200; **Board Cert:** Diagnostic Radiology 1974; **Med School:** SUNY Upstate Med Univ 1969; **Resid:** Diagnostic Radiology, Montefiore Med Ctr 1974

Poplausky, Maurice R MD (DR) - **Spec Exp:** Interventional Radiology; **Hospital:** Hudson Valley Hosp Ctr, Westchester Med Ctr; **Address:** Hudson Valley Hospital, Dept Radiology, 1980 Crompound Rd, Cortland Manor, NY 10567; **Phone:** 914-734-3680; **Board Cert:** Diagnostic Radiology 1995; Vascular & Interventional Radiology 2008; **Med School:** SUNY Buffalo 1990; **Resid:** Diagnostic Radiology, SUNY Downstate Med Ctr 1995; **Fellow:** Vascular & Interventional Radiology, Mass Genl Hosp 1996; **Fac Appt:** Assoc Prof Rad, NY Med Coll

Staeger-Hirsch, Christine N MD (DR) - **Spec Exp:** Breast Imaging; **Address:** Rye Radiology, 30 Rye Ridge Plaza, Rye Brook, NY 10573-2830; **Phone:** 914-253-9200; **Board Cert:** Diagnostic Radiology 2006; **Med School:** NYU Sch Med 2001; **Resid:** Diagnostic Radiology, St Luke's Roosevelt Med Ctr 2006; **Fellow:** Breast Imaging, NYU Med Ctr 2007

Wald, Leonard A MD (DR) - **Spec Exp:** Body Imaging; Women's Imaging; **Hospital:** Northern Westchester Hosp (page 639); **Address:** Mount Kisco Medical Group, 90 S Bedford Rd, Mt Kisco, NY 10549; **Phone:** 914-241-1050; **Board Cert:** Diagnostic Radiology 1985; **Med School:** Albert Einstein Coll Med 1981; **Resid:** Diagnostic Radiology, Montefiore Med Ctr 1985; **Fellow:** Ultrasound/CT/MRI, Thomas Jefferson Univ Hosp 1986

Weiss, Jonathan D MD (DR) - ; **Address:** Westmed Medical Group, Radiology, 210 Westchester Ave, White Plains, NY 10601; **Phone:** 914-682-6430; **Board Cert:** Diagnostic Radiology 1987; **Med School:** Tufts Univ 1983; **Resid:** Diagnostic Radiology, SUNY Downstate Med Ctr 1987; **Fellow:** Interventional Radiology, SUNY Downstate Med Ctr 1988

Endocrinology, Diabetes & Metabolism

Albin, Joan T MD (EDM) - **Spec Exp:** Diabetes; Thyroid Disorders; Polycystic Ovarian Syndrome; **Hospital:** Montefiore New Rochelle Hosp, Lawrence Hosp Ctr; **Address:** 77 Pondfield Rd, Bronxville, NY 10708; **Phone:** 914-793-1500; **Board Cert:** Internal Medicine 1972; Endocrinology, Diabetes & Metabolism 1973; **Med School:** NY Med Coll 1967; **Resid:** Internal Medicine, Metropolitan Hosp 1969; Internal Medicine, Montefiore Med Ctr 1970; **Fellow:** Endocrinology, Diabetes & Metabolism, Mount Sinai Hosp 1971; Endocrinology, Diabetes & Metabolism, Westchester Co Med Ctr 1972; **Fac Appt:** Assoc Prof Med, Albert Einstein Coll Med

Bloomgarden, David K MD (EDM) - **Spec Exp:** Diabetes; Osteoporosis; Thyroid Disorders; Hypogonadism-Male; **Hospital:** White Plains Hosp (page 640); **Address:** Scarsdale Medical Group, 550 Mamaroneck Ave, Ste 101, Harrison, NY 10528; **Phone:** 914-723-8100 x302; **Board Cert:** Internal Medicine 1980; Endocrinology, Diabetes & Metabolism 1983; **Med School:** NYU Sch Med 1977; **Resid:** Internal Medicine, Albert Einstein/Jacobi Med Ctr 1980; **Fellow:** Endocrinology, Diabetes & Metabolism, Albert Einstein 1982

Blum, David MD (EDM) - **Spec Exp:** Diabetes; Osteoporosis; Thyroid Disorders; **Hospital:** Montefiore New Rochelle Hosp; **Address:** Diabetes Center - 5th Floor, 16 Guion Pl, New Rochelle, NY 10801; **Phone:** 914-633-8680; **Board Cert:** Internal Medicine 1977; Endocrinology, Diabetes & Metabolism 1979; **Med School:** Northwestern Univ 1974; **Resid:** Internal Medicine, Mt Sinai Hosp 1977; **Fellow:** Endocrinology, Mt Sinai Hosp 1979; **Fac Appt:** Asst Clin Prof Med, NY Med Coll

Gitler, Ellen S MD (EDM) - **Spec Exp:** Cardiac Rehabilitation; **Hospital:** Burke Rehab Hosp; **Address:** 785 Mamaroneck Ave, White Plains, NY 10605-2523; **Phone:** 914-597-2409; **Board Cert:** Internal Medicine 1980; Endocrinology, Diabetes & Metabolism 1983; **Med School:** Cornell Univ-Weill Med Coll 1977; **Resid:** Internal Medicine, Bronx Muni Hosp 1980; **Fellow:** Endocrinology, Diabetes & Metabolism, Mount Sinai Med Ctr 1982

Hellerman, James MD (EDM) - **Spec Exp:** Thyroid Disorders; Diabetes; Calcium Disorders; **Hospital:** Phelps Meml Hosp Ctr; **Address:** 200 S Broadway, Ste 100, Tarrytown, NY 10591-4504; **Phone:** 914-631-9300; **Board Cert:** Internal Medicine 1979; Endocrinology 1983; **Med School:** Univ Rochester 1976; **Resid:** Internal Medicine, Montefiore Med Ctr 1980; **Fellow:** Endocrinology, Diabetes & Metabolism, Mass Genl Hosp 1984

Kantor, Alan MD (EDM) - **Spec Exp:** Thyroid Disorders; Osteoporosis; Diabetes; Endocrine Tumors; **Hospital:** Northern Westchester Hosp (page 639); **Address:** 1940 Commerce St, Ste 310, Yorktown Heights, NY 10598; **Phone:** 914-245-1111; **Board Cert:** Internal Medicine 1981; Endocrinology, Diabetes & Metabolism 1983; **Med School:** South Africa 1975; **Resid:** Internal Medicine, La Guardia Hosp 1980; Internal Medicine, LI Jewish-Hillside Med Ctr 1981; **Fellow:** Endocrinology, Diabetes & Metabolism, Meml Sloan Kettering Cancer Ctr 1983; **Fac Appt:** Asst Clin Prof Med, NY Med Coll

Kleinbaum, Jerry I MD (EDM) - **Spec Exp:** Diabetes; **Hospital:** Putnam Hosp Ctr, Hudson Valley Hosp Ctr; **Address:** Mount Kisco Medical Group-Endocrinology, 46 Route 6 at Mahopac Ave, Ste 103, Yorktown Heights, NY 10598; **Phone:** 914-864-4170; **Board Cert:** Internal Medicine 1979; Endocrinology 1985; **Med School:** Tufts Univ 1976; **Resid:** Internal Medicine, Montefiore Med Ctr 1980; **Fellow:** Endocrinology, Diabetes & Metabolism, Montefiore Med Ctr 1981

Leibowitz, Jonas MD (EDM) - **Spec Exp:** Diabetes; Osteoporosis; Thyroid Disorders; Nutrition; **Hospital:** Lawrence Hosp Ctr, White Plains Hosp (page 640); **Address:** 770 B McLean Ave, Yonkers, NY 10704; **Phone:** 914-237-3636; **Board Cert:** Internal Medicine 2005; Endocrinology, Diabetes & Metabolism 2007; **Med School:** SUNY Downstate 1992; **Resid:** Internal Medicine, Mt Sinai Med Ctr 1995; **Fellow:** Endocrinology, Mt Sinai Med Ctr 1997; **Fac Appt:** Asst Clin Prof Med, NY Med Coll

Powell, Jeffrey S MD (EDM) - **Hospital:** Northern Westchester Hosp (page 639); **Address:** Mount Kisco Med Group, 90 S Bedford Rd, Mount Kisco, NY 10549; **Phone:** 914-241-1050; **Board Cert:** Internal Medicine 2008; Endocrinology, Diabetes & Metabolism 2010; **Med School:** Albert Einstein Coll Med 1995; **Resid:** Internal Medicine, Columbia-Presby Med Ctr 1998; **Fellow:** Endocrinology, Diabetes & Metabolism, Columbia-Presby Med Ctr 2001

Pretto, Zorayda MD (EDM) - **Hospital:** White Plains Hosp (page 640); **Address:** Mid-Westchester Medical Assocs, 210 Westchester Ave, White Plains, NY 10605; **Phone:** 914-831-4150; **Board Cert:** Internal Medicine 2005; Endocrinology, Diabetes & Metabolism 2006; **Med School:** Panama 1986; **Resid:** Internal Medicine, St John's Episcopal Hosp 1991; **Fellow:** Endocrinology, Diabetes & Metabolism, Beth Israel Hosp 1993

Rudin, Eric A MD (EDM) - **Spec Exp:** Diabetes; **Hospital:** Northern Westchester Hosp (page 639); **Address:** MKMG, Endocrinology, 111 Bedford Rd, Katonah, NY 10549; **Phone:** 914-232-3135; **Board Cert:** Internal Medicine 2003; Endocrinology, Diabetes & Metabolism 2005; **Med School:** Mount Sinai Sch Med 2000; **Resid:** Internal Medicine, Thomas Jefferson Univ Hosp` 2003; **Fellow:** Endocrinology, Diabetes & Metabolism, Montefiore Med Ctr 2005

Stein, Randy MD (EDM) - **Spec Exp:** Diabetes; Osteoporosis; **Hospital:** White Plains Hosp (page 640); **Address:** Westchester Medical Group-Endocrinology, 210 Westchester Ave, White Plains, NY 10604; **Phone:** 914-831-4150; **Board Cert:** Internal Medicine 1981; Endocrinology, Diabetes & Metabolism 1983; **Med School:** Albert Einstein Coll Med 1978; **Resid:** Internal Medicine, Montefiore Med Ctr 1981; **Fellow:** Endocrinology, Diabetes & Metabolism, Montefiore Med Ctr 1983

Weiser, Kenneth R MD (EDM) - **Spec Exp:** Diabetes; Osteoporosis; **Hospital:** White Plains Hosp (page 640); **Address:** Westchester Med Group-Endocrinolgy, 210 Westchester Ave, White Plains, NY 10604; **Phone:** 914-831-4150; **Board Cert:** Internal Medicine 2003; Endocrinology, Diabetes & Metabolism 2005; **Med School:** Albert Einstein Coll Med 1990; **Resid:** Internal Medicine, Jacobi Med Ctr 1993; **Fellow:** Endocrinology, Diabetes & Metabolism, Mt Sinai Med Ctr 1995

Family Medicine

Annabi, Iyad N MD (FMed) *PCP* - **Hospital:** St. John's Riverside Hosp-Andrus Pavil; **Address:** Westchester Family Medicine Practice, 472 Palmer Rd, Yonkers, NY 10701-5207; **Phone:** 914-375-2300; **Board Cert:** Family Medicine 2008; **Med School:** Mexico 1988; **Resid:** Family Medicine, St Joseph Med Ctr 1995

Apuzzo, Thomas R MD (FMed) *PCP* - **Hospital:** Saint Joseph's Med Ctr - Yonkers, St. John's Riverside Hosp-Andrus Pavil; **Address:** 955 Yonkers Ave, Yonkers, NY 10704; **Phone:** 914-237-0994; **Board Cert:** Family Medicine 2009; **Med School:** Italy 1985; **Resid:** Surgery, Caledonian Hosp 1986; Family Medicine, St Joseph's Med Ctr 1989

Gottesfeld, Peter Michael MD (FMed) *PCP* - **Spec Exp:** Aging; Preventive Medicine; ADD/ADHD; **Hospital:** Northern Westchester Hosp (page 639), Hudson Valley Hosp Ctr; **Address:** 101 S Bedford Rd, Ste 412, Mt Kisco, NY 10549-3455; **Phone:** 914-241-7800; **Board Cert:** Family Medicine 2010; **Med School:** UMDNJ-RW Johnson Med Sch 1985; **Resid:** Family Medicine, Thomas Jefferson U Hosp 1988; **Fac Appt:** Assoc Clin Prof FMed, NY Med Coll

Merker, Edward L MD (FMed) *PCP* - **Spec Exp:** Geriatric Care; **Hospital:** Phelps Meml Hosp Ctr; **Address:** 180 Marble Ave, North Star Medical Group, Pleasantville, NY 10570; **Phone:** 914-769-7300 x202; **Board Cert:** Family Medicine 2012; **Med School:** Albert Einstein Coll Med 1981; **Resid:** Family Medicine, Overlook Hosp 1984

Miller, Daniel MD (FMed) *PCP* - **Hospital:** St. John's Riverside Hosp-Andrus Pavil, Saint Joseph's Med Ctr - Yonkers; **Address:** Hudson River HealthCare, 503 S Broadway, Yonkers, NY 10703; **Phone:** 914-965-9771; **Board Cert:** Family Medicine 2007; **Med School:** Univ Cincinnati 1984; **Resid:** Family Medicine, Montefiore Med Ctr 1987; **Fac Appt:** Asst Prof FMed, NY Med Coll

Piccirilli, Dora C MD (FMed) *PCP* - **Hospital:** Phelps Meml Hosp Ctr; **Address:** 180 Marble Ave, North Star Medical Group, Pleasantville, NY 10570; **Phone:** 914-769-7300; **Board Cert:** Family Medicine 2005; **Med School:** SUNY Hlth Sci Ctr 1988; **Resid:** Family Medicine, Overlook Hosp 1991

Sharpe, Arleen S MD (FMed) *PCP* - **Hospital:** Lawrence Hosp Ctr, White Plains Hosp (page 640); **Address:** West Med Group, 73 Market St, Yonkers, NY 10710; **Phone:** 914-693-1660; **Board Cert:** Family Medicine 2005; **Med School:** SUNY Stony Brook 1988; **Resid:** Family Medicine, Montefiore Med Ctr 1991

Strongwater, Richard F MD (FMed) *PCP* - **Spec Exp:** Travel Medicine; **Hospital:** Phelps Meml Hosp Ctr; **Address:** North Star Medical, 180 Marble Ave, Pleasantville, NY 10570; **Phone:** 914-769-7300; **Board Cert:** Family Medicine 2012; **Med School:** SUNY Upstate Med Univ 1981; **Resid:** Family Medicine, Overlook Hosp 1984

Sutton, Ira MD (FMed) *PCP* - **Spec Exp:** Preventive Medicine; Skin Diseases; **Hospital:** White Plains Hosp (page 640), Montefiore New Rochelle Hosp; **Address:** 2 Overhill Rd, Ste 225, Scarsdale, NY 10583; **Phone:** 914-636-0077; **Board Cert:** Family Medicine 2008; **Med School:** Albert Einstein Coll Med 1980; **Resid:** Family Medicine, Brown Univ/Memorial Hosp 1983

Vaidya, Sudhir P MD (FMed) - **Spec Exp:** Primary Care Sports Medicine; Pain Management; Geriatric Rehabilitation; **Hospital:** Burke Rehab Hosp, St. Joseph's Hosp-Nassau; **Address:** Burke Rehab Hosp, 785 Mamaroneck Ave, White Plains, NY 10605; **Phone:** 914-597-2332; **Board Cert:** Family Medicine 2005; Sports Medicine 2011; **Med School:** India 1979; **Resid:** Physical Medicine & Rehabilitation, NHS Hosps-Leicester, Milton Keynes-Bedford 1995; Family Medicine, St Joseph's Hosp 1998; **Fac Appt:** Asst Clin Prof Med, Cornell Univ-Weill Med Coll

Yudin, Howard MD (FMed) *PCP* - **Hospital:** Greenwich Hosp (page 938); **Address:** 18 Rye Ridge Plaza, Rye Brook, NY 10573-2820; **Phone:** 914-251-1261; **Board Cert:** Family Medicine 2008; **Med School:** Univ Montreal 1974; **Resid:** Family Medicine, Jewish Genl Hosp 1976

Gastroenterology

Abemayor, Elie M MD (Ge) - **Spec Exp:** Inflammatory Bowel Disease; Endoscopy; Irritable Bowel Syndrome; Gastroesophageal Reflux Disease (GERD); **Hospital:** Northern Westchester Hosp (page 639); **Address:** 91 Smith Ave, Mt Kisco, NY 10549-2810; **Phone:** 914-241-9026; **Board Cert:** Internal Medicine 1988; Gastroenterology 2005; **Med School:** SUNY Stony Brook 1985; **Resid:** Internal Medicine, NYU-Bellevue Med Ctr 1988; **Fellow:** Gastroenterology, NYU/Manhattan VA Med Ctr 1990; **Fac Appt:** Asst Clin Prof Med, NYU Sch Med

Antonelle, Robert W MD (Ge) - **Spec Exp:** Gastroesophageal Reflux Disease (GERD); Liver & Biliary Disease; Colonoscopy; **Hospital:** White Plains Hosp (page 640); **Address:** White Plains Gastroenterologists, 311 North St, rm 403, White Plains, NY 10605-2232; **Phone:** 914-949-7171; **Board Cert:** Gastroenterology 2006; **Med School:** NY Med Coll 1989; **Resid:** Internal Medicine, Westchester Med Ctr 1992; **Fellow:** Gastroenterology, Westchester Med Ctr 1995

Auerbach, Mitchell E MD (Ge) - **Spec Exp:** Colonoscopy; Crohn's Disease; Ulcerative Colitis; **Hospital:** Saint Joseph's Med Ctr - Yonkers, St. John's Riverside Hosp-Andrus Pavil; **Address:** Westchester Digestive Disease Group, 469 N Broadway, Yonkers, NY 10701-1923; **Phone:** 914-969-1115; **Board Cert:** Gastroenterology 2008; **Med School:** Tufts Univ 1991; **Resid:** Internal Medicine, Mt Sinai Hosp 1994; **Fellow:** Gastroenterology, Mt Sinai Hosp 1996

Byfield, Floyd MD (Ge) - **Hospital:** Phelps Meml Hosp Ctr; **Address:** Westchester Gastroenterology Assocs, 777 N Broadway, Ste 305, North Tarrytown, NY 10591; **Phone:** 914-366-6120; **Board Cert:** Internal Medicine 2006; Gastroenterology 2009; **Med School:** Mount Sinai Sch Med 1993; **Resid:** Internal Medicine, Ny Presby-Cornell Med Ctr 1996; **Fellow:** Gastroenterology, NY Presby-Cornell Med Ctr 1998

Chinitz, Marvin MD (Ge) - **Spec Exp:** Colonoscopy; Inflammatory Bowel Disease; Liver Disease; Gastroesophageal Reflux Disease (GERD); **Hospital:** Northern Westchester Hosp (page 639); **Address:** MKMG, Gastroenterology, 90 S Bedford Rd, Mt Kisco, NY 10549-3422; **Phone:** 914-241-1050; **Board Cert:** Internal Medicine 1981; Gastroenterology 1985; **Med School:** Boston Univ 1978; **Resid:** Internal Medicine, Boston Med Ctr 1981; **Fellow:** Gastroenterology, Montefiore Med Ctr 1984; **Fac Appt:** Assoc Prof Med, Albert Einstein Coll Med

Dworkin, Brad M MD (Ge) - **Spec Exp:** Gastrointestinal Motility Disorders; Nutrition; Inflammatory Bowel Disease; **Hospital:** Westchester Med Ctr; **Address:** 19 Bradhurst Ave, 2550 South, Hawthorne, NY 10595; **Phone:** 914-493-7337; **Board Cert:** Internal Medicine 1979; Gastroenterology 1981; **Med School:** Jefferson Med Coll 1976; **Resid:** Internal Medicine, New York Hosp 1979; **Fellow:** Gastroenterology, Meml Sloan Kettering Cancer Ctr 1981; Nutrition, Meml Sloan Kettering Cancer Ctr 1982; **Fac Appt:** Prof Med, NY Med Coll

Ehrlich, James B MD (Ge) - **Spec Exp:** Esophageal Disorders; Gastroesophageal Reflux Disease (GERD); Gastrointestinal Motility Disorders; **Hospital:** Lawrence Hosp Ctr; **Address:** WestMed Medical Group, 73 Market St, Ste 219, Yonkers, NY 10710; **Phone:** 914-831-6820; **Board Cert:** Internal Medicine 1983; Gastroenterology 1985; **Med School:** Univ Hlth Scis, Chicago Med Sch 1980; **Resid:** Internal Medicine, Univ Illinois Med Ctr 1983; **Fellow:** Gastroenterology, Michael Reese/Univ of Chicago Med Ctr 1985

Fath Jr, Robert MD (Ge) - **Spec Exp:** Colonoscopy; **Hospital:** White Plains Hosp (page 640); **Address:** Scarsdale Medical Group, 550 Mamaroneck Ave, Ste 101, Harrison, NY 10528; **Phone:** 914-723-8100 x309; **Board Cert:** Internal Medicine 1981; Gastroenterology 1983; **Med School:** Univ Miss 1978; **Resid:** Internal Medicine, N Shore Hosp 1981; **Fellow:** Gastroenterology, Meml Sloan-Kettering Cancer Ctr 1983; **Fac Appt:** Med, Cornell Univ-Weill Med Coll

Field, Barry E MD (Ge) - **Spec Exp:** Ulcerative Colitis; Crohn's Disease; **Hospital:** Phelps Meml Hosp Ctr; **Address:** Westchester Gastroenterology, 777 N Broadway Fl 3 - Ste 305, Sleepy Hollow, NY 10591-1040; **Phone:** 914-366-6120; **Board Cert:** Internal Medicine 1976; Gastroenterology 1979; **Med School:** Albert Einstein Coll Med 1972; **Resid:** Internal Medicine, Metropolitan Hosp Ctr 1976; **Fellow:** Gastroenterology, Harbor Genl Hosp 1978

Finegold, Jonathan MD (Ge) - **Spec Exp:** Barrett's Esophagus; Colon Cancer; Inflammatory Bowel Disease/Crohn's; **Hospital:** Lawrence Hosp Ctr; **Address:** WestMed Med Grp, Ridge Hill, 73 Market St, Ste 219, Yonkers, NY 10710; **Phone:** 914-831-6820; **Board Cert:** Internal Medicine 2005; Gastroenterology 2007; **Med School:** Univ Miami Sch Med 1991; **Resid:** Internal Medicine, NY-Presby/Columbia Med Ctr 1994; **Fellow:** Gastroenterology, NY-Presby/Columbia Med Ctr 1997

Geders, Jane MD/PhD (Ge) - **Spec Exp:** Hepatitis C; Nutrition; Colon Cancer Screening; **Hospital:** Northern Westchester Hosp (page 639); **Address:** 90 S Bedford Rd, Mt Kisco, NY 10549; **Phone:** 914-242-1307; **Board Cert:** Gastroenterology 2003; **Med School:** Univ S Fla Coll Med 1987; **Resid:** Internal Medicine, Meml Sloan Kettering Cancer Ctr 1990; **Fellow:** Gastroenterology, Mt Sinai Med Ctr 1992; Hepatology, Mt Sinai Med Ctr 1993

Gendler, Seth MD (Ge) - **Spec Exp:** Pancreatic/Biliary Endoscopy (ERCP); Biliary Disease; Pancreatic Disease; **Hospital:** White Plains Hosp (page 640); **Address:** 1296 North Ave Fl 2, New Rochelle, NY 10804; **Phone:** 914-235-0918; **Board Cert:** Internal Medicine 1986; Gastroenterology 2011; **Med School:** Rush Med Coll 1983; **Resid:** Internal Medicine, St Lukes Hosp 1986; **Fellow:** Gastroenterology, St Lukes Hosp 1988; Endoscopy, Univ Hosp 1989

Genn, David A MD (Ge) - **Spec Exp:** Colon Cancer Screening; Biliary Disease; Gastroesophageal Reflux Disease (GERD); Barrett's Esophagus; **Hospital:** Hudson Valley Hosp Ctr; **Address:** 1985 Crompond Road, Bldg D, Cortlandt Manor, NY 10567-4146; **Phone:** 914-739-2400; **Board Cert:** Gastroenterology 2003; **Med School:** Boston Univ 1988; **Resid:** Internal Medicine, Montefiore Med Ctr 1991; **Fellow:** Gastroenterology, Westchester Med Ctr 1993

Goldblatt, Robert MD (Ge) - **Spec Exp:** Liver Disease; Biliary Disease; Endoscopy; Inflammatory Bowel Disease; **Hospital:** White Plains Hosp (page 640), Greenwich Hosp (page 938); **Address:** 18 Rye Ridge Plaza, Rye Brook, NY 10573-2820; **Phone:** 914-253-9252; **Board Cert:** Internal Medicine 1978; Gastroenterology 1979; **Med School:** Geo Wash Univ 1974; **Resid:** Internal Medicine, Univ FL-Shands Hosp 1977; **Fellow:** Gastroenterology, Yale-New Haven Hosp 1979; **Fac Appt:** Asst Clin Prof Med, Cornell Univ-Weill Med Coll

Gould, Richard B MD (Ge) - **Spec Exp:** Colonoscopy; Gastroscopy; **Hospital:** Lawrence Hosp Ctr, Montefiore Med Ctr-Einstein Campus (page 100); **Address:** 1 Pondfield Rd W, Ste 1R, Bronxville, NY 10708; **Phone:** 914-779-6200; **Board Cert:** Internal Medicine 1975; Gastroenterology 1977; **Med School:** SUNY Upstate Med Univ 1972; **Resid:** Internal Medicine, Montefiore Hosp Med Ctr 1975; **Fellow:** Gastroenterology, Montefiore Hosp Med Ctr 1977; **Fac Appt:** Assoc Clin Prof Med, Columbia P&S

Heier, Stephen K MD (Ge) - **Spec Exp:** Colonoscopy/Polypectomy; Gastric & Esophageal Disorders; Pancreatic/Biliary Endoscopy (ERCP); **Hospital:** Phelps Meml Hosp Ctr; **Address:** Phelps Memorial Hosp, Advanced Endoscopy & Gastroenterology, 755 N Broadway, Ste 530, Sleepy Hollow, NY 10591; **Phone:** 914-366-1190; **Board Cert:** Internal Medicine 1979; Gastroenterology 1981; **Med School:** Albany Med Coll 1976; **Resid:** Internal Medicine, Metro Hosp Ctr 1979; **Fellow:** Gastroenterology, Tufts Univ 1981; **Fac Appt:** Clin Prof Med, NY Med Coll

Hillman, Deborah L MD (Ge) - **Spec Exp:** Women's Health; Irritable Bowel Syndrome; **Hospital:** Northern Westchester Hosp (page 639); **Address:** Mount Kisco Medical Group, 90 S Bedford Rd, Mount Kisco, NY 10549-3412; **Phone:** 914-241-1050; **Board Cert:** Internal Medicine 2002; Gastroenterology 2006; **Med School:** NYU Sch Med 1999; **Resid:** Internal Medicine, Columbia Presby Med Ctr 2002; **Fellow:** Gastroenterology, Montefiore Med Ctr 2005

Jaffe, Alan H MD (Ge) - **Hospital:** White Plains Hosp (page 640); **Address:** WestMed Medical Group, 210 Westchester Ave Fl 2 - Ste 205, White Plains, NY 10604; **Phone:** 914-682-6466; **Board Cert:** Internal Medicine 1977; Gastroenterology 1979; **Med School:** Cornell Univ-Weill Med Coll 1974; **Resid:** Internal Medicine, N Shore U Med Ctr 1977; **Fellow:** Gastroenterology, St Raphael Hosp 1979

Kahn, Oren MD (Ge) - **Spec Exp:** Inflammatory Bowel Disease; Peptic Ulcer Disease; Gastroesophageal Reflux Disease (GERD); Colonoscopy; **Hospital:** Northern Westchester Hosp (page 639); **Address:** Mount Kisco Medical Group, 90 S Bedford Rd, Mount Kisco, NY 10549; **Phone:** 914-241-1050; **Board Cert:** Internal Medicine 2004; Gastroenterology 2007; **Med School:** Albert Einstein Coll Med 1990; **Resid:** Internal Medicine, Mt Sinai Med Ctr 1994; **Fellow:** Gastroenterology, Mt Sinai Med Ctr 1996; **Fac Appt:** Assoc Clin Prof Med, Mount Sinai Sch Med

Katz, Henry J MD (Ge) - **Hospital:** Montefiore Med Ctr-Moses Campus (page 100), St. John's Riverside Hosp-Andrus Pavil; **Address:** 1234 Central Park Ave, Yonkers, NY 10704-1068; **Phone:** 914-793-1600; **Board Cert:** Internal Medicine 1983; Gastroenterology 1985; **Med School:** Albany Med Coll 1980; **Resid:** Internal Medicine, Bellevue Hosp 1983; **Fellow:** Gastroenterology, Montefiore Med Ctr 1985

Kozicky, Orest J MD (Ge) - **Spec Exp:** Colitis; Peptic Ulcer Disease; Gastroesophageal Reflux Disease (GERD); **Hospital:** St. John's Riverside Hosp-Andrus Pavil; **Address:** Westchester Digestive Disease Grp, 469 N Broadway Fl 1st, Yonkers, NY 10701-1923; **Phone:** 914-969-1115; **Board Cert:** Internal Medicine 1985; Gastroenterology 1987; **Med School:** NY Med Coll 1981; **Resid:** Internal Medicine, Jacobi Med Ctr 1985; **Fellow:** Gastroenterology, Montefiore Hosp Med Ctr 1987; **Fac Appt:** Assoc Clin Prof Med, Albert Einstein Coll Med

Kressner, Michael MD (Ge) - **Spec Exp:** Colon Cancer; Inflammatory Bowel Disease; Biliary Disease; **Hospital:** Montefiore New Rochelle Hosp, Montefiore Mt Vernon Hosp; **Address:** 140 Lockwood Ave, Ste 110, New Rochelle, NY 10801-4907; **Phone:** 914-636-5222; **Board Cert:** Internal Medicine 1980; Gastroenterology 1983; **Med School:** SUNY Buffalo 1977; **Resid:** Internal Medicine, Jacobi Med Ctr 1980; **Fellow:** Gastroenterology, Jacobi Med Ctr 1982

Landau, Steven R MD (Ge) - **Spec Exp:** Inflammatory Bowel Disease; Colon Cancer; **Hospital:** White Plains Hosp (page 640); **Address:** 30 Greenridge Ave, White Plains, NY 10605; **Phone:** 914-328-8555; **Board Cert:** Internal Medicine 1984; Gastroenterology 1987; **Med School:** NYU Sch Med 1981; **Resid:** Internal Medicine, Jacobi Med Ctr 1982; Internal Medicine, Montefiore Med Ctr 1984; **Fellow:** Gastroenterology, Mount Sinai Hosp 1986; **Fac Appt:** Asst Prof Med, Columbia P&S

Lebovics, Edward MD (Ge) - **Spec Exp:** Hepatitis B & C; Pancreatic/Biliary Endoscopy (ERCP); Crohn's Disease; Liver Disease; **Hospital:** Westchester Med Ctr; **Address:** NY Med College-Div Gastroenterology, Munger Pavilion, Ste 206, Valhalla, NY 10595; **Phone:** 914-493-7337; **Board Cert:** Internal Medicine 1983; Gastroenterology 1985; **Med School:** NYU Sch Med 1980; **Resid:** Internal Medicine, Jewish Hosp 1983; **Fellow:** Hepatology, Mt Sinai Hosp 1984; Gastroenterology, NY Med Coll 1986; **Fac Appt:** Prof Med, NY Med Coll

Lee, Sang Y MD (Ge) - **Spec Exp:** Liver Disease; **Hospital:** Northern Westchester Hosp (page 639); **Address:** Mount Kisco Medical Group, 111 Bedford Rd, Katonah, NY 10536; **Phone:** 914-232-3135; **Board Cert:** Internal Medicine 2003; Gastroenterology 2007; **Med School:** Tufts Univ 2000; **Resid:** Internal Medicine, Montefiore Med Ctr 2003; **Fellow:** Gastroenterology, Montefiore Med Ctr 2007

Liss, Mark MD (Ge) - **Spec Exp:** Endoscopy; Peptic Acid Disorders; Inflammatory Bowel Disease; **Hospital:** Montefiore New Rochelle Hosp, Montefiore Med Ctr-Moses Campus (page 100); **Address:** 140 Lockwood Ave, Ste 318, New Rochelle, NY 10801; **Phone:** 914-633-0888; **Board Cert:** Internal Medicine 1980; Gastroenterology 1983; **Med School:** Mount Sinai Sch Med 1977; **Resid:** Internal Medicine, Mt Sinai Hosp 1980; **Fellow:** Gastroenterology, Montefiore Med Ctr 1982; **Fac Appt:** Asst Clin Prof Med, Albert Einstein Coll Med

Martin, Christopher MD (Ge) - **Hospital:** Phelps Meml Hosp Ctr; **Address:** 777 N Broadway, Ste 305, Sleepy Hollow, NY 10591; **Phone:** 914-366-6120; **Board Cert:** Internal Medicine 2002; Gastroenterology 2005; **Med School:** Cornell Univ-Weill Med Coll 1999; **Resid:** Internal Medicine, NY Presby Hosp-Cornell 2002; **Fellow:** Gastroenterology, St Luke's-Roosevelt Hosp Ctr 2005

Rosemarin, Jack I MD (Ge) - **Spec Exp:** Colonoscopy; Peptic Acid Disorders; Nutrition; **Hospital:** White Plains Hosp (page 640); **Address:** Digestive Disease & Nutrition Ctr-Westchester, 2 Gannett Drive, Ste L1, White Plains, NY 10604; **Phone:** 914-683-1555; **Board Cert:** Internal Medicine 1982; Gastroenterology 1983; **Med School:** NY Med Coll 1978; **Resid:** Internal Medicine, NY Med Coll Affil Hosp 1981; **Fellow:** Gastroenterology, Yale Affil Hosp 1983

Roston, Alfred D MD (Ge) - **Spec Exp:** Barrett's Esophagus; Gastroesophageal Reflux Disease (GERD); Inflammatory Bowel Disease; Irritable Bowel Syndrome; **Hospital:** White Plains Hosp (page 640); **Address:** Digestive Disease & Nutrition Ctr of Westchester, 2 Gannett Drive, Ste L1, White Plains, NY 10604; **Phone:** 914-683-1555; **Board Cert:** Gastroenterology 2005; **Med School:** NYU Sch Med 1989; **Resid:** Internal Medicine, Mt Sinai Hosp 1992; **Fellow:** Gastroenterology, NY Hosp-Cornell Univ Med 1994; Endoscopy, Brigham & Women's Hospital 1995

Sgouros, Anthony Peter MD (Ge) - **Spec Exp:** Inflammatory Bowel Disease; Gastrointestinal Cancer; **Hospital:** Northern Westchester Hosp (page 639); **Address:** Westchester Health, 60 Goldens Bridge Rd, Katonah, NY 10536; **Phone:** 914-269-9632; **Board Cert:** Internal Medicine 2003; Gastroenterology 2005; **Med School:** Mount Sinai Sch Med 1990; **Resid:** Internal Medicine, NY-Presby/Columbia Univ Med Ctr 1993; **Fellow:** Gastroenterology, Montefiore Med Ctr 1995

Shapiro, Neil H MD (Ge) - **Spec Exp:** Endoscopy; Liver Disease; Inflammatory Bowel Disease; **Hospital:** White Plains Hosp (page 640), Greenwich Hosp (page 938); **Address:** 18 Rye Ridge Plaza, Rye Brook, NY 10573-2820; **Phone:** 914-253-9252; **Board Cert:** Internal Medicine 1978; Gastroenterology 1981; **Med School:** Wayne State Univ 1975; **Resid:** Internal Medicine, Beth Israel Hosp 1978; Gastroenterology, Montefiore Med Ctr 1980; **Fac Appt:** Asst Clin Prof Med, Cornell Univ-Weill Med Coll

Taffet, Sanford L MD (Ge) - **Spec Exp:** Inflammatory Bowel Disease; Colon Cancer; Liver Disease; **Hospital:** Montefiore New Rochelle Hosp, Montefiore Mt Vernon Hosp; **Address:** 140 Lockwood Ave, Ste 110, New Rochelle, NY 10801-4907; **Phone:** 914-636-5222; **Board Cert:** Internal Medicine 1980; Gastroenterology 1981; **Med School:** NY Med Coll 1976; **Resid:** Internal Medicine, Maimonides Med Ctr 1979; **Fellow:** Gastroenterology, Albert Einstein Med Ctr 1981

Torman, Julie MD (Ge) - **Spec Exp:** Colon Cancer Screening; Swallowing Disorders; **Hospital:** Phelps Meml Hosp Ctr; **Address:** 2005 Albany Post Rd, Ste 15, Croton-on-Hudson, NY 10520; **Phone:** 914-271-4212; **Board Cert:** Internal Medicine 1983; Gastroenterology 1989; **Med School:** Univ Nevada 1980; **Resid:** Internal Medicine, Brigham & Womens Hosp 1983; **Fellow:** Gastroenterology, Stanford Univ Med Ctr 1985

Wayne, Peter MD (Ge) - **Spec Exp:** Hepatitis; Pancreatic/Biliary Endoscopy (ERCP); Liver Disease; Colonoscopy; **Hospital:** Saint Joseph's Med Ctr - Yonkers, St. John's Riverside Hosp-Andrus Pavil; **Address:** 469 N Broadway, Yonkers, NY 10701-1923; **Phone:** 914-969-1115; **Board Cert:** Internal Medicine 1979; Gastroenterology 1981; **Med School:** Albert Einstein Coll Med 1976; **Resid:** Internal Medicine, Montefiore Hosp Med Ctr 1979; **Fellow:** Gastroenterology, Mount Sinai Hosp 1981

Wolf, David C MD (Ge) - **Spec Exp:** Liver Failure; Transplant Medicine-Liver; Liver Disease; **Hospital:** Westchester Med Ctr; **Address:** Westchester Medical Ctr, Liver Transplant Ctr, 100 Woods Rd, BHC Lower Level, Valhalla, NY 10595; **Phone:** 914-493-8916; **Board Cert:** Internal Medicine 1988; Gastroenterology 2011; Transplant Hepatology 2006; **Med School:** Columbia P&S 1985; **Resid:** Internal Medicine, NY Presby Hosp 1988; **Fellow:** Gastroenterology, Montefiore Med Ctr 1991; **Fac Appt:** Clin Prof Med, NY Med Coll

Geriatric Medicine

Banc, Tobe E MD (Ger) - **Spec Exp:** Geriatric Care; Preventive Medicine; **Hospital:** Phelps Meml Hosp Ctr; **Address:** 755 N Broadway, Ste 100, Sleepy Hollow, NY 10510; **Phone:** 914-366-3677; **Board Cert:** Internal Medicine 2010; Geriatric Medicine 2012; **Med School:** NYU Sch Med 1993; **Resid:** Internal Medicine, Hartford Hosp 1996; **Fellow:** Geriatric Medicine, Mt Sinai Med Ctr 1998

Devons, Cathryn A MD (Ger) - **Spec Exp:** Alzheimer's Disease; Memory Disorders; Dementia; Osteoporosis; **Hospital:** Phelps Meml Hosp Ctr, Mt Sinai Med Ctr (page 102); **Address:** Phelps Memorial Hosp, Div Geriatrics, 755 N Broadway, Sleepy Hollow, NY 10591; **Phone:** 914-366-3669; **Board Cert:** Geriatric Medicine 2004; **Med School:** Israel 1988; **Resid:** Internal Medicine, Montefiore Med Ctr 1991; **Fellow:** Geriatric Medicine, Mt Sinai Med Ctr 1993; **Fac Appt:** Asst Clin Prof Med, Mount Sinai Sch Med

Escher, Jeffrey E MD (Ger) - **Spec Exp:** Geriatric Care; **Hospital:** Saint Joseph's Med Ctr - Yonkers, Westchester Med Ctr; **Address:** Park Avenue Healthcare Assocs, 3 Barker Ave, White Plains, NY 10601; **Phone:** 914-949-1199; **Med School:** Belgium 1980; **Resid:** Internal Medicine, New Britain Genl Hosp 1983; **Fellow:** Geriatric Medicine, NYU Med Ctr 1985

Grimshaw Jr, Robert S MD (Ger) *PCP* - **Hospital:** Hudson Valley Hosp Ctr; **Address:** 48 Route 6 & Mahopac Ave, Ste 103, Mount Kisco Med Group, Yorktown Heights, NY 10598; **Phone:** 914-962-3180; **Board Cert:** Internal Medicine 1982; Geriatric Medicine 2004; **Med School:** Albert Einstein Coll Med 1979; **Resid:** Internal Medicine, Jacobi Med Ctr 1982; **Fac Appt:** Assoc Prof Med, NY Med Coll

Kalchthaler, Thomas J DO (Ger) *PCP* - **Spec Exp:** Geriatric Care; Frail Elderly; **Hospital:** Saint Joseph's Med Ctr - Yonkers; **Address:** Park Avenue Healthcare Assocs, 3 Barker Ave, White Plains, NY 10601; **Phone:** 914-949-1199; **Board Cert:** Internal Medicine 1976; **Med School:** Chicago Coll Osteo Med 1971; **Resid:** Internal Medicine, Elmhurst Hosp 1974; **Fellow:** Geriatric Medicine, Elmhurst Hosp 1975; **Fac Appt:** Asst Prof Med, NY Med Coll

Martimucci, William A MD (Ger) *PCP* - **Spec Exp:** Geriatric Care; Preventive Medicine; **Hospital:** White Plains Hosp (page 640); **Address:** WestMed Practice Partners, 1 Theall Rd, Rye, NY 10580; **Phone:** 914-848-8700; **Board Cert:** Internal Medicine 1989; **Med School:** Grenada 1985; **Resid:** Internal Medicine, Caledonian Hosp 1988; **Fellow:** Geriatric Medicine, Mt Sinai Med Ctr 1990

Vaughan, Margaret E MD (Ger) - **Hospital:** Northern Westchester Hosp (page 639); **Address:** 111 Bedford Rd, Katonah, NY 10536; **Phone:** 914-232-3135; **Board Cert:** Internal Medicine 2012; Geriatric Medicine 2003; **Med School:** SUNY Upstate Med Univ 1994; **Resid:** Anesthesiology, NY Presby-Cornell Med Ctr 1998; Internal Medicine, St Vincent's Catholic Med Ctr 2001; **Fellow:** Geriatric Medicine, St Vincent's Catholic Med Ctr 2002

Gynecologic Oncology

Gretz, Herbert F MD (GO) - **Spec Exp:** Gynecologic Cancer; Minimally Invasive Surgery; Robotic Surgery; **Hospital:** White Plains Hosp (page 640), Greenwich Hosp (page 938); **Address:** 2 Longview Ave, Ste 302, White Plains, NY 10601; **Phone:** 914-305-2730; **Board Cert:** Obstetrics & Gynecology 2010; Gynecologic Oncology 2010; **Med School:** NY Med Coll 1986; **Resid:** Obstetrics & Gynecology, NYU Med Ctr 1990; **Fellow:** Gynecologic Oncology, Univ Michigan Med Ctr 1993; **Fac Appt:** Assoc Prof ObG, Mount Sinai Sch Med

Tedjarati, Sean S MD (GO) - **Spec Exp:** Uterine Cancer; Ovarian Cancer; Cervical Cancer; **Hospital:** Westchester Med Ctr; **Address:** 19 Bradhurst Ave, rm 2575 South, Hawthorne, NY 10532; **Phone:** 914-493-2181; **Board Cert:** Obstetrics & Gynecology 2012; Gynecologic Oncology 2012; **Med School:** Yale Univ 1994; **Resid:** Family Medicine, Ohio State Univ Med Ctr 1997; Obstetrics & Gynecology, Ohio State Univ Med Ctr 2000; **Fellow:** Gynecologic Oncology, MD Anderson Cancer Ctr 2003; **Fac Appt:** Assoc Prof ObG, NY Med Coll

Wertheim, Iris MD (GO) - **Hospital:** Northern Westchester Hosp (page 639); **Address:** 400 E Main St, Mount Kisco, NY 10549; **Phone:** 914-242-2991; **Board Cert:** Obstetrics & Gynecology 2012; Gynecologic Oncology 2012; **Med School:** Columbia P&S 1989; **Resid:** Obstetrics & Gynecology, Brigham & Women's Hosp 1993; **Fellow:** Gynecologic Oncology, Brigham & Women's Hosp 1996; **Fac Appt:** Asst Prof S, Columbia P&S

Hand Surgery

Fragner, Paul D MD (HS) - **Spec Exp:** Hand & Wrist Surgery; Elbow Surgery; **Hospital:** White Plains Hosp (page 640); **Address:** White Plains Physician Assocs Orthopedic Specialists, 222 Westchester Ave, Ste 101, White Plains, NY 10604; **Phone:** 914-946-1010; **Board Cert:** Orthopaedic Surgery 2006; Hand Surgery 2006; **Med School:** SUNY Upstate Med Univ 1986; **Resid:** Orthopaedic Surgery, SUNY Downstate Med Ctr 1991; **Fellow:** Hand Surgery, Hosp U Penn 1992

Ilan, Doron MD (HS) - **Spec Exp:** Hand & Upper Extremity Surgery; Shoulder Surgery; Arthroscopic Surgery; Rotator Cuff Surgery; **Hospital:** St. John's Riverside Hosp-Dobbs Ferry Pavil, Nyack Hosp; **Address:** Premier Othropedics of Westchester & Rockland, 128 Ashford Ave, Lower Level Dobbs Ferry Hosp, Dobbs Ferry, NY 10522; **Phone:** 914-693-2057; **Board Cert:** Orthopaedic Surgery 2005; Hand Surgery 2007; **Med School:** Tulane Univ 1997; **Resid:** Surgery, NYU-Hosp Joint Diseases 1998; Orthopaedic Surgery, NYU-Hosp Joint Diseases 2002; **Fellow:** Hand Surgery, Stanford Univ Med Ctr

Magill Jr, Richard M MD (HS) - **Spec Exp:** Hand & Upper Extremity Surgery; Microvascular Surgery; Shoulder Surgery; **Hospital:** Westchester Med Ctr, Phelps Meml Hosp Ctr; **Address:** University Orthopaedics, 19 Bradhurst Ave, Ste 1300-N, Hawthorne, NY 10532; **Phone:** 914-789-2733; **Board Cert:** Orthopaedic Surgery 2006; Hand Surgery 2006; **Med School:** Temple Univ 1983; **Resid:** Surgery, Temple Univ Hosp 1985; Orthopaedic Surgery, Maimonides Med Ctr 1992; **Fellow:** Hand Surgery, Duke Univ Med Ctr 1993

Pianka, George MD (HS) - **Spec Exp:** Hand & Wrist Surgery; Hand & Upper Extremity Surgery; Arthroscopic Surgery; Dupuytren's Contracture; **Hospital:** Lenox Hill Hosp (page 106), Phelps Meml Hosp Ctr; **Address:** Hudson Valley Bone & Joint Surgeons, 24 Saw Mill River Rd, Ste 206, Hawthorne, NY 10532; **Phone:** 914-631-7777; **Board Cert:** Orthopaedic Surgery 2013; Hand Surgery 2013; **Med School:** Univ Conn 1984; **Resid:** Orthopaedic Surgery, Lenox Hill Hosp 1989; **Fellow:** Hand Surgery, NYU Hosp For Joint Diseases 1990

Schefer, Alan MD (HS) - **Spec Exp:** Hand & Upper Extremity Surgery; **Hospital:** Northern Westchester Hosp (page 639); **Address:** Mt Kisco Medical Group, 90 S Bedford Rd, Mount Kisco, NY 10549; **Phone:** 914-241-1050; **Board Cert:** Orthopaedic Surgery 2009; Hand Surgery 2009; **Med School:** Hahnemann Univ 1990; **Resid:** Orthopaedic Surgery, Mt Sinai Med Ctr 1995; **Fellow:** Hand Surgery, Stony Brook Univ Hosp-SUNY 1996

Hematology

Lester, Thomas J MD (Hem) - **Spec Exp:** Lymphoma; Breast Cancer; **Hospital:** Northern Westchester Hosp (page 639); **Address:** Mt Kisco Medical Group, 90 S Bedford Rd, Mt Kisco, NY 10549; **Phone:** 914-242-2991; **Board Cert:** Internal Medicine 1982; Hematology 1984; Medical Oncology 1987; **Med School:** UMDNJ-Rutgers Med Sch 1979; **Resid:** Internal Medicine, Mt Sinai Hosp 1982; **Fellow:** Hematology, Mt Sinai Hosp 1984; Medical Oncology, Meml Sloan Kettering Cancer Ctr 1986

Nelson, John C MD (Hem) - **Spec Exp:** Hematologic Malignancies; **Hospital:** Westchester Med Ctr, Phelps Meml Hosp Ctr; **Address:** Hudson Valley Hematology Oncology Assocs, 19 Bradhurst Ave, Ste 2100, Hawthorne, NY 10532; **Phone:** 914-493-8375; **Board Cert:** Internal Medicine 1974; Hematology 1976; **Med School:** Harvard Med Sch 1971; **Resid:** Internal Medicine, Mt Sinai Med Ctr 1974; **Fellow:** Hematology, Westchester Med Ctr 1976; **Fac Appt:** Assoc Prof Med, NY Med Coll

Infectious Disease

Berkey, Peter B MD (Inf) - **Spec Exp:** Immune Deficiency; Tick-borne Diseases; Travel Medicine; **Hospital:** St. John's Riverside Hosp-Andrus Pavil, Saint Joseph's Med Ctr - Yonkers; **Address:** 970 N Broadway, Ste 212, Yonkers, NY 10701-1311; **Phone:** 914-376-1543; **Board Cert:** Internal Medicine 1985; Infectious Disease 1988; **Med School:** Univ Puerto Rico 1980; **Resid:** Internal Medicine, NY Med Coll/Univ Hosp 1984; **Fellow:** Infectious Disease, MD Anderson Cancer Ctr 1988

Kesh, Sandra MD (Inf) - **Spec Exp:** Hospital Acquired Infections; Antibiotic Resistance; Staphylococcal Infections; **Hospital:** White Plains Hosp (page 640), Greenwich Hosp (page 938); **Address:** WestMed Medical Grp, 210 Westchester Ave, White Plains, NY 10604; **Phone:** 914-682-6511; **Board Cert:** Internal Medicine 2003; Infectious Disease 2007; **Med School:** Cornell Univ-Weill Med Coll 2000; **Resid:** Internal Medicine, NY Presby-Cornell Med Ctr 2003; **Fellow:** Infectious Disease, NY Presby-Cornell Med Ctr 2007

Lederman, Jeffrey A MD (Inf) - **Spec Exp:** Travel Medicine; HIV; Lyme Disease; Tuberculosis; **Hospital:** Montefiore New Rochelle Hosp; **Address:** Sound Shore Med Ctr, Infection Control, 16 Guion Pl Fl 2, New Rochelle, NY 10802; **Phone:** 914-637-1657; **Board Cert:** Internal Medicine 2011; Infectious Disease 2000; **Med School:** Jefferson Med Coll 1988; **Resid:** Internal Medicine, Mt Sinai Hosp 1991; **Fellow:** Infectious Disease, Montefiore Med Ctr 1995

Moorjani, Harish MD (Inf) - **Spec Exp:** Lyme Disease; AIDS/HIV; **Hospital:** Montefiore Mt Vernon Hosp, Phelps Meml Hosp Ctr; **Address:** 127 Woodside Ave, Ste 204, Briarcliff Manor, NY 10510; **Phone:** 914-762-2276; **Board Cert:** Internal Medicine 1992; Infectious Disease 1994; **Med School:** India 1986; **Resid:** Internal Medicine, UMDNJ Med Ctr 1992; **Fellow:** Infectious Disease, Stony Brook Univ Med Ctr 1994

Nadelman, Robert MD (Inf) - **Spec Exp:** Tick-borne Diseases; Lyme Disease; **Hospital:** Westchester Med Ctr; **Address:** NY Med Coll, Div Infectious Disease, Munger Pavillion, rm 245, Valhalla, NY 10595; **Phone:** 914-493-8865; **Board Cert:** Internal Medicine 1983; Infectious Disease 1988; **Med School:** Albert Einstein Coll Med 1980; **Resid:** Internal Medicine, Beth Israel Hosp 1983; **Fellow:** Infectious Disease, Beth Israel Hosp 1985; **Fac Appt:** Prof Med, NY Med Coll

Raffalli, John T MD (Inf) - **Spec Exp:** Lyme Disease; Tick-borne Diseases; **Hospital:** Northern Westchester Hosp (page 639); **Address:** Mt Kisco Medical Group, 90 S Bedford Rd, Mount Kisco, NY 10549; **Phone:** 914-241-1050; **Board Cert:** Internal Medicine 2005; Infectious Disease 2005; **Med School:** SUNY Downstate 1989; **Resid:** Internal Medicine, NYU Med Ctr 1992; **Fellow:** Infectious Disease, Meml Sloan Kettering Cancer Ctr 1992; **Fac Appt:** Assoc Clin Prof Med, NY Med Coll

Rush, Thomas MD (Inf) - **Spec Exp:** AIDS/HIV; Lyme Disease; Travel Medicine; **Hospital:** Phelps Meml Hosp Ctr, Putnam Hosp Ctr; **Address:** 127 Woodside Ave, Ste 204, Briarcliff Manor, NY 10510; **Phone:** 914-762-2276; **Board Cert:** Internal Medicine 1981; Infectious Disease 1984; **Med School:** Rush Med Coll 1978; **Resid:** Internal Medicine, Genesee Hosp 1981; **Fellow:** Infectious Disease, Strong Meml Hosp 1983; **Fac Appt:** Asst Clin Prof Med, NY Med Coll

Spicehandler, Debra A MD (Inf) - **Spec Exp:** Viral Infections; Antibiotic Resistance; **Hospital:** Northern Westchester Hosp (page 639); **Address:** 16 Bessel Ln, Chappaqua, NY 10514; **Phone:** 914-238-6330; **Board Cert:** Internal Medicine 1983; Infectious Disease 2007; **Med School:** Univ Cincinnati 1980; **Resid:** Internal Medicine, NYU Med Ctr 1983; **Fellow:** Infectious Disease, NYU Med Ctr 1985

Wormser, Gary P MD (Inf) - **Spec Exp:** Lyme Disease; AIDS/HIV; Diagnostic Problems; **Hospital:** Westchester Med Ctr; **Address:** New York Med Coll, Div Infectious Disease, Munger Pavilion, rm 149, Valhalla, NY 10595; **Phone:** 914-493-8865; **Board Cert:** Internal Medicine 1978; Infectious Disease 1982; **Med School:** Johns Hopkins Univ 1972; **Resid:** Internal Medicine, Mt Sinai Hosp 1975; **Fellow:** Infectious Disease, Mt Sinai Hosp 1977; **Fac Appt:** Prof Med, NY Med Coll

Internal Medicine

Abdoo, Robert A MD (IM) *PCP* - **Hospital:** Hudson Valley Hosp Ctr; **Address:** 3630 Hill Blvd, Ste 402, Jefferson Valley, NY 10535-1506; **Phone:** 914-245-8808; **Board Cert:** Internal Medicine 1982; **Med School:** Univ Rochester 1979; **Resid:** Internal Medicine, Westchester Co Med Ctr 1982; **Fac Appt:** Asst Prof Med, NY Med Coll

Abenavoli, Tancredi J MD (IM) *PCP* - **Hospital:** White Plains Hosp (page 640); **Address:** 446 Westchester Ave, Port Chester, NY 10573; **Phone:** 914-939-1573; **Board Cert:** Internal Medicine 1979; Cardiovascular Disease 1981; **Med School:** NYU Sch Med 1976; **Resid:** Internal Medicine, VA Hosp/NYU Med Ctr 1979; **Fellow:** Cardiovascular Disease, VA Hosp/NYU Med Ctr 1981

Ades, Joseph R MD (IM) *PCP* - **Spec Exp:** Acupuncture; Complementary Medicine; **Hospital:** Phelps Meml Hosp Ctr; **Address:** 150 White Plains Rd, Ste 207, Tarrytown, NY 10591; **Phone:** 914-631-2480; **Board Cert:** Internal Medicine 1985; **Med School:** Albert Einstein Coll Med 1982; **Resid:** Internal Medicine, LAC-USC Med Ctr 1986

Alpert, Barbara MD (IM) *PCP* - **Spec Exp:** Osteoporosis; Lyme Disease; **Hospital:** Northern Westchester Hosp (page 639); **Address:** 90 S Bedford Rd, Mount Kisco, NY 10549; **Phone:** 914-241-1050; **Board Cert:** Internal Medicine 1987; **Med School:** Univ Pennsylvania 1984; **Resid:** Internal Medicine, NY-Cornell Hosp 1987; **Fac Appt:** Asst Clin Prof Med, Mount Sinai Sch Med

Altholz, Jeffrey D MD (IM) *PCP* - **Spec Exp:** Occupational Medicine; Addiction/Substance Abuse; **Hospital:** Phelps Meml Hosp Ctr; **Address:** Westchester Medical Care, 160 S Central Ave, Elmsford, NY 10523; **Phone:** 914-345-3135; **Board Cert:** Internal Medicine 2003; **Med School:** Albert Einstein Coll Med 1986; **Resid:** Internal Medicine, St Vincent Hosp Med Ctr 1989; **Fellow:** Internal Medicine, St Vincent Hosp Med Ctr 1990

Aversa, Alphonse R MD (IM) *PCP* - **Hospital:** Northern Westchester Hosp (page 639); **Address:** Mt Kisco Medical Group, 90 S Bedford Rd, Mount Kisco, NY 10549; **Phone:** 914-241-1050; **Board Cert:** Internal Medicine 1999; **Med School:** SUNY Downstate 1977; **Resid:** Internal Medicine, Kings Co Hosp Ctr 1981

Bennett, Stanford W MD (IM) *PCP* - **Hospital:** Northern Westchester Hosp (page 639); **Address:** 1838 Commerce St, Yorktown Heights, NY 10598; **Phone:** 914-962-3500; **Board Cert:** Internal Medicine 2005; **Med School:** Dominica 2001; **Resid:** Internal Medicine, Stamford Hosp 2005

Beran, Nancy R MD (IM) *PCP* - **Spec Exp:** Women's Health; **Hospital:** Northern Westchester Hosp (page 639); **Address:** Westchester Hlth Int Medicine for Women, 645 Marble Ave, Thornwood, NY 10594; **Phone:** 914-769-1600; **Board Cert:** Internal Medicine 2009; **Med School:** Thomas Jefferson Univ 1995; **Resid:** Internal Medicine, Parkland Meml Hosp 1998

Carosella, Christine MD (IM) *PCP* - **Spec Exp:** Hypertension; Asthma; Cholesterol/Lipid Disorders; **Hospital:** Westchester Med Ctr; **Address:** 19 Bradhurst Ave, Ste 3090 North, Hawthorne, NY 10532; **Phone:** 914-592-2400; **Board Cert:** Internal Medicine 2005; **Med School:** NY Med Coll 1992; **Resid:** Internal Medicine, Westchester Med Ctr 1995; **Fac Appt:** Asst Prof Med, NY Med Coll

Colangelo, Daniel A MD (IM) *PCP* - **Hospital:** White Plains Hosp (page 640); **Address:** 1600 Harrison Ave, Ste G 105, Mamaroneck, NY 10543-3149; **Phone:** 914-698-4466; **Board Cert:** Internal Medicine 2004; **Med School:** NYU Sch Med 1980; **Resid:** Internal Medicine, Lenox Hill Hosp 1983

Croen, Kenneth MD (IM) *PCP* - **Spec Exp:** Infectious Disease; Herpes Simplex; **Hospital:** White Plains Hosp (page 640); **Address:** 600 Mamaroneck Ave, Ste 200, Harrison, NY 10583; **Phone:** 914-723-8100; **Board Cert:** Internal Medicine 1984; Infectious Disease 1988; **Med School:** Albert Einstein Coll Med 1980; **Resid:** Internal Medicine, NY-Presby/Columbia Univ Med Ctr 1983; Infectious Disease, Presby Hosp 1984; **Fellow:** Infectious Disease, Natl Inst Hlth 1989

Dennett, Ronald MD (IM) *PCP* - **Hospital:** Lawrence Hosp Ctr; **Address:** WestMed Med Group, Ridge Hill, 73 Market St Fl 2, Yonkers, NY 10710; **Phone:** 914-831-6840; **Board Cert:** Internal Medicine 1980; **Med School:** Univ VT Coll Med 1977; **Resid:** Internal Medicine, Univ Colorado Hosp 1980; **Fac Appt:** Asst Clin Prof Med, Albert Einstein Coll Med

Engelhardt III, Martin B DO (IM) *PCP* - **Hospital:** Montefiore New Rochelle Hosp; **Address:** North Ridge Medical Group, 1296 North Ave, New Rochelle, NY 10804; **Phone:** 914-235-8224; **Board Cert:** Internal Medicine 2009; **Med School:** Philadelphia Coll Osteo Med 1993; **Resid:** Internal Medicine, Montefiore Med Ctr 1998

Ennis, David T MD (IM) *PCP* - **Hospital:** Northern Westchester Hosp (page 639); **Address:** Westchester Health Assocs, 1838 Commerce St, Yorktown Heights, NY 10598-4400; **Phone:** 914-962-3500; **Board Cert:** Internal Medicine 1986; **Med School:** NY Med Coll 1983; **Resid:** Internal Medicine, Westchester Co Med Ctr 1986

Fazio, Nelson M MD (IM) *PCP* - **Spec Exp:** Skin Diseases; Hypertension; Obesity; Infectious Disease; **Hospital:** Lawrence Hosp Ctr; **Address:** 133 Montgomery Ave, Scarsdale, NY 10583; **Phone:** 914-713-8517; **Board Cert:** Internal Medicine 1986; **Med School:** NY Med Coll 1981; **Resid:** Internal Medicine, Westchester Co Med Ctr 1984; **Fellow:** Infectious Disease, Montefiore Hosp Med Ctr 1994

Fenster, Mitchell MD (IM) *PCP* - **Hospital:** White Plains Hosp (page 640); **Address:** 401 Columbus Ave, Valhalla, NY 10595; **Phone:** 914-769-0268; **Board Cert:** Internal Medicine 1987; **Med School:** Mount Sinai Sch Med 1981; **Resid:** Internal Medicine, NYU-Bellevue Med Ctr 1984

Fiorentino, Thomas MD (IM) - **Spec Exp:** Palliative Care; **Hospital:** St. John's Riverside Hosp-Andrus Pavil, Mt Sinai Med Ctr (page 102); **Address:** 984 N Broadway, Ste 303, Yonkers, NY 10701; **Phone:** 914-969-0770; **Board Cert:** Internal Medicine 1975; Hospice & Palliative Medicine 2008; **Med School:** NY Med Coll 1972; **Resid:** Internal Medicine, Metropolitan Hosp 1976

Glickstein, Shari MD (IM) *PCP* - **Hospital:** White Plains Hosp (page 640); **Address:** 30 Davis Ave, White Plains, NY 10601; **Phone:** 914-328-2355; **Board Cert:** Internal Medicine 1986; **Med School:** Mount Sinai Sch Med 1983; **Resid:** Internal Medicine, Mt Sinai Med Ctr 1986

Goldman, Jack S MD (IM) *PCP* - **Spec Exp:** Colonoscopy/Polypectomy; Liver Disease; Endoscopy; **Hospital:** Saint Joseph's Med Ctr - Yonkers, Montefiore Med Ctr-Moses Campus (page 100); **Address:** 750 McLean Ave, Yonkers, NY 10704; **Phone:** 914-237-8686; **Board Cert:** Internal Medicine 1975; Gastroenterology 1979; **Med School:** Albert Einstein Coll Med 1961; **Resid:** Internal Medicine, Bronx Lebanon Hosp 1963; Internal Medicine, VA Med Ctr 1966; **Fellow:** Gastroenterology, VA Med Ctr 1965

Gross, Jeffrey D MD (IM) *PCP* - **Hospital:** Northern Westchester Hosp (page 639); **Address:** Mt Kisco Medical Group, 90 S Bedford Rd, Mt Kisco, NY 10549; **Phone:** 914-241-1050; **Board Cert:** Internal Medicine 2005; **Med School:** SUNY Hlth Sci Ctr 1992; **Resid:** Internal Medicine, Montefiore Med Ctr 1996

Herzog, David A MD (IM) *PCP* - **Spec Exp:** Cholesterol/Lipid Disorders; Preventive Medicine; **Hospital:** White Plains Hosp (page 640); **Address:** 1 Theall Rd, Ste 204, Rye, NY 10580; **Phone:** 914-848-8700; **Board Cert:** Internal Medicine 1984; **Med School:** Mount Sinai Sch Med 1981; **Resid:** Internal Medicine, St Luke's Hosp 1984

Higgins, William J MD (IM) *PCP* - **Spec Exp:** Alzheimer's Disease; Geriatric Medicine; Preventive Medicine; **Hospital:** Hudson Valley Hosp Ctr; **Address:** Westchester Medical Practice, 2050 Saw Mill River Rd, Ste 1, Yorktown Heights, NY 10598; **Phone:** 914-962-5533; **Board Cert:** Internal Medicine 2002; **Med School:** Geo Wash Univ 1986; **Resid:** Internal Medicine, Lenox Hill Hosp 1989; **Fellow:** Pulmonary Disease, Lenox Hill Hosp 1991

Hopkins, Arthur J MD (IM) *PCP* - **Spec Exp:** Preventive Medicine; **Hospital:** Montefiore Med Ctr-Moses Campus (page 100); **Address:** Montefiore Medical Grp-Cross County, 1010 Central Park Ave, Yonkers, NY 10704; **Phone:** 914-964-4133; **Board Cert:** Internal Medicine 1986; **Med School:** Univ Pennsylvania 1983; **Resid:** Internal Medicine, Hosp Univ Penn 1986; **Fac Appt:** Asst Prof Med, Albert Einstein Coll Med

Indio, Lillian R MD (IM) *PCP* - **Hospital:** St. John's Riverside Hosp-Andrus Pavil; **Address:** Mount Sinai Riverside Medical Group, 1010 N Broadway, Yonkers, NY 10701; **Phone:** 914-965-4424; **Board Cert:** Internal Medicine 2006; **Med School:** Albert Einstein Coll Med 1992; **Resid:** Internal Medicine, Montefiore-Einstein Med Ctr 1995

Isaacs, Ellen S MD (IM) *PCP* - **Spec Exp:** Hypertension; Heart Disease; **Hospital:** St. John's Riverside Hosp-Andrus Pavil, Saint Joseph's Med Ctr - Yonkers; **Address:** 1019 Yonkers Ave, Yonkers, NY 10704; **Phone:** 914-963-9493; **Board Cert:** Internal Medicine 1972; Cardiovascular Disease 1981; **Med School:** NYU Sch Med 1969; **Resid:** Internal Medicine, Bellevue Hosp 1972; **Fellow:** Cardiovascular Disease, St Vincent Hosp Med Ctr 1974; **Fac Appt:** Asst Clin Prof Med, NY Med Coll

Kapoor, Satish MD (IM) *PCP* - **Spec Exp:** Asthma; Emphysema; Preventive Medicine; **Hospital:** Phelps Meml Hosp Ctr; **Address:** 362 N Broadway Fl 2, Sleepy Hollow, NY 10591-1040; **Phone:** 914-631-2070; **Board Cert:** Internal Medicine 1979; **Med School:** India 1972; **Resid:** Internal Medicine, Kingsbrook Jewish Med Ctr 1979; **Fellow:** Pulmonary Disease, Queens Hosp 1981

Karmen, Carol L MD (IM) *PCP* - **Spec Exp:** Preventive Medicine; **Hospital:** Westchester Med Ctr; **Address:** 19 Bradhurst Ave, Ste 3090 North, Hawthorne, NY 10532; **Phone:** 914-592-2400; **Board Cert:** Internal Medicine 2007; **Med School:** Albert Einstein Coll Med 1986; **Resid:** Internal Medicine, Westchester Med Ctr 1990; **Fac Appt:** Assoc Prof Med, NY Med Coll

Krieger, Sharon MD (IM) *PCP* - **Hospital:** Northern Westchester Hosp (page 639); **Address:** Mt Kisco Medical Group, 90 S Bedford Rd, Mt Kisco, NY 10549-3422; **Phone:** 914-241-1050; **Board Cert:** Internal Medicine 2004; **Med School:** Louisiana State U, New Orleans 1991; **Resid:** Internal Medicine, NY Presby-Cornell Med Ctr 1994

Kubersky, Steven MD (IM) *PCP* - **Hospital:** White Plains Hosp (page 640), Lawrence Hosp Ctr; **Address:** WestMed Med Group, Ridge Hill, 73 Market St Fl 2, Yonkers, NY 10710; **Phone:** 914-831-6860; **Board Cert:** Internal Medicine 2002; **Med School:** NYU Sch Med 1988; **Resid:** Internal Medicine, Mount Sinai Med Ctr 1992

Lebofsky, Martin MD (IM) - **Spec Exp:** Kidney Disease; Hypertension; Dialysis Care; **Hospital:** Lawrence Hosp Ctr, Saint Joseph's Med Ctr - Yonkers; **Address:** 1 Stone Pl, Ste 202, Bronxville, NY 10708-3406; **Phone:** 914-337-9004; **Board Cert:** Internal Medicine 1975; Nephrology 1978; **Med School:** Albert Einstein Coll Med 1972; **Resid:** Internal Medicine, Harlem Hosp 1975; **Fellow:** Nephrology, Montefiore Med Ctr 1978

Lechner, Michael MD (IM) *PCP* - **Spec Exp:** Geriatric Medicine; Geriatric Rehabilitation; **Hospital:** Phelps Meml Hosp Ctr; **Address:** 14 Church St, Ste 208, Ossining, NY 10562-4831; **Phone:** 914-631-0866; **Board Cert:** Internal Medicine 1980; **Med School:** Albert Einstein Coll Med 1961; **Resid:** Internal Medicine, Westchester Med Ctr 1964; **Fellow:** Hematology, LI Jewish Med Ctr 1965

Margulis, Steven M MD (IM) *PCP* - **Hospital:** Northern Westchester Hosp (page 639); **Address:** Mt Kisco Medical Group, 90 S Bedford Rd, Mt Kisco, NY 10549; **Phone:** 914-241-1050; **Board Cert:** Internal Medicine 2010; **Med School:** Albert Einstein Coll Med 1997; **Resid:** Internal Medicine, Mt Sinai Med Ctr 2000

Melman, Martin MD (IM) *PCP* - **Spec Exp:** Hypertension; Asthma; Geriatric Medicine; **Hospital:** Phelps Meml Hosp Ctr; **Address:** 87 Grand St, Croton-on-Hudson, NY 10520-2518; **Phone:** 914-271-4845; **Board Cert:** Internal Medicine 1977; **Med School:** NY Med Coll 1974; **Resid:** Internal Medicine, Metropolitan Hosp Ctr 1977; Internal Medicine, Westchester Med Ctr 1978; **Fac Appt:** Asst Clin Prof Med, NY Med Coll

Pappas, Steven MD (IM) *PCP* - **Spec Exp:** Occupational Medicine; Preventive Medicine; **Hospital:** Montefiore New Rochelle Hosp; **Address:** 266 White Plains Rd, Ste 1A, Eastchester, NY 10709; **Phone:** 914-793-1115; **Board Cert:** Internal Medicine 1982; **Med School:** Albert Einstein Coll Med 1978; **Resid:** Internal Medicine, St Luke's Roosevelt Hosp Ctr 1981

Pomerantz, Daniel MD (IM) *PCP* - **Spec Exp:** Palliative Care; Ethics; **Hospital:** Montefiore New Rochelle Hosp; **Address:** Goldstein Ambulatory Care Ctr, 16 Guion Pl, New Rochelle, NY 10802; **Phone:** 914-365-3615; **Board Cert:** Internal Medicine 2003; Hospice & Palliative Medicine 2010; **Med School:** Harvard Med Sch 1990; **Resid:** Internal Medicine, NYU Med Ctr 1994

Ridge, Gerald A MD (IM) *PCP* - **Spec Exp:** Geriatric Medicine; Preventive Medicine; **Hospital:** Lawrence Hosp Ctr, NY-Presby/Columbia Univ Med Ctr, NY (page 104); **Address:** Lawrence Medical Assocs, 685 White Plains Rd, Eastchester, NY 10709; **Phone:** 914-787-4100; **Board Cert:** Internal Medicine 2008; Geriatric Medicine 2008; **Med School:** UCSF 1979; **Resid:** Internal Medicine, Bronx Muni Hosp Ctr 1981; Internal Medicine, Columbia-Presby Med Ctr 1982; **Fellow:** Neurology, New York Hosp 1983; **Fac Appt:** Clin Prof Med, Columbia P&S

Rosch, Elliott MD (IM) *PCP* - **Spec Exp:** Preventive Medicine; Cholesterol/Lipid Disorders; Hypertension; Weight Management; **Hospital:** St. John's Riverside Hosp-Andrus Pavil, Mt Sinai Med Ctr (page 102); **Address:** 1010 N Broadway, Mount Sinai Riverside Medical Group, Yonkers, NY 10701-1303; **Phone:** 914-965-4424; **Board Cert:** Internal Medicine 1981; **Med School:** Univ Pennsylvania 1978; **Resid:** Internal Medicine, Pennsylvania Hosp 1981; **Fac Appt:** Asst Prof Med, Mount Sinai Sch Med

Saltzman-Gabelman, Lori MD (IM) *PCP* - **Hospital:** White Plains Hosp (page 640), Greenwich Hosp (page 938); **Address:** 210 Westchester Ave Fl 2, White Plains, NY 10604-2914; **Phone:** 914-682-0700; **Board Cert:** Internal Medicine 1989; **Med School:** NY Med Coll 1986; **Resid:** Internal Medicine, Westchester Med Ctr 1989

Soltren, Rafael MD (IM) *PCP* - **Spec Exp:** Diabetes; Hypertension; **Hospital:** Phelps Meml Hosp Ctr; **Address:** 100 S Highland Ave, Ossining, NY 10562; **Phone:** 914-941-1277; **Board Cert:** Internal Medicine 1985; **Med School:** Cornell Univ-Weill Med Coll 1981; **Resid:** Internal Medicine, Montefiore Med Ctr 1984

Starke, Charles L MD (IM) *PCP* - **Hospital:** Phelps Meml Hosp Ctr, Westchester Med Ctr; **Address:** 302 W Chappaqua Rd, Briarcliff Manor, NY 10510-1526; **Phone:** 914-762-4460; **Board Cert:** Internal Medicine 1978; **Med School:** Albert Einstein Coll Med 1975; **Resid:** Internal Medicine, Georgetown Univ Hosp 1978; **Fac Appt:** Prof Med, Columbia P&S

Tang, David J MD (IM) *PCP* - **Hospital:** St. John's Riverside Hosp-Andrus Pavil, Mt Sinai Med Ctr (page 102); **Address:** Mount Sinai Riverside Group, 1010 N Broadway, Yonkers, NY 10701; **Phone:** 914-965-4424; **Board Cert:** Internal Medicine 2005; **Med School:** Meharry Med Coll 2002; **Resid:** Internal Medicine, LIJ Med Ctr 2005

Turro, James J MD (IM) *PCP* - **Hospital:** Northern Westchester Hosp (page 639); **Address:** 90 S Bedford Rd, Mt Kisco Medical Group, Mt Kisco, NY 10549; **Phone:** 914-241-1050; **Board Cert:** Internal Medicine 1985; **Med School:** Cornell Univ-Weill Med Coll 1982; **Resid:** Internal Medicine, Bronx Muni Hosp 1986

Warshafsky, Stephen MD (IM) *PCP* - **Spec Exp:** Lyme Disease; Cholesterol/Lipid Disorders; Preventive Cardiology; Preventive Medicine; **Hospital:** Westchester Med Ctr; **Address:** 1055 Saw Mill River Rd, Ste 206, Ardsley, NY 10502; **Phone:** 914-591-0733; **Board Cert:** Internal Medicine 2004; **Med School:** NY Med Coll 1989; **Resid:** Internal Medicine, Westchester Med Ctr 1992; **Fac Appt:** Assoc Clin Prof Med, NY Med Coll

Wolfe, Mary J MD (IM) *PCP* - **Hospital:** Phelps Meml Hosp Ctr; **Address:** 14 Church St, Ossining, NY 10562; **Phone:** 914-941-1334; **Board Cert:** Internal Medicine 1980; **Med School:** Penn State Coll Med 1976; **Resid:** Internal Medicine, Westchester Med Ctr 1979

Wolfson, Robert A MD (IM) *PCP* - **Hospital:** Northern Westchester Hosp (page 639); **Address:** 90 S Bedford Rd, Mt Kisco Medical Group, Mount Kisco, NY 10549; **Phone:** 914-241-1050; **Board Cert:** Internal Medicine 1980; **Med School:** SUNY Downstate 1977; **Resid:** Internal Medicine, Kings Co Hosp 1981

Zarowitz, William MD (IM) *PCP* - **Spec Exp:** Occupational Medicine; Preventive Medicine; **Hospital:** White Plains Hosp (page 640); **Address:** 143 Maple Ave, White Plains, NY 10601; **Phone:** 914-683-8610; **Board Cert:** Internal Medicine 1981; **Med School:** NY Med Coll 1978; **Resid:** Internal Medicine, Montefiore Med Ctr 1981; **Fac Appt:** Assoc Clin Prof Med, NY Med Coll

Interventional Cardiology

Hjemdahl-Monsen, Craig MD (IC) - **Hospital:** NY-Presby/Columbia Univ Med Ctr, NY (page 104); **Address:** 19 Bradhurst Ave, Ste 700, Columbia Doctors Medical Group, Hawthorne, NY 10532; **Phone:** 914-593-7800; **Board Cert:** Internal Medicine 1983; Cardiovascular Disease 1985; Interventional Cardiology 2009; **Med School:** Johns Hopkins Univ 1980; **Resid:** Internal Medicine, Univ Hosp 1983; **Fellow:** Cardiovascular Disease, Mount Sinai Med Ctr 1985; Interventional Cardiology, Mount Sinai Med Ctr 1987; **Fac Appt:** Asst Clin Prof Med, Columbia P&S

Kalapatapu, Kumar S MD (IC) - **Hospital:** NY-Presby/Columbia Univ Med Ctr, NY (page 104), White Plains Hosp (page 640); **Address:** Columbia Doctors Medical Group, 19 Bradhurst Ave, Ste 700, Hawthorne, NY 10532; **Phone:** 914-593-7800; **Board Cert:** Cardiovascular Disease 2008; Interventional Cardiology 2003; **Med School:** India 1985; **Resid:** Internal Medicine, Advocate Christ Med Ctr 1993; **Fellow:** Cardiovascular Disease, St Vincents Med Ctr 1994; Interventional Cardiology, Westchester Med Ctr 1996

Messinger, David MD (IC) - **Spec Exp:** Coronary Angioplasty/Stents; **Hospital:** NY-Presby/Weill Cornell Med Ctr, NY (page 104), Westchester Med Ctr; **Address:** 175 Memorial Hwy, New Rochelle, NY 10801; **Phone:** 914-235-3535; **Board Cert:** Cardiovascular Disease 2005; Interventional Cardiology 2009; **Med School:** Cornell Univ-Weill Med Coll 1987; **Resid:** Internal Medicine, NY-Presby/Weill Cornell Med Ctr 1990; **Fellow:** Cardiovascular Disease, NY-Presby/Weill Cornell Med Ctr 1993; Interventional Cardiology, NY-Presby/Weill Cornell Med Ctr 1994

Weiss, Melvin MD (IC) - **Spec Exp:** Cardiac Imaging; Congestive Heart Failure; Diabetes & Heart Disease; Coronary Artery Disease; **Hospital:** NY-Presby/Columbia Univ Med Ctr, NY (page 104), White Plains Hosp (page 640); **Address:** Columbia Doctors Medical Grp, 19 Bradhurst Ave, Ste 700, Hawthorne, NY 10532-2140; **Phone:** 914-593-7800; **Board Cert:** Internal Medicine 1972; Cardiovascular Disease 1975; **Med School:** SUNY Hlth Sci Ctr 1967; **Resid:** Internal Medicine, New York Hosp 1971; **Fellow:** Cardiovascular Disease, NY-Presby/Columbia Univ Med Ctr 1972; **Fac Appt:** Prof Med, NY Med Coll

Maternal & Fetal Medicine

Berck, David J MD (MF) - **Spec Exp:** Ultrasound; Pregnancy-High Risk; **Hospital:** Northern Westchester Hosp (page 639); **Address:** Mount Kisco Medical Group, 90 S Bedford Rd, Mount Kisco, NY 10549; **Phone:** 914-241-1050; **Board Cert:** Obstetrics & Gynecology 1999; Maternal & Fetal Medicine 2001; **Med School:** Harvard Med Sch 1991; **Resid:** Obstetrics & Gynecology, Mass Genl Hosp 1995; **Fellow:** Maternal & Fetal Medicine, Columbia Presby Med Ctr 1998

Devine, Patricia Ann MD (MF) - **Spec Exp:** Pregnancy-High Risk; Prenatal Diagnosis; Diabetes in Pregnancy; Premature Labor; **Hospital:** Montefiore New Rochelle Hosp; **Address:** Sound Shore Antenatal Testing Lab, 16 Guion Place Fl 4, New Rochelle, NY 10802; **Phone:** 914-365-4263; **Board Cert:** Obstetrics & Gynecology 2010; Maternal & Fetal Medicine 2010; **Med School:** Mount Sinai Sch Med 1987; **Resid:** Obstetrics & Gynecology, Beth Israel Med Ctr 1991; **Fellow:** Maternal & Fetal Medicine, Westchester Co Med Ctr 1993; **Fac Appt:** Assoc Clin Prof ObG, NY Med Coll

Gallousis, Francene MD (MF) - **Hospital:** Northern Westchester Hosp (page 639); **Address:** Northern Westchester Hosp, Maternal/Fetal Dept, 400 E Main St, Mount Kisco, NY 10549; **Phone:** 914-666-1010; **Board Cert:** Obstetrics & Gynecology 2011; Maternal & Fetal Medicine 2011; **Med School:** SUNY Downstate 1990; **Resid:** Obstetrics & Gynecology, Westchester Med Ctr 1994

Lescale, Keith B MD (MF) - **Spec Exp:** Pregnancy-High Risk; Prenatal Diagnosis; Fetal Ultrasound/Obstetrical Imaging; **Hospital:** White Plains Hosp (page 640), Phelps Meml Hosp Ctr; **Address:** Hudson Valley Perinatal Consulting, 600 Mamaroneck Ave, Ste 110, Harrison, NY 10528-1647; **Phone:** 914-670-0500; **Board Cert:** Obstetrics & Gynecology 2012; Maternal & Fetal Medicine 2012; **Med School:** Louisiana State U, New Orleans 1987; **Resid:** Obstetrics & Gynecology, New Orleans/LSU Med Ctr 1991; **Fellow:** Maternal & Fetal Medicine, NY Hosp-Cornell Med Ctr 1994

Mootabar, Hamid MD (MF) - **Spec Exp:** Pregnancy-High Risk; **Hospital:** Lawrence Hosp Ctr, NY-Presby/Columbia Univ Med Ctr, NY (page 104); **Address:** Amniocentesis & Genetics Ctr, 77 Pondfield Rd, Bronxville, NY 10708; **Phone:** 914-337-2102; **Board Cert:** Obstetrics & Gynecology 1975; Maternal & Fetal Medicine 1983; **Med School:** Iran 1966; **Resid:** Obstetrics & Gynecology, Roosevelt Hosp 1973; **Fellow:** Maternal & Fetal Medicine, Roosevelt Hosp 1979; **Fac Appt:** Assoc Clin Prof ObG, Columbia P&S

Medical Oncology

Ahmed, Tauseef MD (Onc) - **Spec Exp:** Bone Marrow Transplant; Lymphoma; Brain Tumors; Genitourinary Cancer; **Hospital:** Westchester Med Ctr; **Address:** 19 Bradhurst Ave, Ste 2100, Hawthorne, NY 10532; **Phone:** 914-493-8375; **Board Cert:** Internal Medicine 1980; Hematology 1982; Medical Oncology 1983; **Med School:** Pakistan 1976; **Resid:** Internal Medicine, Sinai-Grace Hosp 1980; **Fellow:** Medical Oncology, Meml Sloan-Kettering Cancer Ctr 1983; **Fac Appt:** Prof Med, NY Med Coll

Bernhardt, Bernard MD (Onc) - **Spec Exp:** Lung Cancer; Lymphoma; Leukemia-Chronic Lymphocytic; Anemias & Red Blood Cell Disorders; **Hospital:** Montefiore New Rochelle Hosp, Montefiore Med Ctr-Einstein Campus (page 100); **Address:** Advanced Oncology Assocs, 50 Guion Pl, Ste 32, New Rochelle, NY 10801-5512; **Phone:** 914-632-5397; **Board Cert:** Internal Medicine 1968; Hematology 1972; Medical Oncology 1973; **Med School:** Northwestern Univ 1961; **Resid:** Internal Medicine, DC Genl Hosp 1963; Internal Medicine, NY Med Coll 1966; **Fellow:** Hematology, Montefiore Hosp Med Ctr 1968; **Fac Appt:** Clin Prof Med, NY Med Coll

Caron, Philip C MD/PhD (Onc) - **Spec Exp:** Lymphoma; Gastrointestinal Cancer; **Hospital:** Meml Sloan-Kettering Canc Ctr (page 114), Phelps Meml Hosp Ctr; **Address:** Meml Sloan-Kettering at Phelps Meml Hosp, 777 N Broadway, Ste 102, Sleepy Hollow, NY 10591; **Phone:** 914-366-0664; **Board Cert:** Internal Medicine 1989; Medical Oncology 2003; Hematology 2007; **Med School:** NY Med Coll 1986; **Resid:** Internal Medicine, Mt Sinai Hosp 1989; **Fellow:** Hematology & Oncology, Meml Sloan-Kettering Cancer Ctr 1992

Feldman, Stuart P MD (Onc) - **Spec Exp:** Breast Cancer; Lymphoma; **Hospital:** White Plains Hosp (page 640), Greenwich Hosp (page 938); **Address:** 210 Westchester Ave, White Plains, NY 10604-2901; **Phone:** 914-681-5200; **Board Cert:** Internal Medicine 1980; Hematology 1982; Medical Oncology 1985; **Med School:** Geo Wash Univ 1977; **Resid:** Internal Medicine, New York Hosp-Cornell 1980; **Fellow:** Hematology & Oncology, Meml Sloan-Kettering Cancer Ctr 1983; **Fac Appt:** Asst Clin Prof Med, Cornell Univ-Weill Med Coll

Fialk, Mark A MD (Onc) - **Hospital:** White Plains Hosp (page 640), Westchester Med Ctr; **Address:** 600 Mamaroneck Ave Fl 2, Harrison, NY 10528; **Phone:** 914-723-8100; **Board Cert:** Internal Medicine 1976; Medical Oncology 1977; Hematology 1978; **Med School:** Tufts Univ 1973; **Resid:** Internal Medicine, NY Hosp-Cornell Med Ctr 1975; Internal Medicine, Meml Sloan-Kettering Cancer Ctr 1976; **Fellow:** Hematology & Oncology, NY Hosp-Cornell Med Ctr 1978; Infectious Disease, Meml Sloan-Kettering Cancer Ctr 1979; **Fac Appt:** Asst Clin Prof Med, NY Med Coll

Gold, Julie M MD (Onc) - **Hospital:** Northern Westchester Hosp (page 639); **Address:** 400 E Main St, Mount Kisco Medical Group, Mount Kisco, NY 10549-3417; **Phone:** 914-242-2991; **Board Cert:** Internal Medicine 2005; Hematology 2009; Medical Oncology 2009; **Med School:** Cornell Univ-Weill Med Coll 2002; **Resid:** Internal Medicine, NY Presby Hosp-Cornell Med Ctr 2005; **Fellow:** Hematology & Oncology, Brigham & Women's Hosp 2009

Goldberg, Jonathan S MD (Onc) - **Spec Exp:** Breast Cancer; Lymphoma; Gastrointestinal Cancer; Lung Cancer; **Hospital:** Northern Westchester Hosp (page 639), Putnam Hosp Ctr; **Address:** Mount Kisco Medical Group, 90 S Bedford Rd, Mount Kisco, NY 10549; **Phone:** 914-241-1050; **Board Cert:** Internal Medicine 2007; Hematology 2011; Medical Oncology 2011; **Med School:** Mount Sinai Sch Med 1994; **Resid:** Internal Medicine, NY Presby Med Ctr 1997; **Fellow:** Hematology & Oncology, NY Presby Med Ctr 1999

Halaas, Jeffrey L MD (Onc) - **Spec Exp:** Breast Cancer; Leukemia & Lymphoma; Ovarian Cancer; Lung Cancer; **Hospital:** Northern Westchester Hosp (page 639), Putnam Hosp Ctr; **Address:** Mt Kisco Medical Group, 90 S Bedford Rd, Mt Kisco, NY 10549; **Phone:** 914-241-1050; **Board Cert:** Internal Medicine 2002; Medical Oncology 2005; Hematology 2005; **Med School:** Cornell Univ-Weill Med Coll 1999; **Resid:** Internal Medicine, NY-Presby/Weill Cornell Med Ctr 2001; **Fellow:** Hematology & Oncology, Meml Sloan-Kettering Cancer Ctr 2005

Liu, DeLong MD/PhD (Onc) - **Spec Exp:** Lung Cancer; Leukemia; Bone Marrow Transplant; Lymphoma; **Hospital:** Westchester Med Ctr; **Address:** Hudson Valley Hem/Onc Assocs, 19 Bradhurst Ave, Ste 2100, Hawthorne, NY 10532; **Phone:** 914-493-8375; **Board Cert:** Internal Medicine 2006; Medical Oncology 2011; Hematology 2002; **Med School:** China 1984; **Resid:** Internal Medicine, Montefiore Med Ctr 1996; **Fellow:** Hematology & Oncology, Meml Sloan Kettering Cancer Ctr 1998; **Fac Appt:** Prof Med, NY Med Coll

Mills, Nancy Ellyn MD (Onc) - **Spec Exp:** Breast Cancer; Gynecologic Cancer; **Hospital:** Phelps Meml Hosp Ctr, Meml Sloan-Kettering Canc Ctr (page 114); **Address:** Meml Sloan Kettering @ Sleepy Hollow, 777 N Broadway, Ste 102, Sleepy Hollow, NY 10591; **Phone:** 914-366-0664; **Board Cert:** Internal Medicine 2000; Medical Oncology 2003; Hematology 2004; **Med School:** Mount Sinai Sch Med 1987; **Resid:** Internal Medicine, Mt Sinai Med Ctr 1990; **Fellow:** Hematology & Oncology, NYU Med Ctr 1993; **Fac Appt:** Asst Clin Prof Med, Cornell Univ-Weill Med Coll

Phillips, Elizabeth MD (Onc) - **Spec Exp:** Breast Cancer; Hematology; Lymphoma; Leukemia; **Hospital:** Montefiore New Rochelle Hosp, Montefiore Med Ctr-Moses Campus (page 100); **Address:** Advanced Oncology Assocs, 50 Guion Pl, Ste 32, New Rochelle, NY 10801-4914; **Phone:** 914-632-5397; **Board Cert:** Internal Medicine 1974; Hematology 1976; Medical Oncology 1977; **Med School:** Univ Wash 1969; **Resid:** Internal Medicine, Harlem Hosp 1972; Hematology, Montefiore Med Ctr 1973; **Fellow:** Hematology & Oncology, Mem Sloan Kettering Canc Ctr 1976; **Fac Appt:** Assoc Clin Prof Med, NY Med Coll

Provenzano, Anthony F MD (Onc) - **Spec Exp:** Lung Cancer; Breast Cancer; Cancer Genetics; Gastrointestinal Cancer; **Hospital:** Lawrence Hosp Ctr, Montefiore Mt Vernon Hosp; **Address:** 1 Pondfield Rd W, Ste 1, Bronxville, NY 10708-2635; **Phone:** 914-961-3421; **Board Cert:** Internal Medicine 1979; Medical Oncology 1981; **Med School:** Cornell Univ-Weill Med Coll 1976; **Resid:** Internal Medicine, Lenox Hill Hosp 1978; **Fellow:** Medical Oncology, St Vincents Hosp 1979; Medical Oncology, Lenox Hill Hosp 1981; **Fac Appt:** Asst Clin Prof Med, NY Med Coll

Puccio, Carmelo A MD (Onc) - **Spec Exp:** Breast Cancer; Lung Cancer; Solid Tumors; Gynecologic Cancer; **Hospital:** Westchester Med Ctr; **Address:** 19 Bradhurst Ave, Ste 2100, Hawthorne, NY 10532; **Phone:** 914-493-8375; **Board Cert:** Internal Medicine 1984; Medical Oncology 1989; **Med School:** Mexico 1979; **Resid:** Internal Medicine, Maimonides Med Ctr 1984; **Fellow:** Medical Oncology, Westchester Co Med Ctr 1985; **Fac Appt:** Asst Prof Med, NY Med Coll

Rosen, Norman MD (Onc) - **Spec Exp:** Lung Cancer; Breast Cancer; **Hospital:** St. John's Riverside Hosp-Andrus Pavil; **Address:** 984 N Broadway, Ste 311, Yonkers, NY 10701-1308; **Phone:** 914-965-2060; **Board Cert:** Internal Medicine 1975; Medical Oncology 1977; **Med School:** Tufts Univ 1972; **Resid:** Internal Medicine, Montefiore Med Ctr 1975; **Fellow:** Hematology & Oncology, Montefiore Med Ctr 1977; **Fac Appt:** Asst Clin Prof Med, Albert Einstein Coll Med

Sadan, Sara MD (Onc) - **Spec Exp:** Breast Cancer; Gynecologic Cancer; Gastrointestinal Cancer; Lymphoma; **Hospital:** White Plains Hosp (page 640); **Address:** Oncology & Hematology of White Plains, 244 Westchester Ave, Ste 411, White Plains, NY 10604; **Phone:** 914-684-8100; **Board Cert:** Internal Medicine 2002; Medical Oncology 2005; **Med School:** Israel 1984; **Resid:** Internal Medicine, St Luke's-Roosevelt Hosp Ctr 1991; **Fellow:** Hematology & Oncology, Meml Sloan Kettering Cancer Ctr 1994

Saponara, Eduardo M MD (Onc) - **Spec Exp:** Breast Cancer; Hematology; Lymphoma; Multiple Myeloma; **Hospital:** Lawrence Hosp Ctr, Mt Sinai Med Ctr (page 102); **Address:** 77 Pondfield Rd, Bronxville, NY 10708-3809; **Phone:** 914-793-1500; **Board Cert:** Internal Medicine 1977; Hematology 1978; Medical Oncology 1979; **Med School:** Peru 1973; **Resid:** Internal Medicine, Westchester Med Ctr 1976; **Fellow:** Hematology & Oncology, Flower Fifth Ave Hospital/NY Med Coll 1978; Oncology, Mount Sinai Hosp 1979; **Fac Appt:** Asst Clin Prof Onc, NY Med Coll

Schneider, Robert Jay MD (Onc) - **Spec Exp:** Breast Cancer; Genitourinary Cancer; **Hospital:** Northern Westchester Hosp (page 639); **Address:** 101 S Bedford, Ste 202A, Mt Kisco, NY 10549-3456; **Phone:** 914-666-8976; **Board Cert:** Internal Medicine 1979; Medical Oncology 1985; **Med School:** Albert Einstein Coll Med 1975; **Resid:** Internal Medicine, Jacobi Med Ctr 1978; **Fellow:** Medical Oncology, Meml Sloan Kettering Cancer Ctr 1980

Seiter, Karen MD (Onc) - **Spec Exp:** Hematologic Malignancies; Leukemia; Myelodysplastic Syndromes; **Hospital:** Westchester Med Ctr; **Address:** Hudson Valley Hem/Onc Assocs, 19 Bradhurst Ave, Ste 2100, Hawthorne, NY 10532; **Phone:** 914-493-8375; **Board Cert:** Internal Medicine 1988; Medical Oncology 2011; Hematology 2002; **Med School:** NY Med Coll 1985; **Resid:** Internal Medicine, Albert Einstein Hosp 1988; **Fellow:** Hematology & Oncology, Meml Sloan Kettering Cancer Ctr 1991; **Fac Appt:** Prof Med, NY Med Coll

Wasserheit, Carolyn MD (Onc) - **Spec Exp:** Solid Tumors; Breast Cancer; Gynecologic Cancer; **Hospital:** Phelps Meml Hosp Ctr, Meml Sloan-Kettering Canc Ctr (page 114); **Address:** Memorial Sloan Kettering @ Sleepy Hollow, 777 N Broadway, Ste 102, Sleepy Hollow, NY 10591; **Phone:** 914-366-0664; **Board Cert:** Internal Medicine 1988; Medical Oncology 2011; **Med School:** Mount Sinai Sch Med 1985; **Resid:** Internal Medicine, Mount Sinai Med Ctr 1988; **Fellow:** Hematology, Mount Sinai Med Ctr 1990; Medical Oncology, Meml Sloan-Kettering Cancer Ctr 1992

Neonatal-Perinatal Medicine

Brumberg, Heather L MD (NP) - **Spec Exp:** Nutrition; **Hospital:** Westchester Med Ctr; **Address:** WMC, Maria Fareri Chldns Hosp, 100 Woods Rd, rm 2215, Valhalla, NY 10595; **Phone:** 914-493-8558; **Board Cert:** Pediatrics 2007; Neonatal-Perinatal Medicine 2011; **Med School:** Tufts Univ 1996; **Resid:** Pediatrics, Floating Hosp Chldn 1999; **Fellow:** Neonatal-Perinatal Medicine, Yale-New Haven Hosp 2002; **Fac Appt:** Asst Prof ObG, NY Med Coll

Golombek, Sergio G MD (NP) - **Spec Exp:** Prematurity/Low Birth Weight Infants; Lung Disease in Newborns; **Hospital:** Westchester Med Ctr, Children's & Women's Phys.of Westchester (page 638); **Address:** Maria Fareri Children's Hosp, 100 Woods Rd, rm 2215, Valhalla, NY 10595; **Phone:** 914-493-8558; **Board Cert:** Neonatal-Perinatal Medicine 2012; Pediatrics 2008; **Med School:** Argentina 1983; **Resid:** Pediatrics, Dr Ignacio Pirovano Hosp 1987; Pediatrics, Raymond Blank Meml Hosp Chldn 1991; **Fellow:** Neonatal-Perinatal Medicine, Chldns Mercy Hosp 1996; **Fac Appt:** Prof Ped, NY Med Coll

Jaile-Marti, Jesus MD (NP) - **Spec Exp:** Lung Disease in Newborns; Neonatal Nutrition; **Hospital:** White Plains Hosp (page 640), Nyack Hosp; **Address:** White Plains Hosp Ctr, Div Neonatology, Davis Ave at East Post Rd, White Plains, NY 10601; **Phone:** 914-681-2282; **Board Cert:** Pediatrics 2012; Neonatal-Perinatal Medicine 2012; **Med School:** Columbia P&S 1987; **Resid:** Pediatrics, Columbia-Presby Med Ctr 1990; **Fellow:** Neonatology, Columbia-Presby Med Ctr 1993

La Gamma, Edmund F MD (NP) - **Spec Exp:** Neonatal Infections; Prematurity/Low Birth Weight Infants; Necrotizing Enterocolitis; **Hospital:** Westchester Med Ctr, Children's & Women's Phys.of Westchester (page 638); **Address:** Maria Fareri Chldns Hosp, 100 Woods Rd, rm 2215, Valhalla, NY 10595; **Phone:** 914-493-8558; **Board Cert:** Pediatrics 1981; Neonatal-Perinatal Medicine 1981; **Med School:** NY Med Coll 1976; **Resid:** Pediatrics, NY Hosp-Cornell Med Ctr 1978; **Fellow:** Neonatal-Perinatal Medicine, NY Hosp-Cornell Med Ctr 1980; Cardiovascular Disease, UCSF Med Ctr 1981; **Fac Appt:** Prof Ped, NY Med Coll

Stafford Jr, John R MD (NP) - **Spec Exp:** Neonatal Care; **Hospital:** Northern Westchester Hosp (page 639); **Address:** 400 E Main St Fl 3, Mt Kisco, NY 10549-3446; **Phone:** 914-666-1272; **Board Cert:** Pediatrics 2008; Neonatal-Perinatal Medicine 2008; **Med School:** SUNY Downstate 1986; **Resid:** Pediatrics, Columbia-Presby Med Ctr 1989; **Fellow:** Neonatology, Columbia-Presby Med Ctr 1992; **Fac Appt:** Clin Prof Ped, Columbia P&S

Nephrology

Adler, Stephen MD (Nep) - **Spec Exp:** Kidney Failure; Glomerulonephritis; Hypertension; Dialysis Care; **Hospital:** Westchester Med Ctr, White Plains Hosp (page 640); **Address:** Nephrology Assocs of Westchester, 19 Bradhurst Ave, Ste 200N, Hawthorne, NY 10532-2169; **Phone:** 914-493-7701; **Board Cert:** Internal Medicine 1979; Nephrology 1982; **Med School:** NYU Sch Med 1976; **Resid:** Internal Medicine, Mt Sinai Hosp 1979; **Fellow:** Nephrology, Boston Univ Med Ctr 1982; **Fac Appt:** Prof Med, NY Med Coll

Buzzeo, Louis MD (Nep) - **Spec Exp:** Hypertension; Kidney Disease; **Hospital:** Phelps Meml Hosp Ctr; **Address:** 777 N Broadway, Ste 203, Sleepy Hollow, NY 10591-1019; **Phone:** 914-332-9100; **Board Cert:** Internal Medicine 1975; Nephrology 1978; **Med School:** Tufts Univ 1972; **Resid:** Internal Medicine, St Vincent's Hosp & Med Ctr 1975; **Fellow:** Nephrology, NYU Med Ctr 1977

Delaney, Veronica MD/PhD (Nep) - **Spec Exp:** Transplant Medicine-Kidney; Kidney Failure; **Hospital:** Westchester Med Ctr; **Address:** Nephrology Assocs of Westchester, 19 Bradhurst Ave, Ste 200N, Hawthorne, NY 10532; **Phone:** 914-493-7701; **Board Cert:** Internal Medicine 1981; Nephrology 1982; **Med School:** England, UK 1973; **Resid:** Internal Medicine, Dublin Univ Hosps; **Fellow:** Nephrology, Univ Pittsburgh Med Ctr 1983; **Fac Appt:** Assoc Prof Med, NY Med Coll

Garrick, Renee MD (Nep) - **Spec Exp:** Hypertension; Dialysis Care; **Hospital:** Westchester Med Ctr; **Address:** Nephrology Assocs of Westchester, 19 Bradhurst Ave, Ste 200N, Hawthorne, NY 10532; **Phone:** 914-493-7701; **Board Cert:** Internal Medicine 1981; Nephrology 1984; **Med School:** Rush Med Coll 1978; **Resid:** Internal Medicine, Jacobi Med Ctr 1981; **Fellow:** Nephrology, Hosp U Penn 1984; **Fac Appt:** Prof Med, NY Med Coll

Klein, Michael D MD (Nep) - **Spec Exp:** Kidney Disease; **Hospital:** Westchester Med Ctr; **Address:** Nephrology Assocs of Westchester, 19 Bradhurst Ave, Ste 1200N, Hawthorne, NY 10532; **Phone:** 914-493-7701; **Board Cert:** Internal Medicine 2006; Nephrology 2008; **Med School:** Univ IL Coll Med 1993; **Resid:** Internal Medicine, Jacobi Med Ctr 1996; **Fellow:** Nephrology, NY Presby Hosp 1998

Reda, Dominick F MD (Nep) - **Spec Exp:** Hypertension; Kidney Disease; **Hospital:** Saint Joseph's Med Ctr - Yonkers; **Address:** 136 S Broadway, Yonkers, NY 10701; **Phone:** 914-965-0621; **Board Cert:** Internal Medicine 1987; Nephrology 2010; **Med School:** Italy 1983; **Resid:** Internal Medicine, Our Lady of Mercy 1987; **Fellow:** Nephrology, Lincoln Med Ctr 1989; **Fac Appt:** Asst Clin Prof Med, NY Med Coll

Rie, Jonathan MD (Nep) - **Spec Exp:** Hypertension; Kidney Stones; **Hospital:** White Plains Hosp (page 640); **Address:** 33 Davis Ave, White Plains, NY 10605; **Phone:** 914-831-2900; **Board Cert:** Internal Medicine 1988; Nephrology 2010; **Med School:** NY Med Coll 1985; **Resid:** Internal Medicine, Montefiore Med Ctr 1988; **Fellow:** Nephrology, Montefiore Med Ctr 1990

Rosen, Michael A MD (Nep) - **Spec Exp:** Kidney Disease-Pediatric & Adult; **Hospital:** Northern Westchester Hosp (page 639); **Address:** Mt Kisco Medical Group, 90 S Bedford Rd, Mt Kisco, NY 10549; **Phone:** 914-241-1050; **Board Cert:** Internal Medicine 2004; Nephrology 2007; **Med School:** Indiana Univ 2000; **Resid:** Internal Medicine & Pediatrics, Mt Sinai Med Ctr 2004; **Fellow:** Nephrology, Nt Sinai Med Ctr 2008

Saltzman, Martin MD (Nep) - **Spec Exp:** Kidney Disease; Hypertension; **Hospital:** Northern Westchester Hosp (page 639), Putnam Hosp Ctr; **Address:** 90 S Bedford Rd, Mt Kisco, NY 10549; **Phone:** 914-241-1050; **Board Cert:** Internal Medicine 1977; Nephrology 1978; **Med School:** SUNY Downstate 1972; **Resid:** Internal Medicine, Kings County Hosp 1973; Internal Medicine, Harlem Hosp 1974; **Fellow:** Nephrology, Univ Hosp 1976

Neurological Surgery

Benzil, Deborah L MD (NS) - **Spec Exp:** Brain Tumors; Peripheral Nerve Surgery; **Hospital:** Northern Westchester Hosp (page 639), Putnam Hosp Ctr; **Address:** Mount Kisco Medical Group, 90 S Bedford Rd, Mount Kisco, NY 10530; **Phone:** 914-241-1050; **Board Cert:** Neurological Surgery 1997; **Med School:** Univ MD Sch Med 1985; **Resid:** Neurological Surgery, Rhode Island Hosp 1993; **Fac Appt:** Assoc Prof NS, NY Med Coll

De Lotbiniere, Alain MD (NS) - **Spec Exp:** Movement Disorders; Brain Tumors; Pituitary Tumors; Deep Brain Stimulation; **Hospital:** Northern Westchester Hosp (page 639), White Plains Hosp (page 640); **Address:** Brain & Spine Surgeons of New York, 244 Westchester Ave, Ste 310, White Plains, NY 10604; **Phone:** 914-948-6688; **Board Cert:** Neurological Surgery 1994; **Med School:** McGill Univ 1981; **Resid:** Surgery, Royal Victoria Hosp 1983; Neurological Surgery, Royal Victoria Hosp 1988; **Fellow:** Neurological Surgery, Univ Cambridge 1989

Kornel, Ezriel MD (NS) - **Spec Exp:** Spinal Surgery-Minimally Invasive; Brain Tumors; Spinal Cord Tumors; **Hospital:** Northern Westchester Hosp (page 639), White Plains Hosp (page 640); **Address:** Brain & Spine Surgeons of New York, 244 Westchester Ave, Ste 310, White Plains, NY 10604; **Phone:** 914-948-0444; **Board Cert:** Neurological Surgery 1987; **Med School:** Rush Med Coll 1978; **Resid:** Surgery, Washington Hosp Ctr 1979; Neurological Surgery, Geo Wash Univ Hosp 1984; **Fac Appt:** Asst Clin Prof NS, Columbia P&S

Lee, Thomas T MD (NS) - **Spec Exp:** Spinal Surgery; Minimally Invasive Spinal Surgery; Stereotactic Radiosurgery; **Hospital:** St. John's Riverside Hosp-Andrus Pavil, Mt Sinai Med Ctr (page 102); **Address:** 150 White Plains Rd, Ste 110, Tarrytown, NY 10591; **Phone:** 914-631-9207; **Board Cert:** Neurological Surgery 2012; **Med School:** UCLA 1993; **Resid:** Neurological Surgery, Jackson Meml Med Ctr 1999; **Fac Appt:** Asst Clin Prof NS, Mount Sinai Sch Med

Murali, Raj MD (NS) - **Spec Exp:** Trigeminal Neuralgia; Skull Base Surgery; Aneurysm-Cerebral; Pituitary Tumors; **Hospital:** Westchester Med Ctr; **Address:** 19 Bradhurst Ave, rm 2800, Valhalla, NY 10532; **Phone:** 914-345-8111; **Board Cert:** Neurological Surgery 1982; **Med School:** India 1968; **Resid:** Neurological Surgery, Royal Infirm-Univ Edinburgh 1974; Neurological Surgery, NYU Med Ctr 1979; **Fac Appt:** Prof NS, NY Med Coll

Rosner, Saran S MD (NS) - **Spec Exp:** Spinal Surgery; Brain & Spinal Cord Tumors; **Hospital:** Hudson Valley Hosp Ctr; **Address:** 245 Saw Mill River Rd, Hawthorne, NY 10532; **Phone:** 914-741-2666; **Board Cert:** Neurological Surgery 1986; **Med School:** Columbia P&S 1976; **Resid:** Surgery, Johns Hopkins Hosp 1978; Neurological Surgery, Columbia-Presby Med Ctr 1983

Neurology

Ahluwalia, Brij M Singh MD (N) - **Spec Exp:** Dementia; Cerebrovascular Disease; Multiple Sclerosis; **Hospital:** Westchester Med Ctr; **Address:** 19 Bradhurst Ave, Ste 2850, Hawthorne, NY 10532; **Phone:** 914-345-1313; **Board Cert:** Neurology 1974; **Med School:** India 1961; **Resid:** Internal Medicine, Beekman Downtown Hosp 1969; Neurology, Metropolitan Hosp 1972; **Fac Appt:** Prof N, NY Med Coll

Carniciu, Sanda I MD (N) - **Spec Exp:** Electrodiagnosis; Epilepsy; **Hospital:** Phelps Meml Hosp Ctr; **Address:** 245 N Broadway, Ste 102, Sleepy Hollow, NY 10591; **Phone:** 914-631-6888; **Board Cert:** Neurology 2008; Clinical Neurophysiology 2010; Electrodiagnostic Medicine 2000; **Med School:** Romania 1987; **Resid:** Internal Medicine, VA Med Ctr 1994; Neurology, NYU Med Ctr 1997; **Fellow:** Clinical Neurophysiology, NY Presby-Cornell Med Ctr 1998

Dickoff, David J MD (N) - **Spec Exp:** Epilepsy/Seizure Disorders; Neuromuscular Disorders; Parkinson's Disease; Trigeminal Neuralgia; **Hospital:** St. John's Riverside Hosp-Andrus Pavil, Mt Sinai Med Ctr (page 102); **Address:** 984 N Broadway, Ste 509, Yonkers, NY 10701-1308; **Phone:** 914-968-0620; **Board Cert:** Neurology 1987; Electrodiagnostic Medicine 1989; **Med School:** Albany Med Coll 1982; **Resid:** Neurology, Mt Sinai Hosp 1986; **Fellow:** Neuromuscular Disease, Columbia-Presby Med Ctr 1987; **Fac Appt:** Asst Clin Prof N, Mount Sinai Sch Med

Dousmanis, Athanasios G MD (N) - **Spec Exp:** Movement Disorders; **Hospital:** Lawrence Hosp Ctr; **Address:** WestMed Medical Group, Neurology, 73 Market St, Ste 217, Yonkers, NY 10710; **Phone:** 914-831-2970; **Board Cert:** Neurology 2012; **Med School:** Cornell Univ 1997; **Resid:** Internal Medicine, Mount Sinai Med Ctr 1998; Neurology, NY Presbyterian Med Ctr 2001

Duncan, David B MD (N) - **Spec Exp:** Multiple Sclerosis; Neurodegenerative Disorders; **Hospital:** Northern Westchester Hosp (page 639); **Address:** Mt Kisco Medical Group, 90 S Bedford Rd, Mt Kisco, NY 10549; **Phone:** 914-241-1050; **Board Cert:** Neurology 2008; **Med School:** Indiana Univ 1988; **Resid:** Neurology, Univ Kentucky Med Ctr 1992

Gross, Elliott George MD (N) - **Spec Exp:** Alzheimer's Disease; Parkinson's Disease; Headache; Pain-Back & Neck; **Hospital:** Montefiore Med Ctr-Moses Campus (page 100); **Address:** 3020 Westchester, Ste 104, Purchase, NY 10577-2525; **Phone:** 914-251-1010; **Board Cert:** Neurology 1969; **Med School:** Albert Einstein Coll Med 1962; **Resid:** Neurology, Jacobi Med Ctr 1966; **Fellow:** Neurology, Albert Einstein Med Coll 1970; **Fac Appt:** Asst Clin Prof N, Columbia P&S

Jordan, Barry D MD (N) - **Spec Exp:** Brain Injury; Sports Neurology; Concussion; Memory Disorders; **Hospital:** Burke Rehab Hosp; **Address:** Burke Rehabilitation Hosp, 785 Mamaroneck Ave, White Plains, NY 10605; **Phone:** 914-597-2332; **Board Cert:** Neurology 1989; **Med School:** Harvard Med Sch 1981; **Resid:** Neurology, New York Hosp 1986; **Fellow:** Hosp Spec Surgery 1987UCLA Med Ctr 1998; **Fac Appt:** Assoc Prof N, Cornell Univ-Weill Med Coll

Kranzler, L Stephan MD (N) - **Hospital:** White Plains Hosp (page 640); **Address:** 244 Westchester Ave, Ste 315, White Plains, NY 10604; **Phone:** 914-946-9444; **Board Cert:** Neurology 1990; **Med School:** Univ Pennsylvania 1985; **Resid:** Neurology, Neuro Inst/Columbia-Presby Med Ctr 1989

Laban-Grant, Olgica MD (N) - **Spec Exp:** Epilepsy; Epilepsy in Women; **Hospital:** White Plains Hosp (page 640); **Address:** NE Regional Epilepsy Group, 333 Westchester Ave, Ste E104, White Plains, NY 10604; **Phone:** 914-428-9213; **Board Cert:** Neurology 2003; Clinical Neurophysiology 2005; **Med School:** Yugoslavia 1991; **Resid:** Neurology, NYU Med Ctr 2002; **Fellow:** Clinical Neurophysiology, NYU Med Ctr 2003

Marks, Stephen J MD (N) - **Spec Exp:** Stroke; Alzheimer's Disease; Dementia; **Hospital:** Westchester Med Ctr; **Address:** Neurology Assocs of Westchester, 19 Bradhurst Ave, Ste 2850, Hawthorne, NY 10532; **Phone:** 914-345-1313; **Board Cert:** Neurology 1985; Vascular Neurology 2006; **Med School:** NY Med Coll 1980; **Resid:** Neurology, Mt Sinai Hosp 1984; **Fellow:** Stroke, Duke Univ Med Ctr 1985; **Fac Appt:** Prof N, NY Med Coll

Morris, James R MD/PhD (N) - **Spec Exp:** Stroke; Headache; Epilepsy; Parkinson's Disease; **Hospital:** Greenwich Hosp (page 938); **Address:** Neurologic Care, 3020 Westchester Ave, Ste 305, Purchase, NY 10577; **Phone:** 203-629-8029; **Board Cert:** Neurology 2006; **Med School:** Indiana Univ 1990; **Resid:** Neurology, Columbia-Presby Med Ctr 1994; **Fellow:** Clinical Neurophysiology, Columbia-Presby Med Ctr 1995

Reding, Michael MD (N) - **Spec Exp:** Neuro-Rehabilitation; **Hospital:** Burke Rehab Hosp; **Address:** 785 Mamaroneck Ave, White Plains, NY 10605-2523; **Phone:** 914-597-2470; **Board Cert:** Internal Medicine 1976; Neurology 1981; **Med School:** Univ Kansas 1973; **Resid:** Internal Medicine, Univ Nebraska Med Ctr 1976; Neurology, Univ Nebraska Med Ctr 1979; **Fellow:** Neurology, NY Hosp/Cornell 1980; **Fac Appt:** Assoc Prof N, Cornell Univ-Weill Med Coll

Rosenkilde, Carl E MD/PhD (N) - **Hospital:** Northern Westchester Hosp (page 639); **Address:** 91 Smith Ave, Neurology Associates, Mt Kisco, NY 10549-2815; **Phone:** 914-241-1717; **Board Cert:** Neurology 1992; **Med School:** Albert Einstein Coll Med 1985; **Resid:** Neurology, Yale-New Haven Hosp 1989; **Fellow:** Neurology, UCLA Med Ctr 1979

Selman, Jay E MD (N) - **Spec Exp:** Pediatric Neurology; Epilepsy/Seizure Disorders; Headache; Tourette's Syndrome; **Hospital:** Blythedale Children's Hosp, Bronx Lebanon Hosp Ctr; **Address:** Blythedale Chldns Hosp, 95 Bradhurst Ave, Valhalla, NY 10595; **Phone:** 914-831-2480; **Board Cert:** Pediatrics 1978; Sleep Medicine 2007; Neurodevelopmental Disabilities 2012; **Med School:** Univ Tex SW, Dallas 1973; **Resid:** Pediatrics, Jacobi Med Ctr 1975; Neurology, Jacobi Med Ctr 1978; **Fellow:** Child Neurology, Jacobi Med Ctr 1977; **Fac Appt:** Assoc Clin Prof N, Columbia P&S

Silvermann, Ronald M MD (N) - **Spec Exp:** Stroke; **Hospital:** Lawrence Hosp Ctr; **Address:** WestMed Medical Group, Neurology, 73 Market St, Ste 217, Yonkers, NY 10710; **Phone:** 914-831-2970; **Board Cert:** Neurology 1978; **Med School:** Albert Einstein Coll Med 1972; **Resid:** Internal Medicine, Metropolitan Hosp 1973; Neurology, Mount Sinai Med Ctr 1976

Singh, Avtar MD (N) - **Spec Exp:** Stroke; Epilepsy; Headache; **Hospital:** White Plains Hosp (page 640), Westchester Med Ctr; **Address:** 244 Westchester Ave, Ste 315, White Plains, NY 10604; **Phone:** 914-946-9444; **Board Cert:** Neurology 1978; **Med School:** India 1967; **Resid:** Neurology, Metropolitan Hosp Ctr 1976; **Fac Appt:** Assoc Clin Prof N, NY Med Coll

Szabo, Albert MD (N) - **Hospital:** Northern Westchester Hosp (page 639); **Address:** Mt Kisco Medical Group, 90 S Bedford Rd, Mount Kisco, NY 10549; **Phone:** 914-241-1050; **Board Cert:** Neurology 2007; **Med School:** Hungary 1989; **Resid:** Neurology, Mount Sinai Sch Med 1994; **Fellow:** Clinical Neurophysiology, Thomas Jefferson U Hosp 1996; Clinical Neurophysiology, SUNY Hlth Sci Ctr 1997

Tolunsky, Eugene MD (N) - **Hospital:** Northern Westchester Hosp (page 639); **Address:** Mt Kisco Medical Group, 90 S Bedford Rd, Mt Kisco, NY 10549; **Phone:** 914-241-1050; **Board Cert:** Neurology 2002; Clinical Neurophysiology 2003; **Med School:** Univ Pennsylvania 1997; **Resid:** Neurology, Mtr Sinai Hosp 2001; **Fellow:** Neurophysiology, Mt Sinai Hosp 2002

Weintraub, Michael Ira MD (N) - **Spec Exp:** Carpal Tunnel Syndrome; Peripheral Neuropathy; Pain-Back & Neck; Diabetic Neuropathy; **Hospital:** Phelps Meml Hosp Ctr, Putnam Hosp Ctr; **Address:** 325 S Highland Ave, Briarcliff Manor, NY 10510-2093; **Phone:** 914-941-0788; **Board Cert:** Neurology 1972; **Med School:** SUNY Buffalo 1966; **Resid:** Neurology, Yale-New Haven Hosp 1970; **Fac Appt:** Clin Prof N, NY Med Coll

Neuroradiology

Berger, Scott B MD (NRad) - **Spec Exp:** Cerebrovascular Disease; Stroke; **Hospital:** Northern Westchester Hosp (page 639); **Address:** Mount Kisco Medical Group, Radiology, 110 S Bedford Rd, Mount Kisco, NY 10549; **Phone:** 914-241-1050; **Board Cert:** Diagnostic Radiology 2010; Neuroradiology 2010; **Med School:** Cornell Univ-Weill Med Coll 1992; **Resid:** Diagnostic Radiology, Yale-New Haven Hosp 1997; **Fellow:** Neurological Radiology, Yale-New Haven Hosp 1998

Tenner, Michael MD (NRad) - **Spec Exp:** Stroke; Brain & Spinal Tumors; Carotid Artery Stent Placement; **Hospital:** Westchester Med Ctr; **Address:** Westchester Med Ctr, 100 Woods Rd, Valhalla, NY 10595; **Phone:** 914-493-8158; **Board Cert:** Diagnostic Radiology 1967; Neuroradiology 2007; **Med School:** Univ MD Sch Med 1960; **Resid:** Diagnostic Radiology, Univ Maryland Hosp 1962; Diagnostic Radiology, Univ Maryland Hosp 1966; **Fellow:** Neuroradiology, Neurological Inst-Columbia Presby 1968; **Fac Appt:** Prof Rad, NY Med Coll

Nuclear Medicine

Gerard, Perry S MD (NuM) - **Spec Exp:** PET Imaging; CT Scan; Nuclear Imaging; Nuclear Oncology; **Hospital:** Westchester Med Ctr; **Address:** 100 Woods Rd, Valhalla, NY 10595; **Phone:** 914-493-8260; **Board Cert:** Diagnostic Radiology 1987; Nuclear Radiology 1989; Nuclear Cardiology 2008; **Med School:** Dominica 1980; **Resid:** Diagnostic Radiology, Maimonides Med Ctr 1984; **Fellow:** Diagnostic Imaging, Maimonides Med Ctr 1985; **Fac Appt:** Assoc Prof Rad, NY Med Coll

Obstetrics & Gynecology

Armbruster, Robert G MD (ObG) - **Spec Exp:** Colposcopy; Pregnancy-High Risk; **Hospital:** Lawrence Hosp Ctr; **Address:** 73 Market St, Ste 212, Yonkers, NY 10710; **Phone:** 914-337-3229; **Board Cert:** Obstetrics & Gynecology 1984; **Med School:** Washington Univ, St Louis 1977; **Resid:** Obstetrics & Gynecology, UCLA Med Ctr 1979; Obstetrics & Gynecology, NY-Cornell Hosp 1981

Burns, Elisa MD (ObG) - **Spec Exp:** Minimally Invasive Surgery; Robotic Surgery; Colposcopy; **Hospital:** Northern Westchester Hosp (page 639); **Address:** 90 S Bedford Rd, Mt Kisco Medical Group, Mt Kisco, NY 10549-3433; **Phone:** 914-241-1050; **Board Cert:** Obstetrics & Gynecology 2012; **Med School:** Columbia P&S 1982; **Resid:** Obstetrics & Gynecology, Columbia-Presby Hosp 1986

Eilen, Bonnie D MD (ObG) *PCP* - **Hospital:** White Plains Hosp (page 640); **Address:** 210 Westchester Ave Fl 3 - rm 306, White Plains, NY 10601; **Phone:** 914-831-6800; **Board Cert:** Obstetrics & Gynecology 2012; **Med School:** Albert Einstein Coll Med 1977; **Resid:** Obstetrics & Gynecology, Bronx Municipal Hosp 1981; **Fac Appt:** Asst Clin Prof ObG, Albert Einstein Coll Med

Florio, Philip L MD (ObG) *PCP* - **Spec Exp:** Pregnancy-High Risk; Laparoscopic Surgery; Gynecologic Cancer; Colposcopy; **Hospital:** St. John's Riverside Hosp-Andrus Pavil; **Address:** 1022 N Broadway, Yonkers, NY 10701-1303; **Phone:** 914-963-0284; **Board Cert:** Obstetrics & Gynecology 1981; **Med School:** SUNY Upstate Med Univ 1974; **Resid:** Obstetrics & Gynecology, St Barnabas Med Ctr 1978

Gannon, Jennifer B MD (ObG) - **Spec Exp:** Adolescent Gynecology; **Hospital:** Northern Westchester Hosp (page 639); **Address:** 90 S Bedford Rd, Mount Kisco, NY 10549; **Phone:** 914-241-1050; **Board Cert:** Obstetrics & Gynecology 2012; **Med School:** Univ Conn 2001; **Resid:** Obstetrics & Gynecology, Women & Infants Hosp 2005

Giuffrida, Regina MD (ObG) *PCP* - **Spec Exp:** Menopause Problems; Gynecologic Surgery; Gynecology Only; **Hospital:** Northern Westchester Hosp (page 639); **Address:** Mt Kisco Med Grp, 90 S Bedford Rd, Mt Kisco, NY 10549; **Phone:** 914-241-1050; **Board Cert:** Obstetrics & Gynecology 2011; **Med School:** NY Med Coll 1980; **Resid:** Obstetrics & Gynecology, UCSD Med Ctr 1984

Grano, Vanessa A MD (ObG) - **Spec Exp:** Laparoscopic Surgery; Pap Smear Abnormalities; Colposcopy; **Hospital:** Greenwich Hosp (page 938); **Address:** Westchester Medical Grp, 1 Theall Rd, Rye, NY 10580; **Phone:** 914-253-4912; **Board Cert:** Obstetrics & Gynecology 2012; **Med School:** SUNY Downstate 1988; **Resid:** Obstetrics & Gynecology, Columbia-Presby Hosp 1993

Grecco, Dominic M MD (ObG) - **Spec Exp:** Pregnancy-High Risk; Hysterectomy Alternatives; Robotic Surgery; **Hospital:** Northern Westchester Hosp (page 639); **Address:** 59 Kensico Drive, Mount Kisco, NY 10549; **Phone:** 914-241-4900; **Board Cert:** Obstetrics & Gynecology 2012; **Med School:** Grenada 1985; **Resid:** Obstetrics & Gynecology, LI Coll Hosp 1990

Hayworth, Scott D MD (ObG) - **Spec Exp:** Minimally Invasive Surgery; Endometriosis; Menopause Problems; **Hospital:** Northern Westchester Hosp (page 639); **Address:** 90 S Bedford Rd, Mt Kisco, NY 10549-3412; **Phone:** 914-241-1050; **Board Cert:** Obstetrics & Gynecology 2012; **Med School:** Cornell Univ-Weill Med Coll 1984; **Resid:** Obstetrics & Gynecology, Mount Sinai Med Ctr 1988; **Fac Appt:** Asst Clin Prof ObG, Mount Sinai Sch Med

Keller, Adina H MD (ObG) - **Spec Exp:** Robotic Surgery; Minimally Invasive Surgery; Menopause Problems; **Hospital:** Northern Westchester Hosp (page 639); **Address:** 90 S Bedford Rd, Mount Kisco, NY 10549; **Phone:** 914-241-1050; **Board Cert:** Obstetrics & Gynecology 2011; **Med School:** Mount Sinai Sch Med 1993; **Resid:** Obstetrics & Gynecology, Mount Sinai Med Ctr 1997

McGovern, Catherine A MD (ObG) - **Hospital:** White Plains Hosp (page 640); **Address:** 210 Westchester Ave Fl 3 - Ste 306, White Plains, NY 10605; **Phone:** 914-831-6800; **Board Cert:** Obstetrics & Gynecology 2012; **Med School:** Albany Med Coll 1985; **Resid:** Obstetrics & Gynecology, Albany Med Ctr 1989

Meacham, Kevin L MD (ObG) - **Spec Exp:** Pregnancy-High Risk; Laparoscopic Surgery; Gynecologic Surgery; **Hospital:** Montefiore New Rochelle Hosp; **Address:** 2701 Boston Post Rd, Larchmont, NY 10538-3701; **Phone:** 914-833-1000; **Board Cert:** Obstetrics & Gynecology 2012; **Med School:** NY Med Coll 1986; **Resid:** Obstetrics & Gynecology, LIJ Med Ctr 1990

Mendelowitz, Lawrence G MD (ObG) - **Spec Exp:** Pelvic Reconstruction; Laparoscopic Hysterectomy; Gynecologic Surgery; Pregnancy-High Risk; **Hospital:** Phelps Meml Hosp Ctr, Westchester Med Ctr; **Address:** 755 N Broadway, Ste 560, Sleepy Hollow, NY 10591; **Phone:** 914-631-0337; **Board Cert:** Obstetrics & Gynecology 2012; **Med School:** NYU Sch Med 1976; **Resid:** Obstetrics & Gynecology, Bellevue Hosp-NYU 1980

Mieszerski, Laura E MD (ObG) - **Spec Exp:** Adolescent Gynecology; Pregnancy-High Risk; **Hospital:** Hudson Valley Hosp Ctr; **Address:** Hudson Valley Health Ctr, Women's Health, 1037 Main St, Peekskill, NY 10566; **Phone:** 914-734-8790; **Board Cert:** Obstetrics & Gynecology 2009; **Med School:** Albany Med Coll 1992; **Resid:** Obstetrics & Gynecology, UTSA Affil Hosp 1996

Nelson, William S MD (ObG) - **Spec Exp:** Menopause Problems; **Hospital:** Greenwich Hosp (page 938); **Address:** Westchester Medical Group, 1 Theall Rd, Rye, NY 10580; **Phone:** 914-253-4912; **Board Cert:** Obstetrics & Gynecology 1981; **Med School:** Albert Einstein Coll Med 1960; **Resid:** Obstetrics & Gynecology, Maimonides Med Ctr 1965; **Fac Appt:** Asst Clin Prof ObG, Albert Einstein Coll Med

Regard, Monique M MD (ObG) - **Spec Exp:** Pediatric & Adolescent Gynecology Only; Birth Defects-Vaginal; Ovarian Masses in Children/Adolescents; **Hospital:** Westchester Med Ctr, Children's & Women's Phys.of Westchester (page 638); **Address:** Children's/Women's Physicians of Westchester, 503 Grasslands Rd, Ste 200, Valhalla, NY 10595; **Phone:** 914-304-5254; **Board Cert:** Obstetrics & Gynecology 2010; **Med School:** Baylor Coll Med 1989; **Resid:** Obstetrics & Gynecology, Univ Minn Med Ctr 1993; **Fac Appt:** Asst Clin Prof Ped, NY Med Coll

Simpson, Joe Leigh MD (ObG) - **Spec Exp:** Prenatal Diagnosis; Ovarian Failure; Infertility/Genetics; **Address:** March of Dimes Foundation, 1275 Mamaroneck Ave, White Plains, NY 10605; **Phone:** 914-997-4555; **Board Cert:** Obstetrics & Gynecology 2012; Clinical Genetics 1982; **Med School:** Duke Univ 1968; **Resid:** Obstetrics & Gynecology, NY-Presby/Weill Cornell Med Ctr 1973

Ullman, Joel MD (ObG) - **Spec Exp:** Laparoscopic Surgery-Complex; Uro-Gynecology; Vulvar Disease; Vaginal Surgery; **Hospital:** Montefiore New Rochelle Hosp; **Address:** 2071 Boston Post Rd, Larchmont, NY 10538-3701; **Phone:** 914-833-1000; **Board Cert:** Obstetrics & Gynecology 1978; **Med School:** NY Med Coll 1963; **Resid:** Obstetrics & Gynecology, Beth Israel Med Ctr 1969; **Fac Appt:** Asst Clin Prof ObG, Albert Einstein Coll Med

Wysoki, Randee S MD (ObG) - **Hospital:** White Plains Hosp (page 640); **Address:** 210 Westchester Ave, Westmed Medical Group, White Plains, NY 10604; **Phone:** 914-831-6800; **Board Cert:** Obstetrics & Gynecology 2012; **Med School:** Georgetown Univ 1982; **Resid:** Obstetrics & Gynecology, Emory Univ Med Ctr 1986

Ophthalmology

Biser, Seth A MD (Oph) - **Spec Exp:** Corneal Disease & Surgery; Cataract Surgery; Refractive Surgery; **Hospital:** Lawrence Hosp Ctr; **Address:** 654 Gramatan Ave, Fleetwood, NY 10552; **Phone:** 914-664-2300; **Board Cert:** Ophthalmology 2003; **Med School:** Univ Pennsylvania 1997; **Resid:** Ophthalmology, Wilmer Eye Inst 2001; **Fellow:** Refractive Surgery, North Shore Hosp 2002; **Fac Appt:** Asst Clin Prof Oph, NYU Sch Med

Bortz, John G MD (Oph) - **Spec Exp:** Oculoplastic & Orbital Surgery; Neuro-Ophthalmology; Orbital & Eyelid Tumors/Cancer; Eyelid Cosmetic & Reconstructive Surgery; **Hospital:** Westchester Med Ctr; **Address:** 811 N Broadway, White Plains, NY 10603-2403; **Phone:** 914-686-0006; **Board Cert:** Ophthalmology 1989; Internal Medicine 1982; **Med School:** Johns Hopkins Univ 1979; **Resid:** Internal Medicine, St Lukes-Roosevelt Hosp 1982; Ophthalmology, Westchester Co Med Ctr 1987; **Fellow:** Oculoplastic & Reconstructive Surgery, Albany Med Ctr 1988

Brustein, Harris C MD (Oph) - **Spec Exp:** Pediatric Ophthalmology; **Hospital:** Montefiore New Rochelle Hosp; **Address:** 77 Quaker Ridge Rd, Ste 203, New Rochelle, NY 10804-2821; **Phone:** 914-235-0022; **Board Cert:** Ophthalmology 1976; **Med School:** Albert Einstein Coll Med 1970; **Resid:** Ophthalmology, Montefiore Med Ctr 1974; **Fellow:** Pediatric Ophthalmology, Chldns Hosp 1975

Dieck, William MD (Oph) - **Spec Exp:** Cataract Surgery; Glaucoma; Lens Implants-Multifocal; Dry Eye Syndrome; **Hospital:** Northern Westchester Hosp (page 639); **Address:** 185 Kisco Ave, Ste 500, Mt Kisco, NY 10549; **Phone:** 914-666-4939; **Board Cert:** Ophthalmology 1990; **Med School:** NY Med Coll 1983; **Resid:** Internal Medicine, Westchester Co Med Ctr 1985; Ophthalmology, Westchester Co Med Ctr 1988

Fern, Craig MD (Oph) - **Spec Exp:** Retinal Disorders; Retina/Vitreous Surgery; **Hospital:** Northern Westchester Hosp (page 639); **Address:** 105 S Bedford Rd, Ste 311, Mt Kisco, NY 10549; **Phone:** 914-244-3800; **Board Cert:** Ophthalmology 2005; **Med School:** NYU Sch Med 1987; **Resid:** Internal Medicine, Bellevue Med Ctr 1989; Ophthalmology, Bellevue Med Ctr 1993; **Fellow:** Vitreoretinal Disease, UC Davis Med Ctr 1995; **Fac Appt:** Asst Prof Oph, NYU Sch Med

Fleischman, Jay MD (Oph) - **Spec Exp:** Diabetic Eye Disease/Retinopathy; Macular Degeneration; Uveitis; **Hospital:** Montefiore Med Ctr-Moses Campus (page 100), Stamford Hosp (page 939); **Address:** 600 Mamaroneck Ave, Ste 103, Harrison, NY 10528-1613; **Phone:** 914-315-5111; **Board Cert:** Ophthalmology 1980; **Med School:** Columbia P&S 1975; **Resid:** Ophthalmology, Johns Hopkins Hosp 1979; **Fellow:** Retina/Vitreous Surgery, Med Coll of Wisconsin 1980; **Fac Appt:** Assoc Prof Oph, Albert Einstein Coll Med

Forman, Scott MD (Oph) - **Spec Exp:** Botox Therapy; Neuro-Ophthalmology; **Hospital:** Westchester Med Ctr; **Address:** Westchester Med Ctr, Dept Ophthalmology, 95 Grasslands Rd, Valhalla, NY 10595; **Phone:** 914-493-7666; **Board Cert:** Ophthalmology 1989; **Med School:** UMDNJ-RW Johnson Med Sch 1981; **Resid:** Ophthalmology, New York Med Coll Affil Hosp 1987; **Fellow:** Neuro-Ophthalmology, Columbia-Presby Med Ctr 1988; **Fac Appt:** Assoc Prof Oph, NY Med Coll

Glassman, Morris I MD (Oph) - **Spec Exp:** Cataract Surgery; Glaucoma; **Hospital:** Northern Westchester Hosp (page 639), Montefiore Med Ctr-Moses Campus (page 100); **Address:** 1940 Commerce St, Yorktown Heights, NY 10598; **Phone:** 914-962-5506; **Board Cert:** Ophthalmology 1975; **Med School:** NYU Sch Med 1968; **Resid:** Ophthalmology, Jacobi Med Ctr 1974; **Fac Appt:** Asst Clin Prof Oph, Albert Einstein Coll Med

Gordon, James R MD (Oph) - **Spec Exp:** Oculoplastic Surgery; Eyelid Cosmetic & Reconstructive Surgery; **Hospital:** White Plains Hosp (page 640); **Address:** Westchester Eye Assocs, 170 Maple Ave, Ste 402, White Plains, NY 10601; **Phone:** 914-949-9200; **Board Cert:** Ophthalmology 2004; **Med School:** Israel 1996; **Resid:** Ophthalmology, St Vincent's Hosp & Med Ctr 2000

Greenbaum, Allen S MD (Oph) - **Spec Exp:** Laser Refractive Surgery; Cataract Surgery; **Hospital:** White Plains Hosp (page 640); **Address:** Westchester Eye Assocs, 170 Maple Ave, Ste 402, White Plains, NY 10601; **Phone:** 914-949-9200; **Board Cert:** Ophthalmology 1985; **Med School:** Mount Sinai Sch Med 1979; **Resid:** Ophthalmology, Mount Sinai Hosp 1984

Greenberg, Steven C MD (Oph) - **Spec Exp:** Pediatric Ophthalmology; **Hospital:** Putnam Hosp Ctr, White Plains Hosp (page 640); **Address:** WestMed Medical Grp, 1 Theall Rd, Rye, NY 10580; **Phone:** 914-848-8999; **Board Cert:** Ophthalmology 1987; **Med School:** Univ Conn 1982; **Resid:** Ophthalmology, NYU Med Ctr 1986; **Fellow:** Pediatric Ophthalmology, Manhattan EET Hosp 1987

Horowitz, Marc A MD (Oph) - **Spec Exp:** Pediatric Ophthalmology; Strabismus; Retinopathy of Prematurity; Eye Muscle Disorders; **Hospital:** Westchester Med Ctr, White Plains Hosp (page 640); **Address:** 14 Harwood Ct, Ste 209, Scarsdale, NY 10583; **Phone:** 914-723-5511; **Board Cert:** Ophthalmology 1983; **Med School:** Mount Sinai Sch Med 1978; **Resid:** Ophthalmology, St Luke's Roosevelt Hosp Ctr 1982; **Fellow:** Pediatric Ophthalmology, Chldns Hosp 1983; **Fac Appt:** Asst Clin Prof Oph, NY Med Coll

Lederman, Martin E MD (Oph) - **Spec Exp:** Pediatric Ophthalmology; Eye Muscle Disorders; Diagnostic Problems; Tear Duct Problems; **Hospital:** White Plains Hosp (page 640), NY-Presby/Columbia Univ Med Ctr, NY (page 104); **Address:** Lederman & Lederman, 3020 Westchester Ave, Ste 402, Purchase, NY 10577; **Phone:** 914-417-6441; **Board Cert:** Ophthalmology 2005; **Med School:** Albert Einstein Coll Med 1964; **Resid:** Ophthalmology, Albert Einstein Affil Hosp 1968; **Fellow:** Pediatric Ophthalmology, Chldns Hosp Natl Med Ctr 1969; **Fac Appt:** Assoc Prof Oph, Columbia P&S

Lippman, Jay I MD (Oph) - **Spec Exp:** Cataract Surgery; LASIK-Refractive Surgery; Cornea Transplant; **Hospital:** New York Eye & Ear Infirm (page 115); **Address:** 828 Pelhamdale Ave, New Rochelle, NY 10801; **Phone:** 914-636-3600; **Board Cert:** Ophthalmology 1972; **Med School:** Ros Franklin Univ/Chicago Med Sch 1964; **Resid:** Ophthalmology, Montefiore Med Ctr 1970; **Fac Appt:** Clin Prof Oph, NY Med Coll

McKee, Heather C MD (Oph) - **Spec Exp:** Cataract Surgery; Glaucoma; **Hospital:** St. John's Riverside Hosp-Dobbs Ferry Pavil; **Address:** Castellano & McKee, 200 S Broadway, Ste 202, Tarrytown, NY 10591-4504; **Phone:** 914-631-7300; **Board Cert:** Ophthalmology 1981; **Med School:** Duke Univ 1976; **Resid:** Ophthalmology, Strong Meml Hosp 1980; **Fac Appt:** Asst Clin Prof Oph, NY Med Coll

Mignone, Biagio V MD (Oph) - **Spec Exp:** Retinal Disorders; Glaucoma; Cataract Surgery; **Hospital:** Montefiore Mt Vernon Hosp, Lawrence Hosp Ctr; **Address:** Mignone Medical Eye Care, 955 Yonkers Ave, Ste 105, Inter-County Medical Plaza, Yonkers, NY 10704; **Phone:** 914-237-2002; **Board Cert:** Ophthalmology 1980; **Med School:** NY Med Coll 1975; **Resid:** Ophthalmology, UMDNJ Med Ctr 1979; **Fac Appt:** Asst Clin Prof Oph, NY Med Coll

Morello, Robert F MD (Oph) - **Spec Exp:** Geriatric Ophthalmology; **Hospital:** Montefiore New Rochelle Hosp; **Address:** Westchester Eye MDs, 120 Warren St, New Rochelle, NY 10801; **Phone:** 914-633-7214; **Board Cert:** Ophthalmology 1985; **Med School:** Mexico 1976; **Resid:** Internal Medicine, Bronx Lebanon Hosp 1978; Ophthalmology, Bronx Lebanon Hosp 1981

Most, Richard W MD (Oph) - **Spec Exp:** Pediatric Ophthalmology; Strabismus-Adult & Pediatric; Tear Duct Problems; **Hospital:** Northern Westchester Hosp (page 639), Mt Sinai Med Ctr (page 102); **Address:** 101 S Bedford Rd, Bldg 400 - Ste 401, MS 10549, Mt Kisco, NY 10549; **Phone:** 914-241-2206; **Board Cert:** Ophthalmology 1977; Pediatric Ophthalmology 1978; **Med School:** Italy 1971; **Resid:** Pathology, Maimonides Med Ctr 1973; Ophthalmology, Lenox Hill Hosp 1976; **Fellow:** Pediatric Ophthalmology, NYU Med Ctr/Bellevue Hosp 1977; Pediatric Ophthalmology, Chldns Hosp Natl Med Ctr 1978; **Fac Appt:** Assoc Clin Prof Oph, Mount Sinai Sch Med

Phillips, Howard P MD (Oph) - **Spec Exp:** Corneal Disease; **Hospital:** Phelps Meml Hosp Ctr; **Address:** Hudson Valley Eye Associates, 24 Saw Mill River Rd, Ste 202, Hawthorne, NY 10532; **Phone:** 914-345-3937; **Board Cert:** Ophthalmology 1982; **Med School:** NYU Sch Med 1977; **Resid:** Ophthalmology, NYU Med Ctr 1981; **Fellow:** Retina, Bellevue Hosp 1982

Ray, Audell W MD (Oph) - **Spec Exp:** Glaucoma; **Hospital:** Lawrence Hosp Ctr; **Address:** Bronxville Eye Associates, 77 Pondfield Rd, Bronxville, NY 10708-3809; **Phone:** 914-337-8844; **Board Cert:** Ophthalmology 1979; **Med School:** Columbia P&S 1974; **Resid:** Internal Medicine, St Lukes-Roosevelt Hosp 1975; Ophthalmology, Manhattan EE &T Hosp 1978

Salzman, Jacqueline G MD (Oph) - **Spec Exp:** Cataract Surgery; Diabetic Eye Disease; Glaucoma; Laser Surgery; **Hospital:** Phelps Meml Hosp Ctr; **Address:** 200 S Broadway, Ste 211, Tarrytown, NY 10591-4504; **Phone:** 914-332-5394; **Board Cert:** Ophthalmology 1985; **Med School:** NYU Sch Med 1979; **Resid:** Ophthalmology, Bellevue Hosp 1983; **Fellow:** Retina, Bellevue Hosp 1984

Solomon, Ira S MD (Oph) - **Spec Exp:** Glaucoma; Laser Surgery; Microsurgery; **Hospital:** Lawrence Hosp Ctr, Lenox Hill Hosp (page 106); **Address:** Scarsdale Ophthalmology Assocs, 700 White Plains Rd, Ste 343, Scarsdale, NY 10583; **Phone:** 914-725-5400; **Board Cert:** Ophthalmology 1989; **Med School:** Jefferson Med Coll 1982; **Resid:** Internal Medicine, Lenox Hill Hosp 1983; Ophthalmology, Montefiore Med Ctr 1986; **Fellow:** Glaucoma, New York E&E Infirm 1987; **Fac Appt:** Asst Clin Prof Oph, Albert Einstein Coll Med

Solomon, Sherry K MD (Oph) - **Spec Exp:** Diabetic Eye Disease/Retinopathy; Macular Degeneration; Retinitis Pigmentosa; **Hospital:** Lawrence Hosp Ctr, Montefiore New Rochelle Hosp; **Address:** Scarsdale Ophthalmology Assocs, 700 White Plains Rd, Ste 343, Scarsdale, NY 10583; **Phone:** 914-725-5400; **Board Cert:** Ophthalmology 1991; **Med School:** Albert Einstein Coll Med 1986; **Resid:** Internal Medicine, Lenox Hill Hosp 1987; Ophthalmology, Montefiore Hosp Med Ctr 1990; **Fellow:** Retina, NYU Med Ctr 1991

Stein, Mitchell B MD (Oph) - **Spec Exp:** Cataract Surgery; Cornea & External Eye Disease; **Hospital:** Northern Westchester Hosp (page 639); **Address:** 69 S Moger Ave, Mount Kisco, NY 10549-2217; **Phone:** 914-666-2961; **Board Cert:** Internal Medicine 1982; Ophthalmology 2005; **Med School:** Albert Einstein Coll Med 1979; **Resid:** Internal Medicine, Bronx Muni Hosp 1982; Ophthalmology, SUNY-Downstate Med Ctr 1986; **Fellow:** Cornea, Mt Sinai Hosp/Beth Israel Hosp 1987; **Fac Appt:** Asst Clin Prof Med, Albert Einstein Coll Med

Tostanoski, Jean R MD (Oph) - **Spec Exp:** Corneal Disease & Transplant; Refractive Surgery; Cataract Surgery; Glaucoma; **Hospital:** Phelps Meml Hosp Ctr; **Address:** Hudson Valley Eye Assocs, 24 Saw Mill River Rd, Ste 202, Hawthorne, NY 10532; **Phone:** 914-345-3937; **Board Cert:** Ophthalmology 2006; **Med School:** Albert Einstein Coll Med 1989; **Resid:** Ophthalmology, Bronx Lebanon Hosp Ctr 1993; Ophthalmology, Manhattan EE&T Hosp 1994

Zaidman, Gerald W MD (Oph) - **Spec Exp:** Laser Vision Surgery; Cornea Transplant; Cataract Surgery; Corneal Disease-Pediatric; **Hospital:** Westchester Med Ctr; **Address:** Westchester Med Ctr, Dept Ophthalmology, Macy Pavilion, rm 1100, Valhalla, NY 10595; **Phone:** 914-493-1599; **Board Cert:** Ophthalmology 1981; **Med School:** Albert Einstein Coll Med 1975; **Resid:** Ophthalmology, Beth Abraham Hosp 1977; Ophthalmology, Lenox Hill Hosp 1980; **Fellow:** Cornea & Ext Eye Disease, Univ Pittsburgh Affil Hosp 1982; **Fac Appt:** Assoc Prof Oph, NY Med Coll

Orthopaedic Surgery

Asprinio, David E MD (OrS) - **Spec Exp:** Trauma; **Hospital:** Westchester Med Ctr; **Address:** University Orthopaedics, 19 Bradhurst Ave, Ste 1300-N, Hawthorne, NY 10595; **Phone:** 914-789-2734; **Board Cert:** Orthopaedic Surgery 2008; **Med School:** Univ VT Coll Med 1986; **Resid:** Surgery, Rhode Island Hosp 1989; Orthopaedic Surgery, Rhode Island Hosp 1992; **Fellow:** Trauma, Hosp for Special Surg 1993

Bavaro, Nicholas A MD (OrS) - **Spec Exp:** Sports Medicine; Knee Surgery; Hip Surgery; Hip & Knee Replacement; **Hospital:** St. John's Riverside Hosp-Dobbs Ferry Pavil, Nyack Hosp; **Address:** Premier Othopaedics of Westchester & Rockland, Community Hosp-Dobbs Ferry, Lower Level, 128 Ashford Ave, Dobbs Ferry, NY 10522; **Phone:** 914-693-2057; **Board Cert:** Orthopaedic Surgery 2014; **Med School:** NY Med Coll 1993; **Resid:** Orthopaedic Surgery, St Lukes Roosevelt Hosp 1998; Orthopaedic Surgery, Meml Sloan Kettering Cancer Ctr 1996; **Fellow:** Sports Medicine, NYU Hosp for Joint Diseases 1999

Burak, George MD (OrS) - **Spec Exp:** Sports Injuries; Arthritis; **Hospital:** Phelps Meml Hosp Ctr; **Address:** Hudson Valley Bone & Joint Surgeons, 24 Saw Mill River Rd, Ste 206, Hawthorne, NY 10532-1541; **Phone:** 914-631-7777; **Board Cert:** Orthopaedic Surgery 1971; **Med School:** SUNY Upstate Med Univ 1964; **Resid:** Orthopaedic Surgery, Kings County Hosp 1969; **Fac Appt:** Asst Prof OrS, SUNY Downstate

Buschmann, William R MD (OrS) - **Spec Exp:** Foot & Ankle Surgery; **Hospital:** White Plains Hosp (page 640); **Address:** White Plains Physician Assocs Orthopedic Specialists, 222 Westchester Ave, Ste 101, White Plains, NY 10604; **Phone:** 914-946-1010; **Board Cert:** Orthopaedic Surgery 2007; **Med School:** NY Med Coll 1978; **Resid:** Orthopaedic Surgery, Hershey Med Ctr 1983; **Fellow:** Foot & Ankle Surgery, Hosp for Joint Diseases 1984

Cristofaro, Robert L MD (OrS) - **Spec Exp:** Pediatric Orthopaedic Surgery; Pediatric Sports Medicine; Foot & Hip Disorders-Complex Pediatric; Neuromuscular Disorders; **Hospital:** Westchester Med Ctr, Montefiore New Rochelle Hosp; **Address:** Superior Orthopaedic Care, 3010 Westchester Ave, Ste 104, Purchase, NY 10577; **Phone:** 914-967-8708; **Board Cert:** Orthopaedic Surgery 1978; **Med School:** SUNY Downstate 1971; **Resid:** Surgery, Montefiore Hosp 1973; Orthopaedic Surgery, Montefiore Hosp 1976; **Fellow:** Pediatric Orthopaedic Surgery, Rancho Los Amigos Med Ctr 1977; **Fac Appt:** Assoc Clin Prof OrS, NY Med Coll

Cushner, Michael A MD (OrS) - **Hospital:** Beth Israel Med Ctr - Petrie Div (page 94), St. John's Riverside Hosp-Dobbs Ferry Pavil; **Address:** WestMed Medical Group, 73 Market St, Ridge Hill, Yonkers, NY 10801; **Phone:** 914-682-6540; **Board Cert:** Orthopaedic Surgery 2012; **Med School:** Univ MD Sch Med 1993; **Resid:** Orthopaedic Surgery, Med Univ SC 1998; **Fellow:** Trauma, S Tahoe Sports Med Group 1999

Edelson, Charles MD (OrS) - **Spec Exp:** Reconstructive Surgery; Sports Medicine; Joint Replacement; Knee Replacement; **Hospital:** St. John's Riverside Hosp-Andrus Pavil, Saint Joseph's Med Ctr - Yonkers; **Address:** S Westchester Ortho & Sports Med Assocs, 970 N Broadway, Ste 204, Yonkers, NY 10701-1310; **Phone:** 914-476-4343; **Board Cert:** Orthopaedic Surgery 1979; **Med School:** NY Med Coll 1973; **Resid:** Surgery, Montefiore Med Ctr 1975; Orthopaedic Surgery, Montefiore Med Ctr 1979

Gundy, Edward V MD (OrS) - **Spec Exp:** Geriatric Orthopaedic Surgery; Sports Medicine; **Hospital:** White Plains Hosp (page 640), Greenwich Hosp (page 938); **Address:** WESTMED Medical Group, 1 Theall Rd, Rye, NY 10580; **Phone:** 914-682-6540; **Board Cert:** Orthopaedic Surgery 1983; **Med School:** Cornell Univ-Weill Med Coll 1976; **Resid:** Surgery, St Lukes-Roosevelt Hosp 1978; Orthopaedic Surgery, Hosp Special Surg 1981

Holder, Jonathan L MD (OrS) - **Spec Exp:** Sports Medicine; Foot & Ankle Surgery; Joint Replacement; **Hospital:** White Plains Hosp (page 640), Westchester Med Ctr; **Address:** 170 Maple Ave, Ste 109, White Plains, NY 10601; **Phone:** 914-421-0600; **Board Cert:** Orthopaedic Surgery 2013; **Med School:** NY Med Coll 1985; **Resid:** Surgery, Metropolitan Hosp Ctr 1996; Orthopaedic Surgery, Metropolitan Hosp Ctr 1990

Karas, Evan H MD (OrS) - **Spec Exp:** Shoulder Surgery; Sports Medicine; **Hospital:** Northern Westchester Hosp (page 639); **Address:** 90 S Bedford Rd, Mt Kisco, NY 10549; **Phone:** 914-241-1050; **Board Cert:** Orthopaedic Surgery 2010; Orthopaedic Sports Medicine 2011; **Med School:** NYU Sch Med 1991; **Resid:** Orthopaedic Surgery, Mt Sinai Hosp 1996; **Fellow:** Sports Medicine, Univ Penn 1997

Khabie, Victor MD (OrS) - **Spec Exp:** Sports Medicine; Shoulder Surgery; Elbow Surgery; Knee Surgery; **Hospital:** Northern Westchester Hosp (page 639), Putnam Hosp Ctr; **Address:** Somers Orth Surg & Sports Med Grp, 657 E Main St, Ste 3, Mt Kisco, NY 10549; **Phone:** 914-666-5550; **Board Cert:** Orthopaedic Surgery 2010; Orthopaedic Sports Medicine 2008; **Med School:** Harvard Med Sch 1991; **Resid:** Orthopaedic Surgery, Hosp for Joint Dis 1996; **Fellow:** Orthopaedic Sports Medicine, Kerlan-Jobe Ortho Clinic 1997; **Fac Appt:** Asst Clin Prof OrS, NYU Sch Med

Lent, David E MD (OrS) - **Spec Exp:** Knee Replacement; Knee Surgery; Arthroscopic Surgery; **Hospital:** St. John's Riverside Hosp-Andrus Pavil; **Address:** S Westchester Ortho & Sports Med Assocs, 970 N Broadway, Ste 204, Yonkers, NY 10701-1310; **Phone:** 914-476-4343; **Board Cert:** Orthopaedic Surgery 2010; **Med School:** NYU Sch Med 1991; **Resid:** Orthopaedic Surgery, Jacobi Med Ctr 1996

Maddalo, Anthony Vincent MD (OrS) - **Spec Exp:** Sports Medicine; Shoulder & Knee Injuries; Rotator Cuff Surgery; **Hospital:** Phelps Meml Hosp Ctr; **Address:** 24 Saw Mill River Rd, Ste 206, Hawthorne, NY 10532; **Phone:** 914-631-7777; **Board Cert:** Orthopaedic Surgery 2009; **Med School:** NY Med Coll 1981; **Resid:** Orthopaedic Surgery, Lenox Hill Hosp 1986

Mann, Ronald L MD (OrS) - **Spec Exp:** Pediatric Orthopaedic Surgery; Fractures; Sports Medicine; **Hospital:** Northern Westchester Hosp (page 639); **Address:** 1888 Commerce St, Yorktown Heights, NY 10598-4431; **Phone:** 914-962-7712; **Board Cert:** Orthopaedic Surgery 2009; **Med School:** Univ Pennsylvania 1980; **Resid:** Surgery, Mount Sinai Hosp 1982; Orthopaedic Surgery, Mount Sinai Hosp 1985; **Fellow:** Pediatric Orthopaedic Surgery, Hosp for Special Surgery 1986

Nelson Jr, John M MD (OrS) - **Spec Exp:** Pediatric Orthopaedic Surgery; Clubfoot/Foot Deformities in Children; Pediatric Sports Medicine; **Hospital:** Montefiore New Rochelle Hosp, Westchester Med Ctr; **Address:** Superior Orthopaedic Care, 3010 Westchester Ave, Ste 104, Purchase, NY 10577; **Phone:** 914-632-4420; **Board Cert:** Orthopaedic Surgery 2008; **Med School:** Mount Sinai Sch Med 1979; **Resid:** Surgery, Mt Sinai Hosp 1980; Orthopaedic Surgery, Hosp for Joint Diseases 1984; **Fellow:** Pediatric Orthopaedic Surgery, Scottish Rite Chldn's Hosp 1985

Oh, Young Don MD (OrS) - **Spec Exp:** Sports Medicine; Arthroscopic Surgery; Joint Replacement; **Hospital:** White Plains Hosp (page 640), Greenwich Hosp (page 938); **Address:** WESTMED Med Grp, Orthopaedic Surgery, 210 Westchester Ave, White Plains, NY 10604; **Phone:** 914-682-6540; **Board Cert:** Orthopaedic Surgery 2012; **Med School:** NYU Sch Med 1993; **Resid:** Surgery, LIJ Med Ctr 1994; Orthopaedic Surgery, LIJ Med Ctr 1998; **Fellow:** Orthopaedic Sports Medicine, UCLA Med Ctr 1999

Pidoriano, Arthur J MD (OrS) - **Spec Exp:** Sports Medicine; Arthroscopic Surgery; Rotator Cuff Surgery; Knee Ligament Reconstruction; **Hospital:** Hudson Valley Hosp Ctr; **Address:** Mt Kisco Med Grp, 1978 Crompond Rd, Ste 201, Cortlandt Manor, NY 10567; **Phone:** 914-739-2121; **Board Cert:** Orthopaedic Surgery 2008; **Med School:** NY Med Coll 1989; **Resid:** Orthopaedic Surgery, Westchester Med Ctr 1994; **Fellow:** Sports Medicine, Univ Conn Sch Med Affil Hosp 1996

Schlesinger, Iris E MD (OrS) - **Spec Exp:** Pediatric Orthopaedic Surgery; **Hospital:** Westchester Med Ctr, Phelps Meml Hosp Ctr; **Address:** 19 Bradhurst Ave, Ste 1300 N, Hawthorne, NY 10532; **Phone:** 914-789-2731; **Board Cert:** Orthopaedic Surgery 2012; **Med School:** Albany Med Coll 1983; **Resid:** Orthopaedic Surgery, NYU Med Ctr 1988; **Fellow:** Pediatric Orthopaedic Surgery, Hosp Sick Children 1989; **Fac Appt:** Assoc Prof OrS, NY Med Coll

Seebacher, J Robert MD (OrS) - **Spec Exp:** Hip Replacement; Knee Replacement; Arthritis; **Hospital:** Phelps Meml Hosp Ctr; **Address:** Hudson Valley Bone & Joint Surgeons, 24 Saw Mill River Rd, Ste 206, Hawthorne, NY 10532; **Phone:** 914-631-7777; **Board Cert:** Orthopaedic Surgery 1984; **Med School:** Georgetown Univ 1976; **Resid:** Surgery, Mount Sinai Hosp 1978; Orthopaedic Surgery, Hosp for Special Surgery 1981; **Fellow:** Pediatric Orthopaedic Surgery, Hosp for Sick Children 1982

Small, Robert D MD (OrS) - **Spec Exp:** Knee Replacement; Hip Replacement; **Hospital:** White Plains Hosp (page 640); **Address:** White Plains Physician Assocs Orthopedic Specialists, 222 Westchester Ave, Ste 101, White Plains, NY 10604; **Phone:** 914-946-1010; **Board Cert:** Neurology 1985; **Med School:** NY Med Coll 1977; **Resid:** Orthopaedic Surgery, Hosp fpr Joint Diseases 1982; **Fellow:** Hip Surgery, Hosp for Special Surgery 1983

Small, Steven R MD (OrS) - **Spec Exp:** Sports Medicine; **Hospital:** Hudson Valley Hosp Ctr; **Address:** 1978 Crompond Rd Fl 2, Cortland Manor, NY 10567; **Phone:** 914-739-2121; **Board Cert:** Orthopaedic Surgery 2011; **Med School:** NY Med Coll 1979; **Resid:** Orthopaedic Surgery, Westchester Med Ctr 1984

Spencer, Eric M MD (OrS) - **Spec Exp:** Hand Surgery; **Hospital:** St. John's Riverside Hosp-Andrus Pavil; **Address:** S Westchester Ortho & Sports Med Assocs, 970 N Broadway, Ste 204, Yonkers, NY 10701; **Phone:** 914-476-4343; **Board Cert:** Orthopaedic Surgery 2006; **Med School:** Columbia P&S 1998; **Resid:** Orthopaedic Surgery, Lenox Hill Hosp 2002; **Fellow:** Hand Surgery, Hosp for Joint Disease 2003

Voellmicke, Kurt V MD (OrS) - **Spec Exp:** Foot & Ankle Surgery; **Hospital:** Northern Westchester Hosp (page 639); **Address:** Mt Kisco Med Grp, 90 S Bedford Rd, Mount Kisco, NY 10549; **Phone:** 914-241-1050; **Board Cert:** Orthopaedic Surgery 2004; **Med School:** Cornell Univ-Weill Med Coll 1996; **Resid:** Surgery, NY Presby Hosp 2001; Orthopaedic Surgery, Hosp for Special Surgery 2001; **Fellow:** Foot & Ankle Surgery, Hosp for Special Surgery 2002

Weinstein, Richard N MD (OrS) - **Spec Exp:** Shoulder Surgery; Rotator Cuff Surgery; Sports Medicine; Knee Surgery; **Hospital:** White Plains Hosp (page 640); **Address:** 1133 Westchester Ave, Ste N008, White Plains, NY 10604; **Phone:** 914-358-9700; **Board Cert:** Orthopaedic Surgery 2010; Orthopaedic Sports Medicine 2007; **Med School:** NYU Sch Med 1991; **Resid:** Orthopaedic Surgery, Bronx Lebanon Hosp 1996; **Fellow:** Sports Medicine, Univ Conn Hlth Syst 1997; **Fac Appt:** , Albert Einstein Coll Med

Yasgur, David J MD (OrS) - **Spec Exp:** Knee Replacement; Joint Replacement; Sports Medicine; **Hospital:** Northern Westchester Hosp (page 639); **Address:** Mount Kisco Med Grp, 111 Bedford Rd, Katonah, NY 10536; **Phone:** 914-232-3135; **Board Cert:** Orthopaedic Surgery 2010; **Med School:** Cornell Univ 1991; **Resid:** Surgery, Bellevue Hosp Med Ctr 1992; Orthopaedic Surgery, Hosp Joint Diseases 1996; **Fellow:** Knee Reconstruction, ISK Ortho Inst/Beth Israel North Med Ctr 1997

Zelicof, Steven B MD/PhD (OrS) - **Spec Exp:** Joint Reconstruction; Arthritis; Sports Medicine; Hip & Knee Replacement; **Hospital:** Montefiore New Rochelle Hosp, Westchester Med Ctr; **Address:** Specialty Orthopedics, 600 Mamaroneck Ave, Ste 101, Harrison, NY 10528; **Phone:** 914-686-0111; **Board Cert:** Orthopaedic Surgery 2003; **Med School:** Univ Pennsylvania 1983; **Resid:** Surgery, Lenox Hill Hosp 1985; Orthopaedic Surgery, Hosp Special Surg 1989; **Fellow:** Orthopaedic Surgery, Brigham & Women's Hosp 1990; **Fac Appt:** Clin Prof OrS, NY Med Coll

Otolaryngology

Fox, Mark L MD (Oto) - **Spec Exp:** Thyroid Surgery; Salivary Gland Surgery; Head & Neck Cancer; Sinus Surgery; **Hospital:** Lawrence Hosp Ctr, Montefiore New Rochelle Hosp; **Address:** ENT & Allergy Assocs, 1 Elm St, Ste 2A, Tuckahoe, NY 10707; **Phone:** 914-961-2515; **Board Cert:** Otolaryngology 1979; **Med School:** NY Med Coll 1973; **Resid:** Surgery, Metropolitan Hosp Ctr 1974; Otolaryngology, Manhattan EET Hosp 1979; **Fac Appt:** Asst Clin Prof Oto, Columbia P&S

Kase, Steven B MD (Oto) - **Spec Exp:** Sinus Disorders; Pediatric Otolaryngology; **Hospital:** White Plains Hosp (page 640), Mt Sinai Med Ctr (page 102); **Address:** 75 S Broadway Fl 3, White Plains, NY 10601; **Phone:** 914-681-0300; **Board Cert:** Otolaryngology 1981; **Med School:** Loyola Univ-Stritch Sch Med 1976; **Resid:** Surgery, St Francis Hosp 1977; Otolaryngology, NY E&E Infirmary 1980

Kates, Matthew J MD (Oto) - **Spec Exp:** Sinus Disorders/Surgery; Sleep Disorders/Apnea; Balance Disorders; **Hospital:** Montefiore New Rochelle Hosp, Lawrence Hosp Ctr; **Address:** 26 Burling Ln Fl 2, New Rochelle, NY 10801-4914; **Phone:** 914-235-1888; **Board Cert:** Otolaryngology 1992; **Med School:** Cornell Univ-Weill Med Coll 1986; **Resid:** Surgery, St Vincent's Hosp 1988; Otolaryngology, Manhattan EET Hosp 1991

Meiteles, Lawrence Z MD (Oto) - **Spec Exp:** Cochlear Implants; Skull Base Surgery; Otology & Neuro-Otology; Balance Disorders; **Hospital:** Westchester Med Ctr; **Address:** The Balance Ctr, 480 Bedford Rd, Chappaqua, NY 10514; **Phone:** 914-242-8111; **Board Cert:** Otolaryngology 1992; **Med School:** Albert Einstein Coll Med 1986; **Resid:** Otolaryngology, New York Eye & Ear 1991; **Fellow:** Otology & Neurotology, Univ Michigan Med Ctr 1993; **Fac Appt:** Assoc Clin Prof Oto, NY Med Coll

Ryback, Hyman MD (Oto) - **Spec Exp:** Endoscopic Sinus Surgery; Laryngeal Disorders; Snoring/Sleep Apnea; Reconstructive Surgery; **Hospital:** White Plains Hosp (page 640); **Address:** 75 S Broadway Fl 3, White Plains, NY 10601; **Phone:** 914-949-3888; **Board Cert:** Otolaryngology 1977; **Med School:** McGill Univ 1970; **Resid:** Surgery, Jewish Genl Hosp 1973; Otolaryngology, Mount Sinai Hosp 1977

Scott, John C MD (Oto) - **Spec Exp:** Head & Neck Surgery; Facial Plastic Surgery; Thyroid Surgery; Cosmetic Surgery-Face; **Hospital:** Northern Westchester Hosp (page 639); **Address:** Mt Kisco Medical Group, 110 S Bedford Rd Fl 2, Mt Kisco, NY 10549; **Phone:** 914-242-1355; **Board Cert:** Otolaryngology 1994; Facial Plastic & Reconstr Surgery 1997; **Med School:** Univ Mich Med Sch 1988; **Resid:** Otolaryngology, Johns Hopkins Hosp 1993; **Fellow:** Facial Plastic Surgery, Mount Sinai Hosp 1994

Shapiro, Barry M MD (Oto) - **Spec Exp:** Endoscopic Sinus Surgery; Sleep Disorders/Apnea; **Hospital:** Phelps Meml Hosp Ctr, St. John's Riverside Hosp-Andrus Pavil; **Address:** West Med Medical Group, Ridge Hill, 73 Market St, Yonkers, NY 10510-1469; **Phone:** 914-945-0505; **Board Cert:** Otolaryngology 1983; **Med School:** Mount Sinai Sch Med 1978; **Resid:** Surgery, Mount Sinai Med Ctr 1979; Otolaryngology, Mount Sinai Med Ctr 1982; **Fac Appt:** , Mount Sinai Sch Med

Siglock, Timothy J MD (Oto) - **Spec Exp:** Ear Disorders/Surgery; Sinus Surgery; Voice Disorders; **Hospital:** Hudson Valley Hosp Ctr; **Address:** Mount Kisco Medical Group, 3630 Hill Blvd, Ste 202, Jefferson Valley, NY 10535-1502; **Phone:** 914-245-7700; **Board Cert:** Otolaryngology 1986; **Med School:** Belgium 1981; **Resid:** Otolaryngology, New York Eye & Ear Infirm 1986; **Fellow:** Research, House Ear Inst 1987

Stidham, Katrina Ruth MD (Oto) - **Spec Exp:** Cochlear Implants; Balance Disorders; Hearing Loss; Ear Disorders; **Hospital:** Westchester Med Ctr, New York Eye & Ear Infirm (page 115); **Address:** 19 Bradhurst Ave, Ste 3600S, Hawthorne, NY 10532; **Phone:** 914-909-4578; **Board Cert:** Otolaryngology 1999; **Med School:** Duke Univ 1993; **Resid:** Otolaryngology, Stanford Univ Hosp 1998; **Fellow:** Neurotology, CA Inst 2000; **Fac Appt:** Assoc Prof Oto, NY Med Coll

Zalvan, Craig H MD (Oto) - **Spec Exp:** Voice Disorders; Swallowing Disorders; Airway Disorders; Vocal Cord Disorders; **Hospital:** Phelps Meml Hosp Ctr, Westchester Med Ctr; **Address:** Inst Voice & Swallowing Disorders, Phelps Meml Hosp Ctr, 777 N Broadway, Ste 303, North Tarrytown, NY 10591; **Phone:** 914-366-3636; **Board Cert:** Otolaryngology 2012; **Med School:** Albert Einstein Coll Med 1995; **Resid:** Otolaryngology, Manhattan EE&T 1999; Otolaryngology, Ny Presby Columbia Presbyterian Med Ctr 2001; **Fellow:** Laryngology, St Luke's Roosevelt Med Ctr 2002; **Fac Appt:** Assoc Prof Oto, NY Med Coll

Pain Medicine

Kizelshteyn, Grigory MD (PM) - **Spec Exp:** Pain-Back & Neck; Pain-Spine; **Hospital:** St. John's Riverside Hosp-Andrus Pavil; **Address:** Pain Medicine Wellness Ctr of New York, 220 Westchester Ave, Ground Floor, White Plains, NY 10604; **Phone:** 914-289-1507; **Board Cert:** Anesthesiology 1991; Pain Medicine 2004; **Med School:** Russia 1977; **Resid:** Anesthesiology, Westchester Med Ctr 1980; **Fellow:** Pain Medicine, Westchester Med Ctr 1987

Lu, Gabriel P MD/PhD (PM) - **Spec Exp:** Acupuncture; Pain-Back & Neck; **Address:** 112 Penn Rd, Scarsdale, NY 10583; **Phone:** 914-725-4240; **Board Cert:** Anesthesiology 1984; Pain Medicine 1997; **Med School:** China 1968; **Resid:** Surgery, St Lukes Hospital 1976; Anesthesiology, Montefiore Med Ctr 1978; **Fellow:** Anesthesiology, Montefiore Med Ctr 1979; **Fac Appt:** Prof Anes, Albert Einstein Coll Med

Malits, Bella M MD (PM) - **Spec Exp:** Pain-Chronic; Reflex Sympathetic Dystrophy (RSD); **Hospital:** Northern Westchester Hosp (page 639); **Address:** Mt Kisco Med Grp, 34 S Bedford Rd Fl 2 - Ste 201, Mt Kisco, NY 10549; **Phone:** 914-242-4400; **Board Cert:** Anesthesiology 1995; Pain Medicine 2007; **Med School:** NY Med Coll 1990; **Resid:** Anesthesiology, Mt Sinai Med Ctr 1995; **Fellow:** Pain Management, Mt Sinai Med Ctr 1996

Pediatric Cardiology

Bierman, Fredrick Zachary MD (PCd) - **Spec Exp:** Fetal Echocardiography; Kawasaki Disease; Congenital Heart Disease; Echocardiography; **Hospital:** Westchester Med Ctr; **Address:** 19 Bradhurst Ave, Hawthorne, NY 10532; **Phone:** 914-594-4370; **Board Cert:** Pediatrics 1978; Pediatric Cardiology 1981; **Med School:** SUNY Downstate 1973; **Resid:** Pediatrics, Mount Sinai Med Ctr 1976; **Fellow:** Pediatric Cardiology, Harvard Chldns Hosp 1979; **Fac Appt:** Prof Ped, NY Med Coll

Crowe, David MD (PCd) - **Spec Exp:** Congenital Heart Disease; **Hospital:** Northern Westchester Hosp (page 639); **Address:** Northern Westchester Hosp, 480 N Bedford Rd, Chappaqua, NY 10514; **Phone:** 914-458-8800; **Board Cert:** Pediatric Cardiology 2010; **Med School:** NY Med Coll 1994; **Resid:** Pediatrics, NY-Presby/Weill Cornell Med Ctr 1997; **Fellow:** Pediatric Cardiology, NY-Presby/Columbia Univ Med Ctr 2000

Erb, Markus MD (PCd) - **Spec Exp:** Cardiac Catheterization; Atrial Septal Defect; Ventricular Septal Defect; Patent Foramen Ovale; **Hospital:** Westchester Med Ctr; **Address:** NY Medical College, Pediatric Cardiology, 19 Bradhurst Ave, Ste 1400, Hawthorne, NY 10532; **Phone:** 914-594-4370; **Board Cert:** Pediatric Cardiology 2006; Pediatrics 2007; **Med School:** NY Med Coll 1987; **Resid:** Pediatrics, Montefiore Med Ctr 1990; **Fellow:** Pediatric Cardiology, Children's Hosp of Philadelphia 1993; **Fac Appt:** Asst Prof Ped, NY Med Coll

Fish, Bernard G MD (PCd) - **Spec Exp:** Cardiac Imaging; Fetal Echocardiography; **Hospital:** Westchester Med Ctr, Children's & Women's Phys.of Westchester (page 638); **Address:** NY Med Coll, Ped Cardiology, 19 Bradhurst Ave, Ste 1400, Hawthorne, NY 10532; **Phone:** 914-594-4370; **Board Cert:** Pediatrics 1974; Pediatric Cardiology 1975; **Med School:** Univ Chicago-Pritzker Sch Med 1969; **Resid:** Pediatrics, Montefiore Hosp Med Ctr 1971; Pediatric Cardiology, Montefiore Hosp Med Ctr 1973; **Fellow:** Pediatric Cardiology, Yale-New Haven Hosp 1975; **Fac Appt:** Assoc Prof Ped, NY Med Coll

Friedman, Deborah M MD (PCd) - **Spec Exp:** Fetal Cardiology; Echocardiography; Fetal Echocardiography; Congenital Heart Disease; **Hospital:** Westchester Med Ctr, Children's & Women's Phys.of Westchester (page 638); **Address:** New York Med College, Munger Pavillion, rm 509, Valhalla, NY 10595; **Phone:** 914-594-4370; **Board Cert:** Pediatrics 1982; Pediatric Cardiology 1983; Pediatric Critical Care Medicine 2007; **Med School:** Univ Chicago-Pritzker Sch Med 1977; **Resid:** Pediatrics, Bronx Muni Hosp Ctr 1980; **Fellow:** Pediatric Cardiology, NYU Med Ctr 1983; **Fac Appt:** Prof Ped, NY Med Coll

Gewitz, Michael H MD (PCd) - **Spec Exp:** Neonatal Cardiology; Kawasaki Disease; Echocardiography; Heart Failure; **Hospital:** Westchester Med Ctr, Children's & Women's Phys.of Westchester (page 638); **Address:** Maria Fareri Children's Hospital, 100 Woods Rd, Munger Pavilion, Ste 618, Valhalla, NY 10595; **Phone:** 914-594-4370; **Board Cert:** Pediatrics 1979; Pediatric Cardiology 1981; **Med School:** Hahnemann Univ 1974; **Resid:** Pediatrics, Chldns Hosp 1976; Pediatrics, Hosp Sick Chldn 1977; **Fellow:** Pediatric Cardiology, Yale-New Haven Hosp 1980; **Fac Appt:** Prof Ped, NY Med Coll

Issenberg, Henry J MD (PCd) - **Spec Exp:** Fetal Echocardiography; Congenital Heart Disease-Adult & Child; Kawasaki Disease; Arrhythmias-Fetal; **Hospital:** Westchester Med Ctr, Children's & Women's Phys.of Westchester (page 638); **Address:** NY Med College, Dept Ped Cardiology, Munger Pavilion, rm 618, Valhalla, NY 10595; **Phone:** 914-594-4370; **Board Cert:** Pediatrics 1979; Pediatric Cardiology 1979; **Med School:** Emory Univ 1974; **Resid:** Pediatrics, Jacobi Med Ctr 1977; **Fellow:** Pediatric Cardiology, Childrens Med Ctr 1980; **Fac Appt:** Assoc Prof Ped, NY Med Coll

Pediatric Critical Care Medicine

Goltzman, Carey S MD (PCCM) - **Spec Exp:** Respiratory Failure; Sepsis & Septic Shock; **Hospital:** Westchester Med Ctr, Children's & Women's Phys.of Westchester (page 638); **Address:** Marla Fareri Children's Hosp, 100 Woods Rd, Valhalla, NY 10595; **Phone:** 914-493-7513; **Board Cert:** Pediatrics 2007; **Med School:** Mexico 1981; **Resid:** Pediatrics, Westchester Med Ctr 1987; **Fellow:** Pediatric Critical Care Medicine, Henry Ford Hosp 1989; **Fac Appt:** Asst Prof Ped, NY Med Coll

Pediatric Endocrinology

Handelsman, Dan G MD (PEn) - **Hospital:** Phelps Meml Hosp Ctr, Children's & Women's Phys.of Westchester (page 638); **Address:** 755 N Broadway, Ste 500, Sleepy Hollow, NY 10591; **Phone:** 914-366-0015; **Board Cert:** Pediatrics 1973; **Med School:** Albert Einstein Coll Med 1968; **Resid:** Pediatrics, Montefiore Hosp 1971; **Fellow:** Genetics and Metabolism, Montefiore Hosp 1973; **Fac Appt:** Assoc Clin Prof Ped, NY Med Coll

Noto, Richard MD (PEn) - **Spec Exp:** Growth/Development Disorders; Diabetes; Lead Poisoning; Thyroid Disorders; **Hospital:** Westchester Med Ctr, Children's & Women's Phys.of Westchester (page 638); **Address:** Children's Physicians of Westchester, 755 N Broadway, Ste 400, Sleepy Hollow, NY 10591; **Phone:** 914-366-3400; **Board Cert:** Pediatrics 1981; Pediatric Endocrinology 1983; **Med School:** Mount Sinai Sch Med 1976; **Resid:** Pediatrics, Beth Israel Med Ctr 1978; **Fellow:** Pediatric Endocrinology, NY-Presby/Weill Cornell Med Ctr 1979; Pediatric Endocrinology, N Shore Univ Hosp 1981; **Fac Appt:** Asst Prof Ped, NY Med Coll

Romano, Alicia MD (PEn) - **Spec Exp:** Growth/Development Disorders; Diabetes; **Hospital:** Westchester Med Ctr, Children's & Women's Phys.of Westchester (page 638); **Address:** Children's Physicians of Westchester, 755 N Broadway, Ste 400, Sleepy Hollow, NY 10591; **Phone:** 914-366-3400; **Board Cert:** Pediatric Endocrinology 2006; **Med School:** SUNY Stony Brook 1985; **Resid:** Pediatrics, Schneider Chldns Hosp 1988; **Fellow:** Pediatric Endocrinology, Schneider Chldns Hosp 1991; **Fac Appt:** Asst Prof Ped, NY Med Coll

Saenger, Paul MD (PEn) - **Spec Exp:** Short Stature in Children; Turner Syndrome; Sexual Differentiation Disorders; **Hospital:** Winthrop Univ Hosp (page 524); **Address:** 150 Lockwood Ave, Ste 34, New Rochelle, NY 10801; **Phone:** 914-636-5924; **Board Cert:** Pediatrics 1973; Pediatric Endocrinology 1978; **Med School:** Germany 1967; **Resid:** Pediatrics, Montefiore Hosp Med Ctr 1970; Pediatrics, Albert Einstein Coll Med 1971; **Fellow:** Pediatric Endocrinology, Cornell Univ Med Ctr 1975

Pediatric Gastroenterology

Berezin, Stuart MD (PGe) - **Hospital:** Westchester Med Ctr, Children's & Women's Phys.of Westchester (page 638); **Address:** CWPW, Pediatric Gastroenterology Dept, 503 Grasslands Rd, Ste 201, Valhalla, NY 10595; **Phone:** 914-367-0000; **Board Cert:** Pediatrics 1980; Pediatric Gastroenterology 2012; **Med School:** Hahnemann Univ 1976; **Resid:** Pediatrics, MetroHealth Med Ctr 1980; **Fellow:** Gastroenterology, Chldns Hosp 1982; **Fac Appt:** Assoc Prof Ped, NY Med Coll

Birnbaum, Audrey MD (PGe) - **Spec Exp:** Food Allergy; Inflammatory Bowel Disease/Crohn's; **Hospital:** Northern Westchester Hosp (page 639), Westchester Med Ctr; **Address:** 110 S Bedford Rd, Mount Kisco, NY 10549; **Phone:** 914-241-1050; **Board Cert:** Pediatric Gastroenterology 2007; **Med School:** NYU Sch Med 1986; **Resid:** Pediatrics, Mount Sinai Med Ctr 1989; **Fellow:** Pediatric Gastroenterology, Mount Sinai Med Ctr 1991

Halata, Michael MD (PGe) - **Spec Exp:** Inflammatory Bowel Disease; Functional Bowel Disorders; Gastroesophageal Reflux Disease (GERD); **Hospital:** Westchester Med Ctr, Children's & Women's Phys.of Westchester (page 638); **Address:** 503 Grasslands Rd, Ste 201, Valhalla, NY 10595; **Phone:** 914-367-0000; **Board Cert:** Pediatrics 1980; Pediatric Gastroenterology 2012; **Med School:** UMDNJ-NJ Med Sch, Newark 1974; **Resid:** Pediatrics, Westchester Med Ctr 1977; **Fellow:** Pediatric Gastroenterology, Westchester Med Ctr 1980

Pediatric Hematology-Oncology

Cairo, Mitchell S MD (PHO) - **Spec Exp:** Bone Marrow Transplant; Stem Cell Transplant; Leukemia; Lymphoma; **Hospital:** Westchester Med Ctr, Children's & Women's Phys.of Westchester (page 638); **Address:** CWPW, Pediatric Hematology/Oncology Dept, 19 Bradhurst Ave, Hawthorne, NY 10532; **Phone:** 914-493-7997; **Board Cert:** Pediatrics 1980; Pediatric Hematology-Oncology 1982; **Med School:** UCSF 1976; **Resid:** Pediatrics, UCLA Med Ctr 1979; **Fellow:** Pediatric Hematology-Oncology, IU Hlth Hosp 1981; **Fac Appt:** Prof Ped, NY Med Coll

Ozkaynak, Mehmet F MD (PHO) - **Spec Exp:** Bone Marrow Transplant; **Hospital:** Westchester Med Ctr, Children's & Women's Phys.of Westchester (page 638); **Address:** 19 Bradhurst Ave, Hawthorne, NY 10532; **Phone:** 914-493-7997; **Board Cert:** Pediatric Hematology-Oncology 2007; **Med School:** Turkey 1978; **Resid:** Pediatrics, Hacettepe Chldn's Hosp 1982; Pediatrics, Chldn's Hosp 1991; **Fellow:** Hematology & Oncology, Chldn's Hosp 1989; **Fac Appt:** Prof Ped, NY Med Coll

Sandoval, Claudio MD (PHO) - **Hospital:** Westchester Med Ctr, Children's & Women's Phys.of Westchester (page 638); **Address:** 19 Bradhurst Ave, Hawthorne, NY 10532; **Phone:** 914-493-7997; **Board Cert:** Pediatric Hematology-Oncology 2009; **Med School:** NY Med Coll 1987; **Resid:** Pediatrics, Schneider Chldns Hosp 1990; **Fellow:** Pediatric Hematology-Oncology, St Jude Chldns Rsch Hosp 1993

Tugal, Oya L MD (PHO) - **Spec Exp:** Leukemia & Lymphoma; Langerhans Cell Histiocytoma; **Hospital:** Westchester Med Ctr, Children's & Women's Phys.of Westchester (page 638); **Address:** 19 Bradhurst Ave, Ste 1400, Hawthorne, NY 10532; **Phone:** 914-493-7997; **Board Cert:** Pediatrics 1986; Pediatric Hematology-Oncology 1987; **Med School:** Turkey 1974; **Resid:** Pediatrics, Hacettepe Med Ctr 1977; Pediatrics, Westchester Med Ctr 1985; **Fellow:** Allergy & Immunology, Hacettepe Med Ctr 1978; Pediatric Hematology-Oncology, Mount Sinai Hosp 1987; **Fac Appt:** Prof Ped, NY Med Coll

Pediatric Infectious Disease

Li, Karl I-Ming MD (PInf) - **Spec Exp:** Lyme Disease; **Hospital:** Westchester Med Ctr; **Address:** 19 Bradhurst Ave Fl 1 - rm 1400, Hawthorne, NY 10532; **Phone:** 914-493-8333; **Board Cert:** Pediatric Infectious Disease 2012; **Med School:** Univ Mass Sch Med 1979; **Resid:** Pediatrics, Penn State Hershey Med Ctr 1982; Pediatrics, Miami Children's Hosp 1983; **Fellow:** Pediatric Infectious Disease, Univ Pittsburgh Med Ctr 1986

Pediatric Nephrology

Samsonov, Dmitry MD (PNep) - **Spec Exp:** Transplant Medicine-Kidney; Kidney Disease-Chronic; **Hospital:** Westchester Med Ctr; **Address:** Chldn & Women's Physicians, 19 Bradhurst Ave, Hawthorne, NY 10532; **Phone:** 914-493-7583; **Board Cert:** Pediatrics ; Pediatric Nephrology ; **Med School:** Russia 1989; **Resid:** Pediatrics, Hadassah Univ Hosp 1999; Pediatrics, Univ KY Affil Hosp 2010; **Fellow:** Pediatric Nephrology, Chldn's Hosp 2002; Transplant Medicine, Chldn's Hosp 2003; **Fac Appt:** Asst Prof Med, NY Med Coll

Zolotnitskaya, Anna MD (PNep) - **Spec Exp:** Kidney Disease-Chronic; Tranpslant Medicine-Kidney; Nephrotic Syndrome; **Hospital:** Westchester Med Ctr; **Address:** Chldn's & Women's Physicians, 19 Bradhurst Ave, Hawthorne, NY 10532; **Phone:** 914-493-7583; **Board Cert:** Pediatrics 2009; Pediatric Nephrology 2013; **Med School:** Russia 1983; **Resid:** Pediatrics, Soroka Med Ctr 1994; Pediatrics, St Luke's-Roosevelt Hosp 2001; **Fellow:** Pediatric Nephrology, Albert Einstein Affil Hosp 1998

Pediatric Otolaryngology

Bernstein, Joseph M MD (PO) - **Spec Exp:** Airway Disorders; Sleep Apnea; Craniofacial Surgery; **Hospital:** New York Eye & Ear Infirm (page 115), Beth Israel Med Ctr - Petrie Div (page 94); **Address:** 244 Westchester Ave, Ste 215, White Plains, NY 10604; **Phone:** 914-997-9100; **Board Cert:** Otolaryngology 1998; **Med School:** NYU Sch Med 1991; **Resid:** Otolaryngology, NYU Med Ctr 1997; **Fellow:** Pediatric Otolaryngology, Texas Chldns Hosp 1998

deSerres, Lianne M MD (PO) - **Spec Exp:** Airway Disorders; Sinus Disorders; Ear Infections; Sleep Apnea; **Hospital:** Westchester Med Ctr; **Address:** ENT Faculty Practice, 1055 Saw Mill River Rd, Ste 101, Ardsley, NY 10502; **Phone:** 914-693-7636; **Board Cert:** Otolaryngology 1997; **Med School:** Univ NC Sch Med 1990; **Resid:** Otolaryngology, Univ Wash Med Ctr 1996; **Fellow:** Pediatric Otolaryngology, Univ Wash Med Ctr 1998; **Fac Appt:** Assoc Clin Prof Oto, NY Med Coll

Keller, Jeffrey L MD (PO) - **Spec Exp:** Otitis Media; Sinusitis; Sleep Disorders/Apnea; **Hospital:** Northern Westchester Hosp (page 639); **Address:** MKMG, Pediatric Otolaryngology, 110 S Bedford Rd Fl 2, Mount Kisco, NY 10549; **Phone:** 914-241-1050; **Board Cert:** Otolaryngology 1996; **Med School:** Stanford Univ 1990; **Resid:** Otolaryngology, Mount Sinai Med Ctr 1995; **Fellow:** Pediatric Otolaryngology, Chldns Hosp 1996; **Fac Appt:** Asst Prof Oto, Mount Sinai Sch Med

Merer, David M MD (PO) - **Hospital:** Westchester Med Ctr; **Address:** ENT Faculty Practice, 1055 Saw Mill River Rd, Ste 101, Ardsley, NY 10502; **Phone:** 914-693-7636; **Board Cert:** Otolaryngology 1996; **Med School:** Albert Einstein Coll Med 1990; **Resid:** Otolaryngology, Montefiore Med Ctr 1995; **Fellow:** Pediatric Otolaryngology, Montefiore Med Ctr 1996; **Fac Appt:** Assoc Prof Oto, NY Med Coll

Pediatric Pulmonology

Amin, Nikhil S MD (PPul) - **Spec Exp:** Cystic Fibrosis; Asthma; Lung Disorders-Congenital; Primary Ciliary Dyskinesia; **Hospital:** Westchester Med Ctr, Children's & Women's Phys.of Westchester (page 638); **Address:** 19 Bradhurst Ave, Hawthorne, NY 10532; **Phone:** 914-493-7585; **Board Cert:** Pediatric Pulmonology 2009; **Med School:** India 1980; **Resid:** Pediatrics, Baroda Med Coll-SSG Hosp 1984; Pediatrics, NY Med Coll 1988; **Fellow:** Pediatric Pulmonology, NY Med Coll 1994; **Fac Appt:** Assoc Prof Ped, NY Med Coll

Boyer, Joseph T MD (PPul) - **Spec Exp:** Asthma; Cystic Fibrosis; **Hospital:** Westchester Med Ctr, Children's & Women's Phys.of Westchester (page 638); **Address:** 19 Bradhurst Ave, Hawthorne, NY 10532; **Phone:** 914-493-7585; **Board Cert:** Pediatric Pulmonology 2013; **Med School:** SUNY Downstate 1988; **Resid:** Pediatrics, Westchester Co Med Ctr 1991; **Fellow:** Pediatric Pulmonology, Westchester Co Med Ctr 1995

Dozor, Allen J MD (PPul) - **Spec Exp:** Asthma; Cystic Fibrosis; **Hospital:** Westchester Med Ctr, Children's & Women's Phys.of Westchester (page 638); **Address:** CWPW, Pediatric Pulmonology Dept, 19 Bradhurst Ave, Ste 1400, Hawthorne, NY 10532; **Phone:** 914-493-7585; **Board Cert:** Pediatrics 1981; Pediatric Pulmonology 2010; **Med School:** Penn State Coll Med 1977; **Resid:** Pediatrics, St Vincents Hosp & Med Ctr 1980; **Fellow:** Pediatric Pulmonology, Chldns Hosp 1982; **Fac Appt:** Prof Ped, NY Med Coll

Kass, Lewis MD (PPul) - **Spec Exp:** Sleep Disorders/Apnea; **Hospital:** Northern Westchester Hosp (page 639), Norwalk Hosp; **Address:** 103 S Bedford Rd, Ste 111, Mount Kisco, NY 10549; **Phone:** 914-242-0445; **Board Cert:** Pediatrics 2010; Pediatric Pulmonology 2012; Sleep Medicine 2007; **Med School:** SUNY Downstate 1991; **Resid:** Pediatrics, Chldns Med Ctr 1995; **Fellow:** Pediatric Pulmonology, Yale-New Have Hosp 1997

Krishnan, Sankaran MD (PPul) - **Spec Exp:** Cystic Fibrosis; Bronchoscopy; Asthma; **Hospital:** Westchester Med Ctr, Children's & Women's Phys.of Westchester (page 638); **Address:** CWPW, Pediatric Pulmonology Dept, 19 Bradhurst Ave, Ste 1400, Hawthrone, NY 10532; **Phone:** 914-493-7585; **Board Cert:** Pediatrics 2009; Pediatric Pulmonology 2013; **Med School:** India 1990; **Resid:** Pediatrics, Lincoln Med & Mental Hlth Ctr 1994; **Fellow:** Pediatric Pulmonology, Westchester Med Ctr 1997; **Fac Appt:** Asst Prof Ped, NY Med Coll

Lowenthal, Diana MD (PPul) - **Spec Exp:** Asthma; Cystic Fibrosis; Cough; Bronchoscopy; **Hospital:** Westchester Med Ctr, Children's & Women's Phys.of Westchester (page 638); **Address:** 19 Bradhurst Ave, Hawthorne, NY 10532; **Phone:** 914-493-7585; **Board Cert:** Pediatric Pulmonology 2007; **Med School:** Albert Einstein Coll Med 1986; **Resid:** Pediatrics, Albert Einstein Coll Med 1989; **Fellow:** Pulmonary Disease, Mount Sinai Hosp 1992; **Fac Appt:** Asst Prof Ped, NY Med Coll

Pediatric Rheumatology

Chao, Chun T MD (PRhu) - **Spec Exp:** Juvenile Arthritis; Lupus/SLE; Dermatomyositis; Arthritis in Lyme Disease; **Hospital:** Westchester Med Ctr, Children's & Women's Phys.of Westchester (page 638); **Address:** 19 Bradhurst Ave, Hawthorne, NY 10532; **Phone:** 914-594-4835; **Board Cert:** Pediatric Rheumatology 2009; **Med School:** Philippines 1982; **Resid:** Pediatrics, St Lukes-Roosevelt Hosp 1988; Pediatrics, Duke Univ Med Ctr 1990; **Fellow:** Pediatric Rheumatology, Univ Tennessee Med Ctr 1993; **Fac Appt:** Asst Prof Ped, NY Med Coll

Pediatric Surgery

McBride, Whitney J MD (PS) - **Spec Exp:** Neonatal Surgery; Laparoscopic Surgery; **Hospital:** Westchester Med Ctr, Children's & Women's Phys.of Westchester (page 638); **Address:** 19 Bradhurst Ave, Ste 1400, Hawthorne, NY 10532; **Phone:** 914-493-7620; **Board Cert:** Surgery 2011; **Med School:** Univ VT Coll Med 1992; **Resid:** Surgery, Fletcher Allen Hlthcare/Univ VT 1998

Muensterer, Oliver J MD/PhD (PS) - **Spec Exp:** Endoscopic Surgery; Minimally Invasive Surgery; Congenital Anomalies-Gastrointestinal; Trauma; **Hospital:** Westchester Med Ctr; **Address:** Maria Fareri Children's Hospital, Munger Pavilion, rm 321, Valhalla, NY 10595; **Phone:** 914-493-7620; **Board Cert:** Pediatrics 2008; **Med School:** Germany 1995; **Resid:** Surgery, Univ Munich 1999; Pediatrics, Duke Univ Hosp 1999; **Fellow:** Pediatric Surgery, UAB Med Ctr 2002; **Fac Appt:** Prof S, NY Med Coll

Stringel, Gustavo MD (PS) - **Spec Exp:** Minimally Invasive Surgery; Cancer Surgery; Neonatal Surgery; **Hospital:** Westchester Med Ctr, Children's & Women's Phys.of Westchester (page 638); **Address:** CWPW, Pediatric Surgery Dept, 19 Bradhurst Ave, Ste 1400, Hawthorne, NY 10532; **Phone:** 914-493-7620; **Board Cert:** Surgery 2007; Pediatric Surgery 2005; Surgical Critical Care 2007; **Med School:** Mexico 1971; **Resid:** Surgery, Univ Toronto 1977; **Fellow:** Pediatric Surgery, Hosp Sick Chldn 1979; **Fac Appt:** Prof S, NY Med Coll

Zitsman, Jeffrey MD (PS) - **Spec Exp:** Minimally Invasive Surgery; Chest Wall Deformities; Obesity/Bariatric Surgery; **Hospital:** Morgan Stanley Children's Hosp of NY-Presby, NY (page 104), White Plains Hosp (page 640); **Address:** 688 White Plains Rd, Ste 223, Scarsdale, NY 10583; **Phone:** 914-722-6737; **Board Cert:** Surgery 2001; Pediatric Surgery 2005; **Med School:** Tufts Univ 1976; **Resid:** Surgery, Tufts Med Ctr 1981; **Fellow:** Pediatric Surgery, NY-Presby/Columbia Univ Med Ctr 1985; **Fac Appt:** Assoc Clin Prof S, Columbia P&S

Pediatric Urology

Franco, Israel MD (Ped Uro) - **Spec Exp:** Voiding Dysfunction-Pediatric; **Hospital:** Westchester Med Ctr; **Address:** Pediatric Urology Associates, 150 White Plains Rd, Ste 306, Tarrytown, NY 10591; **Phone:** 914-493-8628; **Board Cert:** Urology 2008; Pediatric Urology ; **Med School:** Albert Einstein Coll Med 1983; **Resid:** Urology, New York Med Coll Affil Hosp 1989; **Fellow:** Pediatric Urology, Chldns Meml hosp 1991; **Fac Appt:** Assoc Prof U, NY Med Coll

Reda, Edward F MD (Ped Uro) - **Hospital:** Westchester Med Ctr; **Address:** Pediatric Urology Assocs, 150 White Plains Rd, Ste 306, Tarrytown, NY 10591; **Phone:** 914-493-8628; **Board Cert:** Urology 1984; **Med School:** Mexico 1976; **Resid:** Surgery, Bronx Lebanon Hosp 1979; Urology, Montefiore Med Ctr 1982; **Fellow:** Pediatric Urology, Chldns Hosp 1984; **Fac Appt:** Assoc Prof U, NY Med Coll

Pediatrics

Acker, Peter J MD (Ped) *PCP* - **Spec Exp:** Pediatric Dermatology; Adolescent Medicine; Learning Disorders; **Hospital:** Greenwich Hosp (page 938), Westchester Med Ctr; **Address:** Pediatric Assocs, 26 Rye Ridge Plaza, Rye Brook, NY 10573; **Phone:** 914-251-1100; **Board Cert:** Pediatrics 2009; **Med School:** Israel 1982; **Resid:** Pediatrics, NYU/Bellevue Hosp Ctr 1985; **Fellow:** Ambulatory Pediatrics, NYU/Bellevue Hosp Ctr 1987

Altman, Robin L MD (Ped) *PCP* - **Spec Exp:** Child Abuse; **Hospital:** Westchester Med Ctr, Children's & Women's Phys.of Westchester (page 638); **Address:** CWPW, Pediatrics Dept, 19 Bradhurst Ave, Ste 2400, Hawthorne, NY 10532; **Phone:** 914-593-8850; **Board Cert:** Pediatrics 1987; **Med School:** UMDNJ-RW Johnson Med Sch 1983; **Resid:** Pediatrics, NY-Presby/Columbia Univ Med Ctr 1986; **Fac Appt:** Assoc Prof Ped, NY Med Coll

Amler, David H MD (Ped) *PCP* - **Spec Exp:** Adolescent Medicine; **Hospital:** White Plains Hosp (page 640); **Address:** 15 N Broadway, Ste F, White Plains, NY 10601-2214; **Phone:** 914-948-4422; **Board Cert:** Pediatrics 1982; **Med School:** SUNY Buffalo 1969; **Resid:** Pediatrics, NYU Med Ctr 1972

Bailey, Michele L MD (Ped) *PCP* - **Spec Exp:** Adolescent Medicine; **Hospital:** Montefiore Med Ctr-Wakefield Campus (page 100), Lawrence Hosp Ctr; **Address:** 16 North Broadway, Ste LMG, White Plains, NY 10601; **Phone:** 914-686-1848; **Board Cert:** Pediatrics 2009; **Med School:** West Indies 1989; **Resid:** Pediatrics, Lincoln Med Ctr 1994; **Fac Appt:** Asst Clin Prof Ped, NY Med Coll

Barsh, Elliot B MD (Ped) *PCP* - **Hospital:** Northern Westchester Hosp (page 639); **Address:** Mt Kisco Med Group, 90 S Bedford Rd, Mt Kisco, NY 10549; **Phone:** 914-241-1050; **Board Cert:** Pediatrics 2011; **Med School:** NYU Sch Med 1984; **Resid:** Pediatrics, Montefiore Med Ctr 1987; Pediatrics, Bronx-Lebanon Hosp 1988

Baskind, Lawrence J MD (Ped) *PCP* - **Hospital:** Hudson Valley Hosp Ctr; **Address:** 35 S Riverside Ave, Ste 101, Croton-On-Hudson, NY 10520; **Phone:** 914-271-2424; **Board Cert:** Pediatrics 2010; **Med School:** UMDNJ-NJ Med Sch, Newark 1983; **Resid:** Pediatrics, Univ Hosp-UMDNJ 1987

Berkowitz, Norman MD (Ped) *PCP* - **Hospital:** Greenwich Hosp (page 938), Westchester Med Ctr; **Address:** 26 Rye Ridge Plaza, Rye Brook, NY 10573-2820; **Phone:** 914-251-1100; **Board Cert:** Pediatrics 1972; **Med School:** SUNY Buffalo 1967; **Resid:** Pediatrics, Mount Sinai Med Ctr 1970; **Fellow:** Pediatrics, St Christopher Hosp Chldn 1973

Berman, Morton MD (Ped) *PCP* - **Spec Exp:** Developmental Disorders; **Hospital:** White Plains Hosp (page 640); **Address:** 244 Westchester Ave, Ste 210, White Plains, NY 10604; **Phone:** 914-948-7016; **Board Cert:** Pediatrics 1972; **Med School:** NYU Sch Med 1966; **Resid:** Pediatrics, Bellevue Hosp 1968; Pediatric Neurology, Bellevue Hosp 1971; **Fac Appt:** Asst Clin Prof Ped, NYU Sch Med

Bomback, Fredric MD (Ped) *PCP* - **Spec Exp:** Infectious Disease; Complex Diagnosis; **Hospital:** White Plains Hosp (page 640), NY-Presby/Columbia Univ Med Ctr, NY (page 104); **Address:** Westchester Pediatrics, 99 Fieldstone Drive, Hartsdale, NY 10530; **Phone:** 914-428-2120; **Board Cert:** Pediatrics 1984; **Med School:** NYU Sch Med 1969; **Resid:** Pediatrics, Bronx Muni Hosp 1972; **Fellow:** Genetics and Metabolism, Albert Einstein Coll Med 1976; **Fac Appt:** Clin Prof Ped, Columbia P&S

Bookner, Scott D MD (Ped) *PCP* - **Hospital:** White Plains Hosp (page 640); **Address:** Scarsdale Pediatric Assocs, 7 Popham Rd, Ste 301, Scarsdale, NY 10583; **Phone:** 914-725-0800; **Board Cert:** Pediatrics 2007; **Med School:** SUNY Buffalo 1989; **Resid:** Pediatrics, Chldns Hosp 1992; **Fac Appt:** Asst Clin Prof Ped, NY Med Coll

Collins, Margaret A MD (Ped) *PCP* - **Hospital:** Northern Westchester Hosp (page 639); **Address:** Mt Kisco Med Group, 90 S Bedford Ave, Mt Kisco, NY 10549; **Phone:** 914-241-1050; **Board Cert:** Pediatrics 2013; **Med School:** Geo Wash Univ 1988; **Resid:** Pediatrics, N Shore Univ Hosp 1992; **Fac Appt:** Asst Clin Prof Ped, NY Med Coll

Coven, Barbara MD (Ped) *PCP* - **Hospital:** Greenwich Hosp (page 938), White Plains Hosp (page 640); **Address:** Westchester Med Grp, Dept Pediatrics, 210 Westchester Ave Fl 2, White Plains, NY 10604; **Phone:** 914-682-0731; **Board Cert:** Pediatrics 1986; **Med School:** Boston Univ 1980; **Resid:** Pediatrics, Boston City Hosp 1983; **Fellow:** Psychosomatic Medicine, Chldns Hosp Med Ctr 1983

Cowan, Stephen MD (Ped) - **Spec Exp:** Developmental Disorders; ADD/ADHD; Autism; Complementary Medicine; **Hospital:** Hudson Valley Hosp Ctr; **Address:** 491 Lexington Ave, Mt Kisco, NY 10549; **Phone:** 914-864-1976; **Board Cert:** Pediatrics 2010; **Med School:** Italy 1983; **Resid:** Pediatrics, St Lukes-Roosevelt Hosp Ctr 1987; **Fellow:** Behavioral Pediatrics, Developmental Disabilities Ctr-Roosevelt Hosp 1989

Hartz, Cindi MD (Ped) *PCP* - **Hospital:** Montefiore New Rochelle Hosp; **Address:** 1415 Boston Post Rd, Larchmont, NY 10538; **Phone:** 914-833-1502; **Board Cert:** Pediatrics 2011; **Med School:** Mount Sinai Sch Med 1983; **Resid:** Pediatrics, Mt Sinai Hosp 1986; **Fellow:** Hematology & Oncology, Mt Sinai Hosp 1987

Levinson, William MD (Ped) - **Spec Exp:** Developmental & Behavorial Disorders; ADD/ADHD; Autism; **Hospital:** Westchester Med Ctr; **Address:** 503 Grasslands Rd, Ste 200, Valhalla, NY 10595; **Phone:** 914-304-5250; **Board Cert:** Developmental-Behavioral Pediatrics 2012; **Med School:** Albert Einstein Coll Med 1976; **Resid:** Pediatrics, Bronx Municipal Hosp 1979; **Fellow:** Developmental-Behavioral Pediatrics, Albert Einstein Coll of Med 1980; Developmental-Behavioral Pediatrics, Chldn's Hosp 1982; **Fac Appt:** Assoc Clin Prof Ped, NY Med Coll

Levitt, Miriam MD (Ped) *PCP* - **Spec Exp:** Travel Medicine; **Hospital:** Lawrence Hosp Ctr, Montefiore Med Ctr-Moses Campus (page 100); **Address:** 1 Pondfield Rd, Ste 303, Bronxville, NY 10708-3706; **Phone:** 914-961-3604; **Board Cert:** Pediatrics 1975; **Med School:** Albert Einstein Coll Med 1971; **Resid:** Pediatrics, Montefiore Med Ctr 1973; **Fac Appt:** Asst Clin Prof Ped, Albert Einstein Coll Med

London, Ronald MD (Ped) *PCP* - **Hospital:** Montefiore Med Ctr-Moses Campus (page 100), Montefiore Med Ctr-Einstein Campus (page 100); **Address:** Westmed Medical Grp, 171 Huguenot St, New Rochelle, NY 10801; **Phone:** 718-863-1050; **Board Cert:** Pediatrics 2010; **Med School:** Israel 1984; **Resid:** Pediatrics, Montefiore Med Ctr 1987; **Fellow:** Child Development, Albert Einstein Coll Med Affil Hosp 1988

Lubell, Harry R MD (Ped) *PCP* - **Hospital:** Phelps Meml Hosp Ctr, Westchester Med Ctr; **Address:** 150 White Plains Rd, Ste 101, Tarrytown, NY 10591-2657; **Phone:** 914-332-4141; **Board Cert:** Pediatrics 1969; **Med School:** Ros Franklin Univ/Chicago Med Sch 1964; **Resid:** Pediatrics, Montefiore Med Ctr 1967; **Fellow:** Pediatric Hematology-Oncology, Babies Hosp-Columbia Preby 1970; **Fac Appt:** Assoc Clin Prof Ped, NY Med Coll

Meisler, Susan MD (Ped) *PCP* - **Spec Exp:** Adolescent Medicine; **Hospital:** Montefiore Med Ctr-Einstein Campus (page 100), Montefiore New Rochelle Hosp; **Address:** 145 Hugenot St, Ste 200, New Rochelle, NY 10801-5011; **Phone:** 914-235-1400; **Board Cert:** Pediatrics 2011; **Med School:** SUNY Stony Brook 1984; **Resid:** Pediatrics, Schneider Chldn's Hosp 1987

Proskin, Wendy MD (Ped) *PCP* - **Hospital:** White Plains Hosp (page 640), Greenwich Hosp (page 938); **Address:** WestMed, Pediatrics & Adolescent Med, 210 Westchester Ave, White Plains, NY 10604; **Phone:** 914-682-0731; **Board Cert:** Pediatrics 2010; **Med School:** SUNY Downstate 1999; **Resid:** Pediatrics, Montefiore Med Ctr 2002

Richel, Peter MD (Ped) *PCP* - **Hospital:** Northern Westchester Hosp (page 639); **Address:** 36 Smith Ave, Mt Kisco, NY 10549; **Phone:** 914-666-6655; **Board Cert:** Pediatrics 2008; **Med School:** Dominican Republic 1983; **Resid:** Pediatrics, Chldns Hosp-Albany Med Ctr 1987; **Fellow:** Ambulatory Pediatrics, St Luke's-Roosevelt Hosp Ctr 1988; **Fac Appt:** Asst Clin Prof Ped, Albert Einstein Coll Med

Versfelt, Mary MD (Ped) *PCP* - **Spec Exp:** Chronic Illness; Neonatal Care; Adolescent Medicine; **Hospital:** Greenwich Hosp (page 938), Westchester Med Ctr; **Address:** Pediatric Assocs, 26 Rye Ridge Plaza, Rye Brook, NY 10573; **Phone:** 914-251-1100; **Board Cert:** Pediatrics 1983; **Med School:** Columbia P&S 1978; **Resid:** Pediatrics, NY-Presby/Columbia Univ Med Ctr 1981; **Fac Appt:** Assoc Clin Prof Ped, Columbia P&S

Wager, Marc D MD (Ped) *PCP* - **Spec Exp:** Adolescent Medicine; **Hospital:** Montefiore New Rochelle Hosp; **Address:** Pediatric Grp, 140 Lockwood Ave, Ste 115, New Rochelle, NY 10801; **Phone:** 914-235-3800; **Board Cert:** Pediatrics 1986; **Med School:** Albert Einstein Coll Med 1981; **Resid:** Pediatrics, Jacobi Med Ctr 1984; **Fellow:** Adolescent Medicine, Montefiore Med Ctr 1986; **Fac Appt:** Asst Clin Prof Ped, Albert Einstein Coll Med

Weissbrot, Jay M MD (Ped) *PCP* - **Spec Exp:** Adolescent Medicine; **Hospital:** White Plains Hosp (page 640); **Address:** Westchester Hlth, Pediatrics, 410 N Broadway, White Plains, NY 10603; **Phone:** 914-948-0353; **Board Cert:** Pediatrics 1986; **Med School:** SUNY Downstate 1980; **Resid:** Pediatrics, Brookdale Univ Hosp 1983; **Fellow:** Adolescent Medicine, Brookdale Univ Hosp 1984

Physical Medicine & Rehabilitation

McGowan, Charles E MD (PMR) - **Hospital:** Phelps Meml Hosp Ctr; **Address:** 701 N Broadway, Sleepy Hollow, NY 10591; **Phone:** 914-907-6583; **Board Cert:** Physical Medicine & Rehabilitation 1990; **Med School:** Israel 1983; **Resid:** Surgery, Lincoln Hosp 1985; Physical Medicine & Rehabilitation, Westchester Co Med Ctr 1988; **Fellow:** Electrodiagnosis, Westchester Co Med Ctr 1989

Pechman, Karen M MD (PMR) - **Spec Exp:** Electrodiagnosis; Musculoskeletal Disorders; Amputee Rehabilitation; Pain Management; **Hospital:** Burke Rehab Hosp, White Plains Hosp (page 640); **Address:** 170 Maple Ave, Ste 510, White Plains, NY 10601; **Phone:** 914-683-0020; **Board Cert:** Physical Medicine & Rehabilitation 1987; Electrodiagnostic Medicine 1989; **Med School:** Boston Univ 1980; **Resid:** Physical Medicine & Rehabilitation, Jacobi Med Ctr 1986; **Fellow:** Research, NYU Med Ctr 1982; **Fac Appt:** Asst Clin Prof PMR, Cornell Univ-Weill Med Coll

Pici, Ralph A MD (PMR) - **Spec Exp:** Musculoskeletal Disorders; **Hospital:** Lawrence Hosp Ctr; **Address:** Lawrence Hosp Ctr, Physical Med & Rehab, 55 Palmer Ave Fl 2, Bronxville, NY 10708; **Phone:** 914-787-3374; **Board Cert:** Physical Medicine & Rehabilitation 1974; **Med School:** Italy 1965; **Resid:** Pediatrics, Westchester Med Ctr 1967; Physical Medicine & Rehabilitation, Jacobi Med Ctr 1972

Randolph, Audrey L MD (PMR) - **Spec Exp:** Musculoskeletal Disorders; Pain-Back & Neck; **Hospital:** Westchester Med Ctr; **Address:** 19 Bradhurst Ave, Ste 1700S, Hawthorne, NY 10532; **Phone:** 914-909-4168; **Board Cert:** Physical Medicine & Rehabilitation 1970; **Med School:** Med Coll PA Hahnemann 1964; **Resid:** Physical Medicine & Rehabilitation, NYU Med Ctr 1968; **Fac Appt:** Prof PMR, NY Med Coll

Plastic Surgery

Beran, Samuel J MD (PlS) - **Spec Exp:** Reconstructive Surgery; Liposuction; Breast Augmentation; **Hospital:** White Plains Hosp (page 640), Northern Westchester Hosp (page 639); **Address:** Cosmetic Surgery Assocs, 440 Mamaroneck Ave, Ste 412, Harrison, NY 10528; **Phone:** 914-761-8667; **Board Cert:** Plastic Surgery 2009; **Med School:** Albany Med Coll 1990; **Resid:** Surgery, Thomas Jefferson Univ Hosp 1995; Plastic Surgery, UT Southwestern Med Ctr 1997

Chin, Simon H MD (PlS) - **Spec Exp:** Hand Surgery; Cosmetic Surgery; Plastic & Reconstructive Surgery; **Hospital:** Putnam Hosp Ctr, Northern Westchester Hosp (page 639); **Address:** MKMG, Plastic Surgery, 111 Bedford Rd, Katonah, NY 10536; **Phone:** 914-232-3135; **Board Cert:** Plastic Surgery 2009; Hand Surgery 2010; **Med School:** Vanderbilt Univ 2000; **Resid:** Surgery, Yale-New Haven Hosp 2003; Plastic Surgery, Yale-New Haven Hosp 2006; **Fellow:** Hand Surgery, Univ Washington Med Ctr 2007; Cosmetic Plastic Surgery, NYU Med Ctr 2008

Garvey, Richard Charles MD (PlS) - **Spec Exp:** Facial Plastic Surgery; Breast Reconstruction; **Hospital:** Lawrence Hosp Ctr, Montefiore New Rochelle Hosp; **Address:** Plastic Surgery of Westchester, 500 Mamaroneck Ave, Ste 211, Harrison, NY 10528; **Phone:** 914-771-7373; **Board Cert:** Plastic Surgery 2003; **Med School:** Georgetown Univ 1991; **Resid:** Surgery, Montefiore Med Ctr 1993; Surgery, Kings Co Med Ctr 1996; **Fellow:** Plastic/Reconstructive Surgery, Montefiore Med Ctr 1998

Greenwald, Joshua Adam MD (PlS) - **Spec Exp:** Breast Augmentation; Rhinoplasty; Liposuction & Body Contouring; **Hospital:** White Plains Hosp (page 640); **Address:** Cosmetic Surgery Assocs, 440 Mamaroneck Ave, Ste 412, Harrison, NY 10528; **Phone:** 914-761-8667; **Board Cert:** Plastic Surgery 2005; **Med School:** NYU Sch Med 1995; **Resid:** Surgery, NYU Med Ctr 2001; **Fellow:** Plastic Surgery, Emory Univ Hosp 2004

Khoury, F. Frederic MD (PlS) - **Spec Exp:** Pediatric Plastic Surgery; Cosmetic Surgery-Breast; Cosmetic Surgery-Face; **Hospital:** White Plains Hosp (page 640), Greenwich Hosp (page 938); **Address:** 22 Rye Ridge Plaza, Rye Brook, NY 10573-2820; **Phone:** 914-253-9300; **Board Cert:** Plastic Surgery 2004; **Med School:** Lebanon 1971; **Resid:** Surgery, St Luke's-Roosevelt Hosp Ctr 1976; Plastic Surgery, St Luke's-Roosevelt Hosp Ctr 1979; **Fellow:** Plastic Surgery, St Louis Hosp 1977

Kim, Tae Ho MD (PlS) - **Spec Exp:** Craniofacial Surgery; Pediatric Craniofacial Surgery; **Hospital:** Westchester Med Ctr; **Address:** NY Grp Plastic Surgery, 155 White Plains Rd, Ste 109, Tarrytown, NY 10591; **Phone:** 914-366-6139; **Board Cert:** Plastic Surgery 2003; **Med School:** Univ Pittsburgh 1991; **Resid:** Surgery, UC Irvine Med Ctr 1997; Plastic/Reconstructive Surgery, UMass Meml Med Ctr 1999; **Fellow:** Surgical Research, Chldns Hosp 1996; Pediatric Craniofacial Surgery, Chldns Hosp 2000

Kleinman, Andrew MD (PlS) - **Spec Exp:** Cosmetic Surgery; Breast Augmentation; Eyelid Surgery; **Hospital:** Montefiore New Rochelle Hosp; **Address:** Kleinman Plastic Surgery, 800 Westchester Ave, Ste S-512, Rye Brook, NY 10573; **Phone:** 914-253-0700; **Board Cert:** Plastic Surgery 1989; **Med School:** Univ Rochester 1979; **Resid:** Surgery, Harvard Surg Svcs 1982; **Fellow:** Plastic Surgery, Baylor Coll Med 1985

Newman, Scott E MD (PlS) - **Spec Exp:** Breast Reconstruction & Augmentation; Cosmetic Surgery-Breast; Cosmetic Surgery-Body; Abdominoplasty; **Hospital:** St. John's Riverside Hosp-Andrus Pavil, Montefiore Med Ctr-Einstein Campus (page 100); **Address:** 1 Odell Plaza, Yonkers, NY 10701; **Phone:** 914-423-9000; **Board Cert:** Plastic Surgery 2004; **Med School:** NY Med Coll 1985; **Resid:** Surgery, Westchester Med Ctr 1990; Plastic Surgery, Mt Sinai Med Ctr 1993; **Fac Appt:** Asst Clin Prof PlS, Albert Einstein Coll Med

Palaia, David A MD (PlS) - **Spec Exp:** Cosmetic Surgery-Face; Breast Reconstruction; Rhinoplasty; Reconstructive Surgery; **Hospital:** Northern Westchester Hosp (page 639); **Address:** 400 E Main St, North Bldg, Fl 2, Mt Kisco, NY 10549; **Phone:** 914-242-7610; **Board Cert:** Plastic Surgery 1993; **Med School:** UMDNJ-NJ Med Sch, Newark 1985; **Resid:** Surgery, Montefiore-Weiler Einstein Div 1989; Plastic Surgery, Montefiore-Weiler Einstein Div 1991

Reiffel, Robert S MD (PlS) - **Spec Exp:** Cosmetic & Reconstructive Surgery; Hand Surgery; **Hospital:** White Plains Hosp (page 640); **Address:** 12 Greenridge Ave, Ste 203, White Plains, NY 10605; **Phone:** 914-683-1400; **Board Cert:** Plastic Surgery 1981; **Med School:** Columbia P&S 1972; **Resid:** Surgery, St Lukes-Roosevelt Hosp Ctr 1977; Plastic Surgery, NYU Med Ctr 1979; **Fellow:** Hand Surgery, NYU Med Ctr 1980

Rosenberg, Michael H MD (PlS) - **Spec Exp:** Breast Surgery; **Hospital:** Northern Westchester Hosp (page 639), Westchester Med Ctr; **Address:** Northern Westchester Surgical Services, 400 E Main St Fl 2 North, Mount Kisco, NY 10549; **Phone:** 914-242-7610; **Board Cert:** Surgery 2006; Plastic Surgery 2008; **Med School:** Columbia P&S 1987; **Resid:** Surgery, Columbia Presby Med Ctr 1992; Plastic/Reconstructive Surgery, Columbia Presby Med Ctr 1994; **Fac Appt:** Asst Clin Prof PlS, NY Med Coll

Roth, Douglas A MD (PlS) - **Spec Exp:** Cosmetic Surgery-Face; Cosmetic Surgery-Breast; Facial Plastic & Reconstructive Surgery; Skin Cancer; **Hospital:** Northern Westchester Hosp (page 639), Lenox Hill Hosp (Manh Eye, Ear & Throat Hosp) (page 106); **Address:** Mount Kisco Med Grp, Plastic Surgery, 110 S Bedford Rd, Mount Kisco, NY 10549; **Phone:** 914-242-5647; **Board Cert:** Surgery 2008; Plastic Surgery 2010; **Med School:** NYU Sch Med 1990; **Resid:** Surgery, NYU Med Ctr 1996; Plastic Surgery, NYU Med Ctr 1998; **Fellow:** Microvascular Surgery, NYU Med Ctr 1999; **Fac Appt:** Asst Clin Prof S, Mount Sinai Sch Med

Suzman, Michael S MD (PlS) - **Spec Exp:** Rhinoplasty; Facial Plastic & Reconstructive Surgery; Breast Surgery; **Hospital:** Greenwich Hosp (page 938), White Plains Hosp (page 640); **Address:** WestMed, Plastic Surgery, 1 Theall Rd, Ste 211, Rye, NY 10580; **Phone:** 914-848-8880; **Board Cert:** Plastic Surgery 2003; **Med School:** Cornell Univ 1996; **Resid:** Surgery, NY Presby Hosp 2000; Surgical Oncology, Meml Sloan-Kettering Cancer Ctr 2000; **Fellow:** Plastic Surgery, NY Presby Hosp 2002

Psychiatry

Addonizio, Gerard C MD (Psyc) - **Spec Exp:** Psychotherapy; Psychopharmacology; Depression; Anxiety Disorders; **Hospital:** NY-Presby/Westchester Div, NY (page 104); **Address:** 21 Bloomingdale Rd, White Plains, NY 10605-1504; **Phone:** 914-997-5864; **Board Cert:** Psychiatry 1983; **Med School:** Columbia P&S 1978; **Resid:** Psychiatry, Yale-New Haven Hosp 1982; **Fac Appt:** Prof Psyc, Cornell Univ-Weill Med Coll

Badikian, Arthur V MD (Psyc) - **Spec Exp:** Mood Disorders; Aging; Women's Health-Mental Health; Psychiatry in Cancer; **Hospital:** St. Vincent Cath Med Ctrs - Westchester; **Address:** 600 Mamaroneck Ave, Ste 106, Harrison, NY 10528; **Phone:** 914-948-4277; **Board Cert:** Psychiatry 1981; **Med School:** Univ Fla Coll Med 1976; **Resid:** Psychiatry, Westchester Co Med Ctr 1980; **Fac Appt:** Assoc Prof Psyc, NY Med Coll

Bauman, Jonathan H MD (Psyc) - **Spec Exp:** Mood Disorders; Anxiety Disorders; Personality Disorders; **Hospital:** Four Winds Hosp; **Address:** 800 Cross River Rd, Katonah, NY 10536-3549; **Phone:** 914-763-8151; **Board Cert:** Psychiatry 1978; **Med School:** Georgetown Univ 1974; **Resid:** Psychiatry, Univ VA Med Ctr 1975; Psychiatry, Georgetown Univ Hosp 1977; **Fac Appt:** Asst Prof Psyc, Albert Einstein Coll Med

Bogen, Steven MD (Psyc) - **Spec Exp:** Anxiety & Depression; **Hospital:** Phelps Meml Hosp Ctr; **Address:** Phelps Meml Hosp, Dept Psychiatry, 701 N Broadway, Sleepy Hollow, NY 10591-1096; **Phone:** 914-366-3024; **Board Cert:** Psychiatry 2005; Addiction Psychiatry 2006; **Med School:** SUNY Downstate 1988; **Resid:** Psychiatry, Montefiore Med Ctr 1992

Dulit, Rebecca A MD (Psyc) - **Spec Exp:** Personality Disorders-Borderline; Special Needs-Parental Therapy; Anxiety Disorders; Depression; **Hospital:** NY-Presby/Westchester Div, NY (page 104); **Address:** 45 Popham Rd, Ste D, Scarsdale, NY 10583; **Phone:** 914-722-0608; **Board Cert:** Psychiatry 1991; **Med School:** Mount Sinai Sch Med 1985; **Resid:** Psychiatry, Payne Whitney Clinic-Cornell 1989; **Fellow:** Research, Payne Whitney Clinic-Cornell 1992; **Fac Appt:** Assoc Clin Prof Psyc, Cornell Univ-Weill Med Coll

Gabel, Richard H MD (Psyc) - **Spec Exp:** Psychopharmacology; Psychotherapy; **Hospital:** White Plains Hosp (page 640); **Address:** 12 Greenridge Ave, White Plains, NY 10605; **Phone:** 914-681-0202; **Board Cert:** Psychiatry 1982; **Med School:** NYU Sch Med 1976; **Resid:** Psychiatry, Mass Genl Hosp 1980

Harlam, Dean MD (Psyc) - **Spec Exp:** Depression; Bipolar/Mood Disorders; Psychopharmacology; Schizophrenia; **Hospital:** Saint Joseph's Med Ctr - Yonkers; **Address:** St Vincent's Hosp, 275 North St, Harrison, NY 10528; **Phone:** 914-925-5490; **Board Cert:** Psychiatry 1979; **Med School:** Albert Einstein Coll Med 1972; **Resid:** Psychiatry, Bronx Muni Hosp 1976; **Fellow:** Psychiatry, NY Hosp-Cornell Med Ctr 1977; **Fac Appt:** Assoc Clin Prof Psyc, NY Med Coll

Kahn, Jeffrey P MD (Psyc) - **Spec Exp:** Anxiety & Depression; Psychotherapy; Work/Career Problems; Psychopharmacology; **Hospital:** NY-Presby/Weill Cornell Med Ctr, NY (page 104), NY-Presby/Westchester Div, NY (page 104); **Address:** 45 Popham Rd, Ste 1F, Scarsdale, NY 10583; **Phone:** 914-725-6303; **Board Cert:** Psychiatry 1986; **Med School:** Columbia P&S 1979; **Resid:** Psychiatry, NY Presby/Columbia Med Ctr 1983; **Fellow:** Research, NY Presby/Columbia Med Ctr 1985; **Fac Appt:** Assoc Clin Prof Psyc, Cornell Univ-Weill Med Coll

Klagsbrun, Samuel C MD (Psyc) - **Spec Exp:** Psychiatry in Cancer; Psychiatry in Terminal Illness; **Hospital:** Four Winds Hosp; **Address:** 800 Cross River Rd, Katonah, NY 10536; **Phone:** 914-763-8151 x2222; **Board Cert:** Psychiatry 1977; **Med School:** Ros Franklin Univ/Chicago Med Sch 1962; **Resid:** Psychiatry, Yale-New Haven Hosp 1966; **Fac Appt:** Clin Prof Psyc, Albert Einstein Coll Med

Levin, Andrew P MD (Psyc) - **Spec Exp:** Post Traumatic Stress Disorder; Forensic Psychiatry; Psychopharmacology; Cognitive Psychotherapy; **Hospital:** NY-Presby/Columbia Univ Med Ctr, NY (page 104); **Address:** 141 N Central Ave, Hartsdale, NY 10530-1912; **Phone:** 914-949-7699 x376; **Board Cert:** Psychiatry 1985; Forensic Psychiatry 2006; **Med School:** Univ Pennsylvania 1980; **Resid:** Psychiatry, NY State Psych Inst 1984; **Fellow:** Anxiety Disorder, NY State Psych Inst 1986; **Fac Appt:** Asst Clin Prof Psyc, Columbia P&S

Lew, Arthur MD (Psyc) - **Spec Exp:** Child & Adolescent Psychiatry; Psychoanalysis; **Address:** 225 Lyncroft Rd, New Rochelle, NY 10804-4120; **Phone:** 914-632-9679; **Board Cert:** Psychiatry 1974; Child & Adolescent Psychiatry 1979; **Med School:** SUNY Downstate 1968; **Resid:** Psychiatry, SUNY Downstate Med Ctr 1972; **Fellow:** Child & Adolescent Psychiatry, SUNY Downstate Med Ctr 1975; **Fac Appt:** Clin Prof Psyc, NYU Sch Med

Meyers, Barnett MD (Psyc) - **Spec Exp:** Depression; Geriatric Psychiatry; Psychopharmacology; Psychotherapy; **Hospital:** NY-Presby/Westchester Div, NY (page 104); **Address:** NY-Presby, Psychiatry Dept, 21 Bloomingdale Rd, White Plains, NY 10605; **Phone:** 914-997-5721; **Board Cert:** Psychiatry 1975; Geriatric Psychiatry 2010; **Med School:** NYU Sch Med 1966; **Resid:** Psychiatry, Bronx Muni Hosp 1972; **Fac Appt:** Prof Psyc, Cornell Univ-Weill Med Coll

Milone, Richard D MD (Psyc) - **Spec Exp:** Depression; Psychopharmacology; **Hospital:** Saint Joseph's Med Ctr - Yonkers; **Address:** 275 North St, Harrison, NY 10528; **Phone:** 914-925-5311; **Board Cert:** Psychiatry 1970; **Med School:** Creighton Univ 1963; **Resid:** Psychiatry, St Vincent's Hosp & Med Ctr 1967; **Fac Appt:** Assoc Clin Prof Psyc, NY Med Coll

Neschis, Ronald MD (Psyc) - **Spec Exp:** Geriatric Psychiatry; **Hospital:** Saint Joseph's Med Ctr - Yonkers, Rye Hosp Ctr; **Address:** 18 Linden Ave, Larchmont, NY 10538-4139; **Phone:** 914-834-3470; **Board Cert:** Psychiatry 1972; **Med School:** SUNY Downstate 1963; **Resid:** Psychiatry, Montefiore Hosp Med Ctr 1969

Opler, Lewis A MD (Psyc) - **Spec Exp:** Psychopharmacology; Psychotherapy; **Hospital:** NY-Presby/Columbia Univ Med Ctr, NY (page 104); **Address:** 765 Gramatan Ave, Mount Vernon, NY 10552-1043; **Phone:** 914-668-4799; **Board Cert:** Psychiatry 1983; **Med School:** Albert Einstein Coll Med 1976; **Resid:** Psychiatry, Bronx Muni Hosp 1979; **Fac Appt:** Clin Prof Psyc, Columbia P&S

Perlman, Barry B MD (Psyc) - **Hospital:** Saint Joseph's Med Ctr - Yonkers; **Address:** St Joseph's Med Ctr, Dept Psychiatry, 127 S Broadway, Yonkers, NY 10701-4006; **Phone:** 914-378-7342; **Board Cert:** Psychiatry 1977; **Med School:** Yale Univ 1971; **Resid:** Psychiatry, Mt Sinai Hosp 1975; **Fac Appt:** Assoc Clin Prof Psyc, NY Med Coll

Perry, Bradford MD (Psyc) - **Spec Exp:** Anxiety & Mood Disorders; Psychopharmacology; **Hospital:** NY-Presby/Westchester Div, NY (page 104), White Plains Hosp (page 640); **Address:** 455 Central Park Ave, Ste 214, Scarsdale, NY 10583; **Phone:** 914-472-2167; **Board Cert:** Psychiatry 1989; **Med School:** Univ Miami Sch Med 1984; **Resid:** Psychiatry, NY-Presby/Westchester Div 1988; **Fellow:** Psychiatry, NY-Presby/Columbia Univ Med Ctr 1989; **Fac Appt:** Assoc Clin Prof Psyc, Cornell Univ-Weill Med Coll

Russakoff, L. Mark MD (Psyc) - **Spec Exp:** Anxiety & Mood Disorders; **Hospital:** Phelps Meml Hosp Ctr; **Address:** Phelps Meml Hosp, Psychiatry Dept, 755 N Broadway, Ste 250, Sleepy Hollow, NY 10591; **Phone:** 914-366-3604; **Board Cert:** Psychiatry 1976; **Med School:** SUNY Downstate 1971; **Resid:** Psychiatry, Yale-New Haven Hosp 1975

Sullivan, Timothy B MD (Psyc) - **Spec Exp:** Bipolar/Mood Disorders; Psychotherapy & Psychopharmacology; Schizophrenia; Psychiatry in Physical Illness; **Hospital:** Staten Island Univ Hosp - North (page 106), St. Vincent Cath Med Ctrs - Westchester; **Address:** 30 Glenn St, Ste 305, White Plains, NY 10603; **Phone:** 347-328-2201; **Board Cert:** Internal Medicine 1981; Psychiatry 1986; **Med School:** Dartmouth Med Sch 1977; **Resid:** Internal Medicine, St Vincent's Hosp 1980; Psychiatry, New York Hosp-Westchester 1984; **Fellow:** Hematology & Oncology, St Vincents Hosp 1981; **Fac Appt:** Assoc Prof Psyc, NY Med Coll

Zolkind, Neil A MD (Psyc) - **Spec Exp:** Depression; Anxiety Disorders; **Hospital:** Westchester Med Ctr; **Address:** 150 White Plains Rd, Ste 102, Tarrytown, NY 10591; **Phone:** 914-909-5838; **Board Cert:** Psychiatry 1981; **Med School:** Geo Wash Univ 1976; **Resid:** Psychiatry, UCLA Neuropsych Hosp 1980; **Fac Appt:** Assoc Prof Psyc, NY Med Coll

Pulmonary Disease

Binder, Ralph E MD (Pul) - **Spec Exp:** Asthma; Chronic Obstructive Lung Disease (COPD); Interstitial Lung Disease; **Hospital:** Lawrence Hosp Ctr; **Address:** 329 Whiteplains Rd, Ste 100, Eastchester, NY 10709; **Phone:** 914-337-1610; **Board Cert:** Internal Medicine 1978; Pulmonary Disease 1980; **Med School:** Yale Univ 1975; **Resid:** Internal Medicine, Bronx Muni Hosp 1978; **Fellow:** Pulmonary Disease, Boston Med Ctr 1980; **Fac Appt:** Asst Prof Med, Columbia P&S

Brill, Joseph J MD (Pul) - **Spec Exp:** Sarcoidosis; Chronic Obstructive Lung Disease (COPD); Asthma; **Hospital:** St. John's Riverside Hosp-Andrus Pavil, Saint Joseph's Med Ctr - Yonkers; **Address:** 102 Park Ave, Yonkers, NY 10703; **Phone:** 914-968-1611; **Board Cert:** Internal Medicine 1988; Pulmonary Disease 2012; **Med School:** Mexico 1981; **Resid:** Internal Medicine, Elmhurst City Hosp 1986; **Fellow:** Pulmonary Disease, Mt Sinai 1988

Bures, Sergio MD (Pul) - **Hospital:** Northern Westchester Hosp (page 639); **Address:** 111 Bedford Rd, Katonah, NY 10536; **Phone:** 914-232-3135; **Board Cert:** Internal Medicine 2010; Pulmonary Disease 2005; Critical Care Medicine 2006; **Med School:** Albany Med Coll 1994; **Resid:** Internal Medicine, Tripler Army Med Ctr 1997; **Fellow:** Pulmonary Critical Care Medicine, Meml Sloan Kettering Cancer Ctr

Casino, Joseph E MD (Pul) - **Spec Exp:** Asthma; Sleep Disorders; **Hospital:** Montefiore New Rochelle Hosp; **Address:** 2365 Boston Post Rd, Ste 103, Larchmont, NY 10538; **Phone:** 914-833-2020; **Board Cert:** Internal Medicine 1989; Pulmonary Disease 2010; Critical Care Medicine 2011; **Med School:** Italy 1984; **Resid:** Internal Medicine, New Rochelle Med Ctr 1988; **Fellow:** Pulmonary Critical Care Medicine, RW Johnson Univ Hosp 1991; **Fac Appt:** Asst Clin Prof Med, NY Med Coll

De Matteo, Robert E MD (Pul) - **Spec Exp:** Asthma; Emphysema; Lung Cancer-Early Detection; **Hospital:** St. John's Riverside Hosp-Andrus Pavil, Saint Joseph's Med Ctr - Yonkers; **Address:** 970 N Broadway, Ste 209, Yonkers, NY 10701; **Phone:** 914-965-3366; **Board Cert:** Internal Medicine 1988; Pulmonary Disease 2010; **Med School:** Mexico 1982; **Resid:** Internal Medicine, Mount Sinai/Bronx VA Hosp 1985; **Fellow:** Pulmonary Disease, Westchester Med Ctr 1988

Delorenzo, Lawrence MD (Pul) - **Spec Exp:** Asthma; Emphysema; **Hospital:** Westchester Med Ctr; **Address:** Westchester Med Ctr, Pulmonology Dept, 100 Woods Rd, Macy Pav - rm 1042, Valhalla, NY 10595; **Phone:** 914-493-7518; **Board Cert:** Internal Medicine 1979; Pulmonary Disease 1982; Critical Care Medicine 2009; **Med School:** NY Med Coll 1976; **Resid:** Internal Medicine, Metropolitan Hosp Ctr 1979; **Fellow:** Pulmonary Disease, Metropolitan Hosp Ctr 1981; **Fac Appt:** Assoc Clin Prof Med, NY Med Coll

DiCosmo, Bruno F MD (Pul) - **Spec Exp:** Pulmonary Fibrosis; Bronchoscopy; Lung Cancer; Sleep Disorders; **Hospital:** White Plains Hosp (page 640), Greenwich Hosp (page 938); **Address:** WestMed, Pulmonology, 1 Theall Rd, Rye, NY 10580; **Phone:** 914-848-8777; **Board Cert:** Internal Medicine 2011; Pulmonary Disease 2004; Critical Care Medicine 2005; Sleep Medicine 2011; **Med School:** Univ Conn 1988; **Resid:** Internal Medicine, Univ Conn Hlth Ctr 1991; **Fellow:** Pulmonary Disease, Yale-New Haven Hosp 1994; Critical Care Medicine, Yale-New Haven Hosp 1994; **Fac Appt:** Asst Clin Prof Med, Cornell Univ-Weill Med Coll

Frimer, Richard MD (Pul) - **Hospital:** White Plains Hosp (page 640); **Address:** 170 Maple Ave, Ste G1, White Plains, NY 10601-4710; **Phone:** 914-328-0932; **Board Cert:** Internal Medicine 1983; Pulmonary Disease 1986; Critical Care Medicine 2010; **Med School:** SUNY Buffalo 1980; **Resid:** Internal Medicine, Montefiore Med Ctr 1983; **Fellow:** Pulmonary Disease, NYU Med Ctr 1985

Jacobowitz, Marilyn MD (Pul) - **Spec Exp:** Asthma; Cough; **Hospital:** Northern Westchester Hosp (page 639); **Address:** 90 S Bedford Rd, Mt Kisco, NY 10549-3412; **Phone:** 914-241-1050; **Board Cert:** Internal Medicine 2012; Pulmonary Disease 2004; Critical Care Medicine 2005; **Med School:** NYU Sch Med 1989; **Resid:** Internal Medicine, Mt Sinai Hosp 1992; **Fellow:** Pulmonary Disease, Mt Sinai Hosp 1995

Klares, Scott M MD (Pul) - **Spec Exp:** Critical Care; Asthma; Cough; **Hospital:** Northern Westchester Hosp (page 639); **Address:** MKMG, Pulmonary & Critical Care Med, 90 S Bedford Rd, Mount Kisco, NY 10549; **Phone:** 914-241-1050; **Board Cert:** Internal Medicine 2006; Pulmonary Disease 2007; Critical Care Medicine 2008; **Med School:** NY Med Coll 1992; **Resid:** Internal Medicine, Beth Israel Deaconess Med Ctr 1995; **Fellow:** Pulmonary Critical Care Medicine, Boston Med Ctr 1998; **Fac Appt:** Asst Clin Prof Med, Mount Sinai Sch Med

Lehrman, Gary R MD (Pul) - **Spec Exp:** Sleep Disorders; **Hospital:** Phelps Meml Hosp Ctr; **Address:** 160 N State Rd, Briarcliff Manor, NY 10510-1443; **Phone:** 914-762-8383; **Board Cert:** Internal Medicine 1982; Pulmonary Disease 1986; Critical Care Medicine 2004; Sleep Medicine 2007; **Med School:** NYU Sch Med 1979; **Resid:** Internal Medicine, LI Jewish Med Ctr 1984; **Fellow:** Pulmonary Disease, LIJ Med Ctr/Queens Hosp Affil 1985

Lehrman, Stuart MD (Pul) - **Spec Exp:** Lung Cancer; Asthma; **Hospital:** Westchester Med Ctr; **Address:** Westchester Med Ctr, Macys Pavilon-Pulmonary Lab, 100 Woods Rd, Valhalla, NY 10595; **Phone:** 914-493-7518; **Board Cert:** Internal Medicine 1981; Pulmonary Disease 1984; Critical Care Medicine 2007; Sleep Medicine 2007; **Med School:** SUNY Hlth Sci Ctr 1978; **Resid:** Internal Medicine, Cedars-Sinai Med Ctr 1981; **Fellow:** Pulmonary Disease, Cedars-Sinai Med Ctr 1983; **Fac Appt:** Assoc Clin Prof Med, NY Med Coll

Mandel, Michael MD (Pul) - **Spec Exp:** Sleep Disorders/Apnea; Chronic Obstructive Lung Disease (COPD); Asthma; **Hospital:** Montefiore New Rochelle Hosp; **Address:** 2365 Boston Post Rd, Ste 103, Larchmont, NY 10538; **Phone:** 914-833-2020; **Board Cert:** Internal Medicine 1986; Pulmonary Disease 2010; Critical Care Medicine 2011; Sleep Medicine 2009; **Med School:** Columbia P&S 1983; **Resid:** Internal Medicine, St Lukes Roosevelt Hosp 1987; **Fellow:** Pulmonary Critical Care Medicine, UMDNJ Med Ctr 1989; **Fac Appt:** Asst Prof Med, NY Med Coll

Meixler, Steven M MD (Pul) - **Spec Exp:** Asthma; Emphysema; Cough-Chronic; **Hospital:** White Plains Hosp (page 640); **Address:** WestMed, Pulmonology, 210 Westchester Ave, White Plains, NY 10604; **Phone:** 914-682-6511; **Board Cert:** Internal Medicine 1987; Pulmonary Disease 2010; Critical Care Medicine 2011; **Med School:** Boston Univ 1984; **Resid:** Internal Medicine, VA Med Ctr 1988; **Fellow:** Pulmonary Disease, Bellevue Hosp/NYU 1990

Novitch, Richard MD (Pul) - **Spec Exp:** Pulmonary Rehabilitation; **Hospital:** Burke Rehab Hosp; **Address:** 785 Mamaroneck Ave, White Plains, NY 10605; **Phone:** 914-597-2226; **Board Cert:** Internal Medicine 1987; **Med School:** Mexico 1983; **Resid:** Internal Medicine, UMDNJ Med Ctr 1987; **Fellow:** Pulmonary Disease, UMDNJ Med Ctr 1989; **Fac Appt:** Asst Clin Prof Med, Cornell Univ-Weill Med Coll

Schreiber, Michael E MD (Pul) - **Spec Exp:** Asthma; Emphysema; **Hospital:** St. John's Riverside Hosp-Andrus Pavil, Saint Joseph's Med Ctr - Yonkers; **Address:** 970 N Broadway, Ste 209, Yonkers, NY 10701; **Phone:** 914-423-8517; **Board Cert:** Internal Medicine 1976; Pulmonary Disease 1978; Sleep Medicine 2011; **Med School:** Univ Ariz Coll Med 1973; **Resid:** Internal Medicine, Montefiore Med Ctr 1976; **Fellow:** Pulmonary Disease, NYU Med Ctr 1978; **Fac Appt:** Asst Clin Prof Med, NY Med Coll

Sherling, Bruce E MD (Pul) - **Hospital:** White Plains Hosp (page 640), Greenwich Hosp (page 938); **Address:** Westchester Medical Group, 1 Theall Rd, Rye, NY 10580; **Phone:** 914-848-8777; **Board Cert:** Internal Medicine 1976; Pulmonary Disease 1978; **Med School:** NY Med Coll 1973; **Resid:** Internal Medicine, Metropolitan Hosp Ctr 1974; **Fellow:** Pulmonary Disease, Metropolitan Hosp Ctr 1977; Pulmonary Disease, Lenox Hill Hosp 1978

Volcovici, Guido MD (Pul) - **Spec Exp:** Asthma; Emphysema; **Hospital:** Saint Joseph's Med Ctr - Yonkers; **Address:** 127 S Broadway, Ste 406, Yonkers, NY 10701; **Phone:** 914-968-5446; **Board Cert:** Internal Medicine 1985; Pulmonary Disease 1988; **Med School:** Romania 1962; **Resid:** Internal Medicine, Jewish Hosp 1974; **Fellow:** Pulmonary Disease, VA Med Ctr 1976

Weinberg, Harlan MD (Pul) - **Spec Exp:** Asthma; Critical Care Medicine; **Hospital:** Northern Westchester Hosp (page 639); **Address:** 400 E Main St, Mt Kisco, NY 10549; **Phone:** 914-458-8700; **Board Cert:** Internal Medicine 1984; Pulmonary Disease 1986; **Med School:** Univ Conn 1981; **Resid:** Internal Medicine, McGaw Med Ctr-Northwestern 1984; **Fellow:** Pulmonary Disease, Cedars-Sinai Med Ctr 1986

Radiation Oncology

Fass, Daniel E MD (RadRO) - **Spec Exp:** Prostate Cancer; Breast Cancer; Head & Neck Cancer; **Address:** WestMed, Radiation Oncology, 1 Theall Rd, Ste 107, Rye, NY 10580; **Phone:** 914-848-8950; **Board Cert:** Radiation Oncology 1987; **Med School:** Howard Univ 1983; **Resid:** Radiation Oncology, NYU Med Ctr 1986; **Fellow:** Brachytherapy, Meml Sloan-Kettering Cancer Ctr 1987; **Fac Appt:** Asst Prof RadRO, Cornell Univ-Weill Med Coll

Moorthy, Chitti MD (RadRO) - **Spec Exp:** Prostate Cancer; Breast Cancer; Brain Tumors; Mycosis Fungoides; **Hospital:** Westchester Med Ctr; **Address:** Westchester Med Ctr, Radiation Med, 100 Woods Rd, Macy Pav - rm 1297, Valhalla, NY 10595; **Phone:** 914-493-8561; **Board Cert:** Therapeutic Radiology 1979; **Med School:** India 1974; **Resid:** Surgery, Michael Reese Hosp & Med Ctr 1976; Radiation Oncology, Michael Reese Hosp & Med Ctr 1979; **Fellow:** Brachytherapy, Meml Sloan-Kettering Cancer Ctr 1980; **Fac Appt:** Prof RadRO, NY Med Coll

Stevens, Randy E MD (RadRO) - **Spec Exp:** Breast Cancer; **Hospital:** White Plains Hosp (page 640); **Address:** Dickstein Cancer Ctr, 2 Longview Ave, White Plains, NY 10601; **Phone:** 914-681-2727; **Board Cert:** Internal Medicine 1989; Radiation Oncology 1993; **Med School:** NYU Sch Med 1986; **Resid:** Radiation Oncology, NYU Med Ctr 1992

Tinger, Alfred MD (RadRO) - **Spec Exp:** Prostate Cancer; Breast Cancer; Brain Tumors; Gynecologic Cancer; **Hospital:** Northern Westchester Hosp (page 639); **Address:** 21st Century Oncology, 970 N Broadway, Ste 101 & 111, Yonkers, NY 10701; **Phone:** 914-969-1600; **Board Cert:** Radiation Oncology 2008; **Med School:** SUNY Downstate 1992; **Resid:** Radiation Oncology, Washington Univ Med Ctr 1997

Reproductive Endocrinology

Bennett, Rachel MD (RE) - **Spec Exp:** Infertility-IVF; Hysteroscopic Surgery; Polycystic Ovarian Syndrome; **Hospital:** Northern Westchester Hosp (page 639), Hudson Valley Hosp Ctr; **Address:** Westchester Reproductive Med, 344 E Main St, Ste 403, Mt Kisco, NY 10549; **Phone:** 914-218-8955; **Board Cert:** Obstetrics & Gynecology 2012; Reproductive Endocrinology 2012; **Med School:** Mount Sinai Sch Med 1989; **Resid:** Obstetrics & Gynecology, NY-Presby/Weill Cornell Med Ctr 1993; **Fellow:** Reproductive Endocrinology, Brigham & Womens Hosp 1995; **Fac Appt:** Asst Clin Prof Med, Mount Sinai Sch Med

Klein, Jeffrey MD (RE) - **Spec Exp:** Infertility-IVF; Infertility; Polycystic Ovarian Syndrome; Endometriosis; **Hospital:** White Plains Hosp (page 640); **Address:** Reproductive Med Assocs, 15 N Broadway, Garden Level, Ste G, White Plains, NY 10601; **Phone:** 914-997-6200; **Board Cert:** Obstetrics & Gynecology 2012; Reproductive Endocrinology 2012; **Med School:** Albert Einstein Coll Med 1995; **Resid:** Obstetrics & Gynecology, G Washington Univ Med Ctr 1999; **Fellow:** Reproductive Endocrinology, NY-Presby/Columbia Univ Med Ctr 2001

Lieman, Harry J MD (RE) - **Spec Exp:** Infertility-IVF; Polycystic Ovarian Syndrome; Preimplantation Genetic Diagnosis; **Hospital:** Montefiore Med Ctr-Einstein Campus (page 100); **Address:** Montefiore Inst for Reproductive Med, 141 S Central Ave, Ste 201, Hartsdale, NY 10530; **Phone:** 914-997-1060; **Board Cert:** Obstetrics & Gynecology 2012; Reproductive Endocrinology/Infertility 2012; **Med School:** SUNY Downstate 1990; **Resid:** Obstetrics & Gynecology, Jacobi Med Ctr 1994; **Fellow:** Reproductive Endocrinology/Infertility, UMDNJ Affil Hosp 1996; **Fac Appt:** Assoc Prof ObG, Albert Einstein Coll Med

Stangel, John MD (RE) - **Spec Exp:** Infertility-IVF; Endometriosis; Miscarriage-Recurrent; **Hospital:** Northern Westchester Hosp (page 639), Phelps Meml Hosp Ctr; **Address:** Reproductive Med Assocs, 15 N Broadway, Ste G, White Plains, NY 10601; **Phone:** 914-997-6200; **Board Cert:** Obstetrics & Gynecology 1976; Reproductive Endocrinology 1981; **Med School:** NY Med Coll 1969; **Resid:** Obstetrics & Gynecology, Mount Sinai Med Ctr 1974; **Fellow:** Reproductive Endocrinology, Metropolitan Hosp Ctr 1976

Rheumatology

Barone, Richard P MD (Rhu) - **Spec Exp:** Rheumatoid Arthritis; Lupus/SLE; Psoriatic Arthritis; **Hospital:** Montefiore New Rochelle Hosp; **Address:** 421 Huguenot St Fl 4 - Ste 44, New Rochelle, NY 10801-7004; **Phone:** 914-235-3065; **Med School:** Italy 1971; **Resid:** Internal Medicine, Brooklyn Jewish Hosp & Med Ctr 1974; **Fellow:** Rheumatology, Brooklyn Jewish Hosp & Med Ctr 1976; **Fac Appt:** Assoc Clin Prof Med, NY Med Coll

Berger, Jack J MD (Rhu) - **Spec Exp:** Rheumatoid Arthritis; Psoriatic Arthritis; Spondylitis; Gout; **Hospital:** White Plains Hosp (page 640); **Address:** 210 Westchester Ave, White Plains, NY 10604; **Phone:** 914-682-6532; **Board Cert:** Internal Medicine 1979; Rheumatology 1982; **Med School:** Albert Einstein Coll Med 1976; **Resid:** Internal Medicine, Bellevue Hosp 1979; **Fellow:** Rheumatology, Bellevue Hosp 1981

Burns, Mark R MD (Rhu) - **Spec Exp:** Lupus Nephritis; Rheumatoid Arthritis; **Hospital:** Montefiore New Rochelle Hosp; **Address:** 421 Huguenot St, rm 44, New Rochelle, NY 10801; **Phone:** 914-235-3065; **Board Cert:** Internal Medicine 1980; Rheumatology 1984; **Med School:** UCSF 1977; **Resid:** Internal Medicine, Montefiore Med Ctr 1980; **Fellow:** Rheumatology, Montefiore Med Ctr 1983; **Fac Appt:** Asst Clin Prof Med, Albert Einstein Coll Med

Foto, Frank MD (Rhu) - **Spec Exp:** Rheumatoid Arthritis; Lupus/SLE; Gout; Fibromyalgia; **Hospital:** Phelps Meml Hosp Ctr; **Address:** 310 N Highland Ave, Ste 7, Ossining, NY 10562; **Phone:** 914-762-5555; **Board Cert:** Internal Medicine 1989; Rheumatology 2007; **Med School:** Mexico 1983; **Resid:** Internal Medicine, Nassau Univ Med Ctr 1988; **Fellow:** Rheumatology, Univ Iowa Hosp & Clinics 1991

Lans, David M DO (Rhu) - **Spec Exp:** Rheumatoid Arthritis; Lupus/SLE; Asthma; Osteoporosis; **Hospital:** Lawrence Hosp Ctr, Montefiore New Rochelle Hosp; **Address:** 838 Pelhamdale Ave, New Rochelle, NY 10801-1032; **Phone:** 914-235-5577; **Board Cert:** Internal Medicine 1984; Allergy & Immunology 1987; Rheumatology 1988; **Med School:** Univ Osteo Med & Hlth Sci, Des Moines 1981; **Resid:** Internal Medicine, Downstate Univ Hosp 1985; **Fellow:** Allergy & Immunology, New Eng Med Ctr 1987; Rheumatology, Hosp For Special Surgery 1989; **Fac Appt:** Asst Clin Prof Med, NY Med Coll

Lenci, Margaret MD (Rhu) - **Hospital:** Northern Westchester Hosp (page 639); **Address:** MKMG, Rheumatology, 90 S Bedford Rd, Mount Kisco, NY 10549; **Phone:** 914-241-1050; **Board Cert:** Internal Medicine 1983; Rheumatology 1988; **Med School:** SUNY Downstate 1980; **Resid:** Internal Medicine, Montefiore Med Ctr 1983; **Fellow:** Rheumatology, Montefiore Med Ctr 1988

Marmur, Ronen MD/PhD (Rhu) - **Hospital:** Northern Westchester Hosp (page 639); **Address:** 90 S Bedford Rd, Mount Kisco, NY 10549; **Phone:** 914-241-1050; **Board Cert:** Internal Medicine 2001; Rheumatology 2003; **Med School:** Albert Einstein Coll Med 1998; **Resid:** Internal Medicine, NY-Presby/Weill Cornell Univ Med Ctr 2000; **Fellow:** Rheumatology, NY-Presby/Weill Cornell Univ Med Ctr 2004

Mascarenhas, Bento R MD (Rhu) - **Spec Exp:** Arthritis; Lupus/SLE; Osteoporosis; **Hospital:** Burke Rehab Hosp; **Address:** 785 Mamaroneck Ave, White Plains, NY 10605-2523; **Phone:** 914-948-6405; **Board Cert:** Internal Medicine 1972; Rheumatology 1974; **Med School:** India 1961; **Resid:** Internal Medicine, Westchester Med Ctr 1967; **Fellow:** Internal Medicine, Cornell Univ Med Ctr 1970; Rheumatology, Hosp for Special Surg 1970

Reinitz, Elizabeth MD (Rhu) - **Spec Exp:** Rheumatoid Arthritis; Lupus/SLE; Osteoarthritis; Gout; **Hospital:** White Plains Hosp (page 640); **Address:** Scarsdale Medical Group, 600 Mamaroneck Ave, Ste 200, Harrison, NY 10528; **Phone:** 914-723-8100; **Board Cert:** Internal Medicine 1979; Rheumatology 1982; **Med School:** Albert Einstein Coll Med 1976; **Resid:** Internal Medicine, Boston City Hosp 1979; **Fellow:** Rheumatology, Montefiore Med Ctr 1981

Sloane, Lori E MD (Rhu) - **Spec Exp:** Lupus/SLE; Rheumatoid Arthritis; **Hospital:** Northern Westchester Hosp (page 639); **Address:** Westchester Hlth Assocs, 322 Underhill Ave, Yorktown Heights, NY 10598; **Phone:** 914-962-5501; **Board Cert:** Internal Medicine 1989; **Med School:** SUNY Downstate 1986; **Resid:** Internal Medicine, Jacobi Med Ctr 1989; **Fellow:** Rheumatology, Montefiore Hosp Med Ctr 1991

Yegudin-Ash, Julia MD (Rhu) - **Spec Exp:** Lupus/SLE; Rheumatoid Arthritis; Psoriatic Arthritis; Scleroderma; **Hospital:** Westchester Med Ctr; **Address:** MRA Phys, Endocrinology Rheumatology, 19 Bradhurst Ave, Ste 3070N, Hawthorne, NY 10532; **Phone:** 914-594-4444; **Board Cert:** Rheumatology 2006; **Med School:** SUNY Stony Brook 1987; **Resid:** Internal Medicine, Winthrop Univ Hosp 1990; **Fellow:** Rheumatology, Mass Genl Hosp 1992; Rheumatology, NYU Hosp Joint Diseases 1993; **Fac Appt:** Asst Prof Med, NY Med Coll

Sports Medicine

Cavaliere, Gregg MD (SM) - **Spec Exp:** Rotator Cuff Surgery; Knee Injuries/Ligament Surgery; Shoulder Instability; Arthroscopic Surgery; **Hospital:** Phelps Meml Hosp Ctr, Lenox Hill Hosp (page 106); **Address:** Hudson Vly Bone & Joint Surgeons, 24 Saw Mill River Rd, Ste 260, Hawthorne, NY 10532; **Phone:** 914-631-7777; **Board Cert:** Orthopaedic Surgery 2006; **Med School:** NY Med Coll 1987; **Resid:** Orthopaedic Surgery, Lenox Hill Hosp 1992; **Fellow:** Sports Medicine, NYU Med Ctr 1993

Luks, Howard J MD (SM) - **Spec Exp:** Knee Injuries/ACL; Cartilage Damage; Knee Replacement; **Hospital:** Westchester Med Ctr; **Address:** Univ Orthopaedics, 19 Bradhurst Ave, Ste 1300N, Hawthorne, NY 10532; **Phone:** 914-789-2735; **Board Cert:** Orthopaedic Surgery 2010; **Med School:** NY Med Coll 1991; **Resid:** Orthopaedic Surgery, LIJ Med Ctr 1996; **Fellow:** Orthopaedic Sports Medicine, NYU Hosp Joint Diseases 1997; **Fac Appt:** Asst Prof OrS, NY Med Coll

Shifrin, Seth P MD (SM) - **Spec Exp:** Primary Care Sports Medicine; **Hospital:** Northern Westchester Hosp (page 639); **Address:** MKMG, Sports Med, 110 S Bedford Rd Fl 3, Mount Kisco, NY 10549; **Phone:** 914-241-1050; **Board Cert:** Internal Medicine 2004; Sports Medicine 2005; Pediatrics 2013; **Med School:** Univ Chicago-Pritzker Sch Med 2000; **Resid:** Internal Medicine & Pediatrics, Chldns Hosp 2004; **Fellow:** Primary Care Sports Medicine, MacNeal Hosp 2005

Small, Eric W MD (SM) - **Spec Exp:** Primary Care Sports Medicine; Reflex Sympathetic Dystrophy (RSD); Concussion; Compartment Syndrome; **Hospital:** Northern Westchester Hosp (page 639); **Address:** Family Sports Medicine & Fitness, 666 Lexington Ave, Ste 210, Mt Kisco, NY 10549; **Phone:** 914-666-7900; **Board Cert:** Pediatrics 2002; Sports Medicine 2008; **Med School:** UMDNJ-NJ Med Sch, Newark 1989; **Resid:** Pediatrics, Montefiore-Weiler Einstein Med Ctr 1992; **Fellow:** Pediatric Sports Medicine, McMaster Univ/Hamilton 1994; Sports Medicine, Boston Children's Hosp 1995; **Fac Appt:** Asst Clin Prof Ped, Mount Sinai Sch Med

Surgery

Arthur, Karen MD (S) - **Spec Exp:** Breast Cancer & Surgery; **Hospital:** Northern Westchester Hosp (page 639); **Address:** Northern Westchester Hosp Breast Inst, 400 E Main St, Mount Kisco, NY 10549; **Phone:** 914-242-7640; **Board Cert:** Surgery 2011; **Med School:** Mount Sinai Sch Med 1974; **Resid:** Surgery, Mount Sinai Hosp 1979

Ashikari, Andrew Y MD (S) - **Spec Exp:** Breast Cancer; Breast Disease; Nipple Sparing Mastectomy; **Hospital:** St. John's Riverside Hosp-Dobbs Ferry Pavil; **Address:** St Johns Riverside Hosp, Breast Ctr, 128 Ashford Ave, Dobbs Ferry, NY 10522; **Phone:** 914-693-5025; **Board Cert:** Surgery 2006; **Med School:** Univ Pittsburgh 1991; **Resid:** Surgery, Montefiore Med Ctr 1996; **Fellow:** Surgical Oncology, Univ Chicago Med Ctr 1999; **Fac Appt:** Assoc Prof S, NY Med Coll

Cahan, Anthony C MD (S) - **Spec Exp:** Breast Surgery; Breast Cancer; **Hospital:** Northern Westchester Hosp (page 639); **Address:** Northern Westchester Surgical Svcs, 3010 Westchester Ave, Ste 201, Purchase, NY 10577; **Phone:** 914-517-8220; **Board Cert:** Surgery 2008; **Med School:** Cornell Univ-Weill Med Coll 1982; **Resid:** Surgery, NY-Presby/Weill Cornell Med Ctr 1987; **Fac Appt:** Asst Clin Prof Med, NY Med Coll

Charny, Caleb K MD/PhD (S) - **Hospital:** White Plains Hosp (page 640), Greenwich Hosp (page 938); **Address:** WESTMED Medical Grp, 210 Westchester Ave Fl 3, White Plains, NY 10604; **Phone:** 914-682-6557; **Board Cert:** Surgery 2011; **Med School:** NYU Sch Med 1995; **Resid:** Surgery, New York Hosp 2000

Diflo, Thomas MD (S) - **Spec Exp:** Transplant-Kidney; Transplant-Liver; **Hospital:** Westchester Med Ctr; **Address:** Westchester Medical Ctr, 100 Woods Rd, Taylor Pavilion, Room O-127, Valhalla, NY 10595; **Phone:** 914-493-1169; **Board Cert:** Surgery 2012; Surgical Critical Care 2005; **Med School:** Boston Univ 1984; **Resid:** Surgery, Boston Univ Med Ctr 1991; **Fellow:** Transplant Surgery, New England Deaconess Hosp 1992; **Fac Appt:** Prof S, NY Med Coll

Fou, Adora C MD (S) - **Spec Exp:** Breast Cancer; Breast Disease; **Hospital:** White Plains Hosp (page 640), Greenwich Hosp (page 938); **Address:** Westchester Med Grp, 1 Theall Rd, Ste 103, Rye, NY 10580; **Phone:** 914-848-8960; **Board Cert:** Surgery 2007; **Med School:** Univ Ottawa 2000; **Resid:** Surgery, NY Med Coll Affil Hosps 2005

Gordon, Mark S MD (S) - **Spec Exp:** Breast Cancer; Melanoma; Pancreatic Cancer; Colon Cancer; **Hospital:** White Plains Hosp (page 640); **Address:** White Plains Phys, 2 Longview Ave, Ste 302, White Plains, NY 10601; **Phone:** 914-684-5884; **Board Cert:** Surgery 2006; **Med School:** Northwestern Univ 1982; **Resid:** Surgery, NY Hosp 1987; **Fellow:** Surgical Oncology, Meml Sloan-Kettering Cancer Ctr 1989; **Fac Appt:** Asst Clin Prof S, NY Med Coll

Josephson, Lynn G MD (S) - **Spec Exp:** Breast Cancer & Surgery; **Hospital:** White Plains Hosp (page 640); **Address:** WestMed, Surgery, 1 Theall Rd, Ste 103, Rye, NY 10580; **Phone:** 914-848-8960; **Board Cert:** Surgery 2002; **Med School:** Mount Sinai Sch Med 1977; **Resid:** Surgery, NY-Presby/Columbia Univ Med Ctr 1981

Kaul, Ashutosh MD (S) - **Spec Exp:** Obesity/Bariatric Surgery; Minimally Invasive Surgery; **Hospital:** Westchester Med Ctr; **Address:** Surgical Intensivists, 19 Bradhurst Ave, Ste 1700, Hawthorne, NY 10532; **Phone:** 914-347-0162; **Board Cert:** Surgery 2010; **Med School:** India 1988; **Resid:** Surgery, Bronx Lebanon Hosp 1998; Surgery, St Barnabas Med Ctr 2000; **Fac Appt:** Asst Prof S, NY Med Coll

Lau, Har Chi MD (S) - **Spec Exp:** Laparoscopic Surgery; Hernia; **Hospital:** Phelps Meml Hosp Ctr; **Address:** Hudson Vly Surgical Grp, 777 N Broadway, Ste 204, Sleepy Hollow, NY 10591; **Phone:** 914-631-3660; **Board Cert:** Surgery 2007; **Med School:** Univ Pennsylvania 1992; **Resid:** Surgery, Allegheny Genl Hosp 1998

Lemercier, Maud L MD (S) - **Spec Exp:** Breast Cancer; **Hospital:** Northern Westchester Hosp (page 639); **Address:** MKMG, Surgery, 111 Bedford Rd, Katonah, NY 10536; **Phone:** 914-232-3135; **Board Cert:** Surgery 2006; **Med School:** Temple Univ 1999; **Resid:** Surgery, Univ Conn Hlth Ctr 2005

Rajdeo, Heena P MD (S) - **Spec Exp:** Dialysis Access Surgery; Thyroid & Parathyroid Surgery; Trauma; Laparoscopic Surgery; **Hospital:** Westchester Med Ctr; **Address:** 100 Wood Rd, Taylor Pavilion, Ste E130, Valhalla, NY 10595; **Phone:** 914-372-7196; **Board Cert:** Surgery 2012; **Med School:** India 1969; **Resid:** Surgery, KEM Hosp 1972; Surgery, Westchester Med Ctr 1982; **Fac Appt:** Asst Prof S, NY Med Coll

Rangraj, Madhu S MD (S) - **Spec Exp:** Laparoscopic Surgery; Obesity/Bariatric Surgery; Hernia; **Hospital:** Montefiore New Rochelle Hosp; **Address:** 110 Lockwood Ave, Ste 300, New Rochelle, NY 10801; **Phone:** 914-632-9650; **Board Cert:** Surgery 2009; **Med School:** India 1972; **Resid:** Surgery, New Rochelle Hosp 1978; Surgery, VA Med Ctr 1980

Raniolo, Robert MD (S) - **Spec Exp:** Breast Surgery; Gastrointestinal Surgery; Hernia; **Hospital:** Phelps Meml Hosp Ctr; **Address:** Hudson Vly Surgical Grp, 777 N Broadway, Ste 204, Sleepy Hollow, NY 10591; **Phone:** 914-631-3660; **Board Cert:** Surgery 2007; **Med School:** Mexico 1981; **Resid:** Surgery, Lincoln Hosp 1988

Spanknebel, Kathryn A MD (S) - **Spec Exp:** Breast Cancer; Breast Disease; **Hospital:** Westchester Med Ctr; **Address:** New York Medical College, Dept Surgery, Munger Pavilion, rm 211, Valhalla, NY 10595; **Phone:** 914-594-3304; **Board Cert:** Surgery 2010; **Med School:** Univ VT Coll Med 1992; **Resid:** Surgery, Univ Chicago Hosps 2000; **Fac Appt:** Assoc Prof S, NY Med Coll

Weber, Kaare J MD (S) - **Spec Exp:** Endocrine Surgery; Thyroid Cancer; **Hospital:** White Plains Hosp (page 640); **Address:** White Plains Surgical Assocs, 170 Maple Ave, Ste 502, White Plains, NY 10601; **Phone:** 914-948-1000; **Board Cert:** Surgery 2004; **Med School:** Albert Einstein Coll Med 1997; **Resid:** Surgery, Mount Sinai Med Ctr 2003; **Fellow:** Endocrine Surgery, Rush Univ Med Ctr 2004

Wertkin, Martin G MD (S) - **Spec Exp:** Breast Cancer; Breast Surgery; **Hospital:** St. John's Riverside Hosp-Andrus Pavil, Phelps Meml Hosp Ctr; **Address:** 970 N Broadway, Ste 111, Yonkers, NY 10701; **Phone:** 914-965-2026; **Board Cert:** Surgery 2009; **Med School:** SUNY Hlth Sci Ctr 1972; **Resid:** Surgery, Mt Sinai Med Ctr 1978; **Fac Appt:** Asst Clin Prof S, Mount Sinai Sch Med

Thoracic & Cardiac Surgery

Lafaro, Rocco J MD (T&CS) - **Spec Exp:** Minimally Invasive Cardiac Surgery; **Hospital:** Westchester Med Ctr, Phelps Meml Hosp Ctr; **Address:** Westchester Med Ctr Heart Institute, 100 Woods Way, Valhalla, NY 10595; **Phone:** 914-493-7676; **Board Cert:** Thoracic Surgery 2011; **Med School:** NY Med Coll 1982; **Resid:** Surgery, Metropolitan Hosp Ctr 1984; Surgery, Westchester Med Ctr 1986; **Fellow:** Thoracic Surgery, Bronx Muni Hosp Ctr 1991; Thoracic Surgery, Montefiore Med Ctr 1993

Lansman, Steven L MD/PhD (T&CS) - **Spec Exp:** Coronary Artery Surgery; Heart Valve Surgery; Ventricular Assist Device (LVAD); Transplant-Heart; **Hospital:** Westchester Med Ctr; **Address:** Westchester Med Ctr, Heart Inst, 95 Grasslands Rd, Valhalla, NY 10595; **Phone:** 914-493-8793; **Board Cert:** Thoracic Surgery 2004; **Med School:** SUNY Hlth Sci Ctr 1977; **Resid:** Surgery, Montefiore Med Ctr 1982; **Fellow:** Thoracic Surgery, Univ Hosp 1984; **Fac Appt:** Prof S, NY Med Coll

Merav, Avraham D MD (T&CS) - **Spec Exp:** Minimally Invasive Thoracic Surgery; Lung Surgery; Esophageal Surgery; Cardiothoracic Surgery; **Hospital:** Phelps Meml Hosp Ctr, Westchester Med Ctr; **Address:** 755 N Broadway, Sleepy Hollow, NY 10591; **Phone:** 914-366-2333; **Board Cert:** Surgery 1974; Thoracic Surgery 2004; **Med School:** Switzerland 1964; **Resid:** Surgery, Montefiore Med Ctr 1973; **Fellow:** Cardiothoracic Surgery, Montefiore Med Ctr 1975; **Fac Appt:** Assoc Clin Prof TS, Albert Einstein Coll Med

Sett, Suvro S MD (T&CS) - **Spec Exp:** Pediatric Cardiac Surgery; Congenital Heart Disease; Congenital Heart Disease-Adult; **Hospital:** Westchester Med Ctr; **Address:** 155 Grasslands Rd, Munger Pavilion - Fl 6th, Ste 618, MS 10595, Valhalla, NY 10595; **Phone:** 914-594-3322; **Med School:** Canada 1983; **Resid:** Surgery, Univ Saskatchewan Affil Hosps 1988; Cardiovascular Surgery, Univ British Columbia Affil Hosps 1991; **Fellow:** Pediatric Cardiac Surgery, Hosp for Sick Chld 1993

Spielvogel, David MD (T&CS) - **Spec Exp:** Aneurysm-Aortic; Transplant-Heart; Coronary Artery Surgery; Heart Valve Surgery; **Hospital:** Westchester Med Ctr; **Address:** Westchester Med Ctr, Heart Inst, 95 Grasslands Rd Macy Bldg - rm 114W, Valhalla, NY 10595; **Phone:** 914-493-8793; **Board Cert:** Thoracic Surgery 2009; **Med School:** SUNY Downstate 1990; **Resid:** Surgery, SUNY Downtown Med Ctr 1995; Thoracic Surgery, Mount Sinai Med Ctr 1998; **Fellow:** Cardiac Surgery, Harefield Hosp 1999; **Fac Appt:** Prof S, NY Med Coll

Weiser, Todd MD (T&CS) - **Spec Exp:** Lung Cancer; Esophageal Cancer; Minimally Invasive Surgery; Mediastinal Tumors; **Hospital:** White Plains Hosp (page 640); **Address:** White Plains Phys, 2 Longview Ave, Ste 301, White Plains, NY 10601; **Phone:** 914-681-2750; **Board Cert:** Surgery 2004; Thoracic Surgery 2007; **Med School:** Jefferson Med Coll 1996; **Resid:** Surgery, St Vincent's Hosp & Med Ctr 2003; **Fellow:** Surgical Oncology, Natl Cancer Inst 2000; Thoracic & Cardiac Surgery, Mass Genl Hosp 2005

Urology

Axelrod, Sheldon L MD (U) - **Spec Exp:** Prostate Cancer; Prostate Disease; Robotic Surgery; **Hospital:** Northern Westchester Hosp (page 639); **Address:** MKMG, Urology, 111 Bedford Rd, Katonah, NY 10536; **Phone:** 914-232-3135; **Board Cert:** Urology 2012; **Med School:** Albert Einstein Coll Med 1982; **Resid:** Surgery, Montefiore Med Ctr 1984; Urology, NY-Presby/Columbia Med Ctr 1988

Blair, Bryan P MD (U) - **Hospital:** White Plains Hosp (page 640); **Address:** WestMed, Urology, 210 Westchester Ave, White Plains, NY 10604; **Phone:** 914-682-6470; **Board Cert:** Urology 2013; **Med School:** Tulane Univ 1994; **Resid:** Urology, Natl Naval Med Ctr 2001

Boczko, Judd MD (U) - **Spec Exp:** Prostate Cancer/Robotic Surgery; Robotic Urologic Surgery; **Hospital:** Greenwich Hosp (page 938); **Address:** WestMed, Urology, 210 Westchester Ave, White Plains, NY 10604; **Phone:** 914-682-6470; **Board Cert:** Urology 2008; **Med School:** Albert Einstein Coll Med 1999; **Resid:** Surgery, Montefiore Med Ctr 2001; Urology, Montefiore Med Ctr 2005; **Fellow:** Urologic Surgery, Univ Rochester Strong Meml Hosp 2006; **Fac Appt:** Asst Prof U, NY Med Coll

Breslin, David S MD (U) - **Spec Exp:** Urology-Female; Voiding Dysfunction; Prostate Disease; **Hospital:** Hudson Valley Hosp Ctr; **Address:** MKMG, Urology, 1978 Crompond Rd, Cortlandt Manor, NY 10567; **Phone:** 914-737-8675; **Board Cert:** Urology 2007; **Med School:** Mount Sinai Sch Med 1987; **Resid:** Surgery, Mount Sinai Med Ctr 1989; Urology, Lenox Hill Hosp 1994; **Fellow:** Female Urology, Beth Israel Deaconess Med Ctr 1995; **Fac Appt:** Asst Clin Prof U, NY Med Coll

Choudhury, Muhammad MD (U) - **Spec Exp:** Prostate Cancer; Bladder Cancer; Kidney Cancer; Testicular Cancer; **Hospital:** Westchester Med Ctr, Montefiore New Rochelle Hosp; **Address:** Urology Ctr, 19 Bradhurst Ave, Ste 1900, Hawthorne, NY 10532-2144; **Phone:** 914-347-1900; **Board Cert:** Urology 1982; **Med School:** Bangladesh 1972; **Resid:** Urology, NY-Presby/Columbia Univ Med Ctr 1978; Urology, NY Med Coll 1980; **Fellow:** Urologic Oncology, Roswell Park Cancer Inst 1981; **Fac Appt:** Prof U, NY Med Coll

Eshghi, A. Majid MD (U) - **Spec Exp:** Kidney Stones; Laparoscopic Surgery; **Hospital:** Westchester Med Ctr, Montefiore New Rochelle Hosp; **Address:** 19 Bradhurst Ave, Ste 1900, Hawthorne, NY 10532; **Phone:** 914-347-1900; **Board Cert:** Urology 2005; **Med School:** Iran 1976; **Resid:** Surgery, St Barnabas Med Ctr 1981; Urology, LI Jewish Med Ctr 1986; **Fac Appt:** Prof U, NY Med Coll

Glassman, Charles N MD (U) - **Spec Exp:** Pediatric Urology; **Hospital:** White Plains Hosp (page 640); **Address:** 170 Maple Ave, Ste 104, White Plains, NY 10601-4707; **Phone:** 914-949-7556; **Board Cert:** Urology 1980; **Med School:** Tufts Univ 1973; **Resid:** Surgery, UCSF Med Ctr 1975; Urology, UCSF Med Ctr 1978; **Fellow:** Pediatric Urology, Mayo Clin 1979

Housman, Arno D MD (U) - **Spec Exp:** Kidney Stones; Prostate Cancer; Incontinence; Minimally Invasive Urologic Surgery; **Hospital:** Phelps Meml Hosp Ctr; **Address:** 325 S Highland Ave, Briarcliff Manor, NY 10510; **Phone:** 914-941-0617; **Board Cert:** Urology 2009; **Med School:** SUNY Downstate 1980; **Resid:** Surgery, SUNY Downstate Med Ctr 1983; Urology, Yale-New Haven Hosp 1986

Lerner, Seth E MD (U) - **Spec Exp:** Prostate Cancer/Robotic Surgery; Robotic Urologic Surgery; **Hospital:** White Plains Hosp (page 640); **Address:** 170 Maple Ave, Ste 104, White Plains, NY 10601; **Phone:** 914-949-7556; **Board Cert:** Urology 2005; **Med School:** SUNY Downstate 1988; **Resid:** Surgery, Montefiore-Weiler Einstein Div 1990; Urology, Montefiore-Weler Einstein Div 1994; **Fellow:** Urologic Oncology, Mayo Clinic 1995; **Fac Appt:** Asst Prof U, Albert Einstein Coll Med

Matthews, Gerald J MD (U) - **Spec Exp:** Infertility-Male; Impotence; **Hospital:** Westchester Med Ctr, Montefiore Med Ctr-Wakefield Campus (page 100); **Address:** 19 Bradhurst Ave, Ste 1900, Hawthorne, NY 10532-2144; **Phone:** 914-347-1900; **Board Cert:** Urology 2006; **Med School:** NY Med Coll 1986; **Resid:** Urology, Lenox Hill Hosp 1993; Surgery, St Francis Hosp Med Ctr 1989; **Fellow:** Urology, NY-Presby/Weill Cornell Med Ctr 1995; **Fac Appt:** Assoc Prof U, NY Med Coll

Nogueira, Mark A MD (U) - **Spec Exp:** Robotic Surgery; Prostate Cancer; Urologic Cancer; **Hospital:** Northern Westchester Hosp (page 639); **Address:** 110 S Bedford Rd, Mount Kisco, NY 10549; **Phone:** 914-241-1050; **Board Cert:** Urology 2009; **Med School:** Mount Sinai Sch Med 2001; **Resid:** Urology, SUNY-Buffalo Med Ctr 2006; **Fellow:** Urologic Oncology, Roswell Park Cancer Inst 2007

Owens, George F MD (U) - **Spec Exp:** Prostate Disease; Erectile Dysfunction; Incontinence; Minimally Invasive Surgery; **Hospital:** White Plains Hosp (page 640), Westchester Med Ctr; **Address:** Advn Urology Ctrs NY, 311 North St, Ste 406, White Plains, NY 10605-2232; **Phone:** 914-946-1406; **Board Cert:** Urology 2005; **Med School:** NY Med Coll 1979; **Resid:** Surgery, Montefiore Med Ctr 1981; Urology, Montefiore Med Ctr 1984; **Fellow:** Urology, NY Med Coll Affil Hosp 1985; **Fac Appt:** Assoc Clin Prof U, NY Med Coll

Phillips, John L MD (U) - **Spec Exp:** Robotic Surgery; Prostate Cancer; **Hospital:** Westchester Med Ctr; **Address:** 19 Bradhurst Ave, Ste 1900, Hawthorne, NY 10532-2144; **Phone:** 914-347-1900; **Board Cert:** Urology 2012; **Med School:** Yale Univ 1992; **Resid:** Surgery, Yale-New Haven Hosp 1994; Urology, Yale-New Haven Hosp 1997

Riechers, Roger N MD (U) - **Spec Exp:** Incontinence-Female; Prostate Cancer; **Hospital:** Northern Westchester Hosp (page 639); **Address:** Columbia Dr's Med Grp, 19 Bradhurst Ave, Ste 700, Hawthorne, NY 10532; **Phone:** 914-593-7800; **Board Cert:** Urology 1976; **Med School:** NYU Sch Med 1968; **Resid:** Urology, Mt Sinai Med Ctr 1974

Roberts, Larry P MD (U) - **Spec Exp:** Infertility-Male; Erectile Dysfunction; Incontinence; **Hospital:** Montefiore New Rochelle Hosp; **Address:** 175 Memorial Hwy, Ste 3-2, New Rochelle, NY 10801-5641; **Phone:** 914-235-2929; **Board Cert:** Urology 1981; **Med School:** Univ Miami Sch Med 1974; **Resid:** Surgery, Univ Miami Hosps 1976; Urology, Montefiore Hosp 1979; **Fac Appt:** Asst Clin Prof U, Albert Einstein Coll Med

Schrager, Alan MD (U) - **Spec Exp:** Prostate Disease; Urology-Female; Urologic Cancer; Voiding Dysfunction; **Hospital:** Greenwich Hosp (page 938), Montefiore New Rochelle Hosp; **Address:** 1600 Harrison Ave, Ste 102-G, Mamaroneck, NY 10543-3124; **Phone:** 914-698-8106; **Board Cert:** Urology 1975; **Med School:** Ros Franklin Univ/Chicago Med Sch 1966; **Resid:** Surgery, Maimonides Med Ctr 1970; Urology, SUNY Downstate Med Ctr 1975

Siegel, Judy F MD (U) - **Spec Exp:** Voiding Dysfunction-Female; Voiding Dysfunction-Pediatric; **Hospital:** St. John's Riverside Hosp-Andrus Pavil, Phelps Meml Hosp Ctr; **Address:** Family Urology, 623 Warburton Ave, Hastings-on-Hudson, NY 10706; **Phone:** 914-478-3001; **Board Cert:** Urology 2009; **Med School:** Univ VT Coll Med 1988; **Resid:** Surgery, LI Jewish Med Ctr 1990; Urology, LI Jewish Med Ctr 1994; **Fellow:** Pediatric Urology, Schneider Chldns Hosp 1996

Trauzzi, Stephen J MD (U) - **Spec Exp:** Prostate Disease; **Hospital:** Montefiore New Rochelle Hosp; **Address:** Advanced Urology Ctrs NY, 120 Warren St, New Rochelle, NY 10801; **Phone:** 914-636-2121; **Board Cert:** Urology 2006; **Med School:** Georgetown Univ 1988; **Resid:** Urology, St. Luke's - Roosevelt Hosp Ctr - Roosevelt Div 1995

Weinberg, Jerry MD (U) - **Spec Exp:** Robotic Surgery; Minimally Invasive Surgery; **Hospital:** Northern Westchester Hosp (page 639); **Address:** 666 Lexington Ave, Ste 100, Mount Kisco, NY 10549; **Phone:** 914-666-4346; **Board Cert:** Urology 2010; **Med School:** SUNY Downstate 1983; **Resid:** Surgery, LIJ Med Ctr 1985; **Fellow:** Urology, LIJ Med Ctr 1989

Werner, Michael A MD (U) - **Spec Exp:** Infertility-Male; Sexual Dysfunction; Men's Health; **Hospital:** White Plains Hosp (page 640); **Address:** 2975 Westchester Ave, Purchase, NY 10577; **Phone:** 914-997-4100; **Board Cert:** Urology 2005; **Med School:** UCSF 1986; **Resid:** Surgery, Beth Israel Med Ctr 1989; Urology, Mount Sinai Med Ctr 1993; **Fellow:** Male Infertility, Boston Med Ctr 1994

Vascular & Interventional Radiology

Hamet, Marc R MD (VIR) - **Spec Exp:** Osteoporosis Spine-Vertebroplasty; Uterine Fibroid Embolization; Endovascular Surgery; Carotid Artery Stent Placement; **Hospital:** White Plains Hosp (page 640), Lawrence Hosp Ctr; **Address:** White Plains Hosp Radiology, 41 E Post Rd, White Plains, NY 10601; **Phone:** 914-681-1273; **Board Cert:** Diagnostic Radiology 1995; Vascular & Interventional Radiology 2009; Neuroradiology 2010; **Med School:** Univ MD Sch Med 1991; **Resid:** Diagnostic Radiology, Univ Maryland Med Sys 1995; **Fellow:** Neuroradiology, Univ Maryland Med Sys 1996; Interventional Radiology, Johns Hopkins Hosp 1998

Rozenblit, Grigory N MD (VIR) - **Spec Exp:** Interventional Oncology; Liver Cancer; **Hospital:** Westchester Med Ctr; **Address:** Westchester Medical Ctr, Vascular & Interventional Radiology, 100 Woods Rd, Valhalla, NY 10595; **Phone:** 914-493-7560; **Board Cert:** Diagnostic Radiology 1984; Vascular & Interventional Radiology 2004; **Med School:** Russia 1970; **Resid:** Radiology, St. Luke's Roosevelt Hosp Ctr 1984; **Fellow:** Interventional Radiology, NY Presby-Cornell Med Ctr 1985; **Fac Appt:** Prof Rad, NY Med Coll

Tulla, Carlos A MD (VIR) - **Hospital:** Lawrence Hosp Ctr, White Plains Hosp (page 640); **Address:** Lawrence Hospital, Radiology, 55 Palmer Ave, Bronxville, NY 10708; **Phone:** 914-787-3116; **Board Cert:** Diagnostic Radiology 1986; Vascular & Interventional Radiology 2006; **Med School:** Univ Puerto Rico 1980; **Resid:** Radiology, Univ Puerto Rico 1985; **Fellow:** Interventional Radiology, NYU Med Ctr 1986

Vascular Surgery

Babu, Sateesh C MD (VascS) - **Spec Exp:** Carotid Artery Surgery; Aneurysm-Abdominal Aortic; Lower Limb Arterial Disease; Vein Disorders; **Hospital:** Westchester Med Ctr, Northern Westchester Hosp (page 639); **Address:** Westchester Heart & Vascular, 19 Bradhurst Ave, Ste 3850S, Hawthorne, NY 10532; **Phone:** 914-909-6900; **Board Cert:** Vascular Surgery 2001; **Med School:** India 1969; **Resid:** Surgery, Jewish Meml Hosp 1972; Surgery, Metropolitan Hosp 1975; **Fellow:** Vascular Surgery, Metropolitan Hosp 1977; **Fac Appt:** Clin Prof S, NY Med Coll

Fishman, Eric MD (VascS) - **Spec Exp:** Aneurysm-Aortic; Endovascular Surgery; **Hospital:** White Plains Hosp (page 640), Greenwich Hosp (page 938); **Address:** 1 Theall Rd, Rye, NY 10580; **Phone:** 914-723-7737; **Board Cert:** Surgery 2005; Vascular Surgery 2012; **Med School:** Mount Sinai Sch Med 1997; **Resid:** Surgery, Mount Sinai Med Ctr 2005; Vascular Surgery, Mount Sinai Med Ctr 2011

Goyal, Arun MD (VascS) - **Spec Exp:** Endovascular Surgery; Vein Disorders; Aneurysm; **Hospital:** Westchester Med Ctr; **Address:** 19 Bradhurst Ave, Ste 3750 S, Hawthorne, NY 10532; **Phone:** 914-593-1200; **Board Cert:** Surgery 2006; Vascular Surgery 2008; **Med School:** NY Med Coll 1990; **Resid:** Surgery, Mt Sinai Med Ctr 1995; Vascular Surgery, Mt Sinai Med Ctr 1996; **Fac Appt:** Asst Prof S, NY Med Coll

Karanfilian, Richard MD (VascS) - **Spec Exp:** Varicose Veins; Carotid Artery Surgery; Endovascular Surgery; **Hospital:** Montefiore New Rochelle Hosp; **Address:** 150 Lockwood Ave, Ste 14, New Rochelle, NY 10801; **Phone:** 914-636-1700; **Board Cert:** Surgery 2012; Vascular Surgery 2006; **Med School:** Italy 1977; **Resid:** Surgery, Univ Hosp-UMDNJ 1983; **Fellow:** Vascular Surgery, Univ Hosp-UMDNJ 1985; **Fac Appt:** Assoc Clin Prof S, NY Med Coll

Mateo, Romeo MD (VascS) - **Spec Exp:** Endovascular Surgery; Carotid Artery Surgery; Minimally Invasive Surgery; **Hospital:** Westchester Med Ctr; **Address:** Atrium Laser Vein Ctr, 19 Bradhurst Ave, Ste 3850S, Hawthorne, NY 10532; **Phone:** 914-593-1200; **Board Cert:** Surgery 2010; Vascular Surgery 2010; **Med School:** Brown Univ 1988; **Resid:** Surgery, Rhode Island Hosp 1991; **Fellow:** Vascular Surgery, Cleveland Clin 1993; **Fac Appt:** Asst Prof S, NY Med Coll

Suggs, William D MD (VascS) - **Spec Exp:** Vein Disorders; Wound Healing/Care; Carotid Artery Surgery; **Hospital:** White Plains Hosp (page 640); **Address:** Vascular Assocs, 4 Lyon Pl, Lobby Level, Ste 2, White Plains, NY 10601; **Phone:** 914-948-6633; **Board Cert:** Vascular Surgery 2012; **Med School:** Wake Forest Univ 1983; **Resid:** Surgery, G Washington Univ Hosp 1989; **Fellow:** Vascular Surgery, Emory Univ Hosp 1991; **Fac Appt:** Assoc Prof VascS, Albert Einstein Coll Med

Sun, Lucy MD (VascS) - **Spec Exp:** Endovascular Surgery; Aneurysm-Aortic; **Hospital:** Northern Westchester Hosp (page 639); **Address:** MKMG, Vascular Surgery, 110 S Bedford Rd, Mount Kisco, NY 10549-3412; **Phone:** 914-241-1050; **Board Cert:** Vascular Surgery 2007; **Med School:** SUNY Downstate 1993; **Resid:** Surgery, Univ Iowa Hosps & Clin 1998; Surgery, UCSF Med Ctr 2001; **Fellow:** Vascular Surgery, RWJ Univ Med Ctr 2003

The State of New Jersey

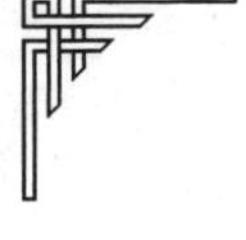

The Best in American Medicine
www.CastleConnolly.com

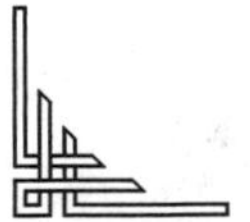
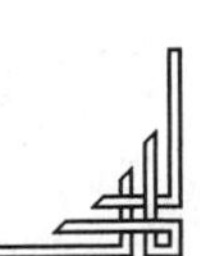

Bergen

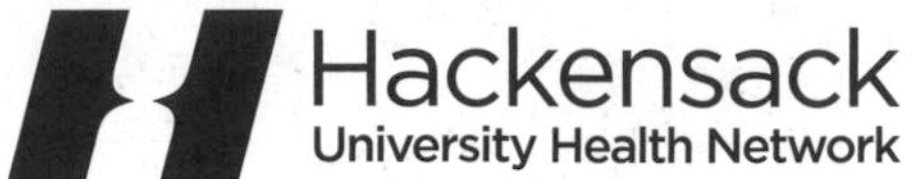

30 Prospect Avenue, Hackensack, NJ 07601 • 551-996-2000
www.HackensackUHN.org

HackensackUMC *(Hackensack University Medical Center)*
HackensackUMC at Pascack Valley
HackensackUMC Mountainside

Year Founded: 2010

Number of beds: 1,268

Number of employees: 9,907

2011 Admissions: 57,805

Number of Hospitals in System: 3

Nursing: Magnet® Recognized for Nursing Excellence

Academic Affiliations: Georgetown University School of Medicine, Saint George's University, Stevens Institute of Technology, Rutgers Medical School

Clinical Affiliations: Georgetown Lombardi Comprehensive Cancer Center, MedStar Georgetown University Hospital, Good Samaritan Regional Medical Center, CentraState Healthcare System, Palisades Medical Center, NYU Langone Medical Center's Division of Pediatric Surgery, MinuteClinic

Strategic Alliance: North Shore-LIJ Health System

• **Network Alliance:** AllSpire Health Partners - seven health systems with a total of 25 hospitals: Atlantic Health System (Morristown, NJ), Hackensack University Health Network (Hackensack, NJ), Lancaster General Health (Lancaster, PA), Lehigh Valley Health Network (Allentown, PA), Meridian Health (Neptune, NJ), Reading Health System (Reading, PA), and WellSpan Health (York, PA).

Hackensack University Health Network (HackensackUHN) is the non-profit, New Jersey-based parent company of HackensackUMC, the HackensackUMC Foundation, Hackensack University HealthPartners Medical Group, and corporate joint venture partners with LHP Hospital Group (Dallas, TX) in ownership of two hospitals: HackensackUMC at Pascack Valley and HackensackUMC Mountainside.

The Network has current clinical collaborations and affiliations with: Georgetown Lombardi Comprehensive Cancer Center, MedStar Georgetown University Hospital, Good Samaritan Regional Medical Center, CentraState Healthcare System, NYU Langone Medical Center's Division of Pediatric Surgery, and Palisades Medical Center. It also formed a strategic alliance with the North Shore-LIJ Health System, and a clinical affiliation with MinuteClinic, the retail healthcare division of CVS Caremark.

• **Hackensack University Medical Groups:** Hackensack University Health Network enjoys various models of employment partnerships with almost 300 physician practices throughout the region. Ranging from sub-specialists to pediatric specialists, these medical groups help to improve efficiency and streamline care. The Hackensack University Medical Group is the largest member of the HackensackAlliance ACO.

• **Accountable Care Organization (ACO):** In April 2012, HackensackAlliance ACO announced it was one of 27 ACOs selected to participate in the Medicare Shared Savings Program (Shared Savings Program) ACO, a multifaceted program sponsored by the Centers for Medicare and Medicaid Services (CMS). As of September 2013, the HackensackAlliance ACO had more than 700 affiliated physicians covering nearly 13,000 lives.

• **United Surgical Partners International:** Hackensack University Health Network entered into a joint venture partnership with community physicians and United Surgical Partners International (USPI) in the acquisition and operation of two ambulatory surgery centers in Bergen County.

For more information, please visit www.HackensackUHN.org.

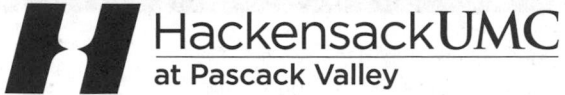

250 Old Hook Road, Westwood, NJ 07675 • 201-383-1035
www.HackensackUMCPV.com

Number of beds: 128

Number of employees: 628 (includes Per Diem)

HackensackUMC at Pascack Valley is a full service 128-bed hospital that serves the Pascack Valley and Northern Valley communities with a caliber of care that is consistent with Hackensack University Health Network's world-class standard. The hospital is a joint venture of the Hackensack University Health Network and the LHP Hospital Group Inc., one of the country's leading private hospital management companies. This state-of-the-art healthcare facility features fully renovated and brand new private rooms at no additional costs to the patient. Services include:

- Bariatric Surgery
- Breast Health Services
- Cancer Services
- Cardiac Services
- Emergency Department
- Imaging and Diagnostics
- Maternity Unit
- Orthopedics and the Center for Joint Replacement
- Surgical Services
- Sleep Center
- Inpatient Therapy Services
- Wound Care

Each all-private, fully-renovated room features a variety of amenities and specialty features for advanced patient care. Special service offerings to help alleviate stress during a patient stay include:

- **Valet parking** – Valet parking is offered at our front main entrance and at our side entrance near labor and delivery. This service is provided free of charge to all patients at HackensackUMC at Pascack Valley.
- **Patient concierge** – Patient concierge is available to all patients from 10 a.m. – 2 p.m., Monday through Friday. Patients can choose from a variety of services including dry-cleaning, prescription and pajama orders, car washes, and more.
- **Room Service** – Room service is offered to our patients as an added convenience. After a long surgery, procedure or delivery our courteous staff will deliver a (medically approved) hot meal to patient rooms at their request from our in-room dining menu.
- **Wi-Fi** – This service is provided to all patients at no additional cost.

HackensackUMC at Pascack Valley proudly offers a number of outreach programs to the local community including Mommy University and the Be Well Community Lecture Series. Mommy University features a series of lectures designed to educate and provide support for new parents or caregivers. These pre and post natal programs are designed to take the mystery out of the birthing process and help expectant parents for one of life's most precious moments, the birth of a child. All lectures are free and conveniently located in the HackensackUMC at Pascack Valley Community Classroom.

The Be Well Community Lecture Series is designed to educate members of the local community about ways to stay well and lead healthier, more fulfilling lives. These seminars are taught by physicians and offered free of charge to the community.

For more information, please call 201-383-1035 or visit www.HackensackUMCPV.com

For more information about Holy Name Medical Center
or for a physician referral, call 1-877-HOLY-NAME.
Please mention "Castle Connolly Guide."

Holy Name Medical Center

718 Teaneck Road
Teaneck, NJ 07666
1-877-HOLY-NAME
(1-877-465-9626)
www.holyname.org

THE HOLY NAME HEALING TRADITION

Holy Name Medical Center (HNMC) is a fully accredited, not-for-profit healthcare facility based in Teaneck, New Jersey, with off-site locations throughout Bergen County, and in Hudson and Passaic counties. Founded and sponsored by the Sisters of St. Joseph of Peace in 1925, the comprehensive 361-bed medical center offers leading-edge medical practice and technology administered in an environment rooted in a tradition of compassion and respect for every patient.

COMPREHENSIVE PROGRAMS AND SERVICES

HNMC provides high-quality health care across a continuum that encompasses education, prevention, early intervention, comprehensive treatment options, rehabilitation and wellness maintenance—from conception through end-of-life.

In addition to patient care, HNMC's School of Nursing is renowned for the education of registered nurses and licensed practical nurses.

PERFORMANCE RECOGNITION

- **Top Performer on Key Quality Measures**
  THE JOINT COMMISSION
- **Best Regional Hospitals**
  US News & World Report
- **Magnet Recognition**
  AMERICAN NURSES CREDENTIALING ASSOCIATION
- **Beacon Award**
  AMERICAN ASSOCIATION OF CRITICAL-CARE NURSES
- **Primary Stroke Care Center**
  THE JOINT COMMISSION
- **American Heart Association/American Stroke Association**
  GOLD PLUS ACHIEVEMENT AWARD
- **"Best Places to Work in Healthcare"**
  MODERN HEALTHCARE MAGAZINE
- **"Best Places to Work in New Jersey"**
  NJ BIZ MAGAZINE

Centers of Excellence

- Bone and Joint Center
- Cardiovascular Services
- Emergency Care Center
- Interventional Institute
- Maternal/Child Health
- Regional Cancer Center

Robotic and Minimally Invasive Surgery

Breast Services

Center for Healthy Living

Center for Sleep Medicine

Post-Acute Services:
- Home Health Care
- Palliative Care
- Community Hospice
- Villa Marie Claire residential hospice
- Adult Medical Day Care

Institute for Clinical Research

Culturally Sensitive Health Care:
- Korean Medical Program
- Hispanic Outreach Program
- Jewish Patient Services

Center for Physical Rehabilitation

HNH Fitness® Medically Based Fitness Center

MS Center

THE VALLEY HOSPITAL

223 North Van Dien Avenue, Ridgewood, NJ 07450
Phone: 201-447-8000 • www.ValleyHealth.com
www.Facebook.com/ValleyHospital • www.Twitter.com/ValleyHospital

Sponsorship: Voluntary Not-for-Profit **Beds:** 451 Acute Care Beds
Accredited by The Joint Commission

■ PROFILE

The Valley Hospital is affiliated with the NewYork-Presbyterian Healthcare System. Valley has been recognized 10 consecutive times under the J.D. Power and Associates Distinguished Hospital Program and is a two-time recipient of the Magnet Award for Nursing Excellence.

Healthgrades has named Valley one of America's 100 Best Hospitals for Cardiac Care, Cardiac Surgery, Coronary Intervention and General Surgery, and recognized the hospital for clinical excellence in cardiac care, cardiac surgery, coronary intervention, gastrointestinal care, general surgery, joint replacement, and orthopedic surgery.

Valley has earned an impressive 11 Disease-Specific Care Certifications for healthcare quality from The Joint Commission: acute myocardial infarction, heart failure, knee replacement, hip replacement, stroke, colorectal cancer, lung cancer, breast cancer, pancreatic cancer, prostate cancer, and uterine-ovarian cancer.

■ MEDICAL STAFF

The Valley Hospital has more than 1,000 physicians on its Active Medical Staff, 92 percent of whom are board certified.

■ CARDIOLOGY

The Valley Heart and Vascular Institute is a leader in the field of cardiology services, including cardiac surgery; coronary angioplasty and other interventional procedures; electrophysiology studies; and cardiac care research. Valley is among only 2.4 percent of hospitals nationwide to receive The Society of Thoracic Surgeons' highest ratings in both coronary artery bypass and aortic valve surgery, and is ranked No. 1 in New Jersey for overall cardiac services by Healthgrades.

■ SURGERY

The Valley Hospital is also known for its comprehensive surgical program, including pioneering advances in surgical oncology, gynecologic oncology, thoracic surgery, and its Center for Minimally Invasive and Robotic Surgery. The hospital has also been designated as a Bariatric Surgery Center of Excellence.

■ ONCOLOGY

Valley is known for its centers specializing in the diagnosis, care and treatment of breast, lung, and prostate cancers; its surgical oncology, neuro-oncology, and gynecologic oncology programs; its comprehensive oncology clinical trials program and its Department of Radiation Oncology, including Tomotherapy. Valley was the first hospital in northern New Jersey to offer Gamma Knife radiosurgery, a noninvasive tool designed to treat cancer and neurological conditions in the brain.

■ WOMEN'S & CHILDREN'S SERVICES

The hospital is well known for its women's and children's services, including the Fertility Center, Maternal-Fetal Medicine program, the Center for Holistic Birth, an enhanced Neonatal Intensive Care Unit, a maternal & child health home care program, and The Kireker Center for Child Development that offers a full spectrum of services.

Physician Referral: Information on physicians affiliated with The Valley Hospital is available by phone at 1-800-VALLEY 1 (1-800-825-5391) or by visiting **www.ValleyMedicalStaff.com.**

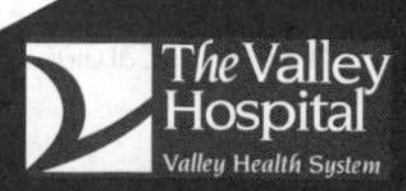

Bergen

Allergy & Immunology

Falk, Theodore MD (A&I) - **Spec Exp:** Asthma; Pediatric Allergy & Immunology; Immunodeficiency Disorders; Chronic Fatigue Syndrome; **Hospital:** Holy Name Med Ctr (page 720), Englewood Hosp & Med Ctr; **Address:** 63 Grand Ave, Ste 100, River Edge, NJ 07661-1930; **Phone:** 201-487-2900; **Board Cert:** Pediatrics 1982; **Med School:** Belgium 1977; **Resid:** Pediatrics, Long Island Jewish Med Ctr 1980; **Fellow:** Allergy & Immunology, Nassau Co Med Ctr 1982

From, Stuart MD (A&I) - **Spec Exp:** Asthma & Allergy; Eczema; Skin Allergies; **Hospital:** Englewood Hosp & Med Ctr; **Address:** 309 Engle St, Ste 2, Englewood, NJ 07631; **Phone:** 201-568-1480; **Board Cert:** Allergy & Immunology 2003; **Med School:** NY Med Coll 1987; **Resid:** Internal Medicine, Montefiore Med Ctr 1990; **Fellow:** Allergy & Immunology, NY-Presby/Weill Cornell Med Ctr 1992

Goodstein, Carolyn E MD (A&I) - **Spec Exp:** Pediatric Allergy & Immunology; Rhinitis; Urticaria; Sinusitis; **Hospital:** Englewood Hosp & Med Ctr, Hackensack Univ Med Ctr (page 718); **Address:** 180 N Dean St, Englewood, NJ 07631; **Phone:** 201-871-4755; **Board Cert:** Internal Medicine 1974; Allergy & Immunology 1980; **Med School:** SUNY Downstate 1964; **Resid:** Internal Medicine, Montefiore Med Ctr 1967; Allergy & Immunology, St Lukes-Roosevelt Hosp 1971

Harish, Ziv MD (A&I) - **Spec Exp:** Asthma & Sinusitis; Hay Fever; Urticaria; Hives; **Hospital:** Englewood Hosp & Med Ctr, Hackensack Univ Med Ctr (page 718); **Address:** 200 Engle St, Ste 18, Englewood, NJ 07631; **Phone:** 201-871-7475; **Board Cert:** Allergy & Immunology 2012; **Med School:** Israel 1983; **Resid:** Pediatrics, Montefiore Med Ctr 1989; **Fellow:** Allergy & Immunology, Montefiore Med Ctr 1991; **Fac Appt:** Clin Prof Med, Albert Einstein Coll Med

Michelis, Mary Ann MD (A&I) - **Spec Exp:** Asthma; Immune Deficiency; **Hospital:** Hackensack Univ Med Ctr (page 718); **Address:** Hackensack Univ Med Ctr, Allergy Asthma, 30 Prospect Ave, rm 3674, Hackensack, NJ 07601; **Phone:** 201-996-2065; **Board Cert:** Internal Medicine 1978; Allergy & Immunology 1981; Diagnostic Lab Immunology 1988; **Med School:** Univ Pittsburgh 1975; **Resid:** Internal Medicine, Lenox Hill Hosp 1978; **Fellow:** Allergy & Immunology, NY-Presby/Weill Cornell Med Ctr 1978; **Fac Appt:** Assoc Clin Prof Med, UMDNJ-NJ Med Sch, Newark

Minikes, Neil I MD (A&I) - **Spec Exp:** Eczema; Food Allergy; Hay Fever; Asthma; **Hospital:** Englewood Hosp & Med Ctr, Hackensack Univ Med Ctr (page 718); **Address:** Allergy & Asthma Ctr, 500 Piermont Rd, Ste 304, Closter, NJ 07624; **Phone:** 201-564-7777; **Board Cert:** Pediatrics 1986; Allergy & Immunology 2011; **Med School:** Columbia P&S 1980; **Resid:** Pediatrics, NY-Presby/Columbia Univ Med Ctr 1983; **Fellow:** Allergy & Immunology, LI Jewish Med Ctr 1990; **Fac Appt:** Asst Clin Prof Ped, Columbia P&S

Perin, Patrick MD (A&I) - **Spec Exp:** Allergy; Asthma; Pediatric Allergy & Immunology; **Hospital:** Holy Name Med Ctr (page 720), St. Joseph's Regl Med Ctr - Paterson; **Address:** Advanced Asthma Allergy Care, 185 Cedar Ln, Ste L2, Teaneck, NJ 07666; **Phone:** 201-836-6400; **Board Cert:** Allergy & Immunology 2003; **Med School:** UC Davis 1987; **Resid:** Pediatrics, Univ Hosp-UMDNJ 1990; **Fellow:** Allergy & Immunology, Thomas Jefferson Univ Hosp 1992

Cardiac Electrophysiology

Mittal, Suneet MD (CE) - **Spec Exp:** Arrhythmias; **Hospital:** Valley Hosp (page 721); **Address:** 223 N Van Dien Ave, Ridgewood, NJ 07450; **Phone:** 201-432-7837; **Board Cert:** Internal Medicine 2004; Cardiovascular Disease 2007; Cardiac Electrophysiology 2008; **Med School:** Boston Univ 1991; **Resid:** Internal Medicine, Hosp U Penn 1994; **Fellow:** Cardiovascular Disease, Hosp U Penn 1996; Cardiac Electrophysiology, Hosp U Penn 1998

Preminger, Mark W MD (CE) - **Spec Exp:** Arrhythmias; Pacemakers/Defibrillators; **Hospital:** Valley Hosp (page 721), St. Luke's - Roosevelt Hosp Ctr - St Luke's Hosp (page 94); **Address:** Valley Hosp, Arrhythmia Dept, 223 N Van Dien Ave, Ridgewood, NJ 07450; **Phone:** 201-432-7837; **Board Cert:** Internal Medicine 1989; Cardiovascular Disease 2011; Cardiac Electrophysiology 2012; **Med School:** Hahnemann Univ 1985; **Resid:** Internal Medicine, N Shore Univ Hosp 1988; **Fellow:** Cardiovascular Disease, NY-Presby/Weill Cornell Med Ctr 1991; Cardiac Electrophysiology, Phildelphia Heart Inst 1992; **Fac Appt:** Assoc Prof Med, Columbia P&S

Simons, Grant R MD (CE) - **Spec Exp:** Arrhythmias; **Hospital:** Englewood Hosp & Med Ctr, Hackensack Univ Med Ctr (page 718); **Address:** Englewood Hosp Arrhythmia Ctr, 350 Engle St, Englewood, NJ 07631; **Phone:** 201-894-3533; **Board Cert:** Cardiovascular Disease 2007; Cardiac Electrophysiology 2008; **Med School:** Duke Univ 1990; **Resid:** Internal Medicine, Brigham & Women's Hosp 1993; **Fellow:** Cardiovascular Disease, Duke Univ Med Ctr 1995; Cardiac Electrophysiology, Duke Univ Med Ctr 1997; **Fac Appt:** Assoc Clin Prof Med, Mount Sinai Sch Med

Cardiovascular Disease

Adibi, Baback MD (Cv) - **Spec Exp:** Cardiac CT Angiography; Coronary Angioplasty/Stents; Cardiac Catheterization; **Hospital:** Hackensack Univ Med Ctr (page 718); **Address:** Bergen Cardiology Assocs, 400 Frank W Burr Blvd, Ste 22, Teaneck, NJ 07666; **Phone:** 201-907-0442; **Board Cert:** Cardiovascular Disease 2005; **Med School:** Univ Pittsburgh 1999; **Resid:** Internal Medicine, Thomas Jefferson Univ Hosp 2002; **Fellow:** Cardiovascular Disease, Thomas Jefferson Univ Hosp 2005

Berkowitz, Walter D MD (Cv) - **Spec Exp:** Arrhythmias; Coronary Artery Disease; Hypertension; **Hospital:** Englewood Hosp & Med Ctr, Hackensack Univ Med Ctr (page 718); **Address:** 2200 Fletcher Ave, Fort Lee, NJ 07024-5005; **Phone:** 201-461-6200; **Board Cert:** Internal Medicine 1969; Cardiovascular Disease 1972; **Med School:** SUNY Downstate 1962; **Resid:** Internal Medicine, Maimonides Hosp 1964; Internal Medicine, Mt Sinai Hosp 1965; **Fellow:** Cardiovascular Disease, Montefiore Med Ctr 1967

Conroy Jr, Daniel P MD (Cv) - **Spec Exp:** Non-Invasive Cardiology; Hypertension; Cholesterol/Lipid Disorders; Diabetes & Heart Disease; **Hospital:** St. Mary's Hosp - Passaic, Hackensack Univ Med Ctr (page 718); **Address:** 358 Valley Brook Ave, Lyndhurst, NJ 07071; **Phone:** 201-460-0142; **Board Cert:** Internal Medicine 1979; Cardiovascular Disease 1981; **Med School:** Mexico 1975; **Resid:** Internal Medicine, St Michaels Med Ctr 1978; **Fellow:** Cardiovascular Disease, St Michaels Med Ctr 1980

Eichman, Gerard MD (Cv) - **Spec Exp:** Coronary Angioplasty/Stents; Cardiac Catheterization; Heart Valve Disease; **Hospital:** Holy Name Med Ctr (page 720), Hackensack Univ Med Ctr (page 718); **Address:** Cardiovascular Assocs, 954 Teaneck Rd, Teaneck, NJ 07666; **Phone:** 201-833-2300; **Board Cert:** Cardiovascular Disease 2005; **Med School:** Dominica 1988; **Resid:** Internal Medicine, Monmouth Med Ctr 1991; **Fellow:** Cardiovascular Disease, Seton Hall Affil Hosp 1992

Eisenberg, Sheldon B MD (Cv) - **Spec Exp:** Nuclear Cardiology; Preventive Cardiology; Coronary Artery Disease; **Hospital:** Valley Hosp (page 721), Hackensack Univ Med Ctr (page 718); **Address:** 333 Old Hook Rd, Ste 200, Westwood, NJ 07675-3200; **Phone:** 201-664-0201; **Board Cert:** Internal Medicine 1979; Cardiovascular Disease 1981; **Med School:** Cornell Univ-Weill Med Coll 1976; **Resid:** Internal Medicine, N Shore Univ Hosp 1979; **Fellow:** Cardiovascular Disease, N Shore Univ Hosp 1981

Erlebacher, Jay A MD (Cv) - **Spec Exp:** Pacemakers; Congestive Heart Failure; Cardiac Stress Testing; Echocardiography; **Hospital:** Englewood Hosp & Med Ctr; **Address:** Englewood Cardiology Consultants, 177 N Dean St, Englewood, NJ 07631; **Phone:** 201-569-4901; **Board Cert:** Internal Medicine 1978; Cardiovascular Disease 1981; **Med School:** SUNY Upstate Med Univ 1975; **Resid:** Internal Medicine, Jacobi Med Ctr 1978; **Fellow:** Cardiovascular Disease, Johns Hopkins Hosp 1980; **Fac Appt:** Asst Clin Prof Med, Cornell Univ-Weill Med Coll

Gardin, Julius M MD (Cv) - **Spec Exp:** Echocardiography; Geriatric Cardiology; Preventive Cardiology; Cholesterol/Lipid Disorders; **Hospital:** Hackensack Univ Med Ctr (page 718); **Address:** Hackensack Univ Med Ctr, Dept Medicine, 30 Prospect Ave, 1 Main, Ste 1647, Hackensack, NJ 07601; **Phone:** 551-996-3500; **Board Cert:** Internal Medicine 1975; Cardiovascular Disease 1977; **Med School:** Univ Mich Med Sch 1972; **Resid:** Internal Medicine, Univ Mich Hosp 1975; **Fellow:** Cardiovascular Disease, Georgetown Univ Hosp 1977; **Fac Appt:** Prof Med, UMDNJ-Univ Med Dent NJ

Goldschmidt, Howard Z MD (Cv) - **Spec Exp:** Heart Valve Disease; Pacemakers; Cardiomyopathy; Atrial Fibrillation; **Hospital:** Valley Hosp (page 721); **Address:** 1200 E Ridgewood Ave, Ridgewood, NJ 07450; **Phone:** 201-670-8660; **Board Cert:** Internal Medicine 1986; Cardiovascular Disease 1989; **Med School:** Columbia P&S 1983; **Resid:** Internal Medicine, Mt Sinai Hosp 1986; **Fellow:** Cardiovascular Disease, Mt Sinai Hosp 1988

Goldweit, Richard S MD (Cv) - **Spec Exp:** Interventional Cardiology; Sleep Disorders/Cardiac Risk; Peripheral Vascular Disease; Cardiac Catheterization; **Hospital:** Englewood Hosp & Med Ctr; **Address:** Englewood Cardiology Consultants, 177 N Dean St, Englewood, NJ 07631; **Phone:** 201-569-4901; **Board Cert:** Internal Medicine 1985; Cardiovascular Disease 1987; Interventional Cardiology 2009; **Med School:** Cornell Univ-Weill Med Coll 1982; **Resid:** Internal Medicine, NY-Presby/Weill Cornell Med Ctr 1985; **Fellow:** Cardiovascular Disease, NY-Presby/Weill Cornell Med Ctr 1987

Hodges, David MD (Cv) - **Spec Exp:** Stress Management; **Hospital:** Englewood Hosp & Med Ctr; **Address:** 200 Grand Ave, Ste 202, Engelwood, NJ 07631; **Phone:** 201-816-9266; **Board Cert:** Internal Medicine 1987; Cardiovascular Disease 2003; **Med School:** NYU Sch Med 1984; **Resid:** Internal Medicine, Boston Med Ctr 1987; Internal Medicine, Beth Israel Deaconess Med Ctr 1989; **Fellow:** Cardiovascular Disease, Brigham & Womens Hosp 1991; **Fac Appt:** Asst Prof Med, Columbia P&S

Jacowitz, Joel MD (Cv) - **Spec Exp:** Echocardiography; Interventional Cardiology; **Hospital:** Valley Hosp (page 721); **Address:** Old Hook Med Assocs, 452 Old Hook Rd, Emerson, NJ 07630; **Phone:** 201-666-3900 x201; **Board Cert:** Internal Medicine 1981; Cardiovascular Disease 1985; Echocardiography 2013; **Med School:** SUNY Downstate 1977; **Resid:** Internal Medicine, Metropolitan Hosp 1980; Internal Medicine, Harlem Hosp 1982; **Fellow:** Cardiovascular Disease, Harlem Hosp 1985; Interventional Cardiology, Dartmouth-Hitchcock Med Ctr 1993; **Fac Appt:** Assoc Clin Prof Med, Seton Hall Univ Sch Hlth & Med Scis

Landers, David B MD (Cv) - **Spec Exp:** Cardiac Catheterization; Coronary Angioplasty/Stents; Angioplasty; Interventional Cardiology; **Hospital:** Hackensack Univ Med Ctr (page 718), Holy Name Med Ctr (page 720); **Address:** 400 Frank Burr Blvd, Teaneck, NJ 07666; **Phone:** 201-928-2300; **Board Cert:** Internal Medicine 1983; Cardiovascular Disease 1987; Interventional Cardiology 2010; **Med School:** Georgetown Univ 1979; **Resid:** Internal Medicine, St Vincents Hosp 1982; **Fellow:** Cardiovascular Disease, Westchester Co Med Ctr 1985; **Fac Appt:** Asst Clin Prof Med, UMDNJ-NJ Med Sch, Newark

Landzberg, Joel S MD (Cv) - **Spec Exp:** Preventive Cardiology; Coronary Artery Disease; Heart Failure; Heart Valve Disease; **Hospital:** Hackensack Univ Med Ctr (page 718), Valley Hosp (page 721); **Address:** Westwood Cardiology Associates, 333 Old Hook Rd, Ste 200, Westwood, NJ 07675-3200; **Phone:** 201-664-0201; **Board Cert:** Internal Medicine 1986; Cardiovascular Disease 1989; Interventional Cardiology 2012; **Med School:** Columbia P&S 1983; **Resid:** Internal Medicine, Vanderbilt Univ Hosp 1986; **Fellow:** Cardiology Research, Moffit Hosp 1987; Cardiovascular Disease, Brigham & Womens Hosp 1991; **Fac Appt:** Assoc Clin Prof Med, UMDNJ-NJ Med Sch, Newark

Lichtstein, Elliott S MD (Cv) - **Spec Exp:** Heart Attack; Congestive Heart Failure; Heart Valve Disease; Heart Failure; **Hospital:** Hackensack Univ Med Ctr (page 718), Valley Hosp (page 721); **Address:** Westwood Cardiology, 333 Old Hook Rd, Ste 200, Westwood, NJ 07675; **Phone:** 201-664-0201; **Board Cert:** Internal Medicine 1984; Cardiovascular Disease 1987; **Med School:** Temple Univ 1981; **Resid:** Internal Medicine, Albany Med Ctr Hosp 1984; **Fellow:** Cardiovascular Disease, LI Jewish Med Ctr 1986

Pumill, Rick MD (Cv) - **Spec Exp:** Coronary Artery Disease; Hypertension; Congestive Heart Failure; **Hospital:** Hackensack Univ Med Ctr (page 718); **Address:** Cross County Cardiology, 103 River Rd Fl 2, Edgewater, NJ 07020; **Phone:** 201-941-8100; **Board Cert:** Internal Medicine 1988; Cardiovascular Disease 2013; **Med School:** Dominica 1984; **Resid:** Internal Medicine, Jersey City Med Ctr 1988; **Fellow:** Cardiovascular Disease, Jersey City Med Ctr 1990

Reison, Dennis S MD (Cv) - **Spec Exp:** Interventional Cardiology; **Hospital:** Valley Hosp (page 721); **Address:** Valley Heart Grp, 1200 E Ridgewood Ave Fl 2, Ridgewood, NJ 07450; **Phone:** 201-670-8660; **Board Cert:** Internal Medicine 1978; Cardiovascular Disease 1981; **Med School:** Stanford Univ 1975; **Resid:** Internal Medicine, NY-Presby/Columbia Univ Med Ctr 1978; **Fellow:** Cardiovascular Disease, Mount Sinai Med Ctr 1979; Cardiovascular Disease, NY-Presby/Columbia Univ Med Ctr 1981; **Fac Appt:** Asst Clin Prof Med, Columbia P&S

Rossakis, Constantine MD (Cv) - **Spec Exp:** Interventional Cardiology; Nuclear Cardiology; **Hospital:** Hackensack Univ Med Ctr (page 718); **Address:** 357 Prospect Ave, Hackensack, NJ 07601; **Phone:** 201-489-3440; **Board Cert:** Internal Medicine 1986; Cardiovascular Disease 1989; Nuclear Cardiology 2009; **Med School:** NYU Sch Med 1983; **Resid:** Internal Medicine, NY-Presby/Weill Cornell Med Ctr 1986; **Fellow:** Cardiovascular Disease, NY-Presby/Weill Cornell Med Ctr 1989; **Fac Appt:** Asst Clin Prof Med, Cornell Univ-Weill Med Coll

Rothman, Howard C MD (Cv) - **Spec Exp:** Cholesterol/Lipid Disorders; Angina; Women's Health; Preventive Medicine; **Hospital:** Hackensack Univ Med Ctr (page 718), Englewood Hosp & Med Ctr; **Address:** Advanced Cardiology Inst, 2200 Fletcher Ave, Fort Lee, NJ 07024-5005; **Phone:** 201-461-6200; **Board Cert:** Internal Medicine 1975; Cardiovascular Disease 1979; **Med School:** Univ Cincinnati 1970; **Resid:** Internal Medicine, NY Hosp-Cornell Med Ctr 1975; **Fellow:** Cardiovascular Disease, NY Hosp-Cornell Med Ctr 1976; **Fac Appt:** Asst Clin Prof Med, Mount Sinai Sch Med

Salerno, William D MD (Cv) - **Spec Exp:** Vein Disorders; Echocardiography; Critical Care Medicine; **Hospital:** Hackensack Univ Med Ctr (page 718); **Address:** Heartcare Ctr, 38 Mayhill St, Saddle Brook, NJ 07663; **Phone:** 201-843-1019; **Board Cert:** Internal Medicine 1987; Cardiovascular Disease 1989; Critical Care Medicine 2011; **Med School:** Mexico 1982; **Resid:** Internal Medicine, Hackensack Univ Med Ctr 1986; Critical Care Medicine, Norwalk Hosp 1987; **Fellow:** Cardiovascular Disease, Hackensack Univ Med Ctr 1989; Interventional Cardiology, Hackensack Univ Med Ctr 1990; **Fac Appt:** Assoc Clin Prof Med, UMDNJ-Rutgers Med Sch

Sotsky, Gerald MD (Cv) - **Spec Exp:** Critical Care Medicine; **Hospital:** Valley Hosp (page 721); **Address:** Valley Heart Grp, 1200 E Ridgewood Ave Fl 2, Ridgewood, NJ 07450; **Phone:** 201-670-8660; **Board Cert:** Internal Medicine 1984; Cardiovascular Disease 1987; **Med School:** Mount Sinai Sch Med 1981; **Resid:** Internal Medicine, Mount Sinai Med Ctr 1984; **Fellow:** Cardiovascular Disease, Mount Sinai Med Ctr 1986

Teichholz, Louis E MD (Cv) - **Spec Exp:** Mitral Valve Disease; Complementary Medicine; Echocardiography; Cholesterol/Lipid Disorders; **Hospital:** Hackensack Univ Med Ctr (page 718); **Address:** Hackensack Univ Med Ctr, Cardiology, 30 Prospect Ave, 4-Main, rm 4655, Hackensack, NJ 07601; **Phone:** 201-996-2314; **Board Cert:** Internal Medicine 1972; Cardiovascular Disease 1975; **Med School:** Harvard Med Sch 1966; **Resid:** Internal Medicine, Brigham & Womens Hosp 1968; **Fellow:** Cardiovascular Disease, Brigham & Womens Hosp 1972; **Fac Appt:** Prof Med, UMDNJ-NJ Med Sch, Newark

Wild, David MD (Cv) - **Hospital:** Holy Name Med Ctr (page 720), Hackensack Univ Med Ctr (page 718); **Address:** Cardiovascular Assocs, 954 Teaneck Rd, Teaneck, NJ 07666; **Phone:** 201-833-2300; **Board Cert:** Cardiovascular Disease 2008; Internal Medicine 2005; **Med School:** UMDNJ-RW Johnson Med Sch 2002; **Resid:** Internal Medicine, Montefiore Med Ctr 2005; **Fellow:** Cardiovascular Disease, St Lukes-Roosevelt Hosp Ctr 2008

Williams, Marcus L MD (Cv) - **Spec Exp:** Cholesterol/Lipid Disorders; Hypertension; Atrial Fibrillation; Coronary Artery Disease; **Hospital:** Chilton Hosp, Valley Hosp (page 721); **Address:** Cardiac Assocs N Jersey, 43 Yawpo Ave, Ste 2, Oakland, NJ 07436; **Phone:** 201-337-0066; **Board Cert:** Internal Medicine 1985; Cardiovascular Disease 1989; **Med School:** Geo Wash Univ 1982; **Resid:** Internal Medicine, NC Meml Hosp 1985; **Fellow:** Cardiovascular Disease, NC Meml Hosp 1988

Child & Adolescent Psychiatry

Kotler, Lisa A MD (ChAP) - **Spec Exp:** Eating Disorders; ADD/ADHD; Depression; Anxiety Disorders; **Hospital:** NYU Langone Med Ctr (page 108); **Address:** NYU Child Study Ctr-Hackensack, 411 Hackensack Ave Fl 7, Hackensack, NJ 07601; **Phone:** 201-465-8111; **Board Cert:** Psychiatry 2008; Child & Adolescent Psychiatry 2009; **Med School:** Yale Univ 1993; **Resid:** Psychiatry, Mt Sinai Med Ctr 1996; **Fellow:** Child & Adolescent Psychiatry, Columbia-Presby Med Ctr 1998; Eating Disorders Research, NY State Psyc Inst-Columbia Presby MC 1999; **Fac Appt:** Asst Clin Prof Psyc, NYU Sch Med

Pincus, Emile I MD (ChAP) - **Spec Exp:** Substance Abuse; Suicide; **Address:** 912 Kinderkamack Rd Fl 2, River Edge, NJ 07661; **Phone:** 201-615-1352; **Board Cert:** Psychiatry 1986; Child & Adolescent Psychiatry 2004; **Med School:** Mount Sinai Sch Med 1978; **Resid:** Psychiatry, St Lukes Hosp Ctr 1979; Psychiatry, Mt Sinai Med Ctr 1982; **Fellow:** Child & Adolescent Psychiatry, New York Hosp-Cornell Med Ctr 1984

Colon & Rectal Surgery

Gallina, Gregory J MD (CRS) - **Spec Exp:** Minimally Invasive Surgery; Colon & Rectal Cancer; Colon Cancer Screening; **Hospital:** Hackensack Univ Med Ctr (page 718), St. Joseph's Regl Med Ctr - Paterson; **Address:** 255 W Spring Valley Ave, Ste 103, Maywood, NJ 07607; **Phone:** 201-525-1031; **Board Cert:** Colon & Rectal Surgery 2011; Colon & Rectal Surgery ; **Med School:** Geo Wash Univ 1992; **Resid:** Surgery, Univ Hosp-UMDNJ 1997; **Fellow:** Colon & Rectal Surgery, SUNY Buffalo Affil Hosp 1998

Helbraun, Mark E MD (CRS) - **Spec Exp:** Colon & Rectal Cancer; **Hospital:** Hackensack Univ Med Ctr (page 718); **Address:** 20 Prospect Ave, Ste 811, Hackensack, NJ 07601; **Phone:** 201-525-1660; **Board Cert:** Colon & Rectal Surgery 1978; **Med School:** Wayne State Univ 1972; **Resid:** Surgery, New York Hosp-Cornell 1977; **Fellow:** Colon & Rectal Surgery, Lahey Clin 1978

Nizin, Joel S MD (CRS) - **Spec Exp:** Colon Cancer; Inflammatory Bowel Disease; **Hospital:** Valley Hosp (page 721), Chilton Hosp; **Address:** 140 Chestnut St, Ste 301, Ridgewood, NJ 07450; **Phone:** 201-689-9100; **Board Cert:** Colon & Rectal Surgery 1987; Surgery 2008; **Med School:** Howard Univ 1978; **Resid:** Surgery, St Luke's Hosp 1983; **Fellow:** Colon & Rectal Surgery, Univ Minn Med Ctr 1984

Waxenbaum, Steven I MD (CRS) - **Spec Exp:** Laparoscopic Surgery; Hemorrhoids; Colon Cancer; **Hospital:** Valley Hosp (page 721), Englewood Hosp & Med Ctr; **Address:** 216 Engle St, Englewood, NJ 07631; **Phone:** 201-567-7615; **Board Cert:** Surgery 2003; Colon & Rectal Surgery 2006; **Med School:** UMDNJ-RW Johnson Med Sch 1988; **Resid:** Surgery, Westchester Med Ctr 1993; **Fellow:** Colon & Rectal Surgery, Lehigh Valley Hosp 1994

White, Ronald A MD (CRS) - **Spec Exp:** Hemorrhoids; Colon & Rectal Cancer; Colonoscopy; **Hospital:** Englewood Hosp & Med Ctr, Valley Hosp (page 721); **Address:** 216 Engle St, Ste 203, Englewood, NJ 07631-2428; **Phone:** 201-567-7615; **Board Cert:** Colon & Rectal Surgery 1988; **Med School:** Boston Univ 1981; **Resid:** Surgery, Montefiore Hosp 1986; **Fellow:** Colon & Rectal Surgery, RW Johnson Med Sch 1987

Critical Care Medicine

Cornell, James S MD/PhD (CCM) - **Spec Exp:** Respiratory Distress Syndrome; Lung Cancer; Chronic Obstructive Lung Disease (COPD); **Hospital:** Valley Hosp (page 721); **Address:** 3100 Broadway Fl 2, Fair Lawn, NJ 07410-2305; **Phone:** 201-796-2255; **Med School:** Cornell Univ-Weill Med Coll 1988; **Resid:** Internal Medicine, New York Hosp-Cornell 1991; Pulmonary Disease, Meml Sloan Kettering Cancer Ctr 1991; **Fellow:** Pulmonary Critical Care Medicine, New York Hosp-Cornell 1994

Dermatology

Andrews, Alan D MD (D) - **Spec Exp:** Skin Cancer; Phototherapy; **Hospital:** NY-Presby/Columbia Univ Med Ctr, NY (page 104), Holy Name Med Ctr (page 720); **Address:** 500 Piermont Rd, Ste 101, Closter, NJ 07624; **Phone:** 201-767-0501; **Board Cert:** Dermatology 1979; **Med School:** Univ VA Sch Med 1972; **Resid:** Dermatology, NCI Affil Hosp 1975; **Fellow:** Dermatology, Columbia P&S 1979

Ashinoff, Robin MD (D) - **Spec Exp:** Mohs' Surgery; Laser Surgery; Cosmetic Dermatology; Melanoma; **Hospital:** Hackensack Univ Med Ctr (page 718), NYU Langone Med Ctr (page 108); **Address:** 360 Essex St, Ste 201, Hackensack, NJ 07601; **Phone:** 201-336-8660; **Board Cert:** Dermatology 2009; **Med School:** NYU Sch Med 1985; **Resid:** Dermatology, NYU Med Ctr 1989; **Fellow:** Mohs Surgery, NYU Med Ctr 1991; Laser Surgery, NYU Med Ctr 1991; **Fac Appt:** Assoc Clin Prof D, NYU Sch Med

Brauner, Gary J MD (D) - **Spec Exp:** Skin Laser Surgery; Black/Asian Skin Care; Cosmetic Dermatology; Hair Removal-Laser; **Hospital:** Englewood Hosp & Med Ctr, Mt Sinai Med Ctr (page 102); **Address:** 1625 Anderson Ave, Ste 201, Fort Lee, NJ 07024; **Phone:** 201-461-5522; **Board Cert:** Dermatology 1972; Dermatopathology 1978; **Med School:** Harvard Med Sch 1967; **Resid:** Dermatology, Jewish Hosp 1968; Dermatology, Mass Genl Hosp 1971; **Fac Appt:** Assoc Clin Prof D, Mount Sinai Sch Med

Corey, Timothy J MD (D) - **Spec Exp:** Psoriasis; Skin Cancer; **Hospital:** Valley Hosp (page 721), NY-Presby/Columbia Univ Med Ctr, NY (page 104); **Address:** 400 Rt 17 S, Ridgewood, NJ 07450; **Phone:** 201-652-4536; **Board Cert:** Dermatology 1979; **Med School:** Columbia P&S 1975; **Resid:** Dermatology, Columbia Presby Med Ctr 1979; **Fac Appt:** Asst Clin Prof D, Columbia P&S

Fishman, Miriam MD (D) - **Spec Exp:** Pediatric Dermatology; Skin Cancer; **Hospital:** Englewood Hosp & Med Ctr; **Address:** 216 Engle St, Ste 104, Englewood, NJ 07631-2428; **Phone:** 201-569-5678; **Board Cert:** Dermatology 2009; **Med School:** NYU Sch Med 1978; **Resid:** Pediatrics, Montefiore Med Ctr 1981; Dermatology, Montefiore Med Ctr 1984

Fried, Sharon Z MD (D) - **Spec Exp:** Skin Cancer; Acne; Psoriasis; **Hospital:** Englewood Hosp & Med Ctr; **Address:** 180 N Dean St, Ste 2 South, Englewood, NJ 07631-2534; **Phone:** 201-569-9800; **Board Cert:** Internal Medicine 1983; Dermatology 2009; **Med School:** NYU Sch Med 1980; **Resid:** Internal Medicine, NYU Med Ctr 1983; Dermatology, SUNY Downstate HSC 1985

Giardina-Beckett, MarieAnn MD (D) - **Spec Exp:** Acne; Botox Therapy; **Hospital:** Meadowlands Hosp Med Ctr, St. Mary's Hosp - Passaic; **Address:** 71 Union Ave, Ste 108, Rutherford, NJ 07070; **Phone:** 201-804-8900; **Board Cert:** Dermatology 2009; **Med School:** NY Med Coll 1986; **Resid:** Dermatology, New York Med Coll 1990

Grodberg, Michele MD (D) - **Spec Exp:** Cosmetic Dermatology; Hair Removal-Laser; Botox Therapy; Facial Rejuvenation; **Hospital:** Englewood Hosp & Med Ctr; **Address:** 106 Grand Ave Fl 3, Englewood, NJ 07631-3574; **Phone:** 201-567-8884; **Board Cert:** Dermatology 2009; **Med School:** NYU Sch Med 1987; **Resid:** Dermatology, NYU Med Ctr 1991

Heldman, Jay MD (D) - **Spec Exp:** Dermatologic Surgery; **Hospital:** Valley Hosp (page 721); **Address:** 23-00 Route 208 S, Fair Lawn, NJ 07410-1559; **Phone:** 201-797-7770; **Board Cert:** Dermatology 1981; **Med School:** Columbia P&S 1977; **Resid:** Dermatology, Mount Sinai Hosp 1981

Morman, Manuel R MD/PhD (D) - **Spec Exp:** Mohs' Surgery; Skin Cancer; Reconstructive Surgery; **Hospital:** St. Mary's Hosp - Passaic; **Address:** 47 Orient Way, Rutherford, NJ 07070-2040; **Phone:** 201-460-0280; **Board Cert:** Dermatology 2009; **Med School:** Jefferson Med Coll 1976; **Resid:** Dermatology, Hosp Univ Penn 1979; **Fellow:** Chemosurgery, Cleveland Clinic 1980

Possick, Paul MD (D) - **Spec Exp:** Skin Cancer; Contact Dermatitis; Eczema; Psoriasis; **Hospital:** NYU Langone Med Ctr (page 108); **Address:** 390 Old Hook Rd Fl 2, Westwood, NJ 07675-2616; **Phone:** 201-666-9550; **Board Cert:** Dermatology 2009; **Med School:** Tufts Univ 1964; **Resid:** Internal Medicine, Montefiore Hosp 1966; Dermatology, Univ Hosp 1968; **Fac Appt:** Asst Prof D, NYU Sch Med

Rapaport, Jeffrey A MD (D) - **Spec Exp:** Cosmetic Dermatology; Scar Revision; Laser Surgery; Skin Laser Surgery; **Hospital:** Holy Name Med Ctr (page 720), Englewood Hosp & Med Ctr; **Address:** 333 Sylvan Ave Fl 2 - Ste 207, Englewood Cliffs, NJ 07632; **Phone:** 201-227-1555; **Board Cert:** Dermatology 1983; **Med School:** Emory Univ 1978; **Resid:** Dermatology, Jefferson Univ Hosp 1982

Scherl, Sharon MD (D) - **Spec Exp:** Acne; Cosmetic Dermatology; Photodynamic Therapy; Tattoo Removal; **Hospital:** Englewood Hosp & Med Ctr; **Address:** 45 Central Ave, Tenafly, NJ 07670; **Phone:** 201-568-8400; **Board Cert:** Dermatology 2010; **Med School:** NY Med Coll 1988; **Resid:** Dermatology, Metropolitian Hosp Ctr 1992

Shin, Helen T MD (D) - **Spec Exp:** Pediatric Dermatology; **Hospital:** Hackensack Univ Med Ctr (page 718); **Address:** 155 Polifly Rd, Ste 101, Hackensack, NJ 07601; **Phone:** 551-996-8697; **Board Cert:** Dermatology 2008; Pediatric Dermatology ; **Med School:** Cornell Univ-Weill Med Coll 1995; **Resid:** Pediatric Surgery, Mt Sinai Med Ctr 1997; Dermatology, NY Presby Hosp/Cornell 2000; **Fellow:** Pediatric Dermatology, NYU Med Ctr 2001

Sweeney, Eugene W MD (D) - **Spec Exp:** Skin Cancer; Pediatric Dermatology; Acne; **Hospital:** Holy Name Med Ctr (page 720), Englewood Hosp & Med Ctr; **Address:** 757 N Teaneck Rd, Teaneck, NJ 07666-4241; **Phone:** 201-837-3939; **Board Cert:** Dermatology 1967; **Med School:** NY Med Coll 1960; **Resid:** Dermatology, Columbia-Presby Med Ctr 1966; **Fac Appt:** Assoc Clin Prof D, Columbia P&S

Weiss, Darryl S MD (D) - **Spec Exp:** Hair Restoration/Transplant; Cosmetic Dermatology; Skin Laser Surgery; **Hospital:** Valley Hosp (page 721); **Address:** 23-00 Route 208 S, Fairlawn, NJ 07410; **Phone:** 201-797-7770; **Board Cert:** Dermatology 1990; **Med School:** Med Coll VA 1986; **Resid:** Dermatology, Jackson Meml Hosp 1990

Diagnostic Radiology

Budin, Joel A MD (DR) - **Spec Exp:** Neuroradiology; **Hospital:** Hackensack Univ Med Ctr (page 718); **Address:** 30 S Newman St, Hackensack, NJ 07601; **Phone:** 201-488-1188; **Board Cert:** Diagnostic Radiology 1975; **Med School:** Columbia P&S 1969; **Resid:** Diagnostic Radiology, Columbia-Presby Med Ctr 1975

Calem-Grunat, Jaclyn A MD (DR) - **Spec Exp:** Breast Imaging; Ultrasound; **Hospital:** Valley Hosp (page 721); **Address:** Radiology Assocs of Ridgewood, 20 Franklin Tpke, Waldwick, NJ 07463; **Phone:** 201-445-8822; **Board Cert:** Diagnostic Radiology 1994; **Med School:** Mount Sinai Sch Med 1988; **Resid:** Internal Medicine, Beeth Israel Med Ctr 1990; Diagnostic Radiology, Harbor-UCLA Med Ctr 1994; **Fellow:** Breast Imaging, UCLA Med Ctr 1995

Goldfischer, Mindy A MD (DR) - **Spec Exp:** Breast Imaging; Ultrasound; **Hospital:** Englewood Hosp & Med Ctr; **Address:** 350 Engle St, Englewood, NJ 07631; **Phone:** 201-894-3480; **Board Cert:** Diagnostic Radiology 1986; **Med School:** NYU Sch Med 1982; **Resid:** Diagnostic Radiology, Montefiore Med Ctr 1986; **Fellow:** Diagnostic Radiology, Thomas Jefferson Univ Hosp 1987

Gross, Joshua David MD (DR) - **Spec Exp:** Breast Imaging; Breast Cancer; **Hospital:** Holy Name Med Ctr (page 720); **Address:** Holy Name Hosp, Breast Imaging, 718 Teaneck Rd, Teaneck, NJ 07666; **Phone:** 201-833-7100; **Board Cert:** Diagnostic Radiology 1984; **Med School:** Albert Einstein Coll Med 1980; **Resid:** Diagnostic Radiology, Einstein/Jacobi Hosp 1984

Krinsky, Glenn MD (DR) - **Spec Exp:** MRI; Musculoskeletal Imaging; Gastrointestinal Imaging; **Hospital:** Valley Hosp (page 721); **Address:** Radiology Assocs of Ridgewood, 20 Franklin Tpke, Waldwick, NJ 07463; **Phone:** 201-445-8822; **Board Cert:** Diagnostic Radiology 1994; **Med School:** NYU Sch Med 1988; **Resid:** Surgical Pathology, Bellevue Hosp 1990; Diagnostic Radiology, Bellevue Hosp 1993; **Fellow:** Magnetic Resonance Imaging, NYU/Bellevue Hosp 1994

Levy, Lauren S MD (DR) - **Spec Exp:** Mammography; Breast MRI; Breast Imaging; **Hospital:** Valley Hosp (page 721); **Address:** Radiology Assocs of Ridgewood, 20 Franklin Tpke, Waldwick, NJ 07463; **Phone:** 201-445-8822; **Board Cert:** Diagnostic Radiology 1996; **Med School:** SUNY Downstate 1991; **Resid:** Diagnostic Radiology, NYU-Bellevue Hosp 1996; **Fellow:** Mammography, NYU-Bellevue Hosp 1997

Liebling, Melissa Schubach MD (DR) - **Spec Exp:** Pediatric Radiology; **Hospital:** Hackensack Univ Med Ctr (page 718); **Address:** Hackensack Univ Med Ctr, Dept Radiology, 30 Prospect Ave, Hackensack, NJ 07601; **Phone:** 201-996-2200; **Board Cert:** Diagnostic Radiology 1992; Pediatric Radiology 2006; **Med School:** Albany Med Coll 1987; **Resid:** Diagnostic Radiology, Columbia-Presby Med Ctr 1992; **Fellow:** Pediatric Radiology, Columbia-Presby/Babies Hosp 1994

Lubat, Edward MD (DR) - **Spec Exp:** Abdominal Imaging; Thoracic Radiology; Musculoskeletal Imaging; Nuclear Medicine; **Hospital:** Valley Hosp (page 721); **Address:** Radiology Assocs, 20 Franklin Tpke, Waldwick, NJ 07463-1749; **Phone:** 201-445-8822; **Board Cert:** Diagnostic Radiology 1989; Nuclear Medicine 1989; **Med School:** Jefferson Med Coll 1982; **Resid:** Diagnostic Radiology, NYU Med Ctr 1988; **Fellow:** Nuclear Medicine, NYU Med Ctr 1985

Panush, David MD (DR) - **Spec Exp:** Neuroradiology; **Hospital:** Hackensack Univ Med Ctr (page 718); **Address:** Hackensack Radiology Group, 30 Prospect Ave, Hackensack, NJ 07601; **Phone:** 201-996-2254; **Board Cert:** Diagnostic Radiology 1990; **Med School:** Albert Einstein Coll Med 1985; **Resid:** Radiology, Montefiore Med Ctr 1990; **Fellow:** Neuroradiology, Yale-New Haven Hosp 1991

Rakow, Joel Ivan MD (DR) - **Spec Exp:** Ultrasound; **Hospital:** Hackensack Univ Med Ctr (page 718); **Address:** Hackensack Univ Med Ctr, Dept Radiology, 30 Prospect Ave, Hackensack, NJ 07601; **Phone:** 551-996-5900; **Board Cert:** Diagnostic Radiology 1986; **Med School:** Albert Einstein Coll Med 1982; **Resid:** Diagnostic Radiology, Montefiore Med Ctr 1986; **Fellow:** Ultrasound, Thomas Jefferson Med Ctr 1987

Rambler, Louis MD (DR) - **Spec Exp:** Ultrasound; **Hospital:** Valley Hosp (page 721); **Address:** Radiology Assocs of Ridgewood, 20 Franklin Tpke, Waldwick, NJ 07463-1749; **Phone:** 201-445-8822; **Board Cert:** Diagnostic Radiology 1977; **Med School:** Cornell Univ-Weill Med Coll 1971; **Resid:** Diagnostic Radiology, Columbia-Presby Med Ctr 1977

Shapiro, Mark Linden MD (DR) - **Hospital:** Englewood Hosp & Med Ctr; **Address:** Englewood Hosp, Dept Radiology, 350 Engle St, Englewood, NJ 07631; **Phone:** 201-894-3480; **Board Cert:** Diagnostic Radiology 1993; **Med School:** SUNY Hlth Sci Ctr 1988; **Resid:** Diagnostic Radiology, North Shore Univ Hosp 1993; **Fellow:** Magnetic Resonance Imaging, Hosp U Penn 1994

Toth, Patrick J MD (DR) - **Spec Exp:** Abdominal Imaging; Thoracic Radiology; Interventional Radiology; Nuclear Radiology; **Hospital:** Hackensack Univ Med Ctr (page 718); **Address:** Hackensack Univ Med Ctr, Dept Radiology, 30 Prospect Ave, Hackensack, NJ 07601; **Phone:** 551-996-5900; **Board Cert:** Diagnostic Radiology 1988; **Med School:** Yale Univ 1982; **Resid:** Surgery, Yale-New Haven Hosp 1984; Diagnostic Radiology, NYU Med Ctr 1987; **Fellow:** Abdominal Imaging, NYU Med Ctr 1988; Interventional Radiology, NYU Med Ctr 1989; **Fac Appt:** Asst Clin Prof Rad, NYU Sch Med

Endocrinology, Diabetes & Metabolism

Cobin, Rhoda H MD (EDM) - **Spec Exp:** Thyroid Disorders; Diabetes; Pituitary Disorders; **Hospital:** Valley Hosp (page 721), Mt Sinai Med Ctr (page 102); **Address:** 75 N Maple Ave, Ste 202, Ridgewood, NJ 07450; **Phone:** 201-444-5552; **Board Cert:** Internal Medicine 1972; Endocrinology, Diabetes & Metabolism 1975; **Med School:** Univ Puerto Rico 1969; **Resid:** Internal Medicine, Beth Israel Med Ctr 1972; **Fellow:** Endocrinology, Diabetes & Metabolism, Mt Sinai Hosp 1974; **Fac Appt:** Clin Prof Med, Mount Sinai Sch Med

Daud-Ahmad, Sameera MD (EDM) - **Spec Exp:** Thyroid Disorders; Diabetes; Polycystic Ovarian Syndrome; **Hospital:** Hackensack Univ Med Ctr (page 718), Valley Hosp (page 721); **Address:** Old Hook Medical Assocs, 452 Old Hook Rd, Emerson, NJ 07630; **Phone:** 201-666-3900; **Board Cert:** Internal Medicine 2007; Endocrinology, Diabetes & Metabolism 2009; **Med School:** Pakistan 2002; **Resid:** Internal Medicine, Loma Linda Univ Med Ctr 2006; Internal Medicine, Overlook Hosp 2007; **Fellow:** Endocrinology, Cleveland Clin 2009

Goldman, Michael MD (EDM) - **Spec Exp:** Thyroid Disorders; Diabetes; Pituitary Disorders; Cholesterol/Lipid Disorders; **Hospital:** Englewood Hosp & Med Ctr; **Address:** 600 E Palisade Ave, Ste 1, Englewood Cliffs, NJ 07632-1826; **Phone:** 201-568-1108; **Board Cert:** Internal Medicine 1980; Endocrinology, Diabetes & Metabolism 1981; **Med School:** NY Med Coll 1973; **Resid:** Internal Medicine, Englewood Hosp 1978; **Fellow:** Endocrinology, Diabetes & Metabolism, Columbia-Presby Med Ctr 1980; **Fac Appt:** Asst Prof Med, Mount Sinai Sch Med

Hochstein, Martin A MD (EDM) - **Spec Exp:** Thyroid Disorders; Thyroid Cancer; Diabetes; Osteoporosis; **Hospital:** Valley Hosp (page 721); **Address:** 1 W Ridgewood Ave, Ste 301, Paramus, NJ 07652; **Phone:** 201-445-1660; **Board Cert:** Internal Medicine 1973; Endocrinology, Diabetes & Metabolism 1975; **Med School:** Univ Louisville Sch Med 1969; **Resid:** Internal Medicine, Maimoides Med Ctr 1971; Internal Medicine, Jacobi Med Ctr 1972; **Fellow:** Endocrinology, Diabetes & Metabolism, Johns Hopkins Med Ctr 1975; **Fac Appt:** Assoc Clin Prof Med, UMDNJ-RW Johnson Med Sch

Schwartz, Joseph J MD (EDM) - **Hospital:** Holy Name Med Ctr (page 720), Englewood Hosp & Med Ctr; **Address:** 229 Engle St, Englewood, NJ 07631; **Phone:** 201-567-3674; **Board Cert:** Internal Medicine 2011; Endocrinology, Diabetes & Metabolism 2003; **Med School:** Albert Einstein Coll Med 1998; **Resid:** Internal Medicine, LIJ Med Ctr 2001; **Fellow:** Endocrinology, Diabetes & Metabolism, Mt Sinai Med Ctr 2003

Tohme, Jack F MD (EDM) - **Spec Exp:** Osteoporosis; Thyroid Disorders; Diabetes; **Hospital:** Valley Hosp (page 721); **Address:** 265 Ackerman Ave, Ste 101, Ridgewood, NJ 07450-4203; **Phone:** 201-444-4363; **Board Cert:** Internal Medicine 1978; Endocrinology, Diabetes & Metabolism 1979; **Med School:** Amer Univ Beirut 1974; **Resid:** Internal Medicine, American Univ Hosp 1976; **Fellow:** Endocrinology, Diabetes & Metabolism, Columbia-Presby Med Ctr 1977; Endocrinology, Diabetes & Metabolism, Barnes Jewish Hosp 1978; **Fac Appt:** Assoc Clin Prof Med, Columbia P&S

Wehmann, Robert MD/PhD (EDM) - **Spec Exp:** Diabetes; Thyroid Disorders; Pituitary Disorders; **Hospital:** Valley Hosp (page 721), Hackensack Univ Med Ctr (page 718); **Address:** 54 Orchard St, Hillsdale, NJ 07642; **Phone:** 201-666-1400; **Board Cert:** Internal Medicine 1977; Endocrinology 1979; **Med School:** Albany Med Coll 1974; **Resid:** Internal Medicine, VA Med Ctr 1976; **Fellow:** Endocrinology, Natl Inst Hlth 1979

Wiesen, Mark MD (EDM) - **Spec Exp:** Diabetes; Thyroid Disorders; Osteoporosis; **Hospital:** Hackensack Univ Med Ctr (page 718), Holy Name Med Ctr (page 720); **Address:** 870 Palisade Ave, Ste 203, Teaneck, NJ 07666; **Phone:** 201-836-5655; **Board Cert:** Internal Medicine 1978; Endocrinology, Diabetes & Metabolism 1981; **Med School:** Columbia P&S 1975; **Resid:** Internal Medicine, Brookdale Hosp 1978; **Fellow:** Endocrinology, Diabetes & Metabolism, Mt Sinai Hosp 1981; **Fac Appt:** Asst Clin Prof Med, UMDNJ-NJ Med Sch, Newark

Family Medicine

Bello, Mary R MD (FMed) *PCP* - **Spec Exp:** Geriatric Care; **Hospital:** Valley Hosp (page 721); **Address:** 400 Franklin Tpke, Ste 106, Mahwah, NJ 07430-3517; **Phone:** 201-327-3333; **Board Cert:** Family Medicine 2010; **Med School:** Dominica 1984; **Resid:** Family Medicine, St Joseph's Hosp 1987; **Fac Appt:** Asst Clin Prof FMed, UMDNJ-NJ Med Sch, Newark

Gross, Harvey MD (FMed) *PCP* - **Spec Exp:** Geriatric Medicine; Dementia; Myasthenia Gravis; **Hospital:** Englewood Hosp & Med Ctr, Holy Name Med Ctr (page 720); **Address:** 370 Grand Ave, Ste 102, Englewood, NJ 07631; **Phone:** 201-567-3370; **Board Cert:** Family Medicine 2005; Geriatric Medicine 2010; **Med School:** Boston Univ 1970; **Resid:** Family Medicine, Southside Hosp 1974; **Fac Appt:** Asst Clin Prof Med, Mount Sinai Sch Med

Karatoprak, Ohan MD (FMed) *PCP* - **Spec Exp:** Nutrition; Asthma; Obesity; Geriatric Medicine; **Hospital:** Holy Name Med Ctr (page 720); **Address:** 420 Deerwood Rd, Fort Lee, NJ 07024-1643; **Phone:** 201-886-8877; **Board Cert:** Family Medicine 2005; Geriatric Medicine 2003; **Med School:** Turkey 1977; **Resid:** Surgery, Brookdale Univ Hosp 1983; Family Medicine, Southside Hosp 1986; **Fac Appt:** Asst Clin Prof FMed, UMDNJ-NJ Med Sch, Newark

Leipsner, George MD (FMed) *PCP* - **Hospital:** Hackensack Univ Med Ctr (page 718); **Address:** 57 W Pleasant Ave, Maywood, NJ 07607-1334; **Phone:** 201-488-2111; **Board Cert:** Family Medicine 2001; **Med School:** Italy 1966; **Resid:** Family Medicine, Hackensack Hosp 1968; **Fac Appt:** Asst Clin Prof FMed, UMDNJ-Rutgers Med Sch

Gastroenterology

Avezzano, Eric S MD (Ge) - **Spec Exp:** Endoscopy; Peptic Acid Disorders; Celiac Disease; Gastroesophageal Reflux Disease (GERD); **Hospital:** Valley Hosp (page 721), Hackensack Univ Med Ctr (page 718); **Address:** Bergen Gastroenterology, 466 Old Hook Rd, Ste 1, Emerson, NJ 07630; **Phone:** 201-967-8221; **Board Cert:** Internal Medicine 1988; Gastroenterology 2011; **Med School:** SUNY Stony Brook 1985; **Resid:** Internal Medicine, G Washington Univ Hosp 1988; **Fellow:** Gastroenterology, Georgetown Univ 1991

Broussard, Crystal N MD (Ge) - **Spec Exp:** Women's Health; **Hospital:** Valley Hosp (page 721), Hackensack Univ Med Ctr (page 718); **Address:** Bergen Gastroenterology, 466 Old Hook Rd, Ste 1, Emerson, NJ 07630; **Phone:** 201-967-8221; **Board Cert:** Internal Medicine 2008; Gastroenterology 2009; **Med School:** Case West Res Univ 1992; **Resid:** Internal Medicine, Johns Hopkins Bayview Med Ctr 1995; **Fellow:** Gastroenterology, Cleveland Clinic 1998

Chessler, Richard K MD (Ge) - **Spec Exp:** Pancreatic Cancer; Endoscopy; Pancreatic/Biliary Endoscopy (ERCP); Colonoscopy; **Hospital:** Englewood Hosp & Med Ctr, Hackensack Univ Med Ctr (page 718); **Address:** 140 Sylvan Ave, Fl 1, Ste 101, rm 1, Englewood Cliffs, NJ 07632-2554; **Phone:** 201-945-6564 x320; **Board Cert:** Internal Medicine 1972; Gastroenterology 1975; **Med School:** Ros Franklin Univ/Chicago Med Sch 1969; **Resid:** Internal Medicine, NY Med Coll/Flower-Fifth Ave Hosp 1972; **Fellow:** Gastroenterology, NY Med Coll/Flower-Fifth Ave Hosp 1974; **Fac Appt:** Asst Clin Prof Med, Mount Sinai Sch Med

DeLillo, Anthony R MD (Ge) - **Spec Exp:** Inflammatory Bowel Disease; Esophageal Disorders; **Hospital:** Valley Hosp (page 721), Hackensack UMC-Pascack Valley (page 719); **Address:** Bergen Gastroenterology, 466 Old Hook Rd, Ste 1, Emerson, NJ 07630; **Phone:** 201-967-8221; **Board Cert:** Gastroenterology 2011; **Med School:** Cornell Univ-Weill Med Coll 1994; **Resid:** Internal Medicine, Mt Sinai Med Ctr 1997; **Fellow:** Gastroenterology, Mt Sinai Med Ctr 1999

Fried, Harry A MD (Ge) - **Hospital:** Englewood Hosp & Med Ctr; **Address:** 333 Old Hook Rd, Ste 101, Westwood, NJ 07675; **Phone:** 201-594-0535; **Board Cert:** Internal Medicine 1989; Gastroenterology 2005; **Med School:** SUNY Downstate 1986; **Resid:** Internal Medicine, St Lukes Hosp 1989; **Fellow:** Gastroenterology, Cooper Hosp 1995

Friedrich, Ivan MD (Ge) - **Spec Exp:** Colonoscopy; Inflammatory Bowel Disease; Constipation; Gastroesophageal Reflux Disease (GERD); **Hospital:** Englewood Hosp & Med Ctr, Holy Name Med Ctr (page 720); **Address:** 420 Grand Ave, Englewood, NJ 07631-4152; **Phone:** 201-569-7044; **Board Cert:** Internal Medicine 1979; Gastroenterology 1981; **Med School:** Albany Med Coll 1976; **Resid:** Internal Medicine, Montefiore Med Ctr 1979; **Fellow:** Gastroenterology, Mt Sinai Med Ctr 1982; **Fac Appt:** Asst Clin Prof Med, Mount Sinai Sch Med

Goldfarb, Joel A MD (Ge) - **Spec Exp:** Colonoscopy/Polypectomy; Colon Cancer; Hepatitis; Liver Disease; **Hospital:** Holy Name Med Ctr (page 720), Englewood Hosp & Med Ctr; **Address:** 1086 Teaneck Rd, Ste 4C, Teaneck, NJ 07666; **Phone:** 201-837-9449; **Board Cert:** Internal Medicine 1978; Gastroenterology 1981; **Med School:** NYU Sch Med 1975; **Resid:** Internal Medicine, NYU Med Ctr 1978; Hepatology, Yale-New Haven Hosp 1979; **Fellow:** Gastroenterology, Columbia-Presby Med Ctr 1981; **Fac Appt:** Asst Clin Prof Med, Mount Sinai Sch Med

Klein, Walter A MD (Ge) - **Spec Exp:** Esophageal Disorders; Gastroesophageal Reflux Disease (GERD); Colon Polyps & Cancer; **Hospital:** Englewood Hosp & Med Ctr; **Address:** The Park Medical Group, 274 County Rd, Ste A, Tenafly, NJ 07670; **Phone:** 201-568-0493; **Board Cert:** Internal Medicine 2010; Gastroenterology 2000; **Med School:** Cornell Univ-Weill Med Coll 1987; **Resid:** Internal Medicine, NY Hosp-Cornell Med Ctr 1990; **Fellow:** Gastroenterology, Temple Univ Hosp 1992; **Fac Appt:** Asst Clin Prof Med, Mount Sinai Sch Med

Levine, Robert S MD (Ge) - **Spec Exp:** Pancreatic/Biliary Endoscopy (ERCP); Pancreatic & Biliary Disease; **Hospital:** Valley Hosp (page 721), Hackensack Univ Med Ctr (page 718); **Address:** Bergen Gastroenterology, 466 Old Hook Rd, Ste 1, Emerson, NJ 07630; **Phone:** 201-967-8221; **Board Cert:** Gastroenterology 2003; **Med School:** Georgetown Univ 1987; **Resid:** Internal Medicine, George Washington Univ 1990; **Fellow:** Gastroenterology, George Washington Univ 1993

Margulis, Stephen J MD (Ge) - **Spec Exp:** Hepatitis; Colonoscopy/Polypectomy; Peptic Ulcer Disease; Inflammatory Bowel Disease; **Hospital:** Valley Hosp (page 721), Hackensack Univ Med Ctr (page 718); **Address:** Bergen Gastroenterology, 466 Old Hook Rd, Ste 1, Emerson, NJ 07630-1368; **Phone:** 201-967-8221; **Board Cert:** Internal Medicine 1984; Gastroenterology 1987; **Med School:** Brown Univ 1981; **Resid:** Internal Medicine, New York Hosp-Cornell 1984; **Fellow:** Gastroenterology, New York Hosp-Cornell 1987

Nikias, George A MD (Ge) - **Spec Exp:** Liver Disease; Endoscopy; **Hospital:** Hackensack Univ Med Ctr (page 718); **Address:** 130 Kinderkamack Rd, Ste 301, River Edge, NJ 07661; **Phone:** 201-489-7772; **Board Cert:** Gastroenterology 2005; **Med School:** NY Med Coll 1989; **Resid:** Internal Medicine, North Shore Univ Hosp 1992; **Fellow:** Gastroenterology, Meml Sloan-Kettering Cancer Ctr 1995; Hepatology, Mayo Clin 1993; **Fac Appt:** Asst Clin Prof Med, UMDNJ-NJ Med Sch, Newark

Panella, Vincent S MD (Ge) - **Spec Exp:** Colon & Rectal Cancer; Hepatitis C; Inflammatory Bowel Disease; Endoscopy; **Hospital:** Englewood Hosp & Med Ctr, Holy Name Med Ctr (page 720); **Address:** Englewood Endoscopic Associates, 420 Grand Ave, Englewood, NJ 07631-4141; **Phone:** 201-569-7044; **Board Cert:** Internal Medicine 1985; Gastroenterology 1987; **Med School:** NY Med Coll 1982; **Resid:** Internal Medicine, North Shore Univ Hosp 1985; **Fellow:** Gastroenterology, Mem Sloan-Kettering Cancer Cntr 1987; **Fac Appt:** Asst Clin Prof Med, Mount Sinai Sch Med

Rahmin, Michael G MD (Ge) - **Spec Exp:** Endoscopy; Hepatitis; **Hospital:** Valley Hosp (page 721); **Address:** 140 Chestnut St, Ste 300, Ridgewood, NJ 07452; **Phone:** 201-444-2600; **Board Cert:** Gastroenterology 2005; **Med School:** NYU Sch Med 1989; **Resid:** Internal Medicine, Mt Sinai Hosp 1992; **Fellow:** Gastroenterology, New York Hosp 1995; Hepatology, Mt Sinai Hosp 1995

Roth, Joseph M MD (Ge) - **Spec Exp:** Endoscopy; Inflammatory Bowel Disease; **Hospital:** St. Mary's Hosp - Passaic, St. Joseph's Regl Med Ctr - Paterson; **Address:** 71 Union Ave, Rutherford, NJ 07070-1272; **Phone:** 201-842-0020; **Board Cert:** Internal Medicine 1984; Gastroenterology 1987; **Med School:** Univ Pittsburgh 1981; **Resid:** Internal Medicine, Lenox Hill Hosp 1984; **Fellow:** Gastroenterology, Univ Conn Hlth Ctr 1986

Rubin, Kenneth MD (Ge) - **Spec Exp:** Gastroesophageal Reflux Disease (GERD); Endoscopy; Inflammatory Bowel Disease; Colon Cancer; **Hospital:** Englewood Hosp & Med Ctr, Mt Sinai Med Ctr (page 102); **Address:** 420 Grand Ave, Englewood, NJ 07631-4152; **Phone:** 201-569-7044; **Board Cert:** Internal Medicine 1978; Gastroenterology 1981; **Med School:** UMDNJ-NJ Med Sch, Newark 1975; **Resid:** Internal Medicine, Bronx Muni Hosp 1979; **Fellow:** Gastroenterology, Mount Sinai Hosp 1981; **Fac Appt:** Asst Clin Prof Med, Mount Sinai Sch Med

Rubinoff, Mitchell J MD (Ge) - **Spec Exp:** Hepatitis; Gastroesophageal Reflux Disease (GERD); **Hospital:** Valley Hosp (page 721); **Address:** 140 Chestnut St, Ste 300, Ridgewood, NJ 07450-2536; **Phone:** 201-444-2600; **Board Cert:** Internal Medicine 1982; Gastroenterology 1985; **Med School:** Mount Sinai Sch Med 1979; **Resid:** Internal Medicine, Columbia-Presby Med Ctr 1982; **Fellow:** Gastroenterology, Columbia-Presby Med Ctr 1985

Spinnell, Mitchell K MD (Ge) - **Hospital:** Englewood Hosp & Med Ctr; **Address:** Advanced Gastro of Bergen County, 140 Sylvan Ave, Ste 101A, Englewood Cliffs, NJ 07632; **Phone:** 201-945-6564; **Board Cert:** Internal Medicine 2009; Gastroenterology 2009; **Med School:** SUNY Buffalo 1991; **Resid:** Internal Medicine, Montefiore Med Ctr 1994; **Fellow:** Gastroenterology, Montefiore Med Ctr 1997

Zingler, Barry M MD (Ge) - **Spec Exp:** Colon Cancer; Hepatitis; Gastroesophageal Reflux Disease (GERD); **Hospital:** Englewood Hosp & Med Ctr, Holy Name Med Ctr (page 720); **Address:** 140 Sylvan Ave, Englewood Cliffs, NJ 07632; **Phone:** 201-945-6564; **Board Cert:** Internal Medicine 1988; Gastroenterology 2011; **Med School:** UMDNJ-Rutgers Med Sch 1985; **Resid:** Internal Medicine, NYU Med Ctr 1988; **Fellow:** Gastroenterology, NYU Med Ctr 1990

Zucker, Ira I MD (Ge) - **Spec Exp:** Colon Cancer; Gastroesophageal Reflux Disease (GERD); Ulcerative Colitis/Crohn's; Hepatitis; **Hospital:** Valley Hosp (page 721), Hackensack Univ Med Ctr (page 718); **Address:** 452 Old Hook Rd, Emerson, NJ 07630; **Phone:** 201-666-3900; **Board Cert:** Internal Medicine 1984; Gastroenterology 1987; **Med School:** Ros Franklin Univ/Chicago Med Sch 1981; **Resid:** Internal Medicine, St Vincents Hosp 1984; **Fellow:** Gastroenterology, St Vincents Hosp 1986

Geriatric Medicine

Chavez, Laura M DO (Ger) - **Spec Exp:** Alzheimer's Disease; **Hospital:** Holy Name Med Ctr (page 720), Hackensack Univ Med Ctr (page 718); **Address:** IMA of Bergen County, 15 Anderson St, Hackensack, NJ 07601; **Phone:** 201-487-3355; **Board Cert:** Internal Medicine 2011; Geriatric Medicine 2004; **Med School:** NY Coll Osteo Med 1998; **Resid:** Internal Medicine, UMDNJ Univ Hosp 2001; **Fellow:** Geriatric Medicine, UMDNJ Univ Hosp 2002

Leifer, Bennett MD (Ger) *PCP* - **Spec Exp:** Dementia; Alzheimer's Disease; **Hospital:** Valley Hosp (page 721); **Address:** 301 Godwin Ave, Midland Park, NJ 07432-1544; **Phone:** 201-444-4526; **Board Cert:** Internal Medicine 2011; **Med School:** SUNY Upstate Med Univ 1986; **Resid:** Internal Medicine, Hartford Hosp 1989; **Fellow:** Geriatric Medicine, Mt Sinai Hosp 1991

Tank, Lisa K MD (Ger) *PCP* - **Spec Exp:** Cancer in the Elderly; **Hospital:** Hackensack Univ Med Ctr (page 718); **Address:** HUMC Div Geriatric Med, 360 Essex St, Ste 401, Hackensack, NJ 07601; **Phone:** 551-996-1140; **Board Cert:** Internal Medicine 2011; Geriatric Medicine 2003; **Med School:** India 1996; **Resid:** Internal Medicine, NY Methodist Hosp 2001; **Fellow:** Geriatric Medicine, Hackensack Univ Med Ctr 2003

Villongco, Raymond M MD (Ger) - **Spec Exp:** Diabetes; Hypertension; **Hospital:** Mt Sinai Med Ctr (page 102), Holy Name Med Ctr (page 720); **Address:** Salus Med P.C., 121 Cedar Ln, Ste 2B, Teaneck, NJ 07666; **Phone:** 201-836-4228; **Board Cert:** Internal Medicine 2004; **Med School:** Philippines 1989; **Resid:** Internal Medicine, Jersey City Med Ctr 1994; **Fellow:** Geriatric Medicine, Mt Sinai Med Ctr 1996; **Fac Appt:** Asst Clin Prof H & PM, Mount Sinai Sch Med

Gynecologic Oncology

Vaidya, Ami MD (GO) - **Spec Exp:** Minimally Invasive Gynecologic Surgery; Robotic Surgery; Gynecologic Cancer; Gynecologic Surgery; **Hospital:** Hackensack Univ Med Ctr (page 718); **Address:** John Theurer Cancer Ctr-Gyn Oncology, 92 2nd St, Hackensack, NJ 07601; **Phone:** 551-996-5811; **Board Cert:** Obstetrics & Gynecology ; Gynecologic Oncology ; Hospice & Palliative Medicine ; **Med School:** Columbia P&S 1999; **Resid:** Obstetrics & Gynecology, NYU Med Ctr 2003; **Fellow:** Gynecologic Oncology, Harvard/Mass Genl Hosp 2006

Hand Surgery

Fakharzadeh, Frederick F MD (HS) - **Hospital:** Hackensack Univ Med Ctr (page 718), Valley Hosp (page 721); **Address:** 22 Madison Ave, Fl 3 Bldg, Paramus, NJ 07652-2721; **Phone:** 201-587-7767; **Board Cert:** Orthopaedic Surgery 2009; Hand Surgery 2009; **Med School:** Columbia P&S 1980; **Resid:** Surgery, Roosevelt Hosp 1982; Orthopaedic Surgery, Columbia-Presby Med Ctr 1985; **Fellow:** Hand Surgery, Thomas Jefferson Univ Hosp 1986

Gurland, Mark MD (HS) - **Spec Exp:** Carpal Tunnel Syndrome; Wrist/Hand Injuries; Arthritis Hand Surgery; **Hospital:** Hackensack Univ Med Ctr (page 718), Englewood Hosp & Med Ctr; **Address:** 216 Engle St, Englewood, NJ 07631-2448; **Phone:** 201-568-4066; **Board Cert:** Orthopaedic Surgery 2009; Hand Surgery 2009; **Med School:** NYU Sch Med 1979; **Resid:** Surgery, Hosp Univ Penn 1980; Orthopaedic Surgery, Hosp for Joint Diseases 1984; **Fellow:** Hand Surgery, Thomas Jefferson Univ Hosp 1985

Miller-Breslow, Anne J MD (HS) - **Spec Exp:** Rheumatoid Arthritis; Wrist/Hand Injuries; Arthroscopic Surgery; Fractures; **Hospital:** Englewood Hosp & Med Ctr; **Address:** Englewood Orthopedic Assocs, 401 S Van Brunt St Fl 3, Englewood, NJ 07631-2904; **Phone:** 201-569-2770; **Board Cert:** Orthopaedic Surgery 2012; Hand Surgery 2012; **Med School:** Harvard Med Sch 1983; **Resid:** Orthopaedic Surgery, Montefiore Med Ctr 1988; **Fellow:** Hand Surgery, New England Med Ctr 1989

Rosenstein, Roger G MD (HS) - **Spec Exp:** Arthritis Hand Surgery; Nerve Compression; Carpal Tunnel Syndrome; **Hospital:** Valley Hosp (page 721), Hackensack Univ Med Ctr (page 718); **Address:** 22 Madison Ave, Ste 301, Paramus, NJ 07652-5474; **Phone:** 201-587-7767; **Board Cert:** Orthopaedic Surgery 1984; Hand Surgery 2010; **Med School:** Columbia P&S 1975; **Resid:** Surgery, St Luke's Roosevelt Hosp Ctr 1977; Orthopaedic Surgery, Columbia-Presby Med Ctr 1980; **Fellow:** Hand Surgery, Thomas Jefferson Univ Hosp 1981; **Fac Appt:** Assoc Clin Prof OrS, UMDNJ-NJ Med Sch, Newark

Hematology

Feldman, Tatyana A MD (Hem) - **Spec Exp:** Lymphoma; **Hospital:** Hackensack Univ Med Ctr (page 718); **Address:** John Pheurer Cancer Ctr, 92 2nd St, Ste 210, Hackensack, NJ 07601; **Phone:** 201-996-5900; **Board Cert:** Internal Medicine 2008; Hematology 2012; Medical Oncology 2012; **Med School:** Ukraine 1992; **Resid:** Internal Medicine, Beth Israel Med Ctr 1998; Internal Medicine, Montefiore Med Ctr 1999; **Fellow:** Hematology & Oncology, NYU Med Ctr 2001

Fernbach, Barry R MD (Hem) - **Hospital:** Valley Hosp (page 721); **Address:** 1 Valley Health Plaza, Paramus, NJ 07652; **Phone:** 201-634-5353; **Board Cert:** Internal Medicine 1974; Medical Oncology 1977; Hematology 1982; **Med School:** Harvard Med Sch 1971; **Resid:** Internal Medicine, Mt Sinai Hosp 1974; Hematology, Mt Sinai Hosp 1976; **Fellow:** Neoplastic Diseases, Mt Sinai Hosp 1977

Israel, Alan M MD (Hem) - **Hospital:** Valley Hosp (page 721); **Address:** 270 Old Hook Rd, Westwood, NJ 07675-3102; **Phone:** 201-666-4949; **Board Cert:** Internal Medicine 1982; Medical Oncology 1985; Hematology 1986; **Med School:** NYU Sch Med 1979; **Resid:** Internal Medicine, Mt Sinai Hosp 1982; **Fellow:** Hematology & Oncology, Meml Sloan Kettering Cancer Ctr 1984; Hematology, LI Jewish Hosp 1986

Rowley, Scott D MD (Hem) - **Spec Exp:** Stem Cell Transplant; Bone Marrow Transplant; Graft vs Host Disease; **Hospital:** Hackensack Univ Med Ctr (page 718); **Address:** John Pheuer Cancer Ctr, 92 2nd St, Ste 230, Hackensack, NJ 07601; **Phone:** 551-996-8297; **Board Cert:** Internal Medicine 1981; Medical Oncology 1983; Hematology 1984; **Med School:** Univ Mass Sch Med 1978; **Resid:** Internal Medicine, Rhode Island Hosp 1981; **Fellow:** Hematology & Oncology, Rhode Island Hosp 1984; **Fac Appt:** Assoc Prof Med, UMDNJ-NJ Med Sch, Newark

Vesole, David H MD/PhD (Hem) - **Spec Exp:** Multiple Myeloma; Stem Cell Transplant; Amyloidosis; Waldenstrom's Macroglobulinemia; **Hospital:** Hackensack Univ Med Ctr (page 718); **Address:** 92 Second St, Hackensack, NJ 07601; **Phone:** 551-996-8704; **Board Cert:** Internal Medicine 1987; **Med School:** Northwestern Univ 1984; **Resid:** Internal Medicine, Univ Iowa Hosp 1987; **Fellow:** Hematology & Oncology, Univ Iowa Hosp 1990; **Fac Appt:** Prof Med, UMDNJ-NJ Med Sch, Newark

Infectious Disease

Birch, Thomas MD (Inf) - **Spec Exp:** AIDS/HIV; Lyme Disease; West Nile Virus; Antibiotic Resistance; **Hospital:** Holy Name Med Ctr (page 720), Englewood Hosp & Med Ctr; **Address:** Birch Tree Med Assocs, 718 Teaneck Rd, Teaneck, NJ 07666; **Phone:** 201-541-6315; **Board Cert:** Internal Medicine 1986; Infectious Disease 2004; **Med School:** Univ Wisc 1983; **Resid:** Internal Medicine, Montefiore Med Ctr 1986; **Fellow:** Infectious Disease, Montefiore Med Ctr 1993

Cicogna, Cristina E MD (Inf) - **Spec Exp:** Infections in Immunocompromised Patients; Hospital Acquired Infections; **Hospital:** Hackensack Univ Med Ctr (page 718); **Address:** 20 Prospect Ave Fl 5 - Ste 507, Hackensack, NJ 07601; **Phone:** 201-487-4088; **Board Cert:** Infectious Disease 2004; **Med School:** Switzerland 1986; **Resid:** Internal Medicine, St Luke's-Roosevelt Hosp 1989; **Fellow:** Infectious Disease, Meml Sloan-Kettering Cancer Ctr 1991; **Fac Appt:** Asst Prof Med, UMDNJ-RW Johnson Med Sch

Desai, Amita J MD (Inf) - **Spec Exp:** Infections in Transplant Patients; Tropical Diseases; Tuberculosis; **Hospital:** Holy Name Med Ctr (page 720); **Address:** Birch Tree Medical Associates, 718 Teaneck Rd, Teaneck, NJ 07666; **Phone:** 201-541-6315; **Board Cert:** Internal Medicine 1987; Infectious Disease 2004; **Med School:** NY Med Coll 1983; **Resid:** Internal Medicine, Montefiore Med Ctr 1986; **Fellow:** Infectious Disease, Mount Sinai Med Ctr 1994

Knackmuhs, Gary G MD (Inf) - **Spec Exp:** Travel Medicine; **Hospital:** Valley Hosp (page 721); **Address:** 947 Lynwood Ave, Ste 2E, Ridgewood, NJ 07450-4407; **Phone:** 201-447-6468; **Board Cert:** Internal Medicine 1979; Infectious Disease 1982; **Med School:** NY Med Coll 1976; **Resid:** Internal Medicine, Mt Sinai Hosp 1979; **Fellow:** Infectious Disease, Montefiore Med Ctr 1981

Kocher, Jeffrey MD (Inf) - **Spec Exp:** Hepatitis B & C; AIDS/HIV; Fungal Infections; Lyme Disease; **Hospital:** Englewood Hosp & Med Ctr; **Address:** 25 Rockwood Pl, Ste 120, Englewood, NJ 07631-4957; **Phone:** 201-568-3335; **Board Cert:** Internal Medicine 1983; Infectious Disease 1986; **Med School:** Cornell Univ-Weill Med Coll 1980; **Resid:** Internal Medicine, New York Hosp 1983; Internal Medicine, St Barnabas Hosp 1984; **Fellow:** Infectious Disease, New York Hosp 1986; **Fac Appt:** Assoc Clin Prof Med, Mount Sinai Sch Med

Sperber, Steven J MD (Inf) - **Hospital:** Hackensack Univ Med Ctr (page 718); **Address:** 20 Prospect Ave, Ste 507, Hackensack, NJ 07601; **Phone:** 201-996-2070; **Board Cert:** Internal Medicine 1985; Infectious Disease 1988; **Med School:** NYU Sch Med 1982; **Resid:** Internal Medicine, SUNY Stony Brook Med Ctr 1985; **Fellow:** Infectious Disease, Univ Va Med Ctr 1988; **Fac Appt:** Assoc Clin Prof Med, UMDNJ-NJ Med Sch, Newark

Tsiouris, Simon J MD (Inf) - **Spec Exp:** Tuberculosis; Travel Medicine; Tropical Diseases; AIDS/HIV; **Hospital:** Valley Hosp (page 721); **Address:** Ridgewooud Infectious Disease Assocs, 947 Linwood Ave, Ste 2E, Ridgewood, NJ 07450; **Phone:** 201-447-6468; **Board Cert:** Infectious Disease 2004; **Med School:** Johns Hopkins Univ 1998; **Resid:** Internal Medicine, NY-Presby/Weill Cornell Med Ctr 2001; **Fellow:** Infectious Disease, NY-Presby/Columbia Univ Med Ctr 2002; **Fac Appt:** Asst Prof Med, Columbia P&S

Weisholtz, Steven J MD (Inf) - **Spec Exp:** AIDS/HIV; Antibiotic Resistance; Travel Medicine; **Hospital:** Englewood Hosp & Med Ctr; **Address:** 25 Rockwood Pl, Ste 120, Englewood, NJ 07631-4957; **Phone:** 201-568-3335; **Board Cert:** Internal Medicine 1981; Infectious Disease 1984; **Med School:** Univ Pennsylvania 1978; **Resid:** Internal Medicine, New York Hosp 1981; **Fellow:** Infectious Disease, New York Hosp 1983; **Fac Appt:** Asst Clin Prof Med, Mount Sinai Sch Med

Internal Medicine

Brunnquell, Stephen MD (IM) *PCP* - **Hospital:** Englewood Hosp & Med Ctr; **Address:** 24 Elm St, Harrington Park, NJ 07640-1902; **Phone:** 201-784-0123; **Board Cert:** Internal Medicine 2012; **Med School:** UMDNJ-NJ Med Sch, Newark 1989; **Resid:** Internal Medicine, Montefiore Med Ctr 1992; **Fac Appt:** Asst Clin Prof Med, Mount Sinai Sch Med

Cacciola, Thomas A MD (IM) *PCP* - **Spec Exp:** Preventive Medicine; Complementary Medicine; **Hospital:** Hackensack Univ Med Ctr (page 718); **Address:** 403 N Farview Ave, Paramus, NJ 07652-4618; **Phone:** 201-261-8386; **Board Cert:** Internal Medicine 1988; **Med School:** Jefferson Med Coll 1983; **Resid:** Internal Medicine, Hackensack Med Ctr 1986; **Fellow:** US Public Hlth Svc 1988

Flanzman, Susan A MD (IM) *PCP* - **Spec Exp:** Women's Health; Anxiety & Depression; Menopause Problems; Nutrition & Obesity; **Hospital:** Valley Hosp (page 721); **Address:** Bergen Medical Assocs, 1 W Ridgewood Ave, Ste 301, Paramus, NJ 07652; **Phone:** 201-445-1660; **Board Cert:** Internal Medicine 2012; **Med School:** Mount Sinai Sch Med 1987; **Resid:** Internal Medicine, Montefiore Med Ctr 1991

Giangola, Joseph MD (IM) - **Spec Exp:** Diabetes; **Hospital:** Hackensack Univ Med Ctr (page 718); **Address:** 810 Main St, Hackensack, NJ 07601-4802; **Phone:** 201-488-5922; **Board Cert:** Internal Medicine 1981; **Med School:** Italy 1978; **Resid:** Internal Medicine, Long Island Coll Hosp 1981; **Fellow:** Diabetes, Joslin Clin 1983

Kushner, Evan G MD (IM) *PCP* - **Spec Exp:** Geriatric Medicine; **Hospital:** Hackensack Univ Med Ctr (page 718), Valley Hosp (page 721); **Address:** Forest Hlthcare Assocs, 277 Forest Ave, Ste 200, Paramus, NJ 07652; **Phone:** 201-986-1881; **Board Cert:** Internal Medicine 1989; Geriatric Medicine 2005; **Med School:** SUNY Upstate Med Univ 1986; **Resid:** Internal Medicine, Univ Hosp 1989

Lan, Vivian E MD (IM) *PCP* - **Spec Exp:** Women's Health; Eating Disorders; **Hospital:** Valley Hosp (page 721), Hackensack Univ Med Ctr (page 718); **Address:** 466 Old Hook Rd, Ste 1, Emerson, NJ 07630; **Phone:** 201-967-8221; **Board Cert:** Internal Medicine 2007; **Med School:** Mount Sinai Sch Med 1994; **Resid:** Internal Medicine, Mt Sinai Med Ctr 1997

Lauricella, Joseph MD (IM) *PCP* - **Spec Exp:** Coronary Artery Disease; **Hospital:** Holy Name Med Ctr (page 720); **Address:** 292 Columbia Ave, Fort Lee, NJ 07024-4124; **Phone:** 201-224-0050; **Board Cert:** Internal Medicine 1985; **Med School:** Mexico 1978; **Resid:** Internal Medicine, Rutgers Univ Med Ctr 1985

Miguel, Eduardo E MD (IM) *PCP* - **Spec Exp:** Rheumatoid Arthritis; **Hospital:** Englewood Hosp & Med Ctr; **Address:** 200 Grand Ave, Ste 202, Englewood, NJ 07631; **Phone:** 201-871-3280; **Board Cert:** Internal Medicine 1982; **Med School:** Paraguay 1966; **Resid:** Internal Medicine, VA Med Ctr 1969; Internal Medicine, NY Polyclinic Hosp 1972; **Fellow:** Rheumatology, Albert Einstein Med Ctr 1973

Pelavin, Martin MD (IM) *PCP* - **Hospital:** Valley Hosp (page 721), Englewood Hosp & Med Ctr; **Address:** 215 Old Tappan Rd, Old Tappan, NJ 07675-7428; **Phone:** 201-666-1000; **Board Cert:** Internal Medicine 1976; **Med School:** NYU Sch Med 1973; **Resid:** Internal Medicine, Montefiore Hosp Med Ctr 1976

Schuster, Joseph C MD (IM) *PCP* - **Hospital:** Holy Name Med Ctr (page 720), Hackensack Univ Med Ctr (page 718); **Address:** 175 Cedar Ln, Teaneck, NJ 07666-4315; **Phone:** 201-692-7766; **Board Cert:** Internal Medicine 1984; **Med School:** Albany Med Coll 1981; **Resid:** Internal Medicine, St Luke's-Roosevelt Hosp Ctr 1982; Internal Medicine, Kings County Hosp 1984

Scibetta, Maria MD (IM) *PCP* - **Hospital:** Valley Hosp (page 721); **Address:** 470 N Franklin Tpke, Ramsey, NJ 07446-2034; **Phone:** 201-327-8765; **Board Cert:** Internal Medicine 2003; **Med School:** UMDNJ-RW Johnson Med Sch 1990; **Resid:** Internal Medicine, Mount Sinai Hosp 1993

Valinoti, Anne Marie MD (IM) - **Spec Exp:** Women's Health; **Hospital:** Valley Hosp (page 721); **Address:** 301 Godwin Avenue, Midland Park, NJ 07432; **Phone:** 201-444-4526; **Board Cert:** Internal Medicine 2004; **Med School:** Columbia P&S 1991; **Resid:** Internal Medicine, New York Hosp 1994

Volpe, Anthony P MD (IM) *PCP* - **Spec Exp:** Hypertension; **Hospital:** Valley Hosp (page 721); **Address:** 466 Old Hook Rd, Ste 14, Emerson, NJ 07630-1368; **Phone:** 201-262-6485; **Board Cert:** Internal Medicine 2005; **Med School:** Mexico 1981; **Resid:** Internal Medicine, Texas Tech Hlth Scis Ctr 1986

Wasserman, Kenneth H MD (IM) *PCP* - **Hospital:** Englewood Hosp & Med Ctr, Holy Name Med Ctr (page 720); **Address:** 177 N Dean St Fl 1, Englewood, NJ 07631; **Phone:** 201-567-1140 x10; **Board Cert:** Internal Medicine 1982; **Med School:** Albert Einstein Coll Med 1979; **Resid:** Internal Medicine, Lenox Hill Hosp 1982

Interventional Cardiology

Angeli, Stephen J MD (IC) - **Spec Exp:** Angioplasty & Stent Placement; Cardiac Catheterization; Coronary Artery Disease; **Hospital:** Holy Name Med Ctr (page 720); **Address:** Cardiovascular Assocs of Teaneck, 954 Teaneck Rd, Teaneck, NJ 07666; **Phone:** 201-833-2300; **Board Cert:** Internal Medicine 1984; Cardiovascular Disease 1987; Interventional Cardiology 2009; **Med School:** SUNY Downstate 1981; **Resid:** Internal Medicine, Kings Co Hosp 1984; **Fellow:** Cardiovascular Disease, St Michael Med Ctr 1986

Syed, Tariqshah M MD (IC) - **Spec Exp:** Cardiac Catheterization; Angiography-Coronary; Angioplasty & Stent Placement; Coronary Artery Disease; **Hospital:** Hackensack Univ Med Ctr (page 718), Holy Name Med Ctr (page 720); **Address:** Holy Name Cardiology Associates, 954 Teaneck Rd, Teaneck, NJ 07666; **Phone:** 201-833-2300; **Board Cert:** Internal Medicine 2004; Cardiovascular Disease 2007; Interventional Cardiology 2008; Echocardiography 2007; **Med School:** Pakistan 1999; **Resid:** Internal Medicine, St. Luke's Roosevelt Hosp Ctr 2004; **Fellow:** Cardiovascular Disease, Mt. Sinai Hosp 2007; Interventional Cardiology, St. Luke's Roosevelt Hosp Ctr 2008

Maternal & Fetal Medicine

Alvarez, Manuel MD (MF) - **Spec Exp:** Multiple Gestation; Pregnancy-High Risk; **Hospital:** Hackensack Univ Med Ctr (page 718), NYU Langone Med Ctr (page 108); **Address:** 20 Prospect Ave, Ste 601, Hackensack, NJ 07601; **Phone:** 201-996-2765; **Board Cert:** Obstetrics & Gynecology 2012; Maternal & Fetal Medicine 2012; **Med School:** Dominican Republic 1981; **Resid:** Obstetrics & Gynecology, St Joseph Hosp 1987; **Fellow:** Maternal & Fetal Medicine, Mount Sinai Med Ctr 1989; Critical Care Obstetrics, Mount Sinai Med Ctr 1990

Frieden, Faith MD (MF) - **Spec Exp:** Prenatal Ultrasound; Prenatal Diagnosis; **Hospital:** Englewood Hosp & Med Ctr; **Address:** 350 Engle St, Englewood, NJ 07631-1808; **Phone:** 201-894-3669; **Board Cert:** Obstetrics & Gynecology 2012; Maternal & Fetal Medicine 2012; **Med School:** Mount Sinai Sch Med 1984; **Resid:** Obstetrics & Gynecology, Beth Israel Med Ctr 1988; **Fellow:** Maternal & Fetal Medicine, Bellevue Hosp 1990; **Fac Appt:** Asst Clin Prof ObG, Mount Sinai Sch Med

Principe, David L MD (MF) - **Spec Exp:** Pregnancy-High Risk; **Hospital:** St. Joseph's Regl Med Ctr - Paterson, Palisades Med Ctr; **Address:** St Joseph's Perinatal Ctr, 1 Broadway, Ste 203, Elmwood Park, NJ 07407; **Phone:** 973-569-6264; **Board Cert:** Obstetrics & Gynecology 2012; Maternal & Fetal Medicine 2012; **Med School:** Grenada 1991; **Resid:** Obstetrics & Gynecology, St Joseph Hosp 1995; **Fellow:** Maternal & Fetal Medicine, Univ Chicago/Chicago Lying in Hosp 1997; Maternal & Fetal Medicine, Yale New Haven Hosp 1998

Zelop, Carolyn M MD (MF) - **Spec Exp:** Prenatal Diagnosis; Fetal Echocardiography; Pregnancy-High Risk; **Hospital:** Valley Hosp (page 721); **Address:** Valley Hospital, 15 Essex Rd, Ste 204, Paramus, NJ 07652; **Phone:** 201-291-6321; **Board Cert:** Obstetrics & Gynecology 2013; Maternal & Fetal Medicine 2013; **Med School:** Tufts Univ 1987; **Resid:** Obstetrics & Gynecology, Brigham and Women's Hosp 1991; **Fellow:** Maternal & Fetal Medicine, Brigham and Women's Hosp 1993

Medical Oncology

Attas, Lewis MD (Onc) - **Spec Exp:** Breast Cancer; Lymphoma; Bleeding/Coagulation Disorders; Gaucher Disease; **Hospital:** Englewood Hosp & Med Ctr, Holy Name Med Ctr (page 720); **Address:** 350 Engle St, Englewood, NJ 07631; **Phone:** 201-568-5250; **Board Cert:** Internal Medicine 1985; Medical Oncology 1987; Hematology 1988; Hospice & Palliative Medicine 2012; **Med School:** Mount Sinai Sch Med 1982; **Resid:** Internal Medicine, Montefiore Hosp Med Ctr 1985; **Fellow:** Hematology & Oncology, North Shore Univ Hosp 1988; **Fac Appt:** Assoc Clin Prof Med, Mount Sinai Sch Med

Condemi, Giuseppe MD (Onc) - **Spec Exp:** Breast Cancer; Prostate Cancer; Colon Cancer; **Address:** Regi Cancer Ctr, 718 Teaneck Rd, Teaneck, NJ 07666; **Phone:** 201-227-6008; **Board Cert:** Internal Medicine 2003; Medical Oncology 2005; **Med School:** Dominica 1998; **Resid:** Internal Medicine, Mt. Sinai Sch Med 2001; **Fellow:** Hematology & Oncology, A Einstein Coll Med 2004

Forte, Francis A MD (Onc) - **Spec Exp:** Breast Cancer; Hematologic Malignancies; Coagulation/Bleeding Disorders; Solid Tumors; **Hospital:** Englewood Hosp & Med Ctr, Holy Name Med Ctr (page 720); **Address:** 350 Engle St Berrie Bldg Fl 1, Englewood, NJ 07631; **Phone:** 201-568-5250; **Board Cert:** Internal Medicine 1971; Hematology 1972; Medical Oncology 1973; **Med School:** Albert Einstein Coll Med 1964; **Resid:** Internal Medicine, Mount Sinai Hosp 1968; **Fellow:** Hematology, Mount Sinai Hosp 1969; **Fac Appt:** Asst Prof Med, Mount Sinai Sch Med

Goldberg, Stuart L MD (Onc) - **Spec Exp:** Leukemia; Stem Cell Transplant; Myelodysplastic Syndromes; **Hospital:** Hackensack Univ Med Ctr (page 718); **Address:** John Theurer Cancer Ctr, HUMC, 92 Second St, Hackensack, NJ 07601; **Phone:** 201-996-3925; **Board Cert:** Internal Medicine 1989; **Med School:** Penn State Coll Med 1986; **Resid:** Internal Medicine, G Washington Univ Hosp 1989; **Fellow:** Hematology & Oncology, G Washington Univ Hosp 1991; Bone Marrow Transplant, Mayo Clin 1992; **Fac Appt:** Assoc Clin Prof Med, UMDNJ-NJ Med Sch, Newark

Goy, Andre MD (Onc) - **Spec Exp:** Lymphoma; Hodgkin's Lymphoma; **Hospital:** Hackensack Univ Med Ctr (page 718); **Address:** 92 2nd St, Hackensack, NJ 07601; **Phone:** 201-996-5900; **Med School:** France 1988; **Resid:** Internal Medicine, Grenoble Univ Med Ctr 1992; **Fellow:** Hematology & Oncology, Grenoble Univ Med Ctr 1993

Harper, Harry MD (Onc) - **Spec Exp:** Lung Cancer; **Hospital:** Hackensack Univ Med Ctr (page 718), Holy Name Med Ctr (page 720); **Address:** John Theurer Cancer Ctr, HUMC, 92 Second St, Hackensack, NJ 07601; **Phone:** 201-996-5087; **Board Cert:** Internal Medicine 1980; Hematology 1982; Medical Oncology 1983; **Med School:** Baylor Coll Med 1977; **Resid:** Internal Medicine, NY-Cornell Med Ctr 1980; **Fellow:** Hematology & Oncology, Meml Sloan-Kettering Cancer Ctr 1983

Jennis, Andrew MD (Onc) - **Spec Exp:** Gastrointestinal Cancer; **Hospital:** Hackensack Univ Med Ctr (page 718); **Address:** John Theurer Cancer Ctr, HUMC, 92 Second St, Hackensack, NJ 07601; **Phone:** 201-996-5900; **Board Cert:** Internal Medicine 1988; Medical Oncology 2011; **Med School:** Columbia P&S 1985; **Resid:** Internal Medicine, Mount Sinai Hosp 1988; **Fellow:** Hematology & Oncology, Beth Israel Hosp 1992

Krutchik, Allan MD (Onc) - **Spec Exp:** Breast Cancer; **Hospital:** St. Joseph's Wayne Hosp, Chilton Hosp; **Address:** John Theurer Cancer Ctr, Bldg C, 795 Franklin Ave, Franklin Lakes, NJ 07417; **Phone:** 201-848-8791; **Board Cert:** Internal Medicine 1976; Medical Oncology 1981; **Med School:** Ros Franklin Univ/Chicago Med Sch 1973; **Resid:** Internal Medicine, Beth Israel Hosp 1976; **Fellow:** Medical Oncology, MD Anderson Cancer Ctr 1978; **Fac Appt:** Asst Clin Prof Med, UMDNJ-NJ Med Sch, Newark

Ligresti, Louise G MD (Onc) - **Spec Exp:** Breast Cancer; **Hospital:** Valley Hosp (page 721), Chilton Hosp; **Address:** One Valley Hlth Plaza, Paramus, NJ 07652; **Phone:** 201-634-5353; **Board Cert:** Medical Oncology 2008; Hematology 2008; **Med School:** SUNY Upstate Med Univ 1991; **Resid:** Internal Medicine, NY Hosp-Cornell Med Ctr 1994; **Fellow:** Hematology & Oncology, Meml Sloan Kettering Cancer Ctr 1995

Pascal, Mark MD (Onc) - **Spec Exp:** Lung Cancer; Breast Cancer; Neuro-Oncology; **Hospital:** Hackensack Univ Med Ctr (page 718), Holy Name Med Ctr (page 720); **Address:** John Theurer Cancer Ctr, HUMC, 92 Second St, Hackensack, NJ 07601; **Phone:** 201-996-5266; **Board Cert:** Internal Medicine 1977; Medical Oncology 1979; **Med School:** Jefferson Med Coll 1973; **Resid:** Pathology, NY Hosp-Cornell Univ Med Ctr 1976; Internal Medicine, NY Hosp-Cornell Univ Med Ctr 1977; **Fellow:** Hematology & Oncology, Meml Sloan-Kettering Cancer Ctr 1979

Pecora, Andrew L MD (Onc) - **Spec Exp:** Stem Cell Transplant; Myelodysplastic Syndromes; Melanoma; Immunotherapy; **Hospital:** Hackensack Univ Med Ctr (page 718); **Address:** 92 2nd St, Hackensack, NJ 07601; **Phone:** 201-996-5900; **Board Cert:** Internal Medicine 1986; Hematology 1988; Medical Oncology 1989; **Med School:** UMDNJ-NJ Med Sch, Newark 1983; **Resid:** Internal Medicine, New York Hosp 1986; **Fellow:** Hematology & Oncology, Meml Sloan Kettering Cancer Ctr 1988; **Fac Appt:** Prof Med, UMDNJ-NJ Med Sch, Newark

Pieczara, Beata K MD (Onc) - **Hospital:** Holy Name Med Ctr (page 720); **Address:** Regional Cancer Ctr at Holy Name, 718 Teaneck Rd, Teaneck, NJ 07666; **Phone:** 201-227-6008; **Board Cert:** Hematology 2003; **Med School:** Poland 1993; **Resid:** Internal Medicine, Bronx Lebanon Hosp 1999; **Fellow:** Hematology & Oncology, Westchester Med Ctr 1999

Rakowski, Thomas MD (Onc) - **Spec Exp:** Breast Cancer; Lung Cancer; Colon Cancer; **Hospital:** Valley Hosp (page 721); **Address:** One Valley Health Plaza, Paramus, NJ 07652; **Phone:** 201-634-5578; **Board Cert:** Internal Medicine 1979; Medical Oncology 1981; **Med School:** SUNY Upstate Med Univ 1976; **Resid:** Internal Medicine, SUNY Hlth Sci Ctr 1979; Hematology & Oncology, NY Presby Hosp-Columbia Campus 1981

Rivera, Yadyra MD (Onc) - **Spec Exp:** Breast Cancer; Colon Cancer; Lung Cancer; **Hospital:** Holy Name Med Ctr (page 720); **Address:** Regional Cancer Ctr at Holy Name, 718 Teaneck Rd, Teaneck, NJ 07666; **Phone:** 201-227-6008; **Board Cert:** Internal Medicine 2005; Medical Oncology 2008; Hematology 2009; **Med School:** Univ del Caribe Escuela Med 1992; **Resid:** Internal Medicine, Cabrini Med Ctr 1995; **Fellow:** Hematology, Cabrini Med Ctr 1997

Schleider, Michael MD (Onc) - **Spec Exp:** Breast Cancer; Colon Cancer; Bleeding/Coagulation Disorders; **Hospital:** Englewood Hosp & Med Ctr, Holy Name Med Ctr (page 720); **Address:** 350 Engle St Berrie Bldg Fl 1, Englewood, NJ 07631; **Phone:** 201-568-5250; **Board Cert:** Internal Medicine 1974; Hematology 1976; Medical Oncology 1977; **Med School:** Univ Pennsylvania 1969; **Resid:** Internal Medicine, New York Hosp 1974; **Fellow:** Hematology & Oncology, New York Hosp 1977

Waintraub, Stanley E MD (Onc) - **Spec Exp:** Breast Cancer; Bleeding/Coagulation Disorders; **Hospital:** Hackensack Univ Med Ctr (page 718); **Address:** 92 2nd St, Hackensack, NJ 07601; **Phone:** 201-996-5864; **Board Cert:** Internal Medicine 1980; Hematology 1982; Medical Oncology 1983; **Med School:** NY Med Coll 1977; **Resid:** Internal Medicine, Metropolitan Hosp Ctr 1980; **Fellow:** Hematology, Montefiore Hosp Med Ctr 1982; Medical Oncology, Meml Sloan Kettering Cancer Ctr 1983

Neonatal-Perinatal Medicine

Carlin, Elizabeth B MD (NP) - **Spec Exp:** Nutrition; **Hospital:** Englewood Hosp & Med Ctr, Mt Sinai Med Ctr (page 102); **Address:** Englewood Hosp & Med Ctr, 350 Engle St, Englewood, NJ 07631-1808; **Phone:** 201-894-3472; **Board Cert:** Neonatal-Perinatal Medicine 2013; **Med School:** Boston Univ 1990; **Resid:** Pediatrics, Boston City Hosp 1993; **Fellow:** Neonatal-Perinatal Medicine, Mt Sinai Med Ctr 1996; **Fac Appt:** Asst Clin Prof Ped, Mount Sinai Sch Med

Giuliano, Michael A MD (NP) - **Hospital:** Hackensack Univ Med Ctr (page 718); **Address:** Hackensack Univ Med Ctr, 30 Prospect Ave Imus Bldg - rm 217, Hackensack, NJ 07601; **Phone:** 551-996-5362; **Board Cert:** Pediatrics 2002; Neonatal-Perinatal Medicine 1987; **Med School:** SUNY Downstate 1981; **Resid:** Pediatrics, New York Hosp 1984; **Fellow:** Neonatal-Perinatal Medicine, New York Hosp/Cornell 1986

Manginello, Frank MD (NP) - **Spec Exp:** Prematurity/Low Birth Weight Infants; Lung Disease in Newborns; Developmental Disorders; **Hospital:** Valley Hosp (page 721); **Address:** Ctr for Child Development, 505 Goffle Rd, Ridgewood, NJ 07450; **Phone:** 201-447-8388; **Board Cert:** Pediatrics 1978; Neonatal-Perinatal Medicine 1979; **Med School:** Georgetown Univ 1973; **Resid:** Pediatrics, Georgetown Univ Hosp 1974; Pediatrics, Georgetown Univ Hosp 1975; **Fellow:** Perinatal Medicine, NY-Presby/Weill Cornell Med Ctr 1977

Perl, Harold MD (NP) - **Spec Exp:** Pulmonary Disease; Jaundice & Bilirubin Metabolism, Sudden Infant Death Syndrome (SIDS); **Hospital:** Hackensack Univ Med Ctr (page 718); **Address:** Hackensack Univ Med Ctr, Dept Pediatrics, 30 Prospect Ave, Imus Bldg, rm 220, Hackensack, NJ 07601-1914; **Phone:** 551-996-5362; **Board Cert:** Pediatrics 1980; Neonatal-Perinatal Medicine 1983; **Med School:** Albert Einstein Coll Med 1975; **Resid:** Pediatrics, Montefiore Med Ctr 1978; **Fellow:** Neonatal-Perinatal Medicine, Montefiore Med Ctr 1980; **Fac Appt:** Asst Clin Prof Ped, UMDNJ-NJ Med Sch, Newark

Nephrology

Fein, Deborah A MD (Nep) - **Spec Exp:** Hypertension; Kidney Disease; Transplant Medicine-Kidney; Lupus Nephritis; **Hospital:** Englewood Hosp & Med Ctr, Holy Name Med Ctr (page 720); **Address:** 177 N Dean St, Ste 207, Englewood, NJ 07631; **Phone:** 201-567-0446; **Board Cert:** Internal Medicine 1983; Nephrology 2004; **Med School:** Tufts Univ 1980; **Resid:** Internal Medicine, Roosevelt Hosp 1983; **Fellow:** Nephrology, NY Hosp 1986

Joseph, Rosy E MD (Nep) - **Hospital:** Hackensack Univ Med Ctr (page 718); **Address:** 360 Essex St Fl 3 - Ste 304, Hackensack, NJ 07601; **Phone:** 201-646-0110; **Board Cert:** Internal Medicine 2008; Nephrology 2009; **Med School:** Columbia P&S 1990; **Resid:** Internal Medicine, NY Hosp 1997; **Fellow:** Nephrology, NY Presby-Columbia Med Ctr 1998

Kozlowski, Jeffrey MD (Nep) - **Spec Exp:** Hypertension; Dialysis Care; Diabetic Kidney Disease; **Hospital:** Valley Hosp (page 721), Hackensack Univ Med Ctr (page 718); **Address:** 44 Godwin Ave, Ste 301, Midland Park, NJ 07432; **Phone:** 201-447-0013; **Board Cert:** Internal Medicine 1981; Nephrology 1984; **Med School:** NYU Sch Med 1978; **Resid:** Internal Medicine, VA Med Ctr 1981; **Fellow:** Nephrology, NYU Med Ctr 1984

Levin, David N MD (Nep) - **Spec Exp:** Hypertension; Dialysis Care; **Hospital:** Holy Name Med Ctr (page 720), Hackensack Univ Med Ctr (page 718); **Address:** 870 Palisade Ave, Ste 202, Teaneck, NJ 07666-3419; **Phone:** 201-836-0897; **Board Cert:** Internal Medicine 1979; Nephrology 1982; **Med School:** UMDNJ-NJ Med Sch, Newark 1976; **Resid:** Internal Medicine, Jacobi Med Ctr 1979; **Fellow:** Nephrology, Albert Einstein Coll Med 1981

Pattner, Austin M MD (Nep) - **Spec Exp:** Hypertension; Dialysis Care; Kidney Disease; **Hospital:** Englewood Hosp & Med Ctr, Hackensack Univ Med Ctr (page 718); **Address:** 177 N Dean St, Ste 207, Englewood, NJ 07631; **Phone:** 201-567-0446; **Board Cert:** Internal Medicine 1974; Nephrology 1976; **Med School:** SUNY Upstate Med Univ 1966; **Resid:** Internal Medicine, Roosevelt Hosp 1969; Internal Medicine, Columbia-Presby Med Ctr 1970; **Fellow:** Nephrology, Columbia-Presby Med Ctr 1972; **Fac Appt:** Asst Prof Med, Mount Sinai Sch Med

Rigolosi, Robert S MD (Nep) - **Spec Exp:** Kidney Disease; Hypertension; Dialysis Care; **Hospital:** Holy Name Med Ctr (page 720), Valley Hosp (page 721); **Address:** Holy Name Med Ctr, 718 Teaneck Rd, Teaneck, NJ 07666-4281; **Phone:** 201-833-3223; **Med School:** Italy 1963; **Resid:** Internal Medicine, Bronx VA Hosp 1967; **Fellow:** Renal Disease, Georgetown Univ Hosp 1969

Salazer, Thomas L MD (Nep) - **Hospital:** Hackensack Univ Med Ctr (page 718), Holy Name Med Ctr (page 720); **Address:** 870 Palisade Ave, Ste 202, Teaneck, NJ 07666; **Phone:** 201-836-0897; **Board Cert:** Internal Medicine 2012; Nephrology 2004; **Med School:** SUNY Stony Brook 1989; **Resid:** Internal Medicine, Mayo Clinic 1992; **Fellow:** Nephrology, Mayo Clinic 1994

Tartini, Albert MD (Nep) - **Spec Exp:** Kidney Disease; Hypertension; Dialysis Care; Anemia; **Hospital:** Valley Hosp (page 721), Holy Name Med Ctr (page 720); **Address:** 400 Franklin Tpke, Ste 208, Mahwah, NJ 07430; **Phone:** 201-833-3223; **Board Cert:** Internal Medicine 1988; Nephrology 2010; **Med School:** Grenada 1984; **Resid:** Internal Medicine, St Joseph Hosp Med Ctr 1988; **Fellow:** Nephrology, Univ Vermont Med Ctr 1990

Weizman, Howard B MD (Nep) - **Spec Exp:** Dialysis Care; Hypertension; **Hospital:** Hackensack Univ Med Ctr (page 718), Valley Hosp (page 721); **Address:** 44 Godwin Ave, Ste 301, Midland Park, NJ 07432-1976; **Phone:** 201-447-0013; **Board Cert:** Internal Medicine 1985; Nephrology 2012; **Med School:** Albert Einstein Coll Med 1982; **Resid:** Internal Medicine, Bronx Muni Hosp 1985; **Fellow:** Nephrology, Mount Sinai Med Ctr 1987

Neurological Surgery

Carpenter, Duncan MD (NS) - **Spec Exp:** Spinal Surgery; Spinal Reconstructive Surgery; **Hospital:** Valley Hosp (page 721); **Address:** 225 Dayton St, Ridgewood, NJ 07450-4407; **Phone:** 201-612-0020; **Board Cert:** Neurological Surgery 1987; **Med School:** Columbia P&S 1978; **Resid:** Surgery, St Lukes Hosp 1980; Neurological Surgery, NY Neuro Inst-Columbia 1985

Fried, Arno H MD (NS) - **Spec Exp:** Epilepsy; Brain Tumors; Head Injury; Pediatric Neurosurgery; **Hospital:** Hackensack Univ Med Ctr (page 718), St. Peter's Univ Hosp; **Address:** 20 Prospect Ave, Ste 905, Hackensack, NJ 07601; **Phone:** 201-996-5251; **Board Cert:** Neurological Surgery 1990; **Med School:** Meharry Med Coll 1980; **Resid:** Neurological Surgery, Albert Einstein Coll Med 1986; Neurological Surgery, Univ Utah 1987; **Fellow:** Pediatric Surgery, Chldns Hosp 1987; **Fac Appt:** Assoc Prof NS, NY Med Coll

Moore, Frank M MD (NS) - **Spec Exp:** Aneurysm-Cerebral; Brain Tumors; Spinal Cord Tumors; Spinal Surgery; **Hospital:** Englewood Hosp & Med Ctr, Mt Sinai Med Ctr (page 102); **Address:** Metropolitan Neurosurgery Assocs, 309 Engle St, Ste 6, Englewood, NJ 07631; **Phone:** 201-569-7737; **Board Cert:** Neurological Surgery 1992; **Med School:** France 1983; **Resid:** Neurological Surgery, Mt Sinai Hosp 1988; **Fac Appt:** Assoc Prof NS, Mount Sinai Sch Med

Roth, Patrick A MD (NS) - **Spec Exp:** Spinal Surgery; Brain Tumors; **Hospital:** Hackensack Univ Med Ctr (page 718), Valley Hosp (page 721); **Address:** 680 Kinderkamack Rd, Ste 300, Oradell, NJ 07649; **Phone:** 201-342-2550; **Board Cert:** Neurological Surgery 1997; **Med School:** Albert Einstein Coll Med 1987; **Resid:** Neurological Surgery, New England Med Ctr 1994; **Fac Appt:** Clin Prof NS, UMDNJ-NJ Med Sch, Newark

Steinberger, Alfred A MD (NS) - **Spec Exp:** Spinal Cord Tumors; Aneurysm; Brain Tumors; Spinal Surgery; **Hospital:** Mt Sinai Med Ctr (page 102), Englewood Hosp & Med Ctr; **Address:** 309 Engle St, Englewood, NJ 07631; **Phone:** 201-569-7737; **Board Cert:** Neurological Surgery 1985; **Med School:** Columbia P&S 1976; **Resid:** Neurological Surgery, Neuro Inst-Columbia-Presby 1982; **Fac Appt:** Asst Clin Prof NS, Mount Sinai Sch Med

Vingan, Roy D MD (NS) - **Spec Exp:** Spinal Surgery; Minimally Invasive Spinal Surgery; **Hospital:** Hackensack Univ Med Ctr (page 718), Valley Hosp (page 721); **Address:** 680 Kinderkamack Rd, Ste 300, Oradell, NJ 07649; **Phone:** 201-342-2550; **Board Cert:** Neurological Surgery 1995; **Med School:** SUNY Downstate 1985; **Resid:** Neurological Surgery, SUNY Hlth Sci Ctr 1992

Neurology

Alweiss, Gary S MD (N) - **Spec Exp:** Electromyography; Carpal Tunnel Syndrome; Headache; **Hospital:** Englewood Hosp & Med Ctr; **Address:** 25 Rockwood Pl, Ste 110, Englewood, NJ 07631; **Phone:** 201-894-5805; **Board Cert:** Neurology 1993; **Med School:** Mount Sinai Sch Med 1988; **Resid:** Neurology, Mount Sinai Med Ctr 1992; **Fellow:** Neuromuscular Disease, Columbia-Presby Med Ctr 1993

Effron, Charles MD (N) - **Spec Exp:** Peripheral Neuropathy; **Hospital:** Mt Sinai Med Ctr (page 102); **Address:** 365 W Passaic St, Rochelle Park, NJ 07662; **Phone:** 201-845-6500; **Board Cert:** Neurology 1989; **Med School:** Brown Univ 1983; **Resid:** Neurology, Mt Sinai Hosp 1987

Fellman, Damon MD (N) - **Spec Exp:** Pediatric Neurology; Vascular Neurology; **Hospital:** Hackensack Univ Med Ctr (page 718); **Address:** Hackensack Neurology Group, 211 Essex St, Ste 202, Hackensack, NJ 07601-3245; **Phone:** 201-488-1515; **Board Cert:** Neurology ; Vascular Neurology ; **Med School:** Univ Cincinnati 1970; **Resid:** Neurology, Mount Sinai Hosp 1974; **Fellow:** Neurology, Johns Hopkins Hosp 1976

Klein, Patricia 25MA03348500 MD (N) - **Spec Exp:** Headache; Dizziness; Stroke; **Address:** 680 Kinderkamack Rd, Ste 302, Oradell, NJ 07649; **Phone:** 201-261-6222; **Board Cert:** Neurology 1980; **Med School:** UMDNJ-NJ Med Sch, Newark 1976; **Resid:** Neurology, UMDNJ 1979; **Fac Appt:** Asst Clin Prof N, UMDNJ-NJ Med Sch, Newark

Levin, Kenneth A MD (N) - **Spec Exp:** Stroke; Alzheimer's Disease; Parkinson's Disease; Epilepsy; **Hospital:** Valley Hosp (page 721); **Address:** 1200 E Ridgewood Ave Fl 2 E Wing, Ridgewood, NJ 07450; **Phone:** 201-444-0868; **Board Cert:** Neurology 1987; **Med School:** Indiana Univ 1982; **Resid:** Neurology, Indiana Univ Med Ctr 1986

Perron, Reed C MD (N) - **Hospital:** Valley Hosp (page 721); **Address:** 1200 E Ridgewood Ave Fl 2 E Wing, Ridgewood, NJ 07450; **Phone:** 201-444-0868; **Board Cert:** Neurology 1974; **Med School:** Univ Rochester 1966; **Resid:** Internal Medicine, Cleveland Clinic 1970; Neurology, Albert Einstein Coll Med 1973

Rabin, Aaron MD/PhD (N) - **Spec Exp:** Parkinson's Disease; Dementia; Peripheral Neuropathy; **Hospital:** Englewood Hosp & Med Ctr; **Address:** 700 E Palisade Ave, Englewood Cliffs, NJ 07632; **Phone:** 201-568-3412; **Board Cert:** Neurology 1981; **Med School:** Albert Einstein Coll Med 1976; **Resid:** Neurology, Albert Einstein Coll Med Affil Hosps 1980; **Fellow:** Neuroelectrophysiology, Neur Inst-Columbia Presby 1981; **Fac Appt:** Asst Clin Prof Med, Mount Sinai Sch Med

Van Engel, Daniel R MD (N) - **Spec Exp:** Electromyography; **Hospital:** Valley Hosp (page 721); **Address:** 1200 E Ridgewood Ave Fl 2 E Wing, Ridgewood, NJ 07450-3957; **Phone:** 201-444-0868; **Board Cert:** Neurology 1980; **Med School:** SUNY Upstate Med Univ 1973; **Resid:** Internal Medicine, North Shore Univ Hosp 1975; Neurology, Bronx Muni Hosp 1978

Van Slooten, David D MD (N) - **Spec Exp:** Electromyography; Headache; Dementia; Brain & Spinal Imaging; **Hospital:** Holy Name Med Ctr (page 720), Valley Hosp (page 721); **Address:** 680 Kinderkamack Rd, Ste 302, Oradell, NJ 07649-1500; **Phone:** 201-261-6222; **Board Cert:** Neurology 1989; Clinical Neurophysiology 2004; **Med School:** UMDNJ-NJ Med Sch, Newark 1984; **Resid:** Neurology, UMDNJ Univ Hosp 1988; **Fellow:** Clinical Neurophysiology, VA Med Ctr 1989

Willner, Joseph H MD (N) - **Spec Exp:** Multiple Sclerosis; Myasthenia Gravis; Peripheral Neuropathy; **Hospital:** Englewood Hosp & Med Ctr; **Address:** 25 Rockwood Pl, Ste 110, Englewood, NJ 07631-4363; **Phone:** 201-894-5805; **Board Cert:** Neurology 1978; **Med School:** NYU Sch Med 1970; **Resid:** Neurology, Columbia-Presby Hosp 1977; **Fac Appt:** Assoc Clin Prof N, Columbia P&S

Neuroradiology

Lerner, Elliot J MD (NRad) - **Spec Exp:** Brain & Spinal Imaging; Head & Neck Imaging; **Hospital:** Valley Hosp (page 721); **Address:** Radiology Assocs of Ridgewood, 20 Franklin Tpke, Waldwick, NJ 07463-1749; **Phone:** 201-445-8822; **Board Cert:** Diagnostic Radiology 1990; Neuroradiology 2004; **Med School:** Brown Univ 1985; **Resid:** Diagnostic Radiology, Hosp Univ Penn 1989; **Fellow:** Neuroradiology, Hosp Univ Penn 1991

Pierce, Sean D MD (NRad) - **Spec Exp:** Neuro-Oncology; **Hospital:** Hackensack Univ Med Ctr (page 718); **Address:** HackensackUMC-Radiology, 30 Prospect Ave, Hackensack, NJ 07601; **Phone:** 551-996-2194; **Board Cert:** Diagnostic Radiology ; Neurotology 2012; **Med School:** Harvard Med Sch 1994; **Resid:** Diagnostic Radiology, Barnes Hosp 1999; **Fellow:** Neurological Radiology, NYU Med Ctr 2001

Nuclear Medicine

Agress Jr, Harry MD (NuM) - **Spec Exp:** PET Imaging; Cancer Detection & Staging; Nuclear Oncology; CT Scan; **Hospital:** Hackensack Univ Med Ctr (page 718); **Address:** Hackensack University Medical Center, 30 Prospect Ave, Hackensack, NJ 07601; **Phone:** 201-996-2196; **Board Cert:** Nuclear Medicine 1976; Diagnostic Radiology 1978; **Med School:** Tufts Univ 1972; **Resid:** Radiology, Columbia- Presby Med Ctr 1978; **Fellow:** Nuclear Medicine, Natl Inst Hlth 1975; **Fac Appt:** Clin Prof Rad, Columbia P&S

Brunetti, Jacqueline C MD (NuM) - **Spec Exp:** PET Imaging; CT Scan; Prostate Cancer-MR Spectroscopy (MRSI); **Hospital:** Holy Name Med Ctr (page 720); **Address:** Holy Name Med Ctr, 718 Teaneck Rd, Teaneck, NJ 07666-4281; **Phone:** 201-833-7225; **Board Cert:** Diagnostic Radiology 1979; Nuclear Medicine 1980; Nuclear Radiology 1980; **Med School:** SUNY Downstate 1975; **Resid:** Diagnostic Radiology, St Vincents Hosp 1979; **Fellow:** Nuclear Medicine, St Vincents Hosp 1980; **Fac Appt:** Assoc Clin Prof Rad, Columbia P&S

Obstetrics & Gynecology

Butler, David G MD (ObG) *PCP* - **Spec Exp:** Gynecologic Surgery; Menopause Problems; **Hospital:** Holy Name Med Ctr (page 720), Englewood Hosp & Med Ctr; **Address:** 420 Grand Ave, Ste 201, Englewood, NJ 07631-4152; **Phone:** 201-871-4040; **Board Cert:** Obstetrics & Gynecology 1972; **Med School:** SUNY Downstate 1965; **Resid:** Obstetrics & Gynecology, St Vincents Hosp 1970

Cavallaro, Barbara A MD (ObG) - **Hospital:** Hackensack Univ Med Ctr (page 718); **Address:** 170 Prospect Ave, Bldg 2, Ste 4, Hackensack, NJ 07601-2255; **Phone:** 201-488-2288; **Board Cert:** Obstetrics & Gynecology 2012; **Med School:** NYU Sch Med 1986; **Resid:** Obstetrics & Gynecology, Mt Sinai Med Ctr 1991

Coven, Roger MD (ObG) - **Hospital:** Valley Hosp (page 721); **Address:** 581 N Franklin Tpke, Ramsey, NJ 07446; **Phone:** 201-447-2200; **Board Cert:** Obstetrics & Gynecology 2013; **Med School:** UMDNJ-NJ Med Sch, Newark 1980; **Resid:** Obstetrics & Gynecology, Thomas Jefferson Univ Hosp 1984

Englert, Christopher A MD (ObG) - **Spec Exp:** Gynecologic Surgery; Laparoscopic Surgery; Robotic Surgery; Vulvar & Vaginal Disorders; **Hospital:** Holy Name Med Ctr (page 720); **Address:** 420 Grand Ave, Ste 201, Englewood, NJ 07631-4141; **Phone:** 201-871-4040; **Board Cert:** Obstetrics & Gynecology 2012; **Med School:** Univ Cincinnati 1985; **Resid:** Obstetrics & Gynecology, Thomas Jefferson Univ Hosp 1990

Faust, Michael G MD (ObG) - **Spec Exp:** Gynecologic Surgery; Menopause Problems; Minimally Invasive Surgery; **Hospital:** Valley Hosp (page 721); **Address:** Valley Ctr for Womens Hlth, 581 N Franklin Tpke, Ramsey, NJ 07446; **Phone:** 201-236-2100; **Board Cert:** Obstetrics & Gynecology 2012; **Med School:** Univ Pittsburgh 1983; **Resid:** Obstetrics & Gynecology, Thomas Jefferson Univ Hosp 1988

Fernandez, Jacinto J MD (ObG) - **Spec Exp:** Women's Health; Uro-Gynecology; **Hospital:** Holy Name Med Ctr (page 720); **Address:** 222 Cedar Ln, Teaneck, NJ 07666; **Phone:** 201-833-7087; **Board Cert:** Obstetrics & Gynecology 1976; **Med School:** Spain 1967; **Resid:** Obstetrics & Gynecology, St. Joseph's Hosp 1975; **Fac Appt:** Prof ObG, Spain

Hurst, Wendy R MD (ObG) - **Spec Exp:** Gynecology Only; Laparoscopic Surgery; Menopause Problems; Adolescent Gynecology; **Hospital:** Englewood Hosp & Med Ctr; **Address:** 370 Grand Ave, Ste 202, Englewood, NJ 07631-4109; **Phone:** 201-894-9599; **Board Cert:** Obstetrics & Gynecology 2012; **Med School:** Tufts Univ 1986; **Resid:** Obstetrics & Gynecology, Hosp Univ Penn - UPHS 1991

Meyer, Monica L MD (ObG) *PCP* - **Spec Exp:** Adolescent Gynecology; Gynecology Only; Menopause Problems; **Hospital:** Valley Hosp (page 721); **Address:** The Women's Grp of Ridgewood, 1 W Ridgewood Ave, Ste 211, Paramus, NJ 07652; **Phone:** 201-251-2323; **Board Cert:** Obstetrics & Gynecology 2012; **Med School:** SUNY Downstate 1991; **Resid:** Obstetrics & Gynecology, Lenox Hill Hosp 1996

Rezvani, Fred F MD (ObG) - **Spec Exp:** Pregnancy-High Risk; Minimally Invasive Surgery; Congenital Anomalies-Gynecologic; **Hospital:** Valley Hosp (page 721); **Address:** 119 Prospect St, Ridgewood, NJ 07450; **Phone:** 201-444-1600; **Board Cert:** Obstetrics & Gynecology 2007; **Med School:** West Indies 1983; **Resid:** Obstetrics & Gynecology, Lincoln Med & Mental Hlth Ctr 1988

Rubenstein, Andrew F MD (ObG) - **Hospital:** Hackensack Univ Med Ctr (page 718); **Address:** 82 E Allendale Rd, Ste 1A, Saddle River, NJ 07458; **Phone:** 201-934-5050; **Board Cert:** Obstetrics & Gynecology 2012; **Med School:** Hahnemann Univ 1990; **Resid:** Obstetrics & Gynecology, Mt Sinai Med Ctr 1995; **Fac Appt:** Assoc Clin Prof ObG, UMDNJ-NJ Med Sch, Newark

Schulze, Ruth J MD (ObG) - **Spec Exp:** Vulvar Disease; Osteoporosis; **Hospital:** Valley Hosp (page 721); **Address:** Women's Total Health, 577 Chestnut Ridge Rd Fl 2, Woodcliff Lake, NJ 07677; **Phone:** 201-391-5770; **Board Cert:** Obstetrics & Gynecology 2012; **Med School:** SUNY Stony Brook 1983; **Resid:** Obstetrics & Gynecology, Baystate Med Ctr 1987

Ophthalmology

Brown, Andrew C MD (Oph) - **Spec Exp:** LASIK-Refractive Surgery; Cataract Surgery; Macular Degeneration; **Hospital:** Hackensack Univ Med Ctr (page 718); **Address:** Brown Eye Care Assocs, 751 Teaneck Rd, Teaneck, NJ 07666; **Phone:** 201-833-0006; **Board Cert:** Ophthalmology 2009; **Med School:** Boston Univ 2002; **Resid:** Ophthalmology, New York Eye & Ear Infirm 2007

Brown, Christopher D MD (Oph) - **Spec Exp:** Corneal Disease; Diabetic Eye Disease/Retinopathy; LASIK-Refractive Surgery; **Hospital:** Englewood Hosp & Med Ctr, Holy Name Med Ctr (page 720); **Address:** Brown Eye Care Assocs, 751 Teaneck Rd, Teaneck, NJ 07666; **Phone:** 201-833-0006; **Med School:** Boston Univ 1996; **Resid:** Ophthalmology, Wills Eye Hosp 2001; **Fellow:** Refractive Surgery, Vision Correction Ctr 2002

Burke, Patricia A MD (Oph) - **Spec Exp:** Corneal Disease; Cataract Surgery; **Hospital:** Holy Name Med Ctr (page 720); **Address:** One Sears Drive, Paramus, NJ 07652; **Phone:** 201-599-0123; **Board Cert:** Ophthalmology 1991; **Med School:** UMDNJ-NJ Med Sch, Newark 1986; **Resid:** Ophthalmology, NY-Presby/Columbia Univ Med Ctr 1990; **Fellow:** Cornea, Lenox Hill Hosp (Manh Eye, Ear & Throat Hosp) 1991

Chin, Patrick K MD (Oph) - **Spec Exp:** Laser Vision Surgery; Cataract Surgery; Refractive Surgery; **Hospital:** Valley Hosp (page 721); **Address:** Westwood Ophthalmology Assocs, 300 Fairview Ave, Westwood, NJ 07675; **Phone:** 201-666-4014; **Board Cert:** Ophthalmology 2007; **Med School:** UMDNJ-NJ Med Sch, Newark 1989; **Resid:** Ophthalmology, NYU Langone Med Ctr 1994; **Fellow:** Ophthalmology, Gimbel Eye Ctr 1995

DeLuca, Joseph A MD (Oph) - **Spec Exp:** Cataract Surgery; Laser Refractive Surgery; Anterior Segment Surgery; Trauma; **Hospital:** Clara Maass Med Ctr; **Address:** 20 Park Ave Fl 1, Lyndhurst, NJ 07071-1012; **Phone:** 201-896-0096; **Board Cert:** Ophthalmology 1991; **Med School:** UMDNJ-Rutgers Med Sch 1985; **Resid:** Ophthalmology, United Hosp Med Ctr 1991; **Fac Appt:** Asst Clin Prof Oph, UMDNJ-NJ Med Sch, Newark

Hersh, Peter S MD (Oph) - **Spec Exp:** LASIK-Refractive Surgery; Cornea Transplant; Keratoconus; **Hospital:** Univ Hosp (Newark); **Address:** The Cornea & Laser Eye Inst-Hersh Vision Grp, Glenpointe Center East, 300 Frank W Burr Blvd, Ste 71, Teaneck, NJ 07666-6704; **Phone:** 201-883-0505; **Board Cert:** Ophthalmology 1987; **Med School:** Johns Hopkins Univ 1982; **Resid:** Internal Medicine, Lenox Hill Hosp 1983; Ophthalmology, Mass Eye & Ear Infirm 1986; **Fellow:** Cornea & Ext Eye Disease, Mass Eye & Ear Infirm 1987; **Fac Appt:** Clin Prof Oph, UMDNJ-NJ Med Sch, Newark

Liva, Douglas MD (Oph) - **Spec Exp:** LASIK-Refractive Surgery; Cataract Surgery; Glaucoma; **Hospital:** Valley Hosp (page 721); **Address:** 1 W Ridgewood Ave, Ste 101 Bldg, Paramus, NJ 07652-2350; **Phone:** 201-444-7770; **Board Cert:** Ophthalmology 1987; **Med School:** Univ Miami Sch Med 1981; **Resid:** Ophthalmology, UMDNJ Affil Hosps 1986

Norden, Richard A MD (Oph) - **Spec Exp:** LASIK-Refractive Surgery; Laser Vision Surgery; **Address:** 1144 E Ridgewood Ave, Ridgewood, NJ 07450-3915; **Phone:** 201-444-2442; **Board Cert:** Ophthalmology 1985; **Med School:** Southern IL Univ 1980; **Resid:** Ophthalmology, UMDNJ Med Ctr 1984; **Fellow:** Cornea & Refractive Surgery, NY Eye & Ear Infirm 1986; **Fac Appt:** Asst Clin Prof Oph, NY Med Coll

Silbert, Glenn MD (Oph) - **Hospital:** Hackensack Univ Med Ctr (page 718), New York Eye & Ear Infirm (page 115); **Address:** 316 State St, Hackensack, NJ 07601-5529; **Phone:** 201-342-8115; **Board Cert:** Ophthalmology 1985; **Med School:** Columbia P&S 1979; **Resid:** Ophthalmology, NYU Langone Med Ctr 1984; **Fac Appt:** Assoc Prof Oph, NY Med Coll

Solomon, Edward MD (Oph) - **Spec Exp:** Cataract Surgery; Laser Surgery; **Hospital:** Valley Hosp (page 721); **Address:** 85 S Maple Ave, Ridgewood, NJ 07450-4500; **Phone:** 201-444-3010; **Board Cert:** Ophthalmology 1976; **Med School:** Tufts Univ 1968; **Resid:** Ophthalmology, NYU Med Ctr 1974

Stabile, John R MD (Oph) - **Spec Exp:** Cataract Surgery; Oculoplastic Surgery; LASIK-Refractive Surgery; **Hospital:** Englewood Hosp & Med Ctr, Holy Name Med Ctr (page 720); **Address:** Tenafly Eye Assocs, 11 Dean Drive, Tenafly, NJ 07670-2764; **Phone:** 201-567-5995; **Board Cert:** Ophthalmology 1981; **Med School:** NY Med Coll 1976; **Resid:** Ophthalmology, St. Luke's - Roosevelt Hosp Ctr - St Luke's Hosp 1980; **Fellow:** Oculoplastic Surgery, NY-Presby/Columbia Univ Med Ctr 1981; **Fac Appt:** Clin Prof Oph, Columbia P&S

Topilow, Harvey W MD (Oph) - **Spec Exp:** Retinal Disorders; Macular Degeneration; Retinopathy of Prematurity; **Hospital:** New York Eye & Ear Infirm (page 115); **Address:** 301 Bridge Plaza N, Fort Lee, NJ 07024; **Phone:** 212-288-3860; **Board Cert:** Ophthalmology 1980; **Med School:** Columbia P&S 1975; **Resid:** Ophthalmology, Albert Einstein Coll Med Affil Hosps 1979; **Fellow:** Vitreoretinal Surgery, Mass Eye & Ear Infirm 1980; **Fac Appt:** Assoc Clin Prof Oph, Albert Einstein Coll Med

Weinberg, Martin R MD (Oph) - **Spec Exp:** Neuro-Ophthalmology; Glaucoma; **Hospital:** Englewood Hosp & Med Ctr, Hackensack Univ Med Ctr (page 718); **Address:** 405 Cedar Ln, Ste 5, Teaneck, NJ 07666-1715; **Phone:** 201-836-8333; **Board Cert:** Ophthalmology 1989; **Med School:** Eastern VA Med Sch 1979; **Resid:** Surgery, Albany Meml Hosp 1981; Ophthalmology, Kings Co Hosp Ctr 1986; **Fellow:** Ocular Pathology, Scheie Eye Inst-Univ Penn 1983; Ocular Oncology, Lenox Hill Hosp (Manh Eye, Ear & Throat Hosp) 1987

Orthopaedic Surgery

Altman, Wayne MD (OrS) - **Spec Exp:** Carpal Tunnel Syndrome; Knee Injuries; Hand & Wrist Injuries; Shoulder Injuries; **Hospital:** St. Mary's Hosp - Passaic, Meadowlands Hosp Med Ctr; **Address:** 85 Orient Way, FL 1, Rutherford, NJ 07070; **Phone:** 201-438-5888; **Board Cert:** Orthopaedic Surgery 2009; **Med School:** UMDNJ-NJ Med Sch, Newark 1978; **Resid:** Orthopaedic Surgery, UMDNJ-NJ Med Sch Affil Hosp 1983; **Fellow:** Hand Surgery, Thomas Jefferson Univ Hosp 1984

Berman, Mark MD (OrS) - **Spec Exp:** Knee Surgery; Shoulder Surgery; Rotator Cuff Surgery; Sports Medicine; **Hospital:** Hackensack Univ Med Ctr (page 718), Holy Name Med Ctr (page 720); **Address:** 920 Main St Fl 2, Hackensack, NJ 07601-3246; **Phone:** 201-489-8250; **Board Cert:** Orthopaedic Surgery 2010; **Med School:** Mount Sinai Sch Med 1981; **Resid:** Surgery, Mt Sinai Med Ctr 1983; Orthopaedic Surgery, SUNY Downstate Med Ctr (Univ Hosp Brooklyn) 1986; **Fellow:** Sports Medicine, Lenox Hill Hosp 1987

Cahill, James W MD (OrS) - **Spec Exp:** Arthroscopic Surgery-Knee; Joint Replacement; Shoulder Arthroscopic Surgery; Cartilage Damage; **Hospital:** Hackensack Univ Med Ctr (page 718), Holy Name Med Ctr (page 720); **Address:** 87 Summit Ave, Hackensack, NJ 07601; **Phone:** 201-489-0022; **Board Cert:** Orthopaedic Surgery 2010; **Med School:** Columbia P&S 1990; **Resid:** Orthopaedic Surgery, Montefiore Med Ctr 1995; **Fellow:** Sports Medicine, NYU Hosp For Joint Dis 1996

Distefano, Michael MD (OrS) - **Spec Exp:** Fractures-Stress; Shoulder & Knee Surgery; Trauma; Sports Medicine; **Hospital:** Hackensack Univ Med Ctr (page 718), Valley Hosp (page 721); **Address:** 140 Route 17 N, Ste 255, Paramus, NJ 07652; **Phone:** 201-261-5501; **Board Cert:** Orthopaedic Surgery 1983; Orthopaedic Sports Medicine 2007; **Med School:** Albert Einstein Coll Med 1977; **Resid:** Orthopaedic Surgery, Montefiore Med Ctr 1981; **Fellow:** Orthopaedic Sports Medicine, Montefiore Med Ctr 2007; **Fac Appt:** Asst Clin Prof OrS, Albert Einstein Coll Med

Doidge, Robert W DO (OrS) - **Spec Exp:** Knee Surgery; Shoulder Surgery; Sports Medicine; **Hospital:** Englewood Hosp & Med Ctr; **Address:** 370 Grand Ave, Ste 100, Englewood, NJ 07631-4109; **Phone:** 201-567-5700; **Board Cert:** Orthopaedic Surgery 2001; **Med School:** Philadelphia Coll Osteo Med 1986; **Resid:** Orthopaedic Surgery, St. John Macomb-Oakland Hosp-Oakland Campus 1992; **Fellow:** Sports Medicine, Michigan State Univ Affil Hosp 1993

Esformes, Ira MD (OrS) - **Spec Exp:** Sports Medicine; Arthroscopic Surgery; Joint Replacement; **Hospital:** Valley Hosp (page 721), Hackensack Univ Med Ctr (page 718); **Address:** 440 Old Hook Rd Fl 2, Emerson, NJ 07630-1325; **Phone:** 201-261-3333; **Board Cert:** Orthopaedic Surgery 1985; Orthopaedic Sports Medicine 2009; **Med School:** Albany Med Coll 1977; **Resid:** Surgery, N Shore Univ Hosp 1979; Orthopaedic Surgery, Hosp For Joint Dis 1983

Gennace, Ronald MD (OrS) - **Hospital:** Clara Maass Med Ctr, Saint Michael's Med Ctr; **Address:** 312 Belleville Tpke, Ste 2A, North Arlington, NJ 07031; **Phone:** 201-997-8777; **Board Cert:** Orthopaedic Surgery 1982; **Med School:** UMDNJ-NJ Med Sch, Newark 1976; **Resid:** Orthopaedic Surgery, St. Joseph's Regl Med Ctr 1982

Hartzband, Mark A MD (OrS) - **Spec Exp:** Knee Replacement; Hip Replacement; **Hospital:** Hackensack Univ Med Ctr (page 718), Holy Name Med Ctr (page 720); **Address:** 10 Forest Ave, Paramus, NJ 07652; **Phone:** 201-291-4040; **Board Cert:** Orthopaedic Surgery 2007; **Med School:** McGill Univ 1978; **Resid:** Surgery, Montefiore Med Ctr 1981; Orthopaedic Surgery, Montefiore Med Ctr 1984

Implicito, Dante A MD (OrS) - **Spec Exp:** Spinal Surgery; **Hospital:** Hackensack Univ Med Ctr (page 718); **Address:** 266 Harristown Rd, Glen Rock, NJ 07452; **Phone:** 201-251-7725; **Board Cert:** Orthopaedic Surgery 2009; **Med School:** UMDNJ-NJ Med Sch, Newark 1990; **Resid:** Orthopaedic Surgery, UMDNJ Med Ctr 1995; **Fellow:** Spine Surgery, St. Marys Hosp 1996

Kelly, Michael A MD (OrS) - **Spec Exp:** Knee Surgery; Knee Replacement; Arthroscopic Surgery; **Hospital:** Hackensack Univ Med Ctr (page 718), Lenox Hill Hosp (page 106); **Address:** 360 Essex St, Ste 303, Hackensack, NJ 07601; **Phone:** 551-996-8867; **Board Cert:** Orthopaedic Surgery 2009; **Med School:** Georgetown Univ 1979; **Resid:** Surgery, St Vincents Hosp 1981; Orthopaedic Surgery, NY-Presby/Columbia Univ Med Ctr 1984; **Fellow:** Knee Surgery, Hosp for Special Surgery 1985

McIlveen, Stephen J MD (OrS) - **Spec Exp:** Joint Replacement; Sports Medicine; Shoulder Surgery; Knee Surgery; **Hospital:** Valley Hosp (page 721), Hackensack Univ Med Ctr (page 718); **Address:** 1 W Ridgewood Ave, Ste 307, Paramus, NJ 07652; **Phone:** 201-670-6702; **Board Cert:** Orthopaedic Surgery 1983; **Med School:** NYU Sch Med 1973; **Resid:** Surgery, NY-Presby/Columbia Univ Med Ctr 1975; Orthopaedic Surgery, NY-Presby/Columbia Univ Med Ctr 1978; **Fellow:** Joint Replacement Surgery, NY-Presby/Columbia Univ Med Ctr 1979; Elbow & Shoulder Surgery, NY-Presby/Columbia Univ Med Ctr 1979; **Fac Appt:** Asst Prof OrS, Columbia P&S

Pizzurro, Joseph MD (OrS) - **Spec Exp:** Hip & Knee Replacement; Joint Replacement; **Hospital:** Valley Hosp (page 721); **Address:** Ridgewood Orthopedic Grp, 85 S Maple Ave Fl 2, Ridgewood, NJ 07450; **Phone:** 201-445-2830; **Board Cert:** Orthopaedic Surgery 1972; **Med School:** St Louis Univ 1963; **Resid:** Surgery, Bronx VA Hosp 1968; Orthopaedic Surgery, Bellevue Hosp Ctr 1971; **Fellow:** Orthopaedic Surgery, Ameri Academy Ortho Surg 1975

Pollock, Roger G MD (OrS) - **Spec Exp:** Rotator Cuff Surgery; Shoulder Injuries; Shoulder Arthroscopic Surgery; **Hospital:** NY-Presby/Columbia Univ Med Ctr, NY (page 104), Valley Hosp (page 721); **Address:** 1 W Ridgewood Ave, Ste 202, Paramus, NJ 07625; **Phone:** 201-612-9774; **Board Cert:** Orthopaedic Surgery 2005; **Med School:** Columbia P&S 1985; **Resid:** Surgery, St. Luke's - Roosevelt Hosp Ctr - Roosevelt Div 1987; Orthopaedic Surgery, NY-Presby/Columbia Univ Med Ctr 1991; **Fellow:** Shoulder Surgery, NY-Presby/Columbia Univ Med Ctr 1992; **Fac Appt:** Asst Prof OrS, Columbia P&S

Salzer Jr, Richard L MD (OrS) - **Spec Exp:** Hip & Knee Replacement; Knee Surgery; Joint Replacement; Minimally Invasive Surgery; **Hospital:** Englewood Hosp & Med Ctr, Palisades Med Ctr; **Address:** Englewood Orthopedic Assocs, 401 S Van Brunt St Fl 3, Englewood, NJ 07631-4800; **Phone:** 201-569-2770; **Board Cert:** Orthopaedic Surgery 1979; **Med School:** Tufts Univ 1973; **Resid:** Surgery, UT Southwestern Med Ctr-St. Paul Campus 1975; Orthopaedic Surgery, Hosp Special Surg 1978

Otolaryngology

Henick, David H MD (Oto) - **Spec Exp:** Nasal & Sinus Surgery; Endoscopic Sinus Surgery; Head & Neck Surgery; **Hospital:** Englewood Hosp & Med Ctr, Hackensack Univ Med Ctr (page 718); **Address:** 301 Bridge Plaza N Fl 3, Fort Lee, NJ 07024-5059; **Phone:** 201-592-8200; **Board Cert:** Otolaryngology 1993; **Med School:** SUNY Buffalo 1987; **Resid:** Otolaryngology, Montefiore Med Ctr 1992; **Fellow:** Head and Neck Surgery, Montefiore Med Ctr 1993; Rhinoplasty & Sinus Surgery, Hosp Univ Penn - UPHS 1994; **Fac Appt:** Asst Clin Prof Oto, UMDNJ-NJ Med Sch, Newark

Ho, Bryan MD (Oto) - **Spec Exp:** Sinus Surgery; Thyroid & Parathyroid Surgery; **Hospital:** Englewood Hosp & Med Ctr, Holy Name Med Ctr (page 720); **Address:** 216 Engle St, Ste 101, Englewood, NJ 07631-2428; **Phone:** 201-816-9800; **Board Cert:** Otolaryngology 1995; **Med School:** Mount Sinai Sch Med 1989; **Resid:** Surgery, Mount Sinai Med Ctr 1991; Otolaryngology, Mount Sinai Med Ctr 1994

Katz, Harry MD (Oto) - **Spec Exp:** Sinus Disorders; **Hospital:** Valley Hosp (page 721); **Address:** 44 Godwin Ave, Ste 300, Midland Park, NJ 07432-1959; **Phone:** 201-445-2900; **Board Cert:** Otolaryngology 1982; **Med School:** NYU Sch Med 1977; **Resid:** Otolaryngology, NYU Langone Med Ctr 1982

Low, Ronald B MD (Oto) - **Spec Exp:** Head & Neck Surgery; Rhinoplasty; Sinus Surgery; **Hospital:** Hackensack Univ Med Ctr (page 718); **Address:** 20 Prospect Ave, Ste 909, Hackensack, NJ 07601-5013; **Phone:** 201-489-6520; **Board Cert:** Otolaryngology 1974; **Med School:** UMDNJ-NJ Med Sch, Newark 1969; **Resid:** Surgery, Montefiore Med Ctr 1971; Otolaryngology, Bellevue Hosp Ctr 1974; **Fac Appt:** Asst Clin Prof Oto

Milgrim, Laurence M MD (Oto) - **Spec Exp:** Facial Plastic Surgery; **Hospital:** Holy Name Med Ctr (page 720), Valley Hosp (page 721); **Address:** 1 Degraw Ave, Teaneck, NJ 07666; **Phone:** 201-837-2174; **Board Cert:** Otolaryngology 1995; Facial Plastic & Reconstr Surgery 2000; **Med School:** UMDNJ-Rutgers Med Sch 1989; **Resid:** Otolaryngology, Montefiore Med Ctr 1995; **Fellow:** Facial Plastic & Reconstr Surgery, Mt Sinai Med Ctr 1995

Rosen, Arie MD (Oto) - **Spec Exp:** Head & Neck Tumors; Sinus Disorders; Facial Plastic Surgery; Ear Surgery; **Hospital:** Hackensack Univ Med Ctr (page 718), Englewood Hosp & Med Ctr; **Address:** 2 S Summit Ave, Hackensack, NJ 07601-1117; **Phone:** 201-996-9200; **Board Cert:** Otolaryngology 1995; **Med School:** Israel 1982; **Resid:** Otolaryngology, Univ Chicago-Pritzker Sch Affil Hosp 1994

Scherl, Michael MD (Oto) - **Spec Exp:** Hearing Loss/Tinnitus; Nasal & Sinus Disorders; **Hospital:** Englewood Hosp & Med Ctr; **Address:** 3541 Old Hook Rd, Westwood, NJ 07675; **Phone:** 201-666-8787; **Board Cert:** Otolaryngology 1987; **Med School:** Albany Med Coll 1982; **Resid:** Surgery, Mount Sinai Med Ctr 1984; Otolaryngology, Mount Sinai Med Ctr 1987; **Fac Appt:** , Mount Sinai Sch Med

Shaari, Christopher MD (Oto) - **Spec Exp:** Sinus Disorders/Surgery; Thyroid & Parathyroid Cancer & Surgery; **Hospital:** Hackensack Univ Med Ctr (page 718); **Address:** 20 Prospect Ave, Ste 712, Hackensack, NJ 07601; **Phone:** 201-342-8060; **Board Cert:** Otolaryngology 1997; **Med School:** Albany Med Coll 1991; **Resid:** Otolaryngology, Mt Sinai Hosp 1996; **Fellow:** Head and Neck Surgery, Mt Sinai Hosp 1997

Surow, Jason B MD (Oto) - **Spec Exp:** Pediatric Otolaryngology; Sinus Disorders; Voice Disorders; **Hospital:** Valley Hosp (page 721), Good Samaritan Regional Med Ctr; **Address:** 690 Kinderkamack Rd, Ste 101, Oradell, NJ 07649; **Phone:** 201-722-9850; **Board Cert:** Otolaryngology 1987; **Med School:** Univ Pennsylvania 1982; **Resid:** Surgery, Hosp Univ Penn - UPHS 1984; Otolaryngology, Hosp Univ Penn - UPHS 1987

Tobias, Geoffrey W MD (Oto) - **Spec Exp:** Rhinoplasty Revision; Nasal Surgery; Nasal Reconstruction; **Hospital:** Englewood Hosp & Med Ctr, Mt Sinai Med Ctr (page 102); **Address:** 214 Engle St, Ste 22, Englewood, NJ 07631; **Phone:** 201-567-6770; **Board Cert:** Otolaryngology 1978; **Med School:** Tufts Univ 1973; **Resid:** Otolaryngology, Mt Sinai Med Ctr 1978

Pain Medicine

Datta, Samyadev MD (PM) - **Spec Exp:** Complex Regional Pain Syndromes; Pain-Cancer; Pain-Back; **Hospital:** Holy Name Med Ctr (page 720); **Address:** Ctr for Pain Management, 294 State St, Ste 1, Hackensack, NJ 07601; **Phone:** 201-488-7246; **Board Cert:** Anesthesiology 1996; Pain Medicine 2009; **Med School:** India 1979; **Resid:** Anesthesiology, NY Presby Hosp 1994

Park, Kenneth H DO (PM) - **Spec Exp:** Pain-Chronic; Pain-Back; Pain-Neuropathic; Pain-Cancer; **Hospital:** Holy Name Med Ctr (page 720); **Address:** 680 Kinderkamack Rd, Ste 207, Oradell, NJ 07649; **Phone:** 201-487-7246; **Board Cert:** Anesthesiology 2007; Pain Medicine 2007; **Med School:** NY Coll Osteo Med 2002; **Resid:** Anesthesiology, Brigham & Women's Hosp 2006; **Fellow:** Pain Medicine, Brigham & Women's Hosp 2007

Ragukonis, Thomas P MD (PM) - ; **Address:** Bergen Pain Mngmt, 37 W Century Rd, Ste 101, Paramus, NJ 07652; **Phone:** 201-634-9000; **Board Cert:** Anesthesiology 1999; Pain Medicine 2000; **Med School:** UMDNJ-NJ Med Sch, Newark 1991; **Resid:** Anesthesiology, NY-Presby/Columbia Univ Med Ctr 1995; **Fac Appt:** Asst Clin Prof Anes, UMDNJ-NJ Med Sch, Newark

Silverman, Robert S MD (PM) - **Hospital:** Valley Hosp (page 721); **Address:** Vally Inst for Pain, 1 Valley Health Plaza, Paramus, NJ 07652; **Phone:** 201-634-5555; **Board Cert:** Anesthesiology 1999; Pain Medicine 2011; **Med School:** NE Ohio Univ 1993; **Resid:** Anesthesiology, Cleveland Clinic 1997; **Fellow:** Pain Medicine, Cleveland Clinic 2000

Pathology

Olsen, Drew A MD (Path) - **Spec Exp:** Gynecologic Pathology; **Hospital:** Holy Name Med Ctr (page 720); **Address:** 718 Teaneck Rd, Teaneck, NJ 07666; **Phone:** 201-833-3246; **Board Cert:** Anatomic & Clinical Pathology ; **Med School:** NY Med Coll 1995; **Resid:** Anatomic & Clinical Pathology, Yale-New Haven Hosp 1999; **Fellow:** Surgical Pathology, Yale-New Haven Hosp 2000

Sanchez, Miguel A MD (Path) - **Spec Exp:** Breast Cancer; Thyroid Cancer; **Hospital:** Englewood Hosp & Med Ctr; **Address:** 350 Engle St, Dean Bldg - Fl LL1, Englewood, NJ 07631-1898; **Phone:** 201-894-3423; **Board Cert:** Anatomic Pathology 1975; Clinical Pathology 1979; Cytopathology 1991; **Med School:** Spain 1969; **Resid:** Pathology, Englewood Hosp 1972; Pathology, Temple Univ 1973; **Fellow:** Pathology, Meml Sloan Kettering Cancer Ctr 1974; Clinical Pathology, St Vincents Hosp 1975; **Fac Appt:** Assoc Prof Path, Mount Sinai Sch Med

Pediatric Allergy & Immunology

Colenda, Maryann MD (PA&I) - **Spec Exp:** Asthma-Adult & Pediatric; Allergy; **Hospital:** Englewood Hosp & Med Ctr, Meadowlands Hosp Med Ctr; **Address:** 811 Abbott Blvd, Fort Lee, NJ 07024-4116; **Phone:** 201-224-2256; **Board Cert:** Pediatrics 1976; Allergy & Immunology 1979; **Med School:** NY Med Coll 1971; **Resid:** Pediatrics, NY-Presby/Columbia Univ Med Ctr 1975; **Fellow:** Allergy & Immunology, NY-Presby/Columbia Univ Med Ctr 1978; **Fac Appt:** Assoc Clin Prof Ped, Columbia P&S

Hicks, Patricia MD (PA&I) - **Spec Exp:** Asthma & Sinusitis; Asthma in Pregnancy; **Hospital:** Valley Hosp (page 721); **Address:** 119 1st St, Ste 5, Hohokus, NJ 07423-1575; **Phone:** 201-444-5277; **Board Cert:** Pediatrics 1978; Allergy & Immunology 2001; **Med School:** Penn State Coll Med 1973; **Resid:** Pediatrics, NY-Presby/Columbia Univ Med Ctr 1977; **Fellow:** Allergy & Immunology, NY-Presby/Columbia Univ Med Ctr 1979

Pediatric Cardiology

Messina, John J MD (PCd) - **Spec Exp:** Critical Care; Interventional Cardiology; Congenital Heart Disease; **Hospital:** St. Joseph's Regl Med Ctr - Paterson; **Address:** 1 Broadway, Ste 203, Elmwood Park, NJ 07407-1844; **Phone:** 973-569-6250; **Board Cert:** Pediatrics 2009; Pediatric Cardiology 2009; **Med School:** West Indies 1986; **Resid:** Pediatrics, St. Joseph's Regl Med Ctr 1989; **Fellow:** Pediatric Cardiology, NY-Presby/Weill Cornell Med Ctr 1992; **Fac Appt:** Asst Prof Ped, Columbia P&S

Solowiejczyk, David E MD (PCd) - **Spec Exp:** Echocardiography; **Hospital:** Morgan Stanley Children's Hosp of NY-Presby, NY (page 104); **Address:** Pediatric Cardiology, 205 Robin Rd, Ste 100, Paramus, NJ 07652; **Phone:** 201-599-0026; **Board Cert:** Pediatric Cardiology 2011; **Med School:** NYU Sch Med 1986; **Resid:** Pediatrics, Mt Sinai Med Ctr 1989; **Fellow:** Cardiovascular Disease, NY Presby Hosp-Columbia Med Ctr 1993; **Fac Appt:** Assoc Prof Ped, Columbia P&S

Tozzi, Robert J MD (PCd) - **Spec Exp:** Hypertrophic Cardiomyopathy; Fetal Echocardiography; Cholesterol/Lipid Disorders; Heart Failure; **Hospital:** Hackensack Univ Med Ctr (page 718); **Address:** 155 Polifly Rd, Fl 1, Ste 106, Hackensack, NJ 07601; **Phone:** 201-487-7617; **Board Cert:** Pediatrics 1987; Pediatric Cardiology 2013; **Med School:** UMDNJ-NJ Med Sch, Newark 1983; **Resid:** Pediatrics, Univ Hosp-UMDNJ 1987; **Fellow:** Pediatric Cardiology, NYU Med Ctr 1988

Pediatric Endocrinology

Aisenberg, Javier E MD (PEn) - **Spec Exp:** Diabetes; Growth Disorders; **Hospital:** Hackensack Univ Med Ctr (page 718); **Address:** 30 Prospect Ave, WFAN Bldg Fl 2 - Ste 251, Hackensack, NJ 07601; **Phone:** 551-996-5329; **Board Cert:** Pediatrics 2008; Pediatric Endocrinology 2010; **Med School:** Argentina 1987; **Resid:** Pediatrics, Bellevue Hosp Ctr 1991; **Fellow:** Pediatric Endocrinology, NY Presby/Cornell Med Ctr 1994

Novogroder, Michael MD (PEn) - **Spec Exp:** Growth/Development Disorders; Pubertal Disorders; Thyroid Disorders; **Hospital:** Englewood Hosp & Med Ctr; **Address:** Metropolitan Pediatric Grp, 704 Palisade Ave, Teaneck, NJ 07666; **Phone:** 201-836-4301; **Board Cert:** Pediatrics 1974; Pediatric Endocrinology 1980; **Med School:** SUNY Hlth Sci Ctr 1969; **Resid:** Pediatrics, Jacobi Med Ctr 1973; **Fellow:** Pediatric Endocrinology, NY-Presby/Weill Cornell Med Ctr 1976; **Fac Appt:** Clin Prof Ped, Columbia P&S

Pediatric Gastroenterology

Jeshion, Wendy MD (PGe) - **Spec Exp:** Inflammatory Bowel Disease/Crohn's; Celiac Disease; Peptic Ulcer Disease; **Hospital:** Hackensack Univ Med Ctr (page 718); **Address:** Joseph M Sazari Chldns Hosp, Ped Gastro, 155 Polifly Rd, Ste 102, Hackensack, NJ 07601; **Phone:** 551-996-8840; **Board Cert:** Pediatric Gastroenterology 2007; **Med School:** Mount Sinai Sch Med 1992; **Resid:** Pediatrics, Chldns Hosp 1995; **Fellow:** Pediatric Gastroenterology, Chldns Hosp 1998

Pediatric Hematology-Oncology

Diamond, Steven H MD (PHO) - **Spec Exp:** Pediatric Cancers; Sickle Cell Disease; Hemophilia; **Hospital:** Hackensack Univ Med Ctr (page 718); **Address:** Hackensack Univ Med Ctr, Div Ped Hem/Onc, 30 Prospect Ave, Hackensack, NJ 07601-1914; **Phone:** 201-996-5437; **Board Cert:** Pediatrics 1979; Pediatric Hematology-Oncology 1980; **Med School:** Univ Pennsylvania 1974; **Resid:** Pediatrics, Mount Sinai Med Ctr 1978; **Fellow:** Pediatric Hematology-Oncology, Beth Israel Med Ctr - Petrie Div 1979; **Fac Appt:** Asst Clin Prof Ped, UMDNJ-NJ Med Sch, Newark

Flug, Frances MD (PHO) - **Spec Exp:** Bleeding/Coagulation Disorders; Sickle Cell Disease; Pediatric Cancers; **Hospital:** Hackensack Univ Med Ctr (page 718), Saint Michael's Med Ctr; **Address:** Hackensack Univ Med Ctr, Div Ped Hem/Onc, 30 Prospect Ave, Hackensack, NJ 07601-2129; **Phone:** 201-996-5437; **Board Cert:** Pediatrics 1984; Pediatric Hematology-Oncology 1984; **Med School:** SUNY Downstate 1979; **Resid:** Pediatrics, NYU Langone Med Ctr 1983; **Fellow:** Pediatric Hematology-Oncology, NYU Langone Med Ctr 1984; **Fac Appt:** Assoc Prof Ped, UMDNJ-NJ Med Sch, Newark

Halpern, Steven L MD (PHO) - **Spec Exp:** Leukemia & Lymphoma; Brain Tumors; Hodgkin's Lymphoma; Hemophilia; **Hospital:** Morristown Med Ctr (page 92), Overlook Med Ctr (page 92); **Address:** 100 Madison Ave, Morristown, NJ 07960; **Phone:** 973-971-6720; **Board Cert:** Pediatrics 1981; Pediatric Hematology-Oncology 1982; **Med School:** Ros Franklin Univ/Chicago Med Sch 1976; **Resid:** Pediatrics, St Christophers Hosp for Children 1979; **Fellow:** Pediatric Hematology-Oncology, Childrens Hosp 1982; **Fac Appt:** Asst Prof Ped, UMDNJ-NJ Med Sch, Newark

Harris, Michael B MD (PHO) - **Spec Exp:** Leukemia & Lymphoma; Bone Tumors; Cancer Survivors-Late Effects of Therapy; **Hospital:** Hackensack Univ Med Ctr (page 718); **Address:** Tomorrows Chldns Inst, JM Sanzari Chldns Hosp, 30 Prospect Ave, Imus 1-TCI, rm PC116, Hackensack, NJ 07601; **Phone:** 201-996-5437; **Board Cert:** Pediatrics 1974; Pediatric Hematology-Oncology 1974; **Med School:** Albert Einstein Coll Med 1969; **Resid:** Pediatrics, Chldns Hosp 1971; **Fellow:** Pediatric Hematology-Oncology, Chldns Hosp 1974; **Fac Appt:** Prof Ped, UMDNJ-NJ Med Sch, Newark

Pediatric Infectious Disease

Boscamp, Jeffrey R MD (PInf) - **Spec Exp:** Fevers of Unknown Origin; Lyme Disease; **Hospital:** Hackensack Univ Med Ctr (page 718); **Address:** Hackensack Univ Med Ctr, 30 Prospect Ave, WFAN Bldg, PC 360, Hackensack, NJ 07601; **Phone:** 551-996-5308; **Board Cert:** Pediatrics 1986; Pediatric Infectious Disease 2009; **Med School:** NY Med Coll 1981; **Resid:** Pediatrics, NY-Presby/Columbia Univ Med Ctr 1984; Internal Medicine, Greenwich Hosp 1985; **Fellow:** Infectious Disease, Montefiore Med Ctr 1987; **Fac Appt:** Assoc Prof Ped, UMDNJ-Univ Med Dent NJ

Piwoz, Julia A MD (PInf) - **Spec Exp:** AIDS/HIV; Congenital Infections; Infections in Transplant Patients; **Hospital:** Hackensack Univ Med Ctr (page 718); **Address:** Joseph M. Sanzari Children's Hosp, 30 Prospect Ave, Don Imus Pediatric Ctr PC360 Bldg, Hackensack, NJ 07601; **Phone:** 201-996 5308; **Board Cert:** Pediatrics 2009; Pediatric Infectious Disease 2007; **Med School:** Hahnemann Univ 1991; **Resid:** Pediatrics, Mt Sinai Med Ctr 1994; **Fellow:** Pediatric Infectious Disease, Mt Sinai Med Ctr 1995; **Fac Appt:** Asst Prof Ped, UMDNJ-NJ Med Sch, Newark

Slavin, Kevin A MD (PInf) - **Spec Exp:** Antibiotic Resistance; Travel Medicine; Infection Control; **Hospital:** Hackensack Univ Med Ctr (page 718); **Address:** Hackensack Univ Med, 30 Prospect Ave, WFAN Bldg, PC 360, Hackensack, NJ 07601; **Phone:** 201-996-5308; **Board Cert:** Pediatrics 2012; Pediatric Infectious Disease 2007; **Med School:** UCLA 1993; **Resid:** Pediatrics, UCSF Med Ctr 1996; **Fellow:** Clinical Pharmacology, UCSF Med Ctr 1997; Pediatric Infectious Disease, UCSF Med Ctr 1999; **Fac Appt:** Asst Prof Ped, UMDNJ-NJ Med Sch, Newark

Pediatric Nephrology

Lieberman, Kenneth V MD (PNep) - **Spec Exp:** Nephrotic Syndrome; Glomerulonephritis; Kidney Failure-Chronic; Hypertension; **Hospital:** Hackensack Univ Med Ctr (page 718); **Address:** 30 Prospect Ave, Hackensack, NJ 07601; **Phone:** 551-996-8228; **Board Cert:** Pediatrics 1981; Pediatric Nephrology 2009; **Med School:** Albert Einstein Coll Med 1977; **Resid:** Pediatrics, Mount Sinai Hosp 1979; **Fellow:** Nephrology, New York Hosp-Cornell 1981; **Fac Appt:** Prof Ped, UMDNJ-NJ Med Sch, Newark

Pediatric Otolaryngology

Respler, Don S MD (PO) - **Spec Exp:** Airway Disorders; Sinus Disorders; Head & Neck Tumors; Sleep Disorders/Apnea; **Hospital:** Hackensack Univ Med Ctr (page 718), Valley Hosp (page 721); **Address:** 2 S Summit Ave, Hackensack, NJ 07601-1117; **Phone:** 201-996-9200; **Board Cert:** Otolaryngology 1986; **Med School:** Mount Sinai Sch Med 1981; **Resid:** Surgery, Beth Israel Med Ctr - Petrie Div 1983; Otolaryngology, UMDNJ-Univ Hosp 1986; **Fellow:** Pediatric Otolaryngology, Chldns Hosp 1988; **Fac Appt:** Asst Clin Prof S, UMDNJ-NJ Med Sch, Newark

Samadi, Sharyar D MD (PO) - **Spec Exp:** Ear Infections; Sinusitis; Tonsil/Adenoid Disorders; Sleep Apnea; **Hospital:** Hackensack Univ Med Ctr (page 718); **Address:** 10 Forest Ave, Ste 100, Paramus, NJ 07652; **Phone:** 201-996-1505; **Board Cert:** Otolaryngology 2012; **Med School:** Johns Hopkins Univ 1996; **Resid:** Otolaryngology, Univ Penn Med Ctr 2001; **Fellow:** Pediatric Otolaryngology, Chldns Hosp of Philadelphia 2003

Pediatric Pulmonology

Kanengiser, Steven MD (PPul) - **Spec Exp:** Asthma; Cough-Chronic; Pneumonia; **Hospital:** Valley Hosp (page 721); **Address:** 505 Goffle Rd, Ridgewood, NJ 07450-4027; **Phone:** 201-447-8026; **Board Cert:** Pediatrics 2003; Pediatric Pulmonology 2009; **Med School:** UCSF 1984; **Resid:** Pediatrics, Children's Hosp 1987; **Fellow:** Pediatric Pulmonology, Westchester Med Ctr 1994; **Fac Appt:** Asst Clin Prof Ped, Columbia P&S

Lee, Donna J MD (PPul) - **Spec Exp:** Pulmonary Infections; Asthma; **Hospital:** Hackensack Univ Med Ctr (page 718); **Address:** Hackensack Univ Med Ctr, DON IMUS Pediatric Ctr, Fl 3, 30 Prospect Ave, Hackensack, NJ 07601; **Phone:** 551-996-5207; **Board Cert:** Pediatrics 2011; Pediatric Pulmonology 2008; **Med School:** UMDNJ-NJ Med Sch, Newark 1993; **Resid:** Pediatrics, Univ Hosp-UMDNJ—Newark 1996; **Fellow:** Pediatric Pulmonology, Columbia P&S/Babies Hosp 1999; **Fac Appt:** Assoc Prof Ped, UMDNJ-NJ Med Sch, Newark

Ngai, Pakkay MD (PPul) - **Spec Exp:** Asthma; Sleep Disorders; **Hospital:** Hackensack Univ Med Ctr (page 718); **Address:** 30 Prospect Ave WFAN Bldg Fl 3, Hackensack, NJ 07601; **Phone:** 201-996-5207; **Board Cert:** Pediatrics 2007; Pediatric Pulmonology 2010; Sleep Medicine 2007; **Med School:** NYU Sch Med 1995; **Resid:** Pediatrics, NY Presby/Columbia Med Ctr 1998; **Fellow:** Pediatric Pulmonology, NY Presby/Columbia Med Ctr 2002

Pediatric Rheumatology

Haines, Kathleen A MD (PRhu) - **Spec Exp:** Juvenile Arthritis; Lupus/SLE; Immune Deficiency; Scleroderma; **Hospital:** Hackensack Univ Med Ctr (page 718), NYU Langone Med Ctr (page 108); **Address:** WFAN Imus Bldg, 30 Prospect Ave, Fl 3, Hackensack, NJ 07601; **Phone:** 551-996-5306; **Board Cert:** Pediatrics 1980; Allergy & Immunology 1981; Pediatric Rheumatology 2007; **Med School:** Albert Einstein Coll Med 1975; **Resid:** Pediatrics, New York Hosp 1977; **Fellow:** Allergy & Immunology, New York Hosp 1980; Rheumatology, NYU Med Ctr 1982; **Fac Appt:** Assoc Prof Ped, UMDNJ-NJ Med Sch, Newark

Kimura, Yukiko MD (PRhu) - **Spec Exp:** Juvenile Arthritis; Lupus/SLE; Dermatomyositis; Vasculitis; **Hospital:** Hackensack Univ Med Ctr (page 718); **Address:** Dan Imus Bldg, 30 Prospect Ave Fl 3, Hackensack, NJ 07601; **Phone:** 201-996-5306; **Board Cert:** Pediatrics 1987; Pediatric Rheumatology 2007; **Med School:** Albert Einstein Coll Med 1982; **Resid:** Pediatrics, Babies Hosp/Columbia Presby 1985; **Fellow:** Pediatric Rheumatology, Babies Hosp/Columbia Presby 1991; **Fac Appt:** Assoc Prof Ped, UMDNJ-NJ Med Sch, Newark

Li, Suzanne MD (PRhu) - **Hospital:** Hackensack Univ Med Ctr (page 718); **Address:** HackensackUMC, 30 Prospect Ave, Hackensack, NJ 07601; **Phone:** 551-996-5306; **Board Cert:** Pediatrics 2011; Pediatric Rheumatology 2011; **Med School:** Columbia P&S 1985; **Resid:** Pediatrics, Columbia Babies Hosp 1988; **Fellow:** Rheumatology, Columbia Babies/NY Presby Hosp 1992; **Fac Appt:** Asst Prof Ped, UMDNJ-Rutgers Med Sch

Pediatric Surgery

Alexander, Frederick MD (PS) - **Spec Exp:** Gastrointestinal Surgery; Thoracic Surgery; Solid Tumors; Congenital Anomalies-Gastrointestinal; **Hospital:** Hackensack Univ Med Ctr (page 718), Valley Hosp (page 721); **Address:** Pediatric Surgical Associates, 30 W Century Rd, Ste 235, Paramas, NJ 07652; **Phone:** 201-225-0029; **Board Cert:** Pediatric Surgery 2010; **Med School:** Columbia P&S 1977; **Resid:** Surgery, Brigham-Womens Hosp 1984; **Fellow:** Pediatric Surgery, Chldns Hosp 1986; **Fac Appt:** Clin Prof S, UMDNJ-NJ Med Sch, Newark

Friedman, David L MD (PS) - **Spec Exp:** Neonatal Surgery; Gastroesophageal Reflux Disease (GERD); Laparoscopic Surgery; **Hospital:** Valley Hosp (page 721), Hackensack Univ Med Ctr (page 718); **Address:** 30 W Century Rd, Ste 235, Paramus, NJ 07652-1433; **Phone:** 201-225-9440; **Board Cert:** Pediatric Surgery 2009; **Med School:** SUNY Downstate 1971; **Resid:** Surgery, SUNY Downstate Med Ctr 1976; **Fellow:** Pediatric Surgery, SUNY Downstate Med Ctr 1977; **Fac Appt:** Asst Prof S, Columbia P&S

Gandhi, Rajinder MD (PS) - **Spec Exp:** Gastrointestinal Surgery; Laparoscopic Surgery; Chest Wall Deformities; **Hospital:** Valley Hosp (page 721); **Address:** 30 W Century Rd, Ste 235, Paramus, NJ 07652; **Phone:** 201-225-9440; **Board Cert:** Surgery 1975; Pediatric Surgery 2007; **Med School:** Burma 1966; **Resid:** Surgery, Montefiore Med Ctr-Einstein Div 1974; **Fellow:** Pediatric Surgery, Columbia-Presby Med Ctr 1976; **Fac Appt:** Assoc Clin Prof S, Columbia P&S

Valda, Victor MD (PS) - **Spec Exp:** Congenital Anomalies; Cancer Surgery; **Hospital:** Hackensack Univ Med Ctr (page 718); **Address:** 30 Prospect Ave, Hackensack, NJ 07601; **Phone:** 201-996-2921; **Board Cert:** Surgery 1974; Pediatric Surgery 2007; **Med School:** Bolivia 1961; **Resid:** Surgery, Mt Zion Hosp 1968; Surgery, Maricopa Med Ctr 1972; **Fellow:** Pediatric Surgery, St Christopher's Hosp 1974

Pediatric Urology

Koo, Harry P MD (Ped Uro) - **Spec Exp:** Congenital Anomalies-Genitourinary; Reconstructive Surgery; Hydronephrosis; **Hospital:** Hackensack Univ Med Ctr (page 718); **Address:** Urology HealthPartners, Hackensack Univ Med Ctr, 360 Essex St, Ste 403, Hackensack, NJ 07601; **Phone:** 551-996-8090; **Board Cert:** Urology 2007; **Med School:** Univ Rochester 1987; **Resid:** Urology, Ny-Presby Hosp/Columbia 1993; **Fellow:** Pediatric Urology, Chldns Hosp 1995; **Fac Appt:** Prof S, UMDNJ-NJ Med Sch, Newark

Tennenbaum, Steven Y MD (Ped Uro) - **Spec Exp:** Hernia; Urinary Reflux/Obstruction; **Hospital:** Holy Name Med Ctr (page 720), Valley Hosp (page 721); **Address:** Chldns Surgical Specialties, 699 Teaneck Rd, Ste 103, Teaneck, NJ 07666; **Phone:** 201-692-9550; **Board Cert:** Urology 2013; **Med School:** Albert Einstein Coll Med 1984; **Resid:** Surgery, Montefiore Med Ctr 1986; Urology, Montefiore Med Ctr 1990; **Fellow:** Pediatric Urology, Chldns Hosp 1991

Pediatrics

Asnes, Russell MD (Ped) *PCP* - **Spec Exp:** Diagnostic Problems; **Hospital:** Englewood Hosp & Med Ctr, Hackensack Univ Med Ctr (page 718); **Address:** Tenafly Pediatrics, 32 Franklin St, Tenafly, NJ 07670; **Phone:** 201-569-2400; **Board Cert:** Pediatrics 2010; **Med School:** Tufts Univ 1963; **Resid:** Pediatrics, Johns Hopkins Hosp 1966; Pediatrics, Johns Hopkins Hosp 1969; **Fellow:** Neonatology, Babies Hosp/Columbia Univ 1970; **Fac Appt:** Clin Prof Ped, Columbia P&S

Berkowitz, Irwin H MD (Ped) *PCP* - **Spec Exp:** Asthma; ADD/ADHD; Parenting Issues; **Hospital:** Valley Hosp (page 721); **Address:** Chestnut Ridge Pediatric Assocs, 595 Chestnut Ridge Rd, Ste 4, Woodcliff Lake, NJ 07677; **Phone:** 201-391-2020; **Board Cert:** Pediatrics 1984; **Med School:** SUNY Downstate 1972; **Resid:** Pediatrics, Lenox Hill Hosp 1976; **Fac Appt:** Asst Clin Prof Ped, NY Med Coll

Buchalter, Maury MD (Ped) *PCP* - **Spec Exp:** Asthma; Infectious Disease; ADD/ADHD; **Hospital:** Hackensack Univ Med Ctr (page 718), Englewood Hosp & Med Ctr; **Address:** Tenafly Pediatrics, 301 Bridge Plaza N, Fort Lee, NJ 07670; **Phone:** 201-592-8787; **Board Cert:** Pediatrics 2010; **Med School:** Mount Sinai Sch Med 1984; **Resid:** Pediatrics, Mt Sinai Hosp 1987; **Fellow:** Infectious Disease, Chldns Hosp 1988

Hages, Harry A MD (Ped) *PCP* - **Hospital:** Englewood Hosp & Med Ctr, Valley Hosp (page 721); **Address:** 215 Old Tappan Rd, Old Tappan, NJ 07675-7000; **Phone:** 201-666-1001; **Board Cert:** Pediatrics 1973; **Med School:** Univ Pittsburgh 1966; **Resid:** Pediatrics, Chldns Hosp 1968; Pediatrics, New York Hosp 1969

Harlow, Paul J MD (Ped) *PCP* - **Spec Exp:** Anemia; Bleeding/Coagulation Disorders; **Hospital:** Hackensack Univ Med Ctr (page 718), Valley Hosp (page 721); **Address:** Pediatric Specialties, 90 Prospect Ave, Ste 1A, Hackensack, NJ 07601; **Phone:** 201-342-4001 x107; **Board Cert:** Pediatrics 1979; Pediatric Hematology-Oncology 1980; **Med School:** SUNY Downstate 1974; **Resid:** Pediatrics, Bronx Municipal Hosp 1977; **Fellow:** Pediatric Hematology-Oncology, Chldn's Hosp 1979

Kanter, Alan MD (Ped) *PCP* - **Spec Exp:** ADD/ADHD; Autism; **Hospital:** Englewood Hosp & Med Ctr, Morgan Stanley Children's Hosp of NY-Presby, NY (page 104); **Address:** 704 Palisade Ave, Teaneck, NJ 07666-3198; **Phone:** 201-836-4301; **Board Cert:** Pediatrics 1977; **Med School:** Albert Einstein Coll Med 1970; **Resid:** Pediatrics, Montefiore Med Ctr 1975; **Fac Appt:** Assoc Clin Prof Ped, Columbia P&S

Kolsky, Neil MD (Ped) *PCP* - **Hospital:** Holy Name Med Ctr (page 720), Hackensack Univ Med Ctr (page 718); **Address:** Pedimedica, 870 Palisade Ave, Ste 201, Teaneck, NJ 07666-3419; **Phone:** 201-692-1661; **Board Cert:** Pediatrics 1972; **Med School:** UMDNJ-NJ Med Sch, Newark 1966; **Resid:** Pediatrics, Johns Hopkins Hosp 1969

Kushner, Susan C MD (Ped) *PCP* - **Spec Exp:** Atopic Dermatitis; Allergic Rhinitis; Asthma; Otitis Media; **Hospital:** Hackensack Univ Med Ctr (page 718), Valley Hosp (page 721); **Address:** Forrest Pediatrics, 299 Forrest Ave Fl 3, Paramus, NJ 07652; **Phone:** 201-267-0888; **Board Cert:** Pediatrics 2011; **Med School:** SUNY Upstate Med Univ 1986; **Resid:** Pediatrics, Schneider Chldns Hosp 1989

Namerow, David MD (Ped) *PCP* - **Spec Exp:** Behavioral Disorders; Adolescent Medicine; **Hospital:** Valley Hosp (page 721), St. Joseph's Regl Med Ctr - Paterson; **Address:** PediatriCare Associates, 2020 Fair Lawn Ave, Fair Lawn, NJ 07410-2319; **Phone:** 201-791-4545; **Board Cert:** Pediatrics 1977; **Med School:** Univ Louisville Sch Med 1972; **Resid:** Pediatrics, Chldn's Hosp 1975; **Fellow:** Adolescent Medicine, Univ MD Hosp 1977; **Fac Appt:** Asst Clin Prof Ped, NY Med Coll

O'Brien, Daryl H MD (Ped) *PCP* - **Hospital:** Valley Hosp (page 721); **Address:** Broadway Pediatric Assocs, 336 Center Ave, Westwood, NJ 07675; **Phone:** 201-664-7444; **Board Cert:** Pediatrics 1986; **Med School:** Dartmouth Med Sch 1979; **Resid:** Pediatrics, Duke Univ Med Ctr 1982

Rabinowitz, Arnold MD (Ped) *PCP* - **Spec Exp:** Allergy; **Hospital:** Hackensack Univ Med Ctr (page 718); **Address:** 22 Madison Ave, Ste 303, Paramus, NJ 07652; **Phone:** 201-291-9797; **Board Cert:** Pediatrics 2011; **Med School:** Mexico 1979; **Resid:** Pediatrics, Brookdale Univ Hosp Med Ctr 1983; **Fellow:** Pediatric Allergy, NY-Presby/Columbia Univ Med Ctr 1985

Schuss, Steven A MD (Ped) *PCP* - **Hospital:** Englewood Hosp & Med Ctr, Hackensack Univ Med Ctr (page 718); **Address:** 197 Cedar Ln, Teaneck, NJ 07666-4301; **Phone:** 201-836-7171; **Board Cert:** Pediatrics 1986; **Med School:** Albert Einstein Coll Med 1979; **Resid:** Pediatrics, Montefiore Med Ctr 1983

Sugarman, Lynn B MD (Ped) *PCP* - **Hospital:** Englewood Hosp & Med Ctr, Hackensack Univ Med Ctr (page 718); **Address:** Tenafly Pediatrics, 32 Franklin St, Tenafly, NJ 07670-2005; **Phone:** 201-569-2400; **Board Cert:** Pediatrics 1981; **Med School:** Harvard Med Sch 1977; **Resid:** Pediatrics, Bronx Muni Hos 1981; **Fellow:** Pediatric Critical Care Medicine, Bronx Muni Hosp 1983

Weiss, Christopher A DO (Ped) - **Hospital:** Hackensack Univ Med Ctr (page 718), Englewood Hosp & Med Ctr; **Address:** Washington Ave Pediatrics, 95 N Washington Ave, Bergenfield, NJ 07621; **Phone:** 201-384-0300; **Board Cert:** Pediatrics 2008; **Med School:** Nova SE Univ, Coll Osteo Med 1996; **Resid:** Pediatrics, Long Island Jewish Med Ctr 2001

Wisotsky, David H MD (Ped) *PCP* - **Hospital:** Englewood Hosp & Med Ctr, Hackensack Univ Med Ctr (page 718); **Address:** Tenafly Pediatrics, 32 Franklin St, Tenafly, NJ 07670; **Phone:** 201-569-2400; **Board Cert:** Pediatrics 2010; **Med School:** Albert Einstein Coll Med 1974; **Resid:** Pediatrics, Bronx Muni Hosp 1978; **Fac Appt:** Asst Clin Prof Ped, Columbia P&S

Physical Medicine & Rehabilitation

Averill, Allison MD (PMR) - **Spec Exp:** Neuro-Rehabilitation; Brain Injury Rehabilitation; Stroke Rehabilitation; **Hospital:** Kessler Inst for Rehab - Saddle Brook; **Address:** Kessler Institute for Rehab, Saddle Brook Campus, 300 Market St, Saddle Brook, NJ 07663; **Phone:** 201-368-6000; **Board Cert:** Physical Medicine & Rehabilitation 2013; **Med School:** UMDNJ RW Johnson Med Sch 1988; **Resid:** Physical Medicine & Rehabilitation, Univ Penn Hosp 1992; **Fac Appt:** Asst Prof PMR, UMDNJ-NJ Med Sch, Newark

Liss, Donald MD (PMR) - **Spec Exp:** Pain-Back; Sports Medicine; Osteoarthritis; **Hospital:** NY-Presby/Columbia Univ Med Ctr, NY (page 104), Englewood Hosp & Med Ctr; **Address:** 500 Grand Ave, Fl 1st, Englewood, NJ 07631-2920; **Phone:** 201-567-2277; **Board Cert:** Physical Medicine & Rehabilitation 1984; **Med School:** Wayne State Univ 1979; **Resid:** Physical Medicine & Rehabilitation, Columbia-Presby Med Ctr 1982; **Fac Appt:** Assoc Clin Prof PMR, Columbia P&S

Liss, Howard MD (PMR) - **Hospital:** NY-Presby/Columbia Univ Med Ctr, NY (page 104), Englewood Hosp & Med Ctr; **Address:** Physical Medicine & Rehabilitation Ctr, 500 Grand Ave Fl 1, Englewood, NJ 07631-2920; **Phone:** 201-567-2277; **Board Cert:** Physical Medicine & Rehabilitation 1982; **Med School:** Wayne State Univ 1977; **Resid:** Physical Medicine & Rehabilitation, NY-Presby/Columbia Univ Med Ctr 1981; **Fac Appt:** Asst Clin Prof PMR, Columbia P&S

Zimmerman, Jerald R MD (PMR) - **Spec Exp:** Post Polio Syndrome/Rehabilitation; Musculoskeletal Disorders; Pain Management; **Hospital:** Englewood Hosp & Med Ctr, Holy Name Med Ctr (page 720); **Address:** 370 Grand Ave, Ste 102, Englewood, NJ 07631; **Phone:** 201-567-3370; **Board Cert:** Physical Medicine & Rehabilitation 1989; **Med School:** Univ IL Coll Med 1982; **Resid:** Orthopaedic Surgery, Univ Minn Med Ctr 1985; Physical Medicine & Rehabilitation, Columbia-Presby Med Ctr 1988; **Fac Appt:** Asst Prof PMR, UMDNJ-NJ Med Sch, Newark

Plastic Surgery

Bikoff, David J MD (PlS) - **Hospital:** Hackensack Univ Med Ctr (page 718); **Address:** 146 Rte 17 N, Fl 3, Hackensack, NJ 07601; **Phone:** 201-488-8584; **Board Cert:** Plastic Surgery 1980; **Med School:** SUNY Downstate 1973; **Resid:** Surgery, Kings Co Hosp 1977; Plastic Surgery, Kings Co Hosp 1979; **Fellow:** Hand Surgery, Kings Co Hosp 1980

Boss Jr, William K MD (PlS) - **Spec Exp:** Cosmetic & Reconstructive Surgery; **Hospital:** Hackensack Univ Med Ctr (page 718); **Address:** Cosmetic Surgery & Rejuvenation Ctr, 305 Route 17, Paramus, NJ 07652; **Phone:** 201-967-1100; **Board Cert:** Plastic Surgery 1984; **Med School:** UMDNJ-NJ Med Sch, Newark 1975; **Resid:** Surgery, UMDNJ Med Ctr 1980; Plastic Surgery, Yale-New Haven Hosp 1982; **Fellow:** Hand & Microvascular Surgery, RK Davies Med Ctr 1983; **Fac Appt:** Asst Clin Prof PlS, UMDNJ-Univ Med Dent NJ

Breslow, Gary D MD (PlS) - **Spec Exp:** Breast Reconstruction; Cosmetic Surgery-Breast; Cosmetic Surgery-Face; **Hospital:** Valley Hosp (page 721); **Address:** Bergen Med Ctr Bldg, 1 W Ridgewood Ave, Ste 110, Paramus, NJ 07652; **Phone:** 201-444-9522; **Board Cert:** Plastic Surgery 2006; **Med School:** NYU Sch Med 1998; **Resid:** Plastic Surgery, Hosp U Penn 2004; **Fellow:** Plastic/Reconstructive Surgery, NYU Med Ctr 2005

D'Amico, Richard A MD (PlS) - **Spec Exp:** Cosmetic Surgery-Face; Liposuction & Body Contouring; Breast Augmentation; Facial Rejuvenation; **Hospital:** Englewood Hosp & Med Ctr, Holy Name Med Ctr (page 720); **Address:** 180 N Dean St, Ste 3N, Englewood, NJ 07631-2534; **Phone:** 201-567-9595; **Board Cert:** Plastic Surgery 1986; **Med School:** NYU Sch Med 1976; **Resid:** Surgery, Tulsa Med Ctr 1979; Surgery, Strong Meml Hosp 1981; **Fellow:** Plastic/Reconstructive Surgery, Columbia-Presby Med Ctr 1983; **Fac Appt:** Asst Clin Prof PlS, Mount Sinai Sch Med

Lipson, David E MD (PlS) - **Spec Exp:** Breast Augmentation; Body Contouring; Facial Rejuvenation; **Hospital:** Valley Hosp (page 721); **Address:** 2300 Route 208 South, Fair Lawn, NJ 07410; **Phone:** 201-797-7770; **Board Cert:** Plastic Surgery 1981; **Med School:** Albert Einstein Coll Med 1971; **Resid:** Surgery, Bellevue/NYU Med Ctr 1976; Plastic Surgery, Bellevue/NYU Med Ctr 1978

Ponamgi, Suri MD (PlS) - **Spec Exp:** Cosmetic & Reconstructive Surgery; **Hospital:** Palisades Med Ctr, Holy Name Med Ctr (page 720); **Address:** 1101 Palisades Ave, Fort Lee, NJ 07024-6329; **Phone:** 201-224-8831; **Board Cert:** Plastic Surgery 1984; **Med School:** India 1970; **Resid:** Surgery, Bronx Lebonon Hosp 1979; Plastic Surgery, NY Methodist Hosp 1982; **Fellow:** Surgery, Bronx Lebonon Hosp 1980

Sternschein, Michael J MD (PlS) - **Spec Exp:** Cosmetic Surgery-Face & Breast; Liposuction & Body Contouring; Laser Surgery; **Hospital:** Hackensack Univ Med Ctr (page 718), Valley Hosp (page 721); **Address:** 1200 E Ridgewood Ave, Fl 2 W Wing, Ridgewood, NJ 07450; **Phone:** 201-444-1188; **Board Cert:** Plastic Surgery 1985; **Med School:** Columbia P&S 1976; **Resid:** Surgery, Columbia-Presby Med Ctr 1980; Plastic Surgery, Columbia-Presby Med Ctr 1982; **Fellow:** Microsurgery, Columbia-Presby Med Ctr 1982

Winters, Richard M MD (PlS) - **Spec Exp:** Cosmetic & Reconstructive Surgery; Rhinoplasty; Cosmetic Surgery-Face & Breast; Breast Reconstruction; **Hospital:** Hackensack Univ Med Ctr (page 718); **Address:** Aesthetic & Reconstructive Surgeons, 20 Prospect Ave, Ste 501, Hackensack, NJ 07601; **Phone:** 201-487-3400; **Board Cert:** Plastic Surgery 2009; **Med School:** Univ Conn 1990; **Resid:** Surgery, Univ Conn Affil Hosp 1995; **Fellow:** Plastic/Reconstructive Surgery, NY-Presby/Weill Cornell Med Ctr 1997; Microsurgery, CA Pacific Med Ctr - Davies Campus 1998

Zubowski, Robert I MD (PlS) - **Spec Exp:** Breast Augmentation; Liposuction & Body Contouring; Cosmetic Surgery-Face; **Hospital:** Valley Hosp (page 721); **Address:** 1 Sears Drive Fl 1, Paramus, NJ 07652; **Phone:** 201-261-7550; **Board Cert:** Plastic Surgery 2003; **Med School:** Mexico 1983; **Resid:** Surgery, Westchester Co Med Ctr 1990; **Fellow:** Plastic Surgery, Cleveland Clinic 1992; **Fac Appt:** Asst Clin Prof S, NY Med Coll

Psychiatry

Chertoff, Harvey R MD (Psyc) - **Spec Exp:** Anxiety & Mood Disorders; Psychoanalysis; **Hospital:** Englewood Hosp & Med Ctr, NY-Presby/Columbia Univ Med Ctr, NY (page 104); **Address:** 205 Engle St, Englewood, NJ 07631-2409; **Phone:** 201-567-4970; **Board Cert:** Psychiatry 1978; **Med School:** Albert Einstein Coll Med 1966; **Resid:** Psychiatry, Columbia Presby Med Ctr 1970; **Fac Appt:** Asst Clin Prof Psyc, Columbia P&S

Farkas, Edward Lewis MD (Psyc) - **Spec Exp:** Depression in the Elderly; Psychotherapy-Men's Issues; Panic Disorder; **Hospital:** Holy Name Med Ctr (page 720); **Address:** 175 Cedar Ln, Ste A, Teaneck, NJ 07666-4315; **Phone:** 201-692-8354; **Board Cert:** Psychiatry 1988; **Med School:** Italy 1979; **Resid:** Psychiatry, Bronx Lebanon Hosp 1981; Psychiatry, St Luke's-Roosevelt Hosp Ctr 1983; **Fellow:** Psychiatry, William Allison White Inst 1983

Gurland, Frances Effron MD (Psyc) - **Spec Exp:** Eating Disorders; ADD/ADHD; **Address:** 216 Engle St, Englewood, NJ 07631; **Phone:** 201-568-4066; **Board Cert:** Psychiatry 2005; **Med School:** SUNY Downstate 1989; **Resid:** Psychiatry, St Lukes-Roosevelt Hosp Ctr 1991; **Fellow:** Child & Adolescent Psychiatry, Mount Sinai Hosp 1994

Narula, Amarjot S MD (Psyc) - **Spec Exp:** Geriatric Psychiatry; Mood Disorders; **Hospital:** Valley Hosp (page 721), Bergen Regl Med Ctr; **Address:** 65 N Maple Ave, Ridgewood, NJ 07450-1600; **Phone:** 201-670-4423; **Board Cert:** Psychiatry 1992; Geriatric Psychiatry 2007; **Med School:** India 1980; **Resid:** Psychiatry, Middletown Psychiatric Ctr 1988; **Fellow:** Psychiatry, Metropolitan Hosp 1989

Rosenfeld, David N MD (Psyc) - **Spec Exp:** Mood Disorders; Anxiety Disorders; Personality Disorders; Geriatric Psychiatry; **Hospital:** Valley Hosp (page 721); **Address:** 265 Ackerman Ave, Ste 202, Ridgewood, NJ 07450-4200; **Phone:** 201-447-5630; **Board Cert:** Psychiatry 2005; **Med School:** UMDNJ-RW Johnson Med Sch 1988; **Resid:** Psychiatry, Mount Sinai Sch Med 1990; Psychiatry, Bergen Pines Co 1994

Samuels, Steven MD (Psyc) - **Spec Exp:** Dementia; Anxiety & Depression; Geriatric Psychiatry; **Hospital:** Englewood Hosp & Med Ctr; **Address:** Psychiatric Medicine Consultants, 60 W Ridgewood Ave Fl 3, Ridgewood, NJ 07450; **Phone:** 201-681-2915; **Board Cert:** Psychiatry 2004; Geriatric Psychiatry 2006; **Med School:** SUNY Buffalo 1989; **Resid:** Psychiatry, St Vincents Hosp & Med Ctr 1993; **Fellow:** Geriatric Psychiatry, Hosp Univ Penn 1995; **Fac Appt:** Asst Prof Psyc, Mount Sinai Sch Med

Shah, Pritesh J MD (Psyc) - **Spec Exp:** Geriatric Psychiatry; **Hospital:** Holy Name Med Ctr (page 720); **Address:** 354 Old Hook Rd, Ste 102, Westwood, NJ 07675; **Phone:** 201-358-0400; **Board Cert:** Psychiatry 2004; **Med School:** India 1985; **Resid:** Psychiatry, Bergen Regl Med Ctr 1991

Wagle, Sharad MD (Psyc) - **Spec Exp:** Anxiety Disorders; Forensic Psychiatry; Geriatric Psychiatry; **Hospital:** Holy Name Med Ctr (page 720); **Address:** 718 Teaneck Rd, Teaneck, NJ 07666; **Phone:** 201-833-3291; **Board Cert:** Psychiatry 2006; **Med School:** India 1972; **Resid:** Psychiatry, Hackensack Univ Med Ctr 1976; Psychiatry, Albert Einstein Coll Med 1978; **Fellow:** Child & Adolescent Psychiatry, Psychoanalytic Inst 1978

Zaidi, Syed A R MD (Psyc) - **Spec Exp:** Addiction Psychiatry; **Hospital:** Holy Name Med Ctr (page 720); **Address:** 294 State St Fl 2, Hackensack, NJ 07601; **Phone:** 201-342-4004; **Board Cert:** Psychiatry 2009; **Med School:** Pakistan 1984; **Resid:** Psychiatry, Temple Univ Hosp 1996; **Fellow:** Geriatric Psychiatry, Mount Sinai Med Ctr 1997

Pulmonary Disease

Barasch, Jeffrey Paul MD (Pul) - **Spec Exp:** Sleep Disorders; Lung Cancer; Asthma; Chronic Obstructive Lung Disease (COPD); **Hospital:** Valley Hosp (page 721); **Address:** Better Breathing, 140 Chestnut St, Ste 200, Ridgewood, NJ 07450; **Phone:** 201-447-3866; **Board Cert:** Sleep Medicine 2007; Pulmonary Disease 1984; Internal Medicine 1982; **Med School:** NYU Sch Med 1979; **Resid:** Internal Medicine, Bellevue Hosp Ctr 1980; Internal Medicine, St. Luke's - Roosevelt Hosp Ctr 1982; **Fellow:** Pulmonary Disease, NYU Med Ctr 1984

Benoff, Brian A MD (Pul) - **Hospital:** Holy Name Med Ctr (page 720), Englewood Hosp & Med Ctr; **Address:** Bergen Pulmonary & Sleep Specialists, 180 N Dean St, Ste 2N, Englewood, NJ 07631; **Phone:** 201-871-8366; **Board Cert:** Internal Medicine 2007; Pulmonary Disease 2009; Critical Care Medicine 2010; Sleep Medicine 2011; **Med School:** Albert Einstein Coll Med 1994; **Resid:** Internal Medicine, Long Island Jewish Med Ctr 1997; **Fellow:** Pulmonary Critical Care Medicine, Long Island Jewish Med Ctr 2000

Brauntuch, Glenn R MD (Pul) - **Spec Exp:** Chronic Obstructive Lung Disease (COPD); Asthma; Lung Cancer; **Hospital:** Englewood Hosp & Med Ctr, Holy Name Med Ctr (page 720); **Address:** Bergen Medical Alliance, 180 Engle St, Englewood, NJ 07631-2507; **Phone:** 201-568-8010; **Board Cert:** Internal Medicine 1981; Pulmonary Disease 1984; **Med School:** Columbia P&S 1978; **Resid:** Internal Medicine, St Lukes-Roosevelt Hosp 1982; **Fellow:** Pulmonary Disease, NYU Med Ctr 1984

Bromberg, Assia MD (Pul) - **Spec Exp:** Asthma; Emphysema; Women's Health; **Hospital:** Valley Hosp (page 721); **Address:** 19-20 Fair Lawn Ave, Fairlawn, NJ 07410; **Phone:** 201-794-1963; **Board Cert:** Internal Medicine 1989; Pulmonary Disease 2004; **Med School:** Israel 1974; **Resid:** Anesthesiology, Chaim Sheba Med Ctr 1981; Internal Medicine, Englewood Hosp 1989; **Fellow:** Pulmonary Disease, Bellevue-NYU Med Ctr 1992

Engler, Mitchell S MD (Pul) - **Spec Exp:** Critical Care; Sleep Disorders; **Hospital:** Holy Name Med Ctr (page 720), Englewood Hosp & Med Ctr; **Address:** Bergen Medical Alliance, 180 Engle St, Englewood, NJ 07631-2507; **Phone:** 201-568-8010; **Board Cert:** Internal Medicine 1981; Pulmonary Disease 1988; Sleep Medicine 2003; **Med School:** Boston Univ 1978; **Resid:** Internal Medicine, St Lukes Hosp 1981; **Fellow:** Pulmonary Disease, St Lukes Hosp 1983

Levine, Selwyn E MD (Pul) - **Spec Exp:** Chronic Obstructive Lung Disease (COPD); Lung Cancer; Asthma; Pneumonia; **Hospital:** Holy Name Med Ctr (page 720), Englewood Hosp & Med Ctr; **Address:** Pulmonary Assocs of Northern NJ, 200 Grand Ave, Ste 102, Englewood, NJ 07631; **Phone:** 201-871-3636; **Board Cert:** Internal Medicine 1985; Pulmonary Disease 1988; **Med School:** NYU Sch Med 1982; **Resid:** Internal Medicine, Bellevue Hosp/NYU Med Ctr 1985; **Fellow:** Pulmonary Disease, Albert Einstein Coll Med 1987

Malovany, Robert MD (Pul) - **Spec Exp:** Exercise Physiology; Interventional Pulmonology; **Hospital:** Englewood Hosp & Med Ctr; **Address:** Bergen Medical Alliance, 180 Engle St, Englewood, NJ 07631-2507; **Phone:** 201-568-8010; **Board Cert:** Internal Medicine 1973; Pulmonary Disease 1976; **Med School:** Jefferson Med Coll 1970; **Resid:** Internal Medicine, Montefiore Med Ctr 1973; **Fellow:** Pulmonary Disease, Montefiore Med Ctr 1975; **Fac Appt:** Asst Clin Prof Med, Mount Sinai Sch Med

Polkow, Melvin MD (Pul) - **Spec Exp:** Asthma; Sarcoidosis; Pulmonary Fibrosis; Lung Cancer; **Hospital:** Hackensack Univ Med Ctr (page 718); **Address:** 211 Essex St, Ste 302, Hackensack, NJ 07601; **Phone:** 201-498-1311; **Board Cert:** Internal Medicine 1980; Pulmonary Disease 1982; Critical Care Medicine 2007; **Med School:** SUNY Downstate 1977; **Resid:** Internal Medicine, Lenox Hill Hosp 1980; **Fellow:** Pulmonary Critical Care Medicine, Univ Hosp 1982; **Fac Appt:** Asst Clin Prof Med, UMDNJ-NJ Med Sch, Newark

Simon, Clifford J MD (Pul) - **Spec Exp:** Asthma; Lung Cancer; Bronchoscopy; **Hospital:** Englewood Hosp & Med Ctr, Holy Name Med Ctr (page 720); **Address:** 180 Engle St, Englewood, NJ 07631-2507; **Phone:** 201-567-2050; **Board Cert:** Internal Medicine 1976; Pulmonary Disease 1980; **Med School:** Cornell Univ-Weill Med Coll 1973; **Resid:** Internal Medicine, Dartmouth Affil Hosps 1975; **Fellow:** Pulmonary Disease, Bellevue Hosp 1977

Radiation Oncology

Dubin, David MD (RadRO) - **Spec Exp:** Breast Cancer; Brachytherapy; Prostate Cancer; **Hospital:** Englewood Hosp & Med Ctr; **Address:** Englewood Hosp, Dept Radiation Oncology, 350 Engle St, Englewood, NJ 07631-1808; **Phone:** 201-894-3125; **Board Cert:** Radiation Oncology 1991; **Med School:** Albert Einstein Coll Med 1986; **Resid:** Radiation Oncology, St Barnabas Hosp 1990

Gejerman, Glen MD (RadRO) - **Spec Exp:** Prostate Cancer; Intensity Modulated Radiotherapy (IMRT); Brachytherapy; Urologic Cancer; **Hospital:** Hackensack Univ Med Ctr (page 718); **Address:** Hackensack University Medical Center, 92 Second St, Hackensack, NJ 07601; **Phone:** 201-996-2464; **Board Cert:** Radiation Oncology 2006; **Med School:** UMDNJ-NJ Med Sch, Newark 1990; **Resid:** Radiation Oncology, Montefiore Med Ctr 1995; **Fac Appt:** Asst Clin Prof RadRO, Albert Einstein Coll Med

Ingenito, Anthony C MD (RadRO) - **Spec Exp:** Brain Tumors; Head & Neck Cancer; Lymphoma; Gastrointestinal Cancer; **Hospital:** Hackensack Univ Med Ctr (page 718); **Address:** Dept Radiation Oncology, 92 Second St, Hackensack, NJ 07601; **Phone:** 201-996-2210; **Board Cert:** Radiation Oncology 2008; **Med School:** UMDNJ-NJ Med Sch, Newark 1991; **Resid:** Anesthesiology, NY-Presby Hosp 1996; Radiation Oncology, NY-Presby Hosp 1996

Vialotti, Charles P MD (RadRO) - **Spec Exp:** Lung Cancer; Palliative Care; **Hospital:** Holy Name Med Ctr (page 720), St. Mary's Hosp - Passaic; **Address:** Holy Name Med Ctr, Regl Cancer Ctr, Rad Onc Dept, 718 Teaneck Rd, Teaneck, NJ 07666; **Phone:** 201-541-5900; **Board Cert:** Therapeutic Radiology 1975; **Med School:** NY Med Coll 1971; **Resid:** Radiology, NYU Med Ctr 1974; **Fellow:** Therapeutic Radiology, NYU Med Ctr 1975

Reproductive Endocrinology

Lesorgen, Philip R MD (RE) - **Spec Exp:** Infertility-IVF; Endometriosis; **Hospital:** Englewood Hosp & Med Ctr, Holy Name Med Ctr (page 720); **Address:** 106 Grand Ave, Ste 400, Englewood, NJ 07631-3570; **Phone:** 201-569-6979; **Board Cert:** Obstetrics & Gynecology 1984; **Med School:** Boston Univ 1977; **Resid:** Obstetrics & Gynecology, LI Jewish Med Ctr 1981; **Fellow:** Reproductive Endocrinology, Thomas Jefferson Univ Hosp 1983; **Fac Appt:** Asst Clin Prof ObG, Seton Hall Univ Sch Hlth & Med Scis

McGovern, Peter G MD (RE) - **Spec Exp:** Infertility-IVF; Fertility Preservation in Cancer; **Hospital:** Univ Hosp (Newark), Hackensack Univ Med Ctr (page 718); **Address:** University Reproductive Assocs, 214 Terrace Ave, Hasbrouck Heights, NJ 07604; **Phone:** 201-288-6330; **Board Cert:** Obstetrics & Gynecology 2012; Reproductive Endocrinology/Infertility 2012; **Med School:** NYU Sch Med 1986; **Resid:** Obstetrics & Gynecology, NYU-Bellevue Hosp Ctr 1990; **Fellow:** Reproductive Endocrinology, UMDNJ-Newark 1992; **Fac Appt:** Prof ObG, UMDNJ-NJ Med Sch, Newark

Miller, Jane E MD (RE) - **Spec Exp:** Infertility-IVF; Laparoscopic Surgery; Hysteroscopic Surgery; **Hospital:** Holy Name Med Ctr (page 720); **Address:** North Hudson IVF Ctr, 385 Sylvan Ave, Ste 12, Englewood Cliffs, NJ 07632; **Phone:** 201-871-1999; **Board Cert:** Obstetrics & Gynecology 2012; Reproductive Endocrinology/Infertility 2012; **Med School:** SUNY Downstate 1978; **Resid:** Obstetrics & Gynecology, Beth Israel Deaconess Med Ctr 1983; Obstetrics & Gynecology, Erlanger Med Ctr 1984; **Fellow:** Reproductive Endocrinology, SUNY Downstate Med Ctr 1989

Weiss, Gerson MD (RE) - **Spec Exp:** Infertility; Menopause Problems; **Hospital:** Hackensack Univ Med Ctr (page 718), Univ Hosp (Newark); **Address:** 214 Terrace Ave, Hasbrouck Heights, NJ 07604-1815; **Phone:** 201-288-6330; **Board Cert:** Obstetrics & Gynecology 2012; Reproductive Endocrinology 2012; **Med School:** NYU Sch Med 1964; **Resid:** Obstetrics & Gynecology, Bellevue Hosp Ctr 1969; **Fellow:** Reproductive Endocrinology, Univ Pittsburgh Affil Hosp 1973; **Fac Appt:** Prof ObG, UMDNJ-NJ Med Sch, Newark

Rheumatology

Chung, Jeff MD (Rhu) - **Spec Exp:** Arthritis; Autoimmune Disease; Inflammatory Arthritis; Musculoskeletal Disorders; **Hospital:** Valley Hosp (page 721); **Address:** Bergen Medical Assocs, 1 W Ridgewood Ave, Ste 301, Paramus, NJ 07652; **Phone:** 201-445-1660; **Board Cert:** Rheumatology 2005; **Med School:** SUNY Downstate 1998; **Resid:** Internal Medicine, Yale-New Haven Hosp 2001; **Fellow:** Rheumatology, Yale-New Haven Hosp 2004

Gonter, Neil J MD (Rhu) - **Spec Exp:** Rheumatoid Arthritis; Gout; Osteoporosis; **Hospital:** Hackensack Univ Med Ctr (page 718), Holy Name Med Ctr (page 720); **Address:** Rheumatology Associates of North Jersey, 1415 Queen Anne Rd, Teaneck, NJ 07666; **Phone:** 201-837-7788; **Board Cert:** Rheumatology 2003; **Med School:** SUNY Upstate Med Univ 1998; **Resid:** Internal Medicine, UMDNJ Univ Hosp 2001; **Fellow:** Rheumatology, SUNY Downstate Med Ctr 2003; **Fac Appt:** Asst Prof Med, Columbia P&S

Guma, Michael DO (Rhu) - **Spec Exp:** Arthritis; Autoimmune Disease; Inflammatory Muscle Disease; Osteoporosis; **Hospital:** Saint Michael's Med Ctr; **Address:** North Jersey Rheumatology Assocs, 312 Belleville Tpke, Ste 3A, North Arlington, NJ 07031; **Phone:** 201-998-2800; **Board Cert:** Internal Medicine 2003; Rheumatology 2004; **Med School:** Kirksville Coll Osteo Med 1989; **Resid:** Internal Medicine, St Michaels Med Ctr 1992; **Fellow:** Rheumatology, St Michaels Med Ctr 1994

Kepecs, Gilbert MD (Rhu) - **Hospital:** Hackensack Univ Med Ctr (page 718), Holy Name Med Ctr (page 720); **Address:** Hackensack Rheumatology, 385 Prospect Ave Fl 2, Hackensack, NJ 07601; **Phone:** 201-498-9060; **Board Cert:** Internal Medicine 1989; Rheumatology 2002; **Med School:** Albert Einstein Coll Med 1986; **Resid:** Internal Medicine, St Lukes Hosp 1989; **Fellow:** Rheumatology, Montefiore Med Ctr 1993; Research, Albert Einstein Coll Med 1995; **Fac Appt:** Asst Clin Prof Med, UMDNJ-NJ Med Sch, Newark

Kopelman, Rima G MD (Rhu) - **Spec Exp:** Rheumatoid Arthritis; Lupus/SLE; Vasculitis; **Hospital:** Valley Hosp (page 721), NY-Presby/Columbia Univ Med Ctr, NY (page 104); **Address:** 301 Godwin Ave, Midland Park, NJ 07432-1544; **Phone:** 201-444-4526; **Board Cert:** Internal Medicine 1980; Rheumatology 1984; **Med School:** Columbia P&S 1977; **Resid:** Internal Medicine, Columbia-Presby Med Ctr 1981; **Fellow:** Rheumatology, Columbia-Presby Med Ctr 1983; **Fac Appt:** Asst Prof Med, Columbia P&S

Leibowitz, Evan H MD (Rhu) - **Spec Exp:** Rheumatoid Arthritis; Gout; Lupus/SLE; **Hospital:** Valley Hosp (page 721); **Address:** Prospect Medical Office, 301 Godwin Ave, Midland Park, NJ 07432; **Phone:** 201-444-4526; **Board Cert:** Rheumatology 2011; **Med School:** UMDNJ-NJ Med Sch, Newark 1996; **Resid:** Internal Medicine, New York Hosp 1999; **Fellow:** Rheumatology, Hosp for Special Surg 2002

Marcus, Ralph E MD (Rhu) - **Spec Exp:** Rheumatoid Arthritis; Osteoporosis; Lupus/SLE; Scleroderma; **Hospital:** Hackensack Univ Med Ctr (page 718), Holy Name Med Ctr (page 720); **Address:** 1415 Queen Anne Rd, Ste 102, 420 Grand Avenue, Englewood, NJ 07631, Teaneck, NJ 07666-3521; **Phone:** 201-837-7788; **Board Cert:** Internal Medicine 1975; Rheumatology 1976; **Med School:** Albert Einstein Coll Med 1969; **Resid:** Internal Medicine, Mount Sinai Hosp 1974; **Fellow:** Rheumatology, Natl Inst Hlth 1972; Rheumatology, Hosp Special Surg 1976; **Fac Appt:** Assoc Clin Prof Med, UMDNJ-RW Johnson Med Sch

Salem, Noel MD (Rhu) - **Hospital:** Englewood Hosp & Med Ctr; **Address:** 285 Engle St, Englewood, NJ 07631-2406; **Phone:** 201-871-0223; **Board Cert:** Internal Medicine 1976; Rheumatology 1998; Geriatric Medicine 2004; **Med School:** SUNY Buffalo 1972; **Resid:** Internal Medicine, US Public Hlth Svc Hosp 1974; **Fellow:** Rheumatology, Columbia-Presby Med Ctr 1976; **Fac Appt:** Asst Prof Med, Mount Sinai Sch Med

Zalkowitz, Alan MD (Rhu) - **Spec Exp:** Rheumatoid Arthritis; Gout; Collagen Vascular Disorders; **Hospital:** Valley Hosp (page 721); **Address:** 31-00 Broadway, Fl 2nd, Fair Lawn, NJ 07410-2331; **Phone:** 201-796-2255; **Board Cert:** Internal Medicine 1977; Rheumatology 1982; **Med School:** Belgium 1970; **Resid:** Internal Medicine, Yale New Haven Hosp 1971; Internal Medicine, Stamford Hosp 1972; **Fellow:** Rheumatology, Mount Sinai Hosp 1974

Sports Medicine

Delfico, Anthony MD (SM) - **Spec Exp:** Arthroscopic Surgery; Shoulder & Knee Surgery; Knee Replacement; **Hospital:** Valley Hosp (page 721); **Address:** Ridgewood Orthopedic Grp, 85 S Maple Ave, Ridgewood, NJ 07450; **Phone:** 201-445-2830; **Board Cert:** Orthopaedic Surgery 2000; **Med School:** UMDNJ-RW Johnson Med Sch 1992; **Resid:** Orthopaedic Surgery, Robert Wood Johnson Univ Hosp 1997; **Fellow:** Sports Medicine, Duke Univ Hosp 1998

Savatsky, Gary MD (SM) - **Spec Exp:** Shoulder & Knee Injuries; **Hospital:** Hackensack Univ Med Ctr (page 718); **Address:** Orthopedic Spine & Sports Med Ctr, 2 Forest Ave, Paramus, NJ 07652; **Phone:** 201-587-1111; **Board Cert:** Orthopaedic Surgery 2007; **Med School:** Columbia P&S 1975; **Resid:** Surgery, St Luke's-Roosevelt Hosp Ctr 1978; Orthopaedic Surgery, Hosp for Special Surg 1980; **Fellow:** Orthopaedic Surgery, Hosp for Special Surg 1983

Surgery

Ahlborn, Thomas N MD (S) - **Spec Exp:** Gastrointestinal Surgery; Laparoscopic Surgery; Breast Surgery; **Hospital:** Valley Hosp (page 721); **Address:** Valley Med Grp, Surgery, 385 S Maple Ave, Ste 202, Glen Rock, NJ 07452; **Phone:** 201-444-5757; **Board Cert:** Surgery 2005; **Med School:** Columbia P&S 1980; **Resid:** Surgery, NY-Presby/Columbia Univ Med Ctr 1985; **Fellow:** Vascular Surgery, NY-Presby/Columbia Univ Med Ctr 1986

Bufalini, Bruno MD (S) - **Spec Exp:** Laparoscopic Surgery; **Hospital:** Englewood Hosp & Med Ctr; **Address:** 200 Grand Ave, Englewood, NJ 07631-4371; **Phone:** 201-871-0303; **Med School:** Italy 1970; **Resid:** Surgery, Englewood Hosp 1977

Christoudias, George MD (S) - **Spec Exp:** Hernia; Laparoscopic Cholecystectomy; Cancer Surgery; **Hospital:** Holy Name Med Ctr (page 720); **Address:** 741 Teaneck Rd, Teaneck, NJ 07666; **Phone:** 201-833-2888; **Med School:** Greece 1969; **Resid:** Surgery, Downstate-Kings Co Med Ctr 1976; **Fellow:** Surgical Oncology, Downstate-Kings Co Med Ctr 1977

Fried, Kenneth S MD (S) - **Spec Exp:** Carotid Artery Surgery; Laparoscopic Surgery; **Hospital:** Englewood Hosp & Med Ctr, Holy Name Med Ctr (page 720); **Address:** 180 N Dean St, Ste 2 South, Englewood, NJ 07631-2541; **Phone:** 201-568-8666; **Board Cert:** Surgery 2004; **Med School:** NYU Sch Med 1978; **Resid:** Surgery, NYU Med Ctr 1983; **Fellow:** Vascular Surgery, NYU Med Ctr 1984

Harris, Michael T MD (S) - **Spec Exp:** Gastrointestinal Surgery; Inflammatory Bowel Disease; **Hospital:** Englewood Hosp & Med Ctr; **Address:** 350 Engle St 2NW Bldg, Englewood, NJ 07639; **Phone:** 201-608-2800; **Board Cert:** Surgery 2003; **Med School:** Columbia P&S 1988; **Resid:** Surgery, Mt Sinai Med Ctr 1994

Licata Jr, Joseph J MD (S) - **Spec Exp:** Laparoscopic Surgery; Breast Surgery; **Hospital:** Valley Hosp (page 721); **Address:** 245 E Main St, Ramsey, NJ 07446; **Phone:** 201-327-0220; **Board Cert:** Surgery 2011; **Med School:** Mexico 1984; **Resid:** Surgery, Westchester Med Ctr 1991

McCain, Donald MD/PhD (S) - **Spec Exp:** Cancer Surgery; Breast Cancer; Gastrointestinal Cancer; Melanoma; **Hospital:** Hackensack Univ Med Ctr (page 718); **Address:** 20 Prospect Ave, Ste 603, Hackensack, NJ 07601; **Phone:** 201-342-1010; **Board Cert:** Surgery 2010; **Med School:** Albert Einstein Coll Med 1991; **Resid:** Surgery, Mt Sinai Med Ctr 1996; **Fellow:** Surgical Oncology, Meml Sloan-Kettering Cancer Ctr 1998

Pereira, Stephen MD (S) - **Spec Exp:** Laparoscopic Abdominal Surgery; **Hospital:** Hackensack Univ Med Ctr (page 718); **Address:** 90 Prospect Ave, Ste 1D, Hackensack, NJ 07601-1918; **Phone:** 201-343-3433; **Board Cert:** Surgery 2007; **Med School:** UMDNJ-RW Johnson Med Sch 1991; **Resid:** Surgery, Northwestern Meml Hosp 1996; **Fellow:** Laparoscopic Surgery, Hackensack Univ Med Ctr 1999; **Fac Appt:** Asst Clin Prof S, UMDNJ-NJ Med Sch, Newark

Poole, John W MD (S) - **Hospital:** Holy Name Med Ctr (page 720); **Address:** 83 Summit Ave, Hackensack, NJ 07601; **Phone:** 201-646-0010; **Board Cert:** Surgery 2008; **Med School:** Univ VA Sch Med 1982; **Resid:** Surgery, Montefiore Med Ctr 1987

Schmidt, Hans J MD (S) - **Spec Exp:** Obesity/Bariatric Surgery; Laparoscopic Abdominal Surgery; **Hospital:** Hackensack Univ Med Ctr (page 718); **Address:** 81 Route 4 W, Ste 401, Paramus, NJ 07652; **Phone:** 201-646-1121; **Board Cert:** Surgery 2008; **Med School:** UMDNJ-NJ Med Sch, Newark 1991; **Resid:** Surgery, Univ Hosp-UMDNJ 1997

Sussman, Barry Clark MD (S) - **Spec Exp:** Laparoscopic Surgery; Breast Surgery; **Hospital:** Englewood Hosp & Med Ctr; **Address:** 375 Engle St, Englewood, NJ 07631-1823; **Phone:** 201-894-0400; **Board Cert:** Surgery 2008; **Med School:** NYU Sch Med 1973; **Resid:** Surgery, NYU Med Ctr 1978; **Fellow:** Vascular Surgery, Englewood Hosp 1979; **Fac Appt:** Asst Clin Prof S, Mount Sinai Sch Med

Yang, Hee K MD (S) - **Spec Exp:** Laparoscopic Surgery; Vascular Surgery; **Hospital:** Holy Name Med Ctr (page 720); **Address:** 464 Hudson Terr, Ste 101, Englewood Cliff, NJ 07632; **Phone:** 201-567-7747; **Board Cert:** Surgery 2006; **Med School:** Rush Med Coll 1989; **Resid:** Surgery, Lenox Hill Hosp 1995

Yiengpruksawan, Anusak MD (S) - **Spec Exp:** Liver & Biliary Surgery; Endoscopic Ultrasound; Robotic Surgery; Minimally Invasive Surgery; **Hospital:** Valley Hosp (page 721), Chilton Hosp; **Address:** Valley Hosp, Surgery Dept, 1 Valley Health Plaza, Paramus, NJ 07652; **Phone:** 201-634-5438; **Board Cert:** Surgery 2011; **Med School:** Japan 1978; **Resid:** Surgery, Harlem Hosp 1989; **Fellow:** Surgical Oncology, Meml Sloan-Kettering Cancer Ctr 1991

Thoracic & Cardiac Surgery

Elmann, Elie M MD (T&CS) - **Spec Exp:** Robotic Cardiac Surgery; Minimally Invasive Cardiac Surgery; Heart Valve Surgery; Atrial Fibrillation; **Hospital:** Hackensack Univ Med Ctr (page 718), Englewood Hosp & Med Ctr; **Address:** Hackensack Univ Med Ctr, Cardiothoracic, 20 Prospect Ave, Ste 900, Hackensack, NJ 07601; **Phone:** 201-996-2261; **Board Cert:** Surgery 2004; Thoracic & Cardiac Surgery 2005; **Med School:** NY Med Coll 1987; **Resid:** Surgery, Cabrini Med Ctr 1992; **Fellow:** Cardiothoracic Surgery, SUNY Downstate Med Ctr 1995; **Fac Appt:** Asst Prof S, UMDNJ-NJ Med Sch, Newark

Klein, James J MD (T&CS) - **Spec Exp:** Aneurysm-Thoracic Aortic; **Hospital:** Englewood Hosp & Med Ctr; **Address:** Englewood Cardiac Surgery Assocs, 350 Engle St, Ste 2500, Englewood, NJ 07631; **Phone:** 201-894-3636; **Board Cert:** Thoracic Surgery 2007; Surgery 2004; **Med School:** SUNY Stony Brook 1990; **Resid:** Surgery, SUNY Downstate Med Ctr 1995; **Fellow:** Thoracic & Cardiac Surgery, Mount Sinai Med Ctr 1998

McCullough, Jock N MD (T&CS) - **Spec Exp:** Heart Valve Surgery; Minimally Invasive Heart Valve Surgery; Coronary Artery Surgery; Cardiac Surgery; **Hospital:** Hackensack Univ Med Ctr (page 718); **Address:** The Heart & Vascular Hosp at Hackensack, 30 Prospect Ave, Hackensack, NJ 07601; **Phone:** 551-996-5388; **Board Cert:** Surgery 2004; Thoracic Surgery 2005; **Med School:** UMDNJ-NJ Med Sch, Newark 1987; **Resid:** Surgery, UMDNJ Affil Hosp 1993; **Fellow:** Cardiothoracic Surgery, Mt Sinai Med Ctr 1996

Park, Bernard J MD (T&CS) - **Spec Exp:** Lung Cancer; Esophageal Cancer; Mediastinal Tumors; Robotic Surgery; **Hospital:** Hackensack Univ Med Ctr (page 718), Hackensack UMC-Pascack Valley (page 719); **Address:** 30 Prospect Ave, Ste 5640, Hackensack, NJ 07601; **Phone:** 551-996-4218; **Board Cert:** Surgery 2011; Thoracic Surgery 2013; **Med School:** Univ Pennsylvania 1993; **Resid:** Surgery, New York Hosp 1996; Surgery, Meml Sloan Kettering Cancer Ctr 2000; **Fellow:** Cardiothoracic Surgery, Meml Sloan Kettering Cancer Ctr 2002; **Fac Appt:** Asst Clin Prof TS, UMDNJ-NJ Med Sch, Newark

Zairis, Ignatios MD (T&CS) - **Spec Exp:** Endovascular Surgery; Minimally Invasive Thoracic Surgery; **Hospital:** Englewood Hosp & Med Ctr, Holy Name Med Ctr (page 720); **Address:** 741 Teaneck Rd, Teaneck, NJ 07666; **Phone:** 201-837-8282; **Board Cert:** Surgery 2011; **Med School:** Greece 1973; **Resid:** Surgery, Kings Co Hosp 1984; Thoracic Surgery, SUNY Hlth Sci Ctr 1983; **Fellow:** Cardiothoracic Surgery, SUNY Hlth Sci Ctr 1984

Zapolanski, Alex MD (T&CS) - **Spec Exp:** Minimally Invasive Heart Valve Surgery; Aortic Surgery; Coronary Artery Surgery; **Hospital:** Valley Hosp (page 721); **Address:** Valley Hosp, Heart Ctr, 223 N Van Dien Ave, Ridgewood, NJ 07450; **Phone:** 201-447-8377; **Board Cert:** Thoracic Surgery 2004; **Med School:** Argentina 1973; **Resid:** Surgery, Cleveland Clin 1979; Cardiothoracic Surgery, Toronto Genl Hosp 1981

Urology

Agarwal, Saurabh MD (U) - **Spec Exp:** Prostate Cancer; Robotic Surgery; **Hospital:** Valley Hosp (page 721); **Address:** 6 Goodwin Ave, Midland Park, NJ 07432; **Phone:** 201-444-7070; **Board Cert:** Urology 2007; **Med School:** Boston Univ 1999; **Resid:** Surgery, Rhode Island Hosp 2000; Urology, Rhode Island Hosp 2004

Ahmed, Mutahar MD (U) - **Spec Exp:** Robotic Surgery; Prostate Cancer; Minimally Invasive Surgery; Kidney Cancer; **Hospital:** Hackensack Univ Med Ctr (page 718), Holy Name Med Ctr (page 720); **Address:** NJ Ctr Prostate Cancer & Urology, 255 W Spring Valley Ave, Ste 101, Maywood, NJ 07607; **Phone:** 201-487-8866; **Board Cert:** Urology 2005; **Med School:** SUNY Hlth Sci Ctr 1997; **Resid:** Surgery, Univ Hosp-UMDNJ 1999; **Fellow:** Urology, Univ Hosp-UMDNJ 2003; **Fac Appt:** Asst Clin Prof U, UMDNJ-NJ Med Sch, Newark

Andronaco, Raymond B MD (U) - **Spec Exp:** Voiding Dysfunction; Incontinence; **Hospital:** Englewood Hosp & Med Ctr; **Address:** Urologic Specialties, 177 N Dean St, South Tower, Ste 305, Englewood, NJ 07631; **Phone:** 201-569-7777; **Board Cert:** Urology 2003; **Med School:** Mexico 1976; **Resid:** Surgery, Beth Israel Med Ctr 1979; Urology, NYU Med Ctr 1983; **Fac Appt:** Asst Clin Prof U, NYU Sch Med

Basralian, Kevin R MD (U) - **Spec Exp:** Infertility-Male; Prostate Benign Disease; Minimally Invasive Surgery; Reconstructive Urologic Surgery; **Hospital:** Hackensack Univ Med Ctr (page 718); **Address:** HUMC, Urology Dept, 360 Essex St, Ste 403, Hackensack, NJ 07601; **Phone:** 551-996-8090; **Board Cert:** Urology 2010; **Med School:** Mexico 1979; **Resid:** Surgery, Lenox Hill Hosp 1982; Urology, Lenox Hill Hosp 1985; **Fellow:** Reconstructive Pelvic Surgery, Univ Edinburgh 1986

Chun, Thomas MD (U) - **Spec Exp:** Prostate Cancer; Kidney Stones; Erectile Dysfunction; **Hospital:** Englewood Hosp & Med Ctr, Holy Name Med Ctr (page 720); **Address:** Urology Ctr, 300 Grand Ave, Ste 202, Englewood, NJ 07631; **Phone:** 201-816-1900; **Board Cert:** Urology 2008; **Med School:** Geo Wash Univ 1991; **Resid:** Surgery, NYU Med Ctr 1993; **Fellow:** Urology, NYU Med Ctr 1997

Esposito, Michael P MD (U) - **Spec Exp:** Laparoscopic Kidney Surgery; Prostate Cancer/Robotic Surgery; Minimally Invasive Urologic Surgery; Adrenal Surgery; **Hospital:** Hackensack Univ Med Ctr (page 718), Monmouth Med Ctr; **Address:** NJ Ctr Prostate Cancer & Urology, 255 W Spring Valley Ave, Ste 101, Maywood, NJ 07607; **Phone:** 201-487-8866; **Board Cert:** Urology 2012; **Med School:** UMDNJ-NJ Med Sch, Newark 1994; **Resid:** Urology, Univ Hosp-UMDNJ 2000; **Fellow:** Minimally Invasive Surgery, Univ Hosp-UMDNJ 2002; Urologic Laparoscopic Surg-Endourology, Royal Infirm/Western Genl Hosp 2003; **Fac Appt:** Asst Clin Prof S, UMDNJ-NJ Med Sch, Newark

Frey, Howard L MD (U) - **Spec Exp:** Prostate Cancer; Bladder Cancer; Kidney Cancer; **Hospital:** Valley Hosp (page 721); **Address:** Urology Grp, 4 Godwin Ave, Midland Park, NJ 07432; **Phone:** 201-444-7070; **Board Cert:** Urology 2013; **Med School:** Johns Hopkins Univ 1977; **Resid:** Surgery, Johns Hopkins Hosp 1979; Urology, UCLA Med Ctr 1983

Hajjar, John H MD (U) - **Spec Exp:** Laparoscopic Surgery; Prostate Surgery; **Hospital:** Valley Hosp (page 721); **Address:** Sovereign Med Grp, Urology, 1401 Broadway Fl 3, Fair Lawn, NJ 07410; **Phone:** 201-791-4544; **Board Cert:** Urology 2011; **Med School:** Georgetown Univ 1981; **Resid:** Surgery, NYU Med Ctr 1983; Urology, NYU-Bellevue/Sloan Ketterin 1987; **Fellow:** Research, NYU Med Ctr 1988

Hensle, Terry W MD (U) - **Spec Exp:** Pediatric Urology; Hypospadias; Urinary Reconstruction; Wilms' Tumor; **Hospital:** Hackensack Univ Med Ctr (page 718); **Address:** 699 Teaneck Rd, Ste 103, Teaneck, NJ 07666; **Phone:** 201-645-3362; **Board Cert:** Urology 1978; **Med School:** Cornell Univ-Weill Med Coll 1968; **Resid:** Surgery, Boston City Hosp 1973; Urology, Mass Genl Hosp 1976; **Fellow:** Pediatric Urology, Mass Genl Hosp 1977; Pediatric Urology, Great Ormond St Hosp 1978; **Fac Appt:** Prof U, Columbia P&S

Katz, Steven A MD (U) - **Spec Exp:** Transfusion Free Surgery; Prostate Cancer; Laparoscopic Surgery; **Hospital:** Englewood Hosp & Med Ctr, Holy Name Med Ctr (page 720); **Address:** Urology Ctr, 300 Grand Ave, Ste 202, Englewood, NJ 07631; **Phone:** 201-816-1900; **Board Cert:** Urology 1978; **Med School:** SUNY Buffalo 1969; **Resid:** Urology, Metropolitan Hosp Ctr 1976

Kerns, John MD (U) - **Spec Exp:** Urologic Cancer; Incontinence; Infertility-Male; **Hospital:** Holy Name Med Ctr (page 720); **Address:** Urologic Specialists, 177 N Dean St, Ste 305, Englewood, NJ 07631; **Phone:** 201-569-7777; **Board Cert:** Urology ; **Med School:** Georgetown Univ 1975; **Resid:** Surgery, Georgetown Univ Hosp 1977; Urology, Georgetown Univ Hosp 1981

Lanteri, Vincent J MD (U) - **Spec Exp:** Prostate Cancer/Robotic Surgery; Urologic Cancer; **Hospital:** Hackensack Univ Med Ctr (page 718), Holy Name Med Ctr (page 720); **Address:** NJ Ctr for Prostate Cancer & Urology, 255 W Spring Valley Ave, Ste 101, Maywood, NJ 07607; **Phone:** 201-487-8866; **Board Cert:** Urology 1982; **Med School:** Mexico 1974; **Resid:** Surgery, UMDNJ Med Ctr 1977; Urology, UMDNJ Med Ctr 1980; **Fellow:** Urologic Oncology, Roswell Park Cancer Inst 1982

Margolis, Eric J MD (U) - **Spec Exp:** Urologic Cancer; Prostate Disease; Robotic Surgery; **Hospital:** Englewood Hosp & Med Ctr; **Address:** Urology Ctr, 300 Grand Ave, Ste 202, Englewood, NJ 07631; **Phone:** 201-816-1900; **Board Cert:** Urology 2008; **Med School:** SUNY Upstate Med Univ 1990; **Resid:** Urologic Surgery, Mount Sinai Med Ctr 1996

Munver, Ravi MD (U) - **Spec Exp:** Robotic Surgery; Urologic Cancer; Minimally Invasive Urologic Surgery; Prostate Cancer; **Hospital:** Hackensack Univ Med Ctr (page 718); **Address:** Hackensack University Medical Center, 360 Essex St, Ste 403, Hackensack, NJ 07601; **Phone:** 551-996-8090; **Board Cert:** Urology 2013; **Med School:** Cornell Univ-Weill Med Coll 1996; **Resid:** Urology, Duke Univ Med Ctr 2002; **Fellow:** Robotic Surgery, New York Hosp-Cornell Med Ctr 2003; **Fac Appt:** Assoc Prof U, UMDNJ-Univ Med Dent NJ

Rosenberg, Gene S MD (U) - **Spec Exp:** Minimally Invasive Surgery; Prostate Cancer-Cryosurgery; Kidney Cancer-Cryosurgery; **Hospital:** Hackensack Univ Med Ctr (page 718), Holy Name Med Ctr (page 720); **Address:** Univ Urology Assocs, 20 Prospect Ave, Ste 719, Hackensack, NJ 07601; **Phone:** 201-343-0082; **Board Cert:** Urology 1982; **Med School:** NYU Sch Med 1974; **Resid:** Pathology, Kings Co Hosp 1976; Urology, Bellevue Hosp 1980

Sadeghi-Nejad, Hossein MD (U) - **Spec Exp:** Erectile Dysfunction; Peyronie's Disease; Prostate Disease; Infertility-Male; **Hospital:** Hackensack Univ Med Ctr (page 718), Univ Hosp (Newark); **Address:** 20 Prospect Ave, rm 711, Hackensack, NJ 07601; **Phone:** 201-342-7977 x214; **Board Cert:** Urology 2009; **Med School:** McGill Univ 1989; **Resid:** Surgery, UCSF Med Ctr 1991; Urology, Boston Univ Med Ctr 1996; **Fellow:** Microsurgery, Boston Univ Med Ctr 1997; Reproductive Medicine, Boston Univ Med Ctr 1997; **Fac Appt:** Prof U, UMDNJ-Rutgers Med Sch

Sawczuk, Ihor S MD (U) - **Spec Exp:** Bladder Cancer; Kidney Cancer; Prostate Cancer/Robotic Surgery; **Hospital:** Hackensack Univ Med Ctr (page 718), NY-Presby/Columbia Univ Med Ctr, NY (page 104); **Address:** Hackensack Univ Med Ctr, Dept Urology, 360 Essex St, Ste 403, Hackensack, NJ 07601; **Phone:** 551-996-8090; **Board Cert:** Urology 2005; **Med School:** Med Coll PA Hahnemann 1979; **Resid:** Surgery, St Vincents Hosp 1981; Urology, Columbia-Presby Med Ctr 1984; **Fellow:** Urologic Oncology, Columbia-Presby Med Ctr 1986; **Fac Appt:** Prof U, UMDNJ-NJ Med Sch, Newark

Siegel, Andrew MD (U) - **Spec Exp:** Urology-Female; Incontinence; Urodynamics; Voiding Dysfunction; **Hospital:** Hackensack Univ Med Ctr (page 718); **Address:** Bergen Urological Assocs, 20 Prospect Ave, Ste 715, Hackensack, NJ 07601; **Phone:** 201-342-6600; **Board Cert:** Urology 2008; Female Pelvic Medicine & Reconstuctive Surgery 2013; **Med School:** Ros Franklin Univ/Chicago Med Sch 1981; **Resid:** Urology, Hosp Univ Penn-UPHS 1987; **Fellow:** Female Urology, UCLA Med Ctr 1988; **Fac Appt:** Asst Clin Prof U, UMDNJ-NJ Med Sch, Newark

Wasserman, Gary D MD (U) - **Spec Exp:** Kidney Stones; Incontinence; Voiding Dysfunction; **Hospital:** Englewood Hosp & Med Ctr, Holy Name Med Ctr (page 720); **Address:** Urology Ctr, 300 Grand Ave, Ste 202, Englewood, NJ 07631; **Phone:** 201-816-1900; **Board Cert:** Urology 2012; **Med School:** Tulane Univ 1985; **Resid:** Surgery, G Washington Univ Hosp 1987; Urology, Tulane Med Ctr 1991

Vascular & Interventional Radiology

Albert, Arthur MD (VIR) - **Spec Exp:** Interventional Radiology; **Hospital:** Hackensack Univ Med Ctr (page 718); **Address:** HackensackUMC-Dept of Radiology, 30 Prospect Ave, Hackensack, NJ 07601; **Phone:** 201-996-2254; **Board Cert:** Diagnostic Radiology ; **Med School:** Penn State Coll Med 1978; **Resid:** Diagnostic Radiology, Hosp Univ Penn 1982; **Fellow:** Vascular & Interventional Radiology, Alexandria Hosp 1983

Rundback, John H MD (VIR) - **Spec Exp:** Angioplasty; Chemoembolization & Tumor Ablation; Peripheral Vascular Disease; **Hospital:** Holy Name Med Ctr (page 720); **Address:** Holy Name Med Ctr, Radiology Dept, 718 Teaneck Rd, Ste 1E, Teaneck, NJ 07666; **Phone:** 201-833-7268; **Board Cert:** Diagnostic Radiology 1992; Vascular & Interventional Radiology 2006; **Med School:** SUNY Downstate 1987; **Resid:** Diagnostic Radiology, Beth Israel Med Ctr 1992; **Fellow:** Interventional Radiology, Washington Hosp Ctr 1993; **Fac Appt:** Assoc Prof Rad, Columbia P&S

Vascular Surgery

Elias, Steven M MD (VascS) - **Spec Exp:** Vein Disorders; Wound Healing/Care; Minimally Invasive Surgery; Varicose Veins; **Hospital:** Englewood Hosp & Med Ctr, NY-Presby/Columbia Univ Med Ctr, NY (page 104); **Address:** Englewood Hosp & Med Ctr, Ctr Vein Disease, 350 Engle St, Englewood, NJ 07631-2541; **Phone:** 201-894-3252; **Board Cert:** Surgery 2007; **Med School:** SUNY Buffalo 1979; **Resid:** Surgery, Millard Filmore Hosp 1981; **Fellow:** Peripheral Vascular Surgery, Englewood Hosp 1985; **Fac Appt:** Asst Prof S, Columbia P&S

Geuder, James W MD (VascS) - **Spec Exp:** Vein Disorders; Carotid Artery Surgery; Aneurysm-Aortic; Endovascular Surgery; **Hospital:** Hackensack Univ Med Ctr (page 718); **Address:** 680 Kinderkamack Rd, Ste 306, Oradell, NJ 07649; **Phone:** 201-262-8346; **Board Cert:** Surgery 2007; Vascular Surgery 2009; **Med School:** Med Coll Wisc 1981; **Resid:** Surgery, Univ Hosp-UMDNJ 1986; **Fellow:** Vascular Surgery, NYU Med Ctr 1988

Kagan, Peter E MD (VascS) - **Spec Exp:** Aneurysm-Abdominal Aortic; Carotid Artery Surgery; Endovascular Surgery; **Hospital:** Hackensack Univ Med Ctr (page 718), Holy Name Med Ctr (page 720); **Address:** North Jersey Surgical Specialists, 83 Summit Ave, Hackensack, NJ 07601; **Phone:** 201-646-0010; **Board Cert:** Surgery 2011; Vascular Surgery 2006; **Med School:** Grenada 1997; **Resid:** Surgery, Univ Hosp-UMDNJ 2002; **Fellow:** Vascular Surgery, Newark Beth Israel Med Ctr 2004

Manno, Joseph MD (VascS) - **Spec Exp:** Arterial Disease; Angioplasty; Limb Sparing Surgery; **Hospital:** Hackensack Univ Med Ctr (page 718), Holy Name Med Ctr (page 720); **Address:** North Jersey Surgical Specialists, 83 Summit Ave, Hackensack, NJ 07601; **Phone:** 201-646-0010; **Board Cert:** Surgery 2009; Vascular Surgery 2012; **Med School:** Oral Roberts Sch Med 1982; **Resid:** Surgery, Univ Hosp-UMDNJ 1987; **Fellow:** Vascular Surgery, Univ Hosp-UMDNJ 1989

Napolitano, Massimo MD (VascS) - **Hospital:** Hackensack Univ Med Ctr (page 718); **Address:** Bergen Surgical Specialists, 20 Prospect Ave, Ste 707, Hackensack, NJ 07601; **Phone:** 201-343-0040; **Board Cert:** Vascular Surgery 2004; Surgery 2012; **Med School:** Italy 1984; **Resid:** Surgery, UMDNJ Affil Hosp 1987; Surgery, Monmouth Med Ctr 1989; **Fellow:** Surgery, Henry Ford Hosp 1992; Vascular Surgery, Henry Ford Hosp 1994

Wolodiger, Fred A MD (VascS) - **Spec Exp:** Arterial Bypass Surgery-Leg; Carotid Artery Surgery; Aneurysm-Aortic; Endovascular Surgery; **Hospital:** Englewood Hosp & Med Ctr; **Address:** Englewood Surgical Assocs, 375 Engle St, Englewood, NJ 07631; **Phone:** 201-894-0400; **Board Cert:** Surgery 2004; Vascular Surgery 2008; **Med School:** SUNY Downstate 1980; **Resid:** Surgery, N Shore Univ Hosp 1985; **Fellow:** Peripheral Vascular Surgery, Englewood Hosp & Med Ctr 1987

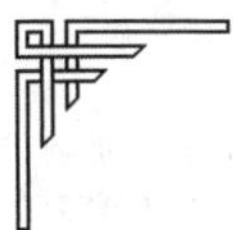

The Best in American Medicine
www.CastleConnolly.com

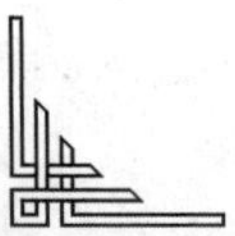

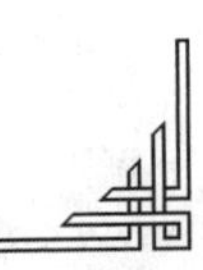

Essex

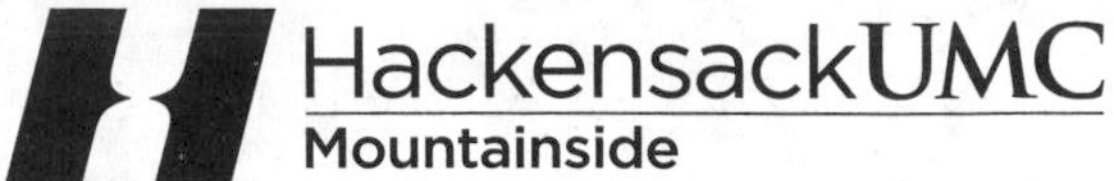

1 Bay Avenue, Montclair, NJ 07042 • 973-429-6000
www.mountainsidehosp.com

Number of beds: 365
Number of employees: 1,660
2012 Admissions: 11,244

Our prestigious affiliation with the Hackensack University Health Network has enhanced the hospital's reputation and paved the way for convenient local access to a larger array of specialized services and medical innovations. This pivotal turning point ensures our ability to grow and uphold our 121-year tradition of service.

With 365 beds and 820,000 square feet, HackensackUMC Mountainside provides a caliber of care within its community hospital setting that rivals the nation's largest and most prestigious facilities. Patients have immediate access to state-of-the-art diagnostic technologies, including high-speed, 3-D CT imaging. Innovative and effective treatment alternatives for an array of diverse conditions are available at specialized centers dedicated to: women's health; cancer care; cardiology; surgery; stroke; chronic kidney disease; wound care; and sleep disorders.

Our surgical center is equipped with the most current generation da Vinci robotics, and more than 200 skilled surgeons successfully perform thousands of procedures at HackensackUMC Mountainside each year. The HackensackUMC Mountainside Center for Advanced Bariatric Surgery, which offers a comprehensive range of laparoscopic options, is a recognized Center of Excellence by the American Society of Metabolic and Bariatric Surgery, and our Breast Health Program was recently awarded Breast Center of Excellence status by the American College of Radiology.

Other distinguished programs include the HackensackUMC Mountainside Cancer Center, which is accredited with commendation by the American College of Surgeons, a distinction awarded to only about one-fourth of all hospital cancer centers nationwide.

- American Society for Metabolic and Bariatric Surgery Center of Excellence
- Joint Commission National Quality Approval
- American College of Radiology for Radiation Oncology and Mammography
- American Heart Association/American Stroke Association Get with the Guidelines Gold Plus Achievement Award
- New Jersey Department of Health and Senior Services-designated Primary Stroke Center
- Federal Drug Administration's Mammography Quality Standards Act for Mammography Services
- American College of Surgeons for the Cancer Center
- College of American Pathologists for laboratory services
- National League for Nursing Accrediting Commission for the Mountainside Nursing School
- Intersocietal Commission for the Accreditation of Echocardiography Laboratories

For more information, please call 973-429-6000 or visit www.Mountainsidehosp.com.

Adolescent Medicine

Johnson, Robert L MD (AM) - **Spec Exp:** AIDS/HIV; Abuse/Neglect; Behavioral Disorders; **Hospital:** Univ Hosp (Newark); **Address:** Univ Hosp, Adolescent Med, 90 Bergen St, Ste 4300, Newark, NJ 07103; **Phone:** 973-972-2100; **Board Cert:** Pediatrics 1977; **Med School:** UMDNJ-NJ Med Sch, Newark 1972; **Resid:** Pediatrics, Martland Hosp 1974; **Fellow:** Adolescent Medicine, NYU Med Ctr 1976; **Fac Appt:** Prof Ped, UMDNJ-NJ Med Sch, Newark

Neal, Wendy P MD (AM) - **Spec Exp:** Adolescent Gynecology; **Hospital:** Chldns Hosp NJ at Newark; **Address:** Pediatric Hlth Ctr, 166 Lyons Ave, Newark, NJ 07112; **Phone:** 973-926-7282; **Board Cert:** Pediatrics 2010; Adolescent Medicine 2011; **Med School:** Tulane Univ 1991; **Resid:** Pediatrics, Montefiore Med Ctr 1994; **Fellow:** Adolescent Medicine, Montefiore Med Ctr 1997

Stanford, Paulette D MD (AM) - **Spec Exp:** AIDS/HIV in Adolescents; Adolescent Gynecology; Adolescent Behavior-High Risk; **Hospital:** Univ Hosp (Newark); **Address:** Univ Hosp, Adolescent Med, 90 Bergen St, Ste 4300, Newark, NJ 07103; **Phone:** 973-972-2100; **Board Cert:** Pediatrics 1984; Adolescent Medicine 2009; **Med School:** UMDNJ-NJ Med Sch, Newark 1975; **Resid:** Pediatrics, UMDNJ-Univ Hosp 1977; **Fellow:** Adolescent Medicine, UMDNJ-Univ Hosp 1979; **Fac Appt:** Prof Ped, UMDNJ-NJ Med Sch, Newark

Allergy & Immunology

Perlman, Donald B MD (A&I) - **Spec Exp:** Asthma; Urticaria; Drug Sensitivity; **Hospital:** Saint Barnabas Med Ctr, Newark Beth Israel Med Ctr; **Address:** Assocs Otolaryngology, 741 Northfield Ave, Ste 104, West Orange, NJ 07052; **Phone:** 973-736-7722; **Board Cert:** Pediatrics 1978; Allergy & Immunology 1979; **Med School:** Mount Sinai Sch Med 1973; **Resid:** Pediatrics, Mount Sinai Med Ctr 1976; **Fellow:** Allergy & Immunology, Duke Univ Hosp 1978; **Fac Appt:** Asst Clin Prof Ped, UMDNJ-NJ Med Sch, Newark

Weiss, Steven J MD (A&I) - **Spec Exp:** Asthma; Sinus Disorders; Drug Sensitivity; **Hospital:** Saint Barnabas Med Ctr; **Address:** 209 S Livingston Ave, Ste 6, Livingston, NJ 07039-4042; **Phone:** 973-992-4171; **Board Cert:** Internal Medicine 1985; Allergy & Immunology 1987; **Med School:** Ros Franklin Univ/Chicago Med Sch 1982; **Resid:** Internal Medicine, St Lukes Roosevelt Hosp 1985; **Fellow:** Allergy & Immunology, St Lukes Roosevelt Hosp 1987; **Fac Appt:** Asst Clin Prof A&I, UMDNJ-Rutgers Med Sch

Cardiac Electrophysiology

Correia, Joaquim J MD (CE) - **Spec Exp:** Arrhythmias; Pacemakers/Defibrillators; Syncope; **Hospital:** Saint Michael's Med Ctr; **Address:** 243 Chestnut St, Ste 2L, Newark, NJ 07105; **Phone:** 973-589-8668; **Board Cert:** Internal Medicine 1989; Cardiac Electrophysiology 2004; Cardiovascular Disease 2013; **Med School:** NYU Sch Med 1986; **Resid:** Internal Medicine, NY-Presby/Columbia Univ Med Ctr 1989; **Fellow:** Cardiovascular Disease, NY-Presby/Columbia Univ Med Ctr 1992; Cardiac Electrophysiology, NY-Presby/Columbia Univ Med Ctr 1993; **Fac Appt:** Asst Prof Med, UMDNJ-NJ Med Sch, Newark

Costeas, Constantinos A MD (CE) - **Spec Exp:** Arrhythmias; Radiofrequency Ablation; Pacemakers; **Hospital:** Saint Michael's Med Ctr, Saint Barnabas Med Ctr; **Address:** NJ Cardiology Assocs, 375 Mount Pleasant Ave Fl 2, West Orange, NJ 07052; **Phone:** 973-731-9598; **Board Cert:** Cardiac Electrophysiology 2008; Cardiovascular Disease 2008; **Med School:** SUNY Stony Brook 1989; **Resid:** Internal Medicine, Stony Brook Univ Med Ctr 1992; **Fellow:** Cardiovascular Disease, St Vincents Hosp 1996; Cardiac Electrophysiology, NY-Presby/Columbia Univ Med Ctr 1998

Roelke, Marc MD (CE) - **Spec Exp:** Pacemakers/Defibrillators; Cardiac Catheterization; **Hospital:** Newark Beth Israel Med Ctr, Saint Barnabas Med Ctr; **Address:** NJ Cardiology Assocs, 375 Mount Pleasant Ave Fl 2, West Orange, NJ 07052; **Phone:** 973-731-9598; **Board Cert:** Cardiovascular Disease 2003; Cardiac Electrophysiology 2006; **Med School:** Columbia P&S 1987; **Resid:** Internal Medicine, Univ Chicago Med Ctr 1990; **Fellow:** Cardiovascular Disease, Mass Genl Hosp 1993; Cardiac Electrophysiology, Mass Genl Hosp 1994

Sauberman, Roy B MD (CE) - **Spec Exp:** Radiofrequency Ablation; Pacemakers/Defibrillators; Syncope; **Hospital:** Saint Barnabas Med Ctr, Jersey City Med Ctr; **Address:** Summit Medical Group, 161 Millburn Ave, Millburn, NJ 07041; **Phone:** 973-467-4220; **Board Cert:** Cardiovascular Disease 2008; Cardiac Electrophysiology 2008; **Med School:** Yale Univ 1990; **Resid:** Internal Medicine, NY-Presby/Weill Cornell Med Ctr 1993; **Fellow:** Cardiovascular Disease, NY-Presby/Columbia Univ Med Ctr 1996; Cardiac Electrophysiology, Beth Israel Med Ctr 1998

Cardiovascular Disease

Klapholz, Marc MD (Cv) - **Spec Exp:** Congestive Heart Failure; Angioplasty; Interventional Cardiology; Pulmonary Hypertension; **Hospital:** Univ Hosp (Newark); **Address:** Univ Hosp, Cardiology Dept, 90 Bergen St, Ste 3500, Newark, NJ 07103; **Phone:** 973-972-2573; **Board Cert:** Internal Medicine 1989; Cardiovascular Disease 2012; Interventional Cardiology 2009; Advanced Heart Failure & Transplant Cardiology 2010; **Med School:** Albert Einstein Coll Med 1986; **Resid:** Internal Medicine, Bronx Muni Hosp 1989; **Fellow:** Cardiovascular Disease, Bronx Muni Hosp 1992; Interventional Cardiology, Montefiore Med Ctr 1995; **Fac Appt:** Prof Med, UMDNJ-NJ Med Sch, Newark

Rogal, Gary J MD (Cv) - **Spec Exp:** Echocardiography; Coronary Artery Disease; Heart Valve Disease; **Hospital:** Saint Barnabas Med Ctr, Newark Beth Israel Med Ctr; **Address:** NJ Cardiology Assocs, 375 Mount Pleasant Ave, West Orange, NJ 07052; **Phone:** 973-731-9442; **Board Cert:** Internal Medicine 1981; Cardiovascular Disease 1983; **Med School:** Geo Wash Univ 1978; **Resid:** Internal Medicine, LI Jewish Med Ctr 1981; **Fellow:** Cardiovascular Disease, Univ Rochester Strong Meml Hosp 1984

Saroff, Alan L MD (Cv) - **Spec Exp:** Heart Valve Disease; Cholesterol/Lipid Disorders; Arrhythmias; Preventive Cardiology; **Hospital:** Hackensack UMC-Mountainside (page 774), NY-Presby/Columbia Univ Med Ctr, NY (page 104); **Address:** Montclair Cardiology Group, 123 Highland Ave, Ste 302, Glen Ridge, NJ 07028-1522; **Phone:** 973-748-9555; **Board Cert:** Internal Medicine 1972; Cardiovascular Disease 1975; **Med School:** SUNY Upstate Med Univ 1965; **Resid:** Internal Medicine, SUNY-Syracuse Med Ctr 1967; Internal Medicine, NY Hosp 1970; **Fellow:** Cardiovascular Disease, Columbia Presby Med Ctr 1972; Cardiac Electrophysiology, Columbia Presby Med Ctr 1973; **Fac Appt:** Assoc Clin Prof Med, Columbia P&S

Shamoon, Fayez E MD (Cv) - **Spec Exp:** Interventional Cardiology; Coronary Artery Disease; Nuclear Cardiology; Angioplasty & Stent Placement; **Hospital:** Saint Michael's Med Ctr, Trinitas Reg Med Ctr (page 914); **Address:** Saint Michaels Med Ctr - Cardiology, 111 Central Ave, Newark, NJ 07102; **Phone:** 973-877-5160; **Board Cert:** Internal Medicine 2006; Cardiovascular Disease 2006; Interventional Cardiology 2009; **Med School:** Jordan 1981; **Resid:** Internal Medicine, Jordan Univ Hosp 1985; Internal Medicine, St Michael's Med Ctr 1992; **Fellow:** Cardiovascular Disease, St Michael's Med Ctr 1995; Interventional Cardiology, St Michael's Med Ctr 1996; **Fac Appt:** Prof Med, Seton Hall Univ Sch Hlth & Med Scis

Wangenheim, Paul M MD (Cv) - **Spec Exp:** Echocardiography; Coronary Angioplasty/Stents; Interventional Cardiology; **Hospital:** Saint Barnabas Med Ctr; **Address:** Consultants Cardiology, 741 Northfield Ave, Ste 205, West Orange, NJ 07052; **Phone:** 973-467-1544; **Board Cert:** Internal Medicine 1985; Cardiovascular Disease 1987; Echocardiography 1997; **Med School:** UMDNJ-NJ Med Sch, Newark 1982; **Resid:** Internal Medicine, Univ Hosp-UMDNJ 1985; **Fellow:** Cardiovascular Disease, Newark Beth Israel Med Ctr 1987

Zucker, Mark J MD (Cv) - **Spec Exp:** Transplant Medicine-Heart; Heart Failure; Pulmonary Hypertension; Amyloid Heart Disease; **Hospital:** Newark Beth Israel Med Ctr, Saint Barnabas Med Ctr; **Address:** NBIMC, Cardiac Transplant Ctr, 201 Lyons Ave, Ste L4, Newark, NJ 07112; **Phone:** 973-926-7205; **Board Cert:** Internal Medicine 1984; Cardiovascular Disease 1987; Advanced Heart Failure & Transplant Cardiology 2010; **Med School:** Northwestern Univ 1981; **Resid:** Internal Medicine, Northwestern Meml Hosp 1984; **Fellow:** Cardiovascular Disease, Northwestern Meml Hosp 1987

Child & Adolescent Psychiatry

Bartlett, Jacqueline MD (ChAP) - **Spec Exp:** Stress Management; ADD/ADHD; Mood Disorders; **Hospital:** Univ Hosp (Newark); **Address:** 183 S Orange Ave, BHSB -rmE1547, Newark, NJ 07103; **Phone:** 973-972-2977; **Board Cert:** Psychiatry 1983; **Med School:** Univ Cincinnati 1971; **Resid:** Pediatrics, Montefiore Hospital 1976; Psychiatry, Columbia-Presby Med Ctr 1981; **Fellow:** Child & Adolescent Psychiatry, Columbia-Presby Med Ctr 1979; **Fac Appt:** Assoc Prof Ped, UMDNJ-NJ Med Sch, Newark

Cammarata, Sandra MD (ChAP) - **Spec Exp:** ADD/ADHD; Bipolar/Mood Disorders; **Hospital:** Hackensack UMC-Mountainside (page 774); **Address:** N Jersey Ctr for Comprehensive Mental Hlth, 14 Smull Ave Fl 2, Caldwell, NJ 07110; **Phone:** 973-618-0100; **Board Cert:** Psychiatry 2007; Child & Adolescent Psychiatry 2007; **Med School:** Italy 1983; **Resid:** Psychiatry, New England Med Ctr 1987; **Fellow:** Child & Adolescent Psychiatry, New England Med Ctr 1989

Child Neurology

Pak, Jayoung MD (ChiN) - **Spec Exp:** Epilepsy/Seizure Disorders; **Hospital:** Univ Hosp (Newark); **Address:** 90 Bergen St, rm 8100, Newark, NJ 07103-2406; **Phone:** 973-972-2922; **Board Cert:** Child Neurology 1993; **Med School:** South Korea 1978; **Resid:** Pediatrics, UMDNJ-Univ Hosp 1991; **Fellow:** Child Neurology, UMDNJ-Univ Hosp 1993; **Fac Appt:** Asst Prof N, UMDNJ-NJ Med Sch, Newark

Clinical Genetics

Desposito, Franklin MD (CG) - **Spec Exp:** Birth Defects; Genetic Disorders; **Hospital:** Univ Hosp (Newark), Saint Barnabas Med Ctr; **Address:** 90 Bergen St, Ste 5400, Newark, NJ 07103; **Phone:** 973-972-3300; **Board Cert:** Pediatrics 1986; Clinical Genetics 1982; Clinical Cytogenetics 1990; Clinical Molecular Genetics 2010; **Med School:** Ros Franklin Univ/Chicago Med Sch 1957; **Resid:** Pediatrics, Long Island Jewish Hosp 1961; **Fellow:** Hematology, Univ Wisc Sch Med 1963; **Fac Appt:** Prof Ped, UMDNJ-NJ Med Sch, Newark

Colon & Rectal Surgery

Gilder, Mark E MD (CRS) - **Spec Exp:** Laparoscopic Surgery; Inflammatory Bowel Disease; **Hospital:** Saint Barnabas Med Ctr, Morristown Med Ctr (page 92); **Address:** Assocs in Colon & Rectal Diseases, 231 Millburn Ave, Millburn, NJ 07041-1718; **Phone:** 973-467-2277; **Board Cert:** Colon & Rectal Surgery 2013; **Med School:** NY Med Coll 1987; **Resid:** Surgery, North Shore Univ Hosp 1992; **Fellow:** Colon & Rectal Surgery, St Francis Hosp 1993

Rothberg, Robert M MD (CRS) - **Spec Exp:** Colon & Rectal Cancer; Colonoscopy; Diverticulitis; **Hospital:** Hackensack UMC-Mountainside (page 774), Saint Barnabas Med Ctr; **Address:** 39 S Fullerton Ave, Montclair, NJ 07042-6303; **Phone:** 973-744-0550; **Board Cert:** Colon & Rectal Surgery 1978; **Med School:** NYU Sch Med 1972; **Resid:** Surgery, Bellevue Hospital Center 1974; Surgery, Hackensack Hosp 1977; **Fellow:** Colon & Rectal Surgery, Muhlenberg Hosp 1978

Dermatology

Connolly, Adrian L MD (D) - **Spec Exp:** Mohs' Surgery; Skin Cancer; **Hospital:** Saint Barnabas Med Ctr; **Address:** 101 Old Short Hills Rd, Ste 503, West Orange, NJ 07052-1023; **Phone:** 973-731-9131; **Board Cert:** Dermatology 2009; **Med School:** UMDNJ-NJ Med Sch, Newark 1975; **Resid:** Dermatology, NYU Med Ctr 1979; **Fellow:** Mohs Surgery, NYU Med Ctr 1980; **Fac Appt:** Asst Clin Prof D, UMDNJ-NJ Med Sch, Newark

Downie, Jeanine B MD (D) - **Spec Exp:** Cosmetic Dermatology; Botox Therapy; Black/Asian Skin Care; Skin Laser Surgery; **Hospital:** Overlook Med Ctr (page 92), Hackensack UMC-Mountainside (page 774); **Address:** 51 Park St, Montclair, NJ 07042; **Phone:** 973-509-6900; **Board Cert:** Dermatology 2006; **Med School:** SUNY Downstate 1992; **Resid:** Pediatrics, New York Hosp 1994; Dermatology, Mt Sinai Med Ctr 1997

Liftin, Alan J MD (D) - **Spec Exp:** Cosmetic Dermatology; Botox Therapy; Facial Rejuvenation; Acne & Rosacea; **Hospital:** Saint Barnabas Med Ctr; **Address:** 22 Old Short Hills Rd, Ste 103, Livingston, NJ 07039-5605; **Phone:** 973-535-5800; **Board Cert:** Dermatology 2009; Anatomic Pathology 1987; Dermatopathology 1989; **Med School:** Mount Sinai Sch Med 1982; **Resid:** Pathology, Mt Sinai Hosp 1985; Dermatology, Mt Sinai Hosp 1990; **Fellow:** Dermatopathology, Hosp Univ Penn 1986

Rozanski, Reuben MD (D) - **Spec Exp:** Cosmetic Dermatology; Acne; Rosacea; **Hospital:** Hackensack UMC-Mountainside (page 774); **Address:** 200 Highland Ave, Glen Ridge, NJ 07028-1528; **Phone:** 973-748-9474; **Board Cert:** Dermatology 1979; Internal Medicine 1974; **Med School:** Boston Univ 1970; **Resid:** Internal Medicine, Montefiore Med Ctr 1973; Dermatology, Albert Einstein Coll Med 1976

Schwartz, Robert A MD (D) - **Spec Exp:** Skin Cancer; Atopic Dermatitis; Tuberous Sclerosis; Rare Skin Disorders; **Hospital:** Univ Hosp (Newark); **Address:** 90 Bergen St, Ste 4400, Newark, NJ 07101; **Phone:** 973-972-1880; **Board Cert:** Dermatology 1978; Clinical & Laboratory Dematologic Immunology 1985; **Med School:** NY Med Coll 1974; **Resid:** Dermatology, Univ Hosp 1977; Dermatology, Roswell Park Meml Inst 1978; **Fellow:** Dermatopathology, NJ Med Sch Affil Hosps 1990; **Fac Appt:** Prof D, UMDNJ-Rutgers Med Sch

Siegel, Eric S MD (D) - **Spec Exp:** Cosmetic Dermatology; Skin Laser Surgery; **Hospital:** Saint Barnabas Med Ctr, Overlook Med Ctr (page 92); **Address:** Millburn Laser Center, 12 E Willow St, Millburn, NJ 07041; **Phone:** 973-376-8500; **Board Cert:** Dermatology 2007; **Med School:** SUNY Downstate 1993; **Resid:** Internal Medicine, Staten Island Univ Hosp 1996; Dermatology, Downstate Med Ctr 1999; **Fac Appt:** Assoc Clin Prof D, SUNY Downstate

Diagnostic Radiology

Byk, Cheryl J MD (DR) - **Spec Exp:** Mammography; Nuclear Medicine; **Address:** 61 Main St, Ste 61 A, West Orange, NJ 07052; **Phone:** 973-669-1989; **Board Cert:** Diagnostic Radiology 1976; Nuclear Radiology 1977; **Med School:** UMDNJ-NJ Med Sch, Newark 1972; **Resid:** Diagnostic Radiology, St Vincent's Hosp 1976; **Fellow:** Nuclear Medicine, St Vincent's Hosp 1977; **Fac Appt:** Asst Clin Prof, Mount Sinai Sch Med

Lee, Huey-Jen MD (DR) - **Spec Exp:** Brain Imaging; Head & Neck Imaging; Spine Neuroradiologic Diagnosis; Brain Tumors; **Hospital:** Univ Hosp (Newark); **Address:** 150 Bergen St, Ste C320, Dept of Radiology, Newark, NJ 07103; **Phone:** 973-972-6900; **Board Cert:** Diagnostic Radiology 1990; Neuroradiology 2004; **Med School:** Taiwan 1976; **Resid:** Pediatrics, Taipei Jen-Ai Hosp 1979; Diagnostic Radiology, Beth Israel Med Ctr 1988; **Fellow:** Neuroradiology, NY Med Coll 1989; **Fac Appt:** Prof Rad, UMDNJ-NJ Med Sch, Newark

Levy, Daniel MD (DR) - **Spec Exp:** Neuroradiology; **Hospital:** Chilton Hosp; **Address:** Montclair Radiology, 116 Park St, Montclair, NJ 07042; **Phone:** 973-746-2525; **Board Cert:** Diagnostic Radiology ; **Med School:** NY Med Coll 1978; **Resid:** Diagnostic Radiology, Mt Sinai Med Ctr 1982; **Fellow:** Neurological Radiology, NY Presby Hosp/Columbia 1983

Moses, Stuart MD (DR) - **Spec Exp:** Nuclear Radiology; MRI; CT Body Scan; Musculoskeletal Imaging; **Hospital:** Chilton Hosp; **Address:** Montclair Radiology, 116 Park St, Montclair, NJ 07042; **Phone:** 973-746-2525; **Board Cert:** Diagnostic Radiology ; Nuclear Radiology ; **Med School:** Mount Sinai Sch Med 1978; **Resid:** Diagnostic Radiology, Mt Sinai Med Ctr 1982; **Fellow:** Nuclear Medicine, Albert Einstein Med Coll 1983

Sanders, Linda M MD (DR) - **Spec Exp:** Breast Imaging; **Hospital:** Saint Barnabas Med Ctr; **Address:** St Barnabas Breast Center, 200 S Orange Ave, Livingston, NJ 07039; **Phone:** 973-322-7800; **Board Cert:** Diagnostic Radiology 1986; **Med School:** Univ Pennsylvania 1982; **Resid:** Diagnostic Radiology, Columbia-Presby Med Ctr 1986; **Fellow:** Mammography, Meml Sloan-Kettering Cancer Ctr 1987

Endocrinology, Diabetes & Metabolism

Baranetsky, Nicholas G MD (EDM) - **Spec Exp:** Thyroid Disorders; Pituitary Disorders; Adrenal Disorders; **Hospital:** Saint Michael's Med Ctr, Clara Maass Med Ctr; **Address:** St Michaels Med Ctr - Endocrinology, 306 Dr Martin Luther King Blvd, Newark, NJ 07102; **Phone:** 973-877-5185; **Board Cert:** Internal Medicine 1977; Endocrinology, Diabetes & Metabolism 1981; **Med School:** NY Med Coll 1974; **Resid:** Internal Medicine, Stamford Hosp 1977; **Fellow:** Endocrinology, Diabetes & Metabolism, VA Med Ctr-Wadsworth 1979; **Fac Appt:** Prof Med, Seton Hall Univ Sch Hlth & Med Scis

Bleich, David MD (EDM) - **Spec Exp:** Diabetes; Metabolic Disorders; Thyroid Disorders; **Hospital:** Univ Hosp (Newark); **Address:** Univ Hosp, Endocrinology Dept, 90 Bergen St, Ste 4500, Newark, NJ 07103; **Phone:** 973-972-2500; **Board Cert:** Internal Medicine 1986; Endocrinology, Diabetes & Metabolism 1989; **Med School:** NY Med Coll 1983; **Resid:** Internal Medicine, Maimonides Med Ctr 1986; **Fellow:** Endocrinology, Diabetes & Metabolism, Brigham & Womens Hosp 1990; Research, Joslin Diabetes Ctr 1992; **Fac Appt:** Assoc Prof Med, UMDNJ-Rutgers Med Sch

Dower, Samuel M MD (EDM) - **Hospital:** Saint Barnabas Med Ctr; **Address:** 200 S Orange Ave, Ste 219, Livingston, NJ 07039; **Phone:** 973-322-7200; **Board Cert:** Internal Medicine 1984; Endocrinology 1987; **Med School:** NYU Sch Med 1981; **Resid:** Internal Medicine, Bronx Muni Hosp 1984; **Fellow:** Endocrinology, Mount Sinai Hosp 1985

Gewirtz, George P MD (EDM) - **Spec Exp:** Diabetes; Thyroid Disorders; Osteoporosis; **Hospital:** Saint Barnabas Med Ctr; **Address:** 200 S Orange Ave, Ste 219, Livingston, NJ 07039; **Phone:** 973-322-7200; **Board Cert:** Internal Medicine 1972; Endocrinology 1975; **Med School:** Harvard Med Sch 1965; **Resid:** Internal Medicine, Bellevue Hosp Ctr 1967; Internal Medicine, Columbia-Presby Med Ctr 1971; **Fellow:** Endocrinology, Diabetes & Metabolism, Mt Sinai Hosp 1973

Sherry, Stephen H MD (EDM) - **Spec Exp:** Thyroid Disorders; Diabetes; Osteoporosis; **Hospital:** Hackensack UMC-Mountainside (page 774); **Address:** 119 Grove St, Montclair, NJ 07042-2629; **Phone:** 973-744-3733; **Board Cert:** Internal Medicine 1979; Endocrinology, Diabetes & Metabolism 1981; **Med School:** Univ Conn 1976; **Resid:** Internal Medicine, New Eng Deaconess 1979; **Fellow:** Endocrinology, Diabetes & Metabolism, New Eng Deaconess 1981; **Fac Appt:** Asst Clin Prof Med, UMDNJ-NJ Med Sch, Newark

Family Medicine

Cirello, Richard MD (FMed) *PCP* - **Hospital:** Hackensack UMC-Mountainside (page 774); **Address:** Town Medical Associates, 271 Grove Ave, Verona, NJ 07044-1730; **Phone:** 973-239-2600; **Board Cert:** Family Medicine 2004; **Med School:** Mexico 1975; **Resid:** Family Medicine, Mountainside Hosp 1979; **Fac Appt:** Asst Clin Prof FMed, UMDNJ-Rutgers Med Sch

Gorman, Robert T MD (FMed) *PCP* - **Hospital:** Hackensack UMC-Mountainside (page 774), Saint Barnabas Med Ctr; **Address:** Town Medical Assocs, 271 Grove Ave, Verona, NJ 07044; **Phone:** 973-239-2600; **Board Cert:** Family Medicine 2005; **Med School:** UMDNJ-NJ Med Sch, Newark 1982; **Resid:** Family Medicine, Mountainside Hosp 1985; **Fac Appt:** Asst Clin Prof FMed, UMDNJ-NJ Med Sch, Newark

Schlam, Everett W MD (FMed) *PCP* - **Spec Exp:** Travel Medicine; **Hospital:** Hackensack UMC-Mountainside (page 774); **Address:** Mountainside Family Practice Assocs, 799 Bloomfield Ave, Verona, NJ 07044; **Phone:** 973-746-7050; **Board Cert:** Family Medicine 2007; Sports Medicine 2011; **Med School:** UMDNJ-RW Johnson Med Sch 1986; **Resid:** Family Medicine, Mountainside Hosp 1989

Gastroenterology

Finkelstein, Warren MD (Ge) - **Spec Exp:** Crohn's Disease; Ulcerative Colitis; Inflammatory Bowel Disease; **Hospital:** Hackensack UMC-Mountainside (page 774); **Address:** The Gastroenterology Group of New Jersey, 123 Highland Ave, Ste 103, Glen Ridge, NJ 07028; **Phone:** 973-429-8800; **Board Cert:** Internal Medicine 1975; Gastroenterology 1983; **Med School:** Med Coll VA 1972; **Resid:** Internal Medicine, Boston City Hosp 1974; Internal Medicine, Boston VA Med Ctr 1975; **Fellow:** Gastroenterology, Mass Genl Hosp 1977; **Fac Appt:** Assoc Clin Prof Med, UMDNJ-NJ Med Sch, Newark

Fiske, Steven C MD (Ge) - **Spec Exp:** Colon Cancer Screening; Colonoscopy; Peptic Acid Disorders; Gastroesophageal Reflux Disease (GERD); **Hospital:** Saint Barnabas Med Ctr, Clara Maass Med Ctr; **Address:** 1500 Pleasant Valley Way, Ste 306, West Orange, NJ 07052-1104; **Phone:** 973-325-5775; **Board Cert:** Internal Medicine 1977; Gastroenterology 1979; **Med School:** NYU Sch Med 1974; **Resid:** Internal Medicine, NYU-Bellevue Hosp Ctr 1976; **Fellow:** Gastroenterology, Harvard /Brigham & Womens Hosp 1978; **Fac Appt:** Assoc Prof Med, Seton Hall Univ Sch Hlth & Med Scis

Kenny, Raymond MD (Ge) - **Spec Exp:** Liver Disease; Hepatitis B & C; Inflammatory Bowel Disease/Crohn's; Ulcerative Colitis; **Hospital:** Hackensack UMC-Mountainside (page 774); **Address:** The Gastroenterology Group of New Jersey, 123 Highland Ave, Ste 103, Glen Ridge, NJ 07028; **Phone:** 973-429-8800; **Board Cert:** Internal Medicine 1984; Gastroenterology 1987; **Med School:** SUNY Stony Brook 1981; **Resid:** Internal Medicine, Mayo Clinic 1984; **Fellow:** Gastroenterology, Univ Penn Med Ctr 1986; **Fac Appt:** Asst Clin Prof Med, UMDNJ-NJ Med Sch, Newark

Mogan, Glen R MD (Ge) - **Spec Exp:** Inflammatory Bowel Disease; Peptic Ulcer Disease; Gastroesophageal Reflux Disease (GERD); **Hospital:** Saint Barnabas Med Ctr; **Address:** 741 N Field Ave, Ste 204, West Orange, NJ 07052-1104; **Phone:** 973-731-8686; **Board Cert:** Internal Medicine 1978; Gastroenterology 1981; **Med School:** SUNY Upstate Med Univ 1975; **Resid:** Internal Medicine, Mount Sinai Hosp 1978; **Fellow:** Gastroenterology, Mount Sinai Hosp 1981; **Fac Appt:** Assoc Clin Prof Med, UMDNJ-Rutgers Med Sch

Spira, Robert S MD (Ge) - **Spec Exp:** Liver Disease; Inflammatory Bowel Disease; Endoscopy; **Hospital:** Saint Michael's Med Ctr, Clara Maass Med Ctr; **Address:** 5 Franklin Ave, Ste 109, Claremont Professional Bldg, Belleville, NJ 07109; **Phone:** 973-759-7240; **Board Cert:** Internal Medicine 1978; Gastroenterology 1981; **Med School:** NYU Sch Med 1975; **Resid:** Internal Medicine, Bellevue Hosp/NYU Med Ctr 1978; **Fellow:** Gastroenterology, VA Med Ctr 1981; **Fac Appt:** Asst Prof Med, UMDNJ-NJ Med Sch, Newark

Geriatric Medicine

Arunachalam, Muthu R MD (Ger) - **Spec Exp:** Palliative Care; **Hospital:** Hackensack UMC-Mountainside (page 774); **Address:** 22 Old Short Hills Rd, Ste 110, Livingston, NJ 07039; **Phone:** 973-994-0899; **Board Cert:** Geriatric Medicine 2004; **Med School:** India 1993; **Resid:** Internal Medicine, Flushing Hosp Med Ctr 1999; **Fellow:** Geriatric Medicine, Flushing Hosp Med Ctr 2000

Schor, Joshua D MD (Ger) - **Spec Exp:** Alzheimer's Disease; **Hospital:** Saint Barnabas Med Ctr; **Address:** Daughters of Israel, 1155 Pleasant Valley Way, West Orange, NJ 07052; **Phone:** 877-209-2041; **Board Cert:** Internal Medicine 1988; Geriatric Medicine 2011; **Med School:** Yale Univ 1985; **Resid:** Internal Medicine, Mass General Hosp 1988; **Fellow:** Geriatric Medicine, Beth Israel Med Ctr 1990

Gynecologic Oncology

Anderson, Patrick S MD (GO) - **Spec Exp:** Gynecologic Cancer; Robotic Surgery; **Hospital:** Holy Name Med Ctr (page 720), Montefiore Med Ctr-Moses Campus (page 100); **Address:** Ctr for Gyn Oncology & Women's Hlth, 120 Irvington Ave, South Orange, NJ 07079; **Phone:** 973-762-7270; **Board Cert:** Obstetrics & Gynecology 2012; Gynecologic Oncology 2012; **Med School:** UMDNJ-NJ Med Sch, Newark 1988; **Resid:** Obstetrics & Gynecology, Montefiore Med Ctr 1995; **Fellow:** Gynecologic Oncology, Montefiore Med Ctr 1998; **Fac Appt:** Asst Clin Prof ObG, Albert Einstein Coll Med

Cracchiolo, Bernadette M MD (GO) - **Hospital:** Univ Hosp (Newark); **Address:** UMDNJ-New Jersey Med Sch, Dept OB/Gyn, 185 S Orange Ave, rm E 506, ACC Level C, Newark, NJ 07101; **Phone:** 973-972-5055; **Board Cert:** Obstetrics & Gynecology 2012; Gynecologic Oncology 2012; Hospice & Palliative Medicine 2008; **Med School:** Univ Hlth Scis, Chicago Med Sch 1991; **Resid:** Obstetrics & Gynecology, Columbia Presby Hosp 1995; **Fellow:** Yale-New Haven Hosp 1997; **Fac Appt:** Asst Prof ObG, UMDNJ-NJ Med Sch, Newark

Denehy, Thad R MD (GO) - **Spec Exp:** Robotic Surgery; Ovarian Cancer; Gynecologic Surgery-Complex; Laparoscopic Surgery; **Hospital:** Saint Barnabas Med Ctr, Overlook Med Ctr (page 92); **Address:** Gyn Cancer & Pelvic Surgery, LLC, 101 Old Short Hills Rd, Ste 400, West Orange, NJ 07052; **Phone:** 973-243-9300; **Board Cert:** Gynecologic Oncology 2012; Obstetrics & Gynecology 2012; **Med School:** Wake Forest Univ 1984; **Resid:** Obstetrics & Gynecology, St Barnabas Med Ctr 1988; **Fellow:** Gynecologic Oncology, Strong Meml Hosp 1990

Taylor, Robert R MD (GO) - **Spec Exp:** Pelvic Reconstruction; Gynecologic Cancer; Laparoscopic Surgery; Robotic Surgery; **Hospital:** Saint Barnabas Med Ctr; **Address:** Gynecologic Cancer & Pelvic Surgery, 101 Old Short Hills Rd, Ste 400, West Orange, NJ 07052; **Phone:** 973-243-9300; **Board Cert:** Obstetrics & Gynecology 2012; Gynecologic Oncology 2012; **Med School:** Uniformed Srvs Univ, Bethesda 1985; **Resid:** Obstetrics & Gynecology, United Naval Med Ctr 1989; **Fellow:** Gynecologic Oncology, Walter Reed Army Med Ctr 1994; **Fac Appt:** Assoc Prof ObG, Uniformed Srvs Univ, Bethesda

Hand Surgery

Tan, Virak MD (HS) - **Spec Exp:** Hand & Upper Extremity Surgery; Microvascular Surgery; Nerve Disorders/Surgery; **Hospital:** Univ Hosp (Newark), Overlook Med Ctr (page 92); **Address:** 90 Bergen St, Ste 1200, Newark, NJ 07103; **Phone:** 973-972-0763; **Board Cert:** Orthopaedic Surgery 2003; Hand Surgery 2004; **Med School:** Univ Pennsylvania 1994; **Resid:** Orthopaedic Surgery, Hosp U Penn 2000; **Fellow:** Hand Surgery, Hosp for Special Surgery 2001; Microvascular Surgery, Chang Gung Meml Hosp 2001; **Fac Appt:** Prof OrS, UMDNJ-NJ Med Sch, Newark

Hematology

Cohen, Alice J MD (Hem) - **Spec Exp:** Bleeding/Coagulation Disorders; **Hospital:** Newark Beth Israel Med Ctr, Saint Barnabas Med Ctr; **Address:** Newark Beth Israel Med Ctr, Div Hem, 201 Lyons Ave, Newark, NJ 07112; **Phone:** 973-926-7230; **Board Cert:** Internal Medicine 1984; Hematology 1986; Medical Oncology 2011; **Med School:** Ros Franklin Univ/Chicago Med Sch 1981; **Resid:** Internal Medicine, NYU-Man VA Med Ctr 1984; **Fellow:** Hematology & Oncology, Geo Wash Univ Med Ctr 1986; Hematology & Oncology, Columbia Presby Med Ctr 1987; **Fac Appt:** Assoc Clin Prof Med, Columbia P&S

Sabnani, Indu MD (Hem) - **Spec Exp:** Lymphoma; **Hospital:** Newark Beth Israel Med Ctr; **Address:** Newark Beth Israel Med Ctr, 2130 Milburn Ave, Ste C11, Maplewood, NJ 07040; **Phone:** 973-762-7676; **Board Cert:** Internal Medicine 1987; Medical Oncology 1989; **Med School:** India 1980; **Resid:** Internal Medicine, United Hosp 1987; **Fellow:** Hematology & Oncology, UMDNJ-Newark 1990

Zauber, N Peter MD (Hem) - **Hospital:** Saint Barnabas Med Ctr; **Address:** 22 Old Short Hills Rd, Ste 108, Livingston, NJ 07039; **Phone:** 973-533-9299; **Board Cert:** Internal Medicine 1976; Hematology 1978; **Med School:** Johns Hopkins Univ 1971; **Resid:** Internal Medicine, New York Hosp 1973; Internal Medicine, Baltimore City Hosp 1976; **Fellow:** Hematology & Oncology, Univ Pittsburgh 1978

Infectious Disease

Slim, Jihad G MD (Inf) - **Spec Exp:** AIDS/HIV; Hepatitis C; Hospital Acquired Infections; Osteomyelitis; **Hospital:** Saint Michael's Med Ctr, Newark Beth Israel Med Ctr; **Address:** Saint Michaels Med Ctr, 111 Central Ave, Newark, NJ 07102; **Phone:** 973-877-5644; **Board Cert:** Internal Medicine 1986; Infectious Disease 1988; **Med School:** Lebanon 1980; **Resid:** Internal Medicine, Broussais Hosp 1983; Internal Medicine, Saint Michael's Med Ctr 1986; **Fellow:** Infectious Disease, Saint Michaels Med Ctr 1988; **Fac Appt:** Asst Prof Med, Seton Hall Univ Sch Hlth & Med Scis

Smith, Leon G MD (Inf) - **Spec Exp:** Fevers of Unknown Origin; Bone/Joint Infections; Hepatitis; Chronic Fatigue Syndrome; **Hospital:** Saint Barnabas Med Ctr; **Address:** 189 Engle St, Roseland, NJ 07068; **Phone:** 973-226-3359; **Board Cert:** Internal Medicine 1963; Infectious Disease 1974; **Med School:** Georgetown Univ 1956; **Resid:** Infectious Disease, Nat Inst Hlth 1959; Internal Medicine, Yale-New Haven Hosp 1962; **Fellow:** Infectious Disease, Yale-New Haven Hosp 1960; **Fac Appt:** Prof Med, UMDNJ-NJ Med Sch, Newark

Smith, Stephen M MD (Inf) - **Spec Exp:** AIDS/HIV; Diagnostic Problems; Hepatitis; Sexually Transmitted Diseases; **Hospital:** Saint Barnabas Med Ctr, Saint Michael's Med Ctr; **Address:** 189 Eagle Rock Ave, Roseland, NJ 07068; **Phone:** 973-226-3359; **Board Cert:** Infectious Disease 2004; **Med School:** Yale Univ 1989; **Resid:** Internal Medicine, Univ Virginia Med Ctr 1991; **Fellow:** Infectious Disease, Natl Inst Allergy & Inf Dis 1993; **Fac Appt:** Asst Prof Med, Seton Hall Univ Sch Hlth & Med Scis

Soroko, Theresa A MD (Inf) - **Spec Exp:** AIDS/HIV; Lyme Disease; Skin/Soft Tissue Infections; **Hospital:** Hackensack UMC-Mountainside (page 774), Clara Maass Med Ctr; **Address:** 199 Broad St, Ste 2A, Bloomfield, NJ 07003-2635; **Phone:** 973-748-4583; **Board Cert:** Internal Medicine 1988; Infectious Disease 2012; **Med School:** Grenada 1985; **Resid:** Internal Medicine, St Michael's Med Ctr 1988; **Fellow:** Infectious Disease, St Michael's Med Ctr 1990; **Fac Appt:** Asst Clin Prof Med, UMDNJ-NJ Med Sch, Newark

Youssef-Bessler, Manal F MD (Inf) - **Spec Exp:** AIDS/HIV; Fevers of Unknown Origin; Staphylococcal infections; **Hospital:** Morristown Med Ctr (page 92), Saint Barnabas Med Ctr; **Address:** 22 Old Short Hills Rd, Ste 106, Livingston, NJ 07039; **Phone:** 973-535-8355; **Board Cert:** Internal Medicine 2003; Infectious Disease 2005; **Med School:** Egypt 1992; **Resid:** Internal Medicine, UMDNJ-Univ Hosp 2003; **Fellow:** Infectious Disease, UMDNJ-Univ Hosp 2005

Internal Medicine

Bains, Yatinder MD (IM) *PCP* - **Spec Exp:** Liver Disease; Inflammatory Bowel Disease; Gastroesophageal Reflux Disease (GERD); **Hospital:** Clara Maass Med Ctr, Jersey City Med Ctr; **Address:** 116 Millburn Ave, Ste 102, Millburn, NJ 07041; **Phone:** 973-376-2121; **Board Cert:** Internal Medicine 2013; Gastroenterology 2003; **Med School:** UMDNJ-NJ Med Sch, Newark 1987; **Resid:** Internal Medicine, Univ Hosp-UMDNJ 1990; **Fellow:** Gastroenterology, Univ Hosp-UMDNJ 1992

Chrisanderson, Donna A MD (IM) - **Spec Exp:** Nutrition; **Hospital:** Saint Barnabas Med Ctr; **Address:** 2040 Millburn Ave, Ste 402, Maplewood, NJ 07040; **Phone:** 973-378-9070; **Board Cert:** Internal Medicine 2004; **Med School:** Med Coll GA 1988; **Resid:** Internal Medicine, Greenwich Hosp 1991; **Fellow:** Internal Medicine, Univ Alabama 1993

De Cosimo, Diana R MD (IM) *PCP* - **Spec Exp:** Women's Health; Geriatric Care; Preventive Medicine; **Hospital:** Univ Hosp (Newark); **Address:** 140 Bergen St, F-Level, Newark, NJ 07103; **Phone:** 973-972-1880; **Board Cert:** Internal Medicine 1977; Cardiovascular Disease 1979; **Med School:** Boston Univ 1974; **Resid:** Internal Medicine, Worcester City Hosp 1977; **Fellow:** Cardiovascular Disease, Univ Mass Med Ctr 1979; **Fac Appt:** Assoc Prof Med, UMDNJ-NJ Med Sch, Newark

Fortunato, Franklin D MD (IM) *PCP* - **Spec Exp:** Asthma; **Hospital:** Hackensack UMC-Mountainside (page 774), Clara Maass Med Ctr; **Address:** 127 Pine St, Montclair, NJ 07042-4835; **Phone:** 973-744-4075; **Board Cert:** Internal Medicine 1978; Pulmonary Disease 1980; **Med School:** UMDNJ-NJ Med Sch, Newark 1975; **Resid:** Internal Medicine, St Michael's Med Ctr 1977; **Fellow:** Pulmonary Disease, St Michael's Med Ctr 1979

Gribbon, John MD (IM) *PCP* - **Spec Exp:** Hypertension; Diabetes; Cholesterol/Lipid Disorders; Diagnostic Problems; **Hospital:** Hackensack UMC-Mountainside (page 774); **Address:** 62 S Fullerton Ave, Montclair, NJ 07042-2686; **Phone:** 973-744-3382; **Board Cert:** Internal Medicine 1980; **Med School:** UMDNJ-NJ Med Sch, Newark 1977; **Resid:** Internal Medicine, UMDNJ-NJ Med Schl 1980; **Fac Appt:** Asst Clin Prof Med, UMDNJ-NJ Med Sch, Newark

Rommer, James A MD (IM) *PCP* - **Spec Exp:** Preventive Medicine; **Hospital:** Saint Barnabas Med Ctr; **Address:** 349 E Northfield Rd, Ste 110, Livingston, NJ 07039-4807; **Phone:** 973-992-2227; **Board Cert:** Internal Medicine 1981; **Med School:** Cornell Univ-Weill Med Coll 1978; **Resid:** Internal Medicine, NY Hosp-Cornell Med Ctr 1981; **Fellow:** Internal Medicine, Johns Hopkins Med Sch 1982; **Fac Appt:** Asst Clin Prof Med, Mount Sinai Sch Med

Russo, John A MD (IM) *PCP* - **Hospital:** Saint Barnabas Med Ctr; **Address:** 1500 Pleasant Valley Way, Ste 302, West Orange, NJ 07052; **Phone:** 973-736-8119; **Board Cert:** Internal Medicine 1988; **Med School:** Mexico 1981; **Resid:** Internal Medicine & Pediatrics, UMDNJ Affil Hosp 1987

Interventional Cardiology

Cohen, Marc MD (IC) - **Hospital:** Newark Beth Israel Med Ctr; **Address:** Newark Beth Israel Med Ctr, 201 Lyons Ave, Ste C2, Newark, NJ 07112; **Phone:** 973-926-7852; **Board Cert:** Internal Medicine 1980; Cardiovascular Disease 1983; Interventional Cardiology 2009; **Med School:** NYU Sch Med 1977; **Resid:** Internal Medicine, Mt Sinai Hosp 1980; **Fellow:** Cardiovascular Disease, Mt Sinai Hosp 1982; **Fac Appt:** Prof Med, Mount Sinai Sch Med

Goldstein, Jonathan E MD (IC) - **Spec Exp:** Cardiac Catheterization; **Hospital:** Saint Michael's Med Ctr, Christ Hosp - Jersey City; **Address:** St Michaels Med Ctr, Cardiology Dept, 111 Central Ave Fl 5, Newark, NJ 07102; **Phone:** 973-877-5430; **Board Cert:** Internal Medicine 1978; Cardiovascular Disease 1981; **Med School:** UMDNJ-NJ Med Sch, Newark 1973; **Resid:** Internal Medicine, Jackson Meml Hosp 1976; **Fellow:** Cardiovascular Disease, Boston Med Ctr 1978; **Fac Appt:** Assoc Prof Med, Seton Hall Univ Sch Hlth & Med Scis

Miller, Kenneth P MD (IC) - **Spec Exp:** Angioplasty & Stent Placement; **Hospital:** Hackensack UMC-Mountainside (page 774), Saint Barnabas Med Ctr; **Address:** 62 S Fullerton Ave, Montclair, NJ 07042-2629; **Phone:** 973-746-8585; **Board Cert:** Internal Medicine 1985; Cardiovascular Disease 1989; Interventional Cardiology 2012; **Med School:** NYU Sch Med 1982; **Resid:** Internal Medicine, Bronx Muni Hosp 1986; **Fellow:** Cardiovascular Disease, Columbia Presby Med Ctr 1989

Maternal & Fetal Medicine

Apuzzio, Joseph MD (MF) - **Spec Exp:** Prenatal Diagnosis; Pregnancy-High Risk; Infectious Disease; **Hospital:** Univ Hosp (Newark); **Address:** UMDNJ Medical School, Dept OB/GYN & Women's Health, 185 S Orange Ave, MSB-rm E506, Newark, NJ 07101; **Phone:** 973-972-5557; **Board Cert:** Obstetrics & Gynecology 2012; Maternal & Fetal Medicine 2012; **Med School:** UMDNJ-NJ Med Sch, Newark 1973; **Resid:** Obstetrics & Gynecology, UMDNJ-Univ Hosp 1976; **Fellow:** Maternal & Fetal Medicine, UMDNJ-Univ Hosp 1982; **Fac Appt:** Prof ObG, UMDNJ-NJ Med Sch, Newark

Gimovsky, Martin MD (MF) - **Spec Exp:** Pregnancy-High Risk; **Hospital:** Newark Beth Israel Med Ctr; **Address:** OB/GYN Ultrasound, 201 Lyons Ave, Newark, NJ 07112; **Phone:** 973-926-4882; **Board Cert:** Obstetrics & Gynecology 2011; Maternal & Fetal Medicine 2011; **Med School:** NYU Sch Med 1976; **Resid:** Obstetrics & Gynecology, Sloane Hosp/Columbia Presby hop 1980; **Fellow:** Maternal & Fetal Medicine, USC Med Ctr 1982; **Fac Appt:** Prof ObG, Mount Sinai Sch Med

Smith Jr, Leon G MD (MF) - **Spec Exp:** Ultrasound; Prenatal Diagnosis; Perinatal Infections; Amniocentesis; **Hospital:** Saint Barnabas Med Ctr, Holy Name Med Ctr (page 720); **Address:** NJ Perinatal Associates, 94 Old Short Hills Rd, East Wing, Ste 402, Livingston, NJ 07039-5672; **Phone:** 973-322-5287; **Board Cert:** Obstetrics & Gynecology 2012; Maternal & Fetal Medicine 2012; **Med School:** Georgetown Univ 1985; **Resid:** Obstetrics & Gynecology, Tulane Univ Hosp 1989; **Fellow:** Maternal & Fetal Medicine, Baylor Univ Hosp 1991

Warren, Wendy B MD (MF) - **Spec Exp:** Pregnancy-High Risk; **Hospital:** Saint Barnabas Med Ctr; **Address:** NJ Perinatal Associates, 94 Old Short Hills Rd, East Wing, Ste 402, Livingston, NJ 07039; **Phone:** 973-322-5287; **Board Cert:** Obstetrics & Gynecology 2012; Maternal & Fetal Medicine 2012; **Med School:** Cornell Univ 1982; **Resid:** Obstetrics & Gynecology, T Jefferson Univ Hosp 1986; **Fellow:** Maternal & Fetal Medicine, Columbia Presby Hosp 1991

Medical Oncology

Leitner, Stuart P MD (Onc) - **Spec Exp:** Urologic Cancer; Breast Cancer; **Hospital:** Saint Barnabas Med Ctr; **Address:** 94 Old Short Hills Rd, SMBC East Wing, Livington, NJ 07039; **Phone:** 973-322-5200; **Board Cert:** Internal Medicine 1982; Medical Oncology 1985; **Med School:** Mount Sinai Sch Med 1979; **Resid:** Internal Medicine, Univ Tex SW Med Ctr 1982; **Fellow:** Medical Oncology, Meml Sloan Kettering Cancer Ctr 1985

Lippman, Alan MD (Onc) - **Hospital:** Clara Maass Med Ctr, Saint Barnabas Med Ctr; **Address:** 36 Newark Ave, Ste 304, Belleville, NJ 07109; **Phone:** 973-751-8880; **Board Cert:** Internal Medicine 1973; Medical Oncology 1975; **Med School:** Hahnemann Univ 1965; **Resid:** Internal Medicine, Newark Beth Israel Med Ctr 1970; **Fellow:** Medical Oncology, Meml Sloan-Kettering Cancer Ctr 1972; **Fac Appt:** Assoc Clin Prof Med, UMDNJ-NJ Med Sch, Newark

Michaelson, Richard MD (Onc) - **Spec Exp:** Breast Cancer; **Hospital:** Saint Barnabas Med Ctr; **Address:** 94 Old Short Hills Rd, SMBC East Wing, Livingston, NJ 07039; **Phone:** 973-322-5200; **Board Cert:** Internal Medicine 1979; Medical Oncology 1981; **Med School:** Univ Pennsylvania 1976; **Resid:** Internal Medicine, Hosp Univ Penn 1979; **Fellow:** Medical Oncology, Meml Sloan Kettering Cancer Ctr 1981

Sagorin, Charles Elliot MD (Onc) - **Hospital:** Hackensack UMC-Mountainside (page 774); **Address:** 70 Park St, Ste 310, Montclair, NJ 07042-2960; **Phone:** 973-783-3300; **Board Cert:** Internal Medicine 1981; Medical Oncology 1983; Hematology 1986; **Med School:** SUNY Downstate 1971; **Resid:** Internal Medicine, Bronx Municipal Hosp 1973; **Fellow:** Hematology, Montefiore Med Ctr 1974; Medical Oncology, Montefiore Med Ctr 1978

Scoppetuolo, Michael MD (Onc) - **Spec Exp:** Sarcoma; Palliative Care; Hematologic Malignancies; Lung Cancer; **Hospital:** Saint Barnabas Med Ctr; **Address:** 94 Short Hills Rd, SMBC East Wing, Livingston, NJ 07039; **Phone:** 973-322-5200; **Board Cert:** Internal Medicine 1982; Medical Oncology 1985; **Med School:** Univ Hlth Scis, Chicago Med Sch 1979; **Resid:** Internal Medicine, Univ Hosp 1982; **Fellow:** Hematology & Oncology, Meml Sloan Kettering Cancer Ctr 1984

Neonatal-Perinatal Medicine

Sun, Shyan-chu MD (NP) - **Spec Exp:** Prematurity/Low Birth Weight Infants; Breathing Disorders; Respiratory Distress Syndrome; **Hospital:** Saint Barnabas Med Ctr; **Address:** Dept Neonatology, 94 Old Short Hills Rd, Livingston, NJ 07039; **Phone:** 973-322-5437; **Board Cert:** Pediatrics 1969; Neonatal-Perinatal Medicine 1975; **Med School:** Taiwan 1961; **Resid:** Pediatrics, Univ London 1967; Pediatrics, Harlem Hosp 1970; **Fellow:** Neonatology, LI Jewish Med Ctr 1972; **Fac Appt:** Clin Prof Ped, UMDNJ-NJ Med Sch, Newark

Nephrology

Byrd, Lawrence H MD (Nep) - **Spec Exp:** Hypertension; Pheochromocytoma; Kidney Tumors; Dialysis Care; **Hospital:** Saint Barnabas Med Ctr, Bayonne Med Ctr; **Address:** 22 Old Short Hills Rd, Ste 212, Livingston, NJ 07039-5605; **Phone:** 973-994-4550; **Board Cert:** Internal Medicine 1977; Nephrology 1978; **Med School:** Med Coll PA 1973; **Resid:** Internal Medicine, Univ Hosp 1976; **Fellow:** Nephrology, New York Hosp-Cornell 1978; **Fac Appt:** Asst Clin Prof Med, UMDNJ-NJ Med Sch, Newark

Grasso, Michael MD (Nep) - **Spec Exp:** Kidney Disease; Hypertension; Dialysis Care; Transplant Medicine-Kidney; **Hospital:** Newark Beth Israel Med Ctr, Saint Barnabas Med Ctr; **Address:** 111 Northfield Ave, Ste 311, West Orange, NJ 07052-4703; **Phone:** 973-325-2103; **Board Cert:** Internal Medicine 1974; Nephrology 1976; **Med School:** Univ MD Sch Med 1970; **Resid:** Internal Medicine, Univ MD Hosp 1974; **Fellow:** Nephrology, Newark Beth Israel Hosp 1976

Mulgaonkar, Shamkant MD (Nep) - **Spec Exp:** Transplant Medicine-Kidney; **Hospital:** Saint Barnabas Med Ctr, Newark Beth Israel Med Ctr; **Address:** St Barnabas Med Ctr, 94 Old Short Hills Rd, Ste 303, Livingston, NJ 07039; **Phone:** 973-322-8216; **Board Cert:** Internal Medicine 1981; Nephrology 1982; **Med School:** India 1975; **Resid:** Internal Medicine, Morristown Meml Hosp 1980; **Fellow:** Nephrology, St Barnabas Med Ctr 1982; **Fac Appt:** Assoc Prof Med, UMDNJ-NJ Med Sch, Newark

Sipzner, Robert J MD (Nep) - **Spec Exp:** Hypertension; Kidney Failure; **Hospital:** Bayonne Med Ctr, Saint Barnabas Med Ctr; **Address:** 22 Old Short Hills Rd, Ste 212, Livingston, NJ 07039; **Phone:** 973-994-4550; **Board Cert:** Internal Medicine 1985; Nephrology 1988; **Med School:** NYU Sch Med 1982; **Resid:** Internal Medicine, SUNY Downstate Med Ctr 1985; **Fellow:** Nephrology, Univ Tenn Hlth Sci Ctr 1987

Neurological Surgery

Heary, Robert F MD (NS) - **Spec Exp:** Spinal Surgery; Spinal Cord Injury; Spinal Deformity; **Hospital:** Univ Hosp (Newark), Overlook Med Ctr (page 92); **Address:** UMDNJ-NJ Med Sch, Div Neurosurg, 90 Bergen St, Ste 8100, Newark, NJ 07101; **Phone:** 973-972-2323; **Board Cert:** Neurological Surgery 2010; **Med School:** Univ Pittsburgh 1986; **Resid:** Surgery, UMDNJ Univ Hosp 1989; Neurological Surgery, UMDNJ Univ Hosp 1994; **Fellow:** Orthopaedic Surgery, Thomas Jefferson Univ Hosp 1995; **Fac Appt:** Prof NS, UMDNJ-NJ Med Sch, Newark

Hubschmann, Otakar R MD (NS) - **Spec Exp:** Spinal Surgery-Complex; Cerebrovascular Neurosurgery; Chiari's Deformity; Brain Tumors; **Hospital:** Saint Barnabas Med Ctr; **Address:** 101 Old Short Hills Rd, Ste 409, West Orange, NJ 07052; **Phone:** 973-322-6732; **Board Cert:** Neurological Surgery 1978; **Med School:** Czech Republic 1967; **Resid:** Surgery, Montefiore Med Ctr 1970; Neurological Surgery, Montefiore Med Ctr 1976; **Fac Appt:** Clin Prof NS, NY Coll Osteo Med

Neurology

Blady, David MD (N) - **Spec Exp:** Parkinson's Disease; Dementia; Multiple Sclerosis; Stroke; **Hospital:** Hackensack UMC-Mountainside (page 774), Clara Maass Med Ctr; **Address:** 230 Sherman Ave, Ste L, Glen Ridge, NJ 07028-1520; **Phone:** 973-743-9555; **Board Cert:** Neurology 1990; **Med School:** SUNY Downstate 1983; **Resid:** Neurology, Bellevue Hosp/NYU Med Ctr 1987

Cook, Stuart D MD (N) - **Spec Exp:** Multiple Sclerosis; Infectious & Demyelinating Diseases; **Hospital:** Univ Hosp (Newark); **Address:** 65 Bergen St, rm 1435, Newark, NJ 07103; **Phone:** 973-972-9181; **Board Cert:** Neurology 1970; **Med School:** Univ VT Coll Med 1962; **Resid:** Neurology, Albert Einstein Coll Med 1968; **Fac Appt:** Prof N, UMDNJ-NJ Med Sch, Newark

Geller, Eric B MD (N) - **Spec Exp:** Epilepsy; **Hospital:** Saint Barnabas Med Ctr; **Address:** St Barnabas Inst Neurolgy/Neurosurgery, 200 S Orange Ave, Ste 101, Livingston, NJ 07039; **Phone:** 973-322-7580; **Board Cert:** Neurology 2005; Clinical Neurophysiology 2006; **Med School:** Brown Univ 1989; **Resid:** Neurology, Harvard Med Sch Prog 1993; **Fellow:** Clinical Neurophysiology, Cleveland Clinic 1995

Marks, David A MD (N) - **Spec Exp:** Epilepsy/Seizure Disorders; Headache; Migraine; **Hospital:** Univ Hosp (Newark); **Address:** 90 Bergen St Fl 8th - Ste 8100, Newark, NJ 07103; **Phone:** 973-972-2550; **Board Cert:** Neurology 1989; **Med School:** South Africa 1983; **Resid:** Neurology, Boston Med Ctr 1988; **Fellow:** Neurophysiology, New England Med Ctr 1989; Epilepsy, Yale-New Haven Hosp 1991; **Fac Appt:** Assoc Prof Med, UMDNJ-NJ Med Sch, Newark

Ruderman, Marvin MD (N) - **Spec Exp:** Neuromuscular Disorders; Peripheral Neuropathy; Myasthenia Gravis; Demyelinating Neuropathy; **Hospital:** Saint Barnabas Med Ctr; **Address:** 1099 Bloomfield Ave, West Caldwell, NJ 07006-7129; **Phone:** 973-439-7000; **Board Cert:** Neurology 1981; **Med School:** Columbia P&S 1976; **Resid:** Neurology, Barnes Hosp 1980; **Fellow:** Neuromuscular Disease, Neuro Inst 1981; **Fac Appt:** Asst Clin Prof N, UMDNJ-NJ Med Sch, Newark

Nuclear Medicine

Lutzker, Letty G MD (NuM) - **Hospital:** Saint Barnabas Med Ctr; **Address:** St Barnabas Med Ctr, Dept Radiology, 94 Old Short Hills Rd, Livingston, NJ 07039-5672; **Phone:** 973-322-5957; **Board Cert:** Diagnostic Radiology 1973; Nuclear Medicine 1974; Nuclear Radiology 1977; **Med School:** Albert Einstein Coll Med 1968; **Resid:** Diagnostic Radiology, Montefiore Med Ctr 1973; **Fac Appt:** Assoc Clin Prof NuM, Albert Einstein Coll Med

Obstetrics & Gynecology

Cooperman, Alan S MD (ObG) - **Spec Exp:** Laparoscopic Surgery; Pelvic Surgery; Colposcopy; **Hospital:** Overlook Med Ctr (page 92), Saint Barnabas Med Ctr; **Address:** 235 Millburn Ave, Ste 101, Millburn, NJ 07041-1738; **Phone:** 973-467-9440; **Board Cert:** Obstetrics & Gynecology 1979; **Med School:** Italy 1968; **Resid:** Obstetrics & Gynecology, Newark Beth Israel Med Ctr 1973

Crane, Stephen E MD (ObG) - **Hospital:** Saint Barnabas Med Ctr; **Address:** 375 Mount Pleasant Ave, Ste 202, West Orange, NJ 07052; **Phone:** 908-277-8800; **Board Cert:** Obstetrics & Gynecology 2011; **Med School:** UMDNJ-NJ Med Sch, Newark 1986; **Resid:** Obstetrics & Gynecology, St Barnabas Med Ctr 1991

Luciani, Richard L MD (ObG) - **Spec Exp:** Laparoscopic Surgery; Pregnancy-High Risk; Endometriosis; **Hospital:** Overlook Med Ctr (page 92), Saint Barnabas Med Ctr; **Address:** 235 Millburn Ave, Ste 101, Millburn, NJ 07041; **Phone:** 973-467-9440; **Board Cert:** Obstetrics & Gynecology 1982; **Med School:** UMDNJ-NJ Med Sch, Newark 1976; **Resid:** Obstetrics & Gynecology, St Barnabas Hosp 1981

Quartell, Anthony C MD (ObG) - **Spec Exp:** Minimally Invasive Surgery; Pelvic Reconstruction; Robotic Surgery; Laparoscopic Surgery-Complex; **Hospital:** Saint Barnabas Med Ctr; **Address:** 316 Eisenhower Pkwy, Ste 202, Livingston, NJ 07039-1718; **Phone:** 973-716-9600; **Board Cert:** Obstetrics & Gynecology 1978; **Med School:** UMDNJ-NJ Med Sch, Newark 1969; **Resid:** Surgery, Univ Hosp 1971; Obstetrics & Gynecology, St Barnabas Med Ctr 1977; **Fac Appt:** Asst Clin Prof ObG, Mount Sinai Sch Med

Ophthalmology

Bhagat, Neelakshi MD (Oph) - **Spec Exp:** Retinal Detachment; Trauma; Diabetic Eye Disease/Retinopathy; Macular Degeneration; **Hospital:** Univ Hosp (Newark); **Address:** NJ, Univ Hosp - Dept Ophthalmology, 90 Bergen St, DOC Bldg - Fl 6th, Newark, NJ 07103; **Phone:** 973-972-2032; **Board Cert:** Ophthalmology 2010; **Med School:** SUNY Stony Brook 1994; **Resid:** Ophthalmology, UMDNJ-NJ Med Sch Affil Hosp 1998; **Fellow:** Retina, Doheny Eye Inst - USC 1999; **Fac Appt:** Asst Prof Oph, UMDNJ-NJ Med Sch, Newark

Cangemi, Francis E MD (Oph) - **Spec Exp:** Diabetic Eye Disease/Retinopathy; Macular Degeneration; Retinal Detachment; Retinopathy of Prematurity; **Hospital:** Clara Maass Med Ctr, Valley Hosp (page 721); **Address:** 36 Newark Ave, Ste 212, Belleville, NJ 07109-4121; **Phone:** 973-751-8808; **Board Cert:** Ophthalmology 1976; **Med School:** NY Med Coll 1969; **Resid:** Internal Medicine, Mayo Clin 1971; Ophthalmology, New York Eye & Ear Infirm 1975; **Fellow:** Retina/Vitreous Surgery, Mass Eye & Ear Infirmary 1972; Vitreoretinal Surgery, Mass Eye & Ear Infirmary 1976; **Fac Appt:** Assoc Clin Prof Oph, UMDNJ-NJ Med Sch, Newark

Caputo, Anthony R MD (Oph) - **Spec Exp:** Pediatric Ophthalmology; Strabismus; **Hospital:** Clara Maass Med Ctr; **Address:** 556 Eagle Rock Ave, Ste 203, Roseland, NJ 07068-1500; **Phone:** 973-228-3111; **Board Cert:** Ophthalmology 1976; **Med School:** Italy 1969; **Resid:** Ophthalmology, UMDNJ-Univ Hosp 1974; **Fellow:** Ophthalmology, Wills Eye Hosp 1975; **Fac Appt:** Prof Oph, UMDNJ-NJ Med Sch, Newark

Cohen, Steven B MD (Oph) - **Spec Exp:** Retina/Vitreous Surgery; Diabetic Eye Disease; Macular Degeneration; **Hospital:** Saint Barnabas Med Ctr; **Address:** Retina-Vitreous Consultants, 349 E Northfield Rd, Ste 100, Livingston, NJ 07039; **Phone:** 973-716-0123; **Board Cert:** Ophthalmology 1984; **Med School:** NYU Sch Med 1978; **Resid:** Ophthalmology, LIJ Med Ctr 1982; **Fellow:** Vitreoretinal Surgery, Univ Chicago Med Ctr 1985

Davidson, Lawrence M MD (Oph) - **Spec Exp:** LASIK-Refractive Surgery; Cataract Surgery; Glaucoma; **Hospital:** Hackensack UMC-Mountainside (page 774), Saint Barnabas Med Ctr; **Address:** 825 Bloomfield Ave Fl 1, Verona, NJ 07044-1300; **Phone:** 973-239-4000; **Board Cert:** Ophthalmology 1975; **Med School:** SUNY Downstate 1969; **Resid:** Ophthalmology, Lenox Hill Hosp (Manh Eye, Ear & Throat Hosp) 1974

Eichler, Joel D MD (Oph) - **Spec Exp:** Diabetic Eye Disease/Retinopathy; Macular Degeneration; Retinal Disorders; **Hospital:** Clara Maass Med Ctr; **Address:** Eye Inst of Essex, 5 Franklin Ave, Ste 209, Belleville, NJ 07109; **Phone:** 973-751-6060; **Board Cert:** Ophthalmology 2004; **Med School:** Geo Wash Univ 1988; **Resid:** Ophthalmology, UMDNJ-NJ Med Sch Affil Hosp 1992; **Fellow:** Vitreoretinal Surgery, Touro Infirm 1993

Frohman, Larry P MD (Oph) - **Spec Exp:** Neuro-Ophthalmology; Sarcoidosis; Vision Loss-Unexplained Loss; **Hospital:** Univ Hosp (Newark); **Address:** NJ, Univ Hosp - Dept Ophthalmology, 90 Bergen St DOC Bldg - Ste 6174, Newark, NJ 07103; **Phone:** 973-972-2065; **Board Cert:** Ophthalmology 1985; **Med School:** Univ Pennsylvania 1980; **Resid:** Ophthalmology, Bellevue Hosp Ctr 1984; **Fellow:** Neuro-Ophthalmology, Bellevue Hosp Ctr 1985; **Fac Appt:** Prof Oph, UMDNJ-NJ Med Sch, Newark

Glatt, Herbert L MD (Oph) - **Spec Exp:** Cataract Surgery-Lens Implant; **Hospital:** Hackensack UMC-Mountainside (page 774), Clara Maass Med Ctr; **Address:** 1025 Broad St, Bloomfield, NJ 07003-2844; **Phone:** 973-338-1001; **Board Cert:** Ophthalmology 1991; **Med School:** Mexico 1979; **Resid:** Ophthalmology, UMDNJ-NJ Med Sch Affil Hosps 1984; **Fac Appt:** Asst Clin Prof Oph, UMDNJ-NJ Med Sch, Newark

Langer, Paul D MD (Oph) - **Spec Exp:** Trauma; Orbital Tumors/Cancer; Thyroid Eye Disease; **Hospital:** Univ Hosp (Newark); **Address:** NJ, Univ Hosp - Dept Ophthalmology, 90 Bergen St DOC Bldg - Ste 6174, Newark, NJ 07103; **Phone:** 973-972-2065; **Board Cert:** Ophthalmology 2005; **Med School:** Johns Hopkins Univ 1989; **Resid:** Ophthalmology, UCSF Med Ctr 1993; **Fellow:** Ophthalmic Plastic Surgery, Univ Utah Affil Hosp 1995; Orbital Surgery, Moorfields Eye Hosp 1995; **Fac Appt:** Asst Prof Oph, UMDNJ-NJ Med Sch, Newark

Turbin, Roger E MD (Oph) - **Spec Exp:** Neuro-Ophthalmology; Orbital Tumors/Cancer; Oculoplastic & Orbital Surgery; **Hospital:** Univ Hosp (Newark), Saint Barnabas Med Ctr; **Address:** NJ, Univ Hosp - Dept Ophthalmology, 90 Bergen St DOC Bldg - Ste 6174, Newark, NJ 07103; **Phone:** 973-972-2065; **Board Cert:** Ophthalmology 2010; **Med School:** Washington Univ, St Louis 1993; **Resid:** Ophthalmology, NYU Langone Med Ctr 1997; **Fellow:** Neuro-Ophthalmology, NY Eye & Ear/Beth Israel 1998; Oculoplastic Surgery, Allegheny Genl Hosp 1999; **Fac Appt:** Asst Prof Oph, UMDNJ-NJ Med Sch, Newark

Wagner, Rudolph S MD (Oph) - **Spec Exp:** Strabismus; Eye Disorders-Congenital; Strabismus; Pediatric Ophthalmology; **Hospital:** Clara Maass Med Ctr, Saint Barnabas Med Ctr; **Address:** Chldns Eye Care Ctr New Jersey, 1 Clara Maass Drive, Belleville, NJ 07109; **Phone:** 973-751-1702; **Board Cert:** Ophthalmology 1983; **Med School:** UMDNJ-NJ Med Sch, Newark 1978; **Resid:** Ophthalmology, UMDNJ-NJ Med Sch Affil Hosp 1982; **Fellow:** Pediatric Ophthalmology, Wills Eye Hosp 1983; **Fac Appt:** Clin Prof Oph, UMDNJ-NJ Med Sch, Newark

Zarbin, Marco A MD/PhD (Oph) - **Spec Exp:** Macular Degeneration; Diabetic Eye Disease/Retinopathy; Eye Trauma; Retinal Detachment; **Hospital:** Univ Hosp (Newark), Saint Barnabas Med Ctr; **Address:** NJ, Univ Hosp - Dept Ophthalmology, 90 Bergen St DOC Bldg - Ste 6174, Newark, NJ 07103-2499; **Phone:** 973-972-2065; **Board Cert:** Ophthalmology 1989; **Med School:** Johns Hopkins Univ 1984; **Resid:** Ophthalmology, Johns Hopkins Hosp 1988; **Fellow:** Vitreoretinal Surgery, Johns Hopkins Hosp 1989; **Fac Appt:** Prof Oph, UMDNJ-NJ Med Sch, Newark

Orthopaedic Surgery

Benevenia, Joseph MD (OrS) - **Spec Exp:** Limb Sparing Surgery; Bone Cancer; Sarcoma-Soft Tissue; **Hospital:** Univ Hosp (Newark); **Address:** 140 Bergen St, Ste ACC1610, Newark, NJ 07103; **Phone:** 973-972-2153; **Board Cert:** Orthopaedic Surgery 2013; **Med School:** UMDNJ-NJ Med Sch, Newark 1984; **Resid:** Orthopaedic Surgery, UMDNJ-NJ Med Sch Hosp 1988; **Fellow:** Orthopaedic Oncology, Case Western Reserve Univ 1991; **Fac Appt:** Prof OrS, UMDNJ-NJ Med Sch, Newark

Berberian, Wayne S MD (OrS) - **Spec Exp:** Bone Infections; Foot & Ankle Deformities; Foot & Ankle Surgery-Complex; Tendon Surgery; **Hospital:** Hackensack Univ Med Ctr (page 718), Univ Hosp (Newark); **Address:** 90 Bergen St, DOC Bldg, Ste 1200, Newark, NJ 07103; **Phone:** 973-972-8464; **Board Cert:** Orthopaedic Surgery 2013; **Med School:** Univ Pennsylvania 1991; **Resid:** Surgery, St Lukes Roosevelt Hosp 1992; Orthopaedic Surgery, UMDNJ Univ Hosp 1998; **Fellow:** Orthopaedic Research, Hosp for Special Surgery 1994; Foot & Ankle Reconstruction, Hahnemann Univ Hosp 1999; **Fac Appt:** Assoc Prof OrS, UMDNJ-Rutgers Med Sch

Chase, Mark D MD (OrS) - **Spec Exp:** Sports Medicine; **Hospital:** Hackensack UMC-Mountainside (page 774); **Address:** Montclair Orthopaedic Grp, 200 Highland Ave, Glen Ridge, NJ 07028-1521; **Phone:** 973-746-2200; **Board Cert:** Orthopaedic Surgery 2012; **Med School:** Boston Univ 1983; **Resid:** Orthopaedic Surgery, Boston Med Ctr 1989

Decter, Edward M MD (OrS) - **Spec Exp:** Knee Reconstruction; Shoulder Reconstruction; Sports Medicine; **Hospital:** Saint Barnabas Med Ctr; **Address:** Ctr for Orthopaedics, 1500 Pleasant Vly Way, Ste 101, West Orange, NJ 07052; **Phone:** 973-669-5600; **Board Cert:** Orthopaedic Surgery 1982; **Med School:** Creighton Univ 1975; **Resid:** Orthopaedic Surgery, NYU Hosp For Joint Dis 1981

Mendes, John F MD (OrS) - **Spec Exp:** Hip & Knee Replacement; Foot & Ankle Surgery; Spinal Disorders; **Hospital:** Hackensack UMC-Mountainside (page 774), Clara Maass Med Ctr; **Address:** Montclair Orthopaedic Group, 200 Highland Ave, Glen Ridge, NJ 07028-1521; **Phone:** 973-746-2200; **Board Cert:** Orthopaedic Surgery 1984; **Med School:** Cornell Univ-Weill Med Coll 1976; **Resid:** Surgery, Bryn Mawr Hosp 1978; Orthopaedic Surgery, Hosp Special Surg 1981; **Fellow:** Orthopaedic Surgery, Pennsylvania Hosp-UPHS 1982

Patterson, Francis R MD (OrS) - **Spec Exp:** Musculoskeletal Tumors; Bone Cancer; Limb Sparing Surgery; **Hospital:** Univ Hosp (Newark); **Address:** 90 Bergen St DOC Bldg - Ste 1200, Newark, NJ 07103; **Phone:** 973-972-1993; **Board Cert:** Orthopaedic Surgery 2012; **Med School:** SUNY Buffalo 1993; **Resid:** Orthopaedic Surgery, SUNY Hlth Sci Ctr 1998; **Fellow:** Musculoskeletal Oncology, Univ Chicago Affil Hosps 1999; **Fac Appt:** Assoc Prof OrS, UMDNJ-NJ Med Sch, Newark

Queler, Seth R MD (OrS) - **Hospital:** Clara Maass Med Ctr; **Address:** 5 Franklin Ave, Ste 202, Belleville, NJ 07109-3521; **Phone:** 973-751-0111; **Board Cert:** Orthopaedic Surgery 2008; **Med School:** Northwestern Univ 2000; **Resid:** Orthopaedic Surgery, UMDNJ Med Ctr 2005; **Fellow:** Foot & Ankle Surgery, Univ PA Hlth Sys 2006

Rosa, Richard MD (OrS) - **Spec Exp:** Joint Replacement; Knee Replacement; Arthroscopic Surgery; Knee Surgery; **Hospital:** Saint Barnabas Med Ctr; **Address:** 741 Northfield Ave, Ste 200, MC 07052, West Orange, NJ 07052; **Phone:** 973-736-9980; **Board Cert:** Orthopaedic Surgery 2007; **Med School:** UMDNJ-NJ Med Sch, Newark 1978; **Resid:** Orthopaedic Surgery, UMDNJ-Univ Hosp 1983; **Fellow:** Joint Replacement Surgery, Hosp for Special Surgery 1984; **Fac Appt:** OrS, UMDNJ-NJ Med Sch, Newark

Sabharwal, Sanjeev MD (OrS) - **Spec Exp:** Pediatric Orthopaedic Surgery; Limb Lengthening (Ilizarov Procedure); Limb Deformities; **Hospital:** Univ Hosp (Newark), Overlook Med Ctr (page 92); **Address:** 90 Bergen St DOC Bldg - Ste 1200, Newark, NJ 07103; **Phone:** 973-972-0246; **Board Cert:** Orthopaedic Surgery 2010; **Med School:** India 1985; **Resid:** Surgery, St Elizabeth Hosp 1988; Orthopaedic Surgery, Univ British Columbia Affil Hosp 1994; **Fellow:** Pediatric Orthopaedic Surgery, Chldns Hosp/Shriners Hosp 1996; Reconstructive Surgery, Md Ctr for Limb Lengthening & Reconstruction 1996; **Fac Appt:** Prof OrS, UMDNJ-NJ Med Sch, Newark

Schob, Clifford J MD (OrS) - **Spec Exp:** Sports Medicine; Shoulder & Knee Surgery; **Hospital:** Overlook Med Ctr (page 92), Saint Barnabas Med Ctr; **Address:** 235 Millburn Ave, Ste 102, Millburn, NJ 07041; **Phone:** 973-258-1177; **Board Cert:** Orthopaedic Surgery 2013; **Med School:** UMDNJ-RW Johnson Med Sch 1982; **Resid:** Surgery, NS-LIJ Hlth Sys 1984; Orthopaedic Surgery, NS-LIJ Hlth Sys 1988; **Fellow:** Sports Medicine, Amer Sports Med Inst 1990

Seidenstein, Michael K MD (OrS) - **Spec Exp:** Arthroscopic Surgery; **Address:** 61-C Main St, West Orange, NJ 07052-5338; **Phone:** 973-736-8080; **Board Cert:** Orthopaedic Surgery 1977; **Med School:** NY Med Coll 1970; **Resid:** Orthopaedic Surgery, Hosp for Joint Diseases 1975; **Fellow:** Hip Surgery, Wrightington Hosp Ctr 1975A-O Fellowship 1978; **Fac Appt:** Asst Prof OrS, UMDNJ-NJ Med Sch, Newark

Otolaryngology

Morrow, Todd A MD (Oto) - **Spec Exp:** Cosmetic Surgery-Face; Rhinoplasty; Laser Surgery; Botox Therapy; **Hospital:** Saint Barnabas Med Ctr, Newark Beth Israel Med Ctr; **Address:** Tomorrow's Face, 741 Northfield Ave, Ste 104, West Orange, NJ 07052; **Phone:** 973-243-0600; **Board Cert:** Otolaryngology 1992; Facial Plastic & Reconstr Surgery 1995; **Med School:** Jefferson Med Coll 1986; **Resid:** Otolaryngology, UMDNJ-Univ Hosp 1991; **Fellow:** Facial Plastic & Reconstr Surgery, Univ Toronto Affil Hosps 1992; **Fac Appt:** Asst Clin Prof Oto, UMDNJ-NJ Med Sch, Newark

Zbar, Lloyd I.S. MD (Oto) - **Spec Exp:** Hearing & Balance Disorders; Nasal & Sinus Disorders; Voice Disorders; **Hospital:** Hackensack UMC-Mountainside (page 774), Overlook Med Ctr (page 92); **Address:** 200 Highland Ave, Ste 250, Glen Ridge, NJ 07028-1528; **Phone:** 973-744-2424; **Board Cert:** Otolaryngology 1970; **Med School:** Queens Univ 1964; **Resid:** Surgery, Beth Israel Deaconess Med Ctr 1966; Otolaryngology, Bellevue Hosp Ctr 1969; **Fellow:** Otolaryngology, Bellevue Hosp Ctr 1970; **Fac Appt:** Assoc Clin Prof Oto, NYU Sch Med

Pain Medicine

Kaufman, Andrew G MD (PM) - **Spec Exp:** Complex Regional Pain Syndromes; Pain-Back & Neck; Pain-Cancer; Pain-Neuropathic; **Hospital:** Univ Hosp (Newark), Overlook Med Ctr (page 92); **Address:** 90 Bergen St, Ste 3400, Newark, NJ 07103; **Phone:** 973-972-2085; **Board Cert:** Anesthesiology 1993; Pain Medicine 2005; **Med School:** Univ VA Sch Med 1988; **Resid:** Anesthesiology, Columbia Presby Med Ctr 1992; **Fellow:** Pain Medicine, Beth Israel Hosp/Brigham & Women's/Chldn's Hosp 1993; **Fac Appt:** Assoc Prof Anes, UMDNJ-NJ Med Sch, Newark

Pathology

Heller, Debra S MD (Path) - **Spec Exp:** Gynecologic Pathology; Pediatric Pathology; Perinatal Pathology; **Hospital:** Univ Hosp (Newark); **Address:** UMDNJ-NJ Med Sch Dept Pathology, 185 S Orange Ave, Newark, NJ 07101; **Phone:** 973-972-0751; **Board Cert:** Anatomic Pathology 1988; Obstetrics & Gynecology 2012; Pediatric Pathology 1999; **Med School:** NY Med Coll 1977; **Resid:** Obstetrics & Gynecology, Beth Israel Med Ctr 1981; Anatomic Pathology, Mt Sinai Med Ctr 1988; **Fellow:** Pediatric Pathology, Mt Sinai Med Ctr 1987; Gynecologic Pathology, Mt Sinai Med Ctr 1989; **Fac Appt:** Prof Path, UMDNJ-NJ Med Sch, Newark

Lara, Jonathan F MD (Path) - **Hospital:** Saint Barnabas Med Ctr; **Address:** St Barnabas Med Ctr, Dept Pathology, 94 Old Short Hills Rd, Livingston, NJ 07039-5672; **Phone:** 973-322-5762; **Board Cert:** Anatomic & Clinical Pathology 1988; Cytopathology 1997; **Med School:** Philippines 1984; **Resid:** Pathology, St Barnabas Med Ctr 1988; **Fellow:** Surgical Pathology, Meml Sloan Kettering Canc Ctr 1989; **Fac Appt:** Asst Clin Prof Path, UMDNJ-NJ Med Sch, Newark

Pediatric Allergy & Immunology

Fost, Arthur MD (PA&I) - **Spec Exp:** Asthma; Sinusitis; Urticaria; **Hospital:** Clara Maass Med Ctr; **Address:** 197 Bloomfield Ave, Verona, NJ 07044-2702; **Phone:** 973-857-0330; **Board Cert:** Pediatrics 1968; Allergy & Immunology 1972; **Med School:** Jefferson Med Coll 1963; **Resid:** Pediatrics, Chldns Hosp 1965; Pediatrics, Hosp Univ Penn 1966; **Fellow:** Allergy & Immunology, St Vincent's Hosp 1968; **Fac Appt:** Assoc Clin Prof Ped, UMDNJ-NJ Med Sch, Newark

Morrison, Susan H MD (PA&I) - **Hospital:** Clara Maass Med Ctr; **Address:** 36 Newark Ave, Ste 322, Belleville, NJ 07109; **Phone:** 973-450-0100; **Board Cert:** Pediatrics 1986; Allergy & Immunology 2008; Pediatric Infectious Disease 2009; **Med School:** UMDNJ-NJ Med Sch, Newark 1981; **Resid:** Pediatrics, Univ Hosp-UMDNJ 1985; **Fellow:** Pediatric Allergy & Immunology, Univ Hosp-UMDNJ 1988; **Fac Appt:** Prof Ped, UMDNJ-NJ Med Sch, Newark

Torre, Arthur J MD (PA&I) - **Spec Exp:** Asthma; Diving Medicine; Rhinitis; Sinusitis; **Hospital:** St. Joseph's Regl Med Ctr - Paterson; **Address:** 25 Hollywood Ave, Fairfield, NJ 07004-1113; **Phone:** 973-882-0880; **Board Cert:** Pediatrics 1975; **Med School:** UMDNJ-NJ Med Sch, Newark 1970; **Resid:** Pediatrics, Martland Hosp 1974; **Fellow:** Pediatric Allergy & Immunology, Martland Hosp 1975; **Fac Appt:** Assoc Clin Prof Ped, UMDNJ-NJ Med Sch, Newark

Pediatric Cardiology

Connor, Thomas M MD (PCd) - **Hospital:** Saint Barnabas Med Ctr; **Address:** 101 Old Short Hills Rd, Ste 104, West Orange, NJ 07052; **Phone:** 973-731-5550; **Board Cert:** Pediatrics 1973; Pediatric Cardiology 1977; **Med School:** Italy 1966; **Resid:** Pediatrics, Westchester Med Ctr 1970; **Fellow:** Pediatric Cardiology, Yale-New Haven Hosp 1972; **Fac Appt:** Assoc Prof Ped, Columbia P&S

Fernandes, John MD (PCd) - **Spec Exp:** Congenital Heart Disease; Fetal Cardiology; Echocardiography; **Hospital:** Saint Barnabas Med Ctr, Morgan Stanley Children's Hosp of NY-Presby, NY (page 104); **Address:** 349 E Northfield Rd, Ste 201, Livingston, NJ 07039-4086; **Phone:** 973-533-1031; **Board Cert:** Pediatric Cardiology 2013; **Med School:** India 1983; **Resid:** Pediatrics, Hahnemann Univ Hosp 1988; **Fellow:** Pediatric Cardiology, NYU Med Ctr 1991; Pediatric Cardiology, Johns Hopkins Hosp 1990; **Fac Appt:** Assoc Clin Prof Ped, Columbia P&S

Langsner, Alan M MD (PCd) - **Spec Exp:** Fetal Echocardiography; Congenital Heart Disease-Adult & Child; Preventive Cardiology; **Hospital:** NYU Langone Med Ctr (page 108); **Address:** NYU Pediatric Cardiology Associates, 160 E 32nd St Fl 3, New York, NY 10016; **Phone:** 212-263-5940; **Board Cert:** Pediatrics 1983; Pediatric Cardiology 2010; **Med School:** Mexico 1977; **Resid:** Pediatrics, Metropolitan Hosp Ctr 1981; **Fellow:** Pediatric Cardiology, NYU Med Ctr 1983; **Fac Appt:** Asst Prof Ped, NYU Sch Med

O'Connor, Brian K MD (PCd) - **Hospital:** Newark Beth Israel Med Ctr, Chldns Hosp NJ at Newark; **Address:** Newark Beth Israel - Chldns Hrt Ctr, 201 Lyons Ave, Ste L-5, Newark, NJ 07112; **Phone:** 973-926-3500; **Board Cert:** Pediatric Cardiology 2010; **Med School:** Georgetown Univ 1985; **Resid:** Pediatrics, New England Med Ctr 1989; **Fellow:** Pediatric Cardiology, Mott Chldns Hosp 1991; Pediatric Cardiology, Chldns Hosp 1995

Putman, Donald C MD (PCd) - **Hospital:** Saint Barnabas Med Ctr, Hackensack UMC-Mountainside (page 774); **Address:** MetroPediatric Cardiology Assocs, 349 E Northfield Rd, Ste 105, Livingston, NJ 07039; **Phone:** 973-597-3333; **Board Cert:** Pediatric Cardiology 2011; **Med School:** Grenada 1989; **Resid:** Pediatrics, Bellevue Hosp Ctr 1993; **Fellow:** Pediatric Cardiology, Bellevue Hosp Ctr 1995

Verma, Rajiv MD (PCd) - **Spec Exp:** Congenital Heart Disease-Adult & Child; Kawasaki Disease; **Hospital:** Newark Beth Israel Med Ctr; **Address:** Newark Beth Israel - Chldns Hrt Ctr, 201 Lyons Ave, Ste L-5, Newark, NJ 07112; **Phone:** 973-926-3500; **Board Cert:** Pediatric Cardiology 2009; **Med School:** Zambia 1984; **Resid:** Pediatrics, NYU Langone Med Ctr 1990; **Fellow:** Pediatric Cardiology, NYU Langone Med Ctr 1994; Interventional Cardiology, Chldns Hosp 1996; **Fac Appt:** Asst Clin Prof Ped, NYU Sch Med

Pediatric Critical Care Medicine

Yeh, Timothy S MD (PCCM) - **Hospital:** Saint Barnabas Med Ctr, Monmouth Med Ctr; **Address:** St Barnabas Med Ctr, 94 Old Short Hills Rd, Fl 4th, rm 4134A, Livingston, NJ 07039; **Phone:** 973-322-5691; **Board Cert:** Pediatrics 1982; Pediatric Critical Care Medicine 2010; **Med School:** UC Davis 1976; **Resid:** Pediatrics, UC Davis Med Ctr 1979; **Fellow:** Pediatric Critical Care Medicine, Chldns Natl Med Ctr 1981; **Fac Appt:** Clin Prof Ped, UMDNJ-NJ Med Sch, Newark

Pediatric Endocrinology

Brenner, Dennis J MD (PEn) - **Spec Exp:** Growth Disorders; Pubertal Disorders; Diabetes; Turner Syndrome; **Hospital:** Saint Barnabas Med Ctr, Newark Beth Israel Med Ctr; **Address:** 375 Mt Pleasant Ave, Ste 105, West Orange, NJ 07052; **Phone:** 973-322-7600; **Board Cert:** Pediatric Endocrinology 2011; **Med School:** SUNY Downstate 1997; **Resid:** Pediatrics, Steven & Alexandra Cohen Chldn's Med Ctr of NY 2000; **Fellow:** Pediatric Endocrinology, Steven & Alexandra Cohen Chldn's Med Ctr of NY 2003; **Fac Appt:** Asst Clin Prof Ped, SUNY Downstate

Sivitz, Jennifer N MD (PEn) - **Spec Exp:** Diabetes; Obesity; **Hospital:** Hackensack Univ Med Ctr (page 718), Newark Beth Israel Med Ctr; **Address:** 30 Prospect Ave WFAN Bldg - rm 251, Hackensack, NJ 07601; **Phone:** 551-996-5329; **Board Cert:** Pediatrics 2013; Pediatric Endocrinology 2009; **Med School:** NY Med Coll 2002; **Resid:** Pediatrics, Long Is Jewish Med Ctr 2005; **Fellow:** Pediatric Endocrinology, Mass Genl Hosp 2007

Pediatric Gastroenterology

Sunaryo, Francis P MD (PGe) - **Spec Exp:** Inflammatory Bowel Disease; Gastroesophageal Reflux Disease (GERD); **Hospital:** Newark Beth Israel Med Ctr, Saint Barnabas Med Ctr; **Address:** Newark Beth Israel Med Ctr, Div Pediatric Gastroenterology, 201 Lyons Ave, Newark, NJ 07112; **Phone:** 973-926-7280; **Board Cert:** Pediatrics 1982; Pediatric Gastroenterology 2012; **Med School:** Indonesia 1973; **Resid:** Pediatrics, N Shore Univ Hosp 1979; **Fellow:** Pediatric Gastroenterology, Chldns Hosp 1982; **Fac Appt:** Asst Prof Ped, UMDNJ-Univ Med Dent NJ

Pediatric Hematology-Oncology

Kamalakar, Peri MD (PHO) - **Hospital:** Newark Beth Israel Med Ctr, Monmouth Med Ctr; **Address:** Valerie Fund Chldns Ctr, 201 Lyons Ave, Ste L5, Newark, NJ 07112-2027; **Phone:** 973-926-7161; **Board Cert:** Pediatrics 1975; Pediatric Hematology-Oncology 1997; **Med School:** India 1967; **Resid:** Pediatrics, Beth Israel Med Ctr 1973; **Fellow:** Pediatric Hematology-Oncology, Chldns Hosp 1976; **Fac Appt:** Asst Clin Prof Ped, UMDNJ-NJ Med Sch, Newark

Pediatric Infectious Disease

Oleske, James M MD (PInf) - **Spec Exp:** AIDS/HIV; Pediatric Allergy & Immunology; Pain Management; **Hospital:** Univ Hosp (Newark); **Address:** Univ Hosp, Pediatric Infectious Disease, 570 S Orange Ave, Ste 572, Newark, NJ 07103; **Phone:** 973-972-5066; **Board Cert:** Pediatrics 1976; Allergy & Immunology 1977; Diagnostic Lab Immunology 1986; Hospice & Palliative Medicine 2007; **Med School:** UMDNJ-NJ Med Sch, Newark 1971; **Resid:** Pediatrics, Martland Hosp 1974; **Fellow:** Pediatric Infectious Disease, Grady Meml Hosp 1976; **Fac Appt:** Prof Ped, UMDNJ-NJ Med Sch, Newark

Pediatric Nephrology

Roberti, M. Isabel MD/PhD (PNep) - **Spec Exp:** Transplant Medicine-Kidney; Kidney Failure; Hypertension; Kidney Stones; **Hospital:** Saint Barnabas Med Ctr; **Address:** SBMC - Pediatric Nephrology, 94 Old Short Hills Rd, Ste 304, Livingston, NJ 07039; **Phone:** 973-322-5264; **Board Cert:** Pediatrics 2010; Pediatric Nephrology 2012; **Med School:** Brazil 1983; **Resid:** Pediatrics, Hosp Sao Paulo 1986; **Fellow:** Pediatric Nephrology, Hosp Sao Paulo 1989; Pediatric Nephrology, Mount Sinai Med Ctr 1995; **Fac Appt:** Assoc Clin Prof Ped, Mount Sinai Sch Med

Pediatric Pulmonology

Aguila, Helen MD (PPul) - **Spec Exp:** Asthma; Tuberculosis; **Hospital:** Univ Hosp (Newark), Columbus Hosp; **Address:** UMDNJ-Univ Hosp-Newark, 90 Bergen St Fl 5th - rm 5100, Dept Ped Pulmonology, Newark, NJ 07103; **Phone:** 973-972-5779; **Board Cert:** Pediatrics 1983; Pediatric Pulmonology 2011; **Med School:** Philippines 1974; **Resid:** Pediatrics, Staten Island Hosp 1979; Pediatrics, Kings Co Hosp/Downstate Med Ctr 1980; **Fellow:** Pediatric Pulmonology, Chldns Hosp Michigan 1983; **Fac Appt:** Asst Prof Ped, UMDNJ-NJ Med Sch, Newark

Bisberg, Dorothy S MD (PPul) - **Spec Exp:** Asthma; Cystic Fibrosis; **Hospital:** Saint Barnabas Med Ctr, Newark Beth Israel Med Ctr; **Address:** 200 S Orange Ave Fl 2 - Ste 225, Pediatric Specialty Center, Livingston, NJ 07039; **Phone:** 973-322-7600 x6; **Board Cert:** Pediatrics 1977; Pediatric Pulmonology 2007; **Med School:** Cornell Univ-Weill Med Coll 1972; **Resid:** Pediatrics, Montefiore Med Ctr 1974; Pediatrics, Bronx Lebanon Hosp 1975; **Fac Appt:** Asst Prof Ped, UMDNJ-NJ Med Sch, Newark

Kottler, William MD (PPul) - **Spec Exp:** Asthma; Cystic Fibrosis; **Hospital:** Saint Barnabas Med Ctr, Overlook Med Ctr (page 92); **Address:** 48 Essex St, Millburn, NJ 07041; **Phone:** 973-218-0900; **Board Cert:** Pediatric Pulmonology 2009; **Med School:** Dominica 1987; **Resid:** Pediatrics, Overlook Hosp 1990; **Fellow:** Pediatric Pulmonology, Newark Beth Israel Hosp 1991; Pediatric Pulmonology, Univ Florida Shands Hosp 1993; **Fac Appt:** Asst Clin Prof Ped, UMDNJ-NJ Med Sch, Newark

Mikkilineni, Sushmita MD (PPul) - **Spec Exp:** Critical Care; Sleep Medicine; **Hospital:** Chldns Hosp NJ at Newark; **Address:** 201 Lyons Ave, Ste L-5, Newark, NJ 07112; **Phone:** 973-926-4273; **Board Cert:** Pediatrics 2009; Pediatric Pulmonology 2007; Pediatric Critical Care Medicine 2010; Sleep Medicine 2007; **Med School:** India 1979; **Resid:** Pediatrics, RW Johnson Univ Hosp 1987; **Fellow:** Pediatric Pulmonary & Critical Care, RW Johnson Univ Hosp 1988; Pediatric Pulmonology, NY-Presby/Columbia Univ Med Ctr 1991; **Fac Appt:** Assoc Prof Ped, UMDNJ-RW Johnson Med Sch

Montalvo-Stanton, Evelyn MD (PPul) - **Spec Exp:** Cystic Fibrosis; Asthma; **Hospital:** Univ Hosp (Newark); **Address:** Univ Hosp, Ped Pulmonary Dept, 90 Bergen St, Ste 5100, Newark, NJ 07103; **Phone:** 973-972-5779; **Board Cert:** Pediatrics 2009; Pediatric Pulmonology 2011; **Med School:** UMDNJ-NJ Med Sch, Newark 1981; **Resid:** Pediatrics, Univ Hosp-UMDNJ 1989; **Fellow:** Pediatric Pulmonology, NY-Presby/Columbia Univ Med Ctr 1993; **Fac Appt:** Asst Prof Ped, UMDNJ-NJ Med Sch, Newark

Pediatric Rheumatology

Chalom, Elizabeth C MD (PRhu) - **Spec Exp:** Juvenile Arthritis; **Hospital:** Saint Barnabas Med Ctr; **Address:** 375 Mount Pleasant Ave, West Orange, NJ 07052; **Phone:** 973-322-7600; **Board Cert:** Pediatrics 2009; Pediatric Rheumatology 2013; **Med School:** Columbia P&S 1991; **Resid:** Pediatrics, Chldns Hosp 1994; **Fellow:** Pediatric Rheumatology, Chldns Hosp 1995; **Fac Appt:** Asst Clin Prof S, UMDNJ-NJ Med Sch, Newark

Pediatric Surgery

Bethel, Colin A MD (PS) - **Spec Exp:** Minimally Invasive Surgery; Neonatal Surgery; **Hospital:** Newark Beth Israel Med Ctr, St. Joseph's Regl Med Ctr - Paterson; **Address:** Pediatric Surgery Group, 2130 Millburn Ave, Ste C-1, Maplewood, NJ 07040; **Phone:** 973-313-3115; **Board Cert:** Surgery 2005; Pediatric Surgery 2007; **Med School:** Columbia P&S 1987; **Resid:** Surgery, Yale-New Haven Hosp 1995; **Fellow:** Pediatric Surgery, Chldns Hosp 1997; **Fac Appt:** Asst Prof S, UMDNJ-NJ Med Sch, Newark

Pediatric Urology

Stock, Jeffrey A MD (Ped Uro) - **Spec Exp:** Robotic Surgery-Pediatric; Minimally Invasive Surgery-Pediatric; Hypospadias; **Hospital:** Newark Beth Israel Med Ctr, Mt Sinai Med Ctr (page 102); **Address:** 101 Old Short Hills Rd, Ste 203, West Orange, NJ 07052-1023; **Phone:** 973-325-7188; **Board Cert:** Urology 2010; Pediatric Urology 2010; **Med School:** Mount Sinai Sch Med 1988; **Resid:** Surgery, UMDNJ- Univ Hosp 1990; Urology, UMDNJ- Univ Hosp 1993; **Fellow:** Pediatric Urology, UCSD Med Ctr 1994; **Fac Appt:** Assoc Clin Prof U, UMDNJ-NJ Med Sch, Newark

Pediatrics

Colyer-Aversa, Lori A MD (Ped) *PCP* - **Spec Exp:** Developmental Disorders; **Hospital:** Hackensack UMC-Mountainside (page 774); **Address:** 399 Hoover Ave, Ste 5, Bloomfield, NJ 07003; **Phone:** 973-748-9500; **Board Cert:** Pediatrics 2007; **Med School:** UMDNJ-Univ Med Dent NJ 1989; **Resid:** Pediatrics, Columbia-Presby Med Ctr 1992

Gruenwald, Laurence D MD (Ped) *PCP* - **Spec Exp:** Asthma; Behavioral Disorders; **Hospital:** Saint Barnabas Med Ctr; **Address:** 90 Millburn Ave, Ste 101, Millburn, NJ 07041-1933; **Phone:** 973-378-7990; **Board Cert:** Pediatrics 1981; **Med School:** UMDNJ-NJ Med Sch, Newark 1975; **Resid:** Pediatrics, Chldns Hosp Natl Med Ctr 1978; **Fac Appt:** Asst Clin Prof Ped, UMDNJ-NJ Med Sch, Newark

Marcus, Richard W MD (Ped) *PCP* - **Spec Exp:** ADD/ADHD; **Hospital:** Clara Maass Med Ctr; **Address:** Nutley Pediatrics Associates, 242 Washington Ave, Ste A, Nutley, NJ 07110-1994; **Phone:** 973-667-6676; **Board Cert:** Pediatrics 1988; **Med School:** UMDNJ-NJ Med Sch, Newark 1982; **Resid:** Pediatrics, Univ Hosp-UMDNJ 1985; **Fac Appt:** Asst Clin Prof Ped, UMDNJ-NJ Med Sch, Newark

Rigtrup, Edward MD (Ped) *PCP* - **Hospital:** Hackensack UMC-Mountainside (page 774), Saint Barnabas Med Ctr; **Address:** 73 Park St, Montclair, NJ 07042-2903; **Phone:** 973-746-7375; **Board Cert:** Pediatrics 1980; **Med School:** NY Med Coll 1975; **Resid:** Pediatrics, Chldns Natl Med Ctr 1978; **Fac Appt:** Assoc Clin Prof Ped, NY Med Coll

Rosenblatt, Joshua MD (Ped) *PCP* - **Spec Exp:** Pain Management; **Hospital:** Newark Beth Israel Med Ctr; **Address:** NBIMC, Pediatrics Dept, 201 Lyons Ave, Newark, NJ 07112; **Phone:** 973-926-7273; **Board Cert:** Pediatrics 2010; **Med School:** UMDNJ-NJ Med Sch, Newark 1984; **Resid:** Pediatrics, Newark Beth Israel Med Ctr 1987; **Fac Appt:** Asst Clin Prof Ped, UMDNJ-NJ Med Sch, Newark

Physical Medicine & Rehabilitation

Bach, John R MD (PMR) - **Spec Exp:** Neuromuscular Disorders; Amyotrophic Lateral Sclerosis (ALS); Post Polio Syndrome/Rehabilitation; **Hospital:** Univ Hosp (Newark); **Address:** 90 Bergen St Fl 3 Ste 3100, Newark, NJ 07103; **Phone:** 973-972-2850; **Board Cert:** Physical Medicine & Rehabilitation 1986; **Med School:** UMDNJ-NJ Med Sch, Newark 1976; **Resid:** Physical Medicine & Rehabilitation, NYU Med Ctr 1980; **Fellow:** Neuromuscular Disease, Univ Hosp 1983; **Fac Appt:** Prof PMR, UMDNJ-NJ Med Sch, Newark

Cole, Jeffrey L MD (PMR) - **Spec Exp:** Pain Management; Neuromuscular Disorders; Electromyography; Electrodiagnosis; **Hospital:** Kessler Inst for Rehab - W Orange; **Address:** Kessler Inst for Rehabilitation, 1199 Pleasant Valley Way, West Orange, NJ 07052; **Phone:** 973-243-6943; **Board Cert:** Physical Medicine & Rehabilitation 1983; Pain Medicine 2003; **Med School:** Mexico 1977; **Resid:** Internal Medicine, NY Hosp-Queens Med Ctr 1979; Physical Medicine & Rehabilitation, Montefiore Med Ctr 1982; **Fellow:** Electrodiagnosis, Booth Meml Med Ctr 1983

Francis, Kathleen D MD (PMR) - **Spec Exp:** Lymphedema; **Address:** Lymphedema Physician Services, 200 S Orange Ave, Ste 111, Livingston, NJ 07039; **Phone:** 973-322-7366; **Board Cert:** Physical Medicine & Rehabilitation 2004; **Med School:** UMDNJ-NJ Med Sch, Newark 1989; **Resid:** Physical Medicine & Rehabilitation, UMDNJ-Kessler Inst Rehab 1993; **Fac Appt:** Asst Clin Prof PMR, UMDNJ-NJ Med Sch, Newark

Kirshblum, Steven C MD (PMR) - **Spec Exp:** Spinal Cord Injury; Spasticity Management; **Hospital:** Kessler Inst for Rehab - W Orange, Saint Barnabas Med Ctr; **Address:** Kessler Institute, 1199 Pleasant Valley Way, West Orange, NJ 07052-1424; **Phone:** 973-731-3600 x2258; **Board Cert:** Physical Medicine & Rehabilitation 1991; Spinal Cord Injury Medicine 2008; **Med School:** Univ Hlth Scis, Chicago Med Sch 1986; **Resid:** Physical Medicine & Rehabilitation, Mount Sinai Med Ctr 1990; **Fac Appt:** Prof PMR, UMDNJ-NJ Med Sch, Newark

Shumko, John Z MD/PhD (PMR) - **Hospital:** Saint Barnabas Med Ctr; **Address:** Sports & Physical Medicine Institute, 200 S Orange Ave, Ste 124, Livingston, NJ 07039; **Phone:** 973-322-7909; **Board Cert:** Physical Medicine & Rehabilitation 2007; **Med School:** UMDNJ-NJ Med Sch, Newark 1992; **Resid:** Physical Medicine & Rehabilitation, Univ Hosp-UMDNJ 1996

Plastic Surgery

Ablaza, Valerie J MD (PlS) - **Spec Exp:** Cosmetic Surgery-Breast; Breast Reconstruction; Liposuction & Body Contouring; **Hospital:** Saint Barnabas Med Ctr, Hackensack UMC-Mountainside (page 774); **Address:** The Plastic Surgery Group, 37 N Fullerton Ave, Montclair, NJ 07042; **Phone:** 973-233-1933; **Board Cert:** Plastic Surgery 2010; **Med School:** Med Coll PA Hahnemann 1989; **Resid:** Surgery, Albert Einstein Med Ctr 1994; Plastic Surgery, New York Hosp 1996; **Fellow:** Breast Surgery, Nashville Plastic Surgery 1997

Cooperman, Ross D MD (PlS) - **Spec Exp:** Reconstructive Surgery; Cosmetic Surgery; **Hospital:** Overlook Med Ctr (page 92); **Address:** 22 Old Short Hills Rd, Ste 101, Livingston, NJ 07039; **Phone:** 973-994-2021; **Board Cert:** Surgery 2008; **Med School:** Geo Wash Univ 2003; **Resid:** Surgery, St Barnabas Med Ctr 2008; **Fellow:** Plastic Surgery, Univ Louisville Hosp 2010

DiBernardo, Barry E MD (PlS) - **Spec Exp:** Laser Surgery; Hair Restoration/Transplant; Cosmetic Surgery-Face & Body; Body Contouring after Weight Loss; **Hospital:** Hackensack UMC-Mountainside (page 774), Clara Maass Med Ctr; **Address:** 29 Park St, Montclair, NJ 07042; **Phone:** 973-509-2000; **Board Cert:** Plastic Surgery 1994; **Med School:** Cornell Univ-Weill Med Coll 1984; **Resid:** Surgery, Mt Sinai Med Ctr 1989; Plastic Surgery, Montefiore Med Ctr 1991; **Fac Appt:** Assoc Clin Prof PlS, UMDNJ-NJ Med Sch, Newark

Granick, Mark S MD (PlS) - **Spec Exp:** Reconstructive Surgery; Cosmetic Surgery; Skin Cancer; Liposuction & Body Contouring; **Hospital:** Univ Hosp (Newark), Newark Beth Israel Med Ctr; **Address:** 140 Bergen St, rm E-1620, Newark, NJ 07103; **Phone:** 973-972-8092; **Board Cert:** Otolaryngology 1982; Plastic Surgery 1985; **Med School:** Harvard Med Sch 1977; **Resid:** Otolaryngology, Mass E&E Hosp 1982; Plastic Surgery, Univ Pittsburgh Med Ctr 1984; **Fac Appt:** Prof PlS, UMDNJ-NJ Med Sch, Newark

LoVerme, Paul J MD (PlS) - **Spec Exp:** Cosmetic Surgery-Face; Liposuction & Body Contouring; Breast Reconstruction & Augmentation; **Hospital:** Hackensack UMC-Mountainside (page 774), Saint Barnabas Med Ctr; **Address:** 825 Bloomfield Ave, Ste 205, Verona, NJ 07044; **Phone:** 973-857-9499; **Board Cert:** Plastic Surgery 1987; **Med School:** UMDNJ-NJ Med Sch, Newark 1978; **Resid:** Surgery, UMDNJ Univ Hosp 1983; Plastic Surgery, Med Coll Hosp 1985; **Fac Appt:** Assoc Clin Prof PlS, UMDNJ-NJ Med Sch, Newark

Rosen, Allen D MD (PlS) - **Spec Exp:** Cosmetic Surgery-Face & Breast; Breast Reconstruction; Liposuction & Body Contouring; Eyelid Surgery; **Hospital:** Saint Barnabas Med Ctr, Hackensack UMC-Mountainside (page 774); **Address:** The Plastic Surgery Group, 37 N Fullerton Ave, Montclair, NJ 07042; **Phone:** 973-233-1933; **Board Cert:** Plastic Surgery 1991; **Med School:** SUNY Buffalo 1983; **Resid:** Surgery, Columbia Presby Med Ctr 1986; Plastic Surgery, Columbia Presby Med Ctr 1988; **Fellow:** Hand Surgery, Columbia Presby Med Ctr 1987; **Fac Appt:** Asst Clin Prof PlS, UMDNJ-NJ Med Sch, Newark

Psychiatry

Caracci, Giovanni MD (Psyc) - **Spec Exp:** Geriatric Psychiatry; Psychopharmacology; Psychotherapy; Post Traumatic Stress Disorder; **Hospital:** Univ Hosp (Newark); **Address:** 183 S Orange Ave, rm F-1555, Newark, NJ 07101; **Phone:** 973-972-7117; **Board Cert:** Psychiatry 1990; **Med School:** Italy 1977; **Resid:** Psychiatry, Metropolitan Hosp 1984; **Fac Appt:** Assoc Prof Psyc, UMDNJ-NJ Med Sch, Newark

Faber, Mark P MD (Psyc) - **Spec Exp:** Child Psychiatry; Anxiety Disorders; Depression; ADD/ADHD; **Hospital:** Saint Barnabas Med Ctr, Hackensack UMC-Mountainside (page 774); **Address:** 594 Valley Rd, Upper Montclair, NJ 07043-1882; **Phone:** 973-746-6711; **Board Cert:** Psychiatry 1993; Child & Adolescent Psychiatry 2005; **Med School:** Dominica 1988; **Resid:** Psychiatry, CT Valley Hosp 1991; **Fellow:** Child & Adolescent Psychiatry, UMDNJ-RW Johnson Sch Med 1994; Sleep Medicine, UMDNJ-RW Johnson Sch Med 1996

Nucci, Annamaria MD/PhD (Psyc) - **Spec Exp:** Psychopharmacology; Relationship Problems; Depression; **Address:** 5 Westview Terr, Cedar Grove, NJ 07009; **Phone:** 973-857-2609; **Board Cert:** Psychiatry 1978; **Med School:** Italy 1971; **Resid:** Psychiatry, VA Hosp-NYU 1973; Psychiatry, Payne Whitney Clin 1976; **Fellow:** Child & Adolescent Psychiatry, NY-Presby/Weill Cornell Med Ctr 1976; **Fac Appt:** Asst Clin Prof Psyc, NY Med Coll

Schleifer, Steven J MD (Psyc) - **Spec Exp:** Depression; Psychoneuroimmunology; Anxiety Disorders; **Hospital:** Univ Hosp (Newark); **Address:** 183 S Orange Ave Bldg BHSB F1430, Newark, NJ 07103; **Phone:** 973-972-5023; **Board Cert:** Psychiatry 1980; **Med School:** Mount Sinai Sch Med 1975; **Resid:** Psychiatry, Mount Sinai Med Ctr 1979; **Fac Appt:** Prof Psyc, UMDNJ-NJ Med Sch, Newark

Zornitzer, Michael R MD (Psyc) - **Spec Exp:** Psychopharmacology; Anxiety & Depression; Psychotherapy; **Hospital:** Saint Barnabas Med Ctr; **Address:** 2 W Northfield Rd, Ste 305, Livingston, NJ 07039-3789; **Phone:** 973-992-6090; **Board Cert:** Psychiatry 1976; **Med School:** SUNY Downstate 1971; **Resid:** Psychiatry, NYU Hosps Ctr 1972; Psychiatry, Albert Einstein Coll of Med 1975; **Fac Appt:** Asst Clin Prof Psyc, NY Coll Osteo Med

Pulmonary Disease

Greenberg, Martin J MD (Pul) - **Spec Exp:** Asthma; Emphysema; **Hospital:** Saint Barnabas Med Ctr; **Address:** 124 East Mt Pleasant Ave, Livingston, NJ 07039; **Phone:** 973-994-4130; **Board Cert:** Internal Medicine 1987; **Med School:** Dominica 1983; **Resid:** Internal Medicine, Univ Hosp UMDNJ 1986; **Fellow:** Pulmonary Disease, Newark Beth Israel 1988

Miller, Richard A MD (Pul) - **Spec Exp:** Sarcoidosis; Asthma; Sleep Medicine; **Hospital:** Saint Michael's Med Ctr; **Address:** St Michaels Medical Center, 111 Central Ave, Newark, NJ 07102; **Phone:** 973-877-5493; **Board Cert:** Internal Medicine 1989; Pulmonary Disease 2003; Critical Care Medicine 2005; **Med School:** NY Med Coll 1983; **Resid:** Internal Medicine, St Michaels Med Ctr 1988; **Fellow:** Pulmonary Critical Care Medicine, St Michaels Med Ctr 1991

Safirstein, Benjamin MD (Pul) - **Spec Exp:** Asthma; Sarcoidosis; **Hospital:** Hackensack UMC-Mountainside (page 774), Saint Michael's Med Ctr; **Address:** 123 Highland Ave, Ste 101, Glen Ridge, NJ 07028; **Phone:** 973-744-9125; **Board Cert:** Internal Medicine 1970; Pulmonary Disease 1974; **Med School:** Ros Franklin Univ/Chicago Med Sch 1965; **Resid:** Internal Medicine, Mount Sinai Hosp 1969; **Fellow:** Pulmonary Disease, Brompton Hosp 1972; **Fac Appt:** Assoc Prof Med, Mount Sinai Sch Med

Shah, Smita MD (Pul) - **Spec Exp:** Asthma; Chronic Obstructive Lung Disease (COPD); Lung Cancer; Pulmonary Hypertension; **Hospital:** Saint Barnabas Med Ctr; **Address:** 96 Millburn Ave, Ste 200-A, Millburn, NJ 07040; **Phone:** 973-763-6800; **Board Cert:** Internal Medicine 1986; Pulmonary Disease 2010; Sleep Medicine 2009; **Med School:** India 1980; **Resid:** Internal Medicine, St Marys Hosp 1986; **Fellow:** Pulmonary Critical Care Medicine, Temple Univ Hosp 1988

Radiation Oncology

Grann, Alison MD (RadRO) - **Spec Exp:** Breast Cancer; Gastrointestinal Cancer; Lung Cancer; **Hospital:** Saint Barnabas Med Ctr; **Address:** St Barnabas, Radiation Onc Dept, 94 Old Short Hills Rd, Livingston, NJ 07039; **Phone:** 973-322-5638; **Board Cert:** Radiation Oncology 2010; **Med School:** Geo Wash Univ 1991; **Resid:** Internal Medicine, Beth Israel Deaconess Med Ctr 1994; Radiation Oncology, Meml Sloan-Kettering Cancer Ctr 1998

Wagman, Raquel T MD (RadRO) - **Spec Exp:** Breast Cancer; **Hospital:** Saint Barnabas Med Ctr; **Address:** St Barnabas Med Ctr, 94 Old Short Hills Rd, Livingston, NJ 07039; **Phone:** 973-322-5630; **Board Cert:** Radiation Oncology 2010; **Med School:** Univ Mich Med Sch 1995; **Resid:** Radiation Oncology, Meml Sloan Kettering Cancer Ctr 2000

Reproductive Endocrinology

Chen, Serena H MD (RE) - **Spec Exp:** Infertility-IVF; Laparoscopic Surgery; Hysteroscopic Surgery; **Hospital:** Saint Barnabas Med Ctr; **Address:** IRMS at St Barnabas, 94 Old Short Hills Rd, East Wing, Ste 403, Livingston, NJ 07039; **Phone:** 973-322-8286; **Board Cert:** Obstetrics & Gynecology 2012; Reproductive Endocrinology 2012; **Med School:** Duke Univ 1988; **Resid:** Obstetrics & Gynecology, Johns Hopkins Hosp 1992; **Fellow:** Reproductive Endocrinology, Johns Hopkins Hosp 1994

Rheumatology

Cannarozzi, Nicholas A MD (Rhu) - **Spec Exp:** Rheumatoid Arthritis; Lupus Nephritis; Osteoporosis; Vasculitis; **Hospital:** Hackensack UMC-Mountainside (page 774); **Address:** 127 Pine St, Montclair, NJ 07042-4835; **Phone:** 973-783-6000; **Board Cert:** Internal Medicine 1980; Rheumatology 1972; **Med School:** Hahnemann Univ 1965; **Resid:** Internal Medicine, Philadelphia Genl Hosp 1967; Internal Medicine, St Michaels Med Ctr 1968; **Fellow:** Rheumatology, Yale-New Haven Hosp 1969; Rheumatology, Yale-New Haven Hosp 1972

Lahita, Robert G MD/PhD (Rhu) - **Spec Exp:** Lupus/SLE; Endocrinology & Joint Disorders; Immunodeficiency Disorders; Vasculitis; **Hospital:** Newark Beth Israel Med Ctr; **Address:** Newark Beth Israel Med Ctr, Rheumatology, 201 Lyons Ave, Fl 4, Newark, NJ 07112; **Phone:** 973-926-7472; **Board Cert:** Internal Medicine 2004; Rheumatology 2007; **Med School:** Jefferson Med Coll 1973; **Resid:** Internal Medicine, New York Hosp-Cornell 1976; **Fellow:** Rheumatology, Rockefeller Hosp 1978; **Fac Appt:** Prof Med, Mount Sinai Sch Med

Simon, Jonathan M MD (Rhu) - **Hospital:** Hackensack UMC-Mountainside (page 774); **Address:** 1018 Broad St, Bloomfield, NJ 07003-2807; **Phone:** 973-338-3383; **Board Cert:** Internal Medicine 1981; Rheumatology 1984; **Med School:** NYU Sch Med 1978; **Resid:** Internal Medicine, UMDNJ Univ Hosp 1981; **Fellow:** Rheumatology, UMDNJ Univ Hosp 1983

Sports Medicine

Gehrmann, Robin M MD (SM) - **Spec Exp:** Cartilage Damage & Transplant; Knee Ligament Reconstruction; Shoulder Injuries; Arthroscopic Surgery; **Hospital:** Univ Hosp (Newark); **Address:** Rutgers-New Jersey Medical School, 90 Bergen St, Ste 1200, Newark, NJ 07103; **Phone:** 973-972-8240; **Board Cert:** Orthopaedic Surgery 2004; Orthopaedic Sports Medicine 2007; **Med School:** Hahnemann Univ 1995; **Resid:** Surgery, UMDNJ Med Ctr 1996; Orthopaedic Surgery, UMDNJ Med Ctr 2000; **Fellow:** Orthopaedic Sports Medicine, Pennsylvania Hosp 2001; **Fac Appt:** Asst Prof OrS, UMDNJ-NJ Med Sch, Newark

Levy, Andrew S MD (SM) - **Spec Exp:** Cartilage Damage & Transplant; Ligament Reconstruction; Shoulder Surgery; **Hospital:** Saint Barnabas Med Ctr, Morristown Med Ctr (page 92); **Address:** 90 Milburn Ave, Ste 204A, Milburn, NJ 07041; **Phone:** 908-598-9199; **Board Cert:** Orthopaedic Surgery 2008; **Med School:** Temple Univ 1987; **Resid:** Orthopaedic Surgery, Albert Einstein Med Ctr 1994; **Fellow:** Sports Medicine, Duke Univ Med Ctr 1995; Shoulder Surgery, Duke Univ Med Ctr 1995

Surgery

Andrei, Valeriu E MD (S) - **Spec Exp:** Obesity/Bariatric Surgery; Laparoscopic Surgery; **Hospital:** Robert Wood Johnson Univ Hosp - New Brunswick, Saint Barnabas Med Ctr; **Address:** Bariatric Assocs, 200 S Orange Ave, Ste 123, Livingston, NJ 07039; **Phone:** 973-322-7265; **Board Cert:** Surgery 2009; **Med School:** Romania 1987; **Resid:** Surgery, Methodist Hosp 1988; **Fellow:** Minimally Invasive Surgery, Mount Sinai Med Ctr 1999

Blackwood, M. Michele MD (S) - **Spec Exp:** Breast Cancer; Breast Surgery; Sentinel Node Surgery; Breast Cancer-High Risk Women; **Hospital:** Saint Barnabas Med Ctr; **Address:** St Barnabas, Ambulatory Care, 200 S Orange Ave, Ste 102, Livingston, NJ 07039; **Phone:** 973-322-7020; **Board Cert:** Surgery 2003; **Med School:** Med Univ SC 1988; **Resid:** Surgery, Stamford Hosp 1993; **Fellow:** Surgical Oncology, Meml Sloan-Kettering Cancer Ctr 1994; **Fac Appt:** Asst Clin Prof S, Columbia P&S

Chamberlain, Ronald S MD (S) - **Spec Exp:** Liver & Biliary Surgery; Cancer Surgery; Laparoscopic Surgery; Pancreatic Cancer; **Hospital:** Saint Barnabas Med Ctr; **Address:** St Barnabas Med Ctr, Surgery, 94 Old Short Hills Rd, Ste 1172, Livingston, NJ 07039; **Phone:** 973-322-5195; **Board Cert:** Surgery 2009; **Med School:** Geo Wash Univ 1991; **Resid:** Surgery, G Washington Univ Hosp 1997; **Fellow:** Surgical Oncology, Natl Cancer Inst 1996; Hepatobiliary Surgery, Meml Sloan-Kettering Canc Ctr 1999; **Fac Appt:** Prof S, UMDNJ-NJ Med Sch, Newark

Deitch, Edwin A MD (S) - **Spec Exp:** Burn Care; Abdominal Wall Reconstruction; Critical Care; **Hospital:** Univ Hosp (Newark); **Address:** 185 S Orange Ave, MSB, rm G506, Newark, NJ 07103; **Phone:** 973-972-6639; **Board Cert:** Surgery 2009; Surgical Critical Care 2006; **Med School:** Univ MD Sch Med 1973; **Resid:** Surgery, US Public Hlth Svc Hosp 1976; Surgery, US Public Hlth Svc Hosp 1978; **Fac Appt:** Prof S, UMDNJ-NJ Med Sch, Newark

Fletcher, H. Stephen MD (S) - **Spec Exp:** Vascular Surgery; Breast Surgery; **Hospital:** Saint Barnabas Med Ctr; **Address:** St Barnabas Med Ctr, Surgery Dept, 200 S Orange Ave, Ste 203, Livingston, NJ 07039; **Phone:** 973-322-7977; **Board Cert:** Surgery 1973; **Med School:** Geo Wash Univ 1967; **Resid:** Surgery, G Washington Univ Med Ctr 1972; **Fac Appt:** Assoc Clin Prof S, UMDNJ-NJ Med Sch, Newark

Huston, Jan A MD (S) - **Spec Exp:** Breast Surgery; Breast Disease; **Hospital:** Saint Michael's Med Ctr, Saint Barnabas Med Ctr; **Address:** Summit Breast Care, UMCHackensack Mountainside Breast Center, Harries Pa Bldg - Fl 2 - Ste 4, 1 Bay Ave, Montclair, NJ 07042; **Phone:** 973-259-3505; **Board Cert:** Surgery 2007; **Med School:** Mich State Univ 1982; **Resid:** Surgery, St Barnabas Hosp 1987; **Fellow:** Vascular Surgery, Lehigh Valley Hosp 1988

Maheshwari, Vivek MD (S) - **Spec Exp:** Gastrointestinal Cancer; Endocrine Tumors; Cancer Surgery; Breast Cancer; **Hospital:** Saint Barnabas Med Ctr, Newark Beth Israel Med Ctr; **Address:** Prof Assocs Surgery, 101 Old Short Hills Rd, Ste 206, West Orange, NJ 07052; **Phone:** 973-731-5005; **Board Cert:** Surgery 2003; **Med School:** India 1992; **Resid:** Surgery, Beth Israel Med Ctr 2002; **Fellow:** Surgical Oncology, UPMC 2004

Petrone, Sylvia J MD (S) - **Spec Exp:** Burn Care; Critical Care; **Hospital:** Saint Barnabas Med Ctr; **Address:** St Barnabas Med Ctr, Burn Ctr, 94 Old Short Hills Rd, Livingston, NJ 07039; **Phone:** 973-322-5924; **Board Cert:** Surgery 2011; Surgical Critical Care 2008; **Med School:** Loyola Univ-Stritch Sch Med 1977; **Resid:** Surgery, Boston Med Ctr 1982; **Fellow:** Burn Surgery, NY-Presby/Weill Cornell Med Ctr 1983

Shack, Robert P MD (S) - **Spec Exp:** Vascular Surgery; **Hospital:** Saint Barnabas Med Ctr; **Address:** 745 Northfield Ave, West Orange, NJ 07052; **Phone:** 973-325-7705; **Board Cert:** Surgery 2005; **Med School:** Jefferson Med Coll 1969; **Resid:** Surgery, Mount Sinai Med Ctr 1975

Shapiro, Michael E MD (S) - **Spec Exp:** Transplant-Kidney; Transplant-Pancreas; Parathyroid Surgery; Dialysis Access Surgery; **Hospital:** Hackensack Univ Med Ctr (page 718); **Address:** 90 Bergen St, Ste 7100, Newark, NJ 07103; **Phone:** 973-972-2400; **Board Cert:** Surgery 2005; **Med School:** Univ Rochester 1977; **Resid:** Surgery, Beth Israel Med Ctr 1983; **Fac Appt:** Assoc Prof S, UMDNJ-NJ Med Sch, Newark

Thoracic & Cardiac Surgery

Burns, Paul G MD (T&CS) - **Spec Exp:** Coronary Artery Surgery; **Hospital:** Saint Barnabas Med Ctr; **Address:** St Barnabas Med Ctr, Cardiothoracic Dept, 94 Old Short Hills Rd, Ste 144, Livingston, NJ 07039; **Phone:** 973-322-2200; **Board Cert:** Thoracic & Cardiac Surgery 2010; **Med School:** Columbia P&S 1989; **Resid:** Surgery, Beth Israel Deaconess Med Ctr 1996; **Fellow:** Cardiothoracic Surgery, NY-Presby/Weill Cornell Med Ctr 1998

Camacho, Margarita T MD (T&CS) - **Spec Exp:** Mechanical Assist Devices; Transplant-Heart; Heart Failure; **Hospital:** Newark Beth Israel Med Ctr; **Address:** NBIMC, Cardiothoracic Surgery Dept, 201 Lyons Ave, Ste G5, Newark, NJ 07112; **Phone:** 973-926-6938; **Board Cert:** Thoracic & Cardiac Surgery 2008; **Med School:** NY Med Coll 1984; **Resid:** Surgery, Lenox Hill Hosp 1989; Cardiothoracic Surgery, Albert Einstein Affil Hosp 1991; **Fellow:** Pediatric Cardiothoracic Surgery, LI Jewish Med Ctr 1992; Transplantation/Mechanical Assist Devices, Cleveland Clin 1994

Forman, Mark MD (T&CS) - **Spec Exp:** Lung Cancer; Lung Surgery; Vascular Surgery; Video Assisted Thoracic Surgery (VATS); **Hospital:** Saint Barnabas Med Ctr, Overlook Med Ctr (page 92); **Address:** 1500 Pleasant Valley Way, Ste 302, West Orange, NJ 07052; **Phone:** 973-324-0988; **Board Cert:** Thoracic & Cardiac Surgery 2007; **Med School:** Tulane Univ 1976; **Resid:** Surgery, LI Jewish Med Ctr 1981; **Fellow:** Cardiothoracic Surgery, Montefiore Med Ctr 1984

Goldenberg, Bruce MD (T&CS) - **Spec Exp:** Minimally Invasive Thoracic Surgery; Cardiac Surgery-Adult; Pacemakers; Arrhythmias; **Hospital:** St. Clare's Hosp-Denville, Hackensack UMC-Mountainside (page 774); **Address:** 30 Chatham Rd, Ste 377, Short Hills, NJ 07078; **Phone:** 973-467-5550; **Board Cert:** Thoracic & Cardiac Surgery 2003; **Med School:** Northwestern Univ 1976; **Resid:** Surgery, NYU Med Ctr 1981; **Fellow:** Thoracic & Cardiac Surgery, NYU Med Ctr 1983; **Fac Appt:** Asst Clin Prof S, UMDNJ-NJ Med Sch, Newark

Saunders, Craig R MD (T&CS) - **Spec Exp:** Cardiac Surgery; Minimally Invasive Surgery; **Hospital:** Newark Beth Israel Med Ctr, Saint Barnabas Med Ctr; **Address:** NBIMC, Cardiothoracic Surgery Dept, 201 Lyons Ave, Ste G5, Newark, NJ 07112; **Phone:** 973-926-6938; **Board Cert:** Thoracic & Cardiac Surgery 2011; **Med School:** Univ Iowa Coll Med 1970; **Resid:** Surgery, Univ Iowa Hosps & Clins 1978; Cardiothoracic Surgery, Cleveland Clin 1980

Urology

Boorjian, Peter C MD (U) - **Spec Exp:** Kidney Stones; Prostate Benign Disease; Urinary Tract Infections; Urologic Cancer; **Hospital:** Hackensack UMC-Mountainside (page 774); **Address:** Montclair Urological Group, 777 Bloomfield Ave, Glen Ridge, NJ 07028; **Phone:** 973-429-0462; **Board Cert:** Urology 1978; **Med School:** SUNY Downstate 1971; **Resid:** Surgery, Med Coll VA 1973; Urology, SUNY Downstate 1976

Ciccone, Patrick N MD (U) - **Spec Exp:** Prostate Cancer; Genitourinary Cancer; **Hospital:** Clara Maass Med Ctr, Saint Barnabas Med Ctr; **Address:** NJ Urology, 36 Newark Ave, Ste 200, Belleville, NJ 07109; **Phone:** 973-759-6180; **Board Cert:** Urology 1975; **Med School:** Georgetown Univ 1967; **Resid:** Surgery, VA Med Ctr 1969; Urology, VA Med Ctr 1972

Katz, Jeffrey I MD (U) - **Spec Exp:** Prostate Disease; Kidney Stones; Urologic Cancer; **Hospital:** Saint Barnabas Med Ctr; **Address:** Urology Grp NJ, 741 Northfield Ave, Ste 206, West Orange, NJ 07052; **Phone:** 973-325-6100; **Board Cert:** Urology 1978; **Med School:** Italy 1970; **Resid:** Surgery, Mount Sinai Hosp 1973; Urology, Montefiore Med Ctr 1976

Linsenmeyer, Todd A MD (U) - **Spec Exp:** Infertility-Male in Spinal Cord Injury; Voiding Dysfunction/Spinal Cord Injury; Urodynamics in Spinal Cord Injury; **Hospital:** Kessler Inst for Rehab - W Orange; **Address:** Kessler Inst Rehab, 1199 Pleasant Valley Way, West Orange, NJ 07052; **Phone:** 973-731-3600 x2274; **Board Cert:** Urology 2005; Physical Medicine & Rehabilitation 1990; **Med School:** Univ Hawaii JA Burns Sch Med 1979; **Resid:** Urology, Tripler AMC 1984; **Fellow:** Physical Medicine & Rehabilitation, Stanford Univ Hosp 1989; **Fac Appt:** Prof S, UMDNJ-NJ Med Sch, Newark

Saidi, James MD (U) - **Spec Exp:** Minimally Invasive Surgery; Prostate Cancer; Robotic Urologic Surgery; **Hospital:** Hackensack UMC-Mountainside (page 774); **Address:** Montclair Urological Group, 777 Bloomfield Ave, Glen Ridge, NJ 07028; **Phone:** 973-429-0462; **Board Cert:** Urology 2012; **Med School:** Univ Tex SW, Dallas 1994; **Resid:** Surgery, NY Presby Hosp/Columbia 1996; Urology, NY Presby Hosp/Columbia 2000

Savatta, Domenico J MD (U) - **Spec Exp:** Robotic Urologic Surgery; Prostate Cancer; Kidney Cancer; Bladder Cancer; **Hospital:** Newark Beth Israel Med Ctr, Saint Barnabas Med Ctr; **Address:** Urology Grp NJ, 375 Mt Pleasant Ave, Ste 250, West Orange, NJ 07052; **Phone:** 732-499-0111; **Board Cert:** Urology 2005; **Med School:** SUNY Stony Brook 1997; **Resid:** Surgery, IU Hlth Hosp 1999; Urologic Surgery, IU Hlth Hosp 2003

Vascular Surgery

Brener, Bruce J MD (VascS) - **Spec Exp:** Endovascular Surgery; Minimally Invasive Vascular Surgery; Carotid Artery Surgery; Aneurysm-Aortic; **Hospital:** Newark Beth Israel Med Ctr, Saint Barnabas Med Ctr; **Address:** Vascular Assocs of NJ, 200 S Orange Ave, Ste 109, Livingston, NJ 07039; **Phone:** 973-322-7233; **Board Cert:** Surgery 1972; Vascular Surgery 2005; **Med School:** Harvard Med Sch 1966; **Resid:** Surgery, Chldns Hosp Med Ctr 1968; Surgery, Peter Bent Brigham Hosp 1972; **Fellow:** Vascular Surgery, Mass Genl Hosp 1973; **Fac Appt:** Assoc Clin Prof S, Columbia P&S

Hertz, Steven MD (VascS) - **Hospital:** Saint Barnabas Med Ctr; **Address:** 1500 Pleasant Valley Way, Ste 302, West Orange, NJ 07052; **Phone:** 973-324-0988; **Board Cert:** Surgery 2001; Vascular Surgery 2012; **Med School:** Albert Einstein Coll Med 1987; **Resid:** Surgery, Mount Sinai Med Ctr 1992; **Fellow:** Vascular Surgery, Hosp U Penn 1993

Patel, Amit V MD (VascS) - **Spec Exp:** Aneurysm-Aortic; Endovascular Surgery; Carotid Artery Surgery; **Hospital:** Morristown Med Ctr (page 92); **Address:** 101 Old Short Hills Rd, Ste 206, Livingston, NJ 07078; **Phone:** 973-540-9700; **Board Cert:** Surgery 2004; Vascular Surgery 2006; **Med School:** Albert Einstein Coll Med 1988; **Resid:** Surgery, Montefiore Med Ctr 1993; **Fellow:** Vascular Surgery, Hosp Univ Penn 1994

Hudson

Hudson

Cardiovascular Disease

Cruz, Merle C MD (Cv) - **Spec Exp:** Heart Disease; **Hospital:** Hoboken Univ Med Ctr - Hoboken; **Address:** 201 St Pauls Ave, Ste 1D, Jersey City, NJ 07306; **Phone:** 201-653-7533; **Board Cert:** Internal Medicine 1983; Cardiovascular Disease 1985; **Med School:** Philippines 1976; **Resid:** Internal Medicine, Jersey City Med Ctr 1982; **Fellow:** Cardiovascular Disease, Brookdale Univ Hosp Med Ctr 1984

Elkind, Barry M MD (Cv) - **Spec Exp:** Non-Invasive Cardiology; Preventive Cardiology; Nutrition; **Hospital:** Bayonne Med Ctr, Newark Beth Israel Med Ctr; **Address:** Assocs Cardiovascular Care, 1061 Avenue C, Bayonne, NJ 07002; **Phone:** 201-858-0800; **Board Cert:** Internal Medicine 1979; Cardiovascular Disease 1981; **Med School:** UMDNJ-NJ Med Sch, Newark 1976; **Resid:** Internal Medicine, Boston Med Ctr 1979; **Fellow:** Cardiovascular Disease, Tufts Med Ctr 1982

Moussa, Ghias M MD (Cv) - **Spec Exp:** Heart Valve Disease; Congestive Heart Failure; **Hospital:** Christ Hosp - Jersey City; **Address:** 1815 Kennedy Blvd, Jersey City, NJ 07305; **Phone:** 201-333-3311; **Board Cert:** Internal Medicine 1989; **Med School:** Syria 1979; **Resid:** Internal Medicine, Jersey City Med Ctr 1989; **Fellow:** Cardiovascular Disease, Jersey City Med Ctr 1991; **Fac Appt:** Assoc Prof Med, UMDNJ-NJ Med Sch, Newark

Child Neurology

McAbee, Gary N DO (ChiN) - **Spec Exp:** Autism; Epilepsy; Headache; **Hospital:** Meadowlands Hosp Med Ctr; **Address:** 6017 Bergenline Ave, West New York, NJ 07093; **Phone:** 201-392-3400; **Board Cert:** Pediatrics 1988; Child Neurology 1988; **Med School:** Univ Osteo Med & Hlth Sci, Des Moines 1980; **Resid:** Pediatrics, NY Med Coll 1982; **Fellow:** Child Neurology, St Louis Chldns Hosp 1985; **Fac Appt:** Prof Ped, UMDNJ-RW Johnson Med Sch

Dermatology

Blank, Ellen MD (D) - **Spec Exp:** Acne; **Hospital:** Mt Sinai Med Ctr (page 102); **Address:** 333 Avenue C, Bayonne, NJ 07002; **Phone:** 201-858-4800; **Board Cert:** Dermatology 1979; **Med School:** Mount Sinai Sch Med 1975; **Resid:** Dermatology, Mount Sinai Hosp 1979

Kopec, Anna V MD (D) - **Spec Exp:** Cosmetic Dermatology; Hair & Nail Disorders; **Hospital:** Bayonne Med Ctr; **Address:** 730 Kennedy Blvd, Bayonne, NJ 07002-1838; **Phone:** 201-858-4300; **Board Cert:** Dermatology 2009; **Med School:** UMDNJ-NJ Med Sch, Newark 1975; **Resid:** Dermatology, Albert Einstein 1979; **Fac Appt:** Assoc Clin Prof D, Albert Einstein Coll Med

Endocrinology, Diabetes & Metabolism

Cam, Jenny Rose G MD (EDM) - **Spec Exp:** Diabetes; Thyroid Disorders; Osteoporosis; Adrenal Disorders; **Hospital:** Hoboken Univ Med Ctr - Hoboken, Christ Hosp - Jersey City; **Address:** 10 Huron Ave, Ste 1P, Jersey City, NJ 07306; **Phone:** 201-656-6003; **Board Cert:** Internal Medicine 1988; Endocrinology, Diabetes & Metabolism 1989; **Med School:** Philippines 1979; **Resid:** Internal Medicine, Interfaith Med Ctr 1987; **Fellow:** Endocrinology, Diabetes & Metabolism, UMDNJ-Univ Hosp 1989

Family Medicine

Levine, Martin S DO (FMed) *PCP* - **Spec Exp:** Primary Care Sports Medicine; Osteopathic Manipulation; **Hospital:** Christ Hosp - Jersey City, Bayonne Med Ctr; **Address:** 789 Avenue C, Bayonne, NJ 07002; **Phone:** 201-339-2620; **Board Cert:** Family Medicine 2007; Geriatric Medicine 2011; **Med School:** Kirksville Coll Osteo Med 1980; **Resid:** Family Medicine, Kennedy Meml Hosp 1983; **Fac Appt:** Prof FMed, Touro Coll Osteopathic Med-NY

Sklower, Jay A DO (FMed) *PCP* - **Spec Exp:** Geriatric Medicine; Diabetes; Cholesterol/Lipid Disorders; **Hospital:** Christ Hosp - Jersey City; **Address:** 600 Pavonia Ave, 2nd Fl, Jersey City, NJ 07306-2929; **Phone:** 201-216-3040; **Board Cert:** Family Medicine 2005; **Med School:** SUNY Stony Brook 1971; **Resid:** Family Medicine, Union Meml Hosp 1973; **Fac Appt:** Assoc Prof Ped

Gastroenterology

Hahn, John C MD (Ge) - **Spec Exp:** Colonoscopy; Peptic Acid Disorders; **Hospital:** Bayonne Med Ctr; **Address:** 534 Avenue E, Ste 1C, Bayonne, NJ 07002; **Phone:** 201-823-0450; **Board Cert:** Internal Medicine 1988; Gastroenterology 2011; **Med School:** UMDNJ-NJ Med Sch, Newark 1985; **Resid:** Internal Medicine, Univ Hosp 1988; **Fellow:** Gastroenterology, Univ Hosp 1990

Prakash, Anaka MD (Ge) - **Spec Exp:** Pancreatic/Biliary Endoscopy (ERCP); Capsule Endoscopy; **Hospital:** Bayonne Med Ctr, Jersey City Med Ctr; **Address:** 534 Ave E, Ste 1A, Bayonne, NJ 07002; **Phone:** 201-858-8444; **Board Cert:** Internal Medicine 1976; Gastroenterology 1977; **Med School:** India 1970; **Resid:** Internal Medicine, St Joseph's Hosp 1975; **Fellow:** Gastroenterology, CMDNJ-Newark 1977

Geriatric Medicine

Brown, Mitchell Lee MD (Ger) *PCP* - **Spec Exp:** Alzheimer's Disease; **Hospital:** Bayonne Med Ctr, Jersey City Med Ctr; **Address:** 758 Broadway, Bayonne, NJ 07002; **Phone:** 201-339-2220; **Board Cert:** Geriatric Medicine 2013; **Med School:** West Indies 1987; **Resid:** Internal Medicine, St Elizabeth Hosp 1990; **Fellow:** Geriatric Medicine, St Vincent's Hosp & Med Ctr 1992

Reisner, Michelle R MD (Ger) *PCP* - **Spec Exp:** Frail Elderly; **Hospital:** Jersey City Med Ctr; **Address:** 196 Jewitt Ave, Jersey City, NJ 07304; **Phone:** 201-332-3354; **Board Cert:** Internal Medicine 1989; Geriatric Medicine 2005; Hospice & Palliative Medicine 2008; **Med School:** South Africa 1983; **Resid:** Internal Medicine, Jersey City Med Ctr 1989; **Fac Appt:** Asst Prof Med, Mount Sinai Sch Med

Internal Medicine

Cardiello, Gary P MD (IM) *PCP* - **Spec Exp:** Diabetes; Hypertension; Hemochromatosis; **Hospital:** Clara Maass Med Ctr, Saint Michael's Med Ctr; **Address:** 744 Broadway, Bayonne, NJ 07002; **Phone:** 201-436-8888; **Board Cert:** Internal Medicine 1986; **Med School:** Italy 1983; **Resid:** Internal Medicine, St Michael's Med Ctr 1986

Condo, Dominick MD (IM) *PCP* - **Spec Exp:** Geriatric Care; **Hospital:** Bayonne Med Ctr, Overlook Med Ctr (page 92); **Address:** 622 Broadway, Bayonne, NJ 07002; **Phone:** 201-436-2800; **Board Cert:** Internal Medicine 1984; **Med School:** Mexico 1980; **Resid:** Internal Medicine, St Michael's Med Ctr 1984

Dedousis, John T MD (IM) *PCP* - **Hospital:** Bayonne Med Ctr; **Address:** 1166 Kennedy Blvd, Bayonne, NJ 07002-3112; **Phone:** 201-339-1133; **Board Cert:** Internal Medicine 2003; **Med School:** Dominica 1985; **Resid:** Internal Medicine, Univ Hosp 1988

Kozel, Joseph M MD (IM) *PCP* - **Spec Exp:** Asthma; Chronic Obstructive Lung Disease (COPD); Lung Cancer; Lung Disease in Pregnancy; **Hospital:** Hoboken Univ Med Ctr - Hoboken, Jersey City Med Ctr; **Address:** 331 Grand St, Fl Ground, Hoboken, NJ 07030; **Phone:** 201-656-3519; **Board Cert:** Internal Medicine 1984; **Med School:** Mexico 1973; **Resid:** Family Medicine, St Mary Hosp 1979; Internal Medicine, St Michaels Med Ctr 1980; **Fellow:** Pulmonary Disease, St Michaels Med Ctr 1982

Mutterperl, Mitchell MD (IM) *PCP* - **Spec Exp:** Hypertension; Cholesterol/Lipid Disorders; Cardiovascular Disease; **Hospital:** Bayonne Med Ctr, Jersey City Med Ctr; **Address:** 19 W 33rd St, Bayonne, NJ 07002-3916; **Phone:** 201-858-0090; **Board Cert:** Internal Medicine 1985; **Med School:** Italy 1981; **Resid:** Internal Medicine, UMDNJ-NJ Med Ctr 1985

Nephrology

Thomsen, Stephen MD (Nep) - **Spec Exp:** Diabetes; Hypertension; Kidney Disease; **Hospital:** Christ Hosp - Jersey City, Hackensack UMC-Mountainside (page 774); **Address:** 510 31st St, Union City, NJ 07087; **Phone:** 201-866-3322; **Board Cert:** Internal Medicine 1981; Nephrology 2006; **Med School:** Italy 1977; **Resid:** Internal Medicine, Mountainside Hosp 1980; **Fellow:** Nephrology, Univ Hosp-UMDNJ 1982

Neurology

Anselmi, Gregory D MD (N) - **Spec Exp:** Migraine; Multiple Sclerosis; Stroke; **Hospital:** Bayonne Med Ctr, Hoboken Univ Med Ctr - Hoboken; **Address:** 1222 Kennedy Blvd, Bayonne, NJ 07002-3822; **Phone:** 201-339-6531; **Board Cert:** Neurology 2009; Vascular Surgery 2009; **Med School:** Italy 1988; **Resid:** Internal Medicine, SUNY/Univ Hosp 1989; **Fellow:** Neurology, St Vincent's Hosp & Med Ctr 1992

Charles, James A MD (N) - **Spec Exp:** Headache; Clinical Neurophysiology; **Hospital:** Bayonne Med Ctr, Holy Name Med Ctr (page 720); **Address:** 956 Kennedy Blvd, Bayonne, NJ 07002; **Phone:** 201-858-2457; **Board Cert:** Neurology 1984; Clinical Neurophysiology 2005; **Med School:** UMDNJ-NJ Med Sch, Newark 1978; **Resid:** Neurology, UMDNJ Med Ctr 1982; **Fac Appt:** Assoc Clin Prof N, UMDNJ-NJ Med Sch, Newark

Sadeghi, Hooshang W MD (N) - **Spec Exp:** Parkinson's Disease; Stroke; Multiple Sclerosis; Dystonia-Cervical; **Hospital:** Bayonne Med Ctr, Jersey City Med Ctr; **Address:** 631 Broadway, FL 3, Bayonne, NJ 07002-3846; **Phone:** 201-823-2888; **Board Cert:** Neurology 1977; **Med School:** Iran 1967; **Resid:** Neurology, UMDNJ Med Ctr 1975; **Fac Appt:** Asst Clin Prof N, UMDNJ-NJ Med Sch, Newark

Obstetrics & Gynecology

Banzon, Manuel B MD (ObG) - **Spec Exp:** Laparoscopic Surgery; Vaginal Surgery; Incontinence; **Hospital:** Meadowlands Hosp Med Ctr; **Address:** 1265 Paterson Plank Rd, Ste 3D, Secaucus, NJ 07094; **Phone:** 201-864-4442; **Board Cert:** Obstetrics & Gynecology 1979; **Med School:** Philippines 1962; **Resid:** Obstetrics & Gynecology, Jersey City Med Ctr 1969

Masson, Lalitha MD (ObG) - **Spec Exp:** Infertility; **Hospital:** Christ Hosp - Jersey City; **Address:** 634 Newark Ave, Main Fl, Jersey City, NJ 07306; **Phone:** 201-963-8554; **Board Cert:** Obstetrics & Gynecology 1973; **Med School:** India 1964; **Resid:** Obstetrics & Gynecology, Jersey City Med Ctr 1969; Obstetrics & Gynecology, St Clares Hosp 1970; **Fellow:** Infertility, UMDNJ-NJ Sch Med Affil Hosps 1971

Uy, Vena MD (ObG) *PCP* - **Hospital:** Christ Hosp - Jersey City, Meadowlands Hosp Med Ctr; **Address:** 142 Palisade Ave, Ste 102, Jersey City, NJ 07306; **Phone:** 201-653-0506; **Board Cert:** Obstetrics & Gynecology 1977; **Med School:** Philippines 1968; **Resid:** Obstetrics & Gynecology, Jersey Shore Univ Med Ctr 1973; **Fellow:** Gynecologic Pathology, Magee-Womens Hosp - UPMC 1974

Ophthalmology

Benedetto, Dominick A MD (Oph) - **Spec Exp:** LASIK-Refractive Surgery; Cataract Surgery; **Hospital:** Bayonne Med Ctr, Morristown Med Ctr (page 92); **Address:** EyeMD Assocs, 124 Avenue B, Bayonne, NJ 07002-2033; **Phone:** 201-436-1150; **Board Cert:** Ophthalmology 1982; **Med School:** Univ Fla Coll Med 1975; **Resid:** Ophthalmology, Wills Eye Hosp 1982

Constad, William H MD (Oph) - **Spec Exp:** Cornea Transplant; Cataract Surgery; Refractive Surgery; **Hospital:** Jersey City Med Ctr; **Address:** 600 Pavonia Ave Fl 6, Jersey City, NJ 07306; **Phone:** 201-963-3937; **Board Cert:** Ophthalmology 1985; **Med School:** Med Coll PA Hahnemann 1980; **Resid:** Ophthalmology, Univ Hosp-UMDNJ 1984; **Fellow:** Cornea, New York Eye & Ear Infirm 1985; **Fac Appt:** Clin Prof Oph, UMDNJ-NJ Med Sch, Newark

Orthopaedic Surgery

Granatir, Charles E MD (OrS) - **Hospital:** Clara Maass Med Ctr; **Address:** 586 Kearny Ave, Kearny, NJ 07032; **Phone:** 201-997-7667; **Board Cert:** Orthopaedic Surgery 2010; **Med School:** Hahnemann Univ 1979; **Resid:** Orthopaedic Surgery, Montefiore Med Ctr 1985

Otolaryngology

Garay, Kenneth F MD (Oto) - **Spec Exp:** Nasal & Sinus Disorders; **Hospital:** Jersey City Med Ctr; **Address:** 377 Jersey Ave, Ste 220, Jersey City, NJ 07302; **Phone:** 201-224-4155; **Board Cert:** Otolaryngology 1982; **Med School:** Temple Univ 1978; **Resid:** Surgery, Abington Meml Hosp 1979; Otolaryngology, NY-Presby/Columbia Univ Med Ctr 1982

Pediatrics

Baker, Azzam A MD (Ped) *PCP* - **Hospital:** Hackensack Univ Med Ctr (page 718), Palisades Med Ctr; **Address:** Riverside Pediatric Group, 714 10th St, Secaucus, NJ 07094-2921; **Phone:** 201-863-3346; **Board Cert:** Pediatrics 2011; **Med School:** Egypt 1972; **Resid:** Pediatrics, Jersey City Med Ctr 1978; **Fellow:** Neonatal-Perinatal Medicine, UMDNJ Univ Hosp 1980

Klos, Andrzej E MD (Ped) *PCP* - **Spec Exp:** Nutrition; Preventive Medicine; **Hospital:** Hoboken Univ Med Ctr - Hoboken, Hackensack Univ Med Ctr (page 718); **Address:** 1327 Willow Ave, Hoboken, NJ 07030; **Phone:** 201-963-5633; **Board Cert:** Pediatrics 2013; **Med School:** Poland 1977; **Resid:** Pediatrics, Jersey City Med Ctr 1994; **Fac Appt:** Asst Clin Prof Ped, UMDNJ-NJ Med Sch, Newark

Oko, Piotr MD (Ped) *PCP* - **Hospital:** Christ Hosp - Jersey City, Hoboken Univ Med Ctr - Hoboken; **Address:** Hoboken Pediatrics, 1327 Willow Ave, Hoboken, NJ 07030; **Phone:** 201-963-5633; **Board Cert:** Pediatrics 2010; **Med School:** Poland 1987; **Resid:** Pediatrics, Jersey City Med Ctr 1995

Skripkus, Aldona J MD (Ped) *PCP* - **Hospital:** Clara Maass Med Ctr; **Address:** 381 Kearny Ave, Kearny, NJ 07032-2603; **Phone:** 201-991-4824; **Board Cert:** Pediatrics 1971; **Med School:** Med Coll PA Hahnemann 1966; **Resid:** Pediatrics, Chldns Hosp 1969

Physical Medicine & Rehabilitation

Filippone, Mark A MD (PMR) - **Spec Exp:** Electrodiagnosis; Electromyography; Pain Management; **Hospital:** Christ Hosp - Jersey City, Hoboken Univ Med Ctr - Hoboken; **Address:** 2012 John F Kennedy Blvd W, Jersey City, NJ 07305-1526; **Phone:** 201-332-6855; **Board Cert:** Physical Medicine & Rehabilitation 1980; **Med School:** Georgetown Univ 1974; **Resid:** Pediatrics, St Vincent's Hosp & Med Ctr 1976; Physical Medicine & Rehabilitation, Bronx Muni Hosp-Einstein 1979; **Fac Appt:** Asst Clin Prof PMR, Albert Einstein Coll Med

Psychiatry

Gewolb, Eric B MD (Psyc) - **Spec Exp:** Anxiety Disorders; Dementia; Bipolar/Mood Disorders; **Hospital:** Bayonne Med Ctr; **Address:** 830 Kennedy Blvd, Bayonne, NJ 07002-2872; **Phone:** 201-339-0200; **Board Cert:** Psychiatry 1979; **Med School:** Tulane Univ 1974; **Resid:** Psychiatry, Mount Sinai Hosp 1978

Jacoby, Jacob H MD/PhD (Psyc) - **Spec Exp:** Psychopharmacology; Mood Disorders; **Hospital:** Bayonne Med Ctr, Saint Barnabas Med Ctr; **Address:** 654 Avenue C, Ste 201, Bayonne, NJ 07002-3899; **Phone:** 201-339-0323; **Board Cert:** Psychiatry 1993; **Med School:** SUNY Buffalo 1980; **Resid:** Psychiatry, Western Psychiatric Inst 1983; **Fellow:** Psychiatry, Montefiore Med Ctr 1984; **Fac Appt:** Assoc Clin Prof Psyc, UMDNJ-NJ Med Sch, Newark

Kurani, Devendra MD (Psyc) - **Spec Exp:** Depression; Anxiety Disorders; Panic Disorder; **Hospital:** Saint Barnabas Med Ctr, Christ Hosp - Jersey City; **Address:** 221 Palisade Ave, Jersey City, NJ 07306; **Phone:** 201-656-3116; **Board Cert:** Psychiatry 1986; **Med School:** India 1975; **Resid:** Psychiatry, Warley Hosp 1981; Psychiatry, Harlem Hosp 1983

Moraille, Pascale MD (Psyc) - **Spec Exp:** Autism; Developmental Disorders; ADD/ADHD; **Hospital:** Hoboken Univ Med Ctr - Hoboken; **Address:** CMHC of Hoboken Univ Med Ctr, 506 Third St, Hoboken, NJ 07030; **Phone:** 201-792-8200; **Board Cert:** Psychiatry 1993; **Med School:** Ponce Med Sch 1988; **Resid:** Psychiatry, UMDNJ-Univ Hosp 1991; **Fellow:** Child & Adolescent Psychiatry, UMDNJ-Univ Hosp 1993

Pulmonary Disease

Elamir, Mazhar E MD (Pul) - **Spec Exp:** Sleep Disorders; Allergy; Asthma; **Hospital:** Christ Hosp - Jersey City, Hackensack Univ Med Ctr (page 718); **Address:** 192 Harrison Ave, Jersey City, NJ 07304; **Phone:** 201-333-5363; **Board Cert:** Internal Medicine 1987; Pulmonary Disease 2004; Sleep Medicine 2011; **Med School:** Egypt 1981; **Resid:** Internal Medicine, Jersey City Med Ctr 1987; **Fellow:** Pulmonary Disease, Interfaith Med Ctr 1990

Radiation Oncology

Goodman, Robert L MD (RadRO) - **Spec Exp:** Breast Cancer; Lymphoma; Prostate Cancer; Brain Tumors; **Hospital:** Saint Barnabas Med Ctr; **Address:** Jersey City Radiation Oncology, 631 Grand St, Jersey City, NJ 07304; **Phone:** 201-942-3999; **Board Cert:** Internal Medicine 1971; Therapeutic Radiology 1974; Medical Oncology 1975; **Med School:** Columbia P&S 1966; **Resid:** Internal Medicine, Beth Israel Hosp 1971; Therapeutic Radiology, Harvard Joint Ctr Rad Therapy 1974; **Fellow:** Hematology, NY-Presby Hosp 1975; **Fac Appt:** Prof RadRO, Univ Pennsylvania

Rheumatology

Scarpa, Nicholas P MD (Rhu) - **Spec Exp:** Lupus/SLE in Pregnancy; Rheumatoid Arthritis; Osteoporosis; **Hospital:** Christ Hosp - Jersey City; **Address:** 600 Pavonia Ave, Fl 5, Ste 1, Jersey City, NJ 07306-2932; **Phone:** 201-216-3050; **Board Cert:** Internal Medicine 1983; Rheumatology 1986; **Med School:** UMDNJ-NJ Med Sch, Newark 1980; **Resid:** Internal Medicine, Hackensack Univ Med Ctr 1983; **Fellow:** Rheumatology, Hosp for Special Surgery 1985; **Fac Appt:** Asst Clin Prof Med, UMDNJ-NJ Med Sch, Newark

Surgery

McGovern Jr, Patrick J MD (S) - **Spec Exp:** Vascular Surgery; Aneurysm-Aortic; Carotid Artery Surgery; **Hospital:** Christ Hosp - Jersey City, Bayonne Med Ctr; **Address:** 17 Nardone Pl, Jersey City, NJ 07306; **Phone:** 201-656-0646; **Board Cert:** Surgery 2003; Vascular Surgery 2008; **Med School:** UMDNJ-NJ Med Sch, Newark 1978; **Resid:** Surgery, UMDNJ-Univ Hosp 1983; **Fellow:** Vascular Surgery, UMDNJ-RWJ Univ Hosp 1984

Sultan, Ronald H MD (S) - **Spec Exp:** Hernia; Thyroid Cancer; Breast Cancer; **Hospital:** Jersey City Med Ctr, Palisades Med Ctr; **Address:** 2255 John F Kennedy Blvd, Jersey City, NJ 07304-1428; **Phone:** 201-434-3305; **Board Cert:** Surgery 2009; **Med School:** NYU Sch Med 1973; **Resid:** Surgery, Bronx Muni Hosp 1977; Surgery, Albert Einstein Med Ctr 1980

Urology

Katz, Herbert I MD (U) - **Spec Exp:** Urologic Cancer; Erectile Dysfunction; Kidney Stones; Prostate Disease; **Hospital:** Bayonne Med Ctr; **Address:** Urology Grp NJ, 534 Ave E, Ste 2A, Bayonne, NJ 07002; **Phone:** 201-823-1303; **Board Cert:** Urology 1981; **Med School:** Temple Univ 1974; **Resid:** Surgery, Abington Meml Hosp 1976; Urology, Montefiore Med Ctr 1979

Shulman, Yale MD (U) - **Spec Exp:** Urologic Cancer; Kidney Stones; Sexual Dysfunction; Incontinence; **Hospital:** Christ Hosp - Jersey City, Englewood Hosp & Med Ctr; **Address:** 2255 Kennedy Blvd, Jersey City, NJ 07304-1428; **Phone:** 201-433-1057; **Board Cert:** Urology 1984; **Med School:** Albert Einstein Coll Med 1976; **Resid:** Surgery, Montefiore Hosp Med Ctr 1978; Urology, NYU Med Ctr 1982; **Fac Appt:** Assoc Clin Prof U, NYU Sch Med

Steigman, Elliot G MD (U) - **Spec Exp:** Kidney Stones; Prostate Benign Disease; **Hospital:** Christ Hosp - Jersey City; **Address:** Sovereign Med Grp, Urology, 142 Palisade Ave, Ste 211, Jersey City, NJ 07306; **Phone:** 201-435-2244; **Board Cert:** Urology 1982; **Med School:** SUNY Downstate 1975; **Resid:** Surgery, Brookdale Hosp Med Ctr 1977; Urology, SUNY Downstate Med Ctr 1980

Vascular & Interventional Radiology

Smith, Peter L MD (VIR) - **Spec Exp:** Varicose Veins; Vein Disorders; **Hospital:** Bayonne Med Ctr; **Address:** Bayonne Med Ctr, Vein Treatment Ctr, 29 E 29 St, Bayonne, NJ 07002; **Phone:** 201-858-4590; **Board Cert:** Diagnostic Radiology 1992; Vascular & Interventional Radiology 2006; **Med School:** Washington Univ, St Louis 1987; **Resid:** Diagnostic Radiology, Mass Genl Hosp 1992; **Fellow:** Vascular & Interventional Radiology, Mass Geml Hosp 1995

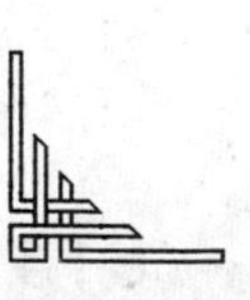

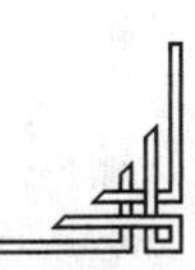

The Best in American Medicine
www.CastleConnolly.com

Mercer

Mercer

Allergy & Immunology

Ricketti, Anthony J MD (A&I) - **Spec Exp:** Asthma in Pregnancy; Allergic Aspergillosis; Eosinophilic Lung Disorders; **Hospital:** St. Francis Med Ctr - Trenton, Robert Wood Johnson Univ Hosp Hamilton; **Address:** Allergy & Pulmonary Assocs, 1542 Kuser Rd, Ste B7, Trenton, NJ 08619; **Phone:** 609-581-1400; **Board Cert:** Internal Medicine 1981; Allergy & Immunology 1983; Pulmonary Disease 1986; Critical Care Medicine 2009; **Med School:** Hahnemann Univ 1978; **Resid:** Internal Medicine, Cleveland Clin Fdn 1981; **Fellow:** Allergy & Immunology, Northwestern Univ Affil Hosp 1983; Pulmonary Disease, Northwestern Univ Affil Hosp 1984; **Fac Appt:** Asst Clin Prof Med, UMDNJ-RW Johnson Med Sch

Winant Jr, John G MD (A&I) - **Spec Exp:** Asthma; Food Allergy; Pediatric Allergy & Immunology; **Hospital:** Univ Med Ctr Princeton at Plainsboro; **Address:** 8 Quakerbridge Plaza, Ste E, Mercerville, NJ 08619; **Phone:** 609-890-8782; **Board Cert:** Pediatrics 1980; Allergy & Immunology 1987; **Med School:** Univ Cincinnati 1975; **Resid:** Pediatrics, Chldns Hosp Med Ctr 1978; **Fellow:** Allergy & Immunology, Chldns Hosp Med Ctr 1980

Cardiovascular Disease

Costin, Andrew MD (Cv) - **Spec Exp:** Nuclear Cardiology; Echocardiography; **Hospital:** Univ Med Ctr Princeton at Plainsboro; **Address:** Princeton Med Grp, 419 N Harrison St, Princeton, NJ 08540; **Phone:** 609-924-9300; **Board Cert:** Internal Medicine 1989; Cardiovascular Disease 2003; Nuclear Cardiology 2007; Echocardiography 2011; **Med School:** Yale Univ 1986; **Resid:** Internal Medicine, NY-Presby/Weill Cornell Med Ctr 1989; **Fellow:** Cardiovascular Disease, Hosp Univ Penn 1993

Mahalingam, Banu MD (Cv) - **Spec Exp:** Heart Disease in Women; Echocardiography; Preventive Cardiology; Nuclear Cardiology; **Hospital:** Univ Med Ctr Princeton at Plainsboro, Robert Wood Johnson Univ Hosp - New Brunswick; **Address:** Cardiac Assocs, 281 Witherspoon St, Ste 210, Princeton, NJ 08542; **Phone:** 609-921-7456; **Board Cert:** Internal Medicine 2008; Cardiovascular Disease 2012; Echocardiography 2013; **Med School:** India 1995; **Resid:** Internal Medicine, RW Johnson Univ Hosp 1998; **Fellow:** Cardiovascular Disease, RW Johnson Univ Hosp 2001

Dermatology

Bagel, Jerry MD (D) - **Spec Exp:** Psoriasis; Atopic Dermatitis; Exfoliate Erythroderma; **Hospital:** Univ Med Ctr Princeton at Plainsboro; **Address:** 59 One Mile Rd, Ste G, East Windsor, NJ 08520-2505; **Phone:** 609-443-4500; **Board Cert:** Dermatology 1985; **Med School:** Mount Sinai Sch Med 1981; **Resid:** Dermatology, Columbia-Presby Med Ctr 1985

Diagnostic Radiology

Choudhri, Ajay MD (DR) - **Hospital:** Capital Health Regl Med Ctr; **Address:** 750 Brunswick Ave, Trenton, NJ 08638; **Phone:** 609-815-7532; **Board Cert:** Diagnostic Radiology ; **Med School:** UMDNJ-NJ Med Sch, Newark 1995; **Resid:** Diagnostic Radiology, Montefiore Med Ctr 2000; **Fellow:** Vascular & Interventional Radiology, Baptist Hosp 2001

Endocrinology, Diabetes & Metabolism

Shelmet, John J MD (EDM) - **Spec Exp:** Diabetes; Metabolic Disorders; **Hospital:** Univ Med Ctr Princeton at Plainsboro; **Address:** 3131 Princeton Pike, Bldg 2B, Ste 104, Lawrenceville, NJ 08648-2526; **Phone:** 609-896-8050; **Board Cert:** Internal Medicine 1984; **Med School:** UMDNJ-RW Johnson Med Sch 1981; **Resid:** Internal Medicine, Middlesex Genl Hosp/Univ Hosp 1984; **Fellow:** Metabolism, Temple Univ 1986; Diabetes, Temple Univ 1986; **Fac Appt:** Clin Prof Med, UMDNJ-RW Johnson Med Sch

Family Medicine

Lansing, Martha MD (FMed) *PCP* - **Spec Exp:** Chronic Illness; Women's Health; Psychosomatic Disorders; **Hospital:** Capital Health Regl Med Ctr, Robert Wood Johnson Univ Hosp - New Brunswick; **Address:** 433 Bellevue Ave, Fl 4th, Trenton, NJ 08618; **Phone:** 609-815-2671; **Board Cert:** Family Medicine 2005; **Med School:** Univ Okla Coll Med 1982; **Resid:** Family Medicine, Univ Tenn 1984; Family Medicine, Williamsport Hosp/Univ Penn 1985; **Fac Appt:** Assoc Prof FMed, UMDNJ-Rutgers Med Sch

Rednor, Jeffrey D DO (FMed) *PCP* - **Spec Exp:** Diabetes; Pain-Back; Preventive Cardiology; **Hospital:** Robert Wood Johnson Univ Hosp Hamilton; **Address:** 1 Washington Blvd, Ste A, Robbinsville, NJ 08691; **Phone:** 609-448-4353; **Board Cert:** Family Medicine 1992; **Med School:** UMDNJ Sch Osteo Med 1989; **Resid:** Family Medicine, Kennedy Meml Hosp 1992

Gastroenterology

Afridi, Shariq A MD (Ge) - **Spec Exp:** Liver Disease; Endoscopy; **Hospital:** Robert Wood Johnson Univ Hosp Hamilton, St. Francis Med Ctr - Trenton; **Address:** 1374 White Horse Square Rd, Yorkshire Bldg - Fl 2, Hamilton, NJ 08690; **Phone:** 609-586-1319; **Board Cert:** Gastroenterology 2003; **Med School:** Pakistan 1986; **Resid:** Internal Medicine, Bridgeport Hosp 1991; **Fellow:** Gastroenterology, Bridgeport Hosp 1993

De Antonio, Joseph R MD (Ge) - **Spec Exp:** Liver Disease; **Hospital:** Capital Health Regl Med Ctr; **Address:** 3100 Princeton Pike, Bldg 4 - Ste C, Lawrenceville, NJ 08648; **Phone:** 609-882-2185; **Board Cert:** Internal Medicine 1989; Gastroenterology 2004; **Med School:** St Louis Univ 1982; **Resid:** Internal Medicine, VA Med Ctr 1989; **Fellow:** Gastroenterology, Bellevue Hosp Ctr 1991

Marin, Geobel A MD (Ge) - **Spec Exp:** Peptic Ulcer Disease; Colonoscopy; Inflammatory Bowel Disease; **Hospital:** Capital Health Med Ctr - Hopewell, Robert Wood Johnson Univ Hosp Hamilton; **Address:** Capital Health Med Ctr at Hopewell, Two Capital Way, Ste 487, Pennington, NJ 08534; **Phone:** 609-818-1900; **Board Cert:** Gastroenterology 1972; Internal Medicine 1977; **Med School:** Columbia P&S 1962; **Resid:** Internal Medicine, Philadelphia Genl Hosp 1966; **Fellow:** Gastroenterology, Philadelphia Genl Hosp 1968

Meirowitz, Robert F MD (Ge) - **Spec Exp:** Inflammatory Bowel Disease; Colon Polyps & Cancer; Colonoscopy; Gastroesophageal Reflux Disease (GERD); **Hospital:** Univ Med Ctr Princeton at Plainsboro; **Address:** Princeton Gastroenterology Assocs, 731 Alexander Rd, Ste 100, Princeton, NJ 08540; **Phone:** 609-924-1422; **Board Cert:** Internal Medicine 1987; Gastroenterology 2012; **Med School:** NY Med Coll 1984; **Resid:** Internal Medicine, RW Johnson Univ Hosp 1988; **Fellow:** Gastroenterology, Univ MD Med Ctr 1990; **Fac Appt:** Asst Clin Prof Med, UMDNJ-RW Johnson Med Sch

Rosner, Bruce P MD (Ge) - **Spec Exp:** Liver Disease; Gastroesophageal Reflux Disease (GERD); Colon Cancer; **Hospital:** St. Francis Med Ctr - Trenton; **Address:** Gastroenterology Associates, 2275 Whitehorse Mercerville Rd, Ste 2, Trenton, NJ 08619-2643; **Phone:** 609-890-0200; **Board Cert:** Internal Medicine 1979; Gastroenterology 1983; **Med School:** Univ Pennsylvania 1976; **Resid:** Internal Medicine, Penn Hosp 1979; **Fellow:** Gastroenterology, Hahnemann Univ 1981

Rubin, Marc R MD (Ge) - **Hospital:** St. Francis Med Ctr - Trenton; **Address:** Gastroenterology Associates, 2275 Whitehorse Mercerville Rd, Ste 2, Trenton, NJ 08619-2643; **Phone:** 609-890-0200; **Board Cert:** Internal Medicine 1977; Gastroenterology 1979; **Med School:** Albert Einstein Coll Med 1974; **Resid:** Internal Medicine, Penn Hosp 1977; **Fellow:** Gastroenterology, Univ Hosp 1979

Hand Surgery

Ark, Jon Wong Tze-Jen MD (HS) - **Spec Exp:** Hand Surgery; Carpal Tunnel Syndrome; Foot & Ankle Surgery; Arthritis Hand Surgery; **Hospital:** Univ Med Ctr Princeton at Plainsboro; **Address:** 325 Princeton Ave, Princeton, NJ 08540; **Phone:** 609-924-8131; **Board Cert:** Orthopaedic Surgery 2007; Hand Surgery 2007; **Med School:** UMDNJ-RW Johnson Med Sch 1987; **Resid:** Orthopaedic Surgery, Columbia-Presby Med Ctr 1992; **Fellow:** Hand Surgery, Mass Genl Hosp 1993; Foot & Ankle Surgery, Jefferson Hosp 1995

Infectious Disease

Aufiero, Patrick MD (Inf) - **Spec Exp:** AIDS/HIV; Lyme Disease; Osteomyelitis; Skin/Soft Tissue Infections; **Hospital:** Robert Wood Johnson Univ Hosp Hamilton, Capital Health Med Ctr - Hopewell; **Address:** 2085 Klockner Rd, Hamilton, NJ 08690; **Phone:** 609-587-4122; **Board Cert:** Internal Medicine 2005; Infectious Disease 2006; **Med School:** Grenada 1984; **Resid:** Internal Medicine, St Michaels Med Ctr 1989; **Fellow:** Infectious Disease, St Michaels Med Ctr 1991

Gekowski, Kathleen MD (Inf) - **Spec Exp:** Travel Medicine; AIDS/HIV; Lyme Disease; **Hospital:** Capital Health Med Ctr - Hopewell, Robert Wood Johnson Univ Hosp Hamilton; **Address:** 1450 Parkside Ave, Ste 4, Ewing, NJ 08638; **Phone:** 609-882-3500; **Board Cert:** Internal Medicine 1979; Infectious Disease 1984; **Med School:** Hahnemann Univ 1976; **Resid:** Internal Medicine, Univ Illinois Hosp 1979; **Fellow:** Infectious Disease, Yale Univ 1982; **Fac Appt:** Assoc Clin Prof Med, UMDNJ-RW Johnson Med Sch

Porwancher, Richard B MD (Inf) - **Spec Exp:** Lyme Disease; AIDS/HIV; Disaster Preparedness; **Hospital:** St. Francis Med Ctr - Trenton, Robert Wood Johnson Univ Hosp Hamilton; **Address:** 1245 Whitehorse-Mercerville Rd, Ste 410-411, Hamilton, NJ 08619-3831; **Phone:** 609-581-2000; **Board Cert:** Internal Medicine 1980; Infectious Disease 1982; **Med School:** Northwestern Univ 1977; **Resid:** Internal Medicine, Med Coll Wisconsin Affil Hosps 1980; **Fellow:** Infectious Disease, VA Med Ctr 1982; **Fac Appt:** Assoc Clin Prof Med

Internal Medicine

Corazza, Douglas P MD (IM) *PCP* - **Hospital:** Univ Med Ctr Princeton at Plainsboro; **Address:** 727 State Road, Princeton, NJ 08540; **Phone:** 609-921-6410; **Board Cert:** Internal Medicine 1988; **Med School:** UMDNJ-Rutgers Med Sch 1985; **Resid:** Internal Medicine, RW Johnson Univ Hosp 1988

Harman, John MD (IM) *PCP* - **Hospital:** Capital Health Med Ctr - Hopewell; **Address:** 2480 Pennington Rd, Ste 108, Pennington, NJ 08534; **Phone:** 609-737-6700; **Board Cert:** Internal Medicine 1972; **Med School:** Univ Pennsylvania 1969; **Resid:** Internal Medicine, Presby Hosp 1972; **Fellow:** Pulmonary Disease, U Penn Hosp 1975

Murray, Simon D MD (IM) *PCP* - **Spec Exp:** Concierge Medicine; Cholesterol/Lipid Disorders; Nutrition; Preventive Medicine; **Hospital:** Univ Med Ctr Princeton at Plainsboro; **Address:** 727 State Rd Fl 2, Princeton, NJ 08540; **Phone:** 609-921-7444; **Board Cert:** Internal Medicine 1985; **Med School:** Philippines 1980; **Resid:** Internal Medicine, UMDNJ/RWJ Univ Hosp 1984; **Fac Appt:** Asst Clin Prof Med, UMDNJ-RW Johnson Med Sch

Schaeffer, Mark A MD (IM) - **Hospital:** Univ Med Ctr Princeton at Plainsboro; **Address:** 800 Bunn Drive, Ste 302, Princeton, NJ 08540; **Phone:** 609-921-1680; **Board Cert:** Internal Medicine 1989; **Med School:** NY Med Coll 1984; **Resid:** Internal Medicine, RW Johnson Univ Hosp 1989

Warren, Ronald MD (IM) - **Spec Exp:** Pulmonary Disease; **Hospital:** Capital Health Regl Med Ctr; **Address:** Pulmonary & Internal Med, 40 Fuld St, Ste 201, Trenton, NJ 08638-5247; **Phone:** 609-695-4422; **Board Cert:** Internal Medicine 1972; **Med School:** Univ Pennsylvania 1968; **Resid:** Internal Medicine, Presby Hosp 1970; Internal Medicine, Grady Meml Hosp 1971; **Fellow:** Pulmonary Disease, Emory Hosps 1972

Yamane, Michael H MD (IM) *PCP* - **Hospital:** Capital Health Med Ctr - Hopewell; **Address:** 2480 Pennington Rd, Ste 104, Pennington, NJ 08534-5227; **Phone:** 609-818-1000; **Board Cert:** Internal Medicine 1984; **Med School:** UCSF 1981; **Resid:** Internal Medicine, Univ Hawaii Med Ctr 1984

Interventional Cardiology

Shanahan, Andrew J MD (IC) - **Spec Exp:** Angioplasty; **Hospital:** Univ Med Ctr Princeton at Plainsboro, Robert Wood Johnson Univ Hosp - New Brunswick; **Address:** Cardiology Assocs of Princeton, 281 Witherspoon St, Ste 210, Princeton, NJ 08542; **Phone:** 609-921-7456; **Board Cert:** Internal Medicine 2005; Cardiovascular Disease 2005; Interventional Cardiology 2011; **Med School:** Med Coll Wisc 1989; **Resid:** Internal Medicine, St Lukes-Roosevelt Hosp 1992; **Fellow:** Cardiovascular Disease, St Lukes-Roosevelt Hosp 1995

Medical Oncology

Grossman, Bernard MD (Onc) - **Hospital:** Capital Health Med Ctr - Hopewell, Robert Wood Johnson Univ Hosp Hamilton; **Address:** Two Capital Way, Ste 220, Pennington, NJ 08534; **Phone:** 609-303-0747; **Board Cert:** Internal Medicine 1977; Medical Oncology 1979; Hematology 1980; Hospice & Palliative Medicine 2010; **Med School:** Temple Univ 1974; **Resid:** Internal Medicine, Albany Meml Hosp 1977; **Fellow:** Hematology & Oncology, George Wash Univ Hosp 1979; Oncology, Fox Chase Cancer Ctr 1980

Lerma, Pauline M MD (Onc) - **Spec Exp:** Breast Cancer; Hematologic Malignancies; **Hospital:** Robert Wood Johnson Univ Hosp Hamilton; **Address:** Cancer Inst NJ-Hamilton, 2575 Klockner Rd, Hamilton, NJ 08690; **Phone:** 609-631-6960; **Board Cert:** Internal Medicine 2006; Medical Oncology 2009; Hematology 2010; **Med School:** Philippines 1992; **Resid:** Internal Medicine, Abington Meml Hosp 1996; **Fellow:** Hematology & Oncology, Hahnemann Univ Hosp 1999; Bone Marrow Transplant, Hahnemann Univ Hosp 2000; **Fac Appt:** Asst Prof Med, UMDNJ-RW Johnson Med Sch

Schaebler, David MD (Onc) - **Hospital:** Capital Health Med Ctr - Hopewell, Robert Wood Johnson Univ Hosp Hamilton; **Address:** Mercer Bucks Hem/Onc, Two Capital Way, Ste 220, Pennington, NJ 08534; **Phone:** 609-303-0747; **Board Cert:** Hospice & Palliative Medicine 2008; Medical Oncology 2003; **Med School:** Jefferson Med Coll 1988; **Resid:** Internal Medicine, Cooper Univ Med Ctr 1991; **Fellow:** Medical Oncology, Fox Chase 1994

Sierocki, John Stanley MD (Onc) - **Spec Exp:** Breast Cancer; Lung Cancer; Lymphoma; Brain Tumors; **Hospital:** Univ Med Ctr Princeton at Plainsboro; **Address:** Princeton Med Grp, 419 N Harrison St, Ste 101, Princeton, NJ 08540-3521; **Phone:** 609-924-9300; **Board Cert:** Internal Medicine 1976; Medical Oncology 1979; **Med School:** Hahnemann Univ 1973; **Resid:** Internal Medicine, Hahnemann Univ Hosp 1976; **Fellow:** Medical Oncology, Meml Sloan-Kettering Cancer Ctr 1978

Yi, Peter I MD (Onc) - **Spec Exp:** Breast Cancer; Lymphoma; Prostate Cancer; Colon Cancer; **Hospital:** Univ Med Ctr Princeton at Plainsboro; **Address:** Princeton HealhCare Center, 419 N Harrison St, Ste 101, Princeton, NJ 08540; **Phone:** 609-924-9300; **Board Cert:** Internal Medicine 1987; Medical Oncology 1989; Hematology 2010; **Med School:** Cornell Univ-Weill Med Coll 1984; **Resid:** Internal Medicine, Brigham & Women's Hosp 1987; **Fellow:** Hematology & Oncology, NY Hosp-Cornell Med Ctr 1990; **Fac Appt:** Asst Clin Prof Med, UMDNJ-RW Johnson Med Sch

Nephrology

Cohen, Barry H MD (Nep) - **Hospital:** Capital Health Med Ctr - Hopewell; **Address:** 40 Fuld St, Ste 401, Trenton, NJ 08638-5247; **Phone:** 609-599-1004; **Board Cert:** Internal Medicine 1971; Nephrology 1974; **Med School:** Hahnemann Univ 1965; **Resid:** Internal Medicine, Hahnemann Univ Hosp 1968; **Fellow:** Nephrology, Hahnemann Univ 1969

Ruddy, Michael MD (Nep) - **Spec Exp:** Hypertension; Renovascular Disease; Diabetic Kidney Disease; Pheochromocytoma; **Hospital:** Univ Med Ctr Princeton at Plainsboro, Robert Wood Johnson Univ Hosp - New Brunswick; **Address:** Princeton Hypertension-Nephrology Assocs, 88 Princeton Hightstown Rd, Ste 203, Princeton Junction, NJ 08550; **Phone:** 609-750-7330; **Board Cert:** Internal Medicine 1977; Nephrology 1980; **Med School:** UMDNJ-NJ Med Sch, Newark 1974; **Resid:** Internal Medicine, UMDNJ-RW Johnson Med Affil Hosp 1977; **Fellow:** Nephrology, NY-Presby/Weill Cornell Med Ctr 1980; **Fac Appt:** Assoc Clin Prof Med, UMDNJ-RW Johnson Med Sch

Sudhakar, Telechery A MD (Nep) - **Spec Exp:** Kidney Disease; **Hospital:** Capital Health Med Ctr - Hopewell, Capital Health Regl Med Ctr; **Address:** 40 Fuld St, Ste 401, Trenton, NJ 08638; **Phone:** 609-599-1004; **Board Cert:** Internal Medicine 1977; Nephrology 1978; **Med School:** India 1971; **Resid:** Internal Medicine, Helene Fuld Med Ctr 1976; **Fellow:** Nephrology, Washington VA Hosp 1978

Wei, Fong MD (Nep) - **Spec Exp:** Hypertension; Kidney Stones; **Hospital:** Univ Med Ctr Princeton at Plainsboro; **Address:** 419 N Harrison St, Princeton, NJ 08540; **Phone:** 609-924-9300; **Board Cert:** Internal Medicine 1976; Nephrology 1976; **Med School:** Tufts Univ 1967; **Resid:** Internal Medicine, Boston City Hosp 1969; Internal Medicine, Bronx Municipal Hosp 1970; **Fellow:** Nephrology, Univ NC Hosp 1972; **Fac Appt:** Assoc Clin Prof Med

Neurological Surgery

Chiurco, Anthony A MD (NS) - **Spec Exp:** Aneurysm-Cerebral; Brain Tumors; Spinal Disc Replacement; **Hospital:** Univ Med Ctr Princeton at Plainsboro, Capital Health Med Ctr - Hopewell; **Address:** 3131 Princeton Pike Bldg 4 - Ste 201, Lawrenceville, NJ 08648; **Phone:** 609-895-8898; **Board Cert:** Neurological Surgery 1977; **Med School:** Jefferson Med Coll 1967; **Resid:** Surgery, Univ Iowa Coll Med 1971; Neurological Surgery, Univ Iowa Coll Med 1975; **Fellow:** Neurological Surgery, Penn Hosp 1976; **Fac Appt:** Asst Clin Prof NS

McLaughlin, Mark R MD (NS) - **Spec Exp:** Spinal Surgery-Complex; Spinal Surgery-Minimally Invasive; Trigeminal Neuralgia; **Hospital:** Univ Med Ctr Princeton at Plainsboro, St. Mary Med Ctr - Langhorne, PA; **Address:** Princeton Brain & Spine Care, 731 Alexander Rd, Ste 200, Princeton, NJ 08540; **Phone:** 609-921-9001; **Board Cert:** Neurological Surgery 2004; **Med School:** Med Coll VA 1992; **Resid:** Neurological Surgery, Univ Pittsburgh Med Ctr 1999; **Fellow:** Spine Surgery, Emory Univ Affil Hosp 2000

Neurology

Kaiser, Paul K MD (N) - **Hospital:** Univ Med Ctr Princeton at Plainsboro, Capital Health Med Ctr - Hopewell; **Address:** 3131 Princeton Pike, Building 3, Ste 202, Lawrenceville, NJ 08648-2526; **Phone:** 609-896-1701; **Board Cert:** Neurology 1993; Vascular Neurology 2009; **Med School:** Jefferson Med Coll 1988; **Resid:** Neurology, Temple Univ Hosp 1992; **Fellow:** Clinical Neurophysiology, Temple Univ Hosp 1993

Kososky, Charles S MD (N) - **Hospital:** St. Francis Med Ctr - Trenton; **Address:** St Francis Med Ctr, Neurosci Inst, 601 Hamilton Ave, Trenton, NJ 08629; **Phone:** 609-599-5792; **Board Cert:** Neurology 1981; **Med School:** UMDNJ-NJ Med Sch, Newark 1975; **Resid:** Internal Medicine, Kings Co Hosp 1975; Neurology, UMDNJ-Univ Hosp 1978

Patchell, Roy A MD (N) - **Spec Exp:** Neuro-Oncology; Brain Tumors; Spinal Tumors; **Hospital:** Capital Health Med Ctr - Hopewell; **Address:** Capital Inst Neurosciences, 2 Capital Way, Ste 456, Pennington, NJ 08534; **Phone:** 609-537-7300; **Board Cert:** Neurology 1984; **Med School:** Univ KY Coll Med 1979; **Resid:** Neurology, Johns Hopkins Hosp 1983; **Fellow:** Neuro-Oncology, Meml Sloan-Kettering Cancer Ctr 1985

Vester, John W MD (N) - **Spec Exp:** Parkinson's Disease; Stroke; Peripheral Neuropathy; Epilepsy/Seizure Disorders; **Hospital:** Univ Med Ctr Princeton at Plainsboro; **Address:** 1000 Herrontown Rd, Princeton, NJ 08540; **Phone:** 609-497-0100; **Board Cert:** Neurology 1979; **Med School:** Georgetown Univ 1973; **Resid:** Internal Medicine, Hartford Hosp 1975; Neurology, Georgetown Univ Hosp 1978

Witte, Arnold S MD (N) - **Spec Exp:** Neuromuscular Disorders; Parkinson's Disease; Electromyography; **Hospital:** Capital Health Med Ctr - Hopewell, Capital Health Regl Med Ctr; **Address:** 2 Princess Rd, Ste 2F, Lawrenceville, NJ 08648; **Phone:** 609-895-9000; **Board Cert:** Internal Medicine 1981; Neurology 1983; **Med School:** Tufts Univ 1977; **Resid:** Internal Medicine, Hosp Univ Penn 1979; Neurology, Hosp Univ Penn 1983

Obstetrics & Gynecology

Brickner, Gary R MD (ObG) *PCP* - **Spec Exp:** Gynecology Only; Menopause Problems; Minimally Invasive Surgery; Weight Management; **Hospital:** Capital Health Med Ctr - Hopewell; **Address:** Brickner-Martell Ctr Women's Hlth, Quakerbridge Plaza Building 1A, Hamilton, NJ 08619-1241; **Phone:** 609-689-9991; **Board Cert:** Obstetrics & Gynecology 1981; **Med School:** Univ Pittsburgh 1975; **Resid:** Obstetrics & Gynecology, Pennsylvania Hosp-UPHS 1980

Ophthalmology

Matossian, Cynthia MD (Oph) - **Spec Exp:** Cataract Surgery; **Hospital:** Capital Health Regl Med Ctr, Doylestown Hosp; **Address:** Two Capital Way, Ste 326, Pennington, NJ 08534; **Phone:** 609-882-8833; **Board Cert:** Ophthalmology 1987; **Med School:** Penn State Coll Med 1981; **Resid:** Ophthalmology, G Washington Univ Hosp 1986

Mulvey, Lauri MD (Oph) - **Spec Exp:** Pediatric Ophthalmology; **Hospital:** Chldns Hosp of Philadelphia; **Address:** CHOP Princeton Specialty Care Ctr, 707 Alexander Rd, Ste 205, Princeton, NJ 08540; **Phone:** 609-520-1717; **Board Cert:** Ophthalmology 1983; **Med School:** Harvard Med Sch 1977; **Resid:** Ophthalmology, Barnes-Jewish Hosp 1981; **Fellow:** Pediatric Ophthalmology, Wills Eye Hosp 1983

Safran, Steven G MD (Oph) - **Spec Exp:** Cataract Surgery; Laser Vision Surgery; Glaucoma; **Hospital:** Capital Health Med Ctr - Hopewell, Robert Wood Johnson Univ Hosp Hamilton; **Address:** 132 Franklin Corner Rd, Ste A-1, Lawrenceville, NJ 08648-2523; **Phone:** 609-896-3931; **Board Cert:** Ophthalmology 2013; **Med School:** SUNY Downstate 1987; **Resid:** Ophthalmology, NYU Langone Med Ctr 1991; **Fellow:** Cornea & Ext Eye Disease, Duke Univ Hosp 1992

Wasserman, Barry N MD (Oph) - **Spec Exp:** Pediatric Ophthalmology; LASIK-Refractive Surgery; Eyelid Surgery; Botox Therapy; **Hospital:** St. Peter's Univ Hosp, Univ Med Ctr Princeton at Plainsboro; **Address:** 100 Canal Pointe Blvd, Ste 112, Princeton, NJ 08540; **Phone:** 609-243-8711; **Board Cert:** Ophthalmology 2009; **Med School:** UMDNJ-NJ Med Sch, Newark 1992; **Resid:** Ophthalmology, UMDNJ-NJ Med Sch Affil Hosps 1996; **Fellow:** Pediatric Ophthalmology, IU Hlth Univ Hosp 1997; **Fac Appt:** Asst Clin Prof Oph, UMDNJ-RW Johnson Med Sch

Wong, Richard H MD (Oph) - **Spec Exp:** Cataract Surgery-Lens Implant; LASIK-Refractive Surgery; **Hospital:** Univ Med Ctr Princeton at Plainsboro; **Address:** Princeton Eye Grp, 419 N Harrison St, Ste 104, Princeton, NJ 08540-3521; **Phone:** 609-921-9437; **Board Cert:** Internal Medicine 1982; Ophthalmology 1987; **Med School:** UMDNJ-NJ Med Sch, Newark 1979; **Resid:** Internal Medicine, Thomas Jefferson Univ Hosp 1982; Ophthalmology, Wills Eye Hosp 1986

Orthopaedic Surgery

Abrams, Jeffrey S MD (OrS) - **Spec Exp:** Shoulder Surgery; Sports Medicine; Arthroscopic Surgery; Rotator Cuff Surgery; **Hospital:** Univ Med Ctr Princeton at Plainsboro; **Address:** Princeton Orthopaedic Assocs, 325 Princeton Ave, Princeton, NJ 08540-1617; **Phone:** 609-924-8131; **Board Cert:** Orthopaedic Surgery 2009; **Med School:** SUNY Upstate Med Univ 1980; **Resid:** Orthopaedic Surgery, Thomas Jefferson Univ Hosp 1985; **Fellow:** Shoulder Surgery, Univ Western Ontario 1986; Sports Medicine, Hughston Sports Med Hosp 1986; **Fac Appt:** Assoc Clin Prof OrS, Seton Hall Univ Sch Hlth & Med Scis

Costa, Leon N MD (OrS) - **Spec Exp:** Arthroscopic Surgery; Joint Replacement; Sports Medicine; **Hospital:** Univ Med Ctr Princeton at Plainsboro, Capital Health Med Ctr - Hopewell; **Address:** 256 Bunn Dr, Ste 2, Princeton, NJ 08540-2859; **Phone:** 609-924-9229; **Board Cert:** Orthopaedic Surgery 2009; **Med School:** Geo Wash Univ 1980; **Resid:** Surgery, Hosp Univ Penn 1982; Orthopaedic Surgery, NY Ortho Hosp/Colum-Presby 1984; **Fellow:** Sports Medicine, NY Ortho Hosp/Colum-Presby 1985

Gomez, William MD (OrS) - **Spec Exp:** Sports Medicine; Arthroscopic Surgery; Arthritis; **Hospital:** Robert Wood Johnson Univ Hosp Hamilton, St. Francis Med Ctr - Trenton; **Address:** Trenton Orthopaedic Grp, 1225 Whitehorse Mercerville Rd, D Bldg - Ste 220, Mercerville, NJ 08619-3876; **Phone:** 609-581-2200; **Board Cert:** Orthopaedic Surgery 2011; **Med School:** Columbia P&S 1982; **Resid:** Surgery, St Vincent's Hosp 1984; Orthopaedic Surgery, NY-Presby/Columbia Univ Med Ctr 1987; **Fellow:** Sports Medicine, UPMC 1988

Grenis, Michael S MD (OrS) - **Spec Exp:** Carpal Tunnel Syndrome; Hand & Wrist Injuries; **Hospital:** Univ Med Ctr Princeton at Plainsboro, Capital Health Med Ctr - Hopewell; **Address:** 256 Bunn Drive, Ste 2, Princeton, NJ 08540; **Phone:** 609-924-9229; **Board Cert:** Orthopaedic Surgery 2013; **Med School:** NY Med Coll 1984; **Resid:** Surgery, Bellevue Hosp Ctr 1985; Orthopaedic Surgery, Bellevue Hosp Ctr 1989; **Fellow:** Hand Surgery, Bellevue Hosp Ctr 1990

Gutowski III, W. Thomas MD (OrS) - **Spec Exp:** Hip Replacement; Knee Replacement; Arthroscopic Surgery; Joint Replacement; **Hospital:** Univ Med Ctr Princeton at Plainsboro; **Address:** Princeton Orthopaedic Assocs, 325 Princeton Ave, Princeton, NJ 08540; **Phone:** 609-924-8131; **Board Cert:** Orthopaedic Surgery 2008; **Med School:** Cornell Univ-Weill Med Coll 1980; **Resid:** Orthopaedic Surgery, Yale-New Haven Hosp 1986

Taitsman, James P MD (OrS) - **Spec Exp:** Sports Medicine; **Hospital:** Capital Health Med Ctr - Hopewell, Robert Wood Johnson Univ Hosp Hamilton; **Address:** 123 Franklin Corner Rd, Ste 114, Lawrenceville, NJ 08648-2526; **Phone:** 609-896-0707; **Board Cert:** Orthopaedic Surgery 1977; **Med School:** Univ Rochester 1971; **Resid:** Surgery, Yale-New Haven Hosp 1973; Orthopaedic Surgery, Yale-New Haven Hosp 1976

Otolaryngology

Brunner, Eugenie MD (Oto) - **Spec Exp:** Cosmetic Surgery-Face; Rhinoplasty; Skin Laser Surgery; Blepharoplasty; **Hospital:** Univ Med Ctr Princeton at Plainsboro; **Address:** 256 Bunn Drive, Ste 4, Princeton, NJ 08540-2859; **Phone:** 609-921-9497; **Board Cert:** Otolaryngology 1997; Facial Plastic & Reconstr Surgery 2002; **Med School:** UMDNJ-RW Johnson Med Sch 1990; **Resid:** Surgery, NYU Langone Med Ctr 1992; Otolaryngology, NYU Langone Med Ctr 1996; **Fellow:** Facial Plastic & Reconstr Surgery, Univ Toronto Affil Hosps 1997

Li, Ronald W MD (Oto) - **Hospital:** Univ Med Ctr Princeton at Plainsboro; **Address:** 800 Bunn Drive, Ste 305, Princeton, NJ 08540; **Phone:** 609-921-1000; **Board Cert:** Otolaryngology 1990; **Med School:** Mount Sinai Sch Med 1984; **Resid:** Otolaryngology, Montefiore Med Ctr 1989

Pain Medicine

Loren, Gary M MD (PM) - **Spec Exp:** Pain-Back; Reflex Sympathetic Dystrophy (RSD); **Hospital:** St. Francis Med Ctr - Trenton; **Address:** 1666 Hamilton Ave, Ste 2, Hamilton Township, NJ 08629; **Phone:** 609-584-9080; **Board Cert:** Anesthesiology 1988; Pain Medicine 2013; **Med School:** Univ Pittsburgh 1984; **Resid:** Anesthesiology, Long Is Jewish Med Ctr 1987; **Fellow:** Pediatrics, Long Is Jewish Med Ctr 1988

Pediatric Gastroenterology

Farhath, Sabeena MD (PGe) - **Spec Exp:** Crohn's Disease; Diarrheal Diseases; Irritable Bowel Syndrome; **Hospital:** Capital Health Med Ctr - Hopewell; **Address:** PedsGastro Ctr, 2123 Klockner Rd, Hamilton, NJ 08690; **Phone:** 609-586-7337; **Board Cert:** Pediatrics 2007; **Med School:** India 1991; **Resid:** Pediatrics, Cooper Univ Hosp 1994; **Fellow:** Pediatric Gastroenterology, Alfred I duPont Hosp Chldn 1997

Pediatrics

Baiser, Dennis MD (Ped) *PCP* - **Spec Exp:** Developmental Disorders; Asthma; **Hospital:** Capital Health Med Ctr - Hopewell, Robert Wood Johnson Univ Hosp Hamilton; **Address:** Hamilton Pediatrics, 3 Hamilton Health Pl, Ste A, Hamilton, NJ 08690; **Phone:** 609-581-4480; **Board Cert:** Pediatrics 1983; **Med School:** NY Med Coll 1978; **Resid:** Pediatrics, Chldns Hosp 1981

Boim, Marilynn MD (Ped) *PCP* - **Hospital:** Capital Health Med Ctr - Hopewell, Robert Wood Johnson Univ Hosp Hamilton; **Address:** Hamilton Pediatrics, 3 Hamilton Health Pl, Ste A, Hamilton, NJ 08690; **Phone:** 609-581-4480; **Board Cert:** Pediatrics 2009; Pediatric Endocrinology 2011; **Med School:** Emory Univ 1982; **Resid:** Pediatrics, Mt Sinai Hosp 1985; **Fellow:** Pediatric Endocrinology, Mt Sinai Hosp 1987

Palsky, Glenn S MD (Ped) *PCP* - **Hospital:** Capital Health Med Ctr - Hopewell, Univ Med Ctr Princeton at Plainsboro; **Address:** Delaware Valley Pediatric Associates, 132 Franklin Corner Rd, Lawrenceville, NJ 08648-2526; **Phone:** 609-896-4141; **Board Cert:** Pediatrics 1978; **Med School:** Penn State Coll Med 1973; **Resid:** Pediatrics, Albany Med Ctr 1977

Raymond, Gerald M MD (Ped) *PCP* - **Hospital:** Univ Med Ctr Princeton at Plainsboro; **Address:** 196 Princeton Heights Town Rd, West Windsor, NJ 08550; **Phone:** 609-799-5335; **Board Cert:** Pediatrics 1987; **Med School:** Penn State Coll Med 1983; **Resid:** Pediatrics, Columbus Chldns Hosp 1986

Physical Medicine & Rehabilitation

Agri, Robyn F MD (PMR) - **Spec Exp:** Acupuncture; Pain Management; **Hospital:** St. Lawrence Rehab Ctr, Capital Health Med Ctr - Hopewell; **Address:** St Lawrence Rehabilitation Ctr, 2381 Lawrenceville Rd, Lawrenceville, NJ 08648-2024; **Phone:** 609-896-9500; **Board Cert:** Physical Medicine & Rehabilitation 1990; **Med School:** SUNY Hlth Sci Ctr 1985; **Resid:** Physical Medicine & Rehabilitation, Hosp Univ Penn 1989

Gribbin, Dorota M MD (PMR) - **Spec Exp:** Industrial Injuries; Sports Injuries; Pain Management; **Hospital:** Robert Wood Johnson Univ Hosp Hamilton, Univ Med Ctr Princeton at Plainsboro; **Address:** 2333 Whitehorse-Mercerville Rd, Ste 8, Mercerville, NJ 08619; **Phone:** 609-588-0540; **Board Cert:** Physical Medicine & Rehabilitation 2013; **Med School:** Poland 1984; **Resid:** Internal Medicine, Beth Israel Med Ctr 1989; Physical Medicine & Rehabilitation, New York Hosp 1992; **Fac Appt:** Asst Clin Prof PMR, Columbia P&S

Plastic Surgery

Drimmer, Marc A MD (PlS) - **Spec Exp:** Cosmetic Surgery; **Hospital:** Univ Med Ctr Princeton at Plainsboro; **Address:** 842 State Rd, Princeton, NJ 08540; **Phone:** 609-924-1026; **Board Cert:** Plastic Surgery 1981; **Med School:** Belgium 1974; **Resid:** Surgery, Beth Israel Med Ctr 1977; Plastic Surgery, Univ Hosp 1979; **Fac Appt:** Asst Clin Prof S, UMDNJ-Rutgers Med Sch

Leach, Thomas A MD (PlS) - **Spec Exp:** Cosmetic Surgery-Face; Cosmetic Surgery-Breast; Liposuction; **Hospital:** Univ Med Ctr Princeton at Plainsboro, Robert Wood Johnson Univ Hosp - New Brunswick; **Address:** 932 State Rd, Princeton, NJ 08540; **Phone:** 609-921-7161; **Board Cert:** Plastic Surgery 1994; **Med School:** UMDNJ-NJ Med Sch, Newark 1985; **Resid:** Surgery, UMDNJ Med Ctr 1990; **Fellow:** Plastic Surgery, UMDNJ Med Ctr 1992

Smotrich, Gary MD (PlS) - **Hospital:** Capital Health Med Ctr - Hopewell, Robert Wood Johnson Univ Hosp Hamilton; **Address:** Lawrenceville Plastic Surgery, 3131 Princeton Pike, Bldg 5 - Ste 205, Lawrenceville, NJ 08648-2300; **Phone:** 609-896-2525; **Board Cert:** Plastic Surgery 1991; **Med School:** Univ Conn 1982; **Resid:** Surgery, Boston Univ Med Ctr 1987; Plastic Surgery, Univ Louisville Hosp 1989

Psychiatry

Leifer, Marvin W MD (Psyc) - **Spec Exp:** Psychopharmacology; Anxiety & Mood Disorders; Depression; Bipolar/Mood Disorders; **Hospital:** Univ Med Ctr Princeton at Plainsboro; **Address:** 42 N Tulane St, Princeton, NJ 08542; **Phone:** 609-683-7929; **Board Cert:** Psychiatry 1977; **Med School:** SUNY Downstate 1970; **Resid:** Psychiatry, Albert Einstein Coll Med Affil Hosp 1974; **Fellow:** Psychopharmacology, Albert Einstein Coll Med Affil Hosp 1976

Schneider, Samuel MD (Psyc) - **Spec Exp:** Mood Disorders; Personality Disorders; Addiction/Substance Abuse; **Hospital:** Univ Med Ctr Princeton at Plainsboro; **Address:** 33 State Rd, Ste J, Princeton, NJ 08540-1304; **Phone:** 609-924-3980; **Board Cert:** Psychiatry 1984; Internal Medicine 1978; **Med School:** Penn State Coll Med 1975; **Resid:** Internal Medicine, MS Hershey Med Ctr 1977; Psychiatry, UMDNJ-RW Johnson Univ Hosp 1982

Pulmonary Disease

Seelagy, Marc M MD (Pul) - **Spec Exp:** Sleep Disorders; Lung Disease; Critical Care Medicine; **Hospital:** St. Francis Med Ctr - Trenton, Robert Wood Johnson Univ Hosp Hamilton; **Address:** Allergy & Pulmonary Associates, 1542 Kuser Rd, Ste B7, Trenton, NJ 08619-3829; **Phone:** 609-581-1400; **Board Cert:** Internal Medicine 1989; Pulmonary Disease 2012; Critical Care Medicine 2003; Sleep Medicine 1995; **Med School:** Univ Chicago-Pritzker Sch Med 1986; **Resid:** Internal Medicine, Univ Colorado Hosp 1989; **Fellow:** Pulmonary Critical Care Medicine, Johns Hopkins Hosp 1993

Radiation Oncology

McKenna, Michael G MD (RadRO) - **Spec Exp:** Prostate Cancer; Breast Cancer; Head & Neck Cancer; **Hospital:** Robert Wood Johnson Univ Hosp Hamilton; **Address:** Cancer Inst NJ-Radiation Oncology, 2575 Klockner Rd, Hamilton, NJ 08690; **Phone:** 609-584-2800; **Board Cert:** Radiation Oncology 1993; **Med School:** Univ Mass Sch Med 1988; **Resid:** Radiation Oncology, Hosp Univ Penn 1992

Reproductive Endocrinology

O'Shaughnessy, Althea MD (RE) - **Spec Exp:** Infertility; **Hospital:** Univ Med Ctr Princeton at Plainsboro, Capital Health Med Ctr - Hopewell; **Address:** Princeton Center for Reproductive Med, 65 S Main St C Bldg - Ste 100, Pennington, NJ 08534; **Phone:** 609-818-1114; **Board Cert:** Obstetrics & Gynecology 2012; Reproductive Endocrinology/Infertility 2012; **Med School:** Univ Rochester 1982; **Resid:** Obstetrics & Gynecology, Univ Conn Hlth Ctr 1986; **Fellow:** Reproductive Endocrinology, Downstate Med Ctr 1988

Rheumatology

Carney, Alexander MD (Rhu) - **Hospital:** Univ Med Ctr Princeton at Plainsboro; **Address:** 8 Quakerbridge Plaza, Ste H, Mercerville, NJ 08619; **Phone:** 609-588-9044; **Board Cert:** Internal Medicine 1972; Rheumatology 1978; **Med School:** Cornell Univ-Weill Med Coll 1966; **Resid:** Internal Medicine, Univ Iowa Hosp 1972; **Fellow:** Rheumatology, Univ Iowa Hosp 1974

Gordon, Richard D MD (Rhu) - **Spec Exp:** Rheumatoid Arthritis; Osteoporosis; Osteoarthritis; **Hospital:** Robert Wood Johnson Univ Hosp Hamilton; **Address:** Professional Ctr at Hamilton, 2121 Klockner Rd, Hamilton, NJ 08690; **Phone:** 609-587-9898; **Board Cert:** Internal Medicine 1978; Rheumatology 1980; **Med School:** Jefferson Med Coll 1975; **Resid:** Internal Medicine, Geo Wash Hosp/VA Hosp 1978; **Fellow:** Rheumatology, St Vincents Hosp 1980

Surgery

Dultz, Rachel P MD (S) - **Spec Exp:** Breast Surgery; Breast Cancer; **Hospital:** Univ Med Ctr Princeton at Plainsboro; **Address:** Breast Surgical Specialist, 300B Princeton Hightstown Rd, Ste 102, East Windsor, NJ 08520; **Phone:** 609-688-2700; **Board Cert:** Surgery 2006; **Med School:** SUNY Downstate 1991; **Resid:** Surgery, RW Johnson Univ Hosp 1997; **Fellow:** Breast Surgery, Baylor Med Ctr 1998; **Fac Appt:** Asst Clin Prof S, UMDNJ-RW Johnson Med Sch

Gannon, Christopher J MD (S) - **Spec Exp:** Liver & Biliary Surgery; Liver Cancer; Pancreatic Cancer; Thyroid Cancer; **Hospital:** Capital Health Med Ctr - Hopewell, Capital Health Regl Med Ctr; **Address:** Two Capital Way, Ste 356, Pennington, NJ 08534; **Phone:** 609-537-6000; **Board Cert:** Surgery 2005; **Med School:** Columbia P&S 1998; **Resid:** Surgery, Univ Maryland Med Ctr 2004; **Fellow:** Surgical Oncology, MD Anderson Cancer Ctr 2007

Thoracic & Cardiac Surgery

Seinfeld, Fredric I MD (T&CS) - **Spec Exp:** Carotid Artery Surgery; Aneurysm; Esophageal Surgery; Cardiovascular Surgery; **Hospital:** St. Francis Med Ctr - Trenton, Univ Med Ctr Princeton at Plainsboro; **Address:** St Francis, Cardiothoracic Surgery, 601 Hamilton Ave, rm 109, Trenton, NJ 08629; **Phone:** 609-599-5308; **Board Cert:** Thoracic & Cardiac Surgery 2005; **Med School:** SUNY Buffalo 1976; **Resid:** Surgery, NYU Med Ctr 1981; Cardiothoracic Surgery, Yale-New Haven Hosp 1984

Urology

Rossman, Barry R MD (U) - **Spec Exp:** Kidney Stones; Incontinence-Female; Prostate Cancer; Erectile Dysfunction; **Hospital:** Univ Med Ctr Princeton at Plainsboro, Robert Wood Johnson Univ Hosp - New Brunswick; **Address:** Urology Grp, 134 Stanhope St, Princeton, NJ 08540; **Phone:** 609-924-6487; **Board Cert:** Urology 2010; **Med School:** Boston Univ 1983; **Resid:** Surgery, Montefiore Med Ctr 1985; Urology, Montefiore Med Ctr 1989; **Fac Appt:** Assoc Clin Prof U, UMDNJ-RW Johnson Med Sch

Vasselli, Anthony J MD (U) - **Hospital:** Univ Med Ctr Princeton at Plainsboro; **Address:** 299 Witherspoon St, Princeton, NJ 08540; **Phone:** 609-252-0575; **Board Cert:** Urology 2006; **Med School:** NY Med Coll 1979; **Resid:** Urology, Albany Meml Hosp 1984

Vukasin, Alexander P MD (U) - **Spec Exp:** Laparoscopic Surgery; Urologic Cancer; Urology-Female; **Hospital:** Univ Med Ctr Princeton at Plainsboro, Robert Wood Johnson Univ Hosp - New Brunswick; **Address:** Urology Grp, 134 Stanhope St, Princeton, NJ 08540; **Phone:** 609-924-6487; **Board Cert:** Urology 2006; **Med School:** Yale Univ 1989; **Resid:** Urology, NY-Presby/Weill Cornell Med Ctr 1995; **Fac Appt:** Asst Clin Prof U, UMDNJ-RW Johnson Med Sch

Middlesex

Middlesex

Addiction Psychiatry

Williams, Jill M MD (AdP) - **Spec Exp:** Addiction/Substance Abuse; Alcohol Abuse; Dual Diagnosis; Smoking Cessation; **Hospital:** Robert Wood Johnson Univ Hosp - New Brunswick; **Address:** 671 Hoes Ln, Piscataway, NJ 08855; **Phone:** 732-235-4402; **Board Cert:** Psychiatry 2008; Addiction Psychiatry 2012; **Med School:** UMDNJ-RW Johnson Med Sch 1993; **Resid:** Psychiatry, Duke Univ Hosp 1997; **Fellow:** Addiction Psychiatry, RW Johnson Univ Hosp 1999; **Fac Appt:** Assoc Prof Psyc, UMDNJ-RW Johnson Med Sch

Adolescent Medicine

Snyder, Barbara K MD (AM) - **Spec Exp:** Eating Disorders; Pediatric Gynecology; **Hospital:** Robert Wood Johnson Univ Hosp - New Brunswick; **Address:** Childrens Health Inst New Jersey, 89 French St, Ste 2230, New Brunswick, NJ 08901; **Phone:** 732-235-7896; **Board Cert:** Pediatrics 1985; Adolescent Medicine 2009; **Med School:** Geo Wash Univ 1979; **Resid:** Pediatrics, Chldns National Med Ctr 1981; Pediatrics, Upstate Med Ctr 1982; **Fellow:** Adolescent Medicine, Univ Rochester 1988; **Fac Appt:** Assoc Prof Ped

Allergy & Immunology

Blum, Jay R MD (A&I) - **Spec Exp:** Rhinitis; Asthma; Hives; Urticaria; **Hospital:** St. Peter's Univ Hosp, Robert Wood Johnson Univ Hosp - New Brunswick; **Address:** 85 Raritan Ave, Highland Park, NJ 08904; **Phone:** 732-846-7861; **Board Cert:** Internal Medicine 1978; Allergy & Immunology 1979; **Med School:** Univ Pennsylvania 1974; **Resid:** Internal Medicine, Beth Israel Med Ctr 1977; **Fellow:** Allergy & Immunology, NY-Presby/Weill Cornell Med Ctr 1979

Kesarwala, Hemant MD (A&I) - **Spec Exp:** Food Allergy; Asthma; Infectious Disease; **Hospital:** St. Peter's Univ Hosp, Robert Wood Johnson Univ Hosp - New Brunswick; **Address:** 3084 Rte 27, Unit 6, Kendall Park, NJ 08824; **Phone:** 732-821-0595; **Board Cert:** Pediatrics 1979; Allergy & Immunology 1979; **Med School:** India 1971; **Resid:** Pediatrics, Lincoln Hosp 1976; **Fellow:** Infectious Disease, RW Johnson Univ Hosp 1978; Allergy & Immunology, Chldns Hosp 1979; **Fac Appt:** Clin Prof Ped, Drexel Univ Coll Med

Leibner, Donald MD (A&I) - **Spec Exp:** Asthma & Allergy; Cough-Chronic; Insect Allergies; Nasal & Sinus Disorders; **Hospital:** Robert Wood Johnson Univ Hosp - New Brunswick, St. Peter's Univ Hosp; **Address:** 579-A Cranbury Rd, Ste 103, East Brunswick, NJ 08816; **Phone:** 732-390-4900; **Board Cert:** Allergy & Immunology 2005; **Med School:** SUNY Downstate 1981; **Resid:** Pediatrics, UMDNJ-Rutgers 1984; **Fellow:** Allergy & Immunology, Long Island Coll Hosp 1986; **Fac Appt:** Asst Clin Prof Ped, Drexel Univ Coll Med

Cardiovascular Disease

Kostis, John B MD (Cv) - **Spec Exp:** Coronary Artery Disease; Hypertension; Cholesterol/Lipid Disorders; **Hospital:** Robert Wood Johnson Univ Hosp - New Brunswick; **Address:** 125 Paterson St, CAB Bldg - Fl 5 - Ste 5200, New Brunswick, NJ 08901; **Phone:** 732-235-7685; **Board Cert:** Internal Medicine 1973; Cardiovascular Disease 1973; **Med School:** Greece 1960; **Resid:** Internal Medicine, Evanglismos Hosp 1964; Internal Medicine, Cumberland Med Ctr 1967; **Fellow:** Cardiovascular Disease, Philadelphia Genl Hosp 1969; **Fac Appt:** Prof Med, UMDNJ-RW Johnson Med Sch

Mermelstein, Erwin MD (Cv) - **Spec Exp:** Cholesterol/Lipid Disorders; Cardiac Catheterization; Congestive Heart Failure; Hypertension; **Hospital:** Robert Wood Johnson Univ Hosp - New Brunswick, St. Peter's Univ Hosp; **Address:** Cardiology Assocs New Brunswick, 593 Cranbury Rd, East Brunswick, NJ 08816; **Phone:** 732-390-3333; **Board Cert:** Internal Medicine 1981; Cardiovascular Disease 1983; **Med School:** Cornell Univ 1978; **Resid:** Internal Medicine, NY-Presby/Weill Cornell Med Ctr 1981; **Fellow:** Cardiovascular Disease, Hosp Univ Penn 1983

Mondrow, Daniel N MD (Cv) - **Spec Exp:** Cardiac Catheterization; Nuclear Stress Testing; Critical Care Medicine; Hypertension; **Hospital:** JFK Med Ctr - Edison, Robert Wood Johnson Univ Hosp - New Brunswick; **Address:** 280 Main St, Metuchen, NJ 08840; **Phone:** 732-494-3177; **Board Cert:** Internal Medicine 1979; Cardiovascular Disease 1985; **Med School:** SUNY Downstate 1976; **Resid:** Internal Medicine, Brookdale Univ Med Ctr 1979; **Fellow:** Cardiovascular Disease, St Vincent Med Ctr 1981

Schanzer, Robert J MD (Cv) - **Spec Exp:** Hypertension; **Hospital:** Robert Wood Johnson Univ Hosp at Rahway, JFK Med Ctr - Edison; **Address:** Advanced Cardiovascular Medicine, 4 Ethel Rd, Ste 405B, Edison, NJ 08820; **Phone:** 732-650-0040; **Board Cert:** Internal Medicine 2009; Cardiovascular Disease 2003; Interventional Cardiology 2004; **Med School:** Albert Einstein Coll Med 1995; **Resid:** Internal Medicine, Mount Sinai Med Ctr 1998; **Fellow:** Cardiovascular Disease, NYU Med Ctr 2001; Interventional Cardiology, NYU Med Ctr 2002

Shell, Roger A MD (Cv) - **Spec Exp:** Coronary Artery Disease; Heart Valve Disease; Cholesterol/Lipid Disorders; Non-Invasive Cardiology; **Hospital:** Robert Wood Johnson Univ Hosp - New Brunswick, St. Peter's Univ Hosp; **Address:** Cardiology Assocs New Brunswick, 593 Cranberry Rd, East Brunswick, NJ 08816; **Phone:** 732-390-3333; **Board Cert:** Internal Medicine 1980; Cardiovascular Disease 1983; **Med School:** UMDNJ-Rutgers Med Sch 1977; **Resid:** Internal Medicine, RW Johnson Univ Hosp 1980; **Fellow:** Cardiovascular Disease, Penn Presby Med Ctr 1982; **Fac Appt:** Asst Clin Prof Med, UMDNJ-RW Johnson Med Sch

Shindler, Daniel M MD (Cv) - **Spec Exp:** Echocardiography; Echocardiography-Transesophageal; Cardiac Tumors/Cancer; **Hospital:** Robert Wood Johnson Univ Hosp - New Brunswick; **Address:** Univ Med Group, 125 Paterson St, Fl 6th, Ste 6100, New Brunswick, NJ 08901; **Phone:** 732-235-7855; **Board Cert:** Internal Medicine 1987; **Med School:** Spain 1979; **Resid:** Internal Medicine, USPHS Hosp 1981; Internal Medicine, RW Johnson Hosp 1984; **Fellow:** Cardiovascular Disease, RW Johnson Hosp 1983; **Fac Appt:** Prof Med, UMDNJ-RW Johnson Med Sch

Child & Adolescent Psychiatry

Shampain, Lawrence R MD (ChAP) - **Spec Exp:** Trauma Psychiatry; Anxiety Disorders; **Hospital:** Somerset Med Ctr, Univ Beh HC-Univ of Med/Dent of NJ; **Address:** 32B Wernik Place, Metuchen, NJ 08840; **Phone:** 732-548-1600; **Board Cert:** Psychiatry 1988; Child & Adolescent Psychiatry 1990; **Med School:** Hahnemann Univ 1982; **Resid:** Psychiatry, Mt Sinai Med Ctr 1985; **Fellow:** Child Psychiatry, UCLA Neuropsych Inst 1987; **Fac Appt:** Assoc Clin Prof Psyc, UMDNJ-RW Johnson Med Sch

Child Neurology

Wollack, Jan B MD (ChiN) - **Spec Exp:** Epilepsy/Seizure Disorders; **Hospital:** Robert Wood Johnson Univ Hosp - New Brunswick; **Address:** 89 French St Fl 2, New Brunswick, NJ 08901; **Phone:** 732-235-7875; **Board Cert:** Pediatrics 1988; Child Neurology 1987; **Med School:** Columbia P&S 1981; **Resid:** Pediatrics, Columbia-Presby Med Ctr 1983; Neurology, Columbia-Presby Med Ctr 1986; **Fac Appt:** Assoc Prof Ped, UMDNJ-RW Johnson Med Sch

Clinical Genetics

Sklower Brooks, Susan MD (CG) - **Spec Exp:** Birth Defects; Inborn Errors of Metabolism; Developmental Disorders; Prenatal Diagnosis; **Hospital:** Robert Wood Johnson Univ Hosp - New Brunswick; **Address:** Child Hlth Inst of NJ, 89 French St, New Brunswick, NJ 08903-2160; **Phone:** 732-235-6230; **Board Cert:** Pediatrics 1979; Clinical Genetics 1982; Clinical Biochemical Genetics 1984; **Med School:** Mount Sinai Sch Med 1975; **Resid:** Pediatrics, Mount Sinai Hosp 1977; **Fellow:** Clinical Genetics, Mount Sinai Hosp 1979; **Fac Appt:** Prof Ped, UMDNJ-RW Johnson Med Sch

Colon & Rectal Surgery

Eisenstat, Theodore E MD (CRS) - **Spec Exp:** Colon Cancer; Inflammatory Bowel Disease; Anorectal Disorders; Hemorrhoids; **Hospital:** Robert Wood Johnson Univ Hosp - New Brunswick, JFK Med Ctr - Edison; **Address:** Robert Wood Johnson Med Group, Clinical Academic Bldg, 125 Paterson St, Ste 4100, New Brunswick, NJ 08901; **Phone:** 732-235-7920; **Board Cert:** Surgery 1974; Colon & Rectal Surgery 1994; **Med School:** NY Med Coll 1968; **Resid:** Surgery, Thomas Jefferson Univ Hosp 1971; Surgery, Pennsylvania Hosp 1973; **Fellow:** Colon & Rectal Surgery, Muhlenberg Med Ctr 1978; **Fac Appt:** Clin Prof S, UMDNJ-RW Johnson Med Sch

Oliver, Gregory C MD (CRS) - **Spec Exp:** Colon & Rectal Cancer; Incontinence-Fecal; Ulcerative Colitis; Crohn's Disease; **Hospital:** JFK Med Ctr - Edison, Overlook Med Ctr (page 92); **Address:** Assoc Colon & Rectal Surgeons, 3900 Park Ave, Ste 101, Edison, NJ 08820; **Phone:** 732-494-6640; **Board Cert:** Colon & Rectal Surgery 1986; **Med School:** Geo Wash Univ 1976; **Resid:** Surgery, Geo Wash Univ Med Ctr 1985; **Fellow:** Colon & Rectal Surgery, UMDNJ-Rutgers 1986; **Fac Appt:** Assoc Clin Prof S, UMDNJ-RW Johnson Med Sch

Rezac, Craig MD (CRS) - **Spec Exp:** Colon & Rectal Cancer; Inflammatory Bowel Disease; Diverticulitis; Pelvic & Perineal Surgery; **Hospital:** Robert Wood Johnson Univ Hosp - New Brunswick; **Address:** 125 Patterson St, Ste 4100, New Brunswick, NJ 08903; **Phone:** 732-235-7920; **Board Cert:** Surgery 2011; Colon & Rectal Surgery 2012; **Med School:** Italy 1995; **Resid:** Surgery, RW Johnson Medical Ctr 2001; **Fellow:** Colon & Rectal Surgery, RW Johnson Med Ctr 2002; Laparoscopic Surgery, Hackensack Med Ctr 2003; **Fac Appt:** Asst Prof S, UMDNJ-RW Johnson Med Sch

Zinkin, Lewis D MD (CRS) - **Spec Exp:** Colon Cancer; Inflammatory Bowel Disease; **Hospital:** Robert Wood Johnson Univ Hosp - New Brunswick, St. Peter's Univ Hosp; **Address:** 620 Cranbury Rd, Ste 111, East Brunswick, NJ 08816; **Phone:** 732-238-2662; **Board Cert:** Colon & Rectal Surgery 1978; **Med School:** UMDNJ-NJ Med Sch, Newark 1970; **Resid:** Surgery, St Vincents Hosp 1977; Colon & Rectal Surgery, Greater Baltimore Med Ctr 1978; **Fac Appt:** Assoc Clin Prof S

Dermatology

Milgraum, Sandy S MD (D) - **Spec Exp:** Skin Laser Surgery; Tattoo Removal; Cosmetic Dermatology; Pediatric Dermatology; **Hospital:** Robert Wood Johnson Univ Hosp - New Brunswick; **Address:** Academic Dermatology Ctr, 81 Brunswick Woods Drive, East Brunswick, NJ 08816-5601; **Phone:** 732-613-0300; **Board Cert:** Dermatology 1986; Pediatric Dermatology 2006; **Med School:** Australia 1983; **Resid:** Dermatology, Univ Mich Hosp 1986; **Fac Appt:** Assoc Prof D, UMDNJ-RW Johnson Med Sch

Vine, John E MD (D) - **Spec Exp:** Mohs' Surgery; Cosmetic Dermatology; Hyperhidrosis/Axillary Curettage; **Hospital:** Univ Med Ctr Princeton at Plainsboro, Robert Wood Johnson Univ Hosp - New Brunswick; **Address:** Medical Arts Pavilion, 4th floor, 5 Plainsboro Rd, Ste 460, Princeton, NJ 08536; **Phone:** 609-799-6222; **Board Cert:** Dermatology 2005; **Med School:** Brown Univ 1992; **Resid:** Dermatology, Meml Hermann Hosp 1996; **Fellow:** Mohs Surgery, Scripps Clinic 1997

Wrone, David A MD (D) - **Spec Exp:** Skin Laser Surgery; Cosmetic Surgery; Mohs' Surgery; Skin Cancer; **Hospital:** Univ Med Ctr Princeton at Plainsboro, Robert Wood Johnson Univ Hosp - New Brunswick; **Address:** 1950 Highway 27, Ste A, North Brunswick, NJ 08902; **Phone:** 609-683-4999; **Board Cert:** Dermatology 2009; **Med School:** Stanford Univ 1996; **Resid:** Dermatology, Univ Wisconsin Med Ctr 1998; Dermatology, Mass Genl Hosp 2001; **Fellow:** Mohs Surgery, UCLA Med Ctr 2002

Diagnostic Radiology

Compito, Gerard A MD (DR) - **Hospital:** Univ Med Ctr Princeton at Plainsboro; **Address:** 3674 Rt 27, Kendall Park, NJ 08824; **Phone:** 732-821-5563; **Board Cert:** Diagnostic Radiology 1990; Neuroradiology 2005; **Med School:** SUNY Upstate Med Univ 1985; **Resid:** Diagnostic Radiology, NY Hosp-Cornell 1990; **Fellow:** Neuroradiology, NY Hosp-Cornell 1992

Epstein, Robert E MD (DR) - **Spec Exp:** MRI; Musculoskeletal Imaging; **Hospital:** Robert Wood Johnson Univ Hosp - New Brunswick; **Address:** University Radiology Group, 579A Cranbury Rd Fl 3, East Brunswick, NJ 08816; **Phone:** 732-390-0040; **Board Cert:** Diagnostic Radiology 1995; **Med School:** Duke Univ 1990; **Resid:** Diagnostic Radiology, Thomas Jefferson Univ Hosp 1995; **Fellow:** Musculoskeletal Imaging, Hosp Univ Penn 1996; **Fac Appt:** Asst Clin Prof Rad, UMDNJ-RW Johnson Med Sch

Ford, Robert R MD (DR) - **Spec Exp:** CT Scan; MRI; Nuclear Medicine; Ultrasound; **Hospital:** Univ Med Ctr Princeton at Plainsboro; **Address:** Princeton Radiology, 3674 Route 27, Kendall Park, NJ 08824; **Phone:** 908-745-9944; **Board Cert:** Diagnostic Radiology 1988; Neuroradiology 2009; **Med School:** UMDNJ-Rutgers Med Sch 1983; **Resid:** Internal Medicine, R W Johnson Univ Hosp 1984; Diagnostic Radiology, NY Hosp-Cornell 1988

Rosenfeld, David L MD (DR) - **Spec Exp:** Pediatric Radiology; **Hospital:** Robert Wood Johnson Univ Hosp - New Brunswick; **Address:** University Radiology Group, 579A Cranbury Rd Fl 3, East Brunswick, NJ 08816; **Phone:** 732-390-0040; **Board Cert:** Diagnostic Radiology 1972; **Med School:** Univ Pittsburgh 1967; **Resid:** Diagnostic Radiology, Montefiore Med Ctr 1971; **Fac Appt:** Clin Prof Rad, UMDNJ-RW Johnson Med Sch

Underberg-Davis, Sharon J MD (DR) - **Spec Exp:** Pediatric Radiology; **Hospital:** Robert Wood Johnson Univ Hosp - New Brunswick; **Address:** Univ Radiology Grp, 579A Cranbury Rd Fl 3, East Brunswick, NJ 08816; **Phone:** 732-390-0040; **Board Cert:** Diagnostic Radiology 1993; Pediatric Radiology 2004; **Med School:** Harvard Med Sch 1988; **Resid:** Diagnostic Radiology, Hosp Univ Penn 1993; **Fellow:** Pediatric Radiology, Chldns Hosp 1995

Endocrinology, Diabetes & Metabolism

Agrin, Richard MD (EDM) - **Spec Exp:** Thyroid Disorders; Parathyroid Disorders; Diabetes; **Hospital:** Robert Wood Johnson Univ Hosp - New Brunswick, Somerset Med Ctr; **Address:** 78 Easton Ave, New Brunswick, NJ 08901; **Phone:** 732-545-1065; **Board Cert:** Internal Medicine 1974; Endocrinology 1977; **Med School:** Univ Pennsylvania 1971; **Resid:** Internal Medicine, USPHS Hosp 1975; **Fellow:** Endocrinology, Boston Univ Hosp 1977; **Fac Appt:** Assoc Clin Prof Med, UMDNJ-RW Johnson Med Sch

Bucholtz, Harvey K MD (EDM) - **Spec Exp:** Diabetes; Thyroid Disorders; Osteoporosis; **Hospital:** JFK Med Ctr - Edison, Newark Beth Israel Med Ctr; **Address:** 2 Lincoln Hwy, Ste 501, Edison, NJ 08820; **Phone:** 732-549-7470; **Board Cert:** Internal Medicine 1973; Endocrinology 1975; **Med School:** SUNY Hlth Sci Ctr 1968; **Resid:** Internal Medicine, Univ Michigan Med Ctr 1971; **Fellow:** Endocrinology, Duke Univ Med Ctr 1975; **Fac Appt:** Asst Clin Prof Med, UMDNJ-NJ Med Sch, Newark

Maman, Arie MD (EDM) - **Spec Exp:** Thyroid Disorders; Diabetes; Pituitary Disorders; **Hospital:** Robert Wood Johnson Univ Hosp - New Brunswick, St. Peter's Univ Hosp; **Address:** D3 Brier Hill Ct, East Brunswick, NJ 08816-3335; **Phone:** 732-613-0707; **Board Cert:** Internal Medicine 1977; Endocrinology, Diabetes & Metabolism 1979; **Med School:** France 1974; **Resid:** Internal Medicine, Jewish Hosp 1977; **Fellow:** Endocrinology, Univ Colorado 1979; **Fac Appt:** Assoc Clin Prof Med, UMDNJ-RW Johnson Med Sch

Schneider, Stephen H MD (EDM) - **Spec Exp:** Diabetes; Nutrition; Cholesterol/Lipid Disorders; **Hospital:** Robert Wood Johnson Univ Hosp - New Brunswick; **Address:** 125 Patterson St, Clinical Academic Bldg Fl 5 - Ste 5100B, New Brunswick, NJ 08901; **Phone:** 732-235-7219; **Board Cert:** Internal Medicine 1975; Endocrinology, Diabetes & Metabolism 1979; **Med School:** Boston Univ 1972; **Resid:** Internal Medicine, Boston Univ Hosp 1975; **Fellow:** Endocrinology, Diabetes & Metabolism, Boston City Hosp 1976; **Fac Appt:** Prof Med, UMDNJ-RW Johnson Med Sch

Spiler, Ira MD (EDM) - **Spec Exp:** Pituitary Disorders; Thyroid Disorders; Calcium Disorders; **Hospital:** Raritan Bay Med Ctr - Perth Amboy, Robert Wood Johnson Univ Hosp - New Brunswick; **Address:** 3 Hospital Plaza, Ste 307, Old Bridge, NJ 08857-3095; **Phone:** 732-360-1122; **Board Cert:** Internal Medicine 1976; Endocrinology, Diabetes & Metabolism 1979; **Med School:** Albert Einstein Coll Med 1971; **Resid:** Internal Medicine, Bronx Municipal Hosp 1973; Internal Medicine, Boston City Hosp 1976; **Fellow:** Endocrinology, Tufts-New England Med Ctr 1978; **Fac Appt:** Assoc Clin Prof Med, UMDNJ-RW Johnson Med Sch

Family Medicine

Metz, John P MD (FMed) *PCP* - **Spec Exp:** Primary Care Sports Medicine; **Hospital:** JFK Med Ctr - Edison; **Address:** 65 James St, Edison, NJ 08818; **Phone:** 732-321-7487; **Board Cert:** Family Medicine 2013; Sports Medicine 2011; **Med School:** Jefferson Med Coll 1994; **Resid:** Family Medicine, Malcolm Grow Med Ctr 1997; **Fellow:** Sports Medicine, Uniformed Srvs U Hlth Scis 2000

Picciano, Anne MD (FMed) *PCP* - **Spec Exp:** Adolescent Medicine; **Hospital:** JFK Med Ctr - Edison; **Address:** 65 James St, JFK Med Ctr Family Practice, Edison, NJ 08818; **Phone:** 732-321-7487; **Board Cert:** Family Medicine 2009; Adolescent Medicine 2003; **Med School:** Univ Pennsylvania 1987; **Resid:** Family Medicine, W Jersey Hlth 1990; **Fac Appt:** Asst Clin Prof FMed, UMDNJ-RW Johnson Med Sch

Swee, David E MD (FMed) *PCP* - **Hospital:** Robert Wood Johnson Univ Hosp - New Brunswick; **Address:** Family Medicine at Monument Square, 317 George St Fl 1 - Ste 100, New Brunswick, NJ 08901; **Phone:** 732-235-8993; **Board Cert:** Family Medicine 2007; **Med School:** Canada 1975; **Resid:** Family Medicine, Somerset Med Ctr 1977; **Fac Appt:** Prof FMed, UMDNJ-RW Johnson Med Sch

Tallia, Alfred F MD (FMed) *PCP* - **Hospital:** Robert Wood Johnson Univ Hosp - New Brunswick; **Address:** Family Med at Monument Square, 317 George St, Fl 1, Ste 100, Rutgers Robert Wood Johnson Medical Group, New Brunswick, NJ 08901-2162; **Phone:** 732-235-8993; **Board Cert:** Family Medicine 2007; **Med School:** UMDNJ-RW Johnson Med Sch 1978; **Resid:** Family Medicine, Thomas Jefferson Univ Hosp 1981; **Fac Appt:** Prof FMed, UMDNJ-RW Johnson Med Sch

Tierney, Peter C MD (FMed) *PCP* - **Hospital:** Univ Med Ctr Princeton at Plainsboro; **Address:** 666 Plainsboro Rd, Ste 1316, Plainsboro, NJ 08536; **Phone:** 609-275-8100; **Board Cert:** Family Medicine 2005; **Med School:** Univ VA Sch Med 1983; **Resid:** Family Medicine, Hunterdon Med Ctr 1986

Winter, Robin O MD (FMed) *PCP* - **Spec Exp:** Geriatric Medicine; **Hospital:** JFK Med Ctr - Edison; **Address:** 65 James St, Edison, NJ 08818; **Phone:** 732-321-7487; **Board Cert:** Family Medicine 2005; Geriatric Medicine 2006; **Med School:** Albert Einstein Coll Med 1978; **Resid:** Family Medicine, Hunterdon Med Ctr 1981; **Fac Appt:** Clin Prof FMed, UMDNJ-RW Johnson Med Sch

Gastroenterology

Hodes, Steven E MD (Ge) - **Hospital:** Raritan Bay Med Ctr - Perth Amboy, JFK Med Ctr - Edison; **Address:** 205 May St, Ste 201, Edison, NJ 08837; **Phone:** 732-661-9225; **Board Cert:** Internal Medicine 1977; Gastroenterology 1979; **Med School:** Albert Einstein Coll Med 1974; **Resid:** Internal Medicine, Montefiore Med Ctr 1977; **Fellow:** Gastroenterology, Mt Sinai-Bronx VA Hosps 1979

Pitchumoni, Capecomorin S MD (Ge) - **Spec Exp:** Pancreatic Disease; Gastroesophageal Reflux Disease (GERD); Pancreatic Cancer; Hepatitis C; **Hospital:** St. Peter's Univ Hosp; **Address:** St Peters Univ Hosp, 254 Easton Ave, CARES Bldg - Fl 4 - Ste 4013, New Brunswick, NJ 08901; **Phone:** 732-745-7939; **Board Cert:** Gastroenterology 1971; Internal Medicine 1977; **Med School:** India 1960; **Resid:** Internal Medicine, Norwalk Hosp 1968; **Fellow:** Gastroenterology, Yale New Haven Hosp 1969Metropolitan Hosp Ctr 1971; **Fac Appt:** Clin Prof Med, India

Plumser, Allan B MD (Ge) - **Spec Exp:** Endoscopy; Pancreatic/Biliary Endoscopy (ERCP); Liver Disease; **Hospital:** Robert Wood Johnson Univ Hosp - New Brunswick, St. Peter's Univ Hosp; **Address:** 465 Cranbury Rd, Ste 102, East Brunswick, NJ 08816; **Phone:** 732-390-1995; **Board Cert:** Internal Medicine 1981; Gastroenterology 1983; **Med School:** NY Med Coll 1978; **Resid:** Internal Medicine, SUNY Stonybrook Med Ctr 1981; **Fellow:** Gastroenterology, SUNY Stonybrook Med Ctr 1983

Geriatric Medicine

Bullock, Richard B MD (Ger) *PCP* - **Spec Exp:** Hypertension; Cholesterol/Lipid Disorders; Dementia; **Hospital:** JFK Med Ctr - Edison; **Address:** 225 May St, Ste E, Edison, NJ 08837-3266; **Phone:** 732-661-2020; **Board Cert:** Internal Medicine 1984; Geriatric Medicine 2010; **Med School:** Mount Sinai Sch Med 1981; **Resid:** Internal Medicine, Mt Sinai Hosp 1984; **Fac Appt:** Asst Clin Prof Med, UMDNJ-RW Johnson Med Sch

Gynecologic Oncology

Goldberg, Michael I MD (GO) - **Spec Exp:** Ovarian Cancer; Uterine Cancer; **Hospital:** St. Peter's Univ Hosp; **Address:** 78 Easton Ave, New Brunswick, NJ 08901-1865; **Phone:** 732-828-3300; **Board Cert:** Obstetrics & Gynecology 1977; Gynecologic Oncology 1980; **Med School:** Italy 1970; **Resid:** Obstetrics & Gynecology, Maimonides Med Ctr 1975; **Fellow:** Gynecologic Oncology, Jackson Meml Hosp 1977; **Fac Appt:** Clin Prof ObG, UMDNJ-RW Johnson Med Sch

Rodriguez, Lorna MD/PhD (GO) - **Spec Exp:** Robotic Surgery; Ovarian Cancer; Cervical Cancer; **Hospital:** Robert Wood Johnson Univ Hosp - New Brunswick; **Address:** Cancer Institute of New Jersey, 195 Little Albany St Fl 1 - rm 1100, New Brunswick, NJ 08903; **Phone:** 732-235-7615; **Board Cert:** Obstetrics & Gynecology 2012; Gynecologic Oncology 2012; **Med School:** Puerto Rico 1979; **Resid:** Obstetrics & Gynecology, Cooper Med Ctr 1983; **Fellow:** Gynecologic Oncology, Univ Michigan 1985; **Fac Appt:** Prof ObG, UMDNJ-RW Johnson Med Sch

Hematology

Karp, George I MD (Hem) - **Spec Exp:** Coagulation/Bleeding Disorders; Anemia; Breast Cancer; **Hospital:** Robert Wood Johnson Univ Hosp - New Brunswick, St. Peter's Univ Hosp; **Address:** Central Jersey Oncology Ctr, 1 Brier Hill Ct, East Brunswick, NJ 08816; **Phone:** 732-390-7750; **Board Cert:** Internal Medicine 1979; Medical Oncology 1981; Hematology 1982; **Med School:** Columbia P&S 1976; **Resid:** Internal Medicine, Univ Chicago Hosps 1978; **Fellow:** Hematology & Oncology, Natl Cancer Inst 1979; Hematology & Oncology, Dana Farber Cancer Inst 1982; **Fac Appt:** Clin Prof Hem & Onc, UMDNJ-RW Johnson Med Sch

Philipp, Claire S MD (Hem) - **Spec Exp:** Bleeding/Coagulation Disorders; **Hospital:** Robert Wood Johnson Univ Hosp - New Brunswick; **Address:** Robert Wood Johnson Med School, 125 Paterson St, CAB5231, New Brunswick, NJ 08901; **Phone:** 732-235-6531; **Board Cert:** Internal Medicine 1981; Hematology 1984; Medical Oncology 1985; **Med School:** Brown Univ 1978; **Resid:** Internal Medicine, Beth Israel Med Ctr 1981; **Fellow:** Hematology & Oncology, NYU Med Ctr 1984; **Fac Appt:** Prof Med, UMDNJ-RW Johnson Med Sch

Strair, Roger MD/PhD (Hem) - **Spec Exp:** Leukemia; Lymphoma; Bone Marrow Transplant; Multiple Myeloma; **Hospital:** Robert Wood Johnson Univ Hosp - New Brunswick; **Address:** Cancer Inst of NJ, 195 Little Albany St, New Brunswick, NJ 08903; **Phone:** 732-235-7464; **Board Cert:** Internal Medicine 1984; Hematology 1986; Medical Oncology 1987; **Med School:** Albert Einstein Coll Med 1981; **Resid:** Internal Medicine, Brigham & Women's Hosp 1984; **Fellow:** Hematology & Oncology, Brigham & Women's Hosp 1988; **Fac Appt:** Assoc Prof Med, UMDNJ-RW Johnson Med Sch

Infectious Disease

Boruchoff, Susan E MD (Inf) - **Spec Exp:** Travel Medicine; AIDS/HIV; Viral Infections; **Hospital:** Robert Wood Johnson Univ Hosp - New Brunswick; **Address:** RWJ Div Infectious Disease/Travel Med, 125 Patterson St Fl 5 - Ste 5100B, New Brunswick, NJ 08901-1928; **Phone:** 732-235-7060; **Board Cert:** Internal Medicine 1985; Infectious Disease 1988; **Med School:** Columbia P&S 1982; **Resid:** Internal Medicine, Geo Wash Univ Hosp 1985; **Fellow:** Infectious Disease, Univ Mass Med Ctr 1988; **Fac Appt:** Prof Med, UMDNJ-RW Johnson Med Sch

Middleton, John R MD (Inf) - **Spec Exp:** AIDS/HIV; Osteomyelitis; **Hospital:** Raritan Bay Med Ctr - Perth Amboy; **Address:** ID Care, 3 Hospital Plaza, Ste 208, Old Bridge, NJ 08857-3093; **Phone:** 732-360-2700; **Board Cert:** Internal Medicine 1973; Infectious Disease 1980; **Med School:** UMDNJ-NJ Med Sch, Newark 1970; **Resid:** Internal Medicine, NY Hosp-Cornell Med Ctr 1973; **Fellow:** Infectious Disease, RWJ Univ Hosp 1977; **Fac Appt:** Assoc Clin Prof Med, UMDNJ-Rutgers Med Sch

Sensakovic, John W MD/PhD (Inf) - **Spec Exp:** Lyme Disease; Fevers of Unknown Origin; Bone Infections; **Hospital:** Saint Michael's Med Ctr, JFK Med Ctr - Edison; **Address:** 113 James St, Edison, NJ 08820; **Phone:** 732-549-3449; **Board Cert:** Internal Medicine 1982; Infectious Disease 1984; **Med School:** UMDNJ-NJ Med Sch, Newark 1977; **Resid:** Internal Medicine, St Michaels Med Ctr 1980; **Fellow:** Infectious Disease, St Michaels Med Ctr 1982; **Fac Appt:** Prof Med, Seton Hall Univ Sch Hlth & Med Scis

Snepar, Richard A MD (Inf) - **Hospital:** Robert Wood Johnson Univ Hosp - New Brunswick, St. Peter's Univ Hosp; **Address:** Highland Park Medical, 579A Cranbury Rd, Ste 102, East Brunswick, NJ 08816; **Phone:** 732-613-0711; **Board Cert:** Internal Medicine 1979; Infectious Disease 1982; **Med School:** Cornell Univ-Weill Med Coll 1976; **Resid:** Internal Medicine, Med Coll PA Affil Hosp 1979; **Fellow:** Infectious Disease, Med Coll PA Affil Hosp 1981; **Fac Appt:** Asst Clin Prof Med, UMDNJ-RW Johnson Med Sch

Weinstein, Melvin P MD (Inf) - **Spec Exp:** Bone/Joint Infections; Infective Endocarditis; Mycobacterial Infections; **Hospital:** Robert Wood Johnson Univ Hosp - New Brunswick; **Address:** 125 Patterson St, Fl 5, New Brunswick, NJ 08901-1928; **Phone:** 732-235-7713; **Board Cert:** Internal Medicine 1975; Infectious Disease 1978; Medical Microbiology 1983; **Med School:** Geo Wash Univ 1970; **Resid:** Internal Medicine, Hartford Hosp 1975; **Fellow:** Infectious Disease, Univ Colo Hosp 1977; **Fac Appt:** Prof Med, UMDNJ-RW Johnson Med Sch

Internal Medicine

Carson, Jeffrey L MD (IM) *PCP* - **Hospital:** Robert Wood Johnson Univ Hosp - New Brunswick; **Address:** 125 Paterson St, Ste 5100, New Brunswick, NJ 08901; **Phone:** 732-235-6968; **Board Cert:** Internal Medicine 1980; **Med School:** Hahnemann Univ 1977; **Resid:** Internal Medicine, Hahnemann Univ Hosp 1980; **Fellow:** Internal Medicine, Univ Penn 1982; **Fac Appt:** Prof Med, UMDNJ-RW Johnson Med Sch

Cassidy, Brian MD (IM) *PCP* - **Hospital:** JFK Med Ctr - Edison; **Address:** 3910 Park Ave, Ste 8, Edison, NJ 08820; **Phone:** 732-767-3130; **Board Cert:** Internal Medicine 1988; **Med School:** Grenada 1985; **Resid:** Internal Medicine, Muhlenberg Med Ctr 1988

DeSilva Jr, Derrick M MD (IM) *PCP* - **Spec Exp:** Complementary Medicine; **Hospital:** Raritan Bay Med Ctr - Perth Amboy; **Address:** 629 Amboy Ave, Fl 2, Edison, NJ 08837; **Phone:** 732-738-8801; **Med School:** Dominican Republic 1982; **Resid:** Internal Medicine, Raritan Bay Med Ctr-Perth Amboy Div 1988

Gil, Constante MD (IM) *PCP* - **Spec Exp:** Hypertension; Stroke; Heart Failure; Diabetes; **Hospital:** Raritan Bay Med Ctr - Perth Amboy; **Address:** 86 New Brunswick Ave, Hopelawn, NJ 08861; **Phone:** 732-826-1609; **Med School:** Dominican Republic 1981; **Resid:** Internal Medicine, Raritan Bay Med Ctr-Perth Amboy Div 1989; **Fac Appt:** Assoc Clin Prof Med, UMDNJ-RW Johnson Med Sch

Guillen, Gregorio MD (IM) *PCP* - **Spec Exp:** Geriatric Medicine; **Hospital:** Raritan Bay Med Ctr - Perth Amboy, JFK Med Ctr - Edison; **Address:** 400 State St, Ste 2, Perth Amboy, NJ 08861; **Phone:** 732-442-6020; **Med School:** Dominican Republic 1982; **Resid:** Internal Medicine, Raritan Bay Med Ctr 1990; **Fellow:** Geriatric Medicine, Univ Florida 1992

Schaer, Teresa M MD (IM) *PCP* - **Spec Exp:** Concierge Medicine; Geriatric Medicine; **Hospital:** St. Peter's Univ Hosp, Robert Wood Johnson Univ Hosp - New Brunswick; **Address:** 12 Stults Rd, Ste 123, Dayton, NJ 08810; **Phone:** 732-230-3272; **Board Cert:** Internal Medicine 1984; Geriatric Medicine 2010; **Med School:** UCSD 1981; **Resid:** Internal Medicine, Bellevue Hosp Ctr 1984; **Fellow:** Geriatric Medicine, Geo Wash Univ Med Ctr 1986; **Fac Appt:** Assoc Clin Prof Med

Interventional Cardiology

Altmann, Dory B MD (IC) - **Spec Exp:** Coronary Artery Disease; Heart Valve Disease; **Hospital:** Robert Wood Johnson Univ Hosp - New Brunswick, St. Peter's Univ Hosp; **Address:** Cardiology Assocs of New Brunswick, 593 Cranbury Rd, East Brunswick, NJ 08816; **Phone:** 732-390-3333; **Board Cert:** Internal Medicine 1989; Cardiovascular Disease 2011; Interventional Cardiology 2009; **Med School:** Yale Univ 1986; **Resid:** Internal Medicine, New England Med Ctr 1989; **Fellow:** Cardiovascular Disease, Mt Sinai Hosp 1992; Interventional Cardiology, Washington Hosp Ctr 1993; **Fac Appt:** Asst Clin Prof Med, UMDNJ-RW Johnson Med Sch

Maternal & Fetal Medicine

MacMillan, William E MD (MF) - **Spec Exp:** Fetal Diagnosis & Therapy; Diabetes in Pregnancy; Reproductive Genetics; Multiple Gestation; **Hospital:** Robert Wood Johnson Univ Hosp - New Brunswick; **Address:** RWJ Med Group, Dept Ob/Gyn, 125 Paterson St, Ste 4200, New Brunswick, NJ 08901; **Phone:** 732-235-6600; **Board Cert:** Obstetrics & Gynecology 2012; Maternal & Fetal Medicine 2012; **Med School:** Univ Wisc 1985; **Resid:** Obstetrics & Gynecology, Univ Wisc Affil Hosp 1989; **Fellow:** Maternal & Fetal Medicine, SUNY Stony Brook 1991; **Fac Appt:** Asst Prof ObG, UMDNJ-RW Johnson Med Sch

Medical Oncology

Aisner, Joseph MD (Onc) - **Spec Exp:** Lung Cancer; Solid Tumors; Thymoma; Mesothelioma; **Hospital:** Robert Wood Johnson Univ Hosp - New Brunswick; **Address:** Cancer Inst of New Jersey, 195 Little Albany St, New Brunswick, NJ 08903-2681; **Phone:** 732-235-7464; **Board Cert:** Internal Medicine 1973; Medical Oncology 1975; **Med School:** Wayne State Univ 1970; **Resid:** Internal Medicine, Georgetown Univ Hosp 1972; **Fellow:** Medical Oncology, Natl Cancer Inst 1975; **Fac Appt:** Prof Med, UMDNJ-RW Johnson Med Sch

DiPaola, Robert S MD (Onc) - **Spec Exp:** Genitourinary Cancer; Prostate Cancer; Urologic Cancer; **Hospital:** Robert Wood Johnson Univ Hosp - New Brunswick; **Address:** Cancer Inst of New Jersey, 195 Little Albany St, New Brunswick, NJ 08903-2681; **Phone:** 732-235-3336; **Board Cert:** Internal Medicine 2011; Medical Oncology 2005; **Med School:** Univ Utah 1988; **Resid:** Internal Medicine, Duke Univ Med Ctr 1991; **Fellow:** Hematology & Oncology, Univ Penn Hosp 1994; **Fac Appt:** Assoc Prof Med, UMDNJ-RW Johnson Med Sch

Nissenblatt, Michael J MD (Onc) - **Spec Exp:** Breast Cancer; Colon Cancer; Lung Cancer; Hereditary Cancer; **Hospital:** Robert Wood Johnson Univ Hosp - New Brunswick, St. Peter's Univ Hosp; **Address:** Central Jersey Oncology Ctr, 1 Brier Hill Ct, East Brunswick, NJ 08816; **Phone:** 732-390-7750; **Board Cert:** Internal Medicine 1976; Medical Oncology 1979; **Med School:** Columbia P&S 1973; **Resid:** Internal Medicine, Johns Hopkins Hosp 1976; **Fellow:** Medical Oncology, Johns Hopkins Hosp 1978; **Fac Appt:** Clin Prof Onc, UMDNJ-RW Johnson Med Sch

Shypula, Gregory J MD (Onc) - **Spec Exp:** Hematology; **Hospital:** Raritan Bay Med Ctr - Perth Amboy, JFK Med Ctr - Edison; **Address:** 1030 St Georges Ave, Ste 307, Avenel, NJ 07001-1330; **Phone:** 732-750-1200; **Board Cert:** Internal Medicine 1989; Medical Oncology 2011; Hematology 2007; **Med School:** Poland 1981; **Resid:** Internal Medicine, T Marciniak Univ 1984; Internal Medicine, Raritan Bay Med Ctr-Perth Amboy Div 1988; **Fellow:** Hematology & Oncology, St Luke's-Roosevelt Hosp Ctr 1992; **Fac Appt:** Assoc Clin Prof Med, Columbia P&S

Toppmeyer, Deborah L MD (Onc) - **Spec Exp:** Breast Cancer; Hereditary Cancer; **Hospital:** Robert Wood Johnson Univ Hosp - New Brunswick; **Address:** Cancer Inst of New Jersey, 195 Little Albany St, New Brunswick, NJ 08903; **Phone:** 732-235-9692; **Board Cert:** Internal Medicine 1988; Medical Oncology 2006; **Med School:** Albany Med Coll 1985; **Resid:** Internal Medicine, Univ Pittsburgh Hlth Ctr Hosp 1988; **Fellow:** Medical Oncology, Dana Farber Cancer Inst 1993; **Fac Appt:** Assoc Prof Med

Neonatal-Perinatal Medicine

Hiatt, I Mark MD (NP) - **Spec Exp:** Respiratory Failure; Prematurity/Low Birth Weight Infants; Ethics; **Hospital:** St. Peter's Univ Hosp; **Address:** St Peter's Univ Hosp, Div Neonatal Med, 254 Easton Ave, New Brunswick, NJ 08902; **Phone:** 732-745-8523; **Board Cert:** Pediatrics 1978; Neonatal-Perinatal Medicine 1979; **Med School:** Cornell Univ-Weill Med Coll 1972; **Resid:** Pediatrics, NY Hosp-Cornell Med Ctr 1975; **Fellow:** Neonatal-Perinatal Medicine, Babies Hosp-Columbia Univ 1977; **Fac Appt:** Prof Ped, Drexel Univ Coll Med

Mehta, Rajeev MD (NP) - **Spec Exp:** Neonatal Critical Care; **Hospital:** Robert Wood Johnson Univ Hosp - New Brunswick; **Address:** RW Johnson Med School, 125 Paterson St, New Brunswick, NJ 08903-1766; **Phone:** 732-235-7036; **Board Cert:** Neonatal-Perinatal Medicine 2008; **Med School:** India 1979; **Resid:** Pediatrics, Queens Park/St Mary's/Dudley Rd Hosps 1985; Pediatrics, Univ Hosp 1990; **Fellow:** Neonatology, Bradford Royal Infirmary 1989; Neonatology, North Shore Univ Hosp 1993; **Fac Appt:** Prof Ped, UMDNJ-RW Johnson Med Sch

Nephrology

Covit, Andrew B MD (Nep) - **Spec Exp:** Hypertension; Kidney Failure; Renovascular Disease; **Hospital:** Robert Wood Johnson Univ Hosp - New Brunswick, St. Peter's Univ Hosp; **Address:** 8 Old Bridge Tpke, South River, NJ 08882; **Phone:** 732-390-4888; **Board Cert:** Internal Medicine 1982; Nephrology 1986; **Med School:** SUNY Downstate 1979; **Resid:** Internal Medicine, NY Hosp 1982; **Fellow:** Nephrology, NY Hosp 1984; **Fac Appt:** Clin Prof Med, UMDNJ-RW Johnson Med Sch

Sherman, Richard A MD (Nep) - **Spec Exp:** Dialysis Care; Electrolyte Disorders; **Hospital:** Robert Wood Johnson Univ Hosp - New Brunswick; **Address:** RWJ Div Nephrology, 125 Patterson St, Ste 5100, New Brunswick, NJ 08901; **Phone:** 732-235-6512; **Board Cert:** Internal Medicine 1978; Nephrology 1980; **Med School:** Albert Einstein Coll Med 1975; **Resid:** Internal Medicine, Metropolitan Hosp 1977; **Fellow:** Nephrology, Albert Einstein 1979; **Fac Appt:** Prof Med, UMDNJ-RW Johnson Med Sch

Neurological Surgery

Lee, Sun H MD/PhD (NS) - **Spec Exp:** Spinal Surgery-Complex; Brain Tumors; Minimally Invasive Surgery; Pituitary Tumors; **Hospital:** Robert Wood Johnson Univ Hosp - New Brunswick; **Address:** University Neuro Assocs, 125 Patterson St, CAB 2100 Bldg Fl 4 - Ste 4011, New Brunswick, NJ 08901; **Phone:** 732-235-7756; **Board Cert:** Neurological Surgery 2012; **Med School:** Korea 1979; **Resid:** Neurological Surgery, Seoul National Univ Hosp 1984; Neurological Surgery, Thos Jefferson Univ Hosp 1998; **Fellow:** Neurological Surgery, Univ Pittsburgh Med Ctr 1999; **Fac Appt:** Assoc Prof NS, UMDNJ-RW Johnson Med Sch

Nosko, Michael G MD/PhD (NS) - **Spec Exp:** Aneurysm-Cerebral; Brain Tumors; Pituitary Tumors; Cerebrovascular Neurosurgery; **Hospital:** Robert Wood Johnson Univ Hosp - New Brunswick, Univ Med Ctr Princeton at Plainsboro; **Address:** University Neuro Assocs, 125 Paterson St Fl 2, New Brunswick, NJ 08901-1962; **Phone:** 732-235-7756; **Board Cert:** Neurological Surgery 1993; **Med School:** Univ Toronto 1982; **Resid:** Neurological Surgery, Univ Alberta Affil Hosp 1991; **Fellow:** Research, Alberta Heritage Fdn Med Rsch 1986; **Fac Appt:** Assoc Prof NS, UMDNJ-RW Johnson Med Sch

Przybylski, Gregory J MD (NS) - **Spec Exp:** Spinal Surgery; Multiple Sclerosis; Vascular Neurosurgery; Spinal Cord Tumors; **Hospital:** JFK Med Ctr - Edison, Jersey Shore Univ Med Ctr; **Address:** NJ Neuroscience Inst, 65 James St Fl 1st, Edison, NJ 08820; **Phone:** 732-321-7010; **Board Cert:** Neurological Surgery 2011; **Med School:** Jefferson Med Coll 1987; **Resid:** Neurological Surgery, Univ Pittsburgh 1994; **Fellow:** Spine Surgery, Hosp St Vincent de Paul/Hosp St Roch 1995; Spine Surgery, Med Coll Wisc 1996; **Fac Appt:** Prof NS, Seton Hall Univ Sch Hlth & Med Scis

Neurology

Belsh, Jerry M MD (N) - **Spec Exp:** Neuromuscular Disorders; Amyotrophic Lateral Sclerosis (ALS); **Hospital:** Robert Wood Johnson Univ Hosp - New Brunswick; **Address:** 125 Paterson St, New Brunswick, NJ 08901; **Phone:** 732-235-7340; **Board Cert:** Neurology 1981; **Med School:** Jefferson Med Coll 1975; **Resid:** Neurology, Hahnemann Univ Hosp 1977; Neurology, SUNY-Dwnst Med Ctr 1979; **Fellow:** Neuromuscular Medicine, Mt Sinai Hosp 1980; **Fac Appt:** Prof N, UMDNJ-RW Johnson Med Sch

Gizzi, Martin S MD/PhD (N) - **Spec Exp:** Neuro-Ophthalmology; Stroke; Progressive Supranuclear Palsy (PSP); Stroke; **Hospital:** JFK Med Ctr - Edison; **Address:** NJ Neuroscience Institute, 65 James St, Edison, NJ 08820-3947; **Phone:** 732-321-7010; **Board Cert:** Neurology 1990; Vascular Neurology 2008; **Med School:** Univ Miami Sch Med 1985; **Resid:** Neurology, Mount Sinai Hosp 1989; **Fellow:** Neuro-Ophthalmology, Mount Sinai Hosp 1991; **Fac Appt:** Prof N, Seton Hall Univ Sch Hlth & Med Scis

Golbe, Lawrence I MD (N) - **Spec Exp:** Parkinson's Disease; Progressive Supranuclear Palsy (PSP); Movement Disorders; **Hospital:** Robert Wood Johnson Univ Hosp - New Brunswick; **Address:** 125 Paterson St, Fl 6, rm 6100, New Brunswick, NJ 08901-2160; **Phone:** 732-235-7733; **Board Cert:** Neurology 1984; **Med School:** NYU Sch Med 1978; **Resid:** Internal Medicine, Hahnemann Univ Hosp 1980; Neurology, Bellevue Hosp 1983; **Fac Appt:** Prof N, UMDNJ-RW Johnson Med Sch

Herman, Martin MD (N) - **Spec Exp:** Epilepsy; Stroke; **Hospital:** JFK Med Ctr - Edison; **Address:** 65 James St, Edison, NJ 08818; **Phone:** 732-321-7010; **Board Cert:** Neurology 1973; **Med School:** Northwestern Univ 1964; **Resid:** Psychiatry, Strong Meml Hosp 1965; Neurology, Univ VA Hlth Sci Ctr 1970; **Fellow:** Clinical Neurophysiology, Columbia-Presby Hosp 1971; **Fac Appt:** Assoc Clin Prof N, Drexel Univ Coll Med

Lazar, Mark H MD (N) - **Spec Exp:** Headache; Pain Management; Acupuncture; Sarcoidosis; **Hospital:** Robert Wood Johnson Univ Hosp - New Brunswick; **Address:** 573 Cranbury Rd, Ste A5, East Brunswick, NJ 08816-4026; **Phone:** 732-254-5101; **Board Cert:** Neurology 1982; **Med School:** NYU Sch Med 1977; **Resid:** Neurology, NYU Med Ctr 1981; **Fellow:** Neurology, NY-Cornell Med Ctr 1982; Clinical Neurophysiology, Columbia-Presby Med Ctr 1983; **Fac Appt:** Assoc Clin Prof N, UMDNJ-RW Johnson Med Sch

Lepore, Frederick E MD (N) - **Spec Exp:** Neuro-Ophthalmology; Botox for Blepharospasm; Migraine; Pseudomotor Cerebri; **Hospital:** Robert Wood Johnson Univ Hosp - New Brunswick; **Address:** Dept Neurology, 125 Paterson St, rm 6210, New Brunswick, NJ 08901-2160; **Phone:** 732-235-7730; **Board Cert:** Neurology 1981; **Med School:** Univ Rochester 1975; **Resid:** Internal Medicine, Univ Michigan Med Ctr 1976; Neurology, Univ Virginia Hlth Sci Ctr 1979; **Fellow:** Neuro-Ophthalmology, Bascom Palmer Eye Inst 1980; **Fac Appt:** Prof N, UMDNJ-RW Johnson Med Sch

Oh, Youn K MD (N) - **Spec Exp:** Headache; Stroke; Seizure Disorders; Parkinson's Disease; **Hospital:** JFK Med Ctr - Edison, Robert Wood Johnson Univ Hosp at Rahway; **Address:** 34-36 Progress St, Ste B3, Edison, NJ 08820-1197; **Phone:** 908-757-6633; **Board Cert:** Neurology 1979; Psychiatry 1981; **Med School:** South Korea 1964; **Resid:** Psychiatry, Harvard Psy Svc/Boston City Hosp 1973; Neurology, UMDNJ-NJ Med Sch 1975; **Fac Appt:** Assoc Clin Prof N, UMDNJ-RW Johnson Med Sch

Rosenberg, Michael L MD (N) - **Spec Exp:** Neuro-Ophthalmology; Neuro-Otology; Balance Disorders; **Hospital:** JFK Med Ctr - Edison; **Address:** New Jersey Neuroscience Institute, 65 James St, Edison, NJ 08818; **Phone:** 732-321-7010; **Board Cert:** Neurology 1983; **Med School:** Baylor Coll Med 1976; **Resid:** Neurology, Letterman AMC 1981; **Fellow:** Neuro-Ophthalmology, Bascom-Palmer Eye Inst 1981; **Fac Appt:** Prof N, Seton Hall Univ Sch Hlth & Med Scis

Sage, Jacob I MD (N) - **Spec Exp:** Parkinson's Disease; Dystonia; **Hospital:** Robert Wood Johnson Univ Hosp - New Brunswick; **Address:** Rutgers RWJ Med School-Dept Neurology, 125 Paterson St Fl 6 - Ste 6100, New Brunswick, NJ 08901-2160; **Phone:** 732-235-7733; **Board Cert:** Neurology 1979; **Med School:** Univ Pittsburgh 1972; **Resid:** Neurology, Univ Pittsburgh Hosps 1978; **Fellow:** Neurological Chemistry, NY Hosp-Cornell 1980; **Fac Appt:** Prof N, UMDNJ-RW Johnson Med Sch

Neuroradiology

Keller, Irwin A MD (NRad) - **Spec Exp:** Brain & Spinal Imaging; Interventional Neuroradiology; Aneurysm-Cerebral; **Hospital:** Robert Wood Johnson Univ Hosp - New Brunswick; **Address:** Univ Radiology Grp, 579-A Cranbury Rd, East Brunswick, NJ 08816-5405; **Phone:** 732-390-0040; **Board Cert:** Diagnostic Radiology 1984; Neuroradiology 2005; **Med School:** NY Med Coll 1980; **Resid:** Diagnostic Radiology, Montefiore Med Ctr 1984; **Fellow:** Neuroradiology, NYU Langone Med Ctr 1986; **Fac Appt:** Assoc Prof Rad, UMDNJ-RW Johnson Med Sch

Roychowdhury, Sudipta MD (NRad) - **Spec Exp:** Interventional Neuroradiology; Pediatric Radiology; **Hospital:** Robert Wood Johnson Univ Hosp - New Brunswick; **Address:** Univ Radiology Grp, 579-A Cranbury Rd, East Brunswick, NJ 08816; **Phone:** 732-390-0040; **Board Cert:** Diagnostic Radiology 1997; Neuroradiology 2010; **Med School:** Northwestern Univ 1992; **Resid:** Diagnostic Radiology, Northwestern Meml Hosp 1997; **Fellow:** Neuroradiology, Hosp Univ Penn - UPHS 1999; **Fac Appt:** Asst Clin Prof Rad, UMDNJ-RW Johnson Med Sch

Schonfeld, Steven MD (NRad) - **Spec Exp:** Spine Imaging & Intervention; Pediatric Neuroradiology; Interventional Neuroradiology; **Hospital:** Robert Wood Johnson Univ Hosp - New Brunswick, St. Peter's Univ Hosp; **Address:** University Radiology Group, 579A Cranbury Rd, Fl 3, East Brunswick, NJ 08816; **Phone:** 732-390-0040; **Board Cert:** Diagnostic Radiology 1982; Neuroradiology 2005; **Med School:** Mount Sinai Sch Med 1978; **Resid:** Diagnostic Radiology, Montefiore Hosp Med Ctr 1982; **Fellow:** Neuroradiology, NYU Med Ctr 1984; **Fac Appt:** Clin Prof Rad, UMDNJ-RW Johnson Med Sch

Obstetrics & Gynecology

Bachmann, Gloria A MD (ObG) - **Spec Exp:** Menopause Problems; Sexual Dysfunction; Pelvic Surgery; Uterine Fibroids; **Hospital:** Robert Wood Johnson Univ Hosp - New Brunswick; **Address:** Womens Hlth Inst, 125 Paterson St CAB Bldg - Ste 2104, New Brunswick, NJ 08901-1962; **Phone:** 732-235-7633; **Board Cert:** Obstetrics & Gynecology 1981; **Med School:** Univ Pennsylvania 1974; **Resid:** Obstetrics & Gynecology, Hosp Univ Penn - UPHS 1979; **Fac Appt:** Prof ObG, UMDNJ-RW Johnson Med Sch

Bochner, Ronnie Z MD (ObG) - **Spec Exp:** Gynecologic Surgery; Laparoscopic Surgery; Uterine Fibroids; Menopause Problems; **Hospital:** Robert Wood Johnson Univ Hosp - New Brunswick; **Address:** RWJ OB/GYN Assocs, 3270 Rt 27, Ste 2200, MS 08824, Kendall Park, NJ 08824-1458; **Phone:** 732-422-8989; **Board Cert:** Obstetrics & Gynecology 2012; **Med School:** Mount Sinai Sch Med 1981; **Resid:** Obstetrics & Gynecology, LI Jewish Med Ctr 1985; **Fac Appt:** Asst Clin Prof ObG, UMDNJ-RW Johnson Med Sch

Davis, Nicole D MD (ObG) - **Spec Exp:** Gynecology Only; **Hospital:** St. Peter's Univ Hosp; **Address:** 620 Cranbury Rd, Ste LL90, East Brunswick, NJ 08816; **Phone:** 732-257-0081; **Board Cert:** Obstetrics & Gynecology 2012; **Med School:** Yale Univ 1988; **Resid:** Obstetrics & Gynecology, NY-Presby/Weill Cornell Med Ctr 1992

Friedman, Alan L MD (ObG) - **Spec Exp:** Pregnancy-High Risk; Infertility; **Hospital:** Univ Med Ctr Princeton at Plainsboro; **Address:** Princeton OB/GYN, 5 Plainsboro Rd, Med Arts Pav, Ste 500, Plainsboro, NJ 08536; **Phone:** 609-936-0700; **Board Cert:** Obstetrics & Gynecology 2012; **Med School:** Univ Chicago-Pritzker Sch Med 1982; **Resid:** Obstetrics & Gynecology, NYU Langone Med Ctr 1987

Rathauser, Robert H MD (ObG) - **Hospital:** Robert Wood Johnson Univ Hosp - New Brunswick; **Address:** RWJ OB/GYN Assocs, 3270 Route 27, Ste 2200, MS 08824, Kendall Park, NJ 08824; **Phone:** 732-422-8989; **Board Cert:** Obstetrics & Gynecology 2012; **Med School:** NYU Sch Med 1979; **Resid:** Obstetrics & Gynecology, LI Jewish Med Ctr 1984; **Fac Appt:** Assoc Prof ObG, UMDNJ-RW Johnson Med Sch

Occupational Medicine

Gochfeld, Michael MD/PhD (OM) - **Spec Exp:** Environmental Medicine; Mercury Toxic Exposure; Chemical Exposure; **Hospital:** Robert Wood Johnson Univ Hosp - New Brunswick; **Address:** EOHSI Clin Ctr, 170 Frelinghuysen Rd, Ste 200, Piscataway, NJ 08854; **Phone:** 848-445-0123; **Board Cert:** Occupational Medicine 1983; **Med School:** Albert Einstein Coll Med 1965; **Resid:** Behavioral Medicine, Rockefeller Univ Affil Hosp 1977; **Fac Appt:** Prof OM, UMDNJ-RW Johnson Med Sch

Kipen, Howard M MD (OM) - **Spec Exp:** Environmental Medicine; Occupational Lung Disease; **Hospital:** Robert Wood Johnson Univ Hosp - New Brunswick; **Address:** EOHSI Clin Ctr, 170 Frelinghuysen Rd, Ste 200, Piscataway, NJ 08854; **Phone:** 848-445-0123; **Board Cert:** Internal Medicine 1982; Occupational Medicine 1986; **Med School:** UCSF 1979; **Resid:** Internal Medicine, Columbia Presby Med Ctr 1982; Occupational Medicine, Mt Sinai Hosp 1984; **Fac Appt:** Prof Med, UMDNJ-RW Johnson Med Sch

Ophthalmology

Blondo, Dennis L MD (Oph) - **Hospital:** Raritan Bay Med Ctr - Old Bridge Div; **Address:** 28 Throckmorton Ln, Old Bridge, NJ 08857-2558; **Phone:** 732-679-6100; **Board Cert:** Ophthalmology 1979; **Med School:** Med Coll VA 1973; **Resid:** Ophthalmology, NYU Langone Med Ctr 1978

Engel, J. Mark MD (Oph) - **Spec Exp:** Pediatric Ophthalmology; **Hospital:** Robert Wood Johnson Univ Hosp - New Brunswick, St. Peter's Univ Hosp; **Address:** Univ Chldns Eye Ctr, 4 Cornwall Ct, East Brunswick, NJ 08816; **Phone:** 732-613-9191; **Board Cert:** Ophthalmology 2013; **Med School:** Loyola Univ-Stritch Sch Med 1986; **Resid:** Internal Medicine, Evanston Hosp 1988; Ophthalmology, Interfaith Med Ctr 1991; **Fellow:** Pediatric Ophthalmology, Lurie Chldn's Hosp-Chicago 1992; **Fac Appt:** Assoc Clin Prof Oph, UMDNJ-NJ Med Sch, Newark

Grabowski, Wayne M MD (Oph) - **Spec Exp:** Diabetic Eye Disease; Laser Vision Surgery; Glaucoma; **Hospital:** Univ Med Ctr Princeton at Plainsboro; **Address:** 5 Centre Drive, Ste 1B, Monroe Township, NJ 08831; **Phone:** 609-409-2777; **Board Cert:** Ophthalmology 1982; **Med School:** Albany Med Coll 1977; **Resid:** Ophthalmology, Albany Med Ctr 1981; **Fellow:** Vitreoretinal Surgery, Wills Eye Hosp 1982

Milite, James P MD (Oph) - **Spec Exp:** Oculoplastic Surgery; Eyelid Tumors/Cancer; Thyroid Eye Disease; **Hospital:** New York Eye & Ear Infirm (page 115); **Address:** Omni Eye Svcs, 485 Route 1 S A Bldg, Iselin, NJ 08830; **Phone:** 732-750-0400; **Board Cert:** Ophthalmology 2006; **Med School:** NYU Sch Med 1990; **Resid:** Ophthalmology, New York Eye & Ear Infirm 1994; **Fellow:** Ocular Pathology, New York Eye & Ear Infirm 1995; Ophthalmic Plastic Surgery, New York Eye & Ear Infirm 1996; **Fac Appt:** Asst Prof Oph, NY Med Coll

Napolitano, Joseph D MD (Oph) - **Spec Exp:** Pediatric Ophthalmology; Strabismus; Eye Muscle Disorders; **Hospital:** Robert Wood Johnson Univ Hosp - New Brunswick; **Address:** OMNI Eye Svcs, 485 Route 1 South, A Bldg - Ste 140, Iselin, NJ 08830; **Phone:** 732-750-0400; **Board Cert:** Ophthalmology 2008; **Med School:** UMDNJ-RW Johnson Med Sch 1987; **Resid:** Ophthalmology, UMDNJ-NJ Med Sch Affil Hosp 1992; **Fellow:** Pediatric Ophthalmology, Chldns Hosp 1993

Prenner, Jonathan L MD (Oph) - **Spec Exp:** Retina/Vitreous Surgery; Macular Degeneration; Retinal Detachment; Diabetic Eye Disease/Retinopathy; **Hospital:** Robert Wood Johnson Univ Hosp - New Brunswick; **Address:** NJ Retina, 10 Plum St Fl 6, New Brunswick, NJ 08901; **Phone:** 732-220-1600; **Board Cert:** Ophthalmology 2003; **Med School:** SUNY Stony Brook 1998; **Resid:** Ophthalmology, Scheie Eye Inst 2002; **Fellow:** Vitreoretinal Surgery & Disease, William Beaumont Hosp 2004; **Fac Appt:** Asst Clin Prof Oph, UMDNJ-RW Johnson Med Sch

Santamaria II, Jaime MD (Oph) - **Spec Exp:** Cataract Surgery; LASIK-Refractive Surgery; **Hospital:** Raritan Bay Med Ctr - Perth Amboy, NY-Presby/Columbia Univ Med Ctr, NY (page 104); **Address:** Santamaria Eye Center, 104 Market St, Perth Amboy, NJ 08861-4412; **Phone:** 732-826-5159; **Board Cert:** Ophthalmology 1979; **Med School:** Columbia P&S 1973; **Resid:** Ophthalmology, Columbia-Presby Med Ctr 1978; **Fellow:** Research, Columbia Physicians & Surgeons 1975; **Fac Appt:** Asst Clin Prof Oph, Columbia P&S

Orthopaedic Surgery

Garfinkel, Matthew J MD (OrS) - **Spec Exp:** Shoulder & Knee Surgery; Arthroscopic Surgery; Sports Medicine; **Hospital:** JFK Med Ctr - Edison; **Address:** Edison-Metuchen Orthopaedic Grp, 10 Parsonage Rd Fl 5 - Ste 500, Edison, NJ 08837-2429; **Phone:** 732-494-6226; **Board Cert:** Orthopaedic Surgery 2005; **Med School:** Cornell Univ-Weill Med Coll 1986; **Resid:** Orthopaedic Surgery, Montefiore/Weiler Einsten Med Ctr 1991; **Fellow:** Sports Medicine, Lankenau Hosp 1992

Lombardi, Joseph S MD (OrS) - **Spec Exp:** Spinal Surgery; Spinal Disc Replacement; **Hospital:** JFK Med Ctr - Edison; **Address:** Edison-Metuchen Orthopaedic Grp, 10 Parsonage Rd Fl 5 - Ste 500, Edison, NJ 08837-2475; **Phone:** 732-494-6226; **Board Cert:** Orthopaedic Surgery 2008; **Med School:** UMDNJ-RW Johnson Med Sch 1978; **Resid:** Orthopaedic Surgery, UMDNJ-Univ Hosp 1983; **Fellow:** Spine Surgery, Long Beach Meml Med Ctr 1984

Piskun, Andrew MD (OrS) - **Spec Exp:** Trauma; Sports Injuries; Arthroscopic Surgery; **Hospital:** Robert Wood Johnson Univ Hosp - New Brunswick, St. Peter's Univ Hosp; **Address:** RWJ Univ Hosp - Dept Orthopaedic Surgery, 1132 S Washington Ave, Piscataway, NJ 08854-3335; **Phone:** 732-752-8484; **Board Cert:** Orthopaedic Surgery 1984; **Med School:** UMDNJ-RW Johnson Med Sch 1977; **Resid:** Orthopaedic Surgery, UMDNJ-RW Johnson Univ Hosp 1982; **Fac Appt:** Asst Clin Prof OrS, UMDNJ-RW Johnson Med Sch

Reich, Steven MD (OrS) - **Spec Exp:** Spinal Surgery; Spinal Disorders; **Hospital:** Robert Wood Johnson Univ Hosp - New Brunswick; **Address:** Affil Orthopaedic Specialists, 2186 Route 27, Ste 1A, North Brunswick, NJ 08902; **Phone:** 732-422-1222; **Board Cert:** Orthopaedic Surgery 2005; **Med School:** Albert Einstein Coll Med 1986; **Resid:** Orthopaedic Surgery, Hosp for Joint Dis 1991; **Fellow:** Spine Surgery, Pennsylvania Hosp 1992; Spine Surgery, Thomas Jefferson Univ Hosp 1992

Swan Jr, Kenneth G MD (OrS) - **Hospital:** Robert Wood Johnson Univ Hosp - New Brunswick; **Address:** 303 George St, Ste 105, New Brunswick, NJ 08901; **Phone:** 732-846-6100; **Board Cert:** Orthopaedic Surgery 2008; Sports Medicine 2011; **Med School:** Cornell Univ-Weill Med Coll 2000; **Resid:** Orthopaedic Surgery, UMDNJ Univ Hosp 2005; **Fellow:** Sports Medicine & Shoulder Surgery, Univ of Colorado 2006

Otolaryngology

Edelman, Bruce A MD (Oto) - **Spec Exp:** Ear Disorders; Sinusitis; **Hospital:** St. Peter's Univ Hosp; **Address:** B3 Cornwall Drive, East Brunswick, NJ 08816; **Phone:** 732-238-0300; **Board Cert:** Otolaryngology 1990; **Med School:** NYU Sch Med 1984; **Resid:** Surgery, Albert Einstein Med Ctr 1986; Otolaryngology, NYU Langone Med Ctr 1990; **Fellow:** Pediatric Otolaryngology, Chldns Hosp 1991

Kay, Scott L MD (Oto) - **Spec Exp:** Facial Nerve Disorders; Otology; Hearing Loss; Sinus Surgery; **Hospital:** Univ Med Ctr Princeton at Plainsboro; **Address:** 7 Schalks Crossing Rd, Ste 324, Plainsboro, NJ 08536; **Phone:** 609-897-0203; **Board Cert:** Otolaryngology 1993; **Med School:** Univ Pennsylvania 1986; **Resid:** Surgery, Mt Sinai Med Ctr 1988; Otolaryngology, NY-Presby/Columbia Univ Med Ctr 1992; **Fellow:** Facial Plastic Surgery, UPMC Shadyside 1993; **Fac Appt:** Prof S

Mazzara, Carl A MD (Oto) - **Spec Exp:** Rhinoplasty; Eyelid Surgery; Cancer Reconstruction; Facial Plastic & Reconstructive Surgery; **Hospital:** JFK Med Ctr - Edison, Overlook Med Ctr (page 92); **Address:** Mazzara Aesthetics, 5 Lincoln Hwy, Ste 4, Edison, NJ 08820; **Phone:** 732-635-1800; **Board Cert:** Otolaryngology 1994; Facial Plastic & Reconstr Surgery 1995; **Med School:** Mount Sinai Sch Med 1988; **Resid:** Otolaryngology, UMDNJ-Univ Hosp 1992; **Fellow:** Facial Plastic & Reconstr Surgery, Inst Facial Plastic Surg 1993

Miller, Andrew J MD (Oto) - **Spec Exp:** Cosmetic Surgery-Face; **Hospital:** JFK Med Ctr - Edison; **Address:** Assocs in Plastic Surgery, 1150 Amboy Ave, Edison, NJ 08837; **Phone:** 732-548-3200; **Board Cert:** Otolaryngology 2000; Facial Plastic & Reconstr Surgery 2002; **Med School:** Baylor Coll Med 1994; **Resid:** Otolaryngology, Tulane Med Ctr 2000

Rosenbaum, Jeffrey M MD (Oto) - **Spec Exp:** Head & Neck Surgery; Cosmetic Surgery-Face; Salivary Gland Surgery; Thyroid & Parathyroid Surgery; **Hospital:** St. Peter's Univ Hosp; **Address:** B3 Cornwall Drive, East Brunswick, NJ 08816; **Phone:** 732-238-0300; **Board Cert:** Otolaryngology 1978; **Med School:** Albany Med Coll 1973; **Resid:** Surgery, Hartford Hosp 1975; Otolaryngology, NYU Langone Med Ctr 1978; **Fellow:** Plastic Surgery, Wayne State Univ Hosp 1979; **Fac Appt:** Assoc Prof Oto, NYU Sch Med

Pain Medicine

Grubb, William R MD (PM) - **Spec Exp:** Complex Regional Pain Syndromes; Pain-Cancer; **Hospital:** Robert Wood Johnson Univ Hosp - New Brunswick; **Address:** NJ Pain Inst, 125 Patterson St Fl 5 - Ste 5100, New Brunswick, NJ 08901; **Phone:** 732-235-7246; **Board Cert:** Anesthesiology 1990; Pain Medicine 2007; **Med School:** Geo Wash Univ 1985; **Resid:** Anesthesiology, G Washington Univ Med Ctr 1989; **Fellow:** Cardiac Anesthesiology, Univ S Fla Coll Med 1994; **Fac Appt:** Asst Prof Anes, UMDNJ-RW Johnson Med Sch

Levin, Alexander MD (PM) - **Spec Exp:** Pain-Chronic; **Hospital:** Robert Wood Johnson Univ Hosp - New Brunswick; **Address:** 561 Cranbury Road Fl Ground, East Brunswick, NJ 08816-5400; **Phone:** 732-651-1300; **Board Cert:** Anesthesiology 1990; Pain Medicine 2007; **Med School:** Russia 1978; **Resid:** Anesthesiology, Westchester Med Ctr 1986; **Fellow:** Pain Medicine, Univ Cincinnati Med Ctr 1988

Pathology

Barnard, Nicola J MD (Path) - **Spec Exp:** Breast Pathology; Surgical Pathology; **Hospital:** Robert Wood Johnson Univ Hosp - New Brunswick; **Address:** RJW Dept Surgical Pathology, 1 Robert Wood Johnson Pl, New Brunswick, NJ 08901; **Phone:** 732-937-8592; **Board Cert:** Anatomic Pathology 1981; **Med School:** England, UK 1975; **Resid:** Anatomic Pathology, Yale-New Haven Hosp 1980; Anatomic Pathology, Beth Israel Deaconess Hosp 1982; **Fellow:** Clinical Pathology, Harvard Univ 1982; **Fac Appt:** Assoc Prof Path, UMDNJ-RW Johnson Med Sch

Pediatric Cardiology

Agarwal, Kishan C MD (PCd) - **Spec Exp:** Echocardiography; Heart Disease in Adolescents; Arrhythmias; **Hospital:** JFK Med Ctr - Edison, Children's Specialized Hosp; **Address:** 450 Plainfield Rd, Edison, NJ 08820-2628; **Phone:** 732-494-9500; **Board Cert:** Pediatrics 1980; Pediatric Cardiology 1983; **Med School:** India 1969; **Resid:** Pediatrics, St John's Episcopal Hosp 1977; Pediatrics, SUNY Downstate Med Ctr 1979; **Fellow:** Pediatric Cardiology, Mayo Clinic 1981; **Fac Appt:** Clin Prof Ped, UMDNJ-RW Johnson Med Sch

Gaffney, Joseph W MD (PCd) - **Spec Exp:** Echocardiography; Fetal Echocardiography; Critical Care; **Hospital:** Robert Wood Johnson Univ Hosp - New Brunswick, Morgan Stanley Children's Hosp of NY-Presby, NY (page 104); **Address:** RWJ Univ Hosp - Dept Ped Cardiology, 125 Paterson St Fl 6 - Ste 6100, Clin Academic Bldg, New Brunswick, NJ 08901; **Phone:** 732-235-7905; **Board Cert:** Pediatric Cardiology 2013; **Med School:** NY Med Coll 1981; **Resid:** Pediatrics, Brookdale Univ Hosp Med Ctr 1985; **Fellow:** Pediatric Cardiology, NY-Presby/Columbia Univ Med Ctr 1987; **Fac Appt:** Assoc Prof Ped, UMDNJ-RW Johnson Med Sch

Kurer, Cheryl C MD (PCd) - **Hospital:** Chldns Hosp of Philadelphia, St. Peter's Univ Hosp; **Address:** St Peters Univ Hosp - CHOP Cardiac Ctr, 254 Easton Ave, Med Offc Bldg Fl 2, New Brunswick, NJ 08901-1766; **Phone:** 732-846-2855; **Board Cert:** Pediatrics 1987; Pediatric Cardiology 2013; **Med School:** Mount Sinai Sch Med 1983; **Resid:** Pediatrics, Mt Sinai Med Ctr 1986; **Fellow:** Pediatric Cardiology, Chldns Hosp 1989; **Fac Appt:** Assoc Clin Prof Ped, Univ Pennsylvania

Pediatric Critical Care Medicine

Anene, Okechukwu P MD (PCCM) - **Hospital:** JFK Med Ctr - Edison; **Address:** Chldns Svc Dept, JFK Med Ctr, 65 James St, Edison, NJ 08820; **Phone:** 732-321-7010; **Board Cert:** Pediatric Critical Care Medicine 2011; Pediatrics 2009; **Med School:** Nigeria 1983; **Resid:** Pediatrics, UMDNJ-New Jersey Med Sch Affil Hosp 1991; **Fellow:** Pediatric Critical Care Medicine, Wayne St Univ Affil Hosp 1995; **Fac Appt:** Assoc Prof Ped, Seton Hall Univ Sch Hlth & Med Scis

Jonna, Siva P MD (PCCM) - **Hospital:** St. Peter's Univ Hosp; **Address:** 254 Easton Ave, rm 5094, New Brunswick, NJ 08901; **Phone:** 732-745-8600 x8152; **Board Cert:** Pediatrics 2013; Pediatric Critical Care Medicine 2013; **Med School:** India 1981; **Resid:** Pediatrics, Howard Univ Hosp 1995; **Fellow:** Pediatric Critical Care Medicine, MedStar Georgetown Univ Hosp 1996

Pediatric Endocrinology

Marshall, Ian MD (PEn) - **Spec Exp:** Adrenal Disorders; Growth Disorders; Pubertal Disorders; **Hospital:** Robert Wood Johnson Univ Hosp - New Brunswick; **Address:** RWJ Univ Hosp, Div Pediatric Endocrinology, 89 French St Fl 2, New Brunswick, NJ 08901; **Phone:** 732-235-6230; **Board Cert:** Pediatric Endocrinology 2011; **Med School:** South Africa 1991; **Resid:** Pediatrics, Steven & Alexandra Cohen Chldn's Med Ctr of NY 1998; **Fellow:** Pediatric Endocrinology, NY Presby Hosp 2002; **Fac Appt:** Asst Prof Ped

Salas, Max MD (PEn) - **Spec Exp:** Growth Disorders; Pubertal Disorders; Diabetes; **Hospital:** St. Peter's Univ Hosp; **Address:** St Peter's Univ Hosp-Ped Endocrinology, 254 Easton Ave Fl 3, New Brunswick, NJ 08901-1766; **Phone:** 732-745-8574; **Board Cert:** Pediatrics 1968; Pediatric Endocrinology 1986; **Med School:** Mexico 1964; **Resid:** Pediatrics, Chldns Hosp 1967; Pediatrics, Chldns Hosp 1968; **Fellow:** Pediatric Endocrinology, Chldns Hosp 1979; Pediatric Endocrinology, N Shore Univ Hosp 1980; **Fac Appt:** Assoc Prof Ped, Drexel Univ Coll Med

Pediatric Gastroenterology

Koniaris, Soula MD (PGe) - **Spec Exp:** Nutrition; **Hospital:** Robert Wood Johnson Univ Hosp - New Brunswick; **Address:** Child Hlth Inst NJ, 89 French St, rm 2226, New Brunswick, NJ 08901; **Phone:** 732-235-7885; **Board Cert:** Pediatric Gastroenterology 2005; **Med School:** Univ Tenn Coll Med 1988; **Resid:** Pediatrics, Montefiore Hosp Med Ctr 1991; **Fellow:** Pediatric Gastroenterology, N Shore Univ Hosp 1994; **Fac Appt:** Asst Prof Ped, UMDNJ-RW Johnson Med Sch

Pediatric Hematology-Oncology

Drachtman, Richard A MD (PHO) - **Spec Exp:** Pediatric Cancers; Sickle Cell Disease; **Hospital:** Robert Wood Johnson Univ Hosp - New Brunswick, Jersey Shore Univ Med Ctr; **Address:** Cancer Inst of New Jersey, 195 Little Albany St, rm 3507, New Brunswick, NJ 08903; **Phone:** 732-235-5437; **Board Cert:** Pediatric Hematology-Oncology 2007; **Med School:** Ros Franklin Univ/Chicago Med Sch 1984; **Resid:** Pediatrics, N Shore Univ Hosp 1988; **Fellow:** Pediatric Hematology-Oncology, Mount Sinai Hosp 1991; **Fac Appt:** Prof Ped, UMDNJ-RW Johnson Med Sch

Pediatric Infectious Disease

Whitley-Williams, Patricia N MD (PInf) - **Spec Exp:** AIDS/HIV; Lyme Disease; Neonatal Infections; Travel Medicine; **Hospital:** Robert Wood Johnson Univ Hosp - New Brunswick; **Address:** RWJ - Div Pediatric Infect Dis, 89 French St Fl 2, New Brunswick, NJ 08903; **Phone:** 732-235-7894; **Board Cert:** Pediatrics 1980; Pediatric Infectious Disease 2012; **Med School:** Johns Hopkins Univ 1975; **Resid:** Pediatrics, Chldns Hosp 1979; **Fellow:** Pediatric Infectious Disease, Boston Med Ctr 1980; **Fac Appt:** Prof Ped, UMDNJ-RW Johnson Med Sch

Pediatric Nephrology

Singh, Anup MD (PNep) - **Spec Exp:** Nephrotic Syndrome; Lupus/SLE; Hypertension in Children; Kidney Stones; **Hospital:** St. Peter's Univ Hosp, Staten Island Univ Hosp - South (page 106); **Address:** St Peter's Univ Hosp, 254 Easton Ave MOB-3, New Brunswick, NJ 08901; **Phone:** 732-565-5489; **Board Cert:** Pediatrics 2007; Pediatric Nephrology 2010; **Med School:** Philippines 1985; **Resid:** Pediatrics, SUNY-Downstate Med Ctr 1991; **Fellow:** Pediatric Nephrology, SUNY-Downstate Med Ctr 1994; **Fac Appt:** Assoc Prof Ped, Drexel Univ Coll Med

Weiss, Lynne S MD (PNep) - **Spec Exp:** Hypertension; Kidney Disease; Kidney Failure-Chronic; **Hospital:** Robert Wood Johnson Univ Hosp - New Brunswick; **Address:** RWJ Univ Hosp - Dept Ped Nephrology, 89 French St Fl 2, New Brunswick, NJ 08901; **Phone:** 732-235-7880; **Board Cert:** Pediatrics 1979; Pediatric Nephrology 1982; **Med School:** Hahnemann Univ 1974; **Resid:** Pediatrics, Michael Reese Hosp & Med Ctr 1978; **Fellow:** Pediatric Nephrology, Michael Reese Hosp & Med Ctr 1980; **Fac Appt:** Prof Ped, UMDNJ-RW Johnson Med Sch

Pediatric Otolaryngology

Traquina, Diana N MD (PO) - **Spec Exp:** Airway Disorders; Ear Disorders; Sinus Disorders; **Hospital:** Robert Wood Johnson Univ Hosp - New Brunswick; **Address:** Univ Otolaryngology Assocs, 181 Somerset St Fl 2, New Brunswick, NJ 08901; **Phone:** 732-247-2401; **Board Cert:** Otolaryngology 1989; **Med School:** Yale Univ 1984; **Resid:** Surgery, Yale-New Haven Hosp 1986; Otolaryngology, Yale-New Haven Hosp 1989; **Fellow:** Pediatric Otolaryngology, Montefiore Med Ctr 1990; **Fac Appt:** Assoc Prof Ped, UMDNJ-RW Johnson Med Sch

Pediatric Rheumatology

Moorthy, Lakshmi MD (PRhu) - **Spec Exp:** Lupus/SLE; Arthritis; **Hospital:** Robert Wood Johnson Univ Hosp - New Brunswick; **Address:** RWJ Univ Hosp, Chld Hlth Inst, 89 French St, Ste 2300, New Brunswick, NJ 08901; **Phone:** 732-235-6230; **Board Cert:** Pediatrics 2008; Pediatric Rheumatology 2012; **Med School:** India 1995; **Resid:** Pediatrics, NY-Presby/Weill Cornell Med Ctr 2000; **Fellow:** Pediatric Rheumatology, Hosp Special Surgery 2003; **Fac Appt:** Asst Prof Ped, UMDNJ-RW Johnson Med Sch

Pediatric Surgery

Gallucci, John MD (PS) - **Spec Exp:** Neonatal Surgery; Thoracic Surgery; **Hospital:** St. Peter's Univ Hosp; **Address:** St Peters Univ Hosp, Surgery, 254 Easton Ave, MOB4, New Brunswick, NJ 08901; **Phone:** 732-565-5482; **Board Cert:** Pediatric Surgery 2009; **Med School:** UMDNJ-RW Johnson Med Sch 1990; **Resid:** Surgery, Cooper Univ Hosp 1997; **Fellow:** Pediatric Surgery, McGill Univ Chldns Hosp 2000

Stafford, Perry MD (PS) - **Spec Exp:** Minimally Invasive Surgery; Neonatal Surgery; Trauma; **Hospital:** Robert Wood Johnson Univ Hosp - New Brunswick; **Address:** RWJ-Pediatric Surgery, 1 Robert Wood Johnson Pl, New Brunswick, NJ 08903; **Phone:** 732-235-7821; **Board Cert:** Surgery 2006; Pediatric Surgery 2009; **Med School:** Univ Fla Coll Med 1979; **Resid:** Surgery, Naval Reg Med Ctr 1984; **Fellow:** Pediatric Surgery, Chldns Hosp 1987; **Fac Appt:** Prof S, UMDNJ-RW Johnson Med Sch

Pediatric Urology

Fleisher, Michael H MD (Ped Uro) - **Hospital:** St. Peter's Univ Hosp, Jersey Shore Univ Med Ctr; **Address:** Pediatric Urology Assocs, 557 Cranbury Rd, Ste 4, East Brunswick, NJ 08816-5400; **Phone:** 732-613-9144; **Board Cert:** Urology 1984; Pediatric Urology 2009; **Med School:** SUNY Downstate 1977; **Resid:** Urology, SUNY Downstate Med Ctr 1982; **Fellow:** Transplant Medicine, Montefiore Hosp Med Ctr 1979; Pediatric Urology, Hosp Sick Chldn 1983; **Fac Appt:** Assoc Clin Prof U

Vates III, Thomas S MD (Ped Uro) - **Hospital:** Robert Wood Johnson Univ Hosp - New Brunswick, Monmouth Med Ctr; **Address:** Pediatric Urology Assocs, 557 Cranbury Rd, Ste 4, East Brunswick, NJ 08816; **Phone:** 732-613-9144; **Board Cert:** Urology 2009; Pediatric Urology 2009; **Med School:** Georgetown Univ 1989; **Resid:** Surgery, RW Johnson Univ Hosp 1991; Urology, RW Johnson Univ Hosp 1995; **Fellow:** Pediatric Urology, Chldns Hosp Michigan 1997

Pediatrics

Yalamanchi, Krishan MD (Ped) - **Spec Exp:** Neurodevelopmental Disabilities; Brain Injury; Pediatric Rehabilitation; **Hospital:** Children's Specialized Hosp, Robert Wood Johnson Univ Hosp - New Brunswick; **Address:** 200 Somerset St, New Brunswick, NJ 08901; **Phone:** 732-258-7065; **Board Cert:** Pediatrics 2011; Neurodevelopmental Disabilities 2004; **Med School:** India 1981; **Resid:** Pediatrics, Newark Beth Israel Med Ctr 1987; **Fac Appt:** Asst Clin Prof Ped, UMDNJ-RW Johnson Med Sch

Physical Medicine & Rehabilitation

Brown, David P DO (PMR) - **Spec Exp:** Sports Medicine; Electrodiagnosis; Electromyography; **Hospital:** JFK Med Ctr - Edison; **Address:** JFK Johnson Rehabilitation Inst, 65 James St, Edison, NJ 08820; **Phone:** 732-321-7070; **Board Cert:** Physical Medicine & Rehabilitation 1990; Sports Medicine 2007; **Med School:** Philadelphia Coll Osteo Med 1985; **Resid:** Physical Medicine & Rehabilitation, Walter Reed AMC 1989

Fantasia, Michele E MD (PMR) - **Spec Exp:** Pediatric Rehabilitation; Spinal Cord Injury-Pediatric; Cerebral Palsy; Neuromuscular Disorders; **Hospital:** Children's Specialized Hosp, Robert Wood Johnson Univ Hosp - New Brunswick; **Address:** Pediatric Phys Med & Rehab, 200 Somerset St, New Brunswick, NJ 08901; **Phone:** 732-258-7065; **Board Cert:** Pediatrics 2007; Physical Medicine & Rehabilitation 2010; Spinal Cord Injury Medicine 2012; Pediatric Rehabilitation Medicine 2004; **Med School:** UMDNJ-NJ Med Sch, Newark 1994; **Resid:** Physical Medicine & Rehabilitation, Univ Hosp-UMDNJ 1999; **Fac Appt:** Asst Prof PMR, UMDNJ-NJ Med Sch, Newark

Greenwald, Brian D MD (PMR) - **Spec Exp:** Stroke Rehabilitation; Brain Injury Rehabilitation; **Hospital:** JFK Med Ctr - Edison; **Address:** JFK Johnson Rehab Inst, 65 James St, Edison, NJ 08818; **Phone:** 732-321-7000 x68121; **Board Cert:** Physical Medicine & Rehabilitation 2010; **Med School:** SUNY Stony Brook 1995; **Resid:** Physical Medicine & Rehabilitation, Univ Hosp 1999; **Fellow:** Physical Medicine & Rehabilitation, Med Coll Va 2000; **Fac Appt:** Assoc Clin Prof PMR, UMDNJ-RW Johnson Med Sch

Plastic Surgery

Borah, Gregory L MD (PlS) - **Spec Exp:** Cosmetic Surgery-Face; Cosmetic Surgery-Breast; Hand Surgery; **Hospital:** Robert Wood Johnson Univ Hosp - New Brunswick, St. Peter's Univ Hosp; **Address:** RWJUH Div Plastic Surgery, 1 Robert Wood Johnson MEB 506, Box 19, New Brunswick, NJ 08901-1928; **Phone:** 732-235-7865; **Board Cert:** Plastic Surgery 2008; **Med School:** Harvard Med Sch 1978; **Resid:** Surgery, Mass Genl Hosp 1983; Plastic Surgery, Yale-New Haven Hosp 1985; **Fac Appt:** Prof PlS, UMDNJ-RW Johnson Med Sch

Herbstman, Robert A MD (PlS) - **Spec Exp:** Breast Cosmetic & Reconstructive Surgery; Liposuction & Body Contouring; Facial Rejuvenation; Minimally Invasive Surgery; **Hospital:** Robert Wood Johnson Univ Hosp - New Brunswick, Riverview Med Ctr; **Address:** 579A Cranbury Rd, Ste 202, East Brunswick, NJ 08816; **Phone:** 732-254-1919; **Board Cert:** Plastic Surgery 1992; **Med School:** Univ Rochester 1982; **Resid:** Surgery, RW Johnson Univ Hosp 1987; Plastic Surgery, Univ Hosp 1989; **Fac Appt:** Asst Clin Prof S, UMDNJ-RW Johnson Med Sch

Kaufman, Matthew R MD (PlS) - **Spec Exp:** Rhinoplasty; Rhinoplasty Revision; Cosmetic Surgery-Breast; Peripheral Nerve Surgery; **Hospital:** Somerset Med Ctr, Jersey Shore Univ Med Ctr; **Address:** 30 Rehill Ave, Ste 3400, Somerville, NJ 08876; **Phone:** 908-927-8993; **Board Cert:** Plastic Surgery 2007; Otolaryngology 2004; **Med School:** SUNY Upstate Med Univ 1998; **Resid:** Surgery, Mount Sinai Med Ctr 1999; Otolaryngology, Mount Sinai Med Ctr 2003; **Fellow:** Plastic Surgery, UCLA Med Ctr 2005; **Fac Appt:** Asst Clin Prof S, Drexel Univ Coll Med

Nini, Kevin T MD (PlS) - **Spec Exp:** Cosmetic Surgery-Face; Cosmetic Surgery-Breast; Liposuction & Body Contouring; **Hospital:** St. Peter's Univ Hosp; **Address:** PSANJ, 78 Easton Ave Fl 2, New Brunswick, NJ 08901; **Phone:** 732-418-0709; **Board Cert:** Plastic Surgery 1994; **Med School:** UMDNJ-RW Johnson Med Sch 1984; **Resid:** Surgery, Hosp Univ Penn 1989; Plastic Surgery, Shands at Univ FL 1991; **Fellow:** Plastic Surgery, Univ Miami Hosp 1992

Wey, Philip D MD (PlS) - **Spec Exp:** Cosmetic Surgery-Face; Breast Cosmetic & Reconstructive Surgery; Liposuction & Body Contouring; **Hospital:** Robert Wood Johnson Univ Hosp - New Brunswick, St. Peter's Univ Hosp; **Address:** 78 Easton Ave, Fl 2, New Brunswick, NJ 08901-1838; **Phone:** 732-418-0709; **Board Cert:** Plastic Surgery 2007; **Med School:** Brown Univ 1986; **Resid:** Surgery, Northwestern Meml Hosp 1990; Plastic Surgery, New York Hosp 1992; **Fellow:** Breast Surgery, NYU/Meml Sloan-Kettering Cancer Ctr 1993; **Fac Appt:** Assoc Clin Prof S, UMDNJ-RW Johnson Med Sch

Psychiatry

Jones Jr, Frank A MD (Psyc) - **Spec Exp:** Depression; Anxiety & Mood Disorders; Psychotherapy; **Address:** 2186 Route 27, Ste 2A, North Brunswick, NJ 08902; **Phone:** 732-422-0800; **Board Cert:** Psychiatry 1977; **Med School:** Case West Res Univ 1972; **Resid:** Psychiatry, Boston State Hosp 1973; Psychiatry, Worcester State Hosp 1975; **Fac Appt:** Clin Prof Psyc, UMDNJ-Rutgers Med Sch

Menza, Matthew A MD (Psyc) - **Spec Exp:** Psychopharmacology; Depression; Anxiety Disorders; **Hospital:** Robert Wood Johnson Univ Hosp - New Brunswick; **Address:** 671 Hoes Ln, Fl 3, Piscataway, NJ 08854; **Phone:** 732-235-7647; **Board Cert:** Psychiatry 1985; **Med School:** Temple Univ 1980; **Resid:** Psychiatry, NYU-Bellevue Hosp 1984; **Fellow:** Psychosomatic Medicine, Mass Genl Hosp 1985; **Fac Appt:** Prof Psyc, UMDNJ-RW Johnson Med Sch

Pulmonary Disease

Goldberg, Jory MD (Pul) - **Spec Exp:** Lung Disease; Asthma; **Hospital:** Univ Med Ctr Princeton at Plainsboro; **Address:** 18 Centre Drive, Ste 103, Monroe Township, NJ 08831-1564; **Phone:** 609-655-1700; **Board Cert:** Internal Medicine 1981; Pulmonary Disease 1984; Critical Care Medicine 2007; **Med School:** Mexico 1976; **Resid:** Internal Medicine, City Hosp Ctr Elmhurst 1979; Internal Medicine, Monmouth Hosp 1980; **Fellow:** Pulmonary Disease, St Barnabas Med Ctr 1981; Pulmonary Disease, Bergen Reg Med Ctr 1982

Goldblatt, Kenneth H MD (Pul) - **Spec Exp:** Asthma; Emphysema; Sarcoidosis; **Hospital:** Univ Med Ctr Princeton at Plainsboro; **Address:** Princeton Healthcare Med Assoc, 5 Plainsboro Rd Fl 3 - Ste 300, Plainsboro, NJ 08536; **Phone:** 609-853-7272; **Board Cert:** Internal Medicine 1975; Pulmonary Disease 1978; **Med School:** NY Med Coll 1972; **Resid:** Internal Medicine, UMDNJ-Rutgers Affil Hosp 1975; **Fellow:** Pulmonary Disease, UMDNJ-Rutgers Affil Hosp 1977; **Fac Appt:** Assoc Prof Med, UMDNJ-RW Johnson Med Sch

Harangozo, Andrea M MD (Pul) - **Hospital:** Robert Wood Johnson Univ Hosp - New Brunswick, St. Peter's Univ Hosp; **Address:** Pulmonary/Intensive Care Specialists NJ, 593 Cranbury Rd, Ste 1-A, East Brunswick, NJ 08816-4029; **Phone:** 732-613-8880; **Board Cert:** Internal Medicine 1989; Pulmonary Disease 2005; Critical Care Medicine 2005; **Med School:** NYU Sch Med 1984; **Resid:** Internal Medicine, RW Johnson Univ Hosp 1987; **Fellow:** Pulmonary Critical Care Medicine, RW Johnson Univ Hosp 1990; **Fac Appt:** Asst Clin Prof Med, UMDNJ-RW Johnson Med Sch

Melillo, Nicholas MD (Pul) - **Spec Exp:** Chronic Obstructive Lung Disease (COPD); Lung Cancer; Asthma; **Hospital:** JFK Med Ctr - Edison; **Address:** 106 James St, Edison, NJ 08820-3945; **Phone:** 732-906-0091; **Board Cert:** Internal Medicine 1983; Pulmonary Disease 1986; Critical Care Medicine 2007; **Med School:** UMDNJ-NJ Med Sch, Newark 1979; **Resid:** Internal Medicine, St Michael's Med Ctr 1983; **Fellow:** Pulmonary Disease, St Michael's Med Ctr 1985; Critical Care Medicine, St Michael's Med Ctr 1986; **Fac Appt:** Assoc Clin Prof Med, Seton Hall Univ Sch Hlth & Med Scis

Riley, David J MD (Pul) - **Spec Exp:** Pulmonary Fibrosis; Interstitial Lung Disease; **Hospital:** Robert Wood Johnson Univ Hosp - New Brunswick; **Address:** RWJ Pulmonary/Critical Care, 125 Patterson St, Ste 5100, New Brunswick, NJ 08901; **Phone:** 732-235-7840; **Board Cert:** Internal Medicine 1980; Pulmonary Disease 1974; **Med School:** Univ MD Sch Med 1968; **Resid:** Internal Medicine, Baltimore City Hosps 1970; Internal Medicine, Johns Hopkins Hosp 1973; **Fellow:** Pulmonary Disease, Hosp Univ Penn 1972; **Fac Appt:** Prof Med, UMDNJ-RW Johnson Med Sch

Sotolongo, Anays MD (Pul) - **Spec Exp:** Sleep Medicine; Sleep & Snoring Disorders; Interventional Pulmonology; Critical Care; **Hospital:** Robert Wood Johnson Univ Hosp - New Brunswick; **Address:** RWJ Medical Group-Pulmonary Disease, 1 Robert Wood Johnson Pl, MEB 568, New Brunswick, NJ 08901; **Phone:** 732-235-7840; **Board Cert:** Internal Medicine 2008; Pulmonary Disease 2008; Critical Care Medicine 2009; Sleep Medicine ; **Med School:** SUNY Buffalo 1992; **Resid:** Internal Medicine, Robert Wood Johnson Univ Hosp 1995; **Fellow:** Pulmonary Critical Care Medicine, Robert Wood Johnson Univ Hosp 1998; **Fac Appt:** Asst Prof Med, UMDNJ-Rutgers Med Sch

Radiation Oncology

Baumann, John MD (RadRO) - **Spec Exp:** Breast Cancer; Cervical Cancer; Prostate Cancer; **Hospital:** Univ Med Ctr Princeton at Plainsboro, Hunterdon Med Ctr; **Address:** Univ Med Ctr Princeton-Dept Rad Onc, One Plainsboro Rd, Plainsboro, NJ 08536; **Phone:** 609-853-6770; **Board Cert:** Radiation Oncology 1981; **Med School:** Harvard Med Sch 1977; **Resid:** Internal Medicine, Walter Reed AMC 1978; Radiation Oncology, Harvard Joint Program 1981

Haas, Alexander MD (RadRO) - **Spec Exp:** Breast Cancer; Prostate Cancer; **Hospital:** St. Peter's Univ Hosp, Robert Wood Johnson Univ Hosp - New Brunswick; **Address:** 254 Easton Ave, New Brunswick, NJ 08901; **Phone:** 732-745-8590; **Board Cert:** Radiation Oncology 1972; **Med School:** Croatia 1962; **Resid:** Diagnostic Radiology, Univ WA Med Ctr 1968; Radiation Oncology, Univ WA Med Ctr 1972; **Fellow:** Neoplastic Diseases, Thomas Jefferson Univ Hosp 1973; **Fac Appt:** Assoc Clin Prof Rad, UMDNJ-RW Johnson Med Sch

Haffty, Bruce G MD (RadRO) - **Spec Exp:** Breast Cancer; Head & Neck Cancer; **Hospital:** Robert Wood Johnson Univ Hosp - New Brunswick; **Address:** The Cancer Institute of New Jersey, 195 Little Albany St, rm 2038, New Brunswick, NJ 08903; **Phone:** 732-253-3939; **Board Cert:** Radiation Oncology 1988; **Med School:** Yale Univ 1984; **Resid:** Therapeutic Radiology, Yale-New Haven Hosp 1985; Radiation Oncology, Yale-New Haven Hosp 1988; **Fac Appt:** Prof RadRO, UMDNJ-RW Johnson Med Sch

Macher, Mark MD (RadRO) - **Hospital:** JFK Med Ctr - Edison; **Address:** JFK Med Ctr, Mid-State Rad Oncology, 65 James St, Edison, NJ 08818; **Phone:** 732-321-7167; **Board Cert:** Radiation Oncology 1986; **Med School:** Howard Univ 1982; **Resid:** Diagnostic Radiology, New York Univ Med Ctr 1985; **Fellow:** Radiation Oncology, Univ Hosp 1986

Soffen, Edward MD (RadRO) - **Spec Exp:** Prostate Cancer; Breast Cancer; Brachytherapy; **Hospital:** Univ Med Ctr Princeton at Plainsboro, CentraState Med Ctr; **Address:** Med Ctr Princeton-Dept Rad Onc, One Plainsboro Rd, Plainsboro, NJ 08536; **Phone:** 609-853-6770; **Board Cert:** Radiation Oncology 1991; **Med School:** Temple Univ 1986; **Resid:** Radiation Oncology, Hosp Univ Penn 1990; **Fac Appt:** Asst Clin Prof RadRO, UMDNJ-RW Johnson Med Sch

Rheumatology

Lichtbroun, Alan S MD (Rhu) - **Spec Exp:** Rheumatoid Arthritis; Sjogren's Syndrome; Fibromyalgia; **Hospital:** Robert Wood Johnson Univ Hosp - New Brunswick, St. Peter's Univ Hosp; **Address:** 63 Brunswick Woods Dr, East Brunswick, NJ 08816-5601; **Phone:** 732-613-1900; **Board Cert:** Internal Medicine 1980; Rheumatology 1984; **Med School:** SUNY Downstate 1977; **Resid:** Internal Medicine, LI Jewish-Hillside Med Ctr 1980; **Fellow:** Rheumatology, Mt Sinai Hosp 1982; **Fac Appt:** Asst Clin Prof Med, UMDNJ-RW Johnson Med Sch

Surgery

August, David A MD (S) - **Spec Exp:** Pancreatic Cancer; Esophageal Cancer; Stomach Cancer; Sarcoma-Soft Tissue; **Hospital:** Robert Wood Johnson Univ Hosp - New Brunswick; **Address:** Cancer Inst of New Jersey, 195 Little Albany St, New Brunswick, NJ 08903; **Phone:** 732-235-7701; **Board Cert:** Surgery 2005; **Med School:** Yale Univ 1980; **Resid:** Surgery, Yale-New Haven Hosp 1986; **Fellow:** Surgical Oncology, Natl Cancer Inst 1984; **Fac Appt:** Prof S, UMDNJ-RW Johnson Med Sch

Chung-Loy, Harold E MD (S) - **Spec Exp:** Laparoscopic Surgery; Breast Surgery; Vascular Surgery; **Hospital:** JFK Med Ctr - Edison, Robert Wood Johnson Univ Hosp at Rahway; **Address:** 98 James St, Ste 202, Edison, NJ 08820-3902; **Phone:** 732-548-1000; **Board Cert:** Surgery 2007; **Med School:** Howard Univ 1980; **Resid:** Surgery, Mount Sinai Hosp 1985

Dasmahapatra, Kumar MD (S) - **Spec Exp:** Cancer Surgery; Breast Surgery; Laparoscopic Surgery; Pancreatic Surgery; **Hospital:** Raritan Bay Med Ctr - Perth Amboy, JFK Med Ctr - Edison; **Address:** Comprehensive Surgical Assocs, 225 May St, Ste A, Edison, NJ 08837; **Phone:** 732-346-5400; **Board Cert:** Surgery 2009; **Med School:** India 1973; **Resid:** Surgery, Grace Hosp 1979; **Fellow:** Surgical Oncology, Roswell Park Meml Inst 1982; **Fac Appt:** Assoc Clin Prof S, UMDNJ-NJ Med Sch, Newark

Goydos, James S MD (S) - **Spec Exp:** Cancer Surgery; Melanoma; Skin Cancer; Sarcoma-Soft Tissue; **Hospital:** Robert Wood Johnson Univ Hosp - New Brunswick, St. Peter's Univ Hosp; **Address:** Cancer Inst NJ, 195 Little Albany St, Ste 3000, New Brunswick, NJ 08901; **Phone:** 732-235-7563; **Board Cert:** Surgery 2004; **Med School:** UMDNJ-RW Johnson Med Sch 1988; **Resid:** Surgery, New Britain Genl Hosp 1993; **Fellow:** Surgical Oncology, UPMC 1995; **Fac Appt:** Prof S, UMDNJ-RW Johnson Med Sch

Jordan III, Lawrence J MD (S) - **Spec Exp:** Laparoscopic Surgery; Endoscopic Surgery; Cancer Surgery; Hernia; **Hospital:** Univ Med Ctr Princeton at Plainsboro; **Address:** Princeton Surgical Assocs, 5 Plainsboro Rd, Ste 400, Princeton, NJ 08536; **Phone:** 609-936-9100; **Board Cert:** Surgery 2009; **Med School:** Cornell Univ-Weill Med Coll 1983; **Resid:** Surgery, NY-Presby/Columbia Univ Med Ctr 1988

Kearney, Thomas J MD (S) - **Spec Exp:** Breast Cancer; **Hospital:** Robert Wood Johnson Univ Hosp - New Brunswick, St. Peter's Univ Hosp; **Address:** Cancer Inst NJ, 195 Little Albany St, Ste 3000, New Brunswick, NJ 08901; **Phone:** 732-235-7563; **Board Cert:** Surgery 2012; **Med School:** Georgetown Univ 1984; **Resid:** Surgery, Cedars-Sinai Med Ctr 1992; **Fellow:** Surgical Oncology, Univ Chicago Med Ctr 1995; **Fac Appt:** Assoc Prof S, UMDNJ-RW Johnson Med Sch

McManus, Susan A MD (S) - **Spec Exp:** Breast Surgery; Cancer Surgery; **Hospital:** St. Peter's Univ Hosp; **Address:** Breast Ctr, 24 Easton Ave, New Brunswick, NJ 08901; **Phone:** 732-846-3300; **Board Cert:** Surgery 2006; **Med School:** Mexico 1979; **Resid:** Surgery, Beth Israel Med Ctr 1985; **Fac Appt:** Asst Clin Prof S, UMDNJ-RW Johnson Med Sch

Trooskin, Stanley Z MD (S) - **Spec Exp:** Minimally Invasive Surgery; Thyroid Cancer; Parathyroid Surgery; Gastrointestinal Surgery; **Hospital:** Robert Wood Johnson Univ Hosp - New Brunswick; **Address:** UMDNJ-RWJ, Surgery Dept, Cab Bldg Fl 4 - Ste 4100, 125 Paterson St, New Brunswick, NJ 08901; **Phone:** 732-235-7763; **Board Cert:** Surgery 2010; **Med School:** Univ Pittsburgh 1975; **Resid:** Surgery, NYU Med Ctr 1980; **Fac Appt:** Prof S

Thoracic & Cardiac Surgery

Heim, John A MD (T&CS) - **Spec Exp:** Cardiothoracic Surgery; Pacemakers; **Hospital:** Univ Med Ctr Princeton at Plainsboro; **Address:** Univ Med Ctr at Princeton, 5 Plainsboro Rd, Ste 260, Plainsboro, NJ 08536; **Phone:** 609-853-7200; **Board Cert:** Thoracic & Cardiac Surgery 2002; **Med School:** UMDNJ-RW Johnson Med Sch 1985; **Resid:** Surgery, Hartford Hosp 1991; **Fellow:** Thoracic Oncology, Meml Sloan-Kettering Cancer Ctr 1992; Cardiothoracic Surgery, Rush Presby-St Lukes Med Ctr 1994; **Fac Appt:** Prof S

Lee, Leonard Y MD (T&CS) - **Spec Exp:** Coronary Artery Surgery; Minimally Invasive Cardiac Surgery; Heart Failure; Gene Therapy-Cardiac Angiogenesis; **Hospital:** Robert Wood Johnson Univ Hosp - New Brunswick; **Address:** RWJ Univ Hosp, Cardiothoracic Surgery, 1 RW Johnson Pl, MED 508, Box 19, New Brunswick, NJ 08903; **Phone:** 732-235-8725; **Board Cert:** Surgery 2011; Thoracic & Cardiac Surgery 2013; **Med School:** UMDNJ-RW Johnson Med Sch 1992; **Resid:** Surgery, St Vincents Hosp 1997; **Fellow:** Thoracic & Cardiac Surgery, NY-Presby/Weill Cornell Med Ctr 2001; **Fac Appt:** Assoc Prof T&CS, UMDNJ-RW Johnson Med Sch

Urology

Richards, Steven L MD (U) - **Spec Exp:** Kidney Stones; Erectile Dysfunction; Prostate Benign Disease; **Hospital:** St. Peter's Univ Hosp, Robert Wood Johnson Univ Hosp - New Brunswick; **Address:** Mid-Jersey Urology, 333 Forsgate Drive, Ste 202, Jamesburg, NJ 08831-1567; **Phone:** 732-561-2058; **Board Cert:** Urology 2009; **Med School:** Albert Einstein Coll Med 1993; **Resid:** Surgery, Montefiore Med Ctr 1995; Urology, Montefiore Med Ctr 1999

Solomon, Michael J MD (U) - **Hospital:** St. Peter's Univ Hosp, Robert Wood Johnson Univ Hosp - New Brunswick; **Address:** GU Surgeons NJ, 579A Cranbury Rd, Ste 105, East Brunswick, NJ 08816; **Phone:** 732-390-8700; **Board Cert:** Urology 1981; **Med School:** Univ Pennsylvania 1973; **Resid:** Surgery, Beth Israel Deaconess Med Ctr 1976; Urology, Lahey Clin 1979; **Fellow:** Pediatric Urology, Mass Genl Hosp 1981; **Fac Appt:** Assoc Clin Prof U, UMDNJ-RW Johnson Med Sch

Weiss, Robert E MD (U) - **Spec Exp:** Bladder Cancer; Kidney Cancer; Testicular Cancer; Robotic Surgery; **Hospital:** Robert Wood Johnson Univ Hosp - New Brunswick; **Address:** 1 Robert Wood Johnson Pl Ste MB588, Dept Urology, New Brunswick, NJ 08901-1928; **Phone:** 732-235-7960; **Board Cert:** Urology 2004; **Med School:** NYU Sch Med 1985; **Resid:** Surgery, Mount Sinai Med Ctr 1987; Urology, Mount Sinai Med Ctr 1991; **Fellow:** Urologic Oncology, Meml Sloan Kettering Cancer Ctr 1994; **Fac Appt:** Assoc Prof U, UMDNJ-RW Johnson Med Sch

Vascular & Interventional Radiology

Censullo, Michael MD (VIR) - **Spec Exp:** Interventional Radiology; **Hospital:** Robert Wood Johnson Univ Hosp - New Brunswick; **Address:** 579A Cranbury Rd, East Brunswick, NJ 08816; **Phone:** 732-390-0040; **Board Cert:** Diagnostic Radiology ; Vascular & Interventional Radiology ; **Med School:** Georgetown Univ 1997; **Resid:** Diagnostic Radiology, Univ TX Hlth Sci Ctr 2000; **Fellow:** Vascular & Interventional Radiology, MD Anderson Cancer Ctr 2003

Denny, Donald F MD (VIR) - **Spec Exp:** Uterine Fibroid Embolization; **Hospital:** Univ Med Ctr Princeton at Plainsboro; **Address:** Princeton Radiology Assocs, 1 Plainsboro Rd, Plainsboro, NJ 08536; **Phone:** 609-497-4310; **Board Cert:** Diagnostic Radiology 1982; Vascular & Interventional Radiology 2005; **Med School:** Hahnemann Univ 1978; **Resid:** Diagnostic Radiology, Yale-New Haven Hosp 1982; **Fellow:** Cardiovascular Radiology, Brigham & Womens Hosp 1983; **Fac Appt:** Assoc Clin Prof Rad, Yale Univ

Nosher, John L MD (VIR) - **Spec Exp:** Endovascular Surgery; Uterine Fibroid Embolization; Interventional Oncology; Liver Cancer; **Hospital:** Robert Wood Johnson Univ Hosp - New Brunswick; **Address:** RW Johnson Univ Hosp, Radiology Dept, 125 Paterson St, MEB 404, Box 19, New Brunswick, NJ 08901; **Phone:** 732-390-0040; **Board Cert:** Diagnostic Radiology 1975; Vascular & Interventional Radiology 2005; **Med School:** Jefferson Med Coll 1970; **Resid:** Diagnostic Radiology, NY-Presby/Columbia Univ Med Ctr 1975; **Fac Appt:** Clin Prof Rad, UMDNJ-RW Johnson Med Sch

Vascular Surgery

Goldman, Kenneth A MD (VascS) - **Spec Exp:** Carotid Artery Surgery; Aneurysm-Aortic; Varicose Veins; Endovascular Surgery; **Hospital:** Univ Med Ctr Princeton at Plainsboro; **Address:** Princeton Surgical Assocs, 5 Plainsboro Rd, Ste 400, Princeton, NJ 08536; **Phone:** 609-936-9100; **Board Cert:** Surgery 2003; Vascular Surgery 2004; **Med School:** NYU Sch Med 1988; **Resid:** Surgery, Bellevue Hosp 1993; **Fellow:** Vascular Surgery, NYU Med Ctr 1994

Graham, Alan M MD (VascS) - **Spec Exp:** Endovascular Surgery; Aneurysm-Abdominal & Thoracic Aortic; Carotid Artery Surgery; Peripheral Vascular Disease; **Hospital:** Robert Wood Johnson Univ Hosp - New Brunswick; **Address:** RWJ Univ Hosp, Vascular Surgery Dept, 125 Paterson St, MEB 541, New Brunswick, NJ 08901; **Phone:** 732-235-8770; **Board Cert:** Vascular Surgery 2006; **Med School:** Canada 1979; **Resid:** Surgery, McGill Univ Med Ctr 1984; **Fellow:** Vascular Surgery, Univ Chicago Med Ctr 1985; **Fac Appt:** Prof VascS, UMDNJ-RW Johnson Med Sch

Monmouth

Monmouth

Allergy & Immunology

Gross, Gary L MD (A&I) - **Spec Exp:** Asthma; Cough-Chronic; Sinus Disorders; Atopic Dermatitis; **Hospital:** Jersey Shore Univ Med Ctr, Monmouth Med Ctr; **Address:** Atlantic Allergy, Asthma, & Immunology, 802 W Park Ave, Ste 213, Ocean Township, NJ 07712; **Phone:** 732-695-2555; **Board Cert:** Allergy & Immunology 1987; Pediatrics 1986; **Med School:** NYU Sch Med 1981; **Resid:** Pediatrics, Chldns Natl Med Ctr 1984; **Fellow:** Allergy & Immunology, Chldns Hosp 1986; **Fac Appt:** Asst Clin Prof Ped, UMDNJ-RW Johnson Med Sch

Hirsch, Andrew C MD (A&I) - **Spec Exp:** Asthma; Sinusitis; Allergic Rhinitis; Eczema; **Hospital:** Riverview Med Ctr, Monmouth Med Ctr; **Address:** 258 Broad Steet, Red Bank, NJ 07701-5623; **Phone:** 732-741-8900; **Board Cert:** Allergy & Immunology 2005; **Med School:** Temple Univ 1988; **Resid:** Pediatrics, New York Hosp 1991; **Fellow:** Allergy & Immunology, Thomas Jefferson Univ Hosp 1993

Picone, Frank J MD (A&I) - **Spec Exp:** Asthma; Sinus Disorders; Allergy; **Hospital:** Riverview Med Ctr, Monmouth Med Ctr; **Address:** Allergy & Asthma Grp, 709 Sycamore Ave, Tinton Falls, NJ 07701; **Phone:** 732-747-8188; **Board Cert:** Pediatrics 1973; Allergy & Immunology 1975; **Med School:** UMDNJ-NJ Med Sch, Newark 1967; **Resid:** Pediatrics, Jackson Meml Hosp 1970; **Fellow:** Allergy & Immunology, Chldns Hosp 1974; **Fac Appt:** Asst Clin Prof Ped, Drexel Univ Coll Med

Sher, Ellen R MD (A&I) - **Spec Exp:** Asthma & Sinusitis; Nasal Allergy; Insect Allergies; Immune Deficiency; **Hospital:** Monmouth Med Ctr, Jersey Shore Univ Med Ctr; **Address:** Atlantic Allergy, Asthma & Immunology, 802 W Park Ave, Ste 213, Ocean Township, NJ 07712; **Phone:** 732-695-2555; **Board Cert:** Internal Medicine 1989; Allergy & Immunology 2003; **Med School:** Georgetown Univ 1986; **Resid:** Internal Medicine, Thomas Jefferson Univ Hosp 1989; **Fellow:** Pulmonary Disease, Thomas Jefferson Univ Hosp 1990; Allergy & Immunology, Natl Jewish Hlth 1992; **Fac Appt:** Asst Clin Prof Med, Drexel Univ Coll Med

Cardiovascular Disease

Beauregard, Lou-Anne M MD (Cv) - **Spec Exp:** Arrhythmias; Heart Disease in Women; Pacemakers; **Hospital:** CentraState Med Ctr; **Address:** Heart Specialists, 901 W Main St, Ste 205, Freehold, NJ 07728; **Phone:** 732-866-0800; **Board Cert:** Internal Medicine 1983; Cardiovascular Disease 1985; Cardiac Electrophysiology 2012; Nuclear Cardiology 2005; **Med School:** Med Coll PA 1980; **Resid:** Internal Medicine, Temple Univ Hosp 1983; **Fellow:** Cardiovascular Disease, Med Coll Penn Affil Hosp 1985; Cardiac Electrophysiology, Cooper Hosp 1986; **Fac Appt:** Assoc Clin Prof Med, UMDNJ-RW Johnson Med Sch

Daniels, Jeffrey S MD (Cv) - **Hospital:** Monmouth Med Ctr, Jersey Shore Univ Med Ctr; **Address:** 215 Brighton Ave, Long Branch, NJ 07740; **Phone:** 732-222-5143; **Board Cert:** Internal Medicine 1983; Cardiovascular Disease 1985; **Med School:** Albany Med Coll 1980; **Resid:** Internal Medicine, Mt Sinai Hosp 1983; **Fellow:** Cardiovascular Disease, Mt Sinai Hosp 1985; **Fac Appt:** Asst Clin Prof Med, Drexel Univ Coll Med

Child Neurology

Barabas, Ronald E MD (ChiN) - **Spec Exp:** Pediatric Neurology; Developmental Disorders; Neurogenetics; Metabolic Disorders; **Hospital:** Monmouth Med Ctr; **Address:** Child Neurology Associates, 3350 Highway 138W, Ste 117, Wall, NJ 07719; **Phone:** 732-556-0200; **Board Cert:** Child Neurology 2007; Clinical Genetics 2010; Neurodevelopmental Disabilities 2007; **Med School:** UMDNJ-Rutgers Med Sch 1986; **Resid:** Pediatrics, Buffalo Chldns Hosp 1988; **Fellow:** Pediatric Neurology, Chldns Hosp of Pittsburgh 1991; Pediatric Metabolism, Chldns Hosp of Philadelphia 1993; **Fac Appt:** Asst Clin Prof Ped, Drexel Univ Coll Med

Colon & Rectal Surgery

Arvanitis, Michael L MD (CRS) - **Spec Exp:** Laparoscopic Surgery; Colon & Rectal Cancer; Ulcerative Colitis; **Hospital:** Monmouth Med Ctr, Riverview Med Ctr; **Address:** Specialty Surgical Assoc, 10 Industrial Way E, Ste 104, Eatontown, NJ 07724; **Phone:** 732-389-1331; **Board Cert:** Sports Medicine 2008; Colon & Rectal Surgery 2008; **Med School:** Hahnemann Univ 1982; **Resid:** Surgery, St Vincent's Hosp 1987; **Fellow:** Colon & Rectal Surgery, Cleveland Clinic 1988; **Fac Appt:** Asst Clin Prof S, Hahnemann Univ

Dermatology

Grossman, Kenneth A MD (D) - **Spec Exp:** Psoriasis; Skin Cancer; Cutaneous Lymphoma; Cosmetic Dermatology; **Hospital:** Riverview Med Ctr; **Address:** 180 White Rd, Ste 103, Little Silver, NJ 07739-1166; **Phone:** 732-842-5222; **Board Cert:** Internal Medicine 1980; Dermatology 1983; **Med School:** SUNY Hlth Sci Ctr 1977; **Resid:** Internal Medicine, Nassau County Med Ctr 1980; Dermatology, Montefiore Med Ctr 1983

Hametz, Irwin MD (D) - **Hospital:** CentraState Med Ctr; **Address:** 77-55 Schanck Rd, Ste B-3, Freehold, NJ 07728; **Phone:** 732-462-9800; **Board Cert:** Dermatology 1978; **Med School:** NY Med Coll 1973; **Resid:** Pediatrics, Long Island Jewish-Hillside Med Ctr 1975; Dermatology, Brown Univ Affil Hosps 1978; **Fac Appt:** Asst Clin Prof Med, UMDNJ-RW Johnson Med Sch

Orsini, William J MD (D) - **Hospital:** Monmouth Med Ctr; **Address:** 223 Monmouth Rd, W Long Branch, NJ 07764; **Phone:** 732-870-2992; **Board Cert:** Internal Medicine 1975; Dermatology 1977; **Med School:** UMDNJ-NJ Med Sch, Newark 1972; **Resid:** Internal Medicine, Monmouth Med Ctr 1975; Dermatology, Albany Med Ctr 1977

Diagnostic Radiology

Chalal, Jeffrey M MD (DR) - **Hospital:** CentraState Med Ctr; **Address:** Freehold Radiology Grp, 901 W Main St, Ground Fl, Freehold, NJ 07728; **Phone:** 732-462-4844; **Board Cert:** Diagnostic Radiology 1982; **Med School:** Univ Pennsylvania 1977; **Resid:** Diagnostic Radiology, Columbia-Presby Med Ctr 1981; **Fellow:** Cross Sectional Imaging, Columbia-Presby Med Ctr 1982

Endocrinology, Diabetes & Metabolism

Nassberg, Barton MD (EDM) - **Spec Exp:** Thyroid Disorders; Diabetes; **Hospital:** Bayshore Community Hosp; **Address:** 723 N Beers St, Ste 2G, Holmdel, NJ 07733-1512; **Phone:** 732-739-0200; **Board Cert:** Internal Medicine 1982; Endocrinology, Diabetes & Metabolism 1985; **Med School:** Belgium 1979; **Resid:** Internal Medicine, Mountainside Hosp 1982; **Fellow:** Endocrinology, Diabetes & Metabolism, MS Hershey Med Ctr 1984

Family Medicine

Bernardo Jr, Salvatore MD (FMed) *PCP* - **Hospital:** CentraState Med Ctr; **Address:** 4255 Rte 9 N, Ste B, Freehold, NJ 07728; **Phone:** 732-683-9897; **Board Cert:** Family Medicine 2009; **Med School:** UMDNJ-NJ Med Sch, Newark 1993; **Resid:** Family Medicine, Somerset Med Ctr 1996; **Fac Appt:** Asst Clin Prof FMed, UMDNJ-NJ Med Sch, Newark

Catanese, Vincent J MD (FMed) *PCP* - **Spec Exp:** Hypertension; Diabetes; Functional Bowel Disorders; **Address:** 733 N Beers St, Ste U3, Holmdel, NJ 07733; **Phone:** 732-264-8484; **Board Cert:** Family Medicine 2005; **Med School:** Penn State Coll Med 1978; **Resid:** Family Medicine, Conemaugh Valley Meml Hosp 1981

Gastroenterology

Binns, Joseph MD (Ge) - **Spec Exp:** Colonoscopy; **Hospital:** Riverview Med Ctr; **Address:** Red Bank Gastroenterology Assocs, 365 Broad St, Ste 1-E, Red Bank, NJ 07701; **Phone:** 732-842-4294; **Board Cert:** Gastroenterology 2003; **Med School:** UMDNJ-RW Johnson Med Sch 1987; **Resid:** Internal Medicine, Pennsylvania Hosp 1990; **Fellow:** Gastroenterology, Graduate Hosp 1992

Fiest, Thomas DO (Ge) - **Spec Exp:** Colitis; Liver Disease; **Hospital:** Monmouth Med Ctr, Jersey Shore Univ Med Ctr; **Address:** Monmouth Gastroenterology, 142 Highway 35, Ste 103, Eatontown, NJ 07724; **Phone:** 732-389-5004; **Board Cert:** Internal Medicine 1989; Gastroenterology 2005; **Med School:** Philadelphia Coll Osteo Med 1985; **Resid:** Internal Medicine, Monmouth Med Ctr 1990; **Fellow:** Gastroenterology, Jersey City Med Ctr 1993

Ludwig, Shelly L MD (Ge) - **Spec Exp:** Inflammatory Bowel Disease; Hepatitis C; Gastroesophageal Reflux Disease (GERD); Endoscopy; **Hospital:** CentraState Med Ctr; **Address:** 901 W Main St, Ste 106, Freehold, NJ 07728; **Phone:** 732-303-3888; **Board Cert:** Internal Medicine 1977; Gastroenterology 1979; **Med School:** Albert Einstein Coll Med 1974; **Resid:** Internal Medicine, LAC-Harbor UCLA Med Ctr 1977; **Fellow:** Gastroenterology, Wadsworth VA Hosp/UCLA 1979; **Fac Appt:** Assoc Clin Prof Med, UMDNJ-RW Johnson Med Sch

Turtel, Penny S MD (Ge) - **Spec Exp:** Inflammatory Bowel Disease; Celiac Disease; Colon Polyps & Cancer; **Hospital:** Monmouth Med Ctr, Jersey Shore Univ Med Ctr; **Address:** Shore Gastroenterology, 1907 Route 35, Ste 1, Oakhurst, NJ 07755-2760; **Phone:** 732-517-0060; **Board Cert:** Internal Medicine 1989; Gastroenterology 2011; **Med School:** Cornell Univ-Weill Med Coll 1986; **Resid:** Internal Medicine, Mount Sinai Hosp 1989; **Fellow:** Gastroenterology, Mount Sinai Hosp 1991

Geriatric Medicine

Israel, Jessica L MD (Ger) - **Spec Exp:** Palliative Care; **Hospital:** Monmouth Med Ctr; **Address:** Monmouth Med Ctr, Dept Geriatrics, 300 Second Ave, Long Branch, NJ 07740; **Phone:** 732-923-7550; **Board Cert:** Geriatric Medicine 2006; **Med School:** Mount Sinai Sch Med 1995; **Resid:** Internal Medicine, Mt Sinai Med Ctr 1998; **Fellow:** Geriatric Medicine, Mt Sinai Med Ctr 2000

Hand Surgery

Lisser, Steven P MD (HS) - **Spec Exp:** Shoulder Surgery; Wrist/Hand Injuries; Ligament Reconstruction; Sports Medicine; **Hospital:** Riverview Med Ctr, Monmouth Med Ctr; **Address:** Orthopaedic, Sports Med & Rehab Ctr, 80 Oak Hill Rd, Red Bank, NJ 07701; **Phone:** 732-741-2313; **Board Cert:** Orthopaedic Surgery 2007; Hand Surgery 2007; Orthopaedic Sports Medicine 2007; **Med School:** Mount Sinai Sch Med 1987; **Resid:** Orthopaedic Surgery, Mt Sinai Med Ctr 1992; **Fellow:** Hand & Microvascular Surgery, Thom Jefferson Univ 1993; Sports Medicine & Shoulder Surgery, Univ Pennsylvania 1994; **Fac Appt:** Asst Clin Prof OrS, Mount Sinai Sch Med

Hematology

Lerner, William A MD (Hem) - **Spec Exp:** Palliative Care; **Hospital:** Jersey Shore Univ Med Ctr, Ocean Med Ctr; **Address:** 1707 Atlantic Ave, Manasquan, NJ 08736-1147; **Phone:** 732-528-0760; **Board Cert:** Internal Medicine 1980; Hematology 1982; Medical Oncology 1983; Hospice & Palliative Medicine 2008; **Med School:** Belgium 1977; **Resid:** Internal Medicine, Albert Einstein Med Ctr 1980; **Fellow:** Hematology & Oncology, NYU Med Ctr 1983

Topilow, Arthur A MD (Hem) - **Spec Exp:** Lymphoma; Multiple Myeloma; **Hospital:** Jersey Shore Univ Med Ctr, Ocean Med Ctr; **Address:** 1707 Atlantic Ave, Manasquan, NJ 08736-1147; **Phone:** 732-528-0760; **Board Cert:** Internal Medicine 1971; Hematology 1972; Medical Oncology 1981; **Med School:** NY Med Coll 1967; **Resid:** Internal Medicine, Flower/NY Metro Hosp 1970; **Fellow:** Hematology, Flower/NY Metro Hosp 1972; **Fac Appt:** Assoc Clin Prof Med, UMDNJ-NJ Med Sch, Newark

Infectious Disease

Eng, Margaret H MD (Inf) - **Spec Exp:** AIDS/HIV; **Hospital:** Monmouth Med Ctr; **Address:** Monmouth Family Hlth Ctr, 300 Second Ave, Long Branch, NJ 07740; **Phone:** 732-923-7930; **Board Cert:** Internal Medicine 1983; Infectious Disease 2010; **Med School:** Albert Einstein Coll Med 1980; **Resid:** Internal Medicine, Kings Co Hosp 1984; **Fellow:** Infectious Disease, Univ Maryland Med Ctr 1986

Internal Medicine

Courtney, Barbara E MD (IM) *PCP* - **Spec Exp:** Geriatric Medicine; **Hospital:** Monmouth Med Ctr; **Address:** Monmouth Med Grp, 370 Highway 35, Ste 201, Red Bank, NJ 07701; **Phone:** 732-842-0290; **Board Cert:** Internal Medicine 1980; Geriatric Medicine 2012; **Med School:** Hahnemann Univ 1977; **Resid:** Internal Medicine, Monmouth Med Ctr 1980; **Fac Appt:** Med

Glowacki, Jan S MD (IM) *PCP* - **Spec Exp:** Preventive Medicine; Diagnostic Problems; **Hospital:** Riverview Med Ctr, Monmouth Med Ctr; **Address:** Fair Haven Internal Medicine, 569 River Rd, Fair Haven, NJ 07704-3262; **Phone:** 732-530-0100; **Board Cert:** Internal Medicine 1980; **Med School:** Jefferson Med Coll 1977; **Resid:** Internal Medicine, Monmouth Med Ctr 1980

Granet, Kenneth M MD (IM) *PCP* - **Hospital:** Monmouth Med Ctr; **Address:** 166 Morris Ave, Long Branch, NJ 07740; **Phone:** 732-229-2020; **Board Cert:** Internal Medicine 1987; **Med School:** SUNY Downstate 1984; **Resid:** Internal Medicine, N Shore Univ Hosp 1987; **Fac Appt:** Asst Clin Prof Med, Drexel Univ Coll Med

Masterson, Raymond M MD (IM) *PCP* - **Spec Exp:** Hypertension; Diabetes; Cholesterol/Lipid Disorders; Peripheral Vascular Disease; **Hospital:** Jersey Shore Univ Med Ctr; **Address:** 700 Highway 71, Ste 9, Sea Girt, NJ 08750-2804; **Phone:** 732-974-0340; **Board Cert:** Internal Medicine 1986; **Med School:** Philippines 1978; **Resid:** Internal Medicine, St Michaels Med Ctr 1982

Maternal & Fetal Medicine

Gonzalez, David MD (MF) - **Spec Exp:** Pregnancy-High Risk; **Hospital:** Monmouth Med Ctr; **Address:** Monmouth Med Group, 73 S Bath Ave, Long Branch, NJ 07740; **Phone:** 732-870-3600; **Board Cert:** Obstetrics & Gynecology 2012; Maternal & Fetal Medicine 2012; **Med School:** Temple Univ 1990; **Resid:** Obstetrics & Gynecology, Univ Hosp-UMDNJ 1994; **Fellow:** Maternal & Fetal Medicine, Univ Hosp-UMDNJ 1996

Medical Oncology

Fitzgerald, Denis B MD (Onc) - **Spec Exp:** Breast Cancer; Lung Cancer; Colon Cancer; Lymphoma, Non-Hodgkin's; **Hospital:** Riverview Med Ctr; **Address:** 180 White Rd, Ste 101, Little Silver, NJ 07739; **Phone:** 732-530-8666; **Board Cert:** Internal Medicine 1981; Medical Oncology 1985; Hematology 1986; **Med School:** SUNY Downstate 1978; **Resid:** Internal Medicine, St Vincents Hosp Med Ctr 1982; **Fellow:** Hematology & Oncology, Univ Rochester 1985

Greenberg, Susan N MD (Onc) - **Spec Exp:** Breast Cancer; Lung Cancer; Palliative Care; **Hospital:** Jersey Shore Univ Med Ctr, Monmouth Med Ctr; **Address:** 39 Sycamore Ave, Little Silver, NJ 07739-1208; **Phone:** 732-576-8610; **Board Cert:** Internal Medicine 1981; Medical Oncology 1983; **Med School:** Med Coll PA Hahnemann 1978; **Resid:** Internal Medicine, Hosp Med Coll Penn 1981; **Fellow:** Hematology & Oncology, Columbia-Presby Med Ctr 1983

Sharon, David J MD (Onc) - **Spec Exp:** Breast Cancer; Lung Cancer; Gastrointestinal Cancer; Hematologic Malignancies; **Hospital:** Monmouth Med Ctr, CentraState Med Ctr; **Address:** The Cancer Ctr - Monmouth Med Ctr, 100 State Highway 36, Ste 1B, West Long Branch, NJ 07764-6205; **Phone:** 732-222-1711; **Board Cert:** Internal Medicine 1980; Medical Oncology 1983; **Med School:** NY Med Coll 1977; **Resid:** Internal Medicine, Beth Israel Med Ctr 1980; **Fellow:** Medical Oncology, Mount Sinai Med Ctr 1982

Walsh, Christina M MD (Onc) - **Spec Exp:** Cancer Genetics; Breast Cancer; **Hospital:** Riverview Med Ctr; **Address:** 180 White Rd, Ste 101, Little Silver, NJ 07739; **Phone:** 732-530-8666; **Board Cert:** Internal Medicine 1980; Hematology 1982; Medical Oncology 1985; **Med School:** Georgetown Univ 1977; **Resid:** Internal Medicine, Georgetown Univ Hosp 1980; **Fellow:** Hematology, Georgetown Univ Hosp 1981; Hematology & Oncology, NYU Med Ctr 1984

Neonatal-Perinatal Medicine

Graff, Michael MD (NP) - **Spec Exp:** Neonatology; **Hospital:** Jersey Shore Univ Med Ctr, Ocean Med Ctr; **Address:** Jersey Shore Univ Med Ctr, Dept Peds, 1945 State Rte 33, Neptune, NJ 07754; **Phone:** 732-776-4283; **Board Cert:** Pediatrics 1981; Neonatal-Perinatal Medicine 1983; **Med School:** Italy 1977; **Resid:** Pediatrics, NYU Med Ctr 1980; **Fellow:** Neonatology, Columbia-Presby Med Ctr 1982; **Fac Appt:** Assoc Clin Prof Ped, UMDNJ-RW Johnson Med Sch

Nephrology

Flis, Raymond S DO (Nep) - **Spec Exp:** Hypertension; Kidney Disease; **Hospital:** Riverview Med Ctr, Monmouth Med Ctr; **Address:** Hypertension & Nephrology Assocs, 6 Industrial Way W, Ste B, Eatontown, NJ 07724-2268; **Phone:** 732-460-1200; **Board Cert:** Internal Medicine 1974; Nephrology 1976; **Med School:** Kirksville Coll Osteo Med 1971; **Resid:** Internal Medicine, Cooper Hosp 1974; **Fellow:** Nephrology, Thomas Jefferson Univ Hosp 1975; Nephrology, Temple Univ Hosp 1976; **Fac Appt:** Assoc Clin Prof Med, Drexel Univ Coll Med

Manning, Eric C MD/PhD (Nep) - **Spec Exp:** Hypertension; Kidney Disease; Dialysis Care; **Hospital:** Robert Wood Johnson Univ Hosp - New Brunswick, Somerset Med Ctr; **Address:** 719 Route 206, Ste 100, Hillsborough, NJ 08844; **Phone:** 908-904-9055; **Board Cert:** Internal Medicine 1989; Nephrology 2012; **Med School:** UC Davis 1985; **Resid:** Internal Medicine, Boston Univ Hosp 1988; **Fellow:** Nephrology, Boston Univ Hosp 1992

Neurological Surgery

Maggio, William W MD (NS) - **Spec Exp:** Epilepsy; Spinal Surgery; Stroke; Brain Tumors; **Hospital:** Jersey Shore Univ Med Ctr, Ocean Med Ctr; **Address:** Meridian Surgical Assocs, 2101 Rte 34, Ste D, Wall Township, NJ 07719; **Phone:** 732-974-0003; **Board Cert:** Neurological Surgery 1993; **Med School:** Penn State Coll Med 1981; **Resid:** Neurological Surgery, Univ Virginia Hlth Sys 1988; **Fellow:** Neurological Surgery, Meml Sloan-Kettering Canc Ctr 1990

Rosenblum, Bruce R MD (NS) - **Spec Exp:** Spinal Surgery; Brain Tumors; Pain-Back & Neck; Chiari's Deformity; **Hospital:** Riverview Med Ctr, Bayshore Community Hosp; **Address:** 160 Ave at the Commons, Ste 2, Shrewsbury, NJ 07702; **Phone:** 732-460-1522; **Board Cert:** Neurological Surgery 1991; **Med School:** Mount Sinai Sch Med 1982; **Resid:** Neurological Surgery, Mount Sinai Med Ctr 1988; **Fellow:** Stroke, Natl Inst Health 1986

Neurology

Gainey, Patrick J MD (N) - **Hospital:** Robert Wood Johnson Univ Hosp - New Brunswick; **Address:** 23 Kilmer Drive Bldg 1 - Ste E, Morganville, NJ 07751; **Phone:** 732-617-0808; **Board Cert:** Neurology 1993; **Med School:** UMDNJ-RW Johnson Med Sch 1988; **Resid:** Neurology, UMDNJ Med Ctr 1990; **Fellow:** Neurology, UMDNJ Med Ctr 1993

Gilson, Noah R MD (N) - **Spec Exp:** Multiple Sclerosis; Headache; Parkinson's Disease; **Hospital:** Monmouth Med Ctr, Riverview Med Ctr; **Address:** Neurology Specialists of Monmouth County, 107 Monmouth Rd, Ste 110, West Long Branch, NJ 07764; **Phone:** 732-935-1850; **Board Cert:** Neurology 1987; Vascular Neurology 2009; **Med School:** Loyola Univ-Stritch Sch Med 1982; **Resid:** Neurology, Mount Sinai Hosp 1986

Holland, Neil R MD (N) - **Spec Exp:** Neuromuscular Disorders; Peripheral Neuropathy; Electrodiagnosis; Spasticity Management; **Hospital:** Monmouth Med Ctr, Riverview Med Ctr; **Address:** 107 Monmouth Rd, Ste 110, West Long Branch, NJ 07764; **Phone:** 732-935-1850; **Board Cert:** Neurology 2010; Clinical Neurophysiology 2011; Vascular Neurology 2009; Neuromuscular Medicine 2008; **Med School:** England, UK 1991; **Resid:** Neurology, Johns Hopkins Univ Hosp 1996; **Fellow:** Clinical Neurophysiology, Johns Hopkins Univ Hosp 1997; **Fac Appt:** Assoc Prof N, Drexel Univ Coll Med

Silbert, Paul J MD (N) - **Spec Exp:** Parkinson's Disease; Migraine; Carpal Tunnel Syndrome; Alzheimer's Disease; **Hospital:** Jersey Shore Univ Med Ctr; **Address:** 2100 Corlies Ave, Ste 5, Neptune, NJ 07753-6116; **Phone:** 732-776-8866; **Board Cert:** Neurology 1980; **Med School:** Jefferson Med Coll 1971; **Resid:** Neurology, Columbia-Presby Med Ctr 1975; **Fellow:** Neurology, Columbia Univ 1976; **Fac Appt:** Asst Clin Prof N, UMDNJ-RW Johnson Med Sch

Neuroradiology

Lu, Stanley MD (NRad) - **Hospital:** Monmouth Med Ctr; **Address:** Monmouth Med Ctr-Neuroradiology, 300 Second Ave Stanley Bldg - Ste 113, Long Branch, NJ 07740; **Phone:** 732-923-6806; **Board Cert:** Diagnostic Radiology 2004; Neuroradiology 2006; **Med School:** NYU Sch Med 1999; **Resid:** Dermatopathology, NYU Langone Med Ctr 2004; **Fellow:** Neurological Radiology, Stanford Univ Hosp & Clins 2005

Obstetrics & Gynecology

Goldstein, Steven A MD (ObG) - **Spec Exp:** Ultrasound; Menopause Problems; Minimally Invasive Surgery; **Hospital:** CentraState Med Ctr, Monmouth Med Ctr; **Address:** 501 Iron Bridge Rd, Ste 4, Freehold, NJ 07728; **Phone:** 732-431-1807; **Board Cert:** Obstetrics & Gynecology 2012; **Med School:** SUNY Downstate 1985; **Resid:** Obstetrics & Gynecology, Robert Wood Johnson Univ Hosp 1990

Martens, Mark G MD (ObG) - **Spec Exp:** Infections in Pregnancy; Vulvar & Vaginal Disorders; Menopause Problems; Viral Infections; **Hospital:** Jersey Shore Univ Med Ctr; **Address:** Jersey Shore Univ Med Ctr, Dept Ob/Gyn, 1944 Rte 33, Ste 101B, Neptune, NJ 07754; **Phone:** 732-776-3797; **Board Cert:** Obstetrics & Gynecology 2012; **Med School:** Geo Wash Univ 1982; **Resid:** Obstetrics & Gynecology, Hartford Hosp 1986; **Fellow:** Ob/Gyn Infectious Diseases, Baylor Coll Med 1987; **Fac Appt:** Prof ObG, UMDNJ-Rutgers Med Sch

Seigel, Mark J MD (ObG) - **Spec Exp:** Adolescent Gynecology; Minimally Invasive Surgery; Menopause Problems; **Hospital:** CentraState Med Ctr, Monmouth Med Ctr; **Address:** 501 Iron Bridge Rd, Ste 4, Freehold, NJ 07728-5305; **Phone:** 732-431-1807; **Board Cert:** Obstetrics & Gynecology 2012; **Med School:** Geo Wash Univ 1980; **Resid:** Obstetrics & Gynecology, NY-Presby/Columbia Univ Med Ctr 1985

Ophthalmology

Engel, Mark L MD (Oph) - **Spec Exp:** Cataract Surgery; Glaucoma; **Hospital:** Bayshore Community Hosp, Riverview Med Ctr; **Address:** 733 N Beers St, Ste U4, Holmdel, NJ 07733-1528; **Phone:** 732-739-0707; **Board Cert:** Ophthalmology 1977; **Med School:** SUNY Downstate 1971; **Resid:** Ophthalmology, SUNY Downstate Med Ctr 1976

Goldberg, Daniel B MD (Oph) - **Spec Exp:** LASIK-Refractive Surgery; Cornea Transplant; Cataract Surgery; Lens Implants; **Address:** Atlantic Eye Physicians, 180 White Rd, Ste 202, Little Silver, NJ 07739-1166; **Phone:** 732-219-9220; **Board Cert:** Ophthalmology 1979; **Med School:** SUNY Downstate 1974; **Resid:** Ophthalmology, SUNY Downstate 1978; **Fellow:** Cornea, Eye & Ear Hosp 1979; **Fac Appt:** Asst Clin Prof Oph, Drexel Univ Coll Med

Kristan, Ronald W MD (Oph) - **Spec Exp:** Cataract Surgery; Oculoplastic Surgery; **Hospital:** Monmouth Med Ctr; **Address:** Atlantic Eye Physicians, 279 Third Ave, Ste 204, Long Branch, NJ 07740; **Phone:** 732-222-7373; **Board Cert:** Ophthalmology ; **Med School:** NYU Sch Med 1980; **Resid:** Ophthalmology, Albany Memorial Hosp 1984; **Fellow:** Oculoplastic Surgery, Albany Memorial Hosp 1985

Talansky, Marvin L MD (Oph) - **Spec Exp:** Cataract Surgery; Diabetic Eye Disease; LASIK-Refractive Surgery; **Hospital:** Jersey Shore Univ Med Ctr, Monmouth Med Ctr; **Address:** Eye Diag & Surgery Ctr, 3333 Fairmont Ave, Asbury Park, NJ 07712; **Phone:** 732-988-4000; **Board Cert:** Ophthalmology 1978; **Med School:** Med Univ SC 1973; **Resid:** Ophthalmology, Storm Eye Inst 1978; **Fellow:** Retina, Storm Eye Inst 1986

Turtel, Lawrence S MD (Oph) - **Spec Exp:** Pediatric Ophthalmology; Strabismus; **Hospital:** Jersey Shore Univ Med Ctr, Monmouth Med Ctr; **Address:** Eye Diag & Surgery Ctr, 3333 Fairmont Ave, Asbury Park, NJ 07712; **Phone:** 732-988-4000; **Board Cert:** Ophthalmology 2013; **Med School:** Columbia P&S 1986; **Resid:** Ophthalmology, St Vincents Hosp 1991; **Fellow:** Pediatric Ophthalmology, Lenox Hill Hosp (Manh Eye, Ear & Throat Hosp) 1992

Orthopaedic Surgery

Bade III, Harry A MD (OrS) - **Spec Exp:** Joint Replacement; Shoulder Arthroscopic Surgery; Hand Surgery; Arthroscopic Surgery-Knee; **Hospital:** Monmouth Med Ctr, Riverview Med Ctr; **Address:** Professional Orthopedics Assoc, 776 Shrewsbury Ave, Ste 201, Tinton Falls, NJ 07724-3006; **Phone:** 732-530-4949; **Board Cert:** Orthopaedic Surgery 1984; Orthopaedic Sports Medicine 2007; **Med School:** Jefferson Med Coll 1976; **Resid:** Surgery, St. Luke's - Roosevelt Hosp Ctr - Roosevelt Div 1978; Orthopaedic Surgery, Hosp for Special Surg 1981; **Fellow:** Shoulder Surgery, Hosp for Special Surg 1982; Hand Surgery, St. Luke's - Roosevelt Hosp Ctr - Roosevelt Div 1983

Grossman, Robert B MD (OrS) - **Spec Exp:** Knee Surgery; **Hospital:** Monmouth Med Ctr, Riverview Med Ctr; **Address:** Shore Orth Group, 35 Gilbert St S, Tinton Falls, NJ 07701-4917; **Phone:** 732-530-1515; **Board Cert:** Orthopaedic Surgery 1978; **Med School:** Univ MD Sch Med 1972; **Resid:** Orthopaedic Surgery, Univ Vermont Med Ctr 1976; **Fellow:** Sports Medicine, Lenox Hill Hosp 1977; **Fac Appt:** Assoc Prof OrS, Hahnemann Univ

Otolaryngology

Rossos, Apostolos A.P. MD (Oto) - **Spec Exp:** Pediatric Otolaryngology; Sinus Disorders; Hearing Disorders; **Hospital:** CentraState Med Ctr, Robert Wood Johnson Univ Hosp Hamilton; **Address:** 501 Iron Bridge Rd, Ste 11, Freehold, NJ 07728-5305; **Phone:** 732-409-2500; **Board Cert:** Otolaryngology 1988; **Med School:** Grenada 1981; **Resid:** Surgery, UMDNJ-Univ Hosp 1983; Otolaryngology, UMDNJ-Univ Hosp 1986

Scaccia, Frank John MD (Oto) - **Spec Exp:** Cosmetic Surgery-Face; Rhinoplasty; Nasal & Sinus Surgery; Reconstructive Surgery; **Hospital:** Riverview Med Ctr, Bayshore Community Hosp; **Address:** Riverside Plastic Surgery & Sinus Ctr, 70 E Front St, Fl 3, Red Bank, NJ 07701; **Phone:** 732-747-5300; **Board Cert:** Otolaryngology 1993; Facial Plastic & Reconstr Surgery 1995; **Med School:** Wake Forest Univ 1985; **Resid:** Surgery, Monmouth Med Ctr 1988; Otolaryngology, Univ Hosp 1992

Shah, Darsit K MD (Oto) - **Spec Exp:** Head & Neck Cancer & Surgery; Thyroid & Parathyroid Surgery; Parotid Gland Tumors; Neuro-Otology; **Hospital:** Monmouth Med Ctr; **Address:** Cen Jersey Otolaryngology, 1131 Broad St, Ste 103, Shrewsbury, NJ 07702; **Phone:** 732-389-3388; **Board Cert:** Otolaryngology 1997; **Med School:** Med Coll PA 1991; **Resid:** Surgery, Mt Sinai Med Ctr 1992; Otolaryngology, Mt Sinai Med Ctr 1996; **Fellow:** Neurotology, Michigan Ear Inst 1997; **Fac Appt:** Asst Clin Prof Oto, Drexel Univ Coll Med

Pain Medicine

Bram, Harris N MD (PM) - **Spec Exp:** Pain-Back & Neck; Complex Regional Pain Syndromes; **Hospital:** Riverview Med Ctr, Kimball Med Ctr; **Address:** NJ Pain Care Specialists, 1806 Highway 35, Ste 305, Oakhurst, NJ 07755; **Phone:** 732-720-0247; **Board Cert:** Anesthesiology 1993; Pain Medicine 2004; **Med School:** Univ Ark 1988; **Resid:** Anesthesiology, Hahnemann Univ Hosp 1992; **Fellow:** Pain Medicine, Thomas Jefferson Univ Hosp 1993

Daknis, Charles MD (PM) - **Spec Exp:** Pain-Spine; Pain-Interventional Techniques; **Hospital:** Monmouth Med Ctr; **Address:** Spine & Pain Ctrs of NY & NJ, 655 Shrewsbury Ave, Ste 202, Shrewsbury, NJ 07702; **Phone:** 732-345-1180; **Board Cert:** Anesthesiology ; Pain Medicine 2007; **Med School:** Hahnemann Univ 1990; **Resid:** Neurological Surgery, Albany Med Ctr 1992; Anesthesiology, Albany Med Ctr 1994; **Fellow:** Pain Medicine, Harvard/Brigham & Women's Hosp 1995

Metzger, Scott E MD (PM) - **Spec Exp:** Pain-Back & Neck; **Hospital:** Riverview Med Ctr; **Address:** Premier Pain Ctrs, 160 Avenue at the Common, Ste 1, Shrewsbury, NJ 07702; **Phone:** 732-380-0200; **Board Cert:** Anesthesiology 1997; Pain Medicine 2009; **Med School:** Boston Univ 1992; **Resid:** Anesthesiology, Johns Hopkins Hosp 1996; **Fellow:** Pain Medicine, Johns Hopkins Hosp 1997

Staats, Peter MD (PM) - **Spec Exp:** Pain-Cancer; Pain-Back; **Hospital:** Riverview Med Ctr, CentraState Med Ctr; **Address:** Premier Pain Centers, 160 Avenue at the Commons, Ste 1, Shrewsbury, NJ 07702; **Phone:** 732-380-0200; **Board Cert:** Anesthesiology 1994; Pain Medicine 2005; **Med School:** Univ Mich Med Sch 1989; **Resid:** Anesthesiology, Johns Hopkins Hosp 1993; **Fellow:** Pain Medicine, Johns Hopkins Hosp 1994

Pediatric Endocrinology

Meyers-Seifer, Cynthia H MD (PEn) - **Spec Exp:** Diabetes; Thyroid Disorders; Growth Disorders; **Hospital:** Jersey Shore Univ Med Ctr, Riverview Med Ctr; **Address:** Meridian Pediatric Assocs, 61 Davis Ave, Ste 1, Neptune, NJ 07753; **Phone:** 732-776-4860; **Board Cert:** Pediatrics 2012; Pediatric Endocrinology 2010; **Med School:** Stanford Univ 1984; **Resid:** Pediatrics, Stanford Univ Hosp & Clins 1986; Pediatrics, Univ Hosp 1987; **Fellow:** Anatomic Pathology, Univ Hosp-SUNY 1989; Pediatric Endocrinology, Yale-New Haven Hosp 1993

Pediatric Infectious Disease

Fisher, Margaret C MD (PInf) - **Hospital:** Monmouth Med Ctr; **Address:** Chldns Hosp at Monmouth Med Ctr, 300 Second Ave Stanley Bldg - rm 209, Long Branch, NJ 07740; **Phone:** 732-923-7250; **Board Cert:** Pediatrics 1980; Pediatric Infectious Disease 2009; **Med School:** UCLA 1975; **Resid:** Pediatrics, St. Christopher's Hosp for Chldn 1978; **Fellow:** Pediatric Infectious Disease, St. Christopher's Hosp for Chldn 1980; **Fac Appt:** Prof Ped, Drexel Univ Coll Med

Pediatric Otolaryngology

Tavill, Michael A MD (PO) - **Hospital:** Monmouth Med Ctr; **Address:** Central Jersey Otolaryngology, 1131 Broad St, Ste 103, Shrewsbury, NJ 07702; **Phone:** 732-389-3388; **Board Cert:** Otolaryngology 1997; **Med School:** Case West Res Univ 1991; **Resid:** Otolaryngology, Hosp Univ Penn 1996; **Fellow:** Pediatric Otolaryngology, Childrens Hosp 1997

Pediatrics

Murphy, Robert D MD (Ped) *PCP* - **Spec Exp:** ADD/ADHD; Asthma; Vaccines; Infectious Disease; **Hospital:** Monmouth Med Ctr; **Address:** Pediatric & Adolescent Med, 223 Monmouth Rd, Ste 2, West Long Branch, NJ 07764; **Phone:** 732-229-4540; **Board Cert:** Pediatrics 1982; **Med School:** Vanderbilt Univ 1977; **Resid:** Pediatrics, Yale-New Haven Hosp 1980

Plastic Surgery

Ashinoff, Russell L MD (PlS) - **Spec Exp:** Breast Reconstruction; Cosmetic Surgery; Lymphedema; Trauma-Reconstructive Plastic Surgery; **Hospital:** Jersey Shore Univ Med Ctr, Ocean Med Ctr; **Address:** Institute for Advanced Reconstruction, 535 Sycamore Ave, Shrewsbury, NJ 07702; **Phone:** 732-741-0970; **Board Cert:** Surgery 2006; Plastic Surgery 2009; **Med School:** SUNY Upstate Med Univ 1999; **Resid:** Surgery, NYU Med Ctr 2005; **Fellow:** Plastic/Reconstructive Surgery, Emory Univ Hosp 2008

Chidyllo, Stephen A MD/DDS (PlS) - **Spec Exp:** Cosmetic Surgery-Face; Cosmetic Surgery-Breast; Body Contouring; Breast Reconstruction; **Hospital:** Jersey Shore Univ Med Ctr, Southern Ocean Med Ctr; **Address:** Central Jersey Plastic Surgery, 107 Monmouth Rd, Ste 106, West Long Branch, NJ 07764; **Phone:** 732-460-9566; **Board Cert:** Plastic Surgery 2003; **Med School:** Hahnemann Univ 1987; **Resid:** Surgery, NY Infirm-Beekman Downtown Hosp 1990; Plastic Surgery, Univ Illinois Med Ctr 1992; **Fellow:** Craniofacial Surgery, Eastern Va Med Sch 1993; **Fac Appt:** Assoc Clin Prof S, Drexel Univ Coll Med

Dudick, Stephen T MD (PlS) - **Spec Exp:** Breast Reconstruction & Augmentation; Cosmetic Surgery; Cleft Palate/Lip; Body Contouring after Weight Loss; **Hospital:** Jersey Shore Univ Med Ctr, Monmouth Med Ctr; **Address:** 252 Broad St, Red Bank, NJ 07701; **Phone:** 732-741-1303; **Board Cert:** Plastic Surgery 1993; **Med School:** Mexico 1975; **Resid:** Surgery, St Vincents Hosp 1981; Plastic Surgery, Indiana Univ Med Ctr 1983

Elkwood, Andrew I MD (PlS) - **Spec Exp:** Cosmetic Surgery-Face; Peripheral Nerve Surgery; Reconstructive Surgery; Limb Surgery/Reconstruction; **Hospital:** Jersey Shore Univ Med Ctr, Riverview Med Ctr; **Address:** Plastic Surgery Ctr, 535 Sycamore Ave, Shrewsbury, NJ 07702; **Phone:** 732-741-0970; **Board Cert:** Surgery 2004; Plastic Surgery 2008; **Med School:** Albany Med Coll 1988; **Resid:** Surgery, NYU Med Ctr 1994; **Fellow:** Plastic/Reconstructive Surgery, NYU Med Ctr 1996

Glicksman, Caroline A MD (PlS) - **Spec Exp:** Breast Reconstruction & Augmentation; Cosmetic Surgery-Breast; Liposuction & Body Contouring; Rhinoplasty; **Hospital:** Jersey Shore Univ Med Ctr; **Address:** 2164 Hwy 35, Bldg A, Sea Girt, NJ 08750; **Phone:** 732-974-2424; **Board Cert:** Plastic Surgery 1994; **Med School:** SUNY Downstate 1985; **Resid:** Surgery, Mt Sinai Hosp 1988; Plastic Surgery, NY Hosp-Cornell Med Ctr 1991; **Fellow:** Cosmetic Plastic Surgery, Mass Genl Hosp-Newton Wellesley Hosp 1992

Hetzler, Peter T MD (PlS) - **Spec Exp:** Breast Cosmetic & Reconstructive Surgery; Liposuction & Body Contouring; Skin Cancer; **Hospital:** Riverview Med Ctr, Monmouth Med Ctr; **Address:** 200 White Rd, Ste 211, Little Silver, NJ 07739-1162; **Phone:** 732-219-0447; **Board Cert:** Plastic Surgery 1991; **Med School:** Univ Mich Med Sch 1981; **Resid:** Surgery, MS Hershey Med Ctr 1986; Plastic/Reconstructive Surgery, MS Hershey Med Ctr 1988; **Fellow:** Microsurgery, York Hosp Trauma Ctr 1988; Cosmetic Plastic Surgery, Manhattan Eye & Ear Hosp 1989

Rose, Michael I MD (PlS) - **Spec Exp:** Body Contouring after Weight Loss; Cosmetic Surgery-Face; Breast Cosmetic & Reconstructive Surgery; Reconstructive Surgery; **Hospital:** Jersey Shore Univ Med Ctr, CentraState Med Ctr; **Address:** The Plastic Surgery Center, 535 Sycamore Ave, Shrewsbury, NJ 07702; **Phone:** 732-741-0970; **Board Cert:** Surgery 2009; Plastic Surgery 2013; **Med School:** NYU Sch Med 1994; **Resid:** Surgery, NYU/Bellevue Med Ctr 2000; **Fellow:** Plastic Surgery, Emory Univ Med Ctr 2002

Samra, Said A MD (PlS) - **Spec Exp:** Reconstructive Surgery; Hand Surgery; Cosmetic Surgery; **Hospital:** Bayshore Community Hosp, Raritan Bay Med Ctr - Perth Amboy; **Address:** 733 N Beers St, Ste U-1, Holmdel, NJ 07733-1528; **Phone:** 732-739-2100; **Board Cert:** Plastic Surgery 1988; **Med School:** Syria 1973; **Resid:** Surgery, UMDNJ-NJ Med Sch 1980; Plastic Surgery, St Barnabas Hosp 1982

Zaccaria, Alan MD (PlS) - **Spec Exp:** Breast Cosmetic & Reconstructive Surgery; Cosmetic Surgery-Face & Body; Botox Therapy; Wound Healing/Care; **Hospital:** Jersey Shore Univ Med Ctr, Monmouth Med Ctr; **Address:** 180 White Rd, Ste 102, Little Silver, NJ 07739; **Phone:** 732-530-8565; **Board Cert:** Plastic Surgery 2005; **Med School:** UMDNJ-RW Johnson Med Sch 1986; **Resid:** Surgery, Monmouth Med Ctr 1991; **Fellow:** Plastic/Reconstructive Surgery, Univ IL Med Ctr 1993

Psychiatry

Rubin, Kenneth J MD (Psyc) - **Spec Exp:** Mood Disorders; Anxiety Disorders; Dementia; **Hospital:** Monmouth Med Ctr; **Address:** 170 Morris Ave, Long Branch, NJ 07740-6660; **Phone:** 732-870-3535; **Board Cert:** Psychiatry 1979; **Med School:** SUNY Downstate 1974; **Resid:** Psychiatry, Kings County Hosp 1977; **Fac Appt:** Assoc Clin Prof Psyc, Drexel Univ Coll Med

Pulmonary Disease

Davis, George C MD (Pul) - **Spec Exp:** Critical Care; Chronic Obstructive Lung Disease (COPD); Sepsis; **Hospital:** Monmouth Med Ctr; **Address:** 279 3rd Ave, Ste 510, Long Branch, NJ 07740; **Phone:** 732-870-0650; **Board Cert:** Internal Medicine 1976; Pulmonary Disease 1980; Critical Care Medicine 2013; **Med School:** Hahnemann Univ 1973; **Resid:** Internal Medicine, Monmouth Med Ctr 1977; **Fellow:** Pulmonary Disease, Monmouth Med Ctr 1979

Reproductive Endocrinology

Damien, Miguel MD (RE) - **Hospital:** Riverview Med Ctr, Monmouth Med Ctr; **Address:** 200 White Rd, Ste 214, Little Silver, NJ 07739; **Phone:** 732-758-6511; **Board Cert:** Obstetrics & Gynecology 2012; Reproductive Endocrinology 2012; **Med School:** Dartmouth Med Sch 1982; **Resid:** Obstetrics & Gynecology, Beth Israel Deaconess Hosp 1986; **Fellow:** Reproductive Endocrinology, Beth Israel Deaconess Hosp 1988; Reproductive Endocrinology, Univ Conn Hlth Ctr 1989

Rheumatology

Schwartzberg, Mori MD (Rhu) - **Spec Exp:** Rheumatoid Arthritis; Spondylitis; Osteoarthritis; **Hospital:** Jersey Shore Univ Med Ctr; **Address:** 3350 Route 138, Wall Township Bldg 1 Fl 2 - Ste 212, Wall Township, NJ 07719; **Phone:** 732-988-5030; **Board Cert:** Internal Medicine 1976; Rheumatology 1978; **Med School:** SUNY Upstate Med Univ 1973; **Resid:** Internal Medicine, Nassau County Med Ctr 1976; **Fellow:** Rheumatology, Albert Einstein Med Ctr 1978; **Fac Appt:** Asst Clin Prof Med, UMDNJ-RW Johnson Med Sch

Wasser, Kenneth B MD (Rhu) - **Spec Exp:** Rheumatoid Arthritis; Lupus Nephritis; Psoriatic Arthritis; **Hospital:** Riverview Med Ctr, Monmouth Med Ctr; **Address:** 43 Gilbert St N, Ste 7, Tinton Falls, NJ 07701; **Phone:** 732-530-7999; **Board Cert:** Internal Medicine 1981; Rheumatology 1982; **Med School:** Case West Res Univ 1977; **Resid:** Internal Medicine, Univ Hosps 1980; **Fellow:** Rheumatology, Univ Hosps 1982

Sports Medicine

Rice, Stephen G MD/PhD (SM) - **Spec Exp:** Primary Care Sports Medicine; Musculoskeletal Injuries; **Hospital:** Jersey Shore Univ Med Ctr; **Address:** Jersey Shore Sports Med Ctr, 51-02 Davis Ave, Ste 02, Neptune, NJ 07753; **Phone:** 732-776-2433; **Board Cert:** Pediatrics 1981; Sports Medicine 2004; **Med School:** NYU Sch Med 1974; **Resid:** Pediatrics, Chldn's Hosp Med Ctr 1977; **Fac Appt:** Clin Prof Ped, UMDNJ-RW Johnson Med Sch

Sclafani, Michael MD (SM) - **Spec Exp:** Knee Injuries/Ligament Surgery; Shoulder Instability; **Hospital:** Jersey Shore Univ Med Ctr; **Address:** Orthopedic Inst, 2315 Route 34 S, Manasquan, NJ 08736; **Phone:** 732-974-0404; **Board Cert:** Orthopaedic Surgery 2007; **Med School:** NYU Sch Med 1988; **Resid:** Orthopaedic Surgery, NYU Med Ctr 1993; **Fellow:** Sports Medicine & Shoulder Surgery, American Sports Med Inst 1994

Surgery

Arbour, Robert MD (S) - **Spec Exp:** Breast Surgery; Colon & Rectal Surgery; Biliary Surgery; Hernia; **Hospital:** Bayshore Community Hosp, Riverview Med Ctr; **Address:** Holmdel Surgical, 668 N Beers St, Ste 102, Holmdel, NJ 07733; **Phone:** 732-847-3300; **Board Cert:** Surgery 1972; **Med School:** UMDNJ-NJ Med Sch, Newark 1965; **Resid:** Surgery, Georgetown Univ Hosp 1971

Borao, Frank J MD (S) - **Spec Exp:** Laparoscopic Abdominal Surgery; Obesity/Bariatric Surgery; Gastroesophageal Reflux Disease (GERD); Critical Care; **Hospital:** Monmouth Med Ctr; **Address:** Specialty Surgical Assocs, 10 Industrial Way E, Ste 104, Eatontown, NJ 07724; **Phone:** 732-389-1331; **Board Cert:** Surgery 2010; **Med School:** UMDNJ-NJ Med Sch, Newark 1994; **Resid:** Surgery, Monmouth Med Ctr 1999; **Fellow:** Laparoscopic Surgery, White Plains Hosp 2000; **Fac Appt:** Asst Prof S, Hahnemann Univ

Goldfarb, Michael A MD (S) - **Spec Exp:** Breast Cancer & Surgery; Telemedicine; **Hospital:** Monmouth Med Ctr; **Address:** Monmouth Med Grp, Surgery, 166 Morris Ave Fl 2, Long Branch, NJ 07740; **Phone:** 732-870-6060; **Board Cert:** Surgery 1973; **Med School:** NYU Sch Med 1967; **Resid:** Surgery, Beth Israel Med Ctr 1972; **Fac Appt:** Prof S, Drexel Univ Coll Med

Johnson Miller, Denise L MD (S) - **Spec Exp:** Breast Cancer; Breast Cancer-High Risk Women; Melanoma; Neuroendocrine Tumors; **Hospital:** Jersey Shore Univ Med Ctr, Ocean Med Ctr; **Address:** Meridian Hlth Breast Surgery Assocs, 1945 Hwy 33, Ackerman 5, Neptune, NJ 07753; **Phone:** 732-776-4594; **Board Cert:** Surgery 2012; **Med School:** Washington Univ, St Louis 1978; **Resid:** Immunology, Univ Texas SW Med Ctr 1982; Surgery, Univ IL Med Ctr 1986; **Fellow:** Surgical Oncology, City of Hope Med Ctr 1988

Thoracic & Cardiac Surgery

Neibart, Richard M MD (T&CS) - **Spec Exp:** Coronary Artery Surgery; Cardiac Surgery; Aortic Surgery; **Hospital:** Jersey Shore Univ Med Ctr; **Address:** Mid-Atlantic Surgical Assocs, 1944 Rte 33, Ste 201, Neptune, NJ 07753; **Phone:** 732-776-4618; **Board Cert:** Thoracic & Cardiac Surgery 2011; **Med School:** Mount Sinai Sch Med 1982; **Resid:** Surgery, St Vincents Hosp 1987; **Fellow:** Thoracic Surgery, Jackson Meml Hosp 1989

Urology

Ebani, Jack MD (U) - **Spec Exp:** Prostate Cancer; Incontinence; **Hospital:** Jersey Shore Univ Med Ctr, Ocean Med Ctr; **Address:** 1820 Corlies Ave, Neptune, NJ 07753; **Phone:** 732-774-4551; **Board Cert:** Urology 2006; **Med School:** SUNY Hlth Sci Ctr 1979; **Resid:** Surgery, N Shore Univ Hosp 1981; Urology, NYU Med Ctr 1985

Geltzeiler, Jules MD (U) - **Spec Exp:** Prostate Cancer; Incontinence; **Hospital:** Monmouth Med Ctr, Jersey Shore Univ Med Ctr; **Address:** NJ Urologic Inst, 10 Industrial Way E, Ste 101, Eatontown, NJ 07724; **Phone:** 732-963-9091; **Board Cert:** Urology 2004; **Med School:** Hahnemann Univ 1979; **Resid:** Surgery, Monmouth Med Ctr 1981; Urology, G Washington Univ Hosp 1984; **Fac Appt:** Asst Clin Prof S, Drexel Univ Coll Med

Litvin, Y. Samuel MD (U) - **Spec Exp:** Infertility; Prostate Disease; **Hospital:** Monmouth Med Ctr, Riverview Med Ctr; **Address:** NJ Urologic Inst, 10 Industrial Way E, Ste 101, Eatontown, NJ 07724; **Phone:** 732-963-9091; **Board Cert:** Urology 2013; **Med School:** UCLA 1986; **Resid:** Surgery, Beth Israel Med Ctr 1988; Urology, Beth Israel Med Ctr 1991; **Fac Appt:** Asst Clin Prof U, Drexel Univ Coll Med

Rose, John G MD (U) - **Hospital:** Riverview Med Ctr, Bayshore Community Hosp; **Address:** Urology Assocs, 595 Shrewsbury Ave, Shrewsbury, NJ 07702; **Phone:** 732-741-5923; **Board Cert:** Urology 1977; **Med School:** Cornell Univ-Weill Med Coll 1968; **Resid:** Surgery, NY-Presby/Weill Cornell Med Ctr 1970; Urology, Univ Virginia Med Ctr 1974; **Fellow:** Urology, Univ Virginia Med Ctr

Rotolo, James MD (U) - **Spec Exp:** Prostate Disease; Urologic Cancer; Kidney Stones; **Hospital:** Ocean Med Ctr, Jersey Shore Univ Med Ctr; **Address:** 2401 Highway 35, Manasquan, NJ 08736; **Phone:** 732-223-7877; **Board Cert:** Urology 2010; **Med School:** Georgetown Univ 1984; **Resid:** Surgery, Georgetown Univ Hosp 1986; Urology, Georgetown Univ Hosp 1990

Morris

Morris

Adolescent Medicine

Clark-Hamilton, Jill MD (AM) - **Spec Exp:** Eating Disorders; Adolescent Gynecology; Behavorial Disorders; **Hospital:** Goryeb Children's Hosp (page 92), Overlook Med Ctr (page 92); **Address:** Goryeb Chldn's Hosp at Morristown, 100 Madison Ave, Morristown, NJ 07962; **Phone:** 973-971-5199; **Board Cert:** Adolescent Medicine 2007; **Med School:** SUNY Upstate Med Univ 1983; **Resid:** Pediatrics, Montefiore Med Ctr 1987; **Fellow:** Adolescent Medicine, Montefiore Med Ctr 1989

Rosenfeld, Walter D MD (AM) - **Spec Exp:** Eating Disorders; **Hospital:** Goryeb Children's Hosp (page 92); **Address:** Goryeb Chldns Hosp, Adolescent Med, 100 Madison Ave, Morristown, NJ 07960; **Phone:** 973-971-5199; **Board Cert:** Pediatrics 1980; Adolescent Medicine 2009; **Med School:** Temple Univ 1975; **Resid:** Pediatrics, NY-Presby/Columbia Univ Med Ctr 1978; **Fellow:** Adolescent Medicine, Chldns Hosp 1979; **Fac Appt:** Prof Ped, UMDNJ-NJ Med Sch, Newark

Allergy & Immunology

Applebaum, Eric MD (A&I) - **Spec Exp:** Asthma; Food Allergy; Sinus Disorders; Rhinitis; **Hospital:** Morristown Med Ctr (page 92), St. Clare's Hosp-Denville; **Address:** 3799 Route 46 E, Parsippany, NJ 07054-1101; **Phone:** 973-335-1700; **Board Cert:** Allergy & Immunology 2003; **Med School:** Albert Einstein Coll Med 1987; **Resid:** Internal Medicine, LI Jewish Med Ctr 1990; **Fellow:** Allergy & Immunology, LI Jewish Med Ctr 1992

Chernack, William J MD (A&I) - **Spec Exp:** Asthma; Sinus Disorders; Insect Allergies; **Hospital:** Morristown Med Ctr (page 92), Morgan Stanley Children's Hosp of NY-Presby, NY (page 104); **Address:** 28 Franklin Pl, Morristown, NJ 07960-5305; **Phone:** 973-538-7271; **Board Cert:** Pediatrics 1975; Allergy & Immunology 1977; **Med School:** NY Med Coll 1970; **Resid:** Pediatrics, Columbia-Presby Med Ctr 1972; **Fellow:** Allergy & Immunology, Columbia-Presby Med Ctr 1974; **Fac Appt:** Asst Clin Prof Ped, Columbia P&S

Kanumury, Sunita MD (A&I) - **Spec Exp:** Asthma; Eczema; Food & Drug Allergy; Sinusitis; **Hospital:** St. Clare's Hosp-Denville, Hackettstown Reg Med Ctr; **Address:** Asthma & Allergy Care, 496 E Main St, Ste 1, Denville, NJ 07834; **Phone:** 973-627-1000; **Board Cert:** Allergy & Immunology 2005; **Med School:** India 1986; **Resid:** Pediatrics, Univ Toledo Med Ctr 1991; **Fellow:** Allergy & Immunology, Univ Hosp-UMDNJ 1993

Cardiac Electrophysiology

Winters, Stephen L MD (CE) - **Spec Exp:** Pacemakers/Defibrillators; Catheter Ablation; Atrial Fibrillation; Syncope; **Hospital:** Morristown Med Ctr (page 92), Overlook Med Ctr (page 92); **Address:** Morristown Meml Hosp, 100 Madison Ave, Morristown, NJ 07962-1956; **Phone:** 973-971-4261; **Board Cert:** Internal Medicine 1982; Cardiovascular Disease 1985; Cardiac Electrophysiology 2012; **Med School:** Mount Sinai Sch Med 1979; **Resid:** Internal Medicine, Mt Sinai Med Ctr 1982; **Fellow:** Cardiovascular Disease, Mt Sinai Med Ctr 1985; Cardiac Electrophysiology, Mt Sinai Med Ctr 1986; **Fac Appt:** Assoc Prof Med, UMDNJ-NJ Med Sch, Newark

Cardiovascular Disease

Blick, Michael D MD (Cv) - **Spec Exp:** Cardiac Catheterization; **Hospital:** St. Clare's Hosp-Dover, Morristown Med Ctr (page 92); **Address:** Lakeland Cardiology, 765 Rte 10 E, Randolph, NJ 07869; **Phone:** 973-989-2566; **Board Cert:** Internal Medicine 1985; Cardiovascular Disease 1987; **Med School:** Geo Wash Univ 1982; **Resid:** Internal Medicine, LI Jewish Med Ctr 1985; **Fellow:** Cardiovascular Disease, Philadelphia Heart Inst 1987

Blum, Mark A MD (Cv) - **Spec Exp:** Interventional Cardiology; Cholesterol/Lipid Disorders; Hypertrophic Cardiomyopathy; Preventive Cardiology; **Hospital:** Morristown Med Ctr (page 92); **Address:** Cardiology Assocs, 95 Madison Ave, Ste A10, Morristown, NJ 07960; **Phone:** 973-889-9001; **Board Cert:** Internal Medicine 1986; Cardiovascular Disease 1989; **Med School:** Mount Sinai Sch Med 1983; **Resid:** Internal Medicine, Montefiore Med Ctr 1985; Internal Medicine, Mount Sinai Med Ctr 1986; **Fellow:** Cardiovascular Disease, Mount Sinai Med Ctr 1988; Interventional Cardiology, Newark Beth Israel Hosp 1989; **Fac Appt:** Asst Clin Prof Med, Mount Sinai Sch Med

Fisch, Arthur P MD (Cv) - **Spec Exp:** Echocardiography; Coronary Artery Disease; Heart Valve Disease; **Hospital:** Morristown Med Ctr (page 92); **Address:** Morristown Cardiology Assocs, 435 South St, Ste 100, Morristown, NJ 07960; **Phone:** 973-267-3944; **Board Cert:** Internal Medicine 1972; Cardiovascular Disease 1975; **Med School:** Boston Univ 1969; **Resid:** Internal Medicine, UCLA Med Ctr 1972; **Fellow:** Cardiovascular Disease, Hosp Univ Penn 1974

Lowell, Barry H MD (Cv) - **Spec Exp:** Interventional Cardiology; Angioplasty; **Hospital:** St. Clare's Hosp-Dover, Morristown Med Ctr (page 92); **Address:** Morris Heart Assocs, 400 Valley Rd, Ste 102, Mount Arlington, NJ 07856; **Phone:** 973-770-7899; **Board Cert:** Internal Medicine 1986; Cardiovascular Disease 1989; Interventional Cardiology 2010; **Med School:** SUNY Stony Brook 1982; **Resid:** Internal Medicine, St Lukes-Roosevelt Hosp Ctr 1985; **Fellow:** Cardiovascular Disease, St Lukes-Roosevelt Hosp Ctr 1989

Raska, Karel MD (Cv) - **Spec Exp:** Preventive Cardiology; Hypertension; Echocardiography; **Hospital:** Morristown Med Ctr (page 92); **Address:** Morristown Cardiology Assocs, 435 South St, Ste 100, Morristown, NJ 07960; **Phone:** 973-267-3944; **Board Cert:** Cardiovascular Disease 2005; **Med School:** Harvard Med Sch 1989; **Resid:** Internal Medicine, Mass Genl Hosp 1992; **Fellow:** Cardiovascular Disease, Johns Hopkins Hosp 1995

Child Neurology

Bennett, Harvey S MD (ChiN) - **Spec Exp:** Concussion; Tourette's Syndrome; Cerebral Palsy; **Hospital:** Goryeb Children's Hosp (page 92), Overlook Med Ctr (page 92); **Address:** Goryeb Chldn's Hosp at Morristown, 100 Madison Ave, Box 24, Morristown, NJ 07960; **Phone:** 973-971-5700; **Board Cert:** Pediatrics 1979; Child Neurology 1991; Neurodevelopmental Disabilities 2009; **Med School:** Albert Einstein Coll Med 1975; **Resid:** Pediatrics, St Christopher's Hosp Chldn 1977; Child Neurology, Montefiore Med Ctr 1980; **Fac Appt:** Clin Prof N, Mount Sinai Sch Med

Desouza, Trevor MD (ChiN) - **Spec Exp:** Epilepsy; Neuromuscular Disorders; Cerebral Palsy; Tourette's Syndrome; **Hospital:** Goryeb Children's Hosp (page 92); **Address:** Advocare Pediatric Neurology Assocs, 25 Lindsley Drive, Ste 205, Morristown, NJ 07960; **Phone:** 973-993-8777; **Board Cert:** Pediatrics 1985; Child Neurology 1989; **Med School:** Kenya 1977; **Resid:** Pediatrics, Bronx-Lebanon Hosp Ctr 1983; **Fellow:** Pediatric Neurology, Montefiore Med Ctr 1986; Neuromuscular Medicine, Montefiore Med Ctr 1987; **Fac Appt:** Asst Prof Ped, UMDNJ-Univ Med Dent NJ

Grossman, Elliot A MD (ChiN) - **Spec Exp:** Migraine; ADD/ADHD; Tourette's Syndrome; Epilepsy; **Hospital:** Saint Barnabas Med Ctr, Morristown Med Ctr (page 92); **Address:** 220 Ridgedale Ave, Ste A3, Florham Park, NJ 07932-1349; **Phone:** 973-966-6333; **Board Cert:** Pediatrics 1987; Child Neurology 1990; **Med School:** Meharry Med Coll 1980; **Resid:** Pediatrics, Bellevue Hosp 1982; Pediatrics, Boston City Hosp 1983; **Fellow:** Pediatric Neurology, Boston City Hosp 1986

Lazar, Lorraine M MD (ChiN) - **Spec Exp:** Epilepsy/Seizure Disorders; **Hospital:** Goryeb Children's Hosp (page 92), Overlook Med Ctr (page 92); **Address:** Goryeb Chldn's Hosp at Morristown, 100 Madison Ave, Morristown, NJ 07962; **Phone:** 973-971-5700; **Board Cert:** Child Neurology 2010; Clinical Neurophysiology 2011; **Med School:** Mount Sinai Sch Med 1993; **Resid:** Neurology, NY Presby Hosp/Cornell 1995; Child Neurology, NY Presby Hosp/Cornell 1997; **Fellow:** Clinical Neurophysiology, NY Presby Hosp/Cornell 1998

Sousa, Rolando MD (ChiN) - **Spec Exp:** Epilepsy; Autism; Neurofibromatosis; **Hospital:** NYU Langone Med Ctr (page 108); **Address:** NJ Pediatric Neurosci Inst, 131 Madison Ave, Ste 140, Morristown, NJ 07960; **Phone:** 973-326-9000; **Board Cert:** Pediatrics 2009; **Med School:** Panama 1990; **Resid:** Pediatrics, Newark Beth Israel Med Ctr 1999; **Fellow:** Child Neurology, NYU Med Ctr 2002; Clinical Neurophysiology, NYU Med Ctr 2003; **Fac Appt:** Asst Clin Prof N, NYU Sch Med

Colon & Rectal Surgery

Moskowitz, Richard L MD (CRS) - **Spec Exp:** Colon & Rectal Cancer; Anorectal Disorders; Inflammatory Bowel Disease; **Hospital:** Morristown Med Ctr (page 92), St. Clare's Hosp-Dover; **Address:** 111 Madison Ave, Ste 312, Morristown, NJ 07960-6083; **Phone:** 973-267-1225; **Board Cert:** Surgery 2005; Colon & Rectal Surgery 1985; **Med School:** Penn State Coll Med 1978; **Resid:** Surgery, LI Jewish-Hillside Med Ctr 1983; Colon & Rectal Surgery, Greater Baltimore Med Ctr 1984; **Fellow:** Colon & Rectal Surgery, St Marks Hosp 1985

Dermatology

Almeida, Laila N MD (D) - **Spec Exp:** Psoriasis; Acne; Skin Cancer; **Hospital:** St. Clare's Hosp-Denville, NY-Presby/Columbia Univ Med Ctr, NY (page 104); **Address:** Dermatology Associates in Morris, 199 Baldwin Rd, Ste 230, Parsippany, NJ 07054-2043; **Phone:** 973-335-2560; **Board Cert:** Internal Medicine 1986; Dermatology 2009; **Med School:** Univ Mich Med Sch 1983; **Resid:** Internal Medicine, Columbia-Presby Hosp 1986; Dermatology, Columbia-Presby Hosp 1989

Cooper, Lauren M MD (D) - **Spec Exp:** Botox Therapy; Facial Rejuvenation; **Hospital:** Morristown Med Ctr (page 92); **Address:** Affil Dermatologists & Surgeons, 182 South St, Ste 1, Morristown, NJ 07960; **Phone:** 973-267-0300; **Board Cert:** Dermatology 1988; **Med School:** NYU Sch Med 1984; **Resid:** Dermatology, Bellevue/NYU Med Ctr 1988

Machler, Brian C MD (D) - **Spec Exp:** Contact Dermatitis; Laser Surgery; Skin Cancer; **Hospital:** Saint Barnabas Med Ctr; **Address:** Center for Dermatology, 128 Columbia Tpke, Ste 200, Florham Park, NJ 07932; **Phone:** 973-736-9535; **Board Cert:** Dermatology 2004; **Med School:** UMDNJ-NJ Med Sch, Newark 1991; **Resid:** Dermatology, Jackson Meml Hosp 1995; **Fac Appt:** Asst Prof D, NYU Sch Med

Diagnostic Radiology

Murphy, Robyn C MD (DR) - **Spec Exp:** Pediatric Radiology; **Hospital:** Morristown Med Ctr (page 92); **Address:** Morristown Meml Hosp, Dept Radiology, 100 Madison Ave, Ste 408, Morristown, NJ 07960; **Phone:** 973-971-5370; **Board Cert:** Diagnostic Radiology 1997; Pediatric Radiology 2010; **Med School:** Med Coll VA 1992; **Resid:** Diagnostic Radiology, Columbia-Presby Med Ctr 1997; **Fellow:** Pediatric Radiology, NY-Presby Hosp 1998

Endocrinology, Diabetes & Metabolism

Nevin, Marie E MD (EDM) - **Hospital:** Morristown Med Ctr (page 92); **Address:** Endocrine Medical Associates, 25 Lindsley Drive, Morristown, NJ 07960; **Phone:** 973-267-9099; **Board Cert:** Internal Medicine 1989; Endocrinology, Diabetes & Metabolism 2013; **Med School:** UMDNJ-NJ Med Sch, Newark 1986; **Resid:** Internal Medicine, Morristown Meml Hosp 1989; **Fellow:** Endocrinology, Mount Sinai Med Ctr 1991

Family Medicine

Holland Jr, Elbridge T MD (FMed) *PCP* - **Hospital:** Overlook Med Ctr (page 92); **Address:** 492 Main St, Chatham, NJ 07928; **Phone:** 973-635-2432; **Board Cert:** Family Medicine 2009; Geriatric Medicine 2007; **Med School:** Univ Chicago-Pritzker Sch Med 1975; **Resid:** Family Medicine, Overlook Hosp 1978; **Fac Appt:** Asst Clin Prof FMed, UMDNJ-NJ Med Sch, Newark

Gastroenterology

Dalena, John M MD (Ge) - **Spec Exp:** Colon Cancer Screening; Endoscopy; Gastroesophageal Reflux Disease (GERD); Inflammatory Bowel Disease; **Hospital:** Morristown Med Ctr (page 92); **Address:** 65 Ridgedale Ave, Cedar Knolls, NJ 07927; **Phone:** 973-401-0500; **Board Cert:** Internal Medicine 1988; Gastroenterology 2011; **Med School:** UMDNJ-NJ Med Sch, Newark 1985; **Resid:** Internal Medicine, Mount Sinai Hosp 1988; **Fellow:** Gastroenterology, UMDNJ-Univ Hosp 1990

Samach, Michael MD (Ge) - **Spec Exp:** Colonoscopy; Gastroesophageal Reflux Disease (GERD); Hepatitis C; **Hospital:** Morristown Med Ctr (page 92); **Address:** 101 Madison Ave, Ste 100, Morristown, NJ 07960; **Phone:** 973-455-0404; **Board Cert:** Internal Medicine 1974; Gastroenterology 1979; **Med School:** NYU Sch Med 1971; **Resid:** Internal Medicine, Montefiore Med Ctr 1974; **Fellow:** Gastroenterology, Montefiore Med Ctr 1978; **Fac Appt:** Asst Clin Prof Med, Mount Sinai Sch Med

Soriano, John G MD (Ge) - **Hospital:** St. Clare's Hosp-Denville, Morristown Med Ctr (page 92); **Address:** 16 Pocono Rd, Ste 201, Denville, NJ 07834; **Phone:** 973-627-4430; **Board Cert:** Internal Medicine 1986; Gastroenterology 2003; **Med School:** Mexico 1981; **Resid:** Internal Medicine, Morristown Meml Hosp 1987; **Fellow:** Gastroenterology, Long Island Coll Hosp 1989

Stein, Lawrence B MD (Ge) - **Spec Exp:** Hepatitis; Gastroesophageal Reflux Disease (GERD); Endoscopy; **Hospital:** Morristown Med Ctr (page 92), Saint Barnabas Med Ctr; **Address:** 101 Madison Ave, Ste 102, Morristown, NJ 07960; **Phone:** 973-410-0960; **Board Cert:** Internal Medicine 1972; Gastroenterology 1973; **Med School:** Univ Minn 1965; **Resid:** Internal Medicine, Bronx Muni Hosp 1967; Internal Medicine, Bronx Muni Hosp 1970; **Fellow:** Gastroenterology, Einstein Med Ctr 1972

Gynecologic Oncology

Heller, Paul B MD (GO) - **Spec Exp:** Gynecologic Cancer; **Hospital:** Morristown Med Ctr (page 92), Overlook Med Ctr (page 92); **Address:** Morristown Meml Hosp, Women's Cancer Ctr, 100 Madison Ave, Morristown, NJ 07962; **Phone:** 973-971-5900; **Board Cert:** Obstetrics & Gynecology 1975; Gynecologic Oncology 1982; **Med School:** NY Med Coll 1968; **Resid:** Obstetrics & Gynecology, Metroplitan Hosp 1971; Obstetrics & Gynecology, Beth Israel Med Ctr 1973; **Fellow:** Gynecologic Oncology, Metropolitan Hosp 1977; **Fac Appt:** Clin Prof ObG, Temple Univ

Tobias, Daniel H MD (GO) - **Spec Exp:** Gynecologic Cancer; Uterine Cancer; Laparoscopic Surgery; **Hospital:** Morristown Med Ctr (page 92), Overlook Med Ctr (page 92); **Address:** Morristown Meml Hosp, Women's Cancer Ctr, 100 Madison Ave, Morristown, NJ 07962; **Phone:** 973-971-5900; **Board Cert:** Obstetrics & Gynecology 2012; Gynecologic Oncology 2012; **Med School:** Univ MO-Kansas City 1992; **Resid:** Obstetrics & Gynecology, Bronx Muni Hosp Ctr 1996; **Fellow:** Gynecologic Oncology, Mt Sinai Med Ctr 1999

Hand Surgery

Ende, Leigh S MD (HS) - **Spec Exp:** Arthritis; Carpal Tunnel Syndrome; Hand & Upper Extremity Surgery; **Hospital:** St. Clare's Hosp-Dover, Newton Med Ctr (page 92); **Address:** 121 Center Grove Rd, Ste 6, Randolph, NJ 07869; **Phone:** 973-366-5565; **Board Cert:** Orthopaedic Surgery 2010; Hand Surgery 2010; **Med School:** Tulane Univ 1978; **Resid:** Orthopaedic Surgery, UMDNJ-Univ Hosp 1983; **Fellow:** Hand Surgery, Columbia Presby Med Ctr 1984

Miller, Jeffrey K MD (HS) - **Spec Exp:** Carpal Tunnel Syndrome; Dupuytren's Contracture; Wrist/Hand Injuries; Elbow Surgery; **Hospital:** Morristown Med Ctr (page 92), Saint Barnabas Med Ctr; **Address:** 111 Madison Ave, Ste 302, Morristown, NJ 07960; **Phone:** 973-538-5200; **Board Cert:** Orthopaedic Surgery 2010; Hand Surgery 2010; **Med School:** Univ Pittsburgh 1981; **Resid:** Surgery, G Washington Univ Hosp 1982; Orthopaedic Surgery, Boston Med Ctr 1986; **Fellow:** Hand Surgery, Thomas Jefferson Univ Hosp 1987

Hematology

Frank, Martin J MD (Hem) - **Hospital:** Chilton Hosp; **Address:** Collins Pavilion, 97 West Pkwy, Pompton Plains, NJ 07444; **Phone:** 973-831-5451; **Board Cert:** Internal Medicine 1985; Medical Oncology 1989; **Med School:** Geo Wash Univ 1982; **Resid:** Hematology, Montefiore Med Ctr 1986

Infectious Disease

Allegra, Donald T MD (Inf) - **Spec Exp:** Tropical Diseases; AIDS/HIV; International Health; Travel Medicine; **Hospital:** St. Clare's Hosp-Denville, Morristown Med Ctr (page 92); **Address:** 765 Rte 10 E, Randolph, NJ 07869; **Phone:** 973-989-0068; **Board Cert:** Infectious Disease 1982; Internal Medicine 1978; **Med School:** Harvard Med Sch 1974; **Resid:** Internal Medicine, Univ Colorado Affil Hosps 1978; **Fellow:** Infectious Disease, Emory Univ Hosp 1981

Krieger, Richard E MD (Inf) - **Spec Exp:** Lyme Disease; Endocarditis; **Hospital:** Chilton Hosp, St. Joseph's Wayne Hosp; **Address:** 765 Route 10 E, Randolph, NJ 07869; **Phone:** 973-989-0068; **Board Cert:** Internal Medicine 1981; Infectious Disease 1984; **Med School:** UMDNJ-NJ Med Sch, Newark 1978; **Resid:** Internal Medicine, Med Coll Penn Hosp 1981; **Fellow:** Infectious Disease, Med Coll Penn Hosp 1983

McManus, Edward J MD (Inf) - **Spec Exp:** Antibiotic Resistance; Wound Healing/Care; **Hospital:** St. Clare's Hosp-Denville, Morristown Med Ctr (page 92); **Address:** 765 Route 10 E, Randolph, NJ 07869; **Phone:** 973-989-0068; **Board Cert:** Internal Medicine 1985; Infectious Disease 1988; Undersea & Hyperbaric Medicine 2011; **Med School:** UMDNJ-NJ Med Sch, Newark 1982; **Resid:** Internal Medicine, Univ Wisconsin Hosp 1986; **Fellow:** Infectious Disease, Nat Inst Health 1989

Internal Medicine

Collum, Robert G MD (IM) *PCP* - **Hospital:** St. Clare's Hosp-Denville; **Address:** 16 Pocono Rd, Ste 317, Denville, NJ 07834; **Phone:** 973-627-2650; **Board Cert:** Internal Medicine 2005; **Med School:** Columbia P&S 1992; **Resid:** Internal Medicine, NY-Presby/Cornell Med Ctr 1995

Pond, William S MD (IM) *PCP* - **Hospital:** Morristown Med Ctr (page 92); **Address:** 95 Madison Ave, Ste A00, Morristown, NJ 07960; **Phone:** 973-538-1388; **Board Cert:** Internal Medicine 1980; **Med School:** Tufts Univ 1977; **Resid:** Internal Medicine, Overlook Hosp 1980

Randazzo, Jean P MD (IM) *PCP* - **Spec Exp:** Women's Health; Arthritis; Hypertension; **Hospital:** Morristown Med Ctr (page 92); **Address:** Internal Med Morristown, 95 Madison Ave, Ste A-00, Morristown, NJ 07960; **Phone:** 973-538-1388; **Board Cert:** Internal Medicine 2013; **Med School:** Tufts Univ 1990; **Resid:** Internal Medicine, Morristown Meml Hosp 1994; **Fac Appt:** Asst Clin Prof Med, UMDNJ-NJ Med Sch, Newark

Scaduto, Philip MD (IM) *PCP* - **Spec Exp:** Hypertension; Diabetes; Geriatric Medicine; Preventive Medicine; **Hospital:** St. Clare's Hosp-Denville; **Address:** 223 W Main St, Boonton, NJ 07005-1166; **Phone:** 973-335-8656; **Board Cert:** Internal Medicine 1986; **Med School:** UMDNJ-NJ Med Sch, Newark 1983; **Resid:** Internal Medicine, UMDNJ-Univ Hosp 1986

Silva, Waldemar MD (IM) - **Hospital:** Chilton Hosp, St. Joseph's Regl Med Ctr - Paterson; **Address:** 488 Newark Pompton Tpke, Pompton Plains, NJ 07444; **Phone:** 973-835-9100; **Board Cert:** Internal Medicine 1987; **Med School:** Harvard Med Sch 1982; **Resid:** Internal Medicine, Bronx Muni Hosp 1985

Storch, Kenneth J MD/PhD (IM) - **Spec Exp:** Nutrition; Diabetes; Cholesterol/Lipid Disorders; **Hospital:** Morristown Med Ctr (page 92), Overlook Med Ctr (page 92); **Address:** Storch Med Nutrition Ctr, 147 Columbia Tpke, Ste 308, Ste 308, Florham Park, NJ 07932; **Phone:** 973-765-9355; **Board Cert:** Internal Medicine 1982; **Med School:** SUNY Downstate 1979; **Resid:** Internal Medicine, Staten Island Hosp 1982; **Fellow:** Nutrition & Metabolism, MIT 1986; Nutrition & Metabolism, New England Deaconess 1988; **Fac Appt:** Asst Clin Prof Med, Mount Sinai Sch Med

Weine, Gary R MD (IM) *PCP* - **Spec Exp:** Hypertension; Cholesterol/Lipid Disorders; **Hospital:** Morristown Med Ctr (page 92); **Address:** 95 Madison Ave, Ste 405, Morristown, NJ 07960-7336; **Phone:** 973-829-9998; **Board Cert:** Internal Medicine 1979; **Med School:** Cornell Univ-Weill Med Coll 1976; **Resid:** Internal Medicine, New York Hosp 1979; **Fac Appt:** Asst Clin Prof Med, UMDNJ-NJ Med Sch, Newark

Maternal & Fetal Medicine

Benito, Carlos W MD (MF) - **Spec Exp:** Pregnancy Loss; Prenatal Diagnosis; Premature Labor; **Hospital:** Morristown Med Ctr (page 92), Overlook Med Ctr (page 92); **Address:** 435 South St, Ste 308, Morristown, NJ 07960; **Phone:** 973-971-7080; **Board Cert:** Obstetrics & Gynecology 2012; Maternal & Fetal Medicine 2012; **Med School:** UMDNJ-RW Johnson Med Sch 1993; **Resid:** Obstetrics & Gynecology, UMDNJ-RWJ Med Ctr 1997; **Fellow:** Maternal & Fetal Medicine, UMDNJ-RWJ Med Ctr 1999; **Fac Appt:** Assoc Prof ObG

Medical Oncology

Adler, Kenneth R MD (Onc) - **Spec Exp:** Breast Cancer; Myeloproliferative Disorders; Lymphoma; **Hospital:** Morristown Med Ctr (page 92); **Address:** Carol G Simon Cancer Ctr, 100 Madison Ave, Box 1089, Morristown, NJ 07962-1089; **Phone:** 973-538-5210; **Board Cert:** Internal Medicine 1976; Hematology 1978; **Med School:** Albany Med Coll 1973; **Resid:** Internal Medicine, Albany Med Ctr 1976; **Fellow:** Hematology & Oncology, Albany Med Ctr 1978; **Fac Appt:** Asst Clin Prof Med, UMDNJ-Rutgers Med Sch

Farber, Charles M MD/PhD (Onc) - **Spec Exp:** Leukemia & Lymphoma; Breast Cancer; Ovarian Cancer; Multiple Myeloma; **Hospital:** Morristown Med Ctr (page 92); **Address:** Carol G Simon Cancer Center, 100 Madison Ave Fl 2, Morristown, NJ 07962-1089; **Phone:** 973-538-5210; **Board Cert:** Medical Oncology 2000; **Med School:** NYU Sch Med 1986; **Resid:** Internal Medicine, NY Hosp 1988; **Fellow:** Hematology & Oncology, NY Hosp 1991; **Fac Appt:** Asst Clin Prof Med, UMDNJ-NJ Med Sch, Newark

Gurubhagavatula, Sarada MD (Onc) - **Spec Exp:** Lung Cancer; **Hospital:** Morristown Med Ctr (page 92), St. Clare's Hosp-Denville; **Address:** Hematology-Oncology Associates, 100 Madison Ave, Fl 2, Box 1089, Morristown, NJ 07962; **Phone:** 973-538-5210; **Board Cert:** Medical Oncology 2004; **Med School:** Johns Hopkins Univ 1998; **Resid:** Internal Medicine, Brigham & Women's Hosp 2001; **Fellow:** Hematology & Oncology, Dana Farber Cancer Inst 2004

Papish, Steven W MD (Onc) - **Spec Exp:** Breast Cancer; Lymphoma; Gynecologic Cancer; **Hospital:** Morristown Med Ctr (page 92), St. Clare's Hosp - Boonton Township NO INPT/ER; **Address:** Carol G Simon Cancer Ctr, 100 Madison Ave Fl 2, Morristown, NJ 07962-1089; **Phone:** 973-538-5210; **Board Cert:** Internal Medicine 1977; Hematology 1980; Medical Oncology 1981; **Med School:** Univ Pennsylvania 1974; **Resid:** Internal Medicine, Geo Wash Univ Med Ctr 1978; **Fellow:** Hematology, New England Med Ctr 1979; Medical Oncology, Dana Farber Canc Inst 1981

Neonatal-Perinatal Medicine

Skolnick, Lawrence MD (NP) - **Spec Exp:** Neonatal Care; **Hospital:** Morristown Med Ctr (page 92), Overlook Med Ctr (page 92); **Address:** 100 Madison Ave, Morristown, NJ 07960-6136; **Phone:** 973-971-5488; **Board Cert:** Pediatrics 1977; Neonatal-Perinatal Medicine 1977; **Med School:** NYU Sch Med 1972; **Resid:** Pediatrics, Albert Einstein 1975; **Fellow:** Neonatal-Perinatal Medicine, Duke Univ Med Ctr 1977; **Fac Appt:** Assoc Clin Prof Ped, UMDNJ-NJ Med Sch, Newark

Nephrology

Fine, Paul L MD (Nep) - **Spec Exp:** Hypertension; Kidney Failure; Dialysis Care; **Hospital:** Morristown Med Ctr (page 92), St. Clare's Hosp-Denville; **Address:** 2 Franklin Pl, Morristown, NJ 07960-5305; **Phone:** 973-267-7673; **Board Cert:** Internal Medicine 1982; Nephrology 1984; **Med School:** Yale Univ 1979; **Resid:** Internal Medicine, New York Hosp 1982; **Fellow:** Nephrology, Kidney Ctr-Cornell Univ Med Ctr 1984; **Fac Appt:** Asst Clin Prof Med, Mount Sinai Sch Med

Lyman, Neil MD (Nep) - **Spec Exp:** Dialysis Care; Kidney Failure; **Hospital:** Saint Barnabas Med Ctr, Clara Maass Med Ctr; **Address:** 83 Hanover Rd, Ste 290, Florham Park, NJ 07932; **Phone:** 973-736-2212; **Board Cert:** Internal Medicine 1976; Nephrology 1980; **Med School:** Albert Einstein Coll Med 1973; **Resid:** Internal Medicine, Mt Sinai Hosp 1976; Nephrology, Mt Sinai Hosp 1979; **Fellow:** Nephrology, Boston Med Ctr 1977; **Fac Appt:** Asst Prof Med, UMDNJ-NJ Med Sch, Newark

Najarian, James MD (Nep) - **Spec Exp:** Hypertension; Kidney Failure; Transplant Medicine-Kidney; Dialysis Care; **Hospital:** Morristown Med Ctr (page 92), St. Clare's Hosp-Denville; **Address:** 121 Center Grove Rd, Ste 1314, Randolph, NJ 07869; **Phone:** 973-361-3737; **Board Cert:** Internal Medicine 1975; Nephrology 2006; **Med School:** Univ Wisc 1972; **Resid:** Internal Medicine, Beth Israel Hosp 1975; **Fellow:** Nephrology, Montefiore Med Ctr 1978

Neurological Surgery

Beyerl, Brian D MD (NS) - **Spec Exp:** Brain Tumors; Stereotactic Radiosurgery; Arteriovenous Malformations; **Hospital:** Morristown Med Ctr (page 92), Overlook Med Ctr (page 92); **Address:** Atlantic Neurosurgical Specialists, 310 Madison Ave, Ste 200, Morristown, NJ 07960; **Phone:** 973-285-7800; **Board Cert:** Neurological Surgery 1990; **Med School:** Johns Hopkins Univ 1980; **Resid:** Surgery, Johns Hopkins Univ Hosp 1981; Neurological Surgery, Mass Genl Hosp 1986; **Fac Appt:** Asst Clin Prof NS, UMDNJ-NJ Med Sch, Newark

Knightly, John J MD (NS) - **Spec Exp:** Spinal Surgery; Stereotactic Radiosurgery; Minimally Invasive Spinal Surgery; Trauma; **Hospital:** Overlook Med Ctr (page 92), Morristown Med Ctr (page 92); **Address:** Atlantic Neurosurgical Specialists, 310 Madison Ave, Ste 300, Morristown, NJ 07960; **Phone:** 973-285-7800; **Board Cert:** Neurological Surgery 1998; **Med School:** UMDNJ-NJ Med Sch, Newark 1985; **Resid:** Neurological Surgery, Bethesda Navval Hosp 1993; **Fellow:** Neurological Surgery, Barrow Neurol Inst 1993

Zampella, Edward J MD (NS) - **Spec Exp:** Stereotactic Radiosurgery; Pain Management; Brain Tumors; **Hospital:** Overlook Med Ctr (page 92), Morristown Med Ctr (page 92); **Address:** Atlantic Neurosurgical Specialists, 310 Madison Ave Fl 2, Morristown, NJ 07960; **Phone:** 973-285-7800; **Board Cert:** Neurological Surgery 1991; Pain Medicine 1997; **Med School:** UAB Sch Med 1982; **Resid:** Neurological Surgery, Univ Alabama Hosp 1988; **Fellow:** Neurology, Natl Hosp Nervous Disorders-Queen Square 1985; **Fac Appt:** Assoc Prof NS, UMDNJ-NJ Med Sch, Newark

Neurology

Fellus, Jonathan L MD (N) - **Spec Exp:** Brain Injury; Neuro-Rehabilitation; **Address:** Advanced Neurocare, 227 Route 206 N Bldg 2 - Ste 101, Flanders, NJ 07836; **Phone:** 732-494-7600; **Board Cert:** Neurology 2009; **Med School:** UMDNJ-RW Johnson Med Sch 1992; **Resid:** Neurology, Penn Hosp 1996; **Fellow:** Neurological Rehabilitation, Kernan Hosp/Univ MD Med Ctr 1997; **Fac Appt:** Asst Clin Prof N, UMDNJ-NJ Med Sch, Newark

Fox, Stuart W MD (N) - **Spec Exp:** Neuromuscular Disorders; Headache; **Hospital:** Morristown Med Ctr (page 92); **Address:** The Neuroscience Center of Northern NJ, 310 Madison Ave, Ste 120, Morristown, NJ 07960-6092; **Phone:** 973-285-1446; **Board Cert:** Internal Medicine ; Neurology ; **Med School:** Cornell Univ-Weill Med Coll 1975; **Resid:** Internal Medicine, Univ Mich Med Ctr 1978; Neurology, Albert Einstein 1981; **Fellow:** Clinical Neurophysiology, LI Jewish-Hillside Hosp 1982; **Fac Appt:** Asst Clin Prof Med, Columbia P&S

Obstetrics & Gynecology

Banks, Judy L MD (ObG) - **Hospital:** Morristown Med Ctr (page 92); **Address:** 256 Columbia Tpke, Ste 212 North, Florham Park, NJ 07932; **Phone:** 973-377-3374; **Board Cert:** Obstetrics & Gynecology 2003; **Med School:** Meharry Med Coll 1975; **Resid:** Obstetrics & Gynecology, Univ Hosp-UMDNJ 1980

Culligan, Patrick J MD (ObG) - **Spec Exp:** Uro-Gynecology; **Hospital:** Overlook Med Ctr (page 92), Morristown Med Ctr (page 92); **Address:** 435 South St, Ste 370, Morristown, NJ 07960; **Phone:** 973-971-7267; **Board Cert:** Obstetrics & Gynecology 2012; **Med School:** Mercer Univ Sch Med 1993; **Resid:** Obstetrics & Gynecology, Greenville Hlth Sys 1998; **Fellow:** Uro-Gynecology, Evanston Hosp 1999; **Fac Appt:** Assoc Clin Prof ObG, UMDNJ-NJ Med Sch, Newark

Dreyfuss, Patricia O MD (ObG) - **Hospital:** St. Clare's Hosp-Denville; **Address:** 115 Route 46 West, D Bldg - Ste 27, Mountain Lakes, NJ 07046; **Phone:** 973-334-3345; **Board Cert:** Obstetrics & Gynecology 1985; **Med School:** UMDNJ-Rutgers Med Sch 1979; **Resid:** Obstetrics & Gynecology, Saint Barnabas Med Ctr 1983

Gluck, Ian J MD (ObG) *PCP* - **Hospital:** Morristown Med Ctr (page 92); **Address:** Lifeline Med Assocs, 59 Franklin St, Morristown, NJ 07960; **Phone:** 973-538-1515; **Board Cert:** Obstetrics & Gynecology 1985; **Med School:** NY Med Coll 1979; **Resid:** Obstetrics & Gynecology, Grady Hlth Sys 1984; **Fac Appt:** Asst Clin Prof ObG, UMDNJ-NJ Med Sch, Newark

Iammatteo, Matthew D MD (ObG) - **Spec Exp:** Pregnancy-High Risk; Hysteroscopic Surgery; Laparoscopic Surgery; **Hospital:** Morristown Med Ctr (page 92); **Address:** Lifeline Med Assocs, 111 Madison Ave, Ste 311, Morristown, NJ 07960; **Phone:** 973-971-9950; **Board Cert:** Obstetrics & Gynecology 2012; **Med School:** Dominica 1985; **Resid:** Obstetrics & Gynecology, St Michaels Med Ctr 1990

Mohr, Robert F MD (ObG) *PCP* - **Spec Exp:** Gynecologic Surgery; Laparoscopic Surgery; Menopause Problems; **Hospital:** Morristown Med Ctr (page 92), St. Clare's Hosp-Denville; **Address:** Lifeline Med Assocs, 390 Route 10, Randolph, NJ 07869; **Phone:** 973-328-1262; **Board Cert:** Obstetrics & Gynecology 2003; **Med School:** Hahnemann Univ 1977; **Resid:** Obstetrics & Gynecology, Northwestern Meml Hosp 1982; **Fac Appt:** Asst Prof ObG, UMDNJ-Univ Med Dent NJ

Steer, Robert L MD (ObG) - **Spec Exp:** Pregnancy-High Risk; Multiple Gestation; **Hospital:** Morristown Med Ctr (page 92), Overlook Med Ctr (page 92); **Address:** 60 Franklin St, Morristown, NJ 07960-5217; **Phone:** 973-993-1919; **Board Cert:** Obstetrics & Gynecology 2012; **Med School:** Cornell Univ-Weill Med Coll 1986; **Resid:** Obstetrics & Gynecology, NY-Presby/Weill Cornell Med Ctr 1991; **Fac Appt:** Clin Prof ObG, Mount Sinai Sch Med

Wallis, Joseph J DO (ObG) - **Spec Exp:** Laparoscopic Surgery; Endoscopy; Infertility; **Hospital:** St. Clare's Hosp-Denville, St. Clare's Hosp-Dover; **Address:** 600 Mt Pleasant Ave, Ste G, Dover, NJ 07801-1629; **Phone:** 973-989-9000; **Board Cert:** Obstetrics & Gynecology 1977; **Med School:** Philadelphia Coll Osteo Med 1970; **Resid:** Internal Medicine, St Michaels Med Ctr 1972; Obstetrics & Gynecology, St Michaels Med Ctr 1976

Ophthalmology

Chen, Lucy L MD (Oph) - **Spec Exp:** Pediatric Ophthalmology; Strabismus; **Hospital:** St. Clare's Hosp-Sussex, Morristown Med Ctr (page 92); **Address:** Advocare Ped Eye Phys, 95 Madison Ave, Ste 301, Morristown, NJ 07960-6092; **Phone:** 973-540-8814; **Board Cert:** Internal Medicine 1988; Ophthalmology 2004; **Med School:** Boston Univ 1985; **Resid:** Internal Medicine, NY-Presby/Columbia Univ Med Ctr 1988; **Fellow:** Pediatric Ophthalmology, Wills Eye Hosp 1992

Kazam, Ezra S MD (Oph) - **Spec Exp:** Glaucoma; Cataract Surgery; Refractive Surgery; **Hospital:** Morristown Med Ctr (page 92); **Address:** 2 Washington Pl, Morristown, NJ 07960-4220; **Phone:** 973-267-8755; **Board Cert:** Ophthalmology 1978; **Med School:** SUNY Downstate 1973; **Resid:** Ophthalmology, Montefiore Med Ctr 1978; **Fac Appt:** Asst Clin Prof Oph, Albert Einstein Coll Med

Pinke, Robert S MD (Oph) - **Spec Exp:** Cataract Surgery; Glaucoma; **Hospital:** St. Clare's Hosp-Dover, St. Clare's Hosp-Denville; **Address:** 66 Sunset Strip, Ste 107, Succasunna, NJ 07876; **Phone:** 973-584-4451; **Board Cert:** Ophthalmology 1989; **Med School:** Mount Sinai Sch Med 1984; **Resid:** Ophthalmology, Methodist Hosp 1989

Sachs, Ronald MD (Oph) - **Spec Exp:** Macular Degeneration; Diabetic Eye Disease/Retinopathy; Retinal Disorders; Retina/Vitreous Surgery; **Hospital:** Morristown Med Ctr (page 92), St. Clare's Hosp-Denville; **Address:** 8 Saddle Rd, Ste 201, Cedar Knolls, NJ 07927; **Phone:** 973-539-3600; **Board Cert:** Ophthalmology 2004; **Med School:** NYU Sch Med 1988; **Resid:** Ophthalmology, Montefiore Med Ctr 1992; **Fellow:** Retina, Albert Einstein Med Ctr 1993

Silverman, Cary M MD (Oph) - **Spec Exp:** LASIK-Refractive Surgery; Cataract Surgery; **Hospital:** Saint Barnabas Med Ctr; **Address:** EyeCare 20/20, 46 Eagle Rock Ave E, East Hanover, NJ 07936; **Phone:** 973-664-7794; **Board Cert:** Ophthalmology 1987; **Med School:** UMDNJ-NJ Med Sch, Newark 1982; **Resid:** Ophthalmology, Hahnemann Univ Hosp 1987; **Fac Appt:** Clin Prof Oph, UMDNJ-RW Johnson Med Sch

Orthopaedic Surgery

Dowling, William J MD (OrS) - **Spec Exp:** Joint Replacement; **Hospital:** Morristown Med Ctr (page 92), Overlook Med Ctr (page 92); **Address:** 111 Madison Ave, Ste 400, Morristown, NJ 07960; **Phone:** 973-971-6895; **Board Cert:** Orthopaedic Surgery 1978; **Med School:** UMDNJ-NJ Med Sch, Newark 1971; **Resid:** Orthopaedic Surgery, UMDNJ-NJ Med Sch Affil Hosp 1977

Montgomery, Kenneth MD (OrS) - **Spec Exp:** Hand Surgery; Shoulder Surgery; Knee Surgery; Rotator Cuff Surgery; **Hospital:** Morristown Med Ctr (page 92); **Address:** TriCounty Orthopaedics, Advanced Med Ctr, 197 Ridgedale Ave, Ste 300, Cedar Knolls, NJ 07927; **Phone:** 973-538-2334; **Board Cert:** Orthopaedic Surgery 2010; Orthopaedic Sports Medicine 2007; **Med School:** UCSF 1990; **Resid:** Orthopaedic Surgery, Hosp Special Surgery 1995; **Fellow:** Sports Medicine, Lenox Hill Hosp 1996; Obstetrics & Anesthesiology, Brigham & Women's Hosp 1997

Rieger, Kenneth J MD (OrS) - **Spec Exp:** Fractures-Pediatric; Scoliosis; Spinal Surgery; **Hospital:** Overlook Med Ctr (page 92), Morristown Med Ctr (page 92); **Address:** 40 Main St, Chatham, NJ 07928; **Phone:** 973-635-0800; **Board Cert:** Orthopaedic Surgery 2009; **Med School:** Columbia P&S 2001; **Resid:** Orthopaedic Surgery, NY Presby Hosp 2006; **Fellow:** Spine Surgery, Leatherman Spine Inst 2007

Rieger, Mark A MD (OrS) - **Spec Exp:** Pediatric Orthopaedic Surgery; Scoliosis; Hip Disorders-Pediatric; Adolescent Sports Medicine; **Hospital:** Morristown Med Ctr (page 92), Saint Barnabas Med Ctr; **Address:** Advocare Orthopedic Ctr, 218 Ridgedale Ave, Ste 104, Cedar Knolls, NJ 07927-2109; **Phone:** 973-538-7700; **Board Cert:** Orthopaedic Surgery 2012; **Med School:** Univ Conn 1983; **Resid:** Orthopaedic Surgery, NS-LIJ Hlth Sys 1988; **Fellow:** Pediatric Orthopaedic Surgery, Nemours/Alfred I. duPont Hosp for Chldn 1989; **Fac Appt:** Asst Clin Prof OrS, NYU Sch Med

Spielman, Joel H MD (OrS) - **Spec Exp:** Spinal Surgery; **Hospital:** St. Clare's Hosp-Dover, St. Clare's Hosp-Denville; **Address:** Ortho Assocs of West Jersey, 600 Mt Pleasant Ave, Dover, NJ 07801-1630; **Phone:** 973-989-0888; **Board Cert:** Orthopaedic Surgery 2005; **Med School:** Albert Einstein Coll Med 1986; **Resid:** Orthopaedic Surgery, Montefiore Med Ctr 1991; **Fellow:** Spine Surgery, Hosp for Special Surg 1993

Taffet, Berton MD (OrS) - **Hospital:** Morristown Med Ctr (page 92); **Address:** 111 Madison Ave Fl 4 - Ste 400, Morristown, NJ 07960; **Phone:** 973-984-0404; **Board Cert:** Orthopaedic Surgery 2011; **Med School:** Albert Einstein Coll Med 1978; **Resid:** Orthopaedic Surgery, Mt Sinai Med Ctr 1983; **Fellow:** Joint Replacement Surgery, Univ Colorado Hosp 1984

Otolaryngology

Fleming, Gregory MD (Oto) - **Spec Exp:** Endoscopic Sinus Surgery; Sleep Disorders/Apnea; **Hospital:** Morristown Med Ctr (page 92), Overlook Med Ctr (page 92); **Address:** Morristown Otolaryngology Grp, 26 Madison Ave, Morristown, NJ 07960; **Phone:** 973-267-1850; **Board Cert:** Otolaryngology 1988; **Med School:** Univ Mass Sch Med 1982; **Resid:** Surgery, UMass Memorial Med Ctr 1984; Otolaryngology, Mass Eye & Ear Infirm 1988

Lachman, Reid MD (Oto) - **Hospital:** Morristown Med Ctr (page 92); **Address:** Advocare ENT Specialists Morristown, 95 Madison Ave, Ste 105, Morristown, NJ 07960-7331; **Phone:** 973-644-0808; **Board Cert:** Otolaryngology 1986; **Med School:** NY Med Coll 1981; **Resid:** Otolaryngology, Albert Einstein Med Ctr 1986

Taylor, Howard MD (Oto) - **Spec Exp:** Hearing Loss; Sinus Surgery; Throat Disorders; Voice Disorders; **Hospital:** Chilton Hosp; **Address:** 51 State Rte 23 S, Riverdale, NJ 07457-1625; **Phone:** 973-831-1220; **Board Cert:** Otolaryngology 1980; **Med School:** Columbia P&S 1976; **Resid:** Otolaryngology, Univ Chicago Affil Hosps 1980; **Fellow:** Facial Plastic Surgery, Med Coll PA Affil Hosps 1981; **Fac Appt:** Asst Clin Prof Oto, UMDNJ-NJ Med Sch, Newark

Pain Medicine

Rudman, Michael E MD (PM) - **Spec Exp:** Pain-Back; Pain-Chronic; Complex Regional Pain Syndromes; **Hospital:** Morristown Med Ctr (page 92); **Address:** NJ Pain Cons, 310 Madison Ave Fl 3 - Ste 301, Morristown, NJ 07960; **Phone:** 908-630-0175; **Board Cert:** Pain Medicine 2007; Anesthesiology 1993; **Med School:** Penn State Coll Med 1988; **Resid:** Anesthesiology, Hosp Univ Penn - UPHS 1993

Pediatric Allergy & Immunology

Barisciano, Lisa MD (PA&I) - **Spec Exp:** Asthma; **Hospital:** Morristown Med Ctr (page 92); **Address:** 15 James St, Ste 4, Florham Park, NJ 07932; **Phone:** 973-503-0600; **Board Cert:** Pediatrics 2009; Allergy & Immunology 2003; **Med School:** UMDNJ-Rutgers Med Sch 1998; **Resid:** Pediatrics, NY-Presby/Weill Cornell Med Ctr 2001; **Fellow:** Allergy & Immunology, NY-Presby/Weill Cornell Med Ctr 2003

Pediatric Cardiology

Donnelly, Christine M MD (PCd) - **Spec Exp:** Fetal Echocardiography; Congenital Heart Disease; Cardiac Catheterization; **Hospital:** Morristown Med Ctr (page 92), Morgan Stanley Children's Hosp of NY-Presby, NY (page 104); **Address:** Goryeb Chldns Hosp-Ped Cardiology, 100 Madison Ave, Morristown, NJ 07962; **Phone:** 973-971-5996; **Board Cert:** Pediatrics 1985; Pediatric Cardiology 1985; **Med School:** Columbia P&S 1978; **Resid:** Pediatrics, NY-Presby/Columbia Univ Med Ctr 1981; **Fellow:** Pediatric Cardiology, NY-Presby/Columbia Univ Med Ctr 1984; **Fac Appt:** Assoc Clin Prof Ped, Columbia P&S

Pediatric Endocrinology

Cerame, Barbara I MD (PEn) - **Spec Exp:** Diabetes; **Hospital:** Goryeb Children's Hosp (page 92), Overlook Med Ctr (page 92); **Address:** Goryeb Chldn's Hosp at Morristown, 100 Madison Ave, Box 53, Morristown, NJ 07960; **Phone:** 973-971-4340; **Board Cert:** Pediatrics 2011; Pediatric Endocrinology 2011; **Med School:** St Louis Univ 1985; **Resid:** Pediatrics, Robert Wood Johnson Univ Hosp 1995; **Fellow:** Pediatric Endocrinology, NY Presby Hosp/Cornell 1998; **Fac Appt:** Asst Prof Ped, UMDNJ-Rutgers Med Sch

Chin, Daisy MD (PEn) - **Spec Exp:** Thyroid Disorders; Growth Disorders; Pubertal Disorders; Diabetes; **Hospital:** Goryeb Children's Hosp (page 92), Overlook Med Ctr (page 92); **Address:** Gorebny Chldn's Hosp at Morristown, 100 Madison Ave, Box 53, Morristown, NJ 07960; **Phone:** 973-971-4340; **Board Cert:** Pediatric Endocrinology 2007; **Med School:** SUNY Downstate 1992; **Resid:** Pediatrics, Columbia Presby Med Ctr 1995; **Fellow:** Pediatric Endocrinology, NYU Med Ctr 1998

Starkman, Harold S MD (PEn) - **Spec Exp:** Diabetes; Growth Disorders; **Hospital:** Goryeb Children's Hosp (page 92), Morristown Med Ctr (page 92); **Address:** Morristown Meml Hosp-Atlantic Hlth, 100 Madison Ave, Morristown, NJ 07962-6136; **Phone:** 973-971-4340; **Board Cert:** Pediatrics 1980; Pediatric Endocrinology 1983; **Med School:** Albert Einstein Coll Med 1976; **Resid:** Pediatrics, Mt Sinai Med Ctr 1978; Pediatrics, NY-Presby/Weill Cornell Med Ctr 1979; **Fellow:** Pediatric Endocrinology, NY-Presby/Weill Cornell Med Ctr 1980; Pediatric Endocrinology, Joslin Diabetes Ctr 1983; **Fac Appt:** Assoc Prof Ped, UMDNJ-NJ Med Sch, Newark

Pediatric Gastroenterology

Rosh, Joel MD (PGe) - **Spec Exp:** Inflammatory Bowel Disease; Celiac Disease; Liver Disease; **Hospital:** Morristown Med Ctr (page 92), Overlook Med Ctr (page 92); **Address:** Dept Peds Gastroenterology & Nutrition, 100 Madison Ave, Morristown, NJ 07960-6136; **Phone:** 973-971-5676; **Board Cert:** Pediatric Gastroenterology 2007; **Med School:** Albert Einstein Coll Med 1986; **Resid:** Pediatrics, Babies Hosp/Columbia-Presby Med Ctr 1989; **Fellow:** Pediatric Gastroenterology, Mount Sinai Med Ctr 1991; **Fac Appt:** Assoc Prof Ped, UMDNJ-NJ Med Sch, Newark

Pediatric Infectious Disease

Baorto, Elizabeth P MD (PInf) - **Spec Exp:** Lyme Disease; **Hospital:** Morristown Med Ctr (page 92); **Address:** Morristown Medical Ctr, Div Pediatric Infectious Disease, 100 Madison Ave, Morristown, NJ 07960; **Phone:** 973-971-6329; **Board Cert:** Pediatrics 2011; Pediatric Infectious Disease 2007; **Med School:** SUNY Downstate 1993; **Resid:** Pediatrics, St Louis Children's Hosp 1996

Pediatric Pulmonology

Atlas, Arthur B MD (PPul) - **Spec Exp:** Asthma; Cystic Fibrosis; Lung Disease; **Hospital:** Morristown Med Ctr (page 92), Overlook Med Ctr (page 92); **Address:** Morristown Meml Hosp, Resp Ctr for Chldn, 100 Madison Ave, Box 107, Morristown, NJ 07962; **Phone:** 973-971-4142; **Board Cert:** Pediatric Pulmonology 2007; **Med School:** Mexico 1982; **Resid:** Pediatrics, St Louis Chldns Hosp 1986; **Fellow:** Allergy & Immunology, St Louis Chldns Hosp 1989; Pediatric Pulmonology, Chldns Hosp/Univ Pittsburgh 1991; **Fac Appt:** Asst Clin Prof Ped, UMDNJ-NJ Med Sch, Newark

Pediatric Urology

Connor, John Patrick MD (Ped Uro) - **Hospital:** Goryeb Children's Hosp (page 92), Overlook Med Ctr (page 92); **Address:** Adult & Pediatric Urology Group, 261 James St, Ste 3A, Morristown, NJ 07960; **Phone:** 973-539-0333; **Board Cert:** Urology 2008; Pediatric Urology 2008; **Med School:** Ireland 1983; **Resid:** Surgery, UCLA Med Ctr 1986; Urology, Columbia-Presby Hosp 1990; **Fellow:** Urologic Oncology, Meml Sloan Kettering 1992; Pediatric Urology, Chldns Hosp Mich 1993; **Fac Appt:** Asst Prof U, Columbia P&S

Pediatrics

Ashton, Julie MD (Ped) *PCP* - **Hospital:** Goryeb Children's Hosp (page 92), Morristown Med Ctr (page 92); **Address:** Franklin Pediatrics, 91 S Jefferson Rd, Whippany, NJ 07981; **Phone:** 973-538-6116; **Board Cert:** Pediatrics 2012; **Med School:** UMDNJ-NJ Med Sch, Newark 1987; **Resid:** Pediatrics, UMDNJ Chldn's Hosp 1990; **Fac Appt:** Asst Clin Prof Ped, UMDNJ-NJ Med Sch, Newark

Gotfried, Fern MD (Ped) *PCP* - **Hospital:** Goryeb Children's Hosp (page 92), Morristown Med Ctr (page 92); **Address:** Franklin Pediatrics, 91 S Jefferson Rd, Ste 200, Whippany, NJ 07981; **Phone:** 973-538-6116; **Board Cert:** Pediatrics 1986; Adolescent Medicine 2009; **Med School:** UMDNJ-Rutgers Med Sch 1980; **Resid:** Pediatrics, Strong Meml Hosp 1983; **Fellow:** Adolescent Medicine, Strong Meml Hosp 1985

Handler, Robert W MD (Ped) *PCP* - **Spec Exp:** Asthma; Allergy; Behavioral Disorders; **Hospital:** Morristown Med Ctr (page 92), St. Clare's Hosp-Denville; **Address:** Advocare Parsippany Pediatrics, 1140 Parsippany Blvd, Ste 102, Parsippany, NJ 07054; **Phone:** 973-263-0066; **Board Cert:** Pediatrics 1980; **Med School:** UMDNJ-NJ Med Sch, Newark 1975; **Resid:** Pediatrics, Chldns Hosp 1978

Lavaia-Marzano, Maria MD (Ped) *PCP* - **Hospital:** Goryeb Children's Hosp (page 92), Overlook Med Ctr (page 92); **Address:** Madison Pediatrics, 435 South St, Ste 200, Morristown, NJ 07960; **Phone:** 973-822-0003; **Board Cert:** Pediatrics 2011; **Med School:** SUNY Downstate 1993; **Resid:** Pediatrics, NY Presby Hosp/Cornell 1996

Lodish, Stephanie R MD (Ped) *PCP* - **Hospital:** Goryeb Children's Hosp (page 92), Overlook Med Ctr (page 92); **Address:** Madison Pediatrics, 435 South St, Ste 200, Morristown, NJ 07960; **Phone:** 973-822-0003; **Board Cert:** Pediatrics 2007; **Med School:** Case West Res Univ 1996; **Resid:** Pediatrics, Chldn's Hosp 1999

Meltzer, Alan J MD (Ped) *PCP* - **Hospital:** Goryeb Children's Hosp (page 92), Overlook Med Ctr (page 92); **Address:** Madison Pediatrics, 435 South St, Ste 200, Morristown, NJ 07960; **Phone:** 973-822-0003; **Board Cert:** Pediatrics 2002; **Med School:** SUNY Downstate 1981; **Resid:** Pediatrics, N Shore Univ Hosp 1984

Scherer, Susan MD (Ped) *PCP* - **Hospital:** Goryeb Children's Hosp (page 92), Overlook Med Ctr (page 92); **Address:** Madison Pediatrics, 435 South St, Ste 200, Morristown, NJ 07940; **Phone:** 973-822-0003; **Board Cert:** Pediatrics 2008; **Med School:** Univ Tex, San Antonio 1997; **Resid:** Pediatrics, Johns Hopkins Hosp 2000

Shaw-Brachfeld, Jennifer MD (Ped) *PCP* - **Spec Exp:** Developmental & Behavioral Disorders; **Hospital:** Overlook Med Ctr (page 92), Saint Barnabas Med Ctr; **Address:** Touchpoint Pediatrics, 17 Watchung Ave, Chatham, NJ 07928; **Phone:** 973-665-0900; **Board Cert:** Pediatrics 2007; Developmental-Behavioral Pediatrics 2010; **Med School:** Univ Conn 1989; **Resid:** Pediatrics, Schneider Chldn's Hosp 1992; **Fellow:** Developmental-Behavioral Pediatrics, Schneider Chldn's Hosp 1994

Suda, Anjuli MD (Ped) *PCP* - **Spec Exp:** Pulmonary Disease; **Hospital:** Chilton Hosp; **Address:** 170 Kinnelon Rd, Ste 28, Kinnelon, NJ 07405; **Phone:** 973-838-0001; **Board Cert:** Pediatrics 1988; **Med School:** India 1976; **Resid:** Pediatrics, St Joseph's Hosp & Med Ctr 1985

Physical Medicine & Rehabilitation

Klecz, Robert J MD (PMR) - **Spec Exp:** Musculoskeletal Disorders; Stroke Rehabilitation; Spasticity Management; Electromyography; **Hospital:** Morristown Med Ctr (page 92); **Address:** Rehab Inst at Morristown Hosp, 95 Mount Kemble Ave, Thebaud Bldg Fl 4, Morristown, NJ 07960; **Phone:** 973-796-3600; **Board Cert:** Physical Medicine & Rehabilitation 2006; **Med School:** Poland 1990; **Resid:** Internal Medicine, UMDNJ Univ Hosp 1992; Physical Medicine & Rehabilitation, UMDNJ-Kessler Inst 1995; **Fac Appt:** Assoc Clin Prof PMR, UMDNJ-Univ Med Dent NJ

Mulford, Gregory J MD (PMR) - **Spec Exp:** Sports Medicine; Electrodiagnosis; **Hospital:** Morristown Med Ctr (page 92), Overlook Med Ctr (page 92); **Address:** Assoc in Rehab Medicine, 95 Mt Kemble Ave, Thebaud Bldg - Fl 4, Morristown, NJ 07960; **Phone:** 973-796-3600; **Board Cert:** Physical Medicine & Rehabilitation 1990; Sports Medicine 2011; **Med School:** UMDNJ-RW Johnson Med Sch 1985; **Resid:** Physical Medicine & Rehabilitation, Columbia-Presby Hosp 1989; **Fac Appt:** Assoc Clin Prof PMR, UMDNJ-Univ Med Dent NJ

Valenza, Joseph P MD (PMR) - **Spec Exp:** Pain Management; Complex Regional Pain Syndromes; Repetitive Strain Injuries; Spinal Cord Injury; **Hospital:** Kessler Inst for Rehab - Chester; **Address:** Kessler Inst for Rehab, Dept Pain Management, 201 Pleasant Hill Rd, Chester, NJ 07930; **Phone:** 973-252-6402; **Board Cert:** Physical Medicine & Rehabilitation 2007; Pain Medicine 2012; **Med School:** SUNY Downstate 1992; **Resid:** Physical Medicine & Rehabilitation, Vet Affairs Med Ctr 1996; **Fac Appt:** Asst Clin Prof PMR, UMDNJ-NJ Med Sch, Newark

Plastic Surgery

Colon, Francisco G MD (PlS) - **Spec Exp:** Cosmetic Surgery-Face & Body; Reconstructive Plastic Surgery; **Hospital:** Saint Barnabas Med Ctr, Morristown Med Ctr (page 92); **Address:** PeerGroup Plastic Surgery Ctr, 124 Columbia Tpke, Florham Park, NJ 07932; **Phone:** 973-822-3000; **Board Cert:** Plastic Surgery 2007; **Med School:** Columbia P&S 1987; **Resid:** Surgery, St Lukes Roosevelt Hosp 1992; Plastic Surgery, Beth Israel Deaconess Med Ctr 1994; **Fellow:** Vascular Surgery, Bet Israel Deaconess Med Ctr 1995

Lange, David J MD (PlS) - **Spec Exp:** Cosmetic Surgery-Breast; Liposuction & Body Contouring; Craniofacial Surgery/Reconstruction; **Hospital:** Saint Barnabas Med Ctr, Morristown Med Ctr (page 92); **Address:** Peer Group, 124 Columbia Tpke, Florham Park, NJ 07932; **Phone:** 973-822-3000; **Board Cert:** Plastic Surgery ; **Med School:** Mexico 1979; **Resid:** Surgery, St Banabas Med Ctr 1985; **Fellow:** Plastic Surgery, St Louis Univ Hosp 1987

Pyo, Daniel J MD (PlS) - **Spec Exp:** Cosmetic Surgery-Breast; Liposuction & Body Contouring; Facial Rejuvenation; **Hospital:** Morristown Med Ctr (page 92), Saint Barnabas Med Ctr; **Address:** Plastic Surgery Ctr of NJ, 131 Madison Ave, Ste 120, Morristown, NJ 07960; **Phone:** 973-540-9055; **Board Cert:** Surgery 2009; Plastic Surgery 2009; **Med School:** Mount Sinai Sch Med 1990; **Resid:** Surgery, Strong Meml Hosp 1995; **Fellow:** Plastic Surgery, Yale-New Haven Hosp 1997

Rafizadeh, Farhad MD (PlS) - **Spec Exp:** Breast Reconstruction; Cosmetic Surgery-Face; Cosmetic Surgery-Breast; Facial Rejuvenation; **Hospital:** Morristown Med Ctr (page 92), Saint Barnabas Med Ctr; **Address:** 101 Madison Ave, Ste 105, Morristown, NJ 07960; **Phone:** 973-267-0928; **Board Cert:** Plastic Surgery 1986; **Med School:** Switzerland 1975; **Resid:** Surgery, St Barnabas Med Ctr 1981; Surgery, Morristown Meml Hosp 1982; **Fellow:** Plastic Surgery, New York Hosp-Cornell Med Ctr 1984

Starker, Isaac MD (PlS) - **Spec Exp:** Cosmetic Surgery-Face & Body; Cosmetic Surgery-Breast; Breast Reconstruction; **Hospital:** Morristown Med Ctr (page 92), Saint Barnabas Med Ctr; **Address:** 124 Columbia Tpke, Florham Park, NJ 07932; **Phone:** 973-822-3000; **Board Cert:** Plastic Surgery 1992; **Med School:** NYU Sch Med 1981; **Resid:** Surgery, St Lukes-Roosevelt Hosp Ctr 1986; Plastic Surgery, Montefiore Med Ctr 1988; **Fellow:** Hand Surgery, St Lukes-Roosevelt Hosp Ctr 1989

Weinstein, Larry MD (PlS) - **Spec Exp:** Breast Cosmetic & Reconstructive Surgery; Cosmetic Surgery-Face; Liposuction & Body Contouring; Facial Rejuvenation; **Hospital:** Morristown Med Ctr (page 92), Overlook Med Ctr (page 92); **Address:** 385 State Rte 24, Ste 3K, Chester, NJ 07930-2910; **Phone:** 908-879-2222; **Board Cert:** Plastic Surgery 1993; **Med School:** Mexico 1979; **Resid:** Surgery, Univ Hosp/Morristown Meml Hosp 1984; Surgical Oncology, Meml Sloan-Kettering Cancer Ctr 1985; **Fellow:** Research, Univ Pittsburgh 1986; Plastic Surgery, SUNY-Brooklyn Med Ctr 1988

Psychiatry

Fennelly, Bryan W MD (Psyc) - **Spec Exp:** Child Psychiatry; ADD/ADHD; Depression; Bipolar/Mood Disorders; **Hospital:** Morristown Med Ctr (page 92); **Address:** 8 Shunpike Rd, Ste 9, Madison, NJ 07940-2740; **Phone:** 973-660-0084; **Board Cert:** Psychiatry 2004; Child & Adolescent Psychiatry 2005; **Med School:** UMDNJ-Univ Med Dent NJ 1989; **Resid:** Psychiatry, NYU Med Ctr 1992; **Fellow:** Child & Adolescent Psychiatry, NYU 1994

Pulmonary Disease

Benton, Marc L MD (Pul) - **Spec Exp:** Asthma & Emphysema; Sleep Disorders/Apnea; Cough; **Hospital:** Morristown Med Ctr (page 92); **Address:** 300 Madison Ave, Fl Third, Madison, NJ 07940; **Phone:** 973-822-2772; **Board Cert:** Internal Medicine 1985; Pulmonary Disease 1988; Critical Care Medicine 2005; Sleep Medicine 2011; **Med School:** Mount Sinai Sch Med 1982; **Resid:** Internal Medicine, Mt Sinai Hosp 1985; **Fellow:** Pulmonary Disease, NYU Med Ctr 1988; **Fac Appt:** Asst Clin Prof Med, Mount Sinai Sch Med

Fiel, Stanley MD (Pul) - **Spec Exp:** Cystic Fibrosis; Chronic Obstructive Lung Disease (COPD); Asthma; Bronchiectasis; **Hospital:** Morristown Med Ctr (page 92), Overlook Med Ctr (page 92); **Address:** 100 Madison Ave, Morristown, NJ 07960; **Phone:** 973-971-7165; **Board Cert:** Internal Medicine 1976; Pulmonary Disease 1978; **Med School:** Med Coll PA 1973; **Resid:** Internal Medicine, Temple Univ Hosp 1976; **Fellow:** Pulmonary Disease, Hosp Univ Penn 1978; **Fac Appt:** Prof Med, Mount Sinai Sch Med

O'Donnell, Timothy DO (Pul) - **Spec Exp:** Asthma; Lung Cancer; Interstitial Lung Disease; **Hospital:** Chilton Hosp, Morristown Med Ctr (page 92); **Address:** 63 Beaver Brook Rd, Ste 301, Lincoln Park, NJ 07035; **Phone:** 973-694-1300; **Board Cert:** Internal Medicine 1989; Pulmonary Disease 2012; Critical Care Medicine 2003; **Med School:** UMDNJ Sch Osteo Med 1985; **Resid:** Internal Medicine, Univ Hosp-UMDNJ 1989; **Fellow:** Pulmonary Critical Care Medicine, UMDNJ-Newark Beth Israel Med Ctr 1992

Radiation Oncology

Wong, James R MD (RadRO) - **Spec Exp:** Prostate Cancer; Head & Neck Cancer; Breast Cancer; Pancreatic Cancer; **Hospital:** Morristown Med Ctr (page 92); **Address:** Morristown Medical Center, Radiation Oncology Dept, 100 Madison Ave, Box 9, Morristown, NJ 07960; **Phone:** 973-971-5329; **Board Cert:** Radiation Oncology 1993; **Med School:** Harvard Med Sch 1986; **Resid:** Radiation Oncology, Harvard Jt Ctr for Rad Therapy 1992; **Fellow:** Radiation Oncology, NY-Presby/Weill Cornell Med Ctr 1997; **Fac Appt:** Assoc Clin Prof RadRO, Columbia P&S

Reproductive Endocrinology

Bergh, Paul A MD (RE) - **Spec Exp:** Infertility-IVF; **Hospital:** Morristown Med Ctr (page 92); **Address:** Reproductive Med Assocs of New Jersey, 140 Allen Rd, Basking Ridge, NJ 07920; **Phone:** 973-971-4600; **Board Cert:** Obstetrics & Gynecology 2012; Reproductive Endocrinology 2012; **Med School:** UMDNJ-RW Johnson Med Sch 1983; **Resid:** Obstetrics & Gynecology, St Barnabas Hosp 1989; **Fellow:** Reproductive Endocrinology, Mount Sinai Med Ctr 1991; **Fac Appt:** Asst Clin Prof ObG, UMDNJ-RW Johnson Med Sch

Rheumatology

Pasik, Deborah MD (Rhu) - **Spec Exp:** Rheumatoid Arthritis; Osteoporosis; Lupus/SLE; **Hospital:** Morristown Med Ctr (page 92); **Address:** 8 Saddle Road, Ste 202, Cedar Knolls, NJ 07927; **Phone:** 973-984-9796; **Board Cert:** Internal Medicine 1985; Rheumatology 1988; **Med School:** Mount Sinai Sch Med 1982; **Resid:** Internal Medicine, Beth Israel Hosp 1985; **Fellow:** Rheumatology, NYU Med Ctr 1988

Sports Medicine

Feldman, David J MD (SM) - **Hospital:** St. Clare's Hosp-Denville; **Address:** 16 Pocono Rd, Ste 100, Denville, NJ 07834; **Phone:** 973-625-5700; **Board Cert:** Orthopaedic Surgery 1979; Orthopaedic Sports Medicine 2007; **Med School:** Boston Univ 1972; **Resid:** Surgery, Mt Sinai Med Ctr 1974; Orthopaedic Surgery, Mt Sinai Med Ctr 1977; **Fellow:** Pediatric Orthopaedic Surgery, Stanford Univ Med Ctr 1978

Surgery

Carter, Mitchel S MD (S) - **Spec Exp:** Laparoscopic Surgery; Laparoscopic Cholecystectomy; Gastroesophageal Reflux Disease (GERD); Hernia; **Hospital:** Morristown Med Ctr (page 92); **Address:** Allied Surgical Grp, 261 James St, Ste 2G, Morristown, NJ 07960; **Phone:** 973-267-6400; **Board Cert:** Surgery 2003; **Med School:** Univ Hlth Scis, Chicago Med Sch 1979; **Resid:** Surgery, Montefiore Med Ctr 1984

Diehl, William L MD (S) - **Spec Exp:** Breast Cancer; Pancreatic Cancer; Gastrointestinal Cancer; Colon Cancer; **Hospital:** Morristown Med Ctr (page 92); **Address:** Allied Surgical Grp, 261 James St, Ste 2G, Morristown, NJ 07960; **Phone:** 973-267-6400; **Board Cert:** Surgery 2009; **Med School:** Mexico 1981; **Resid:** Surgery, Morristown Med Ctr 1986; **Fellow:** Surgical Oncology, Meml Sloan-Kettering Cancer Ctr 1988

Rolandelli, Rolando H MD (S) - **Spec Exp:** Crohn's Disease; Inflammatory Bowel Disease; Gastrointestinal Surgery; Colon & Rectal Surgery; **Hospital:** Morristown Med Ctr (page 92), Overlook Med Ctr (page 92); **Address:** 435 South St, Ste 360, Morristown, NJ 07960; **Phone:** 973-971-7200; **Board Cert:** Surgery 2009; **Med School:** Argentina 1977; **Resid:** Surgery, Central Airforce Hosp 1982; Surgery, Univ Hosp Penn 1990; **Fellow:** Metabolism, Univ Hosp Penn 1984

Strutin, Millard D MD (S) - **Hospital:** St. Clare's Hosp-Denville; **Address:** NW Surgical Assocs, 121 Center Grove Rd, Randolph, NJ 07869; **Phone:** 973-328-1414; **Board Cert:** Surgery 2008; Surgical Critical Care 2012; **Med School:** Italy 1981; **Resid:** Surgery, Univ Hosp-UMDNJ 1986

Whitman, Eric D MD (S) - **Spec Exp:** Melanoma; Endocrine Tumors; Cancer Surgery; Sarcoma; **Hospital:** Morristown Med Ctr (page 92), Overlook Med Ctr (page 92); **Address:** Atlantic Hlth, Melanoma Ctr, 100 Madison Ave, Ste 3502, Morristown, NJ 07960; **Phone:** 973-971-7111; **Board Cert:** Surgery 2002; **Med School:** Penn State Coll Med 1985; **Resid:** Surgery, Hershey Med Ctr 1991; **Fellow:** Surgical Oncology, Natl Inst Hlth 1992

Thoracic & Cardiac Surgery

Brown III, John M MD (T&CS) - **Spec Exp:** Cardiac Surgery-Adult; Heart Valve Surgery; **Hospital:** Morristown Med Ctr (page 92); **Address:** Mid-Atlantic Surgical Assocs, 100 Madison Ave, Morristown, NJ 07960; **Phone:** 973-971-7300; **Board Cert:** Thoracic & Cardiac Surgery 2013; **Med School:** Cornell Univ-Weill Med Coll 1986; **Resid:** Surgery, NY-Presby/Weill Cornell Med Ctr 1991; **Fellow:** Cardiothoracic Surgery, Meml Sloan-Kettering Cancer Ctr 1993

Widmann, Mark D MD (T&CS) - **Spec Exp:** Minimally Invasive Thoracic Surgery; Video Assisted Thoracic Surgery (VATS); **Hospital:** Morristown Med Ctr (page 92), Overlook Med Ctr (page 92); **Address:** North Jersey Thoracic Surgical Assocs, 100 Madison Ave, Ste 4101, Morristown, NJ 07960; **Phone:** 973-644-4844; **Board Cert:** Thoracic & Cardiac Surgery 2007; **Med School:** Yale Univ 1987; **Resid:** Surgery, Yale-New Haven Hosp 1995; **Fellow:** Cardiothoracic Surgery, Univ Iowa Hosps & Clins 1998; **Fac Appt:** Asst Clin Prof S, Columbia P&S

Urology

Chaikin, David C MD (U) - **Spec Exp:** Voiding Dysfunction; Urology-Female; Neuro-Urology; **Hospital:** Morristown Med Ctr (page 92); **Address:** Morristown Urology, 261 James St, Ste 1A, Morristown, NJ 07960; **Phone:** 973-539-1050; **Board Cert:** Urology 2013; Female Pelvic Medicine & Reconstuctive Surgery 2013; **Med School:** Albert Einstein Coll Med 1992; **Resid:** Urology, Hosp Univ Penn 1997; **Fellow:** Female Urology, NY-Presby/Weill Cornell Med Ctr 1999; **Fac Appt:** Asst Clin Prof U, Cornell Univ-Weill Med Coll

Colton, Marc D MD (U) - **Spec Exp:** Prostate Cancer; Urologic Cancer; Kidney Stones; Robotic Urologic Surgery; **Hospital:** St. Clare's Hosp-Denville, Morristown Med Ctr (page 92); **Address:** Morris Urology, 16 Pocono Rd, Ste 205, Denville, NJ 07834; **Phone:** 973-627-0060; **Board Cert:** Urology 2006; **Med School:** Med Coll PA 1989; **Resid:** Surgery, Temple Univ Hosp 1991; Urology, Temple Univ Hosp 1995

Kaynan, Ayal MD (U) - **Spec Exp:** Robotic Surgery; Bladder Cancer; Urologic Cancer; **Hospital:** Morristown Med Ctr (page 92); **Address:** Adult & Pediatric Urology Grp, 261 James St, Ste 3A, Morristown, NJ 07960; **Phone:** 973-539-0333; **Board Cert:** Urology 2011; **Med School:** Duke Univ 1994; **Resid:** Urologic Surgery, Montefiore Med Ctr 2000; **Fellow:** Endourology, Stanford Univ Hosp & Clins 2001

Vascular & Interventional Radiology

Calhoun, Sean K DO (VIR) - **Hospital:** Morristown Med Ctr (page 92); **Address:** 100 Madison Ave, Fl Jeff D, Ste Radiology, Box 31, Morristown, NJ 07962; **Phone:** 973-971-5377; **Board Cert:** Diagnostic Radiology 2001; Vascular & Interventional Radiology 2007; **Med School:** UMDNJ Sch Osteo Med 1996; **Resid:** Diagnostic Radiology, Morristown Meml hosp 2001; **Fellow:** Vascular & Interventional Radiology, Montefiore Med Ctr 2002; **Fac Appt:** Assoc Clin Prof Rad, Mount Sinai Sch Med

Yablonsky, Thaddeus M MD (VIR) - **Spec Exp:** Interventional Radiology; **Hospital:** Morristown Med Ctr (page 92); **Address:** Memorial Radiology Associates, 10 Lanidex Plaza W, Parsippany, NJ 07054; **Phone:** 973-503-5700; **Board Cert:** Diagnostic Radiology ; Vascular & Interventional Radiology 2009; **Med School:** UMDNJ-RW Johnson Med Sch 1990; **Resid:** Diagnostic Radiology, St Vincent's Hosp & Med Ctr 1992; Diagnostic Radiology, Morristown Meml Hosp 1995; **Fellow:** Interventional Radiology, New York Hosp 1996

Vascular Surgery

Kabnick, Lowell MD (VascS) - **Spec Exp:** Varicose Veins; Vein Disorders; **Hospital:** NYU Langone Med Ctr (page 108); **Address:** Summit Med Grp, 95 Madison Ave, Ste 415, Morristown, NJ 07960; **Phone:** 973-538-2000; **Board Cert:** Surgery 2009; **Med School:** Geo Wash Univ 1976; **Resid:** Surgery, NYU Med Ctr 1978; Surgery, Long Island Jewish Med Ctr 1981; **Fellow:** Vascular Surgery, Mount Sinai Med Ctr 1982; **Fac Appt:** Assoc Prof S, NYU Sch Med

Passaic

Passaic

Allergy & Immunology

Klein, Robert Michael MD (A&I) - **Spec Exp:** Asthma; Food Allergy; Urticaria; Hereditary Angioedema; **Hospital:** NY-Presby/Weill Cornell Med Ctr, NY (page 104), NYU Langone Med Ctr (page 108); **Address:** 1005 Clifton Ave, Ste 102, Clifton, NJ 07013-3520; **Phone:** 973-773-7400; **Board Cert:** Pediatrics 1981; **Med School:** NY Med Coll 1976; **Resid:** Pediatrics, Beth Israel Hosp 1979; **Fellow:** Allergy & Immunology, Columbia-Presby Med Ctr 1984; **Fac Appt:** Asst Clin Prof Ped, Columbia P&S

Cardiovascular Disease

Julie, Edward MD (Cv) - **Spec Exp:** Interventional Cardiology; **Hospital:** St. Mary's Hosp - Passaic, St. Joseph's Regl Med Ctr - Paterson; **Address:** 1030 Clifton Ave, Clifton, NJ 07013; **Phone:** 973-778-3777; **Board Cert:** Internal Medicine 1983; Cardiovascular Disease 1987; **Med School:** Albert Einstein Coll Med 1980; **Resid:** Internal Medicine, Mount Sinai Med Ctr 1983; **Fellow:** Cardiovascular Disease, NY-Presby/Weill Cornell Med Ctr 1986

Salimi, Mostafa MD (Cv) - **Hospital:** St. Joseph's Wayne Hosp, St. Joseph's Regl Med Ctr - Paterson; **Address:** Advanced Cardiology, 510 Hamburg Tpke, Ste 201, Wayne, NJ 07470; **Phone:** 973-942-8176; **Board Cert:** Internal Medicine 1973; Cardiovascular Disease 1977; **Med School:** Iran 1964; **Resid:** Internal Medicine, VA Hosp 1970; **Fellow:** Cardiovascular Disease, G Washington Univ Hosp 1972

Siepser, Stuart L MD (Cv) - **Spec Exp:** Coronary Artery Disease; Hypertension; Nuclear Stress Testing; Cholesterol/Lipid Disorders; **Hospital:** Chilton Hosp, Morristown Med Ctr (page 92); **Address:** Cardilogy Assocs, 1777 Hamburg Tpke, Ste 102, Wayne, NJ 07470; **Phone:** 973-831-7455; **Board Cert:** Internal Medicine 1972; Cardiovascular Disease 1975; Nuclear Cardiology 2011; **Med School:** NYU Sch Med 1968; **Resid:** Internal Medicine, NYU Med Ctr 1970; Cardiovascular Disease, NYU Med Ctr 1972; **Fac Appt:** Asst Clin Prof Med, UMDNJ-NJ Med Sch, Newark

Strobeck, John E MD/PhD (Cv) - **Spec Exp:** Congestive Heart Failure; Nuclear Cardiology; Cardiac Imaging; **Hospital:** Valley Hosp (page 721); **Address:** Sovereign Med Grp, Heart & Lung Ctr, 297 Lafayette Ave, Hawthorne, NJ 07506; **Phone:** 973-423-9388; **Board Cert:** Internal Medicine 1979; Cardiovascular Disease 1983; **Med School:** Univ Cincinnati 1974; **Resid:** Internal Medicine, Brigham & Womens Hosp 1976; **Fellow:** Cardiovascular Disease, Albert Einstein Coll Med Affil Hosp 1978

Weiss, E Michael MD (Cv) - **Spec Exp:** Preventive Cardiology; Hypertension; Coronary Artery Disease; Heart Failure; **Hospital:** St. Joseph's Regl Med Ctr - Paterson, St. Mary's Hosp - Passaic; **Address:** 842 Clifton Ave, Ste 5, Clifton, NJ 07013-1881; **Phone:** 973-777-2440; **Board Cert:** Internal Medicine 1984; Cardiovascular Disease 2007; **Med School:** Romania 1980; **Resid:** Internal Medicine, Hackensack Med Ctr 1983; **Fellow:** Cardiovascular Disease, Hackensack Med Ctr 1985; **Fac Appt:** Asst Clin Prof Med, UMDNJ-NJ Med Sch, Newark

Dermatology

Gold, Jonathan A MD (D) - **Spec Exp:** Acne & Rosacea; Eczema; Skin Cancer; **Hospital:** St. Mary's Hosp - Passaic; **Address:** 1033 Clifton Ave, Clifton, NJ 07013; **Phone:** 973-777-6444; **Board Cert:** Dermatology 1987; **Med School:** Canada 1982; **Resid:** Dermatology, McGill Univ Med Ctr 1986; Dermatology, Montefiore Med Ctr 1987; **Fellow:** Dermatologic Pharmacology, NYU Med Ctr 1988

Maier, Herbert MD (D) - **Spec Exp:** Acne; Connective Tissue Disorders; Rosacea; **Hospital:** St. Joseph's Wayne Hosp; **Address:** 220 Hamburg Tpke Fl 2 - Ste 22, Wayne, NJ 07470; **Phone:** 973-595-6338; **Board Cert:** Dermatology 1975; **Med School:** Geo Wash Univ 1967; **Resid:** Dermatology, Mount Sinai Med Ctr 1973

Pollack, Shoshannah S MD (D) - **Hospital:** Chilton Hosp; **Address:** 1777 Hamburg Tpke, Ste 102, Wayne, NJ 07470; **Phone:** 973-835-1823; **Board Cert:** Dermatology 1990; **Med School:** Albert Einstein Coll Med 1986; **Resid:** Dermatology, Montefiore Med Ctr 1990

Tanzer, Floyd R MD (D) - **Spec Exp:** Acne; Eczema; **Hospital:** St. Joseph's Regl Med Ctr - Paterson, Meadowlands Hosp Med Ctr; **Address:** 992 Clifton Ave, Clifton, NJ 07013-3502; **Phone:** 973-365-1800; **Board Cert:** Dermatology 1977; **Med School:** SUNY Downstate 1973; **Resid:** Dermatology, Kings Co Hosp 1977

Endocrinology, Diabetes & Metabolism

Berkowitz, Richard H MD (EDM) - **Spec Exp:** Diabetes; Cholesterol/Lipid Disorders; Thyroid Disorders; **Hospital:** Chilton Hosp; **Address:** 2025 Hamburg Tpke, Ste D, Wayne, NJ 07470-6250; **Phone:** 973-839-5070; **Board Cert:** Internal Medicine 1975; Endocrinology 1977; **Med School:** SUNY Hlth Sci Ctr 1972; **Resid:** Internal Medicine, Montefiore Med Ctr 1974; Internal Medicine, UMDNJ-Univ Hosp 1975; **Fellow:** Endocrinology, Beth Israel Med Ctr 1977

Gastroenterology

Bleicher, Robert MD (Ge) - **Spec Exp:** Inflammatory Bowel Disease; Irritable Bowel Syndrome; Liver Disease; **Hospital:** Chilton Hosp; **Address:** 1825 Route 23 South, Wayne, NJ 07470; **Phone:** 973-633-1484; **Board Cert:** Internal Medicine 1981; Gastroenterology 1983; **Med School:** Columbia P&S 1978; **Resid:** Internal Medicine, Northwestern Meml Hosp 1981; **Fellow:** Gastroenterology, Northwestern Meml Hosp 1983

Farkas, John J MD (Ge) - **Hospital:** St. Joseph's Regl Med Ctr - Paterson, St. Joseph's Wayne Hosp; **Address:** 716 Broad St Fl 1, Clifton, NJ 07013; **Phone:** 973-777-5717; **Board Cert:** Internal Medicine 1989; **Med School:** West Indies 1983; **Resid:** Internal Medicine, St Joseph's Hosp & Med Ctr 1986; **Fellow:** Gastroenterology, St Joseph's Hosp & Med Ctr 1988

Infectious Disease

Najjar, Sessine MD (Inf) - **Spec Exp:** Travel Medicine; **Hospital:** St. Mary's Hosp - Passaic, Valley Hosp (page 721); **Address:** 975 Clifton Ave Fl 2, Clifton, NJ 07013-2722; **Phone:** 973-778-8666; **Board Cert:** Internal Medicine 1979; Infectious Disease 1984; **Med School:** Lebanon 1974; **Resid:** Internal Medicine, Beekman Downtown Hosp 1977; **Fellow:** Infectious Disease, St Michaels Med Ctr 1979

Weiss, Gabriella A MD (Inf) - **Spec Exp:** Chronic Fatigue Syndrome; Lyme Disease; Bone Infections; **Hospital:** St. Mary's Hosp - Passaic; **Address:** 842 Clifton Ave, Clifton, NJ 07013-1800; **Phone:** 973-777-2440; **Board Cert:** Internal Medicine 1985; **Med School:** Romania 1979; **Resid:** Internal Medicine, Hackensack Med Ctr 1984; **Fellow:** Infectious Disease, Hackensack Med Ctr 1985

Internal Medicine

De Giacomo, Frank C MD (IM) *PCP* - **Spec Exp:** Cholesterol/Lipid Disorders; **Hospital:** St. Mary's Hosp - Passaic; **Address:** New Jersey Physicians, 6 Brighton Rd Fl 2, Clifton, NJ 07012; **Phone:** 973-472-2100; **Board Cert:** Internal Medicine 1972; **Med School:** Harvard Med Sch 1965; **Resid:** Internal Medicine, Bellevue Hosp 1968; **Fellow:** Cardiovascular Disease, VA Hosp 1969

Gajdos, Robert MD (IM) *PCP* - **Hospital:** Hackensack UMC-Mountainside (page 774), St. Mary's Hosp - Passaic; **Address:** 1005 Clifton Ave, Clifton, NJ 07013-3520; **Phone:** 973-777-2005; **Board Cert:** Internal Medicine 1989; **Med School:** Grenada 1985; **Resid:** Internal Medicine, Mountainside Hosp 1989

Gold, Jeffrey L MD (IM) *PCP* - **Hospital:** St. Joseph's Regl Med Ctr - Paterson; **Address:** 1135 Broad St, Ste 205, Clifton, NJ 07013-3346; **Phone:** 973-471-8850; **Board Cert:** Internal Medicine 1983; **Med School:** Mexico 1977; **Resid:** Internal Medicine, St Josephs Hosp 1981; **Fac Appt:** Asst Clin Prof Med, UMDNJ-NJ Med Sch, Newark

Jawetz, Harold I MD (IM) - **Spec Exp:** Chronic Obstructive Lung Disease (COPD); Pulmonary Disease; Asthma; **Hospital:** St. Mary's Hosp - Passaic, St. Joseph's Regl Med Ctr - Paterson; **Address:** New Jersey Physicians, 6 Brighton Rd, Clifton, NJ 07012; **Phone:** 973-472-2100; **Board Cert:** Internal Medicine 1974; **Med School:** Albert Einstein Coll Med 1971; **Resid:** Internal Medicine, Montefiore Med Ctr 1974; **Fellow:** Pulmonary Disease, Montefiore Med Ctr 1978

Medical Oncology

Uhm, Kyudong MD (Onc) - **Hospital:** St. Mary's Hosp - Passaic, St. Joseph's Regl Med Ctr - Paterson; **Address:** 1117 Route 46 East, Ste 205, Clifton, NJ 07013; **Phone:** 973-471-0981; **Board Cert:** Internal Medicine 1978; Medical Oncology 1979; Hematology 1980; **Med School:** South Korea 1969; **Resid:** Internal Medicine, Englewood 1977; Hematology, Montefiore Hosp Med Ctr 1978; **Fellow:** Medical Oncology, Montefiore Hosp Med Ctr 1980

Nephrology

Vitting, Kevin E MD (Nep) - **Spec Exp:** Hypertension; Kidney Failure; **Hospital:** St. Joseph's Regl Med Ctr - Paterson, St. Joseph's Wayne Hosp; **Address:** 342 Hamburg Tpke, Ste 201, Wayne, NJ 07470; **Phone:** 973-389-1119; **Board Cert:** Internal Medicine 1985; Nephrology 1988; **Med School:** UMDNJ-RW Johnson Med Sch 1982; **Resid:** Internal Medicine, Lenox Hill Hosp 1985; **Fellow:** Nephrology, Lenox Hill Hosp 1987; **Fac Appt:** Asst Clin Prof Med, Mount Sinai Sch Med

Neurology

Chodosh, Eliot H MD (N) - **Spec Exp:** Stroke; Multiple Sclerosis; **Hospital:** St. Joseph's Wayne Hosp, Chilton Hosp; **Address:** 220 Hamburg Tpke, Ste 16, Wayne, NJ 07470-2193; **Phone:** 973-942-4778; **Board Cert:** Neurology 1987; **Med School:** Mexico 1981; **Resid:** Neurology, Boston Univ Med Ctr 1986; **Fellow:** Cerebrovascular Disease, Boston Univ Med Ctr 1987

Knep, Stanley MD (N) - **Spec Exp:** Electromyography; Parkinson's Disease; Headache; Stroke; **Address:** 905 Allwood Rd, Ste 105, Clifton, NJ 07013; **Phone:** 973-471-3680; **Board Cert:** Neurology 1977; **Med School:** South Africa 1965; **Resid:** Internal Medicine, Johannesburg Hosp 1970; Neurology, Albert Einstein Coll Med 1975; **Fac Appt:** Asst Clin Prof N, Seton Hall Univ Sch Hlth & Med Scis

Padela, Mohammad F MD (N) - **Spec Exp:** Acupuncture; Balance Disorders; Multiple Sclerosis; Parkinson's Disease; **Hospital:** Holy Name Med Ctr (page 720); **Address:** North Jersey Neurology Care, 721 Clifton Ave, Ste 1B, Clifton, NJ 07013; **Phone:** 973-471-3730; **Board Cert:** Neurology 2005; **Med School:** India 1983; **Resid:** Internal Medicine, Univ Hosp-UMDNJ 1992; **Fellow:** Neurology, NY Medical Coll-St Vincent Cath Med Ctrs 1995

Obstetrics & Gynecology

Burns, Les A MD (ObG) *PCP* - **Spec Exp:** Menopause Problems; Pap Smear Abnormalities; Hysterectomy Alternatives; Pregnancy After Age 35; **Hospital:** Chilton Hosp, St. Joseph's Regl Med Ctr - Paterson; **Address:** 1784 Hamburg Tpke, Wayne, NJ 07470-4023; **Phone:** 973-831-9925; **Board Cert:** Obstetrics & Gynecology 2012; **Med School:** Hahnemann Univ 1981; **Resid:** Obstetrics & Gynecology, Danbury Hosp 1986

Ophthalmology

Giliberti, Orazio L MD (Oph) - **Spec Exp:** Laser-Refractive Surgery; Cataract Surgery-Lens Implant; Corneal Disease & Surgery; Glaucoma; **Hospital:** Univ Hosp (Newark), Clara Maass Med Ctr; **Address:** Giliberti Eye and Laser Center, 415 Totowa Rd, Totowa, NJ 07512-2081; **Phone:** 973-595-0011; **Board Cert:** Ophthalmology 1989; **Med School:** Grenada 1982; **Resid:** Ophthalmology, UMDNJ Affil Hosps 1987; **Fellow:** Ophthalmology, Pennsylvania Hosp 1984; Refractive Surgery, Vision Sculpting; **Fac Appt:** Asst Prof Oph, UMDNJ-NJ Med Sch, Newark

Vogel, Mitchell MD (Oph) - **Spec Exp:** Corneal Disease; Refractive Surgery; Uveitis; Cataract Surgery; **Hospital:** St. Mary's Hosp - Passaic, Overlook Med Ctr (page 92); **Address:** New Jersey Vision Assocs, 124 Gregory Ave, Ste 104, Passaic, NJ 07055-4856; **Phone:** 973-779-0808; **Board Cert:** Ophthalmology 2010; **Med School:** Temple Univ 1991; **Resid:** Ophthalmology, Nassau Univ Med Ctr 1996; **Fellow:** Cornea, Univ Tex SW Affil Hosp 1998

Orthopaedic Surgery

Drillings, Gary MD (OrS) - **Spec Exp:** Knee Injuries; Shoulder Injuries; Sports Medicine; **Hospital:** Chilton Hosp; **Address:** 1777 Hamburg Tpke, Ste 305, Wayne, NJ 07470; **Phone:** 973-831-6666; **Board Cert:** Orthopaedic Surgery 2004; **Med School:** SUNY Upstate Med Univ 1985; **Resid:** Orthopaedic Surgery, Northwestern Meml Hosp 1990; **Fellow:** Sports Medicine, Lenox Hill Hosp 1991

Emami, Arash MD (OrS) - **Spec Exp:** Spinal Surgery; Scoliosis; Minimally Invasive Spinal Surgery; Spinal Disc Replacement; **Hospital:** St. Joseph's Regl Med Ctr - Paterson, NYU Hosp For Joint Dis (page 108); **Address:** Univ Spine Ctr, 504 Valley Rd Fl 2 - Ste 203, Wayne, NJ 07470; **Phone:** 973-686-0700; **Board Cert:** Orthopaedic Surgery 2013; **Med School:** Univ Chicago-Pritzker Sch Med 1994; **Resid:** Orthopaedic Surgery, Univ Chicago Affil Hosps 1999; **Fellow:** Spine Surgery, UCSF Med Ctr 2000; **Fac Appt:** Asst Prof OrS, Seton Hall Univ Sch Hlth & Med Scis

Mc Inerney, Vincent K MD (OrS) - **Spec Exp:** Hip Replacement; Minimally Invasive Surgery; Knee Replacement; Shoulder Replacement; **Hospital:** St. Joseph's Regl Med Ctr - Paterson; **Address:** Northland Orthopedics, 504 Valley Rd, Ste 200, Wayne, NJ 07470; **Phone:** 973-694-2690; **Board Cert:** Orthopaedic Surgery 1984; **Med School:** UMDNJ-NJ Med Sch, Newark 1977; **Resid:** Orthopaedic Surgery, St. Joseph's Regl Med Ctr 1982; **Fellow:** Sports Medicine, Mass Genl Hosp 1984

Reicher, Oscar A MD (OrS) - **Spec Exp:** Reconstructive Surgery; Sports Medicine; **Hospital:** Chilton Hosp, St. Joseph's Wayne Hosp; **Address:** 2035 Hamburg Tpke, Ste D, Wayne, NJ 07470; **Phone:** 973-616-0200; **Board Cert:** Orthopaedic Surgery 2007; **Med School:** Univ Pittsburgh 1979; **Resid:** Orthopaedic Surgery, Vanderbilt Univ Med Ctr 1984

Strongwater, Allan M MD (OrS) - **Spec Exp:** Pediatric Orthopaedic Surgery; Cerebral Palsy; Deformity Reconstruction; **Hospital:** St. Joseph's Regl Med Ctr - Paterson; **Address:** St Josephs Chldns Hosp-Dept Ped Ortho Surg, 703 Main St Xavier Bldg - Ste 702, Paterson, NJ 07503; **Phone:** 973-754-2414; **Board Cert:** Orthopaedic Surgery 2007; **Med School:** Rush Med Coll 1978; **Resid:** Orthopaedic Surgery, Yale-New Haven Hosp 1983; Pediatric Orthopaedic Surgery, Hosp Joint Diseases 1984; **Fac Appt:** Clin Prof OrS, NYU Sch Med

Otolaryngology

Cece, John A MD (Oto) - **Spec Exp:** Sinus Surgery; Cosmetic Surgery-Face; Rhinoplasty; **Hospital:** Chilton Hosp, St. Mary's Hosp - Passaic; **Address:** ENT & Allergy Assocs, 1211 Hamburg Tpke, Ste 205, Wayne, NJ 07470; **Phone:** 973-633-0808; **Board Cert:** Otolaryngology 1986; Facial Plastic & Reconstr Surgery 1992; **Med School:** UMDNJ-RW Johnson Med Sch 1981; **Resid:** Otolaryngology, Mt Sinai Med Ctr 1986

La Bagnara Jr, James MD (Oto) - **Spec Exp:** Thyroid & Parathyroid Surgery; Pediatric Otolaryngology; **Hospital:** St. Joseph's Regl Med Ctr - Paterson, St. Joseph's Wayne Hosp; **Address:** 311 Lexington Ave, Paterson, NJ 07502-1010; **Phone:** 973-942-1300; **Board Cert:** Otolaryngology 1978; **Med School:** UMDNJ-NJ Med Sch, Newark 1974; **Resid:** Otolaryngology, UMDNJ-NJ Med Sch Affil Hosp 1978; **Fac Appt:** Assoc Clin Prof Oto, UMDNJ-NJ Med Sch, Newark

Mattel, Stephen F MD (Oto) - **Spec Exp:** Pediatric Otolaryngology; **Hospital:** Chilton Hosp; **Address:** 1211 Hamburg Tpke, Ste 205, Wayne, NJ 07470; **Phone:** 973-633-0808; **Board Cert:** Otolaryngology 1981; **Med School:** NYU Sch Med 1977; **Resid:** Surgery, Mount Sinai Hosp 1978; Otolaryngology, Bellevue Hosp/NYU Med Ctr 1981

Pediatric Hematology-Oncology

Bonilla, Mary Ann MD (PHO) - **Hospital:** St. Joseph's Regl Med Ctr - Paterson; **Address:** SJCH, Hematology-Oncology Dept, 703 Main St, Ste 700, Paterson, NJ 07503; **Phone:** 973-754-3230; **Board Cert:** Pediatrics 1986; Pediatric Hematology-Oncology 2012; **Med School:** Loyola Univ-Stritch Sch Med 1981; **Resid:** Pediatrics, Brookdale Univ Hosp Med Ctr 1984; **Fellow:** Pediatric Hematology-Oncology, Meml Sloan-Kettering Canc Ctr 1988

Pediatric Pulmonology

Nachajon, Roberto MD (PPul) - **Spec Exp:** Asthma; Cystic Fibrosis; Sleep Disorders; Bronchoscopy; **Hospital:** St. Joseph's Regl Med Ctr - Paterson, Mt Sinai Med Ctr (page 102); **Address:** 11 Getty Ave, Paterson, NJ 07503; **Phone:** 973-754-2550; **Board Cert:** Pediatric Pulmonology 2011; Sleep Medicine 2007; **Med School:** Uruguay 1985; **Resid:** Pediatrics, Chldns Hosp Uruguay 1990; Pediatrics, Beth Israel Med Ctr 1993; **Fellow:** Pediatric Pulmonology, Chldns Hosp 1996; **Fac Appt:** Asst Clin Prof Ped, Mount Sinai Sch Med

Pediatric Surgery

Bhattacharyya, Nishith MD (PS) - **Spec Exp:** Cancer Surgery; Minimally Invasive Surgery; Chest Wall Deformities; Pediatric Plastic Surgery; **Hospital:** St. Joseph's Regl Med Ctr - Paterson, Newark Beth Israel Med Ctr; **Address:** 2130 Milburn Ave, Ste C-1, Maplewood, NJ 07470; **Phone:** 973-313-3115; **Board Cert:** Surgery 2004; Pediatric Surgery 2007; **Med School:** India 1984; **Resid:** Surgery, Univ Hawaii Med Ctr 1994; Surgery, Chldns Hosp 1991; **Fellow:** Pediatric Surgery, Chldns Hosp-Ohio 1996; **Fac Appt:** Asst Clin Prof PS, NY Med Coll

Pediatrics

Scofield, Lisa MD (Ped) *PCP* - **Hospital:** St. Joseph's Regl Med Ctr - Paterson, Chilton Hosp; **Address:** 57 Willowbrook Blvd, Ste 421, Wayne, NJ 07470; **Phone:** 973-754-4025; **Board Cert:** Pediatrics 2009; **Med School:** UMDNJ-NJ Med Sch, Newark 1990; **Resid:** Pediatrics, New York Hosp-Cornell 1994

Plastic Surgery

Figlia, Paul M MD (PlS) - **Spec Exp:** Reconstructive Plastic Surgery; Facial Rejuvenation; Breast Augmentation; **Hospital:** JFK Med Ctr - Edison, Saint Barnabas Med Ctr; **Address:** 1500 Pleasant Vly Way, Ste 307, West Orange, NJ 07502; **Phone:** 973-324-5333; **Board Cert:** Plastic Surgery ; **Med School:** UMDNJ-RW Johnson Med Sch 1984; **Resid:** Surgery, St Barnabas Med Ctr 1986; Surgery, Washington Hosp Ctr 1989; **Fellow:** Plastic Surgery, OU Med Ctr 1992

Ganchi, Parham A MD/PhD (PlS) - **Spec Exp:** Cosmetic Surgery-Face & Body; Cosmetic Surgery-Breast; Facial Rejuvenation; Body Contouring; **Hospital:** Chilton Hosp, St. Joseph's Wayne Hosp; **Address:** 246 Hamburg Tpke, Ste 307, Wayne, NJ 07470; **Phone:** 973-942-6600; **Board Cert:** Plastic Surgery 2013; **Med School:** Duke Univ 1994; **Resid:** Surgery, Brigham & Womens Hosp 1999; **Fellow:** Plastic Surgery, Brigham & Womens Hosp 2002

Psychiatry

Hindin, Lee MD (Psyc) - **Spec Exp:** Addiction Psychiatry; **Hospital:** Saint Barnabas Med Ctr; **Address:** Creative Intervention, 1149 Bloomfield Ave, Clifton, NJ 07012; **Phone:** 973-365-2300; **Board Cert:** Psychiatry 1984; **Med School:** UMDNJ-NJ Med Sch, Newark 1977; **Resid:** Psychiatry, UCLA-Neuropsych Inst 1982

Pulmonary Disease

Amoruso, Robert C MD (Pul) - **Spec Exp:** Asthma; Critical Care; **Hospital:** St. Joseph's Regl Med Ctr - Paterson, St. Joseph's Wayne Hosp; **Address:** 999 McBride Ave, Ste 201B, Woodland Park, NJ 07424; **Phone:** 973-256-0287; **Board Cert:** Internal Medicine 1979; Pulmonary Disease 1982; **Med School:** Italy 1975; **Resid:** Internal Medicine, St Joseph's Hosp Med Ctr 1979; **Fellow:** Pulmonary Disease, College Hosp-UMDNJ 1981

Grizzanti, Joseph N DO (Pul) - **Spec Exp:** Lung Cancer; Asthma; Allergy; Immunologic Lung Disease; **Hospital:** Valley Hosp (page 721); **Address:** 297 Lafayette Ave, Hawthorne, NJ 07506; **Phone:** 973-790-4111; **Board Cert:** Internal Medicine 1979; Pulmonary Disease 1982; Allergy & Immunology 1985; **Med School:** Philadelphia Coll Osteo Med 1976; **Resid:** Internal Medicine, UMDNJ-Univ Hosp 1979; **Fellow:** Pulmonary Disease, Montefiore Med Ctr 1981; Allergy & Immunology, Montefiore Med Ctr 1984; **Fac Appt:** Assoc Clin Prof Med, Albert Einstein Coll Med

Radiation Oncology

Cole, Robert J MD (RadRO) - **Spec Exp:** Brachytherapy; Breast Cancer; Prostate Cancer; **Hospital:** St. Mary's Hosp - Passaic, Robert Wood Johnson Univ Hosp - New Brunswick; **Address:** St Mary's Hosp, Dept Oncology, 350 Boulevard, Passaic, NJ 07055; **Phone:** 973-365-5088; **Board Cert:** Therapeutic Radiology 1983; **Med School:** Wake Forest Univ 1979; **Resid:** Radiation Oncology, Univ VA Hlth Sci Ctr 1983

Reproductive Endocrinology

Ransom, Mark X MD (RE) - **Spec Exp:** Infertility-IVF; **Hospital:** St. Joseph's Wayne Hosp, Hackensack Univ Med Ctr (page 718); **Address:** 57 Willowbrook Blvd, Wayne, NJ 07470; **Phone:** 973-754-4055; **Board Cert:** Obstetrics & Gynecology 2012; Reproductive Endocrinology 2012; **Med School:** UMDNJ-RW Johnson Med Sch 1987; **Resid:** Obstetrics & Gynecology, RWJ Univ Hosp 1991; **Fellow:** Reproductive Endocrinology, RWJ Univ Hosp 1993

Rheumatology

Goldberg, Marc A MD (Rhu) - **Spec Exp:** Rheumatoid Arthritis; Osteoporosis; Osteoarthritis; **Hospital:** St. Mary's Hosp - Passaic; **Address:** 6 Brighton Rd, Clifton, NJ 07012; **Phone:** 973-473-2597; **Board Cert:** Internal Medicine 1972; Rheumatology 1976; **Med School:** Med Coll VA 1969; **Resid:** Internal Medicine, Univ Maryland Hosp 1972; Rheumatology, Johns Hopkins Hosp 1973; **Fellow:** Rheumatology, Hosp Univ Penn 1976

Lewko, Michael P MD (Rhu) - **Spec Exp:** Geriatric Rheumatology; Arthritis; Osteoporosis; Rheumatoid Arthritis; **Hospital:** St. Joseph's Regl Med Ctr - Paterson; **Address:** NJ Arthritis & Osteoporosis Ctr, 871 Allwood Rd, Clifton, NJ 07012; **Phone:** 973-405-5163; **Board Cert:** Internal Medicine 1988; Rheumatology 2012; Geriatric Medicine 2004; **Med School:** UMDNJ-Rutgers Med Sch 1985; **Resid:** Internal Medicine, RW Johnson Univ Hosp 1988; **Fellow:** Geriatric Medicine, Roger Williams Med Ctr 1989; Rheumatology, Hosp Univ Penn 1991; **Fac Appt:** Asst Clin Prof Med, Mount Sinai Sch Med

Surgery

Budd, Daniel C MD (S) - **Spec Exp:** Breast Disease; Endocrine Surgery; Hernia; **Hospital:** St. Joseph's Regl Med Ctr - Paterson, Valley Hosp (page 721); **Address:** 707 Broadway, Paterson, NJ 07514; **Phone:** 973-742-3371; **Board Cert:** Surgery 1975; **Med School:** Duke Univ 1969; **Resid:** Surgery, Columbia-Presbyterian Hosp 1974; **Fac Appt:** Assoc Clin Prof S, UMDNJ-NJ Med Sch, Newark

Feigenbaum, Howard MD (S) - **Spec Exp:** Gastrointestinal Surgery; Colon Surgery; Laparoscopic Surgery; Breast Surgery; **Hospital:** Chilton Hosp, St. Joseph's Wayne Hosp; **Address:** 227 Hamburg Tpke, Pompton Lakes, NJ 07442-1838; **Phone:** 973-839-7999; **Board Cert:** Surgery 2009; **Med School:** NYU Sch Med 1971; **Resid:** Surgery, Bellevue Hosp 1977

Thoracic & Cardiac Surgery

Connolly, Mark W MD (T&CS) - **Spec Exp:** Minimally Invasive Cardiac Surgery; Coronary Artery Surgery; **Hospital:** St. Joseph's Regl Med Ctr - Paterson; **Address:** St Josephs, Cardiothoracic Surgery Dept, 703 Main St, Paterson, NJ 07503; **Phone:** 973-754-2486; **Board Cert:** Thoracic & Cardiac Surgery 2011; **Med School:** Northwestern Univ 1982; **Resid:** Surgery, NYU Med Ctr 1988; Cardiothoracic Surgery, Emory Univ Hosp 1991; **Fellow:** Surgical Research, Maimonides Med Ctr 1986

Kaushik, Raj R MD (T&CS) - **Spec Exp:** Minimally Invasive Cardiac Surgery; Atrial Fibrillation; Laser Surgery; **Hospital:** St. Mary's Hosp - Passaic, Hackensack UMC-Mountainside (page 774); **Address:** St Mary's Hosp, Div Cardiac Surgery, 350 Boulevard, Ste 130, Passaic, NJ 07055; **Phone:** 973-365-4567; **Board Cert:** Thoracic Surgery 2009; **Med School:** India 1979; **Resid:** Surgery, Bridgeport Hosp 1985; Cardiothoracic Surgery, Newark Beth Israel Med Ctr 1988; **Fellow:** Cardiac Surgery, Baylor Univ 1989; Cardiac Surgery, Univ W Ontario Med Ctr 1990

Pontoriero, Michael MD (T&CS) - **Hospital:** Clara Maass Med Ctr; **Address:** Cardiovascular Grp, 1401 Broad St, Clifton, NJ 07013; **Phone:** 973-759-9000; **Board Cert:** Thoracic & Cardiac Surgery 2013; Surgery 2010; **Med School:** UMDNJ-NJ Med Sch, Newark 1985; **Resid:** Surgery, Univ Hosp-UMDNJ 1990; **Fellow:** Cardiothoracic Surgery, Tufts Med Ctr 1993

Urology

Levine, Seth P MD (U) - **Spec Exp:** Prostate Cancer; Incontinence; **Hospital:** Chilton Hosp, Valley Hosp (page 721); **Address:** Assocs in Urology, 1777 Hamburg Tpke, Ste 304, Wayne, NJ 07470; **Phone:** 973-616-8400; **Board Cert:** Urology 1980; **Med School:** Tufts Univ 1971; **Resid:** Surgery, Mount Sinai Med Ctr 1973; Urology, Mount Sinai Med Ctr 1978

Somerset

Somerset

Allergy & Immunology

Caucino, Julie A DO (A&I) - **Spec Exp:** Asthma & Allergy; Drug Sensitivity; Sinusitis; **Hospital:** Univ Med Ctr Princeton at Plainsboro; **Address:** Princeton Allergy & Asthma Assoc, 24 Vreeland Drive, Skillnan, NJ 08558; **Phone:** 609-921-2202; **Board Cert:** Allergy & Immunology 2003; **Med School:** Kirksville Coll Osteo Med 1987; **Resid:** Internal Medicine, RW Johnson Univ Hosp 1991; **Fellow:** Allergy & Immunology, Montefiore Med Ctr 1993

Fox, James A MD (A&I) - **Spec Exp:** Asthma; Urticaria; Food Allergy; Hereditary Angioedema; **Hospital:** Somerset Med Ctr, Hunterdon Med Ctr; **Address:** 3461 US Highway 22 E, D Bldg, Branchburg, NJ 08876-6021; **Phone:** 908-725-4777; **Board Cert:** Pediatrics 1981; Allergy & Immunology 1983; **Med School:** Yale Univ 1977; **Resid:** Pediatrics, Bronx Municipal Hosp Ctr 1980; **Fellow:** Allergy & Immunology, Columbia-Presby Med Ctr 1982

Krol, Kristine MD (A&I) - **Spec Exp:** Insect Allergies; Drug Sensitivity; Food Allergy; Asthma; **Hospital:** Staten Island Univ Hosp - South (page 106), Somerset Med Ctr; **Address:** AllerCare, Allergy Asthma, 177 W High St, Somerville, NJ 08876; **Phone:** 908-725-8666; **Board Cert:** Internal Medicine 1987; Allergy & Immunology 2011; **Med School:** SUNY Downstate 1981; **Resid:** Internal Medicine, Staten Island Univ Hosp 1985; **Fellow:** Allergy & Immunology, Mass Genl Hosp 1987; **Fac Appt:** Asst Clin Prof Med, SUNY Downstate

Pedinoff, Andrew J MD (A&I) - **Spec Exp:** Rhinitis; Asthma; Hay Fever; **Hospital:** Univ Med Ctr Princeton at Plainsboro, Robert Wood Johnson Univ Hosp - New Brunswick; **Address:** Princeton Allergy & Asthma Assocs, 24 Vreeland Drive, Skilman, NJ 08558; **Phone:** 609-921-2202; **Board Cert:** Allergy & Immunology 2003; **Med School:** Dominican Republic 1984; **Resid:** Pediatrics, Georgetown Univ Hosp 1987; **Fellow:** Allergy & Immunology, Georgetown Univ Hosp 1989; **Fac Appt:** Asst Clin Prof Ped, UMDNJ-RW Johnson Med Sch

Schulhafer, Edwin MD (A&I) - **Spec Exp:** Asthma; Sinus Disorders; Allergy; Migraine; **Hospital:** Hunterdon Med Ctr, Somerset Med Ctr; **Address:** Allergy, Asthma & Sinus Ctr, 712 Courtyard Drive, Hillsborough, NJ 08844; **Phone:** 908-526-0200; **Board Cert:** Internal Medicine 1988; Allergy & Immunology 2006; **Med School:** UMDNJ-NJ Med Sch, Newark 1983; **Resid:** Internal Medicine, Overlook Hosp 1986; **Fellow:** Allergy & Immunology, Long Island Coll Hosp 1988

Southern, Darrell L MD (A&I) - **Spec Exp:** Asthma & Allergy; Urticaria; Hereditary Angioedema; Food Allergy; **Hospital:** Univ Med Ctr Princeton at Plainsboro; **Address:** 24 Vreeland Drive, Skillman, NJ 08558; **Phone:** 609-921-2202; **Board Cert:** Pediatrics 1976; **Med School:** Columbia P&S 1971; **Resid:** Pediatrics, Columbia-Presby Med Ctr 1974; **Fellow:** Allergy & Immunology, Columbia-Presby Med Ctr 1976

Cardiovascular Disease

Kulkarni, Rachana A MD (Cv) - **Spec Exp:** Nuclear Cardiology; Echocardiography-Transesophageal; Hypertension; **Hospital:** Somerset Med Ctr, Robert Wood Johnson Univ Hosp - New Brunswick; **Address:** Medicor Cardiology, 225 Jackson St, Bridgewater, NJ 08807; **Phone:** 908-526-8668; **Board Cert:** Cardiovascular Disease 2010; Nuclear Cardiology 2012; **Med School:** India 1988; **Resid:** Internal Medicine, RW Johnson Univ Hosp 1995; **Fellow:** Cardiovascular Disease, RW Johnson Univ Hosp 1998

Saulino, Patrick F MD (Cv) - **Spec Exp:** Cardiac Catheterization; Invasive Cardiology; Non-Invasive Cardiology; **Hospital:** Somerset Med Ctr, Robert Wood Johnson Univ Hosp - New Brunswick; **Address:** Medicor, Cardiology, 3322 Rte 22 W, Ste 505, Branchburg, NJ 08876; **Phone:** 908-231-0041; **Board Cert:** Internal Medicine 1984; Cardiovascular Disease 1987; **Med School:** Georgetown Univ 1981; **Resid:** Internal Medicine, Georgetown Univ Hosp 1984; Cardiovascular Disease, Georgetown Univ Hosp 1985; **Fellow:** Cardiovascular Disease, RW Johnson Univ Hosp 1987; Cardiovascular Disease, Georgetown Univ Hosp 1988

Stroh, Jack A MD (Cv) - **Spec Exp:** Angioplasty & Stent Placement; Hypertension; Cholesterol/Lipid Disorders; **Hospital:** Robert Wood Johnson Univ Hosp - New Brunswick, St. Peter's Univ Hosp; **Address:** 75 Veronica Ave, Ste 101, Somerset, NJ 08873-5002; **Phone:** 732-247-7444; **Board Cert:** Internal Medicine 1987; Cardiovascular Disease 1989; Interventional Cardiology 2009; **Med School:** Albert Einstein Coll Med 1984; **Resid:** Internal Medicine, Boston Univ Med Ctr 1987; **Fellow:** Cardiovascular Disease, NYU Med Ctr 1990; **Fac Appt:** Asst Clin Prof Med, UMDNJ-RW Johnson Med Sch

Dermatology

Fox, Alissa B MD (D) - **Spec Exp:** Acne; Psoriasis; **Hospital:** Somerset Med Ctr, Hunterdon Med Ctr; **Address:** 3461 US Highway 22, Branchburg, NJ 08876; **Phone:** 908-725-4777; **Board Cert:** Dermatology 1984; **Med School:** NYU Sch Med 1980; **Resid:** Dermatology, New York Hosp 1984

Pappert, Amy S MD (D) - **Spec Exp:** Contact Dermatitis; **Hospital:** Robert Wood Johnson Univ Hosp - New Brunswick; **Address:** RW Johnson Medical Group, Dept Dermatology, 1 World's Fair Drive, Ste 2400, Somerset, NJ 08873; **Phone:** 732-463-7546; **Board Cert:** Dermatology 2013; **Med School:** UMDNJ-RW Johnson Med Sch 1989; **Resid:** Dermatology, Columbia Presby Med Ctr 1994; **Fellow:** Research, Columbia Presby Med Ctr 1991; **Fac Appt:** Asst Prof D, UMDNJ-RW Johnson Med Sch

Diagnostic Radiology

Greer, Jeannete G MD (DR) - **Spec Exp:** Breast Imaging; **Hospital:** Somerset Med Ctr; **Address:** Somerset Med Ctr, Dept Radiology, 110 Rehill Ave, Somerville, NJ 08876; **Phone:** 732-968-4899; **Board Cert:** Diagnostic Radiology 1994; **Med School:** Harvard Med Sch 1989; **Resid:** Diagnostic Radiology, T Jefferson Univ Hosp 1994; **Fellow:** Breast Imaging, T Jefferson Univ Hosp 1995

Melville, Gordon E MD (DR) - **Spec Exp:** Neuroradiology; MRI; **Hospital:** Somerset Med Ctr; **Address:** Somerset Medical Ctr, Dept Radiology, 100 Rehill Ave, Somerville, NJ 08876; **Phone:** 732-968-4899; **Board Cert:** Diagnostic Radiology 1984; Neuroradiology 2006; **Med School:** Univ NC Sch Med 1979; **Resid:** Diagnostic Radiology, G Washington Univ Hosp 1984; **Fellow:** Neuroradiology, Mass Genl Hosp 1985

Yang, Roger S MD (DR) - **Spec Exp:** Breast Imaging; Women's Imaging; **Hospital:** Somerset Med Ctr; **Address:** Somerset Med Ctr, Dept Radiology, 110 Rehill Ave, Somerville, NJ 08876; **Phone:** 732-968-4899; **Board Cert:** Diagnostic Radiology 1997; **Med School:** Northwestern Univ 1992; **Resid:** Diagnostic Radiology, Univ Hosp 1997; **Fellow:** Women's Imaging, Univ Hosp/Kings Co Hosp 1998; **Fac Appt:** Asst Clin Prof Rad, SUNY Downstate

Family Medicine

Corson, Richard L MD (FMed) *PCP* - **Hospital:** Somerset Med Ctr; **Address:** 313 Courtyard Drive, Hillsborough, NJ 08844; **Phone:** 908-722-9962; **Board Cert:** Family Medicine 2004; **Med School:** UMDNJ-RW Johnson Med Sch 1983; **Resid:** Family Medicine, Somerset Med Ctr 1986

Frisoli, Anthony MD (FMed) *PCP* - **Spec Exp:** Sports Medicine; Geriatric Care; **Hospital:** Somerset Med Ctr; **Address:** Martinsville Family Practice, 1973 Washington Valley Rd, Martinsville, NJ 08836; **Phone:** 732-560-9225; **Board Cert:** Family Medicine 2005; **Med School:** UMDNJ-Rutgers Med Sch 1983; **Resid:** Family Medicine, Somerset Med Ctr 1986

Steckel, Rebecca MD (FMed) *PCP* - **Spec Exp:** Women's Health; Preventive Medicine; **Hospital:** Somerset Med Ctr; **Address:** Franklin Family Practice, 29 Clyde Rd, Ste 101, Somerset, NJ 08873; **Phone:** 732-873-0330; **Board Cert:** Family Medicine 2004; **Med School:** NY Med Coll 1983; **Resid:** Family Medicine, Hackensack UMC 1986; **Fellow:** Obstetrics, OSU Med Ctr 1987; **Fac Appt:** FMed

Ziering, Thomas S MD (FMed) *PCP* - **Spec Exp:** Concierge Medicine; Anxiety & Depression; Gay/Lesbian/Transgender Health; Complementary Medicine; **Hospital:** Morristown Med Ctr (page 92); **Address:** 39 Olcott Sq, Bernardsville, NJ 07924-2317; **Phone:** 908-221-1919; **Board Cert:** Family Medicine 2012; **Med School:** UMDNJ-NJ Med Sch, Newark 1987; **Resid:** Family Medicine, Somerset Med Ctr 1990; **Fac Appt:** Assoc Clin Prof FMed, UMDNJ-RW Johnson Med Sch

Gastroenterology

Accurso, Charles A MD (Ge) - **Spec Exp:** Colon Cancer Screening; Irritable Bowel Syndrome; Gastroesophageal Reflux Disease (GERD); Endoscopy; **Hospital:** Somerset Med Ctr; **Address:** 511 Courtyard Drive, Bldg 500, Digestive Healthcare Ctr, Hillsborough, NJ 08844-2017; **Phone:** 908-218-9222; **Board Cert:** Internal Medicine 1987; Gastroenterology 1989; **Med School:** UMDNJ-NJ Med Sch, Newark 1984; **Resid:** Internal Medicine, Univ Hosp 1987; **Fellow:** Gastroenterology, Univ Hosp/NJ Med Sch 1989; **Fac Appt:** Asst Clin Prof Med, UMDNJ-NJ Med Sch, Newark

Ferges, Mitchell L MD (Ge) - **Spec Exp:** Liver Disease; **Hospital:** St. Peter's Univ Hosp, Robert Wood Johnson Univ Hosp - New Brunswick; **Address:** 33 Clyde Rd, Ste 102, Somerset, NJ 08873; **Phone:** 732-873-9200; **Board Cert:** Internal Medicine 1978; Gastroenterology 1981; **Med School:** UMDNJ-RW Johnson Med Sch 1975; **Resid:** Internal Medicine, UMDNJ Rutgers Affil Hosps 1978; **Fellow:** Gastroenterology, UMDNJ Univ Hosp 1980

Hand Surgery

Coyle Jr, Michael P MD (HS) - **Spec Exp:** Arthritis Hand Surgery; Nerve Compression; Dupuytren's Contracture; Sports Injuries; **Hospital:** Robert Wood Johnson Univ Hosp - New Brunswick, St. Peter's Univ Hosp; **Address:** University Orthopaedic Assocs, 2 Worlds Fair Drive, Somerset, NJ 08873; **Phone:** 732-537-0909; **Board Cert:** Orthopaedic Surgery 2005; Hand Surgery 2010; Orthopaedic Sports Medicine 2007; **Med School:** Columbia P&S 1968; **Resid:** Surgery, UCSF-Moffitt Hosp 1970; Orthopaedic Surgery, NY Orth Hosp 1976; **Fellow:** Hand Surgery, NY Orth Hosp 1977; **Fac Appt:** Clin Prof OrS, UMDNJ-RW Johnson Med Sch

Hematology

Toomey, Kathleen C MD (Hem) - **Spec Exp:** Breast Cancer; **Hospital:** Somerset Med Ctr, St. Peter's Univ Hosp; **Address:** Steepchase Cancer Ctr, 30 Rehill Ave, Ste 2500, Somerville, NJ 08876; **Phone:** 908-927-8700; **Board Cert:** Internal Medicine 1982; Medical Oncology 1987; Hematology 2003; **Med School:** Italy 1978; **Resid:** Internal Medicine, St Peters Med Ctr 1982; **Fellow:** Hematology & Oncology, UMDNJ-Rutgers Med Sch 1985

Infectious Disease

Herman, David J MD (Inf) - **Spec Exp:** Lyme Disease; AIDS/HIV; Travel Medicine; **Hospital:** Univ Med Ctr Princeton at Plainsboro, Somerset Med Ctr; **Address:** 105 Raider Blvd, Ste 101, Hillsborough, NJ 08844; **Phone:** 908-281-0221; **Board Cert:** Internal Medicine 1988; Infectious Disease 2010; **Med School:** Univ MO-Columbia Sch Med 1985; **Resid:** Internal Medicine, Northwestern Univ 1988; **Fellow:** Infectious Disease, Univ Minn 1991; **Fac Appt:** Assoc Clin Prof Med, UMDNJ-RW Johnson Med Sch

Nahass, Ronald G MD (Inf) - **Spec Exp:** HIV; Hepatitis B & C; Diagnostic Problems; Bone Infections; **Hospital:** Robert Wood Johnson Univ Hosp - New Brunswick, Univ Med Ctr Princeton at Plainsboro; **Address:** Infectious Disease Care, 105 Raider Blvd, Ste 101, Hillsborough, NJ 08844-4254; **Phone:** 908-281-0221; **Board Cert:** Internal Medicine 1985; Infectious Disease 1988; **Med School:** UMDNJ-RW Johnson Med Sch 1982; **Resid:** Internal Medicine, RWJ Univ Hosp 1985; **Fellow:** Infectious Disease, RWJ Univ Hosp 1988; **Fac Appt:** Clin Prof Med, UMDNJ-RW Johnson Med Sch

Internal Medicine

Bell, Kevin E MD (IM) *PCP* - **Spec Exp:** Lyme Disease; Hypertension; **Hospital:** Overlook Med Ctr (page 92); **Address:** 10 Mountain Blvd, Warren, NJ 07059-2639; **Phone:** 908-226-9000; **Board Cert:** Internal Medicine 1978; **Med School:** Columbia P&S 1975; **Resid:** Internal Medicine, Univ Wisconsin Med Ctr 1979; **Fac Appt:** Asst Clin Prof Med, Columbia P&S

Bonaventura, Lisa M MD (IM) *PCP* - **Spec Exp:** Concierge Medicine; **Hospital:** Morristown Med Ctr (page 92); **Address:** 2345 Lamington Rd, Ste 104, Bedminster, NJ 07921-2612; **Phone:** 908-781-9661; **Board Cert:** Internal Medicine 1989; **Med School:** Univ Cincinnati 1986; **Resid:** Internal Medicine, Morristown Meml Hosp 1989

Ferrante, Maurice A MD (IM) *PCP* - **Hospital:** Overlook Med Ctr (page 92); **Address:** 8 Mountain Blvd, Warren, NJ 07059; **Phone:** 908-561-8600; **Board Cert:** Internal Medicine 2010; **Med School:** Jefferson Med Coll 1987; **Resid:** Internal Medicine, Univ Maryland Med Ctr 1990

Neiman, Deborah L MD (IM) - **Spec Exp:** Weight Management; **Hospital:** Morristown Med Ctr (page 92), Hunterdon Med Ctr; **Address:** 311 Omni Drive, Hillsborough, NJ 08844; **Phone:** 908-281-0632; **Board Cert:** Internal Medicine 1987; **Med School:** NY Med Coll 1984; **Resid:** Internal Medicine, Morristown Meml Hosp 1987

Sanchez-Catanese, Betty MD (IM) *PCP* - **Hospital:** Somerset Med Ctr; **Address:** 315 E Main St, Somerville, NJ 08876-3109; **Phone:** 908-722-3442; **Board Cert:** Internal Medicine 1987; **Med School:** NY Med Coll 1983; **Resid:** Internal Medicine, Northshore Univ Hosp 1986

Medical Oncology

Casper, Ephraim S MD (Onc) - **Spec Exp:** Gastrointestinal Cancer; Pancreatic Cancer; Sarcoma-Soft Tissue; Solid Tumors; **Hospital:** Meml Sloan-Kettering Canc Ctr (page 114); **Address:** MSKCC at Basking Ridge, 136 Mountainview Blvd, Basking Ridge, NJ 07920; **Phone:** 908-542-3000; **Board Cert:** Internal Medicine 1977; Medical Oncology 1979; **Med School:** Rush Med Coll 1974; **Resid:** Internal Medicine, Rush Univ Med Ctr 1977; **Fellow:** Medical Oncology, Meml Sloan-Kettering Cancer Ctr 1979

Fang, Bruno S MD (Onc) - **Spec Exp:** Lung Cancer; Head & Neck Cancer; Breast Cancer; Colon Cancer; **Hospital:** Robert Wood Johnson Univ Hosp - New Brunswick, St. Peter's Univ Hosp; **Address:** Central Jersey Oncology Ctr, 454 Elizabeth Ave, Ste 240, Somerset, NJ 08873; **Phone:** 732-390-7750; **Board Cert:** Internal Medicine 2006; Hematology 2010; Medical Oncology 2010; **Med School:** Brazil 1991; **Resid:** Internal Medicine, Jackson Meml Hosp 1996; Internal Medicine, VA Med Ctr 1997; **Fellow:** Hematology & Oncology, Natl Cancer Inst/NIH 2000

Hamilton, Audrey M MD (Onc) - **Spec Exp:** Hematologic Malignancies; **Hospital:** Meml Sloan-Kettering Canc Ctr (page 114); **Address:** Meml Sloan Kettering Cancer Ctr, 136 Mountain View Blvd, Basking Ridge, NJ 07920; **Phone:** 908-542-3000; **Board Cert:** Internal Medicine 1986; Hematology 2004; Medical Oncology 2005; **Med School:** Harvard Med Sch 1983; **Resid:** Internal Medicine, Brigham & Womens Hosp 1986; **Fellow:** Hematology & Oncology, NY Hosp-Cornell Med Ctr 1989

Salwitz, James C MD (Onc) - **Spec Exp:** Colon Cancer; Breast Cancer; Lung Cancer; Leukemia & Lymphoma; **Hospital:** Robert Wood Johnson Univ Hosp - New Brunswick, St. Peter's Univ Hosp; **Address:** Central Jersey Oncology Ctr, 454 Elizabeth Ave, Ste 240, Somerset, NJ 08873; **Phone:** 732-390-7750; **Board Cert:** Internal Medicine 1984; Medical Oncology 1987; **Med School:** UMDNJ-Rutgers Med Sch 1981; **Resid:** Internal Medicine, Northwestern Univ/McGaw Med Ctr 1984; **Fellow:** Medical Oncology, NIH-Natl Canc Inst 1987

Nephrology

Kabis, Suzanne M MD (Nep) - **Spec Exp:** Lupus Nephritis; Hypertension; Glomerulonephritis; Kidney Disease in Pregnancy; **Hospital:** Robert Wood Johnson Univ Hosp - New Brunswick, St. Peter's Univ Hosp; **Address:** 1350 Hamilton St, Somerset, NJ 08873; **Phone:** 732-246-2626; **Board Cert:** Internal Medicine 1982; Nephrology 1988; **Med School:** UMDNJ-Rutgers Med Sch 1979; **Resid:** Internal Medicine, NC Meml Hosp 1982; **Fellow:** Nephrology, NC Meml Hosp 1985; **Fac Appt:** Asst Clin Prof Med

Neurology

Friedlander, Devin S MD (N) - **Spec Exp:** Headache; Botox Therapy; **Hospital:** St. Peter's Univ Hosp; **Address:** Princeton & Rutgers Neurology, 77 Veronica Ave, Ste 102, Somerset, NJ 08873-3448; **Phone:** 732-246-1311; **Board Cert:** Neurology 2013; **Med School:** UMDNJ-RW Johnson Med Sch 1989; **Resid:** Neurology, Albert Einstein Coll Med Affil Hosps 1993; **Fellow:** Neurophysiology, Lyons VA Med Ctr 1994

Obstetrics & Gynecology

Sanderson, Rhonda A MD (ObG) - **Spec Exp:** Gynecology Only; **Hospital:** Overlook Med Ctr (page 92); **Address:** 8 Mountain Blvd, Warren, NJ 07059; **Phone:** 908-754-5775; **Board Cert:** Obstetrics & Gynecology 2012; **Med School:** Hahnemann Univ 1980; **Resid:** Obstetrics & Gynecology, Women & Infants Hosp 1985

Ophthalmology

Angrist, Richard C MD (Oph) - **Spec Exp:** Cataract Surgery; Glaucoma; Eyelid/Tear Duct Disorders; Ophthalmic Plastic Surgery; **Hospital:** Robert Wood Johnson Univ Hosp - New Brunswick, Kimball Med Ctr; **Address:** 1527 State Route 27, Ste 2600, Somerset, NJ 08873; **Phone:** 732-246-1050; **Board Cert:** Ophthalmology 1985; **Med School:** Albany Med Coll 1979; **Resid:** Ophthalmology, NY Eye& Ear Infirm 1983; **Fellow:** Ophthalmic Plastic & Reconstructive Surgery, Univ Wisconsin 1984

Salz, Alan G MD (Oph) - **Spec Exp:** LASIK-Refractive Surgery; Cataract Surgery-Lens Implant; **Hospital:** Somerset Med Ctr; **Address:** The Eye Specialists, 31 Monroe St, Bridgewater, NJ 08807; **Phone:** 908-231-1110; **Board Cert:** Ophthalmology 1987; **Med School:** Boston Univ 1981; **Resid:** Ophthalmology, Wills Eye Hosp 1985

Orthopaedic Surgery

Butler, Mark S MD (OrS) - **Spec Exp:** Trauma; Foot & Ankle Surgery; **Hospital:** Robert Wood Johnson Univ Hosp - New Brunswick, St. Peter's Univ Hosp; **Address:** Univ Orthopaedic Assocs, 2 Worlds Fair Drive, Somerset, NJ 08873; **Phone:** 732-537-0909; **Board Cert:** Orthopaedic Surgery 2004; **Med School:** UMDNJ-RW Johnson Med Sch 1984; **Resid:** Orthopaedic Surgery, UMDNJ-RW Johnson Univ Hosp 1989; **Fellow:** Orthopaedic Trauma Surgery, Maryland Inst EMS 1990; Foot & Ankle Surgery, Maryland Inst EMS 1992; **Fac Appt:** Assoc Prof OrS, UMDNJ-RW Johnson Med Sch

D'Agostini Jr, Robert J MD (OrS) - **Spec Exp:** Joint Replacement; Sports Medicine; **Hospital:** Morristown Med Ctr (page 92); **Address:** Tri-Co Orthopedics, 1590 Route 206 N, Bedminster, NJ 07921; **Phone:** 908-234-2002; **Board Cert:** Orthopaedic Surgery 2008; Sports Medicine 2009; **Med School:** UMDNJ-RW Johnson Med Sch 1980; **Resid:** Orthopaedic Surgery, MedStar Georgetown Univ Hosp 1986

Dwyer, James W MD (OrS) - **Spec Exp:** Spinal Surgery; Minimally Invasive Spinal Surgery; Spinal Disc Replacement; Spinal Reconstructive Surgery; **Hospital:** Somerset Med Ctr, Univ Hosp (Newark); **Address:** NJ Spine Inst, 1 Robertson Drive, Ste 11, Bedminster, NJ 07921; **Phone:** 908-722-0822; **Board Cert:** Orthopaedic Surgery 2013; **Med School:** UMDNJ-NJ Med Sch, Newark 1982; **Resid:** Orthopaedic Surgery, UMDNJ Affil Hosps 1989; **Fellow:** Spine Surgery, Seton Med Ctr/St Marys Spine Ctr 1990; **Fac Appt:** Asst Clin Prof OrS, UMDNJ-NJ Med Sch, Newark

Otolaryngology

Lazar, Amy D MD (Oto) - **Spec Exp:** Sinus Disorders; **Hospital:** Somerset Med Ctr; **Address:** ENT and Allergy Associates, 245 US Hwy 22, Fl 3, Bridgewater, NJ 08807; **Phone:** 908-722-1022; **Board Cert:** Otolaryngology 1999; **Med School:** Ros Franklin Univ/Chicago Med Sch 1992; **Resid:** Otolaryngology, Manhattan EE & T Hosp 1995; Otolaryngology, Boston Med Ctr 1998

Pediatric Pulmonology

Turcios, Nelson L MD (PPul) - **Spec Exp:** Breathing Disorders; Cough-Chronic; Cystic Fibrosis; Ciliary Dyskinesia; **Hospital:** Somerset Med Ctr, St. Peter's Univ Hosp; **Address:** 282 E Main St, Pediatric Pulmonology & Cystic Fibrosis, Somerville, NJ 08876; **Phone:** 908-526-5212; **Board Cert:** Pediatrics 1982; Pediatric Pulmonology 2007; **Med School:** El Salvador 1973; **Resid:** Pediatrics, Univ Mississippi Med Ctr 1978; Pediatrics, Univ Maryland Hosp 1980; **Fellow:** Pediatric Pulmonology, Childrens Hosp 1982; **Fac Appt:** Assoc Prof Ped, UMDNJ-NJ Med Sch, Newark

Pediatric Urology

Barone, Joseph G MD (Ped Uro) - **Spec Exp:** Robotic Surgery-Pediatric; Urinary Reconstruction; Incontinence; Hypospadias; **Hospital:** Robert Wood Johnson Univ Hosp - New Brunswick, Univ Med Ctr Princeton at Plainsboro; **Address:** RWJ Dept Urology, 1 Worlds Fair Drive Fl 1, Somerset, NJ 08873; **Phone:** 732-235-7960; **Board Cert:** Urology 2009; Pediatric Urology 2009; **Med School:** UMDNJ-Rutgers Med Sch 1987; **Resid:** Urology, R W Johnson Univ Hosp 1993; **Fellow:** Pediatric Urology, Emory Univ 1994; **Fac Appt:** Assoc Prof S, UMDNJ-RW Johnson Med Sch

Pediatrics

Katz, Andrea G MD (Ped) *PCP* - **Spec Exp:** Developmental & Behavioral Disorders; Chronic Illness; Obesity; **Hospital:** Overlook Med Ctr (page 92); **Address:** 76 Stirling Rd, Ste 201, Warren, NJ 07059; **Phone:** 908-755-5437; **Board Cert:** Pediatrics 2013; **Med School:** NY Med Coll 1988; **Resid:** Pediatrics, NY Hosp-Cornell Med Ctr 1991

Yorke, Eric R MD (Ped) *PCP* - **Hospital:** Somerset Med Ctr, Morristown Med Ctr (page 92); **Address:** Somerset Pediatric Group, 2345 Lamington Rd, Ste 101, Bedminster, NJ 07921; **Phone:** 908-470-1124; **Board Cert:** Pediatrics 2009; **Med School:** Columbia P&S 1982; **Resid:** Pediatrics, Babies Hosp-Columbia 1986

Plastic Surgery

Olson, Robert Martin MD (PlS) - **Spec Exp:** Cleft Palate/Lip; Head & Neck Surgery; Wound Healing/Care; **Hospital:** St. Peter's Univ Hosp, Robert Wood Johnson Univ Hosp - New Brunswick; **Address:** 888 Easton Ave, Ste 6, Somerset, NJ 08873-1898; **Phone:** 732-418-1888; **Board Cert:** Plastic Surgery 1982; **Med School:** Univ Pennsylvania 1974; **Resid:** Surgery, Peter Bent Brigham Hosp 1979; Plastic Surgery, Mayo Clinic 1981; **Fac Appt:** Assoc Prof S, UMDNJ-RW Johnson Med Sch

Perry, Arthur W MD (PlS) - **Spec Exp:** Rhinoplasty; Eyelid Surgery; Liposuction; Abdominoplasty; **Hospital:** Robert Wood Johnson Univ Hosp - New Brunswick, Somerset Med Ctr; **Address:** 3055 Route 27, Franklin Park, NJ 08823-1315; **Phone:** 732-422-9600; **Board Cert:** Plastic Surgery 1989; **Med School:** Albany Med Coll 1981; **Resid:** Surgery, Beth Israel Hosp 1984; Plastic Surgery, Univ Chicago Hosps 1987; **Fellow:** Burn Surgery, New York Hosp-Cornell 1985; Cosmetic Plastic Surgery, Univ Miami/Baker-Gordon Assocs 1987; **Fac Appt:** Assoc Prof PlS, Columbia P&S

Psychiatry

Donnellan, Joseph A MD (Psyc) - **Spec Exp:** Eating Disorders; Obsessive-Compulsive Disorder; **Hospital:** Somerset Med Ctr; **Address:** 422 Courtyard Drive, Hillsborough, NJ 08844; **Phone:** 908-725-5595; **Board Cert:** Psychiatry 1991; **Med School:** UMDNJ-NJ Med Sch, Newark 1986; **Resid:** Psychiatry, UMDNJ Univ Hosp 1990; **Fac Appt:** Asst Clin Prof Psyc, UMDNJ-RW Johnson Med Sch

Rochford, Joseph MD (Psyc) - **Spec Exp:** Depression; Anxiety Disorders; Eating Disorders; **Hospital:** Somerset Med Ctr; **Address:** 407 Omni Drive, Hillsborough, NJ 08844; **Phone:** 908-359-2312; **Board Cert:** Psychiatry 1975; **Med School:** Yale Univ 1969; **Resid:** Psychiatry, Hosp Univ Penn 1973; **Fac Appt:** Assoc Clin Prof Psyc, UMDNJ-RW Johnson Med Sch

Pulmonary Disease

Arno, Louis J MD (Pul) - **Spec Exp:** Critical Care; **Hospital:** Somerset Med Ctr; **Address:** RespaCare, 489 Union Ave, Bridgewater, NJ 08807; **Phone:** 732-356-9950; **Board Cert:** Pulmonary Disease 2006; Critical Care Medicine 2009; **Med School:** Grenada 1986; **Resid:** Internal Medicine, St Michaels Med Ctr 1990; **Fellow:** Pulmonary Disease, St Michaels Med Ctr 1992; Critical Care Medicine, St Michaels Med Ctr 1993

Gerhard, Harvey MD (Pul) - **Hospital:** Morristown Med Ctr (page 92); **Address:** The Pulmonary Group, 416 Mount Airy Rd, Basking Ridge, NJ 07920-2438; **Phone:** 908-766-6605; **Board Cert:** Internal Medicine 1977; **Med School:** Yale Univ 1974; **Resid:** Internal Medicine, Bellevue Hosp Ctr 1977; **Fellow:** Pulmonary Disease, Yale-New Haven Hosp 1979

Radiation Oncology

Braver, Joel K MD (RadRO) - **Spec Exp:** Prostate Cancer; Stereotactic Radiosurgery; Merkel Cell Carcinoma; **Hospital:** Somerset Med Ctr; **Address:** Steeplchase Cancer Center, 30 Rehill Ave, Ste 1100, Somerville, NJ 08876; **Phone:** 908-927-8777; **Board Cert:** Radiation Oncology 2006; **Med School:** UMDNJ-RW Johnson Med Sch 1991; **Resid:** Radiation Oncology, Montefiore Med Ctr 1996

Hug, Eugen B MD (RadRO) - **Spec Exp:** Pediatric Cancers; **Address:** ProCure Proton Therapy Ctr, 103 Cedar Grove Ln, Somerset, NJ 08873; **Phone:** 732-357-2600; **Board Cert:** Radiation Oncology ; **Med School:** Germany 1987; **Resid:** Radiation Oncology, Mass Genl Hosp 1992; **Fellow:** Radiation Oncology, Mass Genl Hosp 1993

Reproductive Endocrinology

Drews, Michael MD (RE) - **Spec Exp:** Infertility-IVF; **Hospital:** Morristown Med Ctr (page 92); **Address:** RMA NJ, 140 Allen Rd, Basking Ridge, NJ 07920; **Phone:** 908-604-7800; **Board Cert:** Obstetrics & Gynecology 2012; Reproductive Endocrinology 2012; **Med School:** Cornell Univ-Weill Med Coll 1986; **Resid:** Obstetrics & Gynecology, N Shore Univ Hosp 1990; **Fellow:** Reproductive Endocrinology, Mount Sinai Med Ctr 1992; **Fac Appt:** Assoc Clin Prof ObG, UMDNJ-RW Johnson Med Sch

Scott, Richard T MD (RE) - **Spec Exp:** Infertility; Infertility-IVF; Fertility Preservation in Cancer; **Hospital:** Morristown Med Ctr (page 92); **Address:** Reproductive Med Assocs of NJ, 140 Allen Rd, Basking Ridge, NJ 07920; **Phone:** 908-604-7800; **Board Cert:** Obstetrics & Gynecology 2012; Reproductive Endocrinology 2012; **Med School:** Univ VA Sch Med 1983; **Resid:** Obstetrics & Gynecology, Wilford Hall USAF Med Ctr 1987; **Fellow:** Reproductive Endocrinology, Jones Inst Reproductive Med 1989; **Fac Appt:** Prof ObG, UMDNJ-RW Johnson Med Sch

Treiser, Susan L MD/PhD (RE) - **Spec Exp:** Infertility; Infertility-IVF; **Hospital:** St. Peter's Univ Hosp; **Address:** IVF NJ Fertility & Gynecology Ctr, 81 Veronica Ave, Somerset, NJ 08873; **Phone:** 732-220-9060; **Board Cert:** Obstetrics & Gynecology 2012; Reproductive Endocrinology 2012; **Med School:** Georgetown Univ 1983; **Resid:** Obstetrics & Gynecology, UMDNJ Med Ctr 1988; **Fellow:** Reproductive Endocrinology, Columbia Presby Med Ctr 1990

Sports Medicine

France, Matthew MD (SM) - **Spec Exp:** Arthroscopic Surgery; Shoulder Injuries; Knee Surgery; **Hospital:** Morristown Med Ctr (page 92); **Address:** 1 Robertson Drive, Ste 11, Bedminster, NJ 07921; **Phone:** 908-234-9800; **Board Cert:** Orthopaedic Surgery 2006; Orthopaedic Sports Medicine 2010; **Med School:** UAB Sch Med 1986; **Resid:** Orthopaedic Surgery, Univ Hosp-UMDNJ 1991; **Fellow:** Sports Medicine & Arthroscopic Surgery, UCSD Med Ctr 2007; Shoulder Surgery, Univ Wash Med Ctr 2009

Surgery

Drascher, Gary MD (S) - **Spec Exp:** Laparoscopic Surgery-Complex; Aneurysm; Carotid Artery Surgery; Vascular Surgery; **Hospital:** Somerset Med Ctr; **Address:** Surgical Assocs Central NJ, 30 Rehill Ave, Ste 3300, Somerville, NJ 08776; **Phone:** 908-927-8994; **Board Cert:** Surgery 2007; **Med School:** Mount Sinai Sch Med 1981; **Resid:** Internal Medicine, St Lukes-Roosevelt Hosp Ctr 1982; Surgery, St Lukes-Roosevelt Hosp Ctr 1987; **Fellow:** Vascular Surgery, Englewood Hosp 1989

Lanfranchi, Angela E MD (S) - **Spec Exp:** Breast Cancer; Breast Surgery; **Hospital:** Somerset Med Ctr; **Address:** Surgical Assocs Central NJ, 30 Rehill Ave, Ste 3300, Somerville, NJ 08776; **Phone:** 908-927-8994; **Board Cert:** Surgery 2012; **Med School:** Georgetown Univ 1975; **Resid:** Family Medicine, Somerset Hosp 1978; Surgery, Stony Brook Univ Med Ctr 1982; **Fellow:** Vascular Surgery, Nassau Hosp 1983

Thoracic & Cardiac Surgery

Caccavale, Robert J MD (T&CS) - **Spec Exp:** Video Assisted Thoracic Surgery (VATS); **Hospital:** Somerset Med Ctr, CentraState Med Ctr; **Address:** Thoracic Grp, 35 Clyde Rd, Ste 104, Somerset, NJ 08873; **Phone:** 732-247-3002; **Board Cert:** Thoracic & Cardiac Surgery 2008; **Med School:** SUNY Buffalo 1981; **Resid:** Surgery, NYU Med Ctr 1984; Surgery, Booth Meml Med Ctr 1986; **Fellow:** Thoracic Surgery, SUNY Downstate Med Ctr 1988; **Fac Appt:** Assoc Clin Prof T&CS, UMDNJ-RW Johnson Med Sch

Urology

Catanese, Anthony J MD (U) - **Spec Exp:** Urologic Cancer; Kidney Cancer; **Hospital:** Somerset Med Ctr, St. Peter's Univ Hosp; **Address:** Partners in Urology, 315 E Main St, Somerville, NJ 08876; **Phone:** 908-722-6900; **Board Cert:** Urology 2009; **Med School:** NY Med Coll 1983; **Resid:** Surgery, NYU Med Ctr 1985; Urology, NYU Med Ctr 1989

The Best in American Medicine
www.CastleConnolly.com

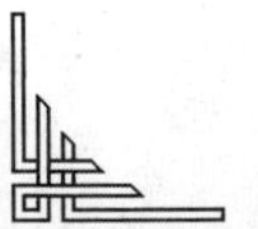
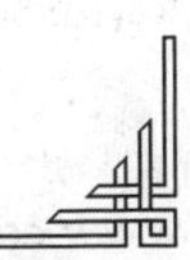

Union

Trinitas Regional Medical Center

225 Williamson Street | Elizabeth, New Jersey 07207
Ph 908.994.5000 | www.TrinitasRMC.org

Caring For You In Every Way

Sponsorship: Trinitas Regional Medical Center is a voluntary not-for-profit Catholic teaching hospital sponsored by the Sisters of Charity of Saint Elizabeth in partnership with Elizabethtown Healthcare Foundation.

Beds: 556

Accredited by The Joint Commission

Medical Staff

Trinitas Regional Medical Center has nearly 500 physicians and over 40 residents on its medical staff. Trinitas is a major clinical site for the Seton Hall School of Health and Medical Sciences' Internal Medicine Residency Program.

Centers of Excellence:

Behavioral Health & Psychiatry: Behavioral Health services at Trinitas are among the most comprehensive in New Jersey and include a full range of inpatient and outpatient psychiatric care for seniors, adults, adolescents and children.

Cancer Care: The Trinitas Comprehensive Cancer Center offers the most advanced medical and radiation technology available, including Rapid Arc radiotherapy, to cancer patients. An interdisciplinary team works with each patient to develop a care plan encompassing the latest diagnostic treatment options, medical technology, clinical trials and integrative therapy.

Cardiology: Trinitas maintains a full-service cardiac facility for the intensive care of patients with heart disease, including elective angioplasty, a cardiac care unit, intermediate coronary care unit, cardiac catheterization lab, non-invasive cardiology services, full-service emergency department, and cardiac rehabilitation services.

Maternal & Child Health: Trinitas offers a Level II Intermediate Care Nursery, a 24-hour in-house pediatrician and obstetrician, and midwifery services. Inpatient care for child/adolescent psychiatric patients is also offered.

Renal Care: Trinitas is committed to patients experiencing kidney failure, and initiated the THRIVE early intervention program to reach high-risk patients.

Seniors Services: The Trinitas commitment to seniors takes many forms, most recently the establishment of the Acute Care for the Elderly (ACE) nursing unit. The Seniors First Membership Program offers special gifts and invitations to special events.

School of Nursing: The third largest school of nursing in the United States, the Trinitas School of Nursing, affiliated with Union County College, is known for an outstanding nursing education program that was recently designated a Center of Excellence in Nursing Education by the National League for Nursing.

Sleep Disorders: The Comprehensive Sleep Disorders Center provides monitored, fully-attended diagnostic sleep studies designed to rule out physical, non-stress related symptoms that may prevent restful sleep in adults and children. Two locations are offered, including the first hotel-based sleep center in New Jersey.

Women's Services: In addition to the latest modalities in digital mammography, breast biopsy, breast MRI, bone density screening and ultrasound, women can visit Trinitas for cosmetic and reconstructive surgery and innovative surgical care using the da Vinci® Robotic Surgical System for female incontinence and prolapse.

Wound Healing/Diabetes Management: The Trinitas Center for Wound Healing and Hyperbaric Medicine has one of the highest heal rates in the nation. Specially-trained certified nurses and physicians treat those with chronic, hard-to-heal wounds. Recognized by the American Diabetes Association, the Diabetes Management Center offers a high quality education program for diabetics.

Adolescent Medicine

Sanders, Leslie MD (AM) - **Spec Exp:** Eating Disorders; **Hospital:** Overlook Med Ctr (page 92), Morristown Med Ctr (page 92); **Address:** Overlook Med Ctr, Eating Disoders Program, 99 Beauvoir Ave, Summit, NJ 07902; **Phone:** 908-522-5757; **Board Cert:** Adolescent Medicine 2012; **Med School:** Albert Einstein Coll Med 1984; **Resid:** Pediatrics, Univ Pittsburgh Med Ctr 1987

Allergy & Immunology

Bielory, Leonard MD (A&I) - **Spec Exp:** Dry Eye Syndrome; Asthma; Eye Allergy; Autoimmune Occular Disorders; **Hospital:** Saint Barnabas Med Ctr; **Address:** 400 Mountain Ave, Springfield, NJ 07081; **Phone:** 973-912-9817; **Board Cert:** Internal Medicine 1984; Allergy & Immunology 1985; Clinical & Laboratory Immunology 1986; **Med School:** UMDNJ-NJ Med Sch, Newark 1980; **Resid:** Internal Medicine, Univ Md Hosp 1982; Hematology, Natl Inst Hlth 1983; **Fellow:** Allergy & Immunology, Natl Inst Hlth 1985; Diagnostic Lab Immunology, Natl Inst Hlth 1985; **Fac Appt:** Prof A&I, UMDNJ-NJ Med Sch, Newark

Brown, David K MD (A&I) - **Spec Exp:** Asthma; Sinus Disorders; Headache; **Hospital:** Overlook Med Ctr (page 92); **Address:** Allergy Diagnostic & Treatment Ctr, 33 Overlook Rd, Ste 307, Summit, NJ 07901; **Phone:** 908-522-9696; **Board Cert:** Internal Medicine 1984; Allergy & Immunology 1987; **Med School:** Med Coll OH 1981; **Resid:** Internal Medicine, Overlook Hosp 1984; **Fellow:** Allergy & Immunology, St Lukes-Roosevelt Hosp 1986

Goodman, Alan J MD (A&I) - **Spec Exp:** Rhinitis; Sinus Disorders; Asthma; **Hospital:** Saint Barnabas Med Ctr; **Address:** 381 Chestnut St, Union, NJ 07083; **Phone:** 908-688-6200; **Board Cert:** Internal Medicine 1985; Allergy & Immunology 2009; **Med School:** SUNY Upstate Med Univ 1982; **Resid:** Internal Medicine, Washington Hosp Ctr 1985; **Fellow:** Allergy & Immunology, St Luke's-Roosevelt Hosp Ctr 1988

LeBenger, Kerry S MD (A&I) - **Spec Exp:** Asthma; Allergy; **Hospital:** Overlook Med Ctr (page 92); **Address:** Summit Med Grp, ENT Allergy, 1 Diamond Hill Rd Fl 2, Lawrence Pav, Berkely Heights, NJ 07922; **Phone:** 908-277-8681; **Board Cert:** Internal Medicine 1983; Allergy & Immunology 1985; **Med School:** NY Med Coll 1980; **Resid:** Internal Medicine, Lenox Hill Hosp 1983; **Fellow:** Allergy & Immunology, NY-Presby/Weill Cornell Med Ctr 1985; **Fac Appt:** Asst Clin Prof Med, UMDNJ-Rutgers Med Sch

Maccia, Clement MD (A&I) - **Spec Exp:** Rhinitis; Asthma; Urticaria; Eczema; **Hospital:** JFK Med Ctr - Edison, Robert Wood Johnson Univ Hosp - New Brunswick; **Address:** Asthma, Sinus & Allergy Ctrs, 19 Holly St, Cranford, NJ 07016; **Phone:** 908-276-0666; **Board Cert:** Pediatrics 1980; Allergy & Immunology 1985; **Med School:** Italy 1971; **Resid:** Pediatrics, Muhlenberg Med Ctr 1974; **Fellow:** Allergy & Immunology, Univ Hosp 1976; **Fac Appt:** Clin Prof A&I, UMDNJ-RW Johnson Med Sch

Mendelson, Joel S MD (A&I) - **Spec Exp:** Infectious Disease; Food Allergy; Urticaria; Eczema; **Hospital:** Saint Barnabas Med Ctr, Chldns Hosp NJ at Newark; **Address:** 1124 Springfield Ave, Mountainside, NJ 07092; **Phone:** 908-233-4477; **Board Cert:** Pediatrics 1987; Allergy & Immunology 2009; Pediatric Infectious Disease 2005; **Med School:** Dominican Republic 1982; **Resid:** Pediatrics, St Lukes-Roosevelt Hosp 1985; **Fellow:** Allergy & Immunology, Univ Hosp-UMDNJ 1987; Infectious Disease, Univ Hosp-UMDNJ 1987; **Fac Appt:** Asst Prof Ped, Grenada

Cardiovascular Disease

Kalischer, Alan L MD (Cv) - **Spec Exp:** Echocardiography; Nuclear Cardiology; Coronary Artery Disease; Arrhythmias; **Hospital:** Overlook Med Ctr (page 92), JFK Med Ctr - Edison; **Address:** Fanwood-Westfield Cardiology, 313 South Ave, Ste 202, Fanwood, NJ 07023; **Phone:** 908-889-1900; **Board Cert:** Internal Medicine 1982; Cardiovascular Disease 1985; Echocardiography 2011; Nuclear Cardiology 2012; **Med School:** NY Med Coll 1977; **Resid:** Internal Medicine, SUNY Downstate Med Ctr 1980; **Fellow:** Cardiovascular Disease, NY-Presby/Columbia Univ Med Ctr 1984; **Fac Appt:** Asst Prof Med, UMDNJ-RW Johnson Med Sch

Sachs, R. Gregory MD (Cv) - **Spec Exp:** Heart Disease; Heart Valve Disease; Congenital Heart Disease-Adult; **Hospital:** Overlook Med Ctr (page 92), Morristown Med Ctr (page 92); **Address:** Summit Med Grp, Cardiology, 1 Diamond Hill Rd Fl 2, Berkeley Heights, NJ 07922; **Phone:** 908-277-8713; **Board Cert:** Internal Medicine 1972; Cardiovascular Disease 1976; **Med School:** Georgetown Univ 1966; **Resid:** Internal Medicine, Georgetown Univ Hosp 1968; **Fellow:** Cardiovascular Disease, Emory Univ Hosp 1970; Cardiovascular Disease, Natl Heart Hosp 1971; **Fac Appt:** Asst Clin Prof Med, Columbia P&S

Sheris, Steven J MD (Cv) - **Spec Exp:** Stress Echocardiography; Nuclear Cardiology; **Hospital:** Overlook Med Ctr (page 92), Morristown Med Ctr (page 92); **Address:** Assocs Cardiovascular Disease, 571 Central Ave, Ste 115, New Providence, NJ 07974; **Phone:** 908-464-4200; **Board Cert:** Internal Medicine 2003; Cardiovascular Disease 2007; Nuclear Cardiology 2003; **Med School:** UMDNJ-Rutgers Med Sch 1988; **Resid:** Internal Medicine, Natl Naval Med Ctr 1994; **Fellow:** Cardiovascular Disease, Georgetown Univ Hosp 1997

Slama, Robert D MD (Cv) - **Spec Exp:** Echocardiography; Preventive Cardiology; Nuclear Cardiology; **Hospital:** Overlook Med Ctr (page 92), Morristown Med Ctr (page 92); **Address:** Summit Med Grp, Cardiology, 1 Diamond Hill Rd, Berkeley Heights, NJ 07922; **Phone:** 908-277-8714; **Board Cert:** Internal Medicine 1974; Cardiovascular Disease 1977; **Med School:** Temple Univ 1971; **Resid:** Internal Medicine, Boston Med Ctr 1973; Internal Medicine, Georgetown Univ Hosp 1974; **Fellow:** Cardiovascular Disease, Boston Med Ctr 1976

Child & Adolescent Psychiatry

Greenberg, Rosalie MD (ChAP) - **Spec Exp:** Bipolar/Mood Disorders; ADD/ADHD; **Hospital:** Overlook Med Ctr (page 92); **Address:** 33 Overlook Rd, Ste 406, Summit, NJ 07901; **Phone:** 908-598-0200; **Board Cert:** Psychiatry 1982; Child & Adolescent Psychiatry 1983; **Med School:** Columbia P&S 1976; **Resid:** Psychiatry, Columbia-Presby Hosp 1980; **Fellow:** Child & Adolescent Psychiatry, Columbia-Presby Hosp 1981; **Fac Appt:** Asst Clin Prof Psyc, Columbia P&S

Child Neurology

Traeger, Eveline C MD (ChiN) - **Spec Exp:** Autism; ADD/ADHD; Learning Disorders; **Hospital:** Children's Specialized Hosp; **Address:** Chldns Specialized Hosp, 150 New Providence Rd, Mountainside, NJ 07092; **Phone:** 908-233-3720; **Board Cert:** Child Neurology 2004; Clinical Genetics 1990; **Med School:** SUNY Buffalo 1984; **Resid:** Child Neurology, Yeshiva Univ 1986; Pediatrics, Jacobi Med Ctr 1988

Colon & Rectal Surgery

Chinn, Bertram T MD (CRS) - **Spec Exp:** Laparoscopic Surgery; Colon & Rectal Cancer; Inflammatory Bowel Disease; Diverticulitis; **Hospital:** Overlook Med Ctr (page 92), Robert Wood Johnson Univ Hosp - New Brunswick; **Address:** Associated Colon & Rectal Surgeons, Overlook Medical Center, 96 Beauvoir Ave, Cancer Ctr Fl 6, Summit, NJ 07902; **Phone:** 732-494-6640; **Board Cert:** Surgery 2002; Colon & Rectal Surgery 2012; **Med School:** Jefferson Med Coll 1987; **Resid:** Surgery, Thomas Jefferson Univ Hosp 1992; **Fellow:** Colon & Rectal Surgery, UMDNJ-RW Johnson Med Ctr 1993; **Fac Appt:** Assoc Clin Prof S, UMDNJ-RW Johnson Med Sch

Groff, Walter L MD (CRS) - **Spec Exp:** Colonoscopy; Rectal Cancer/Sphincter Preservation; **Hospital:** Overlook Med Ctr (page 92), Saint Barnabas Med Ctr; **Address:** 33 Overlook Rd, Ste 412, Summit, NJ 07901-3564; **Phone:** 908-598-0220; **Board Cert:** Colon & Rectal Surgery 1980; **Med School:** Albany Med Coll 1970; **Resid:** Surgery, St Vincent's Hosp 1979; Colon & Rectal Surgery, Muhlenberg Med Ctr 1980; **Fac Appt:** Assoc Prof S, Columbia P&S

Dermatology

Eisenberg, Richard R MD (D) - **Spec Exp:** Skin Cancer; Melanoma; Acne; **Hospital:** Overlook Med Ctr (page 92); **Address:** 40 Stirling Rd, Ste 203, Watchung, NJ 07069; **Phone:** 908-753-4144; **Board Cert:** Internal Medicine 1985; Dermatology 1989; **Med School:** Cornell Univ-Weill Med Coll 1982; **Resid:** Internal Medicine, NY Hosp-Cornell Med Ctr 1985; Dermatology, NY Hosp-Cornell/Meml Sloan Kettering Cancer Ctr 1989

Weinberger, George I MD (D) - **Spec Exp:** Skin Cancer; **Hospital:** Saint Barnabas Med Ctr; **Address:** 190 Greenbrook Rd, North Plainfield, NJ 07060-3903; **Phone:** 908-561-8070; **Board Cert:** Dermatology 1977; **Med School:** UMDNJ-NJ Med Sch, Newark 1973; **Resid:** Dermatology, Henry Ford Hosp 1977

Zirvi, Monib A MD (D) - **Spec Exp:** Cosmetic Dermatology; Skin Cancer; **Hospital:** Morristown Med Ctr (page 92), Overlook Med Ctr (page 92); **Address:** 1 Diamond Hill Rd, Laurence Bldg-2nd Fl, Berkeley Heights, NJ 07922; **Phone:** 908-769-0100; **Board Cert:** Dermatology 2004; **Med School:** Cornell Univ 2000; **Resid:** Dermatology, Univ Penn Affil Hosp 2004

Diagnostic Radiology

Grosso-Rivas, Sue Jane MD (DR) - **Spec Exp:** Breast Imaging; Nuclear Radiology; CT Body Scan; **Hospital:** Overlook Med Ctr (page 92); **Address:** Summit Med Grp, 1 Diamond Hill Rd, Berkeley Heights, NJ 07922; **Phone:** 908-273-4300; **Board Cert:** Diagnostic Radiology 1991; **Med School:** Harvard Med Sch 1985; **Resid:** Diagnostic Radiology, NYU Med Ctr 1990; Internal Medicine, Waterbury Hospital 1986; **Fellow:** Breast Imaging, NYU Med Ctr 1991; Nuclear Medicine, NYU Med Ctr 1991

Endocrinology, Diabetes & Metabolism

Fuhrman, Robert A MD (EDM) - **Spec Exp:** Diabetes; Thyroid Disorders; Osteoporosis; **Hospital:** Overlook Med Ctr (page 92); **Address:** 552 Westfield Ave, Westfield, NJ 07090-3312; **Phone:** 908-654-3377; **Board Cert:** Internal Medicine 1971; Endocrinology, Diabetes & Metabolism 1972; **Med School:** Ros Franklin Univ/Chicago Med Sch 1966; **Resid:** Internal Medicine, Mount Sinai Hosp 1970; Nuclear Medicine, VA Hospital 1970; **Fellow:** Endocrinology, Diabetes & Metabolism, Mount Sinai Hosp 1970

Rosenbaum, Robert L MD (EDM) - **Spec Exp:** Thyroid Disorders; Diabetes; Osteoporosis; **Hospital:** Overlook Med Ctr (page 92); **Address:** Summit Med Grp, One Diamond Hill Rd, Berkeley Heights, NJ 07922-2104; **Phone:** 908-277-8667; **Board Cert:** Internal Medicine 1978; Endocrinology, Diabetes & Metabolism 1981; **Med School:** Columbia P&S 1975; **Resid:** Internal Medicine, Montefiore Hosp Med Ctr 1978; **Fellow:** Endocrinology, Diabetes & Metabolism, Montefiore Hosp Med Ctr 1980; **Fac Appt:** Asst Clin Prof Med, Mount Sinai Sch Med

Selinger, Sharon E MD (EDM) - **Spec Exp:** Diabetes; Thyroid Disorders; Pituitary Disorders; Osteoporosis; **Hospital:** Overlook Med Ctr (page 92); **Address:** Summit Endocrinology & Diabetes, 1 Springfield Ave, Ste 1A, Summit, NJ 07901; **Phone:** 908-273-8300; **Board Cert:** Internal Medicine 1984; Endocrinology, Diabetes & Metabolism 1987; **Med School:** Cornell Univ-Weill Med Coll 1981; **Resid:** Internal Medicine, Montefiore Hosp Med Ctr 1984; **Fellow:** Endocrinology, Diabetes & Metabolism, Bellevue Hosp-NYU Med Ctr 1986

Silverman, Mitchell MD (EDM) - **Spec Exp:** Diabetes; Thyroid Disorders; Adrenal Disorders; **Hospital:** Newark Beth Israel Med Ctr, Saint Barnabas Med Ctr; **Address:** 2333 Morris Ave, Ste B-109, Union, NJ 07083; **Phone:** 908-964-5511; **Board Cert:** Internal Medicine 1983; Endocrinology 1987; **Med School:** Duke Univ 1980; **Resid:** Internal Medicine, Emory Univ Hosp 1983; **Fellow:** Endocrinology, Diabetes & Metabolism, NY Hosp-Meml Sloan-Kettering 1988

Family Medicine

Eisenstat, Steven DO (FMed) *PCP* - **Spec Exp:** Osteoporosis; Hypertension; Alzheimer's Disease; **Hospital:** Overlook Med Ctr (page 92); **Address:** 1050 Galloping Hill Rd, Ste 202, Union, NJ 07083-7980; **Phone:** 908-688-4845; **Board Cert:** Family Medicine 1993; Geriatric Medicine 1991; **Med School:** Ohio State Univ 1984; **Resid:** Family Medicine, Union Hosp 1987; **Fac Appt:** Asst Clin Prof FMed, NY Coll Osteo Med

Podell, Richard N MD (FMed) - **Spec Exp:** Complementary Medicine; Nutrition & Disease Prevention/Control; Fibromyalgia; Chronic Fatigue Syndrome; **Hospital:** Overlook Med Ctr (page 92); **Address:** Medical Arts Center, 11 Overlook Rd, Ste 140, Summit, NJ 07901; **Phone:** 908-273-7770; **Board Cert:** Internal Medicine 1980; Family Medicine 2005; **Med School:** Harvard Med Sch 1969; **Resid:** Internal Medicine, Mt Sinai Hosp 1972; **Fellow:** Nutrition, Harvard Sch Pub Hlth 1973; **Fac Appt:** Clin Prof FMed, UMDNJ-RW Johnson Med Sch

Tabachnick, John F MD (FMed) *PCP* - **Hospital:** Overlook Med Ctr (page 92); **Address:** 563 Westfield Ave, Westfield, NJ 07090; **Phone:** 908-232-5858; **Board Cert:** Family Medicine 2007; **Med School:** Mount Sinai Sch Med 1979; **Resid:** Family Medicine, Overlook Hosp 1982; **Fac Appt:** Asst Clin Prof FMed, UMDNJ Sch Osteo Med

Gastroenterology

Barrison, Adam F MD (Ge) - **Spec Exp:** Endoscopy; **Hospital:** Overlook Med Ctr (page 92); **Address:** Summit Medical Group, 1 Diamond Hill Rd, Berkeley Heights, NJ 07922; **Phone:** 908-227-8940; **Board Cert:** Gastroenterology 2011; **Med School:** NYU Sch Med 1995; **Resid:** Internal Medicine, Beth Israel Hosp 1998; **Fellow:** Gastroenterology, Boston Univ Med Ctr 2001

Ben-Menachem, Tamir MD (Ge) - **Spec Exp:** Endoscopy; Pancreatic/Biliary Endoscopy (ERCP); Endoscopic Ultrasound; **Hospital:** Overlook Med Ctr (page 92); **Address:** Summit Medical Group, 1 Diamond Hill Rd, Berkeley Heights, NJ 07922; **Phone:** 908-277-8940; **Board Cert:** Internal Medicine 2004; Gastroenterology 2007; **Med School:** Israel 1989; **Resid:** Internal Medicine, Henry Ford Hosp 1993; **Fellow:** Gastroenterology, Henry Ford Hosp 1997; **Fac Appt:** Assoc Prof Med

Feit, David MD (Ge) - **Spec Exp:** Hepatitis; **Hospital:** Hackensack Univ Med Ctr (page 718); **Address:** Hackensack Digestive Diseases Assocs, 385 Prospect Ave, Hackensack, NJ 07061; **Phone:** 201-488-3003; **Board Cert:** Internal Medicine 1984; Gastroenterology 1989; **Med School:** Columbia P&S 1981; **Resid:** Internal Medicine, Columbia-Presby Med Ctr 1984; **Fellow:** Gastroenterology, Columbia-Presby Med Ctr 1987

Goldenberg, David MD (Ge) - **Spec Exp:** Inflammatory Bowel Disease/Crohn's; Biliary Disease; Gastroesophageal Reflux Disease (GERD); **Hospital:** JFK Med Ctr - Edison, Somerset Med Ctr; **Address:** Gastroenterology Associates, 1165 Park Ave, Plainfield, NJ 07060-3010; **Phone:** 908-754-2992; **Board Cert:** Internal Medicine 1977; Gastroenterology 1981; **Med School:** NY Med Coll 1974; **Resid:** Internal Medicine, Metropolitan Hosp 1977; **Fellow:** Gastroenterology, Emory Univ Hosp 1980; **Fac Appt:** Asst Clin Prof Med, UMDNJ-NJ Med Sch, Newark

Kerner, Michael B MD (Ge) - **Spec Exp:** Colonoscopy; Biliary Disease; Gastroesophageal Reflux Disease (GERD); Inflammatory Bowel Disease; **Hospital:** Overlook Med Ctr (page 92), Morristown Med Ctr (page 92); **Address:** 25 Morris Ave, Springfield, NJ 07081-1406; **Phone:** 973-467-1313; **Board Cert:** Internal Medicine 1975; Gastroenterology 1977; **Med School:** Wake Forest Univ 1971; **Resid:** Internal Medicine, NYU Med Ctr 1974; **Fellow:** Gastroenterology, Manhattan VA-Bellevue Hosp 1976; **Fac Appt:** Asst Clin Prof Med, Mount Sinai Sch Med

Mahal, Pradeep MD (Ge) - **Spec Exp:** Gastrointestinal Cancer; **Hospital:** Overlook Med Ctr (page 92), Trinitas Reg Med Ctr (page 914); **Address:** 1308 Morris Ave, Ste 202, Union, NJ 07083; **Phone:** 908-851-6767; **Board Cert:** Gastroenterology 1981; Internal Medicine 1978; Medical Oncology 1983; **Med School:** India 1975; **Resid:** Internal Medicine, UMDNJ Univ Hosp 1978; **Fellow:** Medical Oncology, MD Anderson Tumor Inst 1980; Gastroenterology, MD Anderson Tumor Inst 1980

Tempera, Patrick G MD (Ge) - **Spec Exp:** Biliary Disease; Pancreatic Disease; Gastroesophageal Reflux Disease (GERD); **Hospital:** Overlook Med Ctr (page 92), Somerset Med Ctr; **Address:** 1308 Morris Ave, Ste 102, Union, NJ 07083; **Phone:** 908-851-2770; **Board Cert:** Gastroenterology 2004; **Med School:** Grenada 1986; **Resid:** Surgery, Brooklyn Hosp 1987; Internal Medicine, Seton Hall Univ Hosp 1990; **Fellow:** Gastroenterology, Seton Hall Univ Hosp 1992; **Fac Appt:** Assoc Prof Med, Seton Hall Univ Sch Hlth & Med Scis

Geriatric Medicine

Khimani, Karim J MD (Ger) *PCP* - **Hospital:** Trinitas Reg Med Ctr (page 914); **Address:** 240 Williamson St, Ste 306, Elizabeth, NJ 07202; **Phone:** 908-352-5071; **Board Cert:** Internal Medicine 1986; Geriatric Medicine 2003; Hospice & Palliative Medicine 2008; **Med School:** Dominican Republic 1982; **Resid:** Internal Medicine, St Elizabeth Hosp 1985

Solomon, Robert B MD (Ger) *PCP* - **Spec Exp:** Alzheimer's Disease; Osteoporosis; **Hospital:** Trinitas Reg Med Ctr (page 914), Overlook Med Ctr (page 92); **Address:** 744 Galloping Hill Rd, Roselle Park, NJ 07204-1758; **Phone:** 908-241-0044; **Board Cert:** Internal Medicine 1980; Geriatric Medicine 2008; **Med School:** SUNY Hlth Sci Ctr 1977; **Resid:** Internal Medicine, Westchester Med Ctr 1980; **Fellow:** Geriatric Medicine, NY Hosp 1981

Hematology

Kessler, William MD (Hem) - **Hospital:** Trinitas Reg Med Ctr (page 914); **Address:** 225 Williamson St, Elizabeth, NJ 07083; **Phone:** 908-994-8773; **Board Cert:** Internal Medicine 1978; Hematology 1980; **Med School:** Albert Einstein Coll Med 1975; **Resid:** Internal Medicine, UMDNJ-Newark 1978; **Fellow:** Hematology, VA Hosp 1979

Infectious Disease

Farrer, William Eric MD (Inf) - **Spec Exp:** AIDS/HIV; Diabetic Leg/Foot Infections; Travel Medicine; **Hospital:** Trinitas Reg Med Ctr (page 914); **Address:** 240 Williamson St, Ste 502, Elizabeth, NJ 07202; **Phone:** 908-994-5300; **Board Cert:** Internal Medicine 1978; Infectious Disease 1980; **Med School:** Harvard Med Sch 1975; **Resid:** Internal Medicine, Montefiore Med Ctr 1978; **Fellow:** Infectious Disease, Montefiore Med Ctr 1980; **Fac Appt:** Assoc Prof Med, Seton Hall Univ Sch Hlth & Med Scis

Greenman, James L MD (Inf) - **Spec Exp:** AIDS/HIV; Lyme Disease; **Hospital:** Overlook Med Ctr (page 92); **Address:** Medical Diagnostic Associates, 525 Central Ave, Ste C, Westfield, NJ 07090; **Phone:** 908-233-0895; **Board Cert:** Internal Medicine 1985; Infectious Disease 1988; **Med School:** Albert Einstein Coll Med 1982; **Resid:** Internal Medicine, Columbia-Presby Med Ctr 1985; **Fellow:** Infectious Disease, Montefiore Med Ctr 1988

Roland, Robert DO (Inf) - **Spec Exp:** AIDS/HIV; Travel Medicine; Hepatitis C; **Hospital:** Overlook Med Ctr (page 92), Robert Wood Johnson Univ Hosp at Rahway; **Address:** Overlook Hosp Wound Healing Program, 11 Overlook Rd, Bldg II, Ste LL101, Summit, NJ 07901; **Phone:** 908-522-5900; **Board Cert:** Internal Medicine 1990; Infectious Disease 1992; **Med School:** Kirksville Coll Osteo Med 1985; **Resid:** Internal Medicine, Union Hosp 1989; **Fellow:** Infectious Disease, Kennedy Meml Hosp 1991; **Fac Appt:** Asst Clin Prof Med, NY Coll Osteo Med

Internal Medicine

Alterman, Lloyd H MD (IM) - **Spec Exp:** Hypertension; Kidney Disease-Chronic; **Hospital:** Overlook Med Ctr (page 92); **Address:** 1 Diamond Hill Rd, Berkeley Heights, NJ 07922; **Phone:** 908-277-8683; **Board Cert:** Internal Medicine 1980; Nephrology 1982; **Med School:** Wayne State Univ 1977; **Resid:** Internal Medicine, Overlook Hosp 1980; **Fellow:** Nephrology, Montefiore Med Ctr 1982

DiGiacomo, William A MD (IM) *PCP* - **Hospital:** Saint Michael's Med Ctr, Overlook Med Ctr (page 92); **Address:** 2801 Morris Ave, Union, NJ 07083; **Phone:** 908-851-2500; **Board Cert:** Internal Medicine 1978; **Med School:** Mexico 1974; **Resid:** Internal Medicine, St Michaels Med Ctr 1978; **Fac Appt:** Assoc Prof Med, Seton Hall Univ Sch Hlth & Med Scis

Feldman, Jeffrey N MD (IM) - **Spec Exp:** Kidney Disease-Chronic; Cholesterol/Lipid Disorders; Diabetes; Hypertension; **Hospital:** Overlook Med Ctr (page 92); **Address:** 440 Chestnut St, Fl 1, Union, NJ 07083-9306; **Phone:** 908-686-9330; **Board Cert:** Internal Medicine 1979; Nephrology 1982; **Med School:** Hahnemann Univ 1976; **Resid:** Internal Medicine, Bronx Municipal Hosp 1979; **Fellow:** Nephrology, SUNY Hlth Sci Ctr 1981

Goodgold, Abraham MD (IM) *PCP* - **Hospital:** Trinitas Reg Med Ctr (page 914), Robert Wood Johnson Univ Hosp at Rahway; **Address:** union county healthcare associates, 310 W Jersey St, Elizabeth, NJ 07202-1832; **Phone:** 908-351-2222; **Board Cert:** Internal Medicine 1977; **Med School:** NYU Sch Med 1973; **Resid:** Internal Medicine, Montefiore Med Ctr 1976; **Fellow:** Endocrinology, Mt Sinai Med Ctr 1978

Maglaras, Nicholas C MD (IM) - **Hospital:** Trinitas Reg Med Ctr (page 914); **Address:** 236 E Westfield Ave, Ste 5, Roselle Park, NJ 07204; **Phone:** 908-245-8222; **Board Cert:** Internal Medicine 2003; Pulmonary Disease 2006; **Med School:** Grenada 1987; **Resid:** Internal Medicine, Elmhurst Hosp 1990; **Fellow:** Pulmonary Disease, Elmhurst Hosp 1992

Interventional Cardiology

Lux, Michael S MD (IC) - **Hospital:** Overlook Med Ctr (page 92), Morristown Med Ctr (page 92); **Address:** Assocs in Cardiovascular Disease, 211 Mountain Ave, Springfield, NJ 07081-1581; **Phone:** 973-467-0005; **Board Cert:** Internal Medicine 1980; Cardiovascular Disease 1985; **Med School:** NYU Sch Med 1977; **Resid:** Internal Medicine, Johns Hopkins Hosp 1980; **Fellow:** Cardiovascular Disease, Johns Hopkins Hosp 1983; **Fac Appt:** Asst Prof Med, Columbia P&S

Mich, Robert J MD (IC) - **Spec Exp:** Arrhythmias; **Hospital:** Morristown Med Ctr (page 92), Overlook Med Ctr (page 92); **Address:** Assocs in Cardiovascular Disease, 571 Central Ave, Ste 115, New Providence, NJ 07974; **Phone:** 908-464-4200; **Board Cert:** Internal Medicine 1984; Cardiovascular Disease 1985; **Med School:** Johns Hopkins Univ 1979; **Resid:** Internal Medicine, John Hopkins Hosp 1982; **Fellow:** Cardiovascular Disease, Vanderbilt Univ Hosp 1984; Cardiovascular Disease, Mass Genl Hosp 1986

Medical Oncology

Guerin, Bonni L MD (Onc) - **Spec Exp:** Breast Cancer; **Hospital:** Overlook Med Ctr (page 92); **Address:** Medical Diagnostic Assocs, Overlook Oncology Ctr, 99 Beauvoir Ave Fl 5, Summit, NJ 07902; **Phone:** 908-608-0078; **Board Cert:** Internal Medicine 2005; Medical Oncology 2005; **Med School:** SUNY Stony Brook 1988; **Resid:** Internal Medicine, Vanderbilt Univ Med Ctr 1991; **Fellow:** Medical Oncology, UCSD Cancer Ctr 1993

Lowenthal, Dennis A MD (Onc) - **Spec Exp:** Lung Cancer; Lymphoma; Prostate Cancer; Thoracic Cancers; **Hospital:** Overlook Med Ctr (page 92); **Address:** The Carol G. Simon Cancer Center, Overlook Medical Center, 99 Beauvoir Ave, Summit, NJ 07902; **Phone:** 908-608-0078; **Board Cert:** Internal Medicine 1982; Medical Oncology 1985; Hematology 1986; **Med School:** Boston Univ 1979; **Resid:** Internal Medicine, Montefiore Med Ctr 1982; **Fellow:** Hematology, Montefiore Med Ctr 1983; Medical Oncology, Mem Sloan Kettering Cancer Ctr 1986; **Fac Appt:** Asst Clin Prof Med, Mount Sinai Sch Med

Moriarty, Daniel J MD (Onc) - **Spec Exp:** Gastrointestinal Cancer; **Hospital:** Overlook Med Ctr (page 92); **Address:** Med Diagnostic Assocs, 99 Beauvoir Ave Fl 5, Summit, NJ 07902; **Phone:** 908-608-0078; **Board Cert:** Internal Medicine 1982; Medical Oncology 1987; **Med School:** Univ VT Coll Med 1976; **Resid:** Internal Medicine, Cambridge Hosp 1984; **Fellow:** Hematology & Oncology, St Elizabeth Hosp 1987

Wax, Michael MD (Onc) - **Hospital:** Overlook Med Ctr (page 92); **Address:** 1 Diamond Hill Rd, Berkeley Hieghts, NJ 07922; **Phone:** 908-277-8890; **Board Cert:** Internal Medicine 1980; Medical Oncology 1983; **Med School:** Med Coll PA Hahnemann 1977; **Resid:** Internal Medicine, Hosp Med Coll Penn 1980; **Fellow:** Hematology & Oncology, Univ Wash Med Ctr 1980; **Fac Appt:** Asst Clin Prof Med, Mount Sinai Sch Med

Nephrology

Goldstein, Carl S MD (Nep) - **Spec Exp:** Hypertension; Kidney Stones; Kidney Failure; Metabolic Syndrome; **Hospital:** Overlook Med Ctr (page 92); **Address:** 215 North Ave W, Westfield, NJ 07090-1428; **Phone:** 908-232-4321; **Board Cert:** Internal Medicine 1981; Nephrology 1984; **Med School:** Washington Univ, St Louis 1978; **Resid:** Internal Medicine, Univ Minn Med Ctr 1981; **Fellow:** Nephrology, Hosp Univ Penn 1984; **Fac Appt:** Clin Prof Med, Mount Sinai Sch Med

McAnally, James F MD (Nep) - **Spec Exp:** Kidney Disease; Hypertension; Diabetes; **Hospital:** Trinitas Reg Med Ctr (page 914); **Address:** 240 Williamson St, Ste 307, Elizabeth, NJ 07202-3672; **Phone:** 908-994-9200; **Board Cert:** Internal Medicine 1978; Nephrology 1980; **Med School:** UMDNJ-NJ Med Sch, Newark 1975; **Resid:** Internal Medicine, CMDNJ-Newark Affil Hosp 1978; Internal Medicine, Georgetown Univ Hosp 1980; **Fellow:** Nephrology, Georgetown Univ Hosp 1980; **Fac Appt:** Assoc Clin Prof Med, Seton Hall Univ Sch Hlth & Med Scis

Neurological Surgery

Friedlander, Marvin E MD (NS) - **Spec Exp:** Spinal Surgery; **Hospital:** Trinitas Reg Med Ctr (page 914), Overlook Med Ctr (page 92); **Address:** 700 Rahway Ave, Union, NJ 07083; **Phone:** 908-688-1999; **Board Cert:** Neurological Surgery 1994; **Med School:** SUNY Downstate 1982; **Resid:** Neurological Surgery, Kings Co Hosp 1989; **Fellow:** Metabolism, SUNY Downstate Med Ctr 1984

Hodosh, Richard M MD (NS) - **Spec Exp:** Acoustic Neuroma; Neurovascular Surgery; Spinal Surgery; **Hospital:** Overlook Med Ctr (page 92), Morristown Med Ctr (page 92); **Address:** Atlantic Brain & Spine Institute, 99 Beauvoir Ave, MS 07902, Clinical Office MAC 1, ste 405, Summit, NJ 07901; **Phone:** 908-522-4979; **Board Cert:** Neurological Surgery 1980; **Med School:** Univ Cincinnati 1972; **Resid:** Neurological Surgery, Univ Tex Hlth Scis Ctr 1978; **Fellow:** Neuroradiology, Natl Hosp Neur Dis 1975; Neurological Surgery, Kantonsspital 1976; **Fac Appt:** Clin Prof NS, UMDNJ-NJ Med Sch, Newark

Neurology

Bansil, Shalini M MD (N) - **Spec Exp:** Stroke; **Hospital:** Overlook Med Ctr (page 92); **Address:** Overlook Hospital, Director, Stroke Center, 99 Beauvoir Ave, Summit, NJ 07902; **Phone:** 908-522-5545; **Board Cert:** Neurology 1989; Vascular Neurology 2006; **Med School:** India 1981; **Resid:** Neurology, UMDNJ Med Ctr 1989; **Fellow:** Stroke, Beth Israel Med Ctr

Coohill, Lisa M MD (N) - **Spec Exp:** Neurologic Rehabilitation; **Hospital:** Overlook Med Ctr (page 92); **Address:** Summit Medical Grp, 1 Diamond Hill Rd, Bensley Fl 3, Berkshire Heights, NJ 07922; **Phone:** 908-277-8639; **Board Cert:** Neurology 2010; **Med School:** UMDNJ-NJ Med Sch, Newark 1991; **Resid:** Neurology, Univ Hosp-UMDNJ 1995; Neurology, NYU Med Ctr 2002; **Fellow:** Neurological Rehabilitation, NYU Hosp for Joint Diseases 2003

Halperin, John MD (N) - **Spec Exp:** Neuromuscular Disorders; Lyme Disease; Multiple Sclerosis; Neuro-Immunology; **Hospital:** Overlook Med Ctr (page 92), Morristown Med Ctr (page 92); **Address:** Overlook Medical Center, 99 Beauvoir Ave, Department of Neurosciences, Summit, NJ 07902; **Phone:** 908-522-2829; **Board Cert:** Internal Medicine 1978; Neurology 1982; Clinical Neurophysiology 2005; **Med School:** Harvard Med Sch 1975; **Resid:** Internal Medicine, Univ Chicago Hosps 1977; Neurology, Mass Genl Hosp 1980; **Fellow:** Neurology, Mass Genl Hosp 1983; **Fac Appt:** Prof N, Mount Sinai Sch Med

Kurlan, Roger M MD (N) - **Spec Exp:** ADD/ADHD; Tourette's Syndrome; **Hospital:** Overlook Med Ctr (page 92); **Address:** 99 Beauvoir Ave, Summit, NJ 07902; **Phone:** 908-522-6144; **Board Cert:** Neurology 1984; **Med School:** Washington Univ, St Louis 1978; **Resid:** Neurology, Univ Rochester Med Ctr 1983; **Fellow:** Movement Disorders, Univ Rochester 1984

Politsky, Jeffrey M MD (N) - **Spec Exp:** Epilepsy/Seizure Disorders; Critical Care; **Hospital:** Overlook Med Ctr (page 92), Morristown Med Ctr (page 92); **Address:** Atlantic Neuroscience Institute, Overlook Medical Center, 99 Beauvoir Ave, Summit, NJ 07901; **Phone:** 908-522-4990; **Board Cert:** Neurology 2005; Clinical Neurophysiology 2001; **Med School:** Canada 1994; **Resid:** Neurology, Univ British Columbia 1999; **Fellow:** Epilepsy, Harvard Med Sch-Mass Genl Hosp 2001; **Fac Appt:** Assoc Clin Prof N, Mount Sinai Sch Med

Pollock, Jeffrey C MD (N) - **Hospital:** Overlook Med Ctr (page 92); **Address:** 47 Maple St, Ste 104, Summit, NJ 07901; **Phone:** 908-277-2722; **Board Cert:** Neurology 1987; **Med School:** Med Coll GA 1982; **Resid:** Neurology, UMDNJ Med Ctr 1986

Sachs, Stephen M MD (N) - **Spec Exp:** Headache; Stroke; Dementia; Parkinson's Disease; **Hospital:** Robert Wood Johnson Univ Hosp at Rahway, Trinitas Reg Med Ctr (page 914); **Address:** 700 N Broad St, Ste 201, Elizabeth, NJ 07208; **Phone:** 908-354-3994; **Board Cert:** Neurology 1977; **Med School:** Univ Pennsylvania 1971; **Resid:** Internal Medicine, Bellevue Hosp 1973; Neurology, Columbia-Presby Med Ctr 1976

Schanzer, Bernard MD (N) - **Spec Exp:** Stroke; Headache; Multiple Sclerosis; Amyotrophic Lateral Sclerosis (ALS); **Hospital:** Trinitas Reg Med Ctr (page 914), Robert Wood Johnson Univ Hosp at Rahway; **Address:** 700 N Broad St, Ste 201, Elizabeth, NJ 07208; **Phone:** 908-354-3994; **Board Cert:** Neurology 1972; **Med School:** Belgium 1962; **Resid:** Internal Medicine, Maimonides Med Ctr 1965; Neurology, Bronx Muni Med Ctr 1970; **Fac Appt:** Assoc Clin Prof N, UMDNJ-NJ Med Sch, Newark

Neuroradiology

Horner, Neil B MD (NRad) - **Spec Exp:** MRI & CT of Brain & Spine; Spine Imaging & Intervention; Brain Imaging; **Hospital:** Overlook Med Ctr (page 92), Mt Sinai Med Ctr (page 102); **Address:** Overlook Hosp, Dept Radiology, 99 Beauvoir Ave, Summit, NJ 07902; **Phone:** 908-522-2066; **Board Cert:** Diagnostic Radiology 1988; Nuclear Radiology 1989; Neuroradiology 2005; **Med School:** UMDNJ-Rutgers Med Sch 1983; **Resid:** Diagnostic Radiology, NYU Langone Med Ctr 1988; **Fellow:** Neuroradiology, NYU Langone Med Ctr 1989; Nuclear Radiology, NYU Langone Med Ctr 1989; **Fac Appt:** Asst Clin Prof Rad, Mount Sinai Sch Med

Obstetrics & Gynecology

Beim, Robert B MD (ObG) - **Spec Exp:** Laparoscopic Surgery; Minimally Invasive Surgery; Colposcopy; **Hospital:** St. Peter's Univ Hosp, JFK Med Ctr - Edison; **Address:** 190 Greenbrook Rd, N Plainfield, NJ 07060; **Phone:** 908-756-6812; **Board Cert:** Obstetrics & Gynecology 2012; **Med School:** SUNY Upstate Med Univ 1989; **Resid:** Obstetrics & Gynecology, Robert Wood Johnson Univ Hosp 1994; **Fac Appt:** Asst Prof ObG, Drexel Univ Coll Med

Frattarola, Michael A MD (ObG) - **Hospital:** Overlook Med Ctr (page 92); **Address:** 950 W Chestnut St, Ste 102, Union, NJ 07083; **Phone:** 908-688-8545; **Board Cert:** Obstetrics & Gynecology 1984; **Med School:** UMDNJ-NJ Med Sch, Newark 1973; **Resid:** Obstetrics & Gynecology, Univ Hosp-UMDNJ 1976

Hyman, Martin C MD (ObG) - **Spec Exp:** Gynecology Only; **Hospital:** Overlook Med Ctr (page 92); **Address:** 950 W Chestnut St, Ste 102, Union, NJ 07083; **Phone:** 908-688-8545; **Board Cert:** Obstetrics & Gynecology 1983; **Med School:** Mexico 1976; **Resid:** Obstetrics & Gynecology, Newark Beth Israel 1981

Margulis, Elynne B MD (ObG) - **Spec Exp:** Infertility; **Hospital:** Overlook Med Ctr (page 92); **Address:** 522 E Broad St, Westfield, NJ 07090; **Phone:** 908-232-4449; **Board Cert:** Obstetrics & Gynecology 1985; **Med School:** Columbia P&S 1978; **Resid:** Obstetrics & Gynecology, Hosp Univ Penn 1982; **Fac Appt:** Asst Clin Prof ObG, Columbia P&S

Soffer, Jeffrey L MD (ObG) - **Hospital:** Overlook Med Ctr (page 92); **Address:** 522 E Broad St, Westfield, NJ 07090; **Phone:** 908-232-4449; **Board Cert:** Obstetrics & Gynecology 1983; **Med School:** Howard Univ 1975; **Resid:** Obstetrics & Gynecology, Pennsylvania Hosp-UPHS 1980

Ophthalmology

Confino, Joel MD (Oph) - **Spec Exp:** Laser Vision Surgery; Cataract Surgery; Corneal Disease & Transplant; **Hospital:** Overlook Med Ctr (page 92); **Address:** 592 Springfield Ave, Westfield, NJ 07090-1002; **Phone:** 908-789-8999; **Board Cert:** Ophthalmology 1985; **Med School:** Albert Einstein Coll Med 1980; **Resid:** Ophthalmology, Mt Sinai Med Ctr 1984; **Fellow:** Cornea & Ext Eye Disease, UCSD Med Ctr 1985

Natale, Benjamin P DO (Oph) - **Spec Exp:** LASIK-Refractive Surgery; Cataract Surgery; **Hospital:** Saint Barnabas Med Ctr; **Address:** Assoc Eye Phys & Surgeons, 1050 Galloping Hill Rd, Ste 104, Union, NJ 07083-7983; **Phone:** 908-964-7878; **Board Cert:** Ophthalmology 1991; **Med School:** Des Moines Univ 1980; **Resid:** Family Medicine, Union Hosp 1982; Ophthalmology, UMDNJ Affil Hosps 1985; **Fellow:** Refractive Surgery, Newark Eye & Ear Infirm 1986

Orthopaedic Surgery

Barmakian, Joseph T MD (OrS) - **Spec Exp:** Carpal Tunnel Syndrome; Nerve & Tendon Reconstruction; Shoulder Reconstruction; **Hospital:** Overlook Med Ctr (page 92); **Address:** 202 Elmer St, Westfield, NJ 07090-3300; **Phone:** 908-232-7797; **Board Cert:** Orthopaedic Surgery 2013; Hand Surgery 2013; **Med School:** UMDNJ-RW Johnson Med Sch 1984; **Resid:** Surgery, G Washington Univ Hosp 1986; Orthopaedic Surgery, NY-Presby/Columbia Univ Med Ctr 1989; **Fellow:** Hand Surgery, NYU Hosp For Joint Dis 1990

Botwin, Clifford T DO (OrS) - **Spec Exp:** Arthroscopic Surgery; **Hospital:** Overlook Med Ctr (page 92), Bayonne Med Ctr; **Address:** Assoc Orthopaedics, 900 Stuyvesant Ave, Union, NJ 07083-6936; **Phone:** 908-964-6600; **Board Cert:** Orthopaedic Surgery 1982; **Med School:** Kansas City Univ Coll Osteo Med 1971; **Resid:** Orthopaedic Surgery, Delaware Valley Hosp 1976

Drzala, Mark R MD (OrS) - **Spec Exp:** Spinal Surgery; **Hospital:** Hackensack UMC-Mountainside (page 774), Overlook Med Ctr (page 92); **Address:** NJ Spine Specialists, 33 Overlook Rd, Ste 305, Summit, NJ 07901; **Phone:** 908-608-9610; **Board Cert:** Orthopaedic Surgery 2012; **Med School:** UMDNJ-NJ Med Sch, Newark 1991; **Resid:** Orthopaedic Surgery, UMDNJ-NJ Med Sch Affil Hosp 1997; **Fellow:** Spine Surgery, UCSF Med Ctr 1998; **Fac Appt:** Asst Clin Prof OrS, UMDNJ-NJ Med Sch, Newark

Gallick, Gregory S MD (OrS) - **Spec Exp:** Sports Medicine; Knee Reconstruction; Shoulder Reconstruction; **Hospital:** Overlook Med Ctr (page 92); **Address:** 2780 Morris Ave, Ste 2C, Union, NJ 07083; **Phone:** 908-686-6665; **Board Cert:** Orthopaedic Surgery 2009; **Med School:** UMDNJ-Rutgers Med Sch 1980; **Resid:** Surgery, UMDNJ Affil Hosps 1982; Orthopaedic Surgery, UMDNJ Affil Hosps 1985; **Fellow:** Interventional Cardiology, So CA Sports Med 1986

Innella, Robin R DO (OrS) - **Spec Exp:** Sports Medicine; Hip & Knee Replacement; Fractures; **Hospital:** Overlook Med Ctr (page 92); **Address:** Associated Orthopaedics, 900 Stuyvesant Ave Fl 2, Union, NJ 07083; **Phone:** 908-964-6600; **Board Cert:** Orthopaedic Surgery 1991; Sports Medicine 1998; **Med School:** Philadelphia Coll Osteo Med 1982; **Resid:** Orthopaedic Surgery, Kennedy Mem Hosp-Univ Med Ctr 1987; **Fac Appt:** Asst Clin Prof S, NY Coll Osteo Med

Mackessy, Richard P MD (OrS) - **Spec Exp:** Hand Surgery; **Hospital:** Trinitas Reg Med Ctr (page 914), Robert Wood Johnson Univ Hosp at Rahway; **Address:** Union City Orthopaedic Grp, 210 W St Georges Ave, Linden, NJ 07036; **Phone:** 908-486-1111; **Board Cert:** Orthopaedic Surgery 2007; Hand Surgery 2007; **Med School:** UMDNJ-NJ Med Sch, Newark 1978; **Resid:** Surgery, St Vincents Hosp 1980; Orthopaedic Surgery, St. Luke's - Roosevelt Hosp Ctr - St Luke's Hosp 1983; **Fellow:** Hand Surgery, Thomas Jefferson Univ Hosp 1984

Sarokhan, Alan J MD (OrS) - **Spec Exp:** Hip & Knee Replacement; Hand Surgery; **Hospital:** Overlook Med Ctr (page 92), Saint Barnabas Med Ctr; **Address:** 33 Overlook Rd, Med Arts Bldg - Ste 201, Summit, NJ 07901-3562; **Phone:** 908-522-4555; **Board Cert:** Orthopaedic Surgery 2007; **Med School:** Harvard Med Sch 1977; **Resid:** Surgery, Brigham & Women's Hosp 1979; Orthopaedic Surgery, Harvard Affil Hosps 1982; **Fellow:** Hand Surgery, St. Luke's - Roosevelt Hosp Ctr - Roosevelt Div 1984

Otolaryngology

Carniol, Paul J MD (Oto) - **Spec Exp:** Facial Plastic Surgery; Cosmetic Surgery; Skin Cancer; **Hospital:** Overlook Med Ctr (page 92), Univ Hosp (Newark); **Address:** Medical Arts Bldg, 33 Overlook Rd, Ste 401, Summit, NJ 07901; **Phone:** 908-598-1400; **Board Cert:** Otolaryngology 1981; Facial Plastic & Reconstr Surgery 1991; **Med School:** Univ Pennsylvania 1976; **Resid:** Surgery, Hosp of Univ of Pennsylvania 1977; Surgery, North SHore Univ Hosp 1978; **Fellow:** Otolaryngology, Mass Eye & Ear Infirm 1981; Plastic/Reconstructive Surgery, Hosp Univ Penn 1983; **Fac Appt:** Clin Prof Oto, UMDNJ-NJ Med Sch, Newark

Drake III, William MD (Oto) - **Spec Exp:** Endoscopic Sinus Surgery; Head & Neck Surgery; Thyroid & Parathyroid Surgery; **Hospital:** Overlook Med Ctr (page 92); **Address:** 213 Summit Rd, Mountainside, NJ 07092; **Phone:** 908-233-2111; **Board Cert:** Otolaryngology 1995; **Med School:** UMDNJ-NJ Med Sch, Newark 1989; **Resid:** Otolaryngology, Mt Sinai Med Ctr 1995

Kwartler, Jed A MD (Oto) - **Spec Exp:** Acoustic Neuroma; Balance Disorders; Cochlear Implants; Cholesteatoma; **Hospital:** Overlook Med Ctr (page 92); **Address:** Summit Med Grp, 1 Diamond Hill Rd, Berkeley Heights, NJ 07922; **Phone:** 908-277-8681; **Board Cert:** Otolaryngology 1988; Neurotology 2010; **Med School:** UMDNJ-NJ Med Sch, Newark 1983; **Resid:** Surgery, UMDNJ/Univ Hosp 1985; Otolaryngology, UMDNJ/Univ Hosp 1988; **Fellow:** Otology & Neurotology, St Vincent's Hosp & Med Ctr 1990; **Fac Appt:** Assoc Clin Prof Oto, UMDNJ-NJ Med Sch, Newark

Scharf, Richard C DO (Oto) - **Spec Exp:** Sinus Disorders/Surgery; Cosmetic Surgery-Face; Head & Neck Cancer; **Hospital:** Saint Barnabas Med Ctr, Bayonne Med Ctr; **Address:** 505 Chestnut St, Roselle Park, NJ 07204; **Phone:** 908-241-0200; **Board Cert:** Otolaryngology 1993; **Med School:** Univ Hlth Sci, Coll Osteo Med 1986; **Resid:** Otolaryngology, McLaren Flint 1992; **Fac Appt:** Assoc Clin Prof Oto, NY Coll Osteo Med

Pediatric Cardiology

Leichter, Donald A MD (PCd) - **Spec Exp:** Congenital Heart Disease; Fetal Echocardiography; Echocardiography; **Hospital:** Overlook Med Ctr (page 92), Morgan Stanley Children's Hosp of NY-Presby, NY (page 104); **Address:** 47 Maple St, Ste 406, Summit, NJ 07901; **Phone:** 908-522-5566; **Board Cert:** Pediatrics 1988; Pediatric Cardiology 2010; **Med School:** Cornell Univ-Weill Med Coll 1980; **Resid:** Pediatrics, Chldns Natl Med Ctr 1984; **Fellow:** Pediatric Cardiology, NY-Presby/Columbia Univ Med Ctr 1986; **Fac Appt:** Assoc Clin Prof Ped, Columbia P&S

Pediatric Endocrinology

Anhalt, Henry DO (PEn) - **Spec Exp:** Diabetes; Obesity; Growth Disorders; **Address:** 140 Prospect Ave, Ste 2, Hackensack, NJ 07061; **Phone:** 201-996-0777; **Board Cert:** Pediatric Endocrinology 2012; **Med School:** NY Coll Osteo Med 1988; **Resid:** Pediatrics, Winthrop Univ Hosp 1992; **Fellow:** Pediatric Endocrinology, Stanford Univ Hosp & Clins 1995; **Fac Appt:** Assoc Prof Ped, SUNY Hlth Sci Ctr

Pediatric Gastroenterology

Tyshkov, Michael MD (PGe) - **Spec Exp:** Nutrition; Crohn's Disease; Colitis; **Hospital:** Overlook Med Ctr (page 92), Staten Island Univ Hosp - North (page 106); **Address:** Overlook Med Ctr - Kids Tummy, 33 Overlook Rd, Ste 208, Summit, NJ 07901; **Phone:** 908-273-7745; **Board Cert:** Pediatric Gastroenterology 2010; **Med School:** Russia 1977; **Resid:** Pediatrics, Flushing Hosp Med Ctr 1989; **Fellow:** Pediatric Gastroenterology, Westchester Med Ctr 1991; **Fac Appt:** Asst Clin Prof Ped, SUNY Downstate

Pediatric Pulmonology

Kohn, Gary L MD (PPul) - **Hospital:** Overlook Med Ctr (page 92), Morristown Med Ctr (page 92); **Address:** Pulmonary & Allergy Assocs, 1 Livingston Ave, Summit, NJ 07901; **Phone:** 908-934-0555; **Board Cert:** Pediatrics 2012; Pediatric Pulmonology 2008; Pediatric Critical Care Medicine 2010; **Med School:** Ros Franklin Univ/Chicago Med Sch 1994; **Resid:** Pediatrics, U Chicago Hosps 1997; **Fellow:** Pediatric Pulmonology, Chldns Hosp Med Ctr 2000; Pediatric Critical Care Medicine, Schneider Chldns Hosp 2002; **Fac Appt:** Asst Clin Prof Ped, UMDNJ-NJ Med Sch, Newark

Pediatric Surgery

Bergman, Kerry S MD (PS) - **Hospital:** Overlook Med Ctr (page 92), Morristown Med Ctr (page 92); **Address:** Overlook Hospital, 99 Beauvoir Ave, Box 220, Summit, NJ 07902; **Phone:** 908-522-3523; **Board Cert:** Surgery 2007; Pediatric Surgery 2009; **Med School:** Albany Med Coll 1982; **Resid:** Surgery, New England Med Ctr 1988; **Fellow:** Pediatric Surgery, New England Med Ctr 1991

Pediatrics

Ayyanathan, Karpukarasi MD (Ped) *PCP* - **Hospital:** Trinitas Reg Med Ctr (page 914), JFK Med Ctr - Edison; **Address:** Linden Pediatric Grp, 517 Rahway Ave, Elizabeth, NJ 07202-2308; **Phone:** 908-527-1247; **Board Cert:** Pediatrics 1983; **Med School:** India 1975; **Resid:** Pediatrics, St Elizabeth Hosp 1977; Pediatrics, Rahway Hosp 1979

Corbo, Emanuel MD (Ped) *PCP* - **Spec Exp:** Vaccines; Asthma; Otitis Media; Pneumonia; **Hospital:** Overlook Med Ctr (page 92), Trinitas Reg Med Ctr (page 914); **Address:** 443 E Westfield Ave, Roselle Park, NJ 07204-2428; **Phone:** 908-245-2442; **Board Cert:** Pediatrics 2008; **Med School:** Grenada 1985; **Resid:** Pediatrics, Newark Beth Israel Med Ctr 1990; **Fellow:** Pediatric Trauma, Newark Beth Israel Med Ctr 1991

Davis, Kenneth J MD (Ped) *PCP* - **Hospital:** Overlook Med Ctr (page 92), Trinitas Reg Med Ctr (page 914); **Address:** 701 Newark Ave, Ste 212, Elizabeth, NJ 07208-3550; **Phone:** 908-354-9500; **Board Cert:** Pediatrics 1985; **Med School:** Albert Einstein Coll Med 1980; **Resid:** Pediatrics, Bellevue Hosp 1983

Panza, Robert MD (Ped) - **Hospital:** Overlook Med Ctr (page 92); **Address:** Pediatric Associates of Westfield, 566 Westfield Ave, Westfield, NJ 07090; **Phone:** 908-233-7171; **Board Cert:** Pediatrics 2011; **Med School:** Italy 1985; **Resid:** Pediatrics, Overlook Hosp 1988

Panzner, Elizabeth A MD (Ped) *PCP* - **Spec Exp:** Acne; Allergy; Asthma; **Hospital:** Saint Barnabas Med Ctr, Overlook Med Ctr (page 92); **Address:** Union Pediatric Medical Group, 1050 Galloping Hill Rd, Ste 200, Union, NJ 07083-9417; **Phone:** 908-688-9900; **Board Cert:** Pediatrics 2011; **Med School:** Mexico 1984; **Resid:** Pediatrics, UMDNJ-Univ Hosp 1988

Saraiya, Narendra N MD (Ped) *PCP* - **Spec Exp:** Asthma; Anemia; Sickle Cell Disease; **Hospital:** Trinitas Reg Med Ctr (page 914), JFK Med Ctr - Edison; **Address:** 817 Rahway Ave, Elizabeth, NJ 07202; **Phone:** 908-353-5750; **Board Cert:** Pediatrics 1988; **Med School:** India 1971; **Resid:** Pediatrics, NY Methodist Hosp 1980; **Fellow:** Pediatric Hematology-Oncology, Maimonides Med Ctr 1982; Pediatric Hematology-Oncology, Chldns Hosp Buffalo 1984

Physical Medicine & Rehabilitation

Armento, Michael J MD (PMR) - **Spec Exp:** Pediatric Rehabilitation; Cerebral Palsy; Spina Bifida; Spinal Cord Injury-Pediatric; **Hospital:** Children's Specialized Hosp, Newark Beth Israel Med Ctr; **Address:** Chldns Specialized Hosp, 150 New Providence Rd, Mountainside, NJ 07092; **Phone:** 908-301-5502; **Board Cert:** Physical Medicine & Rehabilitation 2003; Pediatric Rehabilitation Medicine 2004; **Med School:** UMDNJ-NJ Med Sch, Newark 1988; **Resid:** Physical Medicine & Rehabilitation, Univ Hosp-UMDNJ 1992; **Fellow:** Pediatric Rehabilitation Medicine, Chldns Specialized Hosp 2004; **Fac Appt:** Assoc Clin Prof Ped, UMDNJ-NJ Med Sch, Newark

Diamond, Martin MD (PMR) - **Spec Exp:** Cerebral Palsy; Neuromuscular Disorders; Electrodiagnosis; Spasticity Management; **Hospital:** Children's Specialized Hosp, Newark Beth Israel Med Ctr; **Address:** Chldns Specialized Hosp, 150 New Providence Rd, Mountainside, NJ 07092; **Phone:** 908-301-5502; **Board Cert:** Pediatrics 1983; Physical Medicine & Rehabilitation 1982; Pediatric Rehabilitation Medicine 2003; **Med School:** Univ Pittsburgh 1975; **Resid:** Pediatrics, Chldns Hosp Natl Med Ctr 1978; Physical Medicine & Rehabilitation, Sinai Hosp 1980; **Fac Appt:** Assoc Clin Prof PMR, UMDNJ-Rutgers Med Sch

Malanga, Gerard A MD (PMR) - **Spec Exp:** Pain-Back & Neck; Sports Injuries; Regenokine Therapy (PRP); Musculoskeletal Imaging; **Hospital:** Overlook Med Ctr (page 92), East Orange Genl Hosp; **Address:** 197 Ridgedale Ave, Ste 210, Cedar Knolls, NJ 07927; **Phone:** 973-998-8301; **Board Cert:** Physical Medicine & Rehabilitation 2013; Pain Medicine 2013; Sports Medicine 2009; **Med School:** UMDNJ-NJ Med Sch, Newark 1983; **Resid:** Physical Medicine & Rehabilitation, UMDNJ Affil Hosp 1992; **Fellow:** Sports Medicine, Mayo Clinic 1993; **Fac Appt:** Clin Prof PMR, UMDNJ-Univ Med Dent NJ

Plastic Surgery

Gardner, James N MD (PlS) - **Spec Exp:** Breast Cosmetic & Reconstructive Surgery; Abdominoplasty; **Hospital:** Overlook Med Ctr (page 92); **Address:** 33 Overlook Rd, Ste 310, Summit, NJ 07901; **Phone:** 908-918-1969; **Board Cert:** Plastic Surgery 2005; **Med School:** UMDNJ-RW Johnson Med Sch 1987; **Resid:** Surgery, UMDNJ Univ Hosp 1992; Plastic Surgery, UMDNJ Univ Hosp 1994

Hyans, Peter MD (PlS) - **Spec Exp:** Cosmetic Surgery-Breast; Breast Reconstruction; Cosmetic Surgery-Face; Liposuction & Body Contouring; **Hospital:** Overlook Med Ctr (page 92), Saint Barnabas Med Ctr; **Address:** Summit Medical Grp, Plastic Surgery Ctr, Lawrence Pavilion, 1 Diamond Hill Rd Fl 1, Berkeley Heights, NJ 07922; **Phone:** 908-277-8759; **Board Cert:** Plastic Surgery 2003; **Med School:** UMDNJ-RW Johnson Med Sch 1986; **Resid:** Surgery, Thomas Jefferson Univ Hosp 1991; Plastic Surgery, Univ Cincinnati Hosp 1993

Tepper, Howard N MD (PlS) - **Spec Exp:** Cosmetic Surgery; Breast Surgery; Hand Surgery; **Hospital:** Overlook Med Ctr (page 92); **Address:** 522 E Broad St, Westfield, NJ 07090-2116; **Phone:** 908-654-6540; **Board Cert:** Plastic Surgery 1983; **Med School:** Albert Einstein Coll Med 1975; **Resid:** Surgery, Montefiore Hosp Med Ctr 1979; Plastic Surgery, Montefiore Hosp Med Ctr 1981; **Fellow:** Hand Surgery, St Luke's-Roosevelt Hosp Ctr 1979

Zeitels, Jerrold R MD (PlS) - **Spec Exp:** Liposuction & Body Contouring; Reconstructive Surgery; Hand Surgery; **Hospital:** Overlook Med Ctr (page 92), Robert Wood Johnson Univ Hosp at Rahway; **Address:** 522 E Broad St, Westfield, NJ 07090-2116; **Phone:** 908-654-6540; **Board Cert:** Plastic Surgery 1989; Hand Surgery 2009; **Med School:** Univ Chicago-Pritzker Sch Med 1980; **Resid:** Surgery, Univ Michigan Med Ctr 1985; Plastic Surgery, Hosp Univ Penn 1987

Psychiatry

Kaplan, Gabriel MD (Psyc) - **Spec Exp:** Psychopharmacology; ADD/ADHD; Depression; **Hospital:** Bergen Regl Med Ctr; **Address:** 535 Morris Ave, Springfield, NJ 07081-1426; **Phone:** 973-376-1020; **Board Cert:** Psychiatry 1987; Child & Adolescent Psychiatry 1989; **Med School:** Argentina 1980; **Resid:** Psychiatry, NY Hosp-Cornell 1986; Child Psychiatry, NY Hosp-Cornell 1988; **Fac Appt:** Assoc Prof Psyc, UMDNJ-NJ Med Sch, Newark

Miller, David G MD (Psyc) - **Spec Exp:** Psychopharmacology; Depression; ADD/ADHD; Bipolar/Mood Disorders; **Address:** 28 Milburn Ave, Ste 5, Springfield, NJ 07081; **Phone:** 973-218-1770; **Board Cert:** Psychiatry 1985; **Med School:** UMDNJ-RW Johnson Med Sch 1980; **Resid:** Psychiatry, Strong Meml Hosp 1984

Richardson, William T MD (Psyc) - **Spec Exp:** Adolescent Psychiatry; Family Therapy; Psychopharmacology; **Hospital:** Overlook Med Ctr (page 92), Morristown Med Ctr (page 92); **Address:** 33 Overlook Rd, Ste 210, Summit, NJ 07901-3570; **Phone:** 908-598-0008; **Board Cert:** Psychiatry 1980; **Med School:** McGill Univ 1967; **Resid:** Psychiatry, Jewish Genl Hosp 1971; Psychiatry, Payne Whitney Clinic 1974; **Fac Appt:** Assoc Clin Prof Psyc, Columbia P&S

Silver, Bennett MD (Psyc) - **Spec Exp:** Child & Adolescent Psychiatry; ADD/ADHD; Anxiety Disorders; **Hospital:** Bergen Regl Med Ctr; **Address:** 535 Morris Ave, Springfield, NJ 07081; **Phone:** 973-376-1020; **Board Cert:** Psychiatry 1979; **Med School:** SUNY Downstate 1974; **Resid:** Psychiatry, Mount Sinai Hosp 1978; **Fellow:** Child & Adolescent Psychiatry, Mount Sinai Hosp 1980

Villafranca, Manuel V MD (Psyc) - **Spec Exp:** Psychopharmacology; Depression; Anxiety Disorders; **Hospital:** Summit Oaks Hosp, Christ Hosp - Jersey City; **Address:** 220 Lenox Ave, Westfield, NJ 07090; **Phone:** 908-232-9369; **Board Cert:** Psychiatry 1982; **Med School:** Philippines 1971; **Resid:** Psychiatry, St Vincents Hosp 1978; **Fellow:** Child & Adolescent Psychiatry, St Vincents Hosp 1980; **Fac Appt:** Asst Clin Prof Psyc, UMDNJ-RW Johnson Med Sch

Pulmonary Disease

Cerrone, Federico MD (Pul) - **Spec Exp:** Sleep Disorders; Asthma; Chronic Obstructive Lung Disease (COPD); **Hospital:** Overlook Med Ctr (page 92), Morristown Med Ctr (page 92); **Address:** 1 Springfield Ave, Summit, NJ 07901; **Phone:** 908-934-0555; **Board Cert:** Internal Medicine 1989; Pulmonary Disease 2012; Critical Care Medicine 2003; Sleep Medicine 2007; **Med School:** Georgetown Univ 1986; **Resid:** Internal Medicine, Bronx Muni Hosp 1989; **Fellow:** Pulmonary Critical Care Medicine, Georgetown Univ Hosp 1992

Hwang, Cheng-hong DO/PhD (Pul) - **Hospital:** Robert Wood Johnson Univ Hosp at Rahway; **Address:** 1457 Raritan Rd, Ste 101, Clark, NJ 07066; **Phone:** 908-272-2270; **Board Cert:** Internal Medicine 1983; Pulmonary Disease 1984; Critical Care Medicine 2005; **Med School:** Des Moines Univ 1978; **Resid:** Internal Medicine, USPHS Hosp 1981; **Fellow:** Pulmonary Disease, UMDNJ-Univ Hosp 1983

Sussman, Robert MD (Pul) - **Spec Exp:** Asthma; Chronic Obstructive Lung Disease (COPD); Pulmonary Fibrosis; Lung Cancer; **Hospital:** Overlook Med Ctr (page 92), Morristown Med Ctr (page 92); **Address:** Pulmonary & Allergy Assocs, 1 Springfield Ave, Summit, NJ 07901; **Phone:** 908-934-0555; **Board Cert:** Internal Medicine 1984; Pulmonary Disease 1988; **Med School:** Albert Einstein Coll Med 1981; **Resid:** Internal Medicine, Montefiore Med Ctr 1984; **Fellow:** Pulmonary Disease, NYU/Bellevue Hosp 1987

Zimmerman, Mark MD (Pul) - **Spec Exp:** Critical Care Medicine; Asthma & Allergy; Chronic Obstructive Lung Disease (COPD); **Hospital:** Overlook Med Ctr (page 92), Morristown Med Ctr (page 92); **Address:** Pulmonary & Allergy Assocs, 1 Springfield Ave, Summit, NJ 07901; **Phone:** 908-934-0555; **Board Cert:** Internal Medicine 1988; Critical Care Medicine 2003; Pulmonary Disease 2012; **Med School:** NYU Sch Med 1985; **Resid:** Internal Medicine, NYU Med Ctr 1988; **Fellow:** Pulmonary Critical Care Medicine, Mount Sinai Med Ctr 1992; **Fac Appt:** Asst Clin Prof Med, Columbia P&S

Radiation Oncology

Schwartz, Louis E MD (RadRO) - **Spec Exp:** Stereotactic Radiosurgery; Prostate Cancer; Brain Tumors; **Hospital:** Overlook Med Ctr (page 92); **Address:** Overlook Hosp, Dept Rad Oncology, 33 Overlook Rd, Ste L05, Medical Arts Ctr 1, Summit, NJ 07901-3561; **Phone:** 908-522-2871; **Board Cert:** Therapeutic Radiology 1979; Pediatrics 1981; **Med School:** SUNY Hlth Sci Ctr 1974; **Resid:** Pediatrics, NY Methodist Hosp 1976; Pediatrics, Chldns Hosp Med Ctr 1977; **Fellow:** Therapeutic Radiology, Columbia-Presby Hosp 1979

Rheumatology

Brodman, Richard R MD (Rhu) - **Spec Exp:** Lupus/SLE; Rheumatoid Arthritis; Osteoporosis; Osteoarthritis; **Hospital:** JFK Med Ctr - Edison; **Address:** 345 Somerset St, Ste 107, North Plainfield, NJ 07060-4774; **Phone:** 908-561-7440; **Board Cert:** Internal Medicine 1976; Rheumatology 1982; **Med School:** SUNY Downstate 1973; **Resid:** Internal Medicine, Rhode Island Hosp 1976; **Fellow:** Rheumatology, Brigham & Womens Hosp 1978; **Fac Appt:** Assoc Clin Prof Med, UMDNJ-RW Johnson Med Sch

Kramer, Neil MD (Rhu) - **Spec Exp:** Rheumatoid Arthritis; Lupus/SLE; Sjogren's Syndrome; Vasculitis; **Hospital:** Overlook Med Ctr (page 92); **Address:** 33 Overlook Rd, Ste 211, Medical Arts Ctr, Summit, NJ 07901; **Phone:** 908-598-7940; **Board Cert:** Internal Medicine 1977; Rheumatology 1980; **Med School:** Univ Pennsylvania 1974; **Resid:** Internal Medicine, Manhattan VA Hosp/NYU Med Ctr 1978; **Fellow:** Rheumatology, NYU Med Ctr 1980; **Fac Appt:** Assoc Clin Prof Med, Mount Sinai Sch Med

Rosenstein, Elliot D MD (Rhu) - **Spec Exp:** Rheumatoid Arthritis; Lupus/SLE; Sjogren's Syndrome; Behcet's Syndrome; **Hospital:** Overlook Med Ctr (page 92), Atl Hlth (page 92); **Address:** 33 Overlook Rd, Ste 211, Summit, NJ 07901; **Phone:** 908-598-7940; **Board Cert:** Internal Medicine 1981; Rheumatology 1984; **Med School:** Mount Sinai Sch Med 1978; **Resid:** Internal Medicine, NYU/Bellevue Hosp 1982; **Fellow:** Rheumatology, NYU/Bellevue Hosp 1984; **Fac Appt:** Assoc Clin Prof Med, Mount Sinai Sch Med

Worth, David MD (Rhu) - **Spec Exp:** Rheumatoid Arthritis; Osteoporosis; **Hospital:** Overlook Med Ctr (page 92); **Address:** 2376 Morris Ave, Union, NJ 07083-5707; **Phone:** 908-686-6616; **Board Cert:** Internal Medicine 1974; Rheumatology 1978; **Med School:** Univ Rochester 1971; **Resid:** Internal Medicine, Montefiore Med Ctr 1975; **Fellow:** Rheumatology, Montefiore Med Ctr 1978

Surgery

Colaco, Rodolfo MD (S) - **Spec Exp:** Hernia; Gallbladder Surgery; Laparoscopic Surgery; Breast Surgery; **Hospital:** Trinitas Reg Med Ctr (page 914); **Address:** 431 Elmora Ave, Elizabeth, NJ 07208; **Phone:** 908-353-4177; **Board Cert:** Surgery 2011; **Med School:** India 1974; **Resid:** Surgery, St Vincent Hosp 1980; Surgery, St Elizabeth Hosp 1983

DiGioia, Julia M MD (S) - **Spec Exp:** Breast Disease; Breast Cancer; **Hospital:** Overlook Med Ctr (page 92), Jersey City Med Ctr; **Address:** Medical Arts Ctr, 33 Overlook Rd, Ste 205, Summit, NJ 07901; **Phone:** 908-522-3200; **Board Cert:** Surgery 2005; **Med School:** Italy 1979; **Resid:** Surgery, Jersey City Med Ctr 1984; **Fac Appt:** Asst Clin Prof S, UMDNJ-NJ Med Sch, Newark

Feteiha, Muhammad S MD (S) - **Spec Exp:** Minimally Invasive Surgery; Obesity/Bariatric Surgery; Colon & Rectal Surgery; **Hospital:** Overlook Med Ctr (page 92), Trinitas Reg Med Ctr (page 914), **Address:** Advanced Surgical Assocs, 155 Morris Ave Fl 2, Springfield, NJ 07081; **Phone:** 973-232-2300; **Board Cert:** Surgery 2009; **Med School:** Tufts Univ 1995; **Resid:** Surgery, Univ Hosp 2000; **Fellow:** Surgery, NY-Presby/Columbia Univ Med Ctr 2001

Frost, James Henry MD (S) - **Spec Exp:** Breast Cancer; Colon Surgery; Laparoscopic Surgery; Vein Disorders; **Hospital:** Overlook Med Ctr (page 92), Trinitas Reg Med Ctr (page 914); **Address:** Advanced Surgical Assocs, 155 Morris Ave Fl 2, Springfield, NJ 07081; **Phone:** 973-232-2300; **Board Cert:** Surgery 2007; **Med School:** Mexico 1982; **Resid:** Surgery, Univ IL Med Ctr 1988

Gumbs, Andrew MD (S) - **Spec Exp:** Gastrointestinal Surgery; Minimally Invasive Surgery; Hepatobiliary Surgery; Pancreatic & Biliary Surgery; **Hospital:** Overlook Med Ctr (page 92); **Address:** Summit Med Grp, Surgery, 1 Diamond Hill Rd Fl 4, Berkeley Heights, NJ 07922; **Phone:** 908-277-8950; **Board Cert:** Surgery 2006; **Med School:** Yale Univ 1998; **Resid:** Surgery, Yale-New Haven Hosp 2005; **Fellow:** Minimally Invasive Surgery, NY-Presby/Columbia Univ Med Ctr 2006; Hepatopancreatobiliary Surgery, Univ Rene Descartes Affil Hosp 2007

Lozner, Jerrold S MD (S) - **Spec Exp:** Breast Cancer & Surgery; Breast Surgery; **Hospital:** Overlook Med Ctr (page 92); **Address:** 1 Diamond Hill Rd, MS 0, Berkeley Heights, NJ 07922; **Phone:** 908-277-8850; **Board Cert:** Surgery 2009; **Med School:** Univ Louisville Sch Med 1971; **Resid:** Surgery, Univ Cincinnati Med Ctr 1976; **Fellow:** Cardiothoracic Surgery, Univ Cincinnati Med Ctr 1978; **Fac Appt:** Assoc Clin Prof S, Columbia P&S

Mandel, Marc S MD (S) - **Spec Exp:** Gallbladder Surgery; Breast Cancer & Surgery; Cancer Surgery; Abdominal Wall Reconstruction; **Hospital:** Overlook Med Ctr (page 92); **Address:** 11 Overlook Rd, Ste 160, Summit, NJ 07901; **Phone:** 908-598-0966; **Board Cert:** Surgery 2009; **Med School:** Albert Einstein Coll Med 1985; **Resid:** Surgery, Montefiore Med Ctr 1988; Surgery, Yale-New Haven Hosp 1990

Nitzberg, Richard S MD (S) - **Spec Exp:** Laparoscopic Surgery; Vein Disorders; Hernia; Vascular Surgery; **Hospital:** Overlook Med Ctr (page 92); **Address:** Summit Med Grp, Surgery, 1 Diamond Hill Rd Fl 4, Berkeley Heights, NJ 07922; **Phone:** 908-277-8950; **Board Cert:** Surgery 2009; Vascular Surgery 2010; **Med School:** Harvard Med Sch 1983; **Resid:** Surgery, NY-Presby/Columbia Univ Med Ctr 1988; **Fellow:** Vascular Surgery, Tufts Med Ctr 1990

Sacco, Margaret M MD (S) - **Spec Exp:** Breast Cancer & Surgery; Breast Disease; **Hospital:** Overlook Med Ctr (page 92), Morristown Med Ctr (page 92); **Address:** Carol G Simon Cancer Ctr, 33 Overlook Rd, MAC-1 Ste 207, Summit, NJ 07901; **Phone:** 908-598-6610; **Board Cert:** Surgery 2011; **Med School:** Hahnemann Univ 1986; **Resid:** Surgery, Univ Hosp-UMDNJ 1991; **Fellow:** Surgical Oncology, Univ Hosp-UMDNJ 1993

Starker, Paul MD (S) - **Spec Exp:** Laparoscopic Surgery; **Hospital:** Overlook Med Ctr (page 92); **Address:** 11 Overlook Rd, Ste 160, Summit, NJ 07901; **Phone:** 908-608-9001; **Board Cert:** Surgery 2006; **Med School:** Columbia P&S 1980; **Resid:** Surgery, NY-Presby/Columbia Univ Med Ctr 1986; **Fellow:** Metabolism, NY-Presby/Columbia Univ Med Ctr 1982; **Fac Appt:** Clin Prof S, Columbia P&S

Urology

Lehrhoff, Bernard J MD (U) - **Spec Exp:** Prostate Cancer; Kidney Stones; Sexual Dysfunction; Bladder Cancer; **Hospital:** Overlook Med Ctr (page 92), Saint Michael's Med Ctr; **Address:** Premier Urology Grp, 275 Orchard St, Westfield, NJ 07090; **Phone:** 908-654-5100; **Board Cert:** Urology 1984; **Med School:** UMDNJ-NJ Med Sch, Newark 1976; **Resid:** Urology, Bellevue Hosp 1982; **Fac Appt:** Asst Clin Prof U, Columbia P&S

Miller, Mark I MD (U) - **Spec Exp:** Kidney Stones; Urology-Female; Urologic Cancer; **Hospital:** Trinitas Reg Med Ctr (page 914); **Address:** Premier Urology Grp, 275 Orchard St, Westfield, NJ 07090; **Phone:** 908-654-5100; **Board Cert:** Urology 2007; **Med School:** Cornell Univ 1991; **Resid:** Urology, NY-Presby/Columbia Univ Med Ctr 1997

Ring, Kenneth S MD (U) - **Spec Exp:** Pediatric Urology; Urologic Cancer; Kidney Stones; **Hospital:** Overlook Med Ctr (page 92); **Address:** Premier Urology Grp, 275 Orchard St, Westfield, NJ 07090; **Phone:** 908-654-5100; **Board Cert:** Urology 2012; **Med School:** Mount Sinai Sch Med 1985; **Resid:** Surgery, Mount Sinai Med Ctr 1987; Urology, NY-Presby/Columbia Univ Med Ctr 1991

Seidman, Barry MD (U) - **Spec Exp:** Sexual Dysfunction; Incontinence; Genitourinary Cancer; **Hospital:** Overlook Med Ctr (page 92); **Address:** 33 Overlook Rd, Ste 408, Summit, NJ 07901; **Phone:** 908-219-4479; **Board Cert:** Urology 2004; **Med School:** Mount Sinai Sch Med 1978; **Resid:** Urology, Mount Sinai Med Ctr 1983

Vascular Surgery

Addis, Michael D MD (VascS) - **Spec Exp:** Endovascular Surgery; Carotid Artery Surgery; **Hospital:** Saint Barnabas Med Ctr, Overlook Med Ctr (page 92); **Address:** The Cardiovascular Care Group, 433 Central Ave, Westfield, NJ 07090; **Phone:** 973-759-9000; **Board Cert:** Surgery 2005; Vascular Surgery 2007; **Med School:** UMDNJ-NJ Med Sch, Newark 1999; **Resid:** Surgery, Mount Sinai Med Ctr 2004; **Fellow:** Vascular Surgery, Mount Sinai Med Ctr 2005

Kumar, Mark MD (VascS) - **Spec Exp:** Endovascular Surgery; **Hospital:** Overlook Med Ctr (page 92), Saint Barnabas Med Ctr; **Address:** The Cardiovascular Care Group, 433 Central Ave, Westfield, NJ 07090; **Phone:** 973-759-9000; **Board Cert:** Surgery 2002; Vascular Surgery 2004; **Med School:** Univ VA Sch Med 1996; **Resid:** Surgery, Saint Barnabas Med Ctr 2001; Vascular Surgery, VA Commonwealth Univ Med Ctr 2002

Sales, Clifford MD (VascS) - **Spec Exp:** Varicose Veins; Aneurysm-Abdominal Aortic; Peripheral Vascular Disease; Carotid Artery Surgery; **Hospital:** Overlook Med Ctr (page 92), Morristown Med Ctr (page 92); **Address:** The Cardiovascular Care Group, 433 Central Ave, Westfield, NJ 07090; **Phone:** 973-759-9000; **Board Cert:** Vascular Surgery 2002; **Med School:** Mount Sinai Sch Med 1986; **Resid:** Surgery, Montefiore Med Ctr 1991; **Fellow:** Vascular Surgery, Montefiore Med Ctr 1993; **Fac Appt:** Asst Clin Prof S, Mount Sinai Sch Med

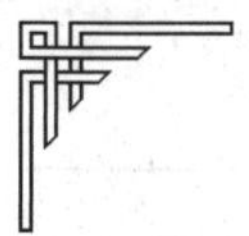

The Best in American Medicine
www.CastleConnolly.com

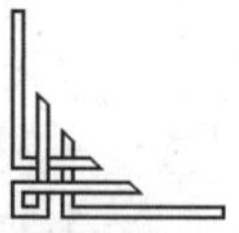
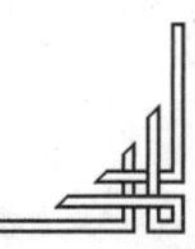

The State of Connecticut

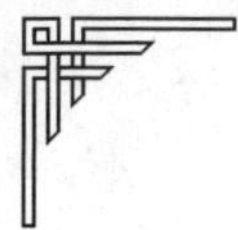

The Best in American Medicine
www.CastleConnolly.com

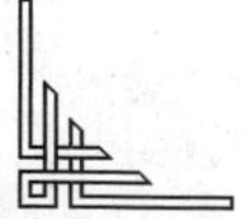
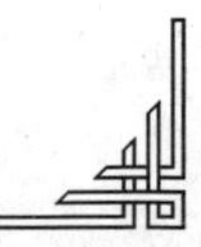

Fairfield

Greenwich Hospital

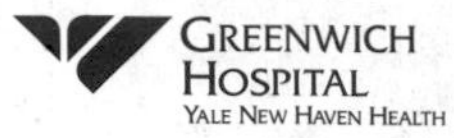

5 Perryridge Road
Greenwich, CT 06830-4697
Tel: 203.863.3000
www.greenwichhospital.org

GENERAL OVERVIEW

Greenwich Hospital is a progressive, regional medical center and teaching institution with an internal medicine residency, serving lower Fairfield and Westchester counties. Care is provided on a beautiful, modern campus designed to create a healing environment for patients and visitors.

ACADEMIC AND CLINICAL AFFILIATIONS

As a member of the Yale New Haven Health System, Greenwich Hospital is a major affiliate of Yale School of Medicine and maintains affiliations with other leading medical providers. Patients have access to a comprehensive range of medical, surgical, diagnostic, ***integrative medicine*** and wellness programs. Greenwich Hospital also offers ***robotic surgery*** and ***hyperbaric medicine and wound healing***. It has a State certified and Joint Commission accredited ***Stroke Center***, and participates in international clinical trials

OUTSTANDING CLINICAL SERVICES

Specialties include oncology care at the hospital's ***Bendheim Cancer Center***; advanced breast care at the ***Breast Center***; a comprehensive Maternity program including ***Level III NICU*** and ***fertility services***; a ***Pediatric Specialty Center***; a ***Weight Loss and Diabetes Center***, expert ***neuroscience and spine services*** and a wide range of ***surgical specialties*** including knee, hip and shoulder joint replacment, plus ***bariatric surgery***.

SERVICE EXCELLENCE

Greenwich Hospital is renowned for service excellence and has been a recipient of Press Ganey's Summit Award for highest ratings in Patient Satisfaction.

Physician Referral:
For a prompt, personal Physician Referral please call Greenwich Hospital at 203-863-3627 or ***visit us online.***

Sponsorship:
Voluntary,
Not-for-profit

Beds:
206

Accreditation:
The Joint Commission

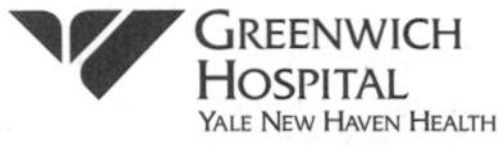

Real Life. Real Care.

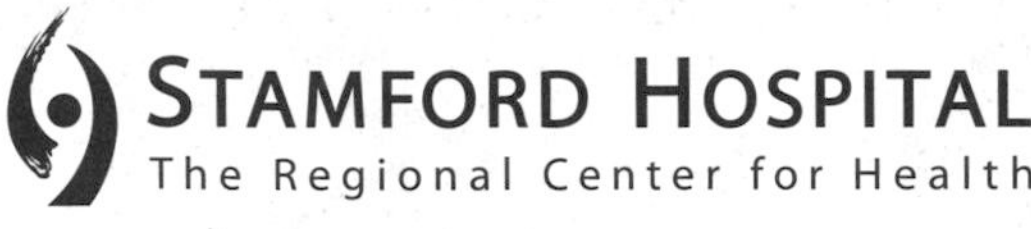

StamfordHospital.org

General Overview

Stamford Hospital provides area residents (Fairfield and Westchester Counties) access to the latest technology with a compassionate, patient-centered care approach in keeping with the Planetree philosophy. Stamford is a Level II trauma center with a nationally recognized adult intensive care unit. Our areas of expertise include:

Cancer Care	StamfordHospital.org/cancer
Heart Services	StamfordHospital.org/heart
Orthopedics	StamfordHospital.org/ortho
Women's Health	StamfordHospital.org/womenshealth

Comprehensive Specialty Centers

Bennett Cancer Center provides compassionate, patient-centered care from diagnosis through post-treatment.

Center for Integrative Medicine and Wellness blends conventional and complementary care for patients.

Center for Robotic Surgery using the *da Vinci* Surgical System, enables surgeons to perform even the most complex and delicate procedures through very small incisions with unmatched precision.

Center for Sleep Medicine offers experts in diagnosing and treating pediatric and adult sleep disorders, including snoring, sleep apnea, insomnia, narcolepsy and restless leg syndrome.

Center for Surgical Weight Loss offers the region's only comprehensive weight management program.

CyberKnife Center, located at the first and only hospital in Fairfield and Westchester Counties, provides the technology to destroy tumors with pinpoint accuracy.

Diabetes & Endocrine Center brings together consultative services and complete clinical care, including comprehensive patient education, medical management and treatment.

Women's Breast Center, first in the nation to receive accreditation from the American College of Surgeons for excellence in breast care. The only breast center in Fairfield County to offer 3-D tomosynthesis to every patient receiving screening mammography.

Academic and Clinical Affiliations

Stamford Hospital is an affiliate of the New York–Presbyterian Healthcare System and a major teaching affiliate of the Columbia University College of Physicians & Surgeons.

Accreditation

Joint Commission on Accreditation of Healthcare Organization (JCAHO)

Beds

305

Sponsorship

Voluntary, Not-for-Profit

For a Physician Referral or more information, please call 1.877.233.9355 or visit StamfordHospital.org /doctor.

Stamford Hospital
30 Shelburne Road
Stamford, CT 06902
203.276.1000

StamfordHospital.org

Fairfield

Adolescent Medicine

Schneider, Marcie B MD (AM) - **Spec Exp:** Eating Disorders; Obesity; Menstrual Disorders; **Hospital:** Greenwich Hosp (page 938); **Address:** Greenwich Adolescent Med Srvs, 239 Glenville Rd, Greenwich, CT 06831; **Phone:** 203-532-1919; **Board Cert:** Pediatrics 1987; Adolescent Medicine 2009; **Med School:** Albert Einstein Coll Med 1983; **Resid:** Pediatrics, Montefiore Med Ctr 1986; **Fellow:** Adolescent Medicine, N Shore Univ Hosp 1988; **Fac Appt:** Assoc Clin Prof Ped, Albert Einstein Coll Med

Zolkowski-Wynne, Joanna MD (AM) - **Spec Exp:** Nutrition; Eating Disorders; Parenting Issues; **Hospital:** Bridgeport Hosp; **Address:** Bridgeport Hosp, 267 Grant St, Bridgeport, CT 06610; **Phone:** 203-384-3064; **Board Cert:** Pediatrics 1985; Adolescent Medicine 2009; **Med School:** SUNY Upstate Med Univ 1980; **Resid:** Pediatrics, Rhode Island Hosp 1983; **Fellow:** Adolescent Medicine, Beth Israel Deaconess Med Ctr 1986; **Fac Appt:** Asst Clin Prof Ped, Yale Univ

Allergy & Immunology

Backman, Kenneth S MD (A&I) - **Spec Exp:** Nasal Allergy; Food Allergy; Asthma; Sinus Disorders; **Hospital:** Bridgeport Hosp, St. Vincent's Med Ctr - Bridgeport; **Address:** Allergy & Asthma Care Fairfield Co, 55 Walls Drive, Ste 405, Fairfield, CT 06824; **Phone:** 203-259-7070; **Board Cert:** Allergy & Immunology 2007; **Med School:** Cornell Univ-Weill Med Coll 1991; **Resid:** Internal Medicine, Univ Chicago Med Ctr 1994; **Fellow:** Allergy & Immunology, Northwestern Meml Hosp 1996

Bell, Jonathan MD (A&I) - **Spec Exp:** Asthma; Insect Allergies; Sinusitis; Hives; **Hospital:** Danbury Hosp; **Address:** Advanced Specialty Care, 107 Newtown Rd, Ste 1B, Danbury, CT 06810; **Phone:** 203-748-7433; **Board Cert:** Pediatrics 1986; Allergy & Immunology 1987; **Med School:** Georgetown Univ 1980; **Resid:** Pediatrics, St Christophers Hosp Chldn 1983; **Fellow:** Pediatric Allergy & Immunology, Chldns Hosp 1987; **Fac Appt:** Asst Clin Prof A&I, NY Med Coll

Bloom, Katherine MD (A&I) - **Spec Exp:** Food Allergy; **Hospital:** St. Vincent's Med Ctr - Bridgeport; **Address:** Allergy & Asthma Care Fairfield Co, 55 Walls Drive, Ste 405, Fairfield, CT 06824; **Phone:** 203-259-7070; **Board Cert:** Allergy & Immunology 2008; Internal Medicine 2006; **Med School:** Albert Einstein Coll Med 2003; **Resid:** Internal Medicine, NY-Presby/Columbia Univ Med Ctr 2006; **Fellow:** Allergy & Immunology, Mount Sinai Med Ctr 2008

Hemmers, Philip H DO (A&I) - **Spec Exp:** Pediatric Allergy & Immunology; Food Allergy; **Hospital:** St. Vincent's Med Ctr - Bridgeport, Norwalk Hosp; **Address:** 4675 Main St, Ste 117, Bridgeport, CT 06606-1813; **Phone:** 203-374-6103; **Board Cert:** Pediatrics 2012; Allergy & Immunology 2007; **Med School:** NY Coll Osteo Med 2001; **Resid:** Pediatrics, Mount Sinai Hosp 2004; **Fellow:** Allergy & Immunology, LI College Hosp 2007

Lee, Richard J MD (A&I) - **Spec Exp:** Pediatric Allergy & Immunology; **Hospital:** Danbury Hosp; **Address:** Advanced Allergy & Asthma Care, 107 Newtown Rd, Ste 1B, Danbury, CT 06810; **Phone:** 203-748-7433; **Board Cert:** Allergy & Immunology 1987; Internal Medicine 1985; **Med School:** Dominican Republic 1980; **Resid:** Internal Medicine, UMDNJ-Rutgers 1983; **Fellow:** Allergy & Immunology, Rhode Island Hosp 1986

Lester, Mitchell R MD (A&I) - **Spec Exp:** Pediatric Allergy & Immunology; Asthma & Allergy; Food Allergy; **Hospital:** Norwalk Hosp, Greenwich Hosp (page 938); **Address:** Fairfield Co Allergy & Asthma, 148 East Ave, Ste 3G, Norwalk, CT 06851; **Phone:** 203-838-4034; **Board Cert:** Pediatrics 1987; Allergy & Immunology 2003; **Med School:** Brown Univ 1983; **Resid:** Pediatrics, Rhode Island Hosp 1987; **Fellow:** Allergy & Immunology, Natl Jewish Hlth Ctr 1994

Lindner, Paul S MD (A&I) - **Spec Exp:** Asthma & Sinusitis; Food & Drug Allergy; Immunodeficiency Disorders; Allergic Rhinitis; **Hospital:** Stamford Hosp (page 939); **Address:** 22 Fifth St, Stamford, CT 06905-5030; **Phone:** 203-978-0072; **Board Cert:** Internal Medicine 1989; Allergy & Immunology 2011; **Med School:** SUNY Buffalo 1985; **Resid:** Internal Medicine, Stamford Hosp 1989; **Fellow:** Allergy & Immunology, Nassau Co Med Ctr 1991; **Fac Appt:** Assoc Clin Prof A&I, Columbia P&S

Litchman, Mark MD (A&I) - **Spec Exp:** Asthma; Immune Deficiency; Lupus/SLE; Vasculitis; **Hospital:** Greenwich Hosp (page 938), Stamford Hosp (page 939); **Address:** 2 1/2 Dearfield Drive, Greenwich, CT 06831-5335; **Phone:** 203-869-2080; **Board Cert:** Internal Medicine 1987; Allergy & Immunology 2011; Rheumatology 1988; **Med School:** Rush Med Coll 1984; **Resid:** Internal Medicine, Greenwich Hosp 1987; **Fellow:** Allergy & Immunology, Yale-New Haven Hosp 1989; Rheumatology, Yale-New Haven Hosp 1989

Matczuk, Agnieszka MD (A&I) - **Spec Exp:** Pediatric Allergy & Immunology; **Hospital:** Greenwich Hosp (page 938); **Address:** 2 1/2 Deerfield Drive, Greenwich, CT 06831; **Phone:** 203-869-2080; **Board Cert:** Pediatrics 2008; Allergy & Immunology 2003; **Med School:** Poland 1993; **Resid:** Pediatrics, Beth Israel Med Ctr 2000; **Fellow:** Allergy & Immunology, Yale-New Haven Hosp 2002

Santilli, John MD (A&I) - **Spec Exp:** Allergy; Sinusitis; **Hospital:** St. Vincent's Med Ctr - Bridgeport; **Address:** 4675 Main St, Ste 117, Bridgeport, CT 06606-1834; **Phone:** 203-374-6103; **Board Cert:** Pediatrics 1973; Allergy & Immunology 1983; **Med School:** Georgetown Univ 1968; **Resid:** Pediatrics, Georgetown Univ Hosp 1971; **Fellow:** Allergy & Immunology, Georgetown Univ Hosp 1973

Sproviero, Joseph MD/PhD (A&I) - **Hospital:** Norwalk Hosp, Greenwich Hosp (page 938); **Address:** Fairfield Co Allergy & Asthma, 148 East Ave, Ste 3G, Norwalk, CT 06851; **Phone:** 203-838-4034; **Board Cert:** Allergy & Immunology 2012; Internal Medicine 1989; **Med School:** Columbia P&S 1985; **Resid:** Internal Medicine, Yale New Haven Hosp 1988; **Fellow:** Allergy & Immunology, Yale-New Haven Hosp 1990; **Fac Appt:** Asst Clin Prof Med, Yale Univ

Veksler-Offengenden, Irena MD (A&I) - **Hospital:** Bridgeport Hosp; **Address:** Allergy & Asthma Care, 55 Walls Drive, Ste 405, Fairfield, CT 06824; **Phone:** 203-259-7070; **Board Cert:** Allergy & Immunology 2005; Internal Medicine 2003; **Med School:** Cornell Univ-Weill Med Coll 2000; **Resid:** Internal Medicine, RWJ-UMDNJ Med Ctr 2003; **Fellow:** Allergy & Immunology, Stony Brook Univ Med Ctr 2005

Cardiac Electrophysiology

Chiravuri, Murali MD/PhD (CE) - **Spec Exp:** Arrhythmias; Atrial Fibrillation; Pacemakers; **Hospital:** Danbury Hosp, Bridgeport Hosp; **Address:** Cardiac Specialists, 25 Germantown Rd, Ste 2B, Danbury, CT 06810; **Phone:** 203-794-0090; **Board Cert:** Internal Medicine 2004; Cardiovascular Disease 2007; Cardiac Electrophysiology 2009; **Med School:** Tufts Univ 2001; **Resid:** Internal Medicine, Brigham & Womens Hosp 2003; **Fellow:** Cardiovascular Disease, Mass Genl Hosp 2007; Cardiac Electrophysiology, Brigham & Womens Hosp 2009

Dhruvakumar, Sandhya MD (CE) - **Spec Exp:** Arrhythmias; Atrial Fibrillation; **Hospital:** Stamford Hosp (page 939); **Address:** Tully Health Ctr, Div Cardiology, 32 Strawberry Hill Court, Stamford, CT 06902; **Phone:** 203-276-2321; **Board Cert:** Internal Medicine 2003; Cardiovascular Disease 2006; Cardiac Electrophysiology 2010; **Med School:** Univ Mass Sch Med 2000; **Resid:** Internal Medicine, Beth Isreal Med Ctr 2003; **Fellow:** Cardiovascular Disease, NY-Presby/Weill Cornell Med Ctr 2006; Cardiac Electrophysiology, Pennsylvania Hosp-UPHS 2008

McPherson, Craig A MD (CE) - **Spec Exp:** Arrhythmias; Pacemakers/Defibrillators; Atrial Fibrillation; **Hospital:** Bridgeport Hosp, Yale-New Haven Hosp; **Address:** Bridgeport Hosp, Dept Electrophysiology, 267 Grant St, Fl 10, Bridgeport, CT 06610; **Phone:** 203-384-3442; **Board Cert:** Internal Medicine 1979; Cardiovascular Disease 1983; Cardiac Electrophysiology 2004; **Med School:** Tufts Univ 1976; **Resid:** Internal Medicine, Tufts-New England Med Ctr 1979; **Fellow:** Cardiovascular Disease, Yale-New Haven Hosp 1982; Cardiac Electrophysiology, Yale-New Haven Hosp 1983; **Fac Appt:** Clin Prof Med, Yale Univ

Pittaro, Michael R MD (CE) - **Spec Exp:** Arrhythmias; **Hospital:** Norwalk Hosp, Stamford Hosp (page 939); **Address:** Cardiology Assocs Fairfield Co, 40 Cross St, Ste 200, Norwalk, CT 06851; **Phone:** 203-845-2160; **Board Cert:** Cardiac Electrophysiology 2012; Cardiovascular Disease 2011; **Med School:** Univ Pennsylvania 1995; **Resid:** Internal Medicine, Barnes-Jewish Hosp 1998; **Fellow:** Cardiovascular Disease, Beth Israel Deaconess Hosp 2000; Cardiac Electrophysiology, Beth Israel Deaconess Hosp 2002

Winslow, Robert D MD (CE) - **Spec Exp:** Arrhythmias; Atrial Fibrillation; Pacemakers; Defibrillators; **Hospital:** Bridgeport Hosp, Danbury Hosp; **Address:** Cardiac Specialists, 1305 Post Rd, Fairfield, CT 06824; **Phone:** 203-292-2000; **Board Cert:** Cardiovascular Disease 2005; Cardiac Electrophysiology 2007; **Med School:** Northwestern Univ-Feinberg Sch Med 1999; **Resid:** Internal Medicine, Brigham & Women's Hosp 2002; **Fellow:** Cardiovascular Disease, Mount Sinai Hosp 2005; Cardiac Electrophysiology, Brigham & Women's Hosp 2007

Cardiovascular Disease

Augenbraun, Charles B MD (Cv) - **Hospital:** Norwalk Hosp; **Address:** Cardio Assocs Fairfield Co, 40 Cross St, Ste 200, Norwalk, CT 06851-4697; **Phone:** 203-845-2160; **Board Cert:** Internal Medicine 1981; Cardiovascular Disease 1985; **Med School:** Univ Pennsylvania 1978; **Resid:** Internal Medicine, Temple Univ Hosp 1981; **Fellow:** Cardiovascular Disease, Hosp Univ Penn 1985

Casale, Linda R MD (Cv) - **Spec Exp:** Non-Invasive Cardiology; Women's Health; Echocardiography; **Hospital:** Bridgeport Hosp, Milford Hosp; **Address:** Cardiac Specialists, 1305 Post Rd, Fairfield, CT 06824; **Phone:** 203-292-2000; **Board Cert:** Cardiovascular Disease 2003; **Med School:** NY Med Coll 1986; **Resid:** Internal Medicine, Montefiore Med Ctr 1989; **Fellow:** Cardiovascular Disease, UCSD Med Ctr 1991

Channamsetty, Venu MD (Cv) - **Spec Exp:** Echocardiography; Nuclear Cardiology; Diagnostic Problems; **Hospital:** St. Vincent's Med Ctr - Bridgeport; **Address:** Cardiology Physicians, PC, 4675 Main St Fl 1, Bridgeport, CT 06606; **Phone:** 203-683-5100; **Board Cert:** Internal Medicine 2004; Cardiovascular Disease 2007; **Med School:** Albany Med Coll 2001; **Resid:** Internal Medicine, Rhode Island Hosp 2004; **Fellow:** Cardiovascular Disease, Westchester Med Ctr 2007

Choi, Joonun MD (Cv) - **Spec Exp:** Coronary Artery Disease; Heart Failure; **Hospital:** Stamford Hosp (page 939); **Address:** Heart Physicians, 80 Mill River St, Ste 1300, Stamford, CT 06902; **Phone:** 203-348-7410; **Board Cert:** Internal Medicine 2003; Cardiovascular Disease 2007; **Med School:** NY Med Coll 2001; **Resid:** Internal Medicine, St Vincent Med Ctr 2004; **Fellow:** Cardiovascular Disease, NY-Presby/Columbia Univ Med Ctr 2007

Copen, David L MD (Cv) - **Spec Exp:** Cardiac Catheterization; Coronary Artery Disease; Congestive Heart Failure; Angioplasty & Stent Replacement; **Hospital:** Danbury Hosp; **Address:** Danbury WCMG, Cardiology, 111 Osborne St Fl 3 - Ste 131, Danbury, CT 06810; **Phone:** 203-739-7155; **Board Cert:** Internal Medicine 1972; Cardiovascular Disease 1975; **Med School:** SUNY Downstate 1969; **Resid:** Internal Medicine, Yale-New Haven Hosp 1972; **Fellow:** Cardiovascular Disease, Mass Genl Hosp 1974; **Fac Appt:** Assoc Clin Prof Med, Yale Univ

Cusack, Evelyn MD (Cv) - **Spec Exp:** Echocardiography; **Hospital:** Stamford Hosp (page 939); **Address:** Stamford Hlth Integrated, Heart Phys, 80 Mill River St, Ste 1300, Stamford, CT 06902; **Phone:** 203-348-7410; **Board Cert:** Cardiovascular Disease 2004; **Med School:** Univ Mass Sch Med 1998; **Resid:** Cardiovascular Disease, Rhode Island Hosp 2001; **Fellow:** Cardiovascular Disease, Westchester Med Ctr 2004; Echocardiography, NY-Presby/Columbia Univ Med Ctr 2005

Fisher, Lawrence I MD (Cv) - **Spec Exp:** Cardiac Catheterization; Pacemakers; Heart Valve Disease; **Hospital:** Danbury Hosp; **Address:** Cardiac Specialists, 25 Germantown Rd, Danbury, CT 06810; **Phone:** 203-794-0090; **Board Cert:** Internal Medicine 1988; Cardiovascular Disease 2011; **Med School:** SUNY Buffalo 1985; **Resid:** Internal Medicine, Bronx Muni Hosp 1988; **Fellow:** Cardiovascular Disease, Albert Einstein Coll Med 1990

Green, Jeffrey A MD (Cv) - **Hospital:** Stamford Hosp (page 939); **Address:** 80 Mill River St, Ste 1300, Stamford, CT 06902; **Phone:** 203-348-7410; **Board Cert:** Cardiovascular Disease 2004; **Med School:** NY Med Coll 1998; **Resid:** Internal Medicine, Montefiore Med Ctr 2001; **Fellow:** Cardiovascular Disease, Montefiore Med Ctr 2004

Heiman, Mark MD (Cv) - **Spec Exp:** Nuclear Cardiology; Cardiac CT Angiography; Clinical Trials; **Hospital:** Stamford Hosp (page 939), St. Vincent's Med Ctr - Bridgeport; **Address:** Cardiology Assocs of Fairfield, 1177 Summer St Fl 5, Stamford, CT 06905; **Phone:** 203-353-1133; **Board Cert:** Internal Medicine 1989; Cardiovascular Disease 2011; **Med School:** Albert Einstein Coll Med 1986; **Resid:** Internal Medicine, Montefiore Med Ctr 1989; **Fellow:** Cardiovascular Disease, Montefiore Med Ctr 1991

Horowitz, Steven F MD (Cv) - **Spec Exp:** Nuclear Cardiology; Preventive Cardiology; Complementary Medicine; **Hospital:** Stamford Hosp (page 939); **Address:** Stamford Hospital, Dept Cardiology, 30 Shelburne Rd Fl 2, Stamford, CT 06904-9317; **Phone:** 203-276-7480; **Board Cert:** Internal Medicine 1975; Cardiovascular Disease 1979; **Med School:** NY Med Coll 1972; **Resid:** Internal Medicine, Beth Israel Hosp 1976; **Fellow:** Cardiovascular Disease, Mt Sinai Hosp 1978; Cardiology Research, Mt Sinai Hosp 1979

Keller, Andrew M MD (Cv) - **Spec Exp:** Echocardiography; Cardiac Imaging; **Hospital:** Danbury Hosp; **Address:** Danbury WCMG, Cardiology, 111 Osborne St Fl 3 - Ste 131, Danbury, CT 06810; **Phone:** 203-739-7155; **Board Cert:** Internal Medicine 1982; Cardiovascular Disease 1985; **Med School:** Ohio State Univ 1979; **Resid:** Internal Medicine, Duke Univ Hosp 1982; **Fellow:** Cardiovascular Disease, UT Southwestern Med Ctr 1985; **Fac Appt:** Assoc Clin Prof Med, Columbia P&S

Kosinski, Edward J MD (Cv) - **Spec Exp:** Angioplasty & Stent Placement; **Hospital:** St. Vincent's Med Ctr - Bridgeport, Bridgeport Hosp; **Address:** Cardiology Physicians, 4675 Main St Fl 1, Bridgeport, CT 06606-4201; **Phone:** 203-683-5100; **Board Cert:** Internal Medicine 1976; Cardiovascular Disease 1979; **Med School:** Wake Forest Univ 1973; **Resid:** Internal Medicine, Columbia-Presby Med Ctr 1976; **Fellow:** Cardiovascular Disease, Peter Bent Brigham Hosp 1978; **Fac Appt:** Assoc Clin Prof Med, Columbia P&S

Kunkes, Steven H MD (Cv) - **Spec Exp:** Cardiovascular Imaging; Diagnostic Problems; **Hospital:** Bridgeport Hosp, Milford Hosp; **Address:** Cardiac Specialists, 1305 Post Rd, Fairfield, CT 06824; **Phone:** 203-292-2000; **Board Cert:** Internal Medicine 1976; Cardiovascular Disease 1979; Geriatric Medicine 2004; **Med School:** Mount Sinai Sch Med 1973; **Resid:** Internal Medicine, Bellevue Hosp Ctr 1976; **Fellow:** Cardiovascular Disease, Mt Sinai Med Ctr 1978; **Fac Appt:** Assoc Clin Prof Med, Yale Univ

Lomnitz, David MD (Cv) - **Spec Exp:** Echocardiography; Nuclear Cardiology; **Hospital:** Norwalk Hosp; **Address:** Cardiology Assocs Fairfield Co, 40 Cross St, Ste 200, Norwalk, CT 06851; **Phone:** 203-845-2160; **Board Cert:** Cardiovascular Disease 2011; Cardiac Electrophysiology 2011; Nuclear Cardiology 2012; **Med School:** Univ Pennsylvania 1995; **Resid:** Internal Medicine, UCSF Med Ctr 1996; **Fellow:** Cardiovascular Disease, NY-Presby/Weill Cornell Med Ctr 2001

Mani, Susan MD (Cv) - **Spec Exp:** Heart Disease in Women; Cholesterol/Lipid Disorders; **Hospital:** Danbury Hosp; **Address:** Danbury WCMG, Cardiology, 111 Osborne St Fl 3 - Ste 131, Danbury, CT 06810; **Phone:** 203-739-7155; **Board Cert:** Cardiovascular Disease 2005; **Med School:** Johns Hopkins Univ 1998; **Resid:** Internal Medicine, Johns Hopkins Hosp 2001; **Fellow:** Cardiovascular Disease, NY-Presby/Columbia Univ Med Ctr 2005

Marshalko, Stephen J MD/PhD (Cv) - **Spec Exp:** Congenital Heart Disease; Coronary Artery Disease; Echocardiography; Mitral Valve Prolapse; **Hospital:** Bridgeport Hosp, St. Vincent's Med Ctr - Bridgeport; **Address:** Advanced Cardiovascular Specialists, 439 Millhill Ave, Bridgeport, CT 06610; **Phone:** 203-334-2100; **Board Cert:** Internal Medicine 2010; Cardiovascular Disease 2003; Interventional Cardiology 2004; **Med School:** Yale Univ 1996; **Resid:** Internal Medicine, Yale-New Haven Hosp 1999; **Fellow:** Cardiovascular Disease, Yale-New Haven Hosp 2000

Meizlish, Jay Lewis MD (Cv) - **Spec Exp:** Interventional Cardiology; Preventive Cardiology; Cholesterol/Lipid Disorders; Nuclear Cardiology; **Hospital:** Bridgeport Hosp, Milford Hosp; **Address:** Cardiac Specialists, 1305 Post Rd, Fairfield, CT 06824; **Phone:** 203-292-2000; **Board Cert:** Internal Medicine 1980; Cardiovascular Disease 1983; Nuclear Medicine 1984; Interventional Cardiology 2010; **Med School:** NYU Sch Med 1977; **Resid:** Internal Medicine, Harbor-UCLA Med Ctr 1980; **Fellow:** Cardiovascular Disease, Yale-New Haven Hosp 1983; Nuclear Medicine, Yale-New Haven Hosp 1984

Michaelson, Stephen MD (Cv) - **Spec Exp:** Congestive Heart Failure; Coronary Artery Disease; **Hospital:** Norwalk Hosp; **Address:** Cardio Assocs Fairfield Co, 40 Cross St, Ste 200, Norwalk, CT 06851; **Phone:** 203-845-2160; **Board Cert:** Internal Medicine 1975; Cardiovascular Disease 1977; **Med School:** SUNY Upstate Med Univ 1972; **Resid:** Internal Medicine, Univ VA Hosp 1975; **Fellow:** Cardiovascular Disease, Yale Univ Sch Med 1977

Neeson, Francis J MD (Cv) - **Spec Exp:** Preventive Cardiology; Echocardiography; **Hospital:** Stamford Hosp (page 939), Greenwich Hosp (page 938); **Address:** 75 Holly Hill Ln, Greenwich, CT 06830; **Phone:** 203-869-6960; **Board Cert:** Internal Medicine 1988; Cardiovascular Disease 2011; **Med School:** NYU Sch Med 1985; **Resid:** Internal Medicine, Bronx Muni Hosp 1988; **Fellow:** Cardiovascular Disease, Montefiore Med Ctr 1991

Pollack, Brian D MD (Cv) - **Spec Exp:** Nuclear Cardiology; Echocardiography; **Hospital:** Danbury Hosp; **Address:** 25 Germantown Rd, Ste 2B, Danbury, CT 06810; **Phone:** 203-794-0090; **Board Cert:** Cardiovascular Disease 2000; Echocardiography 2006; Nuclear Cardiology 2003; **Med School:** Mount Sinai Sch Med 1987; **Resid:** Internal Medicine, Mt Sinai Med Ctr 1990; **Fellow:** Cardiovascular Disease, Westchester Med Ctr 1993

Schmierer, Jeffrey A MD (Cv) - **Spec Exp:** Nutrition; **Hospital:** Danbury Hosp; **Address:** Danbury WCMG, Cardiology, 111 Osborne St Fl 3 - Ste 131, Danbury, CT 06810; **Phone:** 203-739-7155; **Board Cert:** Internal Medicine 1982; Cardiovascular Disease 1985; **Med School:** SUNY Downstate 1979; **Resid:** Internal Medicine, NY-Presby/Weill Cornell Med Ctr 1982; **Fellow:** Cardiovascular Disease, Tufts Med Ctr 1984

Schuster, Edward MD (Cv) - **Hospital:** Stamford Hosp (page 939); **Address:** 32 Strawberry Hill Ct, Stamford, CT 06902; **Phone:** 203-276-2323; **Board Cert:** Internal Medicine 1980; Cardiovascular Disease 1981; **Med School:** Ros Franklin Univ/Chicago Med Sch 1976; **Resid:** Internal Medicine, Duke Univ Med Ctr 1978; **Fellow:** Cardiovascular Disease, Johns Hopkins Hosp 1980

Taikowski, Richard L MD (Cv) - **Spec Exp:** Echocardiography; Congenital Heart Disease-Adult; Nuclear Cardiology; **Hospital:** Bridgeport Hosp, Milford Hosp; **Address:** Cardiac Specialists, 1305 Post Rd, Fairfield, CT 06824; **Board Cert:** Internal Medicine 1988; Cardiovascular Disease 2012; **Med School:** Boston Univ 1985; **Resid:** Internal Medicine, Boston Univ Med Ctr 1988; **Fellow:** Cardiovascular Disease, Mt Sinai Med Ctr 1991

Zarich, Stuart W MD (Cv) - **Spec Exp:** Echocardiography; Heart Disease in Women; Cardiac Catheterization; Mitral Valve Prolapse; **Hospital:** Bridgeport Hosp; **Address:** Northeast Medical Grp, 267 Grant St, Bridgeport, CT 06610; **Phone:** 203-384-3844; **Board Cert:** Internal Medicine 1984; Cardiovascular Disease 1989; **Med School:** SUNY Upstate Med Univ 1981; **Resid:** Internal Medicine, Beth Israel Deaconess Hosp 1984; **Fellow:** Cardiovascular Disease, Beth Israel Deaconess Hosp/Harvard 1988; **Fac Appt:** Asst Clin Prof Med, Yale Univ

Child & Adolescent Psychiatry

Lustbader, Andrew MD (ChAP) - **Spec Exp:** ADD/ADHD; Anxiety & Depression; Parenting Issues; **Hospital:** Yale-New Haven Hosp; **Address:** Therapeutic Ctr Chldn & Families, 215 Main St, Westport, CT 06880; **Phone:** 203-454-2428 x704; **Board Cert:** Child & Adolescent Psychiatry 2012; Psychiatry 2012; Pediatrics 2012; **Med School:** Albert Einstein Coll Med 1991; **Resid:** Psychiatry, Yale-New Haven Hosp 1996; **Fellow:** Child & Adolescent Psychiatry, Yale-New Haven Hosp 1998; **Fac Appt:** Asst Clin Prof ChAP, Yale Univ

Poll, Joan MD (ChAP) - **Spec Exp:** Developmental Disorders; Anxiety Disorders; **Address:** 16 Bushy Ridge Rd, Westport, CT 06880-2105; **Phone:** 203-222-1186; **Board Cert:** Psychiatry 1983; Child & Adolescent Psychiatry 1993; **Med School:** NY Med Coll 1976; **Resid:** Psychiatry, Jacobi Med Ctr 1979; **Fellow:** Child & Adolescent Psychiatry, Yale-New Haven Hosp 1981

Rosenfeld, Alvin A MD (ChAP) - **Spec Exp:** Psychotherapy; Sexual Development Problems; Overscheduled Children; Family Therapy; **Hospital:** NY-Presby/Weill Cornell Med Ctr, NY (page 104); **Address:** 17 Sherwood Pl, Greenwich, CT 06830; **Phone:** 203-861-0700; **Board Cert:** Psychiatry 1976; Child & Adolescent Psychiatry 1978; **Med School:** Harvard Med Sch 1970; **Resid:** Psychiatry, Mass Mental Hlth Ctr 1973; **Fellow:** Child & Adolescent Psychiatry, Beth Israel Hosp 1975

Colon & Rectal Surgery

Bussell, Stuart MD (CRS) - **Spec Exp:** Minimally Invasive Surgery; **Hospital:** Danbury Hosp; **Address:** Danbury, Colon-Rectal Surgery-WCMG, 111 Osborne St Fl 2, Danbury, CT 06810; **Phone:** 203-739-7131; **Board Cert:** Surgery 2012; Colon & Rectal Surgery 2013; **Med School:** Mich State Univ 1996; **Resid:** Surgery, Mich State Univ Hosp 2001; **Fellow:** Colon & Rectal Surgery, Greater Baltimore Med Ctr 2002

Littlejohn, Charles E MD (CRS) - **Spec Exp:** Colon & Rectal Cancer; **Hospital:** Stamford Hosp (page 939), Norwalk Hosp; **Address:** 70 Mill River St, Stamford, CT 06902; **Phone:** 203-323-8989; **Board Cert:** Colon & Rectal Surgery 1985; **Med School:** Dartmouth Med Sch 1978; **Resid:** Surgery, Rochester Genl Hosp 1980; Surgery, UMDNJ Med Ctr 1983; **Fellow:** Colon & Rectal Surgery, UMDNJ Med Ctr 1984

McClane, James M MD (CRS) - **Spec Exp:** Colon & Rectal Cancer; Laparoscopic Surgery; Inflammatory Bowel Disease; Diverticulitis; **Hospital:** Norwalk Hosp; **Address:** Colon & Rectal Surgl Care CT, 30 Stevens St, Ste E, Norwalk, CT 06856; **Phone:** 203-852-2262; **Board Cert:** Colon & Rectal Surgery 2011; **Med School:** Cornell Univ-Weill Med Coll 1995; **Resid:** Surgery, Thomas Jefferson Univ Hosp 2000; **Fellow:** Colon & Rectal Surgery, Cleveland Clin 2001

Thornton, Scott C MD (CRS) - **Spec Exp:** Laparoscopic Surgery; Colon & Rectal Cancer; Minimally Invasive Surgery; Colostomy Avoidance; **Hospital:** Bridgeport Hosp; **Address:** Northeast Med Grp, 1305 Post Rd, Ste 215, Fairfield, CT 06824; **Phone:** 203-255-7088; **Board Cert:** Colon & Rectal Surgery 2012; Surgery 2011; **Med School:** Univ Pittsburgh 1986; **Resid:** Surgery, Univ Conn Sch Med Affil Hosp 1991; **Fellow:** Colon & Rectal Surgery, UMDNJ Med Ctr 1992; **Fac Appt:** Clin Prof S, Yale Univ

Dermatology

Connors, Richard C MD (D) - **Spec Exp:** Skin Cancer; **Hospital:** Greenwich Hosp (page 938); **Address:** 1 Perryridge Rd, Greenwich, CT 06830-4607; **Phone:** 203-622-0808; **Board Cert:** Dermatology 1974; Dermatopathology 1976; **Med School:** Cornell Univ-Weill Med Coll 1967; **Resid:** Dermatology, New York Hosp 1974; **Fellow:** Dermatopathology, NYU Med Ctr 1975; **Fac Appt:** Assoc Clin Prof D, NYU Sch Med

Dietz, Stephanie B MD (D) - **Spec Exp:** Pediatric Dermatology; Acne; Eczema; **Hospital:** Stamford Hosp (page 939), Yale-New Haven Hosp; **Address:** Dermatology Ctr Stamford, 1290 Summer St, Ste 3600, Stamford, CT 06905; **Phone:** 203-325-3576; **Board Cert:** Dermatology 2008; **Med School:** Univ Pennsylvania 1995; **Resid:** Dermatology, NYU Med Ctr 1999

Drugge, Rhett J MD (D) - **Hospital:** Stamford Hosp (page 939); **Address:** 50 Glenbrook Rd, Ste 1C, Stamford, CT 06902-2949; **Phone:** 203-324-5719; **Board Cert:** Dermatology 2013; **Med School:** NY Med Coll 1988; **Resid:** Dermatology, Univ Michigan Med Ctr 1992

Kolenik III, Steven A MD (D) - **Spec Exp:** Skin Cancer; Mohs' Surgery; **Hospital:** Norwalk Hosp, Yale-New Haven Hosp; **Address:** Connecticut Dermatology Group, 761 Main Ave, Ste 102, Norwalk, CT 06851; **Phone:** 203-810-4151; **Board Cert:** Dermatology 2001; **Med School:** Yale Univ 1990; **Resid:** Dermatology, Yale-New Haven Hosp 1994; **Fellow:** Mohs Surgery, Yale-New Haven Hosp 1995; **Fac Appt:** Asst Clin Prof D, Yale Univ

Lipper, Graeme M MD (D) - **Spec Exp:** Pediatric Dermatology; Cosmetic Surgery; Skin Laser Surgery; Botox Therapy; **Hospital:** Danbury Hosp; **Address:** Advanced DermCare, 25 Tamarack Ave, Danbury, CT 06810; **Phone:** 203-797-8990; **Board Cert:** Dermatology 2010; **Med School:** Harvard Med Sch 1997; **Resid:** Dermatology, Mass Genl Hosp 2000; **Fellow:** Cosmetic Surgery, Mass Genl Hosp 2001

Maiocco, Kenneth J MD (D) - **Spec Exp:** Skin Cancer; Dermatologic Surgery; Botox Therapy; **Hospital:** St. Vincent's Med Ctr - Bridgeport, Bridgeport Hosp; **Address:** 4639 Main St, Bridgeport, CT 06606-1873; **Phone:** 203-374-5546; **Board Cert:** Dermatology 1976; **Med School:** Univ Rochester 1967; **Resid:** Surgery, St Vincents Med Ctr 1971; Dermatology, Geisinger Med Ctr 1975

Mayer, Fern E MD (D) - **Spec Exp:** Skin Cancer; Pediatric Dermatology; Immune Deficiency-Skin Disorders; **Hospital:** Stamford Hosp (page 939); **Address:** 132 Morgan St, Stamford, CT 06905; **Phone:** 203-969-0123; **Board Cert:** Dermatology 1990; **Med School:** NYU Sch Med 1986; **Resid:** Dermatology, Downstate Med Ctr 1990

McAleer, Patricia A MD (D) - **Spec Exp:** Acne; Psoriasis; Skin Laser Surgery; Botox Therapy; **Hospital:** Norwalk Hosp; **Address:** Skin Care Physicians of Fairfield County, 13 Park St, Norwalk, CT 06851; **Phone:** 203-847-2400; **Board Cert:** Dermatology 2008; **Med School:** Ros Franklin Univ/Chicago Med Sch 1995; **Resid:** Dermatology, Westchester Med Ctr 1999

Naidorf, Ellen MD (D) - **Spec Exp:** Skin Cancer; Pediatric Dermatology; **Hospital:** Stamford Hosp (page 939), Yale-New Haven Hosp; **Address:** 22 Long Ridge Rd, Stamford, CT 06905-3812; **Phone:** 203-964-1103; **Board Cert:** Dermatology 2009; Pediatrics 1980; **Med School:** Columbia P&S 1975; **Resid:** Pediatrics, Yale-New Haven Hosp 1978; Dermatology, Columbia Presby Hosp 1980

Oestreicher, Mark I MD (D) - **Spec Exp:** Skin Cancer; Hair Loss; Cosmetic Dermatology; **Hospital:** Bridgeport Hosp; **Address:** Adult & Ped Derm Specs, 160 Hawley Ln, Ste 104, Trumbull, CT 06611; **Phone:** 203-377-0639; **Board Cert:** Internal Medicine 1977; Dermatology 1979; **Med School:** Albany Med Coll 1974; **Resid:** Internal Medicine, Albany Meml Hosp 1977; Dermatology, UCLA Med Ctr 1979; **Fac Appt:** Asst Prof D, Yale Univ

Oshman, Robin G MD/PhD (D) - **Spec Exp:** Skin Cancer; Cosmetic Dermatology; Pediatric Dermatology; **Hospital:** Yale-New Haven Hosp, VA Conn Hlthcre Sys-W Haven Campus; **Address:** 101 Long Lots Rd, Westport, CT 06880-5426; **Phone:** 203-454-0743; **Board Cert:** Dermatology 1990; **Med School:** Brown Univ 1985; **Resid:** Dermatology, Mt Sinai Med Ctr 1989; **Fac Appt:** Asst Clin Prof D, Yale Univ

Pesce, Joseph R MD (D) - **Hospital:** St. Vincent's Med Ctr - Bridgeport; **Address:** 4699 Main St, Ste 212, Bridgeport, CT 06606-1830; **Phone:** 203-372-8949; **Board Cert:** Dermatology 1972; **Med School:** Belgium 1967; **Resid:** Dermatology, Dartmouth-Hitchcock Med Ctr 1971

Pruzan-Clain, Debra L MD (D) - **Spec Exp:** Cosmetic Dermatology; Pediatric Dermatology; Skin Cancer; **Hospital:** Stamford Hosp (page 939); **Address:** 1290 Summer St, Ste 3600, Stamford, CT 06905; **Phone:** 203-325-3576; **Board Cert:** Dermatology 1990; **Med School:** Univ Pennsylvania 1986; **Resid:** Dermatology, SUNY Downstate Med Ctr 1990; **Fac Appt:** Asst Prof D, Albert Einstein Coll Med

Sibrack, Laurence A MD/PhD (D) - **Spec Exp:** Skin Cancer; Cosmetic Dermatology; **Hospital:** Danbury Hosp; **Address:** Dermatology Assocs, 73 Sand Pit Rd, Ste 207, Danbury, CT 06810; **Phone:** 203-792-4151; **Board Cert:** Dermatology 1978; **Med School:** Univ Mich Med Sch 1974; **Resid:** Dermatology, Yale-New Haven Hosp 1978; **Fac Appt:** Assoc Clin Prof D, Yale Univ

Whitman, Gail B MD (D) - **Spec Exp:** Pediatric Dermatology; Acne; Skin Laser Surgery; **Hospital:** Norwalk Hosp; **Address:** Skin Care Physicians of Fairfield County, 13 Park St, Norwalk, CT 06851; **Phone:** 203-847-2400; **Board Cert:** Dermatology 1986; **Med School:** UMDNJ-NJ Med Sch, Newark 1980; **Resid:** Pediatrics, Overlook Hosp 1983; Dermatology, NY Presby-Columbia Med Ctr 1986

Diagnostic Radiology

Cohen, Steven M MD (DR) - **Spec Exp:** Ultrasound; Women's Imaging; CT Body Scan; MRI; **Hospital:** Stamford Hosp (page 939), St. Vincent's Med Ctr - Bridgeport; **Address:** Advanced Radiology Consultants, 56 Quarry Rd, Trumbull, CT 06611; **Phone:** 203-696-3672; **Board Cert:** Diagnostic Radiology 1987; **Med School:** NY Med Coll 1983; **Resid:** Internal Medicine, Stamford Hosp 1984; Diagnostic Radiology, Montefiore Med Ctr 1987; **Fellow:** Ultrasound/CT/MRI, Thomas Jefferson Univ Hosp 1989; **Fac Appt:** Asst Prof Rad, Columbia P&S

Donahue, John P MD (DR) - **Spec Exp:** MRI; Women's Imaging; CT Scan; **Address:** Robert Russo MD & Assocs Radiology, 2909 Main St Fl 1, Stratford, CT 06615; **Phone:** 203-683-4570; **Board Cert:** Diagnostic Radiology 1996; **Med School:** Georgetown Univ 1991; **Resid:** Diagnostic Radiology, St Vincents Med Ctr 1996; **Fellow:** Abdominal Imaging, NY-Presby/Columbia Univ Med Ctr 1997

Ehrlich, Conrad MD (DR) - **Spec Exp:** Women's Imaging; Mammography; CT Scan; **Address:** Housatonic Valley Radiology, 67 Sand Pit Rd, Danbury, CT 06810-4032; **Phone:** 203-797-1770; **Board Cert:** Internal Medicine 1979; Nuclear Medicine 1981; Diagnostic Radiology 1983; **Med School:** Boston Univ 1976; **Resid:** Nuclear Medicine, Beth Israel Deaconess Med Ctr 1981; Diagnostic Radiology, Beth Israel Deaconess Med Ctr 1983; **Fellow:** Ultrasound, Beth Israel Deaconess Med Ctr

Ernberg, Lauren MD (DR) - **Hospital:** Norwalk Hosp; **Address:** Norwalk Radiology & Mammography Ctr, 148 East Ave, Ste 1R, Norwalk, CT 06851; **Phone:** 203-838-4886; **Board Cert:** Diagnostic Radiology 2012; **Med School:** Cornell Univ-Weill Med Coll 1997; **Resid:** Diagnostic Radiology, NY-Presby/Weill Cornell Med Ctr 2002; **Fellow:** Musculoskeletal Imaging, Hosp Special Surgery 2003

Fey, Christopher P MD (DR) - **Hospital:** Greenwich Hosp (page 938); **Address:** Greenwich Radiology Group, 49 Lake Ave, Greenwich, CT 06830; **Phone:** 203-869-6220; **Board Cert:** Diagnostic Radiology 1998; Nuclear Medicine 2009; Nuclear Radiology 1999; **Med School:** Yale Univ 1993; **Resid:** Radiology, Beth Israel Deaconess Med Ctr 1998; **Fellow:** Nuclear Medicine, Harvard Univ Affil Hosp 1999

King, Michael H MD (DR) - **Hospital:** Stamford Hosp (page 939); **Address:** Stamford Hosp, Dept Radiology, 30 Shelburne Rd, Stamford, CT 06904; **Phone:** 203-276-7860; **Board Cert:** Diagnostic Radiology 1999; **Med School:** Ros Franklin Univ/Chicago Med Sch 1995; **Resid:** Diagnostic Radiology, Norwalk Hosp 1999; **Fellow:** Radiology, NY Presby Hosp 2000

Lee, Ronald P MD (DR) - **Spec Exp:** MRI; CT Scan; **Hospital:** Norwalk Hosp; **Address:** Norwalk Radiology, 148 East Ave, Ste 1R, Norwalk, CT 06851; **Phone:** 203-851-5645; **Board Cert:** Diagnostic Radiology 1991; **Med School:** NYU Sch Med 1986; **Resid:** Diagnostic Radiology, Bellevue Hosp/NYU Med Ctr 1991; **Fellow:** Magnetic Resonance Imaging, Johns Hopkins Hosp 1992

Mullen, David MD (DR) - **Hospital:** Greenwich Hosp (page 938); **Address:** 49 Lake Ave, Greenwich, CT 06830; **Phone:** 203-869-6220; **Board Cert:** Diagnostic Radiology 1987; **Med School:** Albert Einstein Coll Med 1983; **Resid:** Diagnostic Radiology, Columbia-Presby Med Ctr 1985; **Fellow:** Abdominal Imaging, Columbia-Presby Med Ctr 1986; **Fac Appt:** Asst Clin Prof, Columbia P&S

Riccio, Gioia J MD (DR) - **Spec Exp:** Women's Imaging; Ultrasound; Mammography; **Address:** Robert Russo MD & Assocs Radiology, 4699 Main St, Ste 108, Bridgeport, CT 06606; **Phone:** 203-683-4550; **Board Cert:** Diagnostic Radiology 2000; **Med School:** Puerto Rico 1993; **Resid:** Diagnostic Radiology, St Vincents Med Ctr 1998; **Fellow:** Women's Imaging, Wake Forest Baptist Med Ctr 1999; Mammography, Wake Forest Baptist Med Ctr 1999

Salik, Erez MD (DR) - **Spec Exp:** Interventional Radiology; **Hospital:** Greenwich Hosp (page 938); **Address:** 49 Lake Ave, Ste LL2, Greenwich, CT 06830; **Phone:** 203-863-3960; **Board Cert:** Diagnostic Radiology 2004; **Med School:** Mount Sinai Sch Med 1999; **Resid:** Radiology, NYU Med Ctr 2004; **Fellow:** Vascular & Interventional Radiology, Yale-New Haven Hosp 2005

Endocrinology, Diabetes & Metabolism

Arden-Cordone, Mary MD (EDM) - **Spec Exp:** Osteoporosis; Thyroid Disorders; **Hospital:** Stamford Hosp (page 939); **Address:** Endocrinology Ctr Stamford, 1275 Summer St, Ste A1, Stamford, CT 06905; **Phone:** 203-359-2444; **Board Cert:** Internal Medicine 1992; Endocrinology, Diabetes & Metabolism 2006; **Med School:** NYU Sch Med 1989; **Resid:** Internal Medicine, NY-Presby/Columbia Univ Med Ctr 1992; **Fellow:** Endocrinology, Diabetes & Metabolism, NY-Presby/Columbia Univ Med Ctr 1995

Benaviv-Meskin, Danielle MD (EDM) - **Spec Exp:** Thyroid Disorders; Osteoporosis; Diabetes; **Hospital:** St. Vincent's Med Ctr - Bridgeport; **Address:** PriMed, Endocrinology Dept, 4699 Main St, Ste 101, Bridgeport, CT 06606; **Phone:** 203-371-7048; **Board Cert:** Internal Medicine 2003; Endocrinology, Diabetes & Metabolism 2006; **Med School:** Jefferson Med Coll 2000; **Resid:** Internal Medicine, Montefiore Med Ctr 2004; **Fellow:** Endocrinology, Diabetes & Metabolism, NYU Med Ctr 2006

Goldberg-Berman, Judith C MD/PhD (EDM) - **Spec Exp:** Thyroid Disorders; Osteoporosis; Diabetes; **Hospital:** Greenwich Hosp (page 938); **Address:** 4 Dearfield Drive, Ste 102, Greenwich, CT 06831-5351; **Phone:** 203-622-9160; **Board Cert:** Endocrinology, Diabetes & Metabolism 2000; **Med School:** Cornell Univ-Weill Med Coll 1987; **Resid:** Internal Medicine, NYU/Bellevue Hosp 1990; **Fellow:** Endocrinology, New York Hosp/Meml Sloan Kettering 1993

Rennert, Nancy J MD (EDM) - **Spec Exp:** Diabetes in Minority Populations; Thyroid Disorders; Endocrine Disorders in Pregnancy; **Hospital:** Norwalk Hosp; **Address:** 120 Connecticut Ave, Norwalk, CT 06856; **Phone:** 203-899-1770; **Board Cert:** Internal Medicine 2003; Endocrinology, Diabetes & Metabolism 2003; **Med School:** Univ Pittsburgh 1987; **Resid:** Internal Medicine, Univ Pitt Hlth Ctr 1990; **Fellow:** Endocrinology, Diabetes & Metabolism, Yale-New Haven Hosp 1993

Rich, Glenn MD (EDM) - **Spec Exp:** Calcium Disorders; Diabetes; **Hospital:** Bridgeport Hosp, St. Vincent's Med Ctr - Bridgeport; **Address:** Fairfield Co Med Grp, 15 Corporate Drive, Ste 2-1, Trumbull, CT 06611; **Phone:** 203-459-5100; **Board Cert:** Internal Medicine 1989; Endocrinology, Diabetes & Metabolism 2011; **Med School:** Cornell Univ-Weill Med Coll 1986; **Resid:** Internal Medicine, St Lukes Hospital 1989; **Fellow:** Endocrinology, Diabetes & Metabolism, Brigham & Women's Hosp 1991

Rosa, Joseph MD (EDM) - **Spec Exp:** Diabetes; **Hospital:** St. Vincent's Med Ctr - Bridgeport; **Address:** 4699 Main St, Ste 101, Bridgeport, CT 06606; **Phone:** 203-371-7048; **Board Cert:** Internal Medicine 1987; Endocrinology, Diabetes & Metabolism 1989; **Med School:** Mexico 1982; **Resid:** Internal Medicine, St Vincents Med Ctr 1986; **Fellow:** Endocrinology, Diabetes & Metabolism, Univ Conn Med Ctr 1988; **Fac Appt:** Assoc Prof Med, Columbia P&S

Savino, Robert R DO (EDM) - **Spec Exp:** Diabetes; Hypogonadism-Male; **Hospital:** Danbury Hosp; **Address:** Danbury WCMG, Endocrinology, 25 Germantown Rd, Ste 1A, Danbury, CT 06810; **Phone:** 203-794-5620; **Board Cert:** Endocrinology, Diabetes & Metabolism 2005; **Med School:** NY Coll Osteo Med 1988; **Resid:** Internal Medicine, LIJ Med Ctr 1992; **Fellow:** Endocrinology, Diabetes & Metabolism, Lahey-Hitchcock Med Ctr 1993; Endocrinology, Diabetes & Metabolism, Joslin Diabetes Ctr 1994; **Fac Appt:** Asst Clin Prof Med, Yale Univ

Family Medicine

Acosta, Rodrigo MD (FMed) *PCP* - **Spec Exp:** Geriatric Care; Preventive Medicine; **Hospital:** Stamford Hosp (page 939); **Address:** Stamford Family Prac, 32 Strawberry Hill Ct Fl 4 - Ste 6, Stamford, CT 06902; **Phone:** 203-977-2566; **Board Cert:** Family Medicine 2008; Geriatric Medicine 2012; **Med School:** Univ Tex SW, Dallas 1984; **Resid:** Family Medicine, St. Joseph Med Ctr 1987

Cigno, Thomas MD (FMed) *PCP* - **Hospital:** Danbury Hosp; **Address:** 77 Danbury Rd, Ridgefield, CT 06877; **Phone:** 203-431-6342; **Board Cert:** Family Medicine 2009; **Med School:** Tufts Univ 1986; **Resid:** Family Medicine, St Francis Hosp & Med Ctr 1989

Duchen, Douglas MD (FMed) *PCP* - **Hospital:** St. Vincent's Med Ctr - Bridgeport, Bridgeport Hosp; **Address:** 112 Quarry Rd, Ste 120, Trumbull, CT 06611; **Phone:** 203-372-4065; **Board Cert:** Family Medicine 2011; **Med School:** South Africa 1983; **Resid:** Orthopaedic Surgery, Whittington Hosp 1987; Family Medicine, Brookhaven Meml Hosp 1991

Falkoff, Alan MD (FMed) *PCP* - **Hospital:** Stamford Hosp (page 939); **Address:** High Ridge Family Practice, 30 Buxton Farms Rd, Ste 210, Stamford, CT 06905; **Phone:** 203-322-7070; **Board Cert:** Family Medicine 2007; **Med School:** Grenada 1985; **Resid:** Family Medicine, St Joseph's Med Ctr 1988

Farrell, Matthew M MD (FMed) *PCP* - **Spec Exp:** Primary Care Sports Medicine; **Hospital:** Danbury Hosp; **Address:** 60 Old New Milford Rd, Ste 2A, Brookfield, CT 06804; **Phone:** 203-775-6365; **Board Cert:** Geriatric Medicine 2006; Family Medicine 2007; Sports Medicine 2003; **Med School:** Columbia P&S 1980; **Resid:** Family Medicine, Somerset Med Ctr 1983; **Fac Appt:** Asst Clin Prof FMed, Univ Conn

Filiberto, Cosmo MD (FMed) *PCP* - **Spec Exp:** Geriatric Care; Cholesterol/Lipid Disorders; Preventive Medicine; **Hospital:** St. Vincent's Med Ctr - Bridgeport, Bridgeport Hosp; **Address:** 112 Quarry Rd, Ste 120, Trumbull, CT 06611; **Phone:** 203-372-4065; **Board Cert:** Family Medicine 2006; **Med School:** Italy 1976; **Resid:** Family Medicine, Lutheran Med Ctr 1979; **Fac Appt:** Assoc Prof FMed, Quinnipiac Univ-Netter Sch Med

Greeley, John MD (FMed) *PCP* - **Hospital:** Stamford Hosp (page 939); **Address:** Stamford, Family Med, 1450 Washington Blvd, Ste 103, Stamford, CT 06902; **Phone:** 203-348-2937; **Board Cert:** Family Medicine 2007; **Med School:** Mexico 1977; **Resid:** Family Medicine, St Joseph Med Ctr 1981

Herbert, Joshua MD (FMed) *PCP* - **Hospital:** Stamford Hosp (page 939); **Address:** High Ridge Family Practice, 30 Buxton Farms Rd, Ste 210, Stamford, CT 06905; **Phone:** 203-322-7070; **Board Cert:** Family Medicine 2006; **Med School:** Grenada 1996; **Resid:** Family Medicine, N Shore Univ Hosp 1999

Mallozzi, Angelo MD (FMed) *PCP* - **Hospital:** Stamford Hosp (page 939); **Address:** 32 Strawberry Hill Court, Stamford, CT 06902; **Phone:** 203-977-2566; **Board Cert:** Family Medicine 2008; **Med School:** Italy 1978; **Resid:** Family Medicine, St Joseph's Hosp 1982

Miller, Leslie R DO (FMed) *PCP* - **Hospital:** Bridgeport Hosp, St. Vincent's Med Ctr - Bridgeport; **Address:** 52 Beach Rd, Fairfield, CT 06824; **Phone:** 203-256-9905; **Board Cert:** Family Medicine 2004; **Med School:** NY Coll Osteo Med 1985; **Resid:** Family Medicine, St Francis Hosp 1988; **Fellow:** Preventive Medicine, Yale Univ School of Med 1989

O'Regan, Simon MD (FMed) *PCP* - **Hospital:** Danbury Hosp; **Address:** Danbury, Primary Care, 21 South St, Ridgefield, CT 06877; **Phone:** 203-438-6541; **Board Cert:** Family Medicine 2005; **Med School:** South Africa 1988; **Resid:** Family Medicine, Grott Schuur Hosp 1991

Williams, Ann MD (FMed) *PCP* - **Hospital:** Stamford Hosp (page 939); **Address:** 90 Morgan St, Stamford, CT 06905; **Phone:** 203-359-9997; **Board Cert:** Family Medicine 2008; **Med School:** England, UK 1988; **Resid:** Family Medicine, Stamford Hosp 2008

Gastroenterology

Barenberg, David MD (Ge) - **Hospital:** Danbury Hosp; **Address:** Danbury WCMG, Gastroenterology, 111 Osborne St, Ste 121, Danbury, CT 06810; **Phone:** 203-739-7038; **Board Cert:** Internal Medicine 1983; Gastroenterology 1985; **Med School:** SUNY Downstate 1980; **Resid:** Internal Medicine, NY-Presby/Columbia Univ Med Ctr 1983; **Fellow:** Gastroenterology, Brigham & Womens Hosp 1985

Barro, Jennifer MD (Ge) - **Spec Exp:** Endoscopy; **Hospital:** Greenwich Hosp (page 938); **Address:** Ctr GI Med Fairfield & Westchester, 500 W Putnam Ave, Ste 100, Greenwich, CT 06830; **Phone:** 203-863-2900; **Board Cert:** Internal Medicine 2011; Gastroenterology 2004; **Med School:** Stanford Univ 1998; **Resid:** Internal Medicine, Beth Israel Deaconess Med Ctr 2001; **Fellow:** Gastroenterology, Stanford Univ Hosp & Clins 2004

Bonheim, Nelson MD (Ge) - **Spec Exp:** Inflammatory Bowel Disease; Hepatitis C; Colon Cancer; **Hospital:** Greenwich Hosp (page 938); **Address:** 500 W Putnam Ave, Ste 100, Greenwich, CT 06830; **Phone:** 203-863-2900; **Board Cert:** Internal Medicine 1973; Gastroenterology 1975; **Med School:** Ros Franklin Univ/Chicago Med Sch 1970; **Resid:** Internal Medicine, Bronx Muni Hosp 1973; **Fellow:** Gastroenterology, NY Hosp-Cornell Med Ctr 1975; **Fac Appt:** Assoc Prof Med, Yale Univ

Burns, Bryan MD (Ge) - **Spec Exp:** Inflammatory Bowel Disease; Endoscopic Therapies; Gastroesophageal Reflux Disease (GERD); **Hospital:** St. Vincent's Med Ctr - Bridgeport; **Address:** Fairfield Co Endoscopy Ctr, 888 White Plains Rd, Ste 110, Trumbull, CT 06611; **Phone:** 203-459-4451; **Board Cert:** Internal Medicine 2010; Gastroenterology 2003; **Med School:** Albert Einstein Coll Med 1997; **Resid:** Internal Medicine, NY-Presby/Weill Cornell Med Ctr 2000; **Fellow:** Gastroenterology, Montefiore Med Ctr 2003

Dettmer, Robert M MD (Ge) - **Spec Exp:** Endoscopy; Colonoscopy/Polypectomy; **Hospital:** Stamford Hosp (page 939); **Address:** Tully Ctr, Div Gastroenterology, 32 Strawberry Hill Ct, Ste 41042, Stamford, CT 06902; **Phone:** 203-348-5355; **Board Cert:** Gastroenterology 2010; **Med School:** Albert Einstein Coll Med 1994; **Resid:** Internal Medicine, NY-Presby/Columbia Univ Med Ctr 1998; **Fellow:** Gastroenterology, NY-Presby/Columbia Univ Med Ctr 2000

Grossman, Edward T MD (Ge) - **Spec Exp:** Inflammatory Bowel Disease; Malabsorption; **Hospital:** St. Vincent's Med Ctr - Bridgeport, Bridgeport Hosp; **Address:** 425 Post Rd, Fl 1, Fairfield, CT 06824; **Phone:** 203-292-9000; **Board Cert:** Internal Medicine 1970; Gastroenterology 1973; **Med School:** Albert Einstein Coll Med 1963; **Resid:** Internal Medicine, Bronx Muni Hosp Ctr 1968; **Fellow:** Gastroenterology, NY Hosp-Cornell Med Ctr 1970; **Fac Appt:** Assoc Clin Prof Med, Univ Conn

Gruss, Claudia B MD (Ge) - **Spec Exp:** Colonoscopy; Gastroesophageal Reflux Disease (GERD); Inflammatory Bowel Disease; Nutrition; **Hospital:** Norwalk Hosp; **Address:** Arbor Med Grp, 73 Redding Rd, Georgetown, CT 06829; **Phone:** 203-544-9517; **Board Cert:** Internal Medicine 1980; Gastroenterology 1983; **Med School:** Brown Univ 1977; **Resid:** Internal Medicine, Rhode Island Hosp 1980; **Fellow:** Gastroenterology, Rhode Island Hosp 1982

Hale, William B MD (Ge) - **Spec Exp:** Liver Disease; **Hospital:** Norwalk Hosp; **Address:** Norwalk Hosp, Dept Gastroenterology, 30 Steven St, Ste D, Norwalk, CT 06850; **Phone:** 203-852-2278; **Board Cert:** Internal Medicine 1983; Gastroenterology 1987; **Med School:** Univ Wisc 1980; **Resid:** Internal Medicine, Boston Med Ctr 1984; **Fellow:** Gastroenterology, Boston Med Ctr 1986

Kapel, Robert C MD (Ge) - **Hospital:** Danbury Hosp; **Address:** 2 Glen Hill Rd, Danbury, CT 06810; **Phone:** 203-748-7460; **Board Cert:** Gastroenterology 2005; **Med School:** Cornell Univ 1989; **Resid:** Internal Medicine, Mount Sinai Med Ctr 1993; **Fellow:** Gastroenterology, Univ Miami Hosp 1995

Khaghan, Neda MD (Ge) - **Spec Exp:** Biliary Disease; Capsule Endoscopy; Pancreatic Cancer; **Hospital:** Greenwich Hosp (page 938); **Address:** Ctr GI Med Fairfield & Westchester, 500 W Putnam Ave, Ste 100, Greenwich, CT 06830; **Phone:** 203-863-2900; **Board Cert:** Internal Medicine 2008; Gastroenterology 2011; **Med School:** Mount Sinai Sch Med 1995; **Resid:** Internal Medicine, Mount Sinai Hosp 1998; **Fellow:** Gastroenterology, St. Luke's-Roosevelt Hosp 2001; **Fac Appt:** Asst Prof Med, NY Med Coll

Landau, Alan MD (Ge) - **Hospital:** St. Vincent's Med Ctr - Bridgeport; **Address:** Fairfield Co Endoscopy Center, 888 White Plains Rd, Ste 110, Trumbull, CT 06611; **Phone:** 203-459-4451; **Board Cert:** Internal Medicine 1988; Gastroenterology 2011; **Med School:** Boston Univ 1985; **Resid:** Internal Medicine, St Elizabeths Hosp 1988; **Fellow:** Gastroenterology, VA Med Ctr 1990

Link, Richard J MD (Ge) - **Spec Exp:** Colon Cancer Screening; Gastroesophageal Reflux Disease (GERD); Inflammatory Bowel Disease; **Hospital:** Bridgeport Hosp; **Address:** Fairfield County Int Med & Gastro, 4641 Main St, Ste 1, Bridgeport, CT 06606-1827; **Phone:** 203-374-4966; **Board Cert:** Internal Medicine 1974; Gastroenterology 1989; **Med School:** UMDNJ-NJ Med Sch, Newark 1967; **Resid:** Internal Medicine, St Vincent Hosp 1970; **Fellow:** Gastroenterology, Bridgeport Hosp 1972

Mauer, Kenneth MD (Ge) - **Spec Exp:** Endoscopy; Inflammatory Bowel Disease/Crohn's; Capsule Endoscopy; Colonoscopy; **Hospital:** St. Vincent's Med Ctr - Bridgeport, Mt Sinai Med Ctr (page 102); **Address:** 425 Post Rd, Fairfield, CT 06824; **Phone:** 203-292-9000; **Board Cert:** Internal Medicine 1986; Gastroenterology 1989; **Med School:** NYU Sch Med 1983; **Resid:** Internal Medicine, Bronx Muni Hosp Ctr 1987; **Fellow:** Gastroenterology, Mount Sinai Hosp 1989; **Fac Appt:** Asst Prof Med, Quinnipiac Univ-Netter Sch Med

Meighan, Dennis DO (Ge) - **Hospital:** Norwalk Hosp; **Address:** Norwalk Hosp, Dept Gastroenterology, 30 Stevens St, Ste D, Norwalk, CT 06850-3859; **Phone:** 203-852-2278; **Board Cert:** Internal Medicine 1986; Gastroenterology 1989; **Med School:** Univ New Eng Coll Osteo Med 1982; **Resid:** Internal Medicine, Norwalk Hosp 1986; **Fellow:** Gastroenterology, Norwalk Hosp 1987

Nelson, Alan M MD (Ge) - **Spec Exp:** Swallowing Disorders; Endoscopy; Colon Cancer; **Hospital:** Bridgeport Hosp; **Address:** Fairfield Co Int Med Assocs, 4641 Main St, Ste 1, Bridgeport, CT 06606-1827; **Phone:** 203-374-4966; **Board Cert:** Internal Medicine 1977; Gastroenterology 1979; **Med School:** Georgetown Univ 1974; **Resid:** Internal Medicine, Kings Co Hosp-SUNY Med Ctr 1976; Internal Medicine, Bridgeport Hosp 1977; **Fellow:** Gastroenterology, Yale Univ Affil Hosps 1979; **Fac Appt:** Asst Prof Med, Yale Univ

Soloway, Gregory N MD (Ge) - **Spec Exp:** Colon Cancer Screening; Barrett's Esophagus; Clostridium Difficile Disease; Endoscopic Therapies; **Hospital:** Bridgeport Hosp; **Address:** Gastroenterology Assocs, 2890 Main St Fl 2, Stratford, CT 06614; **Phone:** 203-375-1200; **Board Cert:** Gastroenterology 2004; Internal Medicine 1989; **Med School:** Cornell Univ-Weill Med Coll 1986; **Resid:** Internal Medicine, Montefiore Med Ctr 1989; **Fellow:** Gastroenterology, Montefiore Med Ctr 1993

Spivack, Julie MD (Ge) - **Spec Exp:** Women's Health; Colonoscopy; Gallbladder Disease; **Hospital:** St. Vincent's Med Ctr - Bridgeport; **Address:** Gastroenterology Assocs Fairfield Co, 425 Post Rd, Fairfield, CT 06824; **Phone:** 203-292-9000; **Board Cert:** Gastroenterology 2005; **Med School:** Albert Einstein Coll Med 1990; **Resid:** Internal Medicine, Beth Israel Deaconess Hosp 1993; **Fellow:** Gastroenterology, NY-Presby/Weill Cornell Med Ctr 1995; Hepatobiliary Surgery, Meml Sloan-Kettering Cancer Ctr 1996

Taubin, Howard L MD (Ge) - **Spec Exp:** Celiac Disease; Colon Cancer Screening; Inflammatory Bowel Disease; Peptic Acid Disorders; **Hospital:** Bridgeport Hosp; **Address:** Gastroenterology Assocs, 2890 Main St Fl 2, Stratford, CT 06614; **Phone:** 203-375-1200; **Board Cert:** Internal Medicine 1972; Gastroenterology 1973; **Med School:** Univ VA Sch Med 1965; **Resid:** Internal Medicine, Montefiore Hosp 1967; Internal Medicine, Yale-New Haven Hosp 1970; **Fellow:** Gastroenterology, Yale-New Haven Hosp 1973; **Fac Appt:** Assoc Clin Prof Med, Yale Univ

Whelan, Thomas Patrick MD (Ge) - **Spec Exp:** Food Allergy; Gastroesophageal Reflux Disease (GERD); Barrett's Esophagus; **Hospital:** Danbury Hosp; **Address:** Village Square Internal Med, 2 Elizabeth St, Bethel, CT 06801; **Phone:** 203-791-2221; **Board Cert:** Internal Medicine 1986; Gastroenterology 1989; **Med School:** Univ VT Coll Med 1983; **Resid:** Internal Medicine, Thomas Jefferson Univ Hosp 1986; **Fellow:** Gastroenterology, Temple Univ Hosp 1988

Zwas, Felice R MD (Ge) - **Hospital:** Greenwich Hosp (page 938); **Address:** 500 W Putnam Ave, Ste 100, Greenwich, CT 06830; **Phone:** 203-863-2900; **Board Cert:** Internal Medicine 1983; Gastroenterology 1985; **Med School:** Columbia P&S 1980; **Resid:** Internal Medicine, NY-Presby/Columbia Univ Med Ctr 1983; **Fellow:** Gastroenterology, Beth Israel Deaconess Med Ctr 1985

Geriatric Medicine

Jones, Stephen G MD (Ger) *PCP* - **Spec Exp:** Alzheimer's Disease; **Hospital:** Greenwich Hosp (page 938); **Address:** 5 Perryridge Rd, Greenwich, CT 06830; **Phone:** 203-863-3415; **Board Cert:** Internal Medicine 2012; Geriatric Medicine 2004; **Med School:** SUNY Stony Brook 1985; **Resid:** Geriatric Medicine, SUNY-Stony Brook Hosp 1989; **Fac Appt:** Assoc Clin Prof Med, Yale Univ

Skudlarska, Beata A MD (Ger) - **Spec Exp:** Alzheimer's Disease; Memory Disorders; Dementia; **Hospital:** Bridgeport Hosp; **Address:** Bridgeport Hosp-Ctr for Geriatrics, 95 Armory Rd, Stratford, CT 06614; **Phone:** 203-384-3388; **Board Cert:** Internal Medicine 2005; Geriatric Medicine 2008; Hospice & Palliative Medicine 2010; **Med School:** Poland 1992; **Resid:** Internal Medicine, Univ Missouri Hlth Care 1994; Internal Medicine, Norwalk Hosp 1995; **Fellow:** Geriatric Medicine, Univ Conn Hlth Ctr 1997

Gynecologic Oncology

Shahabi, Shohreh MD (GO) - **Spec Exp:** Hysterectomy Alternatives; Robotic Surgery; **Hospital:** Danbury Hosp; **Address:** Danbury Hosp, Gynecologic Oncology, 24 Hospital Ave, Danbury, CT 06810; **Phone:** 203-739-4900; **Board Cert:** Obstetrics & Gynecology 2007; **Med School:** Bangladesh 1992; **Resid:** Obstetrics & Gynecology, Universite Libre De Bruxelles 1997; Obstetrics & Gynecology, Yale-New Haven Hosp 2003; **Fellow:** Gynecologic Oncology, Montefiore Med Ctr 2006

Hand Surgery

Backe Jr, Henry A MD (HS) - **Hospital:** St. Vincent's Med Ctr - Bridgeport, Bridgeport Hosp; **Address:** Orthopaedic Specialty Group, 75 Kings Highway Cutoff, Fairfield, CT 06824; **Phone:** 203-337-2600; **Board Cert:** Orthopaedic Surgery 2006; Hand Surgery 2006; **Med School:** Temple Univ 1986; **Resid:** Orthopaedic Surgery, Temple Univ Hosp 1991; **Fellow:** Hand Surgery, Hosp for Joint Diseases 1992; Joint Reconstruction, Hosp Special Surgery 1993

Brown, Lionel G MD (HS) - **Spec Exp:** Hand Reconstruction; Carpal Tunnel Syndrome; **Hospital:** Danbury Hosp; **Address:** Danbury Orthopedics, 35 Tamarack Ave, Danbury, CT 06811; **Phone:** 203-792-4263; **Board Cert:** Hand Surgery 2008; **Med School:** UCSF 1964; **Resid:** Surgery, UCSF Med Ctr 1976; **Fellow:** Hand Surgery, UCSF Med Ctr 1975

Crowe, John F MD (HS) - **Spec Exp:** Arthritis; Carpal Tunnel Syndrome; Elbow Surgery; Rotator Cuff Surgery; **Hospital:** Greenwich Hosp (page 938); **Address:** Orthopaedic & Neurosurgery Specialists, 6 Greenwich Office Park, 40 Valley Drive, Greenwich, CT 06831; **Phone:** 203-869-1145 x263; **Board Cert:** Orthopaedic Surgery 1977; **Med School:** Cornell Univ-Weill Med Coll 1971; **Resid:** Surgery, Roosevelt Hosp 1973; Orthopaedic Surgery, Hosp Special Surgery 1976; **Fellow:** Hand Surgery, Roosevelt Hosp 1979

DiGiovanni, Joseph MD (HS) - **Spec Exp:** Wrist Surgery; Carpal Tunnel Syndrome; Pediatric Hand/Arm Surgery; **Hospital:** Danbury Hosp; **Address:** Danbury Orthopedics, 226 White St, Danbury, CT 06810; **Phone:** 203-797-1500 x6626; **Board Cert:** Orthopaedic Surgery 2013; **Med School:** Mount Sinai Sch Med 1994; **Resid:** Orthopaedic Surgery, Mount Sinai Med Ctr 1999; **Fellow:** Hand Surgery, NYU Hosp Joint Diseases 2000

Dowdle, John D MD (HS) - **Spec Exp:** Hand & Wrist Surgery; Elbow Surgery; **Hospital:** Stamford Hosp (page 939); **Address:** 1 Blachley Rd, Stamford, CT 06902; **Phone:** 203-325-8888; **Board Cert:** Orthopaedic Surgery 2009; Hand Surgery 2009; **Med School:** Univ Tex SW, Dallas 1988; **Resid:** Surgery, Johns Hopkins Hosp 1989; Orthopaedic Surgery, Montefiore Med Ctr 1994; **Fellow:** Hand Surgery, Roosevelt Hosp 1995

Kavookjian, Haik G MD (HS) - **Spec Exp:** Hand & Upper Extremity Surgery; **Hospital:** Stamford Hosp (page 939), Norwalk Hosp; **Address:** 555 Newfield Ave, Stamford, CT 06905; **Phone:** 203-358-0661; **Board Cert:** Orthopaedic Surgery 2008; Hand Surgery 2008; **Med School:** NY Med Coll 1985; **Resid:** Orthopaedic Surgery, Boston Med Ctr 1991; **Fellow:** Hand Surgery, NY-Presby/Columbia Univ Med Ctr 1993

Lunt, John MD (HS) - **Spec Exp:** Hand & Upper Extremity Surgery; Trauma; Carpal Tunnel Syndrome; **Hospital:** Danbury Hosp; **Address:** Danbury Orthopedics, 35 Tamarack Ave, Danbury, CT 06811; **Phone:** 203-792-4263; **Board Cert:** Orthopaedic Surgery 2006; Hand Surgery 2006; **Med School:** Columbia P&S 1986; **Resid:** Orthopaedic Surgery, LIJ Med Ctr 1992; **Fellow:** Surgery, NY-Presby/Columbia Univ Med Ctr 1993

Rago, Thomas A MD (HS) - **Spec Exp:** Hand & Wrist Surgery; **Hospital:** St. Vincent's Med Ctr - Bridgeport, Bridgeport Hosp; **Address:** 3101 Main St, Bridgeport, CT 06606; **Phone:** 203-374-5892; **Board Cert:** Orthopaedic Surgery 2007; Hand Surgery 2007; **Med School:** Columbia P&S 1977; **Resid:** Surgery, Roosevelt Hosp 1979; Orthopaedic Surgery, Presby Hosp 1982; **Fellow:** Hand Surgery, Columbia-Presby Med Ctr 1983

Hematology

Bar, Michael H MD (Hem) - **Spec Exp:** Multiple Myeloma; Leukemia & Lymphoma; Bleeding/Coagulation Disorders; Gaucher Disease; **Hospital:** Stamford Hosp (page 939); **Address:** Stamford Hosp, Dept Hematology, 34 Shelburne Rd, Stamford, CT 06902; **Phone:** 203-325-2695; **Board Cert:** Internal Medicine 1986; Medical Oncology 1989; Hematology 2010; **Med School:** Columbia P&S 1983; **Resid:** Internal Medicine, Columbia-Presby Med Ctr 1986; **Fellow:** Hematology & Oncology, UCSF Med Ctr 1990; **Fac Appt:** Asst Clin Prof Med, Columbia P&S

Boyd, D. Barry MD (Hem) - **Spec Exp:** Hematologic Malignancies; Breast Cancer; Complementary Medicine; **Hospital:** Greenwich Hosp (page 938); **Address:** 15 Valley Drive Fl 2, Greenwich, CT 06831; **Phone:** 203-869-2111; **Board Cert:** Internal Medicine 1982; Medical Oncology 1987; **Med School:** Cornell Univ-Weill Med Coll 1979; **Resid:** Internal Medicine, NY Hosp-Cornell Med Ctr 1982; **Fellow:** Hematology & Oncology, NY Hosp-Cornell Med Ctr 1985; **Fac Appt:** Asst Clin Prof Med, Yale Univ

Cohen, Neil S MD (Hem) - **Spec Exp:** Leukemia; **Hospital:** Stamford Hosp (page 939); **Address:** Stamford Hosp, Dept Hematology, 34 Shelburne Rd, Stamford, CT 06902-3658; **Phone:** 203-325-2695; **Board Cert:** Internal Medicine 1983; Medical Oncology 1987; Hematology 1988; **Med School:** NY Med Coll 1980; **Resid:** Internal Medicine, Stamford Hosp 1983; **Fellow:** Hematology & Oncology, UMass Memorial Med Ctr 1987; Hematology & Oncology, N Shore Univ Hosp 1988; **Fac Appt:** Asst Clin Prof Med, Columbia P&S

Duda, E Andrew MD (Hem) - **Hospital:** St. Vincent's Med Ctr - Bridgeport, Bridgeport Hosp; **Address:** Medical Specialists of Fairfield, 425 Post Rd, Fairfield, CT 06824; **Phone:** 203-255-4545; **Board Cert:** Internal Medicine 1988; Medical Oncology 1989; Hematology 2012; **Med School:** Yale Univ 1984; **Resid:** Internal Medicine, Yale-New Haven Hosp 1987; **Fellow:** Hematology & Oncology, Dana Farber Cancer Ctr 1991

Mazur, Eric M MD (Hem) - **Spec Exp:** Bleeding/Coagulation Disorders; Platelet Disorders; **Hospital:** Norwalk Hosp; **Address:** Norwalk Hosp, Div Hematology/Oncology, 34 Maple St, Norwalk, CT 06856; **Phone:** 203-852-2325; **Board Cert:** Hematology 1980; Medical Oncology 1981; Internal Medicine 1978; **Med School:** Johns Hopkins Univ 1975; **Resid:** Internal Medicine, Strong Meml Hosp 1977; Internal Medicine, Yale-New Haven Hosp 1979; **Fellow:** Hematology, Yale Univ Sch Med 1981; **Fac Appt:** Assoc Prof Med, Brown Univ

Infectious Disease

Cipriani, Ralph MD (Inf) - **Spec Exp:** Lyme Disease; Fevers of Unknown Origin; **Hospital:** Stamford Hosp (page 939); **Address:** 1351 Washington Blvd, Stamford, CT 06902; **Phone:** 203-327-1187; **Board Cert:** Infectious Disease 2011; Internal Medicine 2011; **Med School:** Albert Einstein Coll Med 1996; **Resid:** Internal Medicine, Mt Sinai Hosp 1999; **Fellow:** Infectious Disease, Mt Sinai Hosp 2001; **Fac Appt:** Asst Clin Prof Med, NY Med Coll

Herbin, Joseph T MD (Inf) - **Spec Exp:** Lyme Disease; Infectious Disease in Elderly; **Hospital:** St. Vincent's Med Ctr - Bridgeport; **Address:** 2150 Black Rock Tpke, Ste 201, Fairfield, CT 06825; **Phone:** 203-384-0451; **Board Cert:** Internal Medicine 1972; **Med School:** Switzerland 1965; **Resid:** Internal Medicine, St Vincent's Hosp & Med Ctr 1970; **Fellow:** Infectious Disease, Univ VT Affil Hosp 1971; **Fac Appt:** Asst Clin Prof Med, Yale Univ

McLeod, Gavin MD (Inf) - **Spec Exp:** AIDS/HIV; Travel Medicine; Hospital Acquired Infections; Pneumonia; **Hospital:** Greenwich Hosp (page 938); **Address:** 5 Perryridge Rd, Ste 108, Greenwich, CT 06830; **Phone:** 203-869-8838; **Board Cert:** Internal Medicine 1988; Infectious Disease 2013; **Med School:** Univ Conn 1985; **Resid:** Internal Medicine, North Shore Univ Hosp 1988; **Fellow:** Infectious Disease, New England Deaconess Med Ctr 1992; **Fac Appt:** Assoc Clin Prof Med, Columbia P&S

Nee, Paul MD (Inf) - **Spec Exp:** AIDS/HIV; Travel Medicine; Bone/Joint Infections; **Hospital:** Danbury Hosp; **Address:** Danbury, Infectious Disease-WCMG, 33 Germantown Rd Fl 2, Danbury, CT 06810; **Phone:** 203-739-8310; **Board Cert:** Infectious Disease 2009; **Med School:** NY Med Coll 1994; **Resid:** Internal Medicine, Beth Israel Deaconess Hosp 1997; **Fellow:** Infectious Disease, Yale-New Haven Hosp 1999

Parry, Michael F MD (Inf) - **Spec Exp:** Antibiotic Resistance; Lyme Disease; Pneumonia; **Hospital:** Stamford Hosp (page 939); **Address:** 166 W Broad St, Ste 202, Stamford, CT 06902; **Phone:** 203-353-1427; **Board Cert:** Internal Medicine 1974; Infectious Disease 1978; **Med School:** Columbia P&S 1970; **Resid:** Internal Medicine, Columbia-Presby Med Ctr 1974; Internal Medicine, UCSF Med Ctr 1973; **Fellow:** Infectious Disease, Columbia-Presby Med Ctr 1976; **Fac Appt:** Clin Prof Med, Columbia P&S

Sabetta, James MD (Inf) - **Spec Exp:** Lyme Disease; Tropical Diseases; Bone/Joint Infections; Fevers of Unknown Origin; **Hospital:** Greenwich Hosp (page 938); **Address:** 5 Perryridge Rd, Ste 108, Greenwich, CT 06830; **Phone:** 203-869-8838; **Board Cert:** Internal Medicine 1981; Infectious Disease 1984; **Med School:** Brown Univ 1978; **Resid:** Internal Medicine, Rhode Island Hosp 1981; **Fellow:** Infectious Disease, Yale-New Haven Hosp 1984; **Fac Appt:** Assoc Clin Prof Med, Yale Univ

Saul, Zane K MD (Inf) - **Spec Exp:** Lyme Disease; AIDS/HIV; Travel Medicine; **Hospital:** Bridgeport Hosp; **Address:** Int Med & Infectious Dis Assocs, 3241 Main St, Ste B, Stratford, CT 06614; **Phone:** 203-383-4466; **Board Cert:** Internal Medicine 2011; Infectious Disease 2000; **Med School:** Grenada 1985; **Resid:** Internal Medicine, Brooklyn Hosp 1988; **Fellow:** Infectious Disease, Hackensack Univ Med Ctr 1990

Schleiter, Gary S MD (Inf) - **Spec Exp:** Viral Infections; **Hospital:** Danbury Hosp, New Milford Hosp; **Address:** Danbury WCMG, Infectious Disease, 33 Germantown Rd Fl 2, Danbury, CT 06810; **Phone:** 203-739-8310; **Board Cert:** Internal Medicine 1983; Infectious Disease 1986; **Med School:** Wake Forest Univ 1980; **Resid:** Internal Medicine, Univ Conn Hlth Ctr 1983; **Fellow:** Infectious Disease, Univ Mass Med Ctr 1985; **Fac Appt:** Asst Clin Prof Med, Yale Univ

Yee, Arthur MD (Inf) - **Spec Exp:** Lyme Disease; Infections-Respiratory; Hospital Acquired Infections; **Hospital:** Norwalk Hosp; **Address:** 40 Cross St, Ste 400, Norwalk, CT 06851; **Phone:** 203-845-4838; **Board Cert:** Internal Medicine 1986; Infectious Disease 1988; **Med School:** Univ Conn 1982; **Resid:** Internal Medicine, Columbia-Presby Med Ctr 1985; **Fellow:** Infectious Disease, Hosp Univ Penn 1988

Internal Medicine

Altbaum, Robert A MD (IM) *PCP* - **Spec Exp:** Hypertension; Asthma; Osteoporosis; **Hospital:** Norwalk Hosp, Bridgeport Hosp; **Address:** Internal Med Assocs of Westport, 162 Kings Hwy N, Westport, CT 06880-2425; **Phone:** 203-226-0731; **Board Cert:** Internal Medicine 1978; **Med School:** Harvard Med Sch 1975; **Resid:** Internal Medicine, Mass Genl Hosp 1977; Internal Medicine, Yale-New Haven Hosp 1979

Berman, Edward Roy MD (IM) - **Spec Exp:** Occupational Medicine; Geriatric Medicine; **Hospital:** Danbury Hosp; **Address:** 30 Prospect St, Ste 500, Ridgefield, CT 06877; **Phone:** 203-438-0364; **Board Cert:** Internal Medicine 1979; Occupational Medicine 1992; **Med School:** Boston Univ 1976; **Resid:** Internal Medicine, Wayne State Univ Affil Hosp 1978; Internal Medicine, Norwalk Hosp 1979

Bivona, James J MD (IM) *PCP* - **Hospital:** Stamford Hosp (page 939); **Address:** Stamford Primary Care, 1275 Summer St, Ste 105, Stamford, CT 06905; **Phone:** 203-325-2667; **Board Cert:** Internal Medicine 2011; **Med School:** Dominica 1997; **Resid:** Internal Medicine, Stamford Hosp 2000

Blumberg, Joel M MD (IM) *PCP* - **Spec Exp:** Preventive Cardiology; Hypertension; Cholesterol/Lipid Disorders; Echocardiography; **Hospital:** Greenwich Hosp (page 938); **Address:** 55 Holly Hill Ln, MS 0, Greenwich, CT 06830; **Phone:** 203-661-4242; **Board Cert:** Internal Medicine 1972; Cardiovascular Disease 1974; **Med School:** NYU Sch Med 1966; **Resid:** Internal Medicine, Bellevue Hosp 1971; **Fellow:** Cardiovascular Disease, New York Hosp 1973

Costanzo, Joseph V MD (IM) *PCP* - **Hospital:** Stamford Hosp (page 939); **Address:** PrimeCare Med, 80 Mill River St, Ste 2400, Stamford, CT 06902; **Phone:** 203-348-9455; **Board Cert:** Internal Medicine 2010; **Med School:** Harvard Med Sch 1987; **Resid:** Internal Medicine, Jacobi Med Ctr 1990

Couture, Carolyn MD (IM) *PCP* - **Hospital:** Danbury Hosp; **Address:** Fairfield Co Primary Care, 396 Danbury Rd, Wilton, CT 06897; **Phone:** 203-276-4015; **Board Cert:** Internal Medicine 2005; **Med School:** Univ VT Coll Med 1992; **Resid:** Internal Medicine, Univ Rochester Strong Meml Hosp 1995

Dreyer, Neil P MD (IM) *PCP* - **Spec Exp:** Hypertension; Preventive Medicine; **Hospital:** Stamford Hosp (page 939); **Address:** PrimeCare Med, 1351 Washington Blvd Fl 4, Stamford, CT 06902; **Phone:** 203-327-1187; **Board Cert:** Internal Medicine 1980; Nephrology 1974; **Med School:** NYU Sch Med 1967; **Resid:** Internal Medicine, Jacobi Med Ctr 1972; **Fellow:** Nephrology, Montefiore Med Ctr 1974

Fennell, Gail M MD (IM) *PCP* - **Spec Exp:** Concierge Medicine; Hypertension; Cholesterol/Lipid Disorders; Women's Health; **Hospital:** Greenwich Hosp (page 938); **Address:** 75 Holly Hill Ln, Greenwich, CT 06830; **Phone:** 203-413-1130; **Board Cert:** Internal Medicine 2006; **Med School:** Univ Conn 1992; **Resid:** Internal Medicine, Greenwich Hosp 1995

Glazer, Steven MD (IM) *PCP* - **Spec Exp:** Concierge Medicine; **Hospital:** Norwalk Hosp, St. Vincent's Med Ctr - Bridgeport; **Address:** 128 East Ave, Norwalk, CT 06851; **Phone:** 203-852-1300; **Board Cert:** Internal Medicine 2004; **Med School:** Emory Univ 1991; **Resid:** Internal Medicine, Meml Sloan-Kettering Cancer Ctr 1995; **Fellow:** Internal Medicine, NY-Presby/Columbia Univ Med Ctr 1997

Hasapis, Peter G MD (IM) *PCP* - **Spec Exp:** Preventive Medicine; Concierge Medicine; **Hospital:** Norwalk Hosp; **Address:** New Canaan Medical Group, 173 East Ave, New Canaan, CT 06840; **Phone:** 203-972-4218; **Board Cert:** Internal Medicine 2011; **Med School:** Cornell Univ-Weill Med Coll 1997; **Resid:** Internal Medicine, NY-Presby/Weill Cornell Med Ctr 2000

Hoffman, Pamela B MD (IM) *PCP* - **Spec Exp:** Geriatric Care; **Address:** 200 Merritt St, Bridgeport, CT 06606-4201; **Phone:** 203-612-2378; **Board Cert:** Internal Medicine 1983; **Med School:** Univ VA Sch Med 1978; **Resid:** Internal Medicine, St Vincent's Hosp & Med Ctr 1981; **Fellow:** Geriatric Medicine, Jewish Inst Geriatric Care 1983

Horn, Jay A MD (IM) *PCP* - **Hospital:** Norwalk Hosp, Bridgeport Hosp; **Address:** Internal Med Assocs, 162 Kings Hwy N, Westport, CT 06880; **Phone:** 203-226-0731; **Board Cert:** Internal Medicine 1987; **Med School:** Albert Einstein Coll Med 1984; **Resid:** Internal Medicine, Montefiore Med Ctr 1987

Israel, Shara P MD (IM) *PCP* - **Hospital:** Stamford Hosp (page 939); **Address:** PrimeCare Med, 1351 Washington Blvd Fl 4, Stamford, CT 06902; **Phone:** 203-327-1187; **Board Cert:** Internal Medicine 2005; **Med School:** Columbia P&S 1992; **Resid:** Internal Medicine, NY-Presby/Columbia Univ Med Ctr 1995

Klein, Neil C MD (IM) - **Spec Exp:** Inflammatory Bowel Disease/Crohn's; Ulcerative Colitis; **Hospital:** Stamford Hosp (page 939), Norwalk Hosp; **Address:** Shoreline Medical Group, 1450 Washington Blvd, Stamford, CT 06902-2451; **Phone:** 203-327-9321; **Board Cert:** Internal Medicine 1974; Gastroenterology 1975; **Med School:** Cornell Univ-Weill Med Coll 1960; **Resid:** Internal Medicine, Presby/Weill Cornell Med Ctr 1964; **Fellow:** Gastroenterology, Presby/Weill Cornell Med Ctr 1967; **Fac Appt:** Clin Prof Med, Columbia P&S

Mayer, Deborah MD (IM) *PCP* - **Spec Exp:** Diabetes; Hypertension; **Hospital:** St. Vincent's Med Ctr - Bridgeport, Riverview Hosp for Chldrn & Youth; **Address:** 363 Reef Rd, Ste 2E, Fairfield, CT 06824; **Phone:** 203-255-0891; **Board Cert:** Internal Medicine 1981; **Med School:** Columbia P&S 1977; **Resid:** Internal Medicine, Beth Israel Deaconess Med Ctr 1980

Mickley, Diane W MD (IM) - **Spec Exp:** Eating Disorders; **Address:** Wilkins Ctr for Eating Disorders, 7 Riversville Rd Fl 3, Greenwich, CT 06831; **Phone:** 203-531-1909; **Board Cert:** Internal Medicine 1974; **Med School:** Tufts Univ 1971; **Resid:** Internal Medicine, Barnes West County Hosp 1973; Internal Medicine, Montefiore Med Ctr 1974; **Fac Appt:** Assoc Clin Prof Med, Yale Univ

Mickley, Steven P MD (IM) *PCP* - **Hospital:** Greenwich Hosp (page 938); **Address:** Glenville Med Assocs, 7 Riversville Rd Fl 1, Greenwich, CT 06831-3697; **Phone:** 203-531-1808; **Board Cert:** Internal Medicine 1974; **Med School:** Harvard Med Sch 1971; **Resid:** Internal Medicine, Barnes Hosp 1973; Internal Medicine, USPHS 1974; **Fac Appt:** Asst Clin Prof Med, Yale Univ

Miner III, Charles MD (IM) - **Hospital:** Stamford Hosp (page 939), Norwalk Hosp; **Address:** 36 Old Kings Hwy S, Darien, CT 06820-4523; **Phone:** 203-655-8749; **Board Cert:** Internal Medicine 1982; **Med School:** Univ Cincinnati 1979; **Resid:** Internal Medicine, Lenox Hill Hosp 1982

Molloy, Edward M MD (IM) *PCP* - **Spec Exp:** Hypertension; Diabetes; Preventive Medicine; **Hospital:** St. Vincent's Med Ctr - Bridgeport; **Address:** 134 Round Hill Rd, Fl 2, Fairfield, CT 06824; **Phone:** 203-255-0695; **Board Cert:** Internal Medicine 1974; **Med School:** UMDNJ-NJ Med Sch, Newark 1966; **Resid:** Internal Medicine, St Vincent's Hosp & Med Ctr 1972

Olin, Craig H MD (IM) *PCP* - **Spec Exp:** Preventive Medicine; **Hospital:** Stamford Hosp (page 939); **Address:** 5 High Ridge Park, Ste 103, Stamford, CT 06905; **Phone:** 203-276-4644; **Board Cert:** Internal Medicine 2006; **Med School:** NYU Sch Med 1993; **Resid:** Internal Medicine, NY-Presby/Weill Cornell Med Ctr 1996; **Fac Appt:** Asst Clin Prof Med, Columbia P&S

Osnoss, Kenneth MD (IM) *PCP* - **Spec Exp:** Asthma; Lung Disease; **Hospital:** Danbury Hosp; **Address:** Western CT Med Grp-Danbury, 79 Sand Pit Rd, Ste 102, Danbury, CT 06810-6099; **Phone:** 203-749-5700; **Board Cert:** Internal Medicine 1978; Pulmonary Disease 1980; **Med School:** Tufts Univ 1975; **Resid:** Internal Medicine, Hosp Univ Penn 1978; **Fellow:** Pulmonary Disease, Hosp Univ Penn 1980

Puglisi, Jeffrey S MD (IM) *PCP* - **Spec Exp:** Preventive Cardiology; Men's Health; **Hospital:** Greenwich Hosp (page 938); **Address:** Glenville Med Assocs, 7 Riversville Rd, Greenwich, CT 06831; **Phone:** 203-531-1808; **Board Cert:** Internal Medicine 2011; **Med School:** Hahnemann Univ 1998; **Resid:** Internal Medicine, Mount Sinai Med Ctr 2002

Radin, Alan M MD (IM) *PCP* - **Spec Exp:** Geriatric Medicine; **Hospital:** Norwalk Hosp; **Address:** Arbor Med Grp, 195 Danbury Rd, Whitlock Bldg, Ste 210, Wilton, CT 06897-3003; **Phone:** 203-762-3353; **Board Cert:** Internal Medicine 1977; **Med School:** Penn State Coll Med 1974; **Resid:** Internal Medicine, Univ Vermont Med Ctr 1978

Slogoff, Frederick B MD (IM) *PCP* - **Spec Exp:** Preventive Medicine; Cardiovascular Disease; Anxiety & Mood Disorders; **Hospital:** Stamford Hosp (page 939); **Address:** 5 High Ridge Park, Ste 104, Stamford, CT 06905; **Phone:** 203-968-9500; **Board Cert:** Internal Medicine 2009; **Med School:** Mount Sinai Sch Med 1996; **Resid:** Internal Medicine, NY-Presby/Weill Cornell Med Ctr 1999; **Fac Appt:** Clin Prof Med, Columbia P&S

Spano, Frank MD (IM) *PCP* - **Spec Exp:** Preventive Medicine; **Hospital:** Bridgeport Hosp, St. Vincent's Med Ctr - Bridgeport; **Address:** Fairfield County Medical Group, 15 Corporate Drive, Ste 2-1, Trumbull, CT 06611; **Phone:** 203-459-5100; **Board Cert:** Internal Medicine 1987; **Med School:** Albert Einstein Coll Med 1984; **Resid:** Internal Medicine, Jacobi Hosp 1987

Thomas, Byron S MD (IM) *PCP* - **Spec Exp:** Geriatric Care; **Hospital:** Danbury Hosp; **Address:** Danbury WCMG, Primary Care, 79 Sand Pit Rd, Ste 102, Danbury, CT 06810; **Phone:** 203-749-5700; **Board Cert:** Internal Medicine 1978; **Med School:** Univ Pittsburgh 1975; **Resid:** Internal Medicine, Mount Sinai Hosp 1978; **Fac Appt:** Asst Clin Prof Med, Yale Univ

Troy, Cathrine MD (IM) *PCP* - **Hospital:** Stamford Hosp (page 939); **Address:** Stamford Hlth Integrated, Primary Care, 51 Schuyler Ave, Stamford, CT 06902; **Phone:** 203-327-1187; **Board Cert:** Internal Medicine 1983; **Med School:** SUNY Downstate 1980; **Resid:** Internal Medicine, Brookdale Univ Hosp Med Ctr 1983

Walsh, Francis X MD (IM) *PCP* - **Spec Exp:** Kidney Disease; Hypertension; Dialysis Care; **Hospital:** Greenwich Hosp (page 938); **Address:** 31 River Rd, Ste 200, Cos Cob, CT 06807; **Phone:** 203-661-9433; **Board Cert:** Internal Medicine 1972; Nephrology 1974; **Med School:** NY Med Coll 1967; **Resid:** Internal Medicine, Greenwich Hosp 1970; **Fellow:** Nephrology, Duke Univ Med Ctr 1972; **Fac Appt:** Asst Clin Prof Med, Yale Univ

Zucker, Michael MD (IM) *PCP* - **Hospital:** Stamford Hosp (page 939); **Address:** PrimeCare Med, 555 Newfield Ave, Stamford, CT 06905-3330; **Phone:** 203-359-4444; **Board Cert:** Internal Medicine 1988; **Med School:** NYU Sch Med 1985; **Resid:** Internal Medicine, Stamford Hosp 1988

Interventional Cardiology

Driesman, Mitchell H MD (IC) - **Spec Exp:** Cardiac Catheterization; **Hospital:** Bridgeport Hosp; **Address:** Cardiac Specialists, 1305 Post Rd, Fairfield, CT 06824; **Phone:** 203-292-2000; **Board Cert:** Internal Medicine 1980; Cardiovascular Disease 1983; Interventional Cardiology 2009; **Med School:** Brown Univ 1977; **Resid:** Internal Medicine, Tufts-New Eng Med Ctr 1980; **Fellow:** Cardiovascular Disease, Mt Sinai Hosp 1983; **Fac Appt:** Asst Clin Prof Med, Yale Univ

Fishman, Robert F MD (IC) - **Spec Exp:** Carotid Artery Stent Placement; Peripheral Vascular Disease; **Hospital:** Bridgeport Hosp; **Address:** Cardiac Specialists, 1305 Post Rd, Fairfield, CT 06824; **Phone:** 203-292-2000; **Board Cert:** Internal Medicine 1988; Cardiovascular Disease 2011; Interventional Cardiology 2009; **Med School:** Boston Univ 1985; **Resid:** Internal Medicine, Beth Israel Hosp 1988; **Fellow:** Cardiovascular Disease, Beth Israel Hosp 1991

Howes, Christopher J MD (IC) - **Hospital:** Greenwich Hosp (page 938), Yale-New Haven Hosp; **Address:** 55 Holly Hill Ln, Ste 240, Cardiology Svcs of Greenwich, Greenwich, CT 06830; **Phone:** 203-863-4210; **Board Cert:** Internal Medicine 2002; Cardiovascular Disease 2007; Interventional Cardiology 2009; Echocardiography 2011; **Med School:** Albert Einstein Coll Med 1989; **Resid:** Internal Medicine, Yale-New Haven Hosp 1992; **Fellow:** Cardiovascular Disease, Yale-New Haven Hosp 1997; **Fac Appt:** Asst Prof Med, Yale Univ

Jumper, Robert MD (IC) - **Spec Exp:** Peripheral Vascular Disease; Nuclear Cardiology; Echocardiography; **Hospital:** St. Vincent's Med Ctr - Bridgeport; **Address:** Cardiology Assocs Fairfield Co, 115 Technology Drive, Ste C300, Trumbull, CT 06611; **Phone:** 203-445-7093; **Board Cert:** Cardiovascular Disease 2003; Interventional Cardiology 2004; Nuclear Cardiology 2005; Echocardiography 2006; **Med School:** NY Med Coll 1996; **Resid:** Internal Medicine, Jacobi Med Ctr 2000; **Fellow:** Cardiovascular Disease, Montefiore Med Ctr 2003; Interventional Cardiology, Montefiore Med Ctr 2004

Nero, Thomas J MD (IC) - **Spec Exp:** Sports Medicine-Cardiology; Preventive Cardiology; Echocardiography; **Hospital:** Stamford Hosp (page 939), Greenwich Hosp (page 938); **Address:** Cardiology Assocs of Fairfield County, 1177 Summer St Fl 5, Stamford, CT 06905; **Phone:** 203-353-1133; **Board Cert:** Cardiovascular Disease 2011; Interventional Cardiology 2012; **Med School:** Ohio State Univ 1994; **Resid:** Internal Medicine, Beth Israel Med Ctr 1998; **Fellow:** Cardiovascular Disease, Beth Israel Med Ctr 2001; Interventional Cardiology, Beth Israel Med Ctr 2002; **Fac Appt:** Assoc Clin Prof Med, Columbia P&S

Portnay, Edward L MD (IC) - **Spec Exp:** Heart Attack; **Hospital:** Stamford Hosp (page 939); **Address:** Cardiology Assocs Fairfield Co, 117 Summer St Fl 5, Stamford, CT 06905; **Phone:** 203-353-1133; **Board Cert:** Cardiovascular Disease 2005; Interventional Cardiology 2006; **Med School:** Tufts Univ 1997; **Resid:** Internal Medicine, NYU Med Ctr 2001; **Fellow:** Cardiovascular Disease, Yale-New Haven Hosp 2004; Interventional Cardiology, Yale-New Haven Hosp 2005

Selter, Jared MD (IC) - **Spec Exp:** Nuclear Cardiology; Peripheral Vascular Disease; Preventive Cardiology; **Hospital:** St. Vincent's Med Ctr - Bridgeport; **Address:** Cardiology Phys Fairfield Co, 115 Technology Drive, Ste C300, Trumbull, CT 06611; **Phone:** 203-445-7093; **Board Cert:** Cardiovascular Disease 2005; Interventional Cardiology 2006; Nuclear Cardiology 2005; **Med School:** Mount Sinai Sch Med 1998; **Resid:** Internal Medicine, Yale-New Haven Hosp 2001; **Fellow:** Cardiovascular Disease, Yale-New Haven Hosp 2005; Interventional Cardiology, Yale-New Haven Hosp 2006

Warshofsky, Mark MD (IC) - **Spec Exp:** Coronary Artery Disease; Heart Valve Disease; **Hospital:** Danbury Hosp, NY-Presby/Columbia Univ Med Ctr, NY (page 104); **Address:** Western CT Med Grp, 24 Hospital Ave, Fl 7, Danbury, CT 06810; **Phone:** 203-739-7436; **Board Cert:** Cardiovascular Disease 2007; Interventional Cardiology 2009; **Med School:** Geo Wash Univ 1990; **Resid:** Internal Medicine, Columbia-Presby Med Ctr 1993; **Fellow:** Cardiovascular Disease, Columbia-Presby Med Ctr 1996; Interventional Cardiology, Columbia-Presby Med Ctr 1998; **Fac Appt:** Asst Prof Med, Columbia P&S

Wasserman, Hal S MD (IC) - **Spec Exp:** Coronary Angioplasty/Stents; Heart Valve Disease; Coronary Artery Disease; **Hospital:** Danbury Hosp, NY-Presby/Columbia Univ Med Ctr, NY (page 104); **Address:** Western CT Med Grp, 24 Hospital Ave Fl 7, Danbury, CT 06810; **Phone:** 203-739-7600; **Board Cert:** Internal Medicine 1985; Cardiovascular Disease 1987; Interventional Cardiology 2009; **Med School:** Columbia P&S 1982; **Resid:** Internal Medicine, NY Presby/Columbia Univ Med Ctr 1985; **Fellow:** Cardiovascular Disease, NY Presby/Columbia Univ Med Ctr 1987; Interventional Cardiology, NY Presby/Columbia Univ Med Ctr 1988; **Fac Appt:** Assoc Clin Prof Med, Columbia P&S

Maternal & Fetal Medicine

Bobby, Paul D MD (MF) - **Spec Exp:** Pregnancy-High Risk; Prenatal Diagnosis; **Hospital:** Stamford Hosp (page 939); **Address:** Stamford Hosp, Dept Maternal/Fetal Med, 30 Shelburne Rd, Whittingham Pavilion, Stamford, CT 06902; **Phone:** 203-276-7172; **Board Cert:** Obstetrics & Gynecology 2012; Maternal & Fetal Medicine 2012; **Med School:** Boston Univ 1990; **Resid:** Obstetrics & Gynecology, NYU Langone Med Ctr 1995; **Fellow:** Maternal & Fetal Medicine, Montefiore Med Ctr 1997

Bond, Annette L MD (MF) - **Spec Exp:** Pregnancy-High Risk; Multiple Gestation; Prenatal Diagnosis; Hypertension in Pregnancy; **Hospital:** Greenwich Hosp (page 938); **Address:** Greenwich Hospital, 5 Perryridge Rd, rm 1-251, Greenwich, CT 06830; **Phone:** 203-863-3674; **Board Cert:** Obstetrics & Gynecology 2012; Maternal & Fetal Medicine 2012; **Med School:** Harvard Med Sch 1983; **Resid:** Obstetrics & Gynecology, NY Hosp-Cornell Med Ctr 1987; **Fellow:** Perinatal Medicine, NY Hosp-Cornell Med Ctr 1989

Dunston-Boone, Gina A MD (MF) - **Spec Exp:** Amniocentesis; Multiple Gestation; Diabetes in Pregnancy; **Hospital:** Bridgeport Hosp; **Address:** Park Ave Perinatal Specs, 267 Grant St Fl 5, Bridgeport, CT 06610; **Phone:** 203-384-3544; **Board Cert:** Obstetrics & Gynecology 2012; Maternal & Fetal Medicine 2012; **Med School:** Tufts Univ 1985; **Resid:** Obstetrics & Gynecology, NY-Presby/Weill Cornell Med Ctr 1992; **Fellow:** Maternal & Fetal Medicine, Thos Jefferson Univ Hosp 1995

Kim, Matthew J MD (MF) - **Spec Exp:** Fetal Ultrasound; Fetal Echocardiography; **Hospital:** Danbury Hosp; **Address:** Danbury, Maternal & Fetal Med-WCMG, 24 Hospital Ave Fl 2, Danbury, CT 06810; **Phone:** 203-739-7981; **Board Cert:** Obstetrics & Gynecology 2012; Maternal & Fetal Medicine 2012; **Med School:** Baylor Coll Med 1995; **Resid:** Obstetrics & Gynecology, Parkland Hlth & Hosp Sys 1999; **Fellow:** Maternal & Fetal Medicine, UCSD Med Ctr 2002

Laifer, Steven A MD (MF) - **Spec Exp:** Prenatal Diagnosis; **Hospital:** Bridgeport Hosp, Greenwich Hosp (page 938); **Address:** Park Ave Perinatal Specs, 267 Grant St Fl 5, Bridgeport, CT 06610; **Phone:** 203-384-3544; **Board Cert:** Obstetrics & Gynecology 2012; Maternal & Fetal Medicine 2012; **Med School:** SUNY Downstate 1982; **Resid:** Obstetrics & Gynecology, Johns Hopkins Hosp 1988; **Fellow:** Maternal & Fetal Medicine, Magee Womens Hosp 1991; **Fac Appt:** Asst Clin Prof ObG, Yale Univ

Shevell, Tracy MD (MF) - **Spec Exp:** Pregnancy-High Risk; Prenatal Diagnosis; **Hospital:** Stamford Hosp (page 939); **Address:** Advn Obstetrics & Gynecology, 30 Shelburne Rd, Whittingham Pavilion, Stamford, CT 06904; **Phone:** 203-276-7060; **Board Cert:** Obstetrics & Gynecology 2012; Maternal & Fetal Medicine 2012; **Med School:** Albert Einstein Coll Med 1997; **Resid:** Obstetrics & Gynecology, Mt Sinai Med Ctr 2002; **Fellow:** Maternal & Fetal Medicine, NY-Presby-Columbia Univ Med Ctr 2004

Stiller, Robert J MD (MF) - **Spec Exp:** Prenatal Diagnosis; Ultrasound; Pregnancy-High Risk; Infectious Disease in Pregnancy; **Hospital:** Bridgeport Hosp, Greenwich Hosp (page 938); **Address:** Park Ave Perinatal Specs, 267 Grant St Fl 5, Bridgeport, CT 06610; **Phone:** 203-384-3544; **Board Cert:** Obstetrics & Gynecology 2012; Maternal & Fetal Medicine 2012; **Med School:** UMDNJ-Rutgers Med Sch 1979; **Resid:** Obstetrics & Gynecology, Univ Conn Med Ctr 1983; **Fellow:** Maternal & Fetal Medicine, Pennsylvania Hosp-UPHS 1986; **Fac Appt:** Assoc Clin Prof ObG, Yale Univ

Medical Oncology

Abrams, Martin MD (Onc) - **Hospital:** Danbury Hosp; **Address:** Danbury WCMG, Hem/Onc, 95 Locust Ave Stroock Bldg Fl 1, Danbury, CT 06810; **Phone:** 203-739-7029; **Board Cert:** Internal Medicine 1983; Medical Oncology 1985; **Med School:** Tufts Univ 1980; **Resid:** Internal Medicine, St Elizabeths Hosp 1983; **Fellow:** Hematology & Oncology, Boston Med Ctr 1985

Angevine, Anne H MD (Onc) - **Spec Exp:** Lung Cancer; **Hospital:** Stamford Hosp (page 939); **Address:** Bennett Canc Ctr, Hematology-Oncology, 34 Shelburne Rd, Stamford, CT 06902; **Phone:** 203-325-2695; **Board Cert:** Internal Medicine 2003; Medical Oncology 2007; **Med School:** Columbia P&S 2000; **Resid:** Internal Medicine, Brigham & Women's Hosp 2003; **Fellow:** Hematology & Oncology, NY-Presby/Columbia Univ Med Ctr 2004

Cohenuram, Michael K MD (Onc) - **Spec Exp:** Solid Tumors; Hematologic Malignancies; Hematology; **Hospital:** Danbury Hosp, New Milford Hosp; **Address:** WCMG, Med Oncology, 95 Locust Ave, Strook Bldg - Fl 1, Danbury, CT 06810; **Phone:** 203-739-7029; **Board Cert:** Internal Medicine 2003; Medical Oncology 2008; Hematology 2009; **Med School:** Mount Sinai Sch Med 2000; **Resid:** Internal Medicine, Rhode Island Hosp 2003; **Fellow:** Hematology & Oncology, Yale-New Haven Hosp 2008; **Fac Appt:** Asst Clin Prof Med, Univ VT Coll Med

Delprete, Salvatore A MD (Onc) - **Spec Exp:** Lung Cancer; Ovarian Cancer; Melanoma; Colon Cancer; **Hospital:** Stamford Hosp (page 939); **Address:** Bennett Canc Ctr, Hematology-Oncology, 34 Shelburne Rd, Stamford, CT 06902-3658; **Phone:** 203-325-2695; **Board Cert:** Internal Medicine 1981; Medical Oncology 1985; Hematology 1986; **Med School:** SUNY Buffalo 1978; **Resid:** Internal Medicine, Dartmouth-Hitchcock Med Ctr 1981; **Fellow:** Pathology, Dartmouth-Hitchcock Med Ctr 1982; Hematology & Oncology, Dartmouth-Hitchcock Med Ctr 1984

Drucker, Beverly J MD/PhD (Onc) - **Spec Exp:** Breast Cancer; Head & Neck Cancer; Colon & Rectal Cancer; Clinical Trials; **Hospital:** Greenwich Hosp (page 938); **Address:** 77 Lafayette Pl, Ste 200, Greenwich, CT 06830; **Phone:** 203-863-3737; **Board Cert:** Medical Oncology 2009; **Med School:** Columbia P&S 1994; **Resid:** Internal Medicine, NY-Presby/Columbia Univ Med Ctr 1997; **Fellow:** Medical Oncology, Johns Hopkins Hosp 1999

Fischbach, Neal A MD (Onc) - **Spec Exp:** Breast Cancer; Lung Cancer; Colon Cancer; **Hospital:** Bridgeport Hosp, St. Vincent's Med Ctr - Bridgeport; **Address:** Oncology Assocs Bridgeport, 111 Beach Rd Fl 3, Fairfield, CT 06824; **Phone:** 203-255-2766; **Med School:** Harvard Med Sch 1995; **Resid:** Internal Medicine, UCSF Med Ctr 1998; **Fellow:** Hematology & Oncology, UCSF Med Ctr 2002

Folman, Robert S MD (Onc) - **Spec Exp:** Breast Cancer; Lung Cancer; Colon & Rectal Cancer; Genitourinary Cancer; **Hospital:** Bridgeport Hosp, St. Vincent's Med Ctr - Bridgeport; **Address:** Oncology Assocs of Bridgeport, 5520 Park Ave, Ste 203, Trumbull, CT 06611-1351; **Phone:** 203-502-8400; **Board Cert:** Internal Medicine 1975; Medical Oncology 1977; **Med School:** SUNY Buffalo 1972; **Resid:** Internal Medicine, Buffalo Gen Hosp 1975; **Fellow:** Medical Oncology, Meml Sloan Kettering Cancer Ctr 1977; **Fac Appt:** Asst Clin Prof Med, Yale Univ

Frank, Richard C MD (Onc) - **Spec Exp:** Leukemia; Lymphoma; **Hospital:** Norwalk Hosp; **Address:** Norwalk Hosp-Whittingham Canc Ctr, 24 Stevens St, Norwalk, CT 06856; **Phone:** 203-845-4899; **Board Cert:** Medical Oncology 2005; Hematology 2008; **Med School:** SUNY Stony Brook 1985; **Resid:** Internal Medicine, Columbia-Presby Med Ctr 1992; **Fellow:** Hematology & Oncology, Meml Sloan Kettering Cancer Ctr 1996

Hollister Jr, Dickerman MD (Onc) - **Spec Exp:** Breast Cancer; Lung Cancer; Colon Cancer; Leukemia & Lymphoma; **Hospital:** Greenwich Hosp (page 938); **Address:** 77 Lafayette Pl, Ste 200, Greenwich, CT 06830; **Phone:** 203-863-3737; **Board Cert:** Internal Medicine 1978; Hematology 1980; Medical Oncology 1981; **Med School:** Univ VA Sch Med 1975; **Resid:** Internal Medicine, NY-Presby/Weill Cornell Med Ctr 1978; **Fellow:** Hematology & Oncology, NY-Presby/Weill Cornell Med Ctr 1981; **Fac Appt:** Asst Clin Prof Med, Yale Univ

Kloss, Robert MD (Onc) - **Spec Exp:** Breast Cancer; Colon Cancer; Lung Cancer; **Hospital:** Danbury Hosp, New Milford Hosp; **Address:** Danbury WCMG, Hem/Onc, 95 Locust Ave Stroock Bldg Fl 1, Danbury, CT 06810-6010; **Phone:** 203-739-7029; **Board Cert:** Internal Medicine 1979; Medical Oncology 1981; Hospice & Palliative Medicine 2008; **Med School:** Jefferson Med Coll 1976; **Resid:** Internal Medicine, SUNY Buffalo Affil Hosp 1979; **Fellow:** Hematology & Oncology, NY-Presby/Columbia Univ Med Ctr 1981

Lee, Merlin Sung MD (Onc) - **Hospital:** Greenwich Hosp (page 938); **Address:** 77 Lafayette Pl, Ste 200, Greenwich, CT 06830; **Phone:** 203-863-3737; **Board Cert:** Hematology 2012; Medical Oncology 2012; **Med School:** NY Med Coll 1994; **Resid:** Internal Medicine, NY-Presby/Columbia Univ Med Ctr 1997; **Fellow:** Hematology & Oncology, NYU Med Ctr 2001

Lo, K.M. Steve MD (Onc) - **Spec Exp:** Breast Cancer; Lymphoma; **Hospital:** Stamford Hosp (page 939); **Address:** Bennett Canc Ctr, Hematology-Oncology, 34 Shelburne Rd, Stamford, CT 06902-3658; **Phone:** 203-325-2695; **Board Cert:** Internal Medicine 1989; Medical Oncology 2011; Hematology 2012; **Med School:** Harvard Med Sch 1985; **Resid:** Internal Medicine, Brigham & Women's Hosp 1988; **Fellow:** Hematology & Oncology, Dana-Farber Canc Inst 1991; Hematology, Dana-Farber Canc Inst 1992; **Fac Appt:** Asst Clin Prof Med, Columbia P&S

Malefatto, Jerry P MD (Onc) - **Spec Exp:** Breast Cancer; Colon Cancer; Lymphoma; **Hospital:** Bridgeport Hosp, St. Vincent's Med Ctr - Bridgeport; **Address:** Oncology Assocs of Bridgeport, 5520 Park Ave, Ste 203, Trumbull, CT 06611; **Phone:** 203-502-8400; **Board Cert:** Internal Medicine 1979; Medical Oncology 1983; **Med School:** Univ Conn 1976; **Resid:** Internal Medicine, UC Irvine/VA Med Ctr 1980; **Fellow:** Hematology & Oncology, UC Irvine/VA Med Ctr 1983

Tepler, Isidore MD (Onc) - **Spec Exp:** Breast Cancer; Gynecologic Cancer; **Hospital:** Stamford Hosp (page 939); **Address:** Bennett Canc Ctr, Hematology-Oncology, 34 Shelburne Rd, Stamford, CT 06902-3658; **Phone:** 203-325-2695; **Board Cert:** Internal Medicine 1984; Hematology 1986; Medical Oncology 1989; **Med School:** Harvard Med Sch 1980; **Resid:** Internal Medicine, Mass Genl Hosp 1983; **Fellow:** Hematology, Brigham & Women's Hosp 1984; Hematology & Oncology, Dana-Farber Canc Inst 1986; **Fac Appt:** Asst Clin Prof Med, Columbia P&S

Weinstein, Paul L MD (Onc) - **Spec Exp:** Breast Cancer; Lung Cancer; Colon Cancer; **Hospital:** Stamford Hosp (page 939); **Address:** Bennett Canc Ctr, Hematology-Oncology, 34 Shelburne Rd, Stamford, CT 06902-3628; **Phone:** 203-325-2695; **Board Cert:** Internal Medicine 1973; Medical Oncology 1977; Hematology 1978; **Med School:** Ros Franklin Univ/Chicago Med Sch 1970; **Resid:** Internal Medicine, Montefiore Med Ctr 1973; **Fellow:** Hematology & Oncology, Montefiore Med Ctr 1975; **Fac Appt:** Assoc Clin Prof Med, Columbia P&S

Zelkowitz, Richard S MD (Onc) - **Spec Exp:** Breast Cancer; Hematology; Bone Marrow Transplant; **Hospital:** Norwalk Hosp; **Address:** 40 Cross St, Norwalk, CT 06851; **Phone:** 203-845-4890; **Board Cert:** Internal Medicine 1986; Hematology 1988; Medical Oncology 1989; **Med School:** NY Med Coll 1983; **Resid:** Internal Medicine, Westchester Co Med Ctr 1986; **Fellow:** Hematology & Oncology, Brown Univ Hosps 1989

Neonatal-Perinatal Medicine

Herzlinger, Robert A MD (NP) - **Spec Exp:** Neonatology; **Hospital:** Bridgeport Hosp, Yale-New Haven Hosp; **Address:** Bridgeport Hosp, 267 Grant St, Ste 6, Bridgeport, CT 06610-2870; **Phone:** 203-384-3486; **Board Cert:** Pediatrics 1974; Neonatal-Perinatal Medicine 1977; **Med School:** NY Med Coll 1969; **Resid:** Pediatrics, Westchester Co Med Ctr 1971; Pediatrics, Columbia-Presby Med Ctr 1972; **Fellow:** Neonatal-Perinatal Medicine, Columbia-Presby Med Ctr 1973; Neonatal-Perinatal Medicine, Montefiore Med Ctr 1976; **Fac Appt:** Assoc Clin Prof Ped, Yale Univ

Rakos, Gerald B MD (NP) - **Hospital:** Stamford Hosp (page 939); **Address:** Stamford Hosp, Dept Pediatrics, 30 Shelburne Rd, Box 9317, Stamford, CT 06904; **Phone:** 203-276-7085; **Board Cert:** Pediatrics 1985; Neonatal-Perinatal Medicine 1985; **Med School:** SUNY Upstate Med Univ 1980; **Resid:** Pediatrics, UMass Meml Med Ctr 1983; **Fellow:** Neonatology, Montefiore Med Ctr 1985; **Fac Appt:** Asst Clin Prof Ped, Columbia P&S

Theofanidis, Stylianos MD (NP) - **Hospital:** Greenwich Hosp (page 938), Yale-New Haven Hosp; **Address:** Greenwich Hosp, Neonatology Dept, 5 Perryridge Rd, Greenwich, CT 06830; **Phone:** 203-863-3515; **Board Cert:** Neonatal-Perinatal Medicine 2011; **Med School:** Greece 1980; **Resid:** Pediatrics, St Lukes-Roosevelt Hosp 1985; **Fellow:** Neonatal-Perinatal Medicine, NY-Presby/Weill Cornell Med Ctr 1987; **Fac Appt:** Asst Clin Prof Ped, Yale Univ

Nephrology

Brown, Eric Y MD (Nep) - **Spec Exp:** Kidney Disease; Hypertension; Glomerulonephritis; **Hospital:** Stamford Hosp (page 939); **Address:** Stamford Hosp, Dept Nephrology, 30 Commerce Rd, Stamford, CT 06902-4550; **Phone:** 203-324-7666; **Board Cert:** Internal Medicine 1988; Nephrology 2010; **Med School:** Emory Univ 1985; **Resid:** Internal Medicine, Johns Hopkins Hosp 1988; **Fellow:** Nephrology, Yale-New Haven Hosp 1990; **Fac Appt:** Asst Clin Prof Med, Columbia P&S

Chan, Brenda MD (Nep) - **Spec Exp:** Dialysis Care; Kidney Failure-Chronic; Lupus Nephritis; Glomerulonephritis; **Hospital:** Stamford Hosp (page 939), Greenwich Hosp (page 938); **Address:** Stamford Hosp, Dept Nephrology, 30 Commerce Rd, Stamford, CT 06902; **Phone:** 203-324-7666; **Board Cert:** Nephrology 2007; **Med School:** Mount Sinai Sch Med 1990; **Resid:** Internal Medicine, Montefiore Med Ctr-Moses Campus 1993; **Fellow:** Nephrology, Montefiore Med Ctr-Moses Campus 1996

Feintzeig, Irwin D MD (Nep) - **Spec Exp:** Kidney Disease; Hypertension; Dialysis Care; **Hospital:** Bridgeport Hosp, St. Vincent's Med Ctr - Bridgeport; **Address:** Nephrology Assocs, 900 Madison Ave, Ste 209, Bridgeport, CT 06606-5534; **Phone:** 203-335-0195; **Board Cert:** Internal Medicine 1982; Nephrology 1984; **Med School:** Univ Chicago-Pritzker Sch Med 1979; **Resid:** Internal Medicine, Temple Univ Hosp 1982; **Fellow:** Nephrology, Boston Univ Med Ctr 1985; **Fac Appt:** Asst Clin Prof Med, Yale Univ

Fogel, Mitchell A MD (Nep) - **Spec Exp:** Kidney Disease-Chronic; Glomerulonephritis; Dialysis Care; **Hospital:** St. Vincent's Med Ctr - Bridgeport, Bridgeport Hosp; **Address:** Nephrology Assocs, 900 Madison Ave, Ste 209, Bridgeport, CT 06606; **Phone:** 203-335-0195; **Board Cert:** Internal Medicine 1986; Nephrology 1988; **Med School:** Univ Pennsylvania 1982; **Resid:** Internal Medicine, Boston Univ Med Ctr 1985; **Fellow:** Nephrology, Boston Univ Med Ctr 1988; **Fac Appt:** Med

Hines, William H MD (Nep) - **Spec Exp:** Dialysis Care; Hypertension; Kidney Disease; **Hospital:** Stamford Hosp (page 939); **Address:** Stamford Hosp, Dept Nephrology, 30 Commerce Rd, Stamford, CT 06902-4550; **Phone:** 203-324-7666; **Board Cert:** Internal Medicine 1984; Nephrology 1986; **Med School:** Cornell Univ-Weill Med Coll 1981; **Resid:** Internal Medicine, Hosp Univ Penn - UPHS 1984; **Fellow:** Nephrology, Hosp Univ Penn - UPHS 1988; **Fac Appt:** Assoc Clin Prof Med, Columbia P&S

Hunt, William A MD (Nep) - **Spec Exp:** Hypertension; Kidney Disease; **Hospital:** Bridgeport Hosp; **Address:** Nephrology Assocs, 900 Madison Ave, Ste 209, Bridgeport, CT 06606-5534; **Phone:** 203-335-0195; **Board Cert:** Internal Medicine 1984; Nephrology 1986; **Med School:** Yale Univ 1981; **Resid:** Internal Medicine, Univ Hosps Cleveland 1984

Neurological Surgery

Apostolides, Paul J MD (NS) - **Spec Exp:** Minimally Invasive Spinal Surgery; Spinal Surgery; **Hospital:** Greenwich Hosp (page 938), Stamford Hosp (page 939); **Address:** Orthopaedic & Neurosurgery Specialists, 6 Greenwich Office Park, 40 Valley Drive, Greenwich, CT 06831; **Phone:** 203-869-1145; **Board Cert:** Neurological Surgery 2013; **Med School:** Univ Mass Sch Med 1991; **Resid:** Neurological Surgery, Barrow Neuro Inst/St Joseph's Hosp 1998; **Fellow:** Spine Surgery, Barrow Neuro Inst/St Joseph's Hosp 1997

Camel, Mark W MD (NS) - **Spec Exp:** Brain Tumors; Spinal Surgery; Minimally Invasive Spinal Surgery; **Hospital:** Greenwich Hosp (page 938), Stamford Hosp (page 939); **Address:** Orthopaedic & Neurosurgery Specialists, 6 Greenwich Office Park, 40 Valley Drive, Greenwich, CT 06831; **Phone:** 203-869-1145 x616; **Board Cert:** Neurological Surgery 1990; **Med School:** Washington Univ, St Louis 1981; **Resid:** Neurological Surgery, Barnes Jewish Hosp 1986; **Fellow:** Neurological Surgery, Barnes Jewish Hosp 1987; **Fac Appt:** Asst Clin Prof NS, Cornell Univ-Weill Med Coll

Fiore, Amory J MD (NS) - **Spec Exp:** Minimally Invasive Spinal Surgery; Brain Tumors; **Hospital:** Greenwich Hosp (page 938), Stamford Hosp (page 939); **Address:** Orthopaedic and Neurosurgery Specialists, 6 Greenwich Office Park, 40 Valley Drive, Greenwich, CT 06831; **Phone:** 203-869-1145; **Board Cert:** Neurological Surgery 2006; **Med School:** Columbia P&S 1995; **Resid:** Neurological Surgery, NY-Presby/Columbia Univ Med Ctr 2001; **Fellow:** Spine Surgery, Emory Clinic 2002

Ghogawala, Zoher MD (NS) - **Spec Exp:** Minimally Invasive Spinal Surgery; Vascular Neurosurgery; Carotid Artery Surgery; Cerebrovascular Surgery; **Hospital:** Greenwich Hosp (page 938), Lahey Hosp & Med Ctr; **Address:** CSI-Greenwich Neurosurgery, 25 Valley Drive, Greenwich, CT 06831; **Phone:** 203-661-3333; **Board Cert:** Neurological Surgery 2004; **Med School:** Harvard Med Sch 1991; **Resid:** Neurological Surgery, Mass Genl Hosp 1999; **Fac Appt:** Assoc Prof NS, Tufts Univ

Lipow, Kenneth MD (NS) - **Spec Exp:** Spinal Surgery; Brain Tumors; Minimally Invasive Spinal Surgery; **Hospital:** Bridgeport Hosp, St. Vincent's Med Ctr - Bridgeport; **Address:** Connecticut Neurosurgical Specs, 267 Grant St Fl 8, Bridgeport, CT 06610; **Phone:** 203-384-4500; **Board Cert:** Neurological Surgery 1989; **Med School:** Albert Einstein Coll Med 1978; **Resid:** Surgery, Montefiore Med Ctr 1979; Neurological Surgery, Montefiore Med Ctr 1984

Mintz, Abraham MD (NS) - **Spec Exp:** Spinal Surgery; **Hospital:** St. Vincent's Med Ctr - Bridgeport, Bridgeport Hosp; **Address:** 5520 Park Ave, rm 210, Trumbull, CT 06611; **Phone:** 203-372-6460; **Board Cert:** Neurological Surgery 1992; **Med School:** Mexico 1982; **Resid:** Neurological Surgery, Jackson Meml Hosp 1989

Sanderson, Scott MD (NS) - **Spec Exp:** Spinal Tumors; Cerebrovascular Malformations; Spinal Cord Injury; **Hospital:** Danbury Hosp, Norwalk Hosp; **Address:** Neurological Assocs SW CT, 148 East Ave, Ste 3D, Norwalk, CT 06851; **Phone:** 203-853-0003; **Board Cert:** Neurological Surgery 2010; **Med School:** NYU Sch Med 1999; **Resid:** Neurological Surgery, NYU Med Ctr 2005; **Fellow:** Spine Surgery, NYU Med Ctr 2003; **Fac Appt:** Asst Clin Prof NS, NYU Sch Med

Shahid, Syed J MD (NS) - **Spec Exp:** Brain Tumors; Spinal Surgery; Spinal Tumors; **Hospital:** Danbury Hosp, Norwalk Hosp; **Address:** Neurosurgical Assocs, 148 East Ave, Ste 3D, Norwalk, CT 06851; **Phone:** 203-853-0003; **Board Cert:** Neurological Surgery 1983; **Med School:** Pakistan 1972; **Resid:** Surgery, Kings Co Hosp 1977; Neurological Surgery, Kings Co Hosp 1980

Shear, Perry MD (NS) - **Spec Exp:** Spinal Surgery; Pituitary Tumors; Cerebrovascular Surgery; **Hospital:** Bridgeport Hosp, St. Vincent's Med Ctr - Bridgeport; **Address:** Orthopaedic Specialty Grp, 75 Kings Hwy Cutoff, Fl 2, Fairfield, CT 06824; **Phone:** 203-337-2600; **Board Cert:** Neurological Surgery 1996; **Med School:** Univ Toronto 1984; **Resid:** Surgery, Toronto Genl Hosp 1985; Neurological Surgery, Ottawa Civic Hosp 1991

Simon, Scott L MD (NS) - **Spec Exp:** Spinal Surgery; Scoliosis; Stereotactic Radiosurgery; Minimally Invasive Spinal Surgery; **Hospital:** Stamford Hosp (page 939), Greenwich Hosp (page 938); **Address:** Orthopaedic & Neurosurgery Specialists, Tully Ctr, 32 Strawberry Hill Ct, Stamford, CT 06902; **Phone:** 203-487-0363; **Board Cert:** Neurological Surgery 2009; **Med School:** UMDNJ-RW Johnson Med Sch 1998; **Resid:** Neurological Surgery, Hosp Univ Penn - UPHS 2005; **Fellow:** Spine Surgery, Shriners Hosp for Chldn 2004

Zimmerman, Gary A MD (NS) - **Spec Exp:** Spinal Surgery; Cerebrovascular Surgery; Brain Tumors; **Hospital:** Bridgeport Hosp, St. Vincent's Med Ctr - Bridgeport; **Address:** Connecticut Neurosurgical Specs, 267 Grant St Fl 8, Bridgeport, CT 06610-2805; **Phone:** 203-384-4500; **Board Cert:** Neurological Surgery 2011; **Med School:** SUNY Downstate 1990; **Resid:** Neurological Surgery, NY-Presby/Weill Cornell Med Ctr 1996; **Fellow:** Cerebrovascular Disease, Univ Hosp 1997

Neurology

Butler, James B MD (N) - **Spec Exp:** Headache; Migraine; Huntington's Disease; Multiple Sclerosis; **Hospital:** Bridgeport Hosp, Griffin Hosp; **Address:** Neurological Specs, 4 Corporate Drive, Ste 192, Shelton, CT 06484; **Phone:** 203-924-8664; **Board Cert:** Internal Medicine 1982; Neurology 1987; **Med School:** Belgium 1979; **Resid:** Internal Medicine, Hosp St Raphael 1982; Neurology, Yale-New Haven Hosp 1985

Cuzzone, Louis J MD (N) - **Spec Exp:** Migraine; **Hospital:** Norwalk Hosp; **Address:** Neurology Assoc of Norwalk, 637 West Ave, Ste 200, Norwalk, CT 06850; **Phone:** 203-853-5000; **Board Cert:** Neurology 1980; **Med School:** Albert Einstein Coll Med 1975; **Resid:** Neurology, Montefiore Med Ctr 1979; **Fellow:** Electromyography, NYU Med Ctr 1980

Gross, Jeffrey L MD (N) - **Spec Exp:** Multiple Sclerosis; **Hospital:** St. Vincent's Med Ctr - Bridgeport, Milford Hosp; **Address:** Assoc Neurologists of Southern CT, 75 Kings Highway Cutoff Fl 5, Fairfield, CT 06824; **Phone:** 203-333-1133; **Board Cert:** Neurology 1985; **Med School:** Case West Res Univ 1978; **Resid:** Neurology, Hosp Univ Penn 1983; **Fellow:** Neuromuscular Disease, Hosp Univ Penn 1984

Litchman, Charisse D MD (N) - **Spec Exp:** Headache; Migraine; **Hospital:** Stamford Hosp (page 939); **Address:** 1250 Summer St, Ste 202, Stamford, CT 06905; **Phone:** 203-969-7662; **Board Cert:** Neurology 1993; **Med School:** Yale Univ 1988; **Resid:** Neurology, New York Hosp 1992; **Fac Appt:** Asst Clin Prof N, Columbia P&S

McAllister, Peter J MD (N) - **Spec Exp:** Headache; **Hospital:** St. Vincent's Med Ctr - Bridgeport, Bridgeport Hosp; **Address:** Assoc Neurologists of Southern CT, 75 Kings Hwy Cutoff, Fairfield, CT 06430; **Phone:** 203-333-1133; **Board Cert:** Neurology 2007; **Med School:** Univ Conn 1991; **Resid:** Neurology, Med Coll VA Hosps 1995; **Fellow:** Neuromuscular Disease, Med Coll VA Hosps 1996

Nahm, Frederick K MD/PhD (N) - **Spec Exp:** Cerebrovascular Disease; Stroke; **Hospital:** Greenwich Hosp (page 938); **Address:** NeuroCare Health, 49 Lake Ave, Ste LL3, Greenwich, CT 06830; **Phone:** 203-661-9383; **Board Cert:** Neurology 2003; **Med School:** Univ Mich Med Sch 1996; **Resid:** Neurology, Beth Israel Deaconess Med Ctr 2000; **Fellow:** Clinical Neurophysiology, Mass Genl Hosp 2001

Resor, Louise D MD (N) - **Hospital:** Stamford Hosp (page 939); **Address:** 166 W Broad St, Ste 203, Stamford, CT 06902; **Phone:** 203-376-4464; **Board Cert:** Neurology 1979; **Med School:** Washington Univ, St Louis 1974; **Resid:** Neurology, NY-Presby/Columbia Univ Med Ctr 1978; **Fellow:** Neurology, NY-Presby/Columbia Univ Med Ctr 1979

Rusk, Alice H MD (N) - **Spec Exp:** Movement Disorders; Parkinson's Disease; Dystonia; **Hospital:** Greenwich Hosp (page 938), Stamford Hosp (page 939); **Address:** Greenwich Neurology, 25 Valley Drive, Greenwich, CT 06831; **Phone:** 203-869-6446; **Board Cert:** Neurology 2006; **Med School:** Univ Conn 1991; **Resid:** Neurology, NY Hosp-Cornell Med Ctr 1995; **Fellow:** Clinical Neurophysiology, NY-Presby/Columbia Univ Med Ctr 1996

Story, Daryl MD (N) - **Spec Exp:** Stroke; Vascular Neurology; **Hospital:** Norwalk Hosp; **Address:** Neurology Assocs of Norwalk, 637 West Ave, Ste 200, Norwalk, CT 06850; **Phone:** 203-853-5000; **Board Cert:** Neurology 2012; Vascular Neurology 2008; **Med School:** NY Med Coll 1997; **Resid:** Neurology, Yale-New Haven Hosp 2001; **Fellow:** Stroke, Yale-New Haven Hosp 2002

Wirz, Diane MD (N) - **Spec Exp:** Headache; Migraine; **Hospital:** Danbury Hosp; **Address:** Associated Neurologists, 69 Sand Pit Rd, Ste 300, Danbury, CT 06810; **Phone:** 203-748-2551; **Board Cert:** Internal Medicine 1982; Neurology 1986; Headache Medicine 2008; **Med School:** Albany Med Coll 1979; **Resid:** Internal Medicine, Danbury Hosp 1982; Neurology, Univ Conn Hlth Ctr 1985

Neuroradiology

Sullivan, Scott J MD (NRad) - **Hospital:** Greenwich Hosp (page 938); **Address:** Greenwich Hosp-Dept Radiology, 5 Perryridge Rd, Greenwich, CT 06830; **Phone:** 203-863-3960; **Board Cert:** Diagnostic Radiology 1996; Neuroradiology 2004; **Med School:** Georgetown Univ 1991; **Resid:** Radiology, Yale-New Haven Hosp 1995; **Fellow:** Neuroradiology, Yale-New Haven Hosp 1996

Nuclear Medicine

Johns, William D MD (NuM) - **Spec Exp:** PET Imaging; **Hospital:** Danbury Hosp; **Address:** Danbury Hosp, Nuclear Med, 24 Hospital Ave, Danbury, CT 06810; **Phone:** 203-739-7222; **Board Cert:** Internal Medicine 1986; Nuclear Medicine 1988; **Med School:** Univ Conn 1983; **Resid:** Internal Medicine, Danbury Hosp 1986; Nuclear Medicine, Brigham & Womens Hosp 1988

Obstetrics & Gynecology

Ayoub, Thomas V MD (ObG) - **Spec Exp:** Menopause Problems; **Hospital:** Norwalk Hosp; **Address:** Women's Hlth Care New England, 761 Main Ave, Ste 100, Norwalk, CT 06851; **Phone:** 203-644-1100; **Board Cert:** Obstetrics & Gynecology 2012; **Med School:** NYU Sch Med 1980; **Resid:** Obstetrics & Gynecology, Bellevue Hosp 1984

Berger, Robin MD (ObG) - **Spec Exp:** Pregnancy-High Risk; **Hospital:** Bridgeport Hosp; **Address:** Women's Healthcare of Trumball, 5520 Park Ave, Ste 302, Trumbull, CT 06611; **Phone:** 203-374-1018; **Board Cert:** Obstetrics & Gynecology 2012; **Med School:** SUNY Downstate 1983; **Resid:** Obstetrics & Gynecology, Brookdale Hosp 1987

Besser, Gary S MD (ObG) - **Spec Exp:** Laparoscopic Surgery-Complex; Uro-Gynecology; Pelvic Surgery; Robotic Surgery; **Hospital:** Stamford Hosp (page 939), Greenwich Hosp (page 938); **Address:** Obstetrics & Gynecology Assocs, Whittingham Pavilion, 190 W Brand St, Ste G-401, Stamford, CT 06902-3661; **Phone:** 203-325-4321; **Board Cert:** Obstetrics & Gynecology 2012; **Med School:** SUNY Downstate 1982; **Resid:** Obstetrics & Gynecology, Stamford Hosp 1986; **Fac Appt:** Assoc Prof ObG, Columbia P&S

Blair, Emily E DO (ObG) - **Spec Exp:** Pregnancy-High Risk; **Hospital:** Bridgeport Hosp; **Address:** OB/GYN of Fairfield County, 1735 Post Rd, Ste 2A, Fairfield, CT 06824; **Phone:** 203-256-3990; **Board Cert:** Obstetrics & Gynecology 2012; **Med School:** Univ Osteo Med & Hlth Sci, Des Moines 1986; **Resid:** Obstetrics & Gynecology, Bridgeport Hosp 1990; **Fac Appt:** Assoc Prof ObG, Univ Conn

Bruck, Lance MD (ObG) - **Spec Exp:** Minimally Invasive Surgery; Gynecologic Surgery; **Hospital:** Stamford Hosp (page 939); **Address:** Stamford Hosp, Dept Ob/Gyn, 30 Shelburne Rd, Stamford, CT 06902; **Phone:** 203-276-7853; **Board Cert:** Obstetrics & Gynecology 2012; **Med School:** NY Med Coll 1992; **Resid:** Obstetrics & Gynecology, Montefiore Med Ctr 1997

Cahill, Patrick DO (ObG) - **Spec Exp:** Robotic Surgery; **Hospital:** Stamford Hosp (page 939); **Address:** Coastal Ob/Gyn, 999 Summer St, Ste 401, Stamford, CT 06905; **Phone:** 203-353-9099; **Board Cert:** Obstetrics & Gynecology 2012; **Med School:** NY Coll Osteo Med 1996; **Resid:** Obstetrics & Gynecology, Stamford Hosp 2000

Cutcri, Joseph A MD (ObG) - **Spec Exp:** Pregnancy-High Risk; Colposcopy; Ultrasound; **Hospital:** Bridgeport Hosp; **Address:** Shelton OB/GYN, 4 Corporate Drive, Ste 286, Shelton, CT 06484; **Phone:** 203-929-9000; **Board Cert:** Obstetrics & Gynecology 2012; **Med School:** Mexico 1984; **Resid:** Obstetrics & Gynecology, Brooklyn Hosp 1987; Obstetrics & Gynecology, Bridgeport Hosp 1990; **Fac Appt:** Asst Clin Prof ObG, Yale Univ

Deal, Robert Campbell MD (ObG) *PCP* - **Spec Exp:** Laparoscopic Surgery; Menopause Problems; Robotic Surgery; **Hospital:** Bridgeport Hosp; **Address:** Womens Hlth Care, 115 Technology Drive, Ste A100, Trumbull, CT 06611; **Phone:** 203-880-5556; **Board Cert:** Obstetrics & Gynecology 2012; **Med School:** Georgetown Univ 1990; **Resid:** Obstetrics & Gynecology, Bridgeport Hosp 1994; **Fac Appt:** Asst Clin Prof ObG, Yale Univ

Donovan, Leslie MD (ObG) - **Spec Exp:** Adolescent Gynecology; Menopause Problems; Sexually Transmitted Diseases; Gynecology Only; **Hospital:** Greenwich Hosp (page 938); **Address:** Brookside Gynecology, 159 W Putnam Ave, Greenwich, CT 06830; **Phone:** 203-869-7080; **Board Cert:** Obstetrics & Gynecology 2012; **Med School:** Univ Mass Sch Med 1993; **Resid:** Obstetrics & Gynecology, St Joseph's Med Ctr 1999

Ferrucci, Leonard MD (ObG) - **Hospital:** Stamford Hosp (page 939); **Address:** 833 Summer St, Ste 1B, Stamford, CT 06901; **Phone:** 203-325-4665; **Board Cert:** Obstetrics & Gynecology 2012; **Med School:** NY Med Coll 1987; **Resid:** Obstetrics & Gynecology, Stamford Hosp 1990

Ferrucci, Vito MD (ObG) - **Hospital:** Stamford Hosp (page 939); **Address:** 833 Summer St, Ste 1B, Stamford, CT 06901; **Phone:** 203-325-4665; **Board Cert:** Obstetrics & Gynecology 2011; **Med School:** NY Med Coll 1985; **Resid:** Obstetrics & Gynecology, Stamford Hosp 1989

Filor, Caroline MD (ObG) - **Spec Exp:** Robotic Surgery; Minimally Invasive Surgery; Pain-Pelvic; Endometriosis; **Hospital:** Greenwich Hosp (page 938); **Address:** Brookside Gynecology, 159 W Putnam Ave Fl 2, Greenwich, CT 06830; **Phone:** 203-869-7080; **Board Cert:** Obstetrics & Gynecology 2012; **Med School:** NY Med Coll 1998; **Resid:** Obstetrics & Gynecology, Univ Conn Hlth Ctr 2000; Obstetrics & Gynecology, RWJ Univ Hosp 2002

Garrett, Leila MD (ObG) - **Spec Exp:** Menopause Problems; Pap Smear Abnormalities; Sexually Transmitted Diseases; Adolescent Gynecology; **Hospital:** Greenwich Hosp (page 938); **Address:** Greenwich Gynecology, 1 Perryridge Rd, Greenwich, CT 06830; **Phone:** 203-869-8353; **Board Cert:** Obstetrics & Gynecology 2012; **Med School:** Univ Rochester 1990; **Resid:** Obstetrics & Gynecology, Univ VT Coll Med 1994

Geer-Yan, Lisa MD (ObG) *PCP* - **Hospital:** Norwalk Hosp; **Address:** Fairfield Women's Health Center, 140 Sherman St Fl 5, Fairfield, CT 06824; **Phone:** 203-658-8291; **Board Cert:** Obstetrics & Gynecology 2007; **Med School:** SUNY Upstate Med Univ 2001; **Resid:** Obstetrics & Gynecology, Thomas Jefferson Univ Hosp 2005

Ghofrany, Shieva L MD (ObG) - **Hospital:** Stamford Hosp (page 939); **Address:** Coastal OB & GYN, 999 Summer St, Ste 401, Stamford, CT 06905; **Phone:** 203-353-9099; **Board Cert:** Obstetrics & Gynecology 2012; **Med School:** Israel 1999; **Resid:** Obstetrics & Gynecology, Stamford Hosp 2003

Hagberg, Donna J MD (ObG) - **Spec Exp:** Gynecology Only; **Hospital:** Greenwich Hosp (page 938); **Address:** Greenwich Gynecology, One Perryridge Rd, Greenwich, CT 06830; **Phone:** 203-869-8353; **Board Cert:** Obstetrics & Gynecology 2012; **Med School:** Univ Rochester 1989; **Resid:** Internal Medicine, Yale-New Haven Hosp 1990; Obstetrics & Gynecology, Yale-New Haven Hosp 1993

Hines, Brian J MD (ObG) - **Spec Exp:** Uro-Gynecology; Incontinence; Pelvic Organ Prolapse Repair; **Hospital:** Stamford Hosp (page 939), Bridgeport Hosp; **Address:** 1351 Washington Blvd, Ste 201, Stamford, CT 06902; **Phone:** 203-391-6620; **Board Cert:** Obstetrics & Gynecology 2012; **Med School:** Boston Univ 1996; **Resid:** Obstetrics & Gynecology, Mt Sinai Med Ctr 2000; **Fellow:** Uro-Gynecology, NYU Langone Med Ctr 2002; **Fac Appt:** Asst Prof Med, Columbia P&S

Jacobson, Edward MD (ObG) - **Spec Exp:** Gynecology Only; Gynecologic Surgery; **Hospital:** Greenwich Hosp (page 938); **Address:** Greenwich Gynecology, One Perryridge Rd, Greenwich, CT 06830; **Phone:** 203-869-8353; **Board Cert:** Obstetrics & Gynecology 1981; **Med School:** NY Med Coll 1975; **Resid:** Obstetrics & Gynecology, NY-Presby/Cornell Med Ctr 1979

Kerr, Alicia MD (ObG) - **Spec Exp:** Ultrasound; Pregnancy-High Risk; **Hospital:** Norwalk Hosp; **Address:** Womens Hlth CT, 761 Main Ave B Bldg - Ste 100, Norwalk, CT 06851; **Phone:** 203-644-1100; **Board Cert:** Obstetrics & Gynecology 2012; **Med School:** Ohio State Univ 1997; **Resid:** Obstetrics & Gynecology, Stamford Hosp 2001

Kleinman, Gary Eleazar MD (ObG) - **Spec Exp:** Pregnancy-High Risk; Genetic Disorders; **Hospital:** Bridgeport Hosp, Greenwich Hosp (page 938); **Address:** Park Ave Perinatal Specs, 267 Grant St, Bridgeport, CT 06610-2805; **Phone:** 203-384-3544; **Board Cert:** Obstetrics & Gynecology 1984; Maternal & Fetal Medicine 1985; Clinical Genetics 2010; **Med School:** Creighton Univ 1977; **Resid:** Obstetrics & Gynecology, Georgetown Univ Hosp 1981; **Fellow:** Maternal & Fetal Medicine, UCLA Medical Center 1983; Clinical Genetics, LAC Harbor-UCLA Med Ctr 1992

Komarynsky, Irene I MD (ObG) - **Spec Exp:** Maternal & Fetal Medicine; **Hospital:** Stamford Hosp (page 939); **Address:** 166 W Broad St, Ste 301, Stamford, CT 06902; **Phone:** 203-325-9920; **Board Cert:** Obstetrics & Gynecology 2012; **Med School:** Univ Chicago-Pritzker Sch Med 1979; **Resid:** Obstetrics & Gynecology, Hosp Univ Penn - UPHS 1983; **Fellow:** Maternal & Fetal Medicine, Univ IL Med Ctr 1985

Rivera, Jeanette MD (ObG) - **Spec Exp:** Uro-Gynecology; Pelvic Reconstruction; Pelvic Organ Prolapse Repair; **Hospital:** Danbury Hosp; **Address:** Urology Assocs of Danbury, 51-53 Kenosia Ave, Danbury, CT 06810; **Phone:** 203-267-4035; **Board Cert:** Obstetrics & Gynecology 2013; Female Pelvic Medicine & Reconstuctive Surgery 2013; **Med School:** Univ Conn 2000; **Resid:** Obstetrics & Gynecology, NYU Med Ctr 2004; **Fellow:** Uro-Gynecology, NYU Med Ctr 2007

Rohr, Michele MD (ObG) - **Spec Exp:** Pelvic Reconstruction; Pap Smear Abnormalities; Laparoscopic Surgery; Vulvar & Vaginal Disorders; **Hospital:** Greenwich Hosp (page 938); **Address:** Brookside Gynecology, 159 W Putnam Ave Fl 2, Greenwich, CT 06830; **Phone:** 203-869-7080; **Board Cert:** Obstetrics & Gynecology 2012; **Med School:** Washington Univ, St Louis 1996; **Resid:** Obstetrics & Gynecology, Univ Chicago Univ Med Ctr 2000

Samuelson, Robert MD (ObG) - **Spec Exp:** Minimally Invasive Surgery; Robotic Surgery; **Hospital:** Danbury Hosp; **Address:** Danbury, Ob/Gyn-WCMG, 24 Hospital Ave, Danbury, CT 06810; **Phone:** 203-739-4900; **Board Cert:** Obstetrics & Gynecology 2012; **Med School:** Grenada 1985; **Resid:** Obstetrics & Gynecology, Hartford Hosp 1988; **Fellow:** Pelvic Surgery, Lahey Clinic 1991

Schechter, Michael D MD (ObG) - **Hospital:** Greenwich Hosp (page 938); **Address:** Putnam Gynecology & Obstetrics, 500 W Putnam Ave, Greenwich, CT 06830; **Phone:** 203-622-0303; **Board Cert:** Obstetrics & Gynecology 2012; **Med School:** NYU Sch Med 1988; **Resid:** Obstetrics & Gynecology, St Lukes-Roosevelt Hosp 1992

Szeto, Marjorie MD (ObG) - **Spec Exp:** Pregnancy-High Risk; **Hospital:** Norwalk Hosp; **Address:** Avery Ctr for Ob/Gyn, 12 Avery Pl, Westport, CT 06880; **Phone:** 203-227-5125; **Board Cert:** Obstetrics & Gynecology 2012; **Med School:** NYU Sch Med 1985; **Resid:** Obstetrics & Gynecology, Beth Israel Med Ctr 1989

Torbey, Marina C MD (ObG) - **Spec Exp:** Laparoscopic Surgery; Pregnancy-High Risk; **Hospital:** Bridgeport Hosp; **Address:** Women's Healthcare of Trumball, 5520 Park Ave, Ste 302, Trumbull, CT 06611; **Phone:** 203-374-1018; **Board Cert:** Obstetrics & Gynecology 2012; **Med School:** Univ Kansas 1985; **Resid:** Obstetrics & Gynecology, Montefiore-Weiler Med Ctr 1989; **Fac Appt:** Asst Prof ObG, Albert Einstein Coll Med

Ugol, Jay H MD (ObG) - **Hospital:** Norwalk Hosp; **Address:** Women's Hlth Care New England, 761 Main Ave, Ste 100, Norwalk, CT 06851; **Phone:** 203-644-1100; **Board Cert:** Obstetrics & Gynecology 2012; **Med School:** Georgetown Univ 1982; **Resid:** Obstetrics & Gynecology, Univ Colorado Hlth Sci Ctr 1986

Violi, Caterina MD (ObG) - **Spec Exp:** Endometriosis; Pelvic Organ Prolapse Repair; Pregnancy-High Risk; Laparoscopic Surgery-Complex; **Hospital:** Greenwich Hosp (page 938); **Address:** 2 1/2 Dearfield Drive, Ste 101, Greenwich, CT 06831; **Phone:** 203-861-9586; **Board Cert:** Obstetrics & Gynecology 2012; **Med School:** Univ Rochester 1994; **Resid:** Obstetrics & Gynecology, Winthrop Univ Hosp 1998

Weinstein, David B MD (ObG) - **Spec Exp:** Pregnancy-High Risk; **Hospital:** Stamford Hosp (page 939); **Address:** Stamford Hosp, Whittingham Pavilion, 190 W Broad St, Ste G-401, Stamford, CT 06902; **Phone:** 203-325-4321; **Board Cert:** Obstetrics & Gynecology 2013; **Med School:** Univ Hlth Scis, Chicago Med Sch 1969; **Resid:** Obstetrics & Gynecology, New York Hosp 1974

Ophthalmology

Altman, Bruce S MD (Oph) - **Spec Exp:** Glaucoma; **Hospital:** Danbury Hosp; **Address:** Danbury Eye Phys & Surgeons, 69 Sand Pit Rd, Ste 101, Danbury, CT 06810; **Phone:** 203-791-2020; **Board Cert:** Ophthalmology 2003; **Med School:** Univ Pennsylvania 1986; **Resid:** Ophthalmology, Hahnemann Hosp 1991; **Fellow:** Glaucoma, Barnes-Jewish W Co Hosp 1992; Research, Scheie Eye Inst 1988

Conway Jr, Joseph L MD (Oph) - **Spec Exp:** Oculoplastic Surgery; **Hospital:** Greenwich Hosp (page 938); **Address:** Greenwich Ophthalmology Assocs, 4 Dearfield Drive, Greenwich, CT 06831; **Phone:** 203-869-3082; **Board Cert:** Ophthalmology 2006; **Med School:** Penn State Coll Med 1998; **Resid:** Orthopaedic Surgery, Penn State Hershey Med Ctr 2000; Ophthalmology, NYU/Manhattan Eye Ear & Throat Hosp 2003; **Fellow:** Oculoplastic Surgery, NY-Presby/Weill Cornell Med Ctr 2004

DeBroff, Brian M MD (Oph) - **Spec Exp:** Refractive Surgery; Cataract Surgery; Cataract-Pediatric; Anterior Segment Surgery; **Hospital:** Yale-New Haven Hosp, Bridgeport Hosp; **Address:** Eye Surgery Assocs, 495 Hawley Ln, Stratford, CT 06614; **Phone:** 203-375-5819; **Board Cert:** Ophthalmology 2005; **Med School:** Tufts Univ 1989; **Resid:** Ophthalmology, Univ Pittsburg/Eye & Ear Inst 1993; **Fellow:** Anterior Segment - External Disease, Gimbel Eye Ctr 1994; **Fac Appt:** Assoc Clin Prof Oph, Yale Univ

Doctor, Leslie MD (Oph) - **Spec Exp:** Cataract Surgery; Anterior Segment Surgery; Refractive Surgery; **Hospital:** Yale-New Haven Hosp; **Address:** 129 Kings Hwy N, Westport, CT 06880; **Phone:** 203-227-4113; **Board Cert:** Ophthalmology 2008; **Med School:** Ohio State Univ 1989; **Resid:** Ophthalmology, OH State Univ Med Ctr 1993; **Fellow:** Cornea & Ext Eye Disease, OH State Univ Med Ctr 1994

Driesman, Shelley MD (Oph) - **Spec Exp:** Cataract Surgery; Contact Lenses; Glaucoma; **Hospital:** Bridgeport Hosp; **Address:** Ophthalmic Surgeons-Greater Bridgeport, 2371 Black Rock Tpke, Fairfield, CT 06825; **Phone:** 203-371-0141; **Board Cert:** Ophthalmology ; **Med School:** Brown Univ 1980; **Resid:** Ophthalmology, Lenox Hill Hosp 1984

Finlay, Alexis E MD (Oph) - **Spec Exp:** Refractive Surgery; Cataract Surgery; Corneal Disease & Surgery; Lens Implants; **Hospital:** Greenwich Hosp (page 938); **Address:** 38 B Grove St, Lower Floor, Ridgefield, CT 06877; **Phone:** 203-403-3375; **Board Cert:** Ophthalmology 1989; **Med School:** Hahnemann Univ 1981; **Resid:** Ophthalmology, NY Eye and Ear Infirmary 1985; **Fellow:** Ophthalmic Pathology, Johns Hopkins Hosp 1986

Gewirtz, Joan MD (Oph) - **Spec Exp:** Cataract Surgery; Glaucoma; Dry Eye Syndrome; **Hospital:** Stamford Hosp (page 939); **Address:** 70 Mill River St, Ste LL3, Stamford, CT 06902; **Phone:** 203-348-0868; **Board Cert:** Ophthalmology 2010; **Med School:** SUNY Downstate 1980; **Resid:** Ophthalmology, Lenox Hill Hosp 1987; **Fellow:** Ophthalmology, NY-Presby/Weill Cornell Med Ctr 1983

Gladstein, Gina F MD (Oph) - **Spec Exp:** Glaucoma; Cataract Surgery; **Hospital:** Greenwich Hosp (page 938); **Address:** Greenwich Ophthalmology Assocs, 4 Dearfield Drive, Greenwich, CT 06831; **Phone:** 203-869-3082; **Board Cert:** Ophthalmology 1989; **Med School:** Albert Einstein Coll Med 1983; **Resid:** Ophthalmology, Manhattan EE&T Hosp 1987; **Fellow:** Ophthalmology, Manhattan EE&T Hosp 1988

Kaplan, Jeffrey N MD (Oph) - **Spec Exp:** Corneal Disease; Cataract Surgery; Lens Implants; **Hospital:** Bridgeport Hosp; **Address:** Eye Grp of Connecticut, 4699 Main St, Ste 106, Bridgeport, CT 06606; **Phone:** 203-374-8182; **Board Cert:** Ophthalmology 1987; **Med School:** SUNY Stony Brook 1981; **Resid:** Ophthalmology, SUNY Downstate Med Ctr 1985; **Fellow:** Cornea, Dubroff Eye Ctr 1986

Mandava, Suresh MD (Oph) - **Spec Exp:** LASIK-Refractive Surgery; Cataract Surgery; Cornea Transplant; Cornea & External Eye Disease; **Hospital:** Greenwich Hosp (page 938); **Address:** Greenwich Ophthalmology Assocs, 4 Dearfield Drive, Greenwich, CT 06831; **Phone:** 203-869-3082; **Board Cert:** Ophthalmology 2009; **Med School:** Yale Univ 1993; **Resid:** Ophthalmology, Manhattan EE&T 1997; **Fellow:** Cornea & Refractive Surgery, Univ Minnesota Med Ctr 1998

Manjoney, Delia MD (Oph) - **Spec Exp:** Cataract Surgery; Glaucoma; Eyelid Cosmetic Surgery; **Hospital:** St. Vincent's Med Ctr - Bridgeport; **Address:** 2720 Main St Fl 3, Bridgeport, CT 06606; **Phone:** 203-576-6500; **Board Cert:** Pediatrics 1982; Ophthalmology 1988; **Med School:** Univ VT Coll Med 1977; **Resid:** Pediatrics, Parkland Hosp/Chldns Med Ctr 1980; Ophthalmology, Colum Presby Med Ctr/Harkness 1986

Mathias, Stephen Audley MD (Oph) - **Spec Exp:** Pediatric Ophthalmology; Eye Muscle Disorders; **Hospital:** Danbury Hosp; **Address:** 69 Sand Pit Rd, Ste 101, Danbury Eye Physicians, Danbury, CT 06810-4005; **Phone:** 203-791-2020; **Board Cert:** Ophthalmology 1987; **Med School:** Univ Cincinnati 1982; **Resid:** Ophthalmology, Columbia Presby Med Ctr 1986; **Fellow:** Pediatrics, Columbia Presby Med Ctr 1987

Musto, Anthony MD (Oph) - **Spec Exp:** Cataract Surgery-Lens Implant; Eyelid Surgery; Diabetic Eye Disease/Retinopathy; **Hospital:** Bridgeport Hosp; **Address:** Eye Surgery Assocs, 495 Hawley Ln, Stratford, CT 06614; **Phone:** 203-375-5819; **Board Cert:** Ophthalmology 1975; **Med School:** Georgetown Univ 1968; **Resid:** Ophthalmology, USPHS 1971; Ophthalmology, Manhattan EE&T Infirm 1973; **Fac Appt:** Asst Clin Prof Oph, Yale Univ

Ostriker, Glenn E MD (Oph) - **Spec Exp:** Cataract Surgery; Glaucoma; **Hospital:** Stamford Hosp (page 939); **Address:** 71 Strawberry Hill Ave, Ste 116, Stamford, CT 06902; **Phone:** 203-348-6300; **Board Cert:** Ophthalmology 1987; **Med School:** NYU Sch Med 1982; **Resid:** Ophthalmology, NYU Langone Med Ctr 1986; **Fellow:** Neurophysiology, NYU Langone Med Ctr 1983; **Fac Appt:** Assoc Clin Prof Oph, NYU Sch Med

Paul, Matthew D MD (Oph) - **Spec Exp:** Cataract Surgery; **Hospital:** Danbury Hosp; **Address:** Danbury Eye Phys & Surgeons, 69 Sand Pit Rd, Ste 101, Danbury, CT 06810; **Phone:** 203-791-2020; **Board Cert:** Ophthalmology 1985; **Med School:** Columbia P&S 1980; **Resid:** Ophthalmology, NY-Presby/Columbia Univ Med Ctr 1984

Pinke, James MD (Oph) - **Spec Exp:** Cataract Surgery; Glaucoma; Lens Implants; **Hospital:** Griffin Hosp; **Address:** 9 Cots St, Shelton, CT 06484-3866; **Phone:** 203-924-8800; **Board Cert:** Ophthalmology 1983; **Med School:** Tufts Univ 1978; **Resid:** Ophthalmology, Tufts Med Ctr 1982

Piro, Philip A MD (Oph) - **Hospital:** Stamford Hosp (page 939); **Address:** 3070 Main St, Bridgeport, CT 06610; **Phone:** 203-367-7348; **Board Cert:** Ophthalmology 1986; **Med School:** Columbia P&S 1978; **Resid:** Ophthalmology, Johns Hopkins Hosp 1982; **Fellow:** Ophthalmology, Johns Hopkins Hosp 1982; Ophthalmology, LAC & USC Med Ctr 1983

Potter, William S MD (Oph) - **Spec Exp:** Pediatric Ophthalmology; Strabismus-Adult & Pediatric; Lens Implants; Amblyopia; **Hospital:** Greenwich Hosp (page 938), Stamford Hosp (page 939); **Address:** Greenwich Ophthalmology Assocs, 4 Dearfield Drive, Greenwich, CT 06831; **Phone:** 203-869-3082; **Board Cert:** Ophthalmology 1991; **Med School:** NY Med Coll 1985; **Resid:** Ophthalmology, NY E&E Infirmary 1989; **Fellow:** Strabismus, Wills Eye Hosp 1990

Rabinowitz, Stephen M MD (Oph) - **Spec Exp:** Cataract Surgery; Glaucoma; Dry Eye Syndrome; Lens Implants; **Hospital:** Bridgeport Hosp; **Address:** Ophthalmic Surgeons Grtr Bridgeport, 2371 Black Rock Tpke, Fairfield, CT 06825; **Phone:** 203-371-0141; **Board Cert:** Ophthalmology 1990; **Med School:** NYU Sch Med 1984; **Resid:** Ophthalmology, Lenox Hill Hosp 1988; **Fellow:** Cornea & Ext Eye Disease, Bascom Palmer Eye Inst 1989

Reppucci, Vincent S MD (Oph) - **Spec Exp:** Retinal Disorders; Diabetic Eye Disease; Macular Disease/Degeneration; **Hospital:** Danbury Hosp, New York Eye & Ear Infirm (page 115); **Address:** 65 North St, Danbury, CT 06810; **Phone:** 203-792-6291; **Board Cert:** Ophthalmology 1989; **Med School:** Albert Einstein Coll Med 1983; **Resid:** Ophthalmology, NY-Presby/Columbia Univ Med Ctr 1987; **Fellow:** Retina/Vitreous Surgery, NY-Presby/Weill Cornell Med Ctr 1988; **Fac Appt:** Assoc Prof Oph, Cornell Univ-Weill Med Coll

Robbins, Kim P MD (Oph) - **Spec Exp:** Cataract Surgery; **Hospital:** Bridgeport Hosp; **Address:** Robbins Eye Ctr, 4695 Main St, Bridgeport, CT 06606; **Phone:** 203-371-5800; **Board Cert:** Ophthalmology 1985; **Med School:** NY Med Coll 1978; **Resid:** Internal Medicine, Stamford Hosp 1980; Ophthalmology, St Vincents Hosp 1983

Scartozzi, Richard MD (Oph) - **Spec Exp:** Macular Degeneration; Diabetic Eye Disease/Retinopathy; Retinal Detachment; Uveitis; **Hospital:** Danbury Hosp, Yale-New Haven Hosp; **Address:** Danbury Eye Physicians & Surgeons, 69 Sand Pit Rd, Ste 101, Danbury, CT 06810; **Phone:** 203-791-2020; **Board Cert:** Ophthalmology 2007; **Med School:** Johns Hopkins Univ 2002; **Resid:** Ophthalmology, Wills Eye Hosp 2006; **Fellow:** Retina/Vitreous Surgery, LAC-USC Med Ctr 2008

Siderides, Elizabeth MD (Oph) - **Spec Exp:** Cataract Surgery; **Hospital:** Stamford Hosp (page 939); **Address:** Stamford Ophthalmology, 1351 Washington Blvd, Ste 101, Stamford, CT 06902-2453; **Phone:** 203-327-5808; **Board Cert:** Ophthalmology 1991; **Med School:** Columbia P&S 1985; **Resid:** Ophthalmology, NYU Langone Med Ctr 1989; **Fellow:** Medical Retina, NYU Langone Med Ctr 1990

Vietorisz, Esteban MD (Oph) - **Spec Exp:** Corneal & External Eye Disease; Cataract Surgery; Glaucoma; **Hospital:** Stamford Hosp (page 939); **Address:** Stamford Ophthalmology, 1351 Washington Blvd, Ste 101, Stamford, CT 06902; **Phone:** 203-327-5808; **Board Cert:** Ophthalmology 2008; **Med School:** Cornell Univ-Weill Med Coll 1991; **Resid:** Ophthalmology, NY-Presby/Weill Cornell Med Ctr 1997; **Fellow:** Cornea, Duke Univ Hosp 1998

Wasserman, Eric L MD (Oph) - **Spec Exp:** Cataract Surgery; Glaucoma; **Hospital:** Stamford Hosp (page 939); **Address:** Eye Care Ctr, 1275 Summer St, Ste 200, Stamford, CT 06905-5315; **Phone:** 203-978-0800; **Board Cert:** Ophthalmology 1988; **Med School:** NY Med Coll 1979; **Resid:** Ophthalmology, NY Med Coll Affil Hosp 1983; **Fellow:** Anterior Segment - External Disease, John H Sheets Eye Fdn 1984

Weber, Richard B MD (Oph) - **Spec Exp:** Retinal Disorders; **Hospital:** Stamford Hosp (page 939), Greenwich Hosp (page 938); **Address:** 1275 Summer St, Ste 103, Stamford, CT 06905; **Phone:** 203-353-1857; **Board Cert:** Internal Medicine 1979; Ophthalmology 1985; **Med School:** Albert Einstein Coll Med 1976; **Resid:** Internal Medicine, Jacobi Med Ctr 1979; Ophthalmology, Mass Eye & Ear Infirmary 1984; **Fellow:** Retina, Mass Eye & Ear Infirmary 1985

Orthopaedic Surgery

Awad, John N MD (OrS) - **Spec Exp:** Osteoporosis Spine- Kyphoplasty; Spinal Tumors; **Hospital:** Bridgeport Hosp; **Address:** Orthopaedic Specialty Grp, 75 Kings Hway Cutoff Fl 2, Fairfield, CT 06824; **Phone:** 203-337-2600; **Board Cert:** Orthopaedic Surgery 2007; **Med School:** UMDNJ-RW Johnson Med Sch 1999; **Resid:** Orthopaedic Surgery, Johns Hopkins Hosp 2004; **Fellow:** Spine Surgery, New York Univ Med Ctr 2005

Bellapianta, Joseph M MD (OrS) - **Spec Exp:** Sports Medicine; Knee Injuries; Shoulder Injuries; Arthroscopic Surgery; **Hospital:** Greenwich Hosp (page 938); **Address:** Plancher Orthopaedics & Sports Medicine, 31 River Rd, Ste 100, Cos Cob, CT 06807; **Phone:** 203-863-2003; **Board Cert:** Orthopaedic Surgery 2012; **Med School:** Albany Med Coll 2004; **Resid:** Orthopaedic Surgery, Albany Med Ctr 2009; **Fellow:** Sports Medicine, Andrews Inst 2010

Bindelglass, David F MD (OrS) - **Spec Exp:** Arthritis; Minimally Invasive Surgery; Hip Replacement; Knee Replacement; **Hospital:** Bridgeport Hosp; **Address:** Orthopaedic Specialty Grp, 75 Kings Hwy Cutoff Fl 2, Fairfield, CT 06824; **Phone:** 203-337-2600; **Board Cert:** Orthopaedic Surgery 2005; **Med School:** Columbia P&S 1985; **Resid:** Surgery, Beth Israel Hosp 1987; Orthopaedic Surgery, Columbia-Presby Med Ctr 1990; **Fellow:** Joint Replacement Surgery, Kerlan-Jobe Ortho Clin 1991

Bomback, David Aaron MD (OrS) - **Spec Exp:** Scoliosis; **Hospital:** Danbury Hosp; **Address:** CT Neck & Back Specialists, 20 Germantown Rd, Ste 2, Danbury, CT 06810; **Phone:** 203-744-9700; **Board Cert:** Orthopaedic Surgery 2007; **Med School:** Columbia P&S 1999; **Resid:** Orthopaedic Surgery, Yale-New Haven Hosp 2004; **Fellow:** Spine Surgery, Hosp Special Surgery 2005

Boone, Peter S MD (OrS) - **Spec Exp:** Sports Medicine; Knee Replacement; Hip Replacement; **Hospital:** St. Vincent's Med Ctr - Bridgeport; **Address:** Orthopaedic & Sports Medicine Ctr, 888 White Plains Rd, Trumbull, CT 06611; **Phone:** 203-268-2882; **Board Cert:** Orthopaedic Surgery 2005; **Med School:** Univ Pennsylvania 1985; **Resid:** Orthopaedic Surgery, UMDNJ Med Ctr 1991; **Fellow:** Joint Replacement Surgery, IN Univ Med Ctr 1992

Brittis, Dante A MD (OrS) - **Spec Exp:** Sports Medicine; Shoulder & Knee Surgery; Pediatric Sports Medicine; Joint Replacement; **Hospital:** Bridgeport Hosp; **Address:** Orthopaedic Specialty Grp, 75 Kings Hwy Cutoff Fl 2, Fairfield, CT 06824; **Phone:** 203-337-2600; **Board Cert:** Orthopaedic Surgery 2008; **Med School:** NY Med Coll 1987; **Resid:** Orthopaedic Surgery, NY-Presby/Columbia Univ Med Ctr 1993; **Fellow:** Sports Medicine, Lenox Hill Hosp 1994

Brown, David B MD (OrS) - **Spec Exp:** Spinal Surgery; Shoulder Surgery; Rotator Cuff Surgery; **Hospital:** Bridgeport Hosp; **Address:** Orthocare Specialists, 4747 Main St, Bridgeport, CT 06606-1804; **Phone:** 203-372-0649; **Board Cert:** Orthopaedic Surgery 2007; **Med School:** St Louis Univ 1974; **Resid:** Surgery, George Washington Univ Sch Med 1977; Orthopaedic Surgery, Long Island Jewish Med Ctr 1981

Clain, Michael R MD (OrS) - **Spec Exp:** Foot & Ankle Surgery; Sports Medicine; **Hospital:** Greenwich Hosp (page 938); **Address:** Orthopaedic & Neurosurgery Specialists, 6 Greenwich Office Park, 10 Valley Drive, Greenwich, CT 06831; **Phone:** 203-869-1145; **Board Cert:** Orthopaedic Surgery 2004; **Med School:** Columbia P&S 1984; **Resid:** Orthopaedic Surgery, Lenox Hill Hosp 1990; **Fellow:** Foot & Ankle Surgery, Baylor Coll Med 1991

Cunningham, James G MD (OrS) - **Spec Exp:** Arthroscopic Surgery; Shoulder Surgery; Knee Injuries/ACL; Sports Medicine; **Hospital:** Greenwich Hosp (page 938); **Address:** Orthopaedic & Neurosurgery Specialists, 6 Greenwich Office Park, 10 Valley Drive, Greenwich, CT 06831; **Phone:** 203-869-1145; **Board Cert:** Orthopaedic Surgery 2012; Orthopaedic Sports Medicine 2007; **Med School:** NYU Sch Med 1983; **Resid:** Orthopaedic Surgery, Mt Sinai Med Ctr 1988; Surgery, Mt Sinai Med Ctr 1984; **Fellow:** Sports Medicine, New England Baptist Hosp 1989

D'Amico, Joseph M MD (OrS) - **Spec Exp:** Knee Replacement; Hip Replacement; Sports Medicine; **Hospital:** Stamford Hosp (page 939); **Address:** Orthopaedic Assocs, 90 Morgan St Fl 2 - Ste 207, Stamford, CT 06905-5436; **Phone:** 203-325-4087; **Board Cert:** Orthopaedic Surgery 2003; **Med School:** E Tenn State Univ 1982; **Resid:** Orthopaedic Surgery, St. Luke's - Roosevelt Hosp Ctr - St Luke's Hosp 1988

Deluca, Jeffrey V MD (OrS) - **Spec Exp:** Arthroscopic Surgery; Knee Replacement; **Hospital:** Norwalk Hosp; **Address:** Coastal Orthopaedics, 40 Cross St, Ste 300, Norwalk, CT 06851-2439; **Phone:** 203-845-2200; **Board Cert:** Orthopaedic Surgery 2005; **Med School:** Temple Univ 1984; **Resid:** Orthopaedic Surgery, Eastern Virginia Med Sch 1991; **Fellow:** Orthopaedic Trauma Surgery, Boston Med Ctr 1987; Sports Medicine & Arthroscopic Surgery, Washington Ortho & Knee Clin 1992

Ennis Jr, Francis A MD (OrS) - **Spec Exp:** Hip & Knee Replacement; **Hospital:** Greenwich Hosp (page 938); **Address:** Orthopaedic & Neurosurgery Specialists, 6 Greenwich Office Park, 10 Valley Drive, Greenwich, CT 06831; **Phone:** 203-869-1145; **Board Cert:** Orthopaedic Surgery 2007; **Med School:** Duke Univ 1999; **Resid:** Orthopaedic Surgery, Yale-New Haven Hosp 2004; **Fellow:** Reconstructive Surgery, New England Baptist Hosp 2005

FitzGibbons, James J MD (OrS) - **Spec Exp:** Arthroscopic Surgery; Joint Replacement; Sports Medicine; **Hospital:** St. Vincent's Med Ctr - Bridgeport; **Address:** Orthopaedic Specialty Grp, 75 Kings Hwy Cutoff Fl 2, Fairfield, CT 06824-5340; **Phone:** 203-337-2600; **Board Cert:** Orthopaedic Surgery 2011; **Med School:** Loyola Univ-Stritch Sch Med 1992; **Resid:** Orthopaedic Surgery, Northwestern Meml Hosp 1997; **Fellow:** Orthopaedic Sports Medicine, Harvard Univ/Mass Genl Hosp 1998

Henshaw, D. Ross MD (OrS) - **Spec Exp:** Shoulder Surgery; Rotator Cuff Surgery; Sports Medicine; Knee Surgery; **Hospital:** Danbury Hosp; **Address:** Danbury Orthopaedic Assocs, 73 Sand Pit Rd, Ste 204, Danbury, CT 06810; **Phone:** 203-797-1500 x9604; **Board Cert:** Orthopaedic Surgery 2007; Orthopaedic Sports Medicine 2008; **Med School:** Columbia P&S 1998; **Resid:** Orthopaedic Surgery, NY-Presby/Columbia Univ Med Ctr 2003; **Fellow:** Sports Medicine & Shoulder Surgery, Hosp Special Surgery 2005

Hermele, Herbert I MD (OrS) - **Hospital:** Bridgeport Hosp, St. Vincent's Med Ctr - Bridgeport; **Address:** Orthopaedic Specialty Grp, 75 Kings Hwy Cutoff Fl 2, Fairfield, CT 06824-5340; **Phone:** 203-337-2600; **Board Cert:** Orthopaedic Surgery 1975; **Med School:** Albert Einstein Coll Med 1969; **Resid:** Orthopaedic Surgery, Albert Einstein Affil Hosps 1975

Hindman, Steven MD (OrS) - **Spec Exp:** Sports Injuries; Arthritis; Fractures; **Hospital:** Greenwich Hosp (page 938); **Address:** Orthopaedic & Neurosurgery Specialists, 6 Greenwich Office Park, 10 Valley Drive, Greenwich, CT 06831-5151; **Phone:** 203-869-1145; **Board Cert:** Orthopaedic Surgery 2010; **Med School:** Albert Einstein Coll Med 1982; **Resid:** Orthopaedic Surgery, Montefiore Med Ctr 1987

Hughes, Peter W MD (OrS) - **Spec Exp:** Hip Replacement; Knee Replacement; Sports Medicine; **Hospital:** Stamford Hosp (page 939); **Address:** Orthopaedic Assocs, 90 Morgan St Fl 2 - Ste 207, Stamford, CT 06905; **Phone:** 203-325-4087; **Board Cert:** Orthopaedic Surgery 1978; **Med School:** NY Med Coll 1972; **Resid:** Orthopaedic Surgery, Metropolitan Hosp Ctr 1976; **Fellow:** Surgery, Hosp for Special Surg 1977

Kavanagh, Brian MD (OrS) - **Spec Exp:** Hip Replacement; Knee Replacement; Arthritis; **Hospital:** Greenwich Hosp (page 938); **Address:** Orthopaedic & Neurosurgery Specialists, 6 Greenwich Office Park, 10 Valley Drive, Greenwich, CT 06831; **Phone:** 203-869-1145; **Board Cert:** Orthopaedic Surgery 2007; **Med School:** Univ Conn 1979; **Resid:** Orthopaedic Surgery, Mayo Clinic 1984; **Fac Appt:** Asst Clin Prof OrS, Yale Univ

Kramer, David Lawrence MD (OrS) - **Spec Exp:** Spinal Surgery; Trauma; **Hospital:** Danbury Hosp; **Address:** CT Neck & Back Specialists, 20 Germantown Rd, Ste 2, Danbury, CT 06810; **Phone:** 203-744-9700; **Board Cert:** Orthopaedic Surgery 2009; **Med School:** Dartmouth Med Sch 1989; **Resid:** Orthopaedic Surgery, Mass Genl Hosp 1994; Orthopaedic Surgery, Beth Israel Deaconess Med Ctr 1994; **Fellow:** Reconstructive Surgery, Inselspital-Maurice E Muller 1995; Spine Surgery, Thomas Jefferson Univ Hosp 1996

Lynch, Michael M MD (OrS) - **Spec Exp:** Arthroscopic Surgery; Sports Medicine; Knee Replacement; **Hospital:** Stamford Hosp (page 939), Norwalk Hosp; **Address:** Coastal Orthopaedics, 40 Cross St, Ste 300, Norwalk, CT 06851-4646; **Phone:** 203-845-2200; **Board Cert:** Orthopaedic Surgery 2005; **Med School:** Dartmouth Med Sch 1984; **Resid:** Orthopaedic Surgery, Mass Genl Hosp 1990; Pediatric Orthopaedic Surgery, Chldns Hosp 1991; **Fellow:** Sports Medicine, Union Meml Hosp 1992

McGinniss, George H MD (OrS) - **Hospital:** Stamford Hosp (page 939); **Address:** Orthopaedic Surgery & Sports Med, 1290 Summer St Ste 4400, Stamford, CT 06905-5331; **Phone:** 203-323-7331; **Board Cert:** Orthopaedic Surgery 2010; **Med School:** Georgetown Univ 1978; **Resid:** Orthopaedic Surgery, Mt Sinai Med Ctr 1983; **Fellow:** Knee Surgery, Cincinnati Sports Med & Orthopaedic Ctr 1984

Miller, Seth R MD (OrS) - **Spec Exp:** Shoulder Surgery; Rotator Cuff Surgery; Sports Medicine; Shoulder Replacement; **Hospital:** Greenwich Hosp (page 938), NYU Hosp For Joint Dis (page 108); **Address:** Orthopaedic & Neurosurgery Specialists, 6 Greenwich Office Park, 10 Valley Drive, Greenwich, CT 06831; **Phone:** 203-869-1145; **Board Cert:** Orthopaedic Surgery 2012; **Med School:** Mount Sinai Sch Med 1982; **Resid:** Surgery, Mt Sinai Hosp 1985; Orthopaedic Surgery, Columbia-Presby Med Ctr 1988; **Fellow:** Shoulder Surgery, Columbia-Presby Med Ctr 1989; **Fac Appt:** Assoc Prof S, NYU Sch Med

Nocek, David MD (OrS) - **Spec Exp:** Hip & Knee Replacement; Shoulder Injuries; **Hospital:** Greenwich Hosp (page 938); **Address:** Orthopaedic & Neurosurgery Specialists, 6 Greenwich Office Park Fl 3, Greenwich, CT 06631; **Phone:** 203-869-1145; **Board Cert:** Orthopaedic Surgery 2009; **Med School:** NY Med Coll 1981; **Resid:** Orthopaedic Surgery, St Lukes Hosp 1986

Polifroni, Nicholas V MD (OrS) - **Spec Exp:** Sports Medicine; Joint Replacement; **Hospital:** Norwalk Hosp; **Address:** Coastal Orthopaedics, 40 Cross St, Ste 300, Norwalk, CT 06851; **Phone:** 203-845-2200; **Board Cert:** Orthopaedic Surgery 1984; **Med School:** NY Med Coll 1977; **Resid:** Orthopaedic Surgery, Lenox Hill Hosp 1982

Sethi, Paul MD (OrS) - **Spec Exp:** Sports Medicine; Knee Injuries; Shoulder Injuries; Fractures; **Hospital:** Greenwich Hosp (page 938); **Address:** Orthopaedic & Neurosurgery Specialists, 6 Greenwich Office Park, 10 Valley Drive, Greenwich, CT 06831; **Phone:** 203-869-1145; **Board Cert:** Orthopaedic Surgery 2005; Orthopaedic Sports Medicine 2007; **Med School:** Mount Sinai Sch Med 1997; **Resid:** Orthopaedic Surgery, Yale-New Haven Hosp 2002; **Fellow:** Sports Medicine, Kerlan Jobe Ortho Clin 2003; Arthroscopic Surgery, Kerlan Jobe Ortho Clin 2004

Spak, James I MD (OrS) - **Spec Exp:** Sports Medicine; **Hospital:** St. Vincent's Med Ctr - Bridgeport; **Address:** Orthopaedic & Sports Med Ctr, 888 White Plains Rd, Trumbull, CT 06611; **Phone:** 203-268-2882; **Board Cert:** Orthopaedic Surgery 2011; Orthopaedic Sports Medicine 2010; **Med School:** Harvard Med Sch 1992; **Resid:** Orthopaedic Surgery, Brigham & Women's Hosp 1997; **Fellow:** Sports Medicine, Tahoe Fracture & Ortho Cl 1999

Stovell, Peter B MD (OrS) - **Spec Exp:** Joint Replacement; Sports Medicine; **Hospital:** Norwalk Hosp; **Address:** Coastal Orthopaedics, 40 Cross St, Ste 300, Norwalk, CT 06851-5726; **Phone:** 203-845-2200; **Board Cert:** Orthopaedic Surgery 1976; **Med School:** Columbia P&S 1968; **Resid:** Surgery, St Luke's-Roosevelt Hosp Ctr 1970; Orthopaedic Surgery, Hosp for Special Surgery 1975

Troy, Allen I MD (OrS) - **Spec Exp:** Foot & Ankle Surgery; Sports Medicine; **Hospital:** Stamford Hosp (page 939); **Address:** Orthopaedic Assocs, 90 Morgan St Fl 2 - Ste 207, Stamford, CT 06905; **Phone:** 203-325-4087; **Board Cert:** Orthopaedic Surgery 2010; **Med School:** SUNY Downstate 1979; **Resid:** Orthopaedic Surgery, NYU Langone Med Ctr 1984; **Fellow:** Foot & Ankle Surgery, NYU Hosp For Joint Diseases 1985

Wilchinsky, Mark MD (OrS) - **Spec Exp:** Arthroscopic Surgery; Joint Replacement; **Hospital:** St. Vincent's Med Ctr - Bridgeport, Griffin Hosp; **Address:** Orthopaedic & Sports Medicine Ctr, 888 White Plains Rd, Trumbull, CT 06611; **Phone:** 203-268-2882; **Board Cert:** Orthopaedic Surgery 2007; **Med School:** Tulane Univ 1979; **Resid:** Orthopaedic Surgery, Univ Mass Med Ctr 1984; **Fac Appt:** Asst Prof OrS, Univ Mass Sch Med

Otolaryngology

Aferzon, Mark MD (Oto) - **Spec Exp:** Allergy; Nasal & Sinus Disorders; Snoring/Sleep Apnea; Thyroid & Parathyroid Surgery; **Hospital:** Griffin Hosp; **Address:** 2 Ivy Brook Road, Ste 110, Shelton, CT 06484; **Phone:** 203-954-0019; **Board Cert:** Otolaryngology 2013; **Med School:** Brown Univ 1997; **Resid:** Surgery, SUNY Upstate Med Univ 1999; Otolaryngology, Geisinger Med Ctr 2002

Bard, Michael C MD (Oto) - **Spec Exp:** Head & Neck Surgery; Sleep Disorders/Apnea; Sinus Disorders/Surgery; **Hospital:** Danbury Hosp; **Address:** Advanced Specialty Care, ENT, 107 Newtown Rd, Ste 2A, Danbury, CT 06810; **Phone:** 203-830-4700; **Board Cert:** Otolaryngology 1993; **Med School:** Mount Sinai Sch Med 1987; **Resid:** Otolaryngology, Mayo Clin 1992; **Fellow:** Head and Neck Surgery, Inst Laryngology & Otology 1993

Bianchi, Mark S MD (Oto) - **Spec Exp:** Sleep Disorders; Sinus Disorders/Surgery; Hearing Loss; Balance Disorders; **Hospital:** Bridgeport Hosp, Yale-New Haven Hosp; **Address:** Yale Otolaryngology, 2874 Main St, Stratford, CT 06615; **Phone:** 203-459-8330; **Board Cert:** Otolaryngology 1997; Sleep Medicine 2012; **Med School:** Yale Univ 1991; **Resid:** Otolaryngology, Yale-New Haven Hosp 1996; **Fac Appt:** Asst Prof Oto, Yale Univ

Bramwit, Steven A MD (Oto) - **Spec Exp:** Head & Neck Surgery; Nasal & Sinus Disorders; **Hospital:** Stamford Hosp (page 939); **Address:** Stamford ENT, 166 W Broad St, Ste 304, Stamford, CT 06902; **Phone:** 203-348-7797; **Board Cert:** Otolaryngology 2012; **Med School:** Columbia P&S 1995; **Resid:** Surgery, NY-Presby/Columbia Univ Med Ctr 1997; Otolaryngology, NY-Presby/Columbia Univ Med Ctr 2001

Brauer, Richard J MD (Oto) - **Spec Exp:** Head & Neck Surgery; Thyroid Cancer; **Hospital:** Greenwich Hosp (page 938); **Address:** 49 Lake Ave, Ste 205, Greenwich, CT 06830; **Phone:** 203-869-0177; **Board Cert:** Otolaryngology 1981; **Med School:** Hahnemann Univ 1976; **Resid:** Otolaryngology, Bellevue Hosp Ctr 1980; **Fellow:** Head and Neck Surgery, Montefiore Med Ctr 1982

Breda, Stephen D MD (Oto) - **Spec Exp:** Head & Neck Surgery; **Hospital:** St. Vincent's Med Ctr - Bridgeport; **Address:** 4695 Main St, Ste 1, Bridgeport, CT 06606; **Phone:** 203-371-5166; **Board Cert:** Otolaryngology 1988; **Med School:** NYU Sch Med 1983; **Resid:** Otolaryngology, NYU Med Ctr 1988; **Fellow:** Head and Neck Surgery, NYU Med Ctr 1988

Chervin, Bradford S MD (Oto) - **Spec Exp:** Swallowing Disorders; Endoscopy; Sinus Disorders; **Hospital:** Bridgeport Hosp, Norwalk Hosp; **Address:** ENT, Allergy & Facial Plastic Surg Spec, 2600 Post Rd, Southport, CT 06890; **Phone:** 203-256-3338; **Board Cert:** Otolaryngology 2000; **Med School:** Geo Wash Univ 1993; **Resid:** Surgery, Univ of TN Coll of Med 1995; Otolaryngology, Univ of TN Coll of Med 1999

Feldman, Steven MD (Oto) - **Spec Exp:** Throat Disorders; Hearing Disorders; Snoring/Sleep Apnea; **Hospital:** Greenwich Hosp (page 938); **Address:** 4 Dearfield Drive, Ste 104, Greenwich, CT 06831; **Phone:** 203-629-5500; **Board Cert:** Otolaryngology 1998; **Med School:** Albert Einstein Coll Med 1992; **Resid:** Otolaryngology, Montefiore Med Ctr 1994

Gordon, Neil A MD (Oto) - **Spec Exp:** Cosmetic Surgery-Face; **Hospital:** Norwalk Hosp, Yale-New Haven Hosp; **Address:** Split Rock Surgical Assocs, 539 Danbury Rd, Wilton, CT 06897; **Phone:** 203-661-1715; **Board Cert:** Otolaryngology 1996; Facial Plastic & Reconstr Surgery 1998; **Med School:** Albert Einstein Coll Med 1990; **Resid:** Otolaryngology, Yale-New Haven Hosp 1995; **Fellow:** Facial Plastic Surgery, Tulane Univ Med Ctr 1996

Klarsfeld, Jay MD (Oto) - **Spec Exp:** Sinus Disorders; Thyroid & Parathyroid Surgery; **Hospital:** Danbury Hosp, New Milford Hosp; **Address:** Advanced Specialty Care, ENT, 107 Newtown Rd, Ste 2A, Danbury, CT 06810; **Phone:** 203-830-4700; **Board Cert:** Otolaryngology 1986; **Med School:** Mount Sinai Sch Med 1981; **Resid:** Surgery, Mount Sinai Med Ctr 1983; Otolaryngology, Mount Sinai Med Ctr 1986

Klenoff, Bruce H MD (Oto) - **Spec Exp:** Ear Disorders/Surgery; Sinus Disorders/Surgery; Pediatric Otolaryngology; **Hospital:** Stamford Hosp (page 939); **Address:** ENT Ctr - Tully Hlth Ctr, 32 Strawberry Hill Ct, Fl 4 - Ste 4, Stamford, CT 06902; **Phone:** 203-353-0000; **Board Cert:** Otolaryngology 1976; **Med School:** Tufts Univ 1969; **Resid:** Surgery, Steward St Elizabeth's Med Ctr 1973; Otolaryngology, Mass Eye & Ear Infirm 1976

Lane, Edward M MD (Oto) - **Spec Exp:** Gastroesophageal Reflux Disease (GERD); Endoscopic Sinus Surgery; Parathyroid Disorders; Nasal Reconstruction; **Hospital:** Bridgeport Hosp; **Address:** 4675 Main St, Bridgeport, CT 06606-1813; **Phone:** 203-372-0009; **Board Cert:** Otolaryngology 1982; **Med School:** Columbia P&S 1977; **Resid:** Surgery, St Lukes Roosevelt Hosp 1979; Otolaryngology, Columbia-Presby Hosp 1982; **Fellow:** Head and Neck Surgery, UnivTexas MD Anderson Cancer Ctr 1983

Levin, Richard A MD (Oto) - **Spec Exp:** Sinus Disorders; Ear Infections; Facial Plastic & Reconstructive Surgery; **Hospital:** St. Vincent's Med Ctr - Bridgeport, Bridgeport Hosp; **Address:** 1305 Post Rd, Ste 302, Fairfield, CT 06824; **Phone:** 203-259-4700; **Board Cert:** Otolaryngology 1993; **Med School:** Tufts Univ 1987; **Resid:** Otolaryngology, Mount Sinai Hosp 1993; **Fac Appt:** Asst Prof S, Yale Univ

Levine, Steven B MD (Oto) - **Spec Exp:** Sinus Disorders; Allergy & Immunotherapy; Snoring/Sleep Apnea; **Hospital:** Bridgeport Hosp, Norwalk Hosp; **Address:** ENT and Allergy Associates, 160 Hawley Ln, Ste 202, Trumbull, CT 06611; **Phone:** 203-380-3707; **Board Cert:** Otolaryngology 1986; **Med School:** Univ Rochester 1981; **Resid:** Surgery, Hosp Univ Penn 1983; Otolaryngology, Hosp Univ Penn 1986; **Fellow:** Otolaryngology, NY Presby/Cornell Med Ctr 1986; **Fac Appt:** Asst Clin Prof S, Yale Univ

Parker, Andrew J MD (Oto) - **Spec Exp:** Hearing Loss; Sinus Disorders; Voice Disorders; Snoring/Sleep Apnea; **Hospital:** Norwalk Hosp; **Address:** 148 East Ave, Ste 2I, Norwalk, CT 06851; **Phone:** 203-866-8121; **Board Cert:** Otolaryngology 2012; **Med School:** UMDNJ-RW Johnson Med Sch 1995; **Resid:** Otolaryngology, NY Eye & Ear Infirm 2001

Pearl, Adam W MD (Oto) - **Spec Exp:** Head & Neck Surgery; Swallowing Disorders; Voice Disorders; Hearing Loss; **Hospital:** Bridgeport Hosp, St. Vincent's Med Ctr - Bridgeport; **Address:** CT ENT Med & Surgical Specialists, 15 Corporate Drive, Ste 2-8, Trumbull, CT 06611; **Phone:** 203-452-7081; **Board Cert:** Otolaryngology 2013; **Med School:** Mount Sinai Sch Med 1996; **Resid:** Otolaryngology, Mount Sinai Med Ctr 2002

Ross, Douglas MD (Oto) - **Spec Exp:** Head & Neck Surgery; Reconstructive Plastic Surgery; **Hospital:** St. Vincent's Med Ctr - Bridgeport; **Address:** St Vincents Med Ctr, Surgery, 2800 Main St, Bridgeport, CT 06606; **Phone:** 203-576-5435; **Board Cert:** Otolaryngology 1993; **Med School:** Columbia P&S 1986; **Resid:** Otolaryngology, UCLA Med Ctr 1992; **Fellow:** Head and Neck Surgery, UCLA Med Ctr 1993

Salzer, Stephen MD (Oto) - **Spec Exp:** Thyroid & Parathyroid Surgery; Pediatric Otolaryngology; Sinus Disorders/Surgery; Thyroid Cancer; **Hospital:** Greenwich Hosp (page 938), Stamford Hosp (page 939); **Address:** 49 Lake Ave Fl 1, Greenwich, CT 06830-4519; **Phone:** 203-869-2030; **Board Cert:** Otolaryngology 1995; **Med School:** Johns Hopkins Univ 1989; **Resid:** Otolaryngology, Yale-New Haven Hosp 1994; **Fellow:** Otolaryngology, Laennec Hosp 1995

Pain Medicine

Bennett, Steven J DO (PM) - **Spec Exp:** Pain-Chronic; Pain-Cancer; Reflex Sympathetic Dystrophy (RSD); **Hospital:** Greenwich Hosp (page 938); **Address:** Greenwich Pain Consulting Services, 5 Perryridge Rd, Greenwich, CT 06830; **Phone:** 203-863-3448; **Board Cert:** Pain Medicine 2005; **Med School:** NY Coll Osteo Med 1997; **Resid:** Internal Medicine, Lenox Hill Hosp 2000; **Fellow:** Pain Medicine, Meml Sloan Kettering Cancer Ctr 2004

Boolbol, Robert MD (PM) - **Spec Exp:** Pain-Back; Pain-Spine; Pain-Musculoskeletal; **Hospital:** Bridgeport Hosp, Hartford Hosp; **Address:** Pain & Spine Specialists of CT, 5520 Park Ave, Ste 303, Trumball, CT 06611; **Phone:** 203-373-7330; **Board Cert:** Anesthesiology 1994; Pain Medicine 2003; **Med School:** NY Med Coll 1989; **Resid:** Anesthesiology, Univ Chicago Hosps 1992; **Fellow:** Pain Medicine, Univ Chicago Hosps 2002

Pathology

Babkowski, Robert C MD (Path) - **Spec Exp:** Breast Pathology; Gastrointestinal Pathology; Gynecologic Pathology; **Hospital:** Stamford Hosp (page 939); **Address:** Stamford Hosp, Pathology Dept, 30 Shelburne Rd, Stamford, CT 06904; **Phone:** 203-276-7420; **Board Cert:** Anatomic & Clinical Pathology 1996; Cytopathology 1996; **Med School:** Univ Rochester 1990; **Resid:** Anatomic & Clinical Pathology, Univ Rochester Strong Meml Hosp 1995; **Fellow:** Cytopathology, UT MD Anderson Canc Ctr 1996

Pinto, Marguerite MD (Path) - **Spec Exp:** Gynecologic Pathology; Breast Pathology; **Hospital:** Bridgeport Hosp; **Address:** Bridgeport Hosp, Yale Pathology, 267 Grant St Fl 2, Bridgeport, CT 06610; **Phone:** 203-384-3157; **Board Cert:** Pathology 1975; Cytopathology 1989; **Med School:** India 1970; **Resid:** Pathology, Bridgeport Hosp; **Fac Appt:** Asst Prof Path, Yale Univ

Xu, Bo MD/PhD (Path) - **Spec Exp:** Gastrointestinal Pathology; Gynecologic Pathology; Urologic Pathology; **Hospital:** Stamford Hosp (page 939); **Address:** Stamford Hosp, Dept Pathology, 30 Shelburne Rd, Stamford, CT 06904; **Phone:** 203-276-7420; **Board Cert:** Anatomic & Clinical Pathology 2002; Cytopathology 2002; **Med School:** China 1987; **Resid:** Anatomic & Clinical Pathology, Tufts Med Ctr 2000; **Fellow:** Cytopathology, UT MD Anderson Canc Ctr 2001

Pediatric Allergy & Immunology

Burstein, Ora MD (PA&I) - **Spec Exp:** Asthma; **Hospital:** Stamford Hosp (page 939); **Address:** 22 Fifth St Fl 3, Stamford, CT 06905; **Phone:** 203-978-0072; **Board Cert:** Allergy & Immunology 2005; **Med School:** Tufts Univ 1984; **Resid:** Pediatrics, Montefiore Med Ctr-Moses Campus 1987; **Fellow:** Allergy & Immunology, Montefiore Med Ctr-Moses Campus 1989

Pediatric Cardiology

Berkwits, Kieve M MD (PCd) - **Spec Exp:** Congenital Heart Disease; **Hospital:** Bridgeport Hosp, St. Vincent's Med Ctr - Bridgeport; **Address:** Bridgeport Hosp, Pediatric Cardiology, 226 Mill Hill Ave, Bridgeport, CT 06610; **Phone:** 203-384-3783; **Board Cert:** Pediatrics 1986; Pediatric Cardiology 2003; **Med School:** Mexico 1979; **Resid:** Pediatrics, Beth Israel Med Ctr 1983; **Fellow:** Pediatric Cardiology, NY Hosp-Cornell Med Ctr 1985; **Fac Appt:** Asst Clin Prof Ped, Yale Univ

Snyder, Michael S MD (PCd) - **Spec Exp:** Echocardiography; Fetal Echocardiography; **Hospital:** Morgan Stanley Children's Hosp of NY-Presby, NY (page 104), Stamford Hosp (page 939); **Address:** 1500 Boston Post Rd Fl 2, Darien, CT 06820-5936; **Phone:** 203-662-0313; **Board Cert:** Pediatrics 1984; Pediatric Cardiology 1985; **Med School:** Cornell Univ-Weill Med Coll 1979; **Resid:** Pediatrics, NY Hosp 1982; **Fellow:** Pediatric Cardiology, NY Hosp 1984; **Fac Appt:** Assoc Prof Ped, Columbia P&S

Pediatric Gastroenterology

Glassman, Mark MD (PGe) - **Spec Exp:** Inflammatory Bowel Disease/Crohn's; Gastroesophageal Reflux Disease (GERD); Diarrheal Diseases; Food Allergy; **Hospital:** Norwalk Hosp, Children's & Women's Phys.of Westchester (page 638); **Address:** 148 East Ave, Ste 2N, Norwalk, CT 06851; **Phone:** 203-853-7170; **Board Cert:** Pediatrics 1983; Pediatric Gastroenterology 2012; **Med School:** SUNY Buffalo 1978; **Resid:** Pediatrics, Yale-New Haven Hosp 1981; **Fellow:** Gastroenterology & Nutrition, Chldns Hosp 1983; **Fac Appt:** Prof Ped, NY Med Coll

Pediatric Pulmonology

Dworkin, Gregory MD (PPul) - **Spec Exp:** Asthma; Chronic Lung Disease; **Hospital:** Danbury Hosp; **Address:** Danbury WCMG, Child Wellness, 79 Sand Pit Rd, Ste 201, Danbury, CT 06810; **Phone:** 203-790-5437; **Board Cert:** Pediatrics 1987; **Med School:** Albany Med Coll 1982; **Resid:** Pediatrics, Mount Sinai Med Ctr 1986; **Fellow:** Pediatric Pulmonology, Mount Sinai Med Ctr 1989; **Fac Appt:** Asst Clin Prof Ped, NY Med Coll

Hen Jr, Jacob MD (PPul) - **Spec Exp:** Asthma; Critical Care; **Hospital:** Bridgeport Hosp; **Address:** Bridgeport Hosp, Dept Peds, 267 Grant St, Box 5000, Bridgeport, CT 06610-2870; **Phone:** 203-384-3711; **Board Cert:** Pediatrics 1980; Pediatric Pulmonology 2006; Pediatric Critical Care Medicine 2009; **Med School:** UMDNJ-NJ Med Sch, Newark 1975; **Resid:** Pediatrics, UMDNJ-Univ Hosp 1977; **Fellow:** Pediatric Pulmonology, Yale-New Haven Hosp 1981; **Fac Appt:** Assoc Clin Prof Ped, Yale Univ

Sadeghi, Hossein MD (PPul) - **Spec Exp:** Asthma; Cystic Fibrosis; Bronchoscopy; Bronchitis; **Hospital:** Stamford Hosp (page 939), Greenwich Hosp (page 938); **Address:** 32 Strawberry Hill Ct, Ste 11, Tully Ctr, Stamford, CT 06902-2777; **Phone:** 203-276-5949; **Board Cert:** Pediatrics 2010; Pediatric Pulmonology 2006; **Med School:** Australia 1990; **Resid:** Pediatrics, Royal Chldns Hosp 1992; Pediatrics, Med Coll Va Affil Hosp 1995; **Fellow:** Pediatric Pulmonology, Westchester Med Ctr 1998; **Fac Appt:** Asst Clin Prof Ped, Columbia P&S

Pediatrics

Alon, Jamie MD (Ped) *PCP* - **Spec Exp:** Adolescent Medicine; Eating Disorders; **Hospital:** Danbury Hosp; **Address:** Pediatric Assocs Western CT, 41 Germantown Rd, Danbury, CT 06810; **Phone:** 203-744-1680; **Board Cert:** Pediatrics 2009; **Med School:** Cornell Univ-Weill Med Coll 1998; **Resid:** Pediatrics, NY-Presby/Weill Cornell Med Ctr 2001

Beckman, Karen E MD (Ped) *PCP* - **Hospital:** Greenwich Hosp (page 938), Stamford Hosp (page 939); **Address:** Riverside Pediatrics, 35 River Rd, Cos Cob, CT 06807; **Phone:** 203-629-5800; **Board Cert:** Pediatrics 2008; **Med School:** Tufts Univ 1997; **Resid:** Pediatrics, NYU Langone Med Ctr 2000

Chessin, Robert D MD (Ped) *PCP* - **Spec Exp:** Learning Disorders; Developmental Disorders; ADD/ADHD; Autism; **Hospital:** Bridgeport Hosp, St. Vincent's Med Ctr - Bridgeport; **Address:** Pediatric Hlthcare Assocs, 4699 Main St, Ste 215, Commerce Park, Bridgeport, CT 06606-1830; **Phone:** 203-452-8322; **Board Cert:** Pediatrics 1978; **Med School:** Johns Hopkins Univ 1973; **Resid:** Pediatrics, Duke Univ Med Ctr 1976; **Fac Appt:** Assoc Clin Prof Ped, Yale Univ

Cohen, Bruce W MD (Ped) *PCP* - **Spec Exp:** Neonatal Care; Pediatric Gastroenterology; **Hospital:** Danbury Hosp; **Address:** Pediatric Assocs Western CT, 41 Germantown Rd, Ste 201, Danbury, CT 06810-4000; **Phone:** 203-744-1680; **Board Cert:** Pediatrics 2010; **Med School:** UMDNJ-NJ Med Sch, Newark 1992; **Resid:** Pediatrics, N Shore Univ Hosp 1995

Cohen, Elin R MD (Ped) *PCP* - **Spec Exp:** Developmental & Behavioral Disorders; Asthma; **Hospital:** Bridgeport Hosp; **Address:** Black Rock Pediatrics, 1817 Black Rock Tpke, Ste 206, Fairfield, CT 06825; **Phone:** 203-337-5333; **Board Cert:** Pediatrics 2012; **Med School:** Albert Einstein Coll Med 1993; **Resid:** Pediatrics, Montefiore Med Ctr 1996; **Fellow:** Developmental-Behavioral Pediatrics, Yale-New Haven Hosp 1999

Ferguson, Kevin MD (Ped) *PCP* - **Spec Exp:** Asthma; Obesity; Weight Management; **Hospital:** Danbury Hosp; **Address:** Pediatric Assocs Western CT, 41 Germantown Rd, Ste 201, Danbury, CT 06810; **Phone:** 203-744-1680; **Board Cert:** Pediatrics 2009; **Med School:** Jefferson Med Coll 1998; **Resid:** Pediatrics, N Shore Univ Hosp 2001

Freedman, Richard M MD (Ped) *PCP* - **Spec Exp:** Neonatology; **Hospital:** Bridgeport Hosp, Yale-New Haven Hosp; **Address:** Ped Hlthcare Assocs, 4699 Main St, Ste 215, Bridgeport, CT 06606-1830; **Phone:** 203-452-8322; **Board Cert:** Pediatrics 1979; Neonatal-Perinatal Medicine 1981; **Med School:** Boston Univ 1975; **Resid:** Pediatrics, Yale-New Haven Hosp 1979; **Fellow:** Neonatology, Yale-New Haven Hosp 1981; **Fac Appt:** Assoc Clin Prof Ped, Yale Univ

Gropper, David MD (Ped) *PCP* - **Spec Exp:** Allergy; Infectious Disease; **Hospital:** Danbury Hosp; **Address:** Pediatric Assocs Western CT, 41 Germantown Rd, Ste 201, Danbury, CT 06810; **Phone:** 203-744-1680; **Board Cert:** Pediatrics 2011; **Med School:** SUNY Downstate 1986; **Resid:** Pediatrics, Montefiore Med Ctr 1989

Hedrick, David A MD (Ped) *PCP* - **Hospital:** Greenwich Hosp (page 938); **Address:** Children's Medical Group, 42 Sherwood Pl, Greenwich, CT 06830-5633; **Phone:** 203-661-2440; **Board Cert:** Pediatrics 1981; **Med School:** Univ VA Sch Med 1976; **Resid:** Pediatrics, Chldns Hosp 1979

Juan, Paul E MD (Ped) *PCP* - **Spec Exp:** Developmental Disorders; Asthma; **Hospital:** Greenwich Hosp (page 938); **Address:** Valley Pediatrics of Greenwich, 25 Valley Drive Fl 2, Greenwich, CT 06830; **Phone:** 203-622-4301; **Board Cert:** Pediatrics 2009; **Med School:** NY Med Coll 1990; **Resid:** Pediatrics, Med Coll Virginia Hosp 1993

Klenk, Rosemary MD (Ped) *PCP* - **Spec Exp:** ADD/ADHD; Eating Disorders; **Hospital:** Stamford Hosp (page 939), NY-Presby/Columbia Univ Med Ctr, NY (page 104); **Address:** New England Pediatrics, 183 Cherry St, Ste 103, New Canaan, CT 06840; **Phone:** 203-972-5232; **Board Cert:** Pediatrics 1987; **Med School:** Cornell Univ-Weill Med Coll 1980; **Resid:** Pediatrics, NY-Presby/Columbia Univ Med Ctr 1983

Korval, Arnold MD (Ped) *PCP* - **Hospital:** Greenwich Hosp (page 938), Stamford Hosp (page 939); **Address:** Greenwich Pediatric Assocs, 8 W End Ave, Old Greenwich, CT 06870-1642; **Phone:** 203-637-0186; **Board Cert:** Pediatrics 2009; **Med School:** St Louis Univ 1974; **Resid:** Pediatrics, Chldn's Hosp 1978

Levine, Dorothy A MD (Ped) *PCP* - **Spec Exp:** Complex Diagnosis; **Hospital:** Stamford Hosp (page 939), NY-Presby/Columbia Univ Med Ctr, NY (page 104); **Address:** 166 W Broad St, Ste 103, Stamford, CT 06902; **Phone:** 203-323-1770; **Board Cert:** Pediatrics 1985; **Med School:** Albert Einstein Coll Med 1980; **Resid:** Pediatrics, Columbia- Presby Hosp 1983; **Fac Appt:** Asst Clin Prof Ped, Columbia P&S

Magner, Joan A MD (Ped) *PCP* - **Hospital:** Danbury Hosp; **Address:** Ctr Pediatric Med, 107 Newtown Rd, Ste 1D, Danbury, CT 06810; **Phone:** 203-790-0822; **Board Cert:** Pediatrics 1986; **Med School:** Univ Hawaii JA Burns Sch Med 1980; **Resid:** Pediatrics, Chldns Hosp 1984

Marks, Laura MD (Ped) *PCP* - **Spec Exp:** Nutrition; Immune Deficiencies-Primary; **Hospital:** Norwalk Hosp; **Address:** Willows Pediatric Grp, 1563 Post Rd E, Westport, CT 06880; **Phone:** 203-319-3939; **Board Cert:** Pediatrics 2010; **Med School:** Yale Univ 1992; **Resid:** Pediatrics, Yale-New Haven Hosp 1995

Mini, Katherine N MD (Ped) *PCP* - **Hospital:** Greenwich Hosp (page 938); **Address:** Chldns Med Grp, 42 Sherwood Pl, Greenwich, CT 06830-5633; **Phone:** 203-661-2440; **Board Cert:** Pediatrics 2012; **Med School:** Albert Einstein Coll Med 1994; **Resid:** Pediatrics, Yale-New Haven Hosp 1997

Mongillo, Nicholas MD (Ped) *PCP* - **Spec Exp:** AIDS/HIV; Sports Medicine; ADD/ADHD; **Hospital:** Bridgeport Hosp; **Address:** Pedi-Care, 25 Constitution Blvd S, Shelton, CT 06484; **Phone:** 203-924-7334; **Board Cert:** Pediatrics 2013; **Med School:** Grenada 1987; **Resid:** Pediatrics, Bridgeport Hosp 1990

Morelli, Alan H MD (Ped) *PCP* - **Hospital:** Stamford Hosp (page 939); **Address:** New England Pediatrics, 166 W Broad St, Ste 103, Stamford, CT 06902; **Phone:** 203-323-1770; **Board Cert:** Pediatrics 1987; **Med School:** NY Med Coll 1982; **Resid:** Pediatrics, Yale-New Haven Hosp 1985

Perlman, Fern MD (Ped) *PCP* - **Hospital:** Norwalk Hosp; **Address:** Bay Street Pediatrics, 20 Bay St, Westport, CT 06880; **Phone:** 203-227-3674; **Board Cert:** Pediatrics 1981; **Med School:** NY Med Coll 1975; **Resid:** Pediatrics, Lenox Hill Hosp 1978

Rothschild, Rachel MD (Ped) *PCP* - **Spec Exp:** Developmental Disorders; ADD/ADHD; **Hospital:** Danbury Hosp; **Address:** Pediatric Assocs Western CT, 41 Germantown Rd, Ste 201, Danbury, CT 06810; **Phone:** 203-744-1680; **Board Cert:** Pediatrics 2008; **Med School:** Yale Univ 1997; **Resid:** Pediatrics, NY-Presby/Weill Cornell Med Ctr 2000

Schiz, Steven L MD (Ped) *PCP* - **Hospital:** Greenwich Hosp (page 938); **Address:** Children's Medical Group, 42 Sherwood Pl, Greenwich, CT 06830-5633; **Phone:** 203-661-2440; **Board Cert:** Pediatrics 2009; **Med School:** Columbia P&S 1980; **Resid:** Pediatrics, Children's Hosp 1983

Sollinger, Jonathan E MD (Ped) *PCP* - **Spec Exp:** ADD/ADHD; Developmental & Behavioral Disorders; **Hospital:** Norwalk Hosp; **Address:** Willows Pediatric Grp, 1563 Post Rd E, Westport, CT 06880; **Phone:** 203-319-3939; **Board Cert:** Pediatrics 2010; **Med School:** Univ Conn 1999; **Resid:** Pediatrics, Montefiore Med Ctr 2002

Physical Medicine & Rehabilitation

Aaronson, Beth MD (PMR) - **Spec Exp:** Acupuncture; Neurologic Rehabilitation; Cancer Rehabilitation; Lymphedema; **Hospital:** Danbury Hosp; **Address:** Danbury WCMG, Phys Med & Rehab, 33 Germantown Rd Fl 1, Danbury, CT 06810; **Phone:** 203-794-5605; **Board Cert:** Physical Medicine & Rehabilitation 2005; **Med School:** SUNY Stony Brook 1990; **Resid:** Physical Medicine & Rehabilitation, NY-Presby/Columbia Univ Med Ctr 1994

Freedman, Janet MD (PMR) - **Spec Exp:** Acupuncture; Lymphedema; Spasticity Management; **Hospital:** Greenwich Hosp (page 938); **Address:** Greenwich Hosp, Phys Med & Rehab, 5 Perryridge Rd, Greenwich, CT 06830; **Phone:** 203-863-4290; **Board Cert:** Physical Medicine & Rehabilitation 1988; **Med School:** Univ Wisc 1983; **Resid:** Physical Medicine & Rehabilitation, NYU Rusk Inst 1986

Grant, Linda MD (PMR) - **Spec Exp:** Lymphedema; Acupuncture; **Hospital:** Greenwich Hosp (page 938); **Address:** Greenwich Hosp, Physical Med & Rehab, 5 Perryridge Rd, rm 3-3107, Greenwich, CT 06830; **Phone:** 203-863-3290; **Board Cert:** Physical Medicine & Rehabilitation 1990; **Med School:** UMDNJ-Rutgers Med Sch 1985; **Resid:** Physical Medicine & Rehabilitation, NYU Med Ctr 1989

Heftler, Jeffrey M MD (PMR) - **Spec Exp:** Pain Management; Spinal Rehabilitation; **Hospital:** Greenwich Hosp (page 938); **Address:** Orthopaedic & Neurosurgery Specialists, 6 Greenwich Office Park, 40 Valley Drive, Greenwich, CT 06831; **Phone:** 203-869-1145; **Board Cert:** Physical Medicine & Rehabilitation 2012; Pain Medicine 2003; **Med School:** UMDNJ-RW Johnson Med Sch 1997; **Resid:** Physical Medicine & Rehabilitation, Thos Jefferson Univ Med Ctr 2001; **Fellow:** Pain Management, Beth Israel Med Ctr 2002

Richter, Edwin MD (PMR) - **Spec Exp:** Neuro-Rehabilitation; Brain Injury Rehabilitation; Amputee Rehabilitation; Lymphedema; **Hospital:** Stamford Hosp (page 939); **Address:** 166 W Broad St, Ste 305, Stamford, CT 06902; **Phone:** 203-316-0610; **Board Cert:** Physical Medicine & Rehabilitation 1992; **Med School:** NYU Sch Med 1987; **Resid:** Physical Medicine & Rehabilitation, NYU Med Ctr 1991; **Fac Appt:** Asst Clin Prof PMR, NYU Sch Med

Snowball, Halina MD (PMR) - **Spec Exp:** Pain Management; Acupuncture; **Hospital:** Greenwich Hosp (page 938); **Address:** 2015 W Main St, Ste 100, Stamford, CT 06902; **Phone:** 203-863-4588; **Board Cert:** Physical Medicine & Rehabilitation 1990; **Med School:** Univ Fla Coll Med 1985; **Resid:** Physical Medicine & Rehabilitation, Stanford Univ Med Ctr 1989

Plastic Surgery

Attkiss, Keith J MD (PlS) - **Spec Exp:** Breast Cosmetic & Reconstructive Surgery; Liposuction & Body Contouring; **Hospital:** Greenwich Hosp (page 938); **Address:** 2 1/2 Dearfield Drive, Ste 203, Greenwich, CT 06831; **Phone:** 203-862-2700; **Board Cert:** Plastic Surgery 2011; **Med School:** Columbia P&S 1992; **Resid:** Surgery, UC Davis Med Ctr 1997; Plastic Surgery, Yale-New Haven Hosp 2000

Gewirtz, Harold S MD (PlS) - **Spec Exp:** Cosmetic Surgery-Face; Breast Cosmetic & Reconstructive Surgery; Liposuction & Body Contouring; Melanoma; **Hospital:** Stamford Hosp (page 939), Greenwich Hosp (page 938); **Address:** 70 Mill River St, Stamford, CT 06902-3725; **Phone:** 203-325-1381; **Board Cert:** Plastic Surgery 1984; **Med School:** Johns Hopkins Univ 1975; **Resid:** Surgery, UCLA Ronald Reagan Med Ctr 1980; Plastic Surgery, NYU Langone Med Ctr 1982; **Fac Appt:** Asst Clin Prof PlS, Columbia P&S

Goldenberg, David M MD (PlS) - **Spec Exp:** Cosmetic Surgery; Breast Reconstruction; Wound Healing/Care; **Hospital:** Danbury Hosp; **Address:** Advanced Specialty Care, Plastic Surgery, 107 Newtown Rd, Ste 2C, Danbury, CT 06810; **Phone:** 203-791-9661; **Board Cert:** Plastic Surgery 1990; **Med School:** NY Med Coll 1982; **Resid:** Surgery, Montefiore Med Ctr 1986; **Fellow:** Plastic Surgery, Montefiore Med Ctr 1988; **Fac Appt:** Prof S, NY Med Coll

Islam, Sohel MD (PlS) - **Spec Exp:** Hand Surgery; **Hospital:** Danbury Hosp; **Address:** Advanced Specialty Care, Plastic Surgery, 107 Newtown Rd, Ste 2C, Danbury, CT 06810; **Phone:** 203-791-9661; **Board Cert:** Hand Surgery 2011; Plastic Surgery 2011; **Med School:** Cornell Univ-Weill Med Coll 1991; **Resid:** Surgery, St Lukes-Roosevelt Hosp Ctr 1996; Plastic Surgery, Med Coll VA Hosps 2000; **Fellow:** Hand Surgery, Yale-New Haven Hosp 2003

Newman, Fredric A MD (PlS) - **Spec Exp:** Rhinoplasty; Breast Augmentation; Eyelid Surgery; Abdominoplasty; **Hospital:** Greenwich Hosp (page 938), Norwalk Hosp; **Address:** 722 Post Rd, Ste 200, Darien, CT 06820; **Phone:** 203-656-9999; **Board Cert:** Plastic Surgery 1985; **Med School:** SUNY Downstate 1974; **Resid:** Surgery, Beth Israel Med Ctr 1977; Surgery, SUNY Downstate 1979; **Fellow:** Plastic/Reconstructive Surgery, NYU Med Ctr 1981; Plastic Surgery, Jackson Meml Hosp 1982; **Fac Appt:** Asst Prof PlS, NY Med Coll

O'Connell, Joseph B MD (PlS) - **Spec Exp:** Liposuction & Body Contouring; Cosmetic Surgery-Face; Cosmetic Surgery-Breast; **Hospital:** Bridgeport Hosp; **Address:** Plastic Surgery of Southern CT, 208 Post Rd W, Westport, CT 06880; **Phone:** 203-454-0044; **Board Cert:** Plastic Surgery 2007; **Med School:** Cornell Univ-Weill Med Coll 1981; **Resid:** Surgery, St Francis Hosp 1983; Surgery, St Vincents Med Ctr 1986; **Fellow:** Plastic Surgery, New York Hosp 1988

Passaretti, David MD (PlS) - **Spec Exp:** Cosmetic Surgery-Face; Breast Cosmetic & Reconstructive Surgery; Body Contouring after Weight Loss; **Hospital:** Greenwich Hosp (page 938), Stamford Hosp (page 939); **Address:** 722 Post Rd, Ste 200, Darien, CT 06820; **Phone:** 203-656-9999; **Board Cert:** Plastic Surgery 2005; **Med School:** Tufts Univ 1997; **Resid:** Plastic Surgery, Univ Hosps 2005; **Fellow:** Plastic Surgery, Mass Genl Hosp 2006

Raskin, Elsa M MD (PlS) - **Spec Exp:** Eyelid Cosmetic & Reconstructive Surgery; Cosmetic Surgery-Face; Cosmetic Surgery-Breast; **Hospital:** Greenwich Hosp (page 938), Lenox Hill Hosp (page 106); **Address:** 2 1/2 Dearfield Drive, Ste 102, Greenwich, CT 06831-5335; **Phone:** 203-861-6620; **Board Cert:** Plastic Surgery 2012; **Med School:** Switzerland 1987; **Resid:** Ophthalmology, NY Eye & Ear Infirm 1995; Surgery, NYU Med Ctr 1999; **Fellow:** Plastic Surgery, Univ Pittsburgh Med Ctr 1996; Plastic/Reconstructive Surgery, NY Presby Hosp 2001

Rosenstock, Arthur Richard MD (PlS) - **Spec Exp:** Cosmetic Surgery-Face; Eyelid Surgery; Cosmetic Surgery-Breast; **Hospital:** Stamford Hosp (page 939); **Address:** 1290 Summer St, Ste 3100, Stamford, CT 06905-5326; **Phone:** 203-359-1959; **Board Cert:** Plastic Surgery 1985; **Med School:** Belgium 1976; **Resid:** Surgery, Westchester Co Med Ctr 1981; **Fellow:** Plastic/Reconstructive Surgery, Med Coll Virginia 1983; **Fac Appt:** Asst Clin Prof S, Columbia P&S

Sofer, Alfred MD (PlS) - **Spec Exp:** Cosmetic Surgery; Plastic & Reconstructive Surgery; Breast Reconstruction; **Hospital:** St. Vincent's Med Ctr - Bridgeport, Norwalk Hosp; **Address:** Plastic Surgery Ctr of Fairfield, 33 Miller St, Fairfield, CT 06824; **Phone:** 203-336-9862; **Board Cert:** Plastic Surgery 2007; **Med School:** Albany Med Coll 1993; **Resid:** Surgery, Westchester MedCenter 1997; Plastic/Reconstructive Surgery, Med Univ of SC Med Ctr 1999; **Fellow:** Microvascular Surgery, Kleinert Inst 2000

Psychiatry

Abrams, Linus MD (Psyc) - **Spec Exp:** Psychopharmacology; Psychotherapy; **Address:** 4 Dearfield Dr, Greenwich, CT 06831; **Phone:** 203-861-2654; **Board Cert:** Psychiatry 2005; **Med School:** NY Med Coll 1988; **Resid:** Psychiatry, Beth Israel Deaconess Med Ctr 1992

Goldberg, Joseph F MD (Psyc) - **Spec Exp:** Bipolar/Mood Disorders; Psychopharmacology; Anxiety & Depression; Cognitive Psychotherapy; **Hospital:** Mt Sinai Med Ctr (page 102); **Address:** 128 East Avenue, Norwalk, CT 06851; **Phone:** 203-854-9607; **Board Cert:** Psychiatry 2009; **Med School:** Northwestern Univ 1992; **Resid:** Psychiatry, Payne Whitney Clinic 1995; **Fellow:** Psychopharmacology, Payne Whitney Clinic 1998; **Fac Appt:** Clin Prof Psyc, Mount Sinai Sch Med

Hart, Sidney MD (Psyc) - **Spec Exp:** Anxiety Disorders; Mood Disorders; Psychotherapy; **Hospital:** Greenwich Hosp (page 938); **Address:** 282 Railroad Ave, Fl 2, Greenwich, CT 06830; **Phone:** 203-622-1722; **Board Cert:** Psychiatry 1973; **Med School:** Albert Einstein Coll Med 1964; **Resid:** Psychiatry, Bronx Municipal Hosp 1971; **Fellow:** Liaison Psychiatry, Montefiore Hosp Med Ctr 1973

Kalman, Arlene Diane MD (Psyc) - **Spec Exp:** Child & Adolescent Psychiatry; **Hospital:** Danbury Hosp; **Address:** 54 Arrowhead Rd, Brookfield, CT 06804; **Phone:** 203-775-6100; **Board Cert:** Psychiatry 1985; **Med School:** SUNY Downstate 1980; **Resid:** Psychiatry, Bronx Muni Hosp Ctr 1983; **Fellow:** Child & Adolescent Psychiatry, Bronx Muni Hosp Ctr 1985

Lorefice, Laurence S MD (Psyc) - **Spec Exp:** Depression; Bipolar/Mood Disorders; Obsessive-Compulsive Disorder; Anxiety Disorders; **Address:** 1445 E Putnam Ave, Old Greenwich, CT 06870; **Phone:** 203-637-4006; **Board Cert:** Psychiatry 1979; **Med School:** Univ Pennsylvania 1975; **Resid:** Psychiatry, Mass Genl Hosp 1978; **Fellow:** Community Psychiatry, Mass Genl Hosp 1979

Morgan, Charles J MD (Psyc) - **Spec Exp:** Alcohol Abuse; Mood Disorders; Substance Abuse; **Hospital:** Bridgeport Hosp; **Address:** Northeast Medical Group, 226 Mill Hill Ave Fl 3, Bridgeport, CT 06610; **Phone:** 203-384-3897; **Board Cert:** Psychiatry 1990; **Med School:** Cornell Univ-Weill Med Coll 1983; **Resid:** Psychiatry, Yale-New Haven Hosp 1987; **Fac Appt:** Asst Clin Prof Psyc, Yale Univ

Mueller, F. Carl MD (Psyc) - **Spec Exp:** Anxiety & Depression; Obsessive-Compulsive Disorder; Psychopharmacology; **Hospital:** Stamford Hosp (page 939); **Address:** 999 Summer St, Ste 200, Stamford, CT 06905-5513; **Phone:** 203-357-7773; **Board Cert:** Psychiatry 1987; **Med School:** Univ Conn 1982; **Resid:** Psychiatry, Yale-New Haven Hosp 1985; **Fellow:** Psychiatry, Yale-New Haven Hosp 1986; **Fac Appt:** Asst Clin Prof Psyc, Yale Univ

Schechter, Justin O MD (Psyc) - **Spec Exp:** Anxiety Disorders; Mood Disorders; Eating Disorders; Pregnancy & Mood Disorders; **Hospital:** Stamford Hosp (page 939); **Address:** 22 Fifth St Fl 3rd, Stamford, CT 06905-5030; **Phone:** 203-323-7760; **Board Cert:** Psychiatry 1986; Forensic Psychiatry 2008; **Med School:** SUNY Stony Brook 1981; **Resid:** Psychiatry, Yale-New Haven Hosp 1985; **Fac Appt:** Asst Clin Prof Psyc, Yale Univ

Shapiro, Bruce MD (Psyc) - **Spec Exp:** Forensic Psychiatry; Psychopharmacology; Anxiety & Depression; Bipolar/Mood Disorders; **Address:** 666 Glenbrook Rd, River Suite, Stamford, CT 06906; **Phone:** 203-327-4144; **Board Cert:** Psychiatry 1976; **Med School:** NY Med Coll 1972; **Resid:** Psychiatry, Metropolitan Hosp Ctr 1975; **Fac Appt:** Clin Prof Psyc, Columbia P&S

Smith, Joann M MD (Psyc) - **Spec Exp:** Mood Disorders; Anxiety Disorders; Women's Health; **Hospital:** St. Vincent's Med Ctr - Bridgeport; **Address:** 1261 Post Rd, Ste 200-A, Fairfield, CT 06824; **Phone:** 203-255-0770; **Board Cert:** Psychiatry 1980; **Med School:** SUNY Hlth Sci Ctr 1974; **Resid:** Psychiatry, Georgetown Univ Hosp 1979

Sofair, Jane MD (Psyc) - **Spec Exp:** Anxiety & Depression; Women's Health; **Hospital:** Natchaug Hosp; **Address:** CPC Associates, 84 Hospital Ave, Danbury, CT 06810; **Phone:** 203-792-0400; **Board Cert:** Psychiatry 1986; **Med School:** NYU Sch Med 1980; **Resid:** Psychiatry, NYU Med Ctr 1984

Tamerin, John MD (Psyc) - **Spec Exp:** Psychotherapy; Bipolar/Mood Disorders; Substance Abuse; Alcohol Abuse; **Hospital:** NY-Presby/Weill Cornell Med Ctr, NY (page 104), Greenwich Hosp (page 938); **Address:** 27 Stag Ln, Greenwich, CT 06831-3137; **Phone:** 203-661-8282; **Board Cert:** Psychiatry 1970; **Med School:** NYU Sch Med 1963; **Resid:** Psychiatry, Yale-New Haven Hosp 1965; Psychiatry, Mt Sinai Med Ctr 1967; **Fellow:** Child Psychiatry, Natl Rehab Hosp 1969; **Fac Appt:** Assoc Clin Prof Psyc, Cornell Univ-Weill Med Coll

Waynik, Mark MD (Psyc) - **Hospital:** St. Vincent's Med Ctr - Bridgeport; **Address:** The Waynik Group, 52 Beach Rd, Ste 104, Fairfield, CT 06824; **Phone:** 203-254-2000; **Board Cert:** Psychiatry 1987; **Med School:** Mexico 1979; **Resid:** Psychiatry, Inst Living 1984

Pulmonary Disease

Berman, Lewis MD (Pul) - **Hospital:** Norwalk Hosp; **Address:** Norwalk Hosp-Pulmonology, 34 Maple St, Norwalk, CT 06856; **Phone:** 203-852-2392; **Board Cert:** Internal Medicine 2004; Critical Care Medicine 2005; Pulmonary Disease 2004; **Med School:** Albert Einstein Coll Med 1987; **Resid:** Internal Medicine, Univ Hlth Ctr 1990; **Fellow:** Pulmonary Critical Care Medicine, Yale-New Haven Hosp 1994

Bernstein, Michael A MD (Pul) - **Spec Exp:** Sleep Medicine; **Hospital:** Stamford Hosp (page 939); **Address:** Pulmonary Assocs, 190 W Broad St, Stamford, CT 06902; **Phone:** 203-348-2437; **Board Cert:** Internal Medicine 2007; Pulmonary Disease 2009; Critical Care Medicine 2010; Hospice & Palliative Medicine 2012; **Med School:** Duke Univ 2003; **Resid:** Internal Medicine & Pediatrics, Mount Sinai Med Ctr 2007; **Fellow:** Pulmonary Critical Care Medicine, Mount Sinai Med Ctr 2010

Brown, Robert B MD (Pul) - **Hospital:** St. Vincent's Med Ctr - Bridgeport; **Address:** 2800 Main St, Bridgeport, CT 06606; **Phone:** 203-576-5711; **Board Cert:** Internal Medicine 1981; Pulmonary Disease 1984; Critical Care Medicine 2007; **Med School:** SUNY Downstate 1978; **Resid:** Internal Medicine, Westchester Med Ctr 1981; **Fellow:** Pulmonary Disease, NY Med Coll 1984; **Fac Appt:** Asst Prof Med, NY Med Coll

Chronakos, John MD (Pul) - **Spec Exp:** Sleep Disorders; Critical Care Medicine; **Hospital:** Danbury Hosp; **Address:** Danbury WCMG, Pulmonary & Sleep, 33 Germantown Rd Fl 2, Danbury, CT 06810; **Phone:** 203-739-7070; **Board Cert:** Internal Medicine 2011; Pulmonary Disease 2003; Critical Care Medicine 2005; Sleep Medicine 2011; **Med School:** NYU Sch Med 1998; **Resid:** Internal Medicine, NYU Langone Med Ctr 2001; **Fellow:** Pulmonary Disease, Mount Sinai Med Ctr 2004

Fine, Jonathan MD (Pul) - **Spec Exp:** Asthma; **Hospital:** Norwalk Hosp; **Address:** Norwalk Hosp, Div of Pulmonology, 34 Maple St Fl 3, Norwalk, CT 06856; **Phone:** 203-852-2392; **Board Cert:** Internal Medicine 1984; Pulmonary Disease 1986; Critical Care Medicine 2011; **Med School:** Yale Univ 1981; **Resid:** Internal Medicine, Yale-New Haven Hosp 1984; **Fellow:** Pulmonary Disease, Yale-New Haven Hosp 1985; Pulmonary Critical Care Medicine, UCSF Med Ctr 1988

Krinsley, James MD (Pul) - **Spec Exp:** Asthma; Emphysema; Critical Care; **Hospital:** Stamford Hosp (page 939); **Address:** Pulmonary Assocs, 190 W Broad St, Stamford, CT 06902; **Phone:** 203-348-2437; **Board Cert:** Internal Medicine 1983; Pulmonary Disease 1986; Critical Care Medicine 2009; **Med School:** Cornell Univ-Weill Med Coll 1980; **Resid:** Internal Medicine, NYU/VA Med Ctr 1983; **Fellow:** Pulmonary Disease, Yale-New Haven Hosp 1986; **Fac Appt:** Assoc Clin Prof Med, Columbia P&S

Kurtz, Caroline MD (Pul) - **Spec Exp:** Asthma; **Hospital:** Norwalk Hosp; **Address:** 30 Stevens St, Ste C, Norwalk, CT 06850; **Phone:** 203-855-3888; **Board Cert:** Internal Medicine 1988; Pulmonary Disease 2010; Critical Care Medicine 2012; **Med School:** NYU Sch Med 1984; **Resid:** Internal Medicine, Mt Sinai Hosp 1987; **Fellow:** Pulmonary Critical Care Medicine, Mt Sinai Hosp 1990

Marino, A. Michael MD (Pul) - **Spec Exp:** Asthma; Bronchitis; Emphysema; Lung Cancer; **Hospital:** Greenwich Hosp (page 938); **Address:** 5 Perryridge Rd, Greenwich, CT 06830; **Phone:** 203-661-5379; **Board Cert:** Internal Medicine 1972; Pulmonary Disease 1972; **Med School:** Georgetown Univ 1964; **Resid:** Internal Medicine, VA Med Ctr 1967; **Fellow:** Pulmonary Disease, VA Med Ctr 1969; **Fac Appt:** Assoc Clin Prof Med, Yale Univ

McCalley, Stuart W MD (Pul) - **Spec Exp:** Sleep Disorders; Chronic Obstructive Lung Disease (COPD); Asthma; Pulmonary Fibrosis; **Hospital:** Stamford Hosp (page 939), Greenwich Hosp (page 938); **Address:** Greenwich Medical Grp, 75 Holly Hill Ln, Greenwich, CT 06830; **Phone:** 203-869-6960; **Board Cert:** Internal Medicine 1972; Pulmonary Disease 1974; Sleep Medicine 2002; **Med School:** Case West Res Univ 1969; **Resid:** Internal Medicine, Univ Conn Hlth Ctr 1971; Internal Medicine, Univ Vermont Med Ctr 1972; **Fellow:** Pulmonary Disease, Bronx Muni Hosp 1974

Roca, Dominic J MD (Pul) - **Spec Exp:** Sleep Disorders; Allergy; **Hospital:** Stamford Hosp (page 939); **Address:** Stamford Hosp, Pulmonary Assocs, 190 W Broad St, Stamford, CT 06902; **Phone:** 203-348-2437; **Board Cert:** Allergy & Immunology 2008; Pulmonary Disease 2006; Critical Care Medicine 2007; Sleep Medicine 2009; **Med School:** SUNY Downstate 1991; **Resid:** Internal Medicine, NYU Med Ctr 1994; **Fellow:** Allergy & Immunology, Boston Med Ctr 1999; Psychosomatic Medicine, Beth Israel Deaconess Med Ctr 1999

Rudolph, Daniel J MD (Pul) - **Spec Exp:** Asthma; Pneumonia; **Hospital:** Bridgeport Hosp; **Address:** Pulmonary & Int Med Assocs, 15 Corporate Drive, Trumbull, CT 06611; **Phone:** 203-261-3980; **Board Cert:** Internal Medicine 1985; Pulmonary Disease 1988; **Med School:** NYU Sch Med 1982; **Resid:** Internal Medicine, SUNY Stony Brook Med Ctr 1985; **Fellow:** Pulmonary Disease, Montefiore Med Ctr 1988

Sachs, Paul MD (Pul) - **Spec Exp:** Pulmonary Rehabilitation; Asthma; **Hospital:** Stamford Hosp (page 939); **Address:** Pulmonary Assocs, 190 W Broad St, Stamford, CT 06902-3633; **Phone:** 203-348-2437; **Board Cert:** Internal Medicine 1985; Pulmonary Disease 1988; Critical Care Medicine 2009; **Med School:** NYU Sch Med 1982; **Resid:** Internal Medicine, NY Hosp 1985; **Fellow:** Pulmonary Disease, Montefiore Med Ctr 1987

Turetsky, Arthur S MD (Pul) - **Spec Exp:** Sleep Medicine; Asthma; Chronic Obstructive Lung Disease (COPD); Tuberculosis; **Hospital:** Bridgeport Hosp; **Address:** Pulmonary & Int Med Assocs, 15 Corporate Drive, Trumbull, CT 06611; **Phone:** 203-261-3980; **Board Cert:** Internal Medicine 1977; Pulmonary Disease 1980; Sleep Medicine 2009; **Med School:** Albert Einstein Coll Med 1974; **Resid:** Internal Medicine, Einstein Bronx Muncipal Hosp Ctr 1977; Pulmonary Disease, Bronx Municipal Hosp 1980; **Fac Appt:** Asst Clin Prof Med, Albert Einstein Coll Med

Winter, Stephen M MD (Pul) - **Hospital:** Norwalk Hosp; **Address:** Norwalk Hosp, Dept Pulmonology, 34 Maple St Fl 3, Norwalk, CT 06856; **Phone:** 203-852-2392; **Board Cert:** Internal Medicine 1984; Pulmonary Disease 1986; Critical Care Medicine 2007; **Med School:** Cornell Univ-Weill Med Coll 1981; **Resid:** Internal Medicine, NY-Presby/Weill Cornell Med Ctr 1984; **Fellow:** Pulmonary Disease, Yale-New Haven Hosp 1987; **Fac Appt:** Clin Prof Med, Yale Univ

Radiation Oncology

Dowling, Sean MD (RadRO) - **Spec Exp:** Breast Cancer; Gynecologic Cancer; **Hospital:** Stamford Hosp (page 939); **Address:** Stamford Hosp, Dept Radiation Oncology, 34 Shelburne Rd, Stamford, CT 06902; **Phone:** 203-276-7886; **Board Cert:** Internal Medicine 1986; Radiation Oncology 1990; **Med School:** Yale Univ 1983; **Resid:** Internal Medicine, Yale-New Haven Hosp 1986; Radiation Oncology, Yale-New Haven Hosp 1989

Fang, Deborah X MD (RadRO) - **Spec Exp:** Breast Cancer; Gastrointestinal Cancer; **Hospital:** St. Vincent's Med Ctr - Bridgeport; **Address:** 2800 Main St, Bridgeport, CT 06606; **Phone:** 203-576-5085; **Board Cert:** Radiation Oncology 2011; **Med School:** China 1987; **Resid:** Radiation Oncology, Mount Sinai Med Ctr 2001

Iannuzzi, Christopher MD (RadRO) - **Spec Exp:** Breast Cancer; Pancreatic Cancer; Head & Neck Cancer; Prostate Cancer; **Hospital:** St. Vincent's Med Ctr - Bridgeport; **Address:** St Vincents Med Ctr, Rad Oncology Dept, 2800 Main St, Bridgeport, CT 06606; **Phone:** 203-576-5085; **Board Cert:** Radiation Oncology 2011; **Med School:** Mount Sinai Sch Med 1996; **Resid:** Radiation Oncology, Mount Sinai Med Ctr 2001

Masino, Frank A MD (RadRO) - **Spec Exp:** Breast Cancer; Prostate Cancer; Brachytherapy; Stereotactic Radiosurgery; **Hospital:** Stamford Hosp (page 939); **Address:** Stamford Hosp, Therapeutic Radiology, 34 Shelburne Rd, Stamford, CT 06902; **Phone:** 203-276-7886; **Board Cert:** Therapeutic Radiology 1982; **Med School:** Albert Einstein Coll Med 1978; **Resid:** Therapeutic Radiology, Yale-New Haven Hosp 1982

Pathare, Pradip M MD (RadRO) - **Spec Exp:** Breast Cancer; Prostate Cancer; Head & Neck Cancer; Brain Tumors; **Hospital:** Norwalk Hosp; **Address:** Whittingham Cancer Ctr, 24 Stevens St, Norwalk, CT 06856; **Phone:** 203-852-2719; **Board Cert:** Radiology 1980; Therapeutic Radiology 1981; **Med School:** India 1975; **Resid:** Radiology, Misericordia/Lincoln Hosp 1979; Therapeutic Radiology, Yale-New Haven Hosp 1981; **Fac Appt:** Assoc Prof RadRO, Yale Univ

Sanghavi, Seema MD (RadRO) - **Spec Exp:** Breast Cancer; **Hospital:** Danbury Hosp; **Address:** Danbury Hosp, Radiation Oncology, 24 Hospital Ave, Danbury, CT 06810; **Phone:** 203-739-7190; **Board Cert:** Radiation Oncology 2011; **Med School:** Northwestern Univ 1995; **Resid:** Radiation Oncology, Univ WI Hosp & Clins 2001

Spera, John A MD (RadRO) - **Spec Exp:** Breast Cancer; Prostate Cancer; Intensity Modulated Radiotherapy (IMRT); **Hospital:** Danbury Hosp; **Address:** Danbury Hosp, Dept Radiation Oncology, 24 Hospital Ave, Danbury, CT 06810-6099; **Phone:** 203-739-7190; **Board Cert:** Radiation Oncology 1987; **Med School:** Georgetown Univ 1979; **Resid:** Surgery, Hosp Univ Penn 1981; Urology, Hosp Univ Penn 1983; **Fellow:** Radiation Oncology, Hosp Univ Penn 1987

Reproductive Endocrinology

Chacho, Karol J MD (RE) - **Spec Exp:** Endometriosis; Infertility; Menopause Problems; Infertility-IVF; **Hospital:** Bridgeport Hosp, St. Vincent's Med Ctr - Bridgeport; **Address:** 4699 Main St, Ste 210, Bridgeport, CT 06606-1830; **Phone:** 203-372-5282; **Board Cert:** Obstetrics & Gynecology 2012; Reproductive Endocrinology/Infertility 2012; **Med School:** Loyola Univ-Stritch Sch Med 1978; **Resid:** Obstetrics & Gynecology, Michael Reese Hosp Med Ctr 1982; **Fellow:** Reproductive Endocrinology, Michael Reese Hosp Med Ctr 1984

Doyle, Michael B MD (RE) - **Spec Exp:** Infertility-IVF; Endometriosis; **Hospital:** Norwalk Hosp, St. Vincent's Med Ctr - Bridgeport; **Address:** 4920 Main St, Ste 301, Bridgeport, CT 06606-1300; **Phone:** 203-373-1200; **Board Cert:** Obstetrics & Gynecology 2012; **Med School:** UCSF 1985; **Resid:** Obstetrics & Gynecology, Hosp Univ Penn 1989; **Fellow:** Reproductive Endocrinology, Yale-New Haven Hosp 1991

Ginsburg, Frances W MD (RE) - **Spec Exp:** Infertility-IVF; Endometriosis; Menstrual Disorders; **Hospital:** Stamford Hosp (page 939); **Address:** Stamford Hosp, Whittingham Pavilion, 30 Shelburne Rd, Stamford, CT 06904-9317; **Phone:** 203-276-7559; **Board Cert:** Obstetrics & Gynecology 2012; Reproductive Endocrinology 2012; **Med School:** NYU Sch Med 1980; **Resid:** Obstetrics & Gynecology, NYU Langone Med Ctr 1985; **Fellow:** Reproductive Endocrinology, NYU Langone Med Ctr 1988; **Fac Appt:** Asst Clin Prof ObG, Columbia P&S

Hurwitz, Joshua M MD (RE) - **Spec Exp:** Infertility-IVF; Hormonal Disorders; Endometriosis; **Hospital:** Danbury Hosp; **Address:** Reproductive Medicine Asscociates of Ct, 10 Glover Ave, Norwalk, CT 06850; **Phone:** 203-750-7400; **Board Cert:** Obstetrics & Gynecology 2012; Reproductive Endocrinology/Infertility 2012; **Med School:** Jefferson Med Coll 1999; **Resid:** Obstetrics & Gynecology, Thomas Jefferson Univ Hosp 2003; **Fellow:** Reproductive Endocrinology, Albert Einstein Coll Med 2006; **Fac Appt:** Asst Prof ObG, Albert Einstein Coll Med

Leondires, Mark MD (RE) - **Spec Exp:** Endometriosis; Polycystic Ovarian Syndrome; **Hospital:** Danbury Hosp; **Address:** Ctr Advanced Reproductive Med, 10 Glover St, Stamford, CT 06902; **Phone:** 203-750-7400; **Board Cert:** Obstetrics & Gynecology 2012; Reproductive Endocrinology 2012; **Med School:** Univ VT Coll Med 1991; **Resid:** Obstetrics & Gynecology, Maine Med Ctr 1995; **Fellow:** Reproductive Endocrinology, Natl Inst Hlth-Clin Ctr 1999

Murdock, Cynthia MD (RE) - **Spec Exp:** Infertility-IVF; Reproductive Surgery; **Hospital:** Danbury Hosp; **Address:** Reproductive Med Assocs CT, 10 Glover Ave, Norwalk, CT 06850; **Phone:** 203-750-7400; **Board Cert:** Obstetrics & Gynecology 2007; Reproductive Endocrinology/Infertility 2007; **Med School:** Creighton Univ 1995; **Resid:** Obstetrics & Gynecology, Creighton Univ 1999; **Fellow:** Reproductive Endocrinology, Natl Inst Hlth-Clin Ctr 2003

Richlin, Spencer S MD (RE) - **Spec Exp:** Infertility-IVF; Reproductive Surgery; Fertility Preservation; **Hospital:** Norwalk Hosp, Stamford Hosp (page 939); **Address:** RMA of Connecticut, 10 Glover Ave, Norwalk, CT 06850-1202; **Phone:** 203-750-7400; **Board Cert:** Obstetrics & Gynecology 2012; Reproductive Endocrinology/Infertility 2012; **Med School:** USC-Keck School of Medicine 1994; **Resid:** Obstetrics & Gynecology, Stamford Hosp 1999; **Fellow:** Reproductive Endocrinology, Emory Univ Hosp 2002

Williams, Shaun C MD (RE) - **Spec Exp:** Infertility-IVF; Reproductive Surgery; **Hospital:** St. Vincent's Med Ctr - Bridgeport, Bridgeport Hosp; **Address:** RMA of Connecticut, 115 Technology Drive, Ste A203, Trumbull, CT 06611; **Phone:** 203-880-5340; **Board Cert:** Obstetrics & Gynecology 2012; Reproductive Endocrinology/Infertility 2012; **Med School:** Baylor Coll Med 1995; **Resid:** Obstetrics & Gynecology, Univ Texas SW Med Ctr 1999; **Fellow:** Reproductive Endocrinology, Jones Inst for Repro Endocrinology 2002

Witt, Barry R MD (RE) - **Spec Exp:** Infertility-IVF; **Hospital:** Greenwich Hosp (page 938); **Address:** 55 Holly Hill Ln, Ste 270, Greenwich, CT 06830; **Phone:** 203-863-2990; **Board Cert:** Obstetrics & Gynecology 2011; Reproductive Endocrinology 2011; **Med School:** NY Med Coll 1984; **Resid:** Obstetrics & Gynecology, Montefiore-Weiler Einstein Med Ctr 1988; **Fellow:** Reproductive Endocrinology, Tulane Univ Med Ctr 1990; **Fac Appt:** Assoc Prof ObG, NYU Sch Med

Rheumatology

Danehower, Richard L MD (Rhu) - **Spec Exp:** Rheumatoid Arthritis; Temporal Arteritis; Psoriatic Arthritis; Osteoarthritis; **Hospital:** Greenwich Hosp (page 938); **Address:** 49 Lake Ave, Ste 102, Greenwich, CT 06830-4501; **Phone:** 203-869-5715; **Board Cert:** Internal Medicine 1971; Rheumatology 1974; **Med School:** Univ Pennsylvania 1965; **Resid:** Internal Medicine, Univ Michigan Med Ctr 1969; **Fellow:** Rheumatology, Univ Michigan Med Ctr 1970; **Fac Appt:** Asst Clin Prof Med, Yale Univ

Gladstein, Geoffrey S MD (Rhu) - **Spec Exp:** Arthritis; Antiphospholipid Syndrome (APS); Chronic Fatigue Syndrome; Lupus/SLE; **Hospital:** Bridgeport Hosp; **Address:** PriMed Arthritis & Rheumatism Assocs, 5520 Park Ave, Ste 101, Trumbull, CT 06611; **Phone:** 203-371-5873; **Board Cert:** Internal Medicine 1976; Rheumatology 1978; **Med School:** Geo Wash Univ 1973; **Resid:** Internal Medicine, Albany Med Ctr 1976; **Fellow:** Rheumatology, Albany Med Ctr 1978

Miller, Kenneth A MD (Rhu) - **Spec Exp:** Rheumatoid Arthritis; Osteoporosis; Vasculitis; Lupus/SLE; **Hospital:** Danbury Hosp, New Milford Hosp; **Address:** 33 Hospital Ave, Danbury, CT 06810-5954; **Phone:** 203-794-0599; **Board Cert:** Internal Medicine 1978; Rheumatology 1980; **Med School:** Rush Med Coll 1975; **Resid:** Internal Medicine, GW Univ Hosp 1978; **Fellow:** Rheumatology, Worcester City Hosp 1980

Nascimento, Joao MD (Rhu) - **Spec Exp:** Rheumatoid Arthritis; Lupus/SLE; Psoriatic Arthritis; **Hospital:** St. Vincent's Med Ctr - Bridgeport, Bridgeport Hosp; **Address:** 3203 Main St, Bridgeport, CT 06606-4225; **Phone:** 203-371-0009; **Board Cert:** Internal Medicine 1989; Rheumatology 2012; **Med School:** Portugal 1984; **Resid:** Internal Medicine, Bridgeport Hosp 1989; **Fellow:** Rheumatology, Brown Univ Med Ctr 1991

Novack, Stuart N MD (Rhu) - **Spec Exp:** Lupus/SLE; Osteoporosis; Rheumatoid Arthritis; **Hospital:** Norwalk Hosp; **Address:** Norwalk Med Grp, 40 Cross St Fl 4, Norwalk, CT 06851; **Phone:** 203-845-4830; **Board Cert:** Internal Medicine 1971; Rheumatology 1972; **Med School:** SUNY Hlth Sci Ctr 1966; **Resid:** Internal Medicine, Maimonides Med Ctr 1968; Internal Medicine, UCLA Med Ctr 1969; **Fellow:** Rheumatology, UCLA Med Ctr 1970; **Fac Appt:** Assoc Clin Prof Med, Yale Univ

Rose, Roberta MD (Rhu) - **Spec Exp:** Lupus/SLE; Psoriatic Arthritis; Rheumatoid Arthritis; **Hospital:** Norwalk Hosp; **Address:** Norwalk Med Grp, Rheumatology Dept, 40 Cross St Fl 4, Norwalk, CT 06851; **Phone:** 203-845-4829; **Board Cert:** Internal Medicine 1984; Rheumatology 1988; **Med School:** UCSF 1981; **Resid:** Internal Medicine, Mount Sinai Med Ctr 1984; **Fellow:** Rheumatology, NYU Med Ctr 1987

Spiegel, Michael MD (Rhu) - **Hospital:** Danbury Hosp; **Address:** Orthopaedics Assocs, 226 White St, Danbury, CT 06810; **Phone:** 203-702-6630; **Board Cert:** Internal Medicine 1987; Rheumatology 2010; **Med School:** SUNY Downstate 1984; **Resid:** Internal Medicine, St. Francis Hosp 1987; **Fellow:** Rheumatology, Roger Williams Hosp 1987

Surgery

Capasse, Jeanne S MD (S) - **Spec Exp:** Breast Surgery; **Hospital:** Norwalk Hosp; **Address:** Surgical Breast Care of Connecticut, 148 East Ave, Ste 2L, Norwalk, CT 06851; **Phone:** 203-846-8885; **Board Cert:** Surgery 2002; **Med School:** Cornell Univ-Weill Med Coll 1987; **Resid:** Surgery, St Lukes-Roosevelt Hosp Ctr 1992

Choi, Laura Hargie MD (S) - **Spec Exp:** Laparoscopic Surgery; Obesity/Bariatric Surgery; **Hospital:** Danbury Hosp; **Address:** Ctr Weight Loss Surgery, 111 Osborne St Fl 2, Danbury, CT 06810; **Phone:** 203-739-7131; **Board Cert:** Surgery 2004; **Med School:** NYU Sch Med 1998; **Resid:** Surgery, St Lukes-Roosevelt Hosp 2003

Corvo, Philip R MD (S) - **Spec Exp:** Hernia; Gallbladder Surgery; **Hospital:** Stamford Hosp (page 939); **Address:** 32 Strawberry Hill Ct, Ste 41052, Tulley Health Ctr, Stamford, CT 06902; **Phone:** 203-327-6755; **Board Cert:** Surgery 2008; Surgical Critical Care 2009; **Med School:** Univ Conn 1992; **Resid:** Surgery, Stamford Hosp 1997; **Fellow:** Surgical Critical Care, Hartford Hosp 1998; **Fac Appt:** Asst Prof S, Univ Conn

Demestihas, Anthy MD (S) - **Spec Exp:** Breast Surgery; Trauma; Laparoscopic Surgery; **Hospital:** St. Vincent's Med Ctr - Bridgeport; **Address:** 2660 Main St, Ste 110, Southport, CT 06606; **Phone:** 203-332-4744; **Board Cert:** Surgery 2003; **Med School:** Mexico 1986; **Resid:** Surgery, St Vincents Med Ctr 1989; Surgery, Westchester Med Ctr 1992

Dong, Xiang D MD (S) - **Spec Exp:** Gastrointestinal Cancer; Rectal Cancer; Sarcoma; Melanoma; **Hospital:** Stamford Hosp (page 939); **Address:** Fairfield Co Surgical Specialists, 1351 Washington Blvd Fl 6 - Ste 601, Stamford, CT 06902; **Phone:** 203-276-5959; **Board Cert:** Surgery 2005; **Med School:** Duke Univ 1999; **Resid:** Surgery, Drexel Univ Coll Med Affil Hosp 2005; **Fellow:** Surgical Oncology, UPMC 2006

Dwyer, Kevin M MD (S) - **Spec Exp:** Trauma; **Hospital:** Stamford Hosp (page 939); **Address:** Fairfield Co Surgical Specialists, 1351 Washington Blvd Fl 6, Stamford, CT 06902; **Phone:** 203-276-5959; **Board Cert:** Surgery 2011; Surgical Critical Care 2006; **Med School:** Georgetown Univ 1984; **Resid:** Surgery, Army Med Ctr 1991; **Fellow:** Trauma/Critical Care, Inova Fairfax Hosp 1995; Trauma/Critical Care, Univ MD Med Ctr 1996

Floch, Neil MD (S) - **Spec Exp:** Obesity/Bariatric Surgery; Laparoscopic Surgery; **Hospital:** Norwalk Hosp, St. Vincent's Med Ctr - Bridgeport; **Address:** Fairfield Co Bariatric & Surgical, 148 East Ave, Ste 3A, Norwalk, CT 06851; **Phone:** 203-899-0744; **Board Cert:** Surgery 2008; **Med School:** Boston Univ 1992; **Resid:** Surgery, Beth Israel Med Ctr 1997; **Fellow:** Laparoscopic Surgery, Mayo Clin 1998

Garvey, Richard J MD (S) - **Spec Exp:** Breast Surgery; Pediatric Surgery; Laparoscopic Abdominal Surgery; **Hospital:** Bridgeport Hosp; **Address:** Genl Surgeons of Greater Bridgeport, 310 Mill Hill Ave, Bridgeport, CT 06610-2863; **Phone:** 203-366-3211; **Board Cert:** Surgery 2009; **Med School:** Georgetown Univ 1974; **Resid:** Surgery, Boston Univ Med Ctr 1980

Kenler, Andrew S MD (S) - **Spec Exp:** Breast Surgery; Hernia; Laparoscopic Abdominal Surgery; Thyroid Surgery; **Hospital:** Bridgeport Hosp; **Address:** Park Avenue Surgical Assocs, 5520 Park Ave, Ste 207, Trumbull, CT 06611; **Phone:** 203-373-9015; **Board Cert:** Surgery 2006; **Med School:** Cornell Univ-Weill Med Coll 1988; **Resid:** Surgery, Mass Genl Hosp 1991; Surgery, NE Deaconess Hosp 1995; **Fac Appt:** Asst Clin Prof S, Yale Univ

Lazarus, Laura MD (S) - **Spec Exp:** Breast Surgery; Breast Cancer; **Hospital:** Greenwich Hosp (page 938); **Address:** Breast Care Services of Greenwich, 77 Lafayette Pl, Ste 302, Greenwich, CT 06830; **Phone:** 203-863-4250; **Board Cert:** Surgery 2010; **Med School:** Hahnemann Univ 1996; **Resid:** Surgery, LSU Med Ctr 2001; **Fellow:** Breast Surgery, Northwestern Meml Hosp 2002

McWhorter, Philip MD (S) - **Spec Exp:** Cancer Surgery; Gastrointestinal Surgery; **Hospital:** Greenwich Hosp (page 938); **Address:** 77 Lafayette Pl, Ste 301, Greenwich, CT 06830; **Phone:** 203-863-4300; **Board Cert:** Surgery 1997; **Med School:** Cornell Univ-Weill Med Coll 1973; **Resid:** Surgery, New York Hosp 1977

Miller, Kevin D MD (S) - **Spec Exp:** Hepatobiliary Surgery; Trauma; **Hospital:** Stamford Hosp (page 939); **Address:** Fairfield Co Surgical Specialists, 1351 Washington Blvd Fl 6 - Ste 601, Stamford, CT 06902; **Phone:** 203-276-5959; **Board Cert:** Surgery 2010; **Med School:** Columbia P&S 1994; **Resid:** Surgery, Beth Israel Deaconess Hosp 2000

Pass, Helen A MD (S) - **Spec Exp:** Breast Cancer; Breast Disease; Nipple Sparing Mastectomy; **Hospital:** Stamford Hosp (page 939); **Address:** Women's Breast Ctr, Fairfield Co Surgical Specialists, 32 Strawberry Hill Ct, Stamford, CT 06902; **Phone:** 203-276-4255; **Board Cert:** Surgery 2003; **Med School:** Univ Mich Med Sch 1987; **Resid:** Surgery, Univ Texas Affil Hosp 1989; Surgery, MedStar Georgetown Univ Hosp 1994; **Fellow:** Surgical Oncology, NCI/NIH 1992

Passeri, Daniel J MD (S) - **Spec Exp:** Cancer Surgery; Laparoscopic Surgery; **Hospital:** St. Vincent's Med Ctr - Bridgeport, Bridgeport Hosp; **Address:** 888 White Plains Rd Fl 2 - Ste 206, Trumbull, CT 06611-4552; **Phone:** 203-459-2666; **Board Cert:** Surgery 2011; **Med School:** Yale Univ 1975; **Resid:** Surgery, Yale-New Haven Hosp 1980

Petrotos, Athanassios MD (S) - **Spec Exp:** Laparoscopic Surgery; Gallbladder Surgery; **Hospital:** Greenwich Hosp (page 938); **Address:** Surgical Specialists Greenwich, 77 Lafayette Pl, Ste 301, Greenwich, CT 06830; **Phone:** 203-863-4300; **Board Cert:** Surgery 2005; **Med School:** Greece 1991; **Resid:** Surgery, St Lukes-Roosevelt Hosp Ctr 2001

Sarnelle, James A MD (S) - **Hospital:** Stamford Hosp (page 939); **Address:** 90 Morgan St, Ste 304, Stamford, CT 06905-5436; **Phone:** 203-353-8088; **Board Cert:** Surgery 2006; **Med School:** NYU Sch Med 1981; **Resid:** Surgery, Stamford Hosp 1985; **Fellow:** Surgery, Lehigh Valley Hosp 1987

Ward, Barbara A MD (S) - **Spec Exp:** Breast Cancer; Breast Surgery; Breast Disease; **Hospital:** Greenwich Hosp (page 938); **Address:** 77 Lafayette Pl, Ste 302, Greenwich, CT 06830-5426; **Phone:** 203-863-4250; **Board Cert:** Surgery 2011; **Med School:** Temple Univ 1983; **Resid:** Surgery, Yale-New Haven Hosp 1990; **Fellow:** Surgical Oncology, Natl Cancer Inst 1987

Thoracic & Cardiac Surgery

Coady, Michael A MD (T&CS) - **Spec Exp:** Thoracic Aortic Surgery; Heart Valve Surgery; **Hospital:** Stamford Hosp (page 939); **Address:** Stamford Hosp,Heart & Vascular Inst, 32 Strawberry Hill Ct Fl 4, Stamford, CT 06904; **Phone:** 203-276-4415; **Board Cert:** Surgery 2010; Thoracic & Cardiac Surgery 2004; **Med School:** Geo Wash Univ 1993; **Resid:** Surgery, Yale-New Haven Hosp 2000; **Fellow:** Cardiothoracic Surgery, Stanford Univ Hosp & Clin 2003

DiMeo, Albert MD (T&CS) - **Spec Exp:** Coronary Artery Surgery; Heart Valve Surgery; Robotic Surgery; **Hospital:** St. Vincent's Med Ctr - Bridgeport; **Address:** St Vincent's Medical Ctr, Dept Cardiothoracic Surgery, 2800 Main St, Bridgeport, CT 06606; **Phone:** 203-576-5708; **Board Cert:** Surgery 2004; Thoracic Surgery 2006; **Med School:** Univ Pennsylvania 1998; **Resid:** Surgery, NY Presby Hosp 2004; **Fellow:** Thoracic Surgery, NY Presby Hosp 2006

Feng, William C MD (T&CS) - **Hospital:** Stamford Hosp (page 939); **Address:** Stamford Hosp, Heart & Vascular Inst, 32 Strawberry Hill Ct Fl 4, Stamford, CT 06902; **Phone:** 203-276-4415; **Board Cert:** Thoracic Surgery 2010; **Med School:** Brown Univ 1982; **Resid:** Surgery, UAB Hosp 1987; **Fellow:** Cardiothoracic Surgery, Rhode Island Hosp 1989

Lettera, James V MD (T&CS) - **Spec Exp:** Esophageal Surgery; Aneurysm-Aortic; Vascular Surgery; Peripheral Vascular Disease; **Hospital:** Bridgeport Hosp, St. Vincent's Med Ctr - Bridgeport; **Address:** CT Vascular & Thoracic Surgical Assocs, 501 Kings Hwy E, Ste 112, Fairfield, CT 06825; **Phone:** 203-382-1900; **Board Cert:** Thoracic Surgery 2003; **Med School:** Georgetown Univ 1977; **Resid:** Surgery, St Vincent's Hosp Med Ctr 1982; Thoracic Surgery, Jackson Meml Hosp 1984

Squitieri, Rafael P MD (T&CS) - **Spec Exp:** Robotic Surgery; Aneurysm-Aortic; Maze Procedure for Atrial Fibrillation; Heart Valve Surgery; **Hospital:** St. Vincent's Med Ctr - Bridgeport; **Address:** St Vincent's Medical Ctr, Dept Cardiothoracic Surgery, 280 Main St, Bridgeport, CT 06606; **Phone:** 203-576-5708; **Board Cert:** Thoracic Surgery 2002; **Med School:** Mount Sinai Sch Med 1993; **Resid:** Surgery, Morristown Meml Hosp 1998; **Fellow:** Thoracic Surgery, Mt Sinai Med Ctr 2001

Waters, Paul F MD (T&CS) - **Spec Exp:** Lung Cancer; Esophageal Surgery; Thoracic Cancers; **Hospital:** Greenwich Hosp (page 938); **Address:** 77 Lafayette Pl, Ste 302, Greenwich, CT 06830; **Phone:** 203-863-4341; **Board Cert:** Surgery 2004; **Med School:** Univ Toronto 1974; **Resid:** Surgery, Univ Toronto Med Ctr 1979; Thoracic Surgery, Univ Toronto Med Ctr 1980; **Fellow:** Esophageal Surgery, Univ Chicago Hosps 1981

Urology

Andriani, Rudy T MD (U) - **Spec Exp:** Urologic Cancer; Kidney Stones; Incontinence; **Hospital:** Stamford Hosp (page 939); **Address:** 166 W Broad St, Ste 404, Stamford, CT 06902-3661; **Phone:** 203-356-9692; **Board Cert:** Urology 2008; **Med School:** NY Med Coll 1981; **Resid:** Surgery, St Vincent's Med Ctr 1983; Urology, Duke Univ Hosp 1987

Dodds, Peter MD (U) - **Hospital:** Norwalk Hosp; **Address:** Urology Assocs of Norwalk, 12 Elmcrest Terr, Norwalk, CT 06850-3964; **Phone:** 203-853-4200; **Board Cert:** Urology 2004; **Med School:** Columbia P&S 1977; **Resid:** Surgery, Yale-New Haven Hosp 1980; Urology, Yale-New Haven Hosp 1983

Hennessy, William T MD (U) - **Spec Exp:** Pediatric Urology; Urologic Cancer; **Hospital:** Danbury Hosp; **Address:** Urology Assocs, 51-53 Kenosia Ave, Danbury, CT 06810; **Phone:** 203-748-0330; **Board Cert:** Urology 1982; **Med School:** Georgetown Univ 1976; **Resid:** Urology, Hosp Univ Penn 1980; **Fellow:** Pediatric Urology, Chldns Hosp 1982; Urologic Oncology, Meml Sloan-Kettering Cancer Ctr 1982

Muldoon, Lawrence D MD (U) - **Hospital:** St. Vincent's Med Ctr - Bridgeport, Bridgeport Hosp; **Address:** Greater Bridgeport Urology, 425 Post Rd Fl 2, Fairfield, CT 06824; **Phone:** 203-254-1576; **Board Cert:** Urology 2012; **Med School:** Northwestern Univ 1984; **Resid:** Surgery, Univ Hosps 1987; Urology, Univ Hosps 1990

Nurzia, Michael J MD (U) - **Spec Exp:** Prostate Cancer; Prostate Disease; Bladder Cancer; **Hospital:** Stamford Hosp (page 939), Greenwich Hosp (page 938); **Address:** 166 W Broad St, Ste 404, 34 Hoyt St, Stamford, CT 06902; **Phone:** 203-356-9391 x10; **Board Cert:** Urology 2007; **Med School:** Mount Sinai Sch Med 1999; **Resid:** Urology, UMDNJ-RW Johnson Med Ctr 2005

Ranta, Jeffrey A MD (U) - **Spec Exp:** Prostate Cancer; Bladder Cancer; Kidney Stones; **Hospital:** Greenwich Hosp (page 938); **Address:** 49 Lake Ave, Greenwich Med Bldg, Ste 201, Greenwich, CT 06830-4520; **Phone:** 203-869-1285; **Board Cert:** Urology 2004; **Med School:** Georgetown Univ 1979; **Resid:** Surgery, Georgetown Univ Hosp 1981; Urology, Lahey Clinic 1984

Santarosa, Richard P MD (U) - **Spec Exp:** Prostate Cancer; Prostate Disease; Bladder Cancer; Minimally Invasive Urologic Surgery; **Hospital:** Stamford Hosp (page 939), Greenwich Hosp (page 938); **Address:** 166 W Broad St, Ste 404, Stamford, CT 06902; **Phone:** 203-356-9391 x11; **Board Cert:** Urology 2007; **Med School:** Univ Rochester 1989; **Resid:** Surgery, Columbia-Presby Med Ctr 1991; Urology, Columbia-Presby Med Ctr 1995; **Fellow:** Neurourology, Columbia-Presby Med Ctr 1996

Shield, Dennis MD (U) - **Spec Exp:** Prostate Cancer; **Hospital:** Norwalk Hosp; **Address:** Urology Assocs of Norwalk, 12 Elmcrest Terr, Norwalk, CT 06850; **Phone:** 203-853-4200; **Board Cert:** Urology 1978; **Med School:** Yale Univ 1970; **Resid:** Surgery, Yale-New Haven Hosp 1972; Urology, Yale-New Haven Hosp 1976

Viner, Nicholas A MD (U) - **Spec Exp:** Prostate Cancer; Kidney Stones; Bladder Cancer; Vasectomy; **Hospital:** Bridgeport Hosp, St. Vincent's Med Ctr - Bridgeport; **Address:** Urological Assocs of Bridgeport, 160 Hawley Ln, Ste 002, Trumbull, CT 06611-6058; **Phone:** 203-375-3456; **Board Cert:** Urology 1977; **Med School:** Vanderbilt Univ 1968; **Resid:** Surgery, Greenwich Hosp 1970; Urology, Vanderbilt Univ Hosp 1974

Waxberg, Jonathan MD (U) - **Spec Exp:** Prostate Cancer; Erectile Dysfunction; Kidney Stones; Incontinence; **Hospital:** Stamford Hosp (page 939), NY-Presby/Columbia Univ Med Ctr, NY (page 104); **Address:** 35 Hoyt St, Stamford, CT 06905-5602; **Phone:** 203-324-2268; **Board Cert:** Urology 2008; **Med School:** Univ Cincinnati 1980; **Resid:** Urology, Maimonides Med Ctr 1986; **Fac Appt:** Clin Prof U, Univ Cincinnati

Zuckerman, Howard L MD (U) - **Spec Exp:** Incontinence; Prostate Cancer; Pediatric Urology; **Hospital:** Bridgeport Hosp, St. Vincent's Med Ctr - Bridgeport; **Address:** Urological Assocs of Bridgeport, 160 Hawley Ln, Ste 002, Trumbull, CT 06611; **Phone:** 203-375-3456; **Board Cert:** Urology 1977; **Med School:** St Louis Univ 1967; **Resid:** Surgery, VA Commonwealth Univ Med Ctr 1969; Urology, Albert Einstein Med Ctr 1975

Vascular & Interventional Radiology

Hodges, Laura J MD (VIR) - **Spec Exp:** Uterine Fibroid Embolization; **Hospital:** Greenwich Hosp (page 938); **Address:** Greenwich Hospital, Dept Radiology, 49 Lake Ave, Ste LL2, Greenwich, CT 06830; **Phone:** 203-863-3042; **Board Cert:** Diagnostic Radiology 1999; Vascular & Interventional Radiology 2012; **Med School:** Albert Einstein Coll Med 1994; **Resid:** Diagnostic Radiology, Yale-New Haven Hosp 1999; **Fellow:** Vascular & Interventional Radiology, NY-Presby/Cornell Med Ctr 2000

Sandhu, Fatejeet MD (VIR) - **Spec Exp:** Interventional Radiology; **Hospital:** Danbury Hosp; **Address:** Danbury Radiology Assocs, 24 Hospital Ave, Danbury, CT 06810; **Phone:** 203-739-7532; **Board Cert:** Diagnostic Radiology ; Vascular & Interventional Radiology 2006; **Med School:** Emory Univ 1986; **Resid:** Diagnostic Radiology, UCSF Med Ctr 1991; **Fellow:** Body Imaging, UCSF Med Ctr 1992; Interventional Radiology, Emory Univ Hosp 1993

Strauss, Edward B MD (VIR) - **Hospital:** Norwalk Hosp; **Address:** Norwalk Hosp, Radiology, 34 Maple St, Norwalk, CT 06856-3894; **Phone:** 203-852-2715; **Board Cert:** Diagnostic Radiology 1983; Nuclear Medicine 1984; Vascular & Interventional Radiology 2005; **Med School:** Yale Univ 1979; **Resid:** Diagnostic Radiology, Yale-New Haven Hosp 1983; **Fellow:** Nuclear Medicine, Yale-New Haven Hosp 1984

Vascular Surgery

Dietzek, Alan M MD (VascS) - **Spec Exp:** Aneurysm-Aortic; Minimally Invasive Vascular Surgery; Arterial Bypass Surgery-Leg; Carotid Artery Surgery; **Hospital:** Danbury Hosp; **Address:** 41 Germantown Rd, Ste 101, Danbury, CT 06810; **Phone:** 203-794-5680; **Board Cert:** Vascular Surgery 2009; **Med School:** Loyola Univ-Stritch Sch Med 1983; **Resid:** Surgery, LI Jewish Med Ctr 1988; **Fellow:** Vascular Surgery, Montefiore Med Ctr 1990; **Fac Appt:** Asst Clin Prof S, NY Med Coll

Gagne, Paul J MD (VascS) - **Spec Exp:** Endovascular Surgery; Aneurysm-Abdominal Aortic; Carotid Artery Surgery; Vein Disorders; **Hospital:** Norwalk Hosp, Bridgeport Hosp; **Address:** Southern Connecticut Vascular Ctr, 495 Hawley Ln, Ste 2B, Stratford, CT 06614; **Phone:** 203-375-2861; **Board Cert:** Vascular Surgery 2005; **Med School:** NYU Sch Med 1986; **Resid:** Surgery, NYU Med Ctr 1991; **Fellow:** Vascular Surgery, UAMS Med Ctr 1995

Huribal, Marsel MD (VascS) - **Spec Exp:** Endovascular Surgery; Aneurysm-Aortic; Vein Disorders; **Hospital:** Bridgeport Hosp, St. Vincent's Med Ctr - Bridgeport; **Address:** Southern CT Vascular Ctr, 495 Hawley Ln, Ste 2A, Stratford, CT 06614; **Phone:** 203-375-2861; **Board Cert:** Vascular Surgery 2008; **Med School:** Amer Univ Caribbean 1987; **Resid:** Surgery, Bridgeport Hosp 1994; **Fellow:** Vascular Surgery, Millard Filmore Hosp 1996; **Fac Appt:** Asst Clin Prof VascS, Yale Univ

Marsan, Ben U MD (VascS) - **Spec Exp:** Peripheral Vascular Disease; Vein Disorders; Aneurysm-Aortic; Endovascular Surgery; **Hospital:** Norwalk Hosp, Bridgeport Hosp; **Address:** Southern Connecticut Vascular Ctr, 495 Hawley Ln, Ste 2B, Stratford, CT 06614; **Phone:** 203-375-2861; **Board Cert:** Vascular Surgery 2009; **Med School:** Oregon Hlth & Sci Univ 1989; **Resid:** Surgery, Flushing Hosp Med Ctr 1995; **Fellow:** Vascular Surgery, SUNY Buffalo Affil Hosp 1997

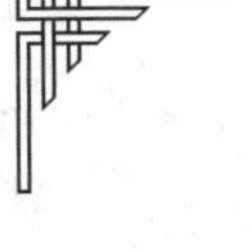

The Best in American Medicine
www.CastleConnolly.com

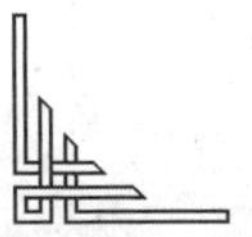

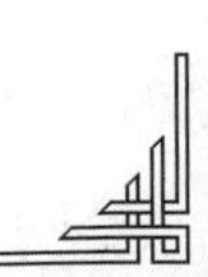

New Haven

New Haven

Addiction Psychiatry

Malison, Robert MD (AdP) - **Spec Exp:** Addiction/Substance Abuse; **Hospital:** Yale-New Haven Hosp; **Address:** Yale, Clin Neuroscience, 34 Park St, New Haven, CT 06519; **Phone:** 203-974-7560; **Board Cert:** Psychiatry 1993; **Med School:** Yale Univ 1987; **Resid:** Psychiatry, Yale-New Haven Hosp 1992; **Fellow:** Addiction Psychiatry, Hosp Univ Penn 1993; **Fac Appt:** Prof Psyc, Yale Univ

Potenza, Marc MD/PhD (AdP) - **Spec Exp:** Addiction/Substance Abuse; Psychotherapy; Women's Health-Mental Health; **Hospital:** Yale-New Haven Hosp; **Address:** Yale, Psychiatry Dept, 34 Park St CMHC Bldg - rm S-104, new Haven, CT 06519; **Phone:** 203-974-7356; **Board Cert:** Psychiatry 2010; **Med School:** Yale Univ 1994; **Resid:** Psychiatry, Yale-New Haven Hosp 1998; **Fellow:** Addiction Psychiatry, Yale-New Haven Hosp 1999; **Fac Appt:** Prof Psyc, Yale Univ

Adolescent Medicine

Ryan, Sheryl MD (AM) - **Spec Exp:** Eating Disorders; Adolescent Gynecology; Behavioral Disorders; **Hospital:** Yale-New Haven Hosp; **Address:** Yale-Primary Care, 789 Howard Ave, New Haven, CT 06520; **Phone:** 203-688-9335; **Board Cert:** Pediatrics ; Adolescent Medicine 2012; **Med School:** Yale Univ 1981; **Resid:** Pediatrics, Chldn's Hosp 1984; **Fellow:** Adolescent Medicine, UCSF Med Ctr 1988; **Fac Appt:** Assoc Prof Ped, Yale Univ

Allergy & Immunology

Adelsberg, Bernard Roy MD (A&I) - **Spec Exp:** Asthma & Allergy; Allergic Rhinitis; Food Allergy; **Hospital:** Yale-New Haven Hosp - St Raphael Campus, Yale-New Haven Hosp; **Address:** CT Med Grp, Allergy, 2416 Whitney Ave Fl 3, Hamden, CT 06518; **Phone:** 203-287-9355; **Board Cert:** Internal Medicine 1975; Allergy & Immunology 1979; Diagnostic Lab Immunology 1986; **Med School:** SUNY Downstate 1972; **Resid:** Internal Medicine, Mount Sinai Med Ctr 1975; **Fellow:** Immunology, Scripps Clin & Rsch 1977

Kaufman, Richard E MD (A&I) - **Spec Exp:** Asthma; Urticaria; Allergy; **Hospital:** Yale-New Haven Hosp; **Address:** Quinninpiac Med, 960 Main St, Branford, CT 06405; **Phone:** 203-488-6358; **Board Cert:** Internal Medicine 1976; Allergy & Immunology 1979; **Med School:** Yale Univ 1971; **Resid:** Internal Medicine, Yale-New Haven Hosp 1976; **Fellow:** Rheumatology/Immunology, Yale-New Haven Hosp 1978; **Fac Appt:** Assoc Clin Prof Med, Yale Univ

Cardiac Electrophysiology

Blitzer, Mark MD (CE) - **Spec Exp:** Atrial Fibrillation; Syncope; **Hospital:** Yale-New Haven Hosp; **Address:** Yale, Arrhythmia Ctr, 330 Orchard St, Ste 210, New Haven, CT 06511; **Phone:** 203-867-5400; **Board Cert:** Cardiovascular Disease 2007; Cardiac Electrophysiology 2009; **Med School:** Harvard Med Sch 1991; **Resid:** Internal Medicine, Brigham & Womens Hosp 1994; **Fellow:** Cardiovascular Disease, NY-Presby/Columbia Univ Med Ctr 1997

Lampert, Rachel Jane MD (CE) - **Spec Exp:** Arrhythmias; Stress Management; Defibrillators; **Hospital:** Yale-New Haven Hosp; **Address:** Yale, Cardiac Electrophysiology, 800 Howard Ave Fl 2, New Haven, CT 06519; **Phone:** 203-785-4126; **Board Cert:** Cardiovascular Disease 2005; Cardiac Electrophysiology 2008; **Med School:** Vanderbilt Univ 1987; **Resid:** Internal Medicine, Bellevue Hosp 1991; **Fellow:** Cardiovascular Disease, Yale-New Haven Hosp 1992; **Fac Appt:** Assoc Prof Med, Yale Univ

Schoenfeld, Mark MD (CE) - **Spec Exp:** Arrhythmias; **Hospital:** Yale-New Haven Hosp - St Raphael Campus; **Address:** Arrhythmia Ctr, 330 Orchard St, Ste 210, New Haven, CT 06511; **Phone:** 203-867-5400; **Board Cert:** Internal Medicine 1982; Cardiovascular Disease 1985; Cardiac Electrophysiology 2012; **Med School:** Harvard Med Sch 1979; **Resid:** Internal Medicine, Mass Genl Hosp 1982; **Fellow:** Cardiovascular Disease, Mass Genl Hosp 1985; Cardiac Electrophysiology, Mass Genl Hosp 1986; **Fac Appt:** Clin Prof Med, Yale Univ

Cardiovascular Disease

Cabin, Henry S MD (Cv) - **Spec Exp:** Interventional Cardiology; Cardiac Catheterization; **Hospital:** Yale-New Haven Hosp; **Address:** Yale Cardiology, 11 Harrison Ave, Branford, CT 06405; **Phone:** 203-483-8300; **Board Cert:** Internal Medicine 1978; Cardiovascular Disease 1983; **Med School:** Yale Univ 1975; **Resid:** Internal Medicine, Yale-New Haven Hosp 1978; **Fellow:** Research, Natl Heart Lung & Blood Inst 1981; Cardiovascular Disease, Yale-New Haven Hosp 1982; **Fac Appt:** Prof Med, Yale Univ

Cleman, Michael W MD (Cv) - **Spec Exp:** Interventional Cardiology; Angioplasty; Cardiac Catheterization; **Hospital:** Yale-New Haven Hosp; **Address:** Yale, Cardiology, 11 Harrison Ave, Branford, CT 06405; **Phone:** 203-483-8300; **Board Cert:** Internal Medicine 1980; Cardiovascular Disease 1985; Interventional Cardiology 2011; **Med School:** Johns Hopkins Univ 1977; **Resid:** Internal Medicine, Shands at Univ Fl 1980; **Fellow:** Cardiovascular Disease, Yale-New Haven Hosp 1981; **Fac Appt:** Prof Med, Yale Univ

Freed, Lisa A MD (Cv) - **Spec Exp:** Heart Disease in Women; Mitral Valve Prolapse; Echocardiography; **Hospital:** Yale-New Haven Hosp, Yale-New Haven Hosp - St Raphael Campus; **Address:** Yale Cardiology Assocs, 2 Devine St, North Haven, CT 06473; **Phone:** 203-789-2272; **Board Cert:** Cardiovascular Disease 2009; **Med School:** Johns Hopkins Univ 1992; **Resid:** Internal Medicine, NY-Presby/Weill Cornell Med Ctr 1995; **Fellow:** Cardiovascular Disease, Mass Genl Hosp 1998; Echocardiography, Framingham Heart Study 1999; **Fac Appt:** Asst Clin Prof Med, Yale Univ

Tuohy IV, Edward R MD (Cv) - **Spec Exp:** Angioplasty & Stent Placement; Peripheral Vascular Disease; **Hospital:** Bridgeport Hosp; **Address:** Cardiac Specialists, 20 Commerce Park, Milford, CT 06460; **Phone:** 203-283-5200; **Board Cert:** Internal Medicine 2008; Cardiovascular Disease 2011; Interventional Cardiology 2012; **Med School:** NYU Sch Med 1995; **Resid:** Internal Medicine, Yale-New Haven Hosp 1998; **Fellow:** Cardiovascular Disease, Yale-New Haven Hosp 2001

Child & Adolescent Psychiatry

Gammon, G. Davis MD (ChAP) - **Hospital:** Yale-New Haven Hosp; **Address:** 33 Edgehill Terrace, Hamden, CT 06517; **Phone:** 203-865-6540; **Board Cert:** Psychiatry 1981; Child & Adolescent Psychiatry 1992; **Med School:** Temple Univ 1976; **Resid:** Psychiatry, Yale-New Haven Hosp 1980; Child Psychiatry, Yale-New Haven Hosp 1984; **Fellow:** Epidemiology, Yale-New Haven Hosp 1983; **Fac Appt:** Asst Clin Prof Psyc, Yale Univ

Leckman, James F MD (ChAP) - **Spec Exp:** Tourette's Syndrome; Obsessive-Compulsive Disorder; Autism; **Hospital:** Yale-New Haven Hosp; **Address:** Yale Child Study Ctr, 230 S Frontage Rd, New Haven, CT 06520; **Phone:** 203-785-7971; **Board Cert:** Psychiatry 1980; Child & Adolescent Psychiatry 1982; **Med School:** Univ New Mexico 1973; **Resid:** Psychiatry, Yale-New Haven Hosp 1979; Child Psychiatry, Yale Chld Stdy Ctr 1980; **Fellow:** Psychiatry, Natl Inst Mental Hlth 1976; **Fac Appt:** Prof Psyc, Yale Univ

Madigan, Janet A MD (ChAP) - **Spec Exp:** Developmental Disorders; Psychotherapy; Psychoanalysis; Attachment Disorders; **Hospital:** Yale-New Haven Hosp; **Address:** 291 Whitney Ave, Ste 203, New Haven, CT 06511; **Phone:** 203-787-5420; **Board Cert:** Psychiatry 1982; Child & Adolescent Psychiatry 1986; **Med School:** NY Med Coll 1977; **Resid:** Psychiatry, Yale-New Haven Hosp 1981; **Fellow:** Child & Adolescent Psychiatry, Yale-New Haven Hosp 1985; Psychoanalysis, Western New England Inst 1986; **Fac Appt:** Asst Clin Prof Psyc, Yale Univ

Child Neurology

Levy, Susan Ruth MD (ChiN) - **Spec Exp:** Epilepsy; Neurophysiology; Headache; **Hospital:** Yale-New Haven Hosp; **Address:** Child Neurology Assocs, 5 Durham Rd, Ste 1-7, Guilford, CT 06437; **Phone:** 203-453-2181; **Board Cert:** Pediatrics 1984; Child Neurology 1986; **Med School:** Wake Forest Univ 1978; **Resid:** Pediatrics, Wake Forest Baptist Hosp 1981; Pediatric Neurology, Univ Mass Med Ctr 1984; **Fellow:** Neurophysiology, Mass Genl Hosp 1985; **Fac Appt:** Clin Prof N, Yale Univ

Ment, Laura R MD (ChiN) - **Spec Exp:** Developmental Disorders; Stroke; **Hospital:** Yale-New Haven Hosp; **Address:** Yale, Ped Neurology, 1 Park St, New Haven, CT 06510; **Phone:** 203-785-5708; **Board Cert:** Pediatrics 1979; Child Neurology 1980; **Med School:** Tufts Univ 1973; **Resid:** Pediatrics, Mass Genl Hosp 1976; **Fellow:** Pediatric Neurology, Mass Genl Hosp 1979; Pediatric Neurology, Hammersmith Hosp 1979; **Fac Appt:** Prof Ped, Yale Univ

Shaywitz, Bennett A MD (ChiN) - **Spec Exp:** Learning Disorders; Dyslexia; Headache; **Hospital:** Yale-New Haven Hosp; **Address:** Yale New Haven Chldns Hosp-Ped Neurology Dept, 1 Park St Fl 2, West Pavilion, New Haven, CT 06510; **Phone:** 203-785-4641; **Board Cert:** Pediatrics 1968; Child Neurology 1973; **Med School:** Washington Univ, St Louis 1963; **Resid:** Pediatrics, Bronx Muni Hosp Ctr 1967; **Fellow:** Child Neurology, Albert Einstein Coll Med 1970; **Fac Appt:** Prof Ped, Yale Univ

Testa, Francine M MD (ChiN) - **Spec Exp:** Epilepsy; **Hospital:** Yale-New Haven Hosp; **Address:** 5 Durham Rd, Ste A-7, Guilford, CT 06437; **Phone:** 203-453-2181; **Board Cert:** Child Neurology 1994; **Med School:** SUNY Downstate 1986; **Resid:** Pediatrics, Yale-New Haven Hosp 1988; Child Neurology, Columbia-Presby Hosp 1991; **Fellow:** Epilepsy, Columbia Univ 1992; **Fac Appt:** Clin Prof N, Yale Univ

Clinical Genetics

Bale, Allen E MD (CG) - **Spec Exp:** Cancer Genetics; **Hospital:** Yale-New Haven Hosp; **Address:** Yale-New Haven, Genetics Dept, 333 Cedar St SHM Bldg - rm 329, New Haven, CT 06510; **Phone:** 203-764-8400; **Board Cert:** Internal Medicine 1983; Clinical Genetics 1987; Clinical Molecular Genetics 2010; **Med School:** Univ Mass Sch Med 1979; **Resid:** Internal Medicine, Western Penn Hosp 1983; **Fellow:** Medical Genetics, Natl Inst Hlth-Clin Ctr 1987; **Fac Appt:** Prof CG, Yale Univ

Mahoney, Maurice J MD (CG) - **Spec Exp:** Fetal Therapy; Prenatal Diagnosis; **Hospital:** Yale-New Haven Hosp; **Address:** Yale Genetics Consultation Serv, 333 Cedar St, rm WWW330, New Haven, CT 06520-8005; **Phone:** 203-785-2661; **Board Cert:** Pediatrics 1967; Clinical Genetics 1982; Clinical Biochemical Genetics 1982; **Med School:** Univ Pittsburgh 1962; **Resid:** Pediatrics, Johns Hopkins Hosp 1965; Pediatrics, Childrens Hosp 1966; **Fellow:** Clinical Genetics, Yale Univ Sch Med 1970; **Fac Appt:** Prof CG, Yale Univ

Seashore, Margretta R MD (CG) - **Spec Exp:** Inherited Metabolic Disorders; Inborn Errors of Metabolism; **Hospital:** Yale-New Haven Hosp; **Address:** 1 Park St, New Haven, CT 06520-8005; **Phone:** 203-785-2660 x1; **Board Cert:** Pediatrics 1970; Clinical Biochemical Genetics 1982; Clinical Genetics 1982; **Med School:** Yale Univ 1965; **Resid:** Pediatrics, Yale-New Haven Hosp 1968; **Fellow:** Clinical Genetics, Yale-New Haven Hosp 1970; **Fac Appt:** Prof CG, Yale Univ

Colon & Rectal Surgery

Longo, Walter E MD (CRS) - **Spec Exp:** Colon & Rectal Cancer; Gastrointestinal Surgery; Inflammatory Bowel Disease; **Hospital:** Yale-New Haven Hosp; **Address:** Yale, Colon & Rectal Surgery Dept, 800 Howard Ave Fl 3, New Haven, CT 06510; **Phone:** 203-785-2616; **Board Cert:** Surgery 2011; Colon & Rectal Surgery 2006; **Med School:** NY Med Coll 1984; **Resid:** Surgery, Yale-New Haven Hosp 1990; **Fellow:** Research, Yale-New Haven Hosp 1988; Colon & Rectal Surgery, Cleveland Clin 1991; **Fac Appt:** Prof S, Yale Univ

Dermatology

Antaya, Richard J MD (D) - **Spec Exp:** Pediatric Dermatology; Laser Surgery; Vascular Malformations/Birthmarks; Genetic Disorders-Skin; **Hospital:** Yale-New Haven Hosp; **Address:** Yale Dermatology Assocs, 2 Church St S, Ste 305, New Haven, CT 06519; **Phone:** 203-789-1249; **Board Cert:** Dermatology 2007; Pediatrics 2007; Pediatric Dermatology 2004; **Med School:** Tufts Univ 1989; **Resid:** Pediatrics, Tripler AMC 1992; Dermatology, Duke Univ Hosp 1998; **Fac Appt:** Prof D, Yale Univ

Bolognia, Jean L MD (D) - **Spec Exp:** Melanoma; Skin Cancer; **Hospital:** Yale-New Haven Hosp; **Address:** Yale, Dermatology Dept, 2 Church St S, Ste 305, New Haven, CT 06519; **Phone:** 203-789-1249; **Board Cert:** Dermatology 2009; **Med School:** Yale Univ 1980; **Resid:** Internal Medicine, Yale-New Haven Hosp 1982; Dermatology, Yale-New Haven Hosp 1985; **Fellow:** Dermatology, Yale-New Haven Hosp 1987; **Fac Appt:** Prof D, Yale Univ

Edelson, Richard L MD (D) - **Spec Exp:** Cutaneous Lymphoma; Immune Deficiency-Skin Disorders; **Hospital:** Yale-New Haven Hosp; **Address:** Yale, Dermatology Dept, 2 Church St S, Ste 305, New Haven, CT 06519; **Phone:** 203-789-1249; **Board Cert:** Dermatology 1977; **Med School:** Yale Univ 1970; **Resid:** Dermatology, Mass Genl Hosp 1972; Dermatology, Natl Inst Hlth-Clin Ctr 1975; **Fac Appt:** Prof D, Yale Univ

Leffell, David J MD (D) - **Spec Exp:** Mohs' Surgery; Melanoma; Cutaneous Lymphoma; Skin Laser Surgery; **Hospital:** Yale-New Haven Hosp; **Address:** Yale, Surgical Dermatology Dept, 40 Temple St, Ste 5A, New Haven, CT 06510; **Phone:** 203-785-3466; **Board Cert:** Internal Medicine 1984; Dermatology 2009; **Med School:** McGill Univ 1981; **Resid:** Internal Medicine, NY-Presby/Weill Cornell Med Ctr 1984; Dermatology, Meml Sloan-Kettering Cancer Ctr 1986; **Fellow:** Dermatology, Yale-New Haven Hosp 1987; Dermatologic Surgery, Univ Michigan Med Ctr 1988; **Fac Appt:** Prof D, Yale Univ

Diagnostic Radiology

Hammers, Lynwood DO (DR) - **Spec Exp:** Ultrasound; **Hospital:** Yale-New Haven Hosp; **Address:** Hammers Healthcare Imaging, 2 Church St S, Ste 110, New Haven, CT 06519; **Phone:** 203-773-8959; **Board Cert:** Diagnostic Radiology 1984; **Med School:** Philadelphia Coll Osteo Med 1979; **Resid:** Diagnostic Radiology, SUNY Downstate Med Ctr 1983; **Fellow:** Ultrasound, Yale-New Haven Hosp 1985; **Fac Appt:** Assoc Clin Prof Rad, Yale Univ

Israel, Gary MD (DR) - **Spec Exp:** CT Body Scan; Pelvic Imaging; Abdominal Imaging; **Hospital:** Yale-New Haven Hosp; **Address:** Yale, Radiology Dept, 20 York St Fl 2, New Haven, CT 06520; **Phone:** 203-688-1010; **Board Cert:** Diagnostic Radiology ; **Med School:** NY Med Coll 1994; **Resid:** Diagnostic Radiology, Montefiore Med Ctr 1999; **Fellow:** Body Imaging, NYU Med Ctr 2000; **Fac Appt:** Prof Rad, Yale Univ

Scoutt, Leslie MD (DR) - **Spec Exp:** Thyroid Cancer; Cardiac CT Angiography; **Hospital:** Yale-New Haven Hosp; **Address:** Yale, Radiology Dept, 20 York St Fl 2, New Haven, CT 06510; **Phone:** 203-785-2385; **Board Cert:** Internal Medicine 1981; Diagnostic Radiology 1985; **Med School:** Univ Rochester 1978; **Resid:** Internal Medicine, Univ Hosp 1981; Diagnostic Radiology, Beth Israel Deaconess Med Ctr 1985; **Fellow:** Ultrasound/CT/MRI, Yale-New Haven Hosp 1986; **Fac Appt:** Prof Rad, Yale Univ

Weinreb, Jeffrey C MD (DR) - **Spec Exp:** MRI; Breast Cancer; Abdominal Imaging; CT Body Scan; **Hospital:** Yale-New Haven Hosp; **Address:** Yale, Diagnostic Radiology Dept, 333 Cedar St, rm MRC165, Box 208042, New Haven, CT 06520-8042; **Phone:** 203-785-5913; **Board Cert:** Diagnostic Radiology 1983; **Med School:** Mount Sinai Sch Med 1978; **Resid:** Diagnostic Radiology, Long Island Jewish Med Ctr 1982; **Fellow:** Ultrasound/CT, Hosp Univ Penn 1983; **Fac Appt:** Prof Rad, Yale Univ

Endocrinology, Diabetes & Metabolism

Inzucchi, Silvio E MD (EDM) - **Spec Exp:** Diabetes; Pituitary Disorders; Growth Hormone Disorder-Adult; Cholesterol/Lipid Disorders; **Hospital:** Yale-New Haven Hosp; **Address:** Yale Diabetes Center, 789 Howard Ave, Dana Clinic Bldg fl 2, New Haven, CT 06520; **Phone:** 203-737-1932; **Board Cert:** Internal Medicine 1988; Endocrinology, Diabetes & Metabolism 2006; **Med School:** Harvard Med Sch 1985; **Resid:** Internal Medicine, Yale-New Haven Hosp 1988; **Fellow:** Endocrinology, Diabetes & Metabolism, Yale-New Haven Hosp 1994; **Fac Appt:** Prof Med, Yale Univ

Mayerson, Adam MD (EDM) - **Spec Exp:** Diabetes; **Hospital:** Yale-New Haven Hosp - St Raphael Campus; **Address:** Endocrine Assocs CT, 200 Orchard St, Ste 207, New Haven, CT 06511; **Phone:** 203-776-4444; **Board Cert:** Internal Medicine 2010; Endocrinology, Diabetes & Metabolism 2011; **Med School:** Albert Einstein Coll Med 1996; **Resid:** Internal Medicine, Yale-New Haven Hosp 1999; **Fellow:** Endocrinology, Diabetes & Metabolism, Yale-New Haven Hosp 2001; **Fac Appt:** Assoc Clin Prof Med, Yale Univ

Wysolmerski, John J MD (EDM) - **Spec Exp:** Bone Disorders-Metabolic; Osteoporosis; Parathyroid Disorders; **Hospital:** Yale-New Haven Hosp; **Address:** Yale, Endocrinology, 789 Howard Ave Dana Bldg Fl 2, New Haven, CT 06519; **Phone:** 203-737-1058; **Board Cert:** Internal Medicine 1989; **Med School:** Yale Univ 1986; **Resid:** Internal Medicine, Tufts Med Ctr 1989; **Fellow:** Endocrinology, Yale-New Haven Hosp 1993; **Fac Appt:** Prof Med, Yale Univ

Gastroenterology

Aslanian, Harry R MD (Ge) - **Spec Exp:** Endoscopic Ultrasound; Esophageal Cancer; Pancreatic Cancer; Rectal Cancer; **Hospital:** Smilow Cancer Hosp at Yale-New Haven; **Address:** Smilow Cancer Hosp, Interventl Endoscopy, 20 York St Fl 4, New Haven, CT 06510; **Phone:** 203-200-5083; **Board Cert:** Gastroenterology 2012; **Med School:** Brown Univ 1996; **Resid:** Internal Medicine, Mayo Clin 1999; **Fellow:** Gastroenterology, Yale-New Haven Hosp 2002; Endoscopy, Yale-New Haven Hosp 2003; **Fac Appt:** Assoc Prof Med, Yale Univ

Dobbins, John Whitby MD (Ge) - **Spec Exp:** Pancreatic & Biliary Disease; Inflammatory Bowel Disease; **Hospital:** Yale-New Haven Hosp, Yale-New Haven Hosp - St Raphael Campus; **Address:** CT Gastroenterology Consultants, 40 Temple St, Ste 4A, New Haven, CT 06510; **Phone:** 203-777-0304; **Board Cert:** Internal Medicine 1973; Gastroenterology 2005; **Med School:** Univ Wash 1968; **Resid:** Internal Medicine, G Washington Univ Hosp 1973; **Fellow:** Gastroenterology, Yale-New Haven Hosp 1976; **Fac Appt:** Clin Prof Med, Yale Univ

Fisher, Rosemarie Louise MD (Ge) - **Spec Exp:** Nutrition; Nutrition in Bowel Disorders; Inflammatory Bowel Disease/Crohn's; Endoscopy; **Hospital:** Yale-New Haven Hosp, St. Mary's Hosp - Waterbury; **Address:** 20 York St, Tompkins Bldg - Ste 236, New Haven, CT 06510; **Phone:** 203-688-1449; **Board Cert:** Internal Medicine 1975; Gastroenterology 1977; **Med School:** Tufts Univ 1971; **Resid:** Internal Medicine, Montefiore Med Ctr 1973; **Fellow:** Gastroenterology, Yale-New Haven Hosp 1975; **Fac Appt:** Prof Med, Yale Univ

Jamidar, Priya A MD (Ge) - **Spec Exp:** Gallbladder Disease; Pancreatic Disease; Gastrointestinal Cancer; Pancreatic/Biliary Endoscopy (ERCP); **Hospital:** Yale-New Haven Hosp; **Address:** Yale, Interventional Endoscopy, 20 York St Fl 4, New Haven, CT 06510; **Phone:** 203-200-5083; **Board Cert:** Internal Medicine 1988; Gastroenterology 2012; **Med School:** Ireland 1984; **Resid:** Internal Medicine, Univ Conn Hlth Ctr 1988; **Fellow:** Gastroenterology, LAC & USC Med Ctr 1990; Gastroenterology, IU Hlth Hosp 1992; **Fac Appt:** Prof Med, Yale Univ

Proctor, Deborah D MD (Ge) - **Spec Exp:** Inflammatory Bowel Disease; Colon Cancer Screening; Endoscopy; **Hospital:** Yale-New Haven Hosp; **Address:** Yale Medical Group, 40 Temple St, Ste 1A, New Haven, CT 06519; **Phone:** 203-785-4138; **Board Cert:** Gastroenterology 2003; **Med School:** Univ Cincinnati 1982; **Resid:** Internal Medicine, Beth Israel Hosp 1990; **Fellow:** Gastroenterology, Beth Israel Hosp 1992; **Fac Appt:** Prof Med, Yale Univ

Zlotoff, Ronald Alan MD (Ge) - **Hospital:** Waterbury Hosp; **Address:** 140 Grandview Ave, Ste L4, Waterbury, CT 06708; **Phone:** 203-755-4515; **Board Cert:** Internal Medicine 1980; Gastroenterology 1983; **Med School:** Univ Okla Coll Med 1977; **Resid:** Internal Medicine, Waterbury Hosp 1980; **Fellow:** Gastroenterology, Johns Hopkins Hosp 1982

Geriatric Medicine

Cooney Jr, Leo M MD (Ger) - **Spec Exp:** Geriatric Functional Assessment; Rheumatology; Mobility Evaluation & Treatment; **Hospital:** Yale-New Haven Hosp; **Address:** Yale-New Haven Hosp, Adler Geriatric Assessment Ctr, 20 York St, New Haven, CT 06510; **Phone:** 203-688-2204; **Board Cert:** Internal Medicine 1974; Rheumatology 1978; **Med School:** Yale Univ 1969; **Resid:** Internal Medicine, Boston Med Ctr 1971; Internal Medicine, Boston Med Ctr 1974; **Fellow:** Rheumatology, Boston Med Ctr 1975; **Fac Appt:** Prof Med, Yale Univ

Gill, Thomas M MD (Ger) - **Spec Exp:** Geriatric Functional Assessment; Memory Disorders; **Hospital:** Yale-New Haven Hosp; **Address:** Yale, Geriatric Med, 874 Howard Ave, New Haven, CT 06519; **Phone:** 203-688-6361; **Board Cert:** Geriatric Medicine 2000; **Med School:** Univ Chicago-Pritzker Sch Med 1987; **Resid:** Internal Medicine, Univ Wash Med Ctr 1990; **Fellow:** Internal Medicine, Yale-New Haven Hosp 1993; Geriatric Medicine, Yale-New Haven Hosp 1994; **Fac Appt:** Prof Med, Yale Univ

Marottoli, Richard MD (Ger) - **Spec Exp:** Geriatric Functional Assessment; **Hospital:** Yale-New Haven Hosp; **Address:** Yale, Geriatric Assessment Ctr, 874 Howard Ave, New Haven, CT 06519; **Phone:** 203-688-6361; **Board Cert:** Internal Medicine ; Geriatric Medicine 2013; **Med School:** Yale Univ 1984; **Resid:** Internal Medicine, Strong Meml Hosp 1987; **Fellow:** Geriatric Medicine, Yale-New Haven Hosp 1990; **Fac Appt:** Assoc Prof Med, Yale Univ

Ott, Casey MD (Ger) *PCP* - **Hospital:** Danbury Hosp; **Address:** Danbury, Primary Care-WCMG, 22 Old Waterbury Rd, Ste 108, Southbury, CT 06488; **Phone:** 203-262-4200; **Board Cert:** Internal Medicine 2005; Geriatric Medicine 2009; **Med School:** Israel 1996; **Resid:** Internal Medicine, Baystate Med Ctr 1999; **Fellow:** Geriatric Medicine, Baystate Med Ctr 2000

Tinetti, Mary E MD (Ger) - **Spec Exp:** Falls in the Elderly; Geriatric Functional Assessment; **Hospital:** Yale-New Haven Hosp; **Address:** Yale-New Haven Hosp, Adler Geriatric Assessment Ctr, 20 York St, New Haven, CT 06510; **Phone:** 203-688-6361; **Board Cert:** Internal Medicine 1981; **Med School:** Univ Mich Med Sch 1978; **Resid:** Internal Medicine, Univ Minnesota Affil Hosp 1981; **Fellow:** Geriatric Medicine, Univ Rochester Affil Hosp 1984; **Fac Appt:** Prof Med, Yale Univ

Walke, Lisa MD (Ger) *PCP* - **Hospital:** Yale-New Haven Hosp; **Address:** Yale, Geriatric Assessment Ctr, 874 Howard Ave, New Haven, CT 06519; **Phone:** 203-688-6163; **Board Cert:** Internal Medicine ; Geriatric Medicine ; **Med School:** Mount Sinai Sch Med 1997; **Resid:** Internal Medicine, Montefiore Med Ctr 2000; **Fellow:** Geriatric Medicine, Yale-New Haven Hosp 2003; **Fac Appt:** Assoc Prof Med, Yale Univ

Geriatric Psychiatry

van Dyck, Christopher H MD (GerPsy) - **Spec Exp:** Alzheimer's Disease; **Hospital:** Yale-New Haven Hosp; **Address:** Yale, Geriatric Med, 874 Howard Ave, New Haven, CT 06510; **Phone:** 203-688-6361; **Board Cert:** Psychiatry 1991; Geriatric Psychiatry 2013; **Med School:** Northwestern Univ 1984; **Resid:** Psychiatry, Yale-New Haven Hosp 1988; **Fellow:** Geriatric Psychiatry, Yale-New Haven Hosp 1990; **Fac Appt:** Prof Psyc, Yale Univ

Gynecologic Oncology

Azodi, Masoud MD (GO) - **Spec Exp:** Laparoscopic Surgery; Ovarian Cancer-Early Detection; Uterine Cancer; Vulvar & Vaginal Cancer; **Hospital:** Smilow Cancer Hosp at Yale-New Haven; **Address:** Smilow Cancer Hosp, Gynecologic Oncology, 25 Park St, Ste B, New Haven, CT 06519; **Phone:** 203-785-4013; **Board Cert:** Gynecologic Oncology 2012; Obstetrics & Gynecology 2012; **Med School:** Wright State Univ 1992; **Resid:** Obstetrics & Gynecology, Aultman Hosp 1996; **Fellow:** Gynecologic Oncology, Yale-New Haven Hosp 1999; **Fac Appt:** Assoc Prof ObG, Yale Univ

Rutherford, Thomas J MD (GO) - **Spec Exp:** Ovarian Cancer; Uterine Cancer; Ovarian Cancer-Early Detection; Cervical Cancer; **Hospital:** Smilow Cancer Hosp at Yale-New Haven; **Address:** Smilow Cancer Hosp, Gynecologic Oncology, 25 Park St, Ste B, New Haven, CT 06519; **Phone:** 203-200-4176; **Board Cert:** Obstetrics & Gynecology 2012; Gynecologic Oncology 2012; **Med School:** Med Coll OH 1989; **Resid:** Obstetrics & Gynecology, Cooper Univ Hosp 1993; **Fellow:** Gynecologic Oncology, Yale-New Haven Hosp 1995; **Fac Appt:** Prof ObG, Yale Univ

Santin, Alessandro MD (GO) - **Spec Exp:** Immunotherapy; Ovarian Cancer; Vulvar & Vaginal Cancer; **Hospital:** Yale-New Haven Hosp; **Address:** Yale Gynecologic Oncology, 35 Park St Fl 1, New Haven, CT 06520; **Phone:** 203-200-4176; **Med School:** Italy 1989; **Resid:** Obstetrics & Gynecology, Univ Brescia Sch Med 1993; **Fellow:** Gynecologic Oncology, UC Irvine Med Ctr 1995; Gynecologic Oncology, UAMS Med Ctr 2000; **Fac Appt:** Prof ObG, Yale Univ

Schwartz, Peter E MD (GO) - **Spec Exp:** Ovarian Cancer; Uterine Cancer; Gynecologic Surgery-Complex; Cervical Cancer; **Hospital:** Smilow Cancer Hosp at Yale-New Haven; **Address:** Smilow Cancer Hosp, Gynecology Oncology, 20 York St, New Haven, CT 06510; **Phone:** 203-785-4014; **Board Cert:** Obstetrics & Gynecology 1973; Gynecologic Oncology 1979; **Med School:** Albert Einstein Coll Med 1966; **Resid:** Obstetrics & Gynecology, Yale-New Haven Hosp 1970; **Fellow:** Gynecologic Oncology, UT MD Anderson Cancer Ctr 1975; **Fac Appt:** Prof ObG, Yale Univ

Silasi, Dan-Arin MD (GO) - **Spec Exp:** Robotic Surgery; **Hospital:** Yale-New Haven Hosp; **Address:** Yale, Gynecologic Oncology, 25 Park St, Ste B, New Haven, CT 06513; **Phone:** 203-737-6214; **Board Cert:** Obstetrics & Gynecology 2012; Gynecologic Oncology 2012; **Med School:** Romania 1993; **Resid:** Otolaryngology, Univ Med & Pharm 1999; Obstetrics & Gynecology, UT Hlth Sci Ctr 2005; **Fellow:** Gynecologic Oncology, Yale-New Haven Hosp 2006; **Fac Appt:** Asst Prof ObG, Yale Univ

Hand Surgery

Swigart, Carrie R MD (HS) - **Spec Exp:** Hand & Wrist Surgery; Elbow Surgery; **Hospital:** Yale-New Haven Hosp; **Address:** 800 Howard Ave, Fl 1, New Haven, CT 06520; **Phone:** 203-785-3851; **Board Cert:** Orthopaedic Surgery 2011; Hand Surgery 2011; **Med School:** Univ Pennsylvania 1991; **Resid:** Surgery, Yale-New Haven Hosp 1992; Orthopaedic Surgery, Yale-New Haven Hosp 1996; **Fellow:** Hand Surgery, St Lukes-Roosevelt Med Ctr 1997; **Fac Appt:** Asst Prof OrS, Yale Univ

Thomson, J Grant MD (HS) - **Spec Exp:** Carpal Tunnel Syndrome; Hand Reconstruction; Microsurgery; Elbow Surgery; **Hospital:** Yale-New Haven Hosp; **Address:** Yale Plastic Surgery, 800 Howard Ave Fl 4, New Haven, CT 06519; **Phone:** 203-737-5130; **Board Cert:** Hand Surgery 2004; Plastic Surgery 2004; **Med School:** McGill Univ 1983; **Resid:** Surgery, Montreal Genl Hosp 1988; Plastic Surgery, Montreal Genl Hosp 1990; **Fellow:** Hand Surgery, Barnes Jewish Hosp 1991; **Fac Appt:** Assoc Prof PlS, Yale Univ

Hematology

Katz, Martin Edward MD (Hem) - **Spec Exp:** Bleeding/Coagulation Disorders; Colon & Rectal Cancer; Leukemia & Lymphoma; **Hospital:** Smilow Cancer Hosp at Yale-New Haven; **Address:** Smilow Cancer Hosp, Hematology Dept, 6 Devine St, Ste 2C, North Haven, CT 06473; **Phone:** 203-407-8002; **Board Cert:** Internal Medicine 1975; Medical Oncology 1977; **Med School:** Univ Pennsylvania 1972; **Resid:** Internal Medicine, Cedars-Sinai Med Ctr 1975; **Fellow:** Hematology, Hosp Univ Penn 1977; **Fac Appt:** Asst Clin Prof Hem & Onc, Yale Univ

Lee, Alfred I MD/PhD (Hem) - **Spec Exp:** Leukemia; Lymphoma; Platelet Disorders; **Hospital:** Smilow Cancer Hosp at Yale-New Haven; **Address:** Smilow Cancer Ctr, 20 York St, New Haven, CT 06520; **Phone:** 203-200-4363; **Board Cert:** Internal Medicine 2007; **Med School:** Yale Univ 2004; **Resid:** Internal Medicine, Brigham & Womens Hosp 2007; **Fellow:** Hematology & Oncology, Dana Farber Cancer Ctr 2008; **Fac Appt:** Asst Prof Med, Yale Univ

Orell, Jeffrey Allan MD (Hem) - **Spec Exp:** Colon Cancer; Lung Cancer; Breast Cancer; **Hospital:** Griffin Hosp, Smilow Cancer Hosp at Yale-New Haven; **Address:** Griffin Hosp, Smilow Cancer Care Ctr, 350 Seymour Ave, Ste 6, Derby, CT 06418; **Phone:** 203-734-1664; **Board Cert:** Hematology 1986; Internal Medicine 1982; Medical Oncology 1985; **Med School:** Columbia P&S 1979; **Resid:** Internal Medicine, Hartford Hosp 1982; **Fellow:** Hematology, Univ Conn Hlth Ctr 1985; **Fac Appt:** Asst Clin Prof Med, Yale Univ

Sabbath, Kert David MD (Hem) - **Hospital:** Smilow Cancer Hosp at Yale-New Haven, St. Mary's Hosp - Waterbury; **Address:** Harold Leever Regl Cancer Ctr, 1075 Chase Pkwy, Ste B, Waterbury, CT 06708; **Phone:** 203-755-6311; **Board Cert:** Internal Medicine 1982; Medical Oncology 1985; Hematology 1986; **Med School:** Boston Univ 1979; **Resid:** Internal Medicine, Boston Med Ctr 1982; **Fellow:** Hematology & Oncology, Mass Genl Hosp 1985; **Fac Appt:** Asst Clin Prof Hem & Onc, Yale Univ

Hospice & Palliative Medicine

Kapo, Jennifer MD (H & PM) - **Spec Exp:** Palliative Care; Pain-Cancer; **Hospital:** Yale-New Haven Hosp; **Address:** Smilow Cancer Hosp, South Frontage & Park Street Fl 8, New Haven, CT 06510; **Phone:** 203-200-4363; **Board Cert:** Internal Medicine 2012; Geriatric Medicine ; Hospice & Palliative Medicine ; **Med School:** Univ Pennsylvania 1997; **Resid:** Internal Medicine, Univ CO Hlth Sci Ctr 2001; **Fellow:** Geriatric Medicine, Hosp Univ Penn 2002; Hospice & Palliative Medicine, Hosp Univ Penn 2003; **Fac Appt:** Assoc Prof Med, Yale Univ

Infectious Disease

Dunne, Dana MD (Inf) - **Spec Exp:** AIDS/HIV; Travel Medicine; **Hospital:** Yale-New Haven Hosp; **Address:** Yale, Infectious Disease Dept, 333 Cedar St, New Haven, CT 06520; **Phone:** 203-785-4140; **Board Cert:** Internal Medicine 1989; Infectious Disease 2013; **Med School:** SUNY Downstate 1986; **Resid:** Internal Medicine, Yale-New Haven Hosp 1990; **Fellow:** Infectious Disease, Yale-New Haven Hosp 1992; **Fac Appt:** Asst Prof Med, Yale Univ

Quagliarello, Vincent J MD (Inf) - **Spec Exp:** Meningitis; Pneumonia; Endocarditis; **Hospital:** Yale-New Haven Hosp; **Address:** Yale Univ Sch Med, 300 Cedar St, TAC S169A, New Haven, CT 06520-8022; **Phone:** 203-785-4140; **Board Cert:** Internal Medicine 1984; Infectious Disease 1988; **Med School:** Washington Univ, St Louis 1980; **Resid:** Internal Medicine, Yale-New Haven Hosp 1984; **Fellow:** Infectious Disease, Univ VA Hlth Sci Ctr 1987; **Fac Appt:** Prof Med, Yale Univ

Internal Medicine

Brenner, Stephen D MD (IM) *PCP* - **Spec Exp:** Preventive Medicine; Hypertension; Diabetes; Cholesterol/Lipid Disorders; **Hospital:** Yale-New Haven Hosp, Yale-New Haven Hosp - St Raphael Campus; **Address:** CT Med Grp, 129 York St, New Haven, CT 06511; **Phone:** 203-789-8888; **Board Cert:** Internal Medicine 1975; **Med School:** SUNY Upstate Med Univ 1970; **Resid:** Internal Medicine, Philadelphia Genl Hosp 1972; Internal Medicine, Roger Williams Med Ctr 1975; **Fac Appt:** Assoc Clin Prof Med, Yale Univ

Concato, John MD (IM) *PCP* - **Spec Exp:** Cancer Prevention; **Hospital:** VA Conn Hlthcre Sys-W Haven Campus; **Address:** VA Med Ctr, Epidemiology, 950 Campbell Ave, MC 151B, West Haven, CT 06516; **Phone:** 203-932-5711 x2993; **Board Cert:** Internal Medicine 1989; **Med School:** NYU Sch Med 1985; **Resid:** Internal Medicine, NYU Med Ctr 1989; **Fellow:** Pulmonary Disease, Yale-New Haven Hosp 1991; Pulmonary Disease, NYU Med Ctr 1992; **Fac Appt:** Prof Med, Yale Univ

Eilbott, David J MD (IM) *PCP* - **Spec Exp:** Diabetes; Infectious Disease; **Hospital:** Yale-New Haven Hosp, Yale-New Haven Hosp - St Raphael Campus; **Address:** Branford Internal Med, 500 E Main St, Ste 212, Branford, CT 06405; **Phone:** 203-481-5665; **Board Cert:** Internal Medicine 1986; **Med School:** Univ Rochester 1981; **Resid:** Internal Medicine, Waterbury Hosp 1985; **Fellow:** Infectious Disease, SUNY Stony Brook 1988; **Fac Appt:** Asst Clin Prof Med, Yale Univ

Ellman, Matthew S MD (IM) *PCP* - **Spec Exp:** Preventive Medicine; **Hospital:** Yale-New Haven Hosp; **Address:** Yale Internal Med Assocs, 800 Howard Ave Fl 3, New Haven, CT 06510; **Phone:** 203-785-7411; **Board Cert:** Internal Medicine 2011; **Med School:** Harvard Med Sch 1987; **Resid:** Internal Medicine, Bellevue Hosp 1990; **Fellow:** Epidemiology, Yale-New Haven Hosp 1993; **Fac Appt:** Assoc Prof Med, Yale Univ

Kernan Jr, Walter N MD (IM) *PCP* - **Spec Exp:** Stroke; Hypertension; **Hospital:** Yale-New Haven Hosp; **Address:** 20 York St, New Haven, CT 06520-1744; **Phone:** 203-688-2984; **Board Cert:** Internal Medicine 1987; **Med School:** Dartmouth Med Sch 1984; **Resid:** Internal Medicine, Johns Hopkins Hosp 1987; **Fellow:** Internal Medicine, Yale New Haven Hosp 1989; **Fac Appt:** Prof Med, Yale Univ

O'Connor, Patrick G MD (IM) *PCP* - **Spec Exp:** Addiction/Substance Abuse; **Hospital:** Yale-New Haven Hosp; **Address:** Yale-New Haven Hosp, Primary Care Ctr, 789 Howard St, New Haven, CT 06520-8093; **Phone:** 203-688-6532; **Board Cert:** Internal Medicine 1986; Addiction Medicine 2009; **Med School:** Albany Med Coll 1982; **Resid:** Internal Medicine, Univ Rochester Med Ctr 1985; Internal Medicine, Univ Rochester Med Ctr 1986; **Fellow:** Internal Medicine, Yale-New Haven Hosp 1988; **Fac Appt:** Prof Med, Yale Univ

Spanolios, Paris MD (IM) *PCP* - **Spec Exp:** Diabetes; Hypertension; Geriatric Medicine; **Hospital:** Milford Hosp; **Address:** Internal Med Milford, 40 Commerce Park, Ste 1, Milford, CT 06460; **Phone:** 203-878-3531; **Board Cert:** Internal Medicine 2008; **Med School:** Johns Hopkins Univ 1995; **Resid:** Internal Medicine, Barnes-Jewish Hosp 1998

Street, Lynn MD (IM) *PCP* - **Hospital:** Yale-New Haven Hosp; **Address:** 100 York St, Ste 2E, New Haven, CT 06511; **Phone:** 203-787-3588; **Board Cert:** Internal Medicine 2013; Geriatric Medicine 2013; **Med School:** Yale Univ 1987; **Resid:** Internal Medicine, Bellevue Hosp 1990; **Fellow:** Epidemiology, RWJ Med Ctr 1992; Geriatric Medicine, Yale-New Haven Hosp 2000

Interventional Cardiology

Henry, Glen MD (IC) - **Spec Exp:** Angiography-Coronary; Cardiac Catheterization; Echocardiography; **Hospital:** Yale-New Haven Hosp; **Address:** Yale Heart & Vascular Ctr, 2 Devine St, North Haven, CT 06473; **Phone:** 203-789-2272; **Board Cert:** Internal Medicine 2004; Cardiovascular Disease 2008; Interventional Cardiology 2010; **Med School:** Med Coll VA 1991; **Resid:** Internal Medicine, Yale-New Haven Hosp 1994; **Fellow:** Cardiovascular Disease, Yale-New Haven Hosp 1996; Interventional Cardiology, Yale-New Haven Hosp 1998

Kett, Kevin Gerard MD (IC) - **Spec Exp:** Nuclear Cardiology; **Hospital:** St. Mary's Hosp - Waterbury; **Address:** Cardiology Assocs, 455 Chase Pkwy, Waterbury, CT 06708-3303; **Phone:** 203-573-1435; **Board Cert:** Internal Medicine 1985; Cardiovascular Disease 1987; **Med School:** SUNY Stony Brook 1982; **Resid:** Internal Medicine, Beth Isreal Deaconess Med Ctr 1985; **Fellow:** Cardiovascular Disease, Beth Isreal Deaconess Med Ctr 1987; Interventional Cardiology, Beth Isreal Deaconess Med Ctr 2000

Maternal & Fetal Medicine

Abdel-Razeq, Sonya MD (MF) - **Spec Exp:** Pregnancy-High Risk; **Hospital:** Yale-New Haven Hosp; **Address:** Yale, Maternal-Fetal Med, 150 Sargent Drive Fl 2, New Haven, CT 06511; **Phone:** 203-785-5682; **Board Cert:** Obstetrics & Gynecology 2013; Maternal & Fetal Medicine 2013; **Med School:** SUNY Buffalo 2001; **Resid:** Obstetrics & Gynecology, SUNY Buffalo Affil Hosp 2005; **Fellow:** Maternal & Fetal Medicine, Yale-New Haven Hosp 2008; Surgical Critical Care, Yale-New Haven Hosp 2009; **Fac Appt:** Asst Prof ObG, Yale Univ

Copel, Joshua A MD (MF) - **Spec Exp:** Prenatal Diagnosis; Fetal Echocardiography; Pregnancy-High Risk; Fetal Diagnosis & Therapy; **Hospital:** Yale-New Haven Hosp; **Address:** Yale Maternal/Fetal Medicine, 150 Sargent Drive Fl 2, New Haven, CT 06511; **Phone:** 203-785-5682; **Board Cert:** Obstetrics & Gynecology 2012; Maternal & Fetal Medicine 2012; **Med School:** Tufts Univ 1979; **Resid:** Obstetrics & Gynecology, Hosp Univ Penn 1983; **Fellow:** Maternal & Fetal Medicine, Yale-New Haven Hosp 1986; **Fac Appt:** Prof ObG, Yale Univ

Magriples, Urania MD (MF) - **Spec Exp:** Pregnancy-High Risk; **Hospital:** Yale-New Haven Hosp; **Address:** Yale, Maternal-Fetal Med, 150 Sargent Drive Fl 2, New Haven, CT 06511; **Phone:** 203-785-5682; **Board Cert:** Obstetrics & Gynecology 2012; Maternal & Fetal Medicine 2012; **Med School:** Mount Sinai Sch Med 1987; **Resid:** Obstetrics & Gynecology, Yale-New Haven Hosp 1991; **Fellow:** Perinatal Medicine, Yale-New Haven Hosp 1994; **Fac Appt:** Assoc Prof ObG, Yale Univ

Paidas, Michael J MD (MF) - **Spec Exp:** Pregnancy-High Risk; Clotting Disorders in Pregnancy; Miscarriage-Recurrent; **Hospital:** Yale-New Haven Hosp; **Address:** Yale Maternal/Fetal Medicine, 150 Sargent Drive Fl 2, New Haven, CT 06511; **Phone:** 203-785-5682; **Board Cert:** Obstetrics & Gynecology 2012; Maternal & Fetal Medicine 2012; **Med School:** Tufts Univ 1987; **Resid:** Obstetrics & Gynecology, Pennsylvania Hosp 1991; **Fellow:** Maternal & Fetal Medicine, Mount Sinai Med Ctr 1993; **Fac Appt:** Prof ObG, Yale Univ

Medical Oncology

Cooper, Dennis L MD (Onc) - **Spec Exp:** Head & Neck Cancer; Bone Marrow Transplant; Leukemia & Lymphoma; **Hospital:** Yale-New Haven Hosp; **Address:** Yale, Hematology/Oncology, 333 Cedar St, New Haven, CT 06520; **Phone:** 203-200-4363; **Board Cert:** Internal Medicine 1983; Medical Oncology 1985; **Med School:** Rush Med Coll 1979; **Resid:** Internal Medicine, Yale-New Haven Hosp 1982; Internal Medicine, UPMC Presby 1983; **Fellow:** Medical Oncology, Yale-New Haven Hosp 1985; **Fac Appt:** Prof Med, Yale Univ

DeVita Jr, Vincent T MD (Onc) - **Spec Exp:** Lymphoma Consultation; Hodgkin's Disease Consultation; **Hospital:** Yale-New Haven Hosp; **Address:** Yale, Cancer Ctr, 333 Cedar St, rm FMP117, New Haven, CT 06520; **Phone:** 203-737-1010; **Board Cert:** Internal Medicine 1974; Hematology 1972; Medical Oncology 1973; **Med School:** Geo Wash Univ 1961; **Resid:** Internal Medicine, Geo Washington Univ Hosp 1963; Internal Medicine, Yale-New Haven Hosp 1966; **Fellow:** Medical Oncology, Natl Cancer Inst 1965; **Fac Appt:** Prof Med, Yale Univ

Foss, Francine M MD (Onc) - **Spec Exp:** Cutaneous T-cell Lymphoma; Stem Cell Transplant; Graft vs Host Disease; Multiple Myeloma; **Hospital:** Smilow Cancer Hosp at Yale-New Haven; **Address:** Smilow Cancer Hosp, Hematology, 35 Park St Fl 7, New Haven, CT 06520; **Phone:** 203-200-4363; **Board Cert:** Internal Medicine 1985; Medical Oncology 1987; **Med School:** Univ Mass Sch Med 1982; **Resid:** Internal Medicine, Brigham & Womens Hosp 1985; **Fellow:** Medical Oncology, Natl Cancer Inst 1988; **Fac Appt:** Prof Med, Yale Univ

Gettinger, Scott MD (Onc) - **Spec Exp:** Thoracic Cancers; Lung Cancer; Thyroid Cancer; Head & Neck Cancer; **Hospital:** Yale-New Haven Hosp; **Address:** Yale, Thoracic Onc, 35 Park St Fl 4, New Haven, CT 06510; **Phone:** 203-200-5864; **Board Cert:** Medical Oncology 2005; **Med School:** SUNY Downstate 1999; **Resid:** Internal Medicine, Beth Israel Med Ctr 2002; **Fellow:** Medical Oncology, Beth Israel Med Ctr 2005; **Fac Appt:** Assoc Prof Onc, Yale Univ

Herbst, Roy S MD/PhD (Onc) - **Spec Exp:** Lung Cancer; Thoracic Cancers; Drug Development; Clinical Trials; **Hospital:** Smilow Cancer Hosp at Yale-New Haven; **Address:** Smilow Cancer Hosp, Thoracic Oncology, 20 York St Fl 4, New Haven, CT 06504; **Phone:** 203-200-5864; **Board Cert:** Medical Oncology 2007; **Med School:** Cornell Univ-Weill Med Coll 1991; **Resid:** Internal Medicine, Brigham & Womens Hosp 1994; **Fellow:** Medical Oncology, Dana Farber Cancer Inst 1996; **Fac Appt:** Prof Med, Univ Tex, Houston

Hochster, Howard S MD (Onc) - **Spec Exp:** Gastrointestinal Cancer; Gynecologic Cancer; Colon & Rectal Cancer; **Hospital:** Smilow Cancer Hosp at Yale-New Haven; **Address:** Smilow Cancer Hosp, GI Cancer Dept, 35 Park St, Ste NP8-202, New Haven, CT 06520; **Phone:** 203-200-4422; **Board Cert:** Internal Medicine 1983; Medical Oncology 1985; Hematology 1986; **Med School:** Yale Univ 1980; **Resid:** Internal Medicine, NYU Med Ctr 1983; **Fellow:** Hematology & Oncology, NYU Med Ctr 1985; Medical Oncology, Jules Bordet Inst 1986; **Fac Appt:** Prof Med, Yale Univ

Lacy, Jill MD (Onc) - **Spec Exp:** Colon & Rectal Cancer; Gastrointestinal Cancer; Pancreatic Cancer; Esophageal Cancer; **Hospital:** Smilow Cancer Hosp at Yale-New Haven; **Address:** Smilow Cancer Hosp, GI Cancer Dept, 35 Park St, Ste NP8-202, New Haven, CT 06520; **Phone:** 203-200-4422; **Board Cert:** Internal Medicine 1982; Medical Oncology 2005; **Med School:** Yale Univ 1978; **Resid:** Internal Medicine, Yale-New Haven Hosp 1981; **Fellow:** Medical Oncology, Yale-New Haven Hosp 1985; **Fac Appt:** Assoc Prof Onc, Yale Univ

Lasala, Johanna MD (Onc) - **Spec Exp:** Breast Cancer; Bleeding/Coagulation Disorders; Leukemia & Lymphoma; Colon & Rectal Cancer; **Hospital:** Smilow Cancer Hosp at Yale-New Haven; **Address:** Yale, Smilow Cancer Ctr, 240 Indian River Rd, Ste A1, Orange, CT 06477; **Phone:** 203-795-1664; **Board Cert:** Hematology 2006; Medical Oncology 2007; **Med School:** Johns Hopkins Univ 1990; **Resid:** Internal Medicine, NY-Presby/Weill Cornell Med Ctr 1993; **Fellow:** Hematology & Oncology, NY-Presby/Weill Cornell Med Ctr 1996

Lilenbaum, Rogerio C MD (Onc) - **Spec Exp:** Thoracic Cancers; Lung Cancer; **Hospital:** Smilow Cancer Hosp at Yale-New Haven; **Address:** Smilow Cancer Hosp, Thoracic Oncology, 20 York St Fl 4, New Haven, CT 06510; **Phone:** 203-200-5864; **Board Cert:** Internal Medicine 2005; Hematology 2008; Medical Oncology 2007; **Med School:** Brazil 1986; **Resid:** Internal Medicine, Univ Hosp 1989; **Fellow:** Hematology & Oncology, Washington Univ Phys 1992; Medical Oncology, UCSD Med Ctr 1994

Lundberg Jr, Walter B MD (Onc) - **Spec Exp:** Lymphoma; Colon Cancer; Lung Cancer; **Hospital:** Smilow Cancer Hosp at Yale-New Haven, Yale-New Haven Hosp - St Raphael Campus; **Address:** Smilow Cancer Hosp, 1450 Chapel St, Ste A, New Haven, CT 06511; **Phone:** 203-867-5420; **Board Cert:** Internal Medicine 1973; Hematology 1974; Blood Banking 1974; Medical Oncology 1975; **Med School:** Columbia P&S 1970; **Resid:** Internal Medicine, NY-Presby/Columbia Univ Med Ctr 1972; Medical Oncology, Yale-New Haven Hosp 1976; **Fellow:** Internal Medicine, Beth Israel Deaconess Med Ctr 1971; Hematology, Natl Inst Hlth 1974; **Fac Appt:** Assoc Clin Prof Med, Yale Univ

Lynch Jr, Thomas J MD (Onc) - **Spec Exp:** Lung Cancer; Thoracic Cancers; **Hospital:** Smilow Cancer Hosp at Yale-New Haven; **Address:** Smilow Cancer Hosp, Thoracic Oncology, 35 Park St Fl 4, New Haven, CT 06510; **Phone:** 203-688-5864; **Board Cert:** Internal Medicine 1989; Medical Oncology 2003; **Med School:** Yale Univ 1986; **Resid:** Internal Medicine, Mass Genl Hosp 1989; **Fellow:** Medical Oncology, Dana Farber Cancer Inst 1991; **Fac Appt:** Assoc Prof Med, Yale Univ

Petrylak, Daniel P MD (Onc) - **Spec Exp:** Testicular Cancer; Prostate Cancer; Bladder Cancer; Kidney Cancer; **Hospital:** Yale-New Haven Hosp, Greenwich Hosp (page 938); **Address:** Yale Smilow Cancer Center, 35 Park St, New Haven, CT 06520; **Phone:** 203-200-4822; **Board Cert:** Internal Medicine 2001; Medical Oncology 2003; **Med School:** Case West Res Univ 1985; **Resid:** Internal Medicine, Jacobi Med Ctr 1988; **Fellow:** Oncology, Meml-Sloan Kettering Cancer Ctr 1991; **Fac Appt:** Prof Onc, Yale Univ

Pusztai, Lajos MD (Onc) - **Spec Exp:** Breast Cancer; **Hospital:** Smilow Cancer Hosp at Yale-New Haven; **Address:** Yale, Breast Cancer, 35 Park St, North Pav 1, New Haven, CT 06510; **Phone:** 203-200-2328; **Board Cert:** Medical Oncology 2011; **Med School:** Hungary 1987; **Resid:** Internal Medicine, St Marys Hosp 1996; **Fellow:** Medical Oncology, UT MD Anderson Cancer Ctr 1999; **Fac Appt:** Prof Med, Yale Univ

Sznol, Mario MD (Onc) - **Spec Exp:** Immunotherapy; Drug Development; Melanoma; **Hospital:** Smilow Cancer Hosp at Yale-New Haven; **Address:** Smilow Cancer Hosp, Melanoma, 333 Cedar St, rm SMP130, New Haven, CT 06520; **Phone:** 203-200-6622; **Board Cert:** Internal Medicine 1985; Medical Oncology 1987; **Med School:** Baylor Coll Med 1982; **Resid:** Internal Medicine, Baylor Coll Med 1985; **Fellow:** Medical Oncology, Mount Sinai Med Ctr 1987; **Fac Appt:** Prof Onc, Yale Univ

Neonatal-Perinatal Medicine

Ehrenkranz, Richard A MD (NP) - **Spec Exp:** Nutrition; Lung Disease in Newborns; Prematurity/Low Birth Weight Infants; **Hospital:** Yale-New Haven Hosp; **Address:** Yale-New Haven Chldn's Hosp, Div of Neonatology, 20 York St, New Haven, CT 06520; **Phone:** 203-688-2320; **Board Cert:** Pediatrics 1977; Neonatal-Perinatal Medicine 1979; **Med School:** SUNY Downstate 1972; **Resid:** Pediatrics, Yale-New Haven Hosp 1975; **Fellow:** Research, Natl Inst Child Hlth & Human Dev 1976; Neonatal-Perinatal Medicine, Yale-New Haven Hosp 1979; **Fac Appt:** Prof Ped, Yale Univ

Gross, Ian MD (NP) - **Spec Exp:** Breathing Disorders; Critical Care; **Hospital:** Yale-New Haven Hosp; **Address:** Yale Sch Med, Dept Pediatrics, 333 Cedar St, PO Box 208064, New Haven, CT 06520-8064; **Phone:** 203-688-2320; **Board Cert:** Pediatrics 1974; Neonatal-Perinatal Medicine 1977; **Med School:** South Africa 1967; **Resid:** Pediatrics, Univ Witwatersrand Affil Hosps 1971; Pediatrics, Chldns Hosp Med Ctr 1974; **Fellow:** Neonatal-Perinatal Medicine, Yale-New Haven Hosp 1977; **Fac Appt:** Prof Ped, Yale Univ

Nephrology

Bia, Margaret MD (Nep) - **Spec Exp:** Transplant Medicine-Kidney; **Hospital:** Yale-New Haven Hosp; **Address:** Yale, Organ Transplant Ctr, 800 Howard Ave Fl 4, New Haven, CT 06520; **Phone:** 203-785-2565; **Board Cert:** Internal Medicine 1975; Nephrology 1978; **Med School:** Cornell Univ-Weill Med Coll 1972; **Resid:** Internal Medicine, Univ Hosp Penn 1975; **Fellow:** Renal Disease, Univ Hosp Penn 1976; **Fac Appt:** Prof Med, Yale Univ

Brewster, Ursula Constant MD (Nep) - **Spec Exp:** Hypertension in Pregnancy; Kidney Disease-Chronic; Dialysis Care; **Hospital:** Yale-New Haven Hosp; **Address:** Yale, Nephrology Dept, 40 Temple St, Ste 1A, New Haven, CT 06510; **Phone:** 203-785-4184; **Board Cert:** Internal Medicine 2011; Nephrology 2004; **Med School:** Dartmouth Med Sch 1998; **Resid:** Internal Medicine, Yale-New Haven Hosp 2001; **Fellow:** Nephrology, Yale-New Haven Hosp 2004; **Fac Appt:** Assoc Prof Med, Yale Univ

Dahl, Neera MD/PhD (Nep) - **Spec Exp:** Kidney Failure; Glomerulonephritis; Lupus Nephritis; **Hospital:** Yale-New Haven Hosp; **Address:** Yale, Nephrology Dept, 40 Temple St, Ste 1A, New Haven, CT 06510; **Phone:** 203-785-4184; **Board Cert:** Internal Medicine 2009; Nephrology 2011; **Med School:** Tufts Univ 1996; **Resid:** Internal Medicine, Beth Israel Deaconess Med Ctr 1999; **Fellow:** Nephrology, Beth Israel Deaconess Med Ctr 2002; **Fac Appt:** Asst Prof Med, Yale Univ

Formica Jr, Richard N MD (Nep) - **Spec Exp:** Transplant Medicine-Kidney; **Hospital:** Yale-New Haven Hosp; **Address:** Yale, Organ Transplant Ctr, 800 Howard Ave Fl 4, New Haven, CT 06520; **Phone:** 203-785-2565; **Board Cert:** Internal Medicine 2007; Nephrology 2009; **Med School:** Boston Univ 1993; **Resid:** Internal Medicine, Boston Med Ctr 1997; **Fellow:** Nephrology, Yale New-Haven Hosp 1997; **Fac Appt:** Assoc Prof S, Yale Univ

Kliger, Alan S MD (Nep) - **Spec Exp:** Kidney Disease; Kidney Disease-Metabolic; **Hospital:** Yale-New Haven Hosp - St Raphael Campus; **Address:** Metabolism Assocs, 136 Sherman Ave, Ste 405, New Haven, CT 06511; **Phone:** 203-787-0117 x307; **Board Cert:** Internal Medicine 1973; Nephrology 1976; **Med School:** SUNY Upstate Med Univ 1970; **Resid:** Internal Medicine, SUNY Upstate Med Ctr 1973; **Fellow:** Nephrology, Georgetown Univ Med Ctr 1975; **Fac Appt:** Clin Prof Med, Yale Univ

Mahnensmith, Rex MD (Nep) - **Spec Exp:** Lupus Nephritis; Polycystic Kidney Disease; **Hospital:** Yale-New Haven Hosp; **Address:** Yale, Nephrology Dept, 40 Temple St, Ste 1A, New Haven, CT 06510; **Phone:** 203-785-4184; **Board Cert:** Internal Medicine 1981; Nephrology 1988; **Med School:** Yale Univ 1977; **Resid:** Internal Medicine, Yale-New Haven Hosp 1981; **Fellow:** Nephrology, Yale-New Haven Hosp 1984; **Fac Appt:** Prof Med, Yale Univ

Neurological Surgery

Abbed, Khalid M MD (NS) - **Spec Exp:** Minimally Invasive Spinal Surgery; Spinal Disorders; Spinal Surgery-Complex; **Hospital:** Yale-New Haven Hosp, Greenwich Hosp (page 938); **Address:** 1 Long Wharf Drive Fl 6, New Haven, CT 06511; **Phone:** 203-785-2807; **Board Cert:** Neurological Surgery 2012; **Med School:** Univ IL Coll Med 1999; **Resid:** Neurological Surgery, Mass Genl Hosp 2005; **Fellow:** Spine Surgery, Cleveland Clinic 2007; **Fac Appt:** Asst Prof NS, Yale Univ

Duncan, Charles C MD (NS) - **Spec Exp:** Pediatric Neurosurgery; Nerve Tumors; Spinal Trauma; **Hospital:** Yale-New Haven Hosp; **Address:** Yale-Chldns Hosp, Ped Neurosurgery, 1 Park St Fl 2, New Haven, CT 06520; **Phone:** 203-785-2809; **Board Cert:** Neurological Surgery 1979; Pediatric Neurological Surgery 2005; **Med School:** Duke Univ 1971; **Resid:** Neurological Surgery, Duke Univ Hosp 1977; **Fac Appt:** Prof NS, Yale Univ

Piepmeier, Joseph MD (NS) - **Spec Exp:** Neuro-Oncology; Brain & Spinal Cord Tumors; **Hospital:** Smilow Cancer Hosp at Yale-New Haven; **Address:** Smilow Cancer Hosp, Neuro-Oncology, 35 Park St Fl 8, New Haven, CT 06520; **Phone:** 203-785-2791; **Board Cert:** Neurological Surgery 1984; **Med School:** Univ Tenn Coll Med 1975; **Resid:** Neurological Surgery, Yale-New Haven Hosp 1982; **Fac Appt:** Prof NS, Yale Univ

Spencer, Dennis D MD (NS) - **Spec Exp:** Epilepsy/Seizure Disorders; Brain Tumors; **Hospital:** Yale-New Haven Hosp; **Address:** Surgical Specialties, 800 Howard Ave, Yale Physicians Bldg, Lower Level, New Haven, CT 06519; **Phone:** 203-785-4891; **Board Cert:** Neurological Surgery 1980; **Med School:** Washington Univ, St Louis 1971; **Resid:** Surgery, Barnes Hosp 1972; Neurological Surgery, Yale-New Haven Hosp 1977; **Fac Appt:** Prof NS, Yale Univ

Waitze, Alan MD (NS) - **Hospital:** Waterbury Hosp, St. Mary's Hosp - Waterbury; **Address:** 500 Chase Pkwy Fl 2, Waterbury, CT 06708; **Phone:** 203-755-6677; **Board Cert:** Neurological Surgery 2004; **Med School:** Hahnemann Univ 1993; **Resid:** Surgery, Emory Univ Hosp 1997; Neurological Surgery, Emory Univ Hosp 2000

Neurology

Baehring, Joachim MD (N) - **Spec Exp:** Neuro-Oncology; Brain Tumors; **Hospital:** Smilow Cancer Hosp at Yale-New Haven; **Address:** Smilow Cancer Hosp, Neuro-Oncology, 35 Park St, New Haven, CT 06520; **Phone:** 203-785-7284; **Board Cert:** Neurology 2011; **Med School:** Germany 1994; **Resid:** Neurology, Hahnemann Univ Hosp 2000; **Fellow:** Neuro-Oncology, Mass General Hosp 2002; **Fac Appt:** Assoc Prof NS, Yale Univ

Duckrow, Robert B MD (N) - **Spec Exp:** Epilepsy; Clinical Neurophysiology; **Hospital:** Yale-New Haven Hosp; **Address:** Yale, Epilepsy, 800 Howard Ave Fl LL, New Haven, CT 06520; **Phone:** 203-785-3565; **Board Cert:** Neurology 1984; Clinical Neurophysiology 2004; **Med School:** Yale Univ 1975; **Resid:** Neurology, Yale-New Haven Hosp 1979; **Fellow:** Metabolic Neurology, Univ Miami Hosp 1981; **Fac Appt:** Assoc Prof N, Yale Univ

Greer, David M MD (N) - **Spec Exp:** Stroke; Cerebrovascular Disease; Neurological Imaging; **Hospital:** Yale-New Haven Hosp; **Address:** Yale Neurology, 800 Howard Ave, Yale Physicians Bldg, Lower Level, New Haven, CT 06519; **Phone:** 203-785-5947; **Board Cert:** Neurology 2010; Vascular Neurology 2008; **Med School:** Univ Fla Coll Med 1995; **Resid:** Neurology, Mass Genl Hosp 1999; **Fellow:** Stroke, Mass Genl Hosp 2001; **Fac Appt:** Prof N, Yale Univ

Hirsch, Lawrence MD (N) - **Spec Exp:** Epilepsy/Seizure Disorders; **Hospital:** Yale-New Haven Hosp; **Address:** Yale, Epilespy Ctr, 800 Howard Ave, New Haven, CT 06510; **Phone:** 203-785-3865; **Board Cert:** Neurology 2006; Clinical Neurophysiology 2007; **Med School:** Yale Univ 1991; **Resid:** Neurology, NY-Presby/Columbia Univ Med Ctr 1995; **Fellow:** Epilepsy, NY-Presby/Columbia Univ Med Ctr 1997; **Fac Appt:** Prof N, Yale Univ

Katz, Amiram MD (N) - **Spec Exp:** Seizure Disorders; Lyme Disease; Sleep Medicine; **Hospital:** Norwalk Hosp, Yale-New Haven Hosp; **Address:** 325 Boston Post Rd, Ste 1B, Orange, CT 06477; **Phone:** 203-795-5425; **Board Cert:** Neurology 1993; **Med School:** Israel 1976; **Resid:** Neurology, Sheba Hosp 1980; Neurology, Tel Aviv Med Ctr 1984; **Fellow:** Clinical Neurophysiology, Cleveland Clin 1988; Epilepsy, Yale-New Haven Hosp 1991; **Fac Appt:** Asst Clin Prof N, Yale Univ

Neuroradiology

Bronen, Richard MD (NRad) - **Spec Exp:** Epilepsy; **Hospital:** Yale-New Haven Hosp; **Address:** Yale, Neuroradiology, 20 York St, New Haven, CT 06510; **Phone:** 203-785-5102; **Board Cert:** Diagnostic Radiology 2010; Neuroradiology 2010; **Med School:** Emory Univ 1980; **Resid:** Diagnostic Radiology, Hahnemann Univ Hosp 1985; **Fellow:** Neuroradiology, Jackson Meml Hosp 1986; Neuroradiology, Yale-New Haven Hosp 1987; **Fac Appt:** Prof Rad, Yale Univ

Errico, Vito MD (NRad) - **Spec Exp:** Spinal Imaging & Intervention; Osteoporosis Spine-Vertebroplasty; Neuro-Oncology; **Hospital:** Milford Hosp; **Address:** Diagnostic Imaging Milford, 30 Commerce Park, Milford, CT 06460; **Phone:** 203-878-2341; **Board Cert:** Diagnostic Radiology 1997; **Med School:** SUNY Stony Brook 1992; **Resid:** Diagnostic Radiology, Stony Brook Univ Med Ctr 1997; **Fellow:** Neuroradiology, Yale-New Haven Hosp 1999

Johnson, Michele MD (NRad) - **Spec Exp:** Head & Neck Cancer; Aneurysm-Cerebral; Interventional Neuroradiology; **Hospital:** Yale-New Haven Hosp; **Address:** Yale, Diag Radiology Dept, 20 York St, New Haven, CT 06510; **Phone:** 203-785-3367; **Board Cert:** Diagnostic Radiology 1983; Neuroradiology 2006; **Med School:** Temple Univ 1979; **Resid:** Diagnostic Radiology, Temple Univ Hosp 1983; **Fellow:** Neuroradiology, Hosp Univ Penn 1985; **Fac Appt:** Assoc Prof Rad, Yale Univ

Sze, Gordon K MD (NRad) - **Spec Exp:** Brain Tumors; Spinal Cord Tumors; Head & Neck Cancer; MRI; **Hospital:** Yale-New Haven Hosp, Yale Med Group; **Address:** Yale, Diagnostic Radiology, 20 York St, New Haven, CT 06510; **Phone:** 203-785-5102; **Board Cert:** Diagnostic Radiology 1985; Neuroradiology 2008; **Med School:** Harvard Med Sch 1981; **Resid:** Diagnostic Radiology, UCSF Med Ctr 1985; **Fellow:** Neuroradiology, UCSF Med Ctr 1986; **Fac Appt:** Prof Rad, Yale Univ

Nuclear Medicine

Cheng, David W MD/PhD (NuM) - **Spec Exp:** PET Imaging; Nuclear Oncology; Thyroid Cancer; Lymphoma; **Hospital:** Yale-New Haven Hosp; **Address:** Smilow Cancer Hosp at Yale, South Frontage Road and Park Street, New Haven, CT 06510; **Phone:** 203-200-5610; **Board Cert:** Nuclear Medicine 2008; **Med School:** Albert Einstein Coll Med 1996; **Resid:** Internal Medicine, Montefiore Med Ctr 1998; Nuclear Medicine, Montefiore Med Ctr 2000; **Fellow:** Nuclear Medicine, Memorial Sloan-Kettering Cancer Center 2001; **Fac Appt:** Assoc Prof Rad, Yale Univ

Obstetrics & Gynecology

Cron, Julia MD (ObG) - **Spec Exp:** Adolescent Gynecology; Pap Smear Abnormalities; **Hospital:** Yale-New Haven Hosp; **Address:** Ob/Gyn & Menopause Phys, 40 Temple St, Ste 7A, New Haven, CT 06510; **Phone:** 203-789-2011; **Board Cert:** Obstetrics & Gynecology 2012; **Med School:** Univ Conn 1999; **Resid:** Obstetrics & Gynecology, John Hopkins Hosp 2003

Fine, Emily A MD (ObG) - **Spec Exp:** Menopause Problems; Vulvar Disease; **Hospital:** Yale-New Haven Hosp; **Address:** 60 Washington Ave, Ste 201, Hamden, CT 06518; **Phone:** 203-230-2939; **Board Cert:** Obstetrics & Gynecology 1984; **Med School:** Yale Univ 1978; **Resid:** Obstetrics & Gynecology, Yale-New Haven Hosp 1982; **Fac Appt:** Asst Clin Prof ObG, Yale Univ

Guess, Marsha Kathleen MD (ObG) - **Spec Exp:** Incontinence; Pelvic Organ Prolapse Repair; Uro-Gynecology; **Hospital:** Yale-New Haven Hosp; **Address:** Yale, Urogyn & Reconstruc Pelvic Surg, 800 Howard Ave Fl 3, New Haven, CT 06510; **Phone:** 203-785-6927; **Board Cert:** Obstetrics & Gynecology 2011; **Med School:** UCLA 1997; **Resid:** Obstetrics & Gynecology, UCLA Med Ctr 2001; **Fellow:** Reconstructive Pelvic Surgery, Montefiore Med Ctr 2004; **Fac Appt:** Asst Prof ObG, Yale Univ

Lynch, Vincent A MD (ObG) - **Spec Exp:** Laparoscopic Surgery; Menopause Problems; Heart Disease in Pregnancy; **Hospital:** Yale-New Haven Hosp; **Address:** Greater New Haven Ob/Gyn, 46 Prince St, Ste 207, New Haven, CT 06519; **Phone:** 203-787-2264; **Board Cert:** Obstetrics & Gynecology 1986; **Med School:** NY Med Coll 1967; **Resid:** Obstetrics & Gynecology, Yale-New Haven Hosp 1972; **Fac Appt:** Clin Prof ObG, Yale Univ

Ophthalmology

Bacal, Darron A MD (Oph) - **Spec Exp:** Pediatric Ophthalmology; Strabismus-Adult & Pediatric; Eye Muscle Disorders; **Hospital:** Yale-New Haven Hosp, Yale-New Haven Hosp - St Raphael Campus; **Address:** EYE Physicians & Surgeons, 202 Cherry St, Milford, CT 06460; **Phone:** 203-878-1236; **Board Cert:** Ophthalmology 2008; **Med School:** Jefferson Med Coll 1992; **Resid:** Ophthalmology, Univ of Maryland Med Ctr 1996; **Fellow:** Pediatric Ophthalmology, Chlldren's Hosp/Scheie Eye Inst 1997

Lesser, Robert L MD (Oph) - **Spec Exp:** Neuro-Ophthalmology; Myasthenia Gravis; Pseudotumor Cerebri; Temporal Arteritis; **Hospital:** Yale-New Haven Hosp, St. Mary's Hosp - Waterbury; **Address:** Eye Care Grp, 40 Temple St, Ste 5B, New Haven, CT 06510; **Phone:** 203-789-2020; **Board Cert:** Ophthalmology 1975; **Med School:** Cornell Univ-Weill Med Coll 1967; **Resid:** Ophthalmology, Yale-New Haven Hosp 1974; **Fellow:** Neuro-Ophthalmology, Bascom Palmer Eye Inst 1972; **Fac Appt:** Clin Prof Oph, Yale Univ

Meskin, Seth W MD (Oph) - **Spec Exp:** Glaucoma; **Hospital:** Yale-New Haven Hosp; **Address:** EYE Physicians & Surgeons, 202 Cherry St, Milford, CT 06460; **Phone:** 203-878-1236; **Board Cert:** Ophthalmology 2005; **Med School:** Jefferson Med Coll 2000; **Resid:** Ophthalmology, New York Eye & Ear Infirm 2004; **Fellow:** Cornea & Ext Eye Disease, New York Eye & Ear Infirm 2005

Shapiro, Martin R MD (Oph) - **Spec Exp:** Glaucoma; Cataract Surgery; **Hospital:** Yale-New Haven Hosp, Milford Hosp; **Address:** EYE Physicians & Surgeons, 202 Cherry St, Milford, CT 06460; **Phone:** 203-878-1236; **Board Cert:** Ophthalmology 1985; **Med School:** Washington Univ, St Louis 1979; **Resid:** Ophthalmology, Barnes Jewish Hosp 1983

Silverstone, Philip J MD (Oph) - **Spec Exp:** Ophthalmic Plastic Surgery; Orbital Surgery; Botox Therapy; **Hospital:** Yale-New Haven Hosp; **Address:** EYE Physicians & Surgeons, 202 Cherry St, Milford, CT 06460; **Phone:** 203-878-1236; **Board Cert:** Ophthalmology 1987; **Med School:** Univ Conn 1980; **Resid:** Internal Medicine, UC-Irvine Med Ctr 1982; Ophthalmology, UC-Irvine Med Ctr 1985; **Fellow:** Ophthalmic Plastic Surgery, NY Eye & Ear Infirmary 1986

Sprotzer, Samuel P MD (Oph) - **Spec Exp:** Refractive Surgery; Cataract Surgery; Glaucoma; **Hospital:** Milford Hosp, Yale-New Haven Hosp; **Address:** EYE Physicians & Surgeons, 202 Cherry St, Milford, CT 06460; **Phone:** 203-878-1236; **Board Cert:** Ophthalmology 1978; **Med School:** NYU Sch Med 1973; **Resid:** Ophthalmology, Yale-New Haven Hosp 1977

Tom, David MD (Oph) - **Spec Exp:** Retinal Disorders; Diabetic Eye Disease/Retinopathy; **Hospital:** Yale-New Haven Hosp, Greenwich Hosp (page 938); **Address:** New England Retina Assocs, 2200 Whitney Ave, Ste 300, Hamden, CT 06518; **Phone:** 203-288-2020; **Board Cert:** Ophthalmology 2008; **Med School:** Geo Wash Univ 1991; **Resid:** Ophthalmology, Yale-New Haven Hosp 1996; **Fellow:** Retinal Surgery, Manhattan EET Hosp 1997; **Fac Appt:** Asst Clin Prof Oph, Yale Univ

Tsai, James C MD (Oph) - **Spec Exp:** Glaucoma; **Hospital:** Yale-New Haven Hosp; **Address:** Yale Eye Ctr, 40 Temple St Fl 3, New Haven, CT 06520-8061; **Phone:** 203-785-2020; **Board Cert:** Ophthalmology 2006; **Med School:** Stanford Univ 1989; **Resid:** Internal Medicine, Cedars-Sinai Med Ctr 1990; Ophthalmology, Doheny Eye Inst/USC 1993; **Fellow:** Glaucoma, Bascom Palmer Eye Inst 1994; Glaucoma, Moorfields Eye Hosp 1995; **Fac Appt:** Prof Oph, Yale Univ

Orthopaedic Surgery

Baumgaertner, Michael R MD (OrS) - **Spec Exp:** Trauma; Hip & Knee Reconstruction; Fractures-Complex & Non Union; **Hospital:** Yale-New Haven Hosp; **Address:** Yale, Orthopaedics & Rehab, 800 Howard Ave Fl 1, New Haven, CT 06519; **Phone:** 203-737-5656; **Board Cert:** Orthopaedic Surgery 2011; **Med School:** UCSD 1982; **Resid:** Orthopaedic Surgery, UCSF Med Ctr 1987; **Fellow:** Plastic Surgery, Univ Mass Med Ctr 1988; Trauma, AO Foundation 1989; **Fac Appt:** Prof OrS, Yale Univ

Beauvais, Paul Joseph MD (OrS) - **Spec Exp:** Trauma; Hand Surgery; Shoulder Surgery; **Hospital:** Waterbury Hosp, St. Mary's Hosp - Waterbury; **Address:** NE Orthopaedic & Hand Surgery, 60 Westwood Ave, Ste 300, Waterbury, CT 06708-2460; **Phone:** 203-755-9166; **Board Cert:** Orthopaedic Surgery 2009; **Med School:** Columbia P&S 1990; **Resid:** Orthopaedic Surgery, NY-Presby/Columbia Univ Med Ctr 1996; **Fellow:** Research, NY-Presby/Columbia Univ Med Ctr 1991

Blaine, Theodore MD (OrS) - **Spec Exp:** Shoulder & Elbow Surgery; Arthroscopic Surgery; Sports Medicine; **Hospital:** Yale-New Haven Hosp; **Address:** Yale, Orthopaedics/Sports Med, 800 Howard Ave, New Haven, CT 06519; **Phone:** 203-737-5656; **Board Cert:** Orthopaedic Surgery 2013; Orthopaedic Sports Medicine 2007; **Med School:** Univ Conn 1993; **Resid:** Orthopaedic Surgery, Strong Meml Hosp 1999; **Fellow:** Sports Medicine, Columbia Univ Med Ctr 2000; Elbow Surgery, Mayo Clin 2000; **Fac Appt:** Assoc Prof OrS, Yale Univ

Flynn Jr, William Francis MD (OrS) - **Spec Exp:** Joint Reconstruction; Sports Medicine; **Hospital:** Waterbury Hosp, St. Mary's Hosp - Waterbury; **Address:** Neurosurgery, Ortho & Spine Specialists, 500 Chase Pkwy, Waterbury, CT 06708; **Phone:** 203-755-4281; **Board Cert:** Orthopaedic Surgery 2006; **Med School:** Cornell Univ 1986; **Resid:** Orthopaedic Surgery, Hosp for Special Surgery 1991; **Fellow:** Joint Reconstruction, Hosp for Special Surgery 1992

Friedlaender, Gary E MD (OrS) - **Spec Exp:** Bone & Soft Tissue Tumors; Limb Surgery/Reconstruction; Fractures-Complex & Non Union; Tissue Banking; **Hospital:** Yale-New Haven Hosp; **Address:** Yale Orthopaedics and Rehabilitation, 800 Howard Ave, Yale Physicians Building YPB 133, Fl 1, New Haven, CT 06519; **Phone:** 203-737-5660; **Board Cert:** Orthopaedic Surgery 1975; **Med School:** Univ Mich Med Sch 1969; **Resid:** Surgery, Michigan Med Ctr 1971; Orthopaedic Surgery, Yale-New Haven Hosp 1974; **Fellow:** Musculoskeletal Oncology, Mass Genl Hosp 1983; **Fac Appt:** Prof OrS, Yale Univ

Grauer, Jonathan N MD (OrS) - **Spec Exp:** Spinal Surgery; Fractures; Pediatric Orthopaedic Surgery; **Hospital:** Yale-New Haven Hosp; **Address:** Yale, Spine Svc, 1 Long Wharf Drive Fl 6, New Haven, CT 06511; **Phone:** 203-737-7463; **Board Cert:** Orthopaedic Surgery 2005; **Med School:** Yale Univ 1997; **Resid:** Orthopaedic Surgery, Yale-New Haven Hosp 2002; **Fellow:** Spine Surgery, Rothman Inst 2003; **Fac Appt:** Assoc Prof OrS, Yale Univ

Jokl, Peter MD (OrS) - **Spec Exp:** Knee Surgery; Sports Medicine; Shoulder Surgery; **Hospital:** Yale-New Haven Hosp; **Address:** Yale Sports Med, Dept Orthopaedics, 800 Howard Ave, New Haven, CT 06519-1369; **Phone:** 203-785-2579; **Board Cert:** Orthopaedic Surgery 1974; **Med School:** Yale Univ 1968; **Resid:** Orthopaedic Surgery, Yale-New Haven Hosp 1972; **Fac Appt:** Prof OrS, Yale Univ

Marsh, James S MD (OrS) - **Spec Exp:** Pediatric Orthopaedic Surgery; **Hospital:** Yale-New Haven Hosp, Yale-New Haven Hosp - St Raphael Campus; **Address:** Family Orthopaedics, 34 York St, Ste 2, Guilford, CT 06437; **Phone:** 203-453-1088; **Med School:** Harvard Med Sch 1981; **Resid:** Orthopaedic Surgery, Stanford Univ Affil Hosp 1986; **Fellow:** Pediatric Orthopaedic Surgery, Mass Genl Hosp 1987; **Fac Appt:** Assoc Prof OrS, Yale Univ

Medvecky, Michael J MD (OrS) - **Spec Exp:** Sports Medicine; Shoulder Surgery; Rotator Cuff Surgery; **Hospital:** Yale-New Haven Hosp; **Address:** 800 Howard Ave Fl 1, New Haven, CT 06520; **Phone:** 203-785-3851; **Board Cert:** Orthopaedic Surgery 2003; Orthopaedic Sports Medicine 2007; **Med School:** NY Med Coll 1995; **Resid:** Surgery, NYU Med Ctr 1996; Orthopaedic Surgery, NYU (Hosp for Joint Diseases) 2000; **Fellow:** Sports Medicine, Cincinnati Sports Med & Ortho ctr 2001

Reznik, Alan MD (OrS) - **Spec Exp:** Pediatric Sports Medicine; Trauma; Shoulder & Knee Reconstruction; Arthroscopic Surgery; **Hospital:** Yale-New Haven Hosp; **Address:** Orthopaedic Grp, 199 Whitney Ave, New Haven, CT 06511; **Phone:** 203-865-6784; **Board Cert:** Orthopaedic Surgery 2012; Pediatric Sports Medicine 2010; **Med School:** Yale Univ 1983; **Resid:** Orthopaedic Surgery, Mount Sinai Med Ctr 1987; **Fellow:** Sports Medicine, UCSD Med Ctr 1989

Smith, Brian Gerard MD (OrS) - **Spec Exp:** Pediatric Orthopaedic Surgery; Spinal Deformity; Scoliosis; Foot Deformities; **Hospital:** Yale-New Haven Hosp, Yale-New Haven Hosp - St Raphael Campus; **Address:** Yale Orthopaedics, 800 Howard Ave, Yale Physicians Bldg, Fl 1, New Haven, CT 06519; **Phone:** 203-737-1616; **Board Cert:** Orthopaedic Surgery 2010; **Med School:** Georgetown Univ 1982; **Resid:** Orthopaedic Surgery, Georgetown Univ Hosp 1987; **Fellow:** Pediatric Orthopaedic Surgery, Children's Hosp 1992; **Fac Appt:** Prof OrS, Yale Univ

Wetmore, Robert S MD (OrS) - **Hospital:** Waterbury Hosp, St. Mary's Hosp - Waterbury; **Address:** 1579 Straits Tpke, Ste E1, Middlebury, CT 06762-1835; **Phone:** 203-758-1760; **Board Cert:** Orthopaedic Surgery 2012; **Med School:** Dartmouth Med Sch 1978; **Resid:** Orthopaedic Surgery, Yale-New Haven Hosp 1983; Orthopaedic Surgery, Yale-New Haven Hosp 1986

Wijesekera, Shirvinda MD (OrS) - **Spec Exp:** Spinal Surgery-Pediatric & Adult; Scoliosis; Spinal Trauma; **Hospital:** Yale-New Haven Hosp; **Address:** Orthopaedic Grp, 199 Whitney Ave, New Haven, CT 06511; **Phone:** 203-865-6784; **Board Cert:** Orthopaedic Surgery 2007; **Med School:** Boston Univ 1998; **Resid:** Orthopaedic Surgery, LAC & USC Med Ctr 2003; **Fellow:** Spine Surgery, UC Davis Med Ctr 2004

Yue, James J MD (OrS) - **Spec Exp:** Spinal Surgery; **Hospital:** Yale-New Haven Hosp; **Address:** Yale Orthopaedics/Spine Service, 800 Howard Ave, New Haven, CT 06519; **Phone:** 203-737-5656; **Board Cert:** Orthopaedic Surgery ; **Med School:** Northwestern Univ 1992; **Resid:** Orthopaedic Surgery, Univ Hosp Cleveland 1997; **Fellow:** Orthopaedic Trauma Surgery, RA Cowley Shock Trauma Hosp 1998; Spine Surgery, Queen's Med Ctr 1998; **Fac Appt:** Assoc Prof OrS, Yale Univ

Otolaryngology

Judson, Benjamin MD (Oto) - **Spec Exp:** Head & Neck Surgery; Skull Base Tumors; **Hospital:** Smilow Cancer Hosp at Yale-New Haven, Yale-New Haven Hosp; **Address:** Yale, Head & Neck Cancer, 35 Park St Fl 4, New Haven, CT 06519; **Phone:** 203-200-4622; **Board Cert:** Otolaryngology ; **Med School:** Jefferson Med Coll 2002; **Resid:** Otolaryngology, Georgetown Univ Hosp 2007; **Fellow:** Head and Neck Surgery, Meml Sloan-Kettering Cancer Ctr 2009; Research, NY-Presby/Weill Cornell Med Ctr 2009; **Fac Appt:** Asst Prof S, Yale Univ

Kveton, John F MD (Oto) - **Spec Exp:** Ear Disorders/Surgery; Cochlear Implants; Acoustic Neuroma; Hearing Loss; **Hospital:** Yale-New Haven Hosp, Yale-New Haven Hosp - St Raphael Campus; **Address:** ENT Med & Surgical Grp, 46 Prince St, Ste 601, New Haven, CT 06519-1634; **Phone:** 203-752-1726; **Board Cert:** Otolaryngology 1982; Neurotology 2004; **Med School:** St Louis Univ 1978; **Resid:** Otolaryngology, Yale-New Haven Hosp 1982; **Fellow:** Neurotology, The Otology Group 1983; **Fac Appt:** Clin Prof Oto, Yale Univ

Michaelides, Elias M MD (Oto) - **Spec Exp:** Neuro-Otology; Hearing Loss; Balance Disorders; Pediatric Otolaryngology; **Hospital:** Yale-New Haven Hosp; **Address:** 800 Howard Ave, Yale Physicians Bldg, Fl 4, New Haven, CT 06519; **Phone:** 203-785-7656; **Board Cert:** Otolaryngology 1999; Neurotology 2008; **Med School:** SUNY Stony Brook 1993; **Resid:** Otolaryngology, Med Coll Va Hosp 1998; **Fellow:** Otology, Michigan Ear Inst 2000; **Fac Appt:** Asst Prof S, Yale Univ

Sasaki, Clarence T MD (Oto) - **Spec Exp:** Head & Neck Cancer; Swallowing Disorders; Zenker Diverticulum; Voice Disorders; **Hospital:** Yale-New Haven Hosp; **Address:** Yale Sch Med, Dept Otolaryngology, 333 Cedar St, Box 208041, New Haven, CT 06520-8041; **Phone:** 203-785-2592; **Board Cert:** Otolaryngology 1973; **Med School:** Yale Univ 1966; **Resid:** Surgery, Mary Hitchcock Hosp 1968; Otolaryngology, Yale-New Haven Hosp 1973; **Fellow:** Head and Neck Surgery, Univ of Milan 1978; Skull Base Surgery, Univ Zurich 1982; **Fac Appt:** Prof Oto, Yale Univ

Takoudes, Thomas MD (Oto) - **Spec Exp:** Snoring/Sleep Apnea; Swallowing Disorders; **Hospital:** Yale-New Haven Hosp; **Address:** ENT Med & Surgl Grp, 31 Broadway, North Haven, CT 06473; **Phone:** 203-234-1324; **Board Cert:** Otolaryngology 2013; **Med School:** Columbia P&S 1996; **Resid:** Otolaryngology, NY-Presby/Columbia Univ Med Ctr 2002; **Fellow:** Pediatric Otolaryngology, NY-Presby/Columbia Univ Med Ctr 2003

Vining, Eugenia M MD (Oto) - **Spec Exp:** Sinus Disorders/Surgery; Skull Base Tumors; Endoscopic Sinus Surgery; **Hospital:** Yale-New Haven Hosp, Yale-New Haven Hosp - St Raphael Campus; **Address:** ENT Medical & Surgical Grp, 46 Prince St, Ste 601, New Haven, CT 06519; **Phone:** 203-752-1726; **Board Cert:** Otolaryngology 1993; **Med School:** Yale Univ 1987; **Resid:** Otolaryngology, Yale-New Haven Hosp 1991; Otolaryngology, Yale-New Haven Hosp 1992; **Fellow:** Sinus Surgery, Univ Penn 1993

Yarbrough, Wendell G MD (Oto) - **Spec Exp:** Head & Neck Cancer; Salivary Gland Tumors; **Hospital:** Yale-New Haven Hosp; **Address:** 800 Howard Ave, Fl 4, New Haven, CT 06519; **Phone:** 203-785-4862; **Board Cert:** Otolaryngology 1995; **Med School:** Univ NC Sch Med 1989; **Resid:** Otolaryngology, Univ NC Hosps 1994; **Fellow:** Surgical Oncology, Univ NC Med Sch 1996

Young, Nwanmegha MD (Oto) - **Spec Exp:** Voice Disorders; Vocal Cord Disorders; Laryngeal Disorders; Swallowing Disorders; **Hospital:** Yale-New Haven Hosp; **Address:** Yale, Otolaryngology, 800 Howard Ave Fl 4, New Haven, CT 06519; **Phone:** 203-785-2593; **Board Cert:** Otolaryngology 2008; **Med School:** UC Davis 1999; **Resid:** Otolaryngology, Barnes-Jewish Hosp 2005; **Fellow:** Neurotology, St Lukes-Roosevelt Hosp 2007; **Fac Appt:** Asst Prof S, Yale Univ

Pain Medicine

Robbins, Michael DO (PM) - **Hospital:** Yale-New Haven Hosp; **Address:** Advanced Diag Pain Treatment Ctrs, 1 Long Wharf, Ste 212, New Haven, CT 06511; **Phone:** 203-624-4208; **Board Cert:** Anesthesiology 1997; Pain Medicine 2009; **Med School:** Philadelphia Coll Osteo Med 1992; **Resid:** Anesthesiology, UPMC St Margaret 1996; **Fellow:** Pain Medicine, Einstein Med Ctr 1997

Saberski, Lloyd MD (PM) - **Spec Exp:** Headache; **Hospital:** Yale-New Haven Hosp, Yale-New Haven Hosp - St Raphael Campus; **Address:** Advanced Diagnostic Pain Treatment Ctr, 1 Long Wharf Drive, Ste 212, New Haven, CT 06511; **Phone:** 203-624-4208; **Board Cert:** Internal Medicine 1985; Anesthesiology 1988; Pain Medicine 2014; **Med School:** NY Med Coll 1982; **Resid:** Internal Medicine, Albany Meml Hosp 1985; Anesthesiology, Albany Meml Hosp 1987; **Fellow:** Pain Medicine, Albany Meml Hosp 1988; **Fac Appt:** Assoc Prof Anes, Yale Univ

Pathology

Chhieng, David Cheung MD (Path) - **Spec Exp:** Pancreatic Cancer; Thyroid Cancer; Cervical Cancer; **Hospital:** Yale-New Haven Hosp; **Address:** Yale, Pathology Dept, 20 York St, Ste CB510, New Haven, CT 06510; **Phone:** 203-737-2658; **Board Cert:** Pathology 1997; Cytopathology 1998; **Med School:** Hong Kong 1987; **Resid:** Pathology, Albany Meml Hosp 1996; **Fellow:** Surgical Pathology, Meml Sloan-Kettering Cancer Ctr 1997; Cytopathology, NYU Med Ctr 1998; **Fac Appt:** Prof Path, Yale Univ

Glusac, Earl MD (Path) - **Spec Exp:** Melanoma; Dermatopathology; **Hospital:** Yale-New Haven Hosp; **Address:** Yale, Dermatopathology, 15 York St, Ste LMP 5031, New Haven, CT 06520; **Phone:** 203-785-4094; **Board Cert:** Pathology ; Dermatopathology ; **Med School:** Mich State Univ 1987; **Resid:** Psychiatry, Cedar-Sinai Med Ctr 1989; Pathology, Cedar-Sinai Med Ctr 1993; **Fellow:** Dermatopathology, Stanford Univ Hosp & Clins 1994; **Fac Appt:** Prof Path, Yale Univ

Jain, Dhanpat MD (Path) - **Spec Exp:** Gastrointestinal Pathology; Liver Cancer; **Hospital:** Yale-New Haven Hosp; **Address:** Yale, Pathology Dept, 200 S Frontage Rd, New Haven, CT 06510; **Phone:** 203-785-2788; **Board Cert:** Anatomic Pathology ; **Med School:** India 1986; **Resid:** Pathology, Yale-New Haven Hosp 1999; **Fac Appt:** Assoc Prof Path, Yale Univ

Morrow, Jon S MD/PhD (Path) - **Spec Exp:** Kidney Cancer; Colon Cancer; Breast Cancer; Hematopathology; **Hospital:** Yale-New Haven Hosp; **Address:** Yale, Pathology, 310 Cedar St, BML 140, New Haven, CT 06510; **Phone:** 203-785-3624; **Board Cert:** Pathology 1980; **Med School:** Yale Univ 1976; **Resid:** Pathology, Yale-New Haven Hosp 1978; **Fellow:** Pathology, Yale-New Haven Hosp 1980; **Fac Appt:** Prof Path, Yale Univ

Rimm, David MD/PhD (Path) - **Spec Exp:** Gastrointestinal Pathology; Breast Cancer; Melanoma; **Hospital:** Yale-New Haven Hosp; **Address:** Yale, Pathology Dept, 310 Cedar St, Ste 116, New Haven, CT 06510; **Phone:** 203-737-4204; **Board Cert:** Anatomic Pathology 1995; Cytopathology 1996; **Med School:** Johns Hopkins Univ 1989; **Resid:** Pathology, Yale-New Haven Hosp 1993; **Fellow:** Cytopathology, Med Coll VA 1994; **Fac Appt:** Prof Path, Yale Univ

Tavassoli, Fattaneh MD (Path) - **Spec Exp:** Breast Pathology; Gynecologic Pathology; **Hospital:** Yale-New Haven Hosp; **Address:** Yale, Pathology Dept, 310 Cedar St, Ste LH222, New Haven, CT 06510; **Phone:** 203-785-5439; **Board Cert:** Anatomic Pathology 2010; **Med School:** St Louis Univ 1972; **Resid:** Pathology, Barnes-Jewish Hosp 1974; **Fellow:** Gynecologic Pathology, St Johns Mercy Hosp 1976; **Fac Appt:** Prof Path, Yale Univ

Pediatric Allergy & Immunology

Randolph, Christopher MD (PA&I) - **Spec Exp:** Asthma; Sinusitis; **Hospital:** Yale-New Haven Hosp; **Address:** Ctr Allergy, Asthma & Immunology, 1389 W Main St, Ste 205, Waterbury, CT 06708; **Phone:** 203-755-7080; **Board Cert:** Pediatrics ; Allergy & Immunology ; **Med School:** Univ Rochester 1980; **Resid:** Pediatrics, Women & Chldns Hosp 1983; **Fellow:** Allergy & Immunology, Buffalo Genl Hosp 1985; **Fac Appt:** Clin Prof Ped, Yale Univ

Pediatric Cardiology

Friedman, Alan H MD (PCd) - **Spec Exp:** Echocardiography; Fetal Echocardiography; Cardiac Imaging; Congenital Heart Disease; **Hospital:** Yale-New Haven Hosp; **Address:** Yale-Chldns Hosp, Ped Cardiology, 1 Park St Fl 2, New Haven, CT 06510; **Phone:** 203-785-2022; **Board Cert:** Pediatric Cardiology 2011; **Med School:** Wayne State Univ 1987; **Resid:** Pediatrics, Chldns Meml Hosp 1991; **Fellow:** Pediatric Cardiology, Yale-New Haven Hosp 1994; **Fac Appt:** Prof Ped, Yale Univ

Hellenbrand, William E MD (PCd) - **Spec Exp:** Interventional Cardiology; **Hospital:** Yale-New Haven Hosp; **Address:** Yale-New Haven Children's Hosp, Pediatric Cardiology, 1 Park St, New Haven, CT 06510; **Phone:** 203-785-2022; **Board Cert:** Pediatrics 1975; Pediatric Cardiology 1977; **Med School:** SUNY Downstate 1970; **Resid:** Pediatrics, Yale-New Haven Hosp 1972; **Fellow:** Pediatric Cardiology, Yale-New Haven Hosp 1976; **Fac Appt:** Prof Ped, Columbia P&S

Pediatric Endocrinology

Boulware, Susan MD (PEn) - **Spec Exp:** Pubertal Disorders; Thyroid Disorders; Adrenal Disorders; **Hospital:** Yale-New Haven Hosp; **Address:** Yale, Pediatric Endocrinology, 1 Long Wharf Drive, rm 503, New Haven, CT 06519; **Phone:** 203-785-4081; **Board Cert:** Pediatric Endocrinology 2007; **Med School:** Univ Tex, San Antonio 1984; **Resid:** Pediatrics, UT Hlth Sci Ctr 1987; **Fellow:** Endocrinology, Yale-New Haven Hosp 1990; **Fac Appt:** Asst Clin Prof Ped, Yale Univ

Carpenter, Thomas O MD (PEn) - **Spec Exp:** Calcium Disorders; Bone Disorders-Metabolic; Thyroid Disorders; Parathyroid Disorders; **Hospital:** Yale-New Haven Hosp; **Address:** Yale-Chldns Hosp, Ped Endocrinology, 1 Long Wharf Drive Fl 3, New Haven, CT 06511; **Phone:** 203-764-9199; **Board Cert:** Pediatrics 1982; Pediatric Endocrinology 1999; **Med School:** UAB Sch Med 1977; **Resid:** Pediatrics, UAB Hosp 1980; **Fellow:** Pediatric Endocrinology, Chldns Hosp 1983; **Fac Appt:** Prof Ped, Yale Univ

Tamborlane, William V MD (PEn) - **Spec Exp:** Diabetes; **Hospital:** Yale-New Haven Hosp; **Address:** Yale Pediatric Endocrinology, 333 Cedar St, rm 3091-LMP, New Haven, CT 06519; **Phone:** 203-764-6747; **Board Cert:** Pediatrics 1978; Pediatric Endocrinology 1986; **Med School:** Georgetown Univ 1972; **Resid:** Pediatrics, Georgetown Univ Hosp 1975; **Fellow:** Pediatric Endocrinology, Yale-New Haven Hosp 1977; **Fac Appt:** Prof Ped, Yale Univ

Pediatric Gastroenterology

Escalera, Sandra MD (PGe) - **Spec Exp:** Ulcerative Colitis; Endoscopy; Liver Disease; **Hospital:** Yale-New Haven Hosp; **Address:** ProHlth Phys, Ped Gastroenterology, 116 Washington Ave Fl 2, North Haven, CT 06473; **Phone:** 203-234-9267; **Board Cert:** Pediatric Gastroenterology ; **Med School:** Puerto Rico 1992; **Resid:** Pediatrics, Stony Brook Univ Med Ctr 1995; **Fellow:** Pediatric Gastroenterology, Yale-New Haven Hosp 1999; **Fac Appt:** Assoc Clin Prof Ped, Yale Univ

Porto, Anthony MD (PGe) - **Spec Exp:** Obesity; Liver Disease; Inflammatory Bowel Disease; **Hospital:** Yale-New Haven Hosp, Greenwich Hosp (page 938); **Address:** Yale, Ped Gastroenterology Dept, 1 Long Wharf Drive Fl 2, New Haven, CT 06511; **Phone:** 203-785-4081; **Board Cert:** Pediatrics 2012; Pediatric Gastroenterology 2007; **Med School:** Tufts Univ 2001; **Resid:** Pediatrics, Chldns Hosp Montefiore 2004; **Fellow:** Pediatric Gastroenterology, NY-Presby/Morgan Stanley Chldns Hosp 2007; **Fac Appt:** Asst Prof Ped, Yale Univ

Pediatric Hematology-Oncology

Kadan-Lottick, Nina S MD (PHO) - **Spec Exp:** Cancer Survivors-Late Effects of Therapy; **Hospital:** Yale-New Haven Hosp; **Address:** Yale Pediatric Hematology/Oncology, 333 Cedar St, LMP 2073, New Haven, CT 06510; **Phone:** 203-785-4640; **Board Cert:** Pediatric Hematology-Oncology 2008; **Med School:** Johns Hopkins Univ 1993; **Resid:** Pediatrics, Johns Hopkins Hosp 1996; **Fellow:** Pediatric Hematology-Oncology, Chldns Hosp 1999; Cancer Epidemiology, Univ Minnesota 2000; **Fac Appt:** Assoc Prof Ped, Yale Univ

Kupfer, Gary MD (PHO) - **Hospital:** Smilow Cancer Hosp at Yale-New Haven; **Address:** Yale, Pediatric Hem/Onc, 789 Howard Ave, New Haven, CT 06519; **Phone:** 203-785-4640; **Board Cert:** Pediatric Hematology-Oncology 2011; **Med School:** Johns Hopkins Univ 1989; **Resid:** Pediatrics, Chldns Hosp 1992; **Fellow:** Pediatric Hematology-Oncology, Chldns Hosp/Dana Farber Cancer Inst 1995; **Fac Appt:** Prof Ped, Yale Univ

McNamara, Joseph M MD (PHO) - **Spec Exp:** Leukemia & Lymphoma; Solid Tumors; **Hospital:** Yale-New Haven Hosp; **Address:** Yale, Ped Hem/Onc Assocs, 405 Church St, Guilford, CT 06437; **Phone:** 203-453-2013; **Board Cert:** Pediatrics 1987; Pediatric Hematology-Oncology 2012; **Med School:** Italy 1982; **Resid:** Pediatrics, Our Lady Mercy Med Ctr 1985; **Fellow:** Pediatric Hematology-Oncology, Schneider Chldns Hosp 1987; **Fac Appt:** Assoc Prof Ped, Yale Univ

Pediatric Infectious Disease

Andiman, Warren A MD (PInf) - **Spec Exp:** AIDS/HIV; Viral Infections; Lyme Disease; Infectious Mononucleosis; **Hospital:** Yale-New Haven Hosp; **Address:** Yale Ped Infectious Disease, 20 York St Fl 2, New Haven, CT 06520-8064; **Phone:** 203-785-4730; **Board Cert:** Pediatrics 1975; **Med School:** Albert Einstein Coll Med 1969; **Resid:** Pediatrics, Babies Hosp-Columbia Presby 1971; **Fellow:** Pediatric Infectious Disease, Yale-New Haven Hosp 1973; **Fac Appt:** Prof Ped, Yale Univ

Baltimore, Robert Samuel MD (PInf) - **Spec Exp:** Neonatal Infections; Hospital Acquired Infections; Tuberculosis; **Hospital:** Yale-New Haven Hosp; **Address:** Yale Pediatric Infectious Diseases, 1 Park St, New Haven, CT 06510; **Phone:** 203-785-4730; **Board Cert:** Pediatrics 1975; Pediatric Infectious Disease 2009; **Med School:** SUNY Buffalo 1968; **Resid:** Pediatrics, Univ Chicago Hosps 1971; **Fellow:** Infectious Disease, Boston Univ Hosp 1976; **Fac Appt:** Prof Ped, Yale Univ

Shapiro, Eugene D MD (PInf) - **Spec Exp:** Lyme Disease; Vaccines; **Hospital:** Yale-New Haven Hosp; **Address:** Yale Univ Sch Med, Dept Pediatrics, 333 Cedar St, Box 208064, New Haven, CT 06520-8064; **Phone:** 203-688-4518; **Board Cert:** Pediatrics 1980; Pediatric Infectious Disease 2009; **Med School:** UCSF 1976; **Resid:** Pediatrics, Chldn's Hosp 1979; **Fellow:** Pediatric Infectious Disease, Chldn's Hosp 1981; Epidemiology, Yale Univ 1983; **Fac Appt:** Prof Ped, Yale Univ

Vazquez, Marietta MD (PInf) - **Spec Exp:** Vaccines; Lyme Disease; Infections-Respiratory; **Hospital:** Yale-New Haven Hosp; **Address:** Yale, Pediatric Infectious Disease, 1 Park St Fl 2, New Haven, CT 06510; **Phone:** 203-737-6018; **Board Cert:** Pediatrics 2012; Pediatric Infectious Disease ; **Med School:** Puerto Rico 1994; **Resid:** Pediatrics, Yale-New Haven Hosp 1997; **Fellow:** Pediatric Infectious Disease, Yale-New Haven Hosp 2000; **Fac Appt:** Assoc Prof Ped, Yale Univ

Pediatric Nephrology

Tufro, Alda MD (PNep) - **Spec Exp:** Hypertension; Kidney Disease; **Hospital:** Yale-New Haven Hosp; **Address:** Yale Chldns Hosp, Ped Nephrology, 1 Park St Fl 2, New Haven, CT 06510; **Phone:** 203-785-4643; **Board Cert:** Pediatrics 2008; Pediatric Nephrology 2009; **Med School:** Argentina 1977; **Resid:** Pediatrics, Hosp Natl Alejandro Posadras 1982; **Fellow:** Pediatric Nephrology, Univ VA Med Ctr 1994; **Fac Appt:** Assoc Prof Ped, Yale Univ

Pediatric Otolaryngology

Baum, Eric D MD (PO) - **Spec Exp:** Head & Neck Surgery; Airway Reconstruction; Ear Disorders/Surgery; **Hospital:** Yale-New Haven Hosp; **Address:** CT Pediatric Otolaryngology, 230 Boston Post Rd, Madison, CT 06443; **Phone:** 203-245-0496; **Board Cert:** Otolaryngology 2014; **Med School:** Univ Pennsylvania 1999; **Resid:** Otolaryngology, Hosp Univ Penn 2002; **Fellow:** Pediatric Otolaryngology, Chldns Hosp 2005

Karas, David E MD (PO) - **Spec Exp:** Sleep Disorders/Apnea; **Hospital:** Yale-New Haven Hosp; **Address:** CT Pediatric Otolaryngology, 230 Boston Post Rd, Madison, CT 06443; **Phone:** 203-245-0496; **Board Cert:** Otolaryngology 1997; **Med School:** Univ Conn 1990; **Resid:** Otolaryngology, Univ Hosp-UMDNJ 1995; **Fellow:** Pediatric Otolaryngology, Chldns Hosp 1996; **Fac Appt:** Asst Prof Ped, Yale Univ

Pediatric Pulmonology

Bazzy-Asaad, Alia MD (PPul) - **Spec Exp:** Asthma; Sleep Disorders; Cystic Fibrosis; **Hospital:** Yale-New Haven Hosp; **Address:** Yale-Chldns Hosp, Ped Pulmonology, 1 Park St Fl 2, New Haven, CT 06510; **Phone:** 203-785-2480; **Board Cert:** Pediatrics 1987; Pediatric Pulmonology 2009; **Med School:** Amer Univ Beirut 1978; **Resid:** Pediatrics, Amer Univ Beirut 1980; **Fellow:** Pediatric Pulmonology, NY-Presby/Columbia Univ Med Ctr 1983; **Fac Appt:** Assoc Prof Ped, Yale Univ

Pediatric Rheumatology

McCarthy, Paul L MD (PRhu) - **Spec Exp:** Lupus/SLE; Juvenile Arthritis; Dermatomyositis; Vasculitis; **Hospital:** Yale-New Haven Hosp; **Address:** Yale New Haven Hosp-Ped Primary Care Ctr, 789 Howard Ave, New Haven, CT 06519; **Phone:** 203-688-2475; **Board Cert:** Pediatrics 1974; Pediatric Rheumatology 2007; **Med School:** Georgetown Univ 1969; **Resid:** Pediatrics, Chldns Hosp 1972; **Fellow:** Ambulatory Pediatrics, Chldns Hosp 1974; **Fac Appt:** Prof Ped, Yale Univ

Pediatric Surgery

Caty, Michael G MD (PS) - **Spec Exp:** Neonatal Surgery; Thoracic Surgery; Gastrointestinal Motility Disorders; Laparoscopic Surgery; **Hospital:** Yale-New Haven Hosp; **Address:** Yale Pediatric Surgery, 310 Cedar St, FMB-131, New Haven, CT 06510; **Phone:** 203-785-2701; **Board Cert:** Pediatric Surgery 2003; **Med School:** Univ Mass Sch Med 1985; **Resid:** Surgery, Univ MI Hosp 1991; **Fellow:** Pediatric Surgery, Boston Chldns Hosp 1993; **Fac Appt:** Prof S, Yale Univ

Cowles, Robert A MD (PS) - **Spec Exp:** Esophageal Surgery; Gastrointestinal Disorders; Hepatobiliary Surgery; **Hospital:** Yale-New Haven Hosp; **Address:** Yale Chldns Hosp, Ped Surgery, 20 York St Fl 2, New Haven, CT 06511; **Phone:** 203-785-2701; **Board Cert:** Pediatric Surgery 2006; **Med School:** Temple Univ 1995; **Resid:** Surgery, Univ Michigan Med Ctr 2002; **Fellow:** Pediatric Surgery, NY-Presby/Columbia Univ Med Ctr 2004; **Fac Appt:** Assoc Prof Ped, Yale Univ

Pediatric Urology

Weiss, Robert M MD (Ped Uro) - **Spec Exp:** Testicular Cancer; Penile Cancer; Bladder Cancer; **Hospital:** Smilow Cancer Hosp at Yale-New Haven; **Address:** Smilow Hosp, Prostate & Urologic Cancer, 20 York St Fl 3, New Haven, CT 06510; **Phone:** 203-785-2815; **Board Cert:** Urology 1970; **Med School:** SUNY Downstate 1960; **Resid:** Surgery, Beth Israel Hosp 1962; Urology, NY-Presby/Columbia Univ Med Ctr 1967; **Fellow:** Pharmacology, NY-Presby/Columbia Univ Med Ctr 1965; **Fac Appt:** Prof U, Yale Univ

Pediatrics

Angoff, Ronald MD (Ped) *PCP* - **Hospital:** Yale-New Haven Hosp - St Raphael Campus, Yale-New Haven Hosp; **Address:** Pediatric & Med Assocs, 200 Orchard St, Ste 108, New Haven, CT 06511; **Phone:** 203-865-3737; **Board Cert:** Pediatrics 1978; **Med School:** Univ Cincinnati 1973; **Resid:** Pediatrics, Yale-New Haven Hosp 1975; **Fellow:** Child Development, Yale-New Haven Hosp 1977; **Fac Appt:** Assoc Prof Ped, Yale Univ

Avni-Singer, A. Joseph MD (Ped) *PCP* - **Spec Exp:** ADD/ADHD; Autism; Developmental & Behavioral Disorders; Learning Disorders; **Hospital:** Yale-New Haven Hosp; **Address:** Child & Adolescent Health Care, One Bradley Rd, Ste 102, Woodbridge, CT 06525; **Phone:** 203-397-1243; **Board Cert:** Pediatrics 2007; Developmental-Behavioral Pediatrics 2010; **Med School:** NYU Sch Med 1989; **Resid:** Pediatrics, Yale-New Haven Hosp 1992; **Fellow:** Developmental-Behavioral Pediatrics, Yale-New Haven Hosp 1995

Canny, Christopher R MD (Ped) *PCP* - **Spec Exp:** Behavioral Disorders; Developmental Disorders; **Hospital:** Yale-New Haven Hosp, Yale-New Haven Hosp - St Raphael Campus; **Address:** Hamden Pediatrics, 9 Washington Ave, Fl 2, Hamden, CT 06518; **Phone:** 203-287-0552; **Board Cert:** Pediatrics 2010; **Med School:** Washington Univ, St Louis 1976; **Resid:** Pediatrics, Yale-New Haven Hosp 1978; **Fellow:** Child Development, Yale Child Study Ctr 1980; **Fac Appt:** Assoc Clin Prof Ped, Yale Univ

Carlson, Andrew J MD (Ped) *PCP* - **Hospital:** Yale-New Haven Hosp, Yale-New Haven Hosp - St Raphael Campus; **Address:** Pediatric & Adolescent Med, 240 Indian River Rd, Ste B1, Orange, CT 06477; **Phone:** 203-795-6025; **Board Cert:** Pediatrics 2009; **Med School:** Univ Conn 1998; **Resid:** Pediatrics, CT Chldns Med Ctr 2001

Gruskay, Jeffrey MD (Ped) *PCP* - **Hospital:** Milford Hosp, Yale-New Haven Hosp; **Address:** Milford Pediatric Grp, 20 Commerce Park, Ste 1, Milford, CT 06460; **Phone:** 203-882-2066; **Board Cert:** Pediatrics 1985; Neonatal-Perinatal Medicine 1987; **Med School:** Yale Univ 1981; **Resid:** Pediatrics, Chldns Hosp 1984; **Fellow:** Neonatal-Perinatal Medicine, Chldns Hosp 1986; **Fac Appt:** Assoc Clin Prof Ped, Yale Univ

Morgan Jr, James L MD (Ped) *PCP* - **Spec Exp:** Sports Medicine; **Hospital:** Yale-New Haven Hosp, Yale-New Haven Hosp - St Raphael Campus; **Address:** Pediatrics & Adolescent Med, 240 Indian River Rd, Ste B1, Orange, CT 06477; **Phone:** 203-795-6025; **Board Cert:** Pediatrics 1983; **Med School:** Med Coll VA 1978; **Resid:** Pediatrics, Chldns Hosp 1982

Robert, Marie F MD (Ped) *PCP* - **Spec Exp:** Infectious Disease; Allergy; **Hospital:** Yale-New Haven Hosp; **Address:** Pediatrics & Adolescent Med, 240 Indian River Rd, Ste B1, Orange, CT 06477; **Phone:** 203-795-6025; **Board Cert:** Pediatrics 1984; **Med School:** McGill Univ 1976; **Resid:** Pediatrics, Chldns Hosp 1978; Allergy & Immunology, Yale-New Haven Hosp 1979; **Fellow:** Infectious Disease, Yale-New Haven Hosp 1984

Shaywitz, Sally E MD (Ped) - **Spec Exp:** Learning Disorders; Dyslexia; **Hospital:** Yale-New Haven Hosp; **Address:** Yale Univ Dept Pediatrics, 333 Cedar St, New Haven, CT 06520-8064; **Phone:** 203-785-4641; **Board Cert:** Pediatrics 1971; **Med School:** Albert Einstein Coll Med 1966; **Resid:** Pediatrics, Albert Einstein Coll Med 1970; **Fellow:** Pediatrics, Bronx Muni Hosp Ctr 1968; Behavioral Pediatrics, Albert Einstein Coll Med 1970; **Fac Appt:** Prof Ped, Yale Univ

Wiesner, Elizabeth Anne MD (Ped) *PCP* - **Spec Exp:** Autism; **Hospital:** Yale-New Haven Hosp, Yale-New Haven Hosp - St Raphael Campus; **Address:** Pediatrics & Adolescent Med, 240 Indian River Rd, Ste B1, Orange, CT 06477; **Phone:** 203-795-6025; **Board Cert:** Pediatrics ; **Med School:** Case West Res Univ 1977; **Resid:** Pediatrics, Yale-New Haven Hosp 1982; **Fellow:** Adolescent Medicine, Yale-New Haven Hosp 1983; **Fac Appt:** Asst Clin Prof Ped, Yale Univ

Physical Medicine & Rehabilitation

Juvan, Luci MD (PMR) - **Spec Exp:** Electrodiagnosis; Musculoskeletal Injuries; Spasticity Management; Stroke; **Hospital:** Gaylord Hosp; **Address:** Gaylord Hosp, Phys Med & Rehab Dept, 50 Gaylord Farm Rd, Wallingford, CT 06492; **Phone:** 203-284-2845; **Board Cert:** Physical Medicine & Rehabilitation 2009; **Med School:** Mount Sinai Sch Med 1994; **Resid:** Physical Medicine & Rehabilitation, Univ Hosp-UMDNJ 1998

Patel, Bhavesh R MD (PMR) - **Spec Exp:** Pain Management; **Address:** Interventional Spine & Sports Med, 1625 Straits Tpke, Ste 205, Middlebury, CT 06762; **Phone:** 203-598-7246; **Board Cert:** Physical Medicine & Rehabilitation 2012; Pain Medicine 2003; **Med School:** Amer Univ Caribbean 1997; **Resid:** Physical Medicine & Rehabilitation, Temple Univ Hosp 2001; **Fellow:** Sports Medicine, Beth Israel Med Ctr 2002; Interventional Spine Medicine, Beth Israel Med Ctr 2002

Rosenblum, David S MD (PMR) - **Spec Exp:** Neuro-Rehabilitation; Spinal Rehabilitation; Multiple Sclerosis; **Hospital:** Gaylord Hosp; **Address:** Gaylord Hosp, Phys Med & Rehab Dept, 50 Gaylord Farm Rd, Wallingford, CT 06492; **Phone:** 203-284-2845; **Board Cert:** Physical Medicine & Rehabilitation ; Spinal Cord Injury Medicine 2008; **Med School:** SUNY Buffalo 1987; **Resid:** Physical Medicine & Rehabilitation, NY-Presby/Columbia Univ Med Ctr 1991; **Fac Appt:** Asst Clin Prof PMR, Yale Univ

Sicklick, Alyse MD (PMR) - **Spec Exp:** Sports Injuries; Stroke Rehabilitation; Brain Injury Rehabilitation; **Hospital:** Gaylord Hosp; **Address:** Gaylord Hosp, Phys Med & Rehab Dept, 50 Gaylord Farm Rd, Wallingford, CT 06492; **Phone:** 203-284-2845; **Board Cert:** Physical Medicine & Rehabilitation 2013; **Med School:** Boston Univ 1988; **Resid:** Physical Medicine & Rehabilitation, NY-Presby/Columbia Univ Med Ctr 1992; **Fac Appt:** Asst Prof EM, Univ Conn

Plastic Surgery

Narayan, Deepak MD (PlS) - **Spec Exp:** Melanoma; Skin Cancer; **Hospital:** Yale-New Haven Hosp; **Address:** Yale, Plastic Surgery Dept, 800 Howard Ave Fl 4, New Haven, CT 06519; **Phone:** 203-785-2571; **Board Cert:** Plastic Surgery 2004; **Med School:** India 1986; **Resid:** Surgery, Yale-New Haven Hosp 1995; Surgery, Univ Conn Hlth Ctr 1997; **Fellow:** Plastic Surgery, Yale-New Haven Hosp 2000; **Fac Appt:** Prof S, Yale Univ

Persing, John A MD (PlS) - **Spec Exp:** Craniofacial Surgery; Vascular Malformations; Cosmetic & Reconstructive Surgery; Velopharyngeal Insufficiency; **Hospital:** Yale-New Haven Hosp; **Address:** Yale Plastic Surgery, 800 Howard Ave Fl 4, New Haven, CT 06520; **Phone:** 203-785-2570; **Board Cert:** Plastic Surgery 2007; Neurological Surgery 1986; **Med School:** Univ VT Coll Med 1974; **Resid:** Surgery, Univ Arizona Med Ctr 1976; Neurological Surgery, Univ Virginia Med Ctr 1982; **Fellow:** Plastic Surgery, Univ Virginia Med Ctr 1984; **Fac Appt:** Prof PlS, Yale Univ

Price, Gary J MD (PlS) - **Spec Exp:** Cosmetic Surgery-Face; Cosmetic Surgery-Breast; Liposuction & Body Contouring; **Hospital:** Yale-New Haven Hosp; **Address:** 5 Durham Rd, Ste 1-8, Guilford, CT 06437; **Phone:** 203-453-6635; **Board Cert:** Plastic Surgery 1986; **Med School:** Penn State Coll Med 1978; **Resid:** Surgery, Yale New-Haven Hosp 1983; Plastic Surgery, Yale New-Haven Hosp 1985; **Fellow:** Hand Surgery, Hartford Hosp 1985; **Fac Appt:** Asst Clin Prof PlS, Yale Univ

Restifo, Richard MD (PlS) - **Spec Exp:** Breast Surgery; Abdominoplasty; Liposuction & Body Contouring; **Hospital:** St. Vincent's Med Ctr - Bridgeport, Yale-New Haven Hosp; **Address:** 59 Elm St, Ste 560, New Haven, CT 06510; **Phone:** 203-772-1444; **Board Cert:** Plastic Surgery 2005; **Med School:** Harvard Med Sch 1986; **Resid:** Surgery, Georgetown Univ Hosp 1991; Plastic Surgery, UPMC 1993

Stahl, Richard S MD (PlS) - **Spec Exp:** Abdominal Wall Reconstruction; Chest Wall Reconstruction; Breast Reconstruction; Chest Wall Deformities; **Hospital:** Yale-New Haven Hosp, Yale-New Haven Hosp - St Raphael Campus; **Address:** 5 Durham Rd, Guilford, CT 06437; **Phone:** 203-458-4440; **Board Cert:** Surgery 2010; Plastic Surgery 1984; **Med School:** Vanderbilt Univ 1976; **Resid:** Surgery, Yale-New Haven Hosp 1981; **Fellow:** Plastic Surgery, Emory Univ Hosp 1983; **Fac Appt:** Clin Prof S, Yale Univ

Psychiatry

Lewis, Dorothy Otnow MD (Psyc) - **Spec Exp:** Dissociative Disorders; Aggression Disorders; Psychoanalysis; **Hospital:** Yale-New Haven Hosp, Bellevue Hosp Ctr; **Address:** 100 York St, 8H, New Haven, CT 06511; **Phone:** 203-624-3933; **Board Cert:** Psychiatry 1972; **Med School:** Yale Univ 1963; **Resid:** Psychiatry, Yale-New Haven Hosp 1967; **Fellow:** Child & Adolescent Psychiatry, Yale-New Haven Hosp 1969; Psychiatric Research, Natl Inst Mental Hlth 1967; **Fac Appt:** Clin Prof Psyc, Yale Univ

Sanacora, Gerard MD/PhD (Psyc) - **Spec Exp:** Depression; Anxiety & Mood Disorders; Stress Management; **Hospital:** Yale New Haven Psychiatric Hosp; **Address:** Yale, Clin Neuroscience, 34 Park St, New Haven, CT 06519; **Phone:** 203-974-7560; **Board Cert:** Psychiatry 2010; **Med School:** SUNY Stony Brook 1994; **Resid:** Psychiatry, Yale-New Haven Hosp 1998; **Fellow:** Neuropsychiatry, Yale-New Haven Hosp 1999; **Fac Appt:** Prof Psyc, Yale Univ

Pulmonary Disease

Friedman, Lloyd Neal MD (Pul) - **Spec Exp:** Tuberculosis; Mycobacterial Infections; Critical Care; **Hospital:** Milford Hosp, Yale-New Haven Hosp; **Address:** Milford Hospital, 300 Seaside Ave, Milford, CT 06460; **Phone:** 203-876-4070; **Board Cert:** Internal Medicine 1983; Pulmonary Disease 1988; Critical Care Medicine 2009; **Med School:** Yale Univ 1979; **Resid:** Internal Medicine, Beth Israel Med Ctr 1980; Internal Medicine, Oregon Hlth Scis Univ 1983; **Fellow:** Pulmonary Intensive Care, Yale-New Haven Hosp 1988; **Fac Appt:** Clin Prof Med, Yale Univ

Pisani, Margaret MD (Pul) - **Spec Exp:** Chronic Obstructive Lung Disease (COPD); Tuberculosis; **Hospital:** Yale-New Haven Hosp; **Address:** Yale, Winchester Chest Clin, 789 Howard Ave, Ste 209FB, New Haven, CT 06519; **Phone:** 203-785-4198; **Board Cert:** Internal Medicine 2009; Critical Care Medicine 2011; Pulmonary Disease 2010; **Med School:** Temple Univ 1994; **Resid:** Internal Medicine, Yale-New Haven Hosp 1997; **Fellow:** Pulmonary Critical Care Medicine, Yale-New Haven Hosp 2000; **Fac Appt:** Assoc Prof Med, Yale Univ

Redlich, Carrie MD (Pul) - **Spec Exp:** Occupational Lung Disease; Lung Disease; **Hospital:** Yale-New Haven Hosp; **Address:** Yale Occupational & Environmental Med, 135 College St Fl 3 - Ste 392, New Haven, CT 06510; **Phone:** 203-785-4197; **Board Cert:** Internal Medicine 1986; Occupational Medicine 1990; **Med School:** Yale Univ 1982; **Resid:** Internal Medicine, Yale-New Haven Hosp 1986; Occupational Medicine, Yale-New Haven Hosp 1987; **Fellow:** Pulmonary Disease, Univ Washington Affil Hosp 1989; **Fac Appt:** Assoc Prof Med, Yale Univ

Rochester, Carolyn L MD (Pul) - **Spec Exp:** Chronic Obstructive Lung Disease (COPD); Emphysema; **Hospital:** VA Conn Hlthcre Sys-W Haven Campus, Yale-New Haven Hosp; **Address:** Winchester Chest Clin, 789 Howard Ave, Fitkin Meml Pavilion, New Haven, CT 06519; **Phone:** 203-785-4163; **Board Cert:** Internal Medicine 1986; Critical Care Medicine 2006; **Med School:** Columbia P&S 1983; **Resid:** Internal Medicine, Columbia Presby Med Ctr 1986; **Fellow:** Pulmonary Disease, Columbia Presby Med Ctr 1988; Critical Care Medicine, Yale New Haven Hosp 1991; **Fac Appt:** Assoc Prof Med, Yale Univ

Tanoue, Lynn MD (Pul) - **Spec Exp:** Lung Cancer; **Hospital:** Yale-New Haven Hosp; **Address:** Smilow Cancer Ctr, Thoracic Oncology, 35 Park St Fl 4, New Haven, CT 06519; **Phone:** 203-688-5864; **Board Cert:** Internal Medicine 1985; Pulmonary Disease 1988; Critical Care Medicine 2012; **Med School:** Yale Univ 1982; **Resid:** Internal Medicine, Yale-New Haven Hosp 1985; **Fellow:** Pulmonary Disease, Yale-New Haven Hosp 1988; Critical Care Medicine, Yale-New Haven Hosp 1988; **Fac Appt:** Assoc Prof Med, Yale Univ

Trow, Terence MD (Pul) - **Spec Exp:** Pulmonary Hypertension; Pulmonary Vascular Disease; **Hospital:** Yale-New Haven Hosp; **Address:** Winchester Chest Clinic, 20 York St, Ste 209FB, New Haven, CT 06510; **Phone:** 203-785-4198; **Board Cert:** Internal Medicine 1989; Critical Care Medicine 2003; Pulmonary Disease 2012; **Med School:** Dartmouth Med Sch 1986; **Resid:** Internal Medicine, New York Hosp 1989; **Fellow:** Pulmonary Critical Care Medicine, Yale-New Haven Hosp 1993; **Fac Appt:** Assoc Prof Med, Yale Univ

Won, Christine H MD (Pul) - **Spec Exp:** Sleep Medicine; **Hospital:** Yale-New Haven Hosp; **Address:** Yale, Pulmonary Disease/Sleep Med, 40 Temple St, Ste 3C, New Haven, CT 06510; **Phone:** 203-785-6760; **Board Cert:** Internal Medicine ; Pulmonary Disease ; Sleep Medicine ; Critical Care Medicine ; **Med School:** Albert Einstein Coll Med 2000; **Resid:** Internal Medicine, Beth Israel Med Ctr 2003; **Fellow:** Pulmonary Critical Care Medicine, Stanford Univ Hosp & Clinics 2006; Sleep Medicine, Stanford Univ Hosp & Clinics 2007; **Fac Appt:** Asst Prof Med, Yale Univ

Radiation Oncology

Chung, Joyce Y MD (RadRO) - **Spec Exp:** Breast Cancer; **Hospital:** Griffin Hosp; **Address:** Griffin Hosp, Ctr Cancer Care, 350 Seymour Ave, Ste 2, Derby, CT 06418; **Phone:** 203-732-1280; **Board Cert:** Radiation Oncology 2009; **Med School:** Georgetown Univ 1993; **Resid:** Radiation Oncology, Yale-New Haven Hosp 1997; **Fac Appt:** Asst Clin Prof RadRO, Yale Univ

Higgins, Susan A MD (RadRO) - **Spec Exp:** Gynecologic Cancer; Vulvar & Vaginal Cancer; Breast Cancer; Gastrointestinal Cancer; **Hospital:** Yale-New Haven Hosp; **Address:** Smilow Cancer Hosp, 35 Park St, Ste LL515, New Haven, CT 06520; **Phone:** 203-785-7033; **Board Cert:** Radiation Oncology 2004; **Med School:** Univ Rochester 1990; **Resid:** Radiology, Yale-New Haven Hosp 1993; **Fac Appt:** Prof RadRO, Yale Univ

Peschel, Richard E MD (RadRO) - **Spec Exp:** Prostate Cancer; Testicular Cancer; **Hospital:** Yale-New Haven Hosp; **Address:** 35 Park St, rm LL-510, MS 06510, New Haven, CT 06510; **Phone:** 203-785-2958; **Board Cert:** Therapeutic Radiology 1982; **Med School:** Yale Univ 1977; **Resid:** Radiation Oncology, Yale-New Haven Hosp 1981; **Fac Appt:** Prof RadRO, Yale Univ

Roberts, Kenneth MD (RadRO) - **Spec Exp:** Pediatric Cancers; Lymphoma; Hodgkin's Lymphoma; **Hospital:** Yale-New Haven Hosp; **Address:** Smilow Cancer Ctr, Radiation Therapy, 15 York St, New Haven, CT 06520-8040; **Phone:** 203-785-2957; **Board Cert:** Internal Medicine 1987; Medical Oncology 1989; Radiation Oncology 1995; **Med School:** Duke Univ 1984; **Resid:** Internal Medicine, Ohio State Univ Hosps 1987; Radiation Oncology, Duke Univ Med Ctr 1992; **Fellow:** Hematology & Oncology, Duke Univ Med Ctr 1989; **Fac Appt:** Assoc Prof Rad, Yale Univ

Wilson, Lynn D MD (RadRO) - **Spec Exp:** Cutaneous T-cell Lymphoma; Lung Cancer; Head & Neck Cancer; **Hospital:** Yale-New Haven Hosp, Yale Med Group; **Address:** Yale Univ Sch Med, Dept Therapeutic Rad, 35 Park St, New Haven, CT 06513; **Phone:** 203-737-1202; **Board Cert:** Radiation Oncology 2004; **Med School:** Geo Wash Univ 1990; **Resid:** Therapeutic Radiology, Yale-New Haven Hosp 1994; **Fac Appt:** Prof RadRO, Yale Univ

Reproductive Endocrinology

Patrizio, Pasquale MD (RE) - **Spec Exp:** Infertility-IVF; Fertility Preservation in Cancer; **Hospital:** Yale-New Haven Hosp; **Address:** Yale Fertility Ctr, Dept OB/GYN, 150 Sargent Drive, New Haven, CT 06511; **Phone:** 203-785-4708; **Board Cert:** Obstetrics & Gynecology 2007; Reproductive Endocrinology 2010; **Med School:** Italy 1983; **Resid:** Obstetrics & Gynecology, Univ Naples 1987; Reproductive Endocrinology, Univ Pisa 1990; **Fellow:** Infertility, UC Irvine Med Ctr 1995; **Fac Appt:** Prof ObG, Yale Univ

Taylor, Hugh S MD (RE) - **Spec Exp:** Infertility-IVF; Endometriosis; Menopause Problems; Uterine/Vaginal Abnormalities; **Hospital:** Yale-New Haven Hosp; **Address:** Yale Univ School Med, Dept OB/GYN, 333 Cedar St, New Haven, CT 06520; **Phone:** 203-785-4708; **Board Cert:** Obstetrics & Gynecology 2012; Reproductive Endocrinology 2012; **Med School:** Univ Conn 1988; **Resid:** Obstetrics & Gynecology, Yale-New Haven Hosp 1997; **Fellow:** Reproductive Endocrinology, Yale-New Haven Hosp 1998; **Fac Appt:** Prof ObG, Yale Univ

Rheumatology

Buckley, Lenore MD (Rhu) - **Spec Exp:** Lupus/SLE; Rheumatoid Arthritis; Inflammatory Arthritis; Osteoporosis; **Hospital:** Yale-New Haven Hosp; **Address:** Yale Interventional Immunology Ctr, 6 Devine St, Ste 2B, North Haven, CT 06473; **Phone:** 203-287-6200; **Board Cert:** Pediatrics ; Internal Medicine ; Pediatric Rheumatology 2008; Rheumatology ; **Med School:** Univ Rochester 1977; **Resid:** Pediatrics, NC Meml Hosp 1982; **Fellow:** Rheumatology, Univ VT Affil Hosp 1984; **Fac Appt:** Prof Med, Yale Univ

Carlson, Elise MD (Rhu) - **Spec Exp:** Fibromyalgia; Lupus/SLE; Gout; **Hospital:** Yale-New Haven Hosp, Milford Hosp; **Address:** 247 Broad St, Milford, CT 06460; **Phone:** 203-878-4312; **Board Cert:** Rheumatology 2004; **Med School:** Univ Conn 1997; **Resid:** Internal Medicine, Univ Conn Hlth Ctr 2001; **Fellow:** Rheumatology, Univ Conn Hlth Ctr 2003

Hutchinson, Gordon J MD (Rhu) - **Spec Exp:** Rheumatoid Arthritis; Lyme Disease; Polymyositis; **Hospital:** Yale-New Haven Hosp - St Raphael Campus, Yale-New Haven Hosp; **Address:** 136 Sherman Ave, Ste 104, New Haven, CT 06511; **Phone:** 203-785-0885; **Board Cert:** Internal Medicine 1980; Rheumatology 1982; **Med School:** Switzerland 1976; **Resid:** Internal Medicine, St Raphael Hosp 1980; **Fellow:** Rheumatology, Yale-New Haven Hosp 1982; **Fac Appt:** Assoc Clin Prof Med, Yale Univ

Liebling, Anne MD (Rhu) - **Spec Exp:** Arthritis; Juvenile Arthritis; Fibromyalgia; **Hospital:** Yale-New Haven Hosp; **Address:** Yale, Ped Rheumatology, 60 Temple St, Ste 6A, New Haven, CT 06510; **Phone:** 203-789-2255; **Board Cert:** Rheumatology 2000; Pediatric Rheumatology 2009; **Med School:** SUNY Downstate 1986; **Resid:** Internal Medicine & Pediatrics, Univ Chicago Med Ctr 1990; **Fellow:** Rheumatology, Univ Chicago Med Ctr 1993; Pediatric Rheumatology, Univ Chicago Med Ctr 1993; **Fac Appt:** Asst Clin Prof Ped, Yale Univ

Schoen, Robert T MD (Rhu) - **Spec Exp:** Rheumatoid Arthritis; Lyme Disease; Osteoporosis; **Hospital:** Yale-New Haven Hosp; **Address:** New Haven Rheumatology, 60 Temple St, Ste 6A, New Haven, CT 06510-2716; **Phone:** 203-789-2255; **Board Cert:** Internal Medicine 1979; Rheumatology 1982; **Med School:** Columbia P&S 1976; **Resid:** Internal Medicine, Yale New Haven Hosp 1979; **Fellow:** Rheumatology, Brigham & Womens Hosp 1981; **Fac Appt:** Clin Prof Med, Yale Univ

Surgery

Barcewicz, Paul MD (S) - **Spec Exp:** Cancer Surgery; Laparoscopic Surgery; Soft Tissue Tumors; Endoscopy; **Hospital:** Yale-New Haven Hosp - St Raphael Campus, Yale-New Haven Hosp; **Address:** Surgl Assocs, 60 Temple St, Ste 5A, New Haven, CT 06510; **Phone:** 203-772-0650 x226; **Board Cert:** Surgery 2012; **Med School:** Univ Rochester 1977; **Resid:** Surgery, Hartford Hosp 1982; **Fellow:** Surgical Oncology, Roswell Park Cancer Ctr 1984; **Fac Appt:** Asst Clin Prof S, Yale Univ

Chagpar, Anees B MD (S) - **Spec Exp:** Breast Cancer & Surgery; Breast Disease; **Hospital:** Smilow Cancer Hosp at Yale-New Haven, Yale Med Group; **Address:** Yale Smilow Cancer Hosp, Breast Ctr, 20 York St, Ste 1A, New Haven, CT 06510; **Phone:** 203-200-2328; **Board Cert:** Surgery 2012; **Med School:** Canada 1996; **Resid:** Surgery, Univ Saskatchewan 2002; **Fellow:** Breast Cancer, MD Anderson Cancer Ctr 2003; **Fac Appt:** Assoc Prof Surg & Onc, Yale Univ

Duffy, Andrew J MD (S) - **Spec Exp:** Laparoscopic Surgery; Gastrointestinal Surgery; Diverticulitis; Colon & Rectal Cancer; **Hospital:** Yale-New Haven Hosp, Yale Med Group; **Address:** Yale, GI Surgery, 40 Temple St, Ste 7B, New Haven, CT 06510; **Phone:** 203-785-6060 x6; **Board Cert:** Surgery 2004; **Med School:** Univ Mass Sch Med 1996; **Resid:** Surgery, UMass Meml Med Ctr 2003; **Fellow:** Minimally Invasive Surgery, NY-Presby/Weill Cornell Med Ctr 2004; **Fac Appt:** Assoc Prof S, Yale Univ

Emre, Sukru MD (S) - **Spec Exp:** Transplant-Liver-Adult & Pediatric; Hepatobiliary Surgery; Liver Cancer; Portal Hypertension; **Hospital:** Yale-New Haven Hosp; **Address:** 330 Cedar St, FMB121 Bldg - Fl 1, FMB 121, New Haven, CT 07520-8062; **Phone:** 203-737-2804; **Med School:** Turkey 1977; **Resid:** Surgery, Univ Istanbul 1982; **Fellow:** Hepatobiliary Surgery, Univ Istanbul 1988; Transplant Surgery, Mount Sinai Med Ctr 1994; **Fac Appt:** Prof S, Yale Univ

Kurtzman, Scott H MD (S) - **Spec Exp:** Breast Cancer & Surgery; Sarcoma; **Hospital:** Waterbury Hosp; **Address:** Alliance Med Grp, Surgery, 1625 Straits Tpke, Ste 200, Middlebury, CT 06762; **Phone:** 203-568-2929; **Board Cert:** Surgery 2009; **Med School:** Albany Med Coll 1981; **Resid:** Surgery, Univ MD Med Ctr 1983; Surgery, Univ Hosp-UMDNJ 1988; **Fellow:** Surgical Oncology, Natl Cancer Inst 1985; Surgical Oncology, Meml Sloan-Kettering Cancer Ctr 1990; **Fac Appt:** Prof S, Univ Conn

Lannin, Donald R MD (S) - **Spec Exp:** Breast Cancer; Breast Surgery; **Hospital:** Smilow Cancer Hosp at Yale-New Haven; **Address:** Smilow Cancer Hosp, Breast Surgery, 20 York St, New Haven, CT 06510; **Phone:** 203-785-2328; **Board Cert:** Surgery 2012; **Med School:** Univ Minn 1974; **Resid:** Surgery, Univ Minn Med Ctr 1982; **Fac Appt:** Prof S, Yale Univ

Nadzam, Geoffrey S MD (S) - **Spec Exp:** Obesity/Bariatric Surgery; **Hospital:** Yale-New Haven Hosp - St Raphael Campus; **Address:** Orchard Surgical Specialists, 330 Orchard St, Ste 309, New Haven, CT 06511; **Phone:** 203-776-4677; **Board Cert:** Surgery 2004; **Med School:** UMDNJ-NJ Med Sch, Newark 1996; **Resid:** Surgery, Stanford Univ Hosp & Clins 2002; **Fellow:** Bariatric Surgery, Stanford Univ Hosp & Clins 2004; Robotic Surgery, Stanford Univ Hosp & Clins 2004; **Fac Appt:** Asst Prof S, Yale Univ

Salem, Ronald R MD (S) - **Spec Exp:** Cancer Surgery; Pancreatic Cancer; Gastrointestinal Cancer; Liver Cancer; **Hospital:** Yale-New Haven Hosp; **Address:** Smilow Cancer Hosp, 35 Park St Fl 8, New Haven, CT 06520; **Phone:** 203-785-3577; **Board Cert:** Surgery 2011; **Med School:** Zimbabwe 1978; **Resid:** Surgery, Hammersmith Hosp 1985; Surgery, New England Deaconess Hosp 1989; **Fac Appt:** Prof S, Yale Univ

Tsangaris, Theodore N MD (S) - **Spec Exp:** Nipple Sparing Mastectomy; Breast Cancer & Surgery; **Hospital:** Yale-New Haven Hosp, Yale Med Group; **Address:** Smilow Cancer Hosp, Yale Breat Ctr, 35 Park St, New Haven, CT 06510; **Phone:** 203-200-2328; **Board Cert:** Surgery 2005; **Med School:** Geo Wash Univ 1983; **Resid:** Surgery, Geo Washington Univ Med Ctr 1989; **Fellow:** Surgical Oncology, Baylor Univ Med Ctr 1990; **Fac Appt:** Assoc Prof S, Yale Univ

Udelsman, Robert MD (S) - **Spec Exp:** Parathyroid Cancer; Adrenal Tumors; Thyroid Cancer; Endocrine Surgery; **Hospital:** Yale-New Haven Hosp; **Address:** Yale-New Haven Hosp, Dept Surgery, 330 Cedar St, Box 208062, New Haven, CT 06520-8062; **Phone:** 203-785-2697; **Board Cert:** Surgery 2009; **Med School:** Geo Wash Univ 1981; **Resid:** Surgery, Natl Inst Hlth 1986; Surgery, Johns Hopkins Hosp 1989; **Fellow:** Gastrointestinal Surgery, Johns Hopkins Hosp 1990; Surgical Oncology, Natl Cancer Inst 1985; **Fac Appt:** Prof S, Yale Univ

Zuckerman, Kaye MD (S) - **Spec Exp:** Breast Surgery; Laparoscopic Surgery; **Hospital:** Yale-New Haven Hosp - St Raphael Campus; **Address:** Surgical Associates of New Haven, 60 Temple St, Ste 5A, Madison, CT 06510; **Phone:** 203-772-0650 x225; **Board Cert:** Surgery 2010; **Med School:** Cornell Univ 1993; **Resid:** Surgery, Univ Pittsburgh Hosp 1995; Surgery, Univ Pittsburgh Hosp 1999; **Fellow:** Research, Univ Pittsburgh Hosp 1997

Thoracic & Cardiac Surgery

Detterbeck, Frank C MD (T&CS) - **Spec Exp:** Lung Cancer; Mediastinal Tumors; Thoracic Cancers; **Hospital:** Yale-New Haven Hosp; **Address:** Yale Sch Medicine, Thoracic Surgery, 330 Cedar St, BB205, New Haven, CT 06520-8062; **Phone:** 203-785-4931; **Board Cert:** Thoracic Surgery 2011; **Med School:** Northwestern Univ 1983; **Resid:** Surgery, Virginia Mason Hosp 1988; **Fellow:** Cardiothoracic Surgery, Univ N Carolina Hosps 1991; **Fac Appt:** Prof S, Yale Univ

Elefteriades, John A MD (T&CS) - **Spec Exp:** Aneurysm-Thoracic Aortic; Ventricular Assist Device (LVAD); **Hospital:** Yale-New Haven Hosp; **Address:** Yale Cardiothoracic Surgery, 330 Cedar St, rm BB 204, New Haven, CT 06520; **Phone:** 203-785-2705; **Board Cert:** Thoracic & Cardiac Surgery 2004; **Med School:** Yale Univ 1976; **Resid:** Surgery, Yale-New Haven Hosp 1981; **Fellow:** Cardiothoracic Surgery, Yale-New Haven Hosp 1983; **Fac Appt:** Prof T&CS, Yale Univ

Federico, John A MD (T&CS) - **Spec Exp:** Lung Cancer; Robotic Surgery; Minimally Invasive Surgery; **Hospital:** Yale-New Haven Hosp - St Raphael Campus, Yale-New Haven Hosp; **Address:** 330 Orchard St, Ste 300, New Haven, CT 06511; **Phone:** 203-787-3488; **Board Cert:** Surgery 2006; **Med School:** Georgetown Univ 1986; **Resid:** Surgery, Maine Med Ctr 1991; **Fellow:** Thoracic Surgery, Frenchay Hosp 1992; Thoracic Surgery, Ottawa Civic Hosp 1993; **Fac Appt:** Asst Clin Prof S, Yale Univ

Hashim, Sabet W MD (T&CS) - **Spec Exp:** Mitral Valve Surgery; Heart Valve Surgery; Maze Procedure for Atrial Fibrillation; **Hospital:** Yale-New Haven Hosp; **Address:** Yale Surgical Specialties, 800 Howard Ave Fl 3, Yale Physician's Bldg, New Haven, CT 06520; **Phone:** 203-785-6214; **Board Cert:** Thoracic & Cardiac Surgery 2013; **Med School:** Lebanon 1975; **Resid:** Surgery, St Lukes Roosevelt Hosp 1979; Cardiothoracic Surgery, Yale-New Haven Hosp 1981; **Fac Appt:** Assoc Prof S, Yale Univ

Kirshbom, Paul M MD (T&CS) - **Spec Exp:** Pediatric Cardiothoracic Surgery; Cardiac Surgery-Neonatal; Congenital Heart Disease; **Hospital:** Yale-New Haven Hosp, CT Chldns Med Ctr; **Address:** Yale-New Haven Childrens Hosp, 1 Park St Fl 2, New Haven, CT 06510; **Phone:** 203-785-2702; **Board Cert:** Thoracic & Cardiac Surgery 2010; Congenital Cardiac Surgery 2009; **Med School:** Johns Hopkins Univ 1991; **Resid:** Surgery, Duke Univ Med Ctr 1998; Cardiothoracic Surgery, Duke Univ Med Ctr 2000; **Fellow:** Pediatric Cardiac Surgery, Childrens Hosp 2002; **Fac Appt:** Prof S, Yale Univ

Kopf, Gary S MD (T&CS) - **Spec Exp:** Cardiac Surgery; Pediatric Cardiothoracic Surgery; Congenital Heart Disease; **Hospital:** Yale-New Haven Hosp; **Address:** Yale Surgical Specialties, 800 Howard Ave Fl 3, Yale Physicians Bldg, New Haven, CT 06520-8039; **Phone:** 203-785-2702; **Board Cert:** Thoracic Surgery 2011; **Med School:** Harvard Med Sch 1970; **Resid:** Surgery, Peter Bent Brigham Hosp 1977; **Fellow:** Cardiothoracic Surgery, Peter Bent Brigham Hosp 1980; **Fac Appt:** Prof S, Yale Univ

Mangi, Abeel A MD (T&CS) - **Spec Exp:** Transplant-Heart; Heart Failure; **Hospital:** Yale-New Haven Hosp; **Address:** Yale Cardiac Surgery, Yale Physicians Bldg, 800 Howard Ave Fl 2, New Haven, CT 06519; **Phone:** 203-785-5252; **Board Cert:** Surgery 2005; Thoracic & Cardiac Surgery 2009; **Med School:** Brown Univ 1997; **Resid:** Surgery, Mass General Hosp 2003; **Fellow:** Research, Brigham & Women's Hosp 2004; Cardiac Surgery, NY Presby-Columbia Med Ctr 2007; **Fac Appt:** Asst Prof S, Yale Univ

Yuh, David D MD (T&CS) - **Spec Exp:** Heart Valve Surgery; Minimally Invasive Cardiac Surgery; Robotic Surgery; **Hospital:** Yale-New Haven Hosp; **Address:** Yale Cardiac Surgery, Yale Physicians Bldg Fl 3, 800 Howard Ave, New Haven, CT 06519; **Phone:** 203-785-3000; **Board Cert:** Thoracic & Cardiac Surgery 2011; **Med School:** Stanford Univ 1991; **Resid:** Surgery, Univ Minn Hosp & Clins 1994; Surgery, Stanford Univ Med Ctr 1996; **Fellow:** Cardiac Surgery, Stanford Univ Med Ctr 1998; **Fac Appt:** Prof S, Yale Univ

Urology

Colberg, John W MD (U) - **Spec Exp:** Prostate Cancer; Bladder Cancer; Kidney Cancer; Testicular Cancer; **Hospital:** Yale-New Haven Hosp; **Address:** Smilow Cancer Hosp, 20 York St, N Pavilion Fl 4, New Haven, CT 06504; **Phone:** 203-785-2815; **Board Cert:** Urology 2001; **Med School:** Washington Univ, St Louis 1985; **Resid:** Surgery, Yale-New Haven Hosp 1987; Urology, Yale-New Haven Hosp 1990; **Fac Appt:** Assoc Prof U, Yale Univ

Flanagan, Michael J MD (U) - **Spec Exp:** Urologic Cancer; Kidney Stones; Infertility-Male; Pediatric Urology; **Hospital:** Waterbury Hosp, St. Mary's Hosp - Waterbury; **Address:** Urology Specialists, 1579 Straits Tpke, Ste 2A, Middlebury, CT 06762; **Phone:** 203-757-8361; **Board Cert:** Urology 2012; **Med School:** UMDNJ-Univ Med Dent NJ 1985; **Resid:** Surgery, Waterbury Hosp 1988; Urology, Temple Univ Hosp 1992

Foster Jr, Harris E MD (U) - **Spec Exp:** Incontinence; Urodynamics; Voiding Dysfunction; Urology-Female; **Hospital:** Yale-New Haven Hosp; **Address:** Smilow Cancer Hosp at Yale New Haven, South Frontage Rd & Park St, 4th Fl, Multispecialty Care Ctr, New Haven, CT 06510; **Phone:** 203-200-4822; **Board Cert:** Urology 2012; **Med School:** Univ Miami Sch Med 1987; **Resid:** Surgery, Univ Michigan Med Ctr 1989; Urology, Univ Michigan Med Ctr 1992; **Fac Appt:** Prof U, Yale Univ

Passarelli, Marianne MD (U) - **Spec Exp:** Urology-Female; Incontinence; **Hospital:** Yale-New Haven Hosp - St Raphael Campus, Yale-New Haven Hosp; **Address:** Urology Grp, 9 Washington Rd, Ste 3A, Hamden, CT 06518; **Phone:** 203-288-4663; **Board Cert:** Urology 2013; **Med School:** Univ VT Coll Med 1986; **Resid:** Surgery, SUNY Hlth Sci Ctr 1988; Urology, SUNY Hlth Sci Ctr 1992

Schulam, Peter G MD/PhD (U) - **Spec Exp:** Prostate Cancer; Kidney Cancer; Kidney Stones; Minimally Invasive Surgery; **Hospital:** Yale-New Haven Hosp; **Address:** Smilow Cancer Hosp, 20 York St, N Pavilion Fl 4 - rm 202B, New Haven, CT 06504; **Phone:** 203-200-4822; **Board Cert:** Urology 2009; **Med School:** Baylor Coll Med 1992; **Resid:** Surgery, Johns Hopkins Hosp 1994; Urology, Johns Hopkins Hosp 1998

Singh, Dinesh MD (U) - **Spec Exp:** Laparoscopic Surgery; Robotic Surgery; Kidney Cancer; Prostate Cancer; **Hospital:** Smilow Cancer Hosp at Yale-New Haven; **Address:** Smilow Hosp, Prostate Urologic Cancer, 35 Park St Fl 4, New Haven, CT 06519; **Phone:** 203-785-2815; **Board Cert:** Urology 2006; **Med School:** Columbia P&S 1997; **Resid:** Surgery, Brigham & Womens Hosp 1999; Urology, Harvard Med Sch 2003; **Fellow:** Research, Dana Farber Cancer Inst 2001; Laparoscopic Surgery, Cleveland Clin 2004; **Fac Appt:** Asst Prof U, Yale Univ

Vascular & Interventional Radiology

Aruny, John E MD (VIR) - **Spec Exp:** Thrombolytic Therapy; Dialysis Access; Vascular Disease; Vein Disorders; **Hospital:** Yale-New Haven Hosp; **Address:** Yale Interventional Radiology, 800 Howard Ave Fl 2, Yale Physicians Bldg, New Haven, CT 06519; **Phone:** 203-785-7026; **Board Cert:** Diag Rad with Spec Comp in Nuc Rad 1989; Vascular & Interventional Radiology 2009; **Med School:** Mexico 1983; **Resid:** Diagnostic Radiology, Westchester Co Med Ctr 1989; **Fellow:** Interventional Radiology, Brigham & Women's Hosp 1992; **Fac Appt:** Assoc Prof Rad, Yale Univ

Pollak, Jeffrey MD (VIR) - **Spec Exp:** Vascular Malformations; Interventional Radiology; Chemoembolization & Tumor Ablation; **Hospital:** Yale-New Haven Hosp; **Address:** Yale Interventional Radiology, 800 Howard Ave Fl 2, New Haven, CT 06520; **Phone:** 203-785-7026; **Board Cert:** Diagnostic Radiology ; Vascular & Interventional Radiology 2006; **Med School:** Columbia P&S 1983; **Resid:** Diagnostic Radiology, Columb-Presby Med Ctr 1988; **Fellow:** Interventional Radiology, Hosp Univ Penn 1989; **Fac Appt:** Prof Rad, Yale Univ

Vascular Surgery

DeNatale, Ralph MD (VascS) - **Hospital:** Yale-New Haven Hosp, Yale-New Haven Hosp - St Raphael Campus; **Address:** CT Vascular Ctr, 280 State St, North Haven, CT 06473; **Phone:** 203-288-2886; **Board Cert:** Vascular Surgery 2009; **Med School:** Italy 1979; **Resid:** Surgery, Hosp St Raphael 1984; Vascular Surgery, Baylor Affil Hosp 1985; **Fellow:** Cardiovascular Surgery, Baylor Affil Hosp 1986; **Fac Appt:** Asst Clin Prof S, Yale Univ

Gusberg, Richard J MD (VascS) - **Spec Exp:** Endovascular Surgery; Aneurysm-Aortic; Renovascular Disease; **Hospital:** VA Conn Hlthcre Sys-W Haven Campus; **Address:** VA Conn Hlthcare System-W Haven Campus, 950 Campbell Ave, West Haven, CT 06516; **Phone:** 203-932-5711; **Board Cert:** Vascular Surgery 2008; **Med School:** Columbia P&S 1970; **Resid:** Surgery, Columbia-Presby Med Ctr 1975; **Fellow:** Vascular Surgery, Columbia-Presby Med Ctr 1976; **Fac Appt:** Prof S, Yale Univ

Sumpio, Bauer E MD/PhD (VascS) - **Spec Exp:** Diabetic Leg/Foot; Endovascular Surgery; Peripheral Vascular Disease; Wound Healing/Care; **Hospital:** Yale-New Haven Hosp; **Address:** Heart & Vascular Ctr, 800 Howard Ave, Yale Physician's Bldg, New Haven, CT 06520; **Phone:** 203-785-6217; **Board Cert:** Vascular Surgery 2009; Surgery 2009; **Med School:** Cornell Univ-Weill Med Coll 1980; **Resid:** Surgery, Yale-New Haven Hosp 1986; **Fellow:** Vascular Surgery, Univ N Carolina Hosp 1987; **Fac Appt:** Prof S, Yale Univ

Sweeney, Thomas F MD (VascS) - **Spec Exp:** Minimally Invasive Vascular Surgery; Varicose Veins; Vein Disorders; **Hospital:** Yale-New Haven Hosp, Yale-New Haven Hosp - St Raphael Campus; **Address:** CT Vascular Ctr, 280 State St, North Haven, CT 06473; **Phone:** 203-288-2886; **Board Cert:** Vascular Surgery 2008; **Med School:** Yale Univ 1973; **Resid:** Surgery, Yale-New Haven Hosp 1977; **Fellow:** Vascular Surgery, Yale-New Haven Hosp 1978; **Fac Appt:** Assoc Clin Prof S, Yale Univ

Section Four

Centers of Excellence

Adolescent Medicine

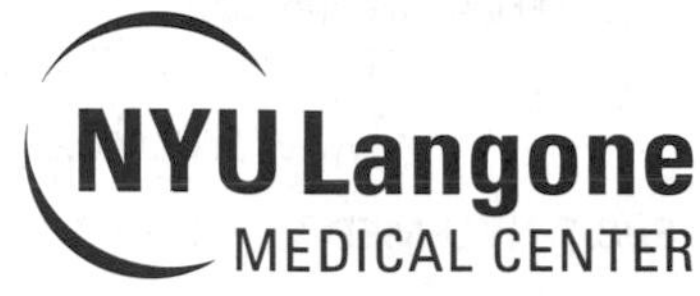

550 First Avenue *(at 31st Street)*
New York, NY 10016

www.NYULMC.org

Hassenfeld Children's Hospital Access Line: **855-NYU-KIDS**

HASSENFELD CHILDREN'S HOSPITAL

Hassenfeld Children's Hospital (HCH) is a full-service specialty children's hospital encompassing all children's health services at NYU Langone Medical Center. At HCH, newborns, children, adolescents and young adults receive the most comprehensive and advanced care possible from a team of pediatricians and pediatric specialists across more than 30 medical and surgical disciplines. With more than 150 full-time pediatric specialists, as well as pediatric nurses, child life specialists and social workers, Hassenfeld Children's Hospital is uniquely equipped to provide innovative pediatric subspecialty care in a highly personalized manner.

A Family-Centered Approach

Integral to the care we provide is a myriad of support services for children and their families. We recognize that the best outcomes are achieved when the child's family is actively involved in every step of care. For that reason, our trained specialists address the needs of not just the patient, but of parents and siblings through ongoing education and communication.

Our pediatric specialties include:

Anesthesia
Cardiology
Cardiothoracic Surgery
Child and Adolescent Psychiatry
and Psychology/Child Study Center
Critical Care
Dermatology
Developmental and Behavioral Pediatrics
Emergency Medicine
Endocrinology
Epilepsy
Gastroenterology
Genetics
Hematology/Oncology
Infectious Diseases
Neonatology
Nephrology
Neurosurgery
Ophthalmology
Orthopaedic Surgery
Otolaryngology
Pathology
Pulmonology
Radiology
Reconstructive Plastic Surgery
Rehabilitation
Rheumatology
Surgery
Urology

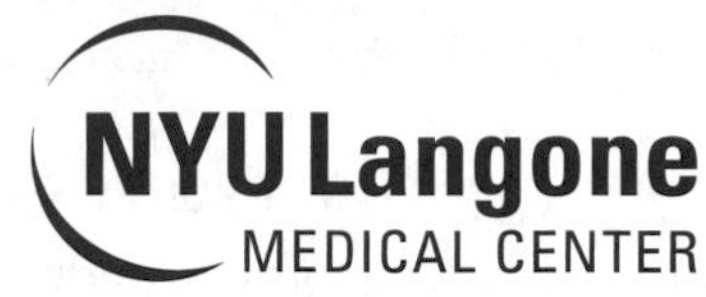

550 First Avenue *(at 31st Street)*
New York, NY 10016

www.NYULMC.org

Physician Referral: **888-7-NYU-MED** *(888-769-8633)*

PSYCHIATRY

NYU Langone's psychiatry team is dedicated to improving the health and well-being of patients by delivering peerless psychiatric services and care. NYU Langone is home to some of the nation's most respected clinical psychiatrists and psychologists, with specialties in psychoanalysis, psychopharmacology, behavioral therapy, child psychiatry, geriatric psychiatry and neuropsychiatry. We specialize in the following areas:

Child and Adolescent Psychiatry

Since 1997, the Child Study Center has treated thousands of children from around the world at its Faculty Group Practices in Manhattan and satellite clinical campuses in New Jersey and Long Island. Through its website, www.AboutOurKids.org, and through professional education programs, parents and practitioners are provided with the tools and knowledge needed to promote children's mental health. We specialize in Anxiety and Mood Disorders, Attention Deficit Hyperactivity and Behavior Disorders, Autism, Asperger's Syndrome and Communication Disorders, Learning Disorders, Tics and Tourette Disorder and more.

Adult Inpatient Services

The inpatient services unit combines comprehensive diagnostic assessment and treatment, including psychopharmacology, neuropsychology, psychotherapies and electroconvulsive therapy.

Adult Outpatient Psychiatry

The outpatient psychiatry program provides expert treatment to individuals suffering from a broad range of mental disorders and emotional problems, including anxiety, depression (including medicine resistant depression), insomnia, manic-depression, reproductive psychiatry, attention-deficit hyperactivity disorder and schizophrenia.

Post-Traumatic Stress Disorder

We offer assessment and treatment of PTSD for victims of sexual and physical assault, natural disasters, terrorism and combat trauma. Treatment includes cognitive behavioral therapy and strategies for the prevention of insomnia, stress, anxiety and depression. Our Military Family Clinic provides compassionate mental healthcare for veterans and their extended family members. The Steven and Alexandra Cohen Veterans Center is dedicated to improving diagnosis and treatment of PTSD and TBI through research.

Memory Impairment

The Pearl Barlow Center for Memory Evaluation and Treatment specializes in treating patients with memory impairments caused by neurological, psychological and physical ailments, as well as memory issues resulting from medication side effects, anxiety, depression and the effects of normal aging from illnesses like Alzheimer's disease.

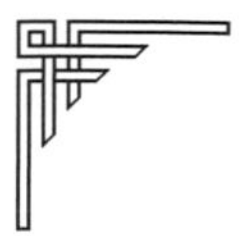

The Best in American Medicine
www.CastleConnolly.com

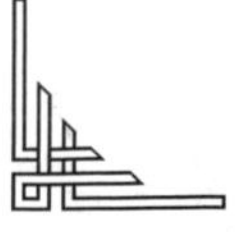
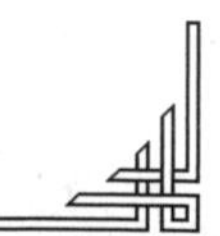

Arthritis and Orthopedics

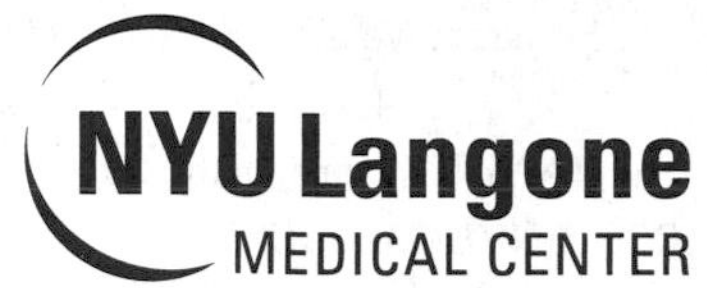

550 First Avenue *(at 31st Street)*
New York, NY 10016
www.NYULMC.org/rheumatology
Physician Referral: **888-7-NYU-MED** *(888-769-8633)*

RHEUMATOLOGY

Rheumatologists at NYU Langone Medical Center are dedicated to the diagnosis and treatment of patients with rheumatic illnesses, particularly autoimmune diseases. *U.S. News & World Report* has repeatedly recognized the Division of Rheumatology as one of the best in the country, ranking #7 nationwide in the 2013-2014 "Best Hospitals" survey. The division provides care at NYU Langone's premier outpatient facility, The Center for Musculoskeletal Care (CMC); the internationally-renowned, inpatient Hospital for Joint Diseases; at NYU Langone's main campus; and at multiple locations in NYU Langone's growing network of community practices throughout the metro New York area.

Arthritis and Autoimmunity: We offer a comprehensive program for the prevention, diagnosis and treatment of all rheumatologic conditions. Patients also have access to complete rheumatologic evaluations, orthopaedic and neurological consultative services, and participation in clinical trials using the most advanced interventional therapies, highly sophisticated diagnostic testing, and complementary medicine.

Behçet's Syndrome: We have the largest North American Behçet's Center for research and the evaluation and treatment of patients with Behçet's Syndrome, a disease that involves inflammation of the blood vessels.

Biological Treatment: Biological treatments for inflammatory arthritis, rheumatoid arthritis, lupus, psoriatic arthritis, vasculitis, and osteoporosis are administered in our comfortable, state-of-the-art infusion center at CMC.

Lupus: The Center for Lupus Care and Research is devoted to the treatment and research of patients with this autoimmune disease. Patients have access to world renowned specialists in lupus, lupus and pregnancy, and related subspecialties.

Osteoporosis: We offer comprehensive care for the prevention, evaluation and treatment of osteoporosis, including state-of-the art bone densitometers, a range of advanced drug therapies, and programs in balance training and exercise.

Psoriatic Arthritis: Patients of our Psoriatic Arthritis Center, a collaborative effort with the Department of Dermatology, are seen by both a rheumatologist and dermatologist who specialize in psoriasis and psoriatic arthritis.

We are also leaders in the research of inflammatory diseases, focusing on the study of drugs, drug delivery systems and protocols, and the roles genes play in the development and treatment of rheumatic diseases, positioning us at the forefront of basic science and translational research, personalized medicine and the genetics of rheumatic diseases. **The Peter D. Seligman Center for Advanced Therapeutics**, renowned for breakthrough research in arthritis and Systematic Lupus Erythematosus, conducts clinical studies using a wide variety of newly developed therapies.

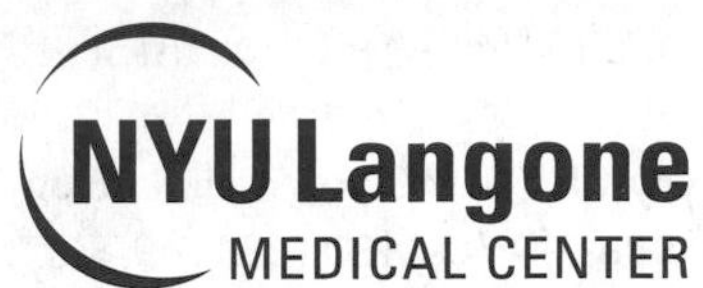

550 First Avenue *(at 31st Street)*
New York, NY 10016
www.NYULMC.org/orthosurgery
Physician Referral: **888-7-NYU-MED** *(888-769-8633)*

ORTHOPAEDIC SURGERY

The Department of Orthopaedic Surgery at NYU Langone Medical Center continues to be recognized as a national leader, **ranked #5 in the nation by *U.S. News & World Report's* 2013-2014 "Best Hospitals" survey**. Our physicians combine extensive experience with cutting-edge research and technology to address bone and joint problems that affect a patient's quality of life. The expertise of our world-class orthopaedists represents the full range of subspecialty areas including **Adult Reconstructive, Sports Medicine and Primary Care Sports Medicine, Spine, Shoulder & Elbow, Foot & Ankle, Hand Surgery, Trauma & Fracture, Orthopaedic Oncology, and Pediatric Orthopaedics**; additional areas of specialization include minimally-invasive surgery and robotic-assisted joint replacement.

Premier Areas of Expertise

Joint Replacement Center physicians evaluate degenerative joint conditions caused by arthritis, injuries, congenital problems and general wear-and-tear to determine the best course of treatment. Our surgeons are experts in knee, hip and shoulder replacements, complex joint revisions, and minimally invasive surgeries, conducting more than 3,000 procedures annually. The experts in our **Hip Center** also specialize in the cutting-edge, minimally invasive anterior total hip replacement technique.

The Spine Center provides conservative care for lower back and neck pain, scoliosis, osteoporosis, problems associated with failed previous surgery, idiopathic disorders, growth disorders, neuromuscular disease, degenerative and congenital conditions, and traumatic deformity. Our surgeons perform over 2,000 procedures a year, including minimally invasive spinal fusions.

Hand Center specialists diagnose and offer operative and non-operative care for a wide range of upper extremity conditions, including fractures, congenital anomalies, soft tissue and skeletal trauma, degenerative and rheumatoid arthritis, sports-related injuries, vascular disorders, tumors and occupational disorders.

Sports Medicine and Primary Care Sports Medicine physicians treat sports-related injuries or conditions of the knee, shoulder, elbow and ankle, using joint preservation techniques as well as surgical procedures. Our patients range from athletes playing at the high school, college and professional levels to recreational athletes/active individuals from every age group.

(continued)

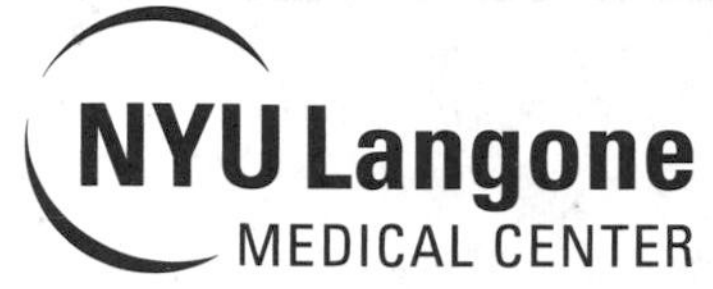

550 First Avenue *(at 31st Street)*
New York, NY 10016
www.NYULMC.org/orthosurgery
Physician Referral: **888-7-NYU-MED** *(888-769-8633)*

ORTHOPAEDIC SURGERY *(continued)*

Specialized Orthopaedic Centers and Services

The Joint Preservation Center provides conservative treatment of joint problems to reduce symptoms, restore function and delay the onset of degenerative arthritis and potential need for a joint replacement.

The Bone Healing Center is staffed by our orthopaedic trauma & fracture specialists, and is a leader in technologies and procedures that help patients recover from complex fracture reconstruction or fracture healing problems.

Harkness Center for Dance Injuries is world-renowned for its orthopaedic and rehabilitation care for dancers, including many subsidized and free services as well as injury prevention screenings and lectures.

The Diabetes Foot and Ankle Center focuses on the prevention and recurrence of foot and ankle problems associated with complications of diabetes.

The Samuels Orthopaedic Immediate Care Center, New York City's only walk-in orthopaedic clinic, is open seven days a week to evaluate and treat urgent bone and joint injuries.

The Concussion Center is a collaborative effort between the Departments of Orthopaedic Surgery, Neurology, and Rehabilitation, providing expert, multidisciplinary evaluation and treatment of individuals who have or are suspected of having a concussion.

The Occupational & Industrial Orthopaedic Center offers care, education, and consulting services in the prevention and treatment of injuries and disorders that arise from the work environment.

Sports Performance Center specialists assist active individuals in reaching their full potential through a state-of-the-art health and fitness evaluation and personalized athletic training plan.

Patient Care Locations

Our physicians and surgeons provide care at multiple NYU Langone locations, including:

- **The Hospital for Joint Diseases**, our internationally-renowned orthopaedic hospital
- **The Center for Musculoskeletal Care (CMC)**, NYU Langone's premier, state-of-the-art, multidisciplinary, bone and joint facility, which houses outpatient orthopaedic and rheumatologic care as well as an infusion center, pain management services, and Rusk Rehab's sports and musculoskeletal rehabilitation services
- CMC's **Outpatient Surgery Center**, where patients undergo minimally invasive, same-day surgery
- **Tisch Hospital**, NYU Langone's flagship hospital at the main campus on First Avenue
- Multiple locations in **NYU Langone's growing network of community practices** in the metro New York area, including Manhattan, Brooklyn, Long Island, Queens, Westchester, and New Jersey

Behavioral Health

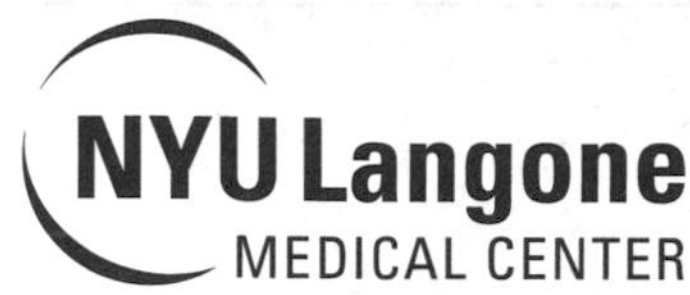

550 First Avenue *(at 31st Street)*
New York, NY 10016

www.NYULMC.org

Physician Referral: **888-7-NYU-MED** *(888-769-8633)*

PSYCHIATRY

NYU Langone's psychiatry team is dedicated to improving the health and well-being of patients by delivering peerless psychiatric services and care. NYU Langone is home to some of the nation's most respected clinical psychiatrists and psychologists, with specialties in psychoanalysis, psychopharmacology, behavioral therapy, child psychiatry, geriatric psychiatry and neuropsychiatry. We specialize in the following areas:

Child and Adolescent Psychiatry

Since 1997, the Child Study Center has treated thousands of children from around the world at its Faculty Group Practices in Manhattan and satellite clinical campuses in New Jersey and Long Island. Through its website, www.AboutOurKids.org, and through professional education programs, parents and practitioners are provided with the tools and knowledge needed to promote children's mental health. We specialize in Anxiety and Mood Disorders, Attention Deficit Hyperactivity and Behavior Disorders, Autism, Asperger's Syndrome and Communication Disorders, Learning Disorders, Tics and Tourette Disorder and more.

Adult Inpatient Services

The inpatient services unit combines comprehensive diagnostic assessment and treatment, including psychopharmacology, neuropsychology, psychotherapies and electroconvulsive therapy.

Adult Outpatient Psychiatry

The outpatient psychiatry program provides expert treatment to individuals suffering from a broad range of mental disorders and emotional problems, including anxiety, depression (including medicine resistant depression), insomnia, manic-depression, reproductive psychiatry, attention-deficit hyperactivity disorder and schizophrenia.

Post-Traumatic Stress Disorder

We offer assessment and treatment of PTSD for victims of sexual and physical assault, natural disasters, terrorism and combat trauma. Treatment includes cognitive behavioral therapy and strategies for the prevention of insomnia, stress, anxiety and depression. Our Military Family Clinic provides compassionate mental healthcare for veterans and their extended family members. The Steven and Alexandra Cohen Veterans Center is dedicated to improving diagnosis and treatment of PTSD and TBI through research.

Memory Impairment

The Pearl Barlow Center for Memory Evaluation and Treatment specializes in treating patients with memory impairments caused by neurological, psychological and physical ailments, as well as memory issues resulting from medication side effects, anxiety, depression and the effects of normal aging from illnesses like Alzheimer's disease.

Birthing Services

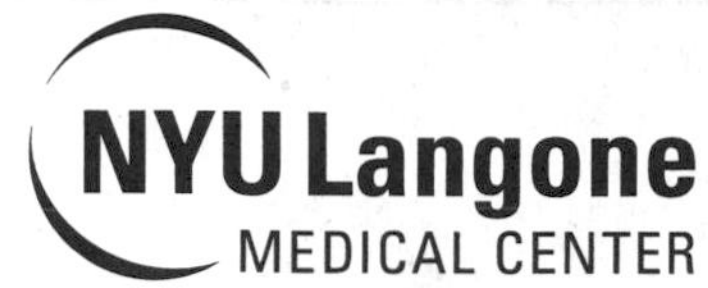

550 First Avenue *(at 31st Street)*
New York, NY 10016

www.NYULMC.org

Physician Referral: **888-7-NYU-MED** *(888-769-8633)*

OBSTETRICS AND GYNECOLOGY

NYU Langone Medical Center provides comprehensive services designed specifically for women, from primary care to highly specialized programs that are supported by sophisticated research and advanced training. We specialize in the following areas:

Obstetrics
We offer a broad range of obstetrical services, including prenatal care that gives equal emphasis to the well-being of the mother and the fetus; fetal monitoring through ultrasound and other techniques; childbirth preparedness and breastfeeding classes.

Maternal-Fetal Medicine
Prenatal care for high-risk pregnancies and detailed consultations before, during and after pregnancy are offered. We specialize in multifetal pregnancies, genetic counseling, women who have miscarried, and preterm deliveries, as well as helping women who have other medical conditions that may complicate a pregnancy, such as diabetes, heart problems, high blood pressure, and lupus. We offer the latest techniques for in-utero diagnosis and treatment and using minimally invasive techniques, our physicians are able to repair a number of life-threatening conditions in a child before it is even born.

Fertility-Related Services
We offer state-of-the-art programs in evaluation of infertility (including the special needs of same-sex couples) egg donation, egg freezing and in-vitro fertilization. Diagnosis and treatment include ovulation induction, assisted reproductive technologies and surgical options that incorporate the latest endoscopic techniques. Preimplantation Genetic Screening (PGS) at the Fertility Center offers tests for aneuploidy (an abnormal number of chromosomes).

Gynecology
In addition to routine gynecological care, we offer pelvic ultrasound; aspiration of breast cysts, colposcopy (a diagnostic evaluation of abnormal pap smears); LEEP (a loop electrosurgical procedure used to diagnose and treat cervical cancer); cryotherapy for vaginal warts; and bone density testing.

Gynecologic Surgery
Minimally invasive gynecologic surgery, including robotic surgery, is offered for a wide range of simple and complex conditions including, resection of endometriosis, hysterectomy, and myomectomy.

Gynecologic Oncology
The NCI-designated NYU Cancer Institute's Women's Cancer Program specializes in the treatment of cervical cancer, endometrial cancer, ovarian cancer, uterine cancer, vaginal cancer and vulvar cancer.

Breast Disease

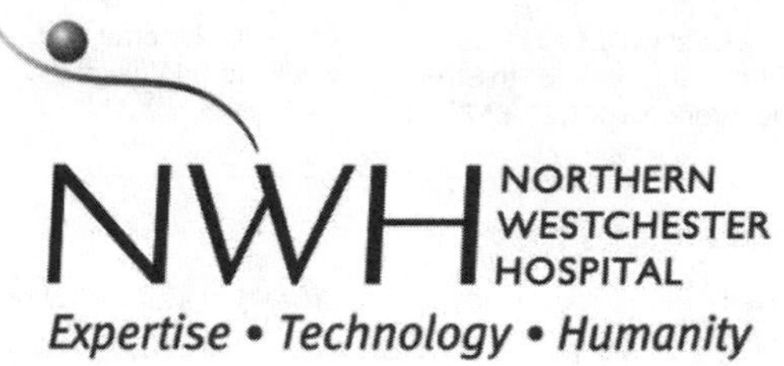

The Breast Institute at Northern Westchester Hospital (NWH) provides an environment of compassion, comfort, and expert medical support. Our staff of dedicated professionals includes oncologists, radiologists, and surgeons with specialized training in using the latest techniques for restoring women to the best possible health. The Breast Institute's Care Team treats your needs—physical, emotional, and spiritual—as our top priorities in one convenient hospital-based location, using innovative, leading-edge technologies.

Northern Westchester Hospital (NWH) provides quality, patient centered care that is close to home through the right combination of medical expertise, leading edge technology, and a commitment to humanity. Over 750 highly skilled physicians, state-of-the-art technology and professional staff of caregivers are all in place to ensure that you and your family receive treatment in a caring, respectful and nurturing environment.

NWH has established extensive internal quality measurements that surpass the standards defined by the Centers for Medicare & Medicaid Services (CMS) and the Hospital Quality Alliance (HQA) National Hospital Quality Measures. Our high quality standards help to ensure that the treatment you receive at NWH is among the best in the nation. For a complete list of our services, please visit www.nwhc.net.

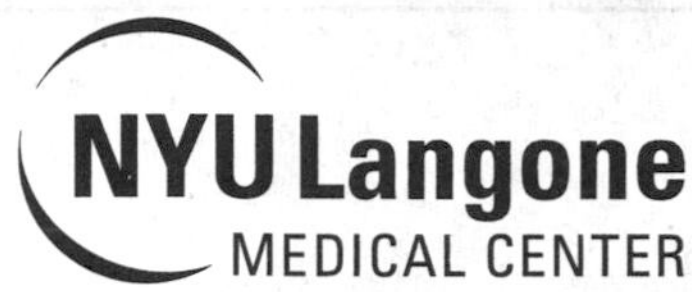

NYU Langone Medical Center
550 First Avenue, New York, NY 10016
www.NYULMC.org

Clinical Cancer Center
160 East 34th Street, New York, NY 10016
www.NYUCI.org

The Stephen D. Hassenfeld Children's Center for Cancer and Blood Disorders
160 East 32nd Street, New York, NY 10016
www.NYULMC.org/hassenfeld

NYU CANCER INSTITUTE

The NYU Cancer Institute is an NCI-designated cancer center providing personalized patient care that is compassionate and state-of-the-art. The Cancer Institute is world-renowned for excellence in cancer-focused research, personalized care, education and community outreach. Its mission is to discover the origins of human cancer and to use that knowledge to eradicate the personal and societal burden of cancer in our community, the nation and the world. For more information about our expert physicians, call 1.888.769.8633.

Patient-Focused Setting
The Clinical Cancer Center is the principal outpatient facility of The Cancer Institute. The Center and its multidisciplinary team of experts provide access to the latest treatment options and clinical trials, along with programs in cancer risk reduction/prevention, screening, diagnostics, genetic counseling and supportive services. In addition, the Center emphasizes the importance of a holistic approach involving integrative health, psychosocial support, survivorship and palliative care. Services are also available at our Ambulatory Care Center on 38th Street in Manhattan, Rego Park, NY, and Lake Success, NY.

Renowned Expertise
The NYU Cancer Institute brings together experts from a variety of disciplines to create collaborative research endeavors and clinical care teams. Our teams are highly skilled in minimally invasive techniques along with video-assisted and robotic surgery. We have created special programs to treat diseases such as breast cancer, brain cancer, melanoma, GI cancer, prostate cancer, hematologic malignancies and lung cancer, as well as translational programs in cancer healthcare disparities; molecularly targeted as well as immune- and stem-cell-based therapies; and the cell signaling pathways involved in cancer.

A Translational Approach
Our scientists and researchers excel in uncovering how cancer develops at the molecular level, and how we can harness that knowledge to reduce the risk of cancer and treat the disease.

Stephen D. Hassenfeld Children's Center for Cancer and Blood Disorders
As part of the Hassenfeld Children's Hospital, the center is a leading pediatric outpatient facility for the treatment of childhood cancers and blood diseases. Its interdisciplinary and family-centered approach combines the most advanced medical treatments with psychosocial and emotional support services.

Cancer Care

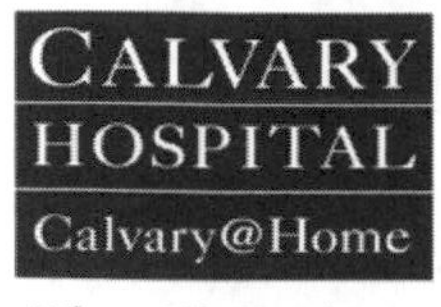

CALVARY HOSPITAL
1740 Eastchester Road
Bronx, NY 10461
Tel: (718) 518-2000
www.calvaryhospital.org

PALLIATIVE CARE INSTITUTE
Calvary's Teaching and Research Arm

The mission of the Palliative Care Institute (PCI), which was founded in 1985, is to transmit, through research and education, Calvary's competence in the care of patients with advanced disease. To date, we have welcomed healthcare professionals from more than 30 countries.

Each year, we train more than 800 medical students, residents, and fellows in palliative care. This includes formalized palliative care observership rotations for residency and fellowship programs throughout the New York area, including Memorial Sloan-Kettering Cancer Center, Mount Sinai School of Medicine, and State University of New York Health Science Center at Brooklyn.

A Model for Excellent Care

Calvary earned a reputation for skillful and compassionate control of patients' symptoms long before palliative and hospice care became popular disciplines.

In 2005, the National Cancer Institute designated Calvary an "international center for training in palliative care" and an alliance was formed between the NCI, Calvary Hospital, and the Middle East Cancer Consortium. Through this alliance, physicians and nurses from Israel, Jordan, Cyprus, Turkey, Egypt, and the Palestinian Authority are sent to Calvary to learn palliative care and increase access to palliative care throughout the Middle East.

Wound Care

The PCI directs Calvary Hospital's Center for Curative and Palliative Wound Care, dedicated to the treatment of complex, intractable wounds related to diabetes, cancer, peripheral vascular disease, and other disorders. For more information about our outstanding wound care services, call (718) 518-2577.

Research Initiatives

The PCI conducts research focusing on wound care, the psychological and emotional impact of terminal illness on patients and families, pain management, and ethical issues concerning end-of-life care.

For more information about Calvary's Palliative Care Institute, please call (718) 518-2147.

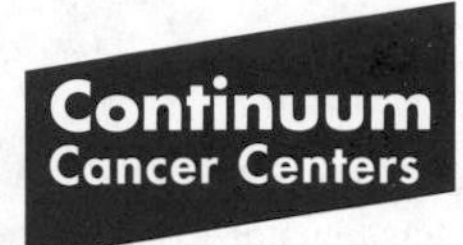

Beth Israel Medical Center
Beth Israel Brooklyn
Roosevelt Hospital
St. Luke's Hospital
NY Eye and Ear Infirmary

Continuum Cancer Centers of New York

Continuum Cancer Centers of New York

212.844.6027

The hospitals of Continuum – Beth Israel Medical Center, Beth Israel Brooklyn, St. Luke's Hospital, Roosevelt Hospital and The New York Eye and Ear Infirmary – are leading providers of cancer care through Continuum Cancer Centers of New York (CCCNY).

We are dedicated to delivering care in ways that are more efficient, more attractive and more convenient for patients. Our cancer patients benefit from system-wide cancer expertise, facilities and resources. Continuum Cancer Centers feature world-renowned cancer specialists, including top-rated surgeons, medical oncologists, radiation oncologists, radiologists, pathologists, and oncology nurses.

Comprehensive diagnostic and treatment services are available for:

- Breast cancer
- Prostate cancer
- Brain cancer
- Thyroid cancer
- Skin cancer
- Lung cancer
- Colorectal cancer
- Gastrointestinal cancer
- Lymphoma/Hodgkin's Disease
- Gynecological cancer
- Head and neck cancer
- Cancer of the central nervous system system

Our services also include prevention programs, expert diagnosis, outpatient treatment, inpatient services and home care. In addition, our research program offers patients access to investigational protocols through a wide number of clinical trials. Our physicians are leaders in both non-invasive and minimally invasive cancer treatments that focus on maximizing both the cure rate and the quality of life.

Supportive Services also play an important role at Continuum Cancer Centers. Our nurses, social workers, psychiatrists, chaplains, pharmacists, rehabilitation therapists and nutritionists all have specialized knowledge and expertise in the field of oncology.

In May 2013, the Commission on Cancer (CoC) of the American College of Surgeons (ACoS) granted Three-Year Network Accreditation with Gold Level Commendation to Continuum Cancer Centers of New York. CCCNY has been recognized by the ACoS/CoC since 2006 and remains the first and only Integrated Network Cancer Program accredited in New York State.

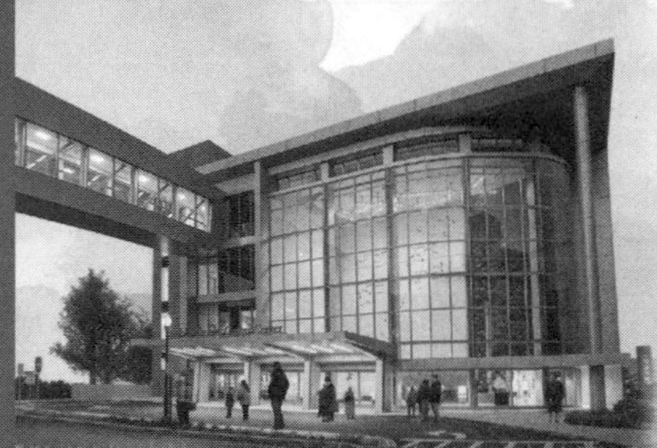

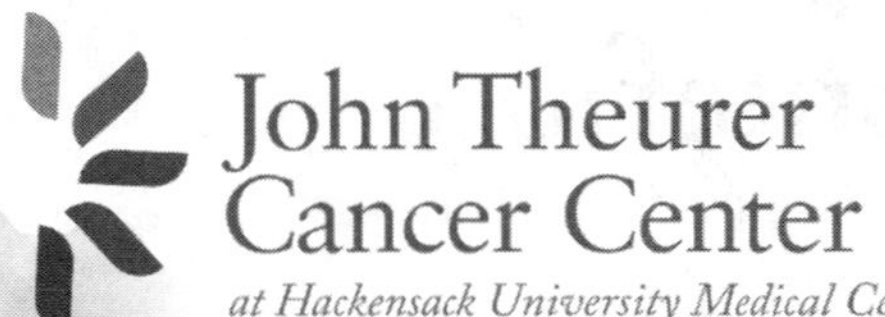

92 Second Street, Hackensack, NJ, 07601 • 551-996-5900
www.jtcancercenter.org

AT JOHN THEURER CANCER CENTER, we believe cancer is hard enough for patients and their loved ones. It is this belief that drives our passion to deliver extraordinary care every day, helping us to become one of the nation's top 50 cancer centers – the only cancer center in New Jersey with this recognition.

Over the past 25 years we have become one of the largest cancer centers in the United States, but we have kept our focus on the unique needs of our patients. Prevention, treatment, and research advances have grown exponentially during this time. We are not only keeping up with the change of pace, we are at the forefront of providing tomorrow's treatment today by:

- Taking multidisciplinary care to a new level with teams of disease-specific experts under one roof
- Delivering personalized medicine focused on novel therapies, participatory treatment, predictive measures and preventive care
- Advancing research through biomarker-driven clinical trials and translational research
- Providing holistic care that includes a wide range of complementary services important to the well-being of our patients that can be easily integrated into their care
- Creating a comforting environment in a new high-tech, high-touch building

We believe our model is the next step towards the future of patient care, changing the cancer care experience one patient at a time.

Innovative Care in a Patient-Centered Environment

In January 2011, we opened a new building that houses 14 specialty divisions, research and support services. This state-of-the-art facility offers a wide range of free resources to help patients become active participants in their treatment and support their fight against cancer. These resources include yoga classes, fitness classes, interactive nutrition classes in the Cooking Studio, art workshops, a patient resource librarian to help patients find credible health information online, and more.

Specialized Practices for Cancer

We are comprised of 14 specialized divisions and Radiation Oncology experts. Division chiefs are supported by medical, research, nursing, nutrition, and psychosocial support for more advanced, focused care.

- Blood and Marrow Stem Cell Transplantation
- Breast Oncology Division
- Gastrointestinal Oncology Division
- Geriatric Oncology Division
- Gynecologic Oncology Division
- Head and Neck Oncology Division
- Leukemia Division
- Lymphoma Division
- Multiple Myeloma Division
- Neurological Oncology Division
- Radiation Oncology Department
- Skin & Sarcoma Division
- Thoracic Oncology Division
- Urologic Oncology Division

Extraordinary Means Cutting Edge Research

Clinical trials and research are the innovation backbone of John Theurer Cancer Center. We have established relationships with cooperative research groups and the pharmaceutical and biotech industry to help bring new therapies into the clinic. This includes expanding our presence in Phase I clinical trials over the next year to provide patients to very early access to novel and promising treatments.

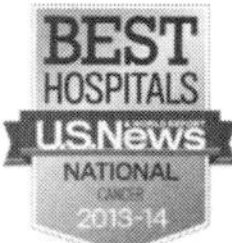

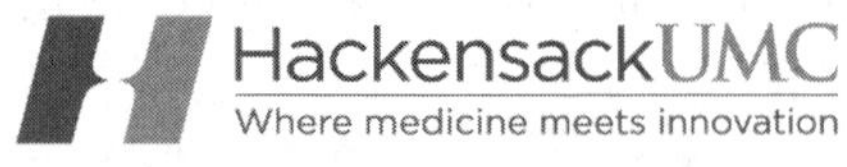

www.HackensackUMC.org

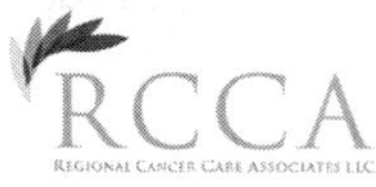

Montefiore
Inspired Medicine

1521 Jarrett Place
Bronx, New York 10461
718-862-8840
www.montefiore.org/cancer

Montefiore Einstein Center for Cancer Care

Each year, thousands of adults and children from around the region benefit from the advanced treatment options offered by the Montefiore Einstein Center for Cancer Care. The Center's commitment to managing all forms of cancer has led to an impressive range of capabilities that include the latest diagnostic and imaging tools, advanced surgical approaches, innovative methods of radiation delivery, and novel medical therapies.

The Center for Cancer Care is one of just four programs in the nation offering regional therapy for melanoma, sarcoma and peritoneal tumors, as well as isolated hepatic perfusion. It is also one of only a handful of programs on the east coast using targeted immunotherapies that zero in on tumors and protect healthy tissue, and one of just two programs in New York State offering high-dose interleukin-2 therapy for advanced-stage melanoma.

To meet the needs of the region's pediatric population, the Center for Cancer Care has partnered with specialists at The Children's Hospital at Montefiore to develop robust treatment programs for sickle cell disease, sarcomas, brain tumors and leukemia. It marked a major milestone in 2013 when, together with CHAM's Blood and Marrow Transplant Program, its physicians performed the first bone marrow transplant to cure sickle cell anemia in a child.

Ranked regionally and recognized as "high performing" by *U.S. News & World Report* in 2012–13, the Center for Cancer Care is committed to treating the whole person and not just the disease. This is exemplified in its Breast Cancer Program, which was recently granted a three-year/full accreditation designation by the National Accreditation Program for Breast Centers. To further demonstrate its commitment to its patients' overall well-being, the Center for Cancer Care has added a full-time psychiatrist and psychological social worker to its team. Through the Caregiver Center, Montefiore provides specialized training and instruction that allows family and friends of cancer patients to assist with their care.

The Center for Cancer Care's diverse research portfolio includes basic, translational and clinical studies that span the full spectrum of cancer care. These include a National Institutes of Health–funded study of inhaled chemotherapy for tobacco-related lung cancer as well as trials studying the use of magnetic resonance imaging–guided high-intensity focused ultrasound to destroy bone tumors, the efficacy of a novel nanomedicine for the treatment of advanced-stage lung cancer and other tumors, and the benefits of using a novel, targeted therapy following the resection of advanced-stage, pancreatic neuroendocrine tumors. Other ongoing research efforts focus on the use of viral therapies for colon cancer, pain management for sickle cell disease, and improved survival of patients with osteosarcoma.

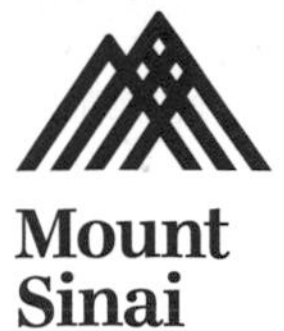

THE MOUNT SINAI MEDICAL CENTER

The Tisch Cancer Institute

One Gustave L. Levy Place
Fifth Avenue and 100th Street
New York, NY 10029-6574

Physician Referral: 1-800-MD-SINAI (637-4624)
www.mountsinai.org

THE TISCH CANCER INSTITUTE is embedded within a renowned medical center that has world-class research facilities, one of the nation's top-ranked hospitals, and an outstanding medical school. Patients have access to the best possible cancer care across a variety of disciplines, including medical, surgical, and radiation treatments; palliative care; behavioral medicine; physical therapy; psychosocial services—and cutting-edge cancer research. For fully integrated, multidisciplinary care, our patients are also treated by the best specialists in every field at Mount Sinai and can receive seamless referrals.

Services and Programs — The Tisch Cancer Institute employs a multidisciplinary treatment approach, providing access to clinical breakthroughs, innovative techniques, leading-edge technologies, and a wide range of diagnostic, therapeutic, and support services for all types of cancer. The Institute treats: breast cancer; hematological malignancies (including multiple myeloma, myelodysplastic syndrome, and myeloproliferative disorders); genitourinary cancers (including prostate, bladder, and kidney); head and neck cancers; thoracic cancer (including lung and esophagus); gynecologic cancers; brain tumors; and other diagnoses. In addition to surgical treatment, the Institute provides radiation and medical oncology therapies, as well as bone marrow transplantation. The Dubin Breast Center, consisting of 15,000 square feet, is a state-of-the-art facility that opened in April 2011 and significantly expands the treatment space for breast cancer patients.

The Tisch Cancer Institute encourages collaboration with colleagues across the Medical Center, drawing upon the knowledge of a vast network of specialists who are outstanding in their fields. These experts consist of award-winning physicians and surgeons specializing in cardiac care, neurology, urology, pediatrics, digestive diseases, obstetrics and gynecology, and other therapeutic areas. Oncologists, surgeons, radiation oncologists, and specialists from across the medical spectrum work together to provide the highest quality care to all cancer patients. Furthermore, Mount Sinai's nursing staff is an important part of the Medical Center's focus on delivering exceptional patient care, and it has received the prestigious Magnet Award for nursing excellence. Mount Sinai is also renowned for its palliative care program, which provides the highest level of care, focusing on the relief of pain, symptoms, and stress in cancer patients in both an inpatient and outpatient setting.

A Heritage of Breakthroughs — Teams of physicians and scientists at The Tisch Cancer Institute at Mount Sinai work together to rapidly translate laboratory research into new patient treatments. Among the advances pioneered at Mount Sinai are the first successful treatment of tumors of the bladder by transurethral electrocoagulation, the first demonstration of how asbestos can cause cancerous changes in the DNA of cells, and the first development of an ultrasound-guided technique to insert radioactive seeds into the prostate to treat prostate cancer.

THE RUTTENBERG TREATMENT CENTER

The Derald H. Ruttenberg Treatment Center, home to the ambulatory cancer program of The Tisch Cancer Institute is now housed in the newly constructed Leon and Norma Hess Center for Science and Medicine.

THE DUBIN BREAST CENTER

The Dubin Breast Center offers the latest, most innovative approaches available for breast health and the treatment of breast cancer.

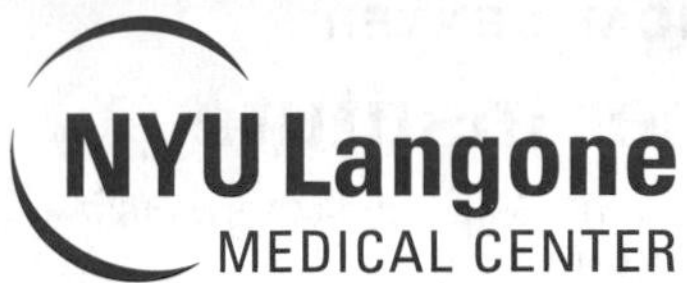

NYU Langone Medical Center
550 First Avenue, New York, NY 10016
www.NYULMC.org

Clinical Cancer Center
160 East 34th Street, New York, NY 10016
www.NYUCI.org

The Stephen D. Hassenfeld Children's Center for Cancer and Blood Disorders
160 East 32nd Street, New York, NY 10016
www.NYULMC.org/hassenfeld

NYU CANCER INSTITUTE

The NYU Cancer Institute is an NCI-designated cancer center providing personalized patient care that is compassionate and state-of-the-art. The Cancer Institute is world-renowned for excellence in cancer-focused research, personalized care, education and community outreach. Its mission is to discover the origins of human cancer and to use that knowledge to eradicate the personal and societal burden of cancer in our community, the nation and the world. For more information about our expert physicians, call 1.888.769.8633.

Patient-Focused Setting
The Clinical Cancer Center is the principal outpatient facility of The Cancer Institute. The Center and its multidisciplinary team of experts provide access to the latest treatment options and clinical trials, along with programs in cancer risk reduction/prevention, screening, diagnostics, genetic counseling and supportive services. In addition, the Center emphasizes the importance of a holistic approach involving integrative health, psychosocial support, survivorship and palliative care. Services are also available at our Ambulatory Care Center on 38th Street in Manhattan, Rego Park, NY, and Lake Success, NY.

Renowned Expertise
The NYU Cancer Institute brings together experts from a variety of disciplines to create collaborative research endeavors and clinical care teams. Our teams are highly skilled in minimally invasive techniques along with video-assisted and robotic surgery. We have created special programs to treat diseases such as breast cancer, brain cancer, melanoma, GI cancer, prostate cancer, hematologic malignancies and lung cancer, as well as translational programs in cancer healthcare disparities; molecularly targeted as well as immune- and stem-cell-based therapies; and the cell signaling pathways involved in cancer.

A Translational Approach
Our scientists and researchers excel in uncovering how cancer develops at the molecular level, and how we can harness that knowledge to reduce the risk of cancer and treat the disease.

Stephen D. Hassenfeld Children's Center for Cancer and Blood Disorders
As part of the Hassenfeld Children's Hospital, the center is a leading pediatric outpatient facility for the treatment of childhood cancers and blood diseases. Its interdisciplinary and family-centered approach combines the most advanced medical treatments with psychosocial and emotional support services.

Trinitas Regional Medical Center

TRINITAS COMPREHENSIVE CANCER CENTER

225 Williamson Street | Elizabeth, New Jersey 07207
Ph 908.994.8000 | www.TrinitasCancerCenter.org

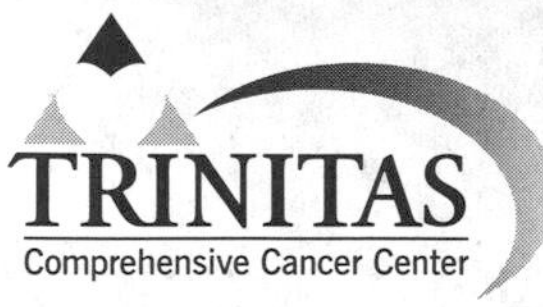

Trinitas Continues its Aggressive Pursuit of Excellence in Cancer Care

As just one of eight healthcare facilities in New Jersey to receive the American College of Surgeons National Accreditation Program for Breast Centers (NAPBC), Trinitas Regional Medical Center has been recognized for its voluntary commitment to providing the best in breast cancer diagnosis and treatment and its compliance with established NAPBC standards. Both the Diagnostic Imaging Center and the Trinitas Comprehensive Cancer Center have received this accreditation for cancer diagnosis and cancer care services.

"When the Trinitas Comprehensive Cancer Center opened its doors in 2005, it did so with the commitment to providing superior, compassionate care to those who use our many services," explains Barry Levinson, MD, Medical Director of the center. "We approach each patient with the utmost of care and direct our attention to giving them not only the best care and treatment but also the best quality of life as they survive cancer. The NAPBC accreditation underscores that commitment and encourages us to maintain the very highest standards for our patients."

Located on the main campus of Trinitas Regional Medical Center in Elizabeth, the Center is the home of the most advanced technology available to cancer patients, including the first Trilogy Linear Accelerator for radiation therapy in New Jersey. The Center is also the site of the state's first AccuBoost breast cancer treatment, and the first RapidArc radiotherapy procedure.

A major quality initiative at the Cancer Center involves a system-wide evaluation of the benefits, risks and efficient management of the increasing number of oral oncology drugs that have become available. These drugs offer a more convenient and less invasive treatment option, but they require a new model for patient education, monitoring, communications and support. Trinitas is well ahead of this curve with the development of in-depth 14-step program that features safeguards, intensive follow-up and a comprehensive system of checks and balances.

Support services include: nutrition/dietician services, genetic counseling, fatigue management, complementary therapies and services, social work, lymphedema management, Look Good – Feel Better, Made for Me boutique, art therapy, pet therapy and pain management.

Trinitas was awarded Comprehensive Cancer Program status by the American College of Surgeons' Commission on Cancer. Further, we are an approved Member of the prestigious Radiation Therapy Oncology Group. Our clinical research program gives many patients access to new treatment approaches that might not otherwise be available.

In 2013, Trinitas joined the Philadelphia-based Jefferson Kimmel Cancer Center Network, bringing Jefferson's many treatment studies to the region.

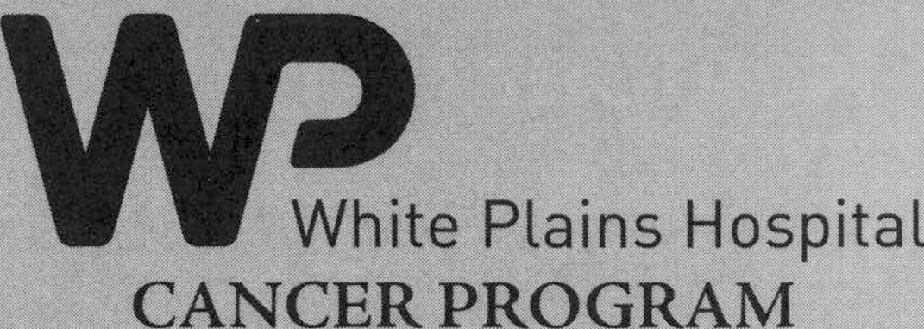

CANCER PROGRAM

2-4 Longview Avenue, White Plains, NY 10601 (914) 681-2700 www.wphospital.org

As the leading cancer facility in the region, the Cancer Program at White Plains Hospital provides patients with the best and most comprehensive care available in an easily accessible setting. Highly specialized clinicians and advanced technology focus on the diagnosis, care and treatment of many types of cancer including breast, prostate, lung, colorectal, gynecologic, thyroid and blood cancers, among others.

The hospital's Breast Program is accredited by the National Accreditation Program for Breast Centers (NAPBC) of the American College of Surgeons. Initially accredited in 1993, the Cancer Program again earned another three-year accreditation with commendation in 2013 from the American College of Surgeons Commission on Cancer, as well as their Outstanding Achievement Award, a recognition given to only 79 other cancer programs in the United States.

DISTINCTIVE FEATURES

· **Radiology and Women's Imaging** at several locations, including two specifically dedicated to the radiological needs of women- the Breast Imaging Center at the hospital's main campus and the Women's Imaging Center in Rye Brook, NY

· **Surgery** including advanced thoracic, colorectal, gynecological, minimally invasive and robotic surgery, oncoplastic techniques and nipple-sparing mastectomy.

· **Medical Oncology** utilizing the most advanced technologies and specifically targeted treatments for maximal efficacy and minimization of toxicity.

· **Radiation Oncology** at the Dickstein Cancer Treatment Center using state-of-the-art therapy and expertise from physicians trained at the finest teaching hospitals in the United States.

· **Clinical Navigators** to explain treatments, procedures and side effects and assistance with physical, psycho-social and financial services, clinical trials and support resources.

· **Cancer Genetics Program** providing guidance on the nature and consequences of various inherited disorders, the probabilities of developing and transmitting the disorders to offspring, methods of early detection, disease management and coping strategies.

· **Research Studies and Expansive Clinical Trials** offering additional options for patients who may not respond to established treatment protocols.

·**Survivorship Program** dedicated to offering a multitude of services and resources both within the Hospital and in the community from the time of diagnosis of cancer, through treatment and beyond.

White Plains Hospital

For more than 120 years, White Plains Hospital has provided advanced, exceptional health care to the people of Westchester County and surrounding areas. Nearly 200,000 patients visit the Hospital each year for a variety of services including emergency care, internal medicine, maternity and high-risk obstetrics, minimally invasive surgery, orthopaedics, oncology and cardiac care, among others.

The Hospital's capabilities for diagnosis and treatment, including state-of-the-art radiology and laboratory services, are second to none and rival those found at many nearby academic medical centers. These resources are combined with highly individualized care provided by the Hospital's more than 900 affiliated physicians and surgeons, many of whom have trained at and the finest medical institutions in the country; and the more than 700 Magnet®- designated nurses with advanced training who provide skilled, compassionate care to their patients, every day.

259 First Street, Mineola, NY 11501
Tel: 1-866-WINTHROP
www.winthrop.org

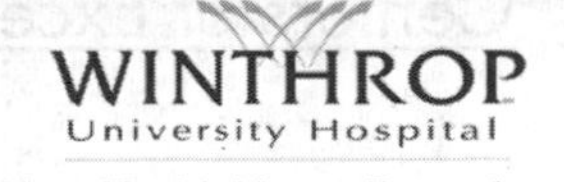

Your Health Means Everything.

CANCER CARE AT WINTHROP-UNIVERSITY HOSPITAL

General Overview
Winthrop-University Hospital's Cancer Care Program is a regional leader in clinical cancer care, offering a full complement of world-class inpatient and outpatient services for adults and children with cancer. Certified by the Commission on Cancer, Winthrop's expert multidisciplinary staff of highly trained professionals utilizes high-tech diagnostics in order to provide a broad spectrum of world-class care options that focus on prevention, leading-edge treatment and support services — all tailored to meet the unique, personal needs of each patient — with a deep sense of compassion.

Approaching care from a curative perspective, Winthrop's cancer specialists seek to maximize benefits for patients, while minimizing potential harm from treatment. They collaborate closely through regular, multidisciplinary treatment-planning conferences to secure the most appropriate treatment for each patient following a definitive diagnosis, and to ensure that National Comprehensive Cancer Network guidelines are followed.

Specialty programs and services include:

- A comprehensive Lung Cancer Program and LI's first Lung Cancer Screening program
- The largest outpatient Pediatric Oncology Program in Nassau County
- Cutting-edge gynecologic oncology services
- Robotic and minimally invasive treatments for pancreatic cancer
- Multidisciplinary, highly proficient urologic cancer services
- A state-of-the-art multidisciplinary, nationally accredited Breast Health Center
- High-level surgical oncology, utilizing the latest robotic technology and techniques
- CyberKnife® stereotactic radiosurgery
- A new, modern Outpatient Infusion Center and Inpatient Oncology/Hematology Unit
- An exceptionally accurate Pathology Department that utilizes advanced cytogenetic and molecular pathology techniques
- Minimally invasive treatment for gastrointestinal and lung cancers
- Neuro-oncology and neurosurgical services, which specialize in the medical and surgical management of brain, spine and central nervous system tumors

Cancer Center for Kids (CCFK)
Winthrop's Cancer Center for Kids (CCFK) meets the complex challenges of children's cancers and blood disorders with a relentless spirit and dedication to improving the lives of patients and their families. The CCFK is Nassau County's largest outpatient facility for treating children with cancer and blood disorders. Skilled and compassionate professionals embody the principles of patient and family-centered care. They not only provide comprehensive, sensitive care, but also help families endure some very tough times with support from the moment of diagnosis through intense treatments and long-term follow-up.

Research
As an academic institution, Winthrop is the site of some of the most current clinical trials and research into cancer, ensuring that patients have access to the latest therapies. The Hospital's cancer specialists and researchers are involved in rigorous basic and clinical studies of a wide variety of cancers, including lung cancer, childhood cancers, blood cancers, breast, colorectal and gynecological cancers.

Cancer Navigator Program
Winthrop's Cancer Navigator Program, the first of its kind on LI, offers individualized assistance to patients, families and caregivers, helping them move seamlessly through the many diagnostic tests, procedures, physician visits and treatments they face after learning they have cancer. Cancer Navigators are nurses and physician assistants who specialize in the care of people with cancer. Services include reducing or eliminating barriers to care, and paving the way for early and timely screenings and diagnostic tests; educating patients about treatment options; identifying and assisting with accessing financial, legal and community support services; connecting patients and families to support groups; and facilitating access to research trials.

Cardiac Electrophysiology

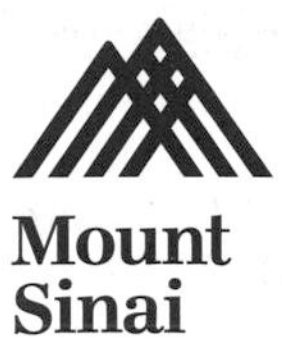

THE MOUNT SINAI MEDICAL CENTER

Cardiac Electrophysiology

One Gustave L. Levy Place
Fifth Avenue and 100th Street
New York, NY 10029-6574

Physician Referral: 1-800-MD-SINAI (637-4624)
www.mountsinai.org

Cardiac Electrophysiology

Ranked #13 in the United States for cardiology and heart surgery by *U.S. News & World Report*, Mount Sinai is a recognized leader in the treatment of abnormal heart rhythms, also known as cardiac electrophysiology. Our clinical leadership, innovative research, and leading-edge therapies continually draws patients from around the world to seek treatment with us.

A major referral destination, our **HELMSLEY CENTER FOR ELECTROPHYSIOLOGY** offers the full range of therapies for all types of arrhythmia, from common arrhythmias such as atrial fibrillation to challenging ones as ventricular tachycardia. We combine technology, technique, and expertise to deliver the highest-quality and most advanced care. Mount Sinai specialists are skilled in performing the most delicate arrhythmia procedures, even those not attempted at most hospitals. Our patients can feel assured they've chosen a center that offers every available treatment for cardiac arrhythmias, as well as experts who can tailor those treatments for the most customized care.

COMBINING SCIENCE WITH PERSONALIZED CARE

The Center for Electrophysiology continues its leadership through various research studies with the goal of developing superior technologies. In fact, Mount Sinai is currently the lead center on several multinational clinical trials exploring new arrhythmia procedures, keeping us on the cutting edge and offering access to the most advanced treatments.

Advancing the Treatment of Arrhythmias

Mount Sinai has been leading the development of new arrhythmia technologies since 1909, when one of our physicians became the first in the United States to use an electrocardiogram. Today the Center for Electrophysiology provides the full spectrum of therapies, including procedures that implant devices for regulating heart rhythms (such as Pacemakers and ICDs) to procedures that use catheters for fixing the source of the abnormal heartbeat (called ablations).

To make ablations safer and more effective, our center was the first in the country to use several breakthrough technologies, including a visually guided laser balloon catheter in 2009 and the TactiCath force-sensing catheter in 2011, as well as a new generation of visually guided catheter in 2012. Vivek Reddy, MD, Director of our Cardiac Arrhythmia Service, was the first physician in the world to use several new ablation techniques, such as the cryoballoon catheter and robotic navigation. Also, Drs. Reddy and Dukkipati were the first in the US to perform a suture-based catheter ligation of the left atrial appendage (to prevent stroke in AF) in 2009.

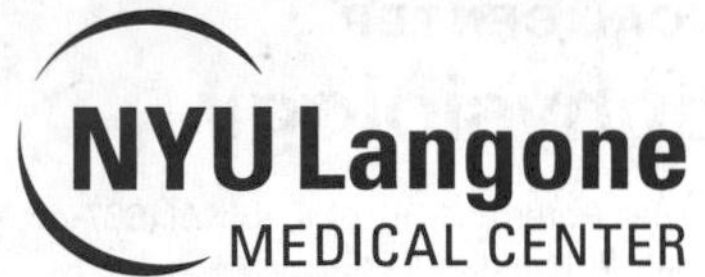

CARDIAC AND VASCULAR INSTITUTE
550 First Avenue *(at 31st Street)*
New York, NY 10016
www.NYULMC.org
Physician Referral: **888-7-NYU-MED** *(888-769-8633)*

CARDIAC AND VASCULAR INSTITUTE

The Cardiac and Vascular Institute (CVI) at NYU Langone Medical Center continues to advance new techniques for repairing heart valves, curing heart rhythm disorders, and treating aortic diseases and congestive heart failure. We care for both adults and children. CVI is consistently ranked among the leading heart and heart surgery centers in *U.S. News & World Report's annual 'Best Hospitals'* rankings.

Cardiac Catheterization CVI offers superior catheter-based diagnosis and evaluation of cardiac health. Our laboratory provides a full range of procedures to evaluate, diagnose, and provide treatment options.

Cardiac Rehabilitation and Prevention The Joan and Joel Smilow Cardiopulmonary Rehabilitation and Prevention Center provides individualized treatment plans through NYU Langone's Rusk Rehabilitation, in a state-of-the-art and comfortable facility.

Cardiac Surgery NYU Langone is a nationally recognized leader in advanced surgical treatments for adult and congenital heart disease. We have world-renowned expertise in mitral valve repair, aortic valve replacement and aortic aneurysm repair, as well as specializing in high-risk and elderly patients.

Cardiology The Leon H. Charney Division of Cardiology is a leader in cardiovascular patient care, biomedical research, and education. We are advancing the field of cardiovascular medicine through a variety of innovative collaborations.

Congenital Heart Disease The pediatric and adult congenital cardiac program treats patients of all ages with inherited and acquired cardiac defects. We have a highly experienced team of specialists in pediatric and adult cardiology, pediatric interventional cardiology, congenital cardiac surgery, neonatal and pediatric cardiac intensive care, pediatric cardiac anesthesiology, nursing, and extracorporeal perfusion.

Heart Failure A multidisciplinary team offers the most advanced care for heart failure including echocardiograms, pacemaker and defibrillator implantations, open heart surgeries, and left ventricular assist devices.

Nuclear Cardiology/Stress The Nuclear Cardiology/Stress Laboratory performs a range of tests that assist cardiologists in the assessment and diagnosis of heart disease.

Vascular Surgery We offer diagnostic and treatment for patients with conditions ranging from arterial aneurysms to deep vein thrombosis, as well as carotid stenosis and limb salvage including minimally invasive vein surgery, endovascular aortic surgery, thoracic aneurysm correction and abdominal aneurysm interventions.

The Best in American Medicine
www.CastleConnolly.com

Cardiovascular Disease

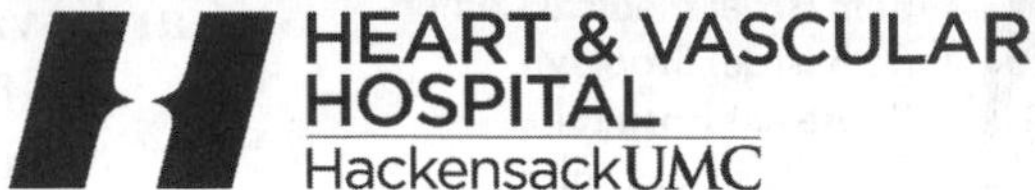

30 Prospect Avenue, Hackensack, NJ 07601 • 551-996-2000

www.HackensackUMC.org

Opened in 2011, Heart & Vascular Hospital at HackensackUMC is one of America's most comprehensive cardiac and vascular care centers, providing a full-range of state-of-the-art invasive and noninvasive services. This "hospital within a hospital" treats all types of cardiac and vascular diseases performed by a world-class team of nurse practitioners, Magnet®-award winning nurses, technicians, specialized personnel, and more than 140 cardiologists, cardiac surgeons, vascular surgeons, and neuro-interventionalists who provide the highest quality of care.

The Heart & Vascular Hospital offers a Cardiac Rehabilitation and Wellness Center as well as designated floors for post-operative patients and specialty areas, including: Neurology/Stroke Recovery, Congestive Heart Failure, Cardiac ICU, Cardiac Surgery ICU, Cardiac Stepdown Unit, and Same Day Admission Rooms/Recovery.

AWARD-WINNING CARE

The Heart & Vascular Hospital has received the following prestigious awards and accolades:

- Ranked #1 in NJ by Healthgrades for Cardiology Services in 2013
- Ranked nationally #33 out of more than 700 hospitals in Cardiology & Heart Surgery by *U.S. News & World Report* in 2013-14
- Designation as an Accredited Chest Pain Center from the Society of Chest Pain Centers
- One of Healthgrades America's 100 Best Hospitals for Cardiac Care™ and Coronary Intervention - 2 Years in a Row
- 2013 *Becker's Hospital Review*'s 100 Hospitals With Great Heart Programs

AWARD-WINNING SERVICES AND PROGRAMS

Hybrid Surgery – The Hybrid Operating Room is one of only a handful of interventional suites in the nation where open or minimally invasive surgical procedures and catheterization can be performed simultaneously.

TAVR - Shortly after it opened, the Hybrid OR was the scene of a procedure that marks a milestone in heart surgery—the transcatheter aortic valve replacement (TAVR). HackensackUMC was the first hospital in northern New Jersey to perform this procedure, and the first in the state to perform this groundbreaking minimally invasive heart valve replacement procedure via transapical delivery.

Stereotaxis Lab – The Heart & Vascular Hospital's Stereotaxis Lab - Northern New Jersey's first - shortens procedures, speeds recovery time, reduces exposure to radiation and helps more patients avoid invasive open heart surgical procedures.

Biplane Angiographic Unit – Our Biplane Angiographic Unit uses a fluoroscopic X-ray machine that images the body's circulatory dynamics from multiple angles to produce virtually unlimited views, which is crucial in obtaining views of critical procedures to treat strokes, aneurysms and brain tumors.

Focus on Patients – The Cardiac Wellness & Rehabilitation program at our Heart & Vascular Hospital is an important resource for area physicians, many of whom refer patients who are at high risk for heart disease or are recovering from heart attacks, cardiac bypass or other cardiovascular procedures.

SPECIFIC PROGRAMS OF EXCELLENCE

In addition to its award-winning cardiovascular care, the Heart & Vascular Hospital is proud to offer the following specific programs of excellence, which distinguish our medical center from the rest:

- Heart Failure Program; Cardiovascular Disease Prevention; Critical Care Medicine; Transcatheter Vascular Surgery Repair; Transcatheter Aortic Valve Replacement; Transcatheter repairs of mitral valve; Minimally Invasive Mitral Valve Repair; and Thoracic Aortic Surgery.

To learn more about our award-winning care at the Heart & Vascular Hospital at HackensackUMC, visit HackensackUMC.org.

For more information about Cardiovascular Services
or for a physician referral, call 1-877-HOLY-NAME.
Please mention "Castle Connolly Guide."

Holy Name Medical Center
Cardiovascular Services

718 Teaneck Road
Teaneck, NJ 07666
1-877-HOLY-NAME
(1-877-465-9626)
www.holyname.org

THE HOLY NAME HEALING TRADITION

Holy Name Medical Center's multidisciplinary team of experts provides accurate diagnosis and gender-specific care for the best cardiac outcomes. Our goal is to detect and treat cardiac disease before it becomes life-threatening, and to provide services along a continuum, so that every patient's care is fluid and streamlined. Prevention initiatives, leading-edge technology, progressive treatments and multi-phase cardiac rehabilitation services—Holy Name puts it all together to keep you healthy when your heart is at risk.

FROM DIAGNOSIS TO REHABILITATION

Holy Name's multidisciplinary cardiac team provides optimal quality of care with experts from all aspects of cardiovascular disease management: board-certified cardiologists and interventional cardiologists, neurologists and emergency medicine physicians, specialized registered nurses and exercise physiologists, registered and certified diagnostic technologists, rehabilitation specialists, and a specially trained support staff.

Holy Name is a leader in the newer, through-the-wrist cardiac catheterization. Patients who undergo radial catheterization experience fewer bleeding complications, less pain, quicker recovery and improved outcomes overall.

Most diagnostic tests and many treatment procedures can be accomplished on an outpatient basis, without an overnight stay in the Medical Center. For patients who require hospitalization with specialized care and monitoring following a medical event, the inpatient continuum of care at Holy Name features award-winning intensive care, intermediate care and telemetry units.

A Recognized Expert in Early Intervention

The Joint Commission "Top Performer on Key Quality Measures" in four areas, including heart attack and heart failure

NJ Department of Health High-Performing Hospital in four out of four measures, including heart attack and heart failure

Advanced Certification—Primary Stroke Center by The Joint Commission

NJ Department of Health Inpatient Quality Indicators find stroke mortality rate significantly below state rate

Beacon Award for Critical Care Excellence awarded to Intensive Care Unit (ICU) and Telemetry Unit, gold and silver status respectively, by the American Association of Critical-Care Nurses

American Heart Association/ American Stroke Association Gold Plus Achievement Award

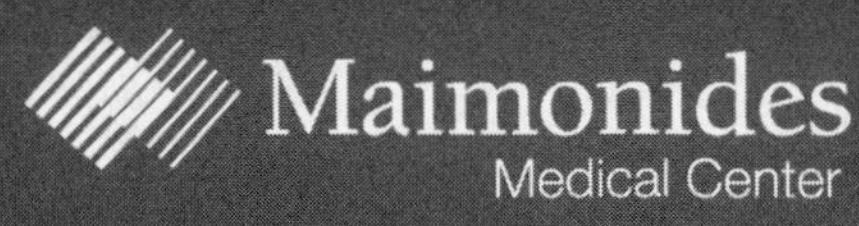

Maimonides Heart & Vascular Center

4802 Tenth Avenue
Brooklyn, New York 11219
Phone: 718.283.7489 • Fax: 718.635.7505
www.maimonidesmed.org/cardiac

The Cardiac Institute and Division of Vascular and Endovascular Surgery were integrated in 2013 to form the Maimonides Heart & Vascular Center.

Heart Services

Having pioneered numerous heart care innovations through the years, the Heart & Vascular Center offers diagnostic studies and therapeutic treatments, procedures and surgeries. It has been ranked by the Centers for Medicare and Medicaid Services among the few hospitals which have achieved excellent ratings in both heart attack and heart failure patient outcomes.

Cardiology

Headed by Jacob Shani, MD, the Department of Cardiology is among the most published and respected in the field, the Maimonides cardiology team continuously sets higher standards for patient care. The division has participated in numerous NIH-sponsored cardiac drug trials, and our Congestive Heart Failure (CHF) Program is among the most effective in the nation.

Interventional Cardiology

Numerous therapeutic devices have been developed and implemented here. Our Electrophysiology Lab has a superb record of achievement in diagnosing and treating arrhythmias. Close collaboration with the Department of Emergency Medicine ensures that chest pain patients are evaluated immediately, and that interventional procedures are used to stop heart attacks in progress whenever necessary.

Cardiothoracic Surgery

The Maimonides Division of Cardiothoracic Surgery has an illustrious history, setting a national standard for advances in cardiothoracic. Under the direction of Greg Ribakove, MD, minimally invasive and robotic heart surgeries, as well as advanced procedures such as LVAD and TAVI, are offered in state-of-the-art facilities, including a hybrid OR. In collaboration with Electrophysiology, Cardiothoracic Surgery has established an Atrial Fibrillation Center of Excellence. Maimonides provides one of the most prestigious cardiothoracic residency programs in the U.S.

Historic Moments

- In 1967, the first successful human heart transplant in the nation was performed at Maimonides.
- The intra-aortic balloon pump was developed here in 1970.
- Surgical techniques that protect the spine during cardiothoracic surgery were perfected here in 1982.
- Revolutionary cardiac catheterization devices were invented here in 1992 and 1997.
- Maimonides was the first hospital in the U.S. to implement fully automatic external cardiac defibrillators in 2001.

The Centers for Medicare and Medicaid Services, an agency of the federal government, recently published the latest data on 30-day mortality rates for hospitals across the country. Maimonides Medical Center achieved better-than-expected results in all three categories measured – heart attack, heart failure and pneumonia – a distinction only 25 hospitals in the U.S. achieved.

Maimonides Medical Center

The right care.
Right here.

www.maimonidesmed.org/cardiac

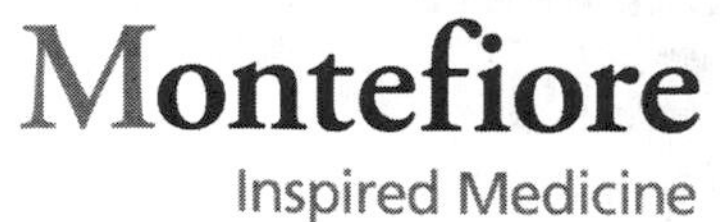

111 East 210th Street
Bronx, New York 10467
718-920-7000
www.montefiore.org/heart

Montefiore Einstein Center for Heart and Vascular Care

The Montefiore Einstein Center for Heart and Vascular Care's proud tradition of innovation and clinical excellence has made it a national leader in adult and pediatric cardiology and cardiovascular surgery. The expertise of its physicians and surgeons spans the full spectrum of cardiovascular care—from novel therapies and interventional treatments to intricate, life-saving procedures.

The Center's Heart Valve Repair Program offers cutting-edge treatments to correct complex valve conditions, including the butterfly procedure for mitral valve regurgitation and transcatheter aortic valve replacement (TAVR) for patients with severe aortic stenosis and at high risk for surgery. The Center's risk-adjusted operative mortality rate for mitral valve repair is among the best in the nation. Montefiore is one of only two centers offering the Perceval S sutureless heart valve (PERCEVAL valve), which reduces patient risk by significantly reducing bypass time.

Through the Center's Heart Failure Program, adults and pediatric patients receive advanced medical and surgical interventions—including ventricular assist devices (LVADs) and heart transplantation. In 2012, the Center performed 28 heart transplants (23 adult and five pediatric) and implanted 28 LVADs. Its one-year survival rate continues to be among the best in the nation, at 97 percent for adults and 100 percent for children. The New York State Department of Health has recognized the Center as a leader among the state's transplant/heart failure programs in achieving appropriate treatment measures and low mortality rates.

In the area of cardiac interventions, the Center possesses an exceptionally low mortality rate and an expanded team that includes renowned electrocardiologists and structural interventionalists.

Nationally ranked by *U.S. News & World Report,* the Center performed more than 9,000 cardiac procedures in 2013 and once again earned the Society of Thoracic Surgeons' prestigious "three-star" ranking for its commitment to surgical excellence, placing Montefiore among the nation's top open-heart surgery programs.

The Center is a leader in basic, translational and clinical research and is supported by more than $10 million in grants, including funding through the National Institutes of Health/National Heart, Lung, and Blood Institute's Cardiothoracic Surgical Trials Network for the 10th consecutive year. The Center is participating in prominent trials exploring the use of stem cells in heart failure patients. Through the LARIAT® trial, the Center is working to provide atrial fibrillation patients with additional options for preventing stroke. Montefiore's Goal to Reduce Readmissions at Montefiore (GRRAM) program exemplifies its commitment to reducing readmission. Within three months of implementing GRRAM, heart patient readmission rates dropped 5 percent.

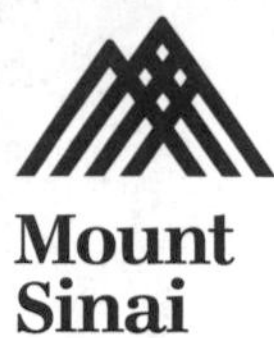

Mount Sinai

THE MOUNT SINAI MEDICAL CENTER
Cardiothoracic Surgery

One Gustave L. Levy Place
Fifth Avenue and 100th Street
New York, NY 10029-6574

Physician Referral: 1-800-MD-SINAI (637-4624)
www.mountsinai.org

THE DEPARTMENT OF CARDIOTHORACIC SURGERY at Mount Sinai is one of the nation's most prestigious programs. **In 2013, *U.S. News & World Report* ranked our cardiology and heart surgery service 13th in the country.** Cardiothoracic surgical patients benefit from an integrated and personalized care plan designed in coordination with expert cardiologists, anesthesiologists, perfusionists, and intensive care physicians. Mount Sinai is a quaternary referral center, meaning its surgeons often operate on the sickest and most complicated patients.

The Mitral Valve Repair Reference Center is one of the largest and most advanced in the nation. The superiority of mitral valve repair over replacement with a mechanical or bioprosthetic valve is now well established. Directed by David H. Adams, MD, Mount Sinai's Mitral Valve Repair Reference Center offers patients one of the highest percentages of successful valve repair in the world. In patients with mitral valve prolapse, our success rate in avoiding valve replacement approaches 100 percent. Our physicians are experts in mitral valve repair for patients with advanced cardiomyopathy. For patients who have associated atrial fibrillation, we offer the latest in concomitant arrhythmia surgery, including the MAZE procedure. Mitral valve repair with minimally invasive approaches is also performed when appropriate. Learn more about our Reference Center at www.mitralvalverepair.org.

The Cardiac Transplant and Assist Program, one of the largest in the nation, is under the direction of Anelechi Anyanwu, MD. We have been involved in the field of mechanical cardiac assistance from its inception, and have experience with most of the available FDA-approved devices. We have also played an active role in multi-institutional studies exploring permanent mechanical heart support.

Transcatheter Aortic Valve Replacement/Implantation (TAVR/TAVI) Program offers breakthrough treatment. Our physicians have been performing TAVR/TAVI for two years, with patients coming from around the world for this treatment. We were the first institution in the country to implant the Medtronic CoreValve Transcatheter Aortic Valve replacement device, and we are the first hospital in New York State able to implant both the Edwards Sapien Valve and the Medtronic CoreValve. These minimally invasive treatments spare patients from open-heart surgery and offer quicker recovery and return to daily activities. Our TAVR/TAVI program is led by Dr. David Adams, the National Co-Principal Investigator of the United States FDA pivotal trial of the Medtronic CoreValve Transcatheter Aortic Valve replacement device, and Dr. Samin Sharma, Director of Clinical Cardiology and Interventional Cardiology.

Pediatric and Congenital Cardiac Surgery Program achieves exceptional results. Led by Dr. Khanh Nguyen, patients from newborns to young adults are cared for in this program, which has achieved outstanding results with challenging problems by incorporating the most advanced techniques available. Part of only three active pediatric heart transplant centers in the state, our program also provides support for very sick hearts in infants and older children, using Extra-Corporeal Membrane Oxygenators (ECMO) or Ventricular Assist Devices (VAD). The care extended to the patient and family is supported by an outstanding multidisciplinary team. Superb post-operative care is provided in a dedicated Pediatric Cardiac Surgical Intensive Care Unit, under the direction of pediatric cardiologists, intensivists, and surgeons.

LEADING SURGEONS, UNPARALLELED POSSIBILITIES

The Department of Cardiothoracic Surgery at Mount Sinai is chaired by David H. Adams, MD, the Marie-Josée and Henry R. Kravis Professor. Dr. Adams is a world-renowned mitral repair surgeon. Anelechi Anyanwu, MD, leads one of the largest ventricular assist device and heart transplant centers in the country. He is also an expert in complex and re-operative valve surgery. Paul Stelzer, MD, is a specialist in aortic root surgery whose experience with the Ross procedure is unmatched, exceeding 20 years and 500 cases. These leaders work in concert with other members of Mount Sinai Heart, which is under the direction of world-renowned cardiologist Valentin Fuster, MD, PhD, to deliver unparalleled possibilities for patients with cardiovascular disease.

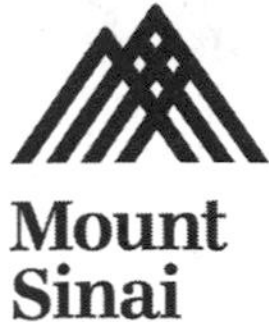

THE MOUNT SINAI MEDICAL CENTER

Mount Sinai Heart-Cardiovascular Health

One Gustave L. Levy Place
Fifth Avenue and 100th Street
New York, NY 10029-6574

Physician Referral: 1-800-MD-SINAI (637-4624)
www.mountsinai.org

At **MOUNT SINAI HEART**, our integrated system of care brings together the world's most accomplished physicians, research scientists, and educators who share the common goal of preventing and treating cardiovascular disease. **In 2013, *U.S. News & World Report* ranked our cardiology and heart surgery service 13th in the nation.**

With access to the latest discoveries and a diversity of the most experienced minds, our doctors ensure that patients receive the best individualized care. The rapid translation of innovative research into prevention, diagnosis, and therapy means that patients receive multidisciplinary treatment of unprecedented quality. Our programs treat patients of all ages – from the unborn fetus, well into the advanced elderly years.

We specialize in consultative cardiology, cardiac catheterization, heart and lung transplantation, cardiovascular surgery, heart failure, pulmonary hypertension, lipid management, and hypertension, as well as:

Noninvasive diagnostic imaging – We offer state-of-the-art echocardiography, nuclear cardiology, PET, CT, and MRI technology.

Coronary artery disease – We are ranked as New York State's safest and busiest center for coronary angioplasty and other catheter-based procedures. We lead many innovative device trials in the development phase before getting final approval for commercial use.

Cardiac rhythm disturbances – We manage all aspects of heart rhythm disorders under the auspices of pioneers in the field, including atrial fibrillation (AFib), the most common abnormal heart rhythm, and ventricular tachycardia, the most common cause of sudden cardiac death, as well as implantable devices, such as pacemakers and defibrillators.

Valvular heart disease – We deliver medical and surgical options, including a leading valve-repair program and long-term follow-up care. We are one of the few centers in the country to provide both types of percutaneous non-surgical aortic valves.

Aortic diseases – We pioneer and advance techniques for stent-graft repair of thoracic and abdominal aortic aneurysms and for surgical correction of the most complex aortic pathology.

Congenital heart disease – Our cardiologists offer minimally invasive approaches to the correction of congenital heart defects in children and adults.

Cardiac failure and transplantation – We take a multidisciplinary team approach to comprehensive, compassionate care for patients with the most advanced forms of heart failure and cardiomyopathy.

Comprehensive cardiac disease prevention and rehabilitation – Our unique synergy provides unparalleled superior patient care and breakthroughs in cardiovascular disease prevention and treatment, while promoting cardiovascular health globally through six projects around the world.

Vascular medicine and surgery – We offer an interdisciplinary approach to disease management, including medical, surgical, catheter-based, and gene therapy techniques for arterial obstruction, limb salvage, venous, and lymphatic diseases. A pioneer in large-artery stenting, Mount Sinai fostered the development of stenting of abdominal aortic aneurysms.

Mount Sinai's Cardiac Catheterization Laboratory – We study the heart with the most precise technologies available, including diagnostic angiography, angioplasty, and biopsy. In a statewide study, our Cath Lab was found to be the safest, with the lowest 30-day risk-adjusted mortality rate for percutaneous coronary intervention (angioplasty), as well as the busiest.

LEADING SURGEONS, UNPARALLELED POSSIBILITIES

Under the direction of internationally renowned cardiologist Valentin Fuster, MD, PhD, Mount Sinai Heart is recognized worldwide for expert evaluation, management, and prevention of cardiovascular disease through integrated patient care, education, and research. Mount Sinai Heart encompasses the Zena and Michael A. Wiener Cardiovascular Institute and the Marie-Josée and Henry R. Kravis Center for Cardiovascular Health at Mount Sinai, both preeminent resources for the study and treatment of heart and blood vessel diseases.

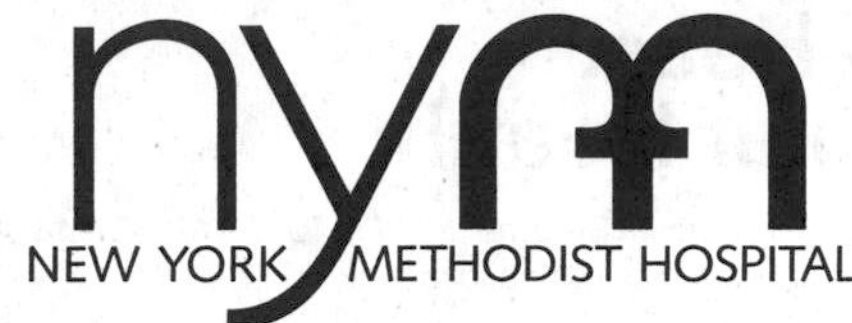

THE INSTITUTE FOR CARDIOLOGY AND CARDIAC SURGERY

New York Methodist Hospital
506 Sixth Street, Brooklyn, N.Y. 11215
Phone 866 84-HEART (866 844-3278)
http://www.nym.org

SPECIALISTS AND MEDICAL SERVICES

The Institute is the Hospital's program for the prevention, diagnosis and treatment of all types of heart disease. The Institute brings together a panel of specialists and a range of services in all areas related to cardiac disease. These services, which range from screening and diagnostic procedures to emergency and ongoing treatment for heart attacks and chronic heart disease, are provided at the Hospital's specialized laboratories and clinical units, on both an inpatient and outpatient basis. New York Methodist houses state-of-the-art diagnostic and surgical facilities, including three cardiac catheterization laboratories and the most modern cardiac surgery suite in the area. The Institute's staff of physicians includes specialists in all areas of cardiology, electrophysiology, interventional cardiology and cardiac surgery.

PROGRAMS OFFERED

The programs and services offered by the Institute include consultative services, a chest pain emergency center (located in the Emergency Department), diagnostic evaluation (including cardiac MRI) and medical treatment for heart disease, interventional cardiology procedures (angioplasty and stents), electrophysiology (pacemakers, implantable defibrillators, ablation, etc.) and cardiac surgery.

***

Referrals to the specialists or to cardiac programs and services can be made through an individual's primary care physician or requested directly through the Institute's referral service. More information (and on-line physician referral) is available at the Hospital's website, http://www.nym.org.

THE NEW YORK METHODIST-CORNELL HEART CENTER

The New York Methodist-Cornell Heart Center is one of only three programs approved to perform cardiac surgery in Brooklyn. It is staffed by physicians from the prestigious Weill Cornell Medical Center of NewYork-Presbyterian Hospital. The Center is located in a state-of-the-art cardiac surgery suite.

Procedures performed at the Center include coronary bypass surgery, off-pump bypass surgery, valve replacement and repair, thoracic aneurysm repair, minimally invasive cardiac surgery and bloodless heart surgery.

CARDIAC AND VASCULAR INSTITUTE

The Cardiac and Vascular Institute (CVI) at NYU Langone Medical Center continues to advance new techniques for repairing heart valves, curing heart rhythm disorders, and treating aortic diseases and congestive heart failure. We care for both adults and children. CVI is consistently ranked among the leading heart and heart surgery centers in *U.S. News & World Report's annual 'Best Hospitals'* rankings.

Cardiac Catheterization CVI offers superior catheter-based diagnosis and evaluation of cardiac health. Our laboratory provides a full range of procedures to evaluate, diagnose, and provide treatment options.

Cardiac Rehabilitation and Prevention The Joan and Joel Smilow Cardiopulmonary Rehabilitation and Prevention Center provides individualized treatment plans through NYU Langone's Rusk Rehabilitation, in a state-of-the-art and comfortable facility.

Cardiac Surgery NYU Langone is a nationally recognized leader in advanced surgical treatments for adult and congenital heart disease. We have world-renowned expertise in mitral valve repair, aortic valve replacement and aortic aneurysm repair, as well as specializing in high-risk and elderly patients.

Cardiology The Leon H. Charney Division of Cardiology is a leader in cardiovascular patient care, biomedical research, and education. We are advancing the field of cardiovascular medicine through a variety of innovative collaborations.

Congenital Heart Disease The pediatric and adult congenital cardiac program treats patients of all ages with inherited and acquired cardiac defects. We have a highly experienced team of specialists in pediatric and adult cardiology, pediatric interventional cardiology, congenital cardiac surgery, neonatal and pediatric cardiac intensive care, pediatric cardiac anesthesiology, nursing, and extracorporeal perfusion.

Heart Failure A multidisciplinary team offers the most advanced care for heart failure including echocardiograms, pacemaker and defibrillator implantations, open heart surgeries, and left ventricular assist devices.

Nuclear Cardiology/Stress The Nuclear Cardiology/Stress Laboratory performs a range of tests that assist cardiologists in the assessment and diagnosis of heart disease.

Vascular Surgery We offer diagnostic and treatment for patients with conditions ranging from arterial aneurysms to deep vein thrombosis, as well as carotid stenosis and limb salvage including minimally invasive vein surgery, endovascular aortic surgery, thoracic aneurysm correction and abdominal aneurysm interventions.

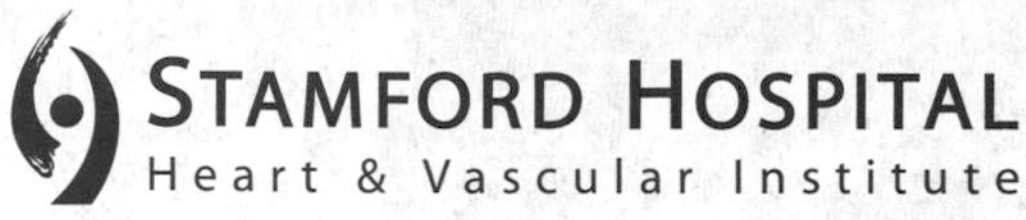

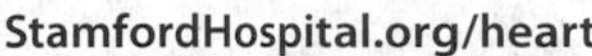

Heart and Vascular Institute

Stamford Hospital's Heart and Vascular Institute is the only comprehensive cardiovascular program to include open heart surgery and elective and primary angioplasty in lower Fairfield County. We offer the finest cardiac services, including cardiovascular screening, diagnostic services, advanced cardiac non-surgical and surgical treatment, cardiac rehabilitation and integrative services and wellness programs.

Nationally Recognized Critical Care Unit

Stamford Hospital's Critical Care Unit has been recognized as one of the best in the country and earned the prestigious, national Codman Award, from the Joint Commission, for development of a life-saving protocol.

Cardiac Catheterization

Our two state-of-the-art Cardiac Catheterization Labs enable diagnosis and treatment of heart conditions and emergency angioplasty to open blocked coronary arteries during heart attacks. Emergency and elective angioplasty are performed for the treatment of acute myocardial infarction (heart attack) and coronary blockages.

Electrophysiology Program

We have the most comprehensive Electrophysiology Program (EP) in lower Fairfield County. We diagnose and treat electrical rhythm disorders of the heart, and offer state-of-the-art diagnostic testing. We are equipped to perform the most complex EP procedures including atrial fibrillation. A new bi-plane lab (imaging which shows two dimensions instead of a flat, one dimensional view), opens in the winter of 2014, the only one of its kind in the area.

Open Heart Surgery

Our expert team is equipped to handle any emergent and non-emergent surgical issue including CABG, valve repairs and replacements and aneurysms using state-of-the-art surgical techniques.

Cardiac Rehabilitation

Located at the Tully Health Center, we help patients with heart disease recover faster and return to full, productive lives. Together with medical and surgical treatment, cardiac rehab includes exercise, education, counseling and behavioral change strategies that lead to a healthier life.

Integrative Cardiology and Wellness Programs

Offered through our Center for Integrative Medicine and Wellness, this program offers multiple lifestyle techniques to complement and support the treatment of heart disease.

Academic and Clinical Affiliations

Stamford Hospital is an affiliate of the New York–Presbyterian Healthcare System and a major teaching affiliate of the Columbia University College of Physicians & Surgeons.

Accreditation

Joint Commission on Accreditation of Healthcare Organization (JCAHO)

Beds

305

Sponsorship

Voluntary, Not-for-Profit

For a Physician Referral or more information, please call 1.877.233.9355 or visit StamfordHospital.org /doctor.

Stamford Hospital
30 Shelburne Road
Stamford, CT 06902
203.276.1000

StamfordHospital.org

259 First Street, Mineola, NY 11501
Tel: 1-866-WINTHROP
www.winthrop.org

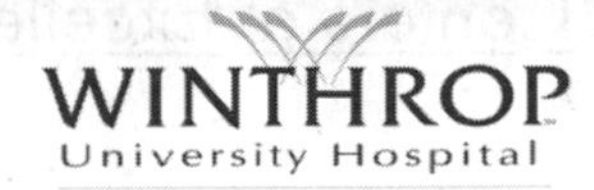

Your Health Means Everything.®

CARDIAC CARE AT WINTHROP-UNIVERSITY HOSPITAL

Winthrop-University Hospital offers a unique and comprehensive multifaceted approach to the prevention and treatment of cardiovascular disease. The program is made up of several centers of excellence, and the cardiovascular specialists of Winthrop-University Hospital bring each patient a focused and individualized level of care not accessible elsewhere.

Winthrop's highly skilled and experienced cardiologists, cardiothoracic surgeons, specialized nurses, physician assistants, cardiology fellows and cardiovascular technologists provide patients and their primary care physicians with a wide range of sophisticated services - including access to consistently outstanding interventional cardiology, cardiac surgery, state-of-the-art computerized diagnostic cardiac catheterization procedures and expert drug-eluding stent placement - as well as innovative electrophysiology used to evaluate and treat all types of heart-rhythm disturbances with the latest generation of implantable electronic devices and pacemakers.

The Pacemaker/Arrhythmia Center

The Pacemaker/Arrhythmia Center at Winthrop is a state-of-the-art facility that offers cutting-edge services with highly skilled clinical cardiac electrophysiologists who specialize in the entire range of heart rhythm diagnostic and herapeutic procedures. The Center offers both inpatient and outpatient services.

Physicians at Winthrop were the first on Long Island to offer a new therapy for patients with Paroxysmal Atrial Fibrillation (PAF) – the Arctic Front® Cardiac CryoAblation Catheter system, the first and only cryoballoon in the United States indicated to treat certain cases of PAF. Approved by the U.S. Food and Drug Administration, the cryoballoon treatment involves a minimally-invasive procedure that efficiently uses freezing to scar or kill the tissue that is causing the erratic electrical signals that cause the irregular heartbeat.

The Women's Cardiovascular Wellness and Prevention Center

Winthrop's Women's Cardiovascular Wellness and Prevention Center is a comprehensive prevention, treatment and recovery 'patient- centric' program designed for those women with cardiovascular disease or at risk for such. The Center provides a full complement of cardiac and wellness services for women, including fitness referrals, patient education, medical screening and counseling.

Thoracic Aortic Vascular Treatment Center

In early 2012, Winthrop became one of only approximately 70 centers in the United States to offer the FDA-approved Edwards Sapien Transcathether Heart Valve (TAVR), one of the newest techniques that allows a heart valve to be replaced without open-heart surgery. Surgeons insert a catheter into an artery in the groin, pass a thin wire through the catheter with the new valve attached, and install the new valve from the inside. Percutaneous valve replacement has proven especially helpful for elderly patients who are not candidates for open-heart surgery. Winthrop is now perhaps the most active TAVR program in the country, and is part of the Partner 2 as well as Partner 3 trial, where it is one of the only 20 centers in the nation.

Hypertrophic Cardiomyopathy Treatment Center

Winthrop-University Hospital's Hypertrophic Cardiomyopathy (HCM) Treatment Center — one of the nation's handful of comprehensive, nationally accredited resources for HCM and the only one on Long Island — treats hundreds of patients and families from the tri-state area and beyond, offering expert, specialized services that address all facets of the disease. The HCM Center is recognized as a national center of excellence by the National Hypertrophic Cardiomyopathy Association.

Child & Adolescent Psychiatry

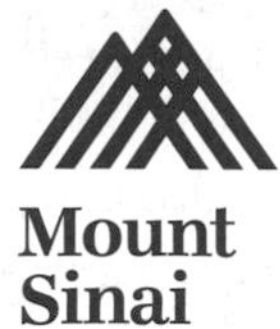

THE MOUNT SINAI MEDICAL CENTER

Division of Child and Adolescent Psychiatry

One Gustave L. Levy Place
Fifth Avenue and 100th Street
New York, NY 10029-6574

Physician Referral: 1-800-MD-SINAI (637-4624)
www.mountsinai.org

Ambulatory Services: The Child, Adolescent and Family Services (CAFS), part of Mount Sinai's Ambulatory Psychiatry Service and certified by the New York State Office of Mental Health, provides outpatient clinic treatment for children and adolescents (from birth through age 18) and their families. The services we offer include:

- Comprehensive evaluation
- Individual, group, and family therapy
- Parent training and support
- Pharmacologic evaluation and ongoing medication management
- Case management services
- Crisis intervention

The CAFS mission is threefold: we provide advanced, accessible clinical care, serve as a training site for educating future child mental health professionals, and advance the field of child and adolescent psychiatry through research. As part of this mission, we make compassionate, comprehensive clinical care accessible to a diverse population of youths and their families with the aim of alleviating symptoms of emotional disturbance and allowing children and adolescents to remain in their natural environments.

We achieve clinical excellence through our use of innovative treatment approaches informed by scientific study and by creating an individualized continuum of care that incorporates the clinical, social and cultural characteristics of the patient and family. We understand that each family has unique strengths, values and goals, and that the best outcomes are possible when families and caregivers are active participants in their child's treatment.

INPATIENT SERVICES

We offer comprehensive evaluation and treatment for a variety of emotional and behavioral problems, including mood disorders, anxiety disorders, psychotic disorders, severe disruptive behavior disorders, such as attention-deficit disorder and conduct disturbances, eating disorders, post-traumatic stress disorder and potential suicide.

SPECIALTY SERVICES

The Division of Child and Adolescent Psychiatry has a prominent role in several of the departmental centers of excellence, including the Seaver Autism Center, ADHD Center, Eating and Weight Disorders Center, Pediatric Mood and Anxiety Disorders Program, OCD Center of Excellence, and the Tics and TD Clinical and Research Program. Each of these programs offer specialty diagnosis and treatment services, and most see patients across their lifespan.

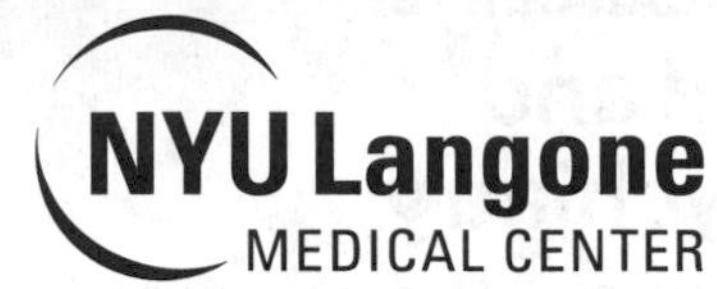

550 First Avenue *(at 31st Street)*
New York, NY 10016

www.NYULMC.org

Hassenfeld Children's Hospital Access Line: **855-NYU-KIDS**

HASSENFELD CHILDREN'S HOSPITAL

Hassenfeld Children's Hospital (HCH) is a full-service specialty children's hospital encompassing all children's health services at NYU Langone Medical Center. At HCH, newborns, children, adolescents and young adults receive the most comprehensive and advanced care possible from a team of pediatricians and pediatric specialists across more than 30 medical and surgical disciplines. With more than 150 full-time pediatric specialists, as well as pediatric nurses, child life specialists and social workers, Hassenfeld Children's Hospital is uniquely equipped to provide innovative pediatric subspecialty care in a highly personalized manner.

A Family-Centered Approach

Integral to the care we provide is a myriad of support services for children and their families. We recognize that the best outcomes are achieved when the child's family is actively involved in every step of care. For that reason, our trained specialists address the needs of not just the patient, but of parents and siblings through ongoing education and communication.

Our pediatric specialties include:

Anesthesia
Cardiology
Cardiothoracic Surgery
Child and Adolescent Psychiatry and Psychology/Child Study Center
Critical Care
Dermatology
Developmental and Behavioral Pediatrics
Emergency Medicine
Endocrinology
Epilepsy
Gastroenterology
Genetics
Hematology/Oncology
Infectious Diseases
Neonatology
Nephrology
Neurosurgery
Ophthalmology
Orthopaedic Surgery
Otolaryngology
Pathology
Pulmonology
Radiology
Reconstructive Plastic Surgery
Rehabilitation
Rheumatology
Surgery
Urology

The Best in American Medicine
www.CastleConnolly.com

Child Neurology

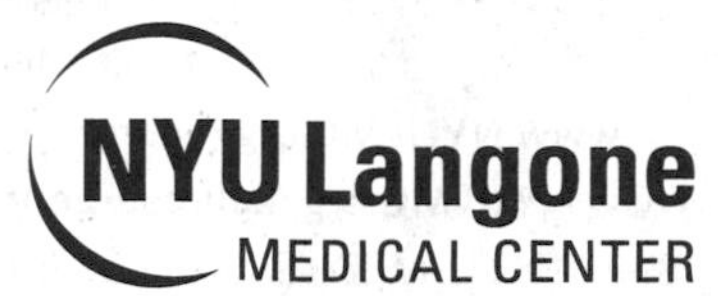

550 First Avenue *(at 31st Street)*
New York, NY 10016
www.NYULMC.org/neurology
www.NYULMC.org/neurosurgery
Physician Referral: **888-7-NYU-MED** *(888-769-8633)*

NEUROLOGY & NEUROSURGERY

NYU Langone Medical Center's Departments of Neurology and Neurosurgery continue to be **ranked among the nation's top 10 in the 2013-2014 U.S. News & World Report's annual survey of "Best Hospitals" in America.**

Patients travel from around the world to consult our renowned specialists for their expertise in the care, treatment, and research of neurological diseases and disorders of the brain, spine and nervous system. These conditions range from migraine headaches, nerve and muscle problems, pain, autism, movement disorders and Alzheimer's disease to stroke, vascular disorders, epilepsy, multiple sclerosis and brain tumors. NYU Langone is home to one of the largest epilepsy centers in the United States, as well as the largest multiple sclerosis program in New York and the first primary stroke center established in New York City.

Neurological Expertise

Autonomic Diseases: Our specialized Center evaluates and treats children and adults with familial dysautonomia and other inherited or acquired autonomic nervous system diseases, including orthostatic hypotension and rare forms of hereditary sensory neuropathy.
Epilepsy: Our Level 4 Comprehensive Epilepsy Center offers the most advanced medical and surgical options. Complementary management approaches complete the comprehensive care plan.
Multiple Sclerosis: The Comprehensive MS Care Center provides state-of-the-art diagnostic evaluations and follow-up care and management.
Neurogenetics: We focus on inherited diseases of the nervous system. Services include diagnosis and management of inherited diseases, biochemical and molecular testing and genetic counseling.
Neuro-oncology: In partnership with the NYU Cancer Institute, our multidisciplinary Brain Tumor Center is one of the nation's leading brain and spinal cord tumor programs, including physicians highly experienced in neuro-oncology, neurosurgery and neuroradiology.
Neuromuscular Diseases: We offer multidisciplinary programs for neuromuscular diseases, including acquired peripheral neuropathy, Charcot Marie Tooth neuropathy, myasthenia gravis, amyotrophic lateral sclerosis, spinal muscular atrophy, post-polio syndrome, muscular dystrophy and Lyme neuroborreliosis.
Parkinson's Disease and Movement Disorders: Our specialized center helps individuals affected by Parkinson's or other movement disorders to achieve the highest possible quality of life. Experts are also available to offer functional neurosurgery for certain conditions that involve involuntary muscle contractions.

(continued)

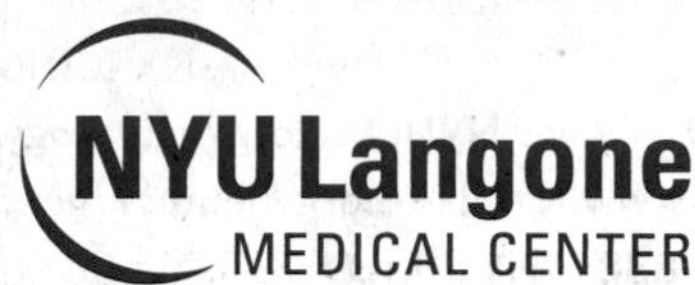

550 First Avenue *(at 31st Street)*
New York, NY 10016
www.NYULMC.org/neurology
www.NYULMC.org/neurosurgery
Physician Referral: **888-7-NYU-MED** *(888-769-8633)*

NEUROLOGY & NEUROSURGERY *(continued)*

Stroke Care: The multidisciplinary, Comprehensive Stroke Care Center provides rapid diagnosis, effective intervention and early rehabilitation for individuals who have had a stroke.
Concussion Center: This multidisciplinary center is a collaborative effort between the Departments of Neurology, Orthopaedic Surgery, and Rehabilitation, providing expert evaluation and treatment of individuals who have or are suspected of having a concussion.

Neurosurgical Expertise

The Department of Neurosurgery at NYU Langone Medical Center offers some of the nation's most skilled and experienced surgeons and advanced, minimally invasive procedures. Patients also benefit from cutting-edge research and a fully integrated approach to medical care.
Brain Tumor: Our neurosurgeons specialize in both malignant and benign brain tumors, including skull base tumors. Expertise includes glioblastoma, ependymoma, hemangioblastoma, other gliomas, meningiomas and vestibular schwannomas (acoustic neuromas).
Cerebrovascular Surgery: The Division of Cerebrovascular Surgery is a premier center for brain aneurysms, giant intracranial aneurysms, brain vascular malformations and cavernomas, and stroke.
Spinal Neurosurgery: The Division of Spine Surgery provides treatment for degenerative spinal diseases, spinal tumors, spinal trauma and spinal infections.
Neuromodulation: This specialized center offers deep brain stimulation (DBS) for Parkinson's, essential tremor, dystonia and obsessive-compulsive disorder, as well as peripheral neurostimulation (PNS) for migraines and other headaches and various types of facial pain.
Hyperhidrosis: The Department offers expertise in the surgical treatment of primary hyperhidrosis (excessive sweating) including Endoscopic Thoracic Sympathectomy.
Neurosurgical Technology: Our neurosurgeons remove deep-seated tumors, vascular malformations and other disease sites using a highly advanced Gamma Knife. Aided by 3-D MRI technology, the Gamma Knife bombards its target with precise doses of radiation, while preserving healthy tissue.

Other Neurosurgical Services

- Facial Pain: provides patients a thorough examination and, if required, nerve injections and minimally invasive surgery.
- Pediatric Neurosurgery: provides treatment to children with brain and spinal cord tumors, congenital and development disorders.
- Peripheral Nerve Surgery: focuses on the diagnosis and treatment of nerve compressions, nerve tremors, Brachial Plexus (nerve fiber) and nerve injuries.
- Neuro-Critical Care: our experts provide care for patients who have an urgent neuro-surgical problem that requires careful monitoring, or is at risk for developing such a problem.

The Best in American Medicine
www.CastleConnolly.com

Clinical Genetics

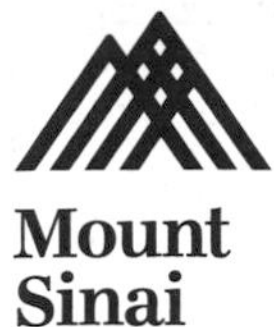

THE MOUNT SINAI MEDICAL CENTER

Genetics and Genomic Sciences

One Gustave L. Levy Place
Fifth Avenue and 100th Street
New York, NY 10029-6574

Physician Referral: 1-800-MD-SINAI (637-4624)
www.mountsinai.org

THE DEPARTMENT OF GENETICS AND GENOMIC SCIENCES at The Mount Sinai Medical Center is one of the largest medical genetics centers in the nation, providing expert diagnostic, therapeutic, and counseling services for patients and families with or at risk for genetics disorders or birth defects. The department performs sophisticated diagnostic tests in its state-of-the-art molecular, biochemical, and cytogenetics laboratories, which are New York State and Clinical Laboratory Improvement Amendments (CLIA) licensed, and certified by the College of American Pathologists (CAP).

The department has more than 50 internationally recognized faculty members, including physicians, counselors, and laboratory geneticists who are certified by the American Board of Medical Genetics or the American Board of Genetic Counseling.

Programs and services offered by the department include:

- Clinical Genetic Disorders Program
- Program for Inherited Metabolic Diseases
- Reproductive Genetic Counseling Program
- Cancer Genetic Counseling Program
- Mount Sinai Center for Jewish Genetic Diseases
- International Center for Fabry Disease
- Mount Sinai Comprehensive Gaucher Disease Treatment Center
- Porphyria Comprehensive Diagnostic and Treatment Center
- Congenital Anomalies and Craniofacial Program
- Cardiovascular Genetics Program
- Niemann Pick Disease Center

GROUNDBREAKING RESEARCH AND NEW FORMS OF TREATMENT

There are more than 10,000 known genetic disorders, and current research is identifying the genetic susceptibilities and causative genes for many of these diseases. The faculty of the Department of Genetics and Genomic Sciences at Mount Sinai is performing research to develop new and improved methods for the diagnosis, prevention, and treatment of rare and common diseases. The Human Genome Project, and advances in gene analysis technology and stem cell biology, have accelerated this research.

Advances In Diagnosis And Disease Treatment – In the past several years, Mount Sinai researchers have identified genes responsible for various genetic diseases and developed new treatments for inherited disorders. The following are some examples and results of this important work:

- We have identified genes involved in over a dozen diseases, most recently a debilitating juvenile arthritis, several dystonias, and an inherited form of obesity. The identification of these genes leads to precise diagnosis, understanding disease pathogenesis, and new treatments for these diseases. We have also recently identified a gene linked to prostate cancer.

- Our researchers helped identify eight genes involved in causing Noonan syndrome, a common genetic disorder that causes congenital heart defects. Affected families can now receive early diagnosis and prevention.

- Research pioneered by the Department of Genetics and Genomic Sciences resulted in the development of a safe, effective, FDA-approved treatment for Fabry disease, an inherited metabolic disorder that can cause kidney failure, heart disease, stroke, and premature death.

- Departmental faculty have developed a treatment for Niemann-Pick Type B disease, a hereditary disorder that results in death in childhood or early adulthood.

Colon & Rectal Surgery

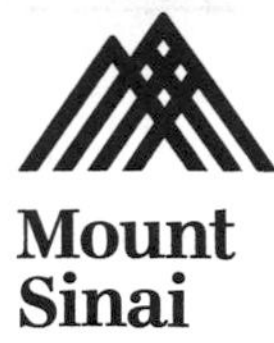

THE MOUNT SINAI MEDICAL CENTER
THE TISCH CANCER INSTITUTE

Colon and Rectal Cancer

One Gustave L. Levy Place
Fifth Avenue and 100th Street
New York, NY 10029-6574

Physician Referral: 1-800-MD-SINAI (637-4624)
www.mountsinai.org

At The Mount Sinai Medical Center's **TISCH CANCER INSTITUTE**, we employ a level of expertise found at only a few medical centers. Our proficiency in delivering the most advanced patient care, pursuing clinical breakthroughs and training tomorrow's specialists is evident in the fact that *U.S. News & World Report* continues to rate us among the best cancer programs and the top medical schools in the country.

Highly skilled in all aspects of colon and rectal cancer, from screening and diagnosis to treatment and follow-up, our experts work with the most advanced technology and take a comprehensive, patient-centered approach to care. Our multidisciplinary team includes medical, surgical and radiation oncologists, radiologists, clinical investigators, specialized nurses, dietitians, and social workers– all dedicated to delivering the best possible care to our patients.

Our specialists who treat colon and rectal cancer include those who concentrate on GI (gastrointestinal) cancers, those who specialize in IBD (inflammatory bowel disease), and those who excel in the resection of colon tumors and metastatic disease in the liver. Our thoracic surgeons are skilled in operating on metastatic colon or rectal cancer that has spread to the lungs, and, although most colon and rectal cancer patients are over the age of 50, we also see younger patients who need specialized, aggressive therapy. We have also have one of the country's largest program utilizing stereotactic body radiation therapy to deliver pinpoint high dose radiation to destroy tumors in the liver.

Our physician-scientists are engaged in a broad range of clinical and basic cancer research initiatives, which can ultimately lead to better cancer prevention, detection and treatment. For these reasons, we remain at the cutting-edge of science and can offer patients access to the newest therapies through clinical trials.

At Mount Sinai, we know that the addressing the complexity of cancer issues requires the highest degree of expert, specialized care. At the same time, we remain focused on a simple guiding principle—to treat the entire person, not just his or her cancer. Patients and their families find that our specialists, range of services, and compassionate approach make Mount Sinai a strong and able ally in their fight against cancer.

Dermatology

THE MOUNT SINAI MEDICAL CENTER
Dermatology

One Gustave L. Levy Place
Fifth Avenue and 100th Street
New York, NY 10029-6574

Physician Referral: 1-800-MD-SINAI (637-4624)
www.mountsinai.org

The Mount Sinai **DEPARTMENT OF DERMATOLOGY** has one of the most comprehensive programs for skin health and the treatment of skin diseases in the nation. In addition to our offices at Mount Sinai Hospital, the department has satellite offices throughout New York City.

Skin Cancer
Our department is at the forefront of research in the treatment and prevention of skin cancer. Our Mohs surgeons, Drs. Hooman Khorasani and David Kriegel perform state-of-the-art surgical treatment and repairs for all types of skin cancer.

Dr. Orit Markowitz uses new imaging techniques for the early diagnosis and prevention of melanoma. We are one of the few dermatology departments with optical coherence tomography (OCT) technology, Molemax technology and Melafind systems. The latter devices are useful for evaluating non-melanoma skin cancers and pigmented lesions and for following and diagnosing melanoma.

Drs. Czernik, Goldenberg, Goldstein, Lamb, Lebwohl, Levitt, Markowitz, Shim-Chang, and Zeichner have expertise in the diagnosis, prevention, and treatment of all skin cancers and have developed many of the treatments currently in use to prevent and treat cancerous and precancerous skin lesions. We also treat one of the largest groups of patients with cutaneous T-cell lymphoma.

General Dermatology
Psoriasis:
Our faculty number among the country's leading experts in psoriasis, including our Department Chairman, Dr. Mark Lebwohl, and Drs. Norman Goldstein, Gary Goldenberg, Jacob Levitt, Annette Czernik and Angela Lamb. Our center includes a state-of- the-art phototherapy unit, an infusion center for intravenous treatments, an excimer laser therapy unit, and a research center where many new therapies available for psoriasis are tested.

Autoimmune and inflammatory skin diseases:
We have one of the largest centers for inflammatory skin diseases where we treat psoriasis, atopic dermatitis and contact dermatitis. Dr. Emma Guttman is doing clinical research in new targeted therapies for severe atopic dermatitis. Dr. Suhail Hadi is one of the most experienced in the use of the excimer laser for psoriasis and vitiligo. Our faculty also includes three renowned acne experts, Drs. Angela Lamb, Joshua Zeichner, and Susan Bershad.

Our bullous disease center is run by Drs. Jacob Levitt and Annette Czernik. We are one of the few dermatology departments in the nation with its own infusion unit, so patients may be treated either as outpatients in the infusion unit or as inpatients at The Mount Sinai Medical Center.

Pediatric and Adolescent Dermatology
Our faculty treats all ages for skin. Dr. Susan Bershad is a board-certified pediatric and adolescent dermatologist. Dr. Lauren Geller is trained in pediatrics and in pediatric dermatology and is board-certified in dermatology. Dr. Emma Guttman is a trailblazer in research on atopic dermatitis and other forms of eczema.

Cosmetic Dermatology Center
We were one of the first programs in the nation to have a procedural dermatology fellowship, which is run by Drs. David Kriegel and Hooman Khorasani. Along with Drs. Marsha Gordon, Heidi Waldorf, Gary Goldenberg, Joshua Zeichner, and Helen Shim-Chang, our team is renowned for noninvasive skin rejuvenation combining topical regimens, soft tissue fillers, botulinum toxin, photodynamic therapy and laser and radio frequency devices. Members of our faculty perform liposuction, blepharoplasty, microdermabrasion, laser hair removal, sclerotherapy, skin tightening procedures, laser removals of tattoos, and pigmented and vascular lesions as well as laser resurfacing such as fraxel and total Fx.

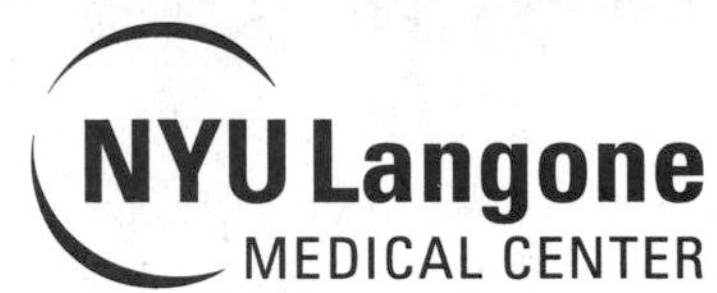

550 First Avenue *(at 31st Street)*
New York, NY 10016

www.NYULMC.org

Physician Referral: **888-7-NYU-MED** *(888-769-8633)*

DERMATOLOGY

The Ronald O. Perelman Department of Dermatology is a national and international leader in dermatology, employing the most advanced science and medicine to diagnose and treat skin disorders. The Department provides high-quality dermatologic care and conducts research into some of the most significant dermatologic problems. We also collaborate with experts from The Cancer Institute at NYU Langone. Services include adult and pediatric medical dermatology, dermatologic/skin cancer surgery and cosmetic dermatology. We specialize in the following areas:

Dermatologic / Skin Cancer Surgery and Cosmetic Dermatology

NYU Langone Medical Center's dermatologists provide specialized care for the treatment of malignant and benign skin lesions and offer cutting-edge therapies for aesthetic and cosmetic concerns.

General Dermatology

Dermatologic associates offer multi-subspecialty dermatology care in private office settings for patients with disorders of the skin, hair, and nails, including inflammatory skin diseases such as psoriasis and lupus, cancers and other skin tumors, hair loss, infections and allergic skin diseases such as eczema, contact dermatitis and hives.

Pediatric and Adolescent Dermatology

The Medical Center also boasts a specialized professional practice dedicated to the treatment of diseases affecting the skin, hair, and nails of infants, children and adolescents. These disorders include acne, atopic dermatitis/eczema, hair loss, hemangiomas, moles, birthmarks, vitiligo and genetic disorders affecting the skin.

Charles C. Harris Skin and Cancer Unit / Dermatology Clinical Trials Unit

The Charles C. Harris Skin and Cancer Unit at the Ambulatory Care Center is an outpatient dermatology teaching center combining unique patient care with superior medical education. Resident and attending physicians provide diagnosis and treatment of skin diseases that include acne, eczema and warts as well as complex medical conditions such as connective tissue disorders, pigmented lesions, skin allergies and skin cancers.

Dermatopathology

Highly trained dermatopathologists at the Medical Center examine skin tissues submitted by physicians from biopsies and surgeries to diagnose skin diseases and malignancies. One of the busiest academic skin pathology units in the country, the Dermatopathology section of the Department also provides consultative services for the review of skin pathology specimens performed elsewhere.

The Best in American Medicine
www.CastleConnolly.com

Diabetes Management/ Wound Care

THE MOUNT SINAI MEDICAL CENTER

The Mount Sinai Diabetes Center

One Gustave L. Levy Place
Fifth Avenue and 100th Street
New York, NY 10029-6574

Physician Referral: 1-800-MD-SINAI (637-4624)
www.mountsinai.org

THE MOUNT SINAI DIABETES CENTER is recognized as an American Diabetes Association "Center of Excellence," and, according to the 2013-2014 "Best Hospitals" edition of *U.S. News & World Report,* ranks among the top programs of its kind in the United States.

As a leader in our field and as part of a world-class academic medical center, we provide highly specialized, state-of-the-art care for people with diabetes and related disorders. We help patients prevent complications by teaching them to take control of their health so they will live well and thrive.

Our Motto: Prevent. Control. Thrive.

We deliver comprehensive, patient-centered care to people with type 1, type 2, gestational (pregnancy related) diabetes, and related disorders. Our team of specialized physicians, registered dieticians, nurse practitioners, and certified diabetes educators work together using state-of-the-art clinical therapies and the latest research to create an individualized treatment program for each patient. In addition, we partner with our patients' primary care providers and specialist care team to ensure they receive the most thorough care possible.

Diabetes is a serious, chronic condition and the possibility of severe complications should not be taken lightly. Our personalized treatment plans help patients manage their condition and lower their risk for dangerous – even life-threatening – complications such as eye-damage (retinopathy), kidney damage (nephropathy), nerve damage (neuropathy), foot problems and cardiovascular disease, just to name a few.

Comprehensive, Multidisciplinary Treatment

We create the best treatment plan for each patient based on age, lifestyle, overall health, type of diabetes and other chronic conditions. We also consult with our colleagues from neurology, ophthalmology, podiatry, vascular surgery, nephrology, cardiology, internal medicine, urology, surgery and other specialties as needed.

The care we deliver to patients is only one side of the equation; the other is empowering them to control their condition. We offer self-management training in meal planning, physical activities, oral and injectable medications, and, if needed, various forms of insulin therapy. Many patients who are initially overwhelmed by their diabetes diagnosis find support when they come to our free diabetes classes.

We routinely treat patients using the latest technological developments and are constantly performing research into diabetes and related endocrine disorders, thus offering opportunities for our patients unlike many others. All our work as researchers, clinicians, and educators has but one goal: to make everyday life better for our patients – every single day of the year.

Diagnostic Radiology

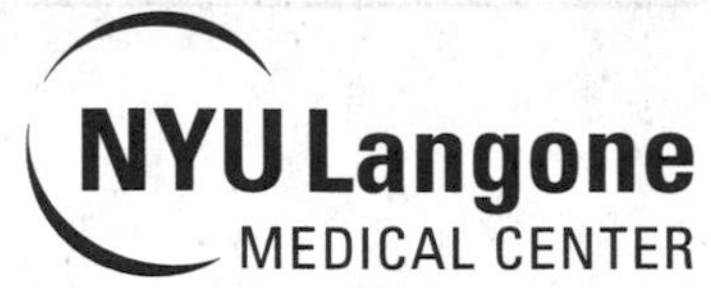

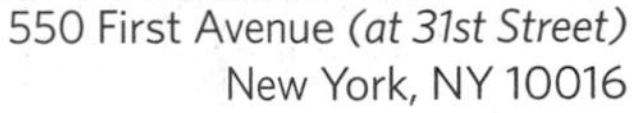

550 First Avenue *(at 31st Street)*
New York, NY 10016

www.NYULMC.org

Physician Referral: **888-7-NYU-MED** *(888-769-8633)*

RADIOLOGY

NYU Langone Radiology is committed to capturing the best images possible with the lowest dose of radiation. As an academic medical center, our radiologists are in a unique position to take the lead in helping to define and advance radiology in today's rapidly evolving technological environment.

Expertise

NYU Langone Medical Center's board certified radiologists and licensed technologists specialize in imaging and are involved in a variety of innovative collaborations and research initiatives. The Department consists of more than 100 sub-specialized academic radiologists, many of them acknowledged leaders and innovators in their fields.

Advanced Technology

NYU Langone uses some of the most advanced imaging equipment in the world, including high and ultra high-field MRI imaging systems (known as 1.5T and 3T magnets). MRI scanners are shorter and wider than ever, making for a more patient-friendly experience. The Center for Biomedical Imaging, an advanced research facility, features a powerful 7T magnet.

Recognition for Safety and Quality

We continually follow a rigorous set of quality standards and maintain accreditation by the American College of Radiology (ACR). Designated by the ACR as a "Breast Imaging Center of Excellence", our team maintains high practice standards in image quality, personnel qualifications, facility equipment, quality control procedures and quality assurance programs.

Patient Focused Approach

We are located in Manhattan, Brooklyn, Queens, and Long Island and participate in many insurance plans. Timely delivery of reports and images allow physicians to view patient exam status, reports and images online. In addition to our convenient hours, weekend, evening and often same-day appointments are available. Language interpretation services are available as needed.

Our Areas of Specialization

Diagnostic services include MRI, CT, ultrasound, PET/CT, X-ray, interventional radiology and nuclear medicine. Sub-specialized radiologists provide diagnostic interpretation in abdominal, biomedical, breast, cardiac, chest, emergency, general, musculoskeletal, neuroradiology, neuro interventional, nuclear medicine, pediatric, vascular interventional, and women's imaging. Specialty procedures include coronary artery disease and virtual colonoscopy screening, stereotactic biopsy capability, minimally invasive techniques including radiofrequency ablation, chemoembolization, radioimmunotherapy, and bone densitometry.

Emergency Services

For more information about the Emergency Care Center or for a physician referral, call 1-877-HOLY-NAME. Please mention "Castle Connolly Guide."

Holy Name Medical Center
Emergency Care Center

718 Teaneck Road
Teaneck, NJ 07666
1-877-HOLY-NAME
(1-877-465-9626)
www.holyname.org

Holy Name Medical Center's George P. Pitkin MD Emergency Care Center is an ultramodern facility that combines an experienced, specialized staff with today's best practices in health care and the highest industry standards for a superior care experience. Accommodating more than 55,000 visits per year, Holy Name's emergency division offers a physical space engineered for efficiency, comfort and privacy, and a care delivery system focused on quality and patient satisfaction.

The Center is staffed by board-certified emergency medicine physicians, physician assistants, nurse practitioners and registered nurses with certification in emergency nursing. In the Pediatric Fast Track, on-site board-certified pediatricians and specialized pediatric nurses provide safe, compassionate care, private rooms and a kid-friendly atmosphere to ensure that a visit to Holy Name's ER is as positive an experience as possible.

Designated by the State of New Jersey as a Medical Coordination Center for large-scale emergency preparedness—the only one in Bergen County—Holy Name's Emergency Care Center is able to manage any mass casualty situation, and has special accommodations and procedures in place for decontamination and radiation detection.

EMERGENCY RESPONDERS IN THE COMMUNITY

Holy Name Medical Center (HNMC) provides pre–Medical Center life support services to our surrounding communities. The first Medical Center–based Basic Life Support (BLS) provider in Bergen County, HNMC also supplies Mobile Intensive Care Units staffed by emergency medical technicians and paramedics trained in CPR, cardiac life support, trauma life support, incident command, HAZMAT and CBRNE (chemical, biological, radiological, nuclear and explosive) response.

Holy Name is the only hospital in the area bringing the Hybrid Ambulance to the community, combining advanced life support (ALS) and basic life support (BLS) in a single mobile intensive care unit. The Medical Center's Special Operations unit provides support to mass-gathering events, patient rescue and all-terrain transport, and EMS branch communications.

To further its commitment to the community it serves, Holy Name EMS professionals also offer emergency medical training for first responders, EMTs, paramedics and other emergency service personnel.

Awards and Accreditations

- Top Performer on Key Quality Measures—from The Joint Commission for excellence in heart attack, heart failure, pneumonia and surgical care
- Magnet Recognition—from the American Nurses Credentialing Center for excellence in patient care
- High-Performing Hospital—from NJ Department of Health for providing "the correct care" for heart attack, heart failure, pneumonia and surgical patients
- Beacon Award for Critical Care Excellence® —from the American Association of Critical-Care Nurses (AACN)
- Primary Stroke Care Certification—from The Joint Commission for excellence in stroke patient care

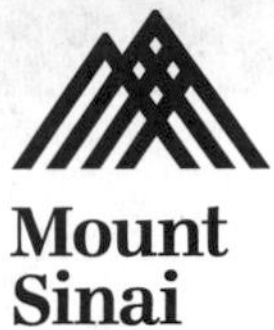

THE MOUNT SINAI MEDICAL CENTER
Emergency Medicine

One Gustave L. Levy Place
Fifth Avenue and 100th Street
New York, NY 10029-6574

Physician Referral: 1-800-MD-SINAI (637-4624)
www.mountsinai.org

The Mount Sinai Medical Center's **DEPARTMENT OF EMERGENCY MEDICINE** delivers the highest level care to more than 100,000 patients a year, offering rapid diagnosis and superior care for the complete array of emergency medical conditions. Patients requiring admission can take comfort knowing that Mount Sinai ranks 14th out of nearly 5,000 hospitals nationwide evaluated by *U.S. News & World Report* staff and holds a spot on the publication's "honor roll" of elite hospitals.

The Department of Emergency Medicine is:

- An officially-designated New York City Department of Emergency Services 911-ambulance receiving hospital.
- A New York State Department of Health-designated primary stroke center and the first Joint Commission-certified primary stroke center in Manhattan.
- A New York State approved hypothermia center for cardiac arrest patients.
- An internationally renowned heart center and a recipient of New York State's highest safety rating for angioplasty for 15 consecutive years.
- Ranked in the top 10 NIH funded emergency departments; An innovator in emergency care and a leader in cutting-edge initiatives to improve quality and services.

Staffed by physicians who are board certified in emergency medicine and award-winning specialty trained nurses, we offer:

- New York City's first emergency department with a separate area created and designed exclusively for geriatric patients.
- Pediatric emergency services, located separate from our adult emergency department and delivered by physicians who are board-certified in pediatric emergency medicine.
- A comprehensive approach to the evaluation and management of critically ill patients to ensure a continuum of high quality care from the emergency department to the Intensive Care Unit.
- Advanced diagnostic equipment, including bedside ultrasound for rapid assessment of basic cardiac function, abdominal pain, and thoracic disorders and to assist in bedside procedures.
- Award-winning and fully implemented electronic medical records, including computerized physician order entry, evidence-based clinical decision support, charting and results retrieval, as well as integration with clinics and inpatient units and health information exchange with participating metropolitan-area hospitals.
- A well-integrated toxicology division staffed by physicians dual boarded in emergency medicine and toxicology that provides bedside consultation service, offering care for a wide scope of clinical poisonings including drug overdoses, drug interactions, and toxic environmental exposures.

The Best in American Medicine
www.CastleConnolly.com

Endocrinology, Diabetes & Metabolism

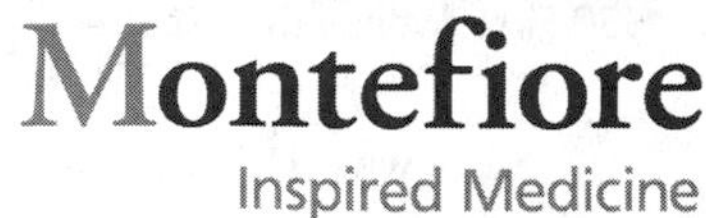

111 East 210th Street
Bronx, New York 10467
1-866-MED-TALK
www.montefiore.org/endocrinology

Clinical Diabetes Center at Montefiore

Diabetes affects more than 14 percent of the Bronx population—a percentage that is among the largest in New York and the nation. Montefiore's commitment to addressing this growing statistic and improving the health of the community has led to unrivaled investments in educational programs, research and outreach.

Montefiore's Clinical Diabetes Center, nationally recognized by *U.S. News & World Report* and designated by the New York Department of Health as a Diabetes Center of Excellence, provides comprehensive care for adults and children with diabetes (types 1 and 2) and endocrine disease. The Center boasts more than 50 full-time endocrinologists supported by a team of 24 dedicated diabetes nurse practitioners—two-thirds of whom are also certified diabetes educators. Together, they emphasize early intervention and ongoing care in both the inpatient and outpatient settings. This includes all three of Montefiore's hospital campuses and 20 integrated primary care clinics in the Bronx, Westchester County and surrounding areas.

Through the **Proactive Managed Information System for Education in Diabetes (PROMISED©),** a multi-site, outpatient diabetes self-management program, the Center is teaching patients how to improve their health through diet and medication, use their insulin pumps and monitor their glucose. PROMISED is nationally recognized by the American Diabetes Association (ADA) for exemplary performance and consistently surpassing national standards.

The Center's Diabetes Disease Management Program is composed of a multidisciplinary team that provides education and works with primary care physicians to coordinate care for those dealing with associated health issues, such as wounds and kidney failure. Telephone monitoring helps select patients keep their diabetes under control.

The Children's Hospital at Montefiore (CHAM) is home to one of only a handful of ADA-recognized pediatric endocrinology programs in New York. Here, diabetes specialists supplement superior clinical care with pioneering research. A prominent example is the Program's National Institutes of Health–funded work to develop an artificial pancreas that provides automated glucose measurement and insulin delivery. Educational events, such as a "Day of Education at the Bronx Zoo" help children in the community learn about healthy eating.

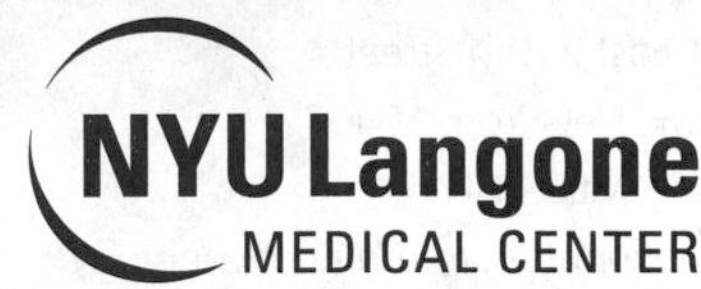

550 First Avenue *(at 31st Street)*
New York, NY 10016
www.NYULMC.org
Physician Referral: **888-7-NYU-MED** *(888-769-8633)*

INTERNAL MEDICINE

Internal medicine physicians at NYU Langone Medical Center are dedicated to treating the whole patient, and not just their disease. Our team addresses both the physical and psychological aspects of health and disease through clear communication and a fully integrated regimen of care. We specialize in the following areas:

Primary and Specialized Healthcare
General Internal Medicine offers a multidisciplinary medical approach to treating illnesses involving the heart, lungs, gastrointestinal tract, joints, bones, muscles, endocrine organs and kidneys. A wide range of laboratory, imaging and advanced diagnostic testing, ranging from throat cultures to the complex mapping of the electrical surface of the heart, is available on-site or by referral. Comprehensive women's healthcare, including cancer screening and osteoporosis prevention and treatment, is also available. We offer a variety of convenient office locations in Manhattan and the surrounding metropolitan area.

Geriatrics
Our geriatric specialists provide comprehensive and multidisciplinary care, consultation and follow-up for elderly patients ranging from prevention and healthy aging to the treatment and care of chronic conditions including dementia, functional impairment and degenerative disorders.

The Best in American Medicine
www.CastleConnolly.com

Family Medicine

THE MOUNT SINAI MEDICAL CENTER

Family Medicine and Community Health

One Gustave L. Levy Place
Fifth Avenue and 100th Street
New York, NY 10029-6574

Physician Referral: 1-800-MD-SINAI (637-4624)
www.mountsinai.org

To expand access to world-class medical care and further our commitment to the communities we serve, The Mount Sinai Medical Center recently established a **DEPARTMENT OF FAMILY MEDICINE AND COMMUNITY HEALTH** in collaboration with the Institute for Family Health, one of the largest networks of community health centers in New York State. Neil S. Calman, MD, President, Co-Founder and Chief Executive Officer of the Institute chairs the Department. Dr. Calman is a visionary in the field of family medicine and his health centers serve as models for others throughout the nation.

The Department's clinical mission to deliver excellent, accessible clinical care to the communities of Central and East Harlem is being carried out expertly under Dr. Calman's direction at the Institute's newly built **Family Health Center of Harlem at Mount Sinai Hospital**. Located at Madison Avenue and 119th Street, the new Center, which spans 37,000 square feet, is home to 35 examination rooms, 14 dental operatories, a 13-room counseling center, program space for pregnant and postpartum nutrition assistance (WIC) and community rooms for health education classes and meetings,

In addition, the Center employs state-of-the-art medical technology, including the Epic electronic medical record system, connecting it to inpatient and specialty care services at Mount Sinai and ensuring our patients continuity and high quality care. The Family Health Center serves people of all ages, from the very young to the very old. Primary care is the heart of the Center and offers physical exams, immunizations, gynecology, health screenings, behavioral health services, dental care, nutrition counseling, care for chronic conditions like diabetes and HIV related illness. It also offers many health education, nutrition and fitness programs.

The new Center is also the home of the **Institute's Harlem Residency in Family Medicine**, a national Teaching Health Center grantee, training a new generation of family physicians, who, along with Dr. Calman and other faculty, are working to eliminate health disparities among the underserved.

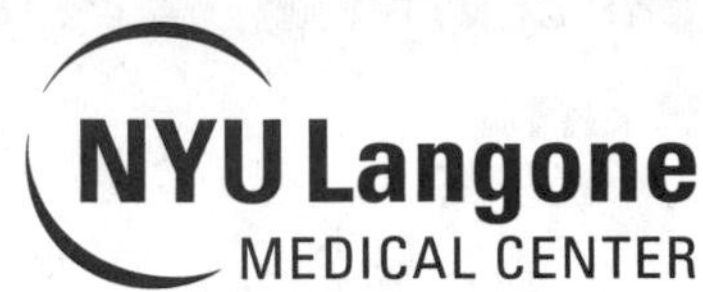

INTERNAL MEDICINE

Internal medicine physicians at NYU Langone Medical Center are dedicated to treating the whole patient, and not just their disease. Our team addresses both the physical and psychological aspects of health and disease through clear communication and a fully integrated regimen of care. We specialize in the following areas:

Primary and Specialized Healthcare
General Internal Medicine offers a multidisciplinary medical approach to treating illnesses involving the heart, lungs, gastrointestinal tract, joints, bones, muscles, endocrine organs and kidneys. A wide range of laboratory, imaging and advanced diagnostic testing, ranging from throat cultures to the complex mapping of the electrical surface of the heart, is available on-site or by referral. Comprehensive women's healthcare, including cancer screening and osteoporosis prevention and treatment, is also available. We offer a variety of convenient office locations in Manhattan and the surrounding metropolitan area.

Geriatrics
Our geriatric specialists provide comprehensive and multidisciplinary care, consultation and follow-up for elderly patients ranging from prevention and healthy aging to the treatment and care of chronic conditions including dementia, functional impairment and degenerative disorders.

The Best in American Medicine
www.CastleConnolly.com

Gastroenterology

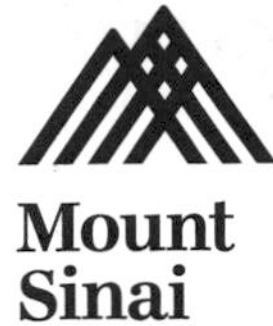

THE MOUNT SINAI MEDICAL CENTER

Gastrointestinal and Surgical Specialties

One Gustave L. Levy Place
Fifth Avenue and 100th Street
New York, NY 10029-6574

Physician Referral: 1-800-MD-SINAI (637-4624)
www.mountsinai.org

Mount Sinai's **DIVISIONS OF GASTROENTEROLOGY, COLON AND RECTAL SURGERY, LIVER DISEASES, PEDIATRIC GASTROENTEROLOGY, AND PEDIATRIC HEPATOLOGY** are renowned for their delivery of patient care, research, and education in diseases of the gastrointestinal (GI) tract. In 2000, the National Institutes of Health (NIH) recognized the importance of Mount Sinai as a research center with a grant for GI/Liver fellowship training. Mount Sinai is the only medical school in New York City to earn this prestigious award.

Mount Sinai's Division of Gastroenterology ranks 9th among all institutions in the country, according to the *U.S. News & World Report's* 2013–2014 "Best Hospitals" issue. Successes include breakthroughs in the medical and surgical management of the inflammatory bowel diseases (IBD): ulcerative colitis, and Crohn's disease. Mount Sinai spearheaded novel therapies for treating severe IBD and helped establish the role of colonoscopy in preventing colon cancer by removing precancerous polyps. More recent innovations include employing a tiny camera within a swallowable capsule to capture images in the stomach and intestines. Mount Sinai offers patients advanced comprehensive and interdisciplinary care; newer agents through clinical trials; services of psychologists and nutritionists; and world-class expertise in endoscopic procedures.

Division of Colon and Rectal Surgery — Continuing a long tradition of expertise in gastrointestinal disorders, Mount Sinai surgeons focus on surgical therapies for all diseases involving the colon, rectum, and anus. Highly skilled in the treatment of Crohn's disease (which was first described at Mount Sinai in 1932), ulcerative colitis, colon and rectal cancer, and diverticulitis, they specialize in the most advanced techniques of rectal surgery with an emphasis on colostomy avoidance. They also employ minimally invasive techniques and cutting-edge technologies for the treatment of hemorrhoids, fistulas, rectal tumors, and fecal incontinence.

Division of Liver Diseases — With a program that is among the largest and most successful in the world, Mount Sinai carries out a diverse portfolio of research projects. Featuring both clinical care and scientific investigations, they involve transplantation; diagnosis and treatment of viral hepatitis, including trials for revolutionary new drugs for Hepatitis B and C; treatment of scarring, or fibrosis; management of primary biliary cirrhosis, an autoimmune disease of bile ducts; treatment of liver cancer; and diagnosis and treatment of genetic liver diseases, including Wilson's disease (copper overload) and hemachromatosis (iron overload).

Division of Pediatric Gastroenterology — The division provides consultation and treatment for the full range of children's digestive and nutritional diseases. The Children's IBD Center offers comprehensive, multidisciplinary, family-centered care for pediatric patients with Crohn's disease and ulcerative colitis, and receives referrals from across the country. The division also provides care to families of infants, children, and teens who have the full range of both complex and common digestive disorders, including celiac disease, gastroesophageal reflux disease, and irritable bowel syndrome. Additionally, the division is involved in both basic science and clinical research, allowing physicians to provide state-of-the-art, evidence-based care.

Division of Pediatric Hepatology — The Transplant Program is one of the largest in the nation and was the first program in New York to perform liver transplants and, later, small bowel transplants. The division is active in clinical research in IBD, focusing on issues of genetic factors, psychosocial interactions, and drug trials in liver disease.

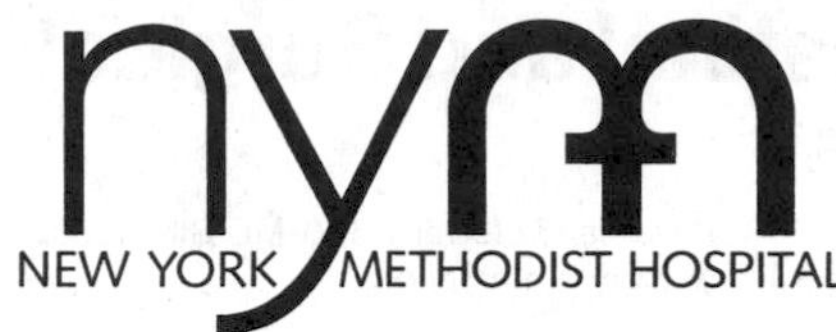

THE INSTITUTE FOR DIGESTIVE AND LIVER DISORDERS

New York Methodist Hospital
506 Sixth Street, Brooklyn, N.Y. 11215
Phone 866 DIGEST-1 (866 344-3781)
http://www.nym.org

SPECIALISTS AND MEDICAL SERVICES

The Institute's panel of physician specialists includes gastroenterologists, hepatologists, surgeons, laparoscopic surgeons, radiologists, medical and radiation oncologists and pathologists. Nutritionists and psychologists are also members of the team. The latest advances in the diagnosis and treatment of the gastrointestinal tract and the liver are available. These include endoscopic ultrasound, pediatric and adult capsule endoscopy and advanced laparoscopic surgery. In addition, the Endoscopy Suite at New York Methodist Hospital enables physicians to perform highly advanced diagnostic and treatment procedures that can detect and determine disorders of the gastrointestinal tract and bile ducts as well as perform the non-surgical removal of bile duct gallstones.

PROGRAMS OFFERED

Among the programs and services offered by the Institute are a Barrett's esophagus program, colorectal cancer program, heartburn (GERD) program, chronic Hepatitis B & C program, liver transplantation evaluation program, ulcer program, bowel disorders program and pediatric gastroenterology program. Gallbladder and pancreatic conditions are also treated.

***

Referrals to the Institute's specialists, programs and services can be made through an individual's primary care physician or requested directly through the Institute's telephone referral service. More information (and on-line physician referral) is available at the Hospital's website, http://www.nym.org.

THE PEDIATRIC GASTROENTEROLOGY PROGRAM

Problems commonly seen by physicians affiliated with the program include regurgitation, colic, constipation, diarrhea, recurrent abdominal pain, jaundice, blood in the stool, failure to thrive and formula intolerances. Children with these disorders present a special challenge because, along with the medical treatment that they receive, they need special care to ensure that their normal growth and development is not disrupted.

Special procedures that can be used to evaluate and diagnose pediatric gastrointestinal disorders include upper and lower endoscopies, liver biopsies and suction rectal biopsies. These procedures are performed by board certified specials in pediatric gastroenterology.

NewYork-Presbyterian

Affiliated with Columbia University College of Physicians and Surgeons and Weill Cornell Medical College

NewYork-Presbyterian Hospital
Columbia University Medical Center
622 West 168th Street
New York, NY 10032

Center for Advanced Digestive Care
NewYork-Presbyterian Hospital
Weill Cornell Medical Center
525 East 68th Street
New York, NY 10065

1-877-NYP-WELL (1-877-697-9355) www.nyp.org/digestive

NewYork-Presbyterian Digestive Disease Services

Since 2010, NewYork-Presbyterian Hospital's gastroenterology program has ranked among the top ten in the nation in the annual "Best Hospitals" survey conducted by *U.S. News & World Report*™. NewYork-Presbyterian's Digestive Disease Services feature a collaborative team approach, an exceptional track record of routine and advanced procedures, prevention programs, and basic science and clinical research aimed at developing novel therapies.

- Interventional endoscopic procedures to treat disorders such as pancreatic cancer, pancreatitis, biliary and pancreatic stones, Barrett's esophagus, and polyps.
- Endoscopic sewing and radiofrequency ablation for gastroesophageal reflux disease (GERD).
- Minimally invasive surgical approaches, including single-incision, endolumenal, "needlescopic" procedures and combined endoscopic laparoscopic surgery (CELS).
- The Center for Liver Disease and Transplantation achieves extraordinary outcomes in living and deceased liver transplant and features laparoscopic removal of living donor liver tissue for select cases.
- Colorectal surgery is enhanced by the state-of-the-art Siemens Artis zeego® medical imaging system. This system provides real-time, more accurate 3-D images of the body and enables surgeons to transition seamlessly from diagnosis to surgical remedy.

Patients benefit from a range of routine diagnostic tests such as endoscopy, colonoscopy, and flexible sigmoidoscopy, as well as laparoscopy to diagnose and stage digestive cancers. Interventional endoscopic approaches are also available, including:

- Endoscopic retrograde cholangiopancreatography (ERCP) to evaluate the ducts of the gallbladder, pancreas, and liver.
- Endoscopic ultrasound (EUS) to diagnose pancreatic disorders and stage esophageal, gastric, and rectal cancers. NewYork-Presbyterian Hospital is one of only a few centers using EUS for needle aspiration of pancreatic cysts and tumors.
- Cholangioscopy to evaluate stones or strictures in the pancreatic or bile ducts.
- Double-balloon and spiral enteroscopy to investigate possible intestinal bleeding.
- Probe-based confocal laser endomicroscopy to enhance the early detection and treatment of cancers and precancerous conditions.
- Endoscopic stenting to relieve obstructions and improve symptoms.

Comprehensive and Compassionate Care

Patients who come to NewYork-Presbyterian Hospital benefit from a personalized multidisciplinary approach to the care of:

- Cancers of the esophagus, liver, pancreas, colon, stomach, and rectum
- Inflammatory bowel diseases (Crohn's disease and ulcerative colitis)
- Liver disease, including fatty liver and cirrhosis and hepatitis B and C
- Esophageal disorders, such as GERD and Barrett's esophagus
- Disorders of the pancreas, gallbladder, and bile ducts
- Celiac disease
- Polyps, particularly in the colon
- Peptic ulcer and other stomach diseases
- Anal and rectal diseases
- Obesity (through weight loss surgery)
- Type 2 diabetes (through metabolic surgery)

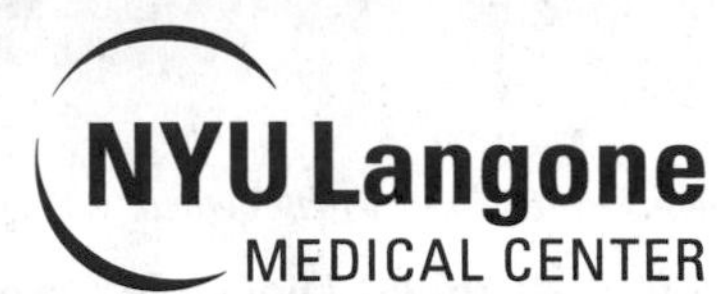

550 First Avenue *(at 31st Street)*
New York, NY 10016

www.NYULMC.org

Physician Referral: **888-7-NYU-MED** *(888-769-8633)*

GASTROENTEROLOGY

NYU Langone Medical Center is dedicated to the diagnosis and treatment of patients with diseases of the gastrointestinal tract. Physicians draw on their extensive knowledge and experience in the diagnosis and management of inflammatory bowel disease, peptic ulcer disease, esophageal disorders, gastrointestinal cancer, and liver, biliary and pancreatic diseases. Laser, laparoscopic, endoscopic, and other minimally invasive options are available, and we specialize in the following areas:

Colorectal Cancer

The Medical Center offers the most advanced screening options available for the diagnosis of colon cancer. Additionally, physicians continue to investigate colorectal cancer in special populations such as women, veterans, immigrants, minorities and patients with HIV, and offer the use of standard and virtual colonoscopy for the detection of colorectal polyps and cancer.

Esophageal Diseases

The Esophageal Disease Center offers patients state-of-the-art diagnosis and treatment of esophageal disorders. The Center focuses on gastroesophageal reflux disease, esophageal motility disorders, Barrett's esophagus, adenocarcinoma of the esophagus and swallowing disorders. It also offers diagnostic studies on esophageal manometry, impedance testing for swallowing, pH catheter and impedance testing for reflux and BRAVO capsule pH testing, as well as such therapies as Barrett's ablation and esophageal dilations.

Gastrointestinal Cancers

Cancer Institute physicians treat patients with all types of gastrointestinal cancers, including those of the esophagus, stomach, colon/rectum, small intestine, liver, pancreas, gallbladder, and biliary tract. They also treat individuals with complex recurring disease, including those originally treated elsewhere. Patients have the opportunity to participate in numerous clinical trials.

Complex Treatments and Diagnosis

Our physicians are highly experienced in the use of enteroscopy and capsule endoscopy for the diagnosis of gastrointestinal bleeding of unknown origin. They have special interest in the diagnosis and treatment of patients with complex pancreatic-biliary disease through the use of ERCP and endoscopic ultrasound.

Liver Lesions and Adrenal Tumors

Our team treats liver lesions with painless radiofrequency ablation and are highly skilled in laproscopic adrenalectomies.

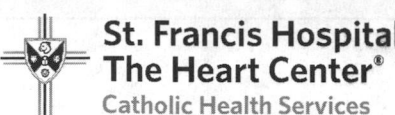

100 Port Washington Blvd.
Roslyn, New York 11576
www.stfrancisheartcenter.com
(516) 562-6000
1-888-HEARTNY

Gastrointestinal and Surgical Services

In a sign of its expanding strengths in non-cardiac care, in 2013-14 St. Francis Hospital was ranked 15th in the nation for the treatment of gastrointestinal disorders and GI surgery by *U.S. News & World Report* and the top hospital on Long Island in this specialty. This specialty has proven to be a pillar of St. Francis' excellent general medical and surgical care, and will continue to be a significant part of the hospital's future.

Innovative Diagnostic Procedures

The physicians in the Department of Gastroenterology at St. Francis Hospital have the skill and expertise to diagnose and treat all forms of gastrointestinal illnesses and employ essential state-of-the-art technologies to diagnose and treat the most difficult of digestive disorders. Headed by Anthony J. Celifarco, M.D., the department provides all forms of endoscopic and non-endoscopic studies on an in-patient or out-patient basis, in addition to consultative services. Procedures offered include colonoscopy, not only for routine colon cancer screening, but also to help diagnose causes of bleeding, diarrhea or constipation. Upper endoscopy is utilized to evaluate causes of abdominal pain, bleeding, weight loss, and difficulties swallowing. The department also performs endoscopic ultrasound (for diagnosis of lesions of the esophagus, stomach, and pancreas that may not be seen on standard endoscopic procedures of the GI tract), endoscopic dilation, stent placement for obstructive lesions, and enteroscopy including Balloon Enteroscopy to help visualize and treat disorders of the small intestine. One of the latest technologies, Capsule Endoscopy, can take images of the entire small intestine to find obscure causes of gastrointestinal bleeding, and help find evidence of undiagnosed disorders such as Crohn's disease. Recently, the Department of Gastroenterology acquired state-of-the-art, high-definition endoscopic equipment. Our center also performs fecal transplantations for treatment of severe Clostridium difficile colitis. In addition, the department now utilizes a carbon dioxide insufflation technique which minimizes discomfort with standard Endoscopic procedures compared to old technology. Acquiring this equipment further demonstrates the department's commitment to remain at the forefront of gastrointestinal endoscopy.

State-of-the-Art Minimally Invasive Surgical Oncology

Chairman of Surgery, Gary R. Gecelter, M.D., a renowned expert in minimally invasive surgery and surgical oncology, and his colleagues specialize in gastrointestinal surgical oncology, particularly colon, esophageal, and pancreatic cancer. Dr. Gecelter oversees the hospital's growing non-cardiac surgical program and has pioneered numerous laparoscopic techniques and is responsible for the development of flexible laparoscopy, which has led to single incision laparoscopic surgery and applies techniques used in gastroenterology. This has aided in allowing the minimally invasive resection of large abdominal tumors and even resection of esophageal cancers without having to make large chest and abdominal incisions. His team is in the forefront of integrating laparoscopy and endoscopy, particularly in the treatment of conditions such as achalasia as well as the surgical management of solid tumors of the GI tract.

St. Francis Hospital Gastroenterology Department
conditions treated:

- Gastroesophageal reflux
- Peptic ulcer disease
- Biliary tract disease
- Disease of the pancreas including pancreatitis and pancreatic cancer
- Liver disease including cirrhosis and hepatitis
- Esophageal varices
- Fecal transplantations for treatment of severe Clostridium difficile disease
- Inflammatory bowel disease including ulcerative colitis and Crohn's disease
- Irritable bowel syndrome
- Colon cancer screening
- GI complications from cardiac surgery
- Celiac disease

Key treatments:

Colonoscopy
Colon cancer, the third most common cancer, is a preventable condition. By using colonoscopy we are able to remove polyps and prevent the disease from occurring.

Gastrointestinal Bleeding
This condition is diagnosed using Gastroscopy, Capsule Endoscopy, Balloon Enteroscopy and Colonoscopy, and frequently can be treated without requiring surgery.

Inflammatory Bowel Disease
This disease is diagnosed based on history, physical examination, laboratory tests, colonoscopy, and capsule endoscopy. Patients are then treated with dietary measures and, if necessary, medication.

Geriatric Medicine

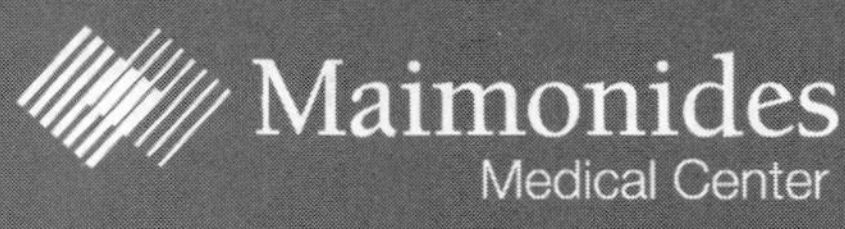

Geriatrics Program

4802 Tenth Avenue
Brooklyn, New York 11219
Phone: 718.283.7071 • Fax: 718.635.6417
www.maimonidesmed.org/geriatrics

Maimonides serves one of the oldest populations in New York State, with one quarter of our patients over the age of 75. The Geriatrics Program at Maimonides is fully equipped to meet the special needs of this growing population. Directed by Barbara Paris, MD, the program encompasses inpatient and outpatient services, featuring the Acute Care for Elderly (ACE) Unit and the Safe at Home program. The staff is focused on the continuity, coordination, quality and dignity of care provided.

Patient Evaluation
ACE Unit services focus on acute medical care and account for the complex needs of hospitalized elderly patients. Special attention is given to the assessment of memory loss and understanding the underlying causes of geriatric syndromes that result in falls, incontinence and frailty. Psychosocial issues affecting elderly patients, such as loneliness and end-of-life care, are also addressed.

Wound Care and Hyperbaric Center
Elderly patients can often have wounds that do not heal easily, which is why we have a dedicated wound care team available. Individualized wound treatment is dependent upon the type and severity of the wound. Treatments include conventional and advanced wound dressings, antibiotic therapy, protective footwear, and hyperbaric oxygen therapy.

Safe at Home Program
The Safe at Home program actively manages the care of the frail elderly so that they may live at home and within their communities. The program is designed to identify patients aged 75 years and older who are at high risk during the transitional period from hospital to home; provide them with coordinated comprehensive care after the transition from hospital to home; actively engage family caregivers and community support networks; increase patient satisfaction with their care during this transitional period; and reduce re-hospitalizations, emergency room visits and nursing home placements.

Outpatient Geriatric Services
Our geriatric team offers comprehensive assessment and primary care services throughout Southern Brooklyn.

Relying heavily on evidence-based medicine, Maimonides Medical Center has been commended for outstanding services by a number of independent rating organizations. Earlier this year, Maimonides was named a Distinguished Hospital for Clinical Excellence by HealthGrades – one of only three hospitals in the metropolitan area; the American Stroke Association bestowed its Gold Plus Achievement Award on the hospital; and the American Hospital Association once again named it a Most Wired hospital.

Maimonides Medical Center
The right care.
Right here.

www.maimonidesmed.org/geriatrics

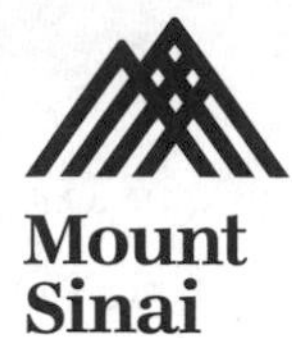

THE MOUNT SINAI MEDICAL CENTER

Geriatrics and Palliative Care

One Gustave L. Levy Place
Fifth Avenue and 100th Street
New York, NY 10029-6574

Physician Referral: 1-800-MD-SINAI (637-4624)
www.mountsinai.org

THE BEST IN CLINICAL CARE

In recognition of the care offered to older patients, The Mount Sinai Medical Center's **BROOKDALE DEPARTMENT OF GERIATRICS AND PALLIATIVE MEDICINE** is cited time and time again among the finest in the nation. In 2013, *U.S. News & World Report* ranked our geriatrics specialty #4 and our medical school program #1 in the United States.

We offer a full spectrum of patient care, including a specialized inpatient care team for the elderly to minimize complications sometimes associated with an older person's hospital stay, a primary care geriatrics practice for older adults living in the community, a hospital-based consultation service for patients throughout Mount Sinai, a number of community-linked programs and partnerships, and a palliative care team dedicated to ensuring the highest quality care and support for patients and families facing serious illnesses.

The Martha Stewart Center for Living, a modern facility designed by renowned architect C.C. Pei, provides clinical care and education for patients and serves as a training ground for physicians. Our newly opened Wiener Family Palliative Care Unit, the only one of its kind in Manhattan, provides inpatient care for patients and families facing serious and life-threatening illness.

Groundbreaking Research—Mount Sinai's researchers continue to advance the understanding, prevention, and treatment of age-related disorders. The extensive research on aging conducted by the Brookdale Department of Geriatrics and Palliative Medicine includes studies on health services, medical decision making and ethical dilemmas, palliative care, the neurobiology of aging, and clinical interventions to promote independence in old age. The department's expertise serves as a renowned educational resource for all Mount Sinai affiliates and other institutions in teaching geriatrics and palliative medicine to medical students, medical residents, geriatrics and palliative care fellows, established physicians, and health profession trainees in other disciplines.

History Of Excellence—The Mount Sinai Medical Center is a pioneer in geriatric medicine. In 1909, a Mount Sinai physician coined the term "geriatrics," and in 1914, he wrote the first textbook on medical care for older adults. Today, the Brookdale Department of Geriatrics and Palliative Medicine continues to break new ground, offering comprehensive care, disease prevention, and the promotion of healthy and productive aging. The department's enhanced expertise in assessing and managing patients with dementia greatly complements its established, interdisciplinary approach to patient care, in which medical staff and social workers address each patient's needs as a team.

THE FIRST FREESTANDING DEPARTMENT OF GERIATRICS AT A U.S. MEDICAL SCHOOL

Mount Sinai's Brookdale Department of Geriatrics and Palliative Medicine was the first freestanding department of geriatrics established by a U.S. medical school, and it continues to be one of the very best. It offers unparalleled inpatient and outpatient care, as well as numerous treatment programs designed to meet the unique needs of older adults. Mount Sinai is also home to world-class researchers dedicated to advancing our understanding of Alzheimer's disease and other common geriatric conditions. At the department's heart are its patients. The geriatricians of The Mount Sinai Medical Center work hard to improve life and longevity for New York's elderly.

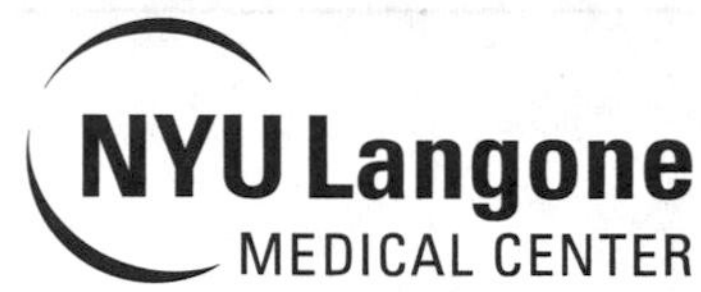

550 First Avenue *(at 31st Street)*
New York, NY 10016

www.NYULMC.org

Physician Referral: **888-7-NYU-MED** *(888-769-8633)*

INTERNAL MEDICINE

Internal medicine physicians at NYU Langone Medical Center are dedicated to treating the whole patient, and not just their disease. Our team addresses both the physical and psychological aspects of health and disease through clear communication and a fully integrated regimen of care. We specialize in the following areas:

Primary and Specialized Healthcare

General Internal Medicine offers a multidisciplinary medical approach to treating illnesses involving the heart, lungs, gastrointestinal tract, joints, bones, muscles, endocrine organs and kidneys. A wide range of laboratory, imaging and advanced diagnostic testing, ranging from throat cultures to the complex mapping of the electrical surface of the heart, is available on-site or by referral. Comprehensive women's healthcare, including cancer screening and osteoporosis prevention and treatment, is also available. We offer a variety of convenient office locations in Manhattan and the surrounding metropolitan area.

Geriatrics

Our geriatric specialists provide comprehensive and multidisciplinary care, consultation and follow-up for elderly patients ranging from prevention and healthy aging to the treatment and care of chronic conditions including dementia, functional impairment and degenerative disorders.

Geriatric Psychiatry

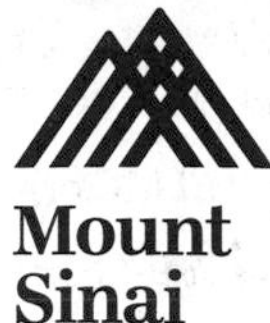

THE MOUNT SINAI MEDICAL CENTER

Geriatric Psychiatry

One Gustave L. Levy Place
Fifth Avenue and 100th Street
New York, NY 10029-6574

Physician Referral: 1-800-MD-SINAI (637-4624)
www.mountsinai.org

THE DIVISION OF GERIATRIC PSYCHIATRY at The Mount Sinai Medical Center delivers effective, compassionate and individualized care to older adults with neuropsychiatric illness and provides therapy, support and guidance to families and caretakers, thereby enhancing the quality of life for all concerned.

Our program includes both an inpatient geriatric psychiatry unit and an outpatient geriatric psychiatry clinic, the latter of which is housed in our beautiful **Martha Stewart Center for Living**. Our staff includes physicians, psychiatric nurses, and licensed clinical social workers, among other professionals, all trained to care for the psychiatric needs of older adults through hands-on, evidence-based care. We also offer participation in clinical research protocols that offer state-of-the-art therapies.

Outpatient Geriatric Psychiatry Clinic

Physicians practicing in our outpatient clinic specialize in treating patients with psychiatric illness and memory problems. Our interdisciplinary team provides psychopharmacology; comprehensive cognitive evaluations for the diagnosis and treatment of memory disorders, including Alzheimer's disease; group therapy for depression and anxiety; and support groups for those suffering from dementia.

Research

Opportunities to participate in research abound. The Division of Geriatric Psychiatry is closely allied with Mount Sinai's **Alzheimer's Disease Research Center**, where physician-scientists study memory problems, such as Alzheimer's disease, and its Brain Stimulation Center of Excellence, where they investigate the treatment of psychiatric disorders with electroconvulsive therapy and deep brain stimulation.

Workshops

We encourage older adults and their caregivers who are interested in learning more about their disease process and other aspects of aging to attend our workshops. We run them in conjunction with staff and patients from Mount Sinai's Martha Stewart Center for Living and Alzheimer's disease Research Center.

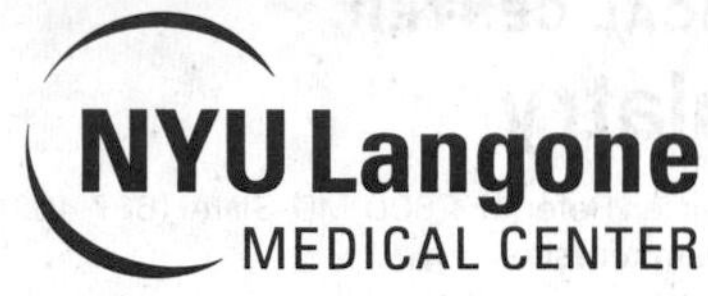

550 First Avenue *(at 31st Street)*
New York, NY 10016

www.NYULMC.org

Physician Referral: **888-7-NYU-MED** *(888-769-8633)*

PSYCHIATRY

NYU Langone's psychiatry team is dedicated to improving the health and well-being of patients by delivering peerless psychiatric services and care. NYU Langone is home to some of the nation's most respected clinical psychiatrists and psychologists, with specialties in psychoanalysis, psychopharmacology, behavioral therapy, child psychiatry, geriatric psychiatry and neuropsychiatry. We specialize in the following areas:

Child and Adolescent Psychiatry

Since 1997, the Child Study Center has treated thousands of children from around the world at its Faculty Group Practices in Manhattan and satellite clinical campuses in New Jersey and Long Island. Through its website, www.AboutOurKids.org, and through professional education programs, parents and practitioners are provided with the tools and knowledge needed to promote children's mental health. We specialize in Anxiety and Mood Disorders, Attention Deficit Hyperactivity and Behavior Disorders, Autism, Asperger's Syndrome and Communication Disorders, Learning Disorders, Tics and Tourette Disorder and more.

Adult Inpatient Services

The inpatient services unit combines comprehensive diagnostic assessment and treatment, including psychopharmacology, neuropsychology, psychotherapies and electroconvulsive therapy.

Adult Outpatient Psychiatry

The outpatient psychiatry program provides expert treatment to individuals suffering from a broad range of mental disorders and emotional problems, including anxiety, depression (including medicine resistant depression), insomnia, manic-depression, reproductive psychiatry, attention-deficit hyperactivity disorder and schizophrenia.

Post-Traumatic Stress Disorder

We offer assessment and treatment of PTSD for victims of sexual and physical assault, natural disasters, terrorism and combat trauma. Treatment includes cognitive behavioral therapy and strategies for the prevention of insomnia, stress, anxiety and depression. Our Military Family Clinic provides compassionate mental healthcare for veterans and their extended family members. The Steven and Alexandra Cohen Veterans Center is dedicated to improving diagnosis and treatment of PTSD and TBI through research.

Memory Impairment

The Pearl Barlow Center for Memory Evaluation and Treatment specializes in treating patients with memory impairments caused by neurological, psychological and physical ailments, as well as memory issues resulting from medication side effects, anxiety, depression and the effects of normal aging from illnesses like Alzheimer's disease.

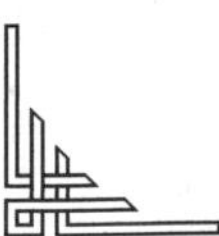

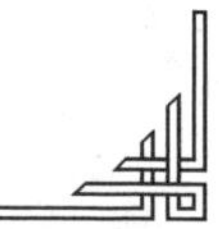

The Best in American Medicine
www.CastleConnolly.com

Gynecologic Oncology

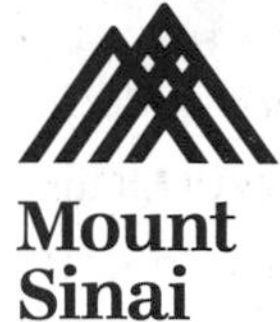

THE MOUNT SINAI MEDICAL CENTER
Gynecologic Oncology

One Gustave L. Levy Place
Fifth Avenue and 100th Street
New York, NY 10029-6574

Physician Referral: 1-800-MD-SINAI (637-4624)
www.mountsinai.org

The Mount Sinai Medical Center's **DIVISION OF GYNECOLOGIC ONCOLOGY** was founded in 1967 before the discipline received official designation as a subspecialty of The American Board of Obstetrics and Gynecology. Since then, we've been at the forefront treating all gynecologic cancers the most common forms of cancer in women after breast, lung, and colon cancers–a fact recognized by *U.S. News & World Report* as it named us among the top medical centers in the country for both cancer and gynecology in its 2013-2014 "Best Hospitals" issue.

Our surgeons were early adaptors of the new robotic surgical systems now in place—years before most centers used the systems. These minimally invasive surgeries offer shorter hospital stays, less scarring, and a faster return to normal activity than other forms of surgery. Approximately 60 percent of our surgeries are now performed using a minimally invasive approach.

To deliver the highest quality, most comprehensive care, we work closely with our colleagues at Mount Sinai's Tisch Cancer Institute as well as with those in diagnostic and interventional radiology, genetics, radiation therapy, palliative care, behavioral medicine, nutrition, and physical therapy. Practicing at the Derald H. Ruttenberg Cancer Center, relocated in 2012 to our beautiful and expansive Leon and Norma Hess Center for Science and Medicine, we manage surgical patients, provide consultations, and administer chemotherapy in a unified and intimate setting designed to ensure patient privacy and comfort. Our nurses are specifically trained in cancer treatment , and we have on-site oncology pharmacists.

ACCESS TO CLINICAL TRIALS

As a member of the Gynecologic Oncology Group (GOG), we offer our patients exposure to national clinical trials for the treatment of gynecologic cancers. Mount Sinai physicians have been pioneers in investigating optimal chemotherapeutic regimens leading to significant improvements in outcomes. Current investigations and clinical trials are available for patients with ovarian, uterine, cervical, and endometrial cancers.

Our services include cancer screening, early detection, therapy, and post-treatment surveillance for cancers of the cervix, fallopian tube, ovary, uterus, vagina and vulva.

Treatments We Provide

We provide a comprehensive range of treatments for gynecologic malignancies and complex benign gynecologic conditions. These include:

- Laser and laparoscopic surgeries
- Lymphadenectomy
- Ovarian cytoreduction and debulking
- Port implantation
- Urologic and bowel surgery

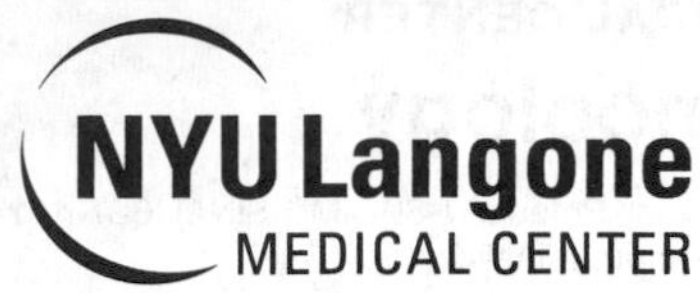

550 First Avenue *(at 31st Street)*
New York, NY 10016

www.NYULMC.org

Physician Referral: **888-7-NYU-MED** *(888-769-8633)*

OBSTETRICS AND GYNECOLOGY

NYU Langone Medical Center provides comprehensive services designed specifically for women, from primary care to highly specialized programs that are supported by sophisticated research and advanced training. We specialize in the following areas:

Obstetrics
We offer a broad range of obstetrical services, including prenatal care that gives equal emphasis to the well-being of the mother and the fetus; fetal monitoring through ultrasound and other techniques; childbirth preparedness and breastfeeding classes.

Maternal-Fetal Medicine
Prenatal care for high-risk pregnancies and detailed consultations before, during and after pregnancy are offered. We specialize in multifetal pregnancies, genetic counseling, women who have miscarried, and preterm deliveries, as well as helping women who have other medical conditions that may complicate a pregnancy, such as diabetes, heart problems, high blood pressure, and lupus. We offer the latest techniques for in-utero diagnosis and treatment and using minimally invasive techniques, our physicians are able to repair a number of life-threatening conditions in a child before it is even born.

Fertility-Related Services
We offer state-of-the-art programs in evaluation of infertility (including the special needs of same-sex couples) egg donation, egg freezing and in-vitro fertilization. Diagnosis and treatment include ovulation induction, assisted reproductive technologies and surgical options that incorporate the latest endoscopic techniques. Preimplantation Genetic Screening (PGS) at the Fertility Center offers tests for aneuploidy (an abnormal number of chromosomes).

Gynecology
In addition to routine gynecological care, we offer pelvic ultrasound; aspiration of breast cysts, colposcopy (a diagnostic evaluation of abnormal pap smears); LEEP (a loop electrosurgical procedure used to diagnose and treat cervical cancer); cryotherapy for vaginal warts; and bone density testing.

Gynecologic Surgery
Minimally invasive gynecologic surgery, including robotic surgery, is offered for a wide range of simple and complex conditions including, resection of endometriosis, hysterectomy, and myomectomy.

Gynecologic Oncology
The NCI-designated NYU Cancer Institute's Women's Cancer Program specializes in the treatment of cervical cancer, endometrial cancer, ovarian cancer, uterine cancer, vaginal cancer and vulvar cancer.

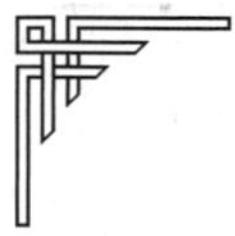

The Best in American Medicine
www.CastleConnolly.com

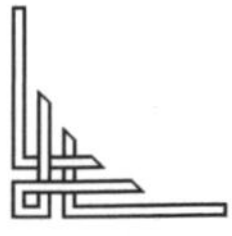
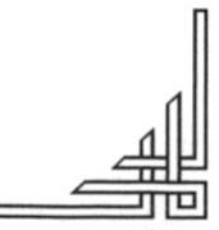

Hand Surgery

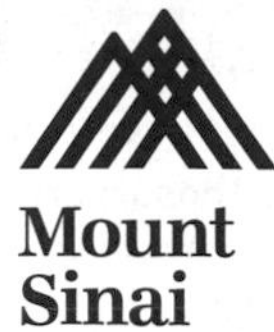

THE MOUNT SINAI MEDICAL CENTER

Hand and Wrist Service

One Gustave L. Levy Place
Fifth Avenue and 100th Street
New York, NY 10029-6574

Physician Referral: 1-800-MD-SINAI (637-4624)
www.mountsinai.org

The Mount Sinai Medical Center's **HAND AND WRIST SERVICE** enjoys a well-earned reputation for excellence in eliminating pain and restoring function for conditions ranging from a finger fracture to carpal tunnel syndrome to complex reconstructions for congenital, neoplastic or traumatic disorders.

Specialists in our Hand and Wrist Service are members of Mount Sinai's Department of Orthopedics and are internationally recognized for their skill in performing in the most advanced diagnostic and therapeutic procedures. They have pioneered new, minimally-invasive treatments for elbow and wrist trauma and common conditions like "tennis elbow".

Sinai offers comprehensive, multidisciplinary and individualized treatments for conditions including:

- Arthroscopic surgery
- Fracture management
- Carpal tunnel release
- Nerve release/reconstruction (e.g., brachial plexus)
- Treatment of stroke and paralysis due to nerve injury
- Tendon release/reconstruction
- Total elbow replacement
- Congenital anomaly reconstruction
- Adult and pediatric elbow treatment
- Vascular disorders of the hand

Multidisciplinary Hand and Wrist Care

Achieving the best outcome requires not only surgical expertise, but also well-orchestrated collaboration among specialists. The Mount Sinai Hand and Wrist Service works closely with anesthesiologists, specialty nurses, rehabilitation therapists, social workers, and pain management physicians—all in an effort to restore function to the fullest extent possible.

We routinely deliver cutting edge treatment services to all our patients. They arise through clinical experience and extensive orthopedic research sources. Our orthopedic research lab investigates both clinical and basic science issues to help solve the problems of orthopedic diseases and bone and soft tissue healing. We continually explore innovative surgical techniques to maximize patients' mobility and outcomes.

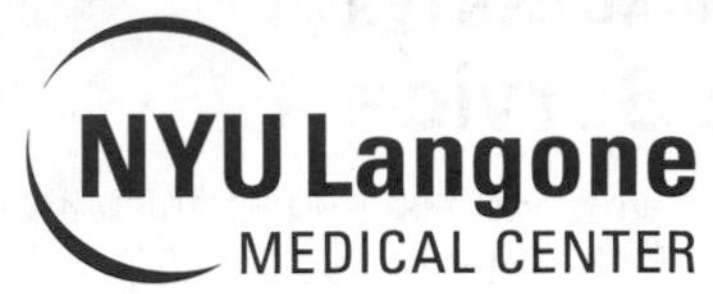

550 First Avenue *(at 31st Street)*
New York, NY 10016
www.NYULMC.org/orthosurgery
Physician Referral: **888-7-NYU-MED** *(888-769-8633)*

ORTHOPAEDIC SURGERY

The Department of Orthopaedic Surgery at NYU Langone Medical Center continues to be recognized as a national leader, **ranked #5 in the nation by *U.S. News & World Report's* 2013-2014 "Best Hospitals" survey**. Our physicians combine extensive experience with cutting-edge research and technology to address bone and joint problems that affect a patient's quality of life. The expertise of our world-class orthopaedists represents the full range of subspecialty areas including **Adult Reconstructive, Sports Medicine and Primary Care Sports Medicine, Spine, Shoulder & Elbow, Foot & Ankle, Hand Surgery, Trauma & Fracture, Orthopaedic Oncology, and Pediatric Orthopaedics**; additional areas of specialization include minimally-invasive surgery and robotic-assisted joint replacement.

Premier Areas of Expertise

Joint Replacement Center physicians evaluate degenerative joint conditions caused by arthritis, injuries, congenital problems and general wear-and-tear to determine the best course of treatment. Our surgeons are experts in knee, hip and shoulder replacements, complex joint revisions, and minimally invasive surgeries, conducting more than 3,000 procedures annually. The experts in our **Hip Center** also specialize in the cutting-edge, minimally invasive anterior total hip replacement technique.

The Spine Center provides conservative care for lower back and neck pain, scoliosis, osteoporosis, problems associated with failed previous surgery, idiopathic disorders, growth disorders, neuromuscular disease, degenerative and congenital conditions, and traumatic deformity. Our surgeons perform over 2,000 procedures a year, including minimally invasive spinal fusions.

Hand Center specialists diagnose and offer operative and non-operative care for a wide range of upper extremity conditions, including fractures, congenital anomalies, soft tissue and skeletal trauma, degenerative and rheumatoid arthritis, sports-related injuries, vascular disorders, tumors and occupational disorders.

Sports Medicine and Primary Care Sports Medicine physicians treat sports-related injuries or conditions of the knee, shoulder, elbow and ankle, using joint preservation techniques as well as surgical procedures. Our patients range from athletes playing at the high school, college and professional levels to recreational athletes/active individuals from every age group.

(continued)

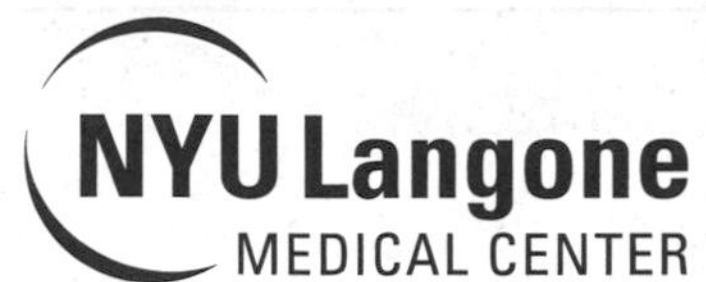

550 First Avenue *(at 31st Street)*
New York, NY 10016
www.NYULMC.org/orthosurgery
Physician Referral: **888-7-NYU-MED** *(888-769-8633)*

ORTHOPAEDIC SURGERY *(continued)*

Specialized Orthopaedic Centers and Services

The Joint Preservation Center provides conservative treatment of joint problems to reduce symptoms, restore function and delay the onset of degenerative arthritis and potential need for a joint replacement.

The Bone Healing Center is staffed by our orthopaedic trauma & fracture specialists, and is a leader in technologies and procedures that help patients recover from complex fracture reconstruction or fracture healing problems.

Harkness Center for Dance Injuries is world-renowned for its orthopaedic and rehabilitation care for dancers, including many subsidized and free services as well as injury prevention screenings and lectures.

The Diabetes Foot and Ankle Center focuses on the prevention and recurrence of foot and ankle problems associated with complications of diabetes.

The Samuels Orthopaedic Immediate Care Center, New York City's only walk-in orthopaedic clinic, is open seven days a week to evaluate and treat urgent bone and joint injuries.

The Concussion Center is a collaborative effort between the Departments of Orthopaedic Surgery, Neurology, and Rehabilitation, providing expert, multidisciplinary evaluation and treatment of individuals who have or are suspected of having a concussion.

The Occupational & Industrial Orthopaedic Center offers care, education, and consulting services in the prevention and treatment of injuries and disorders that arise from the work environment.

Sports Performance Center specialists assist active individuals in reaching their full potential through a state-of-the-art health and fitness evaluation and personalized athletic training plan.

Patient Care Locations

Our physicians and surgeons provide care at multiple NYU Langone locations, including:

- **The Hospital for Joint Diseases**, our internationally-renowned orthopaedic hospital
- **The Center for Musculoskeletal Care (CMC)**, NYU Langone's premier, state-of-the-art, multidisciplinary, bone and joint facility, which houses outpatient orthopaedic and rheumatologic care as well as an infusion center, pain management services, and Rusk Rehab's sports and musculoskeletal rehabilitation services
- CMC's **Outpatient Surgery Center**, where patients undergo minimally invasive, same-day surgery
- **Tisch Hospital**, NYU Langone's flagship hospital at the main campus on First Avenue
- Multiple locations in **NYU Langone's growing network of community practices** in the metro New York area, including Manhattan, Brooklyn, Long Island, Queens, Westchester, and New Jersey

Home Health Care

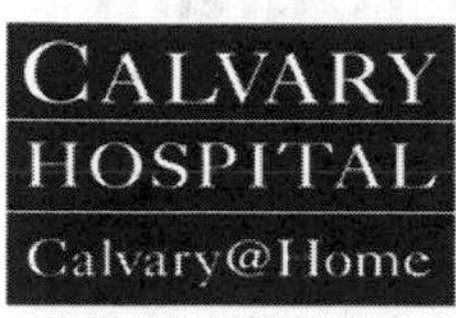

CALVARY HOSPITAL
1740 Eastchester Road
Bronx, NY 10461
Tel: (718) 518-2000
www.calvaryhospital.org

CALVARY@HOME
HOME CARE, HOSPICE, AND NURSING HOME HOSPICE

Calvary@Home, the umbrella for our Home Care, Hospice, and Nursing Home Hospice program, brings compassionate care to patients who can be cared for at home. Our interdisciplinary team includes physicians, nurses, aides, social workers, spiritual care providers, volunteers, bereavement support workers, and other providers as needed. In 2013, The Joint Commission gave Calvary@ Home a Gold Seal of Approval™. Calvary received a 2012 Circle of Life Award® for innovative palliative and end-of-life care. Calvary@Home cares for more than 2,300 patients and families each year.

Certified Home Health Agency
Established in 1985, serves patients with all acute, chronic or life-limiting illnesses. We provide a full range of specialized home healthcare experts to support patients and families. Home care patients approaching the end of life have access to palliative care services such as pain and symptom management, assistance with advance care planning, and psychosocial support. We strive to ensure continuity of care by assigning a core group of caregivers to each patient. Our community health nurses work with the patient's personal physicians to deliver appropriate care. Our home care services are available in Manhattan, the Bronx, Queens, Brooklyn, Staten Island as well as Westchester, Rockland, Putnam, and Nassau counties.

Hospice
Established in 1998, brings comprehensive care to people at home with all end-stage illnesses. Calvary assembles a core group of permanent staff to care for each patient, creating continuity of service for patients and families. Patients who require short-stay inpatient care can be admitted to Calvary in a seamless process. In addition to nurses, physicians and aides, social workers, spiritual counselors, and volunteers make home visits to ensure that physical, psychosocial, emotional and spiritual needs are met. We provide bereavement services for 13 months for families. Staffing exceeds national recommendations. Our hospice services are available in Manhattan, the Bronx, Queens, Brooklyn, as well as Nassau, Westchester and Rockland counties.

Nursing Home Hospice
Brings comprehensive palliative care to nursing home residents suffering from all end-stage illnesses. Provides appropriate care to all dually eligible (Medicare/Medicaid) residents, and bereavement services for loved ones. Through a partnership with Mary Manning Walsh Home in Manhattan, Calvary provides an inpatient level of care for a select number of patients.

Calvary Nursing Home Hospice has contracts with more than 25 facilities in: Manhattan, the Bronx, Queens, Brooklyn, as well as Nassau, Westchester and Rockland Counties.

For information about Calvary@Home, please call 718-518-2465.

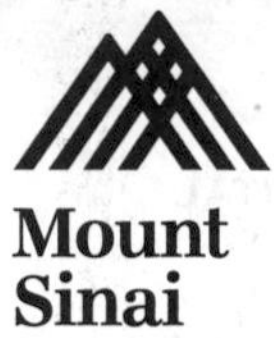

THE MOUNT SINAI MEDICAL CENTER

Visiting Doctors Program

One Gustave L. Levy Place
Fifth Avenue and 100th Street
New York, NY 10029-6574

Physician Referral: 1-800-MD-SINAI (637-4624)
www.mountsinai.org

Since 1995, The Mount Sinai Medical Center's **VISITING DOCTORS PROGRAM** has been delivering high quality, compassionate care to frail, elderly, and ailing adults who are unable to leave their homes. This award-winning program grew out of the collaborative efforts of our Department of Medicine and our Department of Geriatrics and Palliative Medicine. Today, as a health care service and a teaching platform, our program stands as a flagship clinical initiative—the largest academic home-visit program in the nation, with clinicians making more than 6,000 home visits annually to more than 1,100 patients.

The program delivers comprehensive primary and end of life care to an underserved segment of the population—homebound adults, consisting of geriatrics patients, as well as well as those patients with psychiatric, neurologic, complex, and terminal illnesses. We also offer emotional support and counseling to families and caregivers and work closely with home care, visiting nurse, community, and hospice agencies to coordinate care. We are available by phone 24 hours a day, seven days a week, and respond to requests for emergency visits.

The home-based services we provide include:

- Preventive health care
- Diagnosis and treatment of medical conditions
- Prescription of medications, with an emphasis on safety and affordability
- Support to family members and other caregivers
- Referrals for rehabilitation
- Assistance with practical needs, including wheelchairs
- Pain management
- Comprehensive, patient-centered, end-of-life care for the terminally ill

Our Team
Our staff crosses a number of disciplines. Our providers—specializing in internal medicine and/or geriatrics and palliative medicine—manage, coordinate, and deliver personalized, comprehensive care during their home visits. Based on a patient's medical needs, the provider team can consist of:

- Physicians and Nurse Practitioners
- Full-time office-based Registered Nurses
- Certified Clinical Social Workers

THE MOUNT SINAI CHELSEA-VILLAGE HOUSE CALL PROGRAM

In May 2010, the Chelsea-Village Program at St. Vincent's was adopted by The Mount Sinai Visiting Doctors Program and renamed The Mount Sinai Chelsea-Village House Call Program. The Chelsea-Village House Call Program provides in-home, multilingual, interdisciplinary primary medical care to frail and elderly homebound residents in lower Manhattan. With the help of Mount Sinai, the Chelsea-Village House Call Program will continue to serve lower Manhattan's most medically-underserved populations and patients will continue to receive the finest in medical care in the comfort of their own homes and communities with the maximum possible level of independence, health, and quality of life.

Infectious Disease

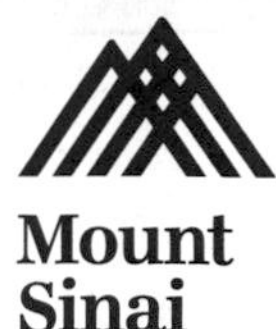

THE MOUNT SINAI MEDICAL CENTER
Infectious Diseases

One Gustave L. Levy Place
Fifth Avenue and 100th Street
New York, NY 10029-6574

Physician Referral: 1-800-MD-SINAI (637-4624)
www.mountsinai.org

Infectious Diseases – The Mount Sinai Medical Center's **DIVISION OF INFECTIOUS DISEASES** boasts an impressive history of achievement, with our physicians treating conditions that are extremely rare or even unheard of in other parts of the country.

In addition to unrivaled inpatient care, we offer comprehensive outpatient services through our Infectious Disease Faculty Practice as well as two specialty clinics. Our physicians diagnose and treat all types of communicable diseases and deliver state-of-the-art care to patients with HIV and other sexually transmitted diseases (STDs), Lyme disease, influenza, hepatitis, human papillomavirus (HPV), as well as food-borne and diarrheal diseases encountered in the U.S. and abroad.

HIV/AIDS Prevention and Treatment – Mount Sinai Hospital was named a "Designated AIDS Center" by the NYSDOH/AIDS Institute in 1989; as such we provide comprehensive inpatient/outpatient primary medical and nursing care, specialty care, case management services, nutritional counseling, health professional education and training and access to clinical trials. In 2010 Mount Sinai Hospital added the Saint Vincent's Hospital HIV program (Chelsea) to its existing Jack Martin Clinic (East Harlem), creating one of the largest HIV service lines in the State. Together the programs provide HIV primary care and case management services to over 3,000 HIV+ individuals living throughout the five boroughs of New York City. Our locations track the current epidemiology of HIV/AIDS as both neighborhoods have the highest incidence/prevalence of HIV/AIDS in the City. Our patient population represents the current face of HIV/AIDS in the City: African American, Hispanic, undocumented, recently incarcerated, women, adolescents, MSM, and mental illness/substance abuse. The programs both have significant linkages to community based organizations that have solidified a bi-directional referral network for HIV primary care and supplemental support services to meet the needs of the client. Our program has a number of specialty projects now in operation, predominantly supported by City, State, and Federal grants. Some of these projects include:

- Prevention with Positives,
- Sexual/Behavioral Health,
- Non Occupational Post Exposure Prophylaxis
- Women, Infants, Children and Youth (WICY)
- HIV Mental Health Services
- Early Intervention Services
- Care Coordination

In addition to those listed above, we have initiatives in the developmental stages to address HIV transmission as it relates to sexually transmitted infections (STI's). STI's are surrogate markers for HIV infection, and NYC is experiencing an epidemic of such conditions.

Antimicrobial Stewardship Program – The Mount Sinai Antimicrobial Stewardship Program strives to improve patient outcomes, to reduce the burden of antimicrobial resistance, and to save healthcare dollars through a collaborative, multidisciplinary, educational and evidence-based approach. This includes ensuring patients receive appropriate antibiotics, at optimal doses, and for the appropriate duration.

Transplant ID Program – Our Transplant Infectious Diseases Program is dedicated to preventing and managing all infectious diseases in solid organ and bone marrow transplant recipients and works in collaboration with Mount Sinai's Recanati-Miller Transplant Institute and our Bone Marrow Transplant Program to produce excellent outcomes.

HIV Hepatitis C Co-Infection Program – As highly active anti-retroviral therapy has improved and extended the lives of people living with HIV/AIDS, the hepatitis C virus (HCV), and the liver disease it can cause, has become an increasing problem. As the only hospital in the state with a division devoted exclusively to the treatment of liver disease, we offer coordinated multidisciplinary care, and transplants when necessary, to patients co-infected with HIV and HCV.

NeuroAIDS Program – We provide compassionate, comprehensive care to HIV-positive patients with neurological disorders including dementia, neuropathy, brain infections, and disorders of the spinal cord and muscle. HIV can affect any part of the nervous system, such as the brain, spinal cord, nerves, or muscle. Symptoms of neurologic disease in HIV-infected individuals may include memory loss, headache, dizziness, weakness, numbness, pain, vision changes, or trouble walking.

Travel Program – The Mount Sinai Travel Medicine Program is a designated Yellow Fever Center and offers official yellow fever vaccine certificates to both adults and children. As an academic center for travel medicine, Mount Sinai serves as a referral center for patients working for the United Nations and Doctors Without Borders. We provide both pre-travel assessments, including all immunizations, health counseling and prescriptions for travel medications, such as anti-malaria medications, and post-travel care, including evaluation and treatment for any travel-acquired health problems. Customized services for business travelers, NGOs, and others are available. Please call us to discuss your particular travel health concerns and needs. We speak English and Spanish.

Internal Medicine

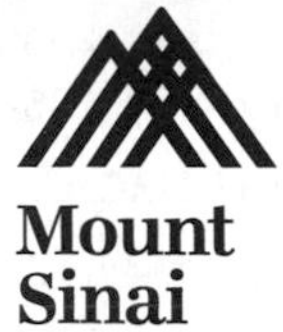

THE MOUNT SINAI MEDICAL CENTER

Internal Medicine

One Gustave L. Levy Place
Fifth Avenue and 100th Street
New York, NY 10029-6574

Physician Referral: 1-800-MD-SINAI (637-4624)
www.mountsinai.org

As the largest and one of the most deeply rooted departments at Mount Sinai, the **DEPARTMENT OF MEDICINE** brings together highly skilled physicians, scientists and educators, all dedicated to delivering advanced treatments in internal medicine and the subspecialties of cardiovascular, infectious, and gastrointestinal diseases; liver, kidney, and lung diseases; and diabetes and immune system disorders.

U.S. News & World Report's **2013-2014 "Best Hospitals"** issue ranks four of our specialties among the best in the nation out of approximately 5,000 hospitals. In addition, our Diabetes Center was ranked among the top 14 programs in the United States. From advanced diagnostic tools to personalized treatment plans and dedicated care centers, our patients benefit from a vast array of expertise and research initiatives including cutting-edge clinical trials.

In addition, we offer the following programs and services:

- Asthma Program
- Center for Inflammatory Bowel Diseases
- Center for Sleep Medicine
- COPD Program
- Diabetes Center
- HIV-Hepatitis C Co-Infection Program
- Kidney Center (Dialysis Program)
- Lung Screening Program
- Ruttenberg Treatment Center (bone marrow transplant, chemotherapy, and other cancer treatments)
- Sarcoidosis Program
- Visiting Doctors and Chelsea-Village House Calls Programs (care for elderly or ailing homebound patients)
- Women's Health Program

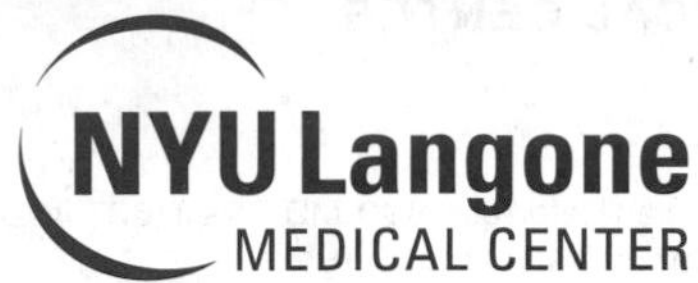

550 First Avenue *(at 31st Street)*
New York, NY 10016

www.NYULMC.org

Physician Referral: **888-7-NYU-MED** *(888-769-8633)*

INTERNAL MEDICINE

Internal medicine physicians at NYU Langone Medical Center are dedicated to treating the whole patient, and not just their disease. Our team addresses both the physical and psychological aspects of health and disease through clear communication and a fully integrated regimen of care. We specialize in the following areas:

Primary and Specialized Healthcare

General Internal Medicine offers a multidisciplinary medical approach to treating illnesses involving the heart, lungs, gastrointestinal tract, joints, bones, muscles, endocrine organs and kidneys. A wide range of laboratory, imaging and advanced diagnostic testing, ranging from throat cultures to the complex mapping of the electrical surface of the heart, is available on-site or by referral. Comprehensive women's healthcare, including cancer screening and osteoporosis prevention and treatment, is also available. We offer a variety of convenient office locations in Manhattan and the surrounding metropolitan area.

Geriatrics

Our geriatric specialists provide comprehensive and multidisciplinary care, consultation and follow-up for elderly patients ranging from prevention and healthy aging to the treatment and care of chronic conditions including dementia, functional impairment and degenerative disorders.

Interventional Cardiology

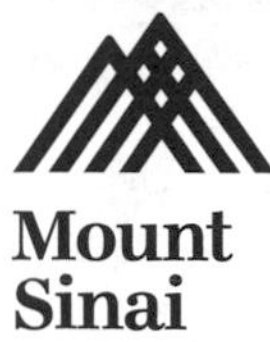

THE MOUNT SINAI MEDICAL CENTER

Interventional Cardiology/ Cath Lab Treatments

One Gustave L. Levy Place
Fifth Avenue and 100th Street
New York, NY 10029-6574

Physician Referral: 1-800-MD-SINAI (637-4624)
www.mountsinai.org

INTERVENTIONAL CARDIOLOGY/ CATH LAB TREATMENTS

Ranked among the top 13 hospitals for heart services by *U.S. News & World Report*, 2013 Mount Sinai Heart is celebrated internationally as a world leader in all facets of cardiology care and research. Our **Cardiac Catheterization Laboratory** ranks among the nation's best and busiest, offering expert diagnosis, state-of-the-art technology, and unparalleled excellence in care and patient safety. It has achieved the highest safety rating among New York State's 54 institutions that perform percutaneous coronary interventions (PCI), a minimally invasive heart procedure commonly known as angioplasty. No other hospital has matched this level of patient safety rating for both emergency and non-emergency cases since public reporting of PCI results began in 1994, per the New York State Department of Health.

Mount Sinai's multidisciplinary interventional cardiology team, patient volume, and procedural offerings continue to expand significantly, as the **Cath Lab** has performed more than 5,500 interventions a year for the last five years. This upward momentum has also drawn an increase in complex cases. Stable interventional growth with declining complications–despite increasing complexity of cases–has been achieved at Mount Sinai Heart through seamless teamwork and dedication to treating each individual patient, taking into account his or her medical history, type and status of condition and lifestyle.

MULTIDISCIPLINARY CARDIAC CATHETERIZATION TEAM

The Cath Lab's multidisciplinary team of interventionalists, nurses, technicians and support staff is committed to continuous quality improvement and providing excellent patient care. Constant communication and adherence of protocols have enabled our team to achieve an unprecedented level of patient safety. Additionally, world-class research physicians have recently joined the team to further our studies of the underlying causes of heart disease and develop targeted tools and procedures to treat its many permutations.

EXCELLENCE IN FULL RANGE OF INTERVENTIONAL CARDIOLOGY PROCEDURES

Patients ranging from pediatrics to geriatrics come to Mount Sinai's Catheterization Laboratory from all over the world for interventional procedures to help restore the pathway to the heart. This includes routine diagnostics and procedures such as angioplasties, and stents (including drug-eluting stents) to the full spectrum of techniques for complex cases. Our team is internationally recognized for our vast expertise in the following complex procedures:

- Rotational atherectomy
- PCI for CTO (chronic total occlusion, or chronic blockage)
- Left main stenting for unprotected left main coronary artery (LMCA) disease
- TAVI/TAVR (transcatheter aortic valve implementation/replacement)
- Balloon valvuloplasty: aortic and mitral

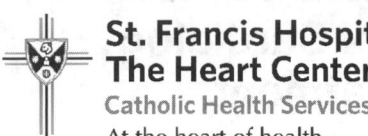

100 Port Washington Blvd.
Roslyn, New York 11576
www.stfrancisheartcenter.com
(516) 562-6000
1-888-HEARTNY

A Leader in Cardiac Care

St. Francis Hospital, The Heart Center® is New York State's only specialty designated cardiac center and is one of the busiest heart centers in the nation. Located in Roslyn, New York, on Long Island's North Shore, St. Francis is ranked among the top 10 hospitals in the United States for cardiology and heart surgery by *U.S. News & World Report*. It is the seventh consecutive year that *U.S. News* has named St. Francis one of the best hospitals in America. In 2013-14, the Hospital was also nationally ranked in ear, nose and throat; gastroenterology and GI surgery; geriatrics; neurology and neurosurgery; orthopedics; pulmonology; and urology.

St. Francis Hospital:

- Has a highly experienced team of physicians and surgeons with one of the largest volumes in the nation for cardiac surgery, interventional cardiology, and arrhythmia procedures

- Offers innovative approaches to cardiac surgery, including minimally invasive procedures and off-pump coronary artery bypass surgery, designed to minimize trauma and reduce surgical complications

- Performs one of the region's highest volumes of catheter-based techniques to correct congenital heart defects such as atrial septal defects (ASDs), ventricular septal defects (VSDs), and patent foramen ovale (PFO)

- Operates a nationally recognized Arrhythmia and Pacemaker Center staffed with electrophysiologists with over a decade of experience in radiofrequency ablation, a permanent cure for certain arrhythmias, including atrial fibrillation

- Maintains a high volume center for the implantation of cardiac pacemakers and defibrillators

- Offers a world-class program in cardiac imaging that fully integrates all technologies, including advanced methods in cardiac MRI, coronary CT angiography, PET/CT and three-dimensional echocardiography

- Has earned the Magnet designation for excellence in nursing services, an honor achieved by only 7 percent of hospitals in the U.S.

- Is a premier center for clinical trials and studies of the application of image-guided methods of diagnosis and treatment of heart disease, such as CoreValve, eValve, CREST, and Symplicity

St. Francis Hospital has outstanding patient satisfaction ratings, and is top-ranked for patients saying they would recommend the Hospital to family and friends.

"Our large cardiac caseload and our growing research program put us in an excellent position to introduce new techniques that can benefit thousands of people in need each year."

–Alan D. Guerci, M.D.
President and Chief Executive Officer
Catholic Health Services of Long Island

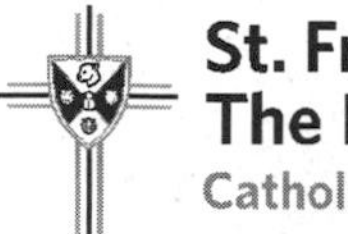

St. Francis Hospital, The Heart Center®

Catholic Health Services

At the heart of health

100 Port Washington Blvd.
Roslyn, New York 11576
www.stfrancisheartcenter.com
(516) 562-6000
1-888-HEARTNY

Noninvasive Cardiac Imaging

Using the latest in noninvasive cardiac imaging technology, St. Francis Hospital's physicians can evaluate blood flow, heart muscle strength, anatomy, and coronary artery blockages, allowing them to more effectively guide a patient's course of treatment.

Among the most recent advances in St. Francis Hospital's range of services are:

Coronary CT Angiography

St. Francis Hospital was the first hospital on Long Island to offer Multidetector Computed Tomography (MDCT) for noninvasive coronary artery imaging. Now, with more advanced technology and personalized design of imaging protocols for each individual, St. Francis can minimize radiation exposure for every patient.

Cardiac MRI

The only center on Long Island with a dedicated Cardiac MRI program and world-class expertise in cardiac MRI, St. Francis Hospital uses MRI to evaluate heart anatomy, function, blood flow, scarring, and inflammation using advanced techniques on two state-of-the-art scanners. Cardiac MRI allows physicians to evaluate effects of heart attack and coronary artery blockages and non-coronary causes of heart failure to determine whether or not patients will benefit from heart surgery or other therapies. World-renowned cardiac MRI authority Nathaniel Reichek, M.D., leads St. Francis Hospital's clinical and research applications of cardiac MRI.

Three-Dimensional Echocardiography

St. Francis Hospital is an internationally recognized leader in three-dimensional echocardiography for quantifying the effects of heart disease. By creating three-dimensional reconstructions of the heart and blood flow within it, this technology provides diagnostic information that surpasses that available with conventional echocardiography in many patients.

Nuclear Imaging

Conventional nuclear imaging involves the injection of nuclear isotopes and imaging by a gamma camera that circles the patient's body, improving the accuracy of stress testing. St. Francis Hospital offers the latest advances in nuclear cardiology, such as positron emission tomography of the heart with CT attenuation correction (PET/CT). The nuclear cardiology laboratory at St. Francis Hospital is also a leader in developing new types of computer analysis to improve the value of all forms of cardiac nuclear imaging, and was among the first facilities in the U.S. to receive accreditation from The Intersocietal Commission for the Accreditation of Nuclear Medicine Laboratories.

Noninvasive Imaging at St. Francis Hospital

Noninvasive imaging services at St. Francis Hospital include:

- Multidetector computed tomographic coronary angiography
- Cardiac MRI
- SPECT/CT nuclear Imaging
- Cardiac PET/CT imaging
- Transesophageal echocardiography
- Three-dimensional echocardiography
- Stress testing with nuclear, echocardiographic or MRI imaging.

The St. Francis Cardiac Imaging Program also supports the Hospital's nationally recognized programs in surgical and interventional cardiology, performing monitoring transesophageal echocardiography during surgical and transarterial valve replacements, catheter treatment of leaky heart valves and minimally invasive treatment to prevent stroke due to cardiac blood clots in atrial fibrillation.

In addition, St. Francis Hospital uses its leading-edge noninvasive imaging technology in its research programs on cardiovascular disease. Drawing on its depth of experience with various imaging modalities, the Hospital has launched a multi-disciplinary effort at its Cardiac Research Institute to improve methods for the diagnosis and treatment of cardiac disease. Past research efforts at the Hospital include The St. Francis Heart Study – a pioneering effort and the largest study of CT calcium scoring to be conducted at any single center – which first demonstrated the value of CT calcium scoring for atherosclerotic plaque detection as a tool in cardiac risk evaluation.

Maternal & Fetal Medicine

For more information about Women's and Children's Health, call 1-877-HOLY-NAME. Please mention "Castle Connolly Guide."

Holy Name Medical Center
Women's and Children's Health

718 Teaneck Road
Teaneck, NJ 07666
1-877-HOLY-NAME
(1-877-465-9626)
www.holyname.org

WOMEN'S AND CHILDREN'S HEALTH DISTINGUISHED FOR SERVICE EXCELLENCE

Consistently recognized for service excellence, Holy Name Medical Center's Women's and Children's Health service features superior medical care with a family-centered focus. At the core of Women's and Children's Health is the Medical Center's staff of specialized physicians and mother-baby nurses, whose expertise fosters the highly positive patient and family experience traditionally associated with Holy Name.

A COMPREHENSIVE PROGRAM OF CARE, EDUCATION AND SUPPORT

Holy Name's beautifully designed BirthPlace offers hotel-like accommodations and amenities, supported by advanced monitoring and infant care technology. The BirthPlace is equipped to address emergencies and cesarean sections with round-the-clock anesthesia coverage, and has an intermediate level II special care nursery with board-certified obstetricians, pediatricians, neonatologists and high-risk specialists available 24/7.

Board-certified perinatologists in Maternal-Fetal Medicine work as consultants with obstetricians to treat women who anticipate or are experiencing a complicated or high-risk pregnancy. They advocate a personalized, hands-on approach to patient care, meeting with the patient at every appointment. The medical team includes perinatal sonographers with advanced training and expertise in perinatal ultrasound, and genetic counselors with extensive training in high-risk pregnancy care.

- Private LDRP suites
- On-unit cesarean-section rooms
- Dedicated nursing staff for labor and delivery, postpartum, and special care nursery
- 24-hour access to board-certified anesthesiologists, obstetrician/gynecologists, pediatricians and neonatologists
- Intermediate level II special care nursery
- Maternal-fetal medicine program and perinatal high-risk services
- Genetic counseling
- Central fetal monitoring and maternal monitoring
- Education classes, support groups and infant care hotline
- State-of-the-art electronic security system
- Participant in National Cord Blood Stem Cell Program (umbilical cord blood storage for future lifesaving interventions)

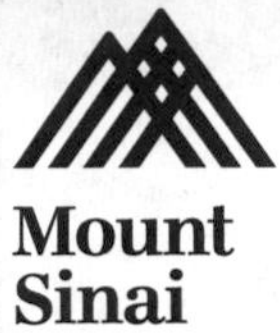

THE MOUNT SINAI MEDICAL CENTER

Maternal Fetal Medicine

One Gustave L. Levy Place
Fifth Avenue and 100th Street
New York, NY 10029-6574

Physician Referral: 1-800-MD-SINAI (637-4624)
www.mountsinai.org

Mount Sinai's **MATERNAL FETAL MEDICINE** team assists expectant mothers with a history of complicated pregnancy or who have special concerns, such as multiple births, diabetes, high blood pressure, and premature labor. Through our state-of-the-art diagnostic services and treatments, including 3-D and 4-D ultrasound, our board-certified specialists in maternal-fetal medicine work in concert with geneticists, neonatologists, pediatric cardiologists and other physicians to help you carry and deliver a healthy baby in a safe and supportive environment.

Our advanced ultrasound-guided procedures enable us to search for genetic, growth, and structural differences in the fetus. While many babies can be treated with medication, Mount Sinai can provide treatment through the womb, which can be lifesaving for both you and you're your child.

Mount Sinai can also help HIV-infected pregnant women realize their goal of delivering a healthy baby.

Our first-trimester Down syndrome screening program and our prenatal genetics counseling program provide comprehensive clinical and laboratory services, such as chorionic villus sampling (CVS) and amniocentesis, to detect chromosomal abnormalities. In the event of a genetic defect, we provide you with comprehensive genetics counseling to help you make informed healthcare decisions regarding your baby.

Mount Sinai employs frequent surveillance of fetal growth, cervical change, and preterm labor when dealing with multiple births. We are highly experienced in multi-fetal reduction and selective termination.

If your baby comes early or has special needs, our **Neonatal Intensive Care Unit (NICU)** is a 35-bed regional perinatal center that cares for the most complex patients. Our NICU specialists include neonatologists, pediatric surgeons, and pediatricians. The unit has more than 65 full-time nurses who specialize in newborn care, as well as social workers, lactation consultants, rehabilitation specialists, and respiratory therapists to provide your little one with the most advanced care possible.

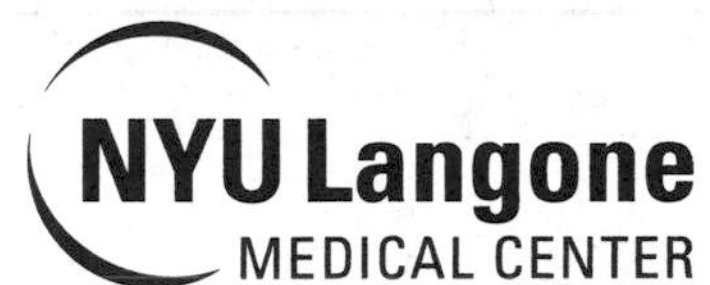

550 First Avenue *(at 31st Street)*
New York, NY 10016

www.NYULMC.org

Physician Referral: **888-7-NYU-MED** *(888-769-8633)*

OBSTETRICS AND GYNECOLOGY

NYU Langone Medical Center provides comprehensive services designed specifically for women, from primary care to highly specialized programs that are supported by sophisticated research and advanced training. We specialize in the following areas:

Obstetrics

We offer a broad range of obstetrical services, including prenatal care that gives equal emphasis to the well-being of the mother and the fetus; fetal monitoring through ultrasound and other techniques; childbirth preparedness and breastfeeding classes.

Maternal-Fetal Medicine

Prenatal care for high-risk pregnancies and detailed consultations before, during and after pregnancy are offered. We specialize in multifetal pregnancies, genetic counseling, women who have miscarried, and preterm deliveries, as well as helping women who have other medical conditions that may complicate a pregnancy, such as diabetes, heart problems, high blood pressure, and lupus. We offer the latest techniques for in-utero diagnosis and treatment and using minimally invasive techniques, our physicians are able to repair a number of life-threatening conditions in a child before it is even born.

Fertility-Related Services

We offer state-of-the-art programs in evaluation of infertility (including the special needs of same-sex couples) egg donation, egg freezing and in-vitro fertilization. Diagnosis and treatment include ovulation induction, assisted reproductive technologies and surgical options that incorporate the latest endoscopic techniques. Preimplantation Genetic Screening (PGS) at the Fertility Center offers tests for aneuploidy (an abnormal number of chromosomes).

Gynecology

In addition to routine gynecological care, we offer pelvic ultrasound; aspiration of breast cysts, colposcopy (a diagnostic evaluation of abnormal pap smears); LEEP (a loop electrosurgical procedure used to diagnose and treat cervical cancer); cryotherapy for vaginal warts; and bone density testing.

Gynecologic Surgery

Minimally invasive gynecologic surgery, including robotic surgery, is offered for a wide range of simple and complex conditions including, resection of endometriosis, hysterectomy, and myomectomy.

Gynecologic Oncology

The NCI-designated NYU Cancer Institute's Women's Cancer Program specializes in the treatment of cervical cancer, endometrial cancer, ovarian cancer, uterine cancer, vaginal cancer and vulvar cancer.

Medical Oncology

For more information about the Regional Cancer Center, call 1-877-HOLY-NAME. Please mention "Castle Connolly Guide."

Holy Name Medical Center
Regional Cancer Center

718 Teaneck Road
Teaneck, NJ 07666
1-877-HOLY-NAME
(1-877-465-9626)
www.holyname.org

Holy Name Medical Center's Regional Cancer Center offers leading-edge diagnosis, staging and treatment services for people with cancer. Holy Name's outstanding team of board-certified specialists cares for patients in an environment that promotes personalized service and ready access to multiple disciplines. The Regional Cancer Center is accredited by the American College of Radiology, the American Society for Radiation Oncology, and the American College of Surgeons Commission on Cancer as a Comprehensive Community Cancer Program—accreditations that ensure access to a broad spectrum of services, and high-quality patient care, safety and technical standards.

A TEAM APPROACH

Individualized treatment plans are formulated not by a single physician, but with input from medical, radiation and surgical oncologists, pathologists and radiologists; specially trained and certified oncology nurses; and other medical specialists who render care in both outpatient and inpatient settings. State-of-the-art noninvasive technologies, including fusion PET/CT, high-resolution CT, PET, MRI, breast MRI, extremity MRI and low-dose mammography, produce exquisitely detailed images for diagnostic and treatment planning purposes.

PATIENT-CENTERED CARE

Holy Name simplifies the logistics associated with cancer therapy with ready access to services and physicians, minimal waiting, and easy parking. Oncology patients needing emergency care related to their diagnosis are admitted directly to the specialized nursing unit, without the delays associated with first visiting the Emergency Care Center.

The Regional Cancer Center features a one-stop concept with the full range of services located in a single convenient setting. Patients can arrange a consultation with their oncologist, receive radiation treatment or chemotherapy, have imaging procedures, biopsies and other tests, and receive physical rehabilitation. They can meet with the Center's oncology-certified dietitian, take part in a support group or seek the assistance of a social worker. Genetic counselors are available to work with patients and their family members.

Accurate diagnosis and staging + Targeted, precision therapy = Fewer complications, minimal side effects and improved outcomes

- PET and fusion PET/CT
- High-resolution CT and MRI
- Breast MRI
- SPECT imaging
- Low-dose digital mammography
- Robotic-assisted surgery
- Intensity-modulated radiation therapy (IMRT)
- Image-guided radiation therapy (IGRT)
- CT-guided prone breast radiation therapy
- Stereotactic body radiotherapy (SBRT)
- High-dose brachytherapy for prostate
- Stereotactic radiosurgery
- Microsphere embolization for liver
- Radiofrequency ablation
- Clinical research trials
- Supportive care, nutrition and pharmacy services, physical rehabilitation, palliative services, and home care
- Genetic counseling

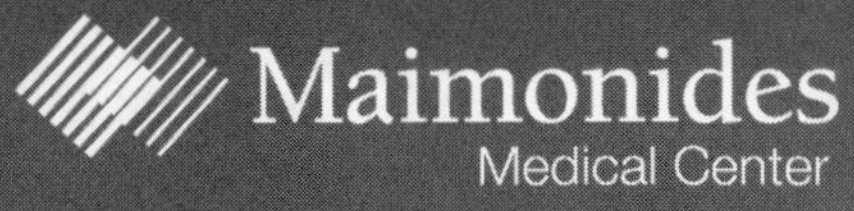

MAIMONIDES CANCER CENTER

6300 Eighth Avenue
Brooklyn, New York 11220
Phone: 718.765.2500 • Fax: 718.765.2574
www.maimonidesmed.org/cancer

The Maimonides Cancer Center offers a fully integrated, multimodal approach to cancer care that includes prevention, education, screening, diagnostics, treatment, palliative care and clinical research. The Lena Cymbrowitz Pavilion contains the following specialty divisions:

Radiation Oncology: equipped with state-of-the art imaging and treatment delivery technologies; offers patients the most precise treatments available, yet does so in an airy, life-affirming environment.

Medical Oncology: provides comprehensive diagnosis, oral drug therapies, intravenous chemotherapy infusions, and biological and hormonal therapies.

Pediatric Oncology: treats children with cancer and diseases of the blood in a child-friendly environment, and features special areas set aside for parent conferences.

Surgical Oncology: provides a convenient location for minor surgical procedures, as well as innovative surgical techniques, such as sentinel node mapping and biopsy, skin/tissue-sparing mastectomy, and nerve-sparing prostatectomy.

Research Center: conducts basic science and genetic research, as well as clinical trials that offer appropriately screened patients, who wish to volunteer, new therapies and medications.

Resource Center: offers access to integrative (complementary) oncology services, dietary advice, as well as psychological and social services.

Located around the block from the Lena Cymbrowitz Pavilion, the newly opened Gilbert Rivera Pavilion houses the **Maimonides Breast Cancer Center**. With a spa-like decor and life-affirming environment, the Center provides digital mammography, sonography, computerized interpretation, digital stereotactic biopsies, breast-specific gamma imaging, and treatment plans tailored to each patient. A genetic counselor is also on-site.

Clinicians at the Maimonides Cancer Center – Brooklyn's only dedicated cancer center – are talented specialists, recruited specifically for their expertise. Our doctors emphasize multimodal care, which means that multiple methods of treatment are available to patients, sometimes simultaneously. Every week, physicians from radiology, surgery, pathology, radiation oncology and medical oncology meet to discuss patient treatment at our case management meetings. The patient's needs, as well as the disease, are considered from many perspectives.

Maimonides Medical Center

The right care.
Right here.

www.maimonidesmed.org/cancer

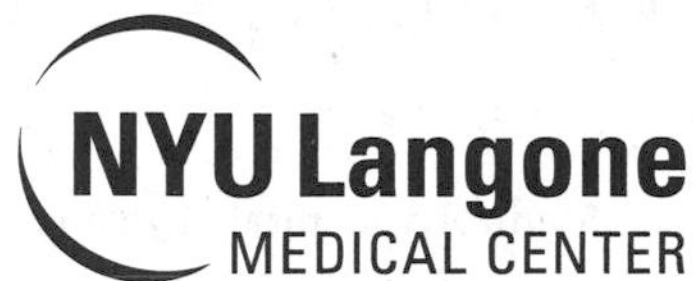

NYU Langone Medical Center
550 First Avenue, New York, NY 10016
www.NYULMC.org

Clinical Cancer Center
160 East 34th Street, New York, NY 10016
www.NYUCI.org

The Stephen D. Hassenfeld Children's Center for Cancer and Blood Disorders
160 East 32nd Street, New York, NY 10016
www.NYULMC.org/hassenfeld

NYU CANCER INSTITUTE

The NYU Cancer Institute is an NCI-designated cancer center providing personalized patient care that is compassionate and state-of-the-art. The Cancer Institute is world-renowned for excellence in cancer-focused research, personalized care, education and community outreach. Its mission is to discover the origins of human cancer and to use that knowledge to eradicate the personal and societal burden of cancer in our community, the nation and the world. For more information about our expert physicians, call 1.888.769.8633.

Patient-Focused Setting
The Clinical Cancer Center is the principal outpatient facility of The Cancer Institute. The Center and its multidisciplinary team of experts provide access to the latest treatment options and clinical trials, along with programs in cancer risk reduction/prevention, screening, diagnostics, genetic counseling and supportive services. In addition, the Center emphasizes the importance of a holistic approach involving integrative health, psychosocial support, survivorship and palliative care. Services are also available at our Ambulatory Care Center on 38th Street in Manhattan, Rego Park, NY, and Lake Success, NY.

Renowned Expertise
The NYU Cancer Institute brings together experts from a variety of disciplines to create collaborative research endeavors and clinical care teams. Our teams are highly skilled in minimally invasive techniques along with video-assisted and robotic surgery. We have created special programs to treat diseases such as breast cancer, brain cancer, melanoma, GI cancer, prostate cancer, hematologic malignancies and lung cancer, as well as translational programs in cancer healthcare disparities; molecularly targeted as well as immune- and stem-cell-based therapies; and the cell signaling pathways involved in cancer.

A Translational Approach
Our scientists and researchers excel in uncovering how cancer develops at the molecular level, and how we can harness that knowledge to reduce the risk of cancer and treat the disease.

Stephen D. Hassenfeld Children's Center for Cancer and Blood Disorders
As part of the Hassenfeld Children's Hospital, the center is a leading pediatric outpatient facility for the treatment of childhood cancers and blood diseases. Its interdisciplinary and family-centered approach combines the most advanced medical treatments with psychosocial and emotional support services.

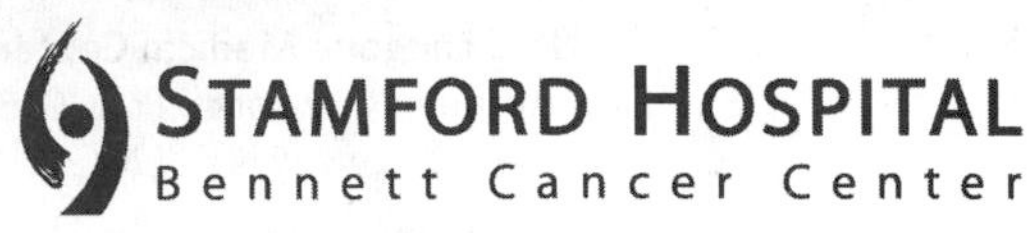

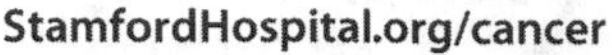

Bennett Cancer Center

Stamford Hospital's Carl & Dorothy Bennett Cancer Center provides compassionate, patient-centered care from diagnosis through post treatment. We are accredited as an Academic Comprehensive Cancer Program and received the outstanding Achievement Award from the American College of Surgeons Commission on Cancer. A multidisciplinary team of physicians, oncology nurses, nurse navigators and radiation therapists, offers advanced surgical, medical and technological services in a warm, caring environment.

Expertise Combined With Comfort
Our physicians' skill, knowledge and expertise are equaled only by their compassion in dealing with our patients. They are represented on the consulting staff of Memorial Sloan-Kettering Cancer Center and teaching faculty of Columbia University College of Physicians and Surgeons. They are also active participants in national research groups. The Center is involved with more clinical trials than any other area hospital.

Genetic Counseling
We offer the only full-time cancer genetic counselor in Fairfield County, ensuring timely delivery of genetic counseling services and superior interaction with other specialists, as well as the most current information in both genetics and oncology.

Treatment Beyond the Disease
We provide chemotherapy and immunotherapy in an outpatient setting, where patients can be treated in private suites with a home-like ambiance or a group room in the company of others. Cancer cases are reviewed by a multidisciplinary team of physicians and staff. This offers patients the benefit of different specialists combining their expertise.

Our Integrative Medicine Program and other support services including the *Transitions: Choices in Recovery* post-treatment survivorship program, offer a wide range of complementary therapies along with stress management, individual, family and group therapy.

Technology That Doesn't Forget Humanity
We are the only hospital in Fairfield and Westchester counties to offer CyberKnife™ stereoatactic radiosurgery to treat tumors with pinpoint accuracy. Additional technology includes simulator and linear accelerator machines with both Intensity Modulated Radiation Therapy and Image-Guided Radiation Therapy. Our diagnostic imaging services include a 64-slice CT scan, ultrasound, nuclear medicine, PET CT and MRI.

Academic and Clinical Affiliations
Stamford Hospital is an affiliate of the New York–Presbyterian Healthcare System and a major teaching affiliate of the Columbia University College of Physicians & Surgeons.

Accreditation
Joint Commission on Accreditation of Healthcare Organization (JCAHO)

Beds
305

Sponsorship
Voluntary, Not-for-Profit

For a Physician Referral or more information, please call 1.877.233.9355 or visit StamfordHospital.org /doctor.

Stamford Hospital
30 Shelburne Road
Stamford, CT 06902
203.276.1000

StamfordHospital.org

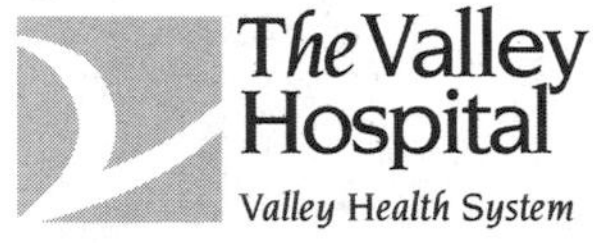

THE VALLEY HOSPITAL

An affiliate of the NewYork-Presbyterian Healthcare System

223 North Van Dien Avenue, Ridgewood, NJ 07450
Phone: 201-447-8000 • www.ValleyHealth.com
www.Facebook.com/ValleyHospital • www.Twitter.com/ValleyHospital

The Daniel & Gloria Blumenthal Cancer Center

Our cancer care experts focus on delivering today's most promising therapies with compassion and dignity. Our multidisciplinary team of board-certified medical, surgical, and radiation oncologists; specialty physicians; Magnet-recognized oncology nurses; and award-winning allied health professionals is dedicated to providing personalized care that meets every person's unique needs and expectations. Our growing clinical and translational research programs offer patients access to new therapies and innovative protocols that are unavailable at other area hospitals. Our outreach educational programs and cancer screenings strive to prevent cancer and/or detect it at an early, treatable stage. Our cancer program has earned six Disease-Specific Care Certifications for healthcare quality from the Joint Commission for colorectal cancer, lung cancer, breast cancer, pancreatic cancer, prostate cancer, and uterine-ovarian cancer.

Diagnostic Imaging and Testing

Our state-of-the-art capabilities help physicians detect, stage, and monitor cancer. Our technology includes low-dose CT scanning, MRI, PET scanning, endoscopic ultrasound, endobronchial ultrasound, and digital mammography.

Powerful Therapies

Our Radiation Oncology Department and specialized centers provide all of the latest advanced modalities of radiation therapy to treat numerous cancers. Our Centers of Excellence include our Breast Center, Gamma Knife Center, Lung Cancer Center, Institute for Brain and Spine Surgery, Melanoma and Skin Cancer Center, and Urologic Oncology Center. Our surgical oncologists and other surgical specialists use the robotic daVinci surgical system, laparoscopic techniques, and other minimally invasive options to offer patients gentler procedures with quicker recoveries. Our ambulatory Medical Infusion Center provides a comfortable site for receiving outpatient chemotherapy and other infusion therapies. Our hyperthermic intraperitoneal chemotherapy (HIPEC) program is the only one in New Jersey and one of the largest in the metropolitan area.

Patient- and Family-Centered Care

At The Valley Hospital, we espouse patient- and family-centered care, which recognizes the impact a diagnosis of cancer can have on the entire family and offers services, education, and guidance for all. Our holistic nursing care and integrative medicine therapies support healing of the mind, body and spirit. Support services, such as nutrition counseling, genetic counseling, social work services, pastoral care, psychosocial counseling, rehabilitation therapy, support groups, home care, and educational programs assist patients during and after cancer care and help to improve their quality of life.

A Dedication to Research

Our oncology research program endeavors to find answers to the complex questions of how cancer develops, how it behaves, why it mutates, and how it can be stopped or controlled. Included among our research are studies in using microRNA to screen for cancer, immune response to lung cancer, a brain cancer vaccine, and stereotactic radiosurgery outcomes.

Cancer Care that is accredited by the American College of Surgeons Commission on Cancer and the American College of Radiology

- Infusion Center and chemotherapy, including NJ's only hyperthermic intraperitoneal chemotherapy program
- Image-guided TomoTherapy
- Intensity-modulated radiation therapy
- Gamma Knife Center
- Stereotactic body radiotherapy
- High-dose-rate afterloading brachytherapy
- Barrett's Esophagus, Breast, Lung, Melanoma and Skin Cancer, and Urologic Oncology Centers
- Gynecologic, radiologic, surgical, thoracic, and urologic oncologists
- Single-port video-assisted thoracic surgery (VATS)
- Minimally invasive breast oncoplastics surgery
- Cancer genetics
- Integrative healing services
- Holistic nursing care
- Home care and hospice

Daniel & Gloria Blumenthal Center, 201-634-5707; www.ValleyFightsCancer.com

Minimally Invasive Surgery

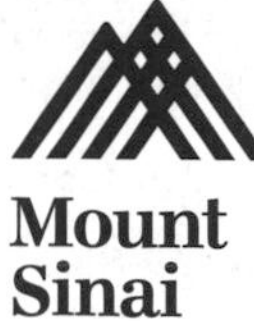

THE MOUNT SINAI MEDICAL CENTER

Minimally Invasive Surgery

One Gustave L. Levy Place
Fifth Avenue and 100th Street
New York, NY 10029-6574

Physician Referral: 1-800-MD-SINAI (637-4624)
www.mountsinai.org

At The Mount Sinai Medical Center, our surgeons perform the most minimally invasive surgical techniques available, combining advanced technology with superior patient care. As a result, patients undergoing these procedures experience less pain, shorter hospital stays, and faster recovery times than ever before.

Although the techniques vary for different procedures, minimally invasive surgical procedures employ video cameras and lens systems to provide anatomic visualization within a specific region of the body. In addition, our surgeons use the **da Vinci Surgical System** to perform robotic procedures for complex benign and malignant conditions.

Minimally Invasive Surgical Procedures Offered:

- Laparoscopic (abdominal) minimally invasive surgery
- Bariatric surgery
- Colorectal surgery
- Gynecologic surgery
- Neurosurgery
- Orthopedic Surgery
- Otolaryngology–Ear, Nose and Throat Surgery
- Thoracic Surgery
- Urologic Surgery
- Vascular Surgery
- Robotic Prostate Surgery

Our surgeons rank as world leaders in the development of new minimally invasive techniques for the treatment of many conditions, and they deliver exceptional patient care. In surveys of leading minimally invasive surgeons in a variety of specialties, Mount Sinai's physicians are consistently ranked at the top of the list.

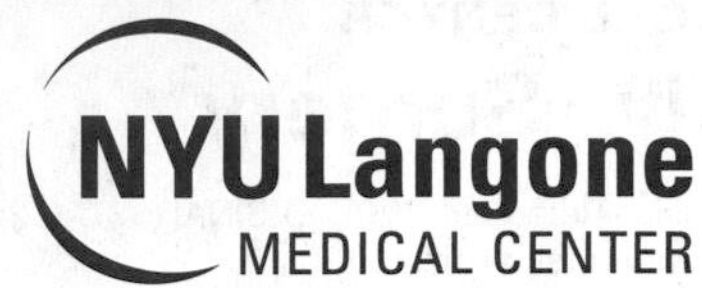

550 First Avenue *(at 31st Street)*
New York, NY 10016
www.NYULMC.org
Physician Referral: **888-7-NYU-MED** *(888-769-8633)*

UROLOGY

Urologists at NYU Langone Medical Center continue to pioneer in the surgical and medical treatment of urological disease and are recognized as a top urology program in the country by U.S. News and World Report.

Smilow Comprehensive Prostate Cancer Center
As part of the NCI-designated NYU Cancer Institute, the Center offers access to a team of uro-oncologic surgeons, radiation oncologists, oncologists and radiologists. Integrative services are available as well.

Benign Prostatic Diseases
Innovative medical and surgical therapies for benign prostatic disease and prostatitis.

Leading Edge Research
We are focused on discovering novel treatments for bladder and prostate cancer, while exploring how cancer markers can be used to determine how cancer treatments are working.

Female Urology and Incontinence
NYU Langone specializes in urological problems unique to women, including recurrent urinary tract infections, pelvic pain, prolapse and sexual dysfunction.

Latest Minimally Invasive Treatments
Advances in prostate imaging and computer biopsy are providing valuable information about tumor location and growth to enable targeted treatment. The latest options are also available to treat kidney stones and other obstructions.

Male Sexual Health
In collaboration with NYU Langone's Fertility Center, urologists use the latest techniques to enable infertile couples to have children. Treatment is also offered to men suffering from erectile dysfunction and low testosterone.

Pediatric Urology and Reconstructive Surgery
Pediatric urologists focus on urinary system disorders in children from birth to early adults.

Robotic Urological Surgery
The Department's robotic surgery program includes prostate and kidney cancers, as well as female incontinence and urinary tract reconstruction.

Urologic Oncology
Because cancer treatment often requires a collaborative approach, urologists work closely with their colleagues at the NYU Cancer Institute to tailor treatments for each patient.

Neonatal-Perinatal Medicine

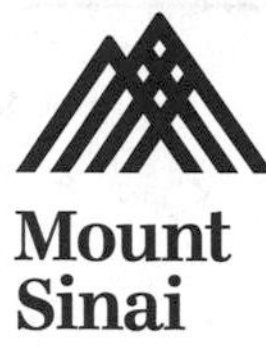

THE MOUNT SINAI MEDICAL CENTER
KRAVIS CHILDREN'S HOSPITAL
Neonatal Medicine

One Gustave L. Levy Place
Fifth Avenue and 100th Street
New York, NY 10029-6574

Physician Referral: 1-800-MD-SINAI (637-4624)
www.kravischildrenshospital.org

INNOVATIVE MEDICINE, FAMILY-CENTERED CARE

Neonatal Medicine

At The Mount Sinai Medical Center's Kravis Children's Hospital, we enjoy a well-earned reputation for excellence in caring for our tiniest and sickest patients–those born prematurely; with birth defects, such as congenital heart disease; liver, intestinal and kidney failure; or with metabolic and genetic conditions.

New York State Designated Level 3 Regional Perinatal Center

Our physicians, board certified in neonatal–perinatal medicine, deliver superior care to these and other infants in our Jo Carole and Ronald S. Lauder Neonatal Intensive Care Unit (NICU), a 35-bed, state-of-the-art, New York State designated Level 3 Regional Perinatal Center. We received this distinction, the highest available, in recognition of our ability to deliver superior care to babies with the most complex conditions and to provide expert consultations to other neonatal units within the region.

We deliver care to more than 800 newborns a year, with our NICU experiencing some of the lowest infection rates in the state. Our medical staff consists of neonatologists, pediatric subspecialists and pediatric surgeons. In addition, our unit staffs 65 full-time nurses who specialize in newborn care, as well as social workers, lactation consultants, rehabilitation specialists and respiratory therapists.

Family-Centered Care

A special feature of our unit is our dedication to delivering family-centered care, which includes:

- Two-full-time social workers, assuring that the help and resources families require during stressful times is consistently available
- Two separate breast milk pumping rooms and facilities for refrigerating and freezing milk
- Regular educational and social programs for parents and a monthly "Sibling Saturday" to accommodate important family needs.

We also offer pre-delivery meetings with the family of a child who might be born with special needs. These meetings are held with experts in different areas of care and include tours of the areas where the baby will receive care. We understand the vital role families play in the care of a sick newborn, and we include them as essential components in our circle of care.

Nephrology

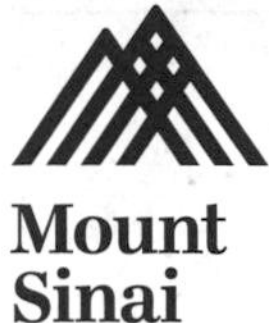

THE MOUNT SINAI MEDICAL CENTER
Nephrology

One Gustave L. Levy Place
Fifth Avenue and 100th Street
New York, NY 10029-6574

Physician Referral: 1-800-MD-SINAI (637-4624)
www.mountsinai.org

Mount Sinai's Department of Nephrology ranks among the best in the nation, according to the 2013-2014 issue of *U.S. News & World Report's* "Americas Best Hospitals."

We have been an international leader in the treatment of kidney disease since we performed the first hemodialysis in the United States in the 1950s. We established New York State's first dialysis center in 1957. We currently operate the largest home dialysis program in New York City, and our **Geriatric Nephrology Program** is the only one of its kind in the country. We have world renowned scientists and physicians to study and treat patients with kidney glomerular disease including diabetic kidney disease.

EXPERT PHYSICIANS

Building on the talent and expertise of our physicians, including Jonathan Winston, MD, Tonia Kim, MD, Mark Swidler, MD, Jaime Uribarri, MD, Joseph Vassalotti, MD, Brian Radbill, MD, and Richard Stein, MD, along with transplantation specialists, Bernd Schroppel, MD, and Vinay Nair, MD, we provide patients with the most advanced and appropriate approach to care. With so much research taking place, we can also offer patients access to experimental treatments often unavailable elsewhere.

Our expertise spans numerous kidney diseases and treatments, including:

- Chronic kidney disease
- Polycystic kidney disease
- Geriatric kidney disease
- Diabetes-related kidney disease
- Glomerular disease
- Hypertensive kidney disease
- HIV-associated nephropathy
- Kidney transplantation
- Hemodialysis
- Peritoneal Dialysis
- Kidney stone

Initiated in 1967, our **kidney transplant program** is now one of the largest and most successful in the country, with our physician-scientists actively investigating new and innovative ways to detect, prevent, and treat rejection.

Under the direction of Barbara Murphy, MD, Chair of Department of Medicine and John He, MD/PhD, the new Division Chief of Nephrology, we are continuing our leadership in patient care, research and education. Proof of our clinical excellence is evident daily in our practice and hospital. Our physicians care for patients referred to us by other nephrologists who recognize the need for our expertise in their most challenging and complex cases.

A Strong Focus on Research

With one of the largest National Institutes of Health research budgets of any nephrology division in the country, we conduct and support numerous clinical trials, and our faculty members have achieved international recognition as authorities on the causes and treatments of all forms of kidney diseases and disorders.

Neurological Surgery

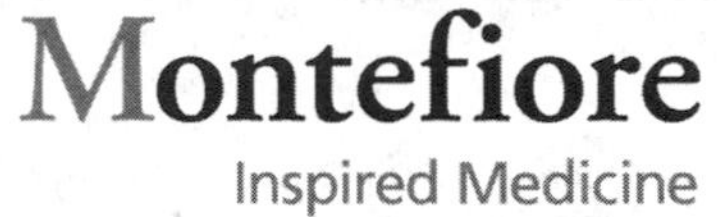

3316 Rochambeau Avenue
Bronx, New York 10467
718-920-7476
www.montefiore.org/neurosurgery

Neurosurgery at Montefiore

Montefiore Medical Center's Department of Neurosurgery brings together state-of-the-art technology and highly experienced specialists to provide exceptional care for children and adults.

Montefiore's neurosurgeons are accomplished in all aspects of neurosurgery and employ the full spectrum of diagnostic and treatment modalities to ensure superior outcomes, including the use of intraoperative computed tomography scanners. Minimally invasive treatment approaches—such as endovascular coiling, stereotactic-guided radiosurgery and microneurosurgery—are also emphasized.

Montefiore's new Neurovascular Program is helping to improve outcomes of patients with disorders related to the blood vessels of the brain—including stroke, carotid artery disease, intracranial aneurysms, and cerebrovascular and arteriovenous malformations. This unique program brings neurosurgeons, neurologists and interventional radiologists together to review cases and administer treatment. The neurovascular team also includes a surgeon who is board certified in both neurosurgery and neurointerventional procedures. This program streamlines care and minimizes the risk of open surgery by using catheter-based approaches as appropriate.

Working in partnership with plastic and reconstructive surgeons, otolaryngologists and other specialists from The Children's Hospital of Montefiore, the Department's pediatric neurosurgeons perform complex craniofacial reconstructions for children with rare facial tumors, traumatic injuries and birth defects—such as craniosyntosis, Apert syndrome and Crouzon syndrome. Using advanced 3D technology to plan reconstructions, the physicians ensure the best outcomes possible for these children. The craniofacial team's commitment to surgical excellence has resulted in reoperative rates of less than 5 percent—substantially lower than the national average—and "return to OR" and relapse rates of less than 1 percent.

CHAM's pediatric neurosurgeons are developing new techniques for safeguarding the nervous system using neurophysiological mapping and monitoring during surgeries to remove tumors. They also specialize in alleviating the painful side effects of hydrocephalus treatment and repairing Chiari malformations.

Montefiore is nationally ranked in neurology and neurosurgery by *U.S. News & World Report.* Its neurosurgeons are involved in clinical research aimed at improving wound closure following spine surgery; the use of chemotherapy for the treatment of malignant brain tumors; understanding the genetics of medulloblastomas, glioblastomas and other cancers of the brain; and the use of special imaging techniques to enhance the treatment of patients with hydrocephalus.

THE MOUNT SINAI MEDICAL CENTER

Neurosurgery

One Gustave L. Levy Place
Fifth Avenue and 100th Street
New York, NY 10029-6574

Physician Referral: 1-800-MD-SINAI (637-4624)
www.mountsinai.org

THE DEPARTMENT OF NEUROSURGERY at Mount Sinai, established in 1914, has earned a distinguished international reputation. Since assuming the position of Chair five years ago, Joshua Bederson, MD, has expanded the department by more than 50 percent through a combination of strategic recruitments, new hospital affiliations, and numerous outreach programs. Neurosurgery is the fastest growing surgical subspecialty at Mount Sinai, performing more than 2,500 procedures a year at The Mount Sinai Hospital. Areas of clinical expertise include the treatment of meningiomas and other skull base tumors, primary and metastatic brain tumors, pituitary adenomas and acoustic neuromas, deep brain stimulation for movement disorders and minimally invasive treatment of spine and spinal cord disorders. The department is a regional leader in endovascular and microsurgical treatment of aneurysms, arteriovenous malformations and stroke, microvascular decompression for trigeminal neuralgia and hemifacial spasm. We are the first medical center in the nation to use the Neurotouch virtual reality brain surgery simulator, which will be used to train our residents, assess skill level and to rehearse upcoming cases.

The Meningioma Program has pioneered endoscopic, minimally invasive surgical approaches for the treatment of meningiomas. Transnasal endoscopic tumor resections and computer-aided navigation help our surgeons achieve even greater precision during surgery. Both tactics reduce risk to the patient and help us avoid critical vascular and intracranial structures. Working with the Minimally Invasive and Endoscopic Skull Base Surgery Program, we unite specialists in neurosurgery, otolaryngology, head and neck cancer, craniofacial surgery, oral and maxillofacial surgery, and microvascular and reconstructive procedures.

The Cerebrovascular Program is composed of an experienced team that provides a complete range of services for the diagnosis and treatment of patients with neurovascular disorders of the brain and spinal cord. Some current treatments include endovascular treatment of aneurysms with coils and/or stents, endovascular treatment of AVMs with liquid acrylics, stereotactic radiosurgical treatment of AVMs, endovascular treatment of stenoses with stents and angioplasty and microsurgical treatment of stenoses and occlusions with bypass. We also specialize in microsurgical treatment of aneurysms and AVMs with clipping and resection. We are the most experienced program in stent-assisted embolization of cerebral aneurysms and stent treatment of carotid artery disease amongst neurovascular centers in New York. The Comprehensive Brain Tumor Program collaborates with The Tisch Cancer Institute and the Departments of Neurology, Radiation Oncology, Radiology, and Pathology to provide comprehensive therapies for primary and metastatic malignant brain tumors. We have pioneered minimally invasive approaches using imaging technology, frameless stereotaxy, awake and asleep brain mapping, and advanced microneurosurgery. Stereotactic radiosurgery, a minimally invasive treatment that does not require open surgery, gene therapy, and clinical trials are also possible options.

The Neurosurgery Spinal Disorders Program offers treatment for all disorders of the spinal column and spinal cord, including degenerative disorders, trauma, infections, congenital disorders (including scoliosis), and tumors. Our neurosurgeons have pioneered endoscopic, minimally invasive approaches for tumor resection and treatment of degenerative diseases. These approaches reduce pain and hospital stays, and facilitate an early return to normal activity.

The Neuroendocrine Program sees more than 200 new pituitary tumor patients each year, more than 300 follow-up patients annually, and has performed more than 2,500 transphenoidal pituitary operations.

The Center for Neuromodulation, a collaboration between the Departments of Neurology and Neurosurgery, uses the latest technology to precisely target areas of abnormal activity in the brain and spinal cord. Our physicians are focused on developing minimally invasive neurosurgical techniques that either modulate neural function, replace lost neuronal populations, or halt the neurodegenerative process altogether. Currently, deep brain stimulation dominates this field, but many technologies with great potential are on the horizon. Our Center for Neuromodulation is currently the highest volume center of its kind in the Northeast.

NewYork-Presbyterian

Affiliated with Columbia University College of Physicians and Surgeons and Weill Cornell Medical College

NewYork-Presbyterian Hospital
Columbia University Medical Center
622 West 168th Street
New York, NY 10032

NewYork-Presbyterian Hospital
Weill Cornell Medical Center
525 East 68th Street
New York, NY 10065

1-877-NYP-WELL (1-877-697-9355) www.nyp.org/neuro

NewYork-Presbyterian Neuroscience

In 2013–2014, NewYork-Presbyterian's neurology and neurosurgery program was ranked 3rd in the nation in the annual "Best Hospitals" survey conducted by *U.S. News & World Report*™. Our Neuroscience Centers offer innovative treatments to improve the quality of life of patients with neurological disorders, including:

- **Stroke:** Our four Stroke Center locations are among the few NYS designated primary stroke centers. Round-the-clock surveillance and state-of-the-art brain monitoring in our Neuro-ICUs minimize damage and maximize the chance for a full recovery.
- **Epilepsy:** Comprehensive Epilepsy Centers use the latest monitoring and imaging tools to locate the source of a patient's seizures and tailor medical and/or surgical treatment.
- **Pediatric neurology/neurosurgery:** Specialists are sensitive to the special needs of children with epilepsy, brain tumors, stroke, craniofacial disorders, vascular anomalies, and movement disorders.
- **Spinal disorders:** Neurosurgeons, rehabilitation medicine physicians, physical therapists, pain management physicians, nurse practitioners, and neurologists personalize a plan of care for patients with neck and back pain and disorders such as scoliosis, disc disease, and compression fractures.
- **Brain and spinal tumors:** Neurosurgeons, neuro-oncologists, radiation oncologists, and others care for patients with brain and spinal tumors. Translational research programs aim to understand the biology of these diseases and develop innovative therapies.
- **Neuro-immune disorders:** Comprehensive care is delivered to patients with multiple sclerosis as well as less common diseases, such as neurosarcoidosis and neuromyelitis optica.
- **Neuro-muscular disorders:** Our multidisciplinary team cares for people with neuromuscular diseases such as ALS (Lou Gehrig's Disease), Guillain-Barre syndrome, muscular dystrophy, myasthenia gravis, myopathy, and neuropathy.
- **Movement disorders:** NewYork-Presbyterian Hospital treats one of the world's largest populations of patients with movement disorders, especially Parkinson's disease. Researchers assess new drugs, imaging techniques, surgical therapies (such as deep brain stimulation), and gene therapy.
- **Memory disorders:** Our programs feature advanced care for patients with Alzheimer's disease or other memory disorders and their families, as well as clinical and laboratory research to better understand these disorders, with the goal of treating them sooner and more effectively.

Highlights:

- Researchers demonstrated that two genes associated with ALS work in tandem to support long-term survival of motor neurons.
- Neurologists, neurosurgeons, and radiologists collaborated to show that intensive medical therapy is more effective than stenting for preventing a second stroke.
- Investigators devised a computer model of the spread of dementia that can be used to predict future disease patterns years before they occur in a patient.
- NewYork-Presbyterian is participating in NeuroNEXT (Network for Excellence in Neuroscience Clinical Trials), an NIH-funded national effort to accelerate the development of therapies for people with neurological diseases.
- Neuro-oncologists are devising innovative approaches, such as the use of microcatheters, to bypass the blood-brain barrier and deliver chemotherapy directly to brain tumors.

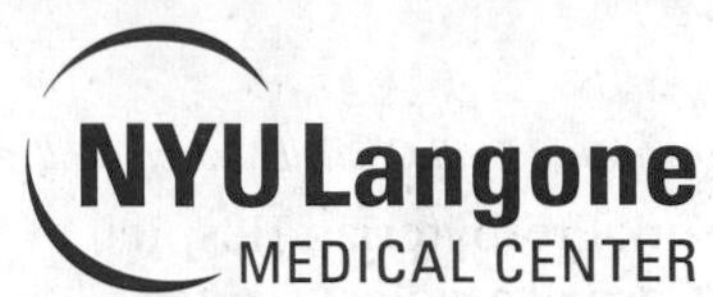

550 First Avenue *(at 31st Street)*
New York, NY 10016
www.NYULMC.org/neurology
www.NYULMC.org/neurosurgery
Physician Referral: **888-7-NYU-MED** *(888-769-8633)*

NEUROLOGY & NEUROSURGERY

NYU Langone Medical Center's Departments of Neurology and Neurosurgery continue to be **ranked among the nation's top 10 in the 2013-2014 U.S. News & World Report's annual survey of "Best Hospitals" in America.**

Patients travel from around the world to consult our renowned specialists for their expertise in the care, treatment, and research of neurological diseases and disorders of the brain, spine and nervous system. These conditions range from migraine headaches, nerve and muscle problems, pain, autism, movement disorders and Alzheimer's disease to stroke, vascular disorders, epilepsy, multiple sclerosis and brain tumors. NYU Langone is home to one of the largest epilepsy centers in the United States, as well as the largest multiple sclerosis program in New York and the first primary stroke center established in New York City.

Neurological Expertise

Autonomic Diseases: Our specialized Center evaluates and treats children and adults with familial dysautonomia and other inherited or acquired autonomic nervous system diseases, including orthostatic hypotension and rare forms of hereditary sensory neuropathy.

Epilepsy: Our Level 4 Comprehensive Epilepsy Center offers the most advanced medical and surgical options. Complementary management approaches complete the comprehensive care plan.

Multiple Sclerosis: The Comprehensive MS Care Center provides state-of-the-art diagnostic evaluations and follow-up care and management.

Neurogenetics: We focus on inherited diseases of the nervous system. Services include diagnosis and management of inherited diseases, biochemical and molecular testing and genetic counseling.

Neuro-oncology: In partnership with the NYU Cancer Institute, our multidisciplinary Brain Tumor Center is one of the nation's leading brain and spinal cord tumor programs, including physicians highly experienced in neuro-oncology, neurosurgery and neuroradiology.

Neuromuscular Diseases: We offer multidisciplinary programs for neuromuscular diseases, including acquired peripheral neuropathy, Charcot Marie Tooth neuropathy, myasthenia gravis, amyotrophic lateral sclerosis, spinal muscular atrophy, post-polio syndrome, muscular dystrophy and Lyme neuroborreliosis.

Parkinson's Disease and Movement Disorders: Our specialized center helps individuals affected by Parkinson's or other movement disorders to achieve the highest possible quality of life. Experts are also available to offer functional neurosurgery for certain conditions that involve involuntary muscle contractions.

(continued)

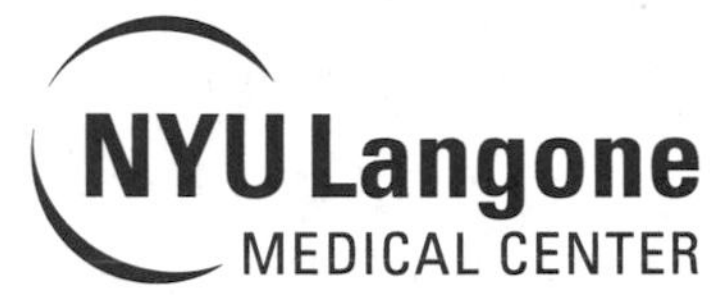

550 First Avenue *(at 31st Street)*
New York, NY 10016
www.NYULMC.org/neurology
www.NYULMC.org/neurosurgery
Physician Referral: **888-7-NYU-MED** *(888-769-8633)*

NEUROLOGY & NEUROSURGERY *(continued)*

Stroke Care: The multidisciplinary, Comprehensive Stroke Care Center provides rapid diagnosis, effective intervention and early rehabilitation for individuals who have had a stroke.
Concussion Center: This multidisciplinary center is a collaborative effort between the Departments of Neurology, Orthopaedic Surgery, and Rehabilitation, providing expert evaluation and treatment of individuals who have or are suspected of having a concussion.

<u>Neurosurgical Expertise</u>

The Department of Neurosurgery at NYU Langone Medical Center offers some of the nation's most skilled and experienced surgeons and advanced, minimally invasive procedures. Patients also benefit from cutting-edge research and a fully integrated approach to medical care.
Brain Tumor: Our neurosurgeons specialize in both malignant and benign brain tumors, including skull base tumors. Expertise includes glioblastoma, ependymoma, hemangioblastoma, other gliomas, meningiomas and vestibular schwannomas (acoustic neuromas).
Cerebrovascular Surgery: The Division of Cerebrovascular Surgery is a premier center for brain aneurysms, giant intracranial aneurysms, brain vascular malformations and cavernomas, and stroke.
Spinal Neurosurgery: The Division of Spine Surgery provides treatment for degenerative spinal diseases, spinal tumors, spinal trauma and spinal infections.
Neuromodulation: This specialized center offers deep brain stimulation (DBS) for Parkinson's, essential tremor, dystonia and obsessive-compulsive disorder, as well as peripheral neurostimulation (PNS) for migraines and other headaches and various types of facial pain.
Hyperhidrosis: The Department offers expertise in the surgical treatment of primary hyperhidrosis (excessive sweating) including Endoscopic Thoracic Sympathectomy.
Neurosurgical Technology: Our neurosurgeons remove deep-seated tumors, vascular malformations and other disease sites using a highly advanced Gamma Knife. Aided by 3-D MRI technology, the Gamma Knife bombards its target with precise doses of radiation, while preserving healthy tissue.

<u>Other Neurosurgical Services</u>

- Facial Pain: provides patients a thorough examination and, if required, nerve injections and minimally invasive surgery.
- Pediatric Neurosurgery: provides treatment to children with brain and spinal cord tumors, congenital and development disorders.
- Peripheral Nerve Surgery: focuses on the diagnosis and treatment of nerve compressions, nerve tremors, Brachial Plexus (nerve fiber) and nerve injuries.
- Neuro-Critical Care: our experts provide care for patients who have an urgent neuro-surgical problem that requires careful monitoring, or is at risk for developing such a problem.

Neurology

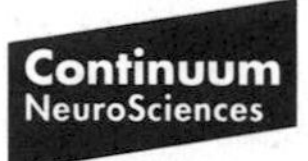

Continuum Health Partners, Inc.

Neurology and Neurosurgery Expertise

800.420.4004

The member hospitals of the Continuum Neurosciences consortium — St. Luke's and Roosevelt Hospitals and Beth Israel Medical Center — are home to many international leaders in neurology, neurosurgery, neuro-radiology and endovascular neurosurgery. Each of the hospitals has clinicians who are nationally and internationally recognized for their accomplishments and attract patients from throughout the United States and other countries who are looking for innovative treatment programs delivered by physicians specializing in both clinical care and research. Our expertise includes treatment for:

- Complex brain tumors, spine and spinal cord; chordomas, meningiomas, acoustic neuromas, trigeminal neuralgia and hemifacial spasms
- Headaches
- Disorders of the brain, spinal cord, peripheral nerves and muscles
- Stroke/cerebrovascular diseases
- Epilepsy and seizures
- Movement disorders (Parkinson's Disease, dystonia and essential tremor)
- Neuro-ophthalmologic conditions
- Neuro-oncology-related illnesses
- Neuro-psychiatry/psychology-based conditions
- Many adult and pediatric neurologic conditions

A few of our Centers of Excellence include:

Beth Israel Medical Center

- The Alan and Barbara Mirken Department of Neurology
- Bachmann-Strauss Dystonia Center of Excellence
- National Parkinson Foundation Center of Excellence
- The Betty and Morton Yarmon Stroke Center
- Internationally respected divisions of adult and pediatric epilepsy
- ALS (Lou Gehrig's disease) Center sponsored by the ALS Association
- Adult Neurosurgery
- Pediatric Neurosurgery
- Peripheral Nerve Center

St. Luke's and Roosevelt Hospitals

- The Hyman-Newman Institute for Neurology and Neurosurgery
- Center for Endovascular Surgery
- The Vascular Birthmarks Institute
- Vascular Malformations Center of NY
- New York Brain Tumor Center
- The Headache Institute
- The Stroke Center
- Adult Neurosurgery
- Pediatric Neurosurgery

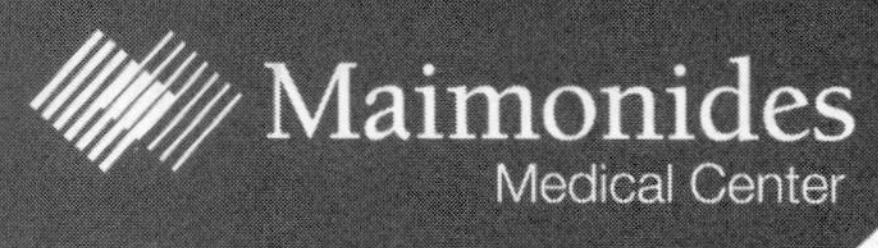

Jaffe Stroke Center

4802 Tenth Avenue
Brooklyn, New York 11219
Phone: 718.283.7670 • Fax: 718.635.7223
www.maimonidesmed.org/stroke

The Jaffe Stroke Center is ranked among the top 5% in the nation, and the top two in New York State. There are several other stroke centers in Brooklyn, but the services at Maimonides are far more advanced than at any other institution.

Steven Rudolph, MD, Director of Jaffe Stroke Center, has been selected as the investigator in two clinical trials for the newest medical stroke therapies. This distinction is bestowed only on the most respected clinicians in the field. These therapies, too, will be able to provide treatment up to nine hours after the onset of symptoms.

After the onset of stroke symptoms, there is a three-hour window of opportunity for the administration of a clot-busting drug. With highly specialized training, experts at certified stroke centers can administer this drug to appropriate patients. But there is a nine-hour window of opportunity for advanced treatment, and Maimonides is one of only a handful of hospitals in the New York metropolitan area with the capability of providing that treatment.

Razvan Buciuc, MD, Director of Interventional Neuroradiology, and his team utilize, where particularly indicated, procedures to access blood vesels in the brain and remove a stroke-causing blood clot. This procedure can greatly reduce stroke damage and, in some cases, has completely reversed all symptoms. Dr. Buciuc is among few in the nation with significant experience utilizing this procedure..

In addition, Maimonides has a multidisciplinary team of stroke experts that includes physicians and nurses from the Department of Emergency Medicine, providing the vital first line of defense in combating stroke. The ER at Maimonides is equipped with telemedicine, an interactive system which allows consultation with a stroke neurologist in real time, even when the doctor is at a remote location.

In our stroke unit and interventional neuroradiology suite, nurses are certified and experienced in these specialties, and they coordinate recovery plans that include numerous technicians and therapists.

The Jaffe Stroke Center at Maimonides Medical Center was awarded the Gold Plus Award for excellence in performance from the American Stroke Association's "Get With the Guidelines" Program. In addition, we have been named to the "Target: Stroke" Honor Roll – one of only 50 hospitals in the U.S. to achieve the recognition.

Maimonides Medical Center

The right care.
Right here.

www.maimonidesmed.org/stroke

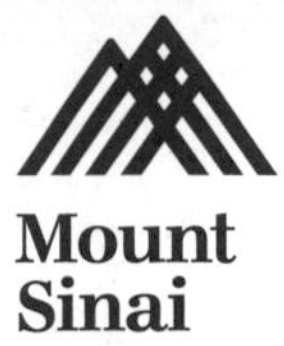

THE MOUNT SINAI MEDICAL CENTER

Neurology

One Gustave L. Levy Place
Fifth Avenue and 100th Street
New York, NY 10029-6574

Physician Referral: 1-800-MD-SINAI (637-4624)
www.mountsinai.org

THE ESTELLE AND DANIEL MAGGIN DEPARTMENT OF NEUROLOGY is renowned for its unique integration of outstanding patient care and cutting-edge research in neurological disease, and can bring the latest advances in treatment to our patients. Our physicians and neuroscientists have made enormous strides in basic and translational research, bringing medical breakthroughs that will change the course of neurological treatment. The department is led by some of the most prominent figures in American neurology, is #3 nationally in the number of academic neurologists trained in our residency program, and receives annual research grants of more than $20 million.

THE ESTELLE AND DANIEL MAGGIN DEPARTMENT OF NEUROLOGY at Mount Sinai provides compassionate, state-of-the-art, interdisciplinary care for disorders of the brain and nervous system. *US News World & Report* recently ranked Mount Sinai Neurology and Neurosurgery as a top program nationwide in recognition of our ability to care for patients with complex diseases of the nervous system.

The Robert and John M. Bendheim Parkinson and Movement Disorders Center is one of the world's leading multidisciplinary centers for clinical care and translational research aimed at Parkinson's disease, dystonia, tremor, Huntington's disease, restless legs syndrome, and others. The Center incorporates a world-renowned deep brain stimulation (DBS) program, and is at the forefront in clinical trials and experimental therapeutics for movement disorders.

The Corinne Goldsmith Dickinson Center for Multiple Sclerosis is an internationally recognized comprehensive center, uniting the efforts of leading physicians and scientists from many disciplines to understand the causes and consequences of MS. The Center provides services in all aspects of diagnosis, disease management, rehabilitation, and patient support, and the opportunity for patients to participate in potentially groundbreaking clinical trials.

The Clinical Program for Cerebrovascular Disorders includes an outstanding team of medical experts who specialize in the most advanced approaches in the evaluation, treatment, and rehabilitation of patients with cerebrovascular diseases. Services include the early diagnosis of stroke, advanced endovascular therapies, a specialized Neurointensive Care Unit, and an advanced inpatient stroke unit. Physicians are available at all times for emergency consultation with referring physicians. The Stroke Center is the first Comprehensive Stroke Center designated by The Joint Commission in New York State.

The NeuroAIDS Program provides diagnosis and treatment for neurological disorders associated with HIV disease. This program is one of the few in the world to treat the various complications of the disease that affect the central and peripheral nervous systems in as many as 70 percent of patients.

The Epilepsy Center provides specific expertise in the diagnosis and treatment of epilepsy and related disorders. The Center encompasses outstanding epileptologists, a new modern inpatient epilepsy monitoring unit, and full outpatient EEG and diagnostic capabilities.

The Center for Headache and Pain Medicine is a multidisciplinary center for the diagnosis and treatment of chronic and acute headaches and other painful disorders of the skull, brain, or face in both adults and children. Specialists in neurology, pain medicine, ENT, ophthalmology, psychiatry, and rehabilitation medicine are available to evaluate and treat individuals with painful disorders.

The Division of Neuromuscular Diseases provides diagnosis, clinical research trials, and compassionate comprehensive care for patients with disorders in neuromuscular transmission, muscle diseases, peripheral nerve problems, and spasticity resulting from stroke or other insults to the central nervous system.

The Center for Cognitive Health provides state-of-the-art diagnosis and treatment for memory disorders, dementias, traumatic brain injury, and other cognitive disorders. Our multidisciplinary team of neurologists, psychiatrists, neuropsychiatrists, neuroscientists, neuropsychologists, and patient care managers bridge the brain-related specialties to provide individualized comprehensive care.

The Eye Movement and Vestibular Disorder Program provides outstanding diagnosis and treatment for visual problems, balance problems, and motion sickness. Our physicians participate in NASA programs, employing technology used to assess these disorders in space, and studying possible treatment applications on earth.

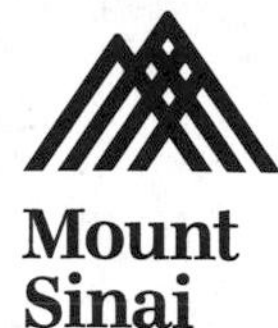

THE MOUNT SINAI MEDICAL CENTER
Neurology

One Gustave L. Levy Place
Fifth Avenue and 100th Street
New York, NY 10029-6574

Physician Referral: 1-800-MD-SINAI (637-4624)
www.mountsinai.org

THE ROBERT AND JOHN M. BENDHEIM PARKINSON AND MOVEMENT DISORDERS CENTER is one of the world's leading multidisciplinary centers for clinical care and translational research aimed at treating Parkinson's disease, dystonia, tremor, and a variety of movement disorders. It houses a world renowned deep-brain stimulation program and offers clinical trials and experimental therapeutics for movement disorders.

Our neurologists excel at diagnosing and treating both hypokinetic and hyperkinetic movement disorders.

- Hypokinetic movement disorders are characterized by an abnormal slowing down or paucity of movement, as with Parkinson's disease.
- Hyperkinetic movement disorders are characterized by excessive, involuntary movements, as with dystonia, Huntington's disease, and tremor disorders.

THE ROBERT AND JOHN M. BENDHEIM PARKINSON AND MOVEMENT DISORDERS CENTER is part of The Mount Sinai Medical Center's Department of Neurology, which is ranked among the top services of its kind in the country, according to *U.S. News & World Report's* "Best Hospitals" issue 2013-2014.

We treat the following conditions:

- Parkinson's disease and parkinsonism syndromes
- Dystonia, including generalized as well as focal dystonias, such as cervical dystonia, blepharospasm, task-related dystonias, and other dystonic disorders
- Essential tremor and other tremor disorders
- Huntington's disease
- Ataxic disorders
- Other hyperkinetic disorders, such as tics and myoclonus
- Pediatric Movement Disorders
- Tics, Stereotypies

Our clinical research is designed to elucidate and better understand the etiology of movement disorders, leading to better treatments and improved quality of life. We are involved in investigator-initiated research studies as well as clinical trials in Parkinson's disease, dystonia, and other movement disorders.

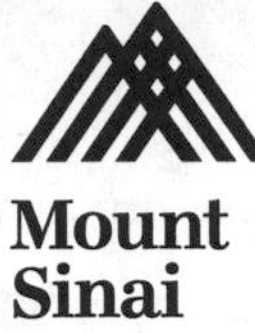

THE MOUNT SINAI MEDICAL CENTER
KRAVIS CHILDREN'S HOSPITAL
Pediatric Neurology

One Gustave L. Levy Place
Fifth Avenue and 100th Street
New York, NY 10029-6574

Physician Referral: 1-800-MD-SINAI (637-4624)
www.kravischildrenshospital.org

INNOVATIVE MEDICINE, FAMILY-CENTERED CARE

The **DIVISION OF PEDIATRIC NEUROLOGY** at The Mount Sinai Medical Center's Kravis Children's Hospital is dedicated to excellence in research, education and innovative, family-centered care. Highly respected within their field, our board certified pediatric neurologists adhere to the highest medical standards while remaining at the forefront of neurological medicine.

We offer outstanding multidisciplinary clinical expertise in evaluating, diagnosing, and treating infants and children with symptoms of neurologic dysfunction, including:

- ADHD
- Learning disabilities
- Autism
- Cerebral Palsy,
- Epilepsy
- Headaches, migraine
- Movement disorders
- Muscular dystrophy
- Myopathy
- Neuropathy
- Neurofibromatosis, neuroectodermal disorders
- Neurodevelopmental disorders
- Tic disorders, Tourette's syndrome
- Tumors of the brain, spinal cord

Committed to the rapid translation of basic science research into life enhancing treatments, our physician-scientists conduct studies in our **Friedman Brain Institute**, which is an interdisciplinary clinical and research hub for defining the mechanisms behind nervous system diseases and for translating those findings into innovative preventative or restorative interventions. The Institute focuses on neural injury and repair, cognitive function and neuropsychiatry. By taking advantage of the growing body of knowledge about brain and spinal cord disorders, we are poised to drive revolutionary advances in the clinic by developing more effective diagnostic tests, treatments and preventions.

Our **Center of Excellence in Neurodevelopmental Disorders** has a particular focus in the areas of autism and related conditions, attention-deficit/hyperactivity disorder, intellectual disabilities and developmental delays, anxiety and mood disorders, and schizophrenia. Our mission, which is realized through collaborative efforts with expert researchers and clinicians, is to discover the causes of these disorders and use that information to guide us on the path to innovative clinical therapies.

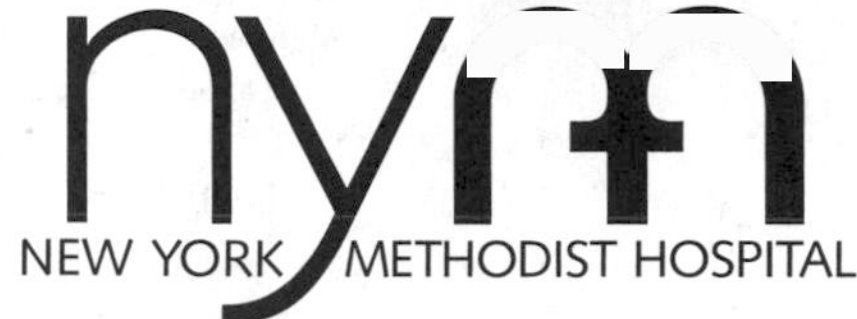

THE INSTITUTE FOR NEUROSCIENCES

New York Methodist Hospital
506 Sixth Street, Brooklyn, N.Y. 11215
Phone: 866 DO-NEURO (866 366-3876)
http://www.nym.org

SPECIALISTS AND MEDICAL SERVICES

The Institute for Neurosciences at New York Methodist Hospital brings together a unique group of specialists and medical services, offering diagnosis and treatment of a broad range of neurological conditions, ranging from frequent headaches to Parkinson's disease to multiple sclerosis.

The Institute's panel of physician specialists includes neurologists, neurosurgeons, psychiatrists, endocrinologists, neuroradiologists, radiation oncologists, physiatrists, geriatricians, psychologists and rehabilitation therapists.

All diagnostic and therapeutic procedures are performed at New York Methodist Hospital or at individual physicians' offices. State-of-the-art equipment to perform computed tomography (CT), magnetic resonance imaging (MRI), and magnetic resonance angiography (MRA) is located in the Hospital's Radiology Department. In addition, equipment and specialists trained to perform neurological diagnostic tests, such as electroencephalography (EEG), electromyography (EMG), and evoked potential examinations are available on the main campus.

The Institute also has a satellite office in Staten Island, located at 1 Harvey Avenue. It can be reached by calling 718 494-4360.

PROGRAMS OFFERED

Special programs and services offered by the Institute include an Alzheimer's disease/memory center, a neuropathy program, pediatric and adult epilepsy programs that offer diagnosis via video EEG, a Parkinson's disease and other movement disorders program, a pituitary program, a multiple sclerosis center, a neuro-oncology service, inpatient and outpatient psychiatry programs, rehabilitation services and a New York State–designated Stroke Center. Neurosurgeons on the Institute's panel perform highly sophisticated procedures, including deep brain stimulation surgery, vascular neurosurgery, skull base surgery and spinal surgery. A stereotactic radiosurgery service is also available at the Hospital's regional radiation oncology center.

***

Referrals to the Institute, its programs and physicians can be made through an individual's primary care physician or requested directly through the Institute's telephone referral service. More information (and on-line physician referral) is available at the Hospital's website, http://www.nym.org.

NYM's Center for Parkinson's Disease and Other Movement Disorders

NYM's Center for Parkinson's Disease and Other Movement Disorders is the only such medical center–based program in the New York City area. The Center simplifies the diagnostic and treatment process for patients by consolidating all services.

Treatment for Parkinson's may include medication, surgery and/or specialized therapies. Some patients may be candidates for deep brain stimulation, a neurosurgical procedure that can have dramatic results. NYM is the only Hospital in Brooklyn where this surgery is performed.

The Center has a patient care coordinator to help patients with appointments, treatment regimens, transportation and coordination with insurance companies. For more information, call 718 246-8820.

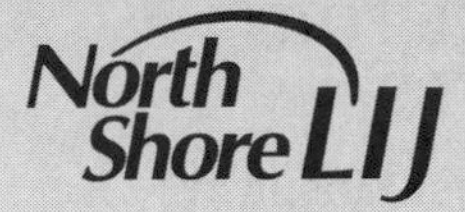

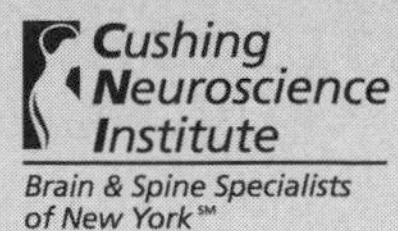

300 Community Drive, 9 Tower
Manhasset, NY 11030
(516) 562-3822
neurocni.com
neuro@nshs.edu

Cushing Neuroscience Institute

North Shore-LIJ's Cushing Neuroscience Institute (CNI) specializes in the diagnosis and treatment of neurological and neurosurgical diseases. CNI combines clinical programs with advanced medicine and surgical techniques, state-of-the art technology and cutting-edge research to bring patients the best possible care.

Award-Winning Care

Our outcomes and capabilities have led to various designations and acknowledgements, including several of our neurosurgeons and neurologists being named as recipients of the **2012 Patients' Choice Awards**. Patients go online to rate different components of the treatment they receive, such as diagnosis accuracy, the amount of time spent with the doctor, the doctor's bedside manner and follow-up care. Only physicians who receive top scores and pass other quality measures are awarded this honor.

Treatments for a Wide Range of Conditions

Our highly skilled and compassionate team of neurospecialists includes neurologists who diagnose and treat conditions that involve the brain, spine, nerves and muscles, as well as surgeons who provide the latest treatment options while contributing to advances in their field. This multidisciplinary team expertly treats patients for brain aneurysms, stroke, brain tumors, brain injuries, movement disorders, epilepsy, neuromuscular disorders and spinal disease.

We are committed to serving our patients and community with a blend of technical expertise and compassion while maintaining the highest ethical standards, and we continually work to discover new and cutting-edge treatments through clinical research.

Our Neuroscience Centers:

- Brain Aneurysm Center
- Brain Tumor Center
- Chiari Institute
- Comprehensive Epilepsy Care Center
- General Neurology
- Headache Center
- Hyperhidrosis Center
- Hypothalamic Hamartoma Center
- Memory Disorders Center
- Movement Disorders Center
- Moyamoya Center of New York
- Multiple Sclerosis Center
- Nerve Disorders Center
- Neurocritical Care Center
- Normal Pressure Hydrocephalus Center
- Pain Center
- Pediatric Neuroscience Center
- Skull Base Center
- Spine Center
- Stroke Center
- Traumatic Brain Injury Center

To find a doctor: **1-888-321-DOCS** or **northshorelij.com**

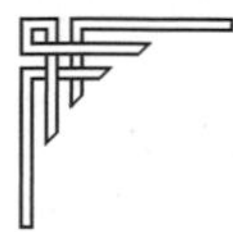

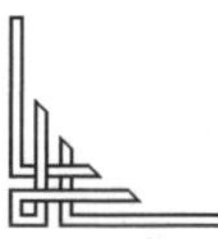
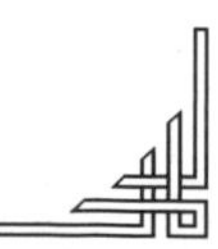

Nuclear Radiology

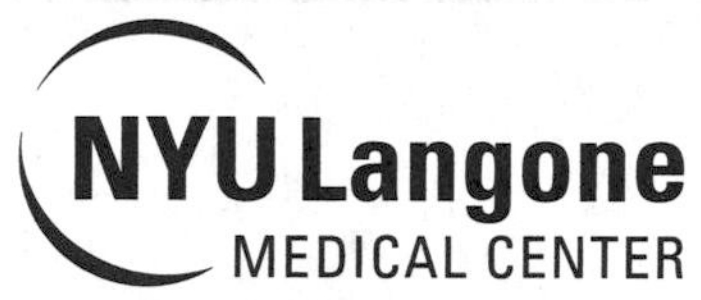

550 First Avenue *(at 31st Street)*
New York, NY 10016

www.NYULMC.org

Physician Referral: **888-7-NYU-MED** *(888-769-8633)*

RADIOLOGY

NYU Langone Radiology is committed to capturing the best images possible with the lowest dose of radiation. As an academic medical center, our radiologists are in a unique position to take the lead in helping to define and advance radiology in today's rapidly evolving technological environment.

Expertise

NYU Langone Medical Center's board certified radiologists and licensed technologists specialize in imaging and are involved in a variety of innovative collaborations and research initiatives. The Department consists of more than 100 sub-specialized academic radiologists, many of them acknowledged leaders and innovators in their fields.

Advanced Technology

NYU Langone uses some of the most advanced imaging equipment in the world, including high and ultra high-field MRI imaging systems (known as 1.5T and 3T magnets). MRI scanners are shorter and wider than ever, making for a more patient-friendly experience. The Center for Biomedical Imaging, an advanced research facility, features a powerful 7T magnet.

Recognition for Safety and Quality

We continually follow a rigorous set of quality standards and maintain accreditation by the American College of Radiology (ACR). Designated by the ACR as a "Breast Imaging Center of Excellence", our team maintains high practice standards in image quality, personnel qualifications, facility equipment, quality control procedures and quality assurance programs.

Patient Focused Approach

We are located in Manhattan, Brooklyn, Queens, and Long Island and participate in many insurance plans. Timely delivery of reports and images allow physicians to view patient exam status, reports and images online. In addition to our convenient hours, weekend, evening and often same-day appointments are available. Language interpretation services are available as needed.

Our Areas of Specialization

Diagnostic services include MRI, CT, ultrasound, PET/CT, X-ray, interventional radiology and nuclear medicine. Sub-specialized radiologists provide diagnostic interpretation in abdominal, biomedical, breast, cardiac, chest, emergency, general, musculoskeletal, neuroradiology, neuro interventional, nuclear medicine, pediatric, vascular interventional, and women's imaging. Specialty procedures include coronary artery disease and virtual colonoscopy screening, stereotactic biopsy capability, minimally invasive techniques including radiofrequency ablation, chemoembolization, radioimmunotherapy, and bone densitometry.

Obstetrics & Gynecology

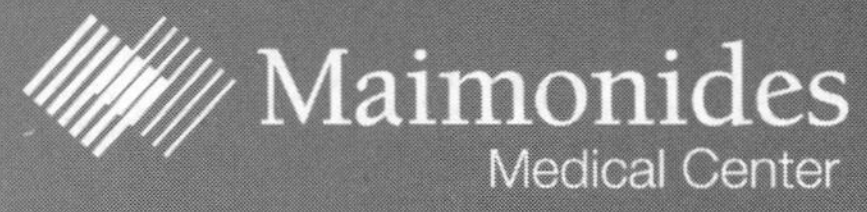

Stella & Joseph Payson Birthing Center

4802 Tenth Avenue
Brooklyn, New York 11219
Phone: 718.283.7048 • Fax: 718.283.7167
www.maimonidesmed.org/obgyn

The Birthing Center features private suites with hardwood floors and a home-like environment. At the same time, physician coverage is provided 24/7 in our advanced Neonatal Intensive Care Unit. Our obstetricians and midwives have found that most families appreciate having both disciplines available to them.

Maimonides provides other unique services for its maternity patients. The largest doula program in the metropolitan area can be found at Maimonides. These fully-trained childbirth assistants are available both before, during and after delivery at no cost to families. And the maternity units utilize an electronic patient record that sets industry standards for patient safety and hospital efficiency.

This combination of family-centered services and advanced technology continues to have enormous appeal to the women served — over 8,000 of them last year alone. Our highly trained staff includes the finest nurses, physicians, midwives and specialists to ensure the safety and comfort of our patients. Several physicians specialize in high-risk pregnancy, including the Chair of Obstetrics & Gynecology, Howard Minkoff, MD.

Women who give birth at Maimonides also have a variety of other services available to them, including:

- A Perinatal Testing Center, directed by Shoshana Haberman, MD, offering amniocentesis, 3-D ultrasound, fetal echocardiograms and other diagnostic exams.
- Neonatologists on-site around-the-clock. The Norma Sutton Center for Neonatology adjoins the Payson Birthing Center and provides the most sophisticated care in a family-friendly environment.

The Stella & Joseph Payson Birthing Center is ranked among the best in the nation for maternity care by HealthGrades, the nation's leading source for independent health care quality information. In recognition of its excellence in obstetrics and pediatrics, Maimonides was designated a Regional Perinatal Center by the New York State Department of Health. More babies are delivered at Maimonides than at any other single-campus hospital in New York State.

Maimonides Medical Center

**The right care.
Right here.**

www.maimonidesmed.org/obgyn

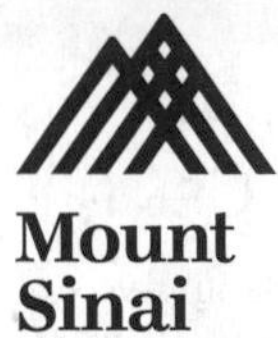

THE MOUNT SINAI MEDICAL CENTER

Gynecology

One Gustave L. Levy Place
Fifth Avenue and 100th Street
New York, NY 10029-6574

Physician Referral: 1-800-MD-SINAI (637-4624)
www.mountsinai.org

At Mount Sinai **OBSTETRICS, GYNECOLOGY AND REPRODUCTIVE SERVICES**, we focus on your reproductive system throughout all phases of life. From yearly wellness physical exams to complex medical and surgical care, the Department of Obstetrics and Gynecology at the Mount Sinai Medical Center offers a full scope of services in all areas of gynecologic care. This includes:

- Abnormal menstruation
- Cancer screening
- Contraception
- Endometriosis
- Menopause
- Pelvic pain
- Preventive and routine gynecologic care
- Sexually-transmitted diseases
- Uterine fibroids
- Oral contraceptives (birth control pills) and other forms of family

We care for young women concerned with irregular cycles, the latest in contraceptive advances, and stress appropriate, preventive gynecologic care. We have a team of highly experienced and caring obstetricians for routine as well as high-risk obstetrical care. As women complete their families, we provide counseling and therapeutic management for midlife women in the peri- and post-menopause. Our outstanding surgeons provide state of the art minimally invasive laparoscopic and robotic procedures for removal of fibroids and ovarian cysts, as well as treatment of endometriosis and irregular heavy vaginal bleeding. We also provide diagnostic and preventive therapy for urinary and fecal incontinence and pelvic floor prolapse.

We also provide comprehensive and innovative support services for patients, including our Perinatal Bereavement Program for women and families experiencing fetal loss. Our services include counseling and guidance to help patients and family members cope with loss, including support groups (in English and Spanish), strategies for coping, community based referrals and facilitation of meaningful rituals sensitive to families' spiritual, cultural and religious beliefs.

We use the least invasive, safest solutions possible to optimize patient outcomes and wellness. Additionally, we offer the latest advances in technological approaches including robotic surgery. Robotic tools allow us to treat a vast majority of patients with a minimally invasive approach. Our robotic system is capable of translating a surgeon's hand movements at a console into real-time procedures inside the patient. This improves surgical precision and instrument range of motion. As a result, we have very low complication rates, decreased lengths of stay, minimal scarring, and high overall satisfaction ratings from our patients. Though not all surgeries can be performed with robotics, we've used this technique in more than 300 pelvic surgeries since 2005.

The Mount Sinai Medical Center in New York City ranks as a top hospital in the United States for gynecologic care, according to *U.S. News & World Report*.

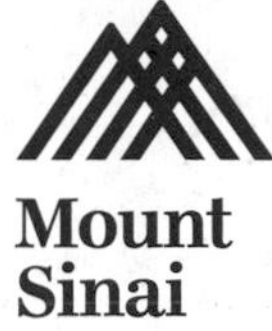

THE MOUNT SINAI MEDICAL CENTER

Obstetrics Programs and Services

One Gustave L. Levy Place
Fifth Avenue and 100th Street
New York, NY 10029-6574

Physician Referral: 1-800-MD-SINAI (637-4624)
www.mountsinai.org

As an expectant mother, you want the very best medical care to ensure that your baby is born healthy and that you stay strong enough to care for your newborn. If prior pregnancies were difficult or you have an underlying medical condition that could impact your pregnancy, you want to rest assured that you are doing everything possible to keep you and your baby healthy. That's why more women come to Mount Sinai's **CENTER FOR MATERNAL AND FETAL MEDICINE** than anywhere else in the greater New York area.

We've welcomed tens of thousands of babies into the world since the first baby was born at Mount Sinai in 1856 and although much has changed in the field of obstetrics since then, one thing has stayed the same—our dedication to providing new families with a nurturing and comfortable environment in which to experience one of life's most precious moments—the birth of your child. Our integrated approach to labor and delivery involves multiple fields—from obstetrics, nursing, and anesthesiology to neonatal intensive care, pediatric surgery, and genetics. Mount Sinai's Jo Carole and Ronald S. Lauder Center for Maternity Care includes the new Alexandra and Steven Cohen Center for Labor and Birth—a state-of-the-art labor and delivery floor that provides safe, modern, and technically advanced care for mother and child in over 6,000 deliveries each year.

Our Jo Carole and Ronald S. Lauder Center for Maternity Care provides:

- 14 labor and delivery rooms
- Four designated ante partum beds
- Three operating rooms
- Mother-baby suites
- General care units
- Level III NICU

We're one of a select few obstetrics practices using progressive technology on our labor and delivery floor. Our doctors are trained in handling high risk births and birthing emergencies on the NOELLE® and newborn HAL® mother and infant simulators, which allows us to take our training and experience to new high-tech levels. NOELLE is a robot simulator that provides trainees a complete birthing experience before, during, and after delivery. With controls that smoothly transition between physiologic states in response to commands from a wireless PC, physicians and trainees can monitor maternal and neonatal vital signs, including blood pressure and oxygen saturation, using real equipment. NOELLE and baby HAL allow our teams to practice birthing drills and the handling of life-threatening complications.

Our obstetrics team includes "The Mount Sinai Midwives," a group of experts in low-risk women's health care, who attend over 500 deliveries per year on Mount Sinai's labor and delivery unit. They provide prenatal, postpartum and well-woman gynecology services to low-risk women at Mount Sinai Hospital in Manhattan, Mount Sinai of Queens, Settlement Health, in East Harlem, and Boriken Health Center in Manhattan. Our midwives offer a broad range of services to support new moms, including breastfeeding assistance, and support groups.

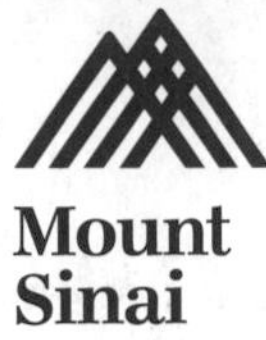

THE MOUNT SINAI MEDICAL CENTER

Obstetrics, Gynecology and Reproductive Science

One Gustave L. Levy Place
Fifth Avenue and 100th Street
New York, NY 10029-6574

Physician Referral: 1-800-MD-SINAI (637-4624)
www.mountsinai.org

Building on more than a century of leadership in providing health care to women, the **DEPARTMENT OF OBSTETRICS, GYNECOLOGY, AND REPRODUCTIVE SCIENCE** at The Mount Sinai Medical Center offers special expertise in:

General obstetrics – Genetic counseling, prenatal care, labor and delivery management, and postpartum care. In addition to our talented physicians, other health care professionals are integrated into our practice, including genetic counselors, nutritionists, social workers, nurse midwives, childbirth educators, and lactation/breastfeeding specialists.

High-risk obstetrics – Advanced techniques in prenatal diagnosis and consultations in the management of complicated pregnancies. Our ultrasound unit is recognized for its expertise in fetal anatomy ultrasound assessments. The latest technology, including 4D imaging, is employed. Antepartum testing, including amniocentesis, chorionic villus sampling, and fetal blood sampling, are all routinely performed at Mount Sinai.

Reproductive endocrinology and infertility – Diagnosis and treatment of both female and male factor infertility. Treatment options for women include fertility medications, intrauterine insemination, in vitro fertilization, intracytoplasmic sperm injection, and ovum donation.

General gynecology – Cancer screening, management of abnormal Pap smears, family planning, and surgical management of fibroids, endometriosis, and other benign gynecologic conditions.

Gynecologic infectious diseases – Treatment and prevention of sexually transmitted infections and consultations on obstetrical and gynecological infections.

Gynecologic oncology – Care for women with cancers of the ovary, uterus, cervix, vulva, and vagina.

Minimally invasive surgery – For many conditions.

Urogynecology and reconstructive pelvic surgery – Lower urinary tract disorders.

INNOVATIVE APPROACHES TO PRENATAL CARE AND THE TREATMENT OF GYNECOLOGIC CANCERS

Known worldwide for excellence and innovative approaches to prenatal diagnosis and fetal therapy, Mount Sinai's Department of Obstetrics, Gynecology, and Reproductive Science has a long tradition of advancing clinical practice through patient-oriented research. Faculty members are pioneering work in diverse areas, including first- and second-trimester screening for fetal chromosomal abnormalities, vaccines for the prevention of sexually transmitted infections, minimally invasive surgical techniques, and new approaches to the diagnosis and treatment of gender-specific cancers.

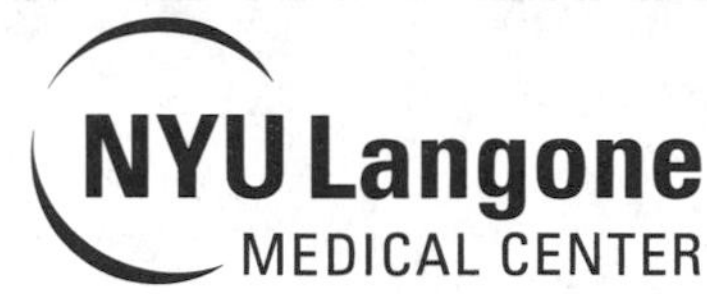

550 First Avenue *(at 31st Street)*
New York, NY 10016

www.NYULMC.org

Physician Referral: **888-7-NYU-MED** *(888-769-8633)*

OBSTETRICS AND GYNECOLOGY

NYU Langone Medical Center provides comprehensive services designed specifically for women, from primary care to highly specialized programs that are supported by sophisticated research and advanced training. We specialize in the following areas:

Obstetrics
We offer a broad range of obstetrical services, including prenatal care that gives equal emphasis to the well-being of the mother and the fetus; fetal monitoring through ultrasound and other techniques; childbirth preparedness and breastfeeding classes.

Maternal-Fetal Medicine
Prenatal care for high-risk pregnancies and detailed consultations before, during and after pregnancy are offered. We specialize in multifetal pregnancies, genetic counseling, women who have miscarried, and preterm deliveries, as well as helping women who have other medical conditions that may complicate a pregnancy, such as diabetes, heart problems, high blood pressure, and lupus. We offer the latest techniques for in-utero diagnosis and treatment and using minimally invasive techniques, our physicians are able to repair a number of life-threatening conditions in a child before it is even born.

Fertility-Related Services
We offer state-of-the-art programs in evaluation of infertility (including the special needs of same-sex couples) egg donation, egg freezing and in-vitro fertilization. Diagnosis and treatment include ovulation induction, assisted reproductive technologies and surgical options that incorporate the latest endoscopic techniques. Preimplantation Genetic Screening (PGS) at the Fertility Center offers tests for aneuploidy (an abnormal number of chromosomes).

Gynecology
In addition to routine gynecological care, we offer pelvic ultrasound; aspiration of breast cysts, colposcopy (a diagnostic evaluation of abnormal pap smears); LEEP (a loop electrosurgical procedure used to diagnose and treat cervical cancer); cryotherapy for vaginal warts; and bone density testing.

Gynecologic Surgery
Minimally invasive gynecologic surgery, including robotic surgery, is offered for a wide range of simple and complex conditions including, resection of endometriosis, hysterectomy, and myomectomy.

Gynecologic Oncology
The NCI-designated NYU Cancer Institute's Women's Cancer Program specializes in the treatment of cervical cancer, endometrial cancer, ovarian cancer, uterine cancer, vaginal cancer and vulvar cancer.

Occupational Medicine

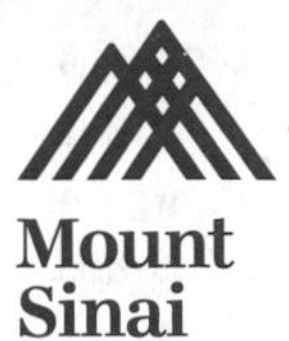

THE MOUNT SINAI MEDICAL CENTER
Occupational Health

One Gustave L. Levy Place
Fifth Avenue and 100th Street
New York, NY 10029-6574

Physician Referral: 1-800-MD-SINAI (637-4624)
www.mountsinai.org

At The Mount Sinai Medical Center, our occupational health professionals take a patient-centered approach to improving and protecting public health. Services offered at our **MOUNT SINAI SELIKOFF CENTERS FOR OCCUPATIONAL HEALTH** demonstrate our commitment to preventing and treating work-related and environmentally induced illnesses and conditions and providing clinical intervention and education to communities and healthcare professionals.

Our services, offered by highly specialized physicians and expert health and social service professionals, are available to workers, labor and community organizations, employers, other health care professionals and agencies. We offer:

- Confidential medical exams for current and retired workers with health problems that may be related to their work
- Treatment for work-related medical conditions
- Medical screenings for groups of workers who have been exposed to work-related hazards
- Social work services to address disease-related personal and family problems, including one-on-one counseling and monthly support groups
- Work-site evaluations to identify possible safety and health hazards, and recommend solutions
- Specialized work-site ergonomic evaluations for workers with musculoskeletal disease who use computers
- Assistance with Workers' Compensation and other benefits
- Training programs and assistance to unions, in order to help make jobs safer and teach workers about the signs and symptoms of occupational disease

The World Trade Center Health Program, Clinical Center of Excellence at Mount Sinai
Through this program, we offer annual monitoring and treatment, including medication, at no cost, to eligible World Trade Center (WTC) workers and volunteers, for both physical and mental health conditions related to their WTC service.

Mount Sinai WTC Health Program staff and affiliated specialists have been providing care to thousands of WTC responders since shortly after the terrorist attacks of 9/11. We continue to see newly enrolled patients on a regular basis at Mount Sinai's main campus in Manhattan, Staten Island, and Hudson Valley Yonkers.

NYU Langone
MEDICAL CENTER

550 First Avenue *(at 31st Street)*
New York, NY 10016
www.NYULMC.org/rusk
Physician Referral: **888-7-NYU-MED** *(888-769-8633)*

RUSK REHABILITATION

Rusk Rehabilitation at NYU Langone Medical Center (Rusk) has been ranked the best rehabilitation program in New York State and among the top ten in the country by *U.S. News & World Report* since 1989. Rusk is internationally renowned for the treatment of adults and children with injuries and disabilities, offering the full continuum of inpatient and outpatient care—physical, occupational, speech/swallowing and vocational therapy, psychology, music and recreational therapy, nutrition, nursing, and social work—for a wide range of conditions. Specialty programs and services include:

The **CARF-Accredited Brain Injury Rehabilitation Program** is tailored for patients who have medical, physical, cognitive, and behavioral changes as a result of a brain injury or neurological illness.

The **CARF-Accredited Stroke Program** offers an interdisciplinary team with specialized training in the medical, nursing or therapeutic care and treatment of stroke patients.

The Concussion Center is a collaborative effort between Rusk Rehabilitation and the Departments of Orthopaedic Surgery and Neurology, providing expert, multidisciplinary evaluation and treatment of individuals who have or are suspected of having a concussion.

Our **Amputee Program** provides specialized limb loss rehabilitation to patients who have undergone amputations.

The Joan and Joel Smilow Cardiac and Pulmonary Rehabilitation & Prevention Center offers a model of transitional care for patients with cardiac and lung conditions.

Orthopaedic/Musculoskeletal Rehabilitation is offered for patients with back, neck, hip, elbow and shoulder disorders, arthritis-related joint pain, conditions affecting the bones, tendon, ligaments and muscles, and for pre- and post-surgical patients.

Sports Injury Rehabilitation addresses the needs of patients with sports-related conditions, including post-operative rehabilitation for patients who require orthopaedic surgery.

Our **Spinal Cord Injury** program offers a comprehensive, patient-centered array of specialized and innovative clinical and educational programs to optimize quality of life.

(continued)

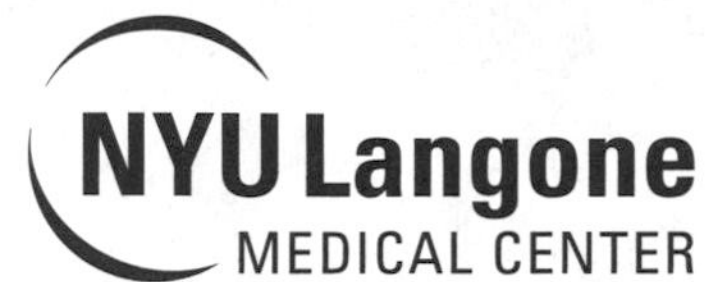

550 First Avenue *(at 31st Street)*
New York, NY 10016
www.NYULMC.org/rusk
Physician Referral: **888-7-NYU-MED** *(888-769-8633)*

RUSK REHABILITATION *(continued)*

The Women's Health Rehab Program addresses issues that uniquely affect women, including pelvic floor muscle dysfunction/pain, urinary incontinence, cancer rehabilitation and lymphedema, and prenatal and postpartum musculoskeletal conditions.

Vestibular Rehabilitation addresses the evaluation and treatment of patients suffering from dizziness and imbalance.

Chest Physical Therapy cares for individuals with lung congestion, secretion retention or areas of lung collapse.

Rehabilitation Psychology provides care to patients with neurological and medical conditions.

Speech-Language Pathology & Swallowing is dedicated to patients with communication disorders due to neurological problems as well as diagnosis and management of swallowing and feeding disorders.

Vocational Services provides disabled individuals with the competencies needed to return to school or work and to lead a productive life.

Patient Care Locations

Our physicians and therapists provide care at multiple NYU Langone locations, including:

- **The Center for Musculoskeletal Care**, NYU Langone's premier, state-of-the-art, multidisciplinary bone and joint facility
- NYU Langone's newly opened, outpatient **Ambulatory Care Center**
- The internationally-renowned, inpatient **Hospital for Joint Diseases**
- **The NYU Langone main campus** on First Avenue
- **The Joan H. Tisch Center for Women's Health**, on the Upper East Side of Manhattan
- Multiple locations in **NYU Langone's growing network of community practices** in the metro New York area

Ophthalmology

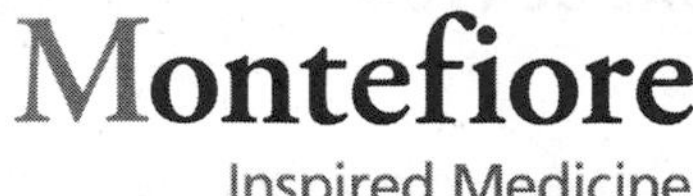

111 East 210th Street
Bronx, New York 10467
718-920-2020
www.montefiore.org/eyes

Ophthalmology and Visual Sciences

Montefiore's Department of Ophthalmology and Visual Sciences provides exceptional care for patients with all forms of ophthalmologic conditions. In addition to its specialty programs in neuro-ophthalmology, retina, refractive surgery (LASIK), uveitis, cornea and glaucoma, the Department provides a full range of surgical and general ophthalmologic services for children and adults.

The Department is the largest ophthalmologic clinical program in New York State and among the largest in the nation, with more than 30 full-time faculty members and annual patient visits exceeding 125,000. It provides care at eight sites throughout the Bronx and Westchester County.

Meeting the vision needs of the region's vast pediatric population is a particular focus of the Department. Led by Norman Medow, MD, FACS, a respected congenital glaucoma and corneal transplant expert and Emeritus Trustee of the Foundation of the American Academy of Ophthalmology, the Department's six pediatric specialists diagnose and treat patients with common conditions such as refractive error or clogged tear ducts as well as urgent or uncommon conditions, including ocular cancers, retinopathy of prematurity, genetic conditions and malformations. Few ophthalmology programs in the nation possess an equal depth and volume of pediatric experience.

To address the high rates of diabetic blindness and glaucoma among adults in the Bronx, the Department offers strong treatment programs that emphasize early diagnosis and intervention. Montefiore's ophthalmologists use the most advanced technology and treatment approaches when caring for patients with these and other vision conditions. An example of such technology is the Trabectome (NeoMedix), a surgical device co-invented by Department Chairman Roy Chuck, MD, PhD, that is used to extract the meshwork tissue in glaucoma cases.

Research is a crucial component of the Department's mission, and its faculty members are widely respected for their pioneering efforts. Recently, the Research to Prevent Blindness Foundation recognized Nicholas Baker, PhD, with its Senior Scientific Investigator Award. The Department has also been awarded an exceptionally competitive R01 grant from the National Institutes of Health (NIH) for work on retinal progenitor and stem cells. The Department's research portfolio includes 11 NIH grants as well as a fully unrestricted grant from Research to Prevent Blindness. Current research endeavors focus on ocular stem cells, information transfers between retinal cells, resistance to retinal ischemia and cataractogenesis, and surgical technique and instrument development.

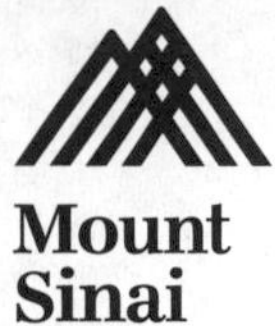

THE MOUNT SINAI MEDICAL CENTER

Ophthalmology

One Gustave L. Levy Place
Fifth Avenue and 100th Street
New York, NY 10029-6574

Physician Referral: 1-800-MD-SINAI (637-4624)
www.mountsinai.org

Specializing in the prevention, diagnosis, and treatment of eye disorders, Mount Sinai's **DEPARTMENT OF OPHTHALMOLOGY** features faculty with wide experience in special eye problems, offers comprehensive eye care services, and houses a state-of-the-art optical shop.

Services include:

- Comprehensive ophthalmology, refractive errors, and cataract surgery
- Corneal and external diseases of the eye
- Refractive surgery
- Retinal disorders (diabetic retinopathy, macular degeneration, inherited retinal diseases, retinal detachment)
- Glaucoma
- Pediatric eye care and strabismus
- Uveitis (inflammation of the eye)
- Neuro-ophthalmic disorders
- Oculplastic surgery, including cosmetic surgery, orbital tumors, and thyroid-related eye problems

Specialized treatments and procedures include:

- LASIK and other refractive surgical procedures
- Cataract surgery, including premium intraocular lenses
- Specialists in dry eye management
- Cosmetic lid treatments, including Botox and Restalayne injections
- Laser surgery
- Management of macular degeneration, including Lucentis and Avastin injections
- Advanced management for severe uveitis, including immunosuppressive drug therapy

INTERNATIONAL LEADERS IN THE FIELD OF UVEITIS

Uveitis, a collection of 30 diseases characterized by inflammation inside the eye, is the 5th leading cause of blindness in the United States. Management of severe uveitis often requires the skilled use of systemically-administered, immunosuppressive drugs, resulting in superior outcomes. Mount Sinai ophthalmologists have been pioneers in these treatments and are internationally recognized for their leadership in the field. A team of three uveitis specialists, augmented by a uveitis training program, offer a comprehensive treatment approach to these diseases.

We offer the full range of sophisticated diagnostic tests for evaluating patient conditions, including spectral domain optical coherence tomography, fluorescein angiography, indocyanine green angiography, autofluorescence, diagnostic ultrasound, electroretinography, visually evoked potential measurements, electro-oculography, corneal topography, confocal microscopy, state-of-the-art perimetry, HRT II imaging, allowing for faster, more accurate diagnosis and help determining the best treatment plan for each patient.

We perform cataract surgery, corneal transplants, refractive, glaucoma, strabismus, laser, ophthalmic plastic and reconstructive surgery, and vitreoretinal surgery for complicated retinal problems. We also offer minimally invasive procedures to treat eye disease, including non-laser refractive surgeries, and small-incision cataract surgery.

LEADERS IN CLINICAL RESEARCH

Mount Sinai ophthalmologists helped pioneer and evaluate new treatments for eye diseases and problems, including glaucoma, uveitis, ocular infections and farsightedness.

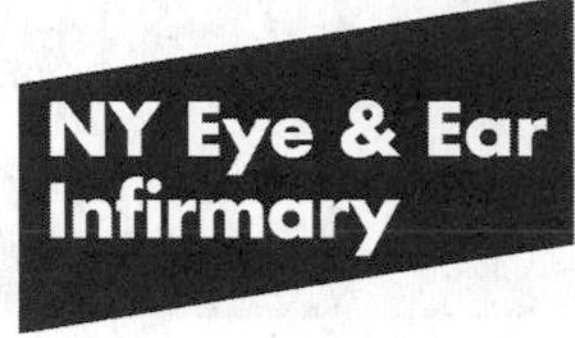

THE NEW YORK EYE AND EAR INFIRMARY

310 East 14th Street
New York, New York 10003
Tel. 212.979.4000 Fax. 212.228.0664
http://www.nyee.edu

PROVIDING EXCEPTIONAL EYE CARE

The Department of Ophthalmology is the region's most comprehensive center for the delivery of primary through tertiary eye care. It is also by far the largest provider of eye care in the metropolitan area—with some 165,000 outpatient visits and 26,000 surgical cases performed each year. 370 board-certified ophthalmologists located throughout New York City and its tri-state area comprise the attending Medical Staff.

IN A HIGHLY SPECIALIZED SETTING

As a specialty hospital, The New York Eye and Ear Infirmary is uniquely qualified to handle the most complicated cases. It serves as a nationwide referral center with a commitment to teaching, research, and high-technology based patient care. Cutting edge ocular imaging instrumentation provides the highest resolution to diagnose diseases of the cornea, anterior segment, retina and optic nerve. Highly experienced staff in state-of-the-art facilities have made The New York Eye and Ear Infirmary's 19 operating rooms a national benchmark in efficiency in eye surgery cases.

FOR PATIENTS OF ALL AGES

The New York Eye and Ear Infirmary's Ophthalmology staff are sensitive to the specific needs of patients of all ages. Senior citizens comprise the vast majority of Nyerere 12,000 cataract patients, as well as those receiving treatment for age-related macular degeneration and glaucoma. Children make up 25 percent of the NYEE patient population, with conditions such as strabismus, acquired and congenital cataract, corneal diseases, glaucoma, and ocular trauma. The Infirmary runs New York's only Pediatric Glaucoma Service and provides urgent care for patients of all ages with traumatic eye injuries through the New York Metropolitan Eye Trauma Center.

Ophthalmology Clinical Services

Ambulatory Care Services
Comprehensive Eye Care
Cornea & External Diseases
Refractive Surgery
Eye Trauma
Glaucoma
Pediatric Glaucoma
Low Vision
Neuro-Ophthalmology
Ophthalmic Pathology
Ophthalmic Oncology
Oculoplastic & Orbital Surgery
Pediatric Ophthalmology & Strabismus
Retina Vitreous
Uveitis/Ocular Immunology

Facilities

Ambulatory Surgery Center
Bendheim Family Retina Center
Einhorn Clinical Trials Area *(supporting more than 100 ophthalmology studies a year)*
Jorge N. Buxton Microsurgical Education Center *(for residents, fellows and attending physicians)*

About The New York Eye and Ear Infirmary

Founded in 1820, it is the nation's first and foremost, continuously operating specialty hospital. More than 10 million people have sought treatment here since its inception.

Physician Referral
1.800.449.HOPE (4673)

The Best in American Medicine
www.CastleConnolly.com

Orthopaedic Surgery

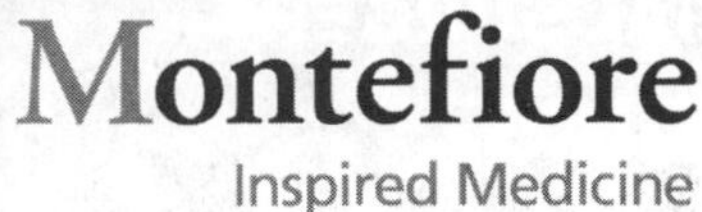

3400 Bainbridge Avenue
Bronx, New York 10467
718 920-2060
www.montefiore.org/surgery-orthopaedic

Orthopaedics at Montefiore

The Department of Orthopaedic Surgery at Montefiore provides state-of-the-art care for adults and children with a range of musculoskeletal problems. Its more than 30 fellowship-trained orthopaedic surgeons and podiatrists are experts in reconstruction and joint replacement surgery, foot and ankle surgery, spine surgery, sports medicine and musculoskeletal tumor surgery, trauma surgery and pediatric orthopaedic surgery. They are supported by a multidisciplinary team that includes physical therapists, rheumatologists, physiatrists, nurse practitioners and social workers.

The Department draws upon the latest technology and research to achieve exceptional outcomes, including arthroscopy for all joints and adductor canal blocks to eliminate postoperative pain.

The Department's Joint Replacement Center is approaching nearly 2,000 procedures annually—making it one of the most active programs in the region. The Center specializes in complex joint replacement procedures, including anterior and posterior hip replacement and minimally invasive knee replacement, and has particular expertise treating elderly patients or those with preexisting medical conditions. As an integral part of their treatment, all patients participate in a class that prepares them—and their family members—for surgery and recovery. This commitment to education has led to superior results and infection rates that are among the lowest in the state.

The Department is developing one of the **strongest divisions of orthopaedic sarcoma surgery** in the nation with orthopaedic surgeons who are specially trained in orthopaedic oncology. In collaboration with the Montefiore Einstein Center for Cancer Care, these surgeons treat adults and children with bone tumors and metastatic cancer, and perform soft-tissue sarcoma reconstruction. Procedures available at Montefiore include osteoarticular allograft bone replacement, tumor endoprostheses and allograft prosthetic composites.

Pediatric orthopaedic surgeons at The Children's Hospital at Montefiore are pioneers in the minimally invasive approach to scoliosis in children. Using just three small incisions and pedicle screws, CHAM surgeons preserve the spinal muscles and nerves while achieving accurate placement rates between 90 and 93 percent on computed tomography scans, among the highest success rates reported.

The Department is actively researching the genetic causes of osteoarthritis, the relationship of diabetes and osteoporosis, and the immune system's response to wear debris from polyethylene and metal-on-metal joint prostheses.

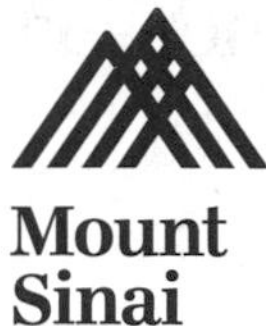

Mount
Sinai

THE MOUNT SINAI MEDICAL CENTER

Orthopaedics

One Gustave L. Levy Place
Fifth Avenue and 100th Street
New York, NY 10029-6574

Physician Referral: 1-800-MD-SINAI (637-4624)
www.mountsinai.org

Beyond its reputation for depth and breadth of expertise, **THE LENI AND PETER W. MAY DEPARTMENT OF ORTHOPAEDICS** at The Mount Sinai Medical Center is known for personalized care. The faculty and staff invest the time to get to know their patients as individuals, ensuring that they receive direct care from superb subspecialty-trained orthopaedists. The faculty share expertise in surgery of the foot and ankle, knee, hip, hand, elbow, shoulder, and spine; total joint replacement; microvascular surgery; cancer surgery; and minimally invasive surgery. Taking a whole-patient approach to care, they work in close collaboration with specialists in geriatrics, neurology, oncology, pathology, and rehabilitation medicine.

Investigation and Innovation – Recent years have seen successive refinements in the techniques of orthopaedic surgery at Mount Sinai, including joint replacement, minimally invasive fracture repair, and microvascular surgery. Faculty members have been instrumental in the design and perfection of hip and shoulder prostheses. Additionally, Mount Sinai has broadened the applications of arthroscopic surgery—the fiber optic technology that first heralded the arrival of minimally invasive surgery.

Mount Sinai orthopaedic bone, spine and tendon scientists are known for their studies of diseases of the skeletal system. Researchers are currently investigating disc degeneration in the spine; rotator cuff degeneration; and the fundamental molecular mechanisms of tendon failure and regeneration.

Use of Cutting-Edge Techniques – Mount Sinai uses innovative, minimally invasive approaches for joint replacement and fracture repair. The Department's prestigious integrated spine program provides a comprehensive spectrum of care from expert, non-operative management by expert spine physiatrists to the latest minimally invasive techniques by Mount Sinai's renowned spine surgeons.

GROUNDBREAKING PROCEDURES ENHANCE QUALITY OF LIFE

Today at Mount Sinai, arthroscopy is used to repair not only the knee, but virtually every joint. Converting what used to be major open surgery to outpatient procedures has dramatically shortened rehabilitation and return to work times. More significantly, it has allowed many more patients to get help for painful, function-limiting conditions. That is the case for many elderly or frail patients who are physically unable to undergo major surgery. The fact that such procedures are now more widely accessible is enhancing the quality of life for many patients and allowing them to lead more active lives.

The Sports Service provides patients with the full spectrum of non-operative and operative treatment including arthroscopic surgery of the hip, shoulder, knee, and elbow. Patients have the ability to return to activities faster and with less pain with this minimally invasive procedure. Our arthroscopists also specialize in cartilage preservation techniques, including cartilage transplantation, allowing patients to preserve their own joints and delaying the need for joint replacement surgery.

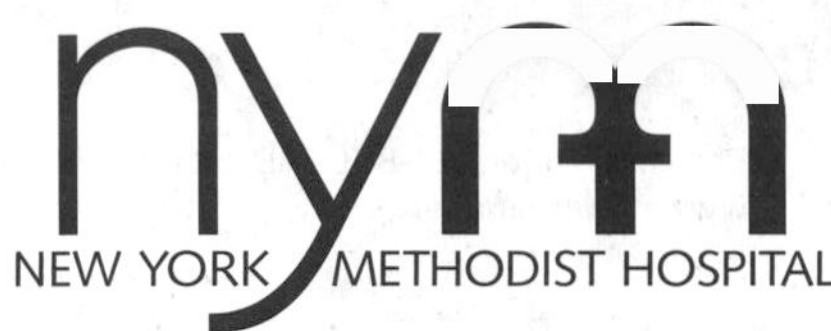

THE INSTITUTE FOR ORTHOPEDIC MEDICINE AND SURGERY

New York Methodist Hospital
506 Sixth Street, Brooklyn, N.Y. 11215
Phone: 866 ORTHO-11 (866 678-4611)
http://www.nym.org.

SPECIALISTS AND MEDICAL SERVICES

The Institute for Orthopedic Medicine and Surgery at New York Methodist Hospital brings together a unique team of specialists, facilities and medical services to provide comprehensive treatment of a broad range of orthopedic disorders.

The Institute's panel of physicians includes specialists in adult and pediatric orthopedic surgery, emergency medicine, rheumatology, podiatric medicine and surgery, endocrinology, sports medicine, pain management, orthopedic oncology and neurosurgery. Other important health care team members include physical and occupational therapists. All diagnostic and therapeutic procedures are performed at New York Methodist Hospital or in the offices of the referred physicians.

PROGRAMS OFFERED

In addition to emergency orthopedic services, programs offered through the Institute include joint replacement, arthroscopic knee surgery and cartilage restoration, medical treatments for arthritis, the geriatric hip fracture program, medical and surgical treatment for hand and shoulder injuries and degenerative conditions, spine surgery, physical therapy and pain management. Podiatric physicians specialize in all foot disorders, including reconstructive foot surgery. In addition, the Institute offers complementary medicine services including chiropractic care, acupuncture and medical massage.

***

Referrals to the Institute, its programs and physicians can be made through an individual's primary care physician or requested directly through the Institute's telephone referral service. More information (and on-line physician referral) is available at the Hospital's website, http://www.nym.org.

The Comprehensive Back and Neck Pain Center

NYM's Comprehensive Back and Neck Pain Center is dedicated to providing patients with the best clinical treatment for disorders of the back and neck. Diagnosis and treatment are centrally coordinated, so that patients avoid duplication of screening and testing procedures, if they need to see more than one specialist.

The Center focuses on conservative treatment, most commonly medication and/or rehabilitation (physical or occupational) therapy. Many other modalities are also available. If surgery is recommended, minimally invasive procedures may be applicable. Treatment decisions are made with consideration for the nature and severity of the condition, as well as the patient's lifestyle and preferences. For information or to make an appointment, call 718 369-BACK (2225).

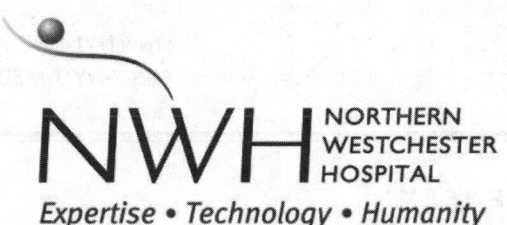

The professionals at The Orthopedic and Spine Institute at Northern Westchester Hospital (NWH) provide high-quality, leading edge orthopedic and spine care through the application of the latest minimally invasive and arthroscopic surgical techniques and advanced technologies. Whether you are recovering from an injury or simply wanting to return to a healthier, more active lifestyle, the experts at the Orthopedic and Spine Institute (OSI) can help. The OSI surgeons are highly experienced, board certified, and have trained at the nation's leading medical schools to treat a complete range of orthopedic, spine, and sports medicine conditions.

Northern Westchester Hospital (NWH) provides quality, patient centered care that is close to home through the right combination of medical expertise, leading edge technology, and a commitment to humanity. Over 750 highly skilled physicians, state-of-the-art technology and professional staff of caregivers are all in place to ensure that you and your family receive treatment in a caring, respectful and nurturing environment.

NWH has established extensive internal quality measurements that surpass the standards defined by the Centers for Medicare & Medicaid Services (CMS) and the Hospital Quality Alliance (HQA) National Hospital Quality Measures. Our high quality standards help to ensure that the treatment you receive at NWH is among the best in the nation. For a complete list of our services, please visit www.nwhc.net.

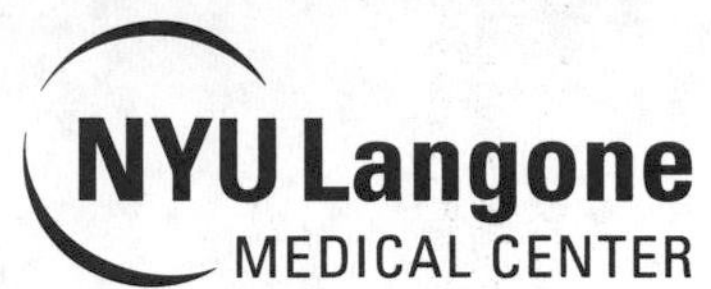

550 First Avenue *(at 31st Street)*
New York, NY 10016
www.NYULMC.org/orthosurgery
Physician Referral: **888-7-NYU-MED** *(888-769-8633)*

ORTHOPAEDIC SURGERY

The Department of Orthopaedic Surgery at NYU Langone Medical Center continues to be recognized as a national leader, **ranked #5 in the nation by *U.S. News & World Report's* 2013-2014 "Best Hospitals" survey**. Our physicians combine extensive experience with cutting-edge research and technology to address bone and joint problems that affect a patient's quality of life. The expertise of our world-class orthopaedists represents the full range of subspecialty areas including **Adult Reconstructive, Sports Medicine and Primary Care Sports Medicine, Spine, Shoulder & Elbow, Foot & Ankle, Hand Surgery, Trauma & Fracture, Orthopaedic Oncology, and Pediatric Orthopaedics**; additional areas of specialization include minimally-invasive surgery and robotic-assisted joint replacement.

<u>Premier Areas of Expertise</u>

Joint Replacement Center physicians evaluate degenerative joint conditions caused by arthritis, injuries, congenital problems and general wear-and-tear to determine the best course of treatment. Our surgeons are experts in knee, hip and shoulder replacements, complex joint revisions, and minimally invasive surgeries, conducting more than 3,000 procedures annually. The experts in our **Hip Center** also specialize in the cutting-edge, minimally invasive anterior total hip replacement technique.

The Spine Center provides conservative care for lower back and neck pain, scoliosis, osteoporosis, problems associated with failed previous surgery, idiopathic disorders, growth disorders, neuromuscular disease, degenerative and congenital conditions, and traumatic deformity. Our surgeons perform over 2,000 procedures a year, including minimally invasive spinal fusions.

Hand Center specialists diagnose and offer operative and non-operative care for a wide range of upper extremity conditions, including fractures, congenital anomalies, soft tissue and skeletal trauma, degenerative and rheumatoid arthritis, sports-related injuries, vascular disorders, tumors and occupational disorders.

Sports Medicine and Primary Care Sports Medicine physicians treat sports-related injuries or conditions of the knee, shoulder, elbow and ankle, using joint preservation techniques as well as surgical procedures. Our patients range from athletes playing at the high school, college and professional levels to recreational athletes/active individuals from every age group.

(continued)

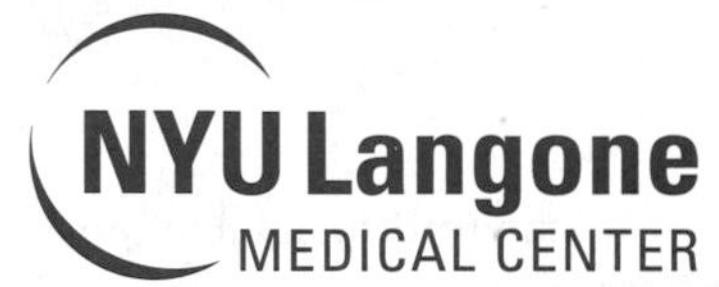

550 First Avenue *(at 31st Street)*
New York, NY 10016
www.NYULMC.org/orthosurgery
Physician Referral: **888-7-NYU-MED** *(888-769-8633)*

ORTHOPAEDIC SURGERY *(continued)*

Specialized Orthopaedic Centers and Services

The Joint Preservation Center provides conservative treatment of joint problems to reduce symptoms, restore function and delay the onset of degenerative arthritis and potential need for a joint replacement.

The Bone Healing Center is staffed by our orthopaedic trauma & fracture specialists, and is a leader in technologies and procedures that help patients recover from complex fracture reconstruction or fracture healing problems.

Harkness Center for Dance Injuries is world-renowned for its orthopaedic and rehabilitation care for dancers, including many subsidized and free services as well as injury prevention screenings and lectures.

The Diabetes Foot and Ankle Center focuses on the prevention and recurrence of foot and ankle problems associated with complications of diabetes.

The Samuels Orthopaedic Immediate Care Center, New York City's only walk-in orthopaedic clinic, is open seven days a week to evaluate and treat urgent bone and joint injuries.

The Concussion Center is a collaborative effort between the Departments of Orthopaedic Surgery, Neurology, and Rehabilitation, providing expert, multidisciplinary evaluation and treatment of individuals who have or are suspected of having a concussion.

The Occupational & Industrial Orthopaedic Center offers care, education, and consulting services in the prevention and treatment of injuries and disorders that arise from the work environment.

Sports Performance Center specialists assist active individuals in reaching their full potential through a state-of-the-art health and fitness evaluation and personalized athletic training plan.

Patient Care Locations

Our physicians and surgeons provide care at multiple NYU Langone locations, including:

- **The Hospital for Joint Diseases**, our internationally-renowned orthopaedic hospital
- **The Center for Musculoskeletal Care (CMC)**, NYU Langone's premier, state-of-the-art, multidisciplinary, bone and joint facility, which houses outpatient orthopaedic and rheumatologic care as well as an infusion center, pain management services, and Rusk Rehab's sports and musculoskeletal rehabilitation services
- CMC's **Outpatient Surgery Center**, where patients undergo minimally invasive, same-day surgery
- **Tisch Hospital**, NYU Langone's flagship hospital at the main campus on First Avenue
- Multiple locations in **NYU Langone's growing network of community practices** in the metro New York area, including Manhattan, Brooklyn, Long Island, Queens, Westchester, and New Jersey

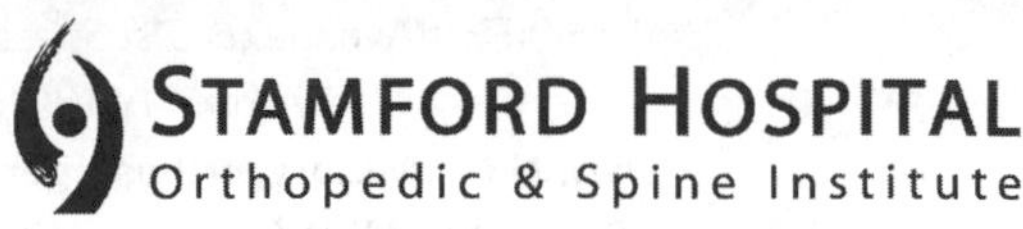

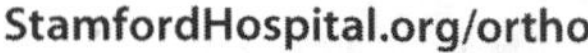

Orthopedic and Spine Institute

Stamford Hospital was the first in the region to earn the Joint Commission certification for our Total Hip and Total Knee Replacement programs in addition to our Spine Fusion Program. We were awarded the Gold Seal of Approval™ for complying with the highest national standards for safety and quality of care. Our doctors and nurses earned this distinction by undergoing a lengthy process of professional review, including on-site evaluations.

Total Joint Replacement

We provide comprehensive orthopedic services, including prevention, assessment, treatment and rehabilitation. Our fellowship-trained surgeons routinely perform total hip and knee replacements, as well as minimally invasive joint replacements and hip fracture surgeries using leading-edge technology to improve patient care and outcomes.

Spine Center

Experts in total spine care, we perform more complex spine surgeries than any other hospital in the region. From acute neck and back pain to spinal instability and deformity, we provide relief to those who may have previously tried non-surgical options. A team of dedicated orthopedic and neurosurgeons, nurses, anesthesiologists, physical therapists and pain-management specialists, are experienced in treating the most challenging spinal conditions.

Sports Medicine

No matter your age or level of play, amateur or seasoned professional, we can help you stay in the game. We combine hands-on evaluation and appropriate diagnostic testing to determine the best plan of care. We provide the latest surgical techniques and are experienced in performing a wide variety of advanced procedures. Our surgeons are fellowship-trained in sports medicine from some of the top programs in the country.

Chelsea Piers Connecticut

Stamford Hospital's Orthopedic and Spine Institute at Chelsea Piers CT, offers: nutritional counseling, integrative medicine, pain management, radiology, sports medicine, spine and general orthopedic care. The only comprehensive 3-D Motion Analysis Program in the region which provides patients with motion and biomechanical analysis. Top optical technologies produce a 3-D avatar you can view at any angle or speed to determine a course of action for performance improvement. Athletes in the Arts is another program which gives athletes and performing artists access to experts in training and injury treatment to excel in their sport or art.

Academic and Clinical Affiliations

Stamford Hospital is an affiliate of the New York–Presbyterian Healthcare System and a major teaching affiliate of the Columbia University College of Physicians & Surgeons.

Accreditation

Joint Commission on Accreditation of Healthcare Organization (JCAHO)

Beds

305

Sponsorship

Voluntary, Not-for-Profit

For a Physician Referral or more information, please call 1.877.233.9355 or visit StamfordHospital.org /doctor.

Stamford Hospital
30 Shelburne Road
Stamford, CT 06902
203.276.1000

StamfordHospital.org

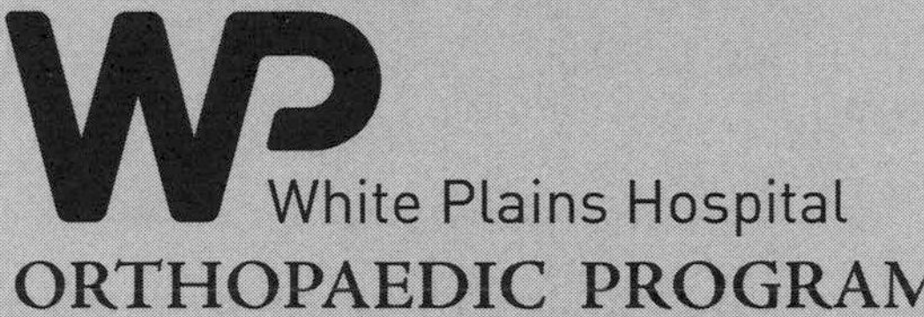

ORTHOPAEDIC PROGRAM

41 East Post Road, White Plains, NY 10601 • Tel: (914) 946-1010 • www.wphospital.org

The orthopaedic surgery program at White Plains Hospital (WPH) is an effective and innovative component of the Hospital's overall clinical offerings. Combining leading-edge technology with a clinical team that seeks the best possible outcome for each patient, the Hospital provides superior patient-oriented and compassionate Orthopaedic care.

The program provides a full range of orthopedic surgical and non-surgical services to relieve pain and improve function. These include highly-specialized and advanced methods of joint replacement surgery, corrective spinal surgery, and the repair of athletic injuries.

Beginning with pre-operative education, continuing through surgery, and including post-operative physical therapy, physicians, nurses and other staff members carry out treatment plans uniquely tailored to each patient's needs.

INPATIENT FACILITIES & AMENITIES: If surgery is indicated, the Hospital's Orthopaedic inpatient unit is an ideal setting that is designed to comfortably accommodate orthopedic patients and minimize the disruption that surgery can cause in their lives. With the professional support of White Plains Hospital and its outstanding doctors, nurses, and rehabilitation staff, surgery is scheduled at optimum times to minimize inpatient hospitalization. The goal is for each patient to resume an active lifestyle as soon as possible.

Patients who do stay overnight recuperate in a bright and modern inpatient unit, with a large number of private rooms, a patient-family lounge and a spacious on-site physical therapy room.

DISTINCTIVE FEATURES:

- Orthopedic specialists, trained at nationally-known academic medical centers.
- More total hip, partial and total knee replacement procedures using minimally-invasive orthopedic surgical techniques are performed at White Plains Hospital than at any other hospital in Westchester County.
- A nursing staff specially certified in orthopedic nursing care and working on an inpatient unit dedicated to orthopedic patients
- Physical therapists, dieticians and other clinical staff who use their specialized training to treat each patient
- Leading-edge radiology services that provide rapid and expert diagnosis
- Advanced methods of post-surgical pain control
- Spacious and modern outpatient physical therapy center in Rye Brook

Procedures Performed

- Minimally-invasive orthopedic surgery
- Arthroscopic surgical repair
- Hip and knee (partial and total) replacement
- Repair of sports injuries
- Hip fracture repair
- Orthopedic trauma repair
- Knee, shoulder, hand and ankle repair
- Spinal surgery including kyphoplasty, a minimally invasive procedure to stabilize spinal fractures and relieve pain
- X-Stop spine surgery procedure for spinal stenosis (narrrowing of the spinal canal)
- Reconstructive orthopedic procedures, including fracture repair

259 First Street, Mineola, NY 11501
Tel: 1-866-WINTHROP
www.winthrop.org

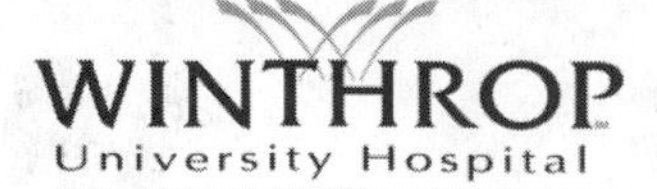

Your Health Means Everything.®

DEPARTMENT OF ORTHOPAEDICS AT WINTHROP-UNIVERSITY HOSPITAL

Winthrop-University Hospital is committed to being a leading center of excellence for orthopaedic surgery on Long Island.

- Dedicated to a highly individualized, multidisciplinary team approach to address the musculoskeletal needs of each patient as a whole person, Winthrop's orthopaedic surgeons address a full range of orthopaedic conditions, using both surgical and non-surgical procedures to relieve pain, discomfort, and maximize each patient's mobility.
- The Winthrop Orthopaedic Team is comprised of specialists who address several specialty areas of orthopaedics including: pediatric orthopaedics, hand and upper extremity surgery, minimally invasive surgery, arthroscopy, sports medicine, trauma and fracture repair, arthritis treatment, joint replacement and reconstruction surgery, spine surgery, and podiatry.
- This combination of advanced treatment options and specialists in virtually every area of adult and pediatric orthopaedic medicine places Winthrop's program at the forefront of orthopaedic care on Long Island.

Robotic Orthopaedic Surgery

A leader in total joint replacement, Winthrop continues to reach new frontiers in total hip replacement surgery, Total Knee replacements and joint replacement revision surgery. The joint replacement team also specializes in performing minimally-invasive, bone-sparing, and tissue-conserving total hip replacements. The department also offers robotically assisted total knee Replacement – a highly accurate approach to knee replacement surgery only offered at Winthrop.

Sports Medicine

Winthrop's comprehensive Sports Medicine Center features orthopaedic surgeons who focus on every joint in the body – from ankles and wrists to knees and hips – for both adults and children. Physicians work with patients individually to attain the highest levels of achievement despite any injury they may have.

Hand Injuries

The hand service treats children and adults with a variety of bone and soft tissue conditions of the hand and upper extremity. Some of the more common conditions include carpal tunnel syndrome, tennis elbow, and trigger finger. The department also specializes in the treatment of deformities, re-implantations, metabolic bone disease, complex fractures, and sports-related injuries.

Pediatric Care

Children's growth plates are delicate and are especially prone to fracture. Because many childhood fractures involve growth plates, it is vital for children to be evaluated quickly when a fracture occurs in order to determine the best course of treatment and avoid growth deformity. Winthrop's Division of Pediatric Orthopaedic Surgery treats pediatric patients from newborn to young adulthood.

Foot and Ankle Treatment

Winthrop's foot and ankle team specializes in a wide range of treatments, which can range from bracing and physical therapy to surgical procedures such as bunion surgery, ankle arthroscopy, complex ligament and tendon reconstructions, total ankle replacements, and osteochondral grafting procedures.

The Best in American Medicine
www.CastleConnolly.com

Otolaryngology

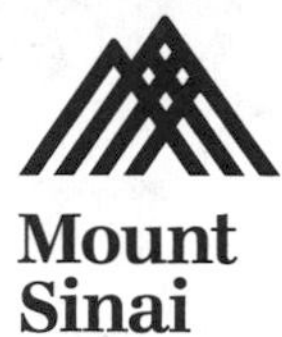

THE MOUNT SINAI MEDICAL CENTER

Hearing and Balance Center

One Gustave L. Levy Place
Fifth Avenue and 100th Street
New York, NY 10029-6574

Physician Referral: 1-800-MD-SINAI (637-4624)
www.mountsinai.org

The Mount Sinai Medical Center boasts one of the oldest and most distinguished otologic services in the United States. A division of the Department of Otolaryngology–Head and Neck Surgery, our excellent outcomes are reflected in the fact that *U.S. News & World Report* continually ranks our otolaryngology service among the best in the country.

At our **CENTER FOR HEARING AND BALANCE**, we provide patients with a full spectrum of treatment for hearing and balance disorders including acoustic neuromas, autoimmune inner ear disease, cholesteteatoma, chronic ear disease, facial nerve disorders, otosclerosis, bone-anchored hearing aids, and cochlear implants.

Dedicated to improving both patient outcomes and the patient experience, our otologic surgeons have pioneered surgical techniques for the management of chronic ear disease and cochlear implantation. They offer the most advanced and effective treatments available today and take a multidisciplinary approach to care, working with specialists from more than a dozen disciplines, to ensure that patients with complex medical conditions have access to the most comprehensive care available anywhere.

Audiology

Professionals in this state-of-the-art facility provide comprehensive diagnostic evaluation and treatment of hearing and balance disorders. Our patients range in age from pediatric to geriatric. Our team of audiologists offers complete diagnostic hearing evaluations, electrophysiological tests of the auditory system, and comprehensive vestibular assessment via Videonystagmography. Our clinical specialists are highly trained in the area of cochlear implantation and offer the latest advances in hearing aid fittings including implantable hearing devices and bone-anchored hearing aids.

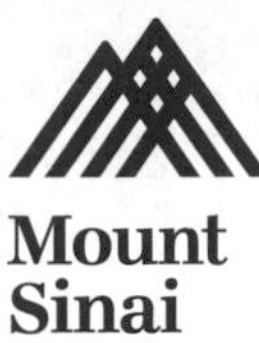

THE MOUNT SINAI MEDICAL CENTER

Otolaryngology – Ear, Nose and Throat

One Gustave L. Levy Place
Fifth Avenue and 100th Street
New York, NY 10029-6574

Physician Referral: 1-800-MD-SINAI (637-4624)
www.mountsinai.org

Mount Sinai's **DEPARTMENT OF OTOLARYNGOLOGY – HEAD AND NECK SURGERY –** ranks as one of the finest in the nation. In 2013, *U.S. News & World Report* ranked us at #10 in the United States, continuing our impressive history of achievement. Since the early nineteenth century, we have pioneered surgical advances in endoscopy, otology, skull-base surgery, laryngology, rhinology, facial plastic surgery, and head and neck oncology and reconstruction. More recently, we have incorporated advanced technology in robotic and endoscopic surgery, basic science research, and translational science programs.

Robotic Head and Neck Surgery – We are a world leader in robotic head and neck surgery. Our surgeons and researchers have published techniques that have changed the paradigm for management of head and neck cancer, allowing for endoscopic surgery without external incisions, shortening hospital stays, and improving outcomes.

THE MULTIDISCIPLINARY HEAD AND NECK ONCOLOGY TEAM— Acclaimed as one of the finest in the country, our multidisciplinary team includes 35 physicians, surgeons, and ancillary staff from 12 departments. We offer top-rated courses, training and research fellowships and enjoy national recognition for expertise in head, neck, and skull-base cancer. Our minimally invasive and endoscopic team includes surgeons and oncologists focused on treating tumors of the oral cavity, jaw, and larynx, while preserving each patient's quality of life. Speech and swallowing rehabilitation therapists work with patients to help them recover, all of which keeps Mount Sinai on the cutting edge of head and neck cancer therapy, reconstruction, and rehabilitation.

Thyroid and Parathyroid Surgery – We are nationally recognized for excellence in clinical care and clinical outcomes research. Our minimally invasive and robotic surgical techniques offer patients surgery through tiny incisions. Cure rates for thyroid cancer using these techniques are higher than 95 percent. Parathyroid surgery is performed using similar techniques and intraoperative parathyroid hormone monitoring.

Otology and Neurotology – Long recognized among the best in the nation, our otologic surgeons have pioneered surgical techniques to manage chronic ear disease and cochlear implantation that have resulted in excellent outcomes.

The Center for Comprehensive Management of Nasal and Sinus Disease – We deliver the most advanced care for patients suffering from allergic and invasive fungal sinusitis, acute and chronic sinusitis, benign and malignant tumors of the sinonasal cavity, cerebrospinal fluid leaks and encephalocele treatment and inflammatory polyp disease.

Endoscopic Laser Surgery of the Larynx and Trachea – Our surgeons and scientists have introduced techniques in laryngeal and tracheal surgery, including endoscopic laser surgery, tracheal transplantation, and reconstructive surgery, allowing removal of malignant disease while preserving voice and swallowing functions.

The Grabscheid Voice Center – Our multidisciplinary group provides professional singers and patients in need with cutting-edge treatments, using endoscopic laser and minimally invasive surgery. We pioneered office-based procedures that offer patients the opportunity to undergo therapy without the need for general anesthesia.

Cranial Base Surgery – Techniques in endoscopic trans-nasal surgery have revolutionized the management of skull base tumors and cerebrospinal leaks. We have developed procedures for accessing the cranial base and frontal lobes of the brain through the nose, delivering excellent outcomes with lower complications rates.

The Sleep Surgery Center – We offer comprehensive management and treatment of obstructive sleep apnea (OSA) and snoring. Collaboration with the divisions of pulmonary medicine, sleep medicine and endocrinology, provides the collective expertise of a multidisciplinary approach, which is necessary to address all conditions in sleep disordered breathing.

Center for Facial Plastic and Reconstructive Surgery – Our plastic surgeons provide expertise in the areas of facial plastic surgery and complex reconstructive surgery. Our team is expert in the areas of congenital and traumatic deformities, skin cancer, and facial nerve paralysis with reanimation. With expertise, they reverse the signs of aging, remove contour irregularities or deformities, and make the overall appearance of the face more natural and youthful.

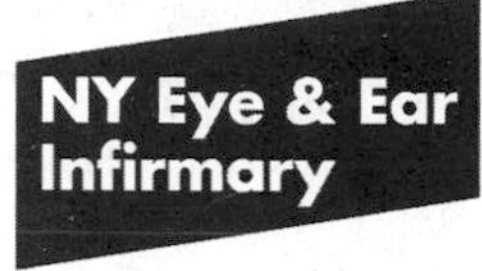

THE NEW YORK EYE AND EAR INFIRMARY

310 East 14th Street
New York, New York 10003
Tel. 212.979.4000 Fax. 212.228.0664
http://www.nyee.edu

PROVIDING EXCEPTIONAL CARE OF THE EAR, NOSE, THROAT, AND HEAD & NECK

Established in 1820 the Department of Otolaryngology/Head & Neck Surgery is the first training program in this specialty in the Western Hemisphere. Over nearly two centuries the department has evolved to be an international referral center for the medical and surgical treatment of diseases of the ear, nose, throat and face.

OUTSTANDING SERVICES:

Ear Institute (Otology – Neuro-otology): Specializing in the care of acute and chronic ear disease including hearing loss, cochlear implantation, dizziness, tinnitus, intra cranial tumors and facial nerve disorders. Our advanced otologic and vestibular diagnostic labs assist physicians in treatment.

Facial Plastic Surgery: Highly specialized and renowned surgeons perform in-office or ambulatory procedures utilizing state-of-the-art technology and techniques to produce outstanding results with minimal incisions, rapid recovery and a natural, youthful appearance.

Facial Paralysis: Comprehensive center treating all causes and offering reconstruction of the paralyzed face.

Head & Neck Oncology: A multi-disciplinary team including board-certified surgeons, medical & radiation oncologists, nutritionists and rehabilitation specialists insure rapid recovery from complex, life-saving surgical procedures and return to daily activities.

Pediatric Otolaryngology: Treating children has long been a priority at the Infirmary. Pediatric care ranges from middle ear infection, tonsil and adenoid disease, and neck masses to complex sinus and airway diseases.

Rhinology and Sinus Surgery Internationally known specialists utilize minimally invasive techniques to treat disorders from sinusitis to intra cranial tumors.

Thyroid Center: A comprehensive program to streamline the diagnosis and treatment of thyroid diseases and cancers. A highly skilled team of surgeons, endocrinologists and radiologists manage the patient's care.

Voice & Swallowing Institute: Combining the expertise of physicians, speech pathologists and a voice physiologist to diagnose and treat voice problems – not only for performing artists but also for teachers, stockbrokers, receptionists, salespeople – anyone for whom voice is an important part of life.

Otolaryngology Clinical Services

General Otolaryngology *plus*
Facial Plastic & Reconstructive Surgery
Cochlear Implantation
Voice & Vocal Dynamics
Head & Neck Oncology
Laryngology
Otology & Neuro-otology
Pediatric Otolaryngology
Rhinology & Sinus Surgery
Swallowing Disorders
Thyroid Center

Facilities

Academic Faculty Practice, *including multiple locations throughout metropolitan NY*
Hearing Aid Dispensary
Vestibular Rehabilitation
Ambulatory Care Services

About The New York Eye and Ear Infirmary

The New York Eye and Ear Infirmary is the nation's first specialty hospital and one of the most experienced in terms of the number of patients it treats and complexity of its cases. Each year the otolaryngology department performs more than 6,000 surgeries and sees more than 70,000 visits from outpatients.

Physician Referral
1.800.449.HOPE (4673)

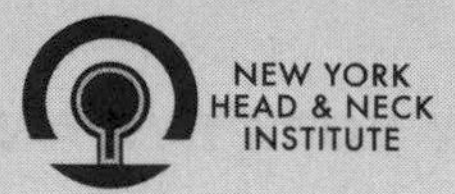

Lenox Hill Hospital (Black Hall)
130 East 77th Street, 10th Floor
(between Lexington & Park Avenues)
New York, NY 10075
(212) 434-4500
nyhni.org

New York Head & Neck Institute (NYHNI)
NYHNI, part of North Shore-LIJ Health System, provides seamless, integrated care across several specialty fields for people with disorders of the head and neck.

We are committed to compassionate treatment and trusted doctor–patient relationships. We share all available information with our patients, empowering them as equal partners when it comes to decisions regarding their care. At NYHNI, our patients always come first.

Award-Winning Care
Our outcomes have led to Lenox Hill's designation by ***U.S. News & World Report*** as one of the nation's top 50 hospitals for ENT.

Many Specialists, One Team
NYHNI consists of 10 centers, each focusing on a type of disorder or anatomical area of the head and neck, allowing us to treat the entire range of these disorders in adults and children. Each center offers medical therapy and the newest minimally invasive surgical techniques to cure the condition or improve the patient's life.

At NYHNI, we use a minimally invasive approach to all procedures, which ensures a faster, more comfortable recovery for the patient.

The physicians, surgeons (more than 100 — and growing) and professional staff of NYHNI all have regional, national or international reputations within their particular head and neck specialty areas. They bring vast experience and training to effectively diagnose and treat head and neck disorders while providing the most advanced patient-centered care.

We have offices in Manhattan, Staten Island and Long Island.

Our Areas of Expertise:

- Aesthetic Plastic Surgery
- Cranial Base Surgery (Skull Base Surgery)
- Facial Reconstruction
- Head and Neck Oncology (Head and Neck Cancer)
- Hearing and Balance (Diseases of the Ear)
- Allergies, Asthma, Nasal and Sinus Disorders
- Sleep Disorders (Obstructive Sleep Apnea)
- Thyroid and Parathyroid Surgery
- Vascular Anomalies
- Voice and Swallowing Disorders

To find a doctor: **1-888-321-DOCS** or visit **nyhni.org**

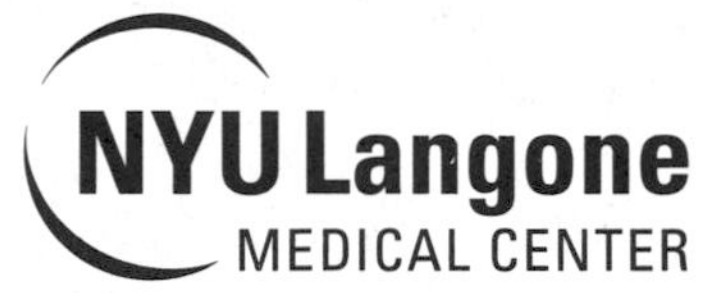

550 First Avenue *(at 31st Street)*
New York, NY 10016

www.NYULMC.org

Physician Referral: **888-7-NYU-MED** *(888-769-8633)*

OTOLARYNGOLOGY

The Department of Otolaryngology at NYU Langone Medical Center provides the highest quality treatment for ear, nose, throat, head and neck disorders, including one of the premier head and neck surgery programs in the country. We specialize in the following areas:

Cochlear Implants

Patients are provided with extensive evaluation, surgical implantation, device mapping, and speech rehabilitation.

Facial Plastic and Reconstructive Surgery

Care is provided to patients requiring facial reconstructive surgery for a wide variety of facial deformities, and to those seeking facial cosmetic surgery. Specialties include functional and aesthetic rhinoplasty, facial rejuvenation surgery, injectable fillers, Botulinum Toxin (Botox) for facial spasm or wrinkles, and chemical peels and microdermabrasion.

General Otolaryngology and Sleep Surgery

Care is provided to adult patients with voice, sleep, allergy and nasal breathing disorders. Additionally, services for children are provided through our pediatric otolaryngologists.

Head and Neck Surgery and Oncology

Care is provided to patients with cancer of the head and neck, including cancer of the larynx, oral cavity, throat, nasal cavity and sinuses, salivary glands and lymph nodes in the neck.

Neurotology/Skull Base Surgery

The Otolaryngology team provides expert care to patients with hearing loss, facial nerve palsy, vertigo and tinnitus, and treats lesions such as acoustic neuromas and skull base meningiomas. Featured services include facial palsy rehabilitation, auditory brainstem implants, cochlear implants, laser surgery and endoscopic anterior and lateral skull base surgery.

Voice and Swallowing Disorders

We treat voice and swallowing disorders, including sore throat, chronic cough, hoarseness, voice loss, swallowing dysfunction, benign growths and cancerous tumors, vocal cord paralysis, the aging voice, recurrent or chronic laryngitis, gastroesophageal reflux, and injuries from overuse and misuse of the voice. Specialized services are available for vocal performers.

Specialized Expertise

Audiology treats patients suffering with hearing or balance disorders; Head and Neck Speech Pathology treats voice, speech or swallowing problems; Rhinology treats all diseases of the paranasal sinuses, nose and related structures; Skull Base Surgery offers a minimally invasive and advanced surgical approach to tumors of the anterior and posterior skull base.

Pain Medicine

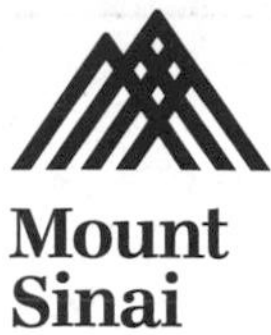

THE MOUNT SINAI MEDICAL CENTER

Pain Management and Integrative Pain

One Gustave L. Levy Place
Fifth Avenue and 100th Street
New York, NY 10029-6574

Physician Referral: 1-800-MD-SINAI (637-4624)
www.mountsinai.org

The Mount Sinai Medical Center's **DIVISION OF PAIN MANAGEMENT AND INTEGRATIVE PAIN** stands on the cutting edge of this vital and rapidly growing field. Our certified pain physicians deliver a blend of traditional and complementary treatment options to eliminate or reduce pain, restore mobility and enhance the quality of our patients' lives.

Committed to both easing pain and identifying and treating its underlying causes, we begin care by conducting diagnostic tests and a complete examination on all patients. This process helps us identify root conditions, determine optimal therapies, and tailor treatment plans to each patient's medical and personal needs. When our outpatients are admitted to Mount Sinai, we continue treating them inside the hospital, delivering uninterrupted care to achieve the best outcomes.

Offering a Range of Pain Management Treatments

Our team of experts range from specialists with decades of experience to those recently trained in the latest techniques at some of our country's top medical centers. All our physicians excel in core pain management, yet each has a different area of special interest, such as kyphoplasty, integrative medicine, and cancer pain management, permitting us to draw from a wide range of medical perspectives and specialties to provide the best possible course of treatment.

Incorporating Complementary Pain Management Techniques

We incorporate both Eastern and Western medicine within our service. We consider each patient's values and preferences to determine what therapies are most likely to succeed. Our resulting approach might incorporate evidence-based therapies, such as medical acupuncture, cupping (the use of suction to promote healing), and yoga, as well as Western treatments. We also incorporate physical therapy as well as dietary changes; for example, we help patients decrease inflammation by making nutritional changes instead of relying on Ibuprofen.

Delivering Successful Pain Management

There are few absolute cures in medicine, and we can't promise to make all patients pain free, but we do offer everyone the best chance at managing pain effectively. Whether it's helping a cancer patient sleep through the night unburdened by pain, or allowing an arthritic patient to participate in activities with grandchildren, our goal is to reduce pain so our patients can enjoy life to the fullest.

Parkinson's Disease

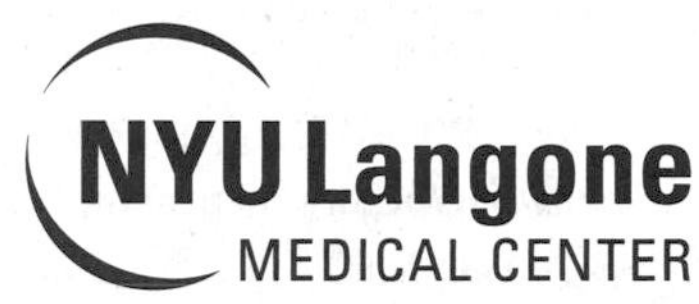

550 First Avenue *(at 31st Street)*
New York, NY 10016
www.NYULMC.org/neurology
www.NYULMC.org/neurosurgery
Physician Referral: **888-7-NYU-MED** *(888-769-8633)*

NEUROLOGY & NEUROSURGERY

NYU Langone Medical Center's Departments of Neurology and Neurosurgery continue to be **ranked among the nation's top 10 in the 2013-2014 U.S. News & World Report's annual survey of "Best Hospitals" in America.**

Patients travel from around the world to consult our renowned specialists for their expertise in the care, treatment, and research of neurological diseases and disorders of the brain, spine and nervous system. These conditions range from migraine headaches, nerve and muscle problems, pain, autism, movement disorders and Alzheimer's disease to stroke, vascular disorders, epilepsy, multiple sclerosis and brain tumors. NYU Langone is home to one of the largest epilepsy centers in the United States, as well as the largest multiple sclerosis program in New York and the first primary stroke center established in New York City.

<u>Neurological Expertise</u>

Autonomic Diseases: Our specialized Center evaluates and treats children and adults with familial dysautonomia and other inherited or acquired autonomic nervous system diseases, including orthostatic hypotension and rare forms of hereditary sensory neuropathy.

Epilepsy: Our Level 4 Comprehensive Epilepsy Center offers the most advanced medical and surgical options. Complementary management approaches complete the comprehensive care plan.

Multiple Sclerosis: The Comprehensive MS Care Center provides state-of-the-art diagnostic evaluations and follow-up care and management.

Neurogenetics: We focus on inherited diseases of the nervous system. Services include diagnosis and management of inherited diseases, biochemical and molecular testing and genetic counseling.

Neuro-oncology: In partnership with the NYU Cancer Institute, our multidisciplinary Brain Tumor Center is one of the nation's leading brain and spinal cord tumor programs, including physicians highly experienced in neuro-oncology, neurosurgery and neuroradiology.

Neuromuscular Diseases: We offer multidisciplinary programs for neuromuscular diseases, including acquired peripheral neuropathy, Charcot Marie Tooth neuropathy, myasthenia gravis, amyotrophic lateral sclerosis, spinal muscular atrophy, post-polio syndrome, muscular dystrophy and Lyme neuroborreliosis.

Parkinson's Disease and Movement Disorders: Our specialized center helps individuals affected by Parkinson's or other movement disorders to achieve the highest possible quality of life. Experts are also available to offer functional neurosurgery for certain conditions that involve involuntary muscle contractions.

(continued)

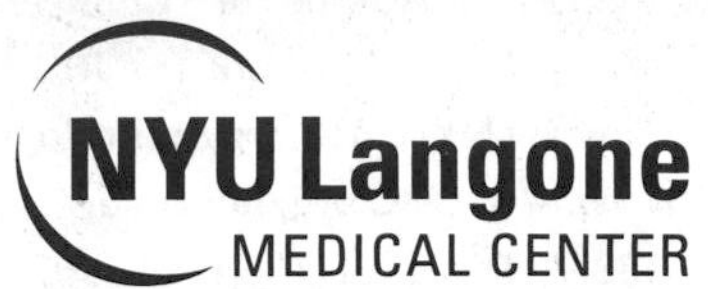

550 First Avenue *(at 31st Street)*
New York, NY 10016
www.NYULMC.org/neurology
www.NYULMC.org/neurosurgery
Physician Referral: **888-7-NYU-MED** *(888-769-8633)*

NEUROLOGY & NEUROSURGERY *(continued)*

Stroke Care: The multidisciplinary, Comprehensive Stroke Care Center provides rapid diagnosis, effective intervention and early rehabilitation for individuals who have had a stroke.
Concussion Center: This multidisciplinary center is a collaborative effort between the Departments of Neurology, Orthopaedic Surgery, and Rehabilitation, providing expert evaluation and treatment of individuals who have or are suspected of having a concussion.

Neurosurgical Expertise

The Department of Neurosurgery at NYU Langone Medical Center offers some of the nation's most skilled and experienced surgeons and advanced, minimally invasive procedures. Patients also benefit from cutting-edge research and a fully integrated approach to medical care.
Brain Tumor: Our neurosurgeons specialize in both malignant and benign brain tumors, including skull base tumors. Expertise includes glioblastoma, ependymoma, hemangioblastoma, other gliomas, meningiomas and vestibular schwannomas (acoustic neuromas).
Cerebrovascular Surgery: The Division of Cerebrovascular Surgery is a premier center for brain aneurysms, giant intracranial aneurysms, brain vascular malformations and cavernomas, and stroke.
Spinal Neurosurgery: The Division of Spine Surgery provides treatment for degenerative spinal diseases, spinal tumors, spinal trauma and spinal infections.
Neuromodulation: This specialized center offers deep brain stimulation (DBS) for Parkinson's, essential tremor, dystonia and obsessive-compulsive disorder, as well as peripheral neurostimulation (PNS) for migraines and other headaches and various types of facial pain.
Hyperhidrosis: The Department offers expertise in the surgical treatment of primary hyperhidrosis (excessive sweating) including Endoscopic Thoracic Sympathectomy.
Neurosurgical Technology: Our neurosurgeons remove deep-seated tumors, vascular malformations and other disease sites using a highly advanced Gamma Knife. Aided by 3-D MRI technology, the Gamma Knife bombards its target with precise doses of radiation, while preserving healthy tissue.

Other Neurosurgical Services

- Facial Pain: provides patients a thorough examination and, if required, nerve injections and minimally invasive surgery.
- Pediatric Neurosurgery: provides treatment to children with brain and spinal cord tumors, congenital and development disorders.
- Peripheral Nerve Surgery: focuses on the diagnosis and treatment of nerve compressions, nerve tremors, Brachial Plexus (nerve fiber) and nerve injuries.
- Neuro-Critical Care: our experts provide care for patients who have an urgent neuro-surgical problem that requires careful monitoring, or is at risk for developing such a problem.

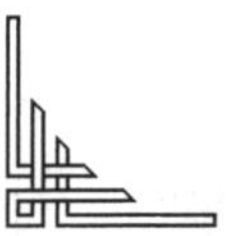
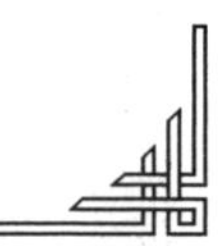

The Best in American Medicine
www.CastleConnolly.com

Pediatric Cardiology

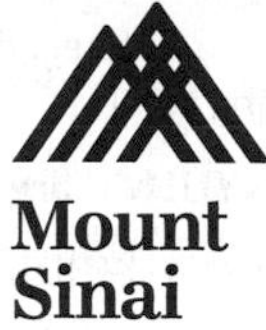

THE MOUNT SINAI MEDICAL CENTER
KRAVIS CHILDREN'S HOSPITAL

Pediatric Cardiology and Cardiac Surgery

One Gustave L. Levy Place
Fifth Avenue and 100th Street
New York, NY 10029-6574

Physician Referral: 1-800-MD-SINAI (637-4624)
www.kravischildrenshospital.org

INNOVATIVE MEDICINE, FAMILY-CENTERED CARE

The **DIVISION OF PEDIATRIC CARDIOLOGY** at Mount Sinai's Kravis Children's Hospital has achieved extraordinary success in diagnosing and treating the most difficult and complex cardiac conditions in fetuses, children, and young adults. We share our accomplishments with Mount Sinai Heart Hospital, globally recognized and pioneering a unique approach to the science and clinical care of patients with cardiovascular diseases. The Heart Hospital developed the Fetal Heart Program to care for newborns with congenital heart disorders and provide support and education to their parents.

As one of only two active pediatric heart transplant centers in New York State, our Congenital and Pediatric Cardiac Surgery program also provides support for very sick hearts in infants and older children, using Extra-Corporeal Membrane Oxygenators (ECMO) or Ventricular Assist Devices (VAD).

We offer a complete range of diagnostic services, including:

- Pediatric and fetal echocardiography
- Exercise testing
- Holter monitoring
- Cardiac MRI
- Electrophysiology
- Cardiovascular genetics

Collaborative, Comprehensive Care
Our interdisciplinary team works closely with referring physicians, and our success in treating patients with a broad range of heart conditions centers on the collaboration of an exceptional team of pediatric specialists, including cardiologists, cardiothoracic surgeons, anesthesiologists, advanced practice nurses and other skilled professionals.

With the Division of Pediatric Cardiology working in concert with the Department of Cardiothoracic Surgery, and Mount Sinai Heart Hospital, our pediatric experts provide the full spectrum of surgical and interventional catheterization treatments for congenital and acquired pediatric heart diseases.

Cardiothoracic Surgery with a Dedicated Post-surgical Cardiac Pediatric ICU
Young patients receive superb postoperative care in our standalone Pediatric Cardiac Surgical Intensive Care Unit (PCICU)—the only one of its kind in New York State. The PCICU is for children with congenital heart disease in need of intensive care for conditions involving the heart, lungs or airways. The PCICU staff of expertly trained doctors, physician assistants and award-winning nursing staff is available around the clock to care for our young patients.

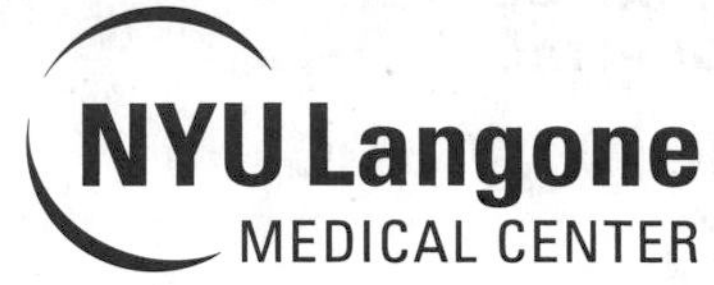

550 First Avenue *(at 31st Street)*
New York, NY 10016

www.NYULMC.org

Hassenfeld Children's Hospital Access Line: **855-NYU-KIDS**

HASSENFELD CHILDREN'S HOSPITAL

Hassenfeld Children's Hospital (HCH) is a full-service specialty children's hospital encompassing all children's health services at NYU Langone Medical Center. At HCH, newborns, children, adolescents and young adults receive the most comprehensive and advanced care possible from a team of pediatricians and pediatric specialists across more than 30 medical and surgical disciplines. With more than 150 full-time pediatric specialists, as well as pediatric nurses, child life specialists and social workers, Hassenfeld Children's Hospital is uniquely equipped to provide innovative pediatric subspecialty care in a highly personalized manner.

A Family-Centered Approach

Integral to the care we provide is a myriad of support services for children and their families. We recognize that the best outcomes are achieved when the child's family is actively involved in every step of care. For that reason, our trained specialists address the needs of not just the patient, but of parents and siblings through ongoing education and communication.

Our pediatric specialties include:

Anesthesia
Cardiology
Cardiothoracic Surgery
Child and Adolescent Psychiatry and Psychology/Child Study Center
Critical Care
Dermatology
Developmental and Behavioral Pediatrics
Emergency Medicine
Endocrinology
Epilepsy
Gastroenterology
Genetics
Hematology/Oncology
Infectious Diseases
Neonatology
Nephrology
Neurosurgery
Ophthalmology
Orthopaedic Surgery
Otolaryngology
Pathology
Pulmonology
Radiology
Reconstructive Plastic Surgery
Rehabilitation
Rheumatology
Surgery
Urology

The Best in American Medicine
www.CastleConnolly.com

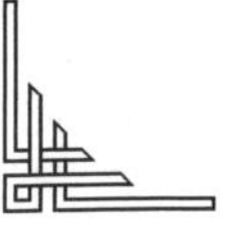
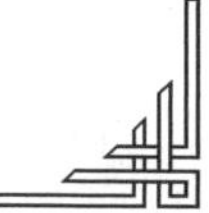

Pediatric Critical Care Medicine

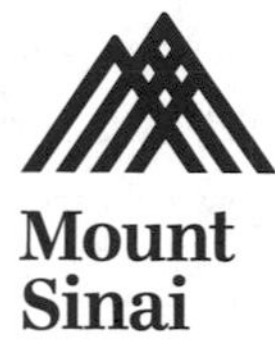

Mount Sinai

THE MOUNT SINAI MEDICAL CENTER
KRAVIS CHILDREN'S HOSPITAL
Pediatric Critical Care

One Gustave L. Levy Place
Fifth Avenue and 100th Street
New York, NY 10029-6574

Physician Referral: 1-800-MD-SINAI (637-4624)
www.kravischildrenshospital.org

INNOVATIVE MEDICINE, FAMILY-CENTERED CARE

The **DIVISION OF CRITICAL CARE MEDICINE** at The Mount Sinai Medical Center's Kravis Children's Hospital delivers quaternary level intensive care to critically ill and injured infants, children, and adolescents. Working with the most advanced diagnostic and therapeutic equipment, the faculty and staff have the training and the tools necessary to achieve optimal outcomes when treating children with serious medical and surgical conditions.

Board certified critical care physicians, together with award-winning nurses and highly skilled ancillary staff, deliver 24-hour care in the newly renovated **Alice Gottesman Bayer Pediatric Intensive Care Unit (PICU)**. The PICU is a state-of-the-art, 14-bed unit that averages 700 admissions per year, approximately one tenth of which are transported from referring hospitals. The PICU is equipped with a treatment room, a designated space for medical procedures and pediatric procedural sedation. Pediatric intensivists work closely with members of the **Division of Pediatric Cardiology** to provide expert critical care for patients in the 6-bed pediatric cardiac/cardiothoracic intensive care unit.

The interdisciplinary critical care team is trained and equipped to provide renal replacement therapy, therapeutic hypothermia, and advanced ventilation support modes, including nitric oxide therapy and high frequency oscillatory ventilation. In conjunction with colleagues in the cardiac/cardiothoracic intensive care unit, extracorporeal membrane oxygenation (ECMO), and ventricular assist device (VAD) support are utilized for the treatment of severe cardiac failure.

Pediatric intensive care unit patients benefit from the contributing expertise of pediatric medical and surgical subspecialists and a multidisciplinary staff which includes pediatric pharmacists, social workers, respiratory therapists, nutritionists, Child Life specialists and rehabilitation specialists. Staff also participates in a pediatric palliative care and pain team consultation service for children being cared for in all areas of Kravis Children's Hospital.

The PICU faculty and staff are committed to improving the health of infants, children, adolescents, and young adults, and look forward to continuing the long and distinguished tradition of excellence in innovative patient care, community involvement, professional education, and research across the translational spectrum.

The Best in American Medicine
www.CastleConnolly.com

Pediatric Emergency Medicine

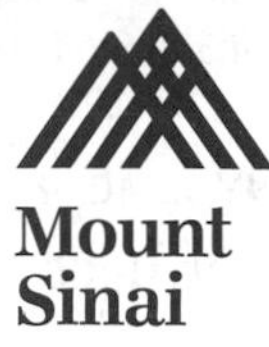

THE MOUNT SINAI MEDICAL CENTER
KRAVIS CHILDREN'S HOSPITAL
Pediatric Emergency Medicine

One Gustave L. Levy Place
Fifth Avenue and 100th Street
New York, NY 10029-6574

Physician Referral: 1-800-MD-SINAI (637-4624)
www.kravischildrenshospital.org

INNOVATIVE MEDICINE, FAMILY-CENTERED CARE

As part of The Mount Sinai Medical Center's Kravis Children's Hospital, which *U.S. News & World Report* consistently ranks among the best in the nation, members of our **DIVISION OF PEDIATRIC EMERGENCY MEDICINE** are dedicated to providing sick and injured infants, children, adolescents, and young adults with the most appropriate care as quickly as possible.

Our physicians are board certified in pediatric emergency medicine and see patients 24-hours a day, seven days a week in our state-of-the-art facility, which is located separate and apart from our adult emergency department, is designed for children's comfort, and has its own access from the waiting room.

We offer the most advanced treatment and technology available for the full range of medical and surgical conditions. Children requiring admission receive the best possible care for even the most complex conditions, and we consult with each child's own pediatrician when appropriate.

Our physicians, award -winning nurses and specially trained staff, understand the special clinical and emotional needs of children and have the right mix of experience, compassion and commitment to provide superior, family-centered care and guidance to young patients and their families.

As part of a major academic medical center, we also provide didactic and bedside teaching of pediatric emergency medicine to both the pediatric and emergency medicine residents and participate in clinical trials to investigate the causes and cures of pediatric illnesses. Some of our current research projects include the treatment of pediatric anaphylaxis, the use of positive airway pressure for patients with asthma, and the use of simulation to augment resident education

Our faculty, staff and trainees are committed to improving the health of infants, children, adolescents and young adults. We look forward to continuing our long and distinguished tradition of excellence in innovative patient care, community involvement, professional education, and research across the translational spectrum.

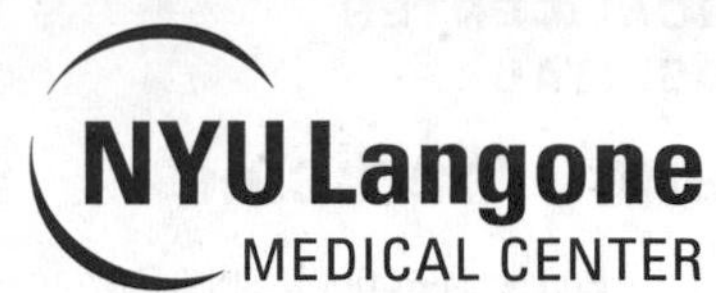

550 First Avenue *(at 31st Street)*
New York, NY 10016

www.NYULMC.org

Hassenfeld Children's Hospital Access Line: **855-NYU-KIDS**

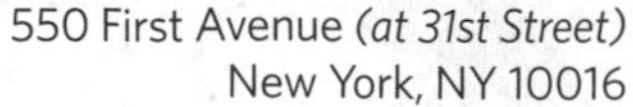

HASSENFELD CHILDREN'S HOSPITAL

Hassenfeld Children's Hospital (HCH) is a full-service specialty children's hospital encompassing all children's health services at NYU Langone Medical Center. At HCH, newborns, children, adolescents and young adults receive the most comprehensive and advanced care possible from a team of pediatricians and pediatric specialists across more than 30 medical and surgical disciplines. With more than 150 full-time pediatric specialists, as well as pediatric nurses, child life specialists and social workers, Hassenfeld Children's Hospital is uniquely equipped to provide innovative pediatric subspecialty care in a highly personalized manner.

A Family-Centered Approach

Integral to the care we provide is a myriad of support services for children and their families. We recognize that the best outcomes are achieved when the child's family is actively involved in every step of care. For that reason, our trained specialists address the needs of not just the patient, but of parents and siblings through ongoing education and communication.

Our pediatric specialties include:

Anesthesia
Cardiology
Cardiothoracic Surgery
Child and Adolescent Psychiatry and Psychology/Child Study Center
Critical Care
Dermatology
Developmental and Behavioral Pediatrics
Emergency Medicine
Endocrinology
Epilepsy
Gastroenterology
Genetics
Hematology/Oncology
Infectious Diseases
Neonatology
Nephrology
Neurosurgery
Ophthalmology
Orthopaedic Surgery
Otolaryngology
Pathology
Pulmonology
Radiology
Reconstructive Plastic Surgery
Rehabilitation
Rheumatology
Surgery
Urology

The Best in American Medicine
www.CastleConnolly.com

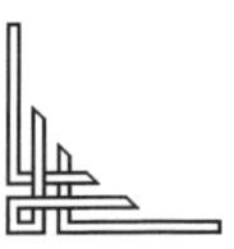
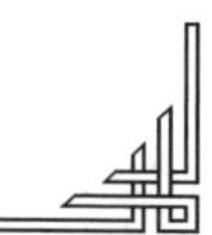

Pediatric Endocrinology

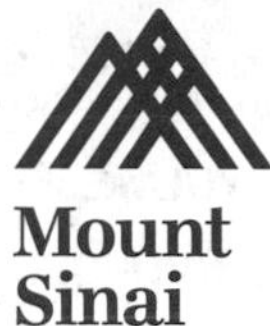

THE MOUNT SINAI MEDICAL CENTER
KRAVIS CHILDREN'S HOSPITAL

Pediatric Diabetes and Endocrinology

One Gustave L. Levy Place
Fifth Avenue and 100th Street
New York, NY 10029-6574

Physician Referral: 1-800-MD-SINAI (637-4624)
www.kravischildrenshospital.org

INNOVATIVE MEDICINE, FAMILY-CENTERED CARE

THE HALL FAMILY CENTER FOR PEDIATRIC ENDOCRINOLOGY AND DIABETES at Kravis Children's Hospital at Mount Sinai is dedicated to excellence in clinical care, education and research – a fact that has led to our being named among the top 25 pediatric diabetes and endocrinology services in America, according to ***The U.S. News & World Report's* 2013-2014 ranking of "Best Children's Hospitals."**

Under the direction of Robert Rapaport, MD, Division Chief, we use a team approach, which is patient and family centered, to manage:

- Diabetes (type 1 and type 2, medication-related, monogenic and pre-diabetes)
- Short stature
- Growth disorders, including growth hormone deficiency, growth in children born small for gestational age, and early and late puberty
- Genetic disorders, including Turner Syndrome and Noonan Syndrome
- Congenital and acquired hypothyroidism and hyperthyroidism
- Hyperparathyroidism
- Congenital adrenal hyperplasia/hypoplasia
- Obesity and other nutritional disorders, including Vitamin D deficiency.

ANNUAL SYMPOSIUM

Our physician-scientists conduct investigations into the causes and treatments of childhood endocrine conditions, and we are committed to translating research into better methods of clinical care. To that end, we hold an annual symposium each November to update pediatricians practicing within the community on the latest advances in pediatric endocrinology and diabetes.

Diabetes – We offer the complete spectrum of high level diagnostic and treatment services, including simulation testing, for children and adolescents and bring families into their circle of care. Since education and support are vital to managing diabetes, we offer a variety of programs for patients and their families, including "Toddlers and Grandparents," "College Prep," for teens entering college, and a free one-week day camp in Central Park in conjunction with the Barton Center for Diabetes Education.

We collaborated with four other medical centers on the **R.O.A.D. (Reduce Obesity and Diabetes) project**, to study and educate middle school children in Harlem. By identifying the metabolic factors that lead from obesity to diabetes, we will develop a protocol for detecting which children will most likely develop diabetes, allowing us to streamline interventions and identify where best to allocate resources.

Endocrine Disorders and Growth – With our faculty leading investigations into both international and multi-center trials, we enjoy a stellar reputation for identifying and treating a host of common and complex endocrine disorders, including growth hormone deficiency, growth in children born small for gestational age, and other disorders caused by Turner or Noonan Syndrome, and congenital hypothyroidism. In addition to offering expert consultations, we employ early screening methods and breakthrough growth hormone therapy that enables children to grow and develop normally.

We also excel at diagnosing and treating children with precocious or delayed puberty and have developed methods to identify and manage these conditions before they appear clinically obvious.

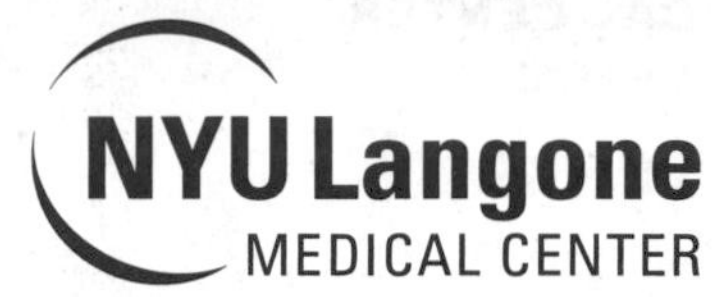

550 First Avenue *(at 31st Street)*
New York, NY 10016

www.NYULMC.org

Hassenfeld Children's Hospital Access Line: **855-NYU-KIDS**

HASSENFELD CHILDREN'S HOSPITAL

Hassenfeld Children's Hospital (HCH) is a full-service specialty children's hospital encompassing all children's health services at NYU Langone Medical Center. At HCH, newborns, children, adolescents and young adults receive the most comprehensive and advanced care possible from a team of pediatricians and pediatric specialists across more than 30 medical and surgical disciplines. With more than 150 full-time pediatric specialists, as well as pediatric nurses, child life specialists and social workers, Hassenfeld Children's Hospital is uniquely equipped to provide innovative pediatric subspecialty care in a highly personalized manner.

A Family-Centered Approach

Integral to the care we provide is a myriad of support services for children and their families. We recognize that the best outcomes are achieved when the child's family is actively involved in every step of care. For that reason, our trained specialists address the needs of not just the patient, but of parents and siblings through ongoing education and communication.

Our pediatric specialties include:

Anesthesia
Cardiology
Cardiothoracic Surgery
Child and Adolescent Psychiatry and Psychology/Child Study Center
Critical Care
Dermatology
Developmental and Behavioral Pediatrics
Emergency Medicine
Endocrinology
Epilepsy
Gastroenterology
Genetics
Hematology/Oncology
Infectious Diseases
Neonatology
Nephrology
Neurosurgery
Ophthalmology
Orthopaedic Surgery
Otolaryngology
Pathology
Pulmonology
Radiology
Reconstructive Plastic Surgery
Rehabilitation
Rheumatology
Surgery
Urology

The Best in American Medicine
www.CastleConnolly.com

Pediatric Gastroenterology

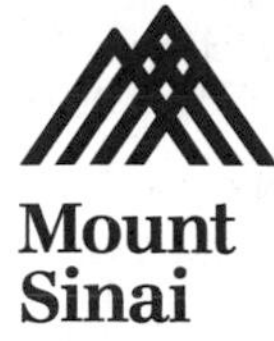

THE MOUNT SINAI MEDICAL CENTER
KRAVIS CHILDREN'S HOSPITAL

Pediatric Gastroenterology

One Gustave L. Levy Place
Fifth Avenue and 100th Street
New York, NY 10029-6574

Physician Referral: 1-800-MD-SINAI (637-4624)
www.kravischildrenshospital.org

INNOVATIVE MEDICINE, FAMILY-CENTERED CARE

In recognition of our tradition of excellence in patient care, research and education, Mount Sinai's Kravis Children's Hospital was named among the country's best in Pediatric Gastroenterology, according to the ***U.S. News and World Report's* 2013-2014 edition of "America's Best Children's Hospitals."**

Under the direction of Keith Benkov, MD, Chief of Pediatric Gastroenterology, we deliver expert consultation and compassionate, evidence-based care to pediatric patients with common and complex digestive disorders, including inflammatory bowel disease, celiac disease, gastroesophageal reflux disease and irritable bowel syndrome.

With a reputation for providing the highest level of innovative and comprehensive care to patients with Crohn's disease and ulcerative colitis, our nationally recognized Children's IBD Center receives referrals from across the country. We are currently following over 600 children and have seen over 2,000 patients with IBD in the last 10 years. The combination of this extensive experience, our focus on basic science and clinical research, and our collaboration with Mount Sinai's internationally renowned adult IBD program, enables us to deliver a unique approach to IBD care in children.

To optimize outcomes, our entire team of healthcare professionals participates in every patient's circle of care. We address each patient's specific needs, including management, nutrition, growth, body image and coping methods for a chronic illness. The center fosters family participation and encourages patients to gather to share ideas. Lectures, discussions and support groups are open to all families.

In addition, we continually strive to advance our knowledge of IBD and its treatments through research. In conjunction with the Department of Pediatric Allergy and Immunology, we are currently investigating the benefits of herbal medicine developed as a complementary therapy for children with Crohn's disease.

IBD runs the spectrum from mild to severe disease. No matter how seriously a child is affected, our ultimate goal is to help every child who comes to us with IBD lead a normal, productive life and achieve all his or her personal aspirations.

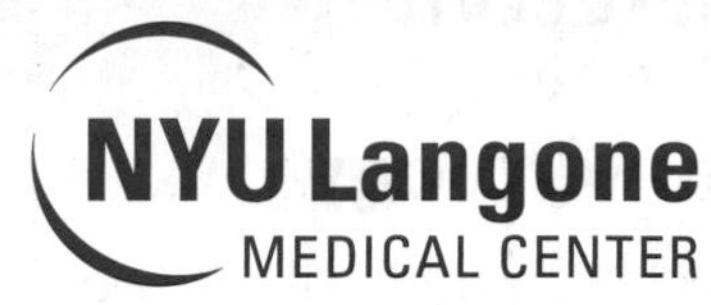

550 First Avenue *(at 31st Street)*
New York, NY 10016

www.NYULMC.org

Hassenfeld Children's Hospital Access Line: **855-NYU-KIDS**

HASSENFELD CHILDREN'S HOSPITAL

Hassenfeld Children's Hospital (HCH) is a full-service specialty children's hospital encompassing all children's health services at NYU Langone Medical Center. At HCH, newborns, children, adolescents and young adults receive the most comprehensive and advanced care possible from a team of pediatricians and pediatric specialists across more than 30 medical and surgical disciplines. With more than 150 full-time pediatric specialists, as well as pediatric nurses, child life specialists and social workers, Hassenfeld Children's Hospital is uniquely equipped to provide innovative pediatric subspecialty care in a highly personalized manner.

A Family-Centered Approach

Integral to the care we provide is a myriad of support services for children and their families. We recognize that the best outcomes are achieved when the child's family is actively involved in every step of care. For that reason, our trained specialists address the needs of not just the patient, but of parents and siblings through ongoing education and communication.

Our pediatric specialties include:

Anesthesia
Cardiology
Cardiothoracic Surgery
Child and Adolescent Psychiatry and Psychology/Child Study Center
Critical Care
Dermatology
Developmental and Behavioral Pediatrics
Emergency Medicine
Endocrinology
Epilepsy
Gastroenterology
Genetics
Hematology/Oncology
Infectious Diseases
Neonatology
Nephrology
Neurosurgery
Ophthalmology
Orthopaedic Surgery
Otolaryngology
Pathology
Pulmonology
Radiology
Reconstructive Plastic Surgery
Rehabilitation
Rheumatology
Surgery
Urology

The Best in American Medicine
www.CastleConnolly.com

Pediatric Hematology-Oncology

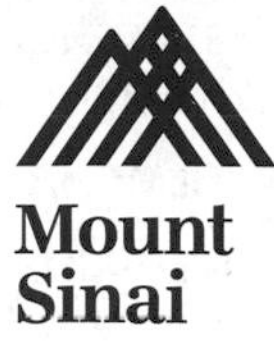

THE MOUNT SINAI MEDICAL CENTER
KRAVIS CHILDREN'S HOSPITAL

Pediatric Hematology/Oncology

One Gustave L. Levy Place
Fifth Avenue and 100th Street
New York, NY 10029-6574

Physician Referral: 1-800-MD-SINAI (637-4624)
www.kravischildrenshospital.org

INNOVATIVE MEDICINE, FAMILY-CENTERED CARE

Named by *U.S. News & World Report* as one of the best in the nation for treating pediatric cancer in its 2012-2013 "Best Children's Hospitals" issue, the Kravis Children's Hospital at Mount Sinai remains dedicated to delivering superior care to all our young patients. Through the efforts of our experienced, child-focused staff, we strive to achieve two goals: curing pediatric cancers and delivering effective, life-sustaining treatment to children with blood diseases.

Physicians in our **DIVISION OF PEDIATRIC HEMATOLOGY/ONCOLOGY** are board certified to treat patients with both hematology and oncology issues and diagnoses, and we maintain membership in both the Children's Oncology Group and the Pediatric Blood and Marrow Transplant Consortium.

We pride ourselves in our ability to provide exemplary clinical care while maintaining a very caring, human touch, one that comes from taking the time to get to know each of our young patients and their specific needs.

Thanks to the size and breadth of our pediatric program, we are able to deliver comprehensive, multidisciplinary care. This means that members of every child's pediatric hematology/oncology team will collaborate with Mount Sinai specialists from other disciplines to develop treatment plans and strategies tailored to his or her individual needs.

In addition, children who require most types of specialized tests or radiological studies (such as CT scans, MRIs or ultrasounds) can have them on-site at The Mount Sinai Medical Center. We assist all patients in setting up these appointments and we maintain constant communication with our patients' parents and caregivers.

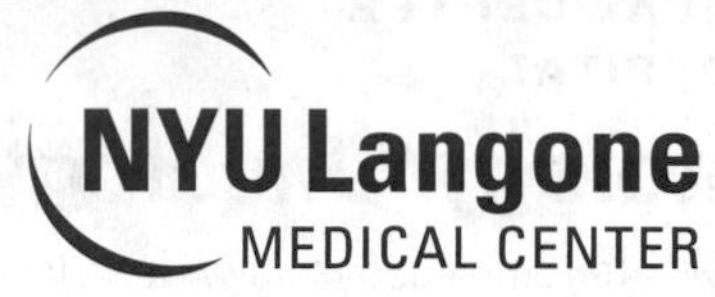

550 First Avenue *(at 31st Street)*
New York, NY 10016
www.NYULMC.org
Hassenfeld Children's Hospital Access Line: **855-NYU-KIDS**

HASSENFELD CHILDREN'S HOSPITAL

Hassenfeld Children's Hospital (HCH) is a full-service specialty children's hospital encompassing all children's health services at NYU Langone Medical Center. At HCH, newborns, children, adolescents and young adults receive the most comprehensive and advanced care possible from a team of pediatricians and pediatric specialists across more than 30 medical and surgical disciplines. With more than 150 full-time pediatric specialists, as well as pediatric nurses, child life specialists and social workers, Hassenfeld Children's Hospital is uniquely equipped to provide innovative pediatric subspecialty care in a highly personalized manner.

A Family-Centered Approach

Integral to the care we provide is a myriad of support services for children and their families. We recognize that the best outcomes are achieved when the child's family is actively involved in every step of care. For that reason, our trained specialists address the needs of not just the patient, but of parents and siblings through ongoing education and communication.

Our pediatric specialties include:

Anesthesia
Cardiology
Cardiothoracic Surgery
Child and Adolescent Psychiatry and Psychology/Child Study Center
Critical Care
Dermatology
Developmental and Behavioral Pediatrics
Emergency Medicine
Endocrinology
Epilepsy
Gastroenterology
Genetics
Hematology/Oncology
Infectious Diseases
Neonatology
Nephrology
Neurosurgery
Ophthalmology
Orthopaedic Surgery
Otolaryngology
Pathology
Pulmonology
Radiology
Reconstructive Plastic Surgery
Rehabilitation
Rheumatology
Surgery
Urology

The Best in American Medicine
www.CastleConnolly.com

Pediatric Infectious Disease

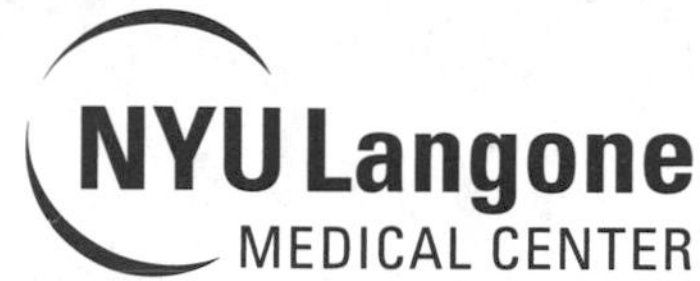

550 First Avenue *(at 31st Street)*
New York, NY 10016

www.NYULMC.org

Hassenfeld Children's Hospital Access Line: **855-NYU-KIDS**

HASSENFELD CHILDREN'S HOSPITAL

Hassenfeld Children's Hospital (HCH) is a full-service specialty children's hospital encompassing all children's health services at NYU Langone Medical Center. At HCH, newborns, children, adolescents and young adults receive the most comprehensive and advanced care possible from a team of pediatricians and pediatric specialists across more than 30 medical and surgical disciplines. With more than 150 full-time pediatric specialists, as well as pediatric nurses, child life specialists and social workers, Hassenfeld Children's Hospital is uniquely equipped to provide innovative pediatric subspecialty care in a highly personalized manner.

A Family-Centered Approach

Integral to the care we provide is a myriad of support services for children and their families. We recognize that the best outcomes are achieved when the child's family is actively involved in every step of care. For that reason, our trained specialists address the needs of not just the patient, but of parents and siblings through ongoing education and communication.

Our pediatric specialties include:

Anesthesia
Cardiology
Cardiothoracic Surgery
Child and Adolescent Psychiatry and Psychology/Child Study Center
Critical Care
Dermatology
Developmental and Behavioral Pediatrics
Emergency Medicine
Endocrinology
Epilepsy
Gastroenterology
Genetics
Hematology/Oncology
Infectious Diseases
Neonatology
Nephrology
Neurosurgery
Ophthalmology
Orthopaedic Surgery
Otolaryngology
Pathology
Pulmonology
Radiology
Reconstructive Plastic Surgery
Rehabilitation
Rheumatology
Surgery
Urology

Pediatric Nephrology

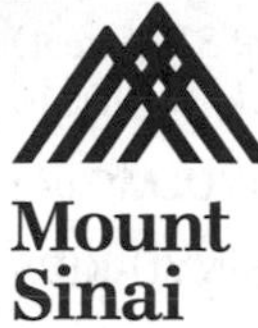

THE MOUNT SINAI MEDICAL CENTER
KRAVIS CHILDREN'S HOSPITAL

Pediatric Nephrology and Hypertension

One Gustave L. Levy Place
Fifth Avenue and 100th Street
New York, NY 10029-6574

Physician Referral: 1-800-MD-SINAI (637-4624)
www.kravischildrenshospital.org

INNOVATIVE MEDICINE, FAMILY-CENTERED CARE

Mount Sinai's Kravis Children's Hospital's **DIVISION OF PEDIATRIC NEPHROLOGY AND HYPERTENSION** is recognized as one of America's best by ***U.S. News & World Report's*** **2013-2014 ranking of "Best Children's Hospitals."**

We are recognized as one of the country's largest and most respected centers for pediatric kidney care and a pioneer in research and education. Under the direction of Jeffrey Saland, MD, Division Chief, we deliver specialized, evidence-based care to children with kidney disease, high blood pressure, urinary tract infections and a wide variety of related conditions, both common and complex.

Our patients benefit from our multidisciplinary team of pediatric nephrologists, urologists, transplantation specialists, psychiatrists, registered nurses, social workers, nutritionists and child life specialists working together to deliver the most effective care. Understanding that children require a special level of support and service, we bring families into their circle of care, and, as our patients become young adults, we help transition them into our excellent adult kidney program.

Our teaching and research programs in pediatric kidney disease serve to drive and maintain our expertise at the highest level. Working closely with our colleagues in diagnostic radiology and pediatric urology, we offer advanced diagnostic services and confident and experienced care for all kidney-related conditions, including:

- Kidney failure
- Dialysis (hemodialysis or peritoneal dialysis)
- Hypertension (high blood pressure)
- Kidney transplant, multiple organ transplant

We are a major referral center for children with high blood pressure, offering state-of-the art diagnostics such as ambulatory blood pressure monitoring (ABPM), a home-based measure that allows us to be sure hypertension is present, and we provide comprehensive treatment plans that include a focus on diet, physical activity, and stress factors.

As a Center of Excellence in Transplantation, we are one of the most sought after pediatric kidney transplant centers in the country. During the past five years, we provided kidney transplants to nearly twice as many children as any other New York hospital, and, even more significant, the outcomes of those transplants were among the best in the country, as verified by the Organ Procurement and Transplantation Network (OPTN) and the Scientific Registry of Transplantation Recipients (SRTR), under contract from the US Department of Health and Human Services.

We offer fast appointments and a streamlined admitting process for admitting physicians.

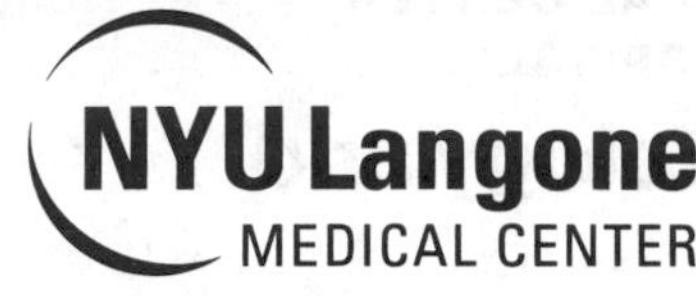

550 First Avenue *(at 31st Street)*
New York, NY 10016

www.NYULMC.org

Hassenfeld Children's Hospital Access Line: **855-NYU-KIDS**

HASSENFELD CHILDREN'S HOSPITAL

Hassenfeld Children's Hospital (HCH) is a full-service specialty children's hospital encompassing all children's health services at NYU Langone Medical Center. At HCH, newborns, children, adolescents and young adults receive the most comprehensive and advanced care possible from a team of pediatricians and pediatric specialists across more than 30 medical and surgical disciplines. With more than 150 full-time pediatric specialists, as well as pediatric nurses, child life specialists and social workers, Hassenfeld Children's Hospital is uniquely equipped to provide innovative pediatric subspecialty care in a highly personalized manner.

A Family-Centered Approach

Integral to the care we provide is a myriad of support services for children and their families. We recognize that the best outcomes are achieved when the child's family is actively involved in every step of care. For that reason, our trained specialists address the needs of not just the patient, but of parents and siblings through ongoing education and communication.

Our pediatric specialties include:

Anesthesia
Cardiology
Cardiothoracic Surgery
Child and Adolescent Psychiatry and Psychology/Child Study Center
Critical Care
Dermatology
Developmental and Behavioral Pediatrics
Emergency Medicine
Endocrinology
Epilepsy
Gastroenterology
Genetics
Hematology/Oncology
Infectious Diseases
Neonatology
Nephrology
Neurosurgery
Ophthalmology
Orthopaedic Surgery
Otolaryngology
Pathology
Pulmonology
Radiology
Reconstructive Plastic Surgery
Rehabilitation
Rheumatology
Surgery
Urology

The Best in American Medicine
www.CastleConnolly.com

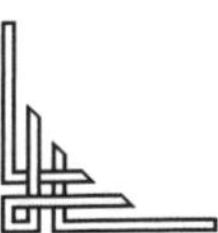

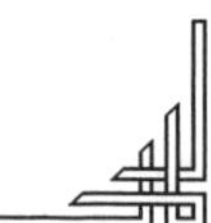

Pediatric Otolaryngology

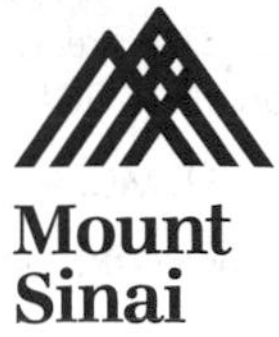

THE MOUNT SINAI MEDICAL CENTER
KRAVIS CHILDREN'S HOSPITAL

Pediatric Otolaryngology

One Gustave L. Levy Place
Fifth Avenue and 100th Street
New York, NY 10029-6574

Physician Referral: 1-800-MD-SINAI (637-4624)
www.kravischildrenshospital.org

INNOVATIVE MEDICINE, FAMILY-CENTERED CARE

The Kravis Children's Hospital at Mount Sinai is dedicated to excellence in clinical care, education and research. Our pediatric otolaryngologists excel at managing common and complex ear, nose and throat (ENT) disorders in children.

Common conditions we treat include:

- Sleep apnea and other nighttime breathing disorders
- Recurrent infections of the ears, throat and sinuses
- Hearing loss related to middle ear fluid
- Feeding problems in newborn infants due to abnormalities of the mouth and tongue

More complex diseases we treat include:

- Congenital abnormalities of the head and neck such as cysts and fistulas
- Blood vessel malformations such as lymphangiomas and hemangiomas
- Disorders of the pediatric larynx and airway
- Sensorineural hearing loss requiring cochlear implantation

Multidisciplinary Pediatric ENT Care

We routinely collaborate and perform joint procedures with pediatric faculty in other subspecialties, such as pulmonology, gastroenterology, genetics, allergy, hematology-oncology, intensive care medicine, and infectious disease. Joint management teams, such as our cleft and craniofacial group, provide additional opportunities for cross-specialty discussion and treatment planning. We also offer pediatric audiology, speech therapy, and swallowing evaluation.

MAGNET STATUS

Mount Sinai Hospital earned Magnet status from the American Nurses Credentialing Center–their highest honor, awarded every five years. Mount Sinai received this status in 2004 and again in 2009, ranking it among the nation's elite hospitals, only 6 percent of which have received this gold standard of nursing excellence designation twice in succession.

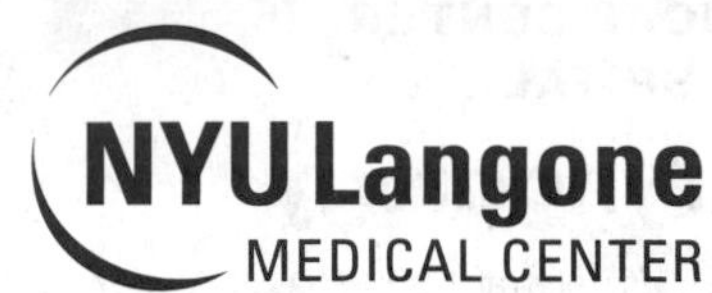

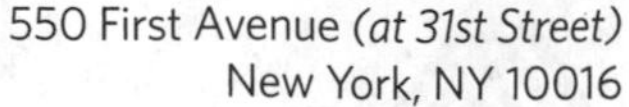

550 First Avenue *(at 31st Street)*
New York, NY 10016

www.NYULMC.org

Hassenfeld Children's Hospital Access Line: **855-NYU-KIDS**

HASSENFELD CHILDREN'S HOSPITAL

Hassenfeld Children's Hospital (HCH) is a full-service specialty children's hospital encompassing all children's health services at NYU Langone Medical Center. At HCH, newborns, children, adolescents and young adults receive the most comprehensive and advanced care possible from a team of pediatricians and pediatric specialists across more than 30 medical and surgical disciplines. With more than 150 full-time pediatric specialists, as well as pediatric nurses, child life specialists and social workers, Hassenfeld Children's Hospital is uniquely equipped to provide innovative pediatric subspecialty care in a highly personalized manner.

A Family-Centered Approach

Integral to the care we provide is a myriad of support services for children and their families. We recognize that the best outcomes are achieved when the child's family is actively involved in every step of care. For that reason, our trained specialists address the needs of not just the patient, but of parents and siblings through ongoing education and communication.

Our pediatric specialties include:

Anesthesia
Cardiology
Cardiothoracic Surgery
Child and Adolescent Psychiatry and Psychology/Child Study Center
Critical Care
Dermatology
Developmental and Behavioral Pediatrics
Emergency Medicine
Endocrinology
Epilepsy
Gastroenterology
Genetics
Hematology/Oncology
Infectious Diseases
Neonatology
Nephrology
Neurosurgery
Ophthalmology
Orthopaedic Surgery
Otolaryngology
Pathology
Pulmonology
Radiology
Reconstructive Plastic Surgery
Rehabilitation
Rheumatology
Surgery
Urology

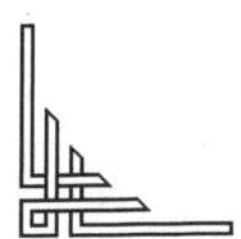

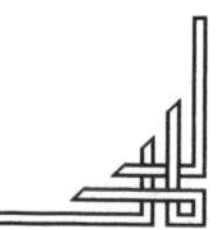

Pediatric Pulmonology

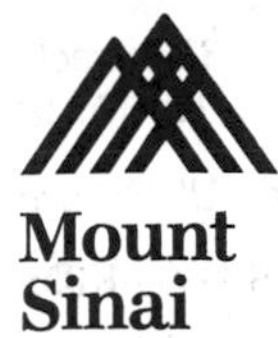

THE MOUNT SINAI MEDICAL CENTER
KRAVIS CHILDREN'S HOSPITAL
Pediatric Pulmonology

One Gustave L. Levy Place
Fifth Avenue and 100th Street
New York, NY 10029-6574

Physician Referral: 1-800-MD-SINAI (637-4624)
www.kravischildrenshospital.org

INNOVATIVE MEDICINE, FAMILY-CENTERED CARE

At Mount Sinai's **DIVISION OF PEDIATRIC PULMONOLOGY**, we are dedicated to treating the full spectrum of children's respiratory illnesses, both common and complex, with a high level of skill and compassion. This dedication has led to our being named among the top pediatric pulmonary services in America, according to ***U.S. News & World Report's*** **2013-2014 ranking of "Best Children's Hospitals."**

Under the direction of Alfin Vicencio, MD, Division Chief, our team of award winning pediatric pulmonologists, nurse practitioners, nurse educators, nutritionists, social workers and respiratory therapists deliver evidence-based care to children with asthma, cystic fibrosis, chronic respiratory failure, bronchopulmonary dysplasia and other respiratory conditions.

Offering medical support and guidance, our **Children's Asthma Center** offers advanced diagnostic and treatment protocols for refractory asthma along with advanced pulmonary function testing, allergy testing, environmental assessment, nutritional evaluation, education, and family services. We teach patients and their parents or guardians to identify asthma triggers and offer a personalized asthma action plan for each patient—a process that has our patients experiencing fewer emergency department visits and hospitalizations, missing less school and enjoying more active lives. In addition, through outreach efforts and care delivered to children from East Harlem—an area with one of the highest asthma rates in the country—we have succeeded in empowering these patients to manage their disease and face the future with confidence.

To significantly enhance our pediatric flexible bronchoscopy service, we recently opened a new **Bronchoscopy Suite** that houses the most advanced technology for both diagnostic capabilities and interventional procedures.

As an accredited **Cystic Fibrosis Foundation Care Center**, we offer the latest therapies and participate in multi-center trials. With our team specially trained in caring for cystic fibrosis patients, we treat all aspects of the disease, ranging from the latest antimicrobial strategies to nutritional optimization. We offer services that include pediatric spirometry, plethysmography, and comprehensive psychosocial support and evaluation.

Our **Chronic Ventilator Program** provides the most advanced and compassionate management of children with chronic respiratory failure as well as those with muscular dystrophies and other conditions that require mechanical ventilation.

Our **Bronchopulmonary Dysplasia Program** offers the highest level of care for premature infants while they are in the hospital and, as outpatients, once they are discharged

FROM BENCH TO BEDSIDE

We have recently recruited Rosalind Wright, MD, MPH, to serve as Vice Chair for Transitional Research and as a member of the Division of Pediatric Pulmonology. Dr. Wright is recognized both nationally and internationally for her investigations into early life events in relation to the development of pediatric asthma and is a welcome addition to our team of physician-scientists.

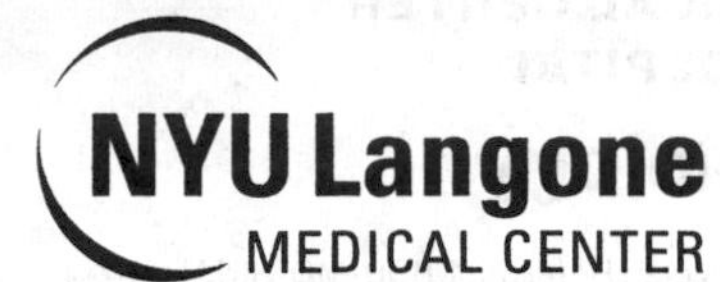

550 First Avenue *(at 31st Street)*
New York, NY 10016
www.NYULMC.org
Hassenfeld Children's Hospital Access Line: **855-NYU-KIDS**

HASSENFELD CHILDREN'S HOSPITAL

Hassenfeld Children's Hospital (HCH) is a full-service specialty children's hospital encompassing all children's health services at NYU Langone Medical Center. At HCH, newborns, children, adolescents and young adults receive the most comprehensive and advanced care possible from a team of pediatricians and pediatric specialists across more than 30 medical and surgical disciplines. With more than 150 full-time pediatric specialists, as well as pediatric nurses, child life specialists and social workers, Hassenfeld Children's Hospital is uniquely equipped to provide innovative pediatric subspecialty care in a highly personalized manner.

A Family-Centered Approach

Integral to the care we provide is a myriad of support services for children and their families. We recognize that the best outcomes are achieved when the child's family is actively involved in every step of care. For that reason, our trained specialists address the needs of not just the patient, but of parents and siblings through ongoing education and communication.

Our pediatric specialties include:

Anesthesia
Cardiology
Cardiothoracic Surgery
Child and Adolescent Psychiatry and Psychology/Child Study Center
Critical Care
Dermatology
Developmental and Behavioral Pediatrics
Emergency Medicine
Endocrinology
Epilepsy
Gastroenterology
Genetics
Hematology/Oncology
Infectious Diseases
Neonatology
Nephrology
Neurosurgery
Ophthalmology
Orthopaedic Surgery
Otolaryngology
Pathology
Pulmonology
Radiology
Reconstructive Plastic Surgery
Rehabilitation
Rheumatology
Surgery
Urology

The Best in American Medicine
www.CastleConnolly.com

Pediatric Radiology

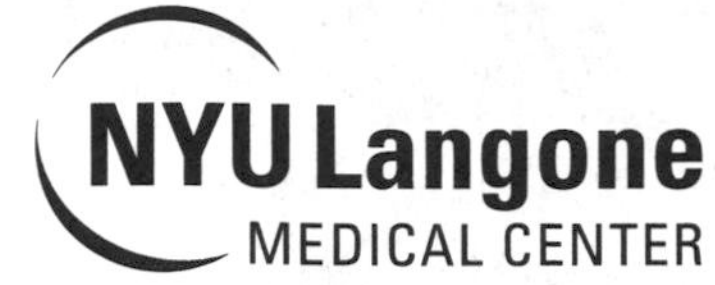

550 First Avenue *(at 31st Street)*
New York, NY 10016

www.NYULMC.org

Hassenfeld Children's Hospital Access Line: **855-NYU-KIDS**

HASSENFELD CHILDREN'S HOSPITAL

Hassenfeld Children's Hospital (HCH) is a full-service specialty children's hospital encompassing all children's health services at NYU Langone Medical Center. At HCH, newborns, children, adolescents and young adults receive the most comprehensive and advanced care possible from a team of pediatricians and pediatric specialists across more than 30 medical and surgical disciplines. With more than 150 full-time pediatric specialists, as well as pediatric nurses, child life specialists and social workers, Hassenfeld Children's Hospital is uniquely equipped to provide innovative pediatric subspecialty care in a highly personalized manner.

A Family-Centered Approach

Integral to the care we provide is a myriad of support services for children and their families. We recognize that the best outcomes are achieved when the child's family is actively involved in every step of care. For that reason, our trained specialists address the needs of not just the patient, but of parents and siblings through ongoing education and communication.

Our pediatric specialties include:

Anesthesia
Cardiology
Cardiothoracic Surgery
Child and Adolescent Psychiatry and Psychology/Child Study Center
Critical Care
Dermatology
Developmental and Behavioral Pediatrics
Emergency Medicine
Endocrinology
Epilepsy
Gastroenterology
Genetics
Hematology/Oncology
Infectious Diseases
Neonatology
Nephrology
Neurosurgery
Ophthalmology
Orthopaedic Surgery
Otolaryngology
Pathology
Pulmonology
Radiology
Reconstructive Plastic Surgery
Rehabilitation
Rheumatology
Surgery
Urology

Pediatric Rheumatology

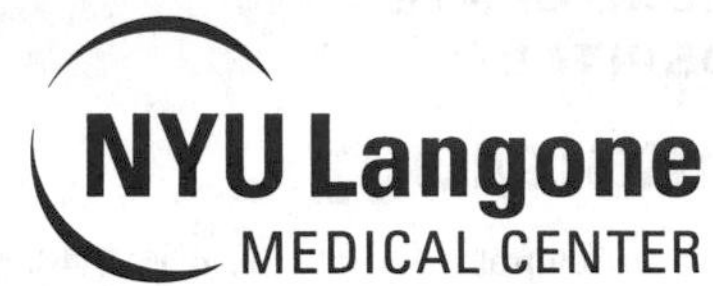

550 First Avenue *(at 31st Street)*
New York, NY 10016

www.NYULMC.org

Hassenfeld Children's Hospital Access Line: **855-NYU-KIDS**

HASSENFELD CHILDREN'S HOSPITAL

Hassenfeld Children's Hospital (HCH) is a full-service specialty children's hospital encompassing all children's health services at NYU Langone Medical Center. At HCH, newborns, children, adolescents and young adults receive the most comprehensive and advanced care possible from a team of pediatricians and pediatric specialists across more than 30 medical and surgical disciplines. With more than 150 full-time pediatric specialists, as well as pediatric nurses, child life specialists and social workers, Hassenfeld Children's Hospital is uniquely equipped to provide innovative pediatric subspecialty care in a highly personalized manner.

A Family-Centered Approach

Integral to the care we provide is a myriad of support services for children and their families. We recognize that the best outcomes are achieved when the child's family is actively involved in every step of care. For that reason, our trained specialists address the needs of not just the patient, but of parents and siblings through ongoing education and communication.

Our pediatric specialties include:

Anesthesia
Cardiology
Cardiothoracic Surgery
Child and Adolescent Psychiatry
  and Psychology/Child Study Center
Critical Care
Dermatology
Developmental and Behavioral Pediatrics
Emergency Medicine
Endocrinology
Epilepsy
Gastroenterology
Genetics
Hematology/Oncology
Infectious Diseases
Neonatology
Nephrology
Neurosurgery
Ophthalmology
Orthopaedic Surgery
Otolaryngology
Pathology
Pulmonology
Radiology
Reconstructive Plastic Surgery
Rehabilitation
Rheumatology
Surgery
Urology

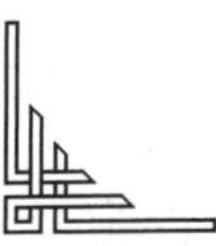
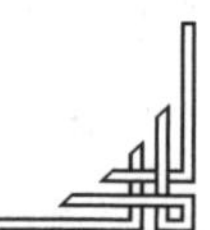

Pediatric Surgery

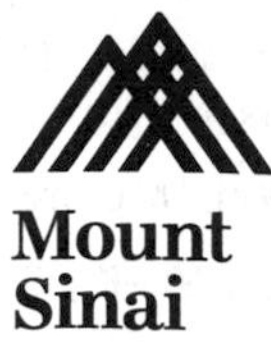

THE MOUNT SINAI MEDICAL CENTER
KRAVIS CHILDREN'S HOSPITAL

Pediatric Surgery

One Gustave L. Levy Place
Fifth Avenue and 100th Street
New York, NY 10029-6574

Physician Referral: 1-800-MD-SINAI (637-4624)
www.kravischildrenshospital.org

INNOVATIVE MEDICINE, FAMILY-CENTERED CARE

The Kravis Children's Hospital at Mount Sinai is dedicated to excellence in pediatric surgery. To achieve that goal we have assembled a care team with the right mix of experience, compassion and commitment to provide superior, family-centered care and guidance to young patients and their families.

We offer comprehensive surgical care for children with both common and complex conditions. Our highly skilled surgeons, board certified in pediatric surgery, are adept at performing the most advanced minimally invasive pediatric surgery techniques. We specialize in neonatal surgery and have extensive experience in the operative management of common conditions such as:

- Anal atresia
- Appendicitis
- Congenital diaphragmatic hernia
- Kidney tumors (Wilms' tumor)
- Pediatric inflammatory bowel disease (IBD)
- Pyloric stenosis

Our care team includes neonatologists, pediatricians, pediatric gastroenterologists, pediatric oncologists, and other skilled professionals. We understand the intense stress that parents experience when their child faces surgery. Our physicians and nurse practitioner work with child life specialists and others to make all procedures, big and small, as comfortable for the child and the family as possible. Our goal is to offer the most advanced care in the most sensitive way possible.

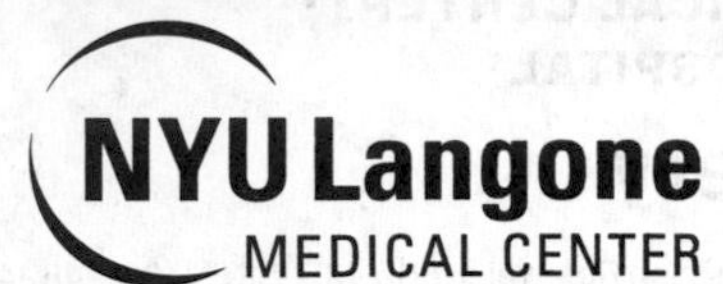

550 First Avenue *(at 31st Street)*
New York, NY 10016

www.NYULMC.org

Hassenfeld Children's Hospital Access Line: **855-NYU-KIDS**

HASSENFELD CHILDREN'S HOSPITAL

Hassenfeld Children's Hospital (HCH) is a full-service specialty children's hospital encompassing all children's health services at NYU Langone Medical Center. At HCH, newborns, children, adolescents and young adults receive the most comprehensive and advanced care possible from a team of pediatricians and pediatric specialists across more than 30 medical and surgical disciplines. With more than 150 full-time pediatric specialists, as well as pediatric nurses, child life specialists and social workers, Hassenfeld Children's Hospital is uniquely equipped to provide innovative pediatric subspecialty care in a highly personalized manner.

A Family-Centered Approach

Integral to the care we provide is a myriad of support services for children and their families. We recognize that the best outcomes are achieved when the child's family is actively involved in every step of care. For that reason, our trained specialists address the needs of not just the patient, but of parents and siblings through ongoing education and communication.

Our pediatric specialties include:

Anesthesia
Cardiology
Cardiothoracic Surgery
Child and Adolescent Psychiatry and Psychology/Child Study Center
Critical Care
Dermatology
Developmental and Behavioral Pediatrics
Emergency Medicine
Endocrinology
Epilepsy
Gastroenterology
Genetics
Hematology/Oncology
Infectious Diseases
Neonatology
Nephrology
Neurosurgery
Ophthalmology
Orthopaedic Surgery
Otolaryngology
Pathology
Pulmonology
Radiology
Reconstructive Plastic Surgery
Rehabilitation
Rheumatology
Surgery
Urology

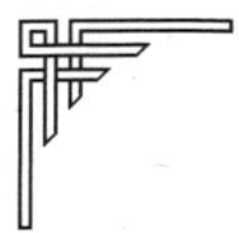

The Best in American Medicine
www.CastleConnolly.com

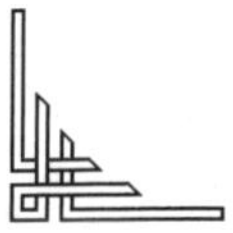
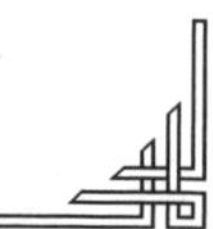

Pediatrics

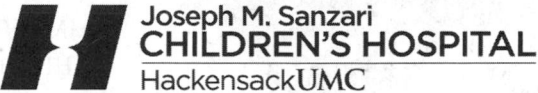

30 Prospect Avenue, Hackensack, NJ 07601 • 551-996-5300

www.HackensackUMC.org

The Joseph M. Sanzari Children's Hospital at HackensackUMC is a state-designated children's hospital and an award-winning facility that has been recognized as one of the top-ranked children's hospitals in New Jersey and in the country. It ranked 29th among the Best Children's Hospitals for Neurology and Neurosurgery in the 2013-14 Best Children's Hospitals rankings by *U.S. News & World Report* — the first hospital in New Jersey to be ranked in any Best Children's Hospitals specialty, and the only hospital in the state to be ranked in Neurology and Neurosurgery.

FACILITY:

As a state-designated children's hospital, The Joseph M. Sanzari Children's Hospital provides comprehensive patient- and family-centered medical and surgical pediatric care in more than 30 specialties, all integrated within a state-of-the-art child-focused facility. The facility offers 24-hour access to leading physicians, nurses, staff and a Pediatric Emergency/Trauma Department. It features a modern facility with children's play and family kitchen areas, and private inpatient rooms with computers, internet access, and flat-screen plasma televisions. Parents are encouraged to take part in their children's treatment and hospitalization and are welcome to stay overnight. The Joseph M. Sanzari Children's Hospital was planned and designed to be a "green" hospital.

SPECIALTIES:

Adolescent medicine, audiology, cardiology, child abuse and neglect, child and adolescent psychiatry, child life, clinical and laboratory immunology, critical care medicine, dermatology, developmental, Pediatric Emergency Department, endocrinology, epilepsy monitoring, gastroenterology, general pediatrics, genetics, hematology-oncology, infectious disease, neonatal-perinatal medicine, nephrology, neurodevelopmental disabilities, neuro oncology, otolaryngology, orthopaedic surgery, pain and palliative medicine, pediatric neurology, pediatric sleep, pediatric surgery, pulmonology, radiology, rehabilitation medicine, rheumatology, social work, and transplant.

SPECIALIZED PROGRAMS:

Audrey Hepburn Children's House; Community CPR and First Aid Training; David Center for Pain and Palliative Care; Sarkis & Siran Gabrellian Child Care and Learning Center; Healthy Futures; Institute for Child Development; Institute for Pediatric Cancer and Blood Disorders; JUDY Center for Down Syndrome; MOLLY Center for Children with Diabetes; SIDS Center of New Jersey; and the Steven and Richard Bader Immunological Institute.

- In 2002, HackensackUMC dedicated the world's first Audrey Hepburn Children's House, a state-designated Regional Diagnostic Center for Child Abuse and Neglect serving Bergen, Passaic, Hudson, Morris, Sussex and Warren counties.
- Our Pediatric Emergency Department is open 24 hours a day, seven days a week, and we provide care for children ranging in age from infancy through the age of 21 years.
- The Institute for Pediatric Cancer and Blood Disorders is home to the Blood and Marrow Transplant Program—the only stem cell transplant program in the state of New Jersey. The institute is also home to Cure and Beyond—the only comprehensive program dedication to childhood cancer survivors in the state.

For more information on any of the services offered at HackensackUMC, please call 551-996-5300, or visit HackensackUMC.org.

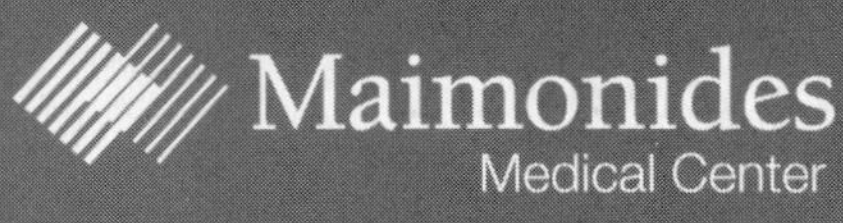

Maimonides Infants & Children's Hospital

4802 Tenth Avenue
Brooklyn, New York 11219
Phone: 718.283.7500 • Fax: 718.635.6149
www.maimonidesmed.org/pediatrics

The Maimonides Infants & Children's Hospital is a NACHRI-certified children's hospital-within-a-hospital. Offering over 30 sub-specialty divisions as well as primary care, the Pediatrics program is unrivaled in the region and serves one of the largest pediatric populations in the nation.

Danielle Laraque, MD, Vice President of the Maimonides Infants & Children's Hospital, leads a family-centered pediatrics program in a state-of-the-art medical environment, where babies, children and adolescents receive the best and most appropriate care. For most children, this involves preventing illness and promoting healthy growth. For those whose problems are more complicated, Maimonides specialists can treat every manner of childhood disorder, no matter how rare or complex. The level and quality of critical care provided is evidenced by the demand for the Maimonides Pediatric Transport Program, through which critically ill children from other hospitals are transferred to Maimonides.

In recognition of its excellence in obstetrics and pediatrics, Maimonides was designated a Regional Perinatal Center by the New York State Department of Health.

Pediatric specialties include:

- Allergy
- Behavioral & Developmental Pediatrics
- Cardiology
- Critical Care Medicine
- Dentistry & Dental Surgery
- Emergency Medicine
- Endocrinology
- Gastroenterology
- Genetics
- Hematology/Oncology
- Immunology
- Infectious Disease
- Neonatology
- Nephrology
- Neurology
- Ophthalmology
- Orthopedic Surgery
- Otolaryngology
- Psychiatry/Psychology
- Pulmonology
- Rheumatology
- Surgery
- Urology

Relying heavily on evidence-based medicine, Maimonides Medical Center has been commended for outstanding services by a number of independent rating organizations. Earlier this year, Maimonides was named a Distinguished Hospital for Clinical Excellence by HealthGrades – one of only three hospitals in the metropolitan area; the American Stroke Association bestowed its Gold Plus Achievement Award on the hospital; and the American Hospital Association once again named it a Most Wired hospital.

Maimonides Medical Center

The right care.
Right here.

www.maimonidesmed.org/pediatrics

Montefiore
Inspired Medicine

3415 Bainbridge Avenue
Bronx, New York 10467
718-741-2450
www.cham.org

Pediatric Services

The Children's Hospital at Montefiore (CHAM) brings leading pediatric specialists together with the latest technology and research to deliver exceptional care to children in the Bronx, Westchester and beyond. Included among CHAM's portfolio of nationally respected clinical programs are:

- The Pediatric Heart Center, a leader in the treatment of patients with both common and rare heart conditions. The Center performed five heart transplants in 2012, with one-year survival rates among the best in the country. It also excels in the use of mechanical assist devices as a bridge to transplant and in cardiac ablation procedures to treat patients with cardiac arrhythmias.
- The Ira Greifer Children's Kidney Center, which is at the forefront of pediatric nephrology, urology and transplant medicine. Eight renal transplants were performed in 2012 with a one-year survival rate of 100 percent.
- CHAM's Division of Gastroenterology and Nutrition, which expertly manages patients with both life-threatening and common gastrointestinal disorders. It is a leader in the care of short bowel syndrome, inflammatory bowel disease and liver disease. The Division boasts one-year liver transplant rates of 100 percent and recently performed its first living-donor transplant.
- The Division of Hematology and Oncology, which is responding to the needs of the community by offering the area's only comprehensive Sickle Cell Program. The Program provides the latest treatment advances and screening methods for sickle cell complications. This year, CHAM physicians marked a major milestone when they performed the Division's first pediatric bone marrow transplant to cure sickle cell anemia. The Division also delivers exceptional care for patients with leukemia, brain tumors, sarcoma, lymphoma and neuroblastoma.
- The Division of Orthopaedics, which is revolutionizing scoliosis treatment through an innovative combination of advanced imaging technologies, minimally invasive surgery and bloodless techniques. The Division's pioneering approach to these cases is reducing postoperative pain, hospital stays and recovery times.
- The Division of Neonatology, which excels in the care of both preterm and critically ill term neonates, achieving exceptional outcomes and shorter length of stays for extremely premature infants. It is the only designated regional perinatal center serving the Bronx.

This year, CHAM expanded both its programs and physical space, including its PICU, which grew to 26 beds. The newly formed Division of Pediatric Hospital Medicine covers 4,000 admissions a year.

CHAM's clinical services are rounded out by one of the finest and busiest pediatric emergency medicine programs in the nation, led by collaborative teams of pediatric general surgeons and subspecialty surgeons, including specialists in pediatric urology, ear/nose/throat, neurosurgery and ophthalmology. CHAM also has an acclaimed pediatric residency and fellowship training program.

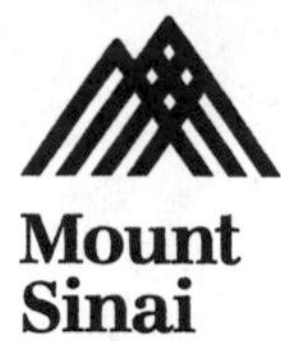

THE MOUNT SINAI MEDICAL CENTER

The Kravis Children's Hospital

One Gustave L. Levy Place
Fifth Avenue and 100th Street
New York, NY 10029-6574

Physician Referral: 1-800-MD-SINAI (637-4624)
www.kravischildrenshospital.org

The **KRAVIS CHILDREN'S HOSPITAL** at The Mount Sinai Medical Center offers the most advanced treatments and technologies available, supported by groundbreaking research, because the health and care of your child is our first priority.

This year the Kravis Children's Hospital saw significant gains in the *U.S. News & World Report* pediatric rankings, which placed it among the country's best children's hospitals in seven of the ten pediatric specialties, as noted in the 2013-2014 edition of the annual "Best Children's Hospitals" report. The seven specialties are: Diabetes and endocrinology (#25), gastroenterology & GI Surgery (#25), nephrology (#26), urology (#28), pulmonology (#36), cancer (#46) and cardiology & heart surgery (#50). Previously, we were ranked in six specialties. The rankings reflect not only double-digit gains within specialties, but also first-time rankings in two new areas GI Surgery and Heart Surgery placing these specialties among the best pediatric programs in the United States.

In all of our services, including 31 subspecialty areas of care, we offer advanced treatments, supported by research, community outreach, and advocacy programs. Our ongoing efforts to recruit the finest physicians and scientists have resulted in our ability to provide fundamental insights into the causes of childhood diseases and to deliver breakthrough treatments.

We have opened a new Pediatric Intensive Care unite (PICU), a 15-bed unit that weds state-of-the-art medical technology with a family-friendly facility for our most critically ill children. Construction is underway on a new 46-bed Neonatal Intensive Care Unit (NICU).

THE ZONE SPACE AT KRAVIS

An especially unique feature of the Kravis Children's Hospital at Mount Sinai is the Zone – a 3,000 square foot state-of-the-art therapeutic and educational play environment for pediatric patients and their families. **The Zone space at Kravis is the only one of its kind in the northeast region of the United States.**

The area is staffed by the Child Life and Creative Arts Therapy Department, a full-time pediatric medical librarian, and numerous consultants and volunteers who share their talents in art, music, cooking, knitting and more. The facility includes a lounge, theatre, family resource center, teen area, full kitchen and performing space. **The Zone features KidsZone TV (KZTV), the first live, interactive broadcast studio in a children's hospital.** The space is also used as a pediatric television programming training site for hospitals across the county and abroad.

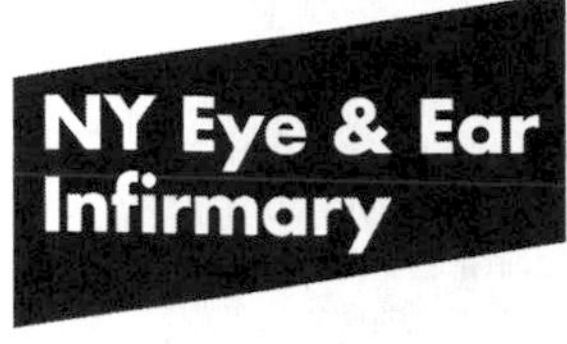

THE NEW YORK EYE AND EAR INFIRMARY

310 East 14th Street
New York, New York 10003
Tel. 212.979.4000 Fax. 212.228.0664
http://www.nyee.edu

PROVIDING EXCEPTIONAL PEDIATRIC SPECIALTY CARE

Pediatric Ophthalmology / Orthoptics: The New York Eye and Ear Infirmary Department of Pediatric Ophthalmology, Adult Strabismus and Orthoptics has a long tradition of being at the forefront of care for children with a wide range of eye and vision disorders and for patients of any age with ocular motility problems. The department offers the full spectrum of therapeutic options including surgery, glasses, prisms, eye patches, medications, and exercises.

Amblyopia (lazy eye) occurs when one or both eyes do not receive normal visual input or the two eyes are not working together and there is competition between the eyes. Treatment may involve glasses, patching, and/or eye drops. Surgery may also be necessary if there is strabismus (ocular misalignment) or an associated structural abnormality such as cataract (a cloudy lens), ptosis (a droopy eyelid), or cloudy cornea.

The Pediatric Ophthalmology department has extensive experience in treating patients with less common conditions such as congenital or developmental cataracts, congenital or developmental glaucoma, pediatric corneal problems, other congenital anomalies of the eyes, developmental anomalies of the visual system, retinopathy of prematurity, ocular infections, tumors and trauma.

Pediatric Otolaryngology: In one of the select specialized hospitals for medical/surgical care of the ears, nose, throat and related structures, medical staff see a great number of routine pediatric problems involving infections of the ears, tonsils and sinuses, in addition to complex and rare conditions such as profound hearing loss, cleft palate, neck masses, vascular anomalies and hemangiomas, and airway disorders.

The hospital also provides superb services in pediatric audiology, speech and language pathology, sleep disorders center, and a pediatric accredited radiology facility.

NYEE's Ear Institute is one of the premiere facilities for diagnostic and therapeutic services for children, teens and adults suffering from hearing loss and congenital defects and conditions related to the ear.

The Institute is a pioneer in cochlear implants, which allow patients, some as young as six months of age, to hear through electrical signals delivered to the auditory nerve. It performs more than 100 implants a year, a large volume for this highly specialized surgery, making it one of the nation's leading providers for cochlear implants. The Ear Institute is distinguished from other hearing centers by its Educator Liaison and Auditory Hearing Habilitation Programs dedicated to assisting children with cochlear implants and/or hearing aids to succeed in school.

Services to Children & Families

The New York Eye and Ear Infirmary is an international leader in restoring the gifts of sight and sound to children. Children comprise more than twenty-five percent of NYEE patients across all specialties. The need for specialized pediatric care continues to rise, as studies prove that early intervention leads to optimal quality of life. NYEE physicians care for children in need of reconstructive surgery to correct congenital defects, or suffering from a comprehensive array of eye, ear, nose and throat disorders, diseases and conditions. NYEE is the best place in the area to get several ophthalmologic subspecialists together to treat children with complex eye disorders and it is a pioneer in cochlear implantations to reverse deafness in infants as young as five months.

Every patient and family receives a thorough evaluation and medical and surgical options are discussed. At the core of every recommendation is a family-centered philosophy with the conviction that physicians and families are partners in making the correct decision to meet each child's needs.

Physician Referral
1.800.449.HOPE (4673)

NewYork-Presbyterian

Affiliated with Columbia University College of Physicians and Surgeons and Weill Cornell Medical College

NewYork-Presbyterian
Morgan Stanley Children's Hospital
Columbia University Medical Center
3959 Broadway
New York, NY 10032

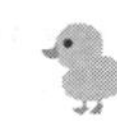

NewYork-Presbyterian
Phyllis and David Komansky
Center for Children's Health
Weill Cornell Medical Center
525 East 68th Street
New York, NY 10065

1-800-245-KIDS (1-800-245-5437) www.nyp.org/kids

Accreditation: The Joint Commission

Overview

The pediatric services of NewYork-Presbyterian Hospital are comprised of NewYork-Presbyterian Morgan Stanley Children's Hospital, which is affiliated with Columbia University College of Physicians and Surgeons, and the NewYork-Presbyterian Phyllis and David Komansky Center for Children's Health, which is affiliated with Weill Cornell Medical College. Together, they serve as one of the nation's premier centers for comprehensive pediatric care. Skilled and experienced physicians, surgeons, nurses and other pediatric healthcare professionals manage some of the most complex medical conditions of children at every stage of development. Their expertise includes general pediatric care and the full range of medical and surgical subspecialties:

- Adolescent Medicine
- Allergy and Immunology
- Anesthesiology
- Blood Disorders
- Blood and Marrow Transplantation
- Cancer
- Cardiology and Cardiac Surgery
- Craniofacial and Plastic Surgery
- Critical Care
- Dermatology
- Digestive Disease
- Ear, Nose and Throat
- Emergency Department, including specialized units for burns and trauma injuries
- Endocrinology, Diabetes and Metabolism
- Epilepsy
- Genetics
- Infectious Diseases
- Kidney Disease
- Liver Disease
- Lung Disease
- Neonatal Medicine
- Neurology and Neurological Surgery
- Nutrition
- Obesity and Bariatric Surgery
- Ophthalmology
- Oral and Maxillofacial Surgery and Pediatric Dentistry
- Organ Transplantation
- Orthopaedic Surgery
- Pain Medicine
- Pediatric Surgery
- Pregnancy and Newborn Services
- Primary Care/General Pediatrics
- Psychiatry
- Radiology
- Rheumatology
- Urology

Highlights at a Glance:

- A national leader in pediatric open-heart surgery with one of the largest pediatric heart transplant programs in the nation.
- A pediatric kidney transplant program, which includes a Living Donor Program and leading edge therapies to help reduce the side effects of anti-rejection drugs.
- Pediatric cardiac surgeons at the forefront of ventricular assist devices for infants and small children as a bridge to recovery or transplantation.
- One of three Level 1-designated Regional Pediatric Trauma Centers in New York State and the only one in New York City.
- A New York State Department of Health-designated Regional Perinatal Center of Expertise for the care of women with high-risk pregnancies.
- One of the largest Type 1 diabetes programs in New York State.
- Outstanding neonatal intensive care programs setting standards of care nationwide for extremely ill newborns.
- The only program in the New York tri-state area that has active programs in both liver and small bowel transplantation.

North Shore LIJ
Steven & Alexandra
Cohen Children's Medical
Center of New York

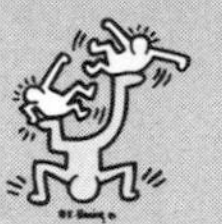

269-01 76th Avenue
New Hyde Park, NY 11040
(516) 734-8300
cohenchildrens.com

Cohen Children's Medical Center

Steven and Alexandra Cohen Children's Medical Center of New York is the largest provider of pediatric health services in New York State, serving children in Brooklyn and Queens, Nassau and Suffolk counties.

Cohen Children's Medical Center, located on Long Island, is a full-service children's hospital dedicated to providing the highest levels of care to children, from newborns to adolescents. Our expert pediatric specialists screen, diagnose and treat a wide variety of injuries and illnesses.

For the seventh year in a row, *U.S. News & World Report* has recognized Cohen Children's Medical Center for superior pediatric care. This year's acknowledgement is for seven different specialties: neonatalogy; gastroenterology and GI surgery; diabetes and endocrinology; urology; orthopaedics; neurosurgery and neurology; and nephrology.

Child-Friendly and Family-Centered Care

Cohen Children's is designed exclusively for children and their families. Caring for children includes providing them with a warm, comforting, homelike setting. That's why every aspect of our spacious open building is child oriented — from the fold-out beds for parents to the fully staffed playrooms on each floor. Our caregivers are dedicated to providing the most skilled treatment for all your child's healthcare needs. Our goal is to help children feel comfortable, safe and stress-free.

At Cohen Children's, family-centered care is an essential part of each child's experience. Our collaborative approach to healthcare involves patients, families and healthcare professionals forming a partnership that benefits everyone.

A Growing Network of Care

State-of-the-art care for children's medical, surgical, psychiatric and dental needs are provided in both inpatient and outpatient settings. Outpatient services are available at our main campus in New Hyde Park and at regional consultation centers in Commack, Hewlett, Bensonhurst, Williamsburg and Flushing.

Our Services Include:

- Adolescent Medicine
- Allergy/Immunology
- Asthma
- Cancer
- Cardiology/Cardiac Surgery
- Craniofacial and Cleft Palate
- Critical Care
- Cystic Fibrosis
- Developmental/ Behavioral Pediatrics
- Emergency Medicine
- Endocrinology/Diabetes
- Epilepsy
- Gastroenterology
- Infectious Diseases
- Neonatology
- Nephrology (Kidney Disease)
- Neurology/Neurosurgery
- Nutritional Disorders
- Ophthalmology
- Orthopaedics
- Otolaryngology (ENT)
- Pediatric/Adolescent Gynecology
- Pediatric Dental Services
- Pulmonology (Lung Disease)
- Rheumatology
- Sleep Study Center
- Surgery
- Trauma
- Urgent Care
- Urology

To find a doctor: **1-888-321-DOCS** or **northshorelij.com**

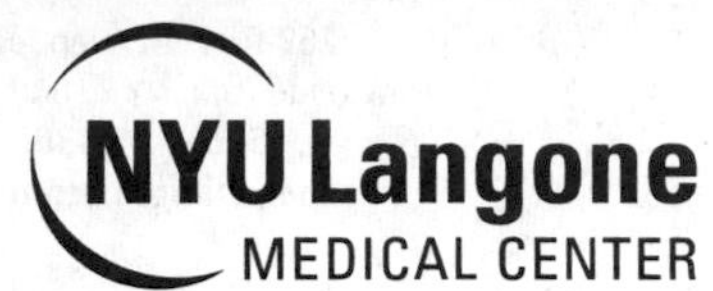

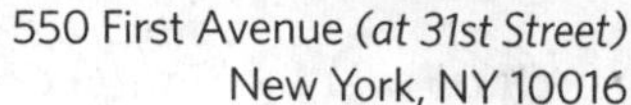

550 First Avenue *(at 31st Street)*
New York, NY 10016

www.NYULMC.org

Hassenfeld Children's Hospital Access Line: **855-NYU-KIDS**

HASSENFELD CHILDREN'S HOSPITAL

Hassenfeld Children's Hospital (HCH) is a full-service specialty children's hospital encompassing all children's health services at NYU Langone Medical Center. At HCH, newborns, children, adolescents and young adults receive the most comprehensive and advanced care possible from a team of pediatricians and pediatric specialists across more than 30 medical and surgical disciplines. With more than 150 full-time pediatric specialists, as well as pediatric nurses, child life specialists and social workers, Hassenfeld Children's Hospital is uniquely equipped to provide innovative pediatric subspecialty care in a highly personalized manner.

A Family-Centered Approach

Integral to the care we provide is a myriad of support services for children and their families. We recognize that the best outcomes are achieved when the child's family is actively involved in every step of care. For that reason, our trained specialists address the needs of not just the patient, but of parents and siblings through ongoing education and communication.

Our pediatric specialties include:

Anesthesia
Cardiology
Cardiothoracic Surgery
Child and Adolescent Psychiatry and Psychology/Child Study Center
Critical Care
Dermatology
Developmental and Behavioral Pediatrics
Emergency Medicine
Endocrinology
Epilepsy
Gastroenterology
Genetics
Hematology/Oncology
Infectious Diseases
Neonatology
Nephrology
Neurosurgery
Ophthalmology
Orthopaedic Surgery
Otolaryngology
Pathology
Pulmonology
Radiology
Reconstructive Plastic Surgery
Rehabilitation
Rheumatology
Surgery
Urology

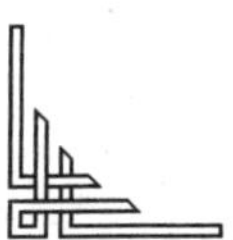

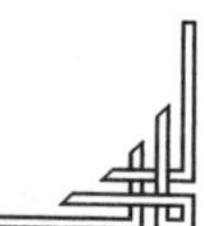

Physical Medicine & Rehabilitation

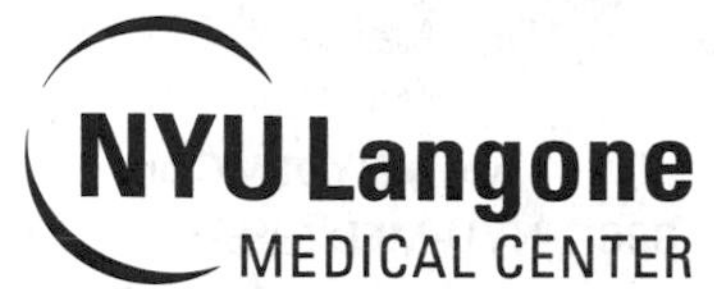

550 First Avenue *(at 31st Street)*
New York, NY 10016
www.NYULMC.org/rusk
Physician Referral: **888-7-NYU-MED** *(888-769-8633)*

RUSK REHABILITATION

Rusk Rehabilitation at NYU Langone Medical Center (Rusk) has been ranked the best rehabilitation program in New York State and among the top ten in the country by *U.S. News & World Report* since 1989. Rusk is internationally renowned for the treatment of adults and children with injuries and disabilities, offering the full continuum of inpatient and outpatient care—physical, occupational, speech/swallowing and vocational therapy, psychology, music and recreational therapy, nutrition, nursing, and social work—for a wide range of conditions. Specialty programs and services include:

The **CARF-Accredited Brain Injury Rehabilitation Program** is tailored for patients who have medical, physical, cognitive, and behavioral changes as a result of a brain injury or neurological illness.

The **CARF-Accredited Stroke Program** offers an interdisciplinary team with specialized training in the medical, nursing or therapeutic care and treatment of stroke patients.

The Concussion Center is a collaborative effort between Rusk Rehabilitation and the Departments of Orthopaedic Surgery and Neurology, providing expert, multidisciplinary evaluation and treatment of individuals who have or are suspected of having a concussion.

Our **Amputee Program** provides specialized limb loss rehabilitation to patients who have undergone amputations.

The Joan and Joel Smilow Cardiac and Pulmonary Rehabilitation & Prevention Center offers a model of transitional care for patients with cardiac and lung conditions.

Orthopaedic/Musculoskeletal Rehabilitation is offered for patients with back, neck, hip, elbow and shoulder disorders, arthritis-related joint pain, conditions affecting the bones, tendon, ligaments and muscles, and for pre- and post-surgical patients.

Sports Injury Rehabilitation addresses the needs of patients with sports-related conditions, including post-operative rehabilitation for patients who require orthopaedic surgery.

Our **Spinal Cord Injury** program offers a comprehensive, patient-centered array of specialized and innovative clinical and educational programs to optimize quality of life.

(continued)

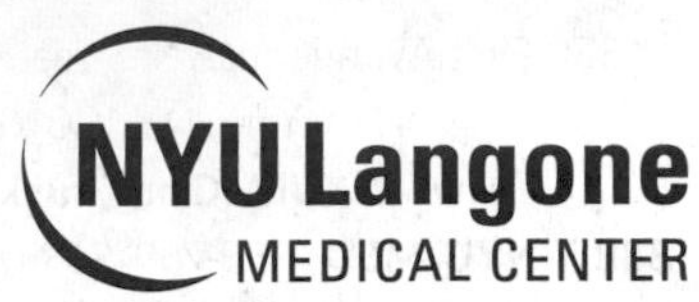

550 First Avenue *(at 31st Street)*
New York, NY 10016
www.NYULMC.org/rusk
Physician Referral: **888-7-NYU-MED** *(888-769-8633)*

RUSK REHABILITATION *(continued)*

The Women's Health Rehab Program addresses issues that uniquely affect women, including pelvic floor muscle dysfunction/pain, urinary incontinence, cancer rehabilitation and lymphedema, and prenatal and postpartum musculoskeletal conditions.

Vestibular Rehabilitation addresses the evaluation and treatment of patients suffering from dizziness and imbalance.

Chest Physical Therapy cares for individuals with lung congestion, secretion retention or areas of lung collapse.

Rehabilitation Psychology provides care to patients with neurological and medical conditions.

Speech-Language Pathology & Swallowing is dedicated to patients with communication disorders due to neurological problems as well as diagnosis and management of swallowing and feeding disorders.

Vocational Services provides disabled individuals with the competencies needed to return to school or work and to lead a productive life.

Patient Care Locations

Our physicians and therapists provide care at multiple NYU Langone locations, including:

- **The Center for Musculoskeletal Care**, NYU Langone's premier, state-of-the-art, multidisciplinary bone and joint facility
- NYU Langone's newly opened, outpatient **Ambulatory Care Center**
- The internationally-renowned, inpatient **Hospital for Joint Diseases**
- **The NYU Langone main campus** on First Avenue
- **The Joan H. Tisch Center for Women's Health**, on the Upper East Side of Manhattan
- Multiple locations in **NYU Langone's growing network of community practices** in the metro New York area

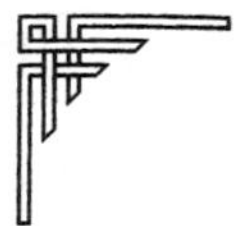

The Best in American Medicine
www.CastleConnolly.com

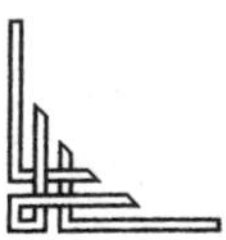

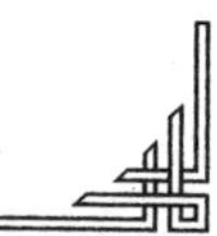

Plastic Surgery

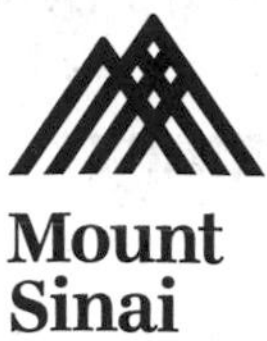

THE MOUNT SINAI MEDICAL CENTER

Plastic and Reconstructive Surgery

One Gustave L. Levy Place
Fifth Avenue and 100th Street
New York, NY 10029-6574

Physician Referral: 1-800-MD-SINAI (637-4624)
www.mountsinai.org

The Mount Sinai Medical Center's **DIVISION OF PLASTIC AND RECONSTRUCTIVE SURGERY** delivers superior, patient-centered care using the safest, most effective procedures available to treat the full spectrum of plastic and reconstructive surgical conditions.

Working together with physicians from other specialties to provide the most comprehensive care, our surgeons excel at correcting abnormalities caused by illness, accidents, and deformities that have been present from birth. Each of our surgeons is certified by the American Board of Plastic Surgery, and all have made significant contributions toward the division's reputation for producing excellent outcomes.

Our Services:

- **Aesthetic (Cosmetic) Surgery**: Abdominoplasty (tummy tuck), blepharoplasty (eyelid reshaping), brachioplasty (arm lift), breast augmentation, face contour, face lift, forehead and brow lift, injectables and fillers, liposuction, rhinoplasty, and skin resurfacing

- **Breast Surgery**: Breast augmentation, breast lift, breast reduction and breast reconstruction

- **Hand Surgery**: Carpal tunnel release, fracture repair, trigger finger release, congenital deformity repair, ganglion and tumor removal, joint replacement, nerve repair, tendon repair, and replantation

- **Reconstructive Surgery/Microsurgery**: Abdominal wall reconstruction, breast reconstruction, body contouring after weight loss surgery, chest wall reconstruction, extremity reconstruction, flap reconstruction, free TRAM (Transverse Rectus Abdominis Muscle) flap, general reconstruction, head and neck reconstruction, perforator TRAM Flap/DIEP (Deep Inferior Epigastric Perforator) flap, Latissimus Dorsi (LD) Myocutaneous Flap, SGAP (Superior Gluteral Artery Pertorator) Flaps, IGAP (In-the-crease-gluteral artery perforator) flap, skin expansion, and microsurgery

- **Vascular Anomalies**: Hemangiomas and vascular malformations

- **Wound Care**

In addition to providing the best surgical care, our surgeons are dedicated to pursuing research and innovation. It is our long-standing mission to discover new ways of approaching plastic surgical problems that will further benefit our patients.

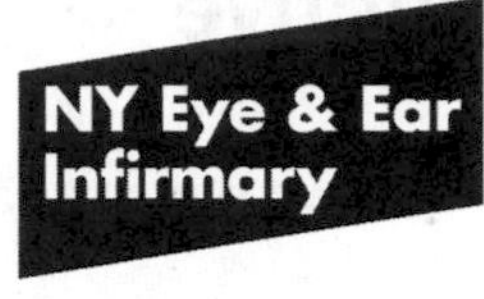

THE NEW YORK EYE AND EAR INFIRMARY

310 East 14th Street
New York, New York 10003
Tel. 212.979.4000 Fax. 212.228.0664
http://www.nyee.edu

PROVIDING EXCEPTIONAL CARE

The Department of Plastic & Reconstructive Surgery is one of the region's most comprehensive centers for surgery which restores the body and spirit. More than 1,500 procedures a year are performed here, and 50 of the most noted board-certified plastic surgeons located throughout New York City and tri-state area comprise the attending medical staff.

IN A HIGHLY SPECIALIZED SETTING

As a specialty hospital, the Infirmary is uniquely qualified to handle the most complicated cases. It serves as a nationwide referral center with a commitment to teaching, research, and high-technology based patient care. Highly experienced staff using state-of-the-art instrumentation have made the Infirmary's 19 operating rooms a national benchmark in efficiency. In addition, private premium patient accommodations are available to assure that the hospital experience is as comfortable and convenient as possible.

FOR PATIENTS OF ALL AGES

The Department treats more than 1,500 patients a year who seek reconstructive surgery of the body as well as facial area as a result of accident, birth defect or cancer, and those who elect cosmetic surgery. It is one of the few hospitals in the region to perform breast reconstruction after mastectomy with microvascular surgery to harvest tissue from patients' lower body to create living, natural, and normal looking breasts, often preferred to artificial implants. State-of-the-art lymph node transfer to cure post-mastectomy lymphedema is also available.

Childhood problems, such as cleft lip and palate and ear deformities also fall under the care of our surgeons.

Innovative cosmetic surgery procedures such as endoscopic and other minimally invasive operations are offered. The Center for Nasal Plastic specializes in closed (no scar) nasal plastic techniques as well as repair of previous nasal surgeries, the secondary nasal plasty. Liposuction using the latest instrumentation and fat grafting by the latest technology is also available as are the latest variants of the abdominoplasty (tummy tuck) operation.

The latest version of a skin tightening Fraxel Re:pair laser enables many patients to avoid a surgical face and eyelid plastic operation.

The hospital has a Post Graduate Cosmetic Surgery Program which offers a year of intensive cosmetic surgery training to surgeons who have completed a formal plastic surgery residency. The program is the largest and most sought-after in the US and also provides a source for affordable cosmetic surgery for the community.

Plastic Surgery Clinical Services

Facial plasty

Eyelid plastic operations

Nasal plastic operations

Breast augmentation
Breast reduction procedures and suspension

Breast reconstruction using patient's own tissue (DIEP, S-GAP, I-GAP and SIEA flap procedures)

Liposuction

Abdominoplasty

Facial resurfacing and dermabrasion

Fraxel laser

Botox

About The New York Eye and Ear Infirmary

Founded in 1820, it is the nation's oldest, continuously operating specialty hospital. Throughout its history, The New York Eye and Ear Infirmary has led clinical advances and research in vision, hearing, speech and restoration of the physical appearance.

Physician Referral
1.800.449.HOPE (4673)

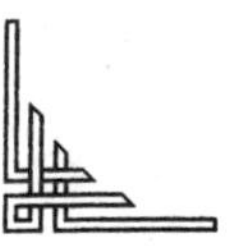
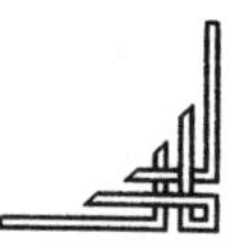

The Best in American Medicine
www.CastleConnolly.com

Preventive Medicine

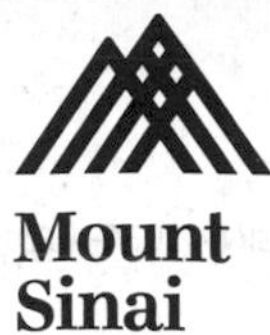

THE MOUNT SINAI MEDICAL CENTER
Preventive Medicine

One Gustave L. Levy Place
Fifth Avenue and 100th Street
New York, NY 10029-6574

Physician Referral: 1-800-MD-SINAI (637-4624)
www.mountsinai.org

Mount Sinai's **DEPARTMENT OF PREVENTIVE MEDICINE** is internationally renowned for excellence in preventive medicine, occupational medicine, and environmental health, community health, and environmental pediatrics. The department is among the largest medical school departments of its kind in the United States. Our mission is to prevent disease, protect the environment, and promote health throughout the communities we serve.

Interdisciplinary research
The Department of Preventive Medicine undertakes interdisciplinary research in:

- Preventive medicine
- Public health
- Epidemiology
- Environmental and occupational medicine
- Social sciences

The department has 7 divisions:

- Behavioral Science and Social Work
- Biostatistics and Data Management
- Environmental Health
- Epidemiology
- International Health
- Occupational Medicine
- Mount Sinai Selikoff Centers for Occupational Health
- Preventive Medicine Residency

Under the direction of Chairman Philip J. Landrigan, MD, the department has strengthened its research base, training programs, and clinical services in environmental, occupational, and preventive medicine, by:

- Being the principal architect of New York's statewide network of Clinical Centers of Excellence in Occupational Medicine – the nation's only state-based network of occupational health clinics.
- Overseeing the creation of the Mount Sinai Irving J. Selikoff Centers for Occupational Health, providing the services of specialized physicians and other health and social service professionals to workers, labor and community organizations, employers and agencies.
- Guiding the development of Mount Sinai's World Trade Center Health Program, established to care for the men and women who responded to the 9/11 attacks and continuing to treat mental and health conditions related to their WTC service.
- Leading development of the Mount Sinai Children's Environmental Health Center to protect children from environmental threats through research, education, and clinical care.

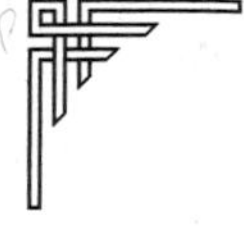

The Best in American Medicine
www.CastleConnolly.com

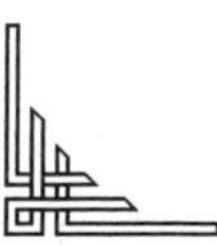
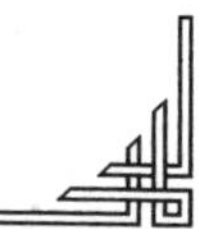

Psychiatry

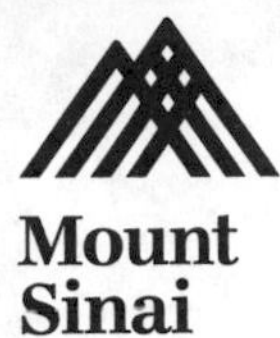

THE MOUNT SINAI MEDICAL CENTER

Psychiatry

One Gustave L. Levy Place
Fifth Avenue and 100th Street
New York, NY 10029-6574

Physician Referral: 1-800-MD-SINAI (637-4624)
www.mountsinai.org

THE DEPARTMENT OF PSYCHIATRY at Mount Sinai strives to bring breakthrough discoveries from neuroscience research to clinical care today. We provide services for children, adolescents, adults, and seniors, offering mental health evaluation and treatment for autism, attention-deficit hyperactivity disorder (ADHD), behavioral disorders, schizophrenia, Alzheimer's disease, mood and anxiety disorders, obsessive-compulsive disorder (OCD), tics and Tourette's Disorder (TD), substance abuse, post-traumatic stress disorder (PTSD), eating disorders, and personality disorders.

Clinical Services – The Department of Psychiatry is organized around key Centers of Excellence that integrate our three missions of clinical care, education and research. We offer a full range of diagnostic and treatment services, including psychotherapy, psychopharmacology, emergency services, electroconvulsive therapy, neuropsychological testing, and management of difficult clinical cases. We also provide mental health services in the Mount Sinai's World Trade Center Medical Monitoring and Treatment Program.

Specialty Programs – The Seaver Autism Center of Excellence offers a comprehensive assessment and treatment program that provides the finest patient care informed by the latest research. Our expert clinical staff is experienced in autism spectrum disorders, specializing in personalized and evidence-based treatment for very young children and high-functioning adults, as well as those individuals considered most difficult to assess and treat. The ADHD Center serves children and adults providing state-of-the-art psychiatric evaluation, psychological testing, behavioral and cognitive-behavioral treatments, and medication management. Our Center for Eating and Weight Disorders serves adults and children, offering innovative and evidence-based treatment for anorexia nervosa, bulimia nervosa, binge eating disorder, and obesity.

TRANSLATING KNOWLEDGE INTO NEW SOLUTIONS

Mount Sinai is at the forefront of unlocking the interactions between biological processes and the myriad states of the human mind. Among our major research programs in psychiatry are the Alzheimer's Disease Research Center, which conducts both basic science and clinical research, and The Seaver Autism Center for Research and Treatment, which is dedicated to unraveling the biological causes of this disorder and to developing innovative treatment strategies. In shedding important new light on mental illness, psychiatrists at Mount Sinai are frequently able to offer experimental interventions for treatment-resistant cases of depression, OCD, and other disorders.

The Mood and Anxiety Disorders Program (MAP) is devoted to understanding the causes of mood and anxiety disorders and aims to advance the latest integrative treatment strategies for patients who suffer from major depression, bipolar disorder, PTSD, panic attacks, generalized anxiety disorder, and social phobia. MAP at Mount Sinai uses state-of-the-art brain imaging, and genetic, and clinical trials methods to enhance our understanding of brain processes associated with these disorders.

The OCD and Tourette's Center of Excellence provides state-of-the-art diagnostic evaluation for children, adolescents and adults with OCD, tics and related disorders. The Center offers comprehensive evaluations, expert consultations, outpatient services, novel and evidence-based treatments, and research studies. We specialize in both behavioral therapy and biological interventions for patients who have not responded to conventional therapies. For adult patients with severe and intractable OCD, we offer Deep Brain Stimulation (DBS).

The Best in American Medicine
www.CastleConnolly.com

Pulmonary Disease

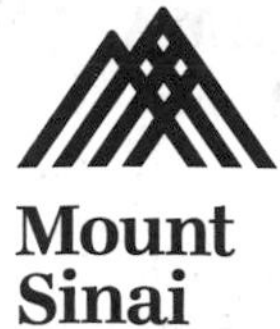

THE MOUNT SINAI MEDICAL CENTER
Pulmonary Medicine

One Gustave L. Levy Place
Fifth Avenue and 100th Street
New York, NY 10029-6574

Physician Referral: 1-800-MD-SINAI (637-4624)
www.mountsinai.org

The mission of Mount Sinai's **DIVISION OF PULMONARY, CRITICAL CARE, AND SLEEP MEDICINE** is to offer state-of-the-art clinical care to patients with all forms of lung disease and critical illness, cutting-edge research that will translate into improved patient care and outcomes, and hands-on training of future leaders in the field.

To achieve this goal, every faculty member is charged with the success of a specific program. Mount Sinai's Pulmonary Division has a long history of providing specialized care and key research in several disease areas that include sarcoidosis and occupational lung diseases. Mount Sinai's Sarcoidosis Service, the largest of its kind in the world, is a Center of Excellence for sarcoidosis research. It is the only site in the United States that performs the diagnostic Kveim-Siltzbach skin test for sarcoidosis, which eliminates the need for more invasive, uncomfortable, and expensive procedures. Through its Pulmonary Physiology Laboratory, Mount Sinai has been instrumental in establishing normal values for various pulmonary function tests and is currently conducting clinical studies of new tests for obesity, sarcoidosis, asthma, and lung cancer.

Pulmonary specialists at Mount Sinai are investigating asthma and emphysema, lung cancer, collagen vascular diseases, pulmonary infections, and occupational lung diseases. Mount Sinai has the largest screening program for workers and anyone in the general population exposed to polluted air at the World Trade Center catastrophe site. Our critical care physicians are experts in treating liver disease and acute and chronic respiratory failure, using the most modern forms of delivery of intensive care and providing compassionate end-of-life care.

The Asthma Program uses a multidisciplinary team approach, focusing on patient education and skill-building to foster self-management.

The Chronic Obstructive Pulmonary Disease Program offers screening, routine state-of-the-art imaging testing, and a coordinated approach of exercise, treatment, and education that improves symptoms and quality of life, for one of the nation's most underdiagnosed conditions.

The Critical Care Medicine Program features state-of-the-art medical intensive care and respiratory care units.

The Interventional Pulmonary Service performs cutting-edge diagnostic and therapeutic procedures for patients with advanced pulmonary diseases.

The Lung Cancer/Thoracic Oncology Service provides specialized care for lung cancer diagnosis and staging and for coordinating multidisciplinary medical care for lung cancer. This is provided as a joint effort with Thoracic Surgery, Radiation Oncology and Medical Oncology.

The Occupational Lung Disorders Program specializes in the diagnosis and management of occupational lung disorders, such as occupational asthma and bronchitis, asbestosis, silicosis, and heavy metal lung injury.

The Pulmonary Fibrosis/Interstitial Lung Disease Program treats patients with chronic inflammatory and scarring disorders of the lungs, including idiopathic pulmonary fibrosis and collagen vascular-associated pulmonary diseases.

The Pulmonary Physiology Laboratory performs the full range of physiological lung function and cardiopulmonary exercise testing for lung disease.

The Pulmonary Rehabilitation Program provides occupational, physical, and cardiopulmonary rehabilitation programs for patients with disabling lung disorders, as well as pre- and post- operative consultation and therapy.

The Sarcoidosis Service, which has passed its 20,000 enrollee count, offers standard care as well as the opportunity to participate in new clinical trials to 60 new enrollees per week.

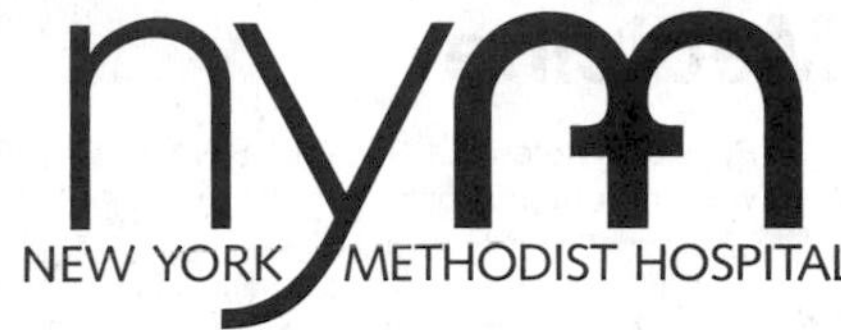

THE INSTITUTE FOR ASTHMA AND OTHER LUNG DISEASES

New York Methodist Hospital
506 Sixth Street, Brooklyn, N.Y. 11215
Phone: 866 ASK-LUNG (866 275-5864)
http://www.nym.org

SPECIALISTS AND MEDICAL SERVICES

The Institute for Asthma and Other Lung Diseases brings together a unique group of specialists and medical services to offer comprehensive diagnosis and treatment of a broad range of lung conditions. The Institute's panel of physician specialists includes both pediatric and adult pulmonologists and allergists. A larger constellation of physicians—medical oncologists, radiologists, radiation oncologists and surgeons—is available as needed. For diagnostic purposes, state-of-the-art specialty facilities—including the interventional bronchoscopy suite, the pulmonary function laboratory, the Pulmonary Hypertension Center and the Sleep Disorders Center—are conveniently located on the Hospital campus. These facilities are used to diagnose and treat a variety of lung disorders and are staffed by registered respiratory therapists, board-certified pulmonary function technologists and exercise physiologists.

PROGRAMS OFFERED

In addition to the treatment of pediatric and adult asthma, physicians affiliated with the Institute diagnose and care for patients with chronic obstructive lung disease (COPD), interstitial lung disease, infectious lung disease, pulmonary hypertension and lung cancer. Highly sophisticated interventional pulmonary services and advanced thoracic surgery procedures are performed at the Hospital, which is a Center of Excellence Epicenter for Robotic Thoracic Surgery.

***

Referrals to the Institute, its programs and physicians can be made through an individual's primary care physician or requested directly through the Institute's telephone referral service. More information (and on-line physician referral) is available at the Hospital's website, http://www.nym.org.

COMPREHENSIVE LUNG CANCER CENTER

New York Methodist Hospital's Comprehensive Lung Cancer Center coordinates and consolidates all services related to the treatment of lung cancer. One of the advantages NYM offers patients is a range of minimally invasive screening, diagnostic and treatment techniques, including a Lung Cancer Screening Program that uses low dose computed tomography.

Treatment options include surgery (both robotic and traditional), radiation and medical oncology, but even patients who are not eligible for surgery, radiation or chemotherapy may benefit from specialized interventional pulmonology treatments.

The Best in American Medicine
www.CastleConnolly.com

Radiation Oncology

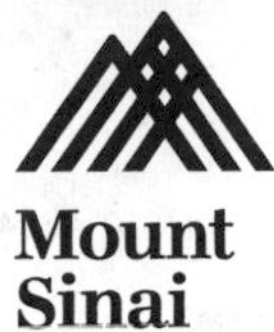

THE MOUNT SINAI MEDICAL CENTER

Radiology

One Gustave L. Levy Place
Fifth Avenue and 100th Street
New York, NY 10029-6574

Physician Referral: 1-800-MD-SINAI (637-4624)
www.mountsinai.org

The **DEPARTMENT OF RADIOLOGY** at Mount Sinai offers patients one of the world's most comprehensive and sophisticated arrays of diagnostic and interventional radiology services. The department uses filmless digital technology that spans high field magnetic resonance imaging (MRI), multi-slice computed tomography (CT), positron emission tomography CT (PET-CT), PET-MRI, single photon emission computed tomography CT (SPECT-CT), advanced ultrasound, conventional radiography, angiography, digital mammography, and state-of-the-art Picture Archiving Communication System (PACS) technology.

Comprehensive Diagnostic Services – Mount Sinai provides the entire range of diagnostic radiology services in a patient-friendly environment. Its nationally renowned radiologic physicians specialize in every area of disease diagnosis, as well as disease prevention and innovative therapeutic approaches. The combination of state-of-the-art imaging equipment with the finest imaging physicians makes Mount Sinai Radiology the place to go for all your imaging needs.

Early Detection Programs – We are committed to special screening approaches for early disease detection. We provide radiological screenings for colon, breast, and lung cancer and atherosclerosis. The early detection programs use a variety of imaging techniques, such as CT and MRI for atherosclerosis, CT for lung and colon cancer, PET for oncology, digital and 3D mammography, MRI, Ultrasound, and computer-aided diagnosis for breast cancer.

Minimally Invasive Procedures – Radiology at Mount Sinai has moved beyond diagnosis to the most sophisticated therapeutic interventions. Interventional radiologists at Mount Sinai perform biopsies, vascular therapies, and uterine artery embolization for fibroids-an alternative to hysterectomy-as well as treatments for aneurysms, atherosclerosis, and many types of cancer. In addition, advanced CT and MR angiography techniques are widely utilized to diagnose vascular diseases in a minimally invasive yet highly accurate manner.

DEVELOPING NEW DIAGNOSTIC TOOLS

Radiology at Mount Sinai is an active center of imaging research and development. Mount Sinai physicians and scientists developed a special form of MRI to diagnose heart disease and atherosclerosis noninvasively and thereby identify patients at greatest risk for stroke and heart attack. We actively collaborate with other disciplines to develop and refine imaging tools that will make prevention and diagnosis increasingly effective. That is the case, for example in neuroscience, where imaging innovations impact our understanding of neurodegenerative conditions, such as Parkinson's disease, multiple sclerosis, stroke, brain tumors, and various psychiatric disorders; cardiovascular disease, assess new therapies for aortic and cerebral artery aneurysms; lung and breast cancer screening; and liver disease, where radiologists, transplant surgeons, and hepatologists collaborate closely to develop optimal therapeutic strategies.

Oncology Imaging – Radiologists work closely with surgeons, oncologists, and other caregivers to optimize the diagnosis and treatment of patients with head and neck, liver, lung, breast, and gastrointestinal cancers. State-of-the-art CT, MRI, ultrasound, SPECT and PET CT are utilized to make the most accurate, least invasive and lowest dose diagnosis.

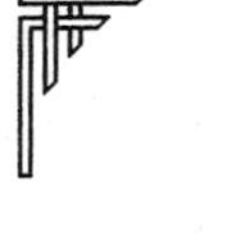

The Best in American Medicine
www.CastleConnolly.com

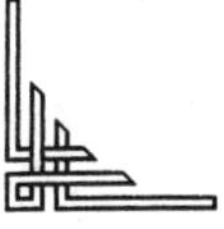
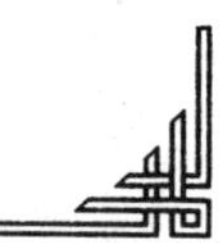

Rehabilitation Medicine

Reproductive Endocrinology

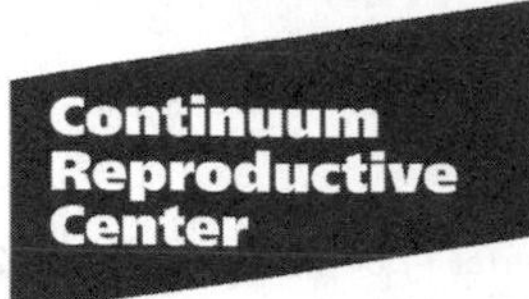

The Continuum Reproductive Center
212.523.7751

The Continuum Reproductive Center (CRC) is one of New York's leading providers of reproductive medicine and fertility care. Our physicians have expertise in many areas of reproductive care including the management of:

- Ovulation Disorders
- Polycystic Ovary Syndrome
- Fallopian Tube Disease
- Fibroid Tumors of the Uterus
- Unexplained Infertility
- Recurrent Pregnancy Loss
- Endometriosis and Pelvic Pain
- Benign Disorders of the Ovaries and Uterus
- Assisted Reproductive Technologies, such as In Vitro Fertilization (IVF)
- Male Factor Infertility

The physicians of the CRC are all double board-certified in both obstetrics and gynecology, and reproductive endocrinology and fertility. Our physicians are well-respected for their clinical and research contributions, have published in peer-review journals, and presented at national and international meetings.

In addition to our physicians, the staff at the CRC is comprised of nurses, medical assistants, and administrators who form an expert, cohesive and professional team with many years of experience in the care of fertility and reproductive endocrinology. Our laboratory is directed by a Ph.D. reproductive physiologist accredited by the American Association of Bioanalysts as a high-complexity laboratory director (HCLD). Our team of embryologists and andrologists possesses a wealth of specialized training and experience in the culture and manipulation of human sperm, eggs and embryos. The result is comprehensive and personalized care with excellent success rates.

We deliver care to patients in the tri-state area, with broader insurance coverage and lower out-of-pocket fees than available from most of our competitors. In addition to our main center in Manhattan, we have a Mount Kisco, NY, office. Please call 914.244.8749 for additional information.

The physicians of the Continuum Reproductive Center are affiliated with St. Luke's and Roosevelt Hospitals, an Academic Affiliate of the Columbia University College of Physicians and Surgeons.

Continuum Reproductive Centers
Manhattan: 425 West 59th Street
Mt. Kisco, NY: 83 South Bedford Road

www.ContinuumFertility.com

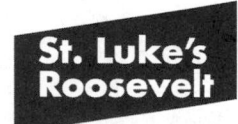

Continuum Health Partners, Inc.

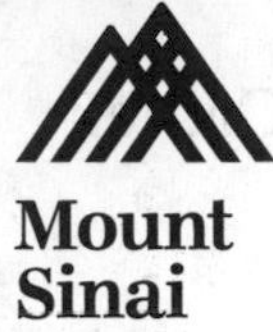

THE MOUNT SINAI MEDICAL CENTER

Reproductive Endocrinology and Infertility

One Gustave L. Levy Place
Fifth Avenue and 100th Street
New York, NY 10029-6574

Physician Referral: 1-800-MD-SINAI (637-4624)
www.mountsinai.org

REPRODUCTIVE ENDOCRINOLOGY AND INFERTILITY

The infertility program at Mount Sinai is based on an affiliation with the Reproductive Medicine Associates of New York, which offers the most advanced services in assisted reproductive technology (ART) to help infertile patients who may require such approaches to achieve a healthy baby. We work closely with each couple to develop treatment protocols using state-of-the-art techniques that are carefully individualized for them. These include:

- In Vitro Fertilization-Embryo Transfer (IVF-ET)
- Gamete intrafallopian transfer (GIFT)
- Embryo Cryopreservation
- Egg Donation
- Gestational Surrogacy
- Intracytoplasmic Sperm Injection (ICSI)
- Assisted Hatching (AH)

In order to determine the proper course of treatment for each couple, we may perform a number of diagnostic tests:

- Preconceptual Counseling
- Transvaginal Ultrasound
- Semen Analysis
- Hormonal Testing
- Endometrial Biopsy
- Post-coital Test
- Hysterosalpingogram
- Basal Body Temperature Charting

The clinical and scientific teams at Mount Sinai and Reproductive Medicine Associates of New York were among the first to help women conceive using previously frozen oocytes (eggs) from egg donors. Effectively, this could halt the biological clock as these eggs could be successfully preserved before egg quantity and quality undergo their natural age-related decline in function.

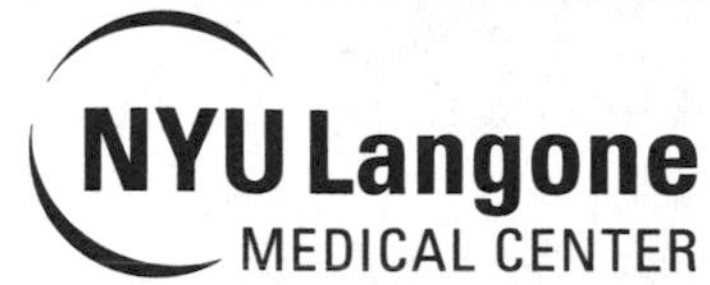

550 First Avenue *(at 31st Street)*
New York, NY 10016

www.NYULMC.org

Physician Referral: **888-7-NYU-MED** *(888-769-8633)*

OBSTETRICS AND GYNECOLOGY

NYU Langone Medical Center provides comprehensive services designed specifically for women, from primary care to highly specialized programs that are supported by sophisticated research and advanced training. We specialize in the following areas:

Obstetrics
We offer a broad range of obstetrical services, including prenatal care that gives equal emphasis to the well-being of the mother and the fetus; fetal monitoring through ultrasound and other techniques; childbirth preparedness and breastfeeding classes.

Maternal-Fetal Medicine
Prenatal care for high-risk pregnancies and detailed consultations before, during and after pregnancy are offered. We specialize in multifetal pregnancies, genetic counseling, women who have miscarried, and preterm deliveries, as well as helping women who have other medical conditions that may complicate a pregnancy, such as diabetes, heart problems, high blood pressure, and lupus. We offer the latest techniques for in-utero diagnosis and treatment and using minimally invasive techniques, our physicians are able to repair a number of life-threatening conditions in a child before it is even born.

Fertility-Related Services
We offer state-of-the-art programs in evaluation of infertility (including the special needs of same-sex couples) egg donation, egg freezing and in-vitro fertilization. Diagnosis and treatment include ovulation induction, assisted reproductive technologies and surgical options that incorporate the latest endoscopic techniques. Preimplantation Genetic Screening (PGS) at the Fertility Center offers tests for aneuploidy (an abnormal number of chromosomes).

Gynecology
In addition to routine gynecological care, we offer pelvic ultrasound; aspiration of breast cysts, colposcopy (a diagnostic evaluation of abnormal pap smears); LEEP (a loop electrosurgical procedure used to diagnose and treat cervical cancer); cryotherapy for vaginal warts; and bone density testing.

Gynecologic Surgery
Minimally invasive gynecologic surgery, including robotic surgery, is offered for a wide range of simple and complex conditions including, resection of endometriosis, hysterectomy, and myomectomy.

Gynecologic Oncology
The NCI-designated NYU Cancer Institute's Women's Cancer Program specializes in the treatment of cervical cancer, endometrial cancer, ovarian cancer, uterine cancer, vaginal cancer and vulvar cancer.

Rheumatology

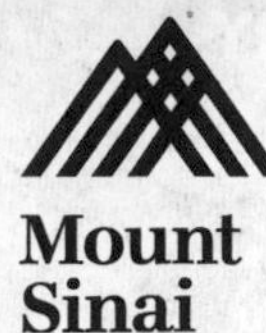

THE MOUNT SINAI MEDICAL CENTER
Rheumatology

One Gustave L. Levy Place
Fifth Avenue and 100th Street
New York, NY 10029-6574

Physician Referral: 1-800-MD-SINAI (637-4624)
www.mountsinai.org

The Mount Sinai Medical Center's **DIVISION OF RHEUMATOLOGY** is dedicated to excellence in patient care, research, and education and serves as a major referral center for disorders such as giant cell arteritis, scleroderma and Sjogren's syndrome.

Our rheumatologists routinely employ the latest, most effective treatments for the full range of rheumatic diseases and related disorders and consult regularly with colleagues from other disciplines to deliver comprehensive care to patients with complications that may affect other organs and systems.

We are one of only four major referral centers for amyloid diseases in the United States and are considered a "Center of Excellence" for the diagnosis and treatment of amyloid diseases, autoinflammatory syndromes, and cryopathies. We also deliver superior care to patients suffering from rheumatoid arthritis, systemic lupus erythematosus, osteoarthritis, Raynaud's disease, other connective tissue disorders, crystal deposition diseases such as gout and pseudogout, complications from inflammatory bowel disease (IBD), chronic renal failure, and diabetes. We are also conducting clinical trials in SLE, Amyloidosis, and Psoriatic arthritis.

As the U.S. population ages, there has been a considerable surge in the incidence and severity of musculoskeletal and autoimmune diseases. Studies, including our own investigations, show that early diagnosis and treatment of rheumatoid arthritis and other autoimmune diseases are crucial to living a productive life, limiting joint and organ damage, helping to avoid complications, and delaying or preventing the need for surgery.

We serve as a resource for the National Amyloidosis Support Group, the South Harlem Lupus Support Group, and the New York Chapter of the National Arthritis Foundation and are committed to providing excellent care and furthering basic knowledge pertinent to rheumatologic diseases.

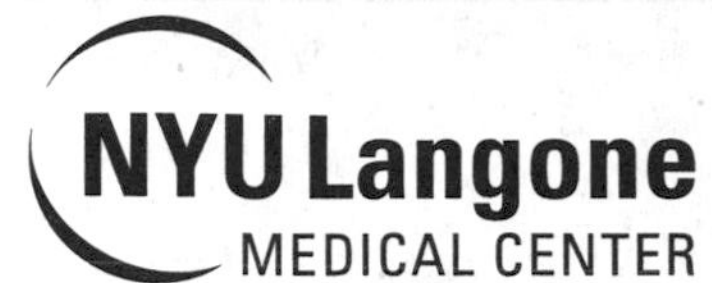

550 First Avenue *(at 31st Street)*
New York, NY 10016
www.NYULMC.org/rheumatology
Physician Referral: **888-7-NYU-MED** *(888-769-8633)*

RHEUMATOLOGY

Rheumatologists at NYU Langone Medical Center are dedicated to the diagnosis and treatment of patients with rheumatic illnesses, particularly autoimmune diseases. *U.S. News & World Report* has repeatedly recognized the Division of Rheumatology as one of the best in the country, ranking #7 nationwide in the 2013-2014 "Best Hospitals" survey. The division provides care at NYU Langone's premier outpatient facility, The Center for Musculoskeletal Care (CMC); the internationally-renowned, inpatient Hospital for Joint Diseases; at NYU Langone's main campus; and at multiple locations in NYU Langone's growing network of community practices throughout the metro New York area.

Arthritis and Autoimmunity: We offer a comprehensive program for the prevention, diagnosis and treatment of all rheumatologic conditions. Patients also have access to complete rheumatologic evaluations, orthopaedic and neurological consultative services, and participation in clinical trials using the most advanced interventional therapies, highly sophisticated diagnostic testing, and complementary medicine.

Behçet's Syndrome: We have the largest North American Behçet's Center for research and the evaluation and treatment of patients with Behçet's Syndrome, a disease that involves inflammation of the blood vessels.

Biological Treatment: Biological treatments for inflammatory arthritis, rheumatoid arthritis, lupus, psoriatic arthritis, vasculitis, and osteoporosis are administered in our comfortable, state-of-the-art infusion center at CMC.

Lupus: The Center for Lupus Care and Research is devoted to the treatment and research of patients with this autoimmune disease. Patients have access to world renowned specialists in lupus, lupus and pregnancy, and related subspecialties.

Osteoporosis: We offer comprehensive care for the prevention, evaluation and treatment of osteoporosis, including state-of-the art bone densitometers, a range of advanced drug therapies, and programs in balance training and exercise.

Psoriatic Arthritis: Patients of our Psoriatic Arthritis Center, a collaborative effort with the Department of Dermatology, are seen by both a rheumatologist and dermatologist who specialize in psoriasis and psoriatic arthritis.

We are also leaders in the research of inflammatory diseases, focusing on the study of drugs, drug delivery systems and protocols, and the roles genes play in the development and treatment of rheumatic diseases, positioning us at the forefront of basic science and translational research, personalized medicine and the genetics of rheumatic diseases. **The Peter D. Seligman Center for Advanced Therapeutics**, renowned for breakthrough research in arthritis and Systematic Lupus Erythematosus, conducts clinical studies using a wide variety of newly developed therapies.

Sleep Disorders

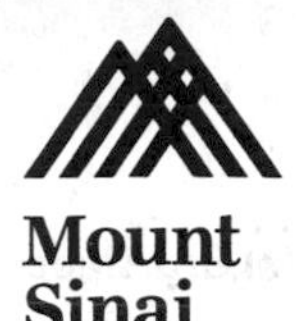

THE MOUNT SINAI MEDICAL CENTER

Sleep Surgery Center

One Gustave L. Levy Place
Fifth Avenue and 100th Street
New York, NY 10029-6574

Physician Referral: 1-800-MD-SINAI (637-4624)
www.mountsinai.org

The **PROGRAM FOR COMPREHENSIVE MANAGEMENT AND TREATMENT OF OBSTRUCTIVE SLEEP APNEA (OSA) AND SNORING** at Mount Sinai's Sleep Surgery Center excels in managing sleep disorders. Working collaboratively with experts from Otolaryngology/Head and Neck Surgery, Pulmonary and Sleep Medicine, Neurology, Endocrine/Nutrition, Oral/Maxillofacial Surgery, and Bariatric Surgery, we provide the collective expertise necessary to address all conditions in sleep disordered breathing.

Obstructive Sleep Apnea and Snoring Causes and Symptoms
OSA is a disorder in which breathing is repeatedly interrupted or decreased during sleep. This is secondary to muscle relaxation in the throat and tongue, closing the airway, preventing airflow, and causing oxygen starvation. The brain responds by sending a survival signal to awaken to a lighter level of sleep, and breathing is restored. This can be repeated hundreds of times each night, so the combination of poor sleep and oxygen starvation may cause daytime sleepiness, deficits in memory, attention, concentration, and depressed mood. There is also an increased risk of automobile accidents, and patients with untreated Sleep Apnea may also be at increased risk for high blood pressure, cardiac arrhythmias, and stroke.

Snoring is a partial obstruction of the airway, usually at the level of the palate and uvula. A narrowed airway passage creates turbulence, which vibrates the tissues of the throat and nose. It is often found in Sleep Apnea patients and is a common source of bed partner complaints.

SLEEP DISORDERS RESEARCH AND EDUCATION

Mount Sinai's Sleep Surgery Center team participates in projects designed to be collaborative and interdisciplinary in nature to take advantage of resources and perspectives unique to each discipline, including Otolaryngology, Bariatric Surgery, Sleep Medicine, and Nutrition. Our mission is to advance education and understanding of sleep disorders and their management among patients and professionals. Additionally, our faculty is routinely involved in lectures to improve the standard-of-care of treatment.

Obstructive Sleep Apnea and Snoring Treatments
Since the cause of airway obstruction varies among patients, and its management depends on the regions contributing to the obstruction of airflow, we create a customized treatment plan for each patient. Our experts stand solidly at the forefront of all surgical and non-surgical treatments for Snoring and OSA. Snoring without the presence of OSA may be treated with oral appliances, radiofrequency technology or pillar implants. For complex OSA cases, we offer the full spectrum of surgical solutions, and, whenever possible, the least invasive option. This includes TransOral Robotic Surgery (TORS) for the tongue base to improve the airway.

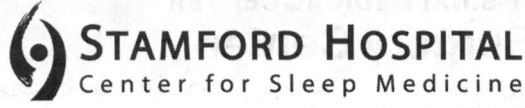

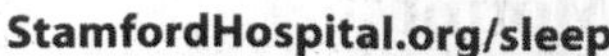

Center for Sleep Medicine

Stamford Hospital's Center for Sleep Medicine is Accredited by the American Academy of Sleep Medicine. All of our physicians are board-certified and highly skilled in diagnosing and treating sleep disorders including: snoring, sleep apnea, insomnia, narcolepsy and restless legs syndrome.

In addition, The Center includes one of Fairfield County's few board-certified sleep specialists trained in pediatric sleep medicine, providing special expertise in the treatment of sleep problems in infancy through teenage years.

Personalized Care

We are one of the state's larger sleep centers, and are able to schedule appointments and sleep studies faster than other facilities.

Located in the Hospital, all rooms are private with their own bath with shower. Each hotel-like room is furnished with a queen-size bed, reclining chair and cable television. Our rooms are large enough to accommodate a caregiver, especially important for pediatric patients.

Sleep Study

Some patients require an overnight sleep study. This non-invasive test monitors heart activity, breathing, oxygenation, position, limb movement, snoring and brain activity. During this painless process, a patient will be free to watch television or read until ready to go to sleep. The sleep study will be conducted throughout the night while the patient sleeps. Patients can leave the following morning for work or whatever their normal routine may be. In special circumstances, a home study can be performed.

Treatment Options

There are numerous treatment options available at the Center for Sleep Medicine—behavior modification, medication and in some instances custom made medical devices. Regardless of your sleep disorder, our physicians are experts in their field and will work with you to achieve a good night's sleep.

Academic and Clinical Affiliations

Stamford Hospital is an affiliate of the New York–Presbyterian Healthcare System and a major teaching affiliate of the Columbia University College of Physicians & Surgeons.

Accreditation

Joint Commission on Accreditation of Healthcare Organization (JCAHO)

Beds

305

Sponsorship

Voluntary, Not-for-Profit

For a Physician Referral or more information, please call 1.877.233.9355 or visit StamfordHospital.org /doctor.

Stamford Hospital
30 Shelburne Road
Stamford, CT 06902
203.276.1000

StamfordHospital.org

Trinitas Regional Medical Center

COMPREHENSIVE SLEEP DISORDERS CENTER

210 WILLIAMSON STREET | ELIZABETH, NEW JERSEY 07207
PH 908.994.8694 | WWW.NJSLEEPDISORDERSCENTER.COM

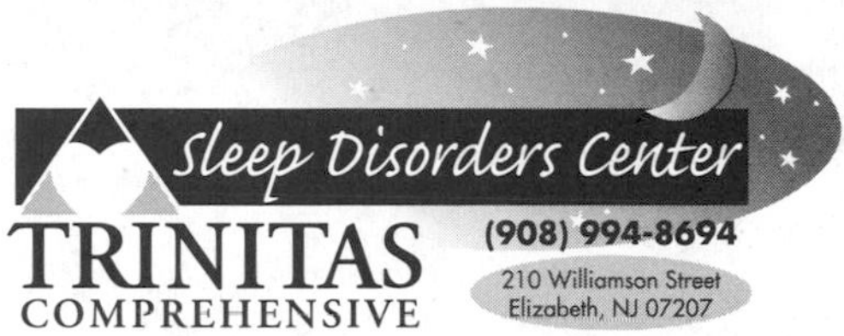

Accredited by The American Academy of Sleep Medicine

Getting a good night's sleep is an essential part of healthy living, but for the millions of Americans who suffer from sleep disorders, getting enough rest can be difficult, if not impossible. Left untreated, sleep disorders can have harmful, even life-threatening effects on health, well-being and safety.

The Comprehensive Sleep Disorders Center at Trinitas Regional Medical Center provides a monitored, fully attended diagnostic sleep study designed to rule out physical, non-stress related symptoms that may prevent restful sleep. The medical director is board certified in Internal Medicine, Critical Care, Sleep Medicine and Pulmonary Medicine. A team of trained sleep specialists supervises each study and coordinates follow-up care with the patient's physician. These professionals can quickly diagnose any sleep problem and, working closely with each patient's primary physician, provide expert treatment and follow-up.

Located within the main campus of Trinitas Regional Medical Center, the state-of-the-art Comprehensive Sleep Disorders Center is designed to diagnose sleep disorders, including insomnia, sleep apnea, restless leg syndrome, snoring and narcolepsy, among others. The private, comfortable testing is performed in home-like suites with soft designer sheets, pillows and a private shower. Studies are provided for adults and children as young as 18 months. Daytime studies are available to meet patient needs.

In 2010, a second sleep center was unveiled in Homewood Suites by Hilton, Cranford. The site is the first hotel-based sleep center in New Jersey.

Both locations offer state-of-the-art diagnostic sleep studies performed by specially trained sleep pulmonologists, registered polysomnographers and licensed, credentialed respiratory therapists.

The Trinitas Comprehensive Sleep Disorders Center is a fully staffed center accredited by The American Academy of Sleep Medicine - the "gold standard" accrediting body for sleep centers - offering the benefits of two distinct locations. With one location on the campus of Trinitas Regional Medical Center, a comprehensive, state-of-the-art medical facility and the other at a nearby nationally known hotel chain, patients who have sleep studies performed at Trinitas receive the high level of attention or treatment that is simply not possible to receive at a neighborhood sleep center.

Sports Medicine

THE MOUNT SINAI MEDICAL CENTER

Sports Medicine

One Gustave L. Levy Place
Fifth Avenue and 100th Street
New York, NY 10029-6574

Physician Referral: 1-800-MD-SINAI (637-4624)
www.mountsinai.org

At The Mount Sinai Medical Center, our board-certified sports medicine specialists are dedicated to helping patients heal from a variety of shoulder, hip, and knee conditions, from a torn ACL to a shoulder dislocation. They are highly experienced in working with all levels of athletes, from recreational to professional, and they excel in the most advanced surgical techniques (both arthroscopic and open) including:

- Anatomic ACL reconstruction
- Meniscal repairs
- Realignment procedures including osteotomies
- Treatment of Patellofemoral (knee cap) disorders
- Multiligament disruption (dislocated knee)
- Cartilage preservation/restoration
- Rotator cuff surgery
- Shoulder stabilization after dislocation
- SLAP and labral repairs
- Hip arthroscopy
- Arthroscopic treatment of hip labral tears
- Arthroscopic treatment of femoroacetabular impingement
- Tennis elbow treatment
- Repair and/or reconstruction of quadriceps and patellar tendon ruptures

Our sports medicine experts are committed to guiding every patient through a treatment plan that is specifically tailored to his or her problem. Each patient is treated individually and we work closely with both our patients and the physical therapists to help them achieve their goals.

ORTHOPAEDIC SURGERY

The Department of Orthopaedic Surgery at NYU Langone Medical Center continues to be recognized as a national leader, **ranked #5 in the nation by *U.S. News & World Report's* 2013-2014 "Best Hospitals" survey**. Our physicians combine extensive experience with cutting-edge research and technology to address bone and joint problems that affect a patient's quality of life. The expertise of our world-class orthopaedists represents the full range of subspecialty areas including **Adult Reconstructive, Sports Medicine and Primary Care Sports Medicine, Spine, Shoulder & Elbow, Foot & Ankle, Hand Surgery, Trauma & Fracture, Orthopaedic Oncology, and Pediatric Orthopaedics**; additional areas of specialization include minimally-invasive surgery and robotic-assisted joint replacement.

Premier Areas of Expertise

Joint Replacement Center physicians evaluate degenerative joint conditions caused by arthritis, injuries, congenital problems and general wear-and-tear to determine the best course of treatment. Our surgeons are experts in knee, hip and shoulder replacements, complex joint revisions, and minimally invasive surgeries, conducting more than 3,000 procedures annually. The experts in our **Hip Center** also specialize in the cutting-edge, minimally invasive anterior total hip replacement technique.

The Spine Center provides conservative care for lower back and neck pain, scoliosis, osteoporosis, problems associated with failed previous surgery, idiopathic disorders, growth disorders, neuromuscular disease, degenerative and congenital conditions, and traumatic deformity. Our surgeons perform over 2,000 procedures a year, including minimally invasive spinal fusions.

Hand Center specialists diagnose and offer operative and non-operative care for a wide range of upper extremity conditions, including fractures, congenital anomalies, soft tissue and skeletal trauma, degenerative and rheumatoid arthritis, sports-related injuries, vascular disorders, tumors and occupational disorders.

Sports Medicine and Primary Care Sports Medicine physicians treat sports-related injuries or conditions of the knee, shoulder, elbow and ankle, using joint preservation techniques as well as surgical procedures. Our patients range from athletes playing at the high school, college and professional levels to recreational athletes/active individuals from every age group.

(continued)

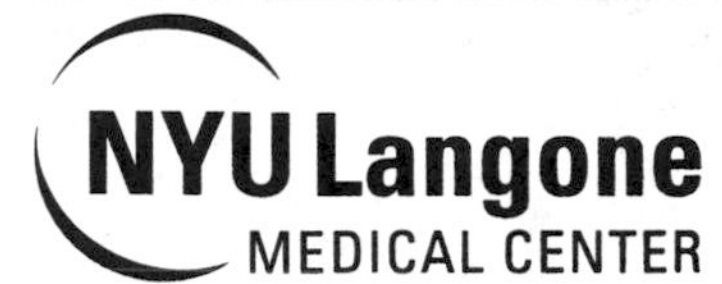

550 First Avenue *(at 31st Street)*
New York, NY 10016
www.NYULMC.org/orthosurgery
Physician Referral: **888-7-NYU-MED** *(888-769-8633)*

ORTHOPAEDIC SURGERY *(continued)*

Specialized Orthopaedic Centers and Services

The Joint Preservation Center provides conservative treatment of joint problems to reduce symptoms, restore function and delay the onset of degenerative arthritis and potential need for a joint replacement.

The Bone Healing Center is staffed by our orthopaedic trauma & fracture specialists, and is a leader in technologies and procedures that help patients recover from complex fracture reconstruction or fracture healing problems.

Harkness Center for Dance Injuries is world-renowned for its orthopaedic and rehabilitation care for dancers, including many subsidized and free services as well as injury prevention screenings and lectures.

The Diabetes Foot and Ankle Center focuses on the prevention and recurrence of foot and ankle problems associated with complications of diabetes.

The Samuels Orthopaedic Immediate Care Center, New York City's only walk-in orthopaedic clinic, is open seven days a week to evaluate and treat urgent bone and joint injuries.

The Concussion Center is a collaborative effort between the Departments of Orthopaedic Surgery, Neurology, and Rehabilitation, providing expert, multidisciplinary evaluation and treatment of individuals who have or are suspected of having a concussion.

The Occupational & Industrial Orthopaedic Center offers care, education, and consulting services in the prevention and treatment of injuries and disorders that arise from the work environment.

Sports Performance Center specialists assist active individuals in reaching their full potential through a state-of-the-art health and fitness evaluation and personalized athletic training plan.

Patient Care Locations

Our physicians and surgeons provide care at multiple NYU Langone locations, including:

- **The Hospital for Joint Diseases**, our internationally-renowned orthopaedic hospital
- **The Center for Musculoskeletal Care (CMC)**, NYU Langone's premier, state-of-the-art, multidisciplinary, bone and joint facility, which houses outpatient orthopaedic and rheumatologic care as well as an infusion center, pain management services, and Rusk Rehab's sports and musculoskeletal rehabilitation services
- CMC's **Outpatient Surgery Center**, where patients undergo minimally invasive, same-day surgery
- **Tisch Hospital**, NYU Langone's flagship hospital at the main campus on First Avenue
- Multiple locations in **NYU Langone's growing network of community practices** in the metro New York area, including Manhattan, Brooklyn, Long Island, Queens, Westchester, and New Jersey

Stroke Care

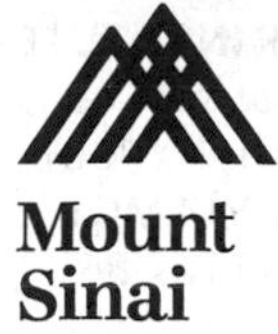

THE MOUNT SINAI MEDICAL CENTER

The Stroke Center

One Gustave L. Levy Place
Fifth Avenue and 100th Street
New York, NY 10029-6574

Physician Referral: 1-800-MD-SINAI (637-4624)
www.mountsinai.org

THE MOUNT SINAI STROKE CENTER provides comprehensive, interdisciplinary care and support to stroke patients and their families. As one of the first stroke centers in New York City, we offer 24/7 availability for emergency consultation and treatment, a specialized neuro-intensive care unit, a state-of-the-art stroke unit, and access to some of the latest clinical trials.

We are a New York State Department of Health-designated primary stroke center and are the first Joint Commission-certified comprehensive stroke center in New York State. Recognized as a leader in stroke research and treatment, our experts have pioneered major advances in medical and interventional therapies for treating and preventing stroke, including innovative neurosurgical and endovascular procedures for the treatment of acute stroke, with the goal of significantly improving the chances that a patient can prevent, or recover optimally, from a stroke.

Several treatments are now available to treat stroke within just a few hours of the onset of acute symptoms. We offer the following advanced treatments for stroke:

- Intravenous clot-busting medication for acute stroke
- Delivery of clot-busting medications directly to the affected cerebral vessel using neuro-endovascular techniques
- Mechanical extraction of the blood clot that is occluding a cerebral vessel
- Carotid endarterectomy and carotid and intracranial stenting for treatment of carotid and cerebral artery stenosis
- A specialized neuro-critical care unit with state-of-the-art monitoring for post-procedure care
- Ongoing evaluation and management of stroke patients in a dedicated, state-of-the-art acute stroke unit

Despite these advances in care, it is clear that there is still much work to be done to reduce the burden of stroke in our community. The Mount Sinai Stroke Center is actively involved in community outreach and in potentially groundbreaking research to optimize chronic disease self-management skills in stroke and transient ischemic attack (TIA) survivors.

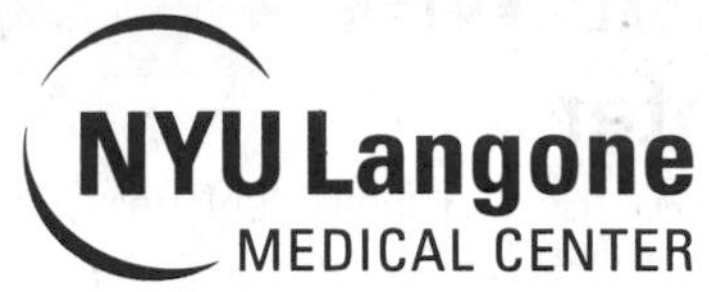

CARDIAC AND VASCULAR INSTITUTE
550 First Avenue *(at 31st Street)*
New York, NY 10016
www.NYULMC.org
Physician Referral: **888-7-NYU-MED** *(888-769-8633)*

CARDIAC AND VASCULAR INSTITUTE

The Cardiac and Vascular Institute (CVI) at NYU Langone Medical Center continues to advance new techniques for repairing heart valves, curing heart rhythm disorders, and treating aortic diseases and congestive heart failure. We care for both adults and children. CVI is consistently ranked among the leading heart and heart surgery centers in *U.S. News & World Report's annual 'Best Hospitals'* rankings.

Cardiac Catheterization CVI offers superior catheter-based diagnosis and evaluation of cardiac health. Our laboratory provides a full range of procedures to evaluate, diagnose, and provide treatment options.

Cardiac Rehabilitation and Prevention The Joan and Joel Smilow Cardiopulmonary Rehabilitation and Prevention Center provides individualized treatment plans through NYU Langone's Rusk Rehabilitation, in a state-of-the-art and comfortable facility.

Cardiac Surgery NYU Langone is a nationally recognized leader in advanced surgical treatments for adult and congenital heart disease. We have world-renowned expertise in mitral valve repair, aortic valve replacement and aortic aneurysm repair, as well as specializing in high-risk and elderly patients.

Cardiology The Leon H. Charney Division of Cardiology is a leader in cardiovascular patient care, biomedical research, and education. We are advancing the field of cardiovascular medicine through a variety of innovative collaborations.

Congenital Heart Disease The pediatric and adult congenital cardiac program treats patients of all ages with inherited and acquired cardiac defects. We have a highly experienced team of specialists in pediatric and adult cardiology, pediatric interventional cardiology, congenital cardiac surgery, neonatal and pediatric cardiac intensive care, pediatric cardiac anesthesiology, nursing, and extracorporeal perfusion.

Heart Failure A multidisciplinary team offers the most advanced care for heart failure including echocardiograms, pacemaker and defibrillator implantations, open heart surgeries, and left ventricular assist devices.

Nuclear Cardiology/Stress The Nuclear Cardiology/Stress Laboratory performs a range of tests that assist cardiologists in the assessment and diagnosis of heart disease.

Vascular Surgery We offer diagnostic and treatment for patients with conditions ranging from arterial aneurysms to deep vein thrombosis, as well as carotid stenosis and limb salvage including minimally invasive vein surgery, endovascular aortic surgery, thoracic aneurysm correction and abdominal aneurysm interventions.

The Best in American Medicine
www.CastleConnolly.com

Surgery

Montefiore
Inspired Medicine

111 East 210th Street
Bronx, New York 10467
718-920-4800
www.montefiore.org/surgery

Surgery at Montefiore

Montefiore's Department of Surgery is at the forefront of innovation and offers the latest technology and treatments to ensure optimal outcomes for its adult and pediatric patients. The Department's five surgical divisions—breast, general, pediatric, transplant, and plastic and reconstructive—are led by renowned surgeons who possess an unparalleled breadth of experience and expertise.

The Department emphasizes the use of minimally invasive surgical approaches as often as possible. Procedures such as single-incision laparoscopic sleeve gastrectomy and Lap Band®, transanal minimally invasive surgery and endoscopic microsurgery, robotic-assisted liver resection and natural orifice transluminal endoscopic surgery are reducing the time that patients spend in the operating room and subsequent recovery.

Montefiore's clinical reputation and exceptional surgical outcomes have made it a magnet for referrals. In 2012 the Department performed 9,299 surgical procedures—nearly a 25 percent increase since 2009. It is also recognized by the American College of Surgeons' National Surgical Quality Improvement Program for exemplary outcomes in several categories, including overall morbidity and mortality.

The Division of General Surgery is a national leader in the use of cutting-edge cancer treatments including hyperthermic intraperitoneal chemotherapy, isolated limb perfusion (for sarcoma or melanoma) and liver perfusion.

The Division of Breast Surgery is accredited by the National Accreditation Program for Breast Centers and is widely recognized for its personalized approach to care. It offers a host of surgical options for the treatment of patients with breast cancer and other breast disorders. These include breast reconstructions, which use state-of-the-art techniques to create replacement breasts that look and feel natural.

Montefiore's Bariatric Surgery Program is designated as a Center of Excellence in Bariatric Surgery by the American College of Surgeons. The Program recently expanded its services to include young adults between ages 18 and 21. To date, the Program has performed more than 700 bariatric procedures.

The Division of Plastic and Reconstructive Surgery's commitment to excellence has placed it at the forefront of craniofacial surgery, pediatric plastic and reconstructive surgery, breast surgery, and microsurgery. This year, the Division will build upon its expertise with the addition of a hand specialist.

The Division of Transplant Surgery performed its first pediatric living-donor liver transplant this year, continuing its tradition of innovation. In 2012, the Division performed close to 200 solid-organ transplants in adults and children, with one-year outcomes in heart, liver and kidney transplant exceeding state and national averages.

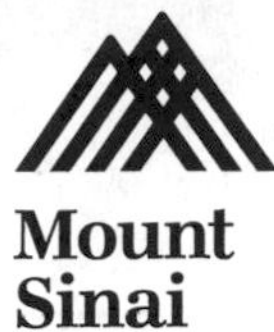

THE MOUNT SINAI MEDICAL CENTER

Surgery

One Gustave L. Levy Place
Fifth Avenue and 100th Street
New York, NY 10029-6574

Physician Referral: 1-800-MD-SINAI (637-4624)
www.mountsinai.org

The **DEPARTMENT OF SURGERY** continues to build upon the legacy of those who have gone before, caring for the very sickest of patients while developing new therapies and training tomorrow's physicians to save and enhance lives. Patients today are experiencing less pain, shorter hospital stays, and faster recovery times than was ever imaginable just 20 years ago.

TOP-RANKING MINIMALLY INVASIVE SURGEONS

In surveys of leading minimally invasive surgeons in a variety of specialties, Mount Sinai's physicians are consistently at the top of the list in surgery of the colon and rectum, liver and bile ducts, thyroid, hernia, chest, and blood vessels.

Colon and Rectal Surgery – Leaders in the treatment of gastrointestinal disorders, our surgeons care for a wide range of diseases, including: inflammatory bowel disease (Crohn's disease and ulcerative colitis), diverticulitis, colon and rectal cancer, and fecal incontinence. We offer many important procedures not commonly available.

General Surgery – The Division of General Surgery specializes in the treatment of abdominal surgical conditions. These include benign and malignant diseases of the gallbladder and gastrointestinal track (stomach, intestine, and colon). Our Comprehensive Hernia Center offers state-of-the-art repair of inguinal, ventral and hiatal hernias. We use minimally invasive and evidence-based surgery to deliver the highest standard of care to our patients.

Laparoscopic and Minimally Invasive Surgery – Mount Sinai surgeons rank as some of the world's most respected and innovative surgeons, performing more laparoscopic procedures than surgeons at any other hospital in New York.

Metabolic, Endocrine and Minimally Invasive Surgery – This division was formed to serve as the backbone for several disease-specific multidisciplinary programs. Ours is a truly novel metabolic surgery program that brings together traditional endocrine, bariatric and laparoscopic techniques to treat diseases of metabolism and the endocrine system.

Bariatric Surgery – The latest minimally invasive techniques are used to perform laparoscopic gastric bypass, lap band placement, duodenal switch, and sleeve gastrectomy.

Pediatric Surgery – Surgeries involving children can be met with even more apprehension than those for adults. Fortunately, Mount Sinai surgeons offer a full range of pediatric surgical procedures in a family-focused, child-sensitive environment.

Plastic and Reconstructive Surgery – Surgical care from aesthetic to complex reconstruction is offered for benign and malignant disease, as well as for deformities that are either congenital or acquired. The aim is to restore function and correct deformities caused by birth defects, aging, accident, or illness.

Surgical Oncology – Our surgeons provide expert care for both minimally invasive and open complex malignancies. Patients are seen promptly and are cared for by a multidisciplinary team of medical and surgical experts, enabling them to benefit from the opinions of dozens of nationally renowned doctors.

Vascular Surgery – Mount Sinai is a recognized world leader in the development of new minimally invasive techniques for the treatment of aortic aneurysms, carotid stenosis for the prevention of stroke and lower extremity ischemia. Mount Sinai performs research in areas ranging from stem cell therapy to specialized vascular devices. Our research serves to advance the field of vascular surgery. A wide array of advanced patient services is available, ensuring that conditions are managed successfully.

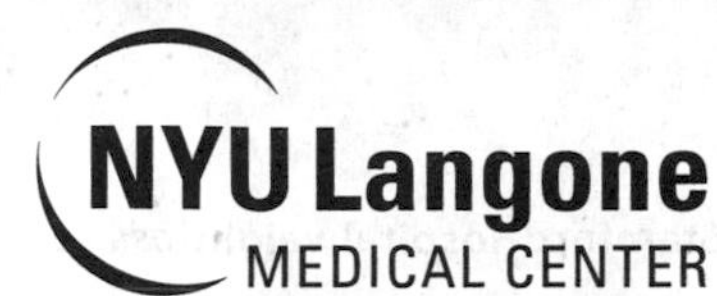

550 First Avenue *(at 31st Street)*
New York, NY 10016
www.NYULMC.org
Physician Referral: **888-7-NYU-MED** *(888-769-8633)*

NYU LANGONE MEDICAL CENTER

NYU Langone Medical Center—a world-class, patient-centered, integrated, academic medical center—is one of the nation's premier destinations for excellence in patient care, biomedical research, and medical education. Located in the heart of Manhattan, NYU Langone is composed of Tisch Hospital, its flagship acute care facility; the Hospital for Joint Diseases, a dedicated in-patient orthopaedic hospital; Hassenfeld Children's Hospital, a comprehensive pediatric hospital supporting a full array of children's health services; Rusk Rehabilitation, the #1 rehab program in New York since *U.S. News & World Report* began its hospital rankings in 1989; and a growing ambulatory care network with locations throughout Manhattan, the outer boroughs, and the tri-state area, bringing services directly to where its patients live and work.

In a culture where treating the whole person and not simply the disease is the norm, NYU Langone Medical Center is renowned for clinical excellence across a wide array of specialties, including cancer, cardiology, cardiac and vascular surgery, musculoskeletal (including orthopaedics and rehabilitation), neurosurgery and children's services.

An integral part of NYU Langone, NYU School of Medicine has trained thousands of physicians and scientists who have helped to shape the course of medical history and enrich the lives of countless people since 1841. NYU Langone's tri-fold mission to serve, teach, and discover is achieved 365 days a year. For more information, go to www.NYULMC.org, Facebook, Twitter, and YouTube.

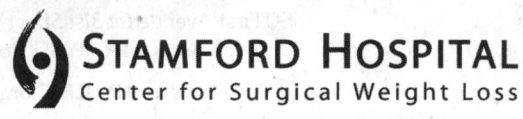

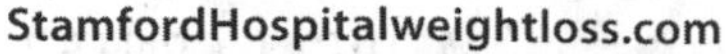

Center for Surgical Weight Loss

At Stamford Hospital's Center for Surgical Weight Loss, patients benefit from a comprehensive program led by a team of weight management specialists. Our highly skilled on-site team consisting of board certified bariatric surgeons, nurse practitioner, registered dietitian, psychologist, and exercise physiologist provide patients with individualized, patient-centered care.

Surgical Procedures

Grounded in the Center's philosophy of providing high-quality individualized care, patients have numerous options for bariatric surgery: gastric bypass, sleeve gastrectomy, gastric banding and duodenal switch, all of which are performed through thumb-nail sized incisions. These laparoscopic procedures result in less pain and scarring, fewer complications and a quicker recovery. Bariatric surgery has been demonstrated to not only reduce weight, but to have profound benefits on metabolic illnesses associated with obesity, such as diabetes and high cholesterol.

Surgical Preparatory Program

Preparing for surgery is a multi-faceted endeavor. The surgical preparatory program includes medical and psychological evaluation, optimization of existing medical conditions prior to surgery, and patient education and counseling in both the individual and group setting.

Patient Care

Patients are cared for by an interprofessional team at all points of care beginning with the first office consultation, extending to in-hospital follow-up by the bariatric team, and then further extending to lifelong follow-up to monitor progress and provide support.

Integrated Approach

The Center for Surgical Weight Loss partners with the Center for Integrative Medicine and Wellness to avail patients to integrative therapies including acupuncture, acupressure and stress management. Patients are offered a 90-day complimentary membership to the Health and Fitness Institute at the Tully Health Center, a state-of-the-art facility, to assist patients in achieving weight loss and fitness goals.

Non-surgical Options for Weight Loss

For those individuals interested in a non-surgical approach to weight loss, the Center offers multiple treatment modalities including dietary counseling, behavior modification, medications and meal replacements.

Academic and Clinical Affiliations

Stamford Hospital is an affiliate of the New York–Presbyterian Healthcare System and a major teaching affiliate of the Columbia University College of Physicians & Surgeons.

Accreditation

Joint Commission on Accreditation of Healthcare Organization (JCAHO)

Beds

305

Sponsorship

Voluntary, Not-for-Profit

For a Physician Referral or more information, please call 1.877.233.9355 or visit StamfordHospital.org /doctor.

Stamford Hospital
30 Shelburne Road
Stamford, CT 06902
203.276.1000

StamfordHospital.org

The Best in American Medicine
www.CastleConnolly.com

Therapeutic Radiology

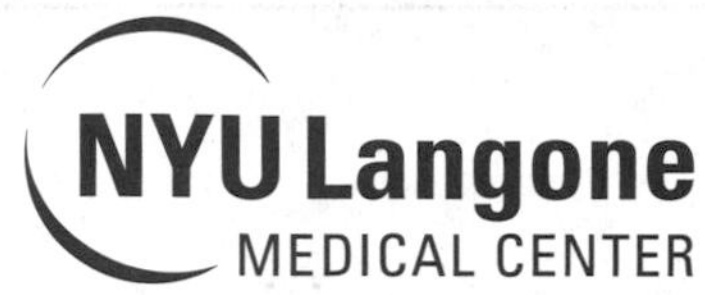

550 First Avenue *(at 31st Street)*
New York, NY 10016

www.NYULMC.org

Physician Referral: **888-7-NYU-MED** *(888-769-8633)*

RADIOLOGY

NYU Langone Radiology is committed to capturing the best images possible with the lowest dose of radiation. As an academic medical center, our radiologists are in a unique position to take the lead in helping to define and advance radiology in today's rapidly evolving technological environment.

Expertise

NYU Langone Medical Center's board certified radiologists and licensed technologists specialize in imaging and are involved in a variety of innovative collaborations and research initiatives. The Department consists of more than 100 sub-specialized academic radiologists, many of them acknowledged leaders and innovators in their fields.

Advanced Technology

NYU Langone uses some of the most advanced imaging equipment in the world, including high and ultra high-field MRI imaging systems (known as 1.5T and 3T magnets). MRI scanners are shorter and wider than ever, making for a more patient-friendly experience. The Center for Biomedical Imaging, an advanced research facility, features a powerful 7T magnet.

Recognition for Safety and Quality

We continually follow a rigorous set of quality standards and maintain accreditation by the American College of Radiology (ACR). Designated by the ACR as a "Breast Imaging Center of Excellence", our team maintains high practice standards in image quality, personnel qualifications, facility equipment, quality control procedures and quality assurance programs.

Patient Focused Approach

We are located in Manhattan, Brooklyn, Queens, and Long Island and participate in many insurance plans. Timely delivery of reports and images allow physicians to view patient exam status, reports and images online. In addition to our convenient hours, weekend, evening and often same-day appointments are available. Language interpretation services are available as needed.

Our Areas of Specialization

Diagnostic services include MRI, CT, ultrasound, PET/CT, X-ray, interventional radiology and nuclear medicine. Sub-specialized radiologists provide diagnostic interpretation in abdominal, biomedical, breast, cardiac, chest, emergency, general, musculoskeletal, neuroradiology, neuro interventional, nuclear medicine, pediatric, vascular interventional, and women's imaging. Specialty procedures include coronary artery disease and virtual colonoscopy screening, stereotactic biopsy capability, minimally invasive techniques including radiofrequency ablation, chemoembolization, radioimmunotherapy, and bone densitometry.

Thoracic & Cardiac Surgery

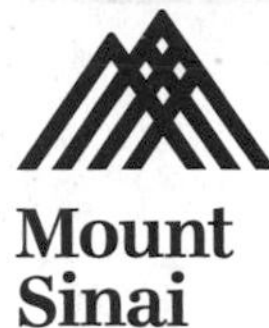

THE MOUNT SINAI MEDICAL CENTER

Thoracic Surgery

One Gustave L. Levy Place
Fifth Avenue and 100th Street
New York, NY 10029-6574

Physician Referral: 1-800-MD-SINAI (637-4624)
www.mountsinai.org

THORACIC SURGERY at The Mount Sinai Medical Center is known for its state-of-the-art surgery, multidisciplinary team approach to treatment, and commitment to compassionate patient care. Protocol-driven therapy ensures that Mount Sinai patients are given access to many clinical trials.

The Division of Thoracic Surgery at Mount Sinai engages in multidisciplinary collaboration, partnering with medical oncology, radiation oncology, pulmonary medicine, diagnostic and interventional radiology, gastroenterology, neurology, and anesthesiology, so patients can benefit from the insights of multiple experts across different specialties. This coordination among teams ensures seamless delivery of high-quality care to patients.

LEADING SURGEONS, PIONEERING RESEARCH

Led by Raja M. Flores, the Division of Thoracic Surgery is internationally recognized as a leader in thoracic surgery drawing patients from across the globe to seek our expertise.

Dr. Flores is a recognized leader in the treatment of mesothelioma and one of the first physicians in the world to use robotic surgery to treat lung and esophageal cancer. Dr. Flores established VATS lobectomy as the gold standard in the surgical treatment of lung cancer. He is one of the foremost educators of other surgeons about the VATS lobectomy.

Our award-winning physicians have consistently contributed to the evolution of this field through their efforts to bring about new technologies and therapies.

With an integrated approach to clinical care and research, our team of dedicated thoracic surgeons are experts in the treatment of all primary cancers of the chest, lung, esophagus, mediastinum, and airway, and all metastatic tumors of the chest. We also diagnose and treat patients who are affected by benign esophageal disorders such as gastroesophageal reflux disease, achalasia, and motility disorders.

Minimally Invasive Care: Minimally invasive interventions are preferred whenever possible, allowing less tissue damage, faster recovery time, and less scarring than open surgery. Mount Sinai's Division of Thoracic Surgery offers state-of-the-art assessment and treatment approaches, including thoracoscopy, rigid and flexible bronchoscopy, and endoscopic laser resection in the diagnosis and management of thoracic conditions. The division has led the national trials for VATS (video-assisted thoracoscopic surgery) lobectomy, a procedure using three small incisions, which is now the surgical approach of choice, particularly for patients with early-stage lung cancer.

Personalized and Targeted Therapy: A unique part of our division is the integration and application of groundbreaking scientific research into the clinical care of our patients. These research efforts are being carried out in the Thoracic Surgery Translational Laboratory. Mount Sinai's thoracic surgeons and physician-scientists are conducting state-of-the-art translational thoracic research, including genomic analysis of tumors to better understand and predict behavior, in order to develop more directed, personalized, therapeutic approaches to treatment with novel targeted therapies.

Lung and Esophageal Cancer: Mount Sinai is New York City's leading center for comprehensive screening for lung and esophageal cancer, including CT scans for early detection, advanced endoscopic techniques, PET scans, and innovative MRI technology with ultrasensitive resolution. Our team is unique in our abilities to screen for cancers in people at risk, treat early cancers less invasively, and provide the most advanced protocol driven treatments available. Our approach to lung cancer care focuses on patients first, providing not only VATS and advanced minimally invasive techniques, but also an ability to treat advanced and challenging cases that require skills and expertise found in few other medical centers.

Mesothelioma: Irving J. Selikoff, MD, was the first to determine the association between mesothelioma and asbestos exposure. His tireless research efforts at Mount Sinai led to the Selikoff Center for Occupational and Environmental Medicine. This tradition of cutting-edge developments continues with Raja M. Flores' work using different modalities in the treatment of mesothelioma, such as the extrapleural pneumonectomy and pleurectomy/decortication procedures. The Division of Thoracic Surgery is also currently involved in several ongoing studies with the goal of discovering new treatments for mesothelioma. Mount Sinai performs research in areas ranging from stem cell therapy to specialized vascular devices. Our research serves to advance the field of vascular surgery. A wide array of advanced patient services is available, ensuring that conditions are managed successfully.

Transplantation

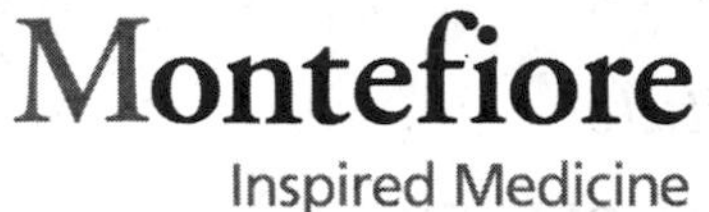

111 East 210th Street
Bronx, New York 10467
Heart: 718-920-6515
Liver: 888-795-4837
Kidney: 877-287-3536
www.montefiore.org/transplant

Montefiore Einstein Center for Transplantation

The Montefiore Einstein Center for Transplantation is a high-volume multi-organ transplant center, one of the busiest and oldest in the United States. Its physicians perform heart, liver, kidney and pancreas transplants in adults and children, and they also perform comprehensive organ failure management. The Center's physicians also perform innovative surgical procedures, including living-donor liver transplantation, split liver transplants, dual kidney transplants and combined kidney pancreas transplantation for selected patients. In partnership with the Montefiore Einstein Center for Cancer Care, the Center also provides multidisciplinary management of liver cancer—a major complication of chronic liver disease.

The Center specializes in meticulous organ failure management to evaluate and facilitate transplantation. Despite long waiting times in the Northeast for donor organs, the Center utilizes every available strategy to shorten waiting time and maintain health while waiting for a donor organ. Pre-transplant health maintenance is crucial to successful outcomes in transplantation. We employ a broad range of transplant specialists to care for patients before and after transplant, including a full psychosocial team, financial counselors, nutritionists, pharmacists, nurse practitioners and physical therapists. In 2012, the Center performed close to 200 solid organ transplants, including 30 liver transplants, 137 kidney transplants and 28 heart transplants. The Center has consistently achieved superlative outcomes, equal to or better than national benchmarks.

The Center works closely with a full-time organ donor liaison to promote living and deceased donor transplantation in the local community. A major focus of the Center is identifying strategies to overcome social, economic and linguistic barriers to transplant that are prevalent in the organ failure population. One successful strategy is the Center's Helping Hands program, which provides transplant patients with assistance before and after transplant surgery when family social support is limited.

The Center's commitment to advancing the field has led to a dynamic partnership with the Marion Bessin Liver Research Center at Albert Einstein College of Medicine. Investigators at the Bessin Center work with the clinical transplant team to promote pioneering work in the area of liver disease. These efforts include a newly opened trial studying the use of the extracorporeal liver-assist device (ELAD) to support patients with acute liver failure who are at a high risk of death without transplant. Other research endeavors focus on novel therapeutic agents for hepatitis C and the use of systemic therapy—combining chemotherapy and radioembolization—to treat patients with liver tumors.

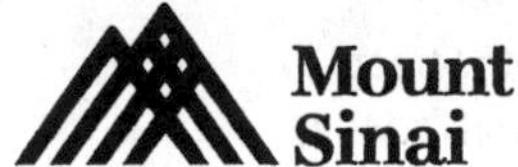

Recanati/Miller Transplantation Institute

THE MOUNT SINAI MEDICAL CENTER

Transplantation

One Gustave L. Levy Place
Fifth Avenue and 100th Street
New York, NY 10029-6574

Physician Referral: 1-800-MD-SINAI (637-4624)
www.mountsinai.org

Scientific breakthroughs, technological advances, and improved clinical therapies make it possible to save more lives through organ transplantation than ever before. The Mount Sinai Medical Center's **RECANATI MILLER/ TRANSPLANTATION INSTITUTE** (RMTI) has been a world leader in these advances. The RMTI brings together clinical programs in adult and pediatric liver, kidney, pancreas, and intestinal transplantation. It is one of the largest transplant centers in the United States and performs more than 350 transplant procedures annually. In addition, RMTI surgeons also perform complex hepatobiliary surgical procedures.

History of Achievement – The kidney transplant program was instituted at Mount Sinai in 1967 and is now one of the largest adult and pediatric programs in the nation, having performed more than 3,000 transplants. The first liver transplant to be performed in New York State was in 1988 at Mount Sinai. There have been many other firsts in the program's history, including the first pediatric liver transplant and the first adult-to-adult living-donor liver transplant in New York State.

Tradition of Excellence – Mount Sinai is one of the few hospitals in the country that offers comprehensive, multi-organ transplant services for both children and adults. Our physicians are able to accept and care for the sickest and most complex patients.

INNOVATIVE PROGRAMS

- **Recipients with HIV** – Since 2001, the RMTI has been one of the only centers in the nation to transplant carefully selected kidney and liver patients with HIV.

- **Living Donor Program** – Mount Sinai has an active living-donor program. The newly endowed Zweig Family Center for Living Donation is the first multi-organ living donor center where dedicated resources ensure the well-being of these heroes who give one, or a part, of their own organs to save another person's life. We also participate in local and national paired-exchange and donor-chain initiatives. RMTI has performed over 1500 living donor kidney transplants and over 250 living donor liver transplants.

- **Multi-organ Transplantation and Intestinal Rehabilitation Program** – We have performed many combined transplant procedures. Our rehabilitation program offers patients with intestinal failure the opportunity, when possible, to avoid transplantation through medical and/or surgical interventions.

- **Translational Research** – Our scientists are actively investigating new and innovative ways to detect, prevent and treat rejection. We have nationally-recognized and well-funded transplant, genomic, and proteomic projects.

The Best in American Medicine
www.CastleConnolly.com

Urology

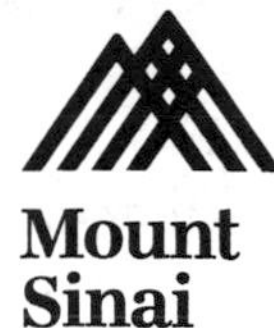

THE MOUNT SINAI MEDICAL CENTER

Urogynecology

One Gustave L. Levy Place
Fifth Avenue and 100th Street
New York, NY 10029-6574

Physician Referral: 1-800-MD-SINAI (637-4624)
www.mountsinai.org

Urogynecology: Incontinence and Pelvic Organ Prolapse

Millions of women of all ages suffer from incontinence or overactive bladder in silence and embarrassment, not knowing where to turn for help. By turning to the experts at Mount Sinai, women who have suffered the physical and emotional effects of pelvic floor disorders such as urinary incontinence, pelvic organ prolapse, overactive bladder, stress incontinence, vaginal laxity, labial enlargement, mesh complications, and complications from previous surgery have had their lives restored.

Urinary incontinence affects millions of women. Some women have leakage every day, others occasionally. Incontinence is sometimes easily diagnosed based on a personal history and physical exam. Patients who only leak with a cough or laugh or who demonstrate leakage with a full bladder most likely have SUI. Other patients may need further testing to find the cause of their leakage.

Our urogynecologists (surgeons who are trained in the treatment of pelvic floor disorders) use a wide variety of conservative treatment options including dietary changes, pelvic floor muscle exercises, medication, biofeedback, counseling, physical therapy and electrical stimulation. We also use an Interstim Sacral Nerve Root Stimulator, a tiny pacemaker for the bladder which is placed in the lower back to control urinary urgency and frequency.

For women whose quality of life is bad enough, surgery to reconstruct the vaginal supportive tissues is an option. We treat patients utilizing the latest technology as a matter of course and minimally-invasive techniques—including the use of Robotics—whenever possible. We also provide religious and culturally-sensitive care to a large number of Orthodox Jewish women.

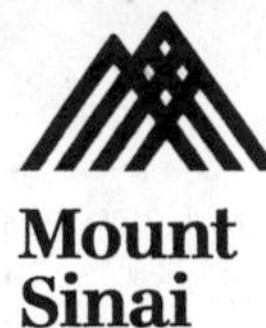

Mount Sinai

THE MOUNT SINAI MEDICAL CENTER

Urology

One Gustave L. Levy Place
Fifth Avenue and 100th Street
New York, NY 10029-6574

Physician Referral: 1-800-MD-SINAI (637-4624)
www.mountsinai.org

THE MILTON AND CARROLL PETRIE DEPARTMENT OF UROLOGY at The Mount Sinai Medical Center offers the latest technologic advances for the diagnosis and treatment of urologic diseases and conditions while supporting a translational and clinical research program.

Prostate Cancer: The Department of Urology's Barbara and Maurice Deane Health and Research Center is at the forefront of diagnosis, treatment and management of localized and advanced prostate cancer. Our surgeons are among the few trained in open, laparoscopic, and robotic surgery. The Robotics Prostatectomy program is one of the world's busiest, with over 4,000 surgeries to date. For men with low grade cancer, we oversee structured and personalized active surveillance. Our research focus is on multi-modal and novel therapies for advanced cancer; our work led to the approval of Provenge®, a cellular immunotherapeutic treatment.

Bladder Cancer: As recognized leaders in the assessment and treatment of all forms of bladder cancer, Mount Sinai urologic oncologists are successfully using tumor markers and new diagnostic techniques. Our surgeons employ robotic and laparoscopic surgery to perform cystectomies (removal of bladder) resulting in minimal impact on quality of life.

Kidney Cancer: Mount Sinai specialists helped pioneer robotic partial nephrectomy for the treatment of small kidney cancers. Other minimally invasive options such as cryoablation (freezing) or radiofrequency ablation (heating) are offered as a means to treat small cancers while preserving maximum kidney function.

Benign Prostatic Hyperplasia (BPH): The Deane Center offers the latest minimally invasive technologies and treatments for BPH, including Holium Laser Enucleation, Greenlight ™ Laser Photoselective Vaporization of the Prostate and bipolar cautery vaporization (Button TURP) in addition to TURP for symptoms of an enlarged prostate. Many of these procedures can be performed on an ambulatory basis.

Reconstructive Urology, Female Urology and Voiding Dysfunction: The Department of Urology provides comprehensive resources for the evaluation and treatment of urinary incontinence, neuro-urologic problems (e.g., spinal cord injury, multiple sclerosis) and pelvic pain syndrome for both men and women. Our specialists are among the few in the country with advanced training in urethral reconstruction. A state-of-the-art continence center provides the convenience of on-site diagnosis and treatment.

THE BARBARA AND MAURICE DEANE PROSTATE HEALTH AND RESEARCH CENTER offers a multidisciplinary approach for the assessment and treatment of all aspects of prostate disease, including cancer, benign enlargement, and inflammation. The Center strives to empower the patient and his family and help them better understand various prostate conditions so they can choose the most appropriate treatment for lasting benefits.

Mount Sinai offers a comprehensive Minimally Invasive Urologic Surgery Program and is a recognized leader in the greater New York area for performing complex and laparoscopic procedures to treat urologic cancers. Areas of focus also include the treatment and management of stone disease and reconstructive procedures for various urologic cancers and anatomic abnormalities.

Erectile Dysfunction and Infertility: The Mount Sinai Sexual Health Program uses the most advanced techniques available to evaluate the causes of erectile dysfunction. Treatment options are extensive and effective. Importantly, patients and their partners receive the guidance they need to make the appropriate personal decision regarding treatment.

Kidney Stones: Mount Sinai's specialists utilize minimally invasive procedures to treat kidney stones, including laser and ultrasonic lithotripsy techniques. Medical and surgical care is highly customized based on type of stone and stone burden.

Infertility: Mount Sinai's state-of-the-art use of medications, in vitro fertilization techniques and microsurgical repairs have resulted in high success rates.

Pediatric Urology: Mount Sinai excels in treating urologic problems in newborns, infants, children and adolescents, The Division of Pediatric Urology is the highest ranked pediatric urology service in New York City by US News and World Report and noted as "superior" for numerous clinical and family services. Minimally invasive procedures are utilized whenever possible, including robotic assisted surgery.

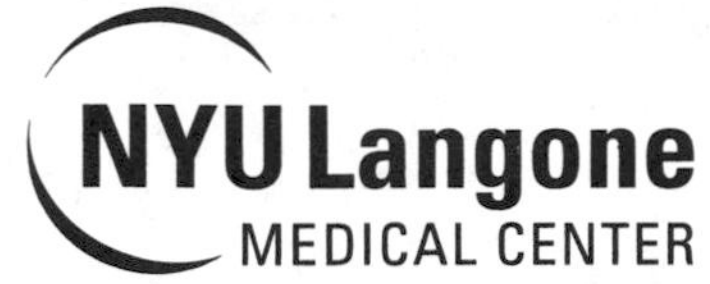

550 First Avenue *(at 31st Street)*
New York, NY 10016

www.NYULMC.org

Physician Referral: **888-7-NYU-MED** *(888-769-8633)*

UROLOGY

Urologists at NYU Langone Medical Center continue to pioneer in the surgical and medical treatment of urological disease and are recognized as a top urology program in the country by U.S. News and World Report.

Smilow Comprehensive Prostate Cancer Center
As part of the NCI-designated NYU Cancer Institute, the Center offers access to a team of uro-oncologic surgeons, radiation oncologists, oncologists and radiologists. Integrative services are available as well.

Benign Prostatic Diseases
Innovative medical and surgical therapies for benign prostatic disease and prostatitis.

Leading Edge Research
We are focused on discovering novel treatments for bladder and prostate cancer, while exploring how cancer markers can be used to determine how cancer treatments are working.

Female Urology and Incontinence
NYU Langone specializes in urological problems unique to women, including recurrent urinary tract infections, pelvic pain, prolapse and sexual dysfunction.

Latest Minimally Invasive Treatments
Advances in prostate imaging and computer biopsy are providing valuable information about tumor location and growth to enable targeted treatment. The latest options are also available to treat kidney stones and other obstructions.

Male Sexual Health
In collaboration with NYU Langone's Fertility Center, urologists use the latest techniques to enable infertile couples to have children. Treatment is also offered to men suffering from erectile dysfunction and low testosterone.

Pediatric Urology and Reconstructive Surgery
Pediatric urologists focus on urinary system disorders in children from birth to early adults.

Robotic Urological Surgery
The Department's robotic surgery program includes prostate and kidney cancers, as well as female incontinence and urinary tract reconstruction.

Urologic Oncology
Because cancer treatment often requires a collaborative approach, urologists work closely with their colleagues at the NYU Cancer Institute to tailor treatments for each patient.

Vascular & Interventional Radiology

For more information about the Interventional Institute or for a physician referral, call 1-877-HOLY-NAME. Please mention "Castle Connolly Guide."

Holy Name Medical Center
Interventional Institute

718 Teaneck Road
Teaneck, NJ 07666
1-877-HOLY-NAME
(1-877-465-9626)
www.holyname.org

A REVOLUTIONARY, NONSURGICAL APPROACH

The Interventional Institute at Holy Name Medical Center offers innovative, nonsurgical treatment options for a broad spectrum of illnesses, from vascular conditions and gynecologic health problems to osteoporosis and cancer.

A dynamic field whose treatment techniques are adaptable to many different medical problems, interventional radiology is a rapidly growing medical specialty devoted to advancing patient care through minimally invasive, targeted treatments that are performed with the assistance of imaging guidance.

Under the leadership of John H. Rundback, MD, an internationally recognized specialist in the field of interventional radiology (IR), board-certified interventionalist physicians insert narrow catheters and miniature instruments through tiny incisions, and navigate them directly to the treatment site. Often performed on an outpatient basis, IR carries fewer risks than surgery, with less discomfort and faster recovery. Most important, treatment results are comparable to those of traditional approaches.

TREAT A WIDE VARIETY OF MEDICAL PROBLEMS

This revolutionary branch of medicine can shrink uterine fibroid tumors that once necessitated a hysterectomy, clear a life-threatening blood clot in a deep leg vein, eliminate leg pain and amputation risk from plaque buildup in the peripheral arteries, resolve unsightly varicose veins, stabilize painful spine fractures due to osteoporosis, and deliver chemotherapy directly to cancer cells.

Services of the Interventional Institute at Holy Name Medical Center:

- Peripheral artery disease (PAD) treatment
- Limb salvage
- Chemoembolization and transcatheter chemoembolization
- Radiofrequency ablation (RFA)
- Ablation of nonresectable lung cancers
- Uterine fibroid embolization
- Fallopian tube recanalization
- Pelvic congestion syndrome
- Deep vein thrombosis (DVT) treatment
- Endovenous laser treatment for varicose veins
- Kyphoplasty and vertebroplasty for osteoporosis
- Microsphere radioembolization

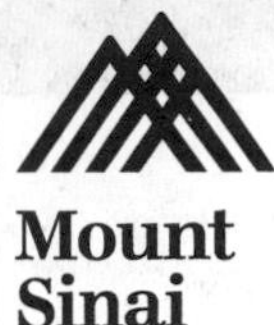

THE MOUNT SINAI MEDICAL CENTER
Interventional Radiology

One Gustave L. Levy Place
Fifth Avenue and 100th Street
New York, NY 10029-6574

Physician Referral: 1-800-MD-SINAI (637-4624)
www.mountsinai.org

The Mount Sinai Medical Center's **DIVISION OF VASCULAR AND INTERVENTIONAL RADIOLOGY** is an acknowledged leader in its growing field. Our experts have developed innovative noninvasive therapies to target cancer and other diseases and routinely use the most advanced technology to offer the safest, most minimally invasive procedures. Our unrivaled expertise draws patients from New York and around the country, as well as Canada, South America, and Europe.

Our interventional radiologists were among the first in the nation to perform diagnostic angiography, percutaneous nephrostomy, non-surgical treatment for uterine fibroids, and transarterial therapy for liver cancer. We were among the first to employ drug-eluting (coated) stents to treat peripheral arterial disease and restore circulation to the legs, and we are one of only a few hospitals with a dedicated Fibroid Care Center offering women the full range of minimally invasive therapies for symptomatic uterine fibroids.

Advanced Multidisciplinary Approach

Our physicians collaborate with colleagues across disciplines and specialties so patients benefit from the insights of multiple experts. We deliver the highest level care for:

- Liver disease
- Uterine fibroid embolization
- Liver cancer
- Deep vein thrombosis (DVT)
- Varicose veins
- End stage renal disease/hemodialysis
- Kidney cancer
- Peripheral arterial disease
- Vascular anomalies and malformations

Our **Translational and Molecular Imaging Institute**, a state-of-the-art, 25,000 square foot imaging research facility, which formally opened in 2012 in our new **Center for Science and Medicine**, serves as the hub for basic and clinical research programs in neurologic, oncologic, cardiovascular, abdominal imaging and other specialties. It is also the center for nanomedicine at Mount Sinai, exploring nanotechnology-based techniques for medical diagnostics and drug delivery.

NYU Langone
MEDICAL CENTER

CARDIAC AND VASCULAR INSTITUTE
550 First Avenue *(at 31st Street)*
New York, NY 10016
www.NYULMC.org
Physician Referral: **888-7-NYU-MED** *(888-769-8633)*

CARDIAC AND VASCULAR INSTITUTE

The Cardiac and Vascular Institute (CVI) at NYU Langone Medical Center continues to advance new techniques for repairing heart valves, curing heart rhythm disorders, and treating aortic diseases and congestive heart failure. We care for both adults and children. CVI is consistently ranked among the leading heart and heart surgery centers in *U.S. News & World Report's annual 'Best Hospitals'* rankings.

Cardiac Catheterization CVI offers superior catheter-based diagnosis and evaluation of cardiac health. Our laboratory provides a full range of procedures to evaluate, diagnose, and provide treatment options.

Cardiac Rehabilitation and Prevention The Joan and Joel Smilow Cardiopulmonary Rehabilitation and Prevention Center provides individualized treatment plans through NYU Langone's Rusk Rehabilitation, in a state-of-the-art and comfortable facility.

Cardiac Surgery NYU Langone is a nationally recognized leader in advanced surgical treatments for adult and congenital heart disease. We have world-renowned expertise in mitral valve repair, aortic valve replacement and aortic aneurysm repair, as well as specializing in high-risk and elderly patients.

Cardiology The Leon H. Charney Division of Cardiology is a leader in cardiovascular patient care, biomedical research, and education. We are advancing the field of cardiovascular medicine through a variety of innovative collaborations.

Congenital Heart Disease The pediatric and adult congenital cardiac program treats patients of all ages with inherited and acquired cardiac defects. We have a highly experienced team of specialists in pediatric and adult cardiology, pediatric interventional cardiology, congenital cardiac surgery, neonatal and pediatric cardiac intensive care, pediatric cardiac anesthesiology, nursing, and extracorporeal perfusion.

Heart Failure A multidisciplinary team offers the most advanced care for heart failure including echocardiograms, pacemaker and defibrillator implantations, open heart surgeries, and left ventricular assist devices.

Nuclear Cardiology/Stress The Nuclear Cardiology/Stress Laboratory performs a range of tests that assist cardiologists in the assessment and diagnosis of heart disease.

Vascular Surgery We offer diagnostic and treatment for patients with conditions ranging from arterial aneurysms to deep vein thrombosis, as well as carotid stenosis and limb salvage including minimally invasive vein surgery, endovascular aortic surgery, thoracic aneurysm correction and abdominal aneurysm interventions.

Vascular Surgery

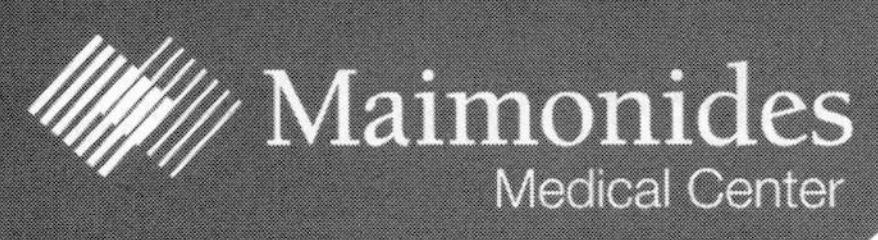

HEART &
VASCULAR CENTER
4802 Tenth Avenue
Brooklyn, New York 11219
Phone: 718.283.7957 • Fax: 718.283.8599
www.maimonidesmed.org/vascular

The Division of Vascular and Endovascular Surgery and Cardiac Institute and were integrated in 2013 to form the Maimonides Heart & Vascular Center.

Vascular Services

Vascular & Endovascular Surgery, now part of the Maimonides Heart & Vascular Center, offer comprehensive diagnostic, clinical and surgical services for patients with vascular disease and associated conditions. Under the direction of Robert Rhee, MD, our vascular team is renowned for its services in wound care, limb salvage, aneurysm repair, blocked arteries, varicose veins and chronic lower limb ischemia, as well as balloon angioplasties, stents and carotid artery dissections.

In addition to traditional open surgery, Maimonides places a focus on therapeutic options based on minimally invasive, endovascular and catheter-directed techniques. Our team of physicians is board-certified, highly-experienced and makes use of innovative technologies, such as our new hybrid OR. At Maimonides, specialists can combine both surgical and catheter techniques to maximize care.

Vascular Diagnostic Laboratory

Accredited by the Intersocietal Commission for the Accreditation of Vascular Laboratories, the Vascular Diagnostic Laboratory at Maimonides performs screening, diagnostic and post-operative non-invasive imaging using state-of-the-art ultrasound and Doppler machines. We offer sophisticated ultrasound examinations, eliminating the need for invasive angiograms. Precise determinations of blood flow to vital organs and limbs are obtained and serve as the basis for further treatment. These findings are reported within 24 hours, enabling physicians to make timely and informed decisions about the future course of therapy for their patients.

We offer a range of diagnostic services, including:

- Ultrasound Vascular Diagnostic Testing
- Arteriograms
- Magnetic Resonance Angiography
- Plethysmography
- Pulse Volume Recordings
- Transcutaneous Oximetry
- Venograms
- Duplex Ultrasound
- Venous Reflux Evaluation and Venous DVT Studies
- Vein Mapping
- Aortic Aneurysm Studies

Vascular services has received accreditation by the Intersocietal Commission for the Accreditation of Vascular Laboratories, which assures patients that they are receiving the highest standard of care possible at the Vascular Diagnostics Laboratory. Every staff member is committed to excellence in all aspects of service. Our experienced technicians perform precise diagnostic imaging and are leaders in their fields.

Maimonides Medical Center

**The right care.
Right here.**

www.maimonidesmed.org/vascular

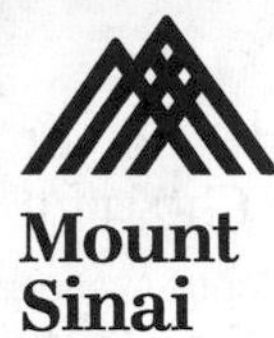

THE MOUNT SINAI MEDICAL CENTER

Vascular Surgery

One Gustave L. Levy Place
Fifth Avenue and 100th Street
New York, NY 10029-6574

Physician Referral: 1-800-MD-SINAI (637-4624)
www.mountsinai.org

THE DIVISION OF VASCULAR SURGERY at The Mount Sinai Medical Center is committed to delivering unrivaled patient care and embracing the safest and most effective treatment innovations. Past decades have seen dramatic advances in the treatment of vascular disease, and our surgeons have contributed to this progress by developing new techniques in aneurysm repair and stroke prevention designed to minimize discomfort and improve outcomes.

Peter L. Faries, MD, Chief of the Division of Vascular Surgery, and Michael L. Marin, MD, Chairman of the Department of Surgery, have assembled a team of internationally recognized surgeons dedicated to clinical excellence and comprehensive patient care.

What We Treat

- **Aneurysmal Disease:** We excel in diagnosing and treating aneurysmal disease and offer the most advanced and minimally invasive treatments available to repair aortic aneurysms, thoracic aortic aneurysms and aneurysms of other blood vessels.

- **Carotid Disease and Stroke Prevention:** Having helped pioneer their development, we are proficient in both carotid endarterectomy surgery and carotid stenting. This level of expertise allows us to offer unbiased counseling and tailor the most advanced procedures to the specific needs of each patient.

- **Dialysis Access:** When patients require dialysis, we are adept at providing access points. The three points of access are through a catheter, through an arteriovenous (AV) graft, or an arteriovenous (AV) fistula.

- **Peripheral Vascular Disease:** We are highly skilled in restoring blood flow to the legs and correcting the symptoms of peripheral vascular disease (PVD), through both minimally invasive and traditional techniques.

- **Venous Disease:** We offer multiple treatment options (both surgical and non-surgical) for varicose and spider veins.

Because our expertise encompasses a broad array of patient services, nearly every patient condition can be managed successfully. Our vascular surgeons, together with our award-winning nurses and ancillary staff, are dedicated to achieving unsurpassed quality in patient care. Our emphasis on comprehensive caring for both the mental and physical health of our patients has resulted in more effective therapy. We pride ourselves on providing the highest level of compassion and communication with our patients and families, serving as a model for medical centers worldwide.

The Best in American Medicine
www.CastleConnolly.com

Women's Health

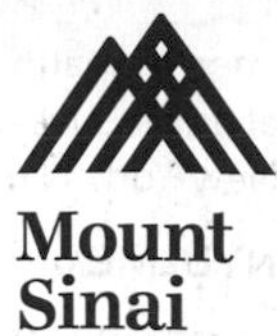

THE MOUNT SINAI MEDICAL CENTER

Women's Health Services

One Gustave L. Levy Place
Fifth Avenue and 100th Street
New York, NY 10029-6574

Physician Referral: 1-800-MD-SINAI (637-4624)
www.mountsinai.org

The Mount Sinai Medical Center's **WOMEN'S HEALTH SERVICES** represent the depth and breadth of women's health care—from preventive care and routine gynecologic services and cancer screenings to cardiology, complex surgeries, genetic screening and more—placing us among the very best in providing comprehensive health care to women throughout every stage of life.

About Mount Sinai Women's Health Services

We are committed to comprehensive, multidisciplinary preventive care for women. The goal of our women's health services is to promote primary care and prevention through health education and screening.

Consistently ranked among the nation's best hospitals by *U.S. News & World Report*, Mount Sinai offers a wide range of women's health care services including, but not limited to:

- Gynecology
- Primary care
- Gastroenterology
- Cardiovascular services
- Dermatology
- Breast health
- Cancer screening
- Genetic counseling
- Endocrinology

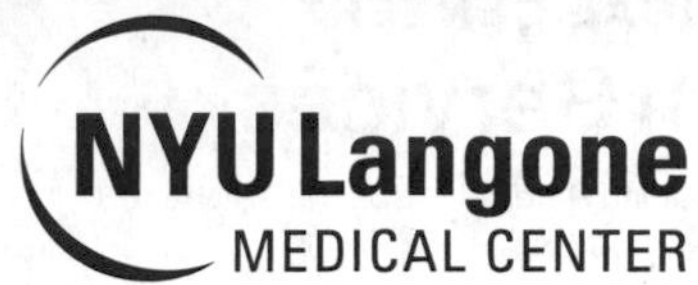

Joan H. Tisch Center for Women's Health
207 East 84th Street *(at 3rd Avenue)*
New York, NY
www.NYULMC.org
646-754-3300
Physician Referral: **888-7-NYU-MED** *(888-769-8633)*

THE JOAN H. TISCH CENTER FOR WOMEN'S HEALTH

About the Joan H. Tisch Center for Women's Health

Because many diseases and conditions impact women differently than men, NYU Langone Medical Center has created the Joan H. Tisch Center for Women's Health. Offering a comprehensive array of primary and specialty care, the Joan H. Tisch Center for Women's Health is New York City's premier destination for healthcare services tailored to the special needs of women. Conveniently located in the heart of Manhattan's Upper East Side, the Center combines NYU Langone's tradition of excellence with a multidisciplinary approach to providing individuals with the best possible medical care. At the Joan H. Tisch Center for Women's Health, the goal is maintaining excellent health and the vehicle is a caring, nurturing environment which understands that women are more than a collection of symptoms and medical conditions.

Expert Staff

Primary and specialty care physicians at the Joan H. Tisch Center for Women's Health have been carefully chosen for their ability to deliver quality, compassionate care to women. These healthcare professionals are focused on the holistic needs of patients in a state-of-the-art setting that relies heavily on teamwork. As part of a major academic medical institution, the Center is able to draw on additional healthcare resources and innovative research, when the need arises.

Comprehensive Range of Services

The Joan H. Tisch Center for Women's Health offers a wide range of primary and specialty medical care geared to women at a single location. Specialty services include breast health, cardiology, dermatology, endocrinology, ear/nose/throat, gastroenterology, gynecology, gynecologic oncology, internal medicine, neurology, orthopaedics, Rusk Rehabilitation, plastic surgery, psychiatry and psychology, pulmonology, radiology, rheumatology, urology, vascular surgery and women's imaging.

Technology

The Joan H. Tisch Center for Women's Health has incorporated sophisticated technology into all levels of the patient experience. This ranges from the Center's informative website to its use of Epic, the Medical Center's up-to-the-minute electronic medical records system. In addition, patients can confidentially view their medical records and test results, as well as make appointments, request prescriptions and communicate with their physicians, through NYULangoneHealth, a secure online service.

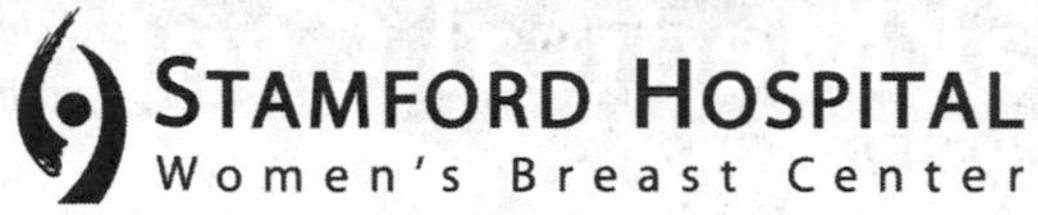

StamfordHospital.org/womenshealth

Women's Breast Center

The Women's Breast Center offers compassionate, convenient and comprehensive breast care supported by the most advanced technology in a setting designed to make every patient feel as relaxed and comfortable as possible.

Advanced Technology

The only breast center in the region and among the first in the country, to offer 3-D tomosynthesis for every patient receiving screening mammography. Research shows, 3-D tomosynthesis increases the cancer detection rate by 27% over digital mammography, and decreases the recall rate by 20-40%, which results in less anxiety and fewer diagnostic mammograms.

Multi-disciplinary Team Approach

Our expert team is comprised of fellowship-trained female breast surgeons, reconstructive plastic surgeons, breast imaging fellowship-trained radiologists, breast pathologists, medical and radiation oncologists, nurse navigator and genetic counselor. The team meets on a weekly basis to discuss the best possible individualized treatment for each patient.

Personalized Care

In the event a problem is identified, our patients will have immediate follow up testing, see a surgeon within 24–26 hours and have the support of a dedicated nurse navigator to guide them through the process, from diagnosis through treatment and beyond. We work closely with the Integrative Medicine and Wellness team and the Bennett Cancer Center, in providing support services. All patients seen during normal business hours will receive their results prior to leaving the Center. Evening and weekend patients will receive their results the next business day. To schedule a mammogram today, call 203.276.PINK.

Academic and Clinical Affiliations

Stamford Hospital is an affiliate of the New York–Presbyterian Healthcare System and a major teaching affiliate of the Columbia University College of Physicians & Surgeons.

Accreditation

Joint Commission on Accreditation of Healthcare Organization (JCAHO)

Beds

305

Sponsorship

Voluntary, Not-for-Profit

For a Physician Referral or more information, please call 1.877.233.9355 or visit StamfordHospital.org /doctor.

Stamford Hospital
30 Shelburne Road
Stamford, CT 06902
203.276.1000

StamfordHospital.org

Trinitas Regional Medical Center

WOMEN'S SERVICES

225 Williamson Street | Elizabeth, New Jersey 07207
Ph 908.994.5138 | www.TrinitasRMC.org

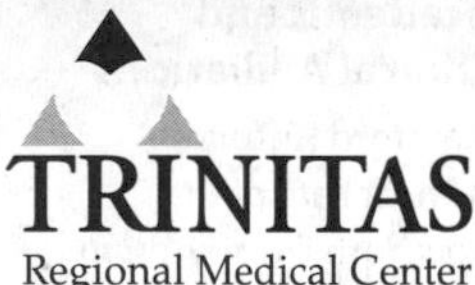

Trinitas Regional Medical Center offers a number of advanced services just for women that range from the latest in imaging and diagnostic technology, to state-of-the-art, minimally invasive procedures used for hysterectomies and in the treatment of incontinence and prolapse.

Women's Imaging Center

Our new, technologically advanced, FDA-approved and MQSA (Mammography Quality Standards Act) certified facility provides the services - digital mammography, stereotactic needle biopsy, ultrasound and bone densitometry - that are essential in addressing women's concerns.

The staff in the Women's Imaging Center has had specialized training, and they will work with you and your physician to provide services in a comfortable and professional environment. State-of-the-art digital mammography equipment further enhances the diagnostic quality of the images of the breast tissue and the accuracy of the interpretation of the mammogram. All studies are interpreted by Board Certified Radiologists.

Procedures may be scheduled by calling 908-994-5984.

Treatment for Incontinence and Prolapse

Trinitas is a pioneer in the latest, minimally invasive procedures for the treatment of female incontinence and vaginal prolapse. A new approach to prolapse includes a single-incision approach that shortens surgical time, minimizes tissue trauma and reduces recovery time. The treatment of incontinence is also accomplished with highly effective, minimally invasive techniques, many performed for the first time in New Jersey at Trinitas Regional Medical Center. Single-incision techniques involve the placement of an internal supporting sling that is highly effective in eliminating stress incontinence. Procedures are commonly performed on an outpatient basis using the da Vinci Surgical System.

Minimally Invasive Hysterectomy

Trinitas Regional Medical Center offers a non-surgical option for women who undergo hysterectomy to treat excessive menstrual or uterine bleeding. Endometrial Ablation involves removing only the lining of a woman's uterus using warmed water.

In the event that surgery is necessary, Trinitas now offers a precise, minimally invasive option for hysterectomy through the use of the da Vinci® Surgical System. The da Vinci system provides surgeons with an alternative to both traditional open surgery and conventional laparoscopy, putting a surgeon's hands at the controls of a state-of-the-art robotic platform. The da Vinci® Surgical System enables surgeons to perform even the most complex and delicate procedures through very small incisions with unmatched precision. Benefits for patients include significantly less pain, less blood loss, less scarring, shorter recovery time, a faster return to normal daily activities and, in many cases, better clinical outcomes.

The Best in American Medicine
www.CastleConnolly.com

Wound Care

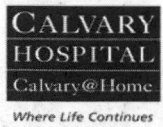

CALVARY HOSPITAL
1740 Eastchester Road
Bronx, NY 10461
Tel: (718) 518-2000
www.calvaryhospital.org

CENTER FOR CURATIVE AND PALLIATIVE WOUND CARE

Founded in 1899, Calvary Hospital is the nation's only acute care specialty hospital dedicated to caring for inpatients with advanced cancer. We serve people of all faith traditions in a restraint-free environment that offers 24/7 visiting hours and extensive bereavement support for families and friends. In addition to inpatient care, we offer outpatient care, home care, hospice, nursing home hospice, and wound care. All Calvary care is guided by our core values of compassion, respect for the dignity of every patient, and non-abandonment of patients and families.

Calvary Wound Care: A Proud Tradition
In the course of caring for people with advanced cancer, Calvary has developed outstanding expertise in the care of complex, intractable wounds. We extend this care to people in the community through our outpatient clinic. In 2004, we established the Center for Curative and Palliative Wound Care, where we treat patients with chronic wounds secondary to diabetes, neuropathy, chronic venous insufficiency, immobility, lymphedema, peripheral vascular disease, cancer, and other inflammatory or hematological disorders that can cause wounds. Since its inception, Calvary's Wound Care Center has recorded more than 42,000 patient visits.

A Personalized Approach
Our personalized approach to wound management goes beyond established curative protocols to address the larger goals of patient care, by seeking to enhance quality of life for patients and families. We strive to relieve the suffering of patients when wounds do not respond to standard interventions, or when demands of treatment are beyond their tolerance or stamina.

The Center for Curative and Palliative Wound Care offers treatment options for chronic wounds such as:

Venous Ulcers	Diabetic Foot Ulcers	Arterial Ulcers
Pressure Ulcers	Inflammatory Wounds	Vasculitic Ulcers
Lymphedema	Sickle Cell Ulcers	Fungating Tumors
Post-op Wounds	Wound Infection	Wounds from Radiation or Chemotherapy

Wound care personnel are available to consult with nursing homes and long-term care facilities on request. Specially trained visiting nurses and therapists provide expert wound care services for patients at home.

We are a community resource for Bronx residents, where the prevalence of Type 2 Diabetes is the highest in New York and among the highest in the country.

Support for Families
Family members often serve as caregivers. Our physicians and nurses strive to build a foundation of trust and open communication with patients and families. We teach family members to clean wounds and change dressings, and we are always available to answer questions or offer guidance about wound care.

Research is integral to the mission of the Center, which is now pursuing a number of protocols focusing on novel treatments for wounds related to diabetes and other disorders.

For information or to refer a patient to the Wound Care Center, please call (718) 518-2577.

Trinitas Regional Medical Center

CENTER FOR WOUND HEALING & HYPERBARIC MEDICINE

240 WILLIAMSON STREET, SUITE 104 | ELIZABETH, NEW JERSEY 07207
PH 908.994.5480 | WWW.WOUNDHEALINGCENTER.ORG

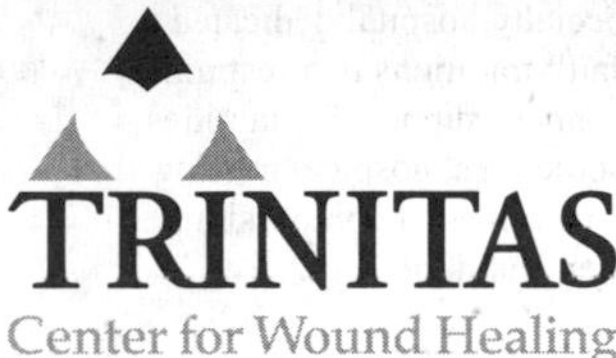

AWARD-WINNING CARE FOR HARD-TO-HEAL WOUNDS

At the Center for Wound Healing & Hyperbaric Medicine, our unique team of highly trained physicians, nurses and foot specialists can help sufferers get their lives back. We specialize in non-healing wounds - those that have resisted healing after months and even years of traditional treatment. This is accomplished with a success rate that is consistently 90% and above, and the vast majority of our patients leave the Center completely healed in an average of just 28 days.

The treatment options offered at the Center include the Vacuum-Assisted Closure (VAC) Therapy System, Hyperbaric Oxygen Therapy, and Apligraf cultured living skin.

Wounds don't heal for a variety of reasons. Diabetes, smoking, poor circulation, heart problems, poor nutrition and many medications may prevent healing. As one of the nation's leading centers for wound healing, we see a complex array of hard-to-heal wounds in patients from all races, nationalities and economic backgrounds. Hard-to-heal wounds come in all shapes and sizes, and can affect many parts of the body.

The five main types of wounds treated at Trinitas are pressure ulcers, venous ulcers, diabetic ulcers, arterial ulcers and trauma wounds. Our approach to wound healing is holistic in that we look at the entire person, not just the wound. How is the wound affecting the patient's life? What other lifestyle factors might hinder successful wound healing? What genetic factors contribute to the patient's overall well-being?

By using well-researched, proven techniques, our multi-disciplinary team provides healing and relief for patients who previously thought their wounds were irreparable or would ultimately result in amputation.

The Center for Wound Healing & Hyperbaric Medicine, named by Praxis Clinical Services as "Center of the Year," was the first in the state to use such innovative technologies as the Apligraf living skin device. The expertise of the Center's physicians in pioneering wound closure technologies such as the Vacuum Assisted Closure (VAC) was shared recently at a number of national wound healing conferences. The Center ranks as one of the top Centers for Wound Healing in the nation.

In 2011, the Center received the Robert Warriner III, MD, "Center of Excellence" award from Diversified Clinical Services (DCS) in recognition of its excellent clinical results. The award salutes Trinitas for exceeding DCS's benchmarks in Healing Outcomes, Patient Satisfaction, Outlier Management, and Clinical Performance. In attaining this recognition, Trinitas is in the top 15 percent of the 340 wound care centers managed by DCS.

SECTION FIVE

Appendices

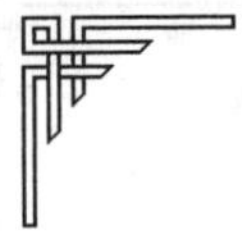

The Best in American Medicine
www.CastleConnolly.com

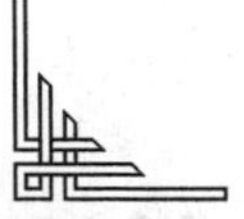
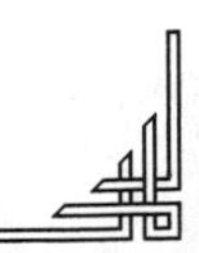

Appendix A:
Medical Boards

Intro to ABMS and Osteopathic Specialties

The following pages contain descriptions of the "official" medical specialties, approved by the American Board of Medical Specialists (for M.D.s) or by the American Osteopathic Association (for D.O.s). These are important because they are the only specialties recognized by the official governing boards. There may be physicians who call themselves one kind of specialist or another, but they may not be certified by the "official" boards. There are, in fact, over 100 such "self-designated" boards, some simply groups of physicians interested in a given area of medicine with no qualifications for membership to other groups with very specific qualifications for membership.

It is important for the medical consumer to seek out physicians certified by the ABMS or AOA to assure their doctor has had the appropriate training and passed the board certification exam.

ABMS

The ABMS is an organization of ABMS approved medical specialty boards. The mission of the ABMS is to maintain and improve the quality of medical care by assisting the Member Boards in their efforts to develop and utilize professional and educational standards for the evaluation and certification of physician specialists. The intent of certification of physicians is to provide assurance to the public that a physician specialist certified by a Member Board of the ABMS has successfully completed an approved educational program and evaluation process which includes an examination designed to assess the knowledge, skills, and experience required to provide quality patient care in that specialty. The ABMS serves to coordinate the activities of its Member Boards and to provide information to the public, the government, the profession and its Members concerning issues involving specialization and certification in medicine.

Following is a list of the addresses of the various medical specialty boards approved by the ABMS. Note that there are 24 board organizations for 25 medical specialties. Psychiatry and Neurology share the same board.

To find out if a physician is certified, consumers can call the individual boards which may charge a fee for the information, or they can contact the ABMS at 866-275-2267 (no fee) or www.abms.org.

American Board of Allergy and Immunology
111 South Independence Mall East
Suite 701
Philadelphia, PA 19106
(215) 592-9466, (866) 264-5568

General Certification in Allergy and Immunology. Certifications awarded since 1989 are valid for 10 years. For those certified prior to 1989 there is no recertification requirement.

American Board of Anesthesiology
4208 Six Forks Rd, Ste 1500
Raleigh, NC 27609-5735
(866) 999-7501

General Certification in Anesthesiology; with Special and Added Qualifications in Critical Care Medicine, Hospice & Palliative Medicine, Pain Medicine and Pediatric Anesthesiology. Certifications awarded since 2000 are valid for 10 years.

American Board of Colon and Rectal Surgery
20600 Eureka Road, Suite 600
Taylor, MI 48180
(734) 282-9400

General Certification in Colon and Rectal Surgery. Certifications awarded since 1990 are valid for 10 years.

American Board of Dermatology
Henry Ford Health System
1 Ford Place
Detroit, MI 48202-3450
(313) 874-1088

General Certification in Dermatology; with Special Qualifications in Dermatopathology, and Pediatric Dermatology. Certifications awarded since 1991 are valid for 10 years.

American Board of Emergency Medicine
3000 Coolidge Road
East Lansing, MI 48823-6319
(517) 332-4800

General Certification in Emergency Medicine; with Special and Added Qualifications in Critical Care Medicine, Emergency Medical Services, Hospice & Palliative Medicine, Medical Toxicology, Pediatric Emergency Medicine, Sports Medicine and Undersea and Hyperbaric Medicine. Certifications awarded since 1980 are valid for 10 years.

American Board of Family Practice
1648 McGrathiana Parkway, Suite 550
Lexington, KY 40511
(859) 269-5626, (888) 995-5700

General Certification in Family Practice; with Added Qualifications in Adolescent Medicine, Geriatric Medicine, Hospice & Palliative Medicine, Sleep Medicine and Sports Medicine. Certifications awarded since 1970 are valid for 7 years.

American Board of Internal Medicine
510 Walnut Street, Suite 1700
Philadelphia, PA 19106-3699
(215) 446-3500, (800) 441-ABIM

General Certification in Internal Medicine; with Special Qualifications in Cardiovascular Disease, Endocrinology, Diabetes and Metabolism, Gastroenterology, Hematology, Infectious Disease, Medical Oncology, Nephrology, Pulmonary Disease, and Rheumatology; and Added Qualifications in Adolescent Medicine, Advanced Heart Failure & Transplant Cardiology, Clinical Cardiac Electrophysiology, Critical Care Medicine, Geriatric Medicine, Hospice & Palliative Medicine, Interventional Cardiology, Sleep Medicine, Sports Medicine and Transplant Hepatology. Certifications awarded since 1990 are valid for 10 years.

American Board of Medical Genetics
9650 Rockville Pike
Bethesda, MD 20814-3998
(301) 634-7315

General Certification in Clinical Genetics (MD), Clinical Biochemical Genetics, Clinical Cytogenetics and Clinical Molecular Genetics; with Added Qualifications in Medical Biochemical Genetics, Molecular Genetic Pathology. Certifications awarded since 2002 are valid for 2 years.

American Board of Neurological Surgery
245 Amity Road, Suite 208
Woodbridge, CT 06525
(203) 397-2267

General Certification in Neurological Surgery. Certifications awarded since 1999 are valid for 10 years.

American Board of Nuclear Medicine
4555 Forest Park Boulevard, Suite 119
St. Louis, MO 63108
(314) 367-2225

General Certification in Nuclear Medicine. Certifications awarded since 1992 are valid for 10 years.

American Board of Obstetrics and Gynecology
2915 Vine Street
Dallas, TX 75204
(214) 871-1619

General Certification in Obstetrics and Gynecology; with Special Qualifications in Gynecologic Oncology, Maternal and Fetal Medicine, Reproductive Endocrinology/Infertility; and Added Qualifications in Female Pelvic Medicine & Reconstructive Surgery, Hospice & Palliative Medicine and Critical Care Medicine. Certifications awarded since 1986 are valid for 6 years.

American Board of Ophthalmology
111 Presidential Boulevard, Suite 241
Bala Cynwyd, PA 19004-1075
(610) 664-1175

General certification in Ophthalmology. Certifications awarded since 1992 are valid for 10 years. For those certified prior to 1992 there is no recertification requirement.

American Board of Orthopaedic Surgery
400 Silver Cedar Court
Chapel Hill, NC 27514
(919) 929-7103

General Certification in Orthopaedic Surgery; with Added Qualification in Hand Surgery and Orthopaedic Sports Medicine. Certifications awarded since 1986 are valid for 10 years.

American Board of Otolaryngology

5615 Kirby Drive, Suite 600
Houston, TX 77005
(713) 850-0399

General Certification in Otolaryngology; with Added Qualifications in Neurotology, Pediatric Otolaryngology, Plastic Surgery within the Head and Neck and Sleep Medicine. Certifications awarded since 2002 are valid for 10 years.

American Board of Pathology

4830 Kennedy Boulevard
Suite 690
Tampa, FL 33609
(813) 286-2444

General Certification in Anatomic and Clinical Pathology, Anatomic Pathology and Clinical Pathology; with Special Qualifications in Blood Banking/Transfusion Medicine, Chemical Pathology, Dermatopathology, Forensic Pathology, Hematology, Medical Microbiology, Molecular Genetic Pathology, Neuropathology and Pediatric Pathology; and Added Qualifications in Clinical Informatics and Cytopathology. Certifications awarded since 1997 are valid for 10 years.

American Board of Pediatrics

111 Silver Cedar Court
Chapel Hill, NC 27514-1651
(919) 929-0461

General Certification in Pediatrics; with Special Qualifications in Adolescent Medicine, Developmental-Behavioral Pediatrics, Neonatal-Perinatal Medicine, Pediatric Cardiology, Pediatric Critical Care Medicine, Pediatric Emergency Medicine, Pediatric Endocrinology, Pediatric Gastroenterology, Pediatric Hematology-Oncology, Pediatric Infectious Diseases, Pediatric Nephrology, Pediatric Pulmonology, and Pediatric Rheumatology; and Added Qualifications in Child Abuse Pediatrics, Hospice & Palliative Medicine, Medical Toxicology, Neurodevelopmental Disabilities, Pediatric Transplant Hepatology, Sleep Medicine and Sports Medicine. Certifications awarded since 1988 valid for 7 years.

American Board of Physical Medicine and Rehabilitation
3015 Allegro Park Lane, S.W.
Rochester, MN 55902-4139
(507) 282-1776

General Certification in Physical Medicine and Rehabilitation; with Special Qualifications in Pain Medicine, Pediatric Rehabilitation Medicine, and Spinal Cord Injury Medicine; and Added Qualifications in Brain Injury Medicine, Hospice & Palliative Medicine, Neuromuscular Medicine and Sports Medicine. Certifications awarded since 1993 are valid for 10 years.

American Board of Plastic Surgery
Seven Penn Center, Suite 400
1635 Market Street
Philadelphia, PA 19103-2204
(215) 587-9322

General Certification in Plastic Surgery; with Added Qualifications in Hand Surgery and Head & Neck Surgery. Certifications awarded since 1995 are valid for 10-years.

American Board of Preventive Medicine
111 W. Jackson, Suite 1110
Chicago, IL 60604
(312) 939-ABPM [2276]

General Certification in Aerospace Medicine, Occupational Medicine and Public Health and General Preventive Medicine; with Added Qualifications in Clinical Informatics, Medical Toxicology and Undersea and Hyperbaric Medicine. Certifications awarded since 1997 are valid for 10 years.

American Board of Psychiatry and Neurology
2150 E. Lake Cook Road, Suite 900
Buffalo Grove, IL 60089
(847) 229-6500

General Certification in Psychiatry, Neurology and Neurology with Special Qualification in Child Neurology; with Special Qualifications in Child and Adolescent Psychiatry, Epilepsy, Hospice & Palliative Medicine, Pain Medicine and Sleep Medicine; and Added Qualifications in Addiction Psychiatry, Brain Injury Medicine, Clinical Neurophysiology, Epilepsy, Forensic Psychiatry, Geriatric Psychiatry, Hospice & Palliative Medicine, Neurodevelopmental Disabilities, Psychosomatic Medicine and Vascular Neurology. Certifications awarded since 1994 are valid for 10 years.

American Board of Radiology
5441 E. Williams Circle
Tucson, AZ 85711
(520) 790-3200

General Certification in Diagnostic Radiology, Medical Physics or Radiation Oncology; with Special Competency in Nuclear Radiology; and Added Qualifications in Hospice & Palliative Medicine, Neuroradiology, Pediatric Radiology and Vascular and Interventional Radiology. Radiological Physics is a non-clinical certification. Certificates are valid for 10 years.

American Board of Surgery
1617 John F. Kennedy Boulevard, Suite 860
Philadelphia, PA 19103-1847
(215) 568-4000

General Certification in Surgery and Vascular Surgery; with Special Qualifications in Pediatric Surgery and Surgery of the Hand; and Added Qualifications in Complex General Surgical Oncology, Hospice & Palliative Medicine and Surgical Critical Care. Certifications awarded since 1976 are valid for 10 years.

American Board of Thoracic Surgery
633 North St. Clair Street, Suite 2320
Chicago, IL 60611
(312) 202-5900

General Certification in Thoracic and Cardiac Surgery; and Added Qualifications in Congenital Cardiac Surgery. Certifications awarded since 1976 are valid for 10 years.

American Board of Urology
600 Peter Jefferson Parkway, Suite 150
Charlottesville, VA 22911
(434) 979-0059

General Certification in Urology; and Added Qualifications in Pediatric Urology. Certifications awarded as of 1985 are valid for 10 years.

Osteopathic

The American Osteopathic Association (AOA) is a member association representing more than 78,000 osteopathic physicians (D.O.s). The AOA serves as the primary certifying body for D.O.s, and is the accrediting agency for all osetopathic medical colleges and healthcare facilities. The AOA's mission is to advance the philosophy and practice of osteopathic medicine by promoting excellence in education, research, and the delivery of quality, cost-effective healthcare within a distinct, unified profession.

American Osteopathic Association
142 E Ontario Street
Chicago, IL 60611

Consumers may call the American Osteopathic Association at (800) 621-1773 or visit the website, www.osteopathic.org, for general certification information.

American Osteopathic Board of Anesthesiology

General certification in Anesthesiology; with Added Qualifications in Critical Care Medicine, and Pain Management. Certifications awarded since 2004 are valid for 10 years. For those certified prior to 2004 there is no recertification requirement.

American Osteopathic Board of Dermatology

General certification in Dermatology; with Added Qualifications in Dermatopathology and Mohs'-Micrographic Surgery. Certifications awarded since 2004 are valid for 10 years.

American Osteopathic Board of Emergency Medicine

General certification in Emergency Medicine; with Added Qualifications in Emergency Medical Services, Medical Toxicology, and Sports Medicine. Certifications awarded since 1994 are valid for 10 years.

American Osteopathic Board of Family Physicians

General certification in Family Practice and Osteopathic Manipulative Treatment (OMT); with Added Qualifications in Geriatric Medicine, Hospice & Palliative Medicine, Sleep Medicine, Sports Medicine and Undersea & Hyperbaric Medicine. Certifications awarded since March 1,1997 are valid for 8 years.

American Osteopathic Board of Internal Medicine

General certification in Internal Medicine; with Special Qualifications in Allergy/Immunology, Cardiology, Endocrinology, Gastroenterology, Hematology, Infectious Disease, Nephrology, Oncology, Pulmonary Disease, Rheumatology; with Added Qualifications in Addiction Medicine, Critical Care Medicine, Clinical Cardiac Electrophysiology, Hospice & Palliative Medicine, Geriatric Medicine, Interventional Cardiology, Sleep Medicine, Sports Medicine and Undersea & Hyperbaric Medicine. Certifications awarded since 1993 are valid for 10 years.

American Osteopathic Board of Neurology and Psychiatry

General certification in Neurology and Psychiatry; with Special Qualifications in Child/Adolescent Psychiatry and Child/Adolescent Neurology; with Added Qualifications in Addiction Medicine, Geriatric Psychiatry, Hospice & Palliative Medicine, Neurophysiology, and Sleep Medicine. Certifications awarded since 1995 are valid for 10 years.

American Osteopathic Board of Neuromusculoskeletal Medicine

General certification in Neuromusculoskelatal Medicine & Osteopathic Manipulative Medicine; with Added qualifications in Sports Medicine.

American Osteopathic Board of Nuclear Medicine

General certification in Nuclear Medicine. Certifications awarded since 1995 are valid for 10 years. This certification is no longer issued.

American Osteopathic Board of Obstetrics and Gynecology

General certification in Obstetrics and Gynecology; with Special Qualifications in Gynecologic Oncology; Maternal and Fetal Medicine and Reproductive Endocrinology. Certifications awarded since June 2002 are valid for 6 years.

American Osteopathic Board of Ophthalmology and Otolaryngology - Head & Neck Surgery

General certification in Ophthalmology, Otolaryngology, Facial Plastic Surgery and Otolaryngology/Facial Plastic Surgery; with Added Qualifications in Otolaryngic Allergy and Sleep Medicine. Certifications awarded in Ophthalmology since 2000 are valid for 10 years. For those certified prior to 2000 there is no recertification requirement. Certifications awarded in Otolaryngology and/or Otolaryngology/Facial Plastic Surgery since 2002 are valid for 10 years.

American Osteopathic Board of Orthopaedic Surgery

General certification in Orthopaedic Surgery; with Added Qualifications in Hand Surgery. Certifications awarded since 1994 are valid for 10 years.

American Osteopathic Board of Pathology

General certification in Laboratory Medicine, Anatomic Pathology and Anatomic Pathology and Laboratory Medicine; with Special Qualifications in Forensic Pathology; and with Added Qualifications in Dermatopathology. Certifications awarded since 1995 are valid for 10 years.

American Osteopathic Board of Pediatrics

General certification in Pediatrics with Special Qualifications in Adolescent and Young Adult Medicine, Neonatology, Pediatric Allergy/Immunology and Pediatric Endocrinology; with Added Qualifications in Sports Medicine. Certifications awarded since 1995 are valid for 7 years.

American Osteopathic Board of Physical Medicine and Rehabilitation Medicine

General certification in Physical Medicine and Rehabilitation; with Added Qualifications in Hospice & Palliative Medicine and Sports Medicine. Certifications awarded since 2004 are valid
for 10 years.

American Osteopathic Board of Preventive Medicine

General certification in Preventive Medicine/Aerospace Medicine, Preventive Medicine/Occupational-Environmental Medicine and Preventive Medicine/Public Health; with Added Qualifications in Undersea & Hyperbaric Medicine. Certifications awarded since 1994 are valid for 10 years.

American Osteopathic Board of Proctology

General certification in Proctology. Certifications awarded since 2004 are valid for 10 years.

American Osteopathic Board of Radiology

General certification in Diagnostic Radiology and Radiation Oncology; with Added Qualifications in Angiography & Interventional Radiology, Neuroradiology, Pediatric Radiology and Vascular & Interventional Radiology. Certifications awarded since 2002 are valid for 10 years.

American Osteopathic Board of Surgery

General certification in General Vascular Surgery, Surgery, Neurological Surgery, Plastic and Reconstructive Surgery, Thoracic Cardiovascular Surgery, Urological Surgery; with Added Qualifications in Surgical Critical Care. Certifications awarded since 1997 are valid for 10 years.

Appendix B:
Self-Designated Medical Specialties

This list of self-designated medical specialty groups was obtained from the American Board of Medical Specialties. However, it is important to point out that these groups are not recognized by the ABMS, the governing board for the recognized twenty-four medical specialty boards (listed in Appendix A).

The organizations listed below range from highly organized groups that are attempting to formalize training and certification in their field to informal groups interested in a particular aspect of medicine.

If you wish to obtain information from any of these groups you will have to do some detective work. Because so many are informal, the location, phone and mailing addresses change frequently, depending upon the person who is functioning as secretary or administrator.

The best way to track down one of these groups is to consult the doctor listings to find a doctor who has expressed a special interest in that field, and call his or her office. You might also call a nearby academic health center in the area to see if they have a faculty or staff member known to be involved in that particular medical interest. If that fails, take the same approach with your community hospital.

A

Abdominal Surgeons
Acupuncture Medicine
Addiction Medicine
Addictionology
Adolescent Psychiatry
Aesthetic Plastic Surgery
Alcoholism and Other Drug Dependencies (AMSAODD)
Algology (Chronic Pain)
Alternative Medicine
Ambulatory Anesthesia
Ambulatory Foot Surgery
Anesthesia
Arthroscopic Surgery
Arthroscopy (Board of North America)

B

Bariatric Medicine
Bionic Psychology
Bloodless Medicine & Surgery

C

Chelation Therapy
Chemical Dependence
Clinical Chemistry
Clinical Ecology
Clinical Medicine and Surgery
Clinical Neurology
Clinical Neurophysiology
Clinical Neurosurgery
Clinical Nutrition
Clinical Orthopaedic Surgery
Clinical Pharmacology
Clinical Polysomnography
Clinical Psychiatry
Clinical Psychology
Clinical Toxicology
Cosmetic Plastic Surgery
Cosmetic Surgery
Council of Non-Board Certified Physicians
Critical Care in Medicine & Surgery

D

Disability Analysis
Disability Evaluating Physicians

E

Electrodiagnostic Medicine
Electroencephalography
Electromyography & Electrodiagnosis
Environmental Medicine
Epidemiology (College)
Eye Surgery

F

Facial Cosmetic Surgery
Facial Plastic & Reconstructive Surgery
Family Practice, Certification
Forensic Examiners
Forensic Psychiatry
Forensic Toxicology

H

Hand Surgery
Head, Facial & Neck Pain & TMJ Orthopaedics
Health Physics
Homeopathic Physicians
Homeotherapeutics
Hypnotic Anesthesiology, National Board for

I

Independent Medical Examiners
Industrial Medicine & Surgery
Insurance Medicine
International Cosmetic & Plastic Facial Reconstructive Standards
Interventional Radiology

L

Laser Surgery
Law in Medicine
Longevity Medicine/Surgery

M

Malpractice Physicians
Maxillofacial Surgeons
Medical Accreditation (American Federation for)
Medical Hypnosis
Medical Laboratory Immunology
Medical-Legal Analysis of Medicine & Surgery
Medical Legal & Workers
  Comp. Medicine & Surgery
Medical-Legal Consultants
Medical Management
Medical Microbiology
Medical Preventics (Academy)
Medical Psychotherapists
Medical Toxicology
Microbiology (Medical Microbiology)
Military Medicine
Mohs' Micrographic Surgery &
  Cutaneous Oncology

N

NeuroImaging
Neurologic & Orthopaedic Dental
  Medicine and Surgery
Neurological & Orthopaedic Medicine
Neurological & Orthopaedic Surgery
Neurological Microsurgery
Neurology
Neuromuscular Thermography
Neuro-Orthopaedic Dental Medicine
Neuro-Orthopaedic Electrodiagnosis
Neuro-Orthopaedic Laser Surgery
Neuro-Orthopaedic Psychiatry
Neuro-Orthopaedic Thoracic Medicine
Neurorehabilitation
Nutrition

O

Orthopaedic Medicine
Orthopaedic Microneurosurgery
Otorhinolaryngology

P

Pain Management (American Academy of)
Pain Management Specialties
Pain Medicine
Palliative Medicine
Percutaneous Diskectomy
Plastic Esthetic Surgeons
Prison Medicine
Professional Disability Consultants
Psychiatric Medicine
Psychiatry (American National Board of)
Psychoanalysis (American Examining
  Board in)
Psychological Medicine (International)

Q

Quality Assurance & Utilization Review

R

Radiology & Medical Imaging
Rheumatologic Surgery
Rheumatological & Reconstructive Medicine
Ringside Medicine & Surgery

S

Skin Specialists
Sleep Medicine (Polysomnography)
Spinal Cord Injury
Spinal Surgery
Sports Medicine
Sports Medicine/Surgery

T

Toxicology
Trauma Surgery
Traumatologic Medicine & Surgery
Tropical Medicine

U

Ultrasound Technology
Urologic Allied Health Professionals
Urological Surgery

W

Weight Reduction Medicine

APPENDIX C:
Hospital Listings

The following is an alphabetical listing of all hospitals that have at least one Castle Connolly Top Doctor in this guide. Institutions listed in **Bold** are profiled in this Guide in association with Castle Connolly's Partnership for Excellence program. The abbreviations as they appear in the listings are in italics below. Due to the many changes taking place in the hospital industry, the names on this list may have changed subsequent to publication of this guide.

Bayonne Medical Center (201) 858-5000
Bayonne Med Ctr
29 E 29th St Bayonne, NJ 07002 HUDSON

Bayshore Community Hospital (732) 739-5900
Bayshore Community Hosp
727 N Beers St Holmdel, NJ 07733 MONMOUTH

Bellevue Hospital Center (212) 562-1000
Bellevue Hosp Ctr
462 First Avenue New York, NY 10016 NEW YORK

Bergen Regional Medical Center (201) 967-4000
Bergen Regl Med Ctr
230 East Ridgewood Avenue Paramus, NJ 07652 BERGEN

Beth Israel Medical Center - Kings Highway Division (718) 252-3000
Beth Israel Med Ctr- Kings Hwy Div
3201 Kings Highway Brooklyn, NY 11234 KINGS

Beth Israel Medical Center - Milton & Caroll Petrie Division (212) 420-2000
Beth Israel Med Ctr - Petrie Div
First Avenue at 16th Street New York, NY 10003 NEW YORK

Blythedale Children's Hospital (914) 592-7555
Blythedale Children's Hosp
95 Bradhurst Avenue Valhalla, NY 10595 WESTCHESTER

Bridgeport Hospital (203) 384-3000
Bridgeport Hosp
267 Grant St Bridgeport, CT 06610 FAIRFIELD

Bronx Lebanon Hospital Center Bronx Lebanon Hosp Ctr 1276 Fulton Ave	Bronx, NY 10457	(718) 590-1800 BRONX
Bronx Psychiatric Center Bronx Psych Ctr 1500 Waters Place	Bronx, NY 10461	(718) 931-0600 BRONX
Brookdale University Hospital Medical Center Brookdale Univ Hosp Med Ctr One Brookdale Plaza	Brooklyn, NY 11212	(718) 240-5000 KINGS
Brookhaven Memorial Hospital & Medical Center Brookhaven Meml Hosp & Med Ctr 101 Hospital Road	Patchogue, NY 11772	(631) 654-7100 SUFFOLK
Brooklyn Hospital Center Brooklyn Hosp Ctr 121 DeKalb Avenue	Brooklyn, NY 11201	(718) 250-8000 KINGS
Burke Rehabilitation Hospital Burke Rehab Hosp 785 Mamaroneck Avenue	White Plains, NY 10605	(914) 597-2500 WESTCHESTER
Capital Health Medical Center - Hopewell Capital Health Med Ctr - Hopewell One Capital Way	Pennington, NJ 08534	(609) 303-4000 MERCER
Capital Health Regional Medical Center Capital Health Regl Med Ctr 750 Brunswick Avenue	Trenton, NJ 08638-4174	(609) 394-6000 MERCER
CentraState Medical Center CentraState Med Ctr 901 West Main Street	Freehold, NJ 07728	(732) 431-2000 MONMOUTH
Children's Hospital at Montefiore Chldns Hosp at Montefiore 3415 Bainbridge Ave	Bronx, NY 10467	(718) 741-2426 BRONX
Children's Hospital of NJ at Newark Chldns Hosp NJ at Newark 201 Lyons Ave N New Jersey	Newark, NJ 07112	(973) 926-7000 ESSEX
Children's Hospital of Philadelphia Chldns Hosp of Philadelphia 34th St & Civic Center Blvd	Philadelphia, PA 19104	(215) 590-1000 PHILADELPHIA

Children's Specialized Hospital (908) 233-3720
Children's Specialized Hosp
150 New Providence Rd | Mountainside, NJ 07092 | UNION

Chilton Hospital (973) 831-5000
Chilton Hosp
97 West Parkway | Pompton Plains, NJ 07444 | MORRIS

Christ Hospital - Jersey City (201) 795-8200
Christ Hosp - Jersey City
176 Palisade Avenue | Jersey City, NJ 07306 | HUDSON

Clara Maass Medical Center (973) 450-2000
Clara Maass Med Ctr
One Clara Maass Drive | Belleville, NJ 07109 | ESSEX

Coney Island Hospital (718) 616-3000
Coney Island Hosp
2601 Ocean Parkway | Brooklyn, NY 11235 | KINGS

Danbury Hospital (203) 739-7000
Danbury Hosp
24 Hospital Avenue | Danbury, CT 06810 | FAIRFIELD

Eastern Long Island Hospital (631) 477-1000
Eastern Long Island Hosp
201 Manor Place | Greenport, NY 11944 | SUFFOLK

Elmhurst Hospital Center (718) 334-4000
Elmhurst Hosp Ctr
79-01 Broadway | Elmhurst, NY 11373 | QUEENS

Englewood Hospital & Medical Center (201) 894-3000
Englewood Hosp & Med Ctr
350 Engle Street | Englewood, NJ 07631 | BERGEN

Flushing Hospital Medical Center (718) 670-5000
Flushing Hosp Med Ctr
4500 Parsons Blvd | Flushing, NY 11355 | QUEENS

Forest Hills Hospital (718) 830-4000
Forest Hills Hosp
102-01 66th Rd | Forest Hills, NY 11375 | QUEENS

Four Winds Hospital (914) 763-8151
Four Winds Hosp
800 Cross River Road | Katonah, NY 10536 | WESTCHESTER

Franklin Hospital (516) 256-6000
Franklin Hosp
900 Franklin Avenue Valley Stream, NY 11580 NASSAU

Gaylord Hospital (203) 284-2800
Gaylord Hosp
50 Gaylord Farm Rd, PO Box 400 Wallingford, CT 06492-0400 NEW HAVEN

Glen Cove Hospital (516) 674-7300
Glen Cove Hosp
101 St Andrew's Ln Glen Cove, NY 11542 NASSAU

Good Samaritan Hospital Medical Center - West Islip (631) 376-4444
Good Samaritan Hosp Med Ctr - West Islip
1000 Montauk Highway West Islip, NY 11795 SUFFOLK

Good Samaritan Regional Medical Center (845) 368-5000
Good Samaritan Regional Med Ctr
255 Lafayette Ave Suffern, NY 10901 ROCKLAND

Goryeb Children's Hospital (973) 971-6700
Goryeb Children's Hosp
100 Madison Ave Morristown, NJ 07960 MORRIS

Gracie Square Hospital (212) 988-4400
Gracie Square Hosp
420 E 76th St New York, NY 10021 NEW YORK

Greenwich Hospital (203) 863-3000
Greenwich Hosp
5 Perryridge Rd Greenwich, CT 06830 FAIRFIELD

Griffin Hospital (203) 735-7421
Griffin Hosp
130 Division St Derby, CT 06418-1377 NEW HAVEN

Hackensack University Medical Center (551) 996-2000
Hackensack Univ Med Ctr
30 Prospect Avenue Hackensack, NJ 07601 BERGEN

Hackensack University Medical Center-Mountainside (973) 429-6000
Hackensack UMC-Mountainside
1 Bay Ave Montclair, NJ 07042 ESSEX

Harlem Hospital Center (212) 939-1000
Harlem Hosp Ctr
506 Lenox Avenue New York, NY 10037 NEW YORK

Helen Hayes Hospital (845) 786-4000
Helen Hayes Hosp
51-55 Route 9W N West Haverstraw, NY 10993 ROCKLAND

Hoboken University Medical Center (201) 418-1000
Hoboken Univ Med Ctr - Hoboken
308 Willow Ave Hoboken, NJ 07030 HUDSON

Holy Name Medical Center (201) 833-3000
Holy Name Med Ctr
718 Teaneck Road Teaneck, NJ 07666-4281 BERGEN

Hospital for Special Surgery (212) 606-1000
Hosp For Special Surgery
535 East 70th Street New York, NY 10021 NEW YORK

Hudson Valley Hospital Center (914) 737-9000
Hudson Valley Hosp Ctr
1980 Crompond Road Cortland Manor, NY 10567 WESTCHESTER

Hunterdon Medical Center (908) 788-6100
Hunterdon Med Ctr
2100 Wescott Dr Flemington, NJ 08822-4604 HUNTERDON

Huntington Hospital (631) 351-2000
Huntington Hosp
270 Park Avenue Huntington, NY 11743 SUFFOLK

Jacobi Medical Center (718) 918-5000
Jacobi Med Ctr
1400 Pelham Parkway South Bronx, NY 10461 BRONX

Jamaica Hospital Medical Center (718) 206-6000
Jamaica Hosp Med Ctr
8900 Van Wyck Expressway Jamaica, NY 11418 QUEENS

James J. Peters VA Medical Center-Bronx (718) 584-9000
James J. Peters VA Med Ctr-Bronx
130 W Kingsbridge Rd Bronx, NY 10468 BRONX

Jersey City Medical Center (201) 915-2000
Jersey City Med Ctr
355 Grand Street Jersey City, NJ 07302 HUDSON

Jersey Shore University Medical Center (732) 775-5500
Jersey Shore Univ Med Ctr
1945 Route 33 Neptune, NJ 07753 MONMOUTH

JFK Medical Center - Edison (732) 321-7000
JFK Med Ctr - Edison
65 James St Edison, NJ 08820 MIDDLESEX

John T Mather Memorial Hospital (631) 473-1320
John T Mather Meml Hosp
75 N Country Rd Port Jefferson, NY 11777 SUFFOLK

Kessler Institute for Rehabiitation - Saddle Brook (201) 368-6000
Kessler Inst for Rehab - Saddle Brook
300 Market St Saddle Brook, NJ 07663 BERGEN

Kessler Institute for Rehabilitation - Chester (973) 252-6300
Kessler Inst for Rehab - Chester
201 Pleasant Hill Rd Chester, NJ 07930 MORRIS

Kessler Institute for Rehabilitation - West Orange (973) 731-3600
Kessler Inst for Rehab - W Orange
1199 Pleasant Valley Way West Orange, NJ 07052-1499 ESSEX

Kings County Hospital Center (718) 245-3131
Kings Co Hosp Ctr
451 Clarkson Avenue Brooklyn, NY 11203 KINGS

Kingsbrook Jewish Medical Center (718) 604-5000
Kingsbrook Jewish Med Ctr
585 Schenectady Avenue Brooklyn, NY 11203 KINGS

Lawrence Hospital Center (914) 787-1000
Lawrence Hosp Ctr
55 Palmer Avenue Bronxville, NY 10708 WESTCHESTER

Lenox Hill Hospital (212) 434-2000
Lenox Hill Hosp
100 East 77th Street New York, NY 10021 NEW YORK

Lenox Hill Hospital (Manhattan Eye, Ear & Throat Hosp) (212) 838-9200
Lenox Hill Hosp (Manh Eye, Ear & Throat Hosp)
210 East 64th Street New York, NY 10021 NEW YORK

Lincoln Medical & Mental Health Center (718) 579-5000
Lincoln Med & Mental Hlth Ctr
234 East 149th St Bronx, NY 10451 BRONX

Long Beach Medical Center (516) 897-1000
Long Beach Med Ctr
455 East Bay Drive Long Beach, NY 11561 NASSAU

Long Island Jewish Medical Center (718) 470-7000
Long Is Jewish Med Ctr
270-05 76th Avenue New Hyde Park, NY 11040 NASSAU

Lutheran Medical Center - Brooklyn (718) 630-7000
Lutheran Med Ctr - Brooklyn
150 55th Street Brooklyn, NY 11220 KINGS

Maimonides Medical Center (718) 283-6000
Maimonides Med Ctr
4802 Tenth Avenue Brooklyn, NY 11219 KINGS

Meadowlands Hospital Medical Center (201) 392-3100
Meadowlands Hosp Med Ctr
55 Meadowland Parkway Secaucus, NJ 07094 HUDSON

Memorial Sloan-Kettering Cancer Center (212) 639-2000
Meml Sloan-Kettering Canc Ctr
1275 York Avenue New York, NY 10021 NEW YORK

Mercy Medical Center - Rockville Centre (516) 705-2525
Mercy Med Ctr - Rockville Centre
1000 North Village Avenue Rockville Centre, NY 11570 NASSAU

Metropolitan Hospital Center - NY (212) 423-6262
Metropolitan Hosp Ctr - NY
1901 First Avenue New York, NY 10029 NEW YORK

Milford Hospital (203) 876-4000
Milford Hosp
300 Seaside Ave Milford, CT 06460 NEW HAVEN

Monmouth Medical Center (732) 222-5200
Monmouth Med Ctr
300 2nd Ave Long Branch, NJ 07740-6300 MONMOUTH

Montefiore Medical Center-Einstein Campus (718) 904-2000
Montefiore Med Ctr-Einstein Campus
1825 Eastchester Road Bronx, NY 10461 BRONX

Montefiore Medical Center-Moses Campus (718) 920-4321
Montefiore Med Ctr-Moses Campus
111 East 210 Street Bronx, NY 10467 BRONX

Montefiore Medical Center-Wakefield Campus (718) 920-9000
Montefiore Med Ctr-Wakefield Campus
600 E 233rd St Bronx, NY 10466 BRONX

Montefiore Mount Vernon Hospital (914) 664-8000
Montefiore Mt Vernon Hosp
12 N Seventh Ave Mount Vernon, NY 10550 WESTCHESTER

Montefiore New Rochelle Hospital (914) 632-5000
Montefiore New Rochelle Hosp
16 Guion Pl New Rochelle, NY 10801 WESTCHESTER

Montefiore Westchester Square (718) 430-7300
Montefiore Westchester Sq
2475 St Raymond Ave Bronx, NY 10461 BRONX

Morgan Stanley Children's Hospital of NewYork-Presbyterian, NY (212) 305-5437
Morgan Stanley Children's Hosp of NY-Presby, NY
3959 Broadway New York, NY 10032 NEW YORK

Morristown Medical Center (973) 971-5000
Morristown Med Ctr
100 Madison Avenue Morristown, NJ 07960-6095 MORRIS

Mount Sinai Hospital of Queens (718) 932-1000
Mount Sinai Hosp of Queens
25-10 30th Avenue Long Island City, NY 11102 QUEENS

Mount Sinai Medical Center (212) 241-6500
Mt Sinai Med Ctr
One Gustave L. Levy Pl New York, NY 10029 NEW YORK

Nassau University Medical Center (516) 572-0123
Nassau Univ Med Ctr
2201 Hempstead Tpke East Meadow, NY 11554 NASSAU

Natchaug Hospital (860) 456-1311
Natchaug Hosp
189 Storrs Rd, PO Box 260 Mansfield Center, CT 06250 TOLLAND

New York Community Hospital (718) 692-5300
New York Comm Hosp
2525 Kings Highway Brooklyn, NY 11229 KINGS

New York Eye & Ear Infirmary (212) 979-4000
New York Eye & Ear Infirm
310 East 14th Street New York, NY 10003 NEW YORK

New York Hospital Queens (718) 670-2000
NY Hosp Queens
56-45 Main Street Flushing, NY 11355 QUEENS

New York Methodist Hospital (718) 780-3000
New York Methodist Hosp
506 Sixth Street Brooklyn, NY 11215 KINGS

New York State Psychiatric Institute (212) 543-5000
NY State Psychiatric Inst
1051 Riverside Dr New York, NY 10032 NEW YORK

Newark Beth Israel Medical Center (973) 926-7000
Newark Beth Israel Med Ctr
201 Lyons Ave Newark, NJ 07112 ESSEX

NewYork-Presbyterian/Columbia University Medical Center, NY (212) 305-2500
NY-Presby/Columbia Univ Med Ctr, NY
622 W 168th St New York, NY 10032 NEW YORK

NewYork-Presbyterian/Lower Manhattan Hospital (212) 312-5000
NY-Presby/Lower Manhattan Hosp
170 William Street New York, NY 10038 NEW YORK

NewYork-Presbyterian/The Allen Hospital, NY (212) 932-4000
NY-Presby Hosp/The Allen Hosp
5141 Broadway New York, NY 10034 NEW YORK

NewYork-Presbyterian/Weill Cornell Medical Center, NY (212) 746-5454
NY-Presby/Weill Cornell Med Ctr, NY
525 E 68th St New York, NY 10021 NEW YORK

NewYork-Presbyterian/Westchester Division, NY (914) 682-9100
NY-Presby/Westchester Div, NY
21 Bloomingdale Rd White Plains, NY 10605 WESTCHESTER

North Shore University Hospital (516) 562-0100
N Shore Univ Hosp
300 Community Dr Manhasset, NY 11030 NASSAU

North Shore-LIJ Health System (516) 465-2550
NS-LIJ Hlth Sys
125 Community Drive Great Neck, NY 11021 NASSAU

Northern Westchester Hospital (914) 666-1200
Northern Westchester Hosp
400 East Main Street Mount Kisco, NY 10549 WESTCHESTER

Norwalk Hospital (203) 852-2000
Norwalk Hosp
34 Maple Street Norwalk, CT 06856 FAIRFIELD

Nyack Hospital		(845) 348-2000
Nyack Hosp		
160 North Midland Avenue	Nyack, NY 10960	ROCKLAND
NYU Hospital for Joint Diseases		(212) 598-6000
NYU Hosp For Joint Dis		
301 East 17th Street	New York, NY 10003	NEW YORK
NYU Langone Medical Center		(212) 263-7300
NYU Langone Med Ctr		
550 First Avenue	New York, NY 10016	NEW YORK
NYU Rusk Institute		(212) 263-1999
NYU Rusk Inst		
400 East 34th Street	New York, NY 10016	NEW YORK
Ocean Medical Center		(732) 840-2200
Ocean Med Ctr		
425 Jack Martin Blvd	Brick, NJ 08724	OCEAN
Overlook Medical Center		(908) 522-2000
Overlook Med Ctr		
99 Beauvoir Ave	Summit, NJ 07901	UNION
Palisades Medical Center		(201) 854-5000
Palisades Med Ctr		
7600 River Road	North Bergen, NJ 07047	HUDSON
Peconic Bay Medical Center		(631) 548-6000
Peconic Bay Med Ctr		
1300 Roanoke Avenue	Riverhead, NY 11901	SUFFOLK
Phelps Memorial Hospital Center		(914) 366-3000
Phelps Meml Hosp Ctr		
701 N Broadway	Sleepy Hollow, NY 10591	WESTCHESTER
Plainview Hospital		(516) 719-3000
Plainview Hosp		
888 Old Country Rd	Plainview, NY 11803	NASSAU
Putnam Hospital Center		(845) 279-5711
Putnam Hosp Ctr		
670 Stoneleigh Ave	Carmel, NY 10512	PUTNAM
Queens Hospital Center - Jamaica		(718) 883-3000
Queens Hosp Ctr - Jamaica		
82-68 164th Street	Jamaica, NY 11432	QUEENS

Raritan Bay Medical Center - Old Bridge Division (732) 360-1000
Raritan Bay Med Ctr - Old Bridge Div
One Hospital Plaza Old Bridge, NJ 08857 MIDDLESEX

Raritan Bay Medical Center - Perth Amboy Division (732) 442-3700
Raritan Bay Med Ctr - Perth Amboy
530 New Brunswick Avenue Perth Amboy, NJ 08861-3654 MIDDLESEX

Richmond University Medical Center (718) 818-1234
Richmond Univ Med Ctr
355 Bard Ave Staten Island, NY 10310-1699 RICHMOND

Riverview Medical Center (732) 741-2700
Riverview Med Ctr
1 Riverview Plaza Red Bank, NJ 07701 MONMOUTH

Robert Wood Johnson University Hospital - Hamilton (609) 586-7900
Robert Wood Johnson Univ Hosp Hamilton
1 Hamilton Health Pl Hamilton, NJ 08690 MERCER

Robert Wood Johnson University Hospital - New Brunswick (732) 828-3000
Robert Wood Johnson Univ Hosp - New Brunswick
1 Robert Wood Johnson Pl New Brunswick, NJ 08903 MIDDLESEX

Robert Wood Johnson University Hospital at Rahway (732) 381-4200
Robert Wood Johnson Univ Hosp at Rahway
865 Stone St Rahway, NJ 07065 UNION

Rockland Psychiatric Center (845) 359-1000
Rockland Psych Ctr
140 Old Orangeburg Rd Orangeburg, NY 10962-1196 ROCKLAND

Saint Barnabas Medical Center (973) 322-5000
Saint Barnabas Med Ctr
94 Old Short Hills Rd Livingston, NJ 07039-5672 ESSEX

Saint Joseph's Medical Center - Yonkers (914) 378-7000
Saint Joseph's Med Ctr - Yonkers
127 South Broadway Yonkers, NY 10701 WESTCHESTER

Saint Michael's Medical Center (973) 877-5000
Saint Michael's Med Ctr
111 Central Avenue Blvd Newark, NJ 07102 ESSEX

Saint Vincent Catholic Medical Centers - St. Vincent's Westchester (914) 967-6500
St. Vincent Cath Med Ctrs - Westchester
275 North Street Harrison, NY 10528 WESTCHESTER

Silver Hill Hospital (203) 966-3561
Silver Hill Hosp
208 Valley Rd New Canaan, CT 06840-3899 FAIRFIELD

Smilow Cancer Hospital at Yale-New Haven (203) 688-4242
Smilow Cancer Hosp at Yale-New Haven
20 York St New Haven, CT 06510 NEW HAVEN

Somerset Medical Center (908) 685-2200
Somerset Med Ctr
110 Rehill Ave Somerville, NJ 08876 SOMERSET

South Nassau Communities Hospital (516) 632-3000
South Nassau Comm Hosp
1 Healthy Way Oceanside, NY 11572 NASSAU

Southampton Hospital (631) 726-8200
Southampton Hosp
240 Meeting House Ln Southampton, NY 11968 SUFFOLK

Southside Hospital (631) 968-3000
Southside Hosp
301 E Main St Bay Shore, NY 11706 SUFFOLK

St. Barnabas Hospital - Bronx (718) 960-9000
St. Barnabas Hosp - Bronx
4422 Third Avenue Bronx, NY 10457 BRONX

St. Catherine's of Siena Medical Center (631) 862-3000
St. Catherine's of Siena Med Ctr
50 Rt 25A Smithtown, NY 11787 SUFFOLK

St. Charles Hospital (631) 474-6000
St. Charles Hosp
200 Belle Terre Rd Port Jefferson, NY 11777 SUFFOLK

St. Clare's Hospital-Denville (973) 625-6000
St. Clare's Hosp-Denville
25 Pocono Road Denville, NJ 07834 MORRIS

St. Clare's Hospital-Dover (973) 625-6000
St. Clare's Hosp-Dover
400 W Blackwell St Dover, NJ 07801 MORRIS

St. Clare's Hospital-Sussex (973) 702-2600
St. Clare's Hosp-Sussex
20 Walnut St Sussex, NJ 07461 SUSSEX

St. Francis Hospital - The Heart Center (516) 562-6000
St. Francis Hosp - The Heart Ctr
100 Port Washington Boulevard Roslyn, NY 11576 NASSAU

St. Francis Medical Center - Trenton (609) 599-5000
St. Francis Med Ctr - Trenton
601 Hamilton Avenue Trenton, NJ 08629 MERCER

St. John's Episcopal Hospital - Queens (718) 869-7000
St. John's Episcopal Hosp - Queens
327 Beach 19th Street Far Rockaway, NY 11691 QUEENS

St. John's Riverside Hospital-Andrus Pavilion (914) 964-4444
St. John's Riverside Hosp-Andrus Pavil
967 N Broadway Yonkers, NY 10701 WESTCHESTER

St. John's Riverside Hospital-Dobbs Ferry Pavilion (914) 693-0700
St. John's Riverside Hosp-Dobbs Ferry Pavil
128 Ashford Ave Dobbs Ferry, NY 10522 WESTCHESTER

St. Joseph's Hospital-Nassau (516) 579-6000
St. Joseph's Hosp-Nassau
4295 Hempstead Turnpike Bethpage, NY 11714 NASSAU

St. Joseph's Regional Medical Center - Paterson (973) 754-2000
St. Joseph's Regl Med Ctr - Paterson
703 Main St Paterson, NJ 07503 PASSAIC

St. Joseph's Wayne Hospital (973) 942-6900
St. Joseph's Wayne Hosp
224 Hamburg Turnpike Wayne, NJ 07470 PASSAIC

St. Lawrence Rehabilitation Center (609) 896-9500
St. Lawrence Rehab Ctr
2381 Lawrencville Rd Lawrencville, NJ 08648 MERCER

St. Luke's - Roosevelt Hospital Center - Roosevelt Division (212) 523-4000
St. Luke's - Roosevelt Hosp Ctr - Roosevelt Div
1000 Tenth Avenue New York, NY 10019 NEW YORK

St. Luke's - Roosevelt Hospital Center - St Luke's Hospital (212) 523-4000
St. Luke's - Roosevelt Hosp Ctr - St Luke's Hosp
1111 Amsterdam Ave New York, NY 10025 NEW YORK

St. Luke's-Cornwall Hospital of Newburgh (845) 561-4400
St. Luke's Newburgh
70 Dubois St Newburgh, NY 12550 ORANGE

St. Mary's Hospital - Passaic (973) 365-4300
St. Mary's Hosp - Passaic
350 Boulevard Passaic, NJ 07055 PASSAIC

St. Mary's Hospital - Waterbury (203) 709-6000
St. Mary's Hosp - Waterbury
56 Franklin St Waterbury, CT 06706-1200 NEW HAVEN

St. Mary's Hospital For Children (718) 281-8800
St. Mary's Hosp for Chldn
29-01 216th St Bayside, NY 11360-2899 QUEENS

St. Peter's University Hospital (732) 745-8600
St. Peter's Univ Hosp
254 Easton Ave New Brunswick, NJ 08901-1780 MIDDLESEX

St. Vincent's Medical Center - Bridgeport (203) 576-6000
St. Vincent's Med Ctr - Bridgeport
2800 Main St Bridgeport, CT 06606 FAIRFIELD

Stamford Hospital (203) 276-1000
Stamford Hosp
30 Shelburne Rd Stamford, CT 06902 FAIRFIELD

Staten Island University Hospital - North (718) 226-9000
Staten Island Univ Hosp - North
475 Seaview Avenue Staten Island, NY 10305 RICHMOND

Staten Island University Hospital - South (718) 226-2000
Staten Island Univ Hosp - South
375 Seguine Avenue Staten Island, NY 10309 RICHMOND

Steven and Alexandra Cohen Children's Medical Center of New York (718) 470-3000
Steven & Alexandra Cohen Chldn's Med Ctr of NY
269-01 76th Ave New Hyde Park, NY 11040 NASSAU

Stony Brook University Medical Center (631) 444-4000
Stony Brook Univ Med Ctr
101 Nicolls Rd Stony Brook, NY 11794-8410 SUFFOLK

Summit Oaks Hospital (908) 522-7000
Summit Oaks Hosp
19 Prospect St Summit, NJ 07902 UNION

SUNY Downstate Medical Center (University Hospital of Brooklyn) (718) 270-1000
SUNY Downstate Med Ctr (Univ Hosp Brooklyn)
450 Clarkson Ave Brooklyn, NY 11203 KINGS

Syosset Hospital (516) 496-6500
Syosset Hosp
221 Jericho Tpke Syosset, NY 11791-4536 NASSAU

Trinitas Regional Medical Center (908) 994-5000
Trinitas Reg Med Ctr
225 Williamson St Elizabeth, NJ 07207 UNION

University Hospital (Newark) (973) 972-4300
Univ Hosp (Newark)
150 Bergen St Newark, NJ 07103-2406 ESSEX

University Medical Center of Princeton at Plainsboro (609) 853-7000
Univ Med Ctr Princeton at Plainsboro
One Plainsboro Rd Plainsboro, NJ 08536 MIDDLESEX

VA Connecticut Healthcare System-West Haven Campus (203) 932-5711
VA Conn Hlthcre Sys-W Haven Campus
950 Campbell Ave West Haven, CT 06516 NEW HAVEN

VA NY Harbor Healthcare System-Brooklyn Campus (718) 630-6600
VA NY Harbor Hlthcr Sys-Brooklyn Campus
800 Poly Pl Bay Ridge, NY 11209 KINGS

VA NY Harbor Healthcare System-Manhattan Campus (212) 686-7500
VA NY Harbor Hlthcare Sys-Manhattan Campus
423 E 23rd St New York, NY 10010 NEW YORK

Valley Hospital (201) 447-8000
Valley Hosp
223 N Van Dien Ave Ridgewood, NJ 07450-2736 BERGEN

Waterbury Hospital (203) 573-6000
Waterbury Hosp
60 Robbins St Waterbury, CT 06721 NEW HAVEN

Westchester Medical Center (914) 493-7000
Westchester Med Ctr
100 Woods Rd Valhalla, NY 10595 WESTCHESTER

White Plains Hospital (914) 681-0600
White Plains Hosp
Davis Ave at E Post Rd White Plains, NY 10601 WESTCHESTER

Winthrop University Hospital (516) 663-0333
Winthrop Univ Hosp
259 1st St Mineola, NY 11501 NASSAU

Woodhull Medical & Mental Health Center (718) 963-8000
Woodhull Med & Mental Hlth Ctr
760 Broadway Brooklyn, NY 11206 KINGS

Wyckoff Heights Medical Center (718) 963-7272
Wyckoff Heights Med Ctr
374 Stockholm Street Brooklyn, NY 11237 KINGS

Yale New Haven Psychiatric Hospital (203) 688-9907
Yale New Haven Psychiatric Hosp
184 Liberty St New Haven, CT 06519 NEW HAVEN

Yale-New Haven Hospital (203) 688-4242
Yale-New Haven Hosp
20 York St New Haven, CT 06510 NEW HAVEN

Yale-New Haven Hospital St Raphael Campus (203) 789-3000
Yale-New Haven Hosp - St Raphael Campus
1450 Chapel Street New Haven, CT 06511 NEW HAVEN

Zucker Hillside Hospital (718) 470-8100
Zucker Hillside Hosp
75-59 263rd St Glen Oaks, NY 11004 QUEENS

Appendix D:
Selected Resources

GENERAL RESOURCES

American Ambulance Association (AAA)

The American Ambulance Association represents emergency and non-emergency medical transportation providers, advocating high quality pre-hospital care and keeping these providers aware of legislation and news that may affect them.

8400 Westpark Drive
Second Floor
McLean, VA 22102

800-523-4447
703-610-9018
fax 703-610-0210
www.the-aaa.org/

America's Health Insurance Plans (AHIP)

America's Health Insurance Plans is a national trade association representing nearly 1,300 member companies providing health benefits to more than 200 million Americans.

601 Pennsylvania Ave, NW
South Building Suite 500
Washington, DC 20004

202-778-3200
fax: 202-331-7487
www.ahip.org/

American Board of Medical Specialties (ABMS)

The ABMS is the authoritative body for the recognition of medical specialties, coordinating 24 medical specialty boards (including 25 medical specialties) and providing information on the board certification of doctors.

222 N LaSalle St, Ste 1500
Chicago, IL 60601

312-436-2600
fax 312-436-2700
www.abms.org

American Hospital Association (AHA)

A national health advocacy organization, the AHA represents hospitals and healthcare networks in legislative and regulatory matters. In 1973 the AHA adopted the Patient Bill of Rights to help patients understand their rights and responsibilities.

155 N Wacker Drive
Chicago, IL 60606

800-424-4301 or 312-422-3000
fax 312-422-4796
www.aha.org/

325 7th St. NW
Washington, DC 20004

800-424-4301 or 202-638-1100
fax 202-626-3245

American Medical Association (AMA)

The AMA is an association that maintains information on physicians practicing throughout the nation. Healthcare consumers can use their database to check the location, licensing, education and specialty of many doctors in the United States.

330 N. Wabash Ave
Chicago, IL 60611

800-621-8335
www.ama-assn.org/

CENTER FOR MEDICAL CONSUMERS

Provides volume and outcome data on certain medical procedures performed in New York state.

239 Thompson St.
New York, NY 10012

212-674-7105
fax 212-674-7100

CenterForMedicalConsumers@gmail.com

www.medicalconsumers.org

CENTERS FOR DISEASE CONTROL AND PREVENTION (CDC)

Part of the Department of Health and Human Services, the CDC's mission is to prevent and manage diseases and illnesses. Its website contains information on a range of illnesses and the research being pursued to manage them. It also provides free faxed reports on disease risk and prevention in various parts of the world.

Public Inquiries/MASO
Mailstop E11
1600 Clifton Road
Atlanta, GA 30333

1-800-CDC-INFO

toll free number for international travelers 877 FYI-TRIP or 404-639-3534
fax information service for international travelers 888-232-3299
www.cdc.gov/netinfo.htm

THE CENTERWATCH CLINICAL TRIALS LISTING SERVICE

Profiles centers conducting clinical research by therapeutic area and geographic region, including more than 41,000 international industry and government-sponsored clinical trials and new FDA approved drug therapies, as well as 5,200 clinical trials that are actively recruiting patients.

10 Winthrop Square, Fl 5
Boston, MA 02110

617-948-5100
fax 617-948-5101
www.centerwatch.com

HEALTH CARE CHOICES

Provides information on volume and outcomes of certain medical procedures performed in hospitals in various states throughout the country.

P.O. Box 21039
Columbus Circle Station
New York, NY 10023

212-724-9395
www.healthcarechoices.org

INTERNATIONAL ASSOCIATION FOR MEDICAL ASSISTANCE TO TRAVELLERS (IAMAT)

IAMAT is a non-profit organization that disseminates information on health and sanitary conditions worldwide. Membership is free but donations are appreciated. Members will receive a membership card making them eligible to access English speaking physicians all over the world. The organization also provides information on immunization requirements, malaria, and other tropical diseases, and sanitary and climactic conditions around the world. For information, send request in writing.

1623 Military Road #279
Niagra Falls, NY 14304-1745

716-754-4883
www.iamat.org

JOINT COMMISSION ON ACCREDITATION OF HEALTHCARE ORGANIZATIONS

The Joint Commission (JCAHO) is an independent, not-for-profit organization, which evaluates the quality and safety of care for nearly 17,000 health care organizations. To maintain and earn accreditation, organizations must have an extensive on-site review by a team of JCAHO health care professionals, at least once every three years. JCAHO is governed by a board that includes physicians, nurses, and consumers. JCAHO sets the standards by which health care quality is measured in America and around the world.

One Renaissance Boulevard
Oakbrook Terrace, IL 60181

630-792-5800
fax 630-792-5005
www.jointcommission.org

Medic Alert Foundation

The Medic Alert Foundation (a non-profit organization) provides an "ID tag" engraved with personal medical facts, as well as a 24-hour emergency response center which can release additional personal medical details. Membership is $45/year and members need to purchase the "ID tag" which sells for as low as $35.

2323 Colorado Avenue
Turlock, CA 95382

888-633-4298
Fax 209-669-2450
www.medicalert.org

Medline

One Medline Place
Mundelein, IL 60060

1-800-MEDLINE (800-633-5463)
fax 1-800-351-1512
www.medline.com

A medical database including millions of medical references and abstracts from thousands of scientific and medical journals.

The National Cancer Institute (NCI)

Part of the NIH, the NCI sponsors cancer clinical trials at more than 100 sites in the United States. Trials are carried out in major medical research centers, such as teaching hospitals, as well as in community hospitals, specialized medical clinics and even in doctors' offices.

Clinical Studies Support Center (CSSC)
9609 Medical Center Drive
GB 9609 MSC 9760
Bethesda, MD 20892

800-4-CANCER (800-422-6237)
www.nci.nih.gov
www.cancer.gov
cancergovstaff@mail.nih.gov

National Center for Complementary and Alternative Medicine Clearinghouse (NCCAMC)

The NCCAMC facilitates the evaluation of alternative medical treatment modalities to help determine their effectiveness and bring alternative medicine into mainstream medicine. This agency does not provide referrals.

9000 Rockville Pike
Bethesda, MD 20892

888-644-6226
fax 866-464-3616
www.nccam.nih.gov
info@nccam.nih.gov

National Consumers League (NCL)

NCL is a private, nonprofit consumer advocacy organization. NCL strives to investigate, educate, and advocate on a variety of issues including healthcare. Membership is $35 annually, but individuals can also write to the organization for a list of publications that non-members can purchase.

1701 K Street, NW, Suite 1200
Washington, DC 20006

202-835-3323
fax 202-835-0747
www.nclnet.org
info@nclnet.org

The National Institutes of Health (NIH)

An organization operated by the U.S. government, the NIH operates its own hospital at which the care provided is usually related to clinical studies its researchers are undertaking. Information about the Warren G. Magnuson Clinical Center is also available.

Patient Recruitment Referral Center
9000 Rockville Pike
Bethesda, MD 20892

800-411-1222 or 301-496-4000
www.nih.gov
www.clinicaltrials.gov
nihinfo@od.nih.gov

NATIONAL INSURANCE INFORMATION INSTITUTE

The National Insurance Information Institute Helpline advises consumers on how to choose an insurance company or broker. It also offers an analysis of life insurance and assists in insurance complaints.

110 William Street
New York, NY 10038

800-942-4242 or 212-346-5500
www.iii.org

THE PATIENT ADVOCATE FOUNDATION

A national non-profit organization that provides consultation, referrals and case management to patients to ensure that they are not denied access to healthcare, insurance coverage, employment and public assistance programs during an illness. In particular, the organization maintains comprehensive information on cancer treatment options that are available to consumers through a separate website: www.oncology.com.

421 Butler Farm Rd
Hampton, VA 23666

800-532-5274
fax 757-873-8999
www.patientadvocate.org/
help@patientadvocate.org

PEOPLE'S MEDICAL SOCIETY

The People's Medical Society, a nonprofit organization, is focused on educating the healthcare consumer about healthcare issues and medical rights. Their website provides information on useful books and publications as well as the latest healthcare developments.

P.O. Box 868
Allentown, PA 18105

610-770-1670
www.peoplesmed.org
cbi@peoplesmed.org

PERSONS UNITED LIMITING SUBSTANDARDS AND ERRORS IN HEALTHCARE (P.U.L.S.E.)

A support group for the survivors of medical malpractice and substandard healthcare, this nonprofit group also advocates patient education and patient-doctor communication.

PO Box 353
Wantagh, NY 11793-0353

800-96-pulse (800-967-8573) or
516-579-4711
fax: 516-520-8105
www.PULSEamerica.org
www.PULSEofNY.org
pulse516@aol.com
719-250-1286
PULSECOLO@YAHOO.COM

PUBLIC CITIZEN'S HEALTH AND RESEARCH GROUP

A non-profit organization, the Public Citizen's Group acts as a watchdog agency by advocating accountability and the open use of doctors' disciplinary backgrounds.

1600 20th Street NW
Washington, DC 20009

202-588-1000
www.citizen.org/hrg/

VERITAS MEDICINE

An organization that allows individuals to perform confidential, personalized searches of their clinical trials database and to access information on new treatment and drug options. The text is submitted by Harvard-affiliated doctors.

11 Cambridge Center
Cambridge, MA 02142

617-234-1500

Appendix E:
State Agencies

While there is a wealth of information available through these state agencies, much of it is not user-friendly. Complicated contractual agreements and other legal documents contain information that might prove to be valuable, providing a consumer can locate it and then review it with some understanding. Often a department will suggest that a consumer visit the office for guidance in reviewing the documents. However, some of these agencies provide useful information on doctors, hospitals, and HMOs. They may also offer statistical reports and consumer-oriented studies.

CONNECTICUT

Doctors

Department of Public Health State of Connecticut
Practitioner Licensing and Investigations Section
410 Capitol Avenue, MS#12MQA
P.O. Box 340308
Hartford, CT 06134-0308
(860) 509-8000
www.dph.state.ct.us
Attn: Physician renewal of verification

Department of Public Health State of Connecticut
Legal Office
410 Capitol Avenue, MS#12LEG
P.O. Box 340308
Hartford, CT 06134-0308
(860) 509-7600

Hospitals

Department of Public Health State of Connecticut
Facilities Licensing and Investigations Section
410 Capitol Avenue, MS#12HSR
P.O. Box 340308
Hartford, CT 06134-0308
(860) 509-7400

HMOs

Department of Insurance (Location address)
153 Market Street, 7th Floor
Hartford, CT 06103-0816
(860) 297-3800

Department of Insurance (Mailing address)
P.O. Box 816
Hartford, CT 06142-0816
(860) 297-3800

www.ct.gov/cid/site/default.asp

Office of Health Care Access
410 Capitol Avenue, MS#13HCA
P.O. Box 340308
Hartford, CT 06134-0308
800-797-9688

TDD 860-418-7001

www.ct.gov/ohca/site/default.asp

NEW JERSEY

Doctors

New Jersey State Board of Medical Examiners (Location address)
140 East Front Street, 2nd Floor
Trenton, NJ 08608
(609) 826-7100

New Jersey State Board of Medical Examiners (Mailing address)
P.O. Box 183
Trenton, NJ 08625-0360

http://www.state.nj.us/lps/ca/bme/index.html
bme@dca.lps.state.nj.us

Hospitals

Department of Health
Division of Health Facilities Evaluation and Licensing
P.O. Box 360
120 S Stockton Street
Trenton, NJ 08625-0360
(609) 292-7837

http://www.nj.gov/health/

HMOs

Department of Health
Division of Health Facilities Evaluation and Licensing
P.O. Box 360
120 S Stockton Street
Trenton, NJ 08625-0360
(609) 292-7837

Department of Health
Office of Managed Care
20 West State St, 11th Fl
P.O. Box 325
Trenton, NJ 08625
(609) 292-5427

http://www.state.nj.us/dobi/managed.htm

Department of Banking & Insurance (Location address)
Division of Insurance, Life and Health Division
Managed Healthcare Bureau
20 West State St
P.O. Box 325
Trenton, NJ 08625
(609) 292-7272

http://www.state.nj.us/dobi/

Department of Banking & Insurance (Mailing address)
Division of Insurance, Life and Health Division
Managed Healthcare Bureau
20 West State St
P.O. Box 325
Trenton, NJ 08625
(609) 292-7272

Office of Managed Care Hotline: 1-888-393-1062
Office of managed Care Fax: (609) 633-0807
Consumer Protection Services Main Line: (609) 292-7272

NEW YORK

Doctors

New York State Department of Health
Office of Professional Medical Conduct
433 River Street, Suite 303
Troy, NY 12180
(518) 402-0836
www.health.state.ny.us
opmc@health.state.ny.us

New York State Education Department
Division of Professional Licensing Services
State Education Building - 2nd floor
89 Washington Avenue
Albany, NY 12234
(518) 474-3817
http://www.op.nysed.gov/home.html

op4info@mail.nysed.gov

Hospitals

Office of Health Systems Management
Corning Tower, Fl 14
Empire State Plaza
Albany, NY 12237
(518) 474-7028

New York State Department of Health
Bureau of Biometrics
Corning Tower, Room 2348
Empire State Plaza
Albany, NY 12237
(518) 474-3189

HMOs

New York State Insurance Department
Health Bureau
99 Washington Ave.
Albany, NY 12257
(518) 474-6272

New York State Insurance Department
Life Policy Bureau
1 Commerce Plaza, Suite 1910
Albany, NY 12257
(518) 474-4552

New York State Department of Health
Office of Managed Care
Corning Tower, Room 1911
Albany, NY 12237
(518) 473-4178

New York State Department of Health
Records Access Office
Corning Tower, Room 2364
Empire State Plaza
Albany, NY 12237
(518) 486-9144

Appendix F:
Sources of Quality Data on Hospitals

U.S. NEWS AND WORLD REPORT

U.S. News & World Report, www.usnews.com/health, has been the nation's leading source of information on hospital rankings since 1990. The Best Hospitals rankings evaluate medical centers on their competence in high-stakes situations. Their annual feature on Best Hospitals has become the standard in the field where rankings are concerned and is heavily anticipated and utilized by consumers and members of the health care profession.

WWW.WHYNOTTHEBEST.ORG

WhyNotTheBest.org was created and is maintained by The Commonwealth Fund, a private foundation working toward a high performance health system. It is a free resource for health care professionals and consumers interested in tracking performance on various measures of health care quality. It enables organizations to compare their performance against that of peer organizations, against a range of benchmarks and over a given period of time. Case studies and improvement tools spotlight successful improvement strategies of the nation's top performers. A regional map shows performance at the county, state and national levels. This site also includes process-of-care measures, patient satisfaction measures, readmission rates, mortality rates and average reimbursement rates. All of these performance measures are publicly reported on the Centers for Medicare and Medicaid Services website, Hospital Compare, and include data from nearly all U.S. hospitals.

THE LEAPFROG GROUP

The Leapfrog Group, http://www.leapfroggroup.org/cp, started in 1998 by a group of large employers. The Leapfrog Hospital Survey compares hospitals' performance on the national standards of safety, quality and efficiency - areas of healthcare that are most relevant to consumers. Hospitals that participate in The Leapfrog Hospital Survey achieve hospital-wide improvements that translate into saving millions of lives and cutting costs for hospitals and consumers. Leapfrog's survey results are later used to inform key employees on purchasing strategies.

Appendix F

HOSPITAL COMPARE

The Hospital Compare website was created through the efforts of the Centers for Medicare & Medicaid Services (CMS), an agency of the U.S. Department of Health and Human Services (DHHS), along with the Hospital Quality Alliance (HQA). The HQA was established to promote reporting on hospital quality of care. The HQA consists of organizations that represent consumers, hospitals, doctors and nurses, employers, accrediting organizations and Federal agencies. The information on this website can be used by patients requiring hospital care. This information helps the consumer and health care providers to compare the quality of care provided in participating hospitals. This information not only helps one to make good decisions about health care, but also encourages hospitals to improve the quality of the care that they provide to their communities. This website can be found at: http://www.hospitalcompare.hhs.gov/hospital-search.aspx or http://bit.ly/jdvCzW

Section Six

Indices

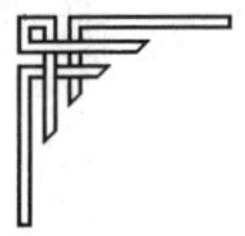

The Best in American Medicine
www.CastleConnolly.com

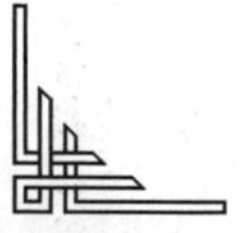
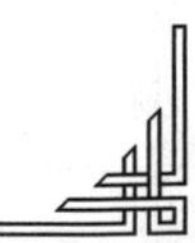

Subject Index

A

B

C

D

E

F

G

H

I

J

L

M

N

O

P

Q

R

S

T

U

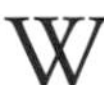

W

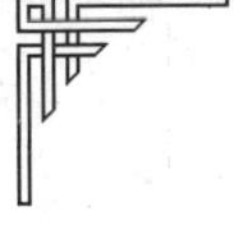

The Best in American Medicine
www.CastleConnolly.com

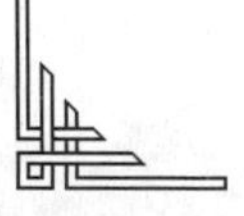
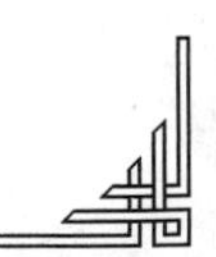

Specialty & Special Expertise Index

This index lists the areas that the physicians listed in the Guide have identified as their "special expertise." They are specific elements of disease, procedures, techniques and treatments for which these physicians are best known and are referred patients. Each doctor's medical specialty is also included.

Specialty & Special Expertise Index

Allergy & Immunotherapy

Alzheimer's Disease

Amblyopia

Amniocentesis

Amputee Rehabilitation

Amyloid Heart Disease

Amyloidosis

Amyloidosis/Joint Disease

Amyotrophic Lateral Sclerosis (ALS)

Anal Cancer

Anal Disorders & Reconstruction

Anal Sphincter Repair

Anaphylaxis

Anemia

Spec	Name	St	Pg
PHO	Viswanathan, K	NY	472

Anemia in Chronic Kidney Disease

Spec	Name	St	Pg
Nep	DeFabritus, A	NY	227

Anemia-Aplastic

Spec	Name	St	Pg
Hem	Castro-Malaspina, H	NY	188
Hem	Isola, L	NY	189
Hem	Schuster, M	NY	617

Anemia-Cancer Related

Spec	Name	St	Pg
Hem	Wisch, N	NY	192

Anemias & Red Blood Cell Disorders

Spec	Name	St	Pg
Onc	Bernhardt, B	NY	672

Aneurysm

Spec	Name	St	Pg
NRad	Pile-Spellman, J	NY	557
NS	Steinberger, A	NJ	745
S	Drascher, G	NJ	911
S	Vitale, G	NY	587
T&CS	Girardi, L	NY	383
T&CS	Seinfeld, F	NJ	827
VascS	Ascher, E	NY	484
VascS	Goyal, A	NY	713
VascS	Pollina, R	NY	636
VascS	Teodorescu, V	NY	400

Aneurysm-Abdominal & Thoracic Aortic

Spec	Name	St	Pg
VascS	Cayne, N	NY	397
VascS	Graham, A	NJ	854
VascS	Lipsitz, E	NY	437
VascS	Morrissey, N	NY	399

Aneurysm-Abdominal Aortic

Spec	Name	St	Pg
T&CS	Plestis, K	NY	385
VascS	Adelman, M	NY	397
VascS	Arnold, T	NY	636
VascS	Babu, S	NY	713
VascS	D'Ayala, M	NY	484
VascS	Faries, P	NY	398
VascS	Faust, G	NY	592
VascS	Gagne, P	CT	996
VascS	Green, R	NY	398
VascS	Grossi, R	NY	398
VascS	Jacobowitz, G	NY	398
VascS	Kagan, P	NJ	771
VascS	McKinsey, J	NY	399
VascS	Rockman, C	NY	400
VascS	Sales, C	NJ	933
VascS	Todd, G	NY	400

Aneurysm-Aortic

Spec	Name	St	Pg
S	McGovern, P	NJ	812
T&CS	DeAnda, A	NY	382
T&CS	Girardi, L	NY	383
T&CS	Lettera, J	CT	994
T&CS	Loulmet, D	NY	384
T&CS	Michler, R	NY	437
T&CS	Plestis, K	NY	385
T&CS	Pogo, G	NY	588
T&CS	Spielvogel, D	NY	710
T&CS	Squitieri, R	CT	994
T&CS	Stewart, A	NY	386
T&CS	Taylor, J	NY	636
VascS	Benvenisty, A	NY	397
VascS	Brener, B	NJ	804
VascS	Carroccio, A	NY	397
VascS	Chaudhry, S	NY	592
VascS	Deitch, J	NY	521
VascS	Dietzek, A	CT	996
VascS	Ellozy, S	NY	398
VascS	Fishman, E	NY	713
VascS	Geuder, J	NJ	770
VascS	Giangola, G	NY	398
VascS	Goldman, K	NJ	854
VascS	Gusberg, R	CT	1034
VascS	Harrington, E	NY	398
VascS	Harrington, M	NY	398
VascS	Huribal, M	CT	996
VascS	Maldonado, T	NY	399
VascS	Marin, M	NY	399
VascS	Marsan, B	CT	997
VascS	Mendes, D	NY	399
VascS	Patel, A	NJ	804
VascS	Purtill, W	NY	592
VascS	Rodino, W	NY	521
VascS	Schanzer, H	NY	400
VascS	Schneider, D	NY	400
VascS	Stein, J	NY	400
VascS	Sun, L	NY	713
VascS	Wolodiger, F	NJ	771
VIR	Rosen, R	NY	395

Aneurysm-Cerebral

Spec	Name	St	Pg
NRad	Bello, J	NY	421
NRad	Berenstein, A	NY	243
NRad	Gobin, Y	NY	244
NRad	Johnson, M	CT	1016
NRad	Keller, I	NJ	842
NRad	Meyers, P	NY	245
NS	Bederson, J	NY	229
NS	Brisman, J	NY	553
NS	Chiurco, A	NJ	822
NS	Flamm, E	NY	419
NS	Holtzman, R	NY	554
NS	Jafar, J	NY	231
NS	Langer, D	NY	231
NS	Moore, F	NJ	745
NS	Murali, R	NY	677
NS	Nosko, M	NJ	840
NS	Patel, A	NY	232
NS	Riina, H	NY	232
NS	Solomon, R	NY	233
NS	Stieg, P	NY	233
NS	Woo, H	NY	621

Aneurysm-Thoracic Aortic

Spec	Name	St	Pg
T&CS	Abrol, S	NY	483
T&CS	Elefteriades, J	CT	1031
T&CS	Hartman, A	NY	635
T&CS	Klein, J	NJ	767
T&CS	Stelzer, P	NY	386
T&CS	Tranbaugh, R	NY	386

Angina

Spec	Name	St	Pg
Cv	Lucariello, R	NY	405
Cv	Rothman, H	NJ	726
Cv	Schulman, I	NY	137
Cv	Siskind, S	NY	490
Cv	Sklaroff, H	NY	138
Cv	Tartaglia, J	NY	648

Angiography-Coronary

Spec	Name	St	Pg
Cv	Pappas, T	NY	532
Cv	Zaloom, R	NY	447
IC	Abittan, M	NY	548
IC	Henry, G	CT	1010
IC	Moses, J	NY	209
IC	Syed, T	NJ	740

Angioplasty

Spec	Name	St	Pg
Cv	Cleman, M	CT	1002
Cv	Coppola, J	NY	131
Cv	Green, S	NY	530
Cv	Klapholz, M	NJ	777
Cv	Landers, D	NJ	725
Cv	Lowell, B	NJ	874
Cv	Sherman, W	NY	138
IC	Brogno, D	NY	597
IC	Shanahan, A	NJ	820
VascS	Manno, J	NJ	771
VIR	Crystal, K	NY	591
VIR	Rundback, J	NJ	770

Angioplasty & Restenosis

Spec	Name	St	Pg
IC	Feit, F	NY	208

Angioplasty & Stent Placement

Spec	Name	St	Pg
Cv	Dangas, G	NY	131
Cv	Jauhar, R	NY	531
Cv	Kosinski, E	CT	944
Cv	Shamoon, F	NJ	777
Cv	Stroh, J	NJ	904
Cv	Tuohy, E	CT	1002
IC	Angeli, S	NJ	740
IC	Brener, S	NY	458
IC	Kodali, S	NY	208
IC	Lawson, W	NY	619
IC	Malpeso, J	NY	513
IC	Miller, K	NJ	785
IC	Moreno, P	NY	209

Arthritis Hand Surgery

Arthritis in Lyme Disease

Arthritis-Hip & Knee

Arthroplasty Imaging

Arthroscopic Surgery

Arthroscopic Surgery-Hip

Arthroscopic Surgery-Knee

Arthroscopic Surgery-Shoulder

Asbestos-related Lung Disease

Asperger's Syndrome

Asthma

Specialty & Special Expertise Index

Specialty & Special Expertise Index

Breast Cancer & Surgery

Breathing Disorders

Bronchiectasis

Bronchiolitis Obliterans

Bronchitis

Bronchoscopy

Brugada Syndrome

Burn Care

Burns-Reconstructive Plastic Surgery

C

Calcium Disorders

Cancer Detection & Staging

Cancer Genetics

Cancer Imaging

Cancer Immune Therapy

Cancer in the Elderly

Cancer Prevention

Cancer Reconstruction

Cataract Surgery-Lens Implant

Cataract-Pediatric

Catheter Ablation

Celiac Disease

Central Nervous System Cancer

Cerebral Palsy

Colonoscopy/Polypectomy

Colostomy Avoidance

Colposcopy

Coma

Compartment Syndrome

Complementary Medicine

Complex Diagnosis

Complex Regional Pain Syndromes

Concierge Medicine

Concussion

Congenital Anomalies

Congenital Anomalies-Gastrointestinal

Congenital Anomalies-Genitourinary

Specialty & Special Expertise Index

Specialty & Special Expertise Index

Specialty & Special Expertise Index

Depression in the Elderly

Depression-Consultation

Depression-TMS Therapy

Dermatologic Surgery

Dermatology

Diabetes

Diabetes & Heart Disease

Diabetes in Minority

Specialty & Special Expertise Index

Endometrial Cancer

Endometriosis

Endoscopic Sinus Surgery

Endoscopic Surgery

Endoscopic Therapies

Endoscopic Ultrasound

Endoscopy

Endoscopy & Colonoscopy

Endourology

Endovascular Neurosurgery

Endovascular Stent Grafts

Endovascular Surgery

Endovascular Therapy

Endscopic Ultrasound

Enteroscopy-Small Bowel

Environmental Health in Children

Environmental Medicine

Specialty & Special Expertise Index

F

Gastroesophageal Reflux Disease (GERD)

Geriatric Ophthalmology

Geriatric Orthopaedic Surgery

Geriatric Psychiatry

Geriatric Rehabilitation

Geriatric Rheumatology

Gestational Trophoblastic Disease

Giant Cell Arteritis

Glaucoma

Specialty & Special Expertise Index

Inflammatory Bowel Disease-Consult

Inflammatory Bowel Disease/Crohn's

Inflammatory Muscle Disease

Inherited Metabolic Disorders

Insect Allergies

Intensity Modulated Radiotherapy (IMRT)

Internal Medicine

International Health

Interstitial Cystitis

Interstitial Lung Disease

Interventional Cardiology

J

K

Laparoscopic Surgery-Advanced

Laparoscopic Surgery-Complex

Laryngeal & Voice Disorders

Laryngeal Cancer

Laryngeal Disorders

Laser Hair Removal

Laser Refractive Surgery

Laser Surgery

Laser Vision Surgery

Laser-Refractive Surgery

LASIK-Refractive Surgery

Lead Poisoning

Learning Disorders

Lens Implants

Lens Implants-Multifocal

Leukemia

Leukemia & Lymphoma

Leukemia-Chronic Lymphocytic

Liaison Psychiatry

Ligament Reconstruction

Limb Deformities

Limb Lengthening

Limb Lengthening (Ilizarov Procedure)

Limb Sparing Surgery

Specialty & Special Expertise Index

Lyme Disease-Neuro Complications

Lymph Node Pathology

Lymphedema

Lymphoma

Lymphoma Consultation

Lymphoma, Non-Hodgkin's

Lysosomal Diseases

M

Macular Degeneration

Specialty & Special Expertise Index

Medications in the Elderly

Melanoma

Melanoma Early Detection/Prevention

Melanoma-Choroidal (eye)

Melanoma-Head & Neck

Memory Disorders

Men's Health

Meniere's Disease

Meningioma

Meningitis

Menopause Problems

Menstrual Disorders

Mental Retardation

Mercury Toxic Exposure

Merkel Cell Carcinoma

Mesothelioma

Metabolic Disorders

Metabolic Genetic Disorders

Metabolic Syndrome

Metastatic Cancer

Microsurgery

Microvascular Surgery

Migraine

Minimally Invasive Cardiac Surgery

Minimally Invasive Gynecologic Surgery

Minimally Invasive Heart Valve Surgery

Minimally Invasive Knee

Specialty & Special Expertise Index

Neuromuscular Disorders

Specialty & Special Expertise Index

Opiate Addiction

Optic Nerve Disorders

Oral Cancers

Orbital & Eyelid Tumors/Cancer

Orbital Diseases

Orbital Surgery

Orbital Tumors/Cancer

Orthopaedic Imaging

Orthopaedic Surgery

P

Specialty & Special Expertise Index

Specialty & Special Expertise Index

Pediatric Infections

Pediatric Infectious Disease

Pediatric Nephrology

Pediatric Neurology

Pediatric Neuroradiology

Pediatric Neurosurgery

Pediatric Ophthalmology

Pediatric Orthopaedic Cancers

Pediatric Orthopaedic Surgery

Pediatric Urology

Pediatrics

Pituitary Disorders

Pituitary Tumors

Plasmapheresis

Plastic & Reconstructive Surgery

Plastic Surgery

Platelet Disorders

Pneumonia

Poison Control

Polycystic Kidney Disease

Polycystic Ovarian Syndrome

Polycythemia Rubra Vera

Primary Care Sports Medicine

Primary Ciliary Dyskinesia

PRK-Refractive Surgery

Progressive Supranuclear Palsy (PSP)

PROSE Contact Lens

Prostate Benign Disease

Prostate Cancer

Prostate Cancer-Cryosurgery

Prostate Cancer-MR Spectroscopy (MRSI)

Prostate Cancer/Robotic Surgery

Prostate Disease

Prostate Surgery

PRP (Platelet Rich Plasma)

Pseudomotor Cerebri

Pseudotumor Cerebri

Pseudoxanthoma Elasticum

Psoriasis

Psoriasis/Eczema

Psoriatic Arthritis

Psychiatry in Cancer

Psychiatry in Head & Neck Cancer

Psychiatry in Physical Illness

Psychiatry in Terminal Illness

Psychiatry of Prostate Cancer

Psychoanalysis

Psychodynamic Psychotherapy

Psychoneuroimmunology

Psychopharmacology

Psychopharmacology-Consultation

Psychosomatic Disorders

Psychotherapy

Psychotherapy & Psychopharmacology

Psychotherapy-Men's Issues

Pubertal Disorders

Pulmonary Complications-Neurodisability

Pulmonary Disease

Pulmonary Disease/Immunocompromised

Pulmonary Embolism

Pulmonary Fibrosis

Pulmonary Hypertension

Pulmonary Infections

Specialty & Special Expertise Index

Rheumatologic Diseases of the Lung

Rheumatology

Specialty & Special Expertise Index

Specialty & Special Expertise Index

Specialty & Special Expertise Index

Specialty & Special Expertise Index

Specialty & Special Expertise Index

Stroke Rehabilitation

Substance Abuse

Substance Abuse Effects in Newborn

Substance Abuse in ADHD Patients

Sudden Death Prevention

Sudden Infant Death Syndrome (SIDS)

Suicide

Surgery

Surgical Pathology

Swallowing Disorders

Specialty & Special Expertise Index

Specialty & Special Expertise Index

Specialty & Special Expertise Index

Specialty & Special Expertise Index

Z

The Best in American Medicine
www.CastleConnolly.com

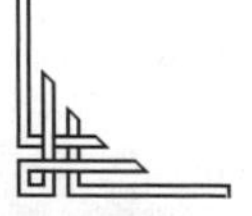
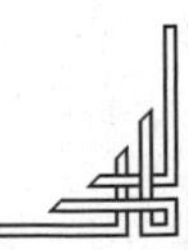

Alphabetical Listing of Doctors

Name	Specialty	Pg
A		
Aaronson, Beth (CT)	PMR	984
Abbed, Khalid (CT)	NS	1014
Abdel-Razeq, Sonya (CT)	MF	1010
Abdoo, Robert (NY)	IM	666
Abelow, Arthur (NY)	Ge	411
Abemayor, Elie (NY)	Ge	658
Abenavoli, Tancredi (NY)	IM	666
Aberg, Judith (NY)	Inf	193
Abittan, Meyer (NY)	IC	548
Ablaza, Valerie (NJ)	PlS	798
Abott, Michael (NY)	Pul	477
Abou-Fayssal, Nada (NY)	N	462
Abramowitz, Avram (NY)	Onc	497
Abrams, Jeffrey (NJ)	OrS	823
Abrams, Linus (CT)	Psyc	986
Abrams, Martin (CT)	Onc	963
Abramson, David (NY)	Oph	253
Abramson, Sara (NY)	DR	157
Abright, A. Reese (NY)	ChAP	140
Abrol, Sunil (NY)	T&CS	483
Abu-Rustum, Nadeem (NY)	GO	182
Abularrage, Joseph (NY)	Ped	501
Accacha, Siham (NY)	PEn	569
Accardi, Frank (NY)	Oph	254
Accurso, Charles (NJ)	Ge	905
Acker, Peter (NY)	Ped	695
Ackerman, Jacob (NY)	Oph	465
Ackert, John (NY)	Ge	168
Acosta, Rodrigo (CT)	FMed	950
Acquista, Angelo (NY)	Pul	352
Adams, David (NY)	T&CS	381
Adams, Francis (NY)	Pul	352
Adams, Marc (NY)	RadRO	519
Addis, Michael (NJ)	VascS	933
Addonizio, Gerard (NY)	Psyc	700
Addonizio, Linda (NY)	PCd	303
Addrizzo-Harris, Doreen (NY)	Pul	352
Adelman, Mark (NY)	VascS	397
Adelman, Ronald (NY)	Ger	180
Adelsberg, Bernard (CT)	A&I	1001
Ades, Joseph (NY)	IM	666
Adesman, Andrew (NY)	Ped	573
Adibi, Baback (NJ)	Cv	724
Adler, Edward (NY)	OrS	269
Adler, Harry (NY)	S	481
Adler, Howard (NY)	Ge	168
Adler, Jack (NY)	Pul	352
Adler, Kenneth (NJ)	Onc	879
Adler, Lenard (NY)	Psyc	338
Adler, Ronald (NY)	DR	157
Adler, Stephen (NY)	Nep	675
Adlersberg, Jay (NY)	Rhu	364
Aferzon, Mark (CT)	Oto	978
Afridi, Shariq (NJ)	Ge	818
Agarwal, Chhavi (NY)	PEn	426
Agarwal, Kishan (NJ)	PCd	846
Agarwal, Nanakram (NY)	S	435
Agarwal, Saurabh (NJ)	U	768
Agdere, Levon (NY)	PEn	471
Aghajanian, Carol (NY)	Onc	212
Agin, Carole (NY)	PM	566
Agress, Harry (NJ)	NuM	747
Agri, Robyn (NJ)	PMR	825
Agrin, Richard (NJ)	EDM	834
Aguila, Helen (NJ)	PPul	795
Agus, Bertrand (NY)	Rhu	364
Agus, Saul (NY)	Ge	168
Aharon, Raphael (NY)	Oph	499
Ahlborn, Thomas (NJ)	S	766
Ahluwalia, Brij M Singh (NY)	N	677
Ahmad, Christopher (NY)	OrS	270
Ahmed, Mutahar (NJ)	U	768
Ahmed, Tauseef (NY)	Onc	672
Ahmed Hosny, M Amr (NY)	PM	297
Ahn, Christina (NY)	PlS	329
Ahn, Jung (NY)	PMR	325
Aisenberg, James (NY)	Ge	168
Aisenberg, Javier (NJ)	PEn	754
Aisner, Joseph (NJ)	Onc	839
Ajl, Stephen (NY)	Ped	474
Akhund, Birjis (NY)	Onc	620
Akin, Oguz (NY)	DR	157
Akinboboye, Olakunle (NY)	Cv	490
Akman, Cigdem (NY)	ChiN	142

Alphabetical Listing of Doctors

Name	Specialty	Pg
Al-Aswad, Lama (NY)	Oph	254
Albert, Arthur (NJ)	VIR	770
Albin, Joan (NY)	EDM	655
Albom, Michael (NY)	D	148
Alderman, Elizabeth (NY)	AM	403
Aldrich, Thomas (NY)	Pul	433
Aledo, Alexander (NY)	PHO	309
Aledort, Louis (NY)	Hem	188
Alexander, Frederick (NJ)	PS	757
Alexiades, Michael (NY)	OrS	270
Alfonso, Antonio (NY)	S	481
Ali, Yousaf (NY)	Rhu	365
Alizadeh, Kaveh (NY)	PlS	576
Allegra, Donald (NJ)	Inf	877
Allen, Answorth (NY)	OrS	270
Allen, Jeffrey (NY)	ChiN	143
Allen, Peter (NY)	S	372
Allen, Robert (NY)	PlS	329
Allen, Steven (NY)	Hem	544
Allendorf, Dennis (NY)	Ped	319
Almeida, Laila (NJ)	D	875
Almeleh, Jack (NY)	Psyc	338
Almeyda, Elizabeth (NY)	PlS	329
Alon, Jamie (CT)	Ped	982
Alper, Kenneth (NY)	Psyc	338
Alpert, Barbara (NY)	IM	666
Altbaum, Robert (CT)	IM	957
Altchek, David (NY)	SM	370
Alterman, Lloyd (NJ)	IM	921
Altholz, Jeffrey (NY)	IM	666
Altman, Bruce (CT)	Oph	972
Altman, Robin (NY)	Ped	695
Altman, Wayne (NJ)	OrS	750
Altmann, Dory (NJ)	IC	838
Altmann, Karen (NY)	PCd	304
Altorki, Nasser (NY)	T&CS	381
Altschul, Larry (NY)	Cv	608
Altus, Jonathan (NY)	Pul	580
Alvarez, Manuel (NJ)	MF	740
Alweiss, Gary (NJ)	N	745
Amer, Jeffrey (NY)	Ped	573
Ames, Richard (NY)	Nep	226
Amin, Hossam (NY)	Pul	477
Amin, Mahendra (NY)	IM	496
Amin, Milan (NY)	Oto	287
Amin, Nikhil (NY)	PPul	693
Amin, Ravindra (NY)	GerPsy	453
Amin, Snehal (NY)	D	148
Amis, E Stephen (NY)	DR	408
Amler, David (NY)	Ped	695
Amodio, John (NY)	DR	449
Amorosi, Edward (NY)	Hem	188
Amoruso, Robert (NJ)	Pul	898
Amory, Spencer (NY)	S	372
Anandasabapathy, Sharmila (NY)	Ge	168
Andaz, Shahriyour (NY)	T&CS	587
Andersen, Holly (NY)	Cv	129
Anderson, Patrick (NJ)	GO	782
Anderson, Richard (NY)	NS	229
Andiman, Warren (CT)	PInf	1023
Andrade, Joseph (NY)	Ped	428
Andrei, Valeriu (NJ)	S	801
Andrews, Alan (NJ)	D	728
Andriani, Rudy (CT)	U	995
Andriola, Mary (NY)	ChiN	610
Andronaco, Raymond (NJ)	U	768
Anene, Okechukwu (NJ)	PCCM	846
Angeli, Stephen (NJ)	IC	740
Angevine, Anne (CT)	Onc	963
Angevine, Peter (NY)	NS	229
Angioletti, Louis (NY)	Oph	254
Angoff, Ronald (CT)	Ped	1025
Angrist, Richard (NJ)	Oph	908
Anhalt, Henry (NJ)	PEn	927
Annabi, Iyad (NY)	FMed	657
Anselmi, Gregory (NJ)	N	809
Antaya, Richard (CT)	D	1004
Anto, Maliakal (NY)	Cv	528
Anton, John (NY)	PlS	631
Antonelle, Robert (NY)	Ge	658
Antonescu, Cristina (NY)	Path	300
Antony, Michael (NY)	Ge	411
Anyane-Yeboa, Kwame (NY)	CG	144
Apatoff, Brian (NY)	N	234
Aponte, Alex (NY)	FMed	614
Apostolides, Paul (CT)	NS	966
Appel, David (NY)	Pul	433
Appel, Gerald (NY)	Nep	226
Appelbaum, Jeffrey (NY)	N	499
Appelbaum, Paul (NY)	Psyc	338

Name	Specialty	Pg
Applebaum, Eric (NJ)	A&I	873
April, Max (NY)	PO	314
Aprile, Georgette (NY)	D	535
Apuzzio, Joseph (NJ)	MF	786
Apuzzo, Thomas (NY)	FMed	657
Aranoff, Shera (NY)	D	148
Arbour, Robert (NJ)	S	868
Arcasoy, Selim (NY)	Pul	352
Arcati, Anthony (NY)	FMed	539
Arcati, Robert (NY)	FMed	539
Arden, Martha (NY)	AM	526
Arden-Cordone, Mary (CT)	EDM	949
Arena, Francis (NY)	Onc	550
Arens, Raanan (NY)	PPul	428
Argenziano, Michael (NY)	T&CS	381
Argilla, Michael (NY)	PCd	304
Aries, Philip (NY)	Oph	623
Ark, Jon (NJ)	HS	819
Arkow, Stan (NY)	Psyc	338
Arlievsky, Nina (NY)	PInf	600
Armbruster, Robert (NY)	ObG	679
Armenakas, Noel (NY)	U	387
Armento, Michael (NJ)	PMR	928
Arnell, Tracey (NY)	CRS	145
Arno, Louis (NJ)	Pul	910
Arnold, Thomas (NY)	VascS	636
Arnon, Rica (NY)	PCd	304
Arnstein, Ellis (NY)	Ped	428
Aron, Alan (NY)	ChiN	143
Aronne, Louis (NY)	IM	198
Aronoff, Michael (NY)	Psyc	339
Aronson, Thomas (NY)	Psyc	631
Arpadi, Stephen (NY)	Ped	319
Arthur, Karen (NY)	S	707
Arunachalam, Muthu (NJ)	Ger	782
Aruny, John (CT)	VIR	1033
Arvan, Glenn (NY)	OrS	625
Arvanitis, Michael (NJ)	CRS	858
Asarian, Armand (NY)	CRS	448
Asbell, Penny (NY)	Oph	254
Ascher, Enrico (NY)	VascS	484
Ascher-Walsh, Charles (NY)	ObG	247
Ascherman, Jeffrey (NY)	PlS	329
Ashamalla, Hani (NY)	RadRO	479
Ashany, Dalit (NY)	Rhu	365
Ashikari, Andrew (NY)	S	707
Ashinoff, Robin (NJ)	D	728
Ashinoff, Russell (NJ)	PlS	866
Ashley, Richard (NY)	U	589
Ashton, Julie (NJ)	Ped	885
Aslanian, Harry (CT)	Ge	1005
Asnes, Russell (NJ)	Ped	758
Asnis, Deborah (NY)	Inf	495
Asnis, Gregory (NY)	Psyc	432
Asnis, Stanley (NY)	OrS	562
Asprinio, David (NY)	OrS	685
Aston, Sherrell (NY)	PlS	329
Astrow, Alan (NY)	Onc	459
Atakent, Pinar (NY)	PMR	475
Athanasian, Edward (NY)	HS	185
Atlas, Arthur (NJ)	PPul	885
Atlas, Mark (NY)	PHO	570
Atluru, Vijaya (NY)	ChiN	533
Attas, Lewis (NJ)	Onc	741
Attia, Evelyn (NY)	Psyc	339
Attiyeh, Fadi (NY)	S	372
Attkiss, Keith (CT)	PlS	985
Attubato, Michael (NY)	IC	208
Auerbach, Mitchell (NY)	Ge	658
Aufiero, Patrick (NJ)	Inf	819
Augenbraun, Charles (CT)	Cv	943
Augenbraun, Michael (NY)	Inf	455
August, David (NJ)	S	852
August, Phyllis (NY)	Nep	226
Auguste, Louis (NY)	S	585
Auran, James (NY)	Oph	254
Austin, John (NY)	DR	157
Austin, Kenneth (NY)	OrS	600
Averill, Allison (NJ)	PMR	759
Aversa, Alphonse (NY)	IM	666
Avezzano, Eric (NJ)	Ge	733
Aviv, Jonathan (NY)	Oto	287
Avni-Singer, A. (CT)	Ped	1025
Avram, Marc (NY)	D	148
Avruskin, Theodore (NY)	PEn	471
Avvento, Louis (NY)	Hem	617
Awad, John (CT)	OrS	975
Axelrod, Deborah (NY)	S	372
Axelrod, Felicia (NY)	Ped	319
Axelrod, Sheldon (NY)	U	710

Alphabetical Listing of Doctors

Name	Specialty	Pg
Ayoub, Thomas (CT)	ObG	969
Ayyanathan, Karpukarasi (NJ)	Ped	927
Azhar, Salman (NY)	N	462
Azodi, Masoud (CT)	GO	1007

B

Name	Specialty	Pg
Babitz, Lisa (NY)	Ger	180
Babkowski, Robert (CT)	Path	981
Babu, Sateesh (NY)	VascS	713
Bacal, Darron (CT)	Oph	1017
Bacall, Charles (NY)	ObG	247
Baccash, Emil (NY)	Ger	453
Bach, John (NJ)	PMR	797
Bacha, Emile (NY)	T&CS	381
Bachmann, Gloria (NJ)	ObG	842
Backe, Henry (CT)	HS	955
Backman, Kenneth (CT)	A&I	941
Badani, Ketan (NY)	U	387
Bade, Harry (NJ)	OrS	864
Badikian, Arthur (NY)	Psyc	700
Baehring, Joachim (CT)	N	1015
Bagel, Jerry (NJ)	D	817
Bailey, Michele (NY)	Ped	695
Bailine, Samuel (NY)	Psyc	578
Bains, Manjit (NY)	T&CS	382
Bains, Yatinder (NJ)	IM	784
Baiocco, Peter (NY)	Ge	168
Baiser, Dennis (NJ)	Ped	825
Bajorin, Dean (NY)	Onc	212
Baker, Azzam (NJ)	Ped	810
Baker, Daniel (NY)	PlS	329
Baker, David (NY)	ObG	622
Bakshi, Sanjay (NY)	PM	297
Balcer, Laura (NY)	N	234
Baldwin, Hilary (NY)	D	448
Bale, Allen (CT)	CG	1003
Balk, Sophie (NY)	Ped	428
Balkin, Michael (NY)	EDM	613
Balot, Barry (NY)	IM	618
Baltimore, Robert (CT)	PInf	1023
Banc, Tobe (NY)	Ger	662
Bangaru, Babu (NY)	PGe	307
Bank, David (NY)	D	651
Bank, Matthew (NY)	S	586
Banks, Judy (NJ)	ObG	881
Bansal, Rajendra (NY)	Oph	254
Bansil, Shalini (NJ)	N	923
Banzon, Manuel (NJ)	ObG	809
Baorto, Elizabeth (NJ)	PInf	884
Bar, Michael (CT)	Hem	956
Bar-Chama, Natan (NY)	U	387
Barabas, Ronald (NJ)	ChiN	858
Barakat, Richard (NY)	GO	182
Baram, Daniel (NY)	Pul	632
Baranetsky, Nicholas (NJ)	EDM	780
Barasch, Jeffrey (NJ)	Pul	762
Barbasch, Avi (NY)	Onc	212
Barbuto, Joseph (NY)	Psyc	339
Barcewicz, Paul (CT)	S	1030
Bard, Michael (CT)	Oto	978
Barenberg, David (CT)	Ge	952
Barie, Philip (NY)	S	373
Barile, Gaetano (NY)	Oph	254
Barisciano, Lisa (NJ)	PA&I	883
Barker, Barbara (NY)	Oph	254
Barley, Christopher (NY)	IM	198
Barmakian, Joseph (NJ)	OrS	925
Barnard, Nicola (NJ)	Path	846
Barone, Clement (NY)	DR	158
Barone, Joseph (NJ)	Ped Uro	909
Barone, Richard (NY)	Rhu	705
Barrett, Leonard (NY)	T&CS	588
Barrison, Adam (NJ)	Ge	919
Barro, Jennifer (CT)	Ge	952
Barron, Otis (NY)	HS	185
Barsh, Elliot (NY)	Ped	695
Bartell, Abraham (NY)	ChAP	140
Bartlett, Jacqueline (NJ)	ChAP	778
Bartolomeo, Robert (NY)	Ge	540
Basch, Samuel (NY)	Psyc	339
Baselga, Jose (NY)	Onc	212
Bashevkin, Michael (NY)	Onc	459
Baskin, David (NY)	IM	198
Baskin, Martin (NY)	Pul	353
Baskind, Lawrence (NY)	Ped	695
Basner, Robert (NY)	Pul	353
Basralian, Kevin (NJ)	U	768
Bassett, Clifford (NY)	A&I	126

Name	Specialty	Pg
Bastawros, Mary (NY)	Ped	517
Basuk, Pamela (NY)	D	611
Basuk, Paul (NY)	Ge	169
Baum, Eric (CT)	PO	1024
Bauman, Jonathan (NY)	Psyc	700
Bauman, Phillip (NY)	OrS	270
Baumann, John (NJ)	RadRO	851
Baumgaertner, Michael (CT)	OrS	1018
Bavaro, Nicholas (NY)	OrS	685
Bazzy-Asaad, Alia (CT)	PPul	1024
Beauregard, Lou-Anne (NJ)	Cv	857
Beauvais, Paul (CT)	OrS	1018
Beccia, David (NY)	U	636
Becker, Alfred (NY)	Rhu	602
Becker, David (NY)	D	148
Becker, Ina (NY)	ChAP	140
Beckman, Karen (CT)	Ped	982
Bederson, Joshua (NY)	NS	229
Bednarek, Karl (NY)	Ge	169
Beer, Jeffry (NY)	PMR	575
Behm, Dutsi (NY)	IM	456
Behr, Raymond (NY)	Psyc	578
Beim, Robert (NJ)	ObG	924
Belamarich, Peter (NY)	Ped	429
Beldner, Steven (NY)	HS	185
Belenkov, Elliot (NY)	Onc	213
Belilos, Elise (NY)	Rhu	584
Bell, David (NY)	AM	124
Bell, Jonathan (CT)	A&I	941
Bell, Kevin (NJ)	IM	906
Bellapianta, Joseph (CT)	OrS	975
Bellemare, Sarah (NY)	S	435
Bello, Jacqueline (NY)	NRad	421
Bello, Mary (NJ)	FMed	733
Bellucci, Alessandro (NY)	Nep	552
Belmont, H. Michael (NY)	Rhu	365
Belok, Lennart (NY)	N	234
Belostotsky, Olga (NY)	Rhu	365
Belsh, Jerry (NJ)	N	841
Belsito, Donald (NY)	D	148
Ben-Menachem, Tamir (NJ)	Ge	919
Benaviv-Meskin, Danielle (CT)	EDM	950
Benchimol, Corinne (NY)	PNep	313
Bendo, John (NY)	OrS	270
Benedetto, Dominick (NJ)	Oph	810
Benedict, Leonard (NY)	ObG	557
Benedicto, Milagros (NY)	ObG	499
Benevenia, Joseph (NJ)	OrS	791
Beniaminovitz, Ainat (NY)	Cv	595
Benisovich, Vladimir (NY)	Onc	497
Benito, Carlos (NJ)	MF	879
Benjamin, John (NY)	Psyc	579
Benkov, Keith (NY)	PGe	308
Bennett, Harvey (NJ)	ChiN	874
Bennett, Rachel (NY)	RE	705
Bennett, Stanford (NY)	IM	666
Bennett, Steven (CT)	PM	980
Benoff, Brian (NJ)	Pul	762
Benowitz, Joel (NY)	S	586
Benson, Mitchell (NY)	U	387
Bent, John (NY)	PO	427
Benton, Marc (NJ)	Pul	887
Benvenisty, Alan (NY)	VascS	397
Benzil, Deborah (NY)	NS	676
Beran, Nancy (NY)	IM	667
Beran, Samuel (NY)	PlS	698
Berbari, Nicholas (NY)	IM	546
Berberian, Wayne (NJ)	OrS	791
Berck, David (NY)	MF	671
Berdoff, Russell (NY)	Cv	130
Berenstein, Alejandro (NY)	NRad	243
Berezin, Marc (NY)	SM	602
Berezin, Stuart (NY)	PGe	691
Berger, Bernard (NY)	D	611
Berger, Jack (NY)	Rhu	706
Berger, Jeffrey (NY)	H & PM	545
Berger, Judith (NY)	Inf	415
Berger, Marvin (NY)	Cv	130
Berger, Robin (CT)	ObG	969
Berger, Scott (NY)	NRad	679
Bergh, Paul (NJ)	RE	888
Bergman, Donald (NY)	EDM	163
Bergman, Kerry (NJ)	PS	927
Bergman, Michael (NY)	Pul	477
Bergmann, Steven (NY)	Cv	130
Bergtraum, Marcia (NY)	ChiN	534
Berke, Andrew (NY)	IC	548
Berke, Stanley (NY)	Oph	559
Berkey, Peter (NY)	Inf	665
Berkowitz, Eric (NY)	D	148

Alphabetical Listing of Doctors

Name	Specialty	Pg
Berkowitz, Howard (NY)	Psyc	476
Berkowitz, Irwin (NJ)	Ped	758
Berkowitz, Leonard (NY)	Inf	455
Berkowitz, Norman (NY)	Ped	695
Berkowitz, Rhonda (NY)	D	651
Berkowitz, Richard (NY)	MF	210
Berkowitz, Richard (NJ)	EDM	894
Berkowitz, Walter (NJ)	Cv	724
Berkwits, Kieve (CT)	PCd	981
Berlin, Scott (NY)	ObG	622
Berman, Alvin (NY)	ObG	247
Berman, Daniel (NY)	Inf	415
Berman, David (NY)	Oph	465
Berman, Edward (CT)	IM	958
Berman, Ellin (NY)	Onc	213
Berman, Lewis (CT)	Pul	988
Berman, Mark (NJ)	OrS	750
Berman, Morton (NY)	Ped	696
Berman, Russell (NY)	S	373
Berman, Sheldon (NY)	Psyc	579
Berman, Steven (NY)	U	387
Bernardini, Dennis (NY)	Pul	632
Bernardo, Salvatore (NJ)	FMed	859
Bernasko, James (NY)	MF	619
Bernhardt, Bernard (NY)	Onc	672
Bernik, Stephanie (NY)	S	373
Bernik, Thomas (NY)	VascS	397
Bernstein, Brett (NY)	Ge	169
Bernstein, Chaim (NY)	Pul	477
Bernstein, Charles (NY)	D	510
Bernstein, David (NY)	Ge	540
Bernstein, Harvey (NY)	Ped	629
Bernstein, Joseph (NY)	PO	693
Bernstein, Larry (NY)	A&I	403
Bernstein, Michael (NY)	S	481
Bernstein, Michael (CT)	Pul	988
Bernstein, Neil (NY)	CE	127
Bernstein, Robert (NY)	D	148
Bernstein, William (NY)	Ped	600
Berry, Richard (NY)	D	448
Berson, Barry (NY)	DR	158
Berson, Diane (NY)	D	149
Besser, Gary (CT)	ObG	969
Besser, Louis (NY)	Cv	509
Besser, Walter (NY)	OrS	500
Bessey, Palmer (NY)	S	373
Bessler, Marc (NY)	S	373
Bethel, Colin (NJ)	PS	796
Better, Donna (NY)	PCd	567
Bevelaqua, Frederick (NY)	Pul	353
Beyda, Allan (NY)	IM	496
Beyda, Bernadette (NY)	D	491
Beyerl, Brian (NJ)	NS	880
Bhagat, Neelakshi (NJ)	Oph	789
Bhansali, Rohan (NY)	Cv	529
Bharathan, Thayyullathil (NY)	IM	456
Bhatt, Anjani (NY)	EDM	538
Bhatt, Ashok (NY)	Psyc	579
Bhattacharyya, Nishith (NJ)	PS	898
Bhora, Faiz (NY)	T&CS	382
Bia, Margaret (CT)	Nep	1013
Biagiotti, Wendy (NY)	FMed	410
Bialer, Martin (NY)	CG	534
Bialer, Philip (NY)	Psyc	339
Biancaniello, Thomas (NY)	PCd	627
Bianchi, Mark (CT)	Oto	978
Bianco, Angela (NY)	MF	210
Bickers, David (NY)	D	149
Bielory, Leonard (NJ)	A&I	916
Bierman, Fredrick (NY)	PCd	689
Bigliani, Louis (NY)	OrS	270
Bikoff, David (NJ)	PlS	760
Bilezikian, John (NY)	EDM	163
Bilfinger, Thomas (NY)	T&CS	635
Billett, Henny (NY)	Hem	415
Bilsky, Mark (NY)	NS	229
Bindelglass, David (CT)	OrS	975
Binder, Ralph (NY)	Pul	702
Binns, Joseph (NJ)	Ge	859
Birch, Thomas (NJ)	Inf	737
Birnbaum, Audrey (NY)	PGe	691
Birnbaum, Henry (NY)	PMR	325
Birnbaum, Jeffrey (NY)	AM	443
Birns, Douglas (NY)	U	387
Biro, David (NY)	D	448
Bisaga, Adam (NY)	AdP	642
Bisberg, Dorothy (NJ)	PPul	795
Biser, Seth (NY)	Oph	681
Bitan, Fabien (NY)	OrS	270
Bitton, Rachelle (NY)	EDM	538

Name	Specialty	Pg
Biviano, Angelo (NY)	CE	128
Biviano, Bernard (NY)	S	504
Bivona, James (CT)	IM	958
Blackwood, M. Michele (NJ)	S	801
Blady, David (NJ)	N	788
Blaine, Theodore (CT)	OrS	1018
Blair, Bryan (NY)	U	710
Blair, Emily (CT)	ObG	969
Blair, Lester (NY)	Pul	353
Blaivas, Jerry (NY)	U	387
Blake, James (NY)	Cv	130
Blanck, Richard (NY)	N	555
Blanco, Jody (NY)	ObG	247
Blank, Ellen (NJ)	D	807
Blank, Stephanie (NY)	GO	183
Blatter, Brett (NY)	Psyc	339
Blau, Sheldon (NY)	Rhu	584
Blaufox, Andrew (NY)	PCd	567
Blei, Francine (NY)	PHO	309
Bleich, David (NJ)	EDM	780
Bleicher, Robert (NJ)	Ge	894
Bleiweiss, Ira (NY)	Path	300
Blick, Michael (NJ)	Cv	874
Blitzer, Andrew (NY)	Oto	287
Blitzer, Mark (CT)	CE	1001
Blondo, Dennis (NJ)	Oph	843
Bloom, Katherine (CT)	A&I	941
Bloom, Norman (NY)	S	373
Bloom, Patricia (NY)	Ger	180
Bloomfield, Diane (NY)	Ped	429
Bloomgarden, David (NY)	EDM	655
Bloomgarden, Zachary (NY)	EDM	163
Blum, Alan (NY)	Pul	580
Blum, Conrad (NY)	EDM	163
Blum, Daniel (NY)	IM	496
Blum, David (NY)	EDM	656
Blum, Jay (NJ)	A&I	831
Blum, Mark (NJ)	Cv	874
Blum, Ronald (NY)	Onc	213
Blumberg, Joel (CT)	IM	958
Blume, Ralph (NY)	Rhu	365
Blumenfeld, Jon (NY)	Nep	226
Blumenthal, David (NY)	Cv	130
Blumstein, Meyer (NY)	Ge	540
Boachie-Adjei, Oheneba (NY)	OrS	271
Bobby, Paul (CT)	MF	962
Bobroff, Lewis (NY)	DR	596
Bochner, Bernard (NY)	U	388
Bochner, Ronnie (NJ)	ObG	843
Bockman, Richard (NY)	EDM	163
Boczko, Judd (NY)	U	710
Boczko, Stanley (NY)	U	388
Bodenstein, Lawrence (NY)	PS	316
Bodis-Wollner, Ivan (NY)	N	462
Bodner, Staci (NY)	Ped	319
Bodner, William (NY)	RadRO	434
Bogen, Steven (NY)	Psyc	700
Bogin, Marc (NY)	Cv	509
Boim, Marilynn (NJ)	Ped	825
Boland, Patrick (NY)	OrS	271
Bolognia, Jean (CT)	D	1004
Bomback, David (CT)	OrS	975
Bomback, Fredric (NY)	Ped	696
Bonagura, Vincent (NY)	PA&I	567
Bonaventura, Lisa (NJ)	IM	906
Bond, Annette (CT)	MF	962
Bondi, Elliott (NY)	Pul	477
Bone, Stanley (NY)	Psyc	339
Bonheim, Nelson (CT)	Ge	952
Bonilla, Mary Ann (NJ)	PHO	897
Boniuk, Vivien (NY)	Oph	559
Boockvar, John (NY)	NS	229
Bookner, Scott (NY)	Ped	696
Boolbol, Robert (CT)	PM	980
Boolbol, Susan (NY)	S	373
Boone, Peter (CT)	OrS	975
Boorady, Roy (NY)	ChAP	140
Boorjian, Peter (NJ)	U	803
Borah, Gregory (NJ)	PlS	849
Borao, Frank (NJ)	S	868
Borbely, Antal (NY)	Psyc	339
Borcich, Anthony (NY)	Ge	169
Borek, Mark (NY)	Cv	608
Borer, Jeffrey (NY)	Cv	444
Borg, Morton (NY)	PCd	304
Borgen, Patrick (NY)	S	481
Borkowsky, William (NY)	PInf	312
Borriello, Raffaele (NY)	S	481
Bortz, John (NY)	Oph	682
Boruchoff, Susan (NJ)	Inf	837

Alphabetical Listing of Doctors

Name	Specialty	Pg
Boscamp, Jeffrey (NJ)	PInf	755
Bosco, Joseph (NY)	OrS	271
Bosl, George (NY)	Onc	213
Boss, William (NJ)	PlS	760
Bosso, John (NY)	A&I	595
Bostrom, Mathias (NY)	OrS	271
Bosworth, Jay (NY)	RadRO	582
Botwin, Clifford (NJ)	OrS	925
Botwinick, Nelson (NY)	HS	186
Boulware, Susan (CT)	PEn	1022
Bourla, Steven (NY)	Nep	552
Boxer, Harriet (NY)	NP	552
Boxer, Mitchell (NY)	A&I	526
Boxer, William (NY)	IM	198
Boyd, D. Barry (CT)	Hem	956
Boyer, Joseph (NY)	PPul	693
Boyle, Jay (NY)	Oto	287
Brademas, Mary Ellen (NY)	D	149
Bradley, Thomas (NY)	Onc	550
Brady, Mary (NY)	S	373
Bram, Harris (NJ)	PM	865
Bramwit, Steven (CT)	Oto	979
Brancaccio, Ronald (NY)	D	448
Brancaccio, William (NY)	DR	612
Brand, Howard (NY)	EDM	613
Brandeis, Steven (NY)	CRS	145
Brandt, Fredric (NY)	D	149
Brandt, Lawrence (NY)	Ge	411
Brannagan, Thomas (NY)	N	234
Branovan, Daniel (NY)	Oto	469
Brathwaite, Collin (NY)	S	586
Brauer, Richard (CT)	Oto	979
Brauner, Gary (NJ)	D	728
Braunstein, Richard (NY)	Oph	255
Brauntuch, Glenn (NJ)	Pul	762
Brause, Barry (NY)	Inf	193
Braver, Joel (NJ)	RadRO	910
Brecher, Rubin (NY)	Oph	465
Breda, Stephen (CT)	Oto	979
Breen, William (NY)	Cv	529
Breglio, Keith (NY)	PGe	308
Bregman, Zachary (NY)	IM	198
Breidbart, David (NY)	Pul	580
Breitbart, Arnold (NY)	PlS	576
Breitbart, William (NY)	Psyc	340
Brener, Bruce (NJ)	VascS	804
Brener, Sorin (NY)	IC	458
Brenner, Dennis (NJ)	PEn	794
Brenner, Ronald (NY)	Psyc	340
Brenner, Stephen (CT)	IM	1009
Brenner, Steven (NY)	RE	583
Brentjens, Renier (NY)	Onc	213
Breslin, David (NY)	U	710
Breslow, Gary (NJ)	PlS	760
Bressman, Susan (NY)	N	235
Brett, Elise (NY)	EDM	163
Brewer, Marlon (NY)	IM	496
Brewster, Ursula (CT)	Nep	1013
Brick, David (NY)	PCd	304
Brickman, Alan (NY)	EDM	450
Brickner, Gary (NJ)	ObG	823
Brief, Rochelle (NY)	PMR	601
Brightman, Rebecca (NY)	ObG	247
Brill, Joseph (NY)	Pul	702
Brill, Paula (NY)	DR	158
Brillon, David (NY)	EDM	164
Briner, William (NY)	SM	585
Brisman, Jonathan (NY)	NS	553
Brisson, Paul (NY)	OrS	271
Brittis, Dante (CT)	OrS	975
Britton, Carolyn (NY)	N	235
Brodherson, Michael (NY)	U	388
Brodie, Jonathan (NY)	Psyc	340
Brodman, Michael (NY)	ObG	247
Brodman, Richard (NJ)	Rhu	930
Brody, Samuel (NY)	Ger	494
Brogno, David (NY)	IC	597
Bromberg, Assia (NJ)	Pul	762
Bromley, Gary (NY)	PlS	329
Bronen, Richard (CT)	NRad	1015
Bronheim, Harold (NY)	Psyc	340
Bronin, Andrew (NY)	D	651
Bronson, Michael (NY)	OrS	271
Bronson, Richard (NY)	RE	633
Bronster, David (NY)	N	235
Broumand, Stafford (NY)	PlS	330
Broussard, Crystal (NJ)	Ge	733
Brovender, Bruce (NY)	Ped	319
Brown, Andrew (NJ)	Oph	748
Brown, Andrew (NY)	PMR	325

Name	Specialty	Pg
Brown, Arthur (NY)	Inf	193
Brown, Carol (NY)	GO	183
Brown, Christopher (NJ)	Oph	748
Brown, David (NJ)	PMR	849
Brown, David (NJ)	A&I	916
Brown, David (CT)	OrS	976
Brown, David (NY)	Cv	608
Brown, Eric (CT)	Nep	965
Brown, Jeffrey (NY)	NS	553
Brown, Jessica (NY)	RE	361
Brown, Jocelyn (NY)	Ped	319
Brown, John (NJ)	T&CS	889
Brown, Karen (NY)	VIR	394
Brown, Kevin (NY)	Oto	287
Brown, Lionel (CT)	HS	955
Brown, Marc (NY)	DR	158
Brown, Mitchell (NJ)	Ger	808
Brown, Richard (NY)	Psyc	340
Brown, Robert (CT)	Pul	988
Brown, Robert (NY)	Ge	169
Browner-Elhanan, Karen (NY)	AM	642
Bruce, Jeffrey (NY)	NS	229
Bruck, Lance (CT)	ObG	969
Bruckner, Howard (NY)	Onc	417
Bruckstein, Alex (NY)	Ge	512
Bruckstein, Robert (NY)	D	535
Brumberg, Heather (NY)	NP	674
Brunckhorst, Keith (NY)	Onc	213
Brunetti, Jacqueline (NJ)	NuM	747
Brunner, Eugenie (NJ)	Oto	824
Brunnquell, Stephen (NJ)	IM	738
Bruno, Anthony (NY)	U	589
Bruno, Peter (NY)	IM	198
Brustein, Harris (NY)	Oph	682
Brustman, Lois (NY)	ObG	247
Bryce, Thomas (NY)	PMR	325
Buchalter, Maury (NJ)	Ped	758
Buchbinder, Ellen (NY)	A&I	126
Buchman, Myron (NY)	ObG	247
Buchness, Mary Ruth (NY)	D	149
Bucholtz, Harvey (NJ)	EDM	834
Buckley, Lenore (CT)	Rhu	1029
Buckner, Cary (NY)	N	462
Budd, Daniel (NJ)	S	899
Budin, Joel (NJ)	DR	730
Budman, Cathy (NY)	Psyc	579
Budman, Daniel (NY)	Onc	550
Bufalini, Bruno (NJ)	S	766
Bukberg, Judith (NY)	Psyc	340
Bukberg, Phillip (NY)	EDM	164
Bulgarelli, Christopher (NY)	Psyc	340
Bullock, Richard (NJ)	Ger	836
Buly, Robert (NY)	OrS	271
Burak, George (NY)	OrS	685
Bures, Sergio (NY)	Pul	702
Burke, Karen (NY)	D	149
Burke, Patricia (NJ)	Oph	748
Burkes, Lynn (NY)	ChAP	140
Burns, Bryan (CT)	Ge	952
Burns, Elisa (NY)	ObG	680
Burns, Les (NJ)	ObG	896
Burns, Mark (NY)	Rhu	706
Burns, Paul (NY)	PM	600
Burns, Paul (NJ)	T&CS	802
Burschtin, Omar (NY)	Pul	353
Burstein, Ora (CT)	PA&I	981
Burstin, Harris (NY)	Ped	319
Burton, Daniel (NY)	A&I	126
Buscaglia, Jonathan (NY)	Ge	615
Busch-Devereaux, Erna (NY)	S	634
Buschmann, William (NY)	OrS	685
Bush, Jacqueline (NY)	MF	459
Bush, Michael (NY)	IM	198
Busillo, Christopher (NY)	Inf	193
Bussel, James (NY)	PHO	309
Bussell, Stuart (CT)	CRS	946
Buterman, Irving (NY)	ObG	248
Butler, David (NJ)	ObG	747
Butler, James (CT)	N	967
Butler, Mark (NJ)	OrS	908
Butt, Ahmar (NY)	IM	456
Buxton, Douglas (NY)	Oph	255
Buyon, Jill (NY)	Rhu	365
Buzzeo, Louis (NY)	Nep	675
Byfield, Floyd (NY)	Ge	658
Byk, Cheryl (NJ)	DR	780
Byrd, Lawrence (NJ)	Nep	787

Alphabetical Listing of Doctors

Name	Specialty	Pg
C		
Cabaniss, Deborah (NY)	Psyc	340
Cabin, Henry (CT)	Cv	1002
Caccavale, Robert (NJ)	T&CS	911
Caccese, William (NY)	Ge	540
Cacciola, Thomas (NJ)	IM	739
Cafferty, Maureen (NY)	N	235
Cahan, Anthony (NY)	S	707
Cahill, James (NJ)	OrS	750
Cahill, John (NY)	PrM	338
Cahill, Linda (NY)	Ped	429
Cahill, Patrick (CT)	ObG	969
Cairo, Mitchell (NY)	PHO	692
Calem-Grunat, Jaclyn (NJ)	DR	730
Calhoun, Sean (NJ)	VIR	890
Caligiuri, Daniel (NY)	HS	495
Caligor, Eve (NY)	Psyc	340
Callahan, Eileen (NY)	Ger	180
Callahan, Lisa (NY)	SM	370
Calman, Neil (NY)	FMed	167
Cam, Jenny Rose (NJ)	EDM	807
Camacho, Fernando (NY)	Onc	417
Camacho, Margarita (NJ)	T&CS	802
Camel, Mark (CT)	NS	966
Cammarata, Sandra (NJ)	ChAP	778
Cammisa, Frank (NY)	OrS	272
Campagna, Robert (NY)	Cv	130
Campbell, Deborah (NY)	NP	418
Campolattaro, Brian (NY)	Oph	255
Cancellieri, Russell (NY)	A&I	607
Cangemi, Francis (NJ)	Oph	789
Cannarozzi, Nicholas (NJ)	Rhu	800
Canny, Christopher (CT)	Ped	1025
Cantor, Michael (NY)	Ge	169
Capasse, Jeanne (CT)	S	992
Caplivski, Daniel (NY)	Inf	193
Capobianco, Luigi (NY)	FMed	540
Capozzi, James (NY)	OrS	562
Cappucci, Roger (NY)	Cv	644
Caprio, Martha (NY)	NP	225
Caputo, Anthony (NJ)	Oph	789
Caputo, Thomas (NY)	GO	183
Caracci, Giovanni (NJ)	Psyc	799
Cardiello, Gary (NJ)	IM	808
Cardoso, Erico (NY)	NS	461
Carew, John (NY)	Oto	287
Carey, Dennis (NY)	PEn	569
Carlin, Elizabeth (NJ)	NP	743
Carlson, Andrew (CT)	Ped	1025
Carlson, Elise (CT)	Rhu	1029
Carlson, Gabrielle (NY)	ChAP	609
Carlson, Harold (NY)	EDM	613
Carlson, Michelle (NY)	HS	186
Carmine, Linda (NY)	AM	526
Carney, Alexander (NJ)	Rhu	827
Carniciu, Sanda (NY)	N	677
Carniol, Paul (NJ)	Oto	926
Caron, Philip (NY)	Onc	672
Carosella, Christine (NY)	IM	667
Carpenter, Duncan (NJ)	NS	744
Carpenter, Thomas (CT)	PEn	1022
Carr-Locke, David (NY)	Ge	169
Carrasquillo, Jorge (NY)	NuM	245
Carroccio, Alfio (NY)	VascS	397
Carroll, William (NY)	PHO	309
Carson, Jeffrey (NJ)	IM	838
Carsons, Steven (NY)	Rhu	584
Carter, Mitchel (NJ)	S	888
Caruana, Salvatore (NY)	Oto	288
Carucci, John (NY)	D	149
Caruso, Rocco (NY)	Onc	620
Carver, Alan (NY)	N	235
Casale, Linda (CT)	Cv	943
Casale, Pasquale (NY)	Ped Uro	318
Casden, Andrew (NY)	OrS	272
Case, David (NY)	IM	199
Casino, Joseph (NY)	Pul	702
Casper, Daniel (NY)	Oph	255
Casper, Ephraim (NJ)	Onc	907
Casper, Theodore (NY)	Pul	433
Cassell, Lauren (NY)	S	374
Cassidy, Brian (NJ)	IM	838
Casson, Ira (NY)	N	499
Castellano, Bartolomeo (NY)	Oto	516
Castellano, Michael (NY)	Pul	518
Castro-Magana, Mariano (NY)	PEn	569
Castro-Malaspina, Hugo (NY)	Hem	188
Catalano, Louis (NY)	HS	186
Catallozzi, Marina (NY)	AM	124

Name	Specialty	Pg
Catanese, Anthony (NJ)	U	911
Catanese, James (NY)	Cv	644
Catanese, Vincent (NJ)	FMed	859
Caty, Michael (CT)	PS	1024
Caucino, Julie (NJ)	A&I	903
Cavaliere, Gregg (NY)	SM	707
Cavallaro, Barbara (NJ)	ObG	747
Cayne, Neal (NY)	VascS	397
Cece, John (NJ)	Oto	897
Ceisler, Emily (NY)	Oph	255
Cemaletin, Nevber (NY)	Cv	130
Censullo, Michael (NJ)	VIR	854
Cerame, Barbara (NJ)	PEn	884
Cerrone, Federico (NJ)	Pul	930
Cerulli, Maurice (NY)	Ge	541
Cervia, Joseph (NY)	Inf	545
Chabot, John (NY)	S	374
Chacho, Karol (CT)	RE	990
Chachoua, Abraham (NY)	Onc	213
Chadda, Kul (NY)	Cv	529
Chadha, Jang B S (NY)	Pul	502
Chadha, Manjeet (NY)	RadRO	358
Chagpar, Anees (CT)	S	1030
Chai, Emily (NY)	H & PM	192
Chaiken, Barry (NY)	Oph	255
Chaikin, David (NJ)	U	889
Chaim, Joshua (NY)	DR	158
Chalal, Jeffrey (NJ)	DR	858
Chalas, Eva (NY)	GO	543
Chalom, Elizabeth (NJ)	PRhu	796
Chamberlain, Ronald (NJ)	S	801
Chan, Brenda (CT)	Nep	965
Chan, Siu-Pun (NY)	PPul	517
Chandler, Michael (NY)	A&I	126
Chandra, Prasanta (NY)	MF	459
Chandrasekhar, Sujana (NY)	Oto	288
Chang, Benjamin (NY)	Pul	602
Chang, Christine (NY)	Ger	180
Chang, Peter (NY)	RE	361
Chang, Peter (NY)	Ge	169
Chang, Stanley (NY)	Oph	255
Channamsetty, Venu (CT)	Cv	943
Chao, Chun (NY)	PRhu	694
Chao, K.S. Clifford (NY)	RadRO	358
Chapman, Mark (NY)	Ge	170
Chapman, Paul (NY)	Onc	213
Chapnick, Edward (NY)	Inf	455
Charap, Mitchell (NY)	IM	199
Charap, Peter (NY)	IM	199
Charles, James (NJ)	N	809
Charles, Norman (NY)	Oph	255
Charney, Jonathan (NY)	N	235
Charney, Richard (NY)	Cv	644
Charnoff, Judah (NY)	Cv	444
Charny, Caleb (NY)	S	708
Charytan, Chaim (NY)	Nep	418
Chase, Mark (NJ)	OrS	791
Chaudhry, M Rashid (NY)	Oto	469
Chaudhry, Saqib (NY)	VascS	592
Chavez, Laura (NJ)	Ger	735
Chawla, Anupama (NY)	PGe	627
Chazotte, Cynthia (NY)	MF	417
Chehade, Mirna (NY)	PGe	308
Chen, Chun (NY)	NS	229
Chen, Constance (NY)	PlS	330
Chen, Jonathan (NY)	T&CS	382
Chen, Lucy (NJ)	Oph	882
Chen, Serena (NJ)	RE	800
Chen, Timothy (NY)	Cv	529
Cheng, David (CT)	NuM	1016
Chengot, Mathew (NY)	Cv	608
Chern, Relly (NY)	Oph	256
Chernack, William (NJ)	A&I	873
Chernobilsky, Lev (NY)	Ped	629
Cherofsky, Alan (NY)	PlS	518
Cherry, Sabrina (NY)	Psyc	341
Chertoff, Harvey (NJ)	Psyc	761
Chervin, Bradford (CT)	Oto	979
Chesner, Michael (NY)	Cv	529
Chess, Jeremy (NY)	Oph	422
Chessin, Robert (CT)	Ped	982
Chessler, Richard (NJ)	Ge	733
Cheung, Nai-Kong (NY)	PHO	309
Chhieng, David (CT)	Path	1021
Chi, Dennis (NY)	GO	183
Chianese, Maurice (NY)	Ped	573
Chiariello, Mario (NY)	S	481
Chideckel, Norman (NY)	VascS	397
Chidyllo, Stephen (NJ)	PlS	866
Chin, Daisy (NJ)	PEn	884

Alphabetical Listing of Doctors

Name	Specialty	Pg
Chin, Jean (NY)	ObG	248
Chin, Patrick (NJ)	Oph	748
Chin, Simon (NY)	PlS	698
Chinitz, Larry (NY)	CE	128
Chinitz, Marvin (NY)	Ge	659
Chinn, Bertram (NJ)	CRS	918
Chiravuri, Murali (CT)	CE	942
Chiriboga-Klein, Claudia (NY)	ChiN	143
Chiu, David (NY)	PlS	330
Chiurco, Anthony (NJ)	NS	822
Chodosh, Eliot (NJ)	N	895
Choi, Janet (NY)	RE	361
Choi, Joonun (CT)	Cv	943
Choi, Laura (CT)	S	992
Choi, Mihye (NY)	PlS	330
Cholst, Ina (NY)	RE	361
Chou, Shyan-Yih (NY)	Nep	460
Choudhri, Ajay (NJ)	DR	817
Choudhri, Tanvir (NY)	NS	230
Choudhury, Muhammad (NY)	U	710
Choueka, Jack (NY)	HS	454
Chrisanderson, Donna (NJ)	IM	784
Christoudias, George (NJ)	S	766
Chronakos, John (CT)	Pul	988
Chuang, Linus (NY)	GO	183
Chun, Audrey (NY)	Ger	180
Chun, Thomas (NJ)	U	768
Chung, Henry (NY)	Psyc	341
Chung, Jeff (NJ)	Rhu	764
Chung, Joyce (CT)	RadRO	1028
Chung, Wendy (NY)	CG	145
Chung-Loy, Harold (NJ)	S	852
Ciccone, Patrick (NJ)	U	803
Cicogna, Cristina (NJ)	Inf	738
Cigno, Thomas (CT)	FMed	950
Cioffi, George (NY)	Oph	256
Cioroiu, Michael (NY)	S	374
Cipriani, Ralph (CT)	Inf	956
Cirello, Richard (NJ)	FMed	781
Citron, Marc (NY)	Onc	550
Clain, Michael (CT)	OrS	976
Clark, Richard (NY)	D	611
Clark, Sheryl (NY)	D	149
Clark-Hamilton, Jill (NJ)	AM	873
Cleman, Michael (CT)	Cv	1002
Close, Lanny (NY)	Oto	288
Coady, Michael (CT)	T&CS	994
Cobelli, Neil (NY)	OrS	423
Cobin, Rhoda (NJ)	EDM	731
Coco, Maria (NY)	Nep	418
Coffey, Barbara (NY)	ChAP	140
Cofsky, Richard (NY)	Inf	455
Cohall, Alwyn (NY)	AM	124
Cohen, Alice (NJ)	Hem	783
Cohen, Anders (NY)	NS	461
Cohen, Arnold (NY)	Psyc	341
Cohen, Barry (NY)	IM	456
Cohen, Barry (NJ)	Nep	821
Cohen, Ben (NY)	Oph	256
Cohen, Bradley (NY)	S	634
Cohen, Bruce (CT)	Ped	982
Cohen, Burton (NY)	DR	158
Cohen, Carl (NY)	GerPsy	453
Cohen, Charmian (NY)	EDM	409
Cohen, Daniel (NY)	Rhu	584
Cohen, Daniel (NY)	N	621
Cohen, David (NY)	Nep	226
Cohen, David (NY)	D	149
Cohen, Elin (CT)	Ped	982
Cohen, Jean-Marc (NY)	Path	300
Cohen, Joel (NY)	N	420
Cohen, Jonathan (NY)	Ge	170
Cohen, Lawrence (NY)	Ge	170
Cohen, Lee (NY)	ChAP	648
Cohen, Leeber (NY)	Oph	256
Cohen, Marc (NJ)	IC	785
Cohen, Martin (NY)	CE	643
Cohen, Martin (NY)	Cv	404
Cohen, Michael (NY)	Pul	580
Cohen, Michael (NY)	Cv	130
Cohen, Michel (NY)	Ped	319
Cohen, Neil (NY)	EDM	511
Cohen, Neil (CT)	Hem	956
Cohen, Richard (NY)	IM	199
Cohen, Robert (NY)	IM	199
Cohen, Seth (NY)	Ge	170
Cohen, Seymour (NY)	Onc	214
Cohen, Steven (CT)	DR	948
Cohen, Steven (NY)	D	407
Cohen, Steven (NJ)	Oph	789

Name	Specialty	Pg
Cohenuram, Michael (CT)	Onc	963
Cohn, Symra (NY)	IM	199
Cohn, William (NY)	Ge	615
Coit, Daniel (NY)	S	374
Colaco, Rodolfo (NJ)	S	931
Colangelo, Daniel (NY)	IM	667
Colberg, John (CT)	U	1032
Cole, Jeffrey (NJ)	PMR	797
Cole, Robert (NJ)	RadRO	899
Cole, William (NY)	Cv	131
Coleman, Donald (NY)	Oph	256
Coleman, Jonathan (NY)	U	388
Coleman, Morton (NY)	Onc	214
Colen, Helen (NY)	PlS	330
Colenda, Maryann (NJ)	PA&I	753
Coll, Raymond (NY)	N	235
Collins, Eric (NY)	AdP	123
Collins, Margaret (NY)	Ped	696
Collum, Robert (NJ)	IM	878
Coloka-Kump, Rodika (NY)	FMed	410
Colon, Francisco (NJ)	PlS	886
Colton, Marc (NJ)	U	889
Colyer-Aversa, Lori (NJ)	Ped	797
Compito, Catherine (NY)	OrS	272
Compito, Gerard (NJ)	DR	834
Comrie, Millicent (NY)	ObG	464
Concato, John (CT)	IM	1009
Condemi, Giuseppe (NJ)	Onc	741
Condo, Dominick (NJ)	IM	808
Confino, Joel (NJ)	Oph	925
Connery, Cliff (NY)	T&CS	382
Connolly, Adrian (NJ)	D	779
Connolly, Mark (NJ)	T&CS	900
Connor, Bradley (NY)	Ge	170
Connor, John (NJ)	Ped Uro	885
Connor, Thomas (NJ)	PCd	793
Connors, Richard (CT)	D	947
Conroy, Daniel (NJ)	Cv	724
Constad, William (NJ)	Oph	810
Constantiner, Arturo (NY)	IM	199
Constantinescu, Andrei (NY)	PPul	315
Constantinides, Minas (NY)	Oto	288
Conte, Charles (NY)	S	586
Conway, Edward (NY)	PCCM	306
Conway, Joseph (CT)	Oph	972
Coohill, Lisa (NJ)	N	923
Cook, Perry (NY)	Hem	188
Cook, Stuart (NJ)	N	788
Cook-Bolden, Fran (NY)	D	150
Cooney, Leo (CT)	Ger	1006
Cooper, Arthur (NY)	PS	317
Cooper, Dennis (CT)	Onc	1011
Cooper, Jay (NY)	RadRO	479
Cooper, Jerome (NY)	Cv	644
Cooper, Kimberly (NY)	U	388
Cooper, Lauren (NJ)	D	875
Cooper, Robert (NY)	Ge	170
Cooper, Rubin (NY)	PCd	567
Cooper, Seymour (NY)	Ped	573
Cooper, Stanley (NY)	VIR	591
Cooperman, Alan (NJ)	ObG	788
Cooperman, Ross (NJ)	PlS	798
Copel, Joshua (CT)	MF	1011
Copen, David (CT)	Cv	943
Coplan, Jeremy (NY)	Psyc	476
Coppa, Gene (NY)	S	586
Copperman, Alan (NY)	RE	361
Coppola, John (NY)	Cv	131
Corapi, Mark (NY)	IM	546
Corazza, Douglas (NJ)	IM	819
Corbo, Emanuel (NJ)	Ped	928
Cordasco, Frank (NY)	OrS	272
Cordeiro, Peter (NY)	PlS	330
Cordero, Evelyn (NY)	FMed	410
Coren, Charles (NY)	PS	572
Corey, Timothy (NJ)	D	729
Corn, Beth (NY)	A&I	126
Cornell, Charles (NY)	OrS	272
Cornell, James (NJ)	CCM	728
Corpuz, Marilou (NY)	Inf	415
Correia, Joaquim (NJ)	CE	776
Corriel, Robert (NY)	A&I	527
Corson, Richard (NJ)	FMed	905
Cortes, Engracio (NY)	Onc	498
Corvo, Philip (CT)	S	992
Cosgrove, John (NY)	S	634
Cosman, Felicia (NY)	EDM	596
Cossari, Alfred (NY)	Oph	623
Costa, Leon (NJ)	OrS	824
Costantino, Peter (NY)	Oto	288

Alphabetical Listing of Doctors

Name	Specialty	Pg
Costanzo, Joseph (CT)	IM	958
Costeas, Constantinos (NJ)	CE	776
Costin, Andrew (NJ)	Cv	817
Coupey, Susan (NY)	AM	403
Courtney, Barbara (NJ)	IM	860
Couture, Carolyn (CT)	IM	958
Coven, Barbara (NY)	Ped	696
Coven, Roger (NJ)	ObG	747
Covey, Alexander (NY)	IM	618
Covey, Anne (NY)	VIR	394
Covit, Andrew (NJ)	Nep	840
Cowan, Stephen (NY)	Ped	696
Cowles, Robert (CT)	PS	1024
Cox, Kathryn (NY)	ObG	248
Coyle, Michael (NJ)	HS	905
Coyle, Patricia (NY)	N	621
Cracchiolo, Bernadette (NJ)	GO	782
Cracco, Joan (NY)	ChiN	447
Craig, Edward (NY)	OrS	272
Cramer, Marvin (NY)	Cv	529
Crane, Michael (NY)	PrM	338
Crane, Richard (NY)	Rhu	365
Crane, Stephen (NJ)	ObG	789
Crasta, Jovita (NY)	Psyc	579
Crawford, Bernard (NY)	T&CS	382
Crawford, James (NY)	Path	566
Cristofaro, Robert (NY)	OrS	685
Croen, Kenneth (NY)	IM	667
Croll, James (NY)	Nep	419
Cron, Julia (CT)	ObG	1016
Cross, Jennifer (NY)	Ped	320
Crowe, David (NY)	PCd	689
Crowe, John (CT)	HS	955
Cruz, Merle (NJ)	Cv	807
Crystal, Howard (NY)	N	462
Crystal, Kenneth (NY)	VIR	591
Culliford, Alfred (NY)	T&CS	382
Culligan, Patrick (NJ)	ObG	881
Cunha, Burke (NY)	Inf	545
Cunningham, James (CT)	OrS	976
Cunningham-Rundles, Charlotte (NY)	A&I	126
Cunningham-Rundles, Ward (NY)	IM	199
Cuomo, Frances (NY)	OrS	272
Curtin, John (NY)	GO	183
Cusack, Evelyn (CT)	Cv	944
Cushner, Fred (NY)	OrS	273
Cushner, Michael (NY)	OrS	685
Cusumano, Barbara (NY)	Ped	629
Cusumano, Stephen (NY)	IM	547
Cuteri, Joseph (CT)	ObG	969
Cutolo, Louis (NY)	PlS	518
Cuzzone, Louis (CT)	N	967
Cykiert, Robert (NY)	Oph	256
Cynamon, Jacob (NY)	VIR	437
Cziner, David (NY)	Cv	644

D

Name	Specialty	Pg
D'Agostini, Robert (NJ)	OrS	908
D'Agostino, Richard (NY)	OrS	562
D'Agostino, Ronald (NY)	Cv	529
D'Alessandro, David (NY)	T&CS	436
D'Alton, Mary (NY)	MF	210
D'Amico, Donald (NY)	Oph	256
D'Amico, Joseph (CT)	OrS	976
D'Amico, Richard (NJ)	PlS	760
D'Anna, John (NY)	S	519
D'Aversa, Gerard (NY)	Oph	559
D'Ayala, Marcus (NY)	VascS	484
D'Esposito, Robert (NY)	U	589
Dabney, Lisa (NY)	ObG	248
DaCosta, Noshir (NY)	Onc	620
Dagum, Alexander (NY)	PlS	631
Dahl, Neera (CT)	Nep	1014
Daknis, Charles (NJ)	PM	865
Dalena, John (NJ)	Ge	876
Dalton, Jack (NY)	RadRO	503
Daluiski, Aaron (NY)	HS	186
Daly, Jane (NY)	Onc	498
Damien, Miguel (NJ)	RE	867
Danehower, Richard (CT)	Rhu	991
Dangas, George (NY)	Cv	131
Daniels, Jeffrey (NJ)	Cv	857
Danziger, Stephen (NY)	D	448
Dar, Pe'er (NY)	ObG	421
Daras, Michael (NY)	N	235
Das, Seshadri (NY)	EDM	511
Dasgupta, Indira (NY)	PHO	426

Name	Specialty	Pg
Dasmahapatra, Kumar (NJ)	S	852
Datta, Rajiv (NY)	S	586
Datta, Samyadev (NJ)	PM	753
Daud-Ahmad, Sameera (NJ)	EDM	732
Daum, Fredric (NY)	PGe	569
Davenport, Deborah (NY)	ObG	622
David, Sami (NY)	RE	361
Davidson, Dennis (NY)	NP	621
Davidson, Lawrence (NJ)	Oph	789
Davies, Terry (NY)	EDM	164
Davis, George (NJ)	Pul	867
Davis, Ira (NY)	D	651
Davis, Jessica (NY)	CG	145
Davis, Joyce (NY)	D	150
Davis, Kenneth (NJ)	Ped	928
Davis, Nicole (NJ)	ObG	843
Davis, Owen (NY)	RE	361
Davis, Raphael (NY)	NS	621
Dayal, Ashlesha (NY)	MF	417
Dayan, Alan (NY)	Oph	256
De Antonio, Joseph (NJ)	Ge	818
De Carlo, Regina (NY)	ChiN	510
De Cosimo, Diana (NJ)	IM	785
De Giacomo, Frank (NJ)	IM	895
De Lotbiniere, Alain (NY)	NS	676
De Matteo, Robert (NY)	Pul	702
De Pietro, William (NY)	D	535
Deal, Robert (CT)	ObG	969
DeAnda, Abelardo (NY)	T&CS	382
DeAngelis, Lisa (NY)	N	235
DeAraujo, Maria (NY)	PMR	431
DeBroff, Brian (CT)	Oph	972
Decter, Edward (NJ)	OrS	791
Decter, Julian (NY)	Onc	214
Dedousis, John (NJ)	IM	809
DeFabritus, Albert (NY)	Nep	227
Degen, Jeffrey (NY)	NS	598
Deitch, Edwin (NJ)	S	801
Deitch, Jonathan (NY)	VascS	521
Deitz, Marcia (NY)	D	448
Del Pizzo, Joseph (NY)	U	388
DeLacure, Mark (NY)	Oto	288
Deland, Jonathan (NY)	OrS	273
Delaney, Brian (NY)	FMed	410
Delaney, Veronica (NY)	Nep	675

Name	Specialty	Pg
Delano, Barbara (NY)	Nep	460
DeLeo, Vincent (NY)	D	150
Delerme, Milton (NY)	Oph	257
Delfico, Anthony (NJ)	SM	765
DeLillo, Anthony (NJ)	Ge	733
Della Rocca, Robert (NY)	Oph	257
Delorenzo, Lawrence (NY)	Pul	703
Delprete, Salvatore (CT)	Onc	963
DeLuca, Albert (NY)	Cv	644
Deluca, Jeffrey (CT)	OrS	976
DeLuca, Joseph (NJ)	Oph	749
Demar, Leon (NY)	D	150
DeMatteo, Ronald (NY)	S	374
Demento, Frank (NY)	D	535
Demestihas, Anthy (CT)	S	992
Demetis, Spiro (NY)	Pul	478
DeNatale, Ralph (CT)	VascS	1033
Denehy, Thad (NJ)	GO	783
Dennett, Ronald (NY)	IM	667
Denny, Donald (NJ)	VIR	854
Denoto, George (NY)	S	586
DePalo, Louis (NY)	Pul	353
Derespinis, Patrick (NY)	Oph	515
DeRose, Joseph (NY)	T&CS	436
Dershaw, D David (NY)	DR	158
Dervan, John (NY)	Cv	608
Desai, Amita (NJ)	Inf	738
deSerres, Lianne (NY)	PO	693
DeSilva, Derrick (NJ)	IM	838
Desnick, Robert (NY)	CG	145
Desouza, Trevor (NJ)	ChiN	874
Desposito, Franklin (NJ)	CG	778
Detterbeck, Frank (CT)	T&CS	1031
Dettmer, Robert (CT)	Ge	952
Deutsch, Adam (NY)	Cv	131
Deutsch, James (NY)	Oph	466
Devanand, Davangere (NY)	GerPsy	182
Devereux, Richard (NY)	Cv	131
Devine, Patricia (NY)	MF	671
Devinsky, Orrin (NY)	N	236
DeVita, Gregory (NY)	PlS	576
DeVita, Maria (NY)	Nep	227
DeVita, Vincent (CT)	Onc	1011
DeVito, Bethany (NY)	Ge	541
DeVivo, Darryl (NY)	ChiN	143

Alphabetical Listing of Doctors

Name	Specialty	Pg
Devons, Cathryn (NY)	Ger	663
Dhalla, Satish (NY)	IM	199
Dharmarajan, Thiruvinvamvalai (NY)	Ger	413
Dhruvakumar, Sandhya (CT)	CE	942
Di Buono, Mark (NY)	Psyc	518
Di Giacinto, George (NY)	NS	230
Di Leo, Frank (NY)	Oph	624
Diamant, Esther (NY)	Ped	600
Diamond, Ezriel (NY)	RadRO	582
Diamond, Martin (NJ)	PMR	928
Diamond, Sharon (NY)	ObG	248
Diamond, Steven (NJ)	PHO	754
Diaz, Michael (NY)	Hem	189
DiBernardo, Barry (NJ)	PlS	798
Dickler, Maura (NY)	Onc	214
Dickoff, David (NY)	N	677
DiCosmo, Bruno (NY)	Pul	703
Dieck, William (NY)	Oph	682
Diehl, William (NJ)	S	889
Dieterich, Douglas (NY)	Ge	170
Dietz, Stephanie (CT)	D	947
Dietzek, Alan (CT)	VascS	996
DiFabrizio, Larry (NY)	Pul	353
Diflo, Thomas (NY)	S	708
DiGiacomo, William (NJ)	IM	921
DiGioia, Julia (NJ)	S	931
DiGiovanni, Joseph (CT)	HS	955
DiGregorio, Vincent (NY)	PlS	576
Diktaban, Theodore (NY)	PlS	330
Dillard, James (NY)	PMR	325
Dillon, Robert (NY)	U	388
Dilmanian, Hajir (NY)	Cv	444
Dimaio, Mary (NY)	PPul	315
DiMango, Angela (NY)	Pul	353
Dimango, Emily (NY)	Pul	354
DiMeo, Albert (CT)	T&CS	994
Dines, David (NY)	OrS	562
Dinkin, Marc (NY)	N	236
Dinlenc, Caner (NY)	U	388
DiPaola, Robert (NJ)	Onc	839
Disa, Joseph (NY)	PlS	331
Distefano, Michael (NJ)	OrS	750
Ditchek, Alan (NY)	IM	456
Diuguid, David (NY)	Hem	189
Divgi, Chaitanya (NY)	NuM	245
Diwan, Sudhir (NY)	PM	298
Dobbins, John (CT)	Ge	1006
Doctor, Leslie (CT)	Oph	972
Doctor, Naishad (NY)	PlS	576
Dodds, Peter (CT)	U	995
Dodick, Jack (NY)	Oph	257
Doidge, Robert (NJ)	OrS	750
Dolgin, Stephen (NY)	PS	572
Dolinsky, Jason (NY)	IM	200
Dolitsky, Charisse (NY)	D	535
Dolitsky, Jay (NY)	PO	314
Donahue, Bernadine (NY)	RadRO	479
Donahue, John (CT)	DR	948
Donath, Joseph (NY)	Pul	580
Dong, Xiang (CT)	S	993
Donnellan, Joseph (NJ)	Psyc	910
Donnelly, Christine (NJ)	PCd	884
Donovan, Leslie (CT)	ObG	969
Dor, Nathan (NY)	ObG	464
Dosik, David (NY)	Onc	459
Dosik, Harvey (NY)	Hem	454
Dottino, Peter (NY)	GO	183
Douglas, Carolyn (NY)	Psyc	341
Douros, Stella (NY)	Oph	466
Dousmanis, Athanasios (NY)	N	677
Dowdle, John (CT)	HS	955
Dower, Samuel (NJ)	EDM	780
Dowling, Sean (CT)	RadRO	989
Dowling, Thomas (NY)	OrS	625
Dowling, William (NJ)	OrS	882
Downey, Robert (NY)	T&CS	382
Downie, Jeanine (NJ)	D	779
Doyle, Michael (CT)	RE	990
Doyle, Werner (NY)	NS	230
Dozor, Allen (NY)	PPul	693
Drachtman, Richard (NJ)	PHO	847
Draizin, Dennis (NY)	Oto	564
Drake, William (NJ)	Oto	926
Drascher, Gary (NJ)	S	911
Drayer, Burton (NY)	NRad	244
Dreifuss, Ronald (NY)	VIR	395
Dresdale, Robert (NY)	Cv	529
Dresner, Lisa (NY)	S	481
Drews, Michael (NJ)	RE	910

Name	Specialty	Pg
Drexler, Ellen (NY)	N	462
Dreyer, Neil (CT)	IM	958
Dreyfuss, Patricia (NJ)	ObG	881
Driesman, Mitchell (CT)	IC	960
Driesman, Shelley (CT)	Oph	972
Drillings, Gary (NJ)	OrS	896
Drimmer, Marc (NJ)	PlS	825
Droesch, James (NY)	ObG	622
Droller, Michael (NY)	U	388
Drooker, Martin (NY)	Psyc	341
Dropkin, Lloyd (NY)	Oto	288
Drucker, Beverly (CT)	Onc	963
Drucker, David (NY)	OrS	516
Drugge, Rhett (CT)	D	947
Drusin, Ronald (NY)	Cv	131
Drzala, Mark (NJ)	OrS	925
Dubin, David (NJ)	RadRO	763
Dubner, Sanford (NY)	PlS	576
Dubois, Nicholas (NY)	Cv	131
Duboys, Elliot (NY)	PlS	631
Duchen, Douglas (CT)	FMed	951
Duchnowska, Alicja (NY)	Ped	517
Duckrow, Robert (CT)	N	1015
Duda, E Andrew (CT)	Hem	956
Dudick, Stephen (NJ)	PlS	866
Duffy, Andrew (CT)	S	1030
Dulit, Rebecca (NY)	Psyc	700
Dultz, Rachel (NJ)	S	827
Duncan, Charles (CT)	NS	1014
Duncan, David (NY)	N	677
Dunkel, Ira (NY)	PHO	310
Dunne, Dana (CT)	Inf	1009
Dunston-Boone, Gina (CT)	MF	962
Durante, Anthony (NY)	Oto	564
Duva, Joseph (NY)	Ge	615
Dweck, Monica (NY)	Oph	466
Dworkin, Brad (NY)	Ge	659
Dworkin, Gregory (CT)	PPul	982
Dwyer, James (NJ)	OrS	908
Dwyer, Kevin (CT)	S	993

E

Name	Specialty	Pg
Eastham, James (NY)	U	389
Ebani, Jack (NJ)	U	869
Ebarb, Raymond (NY)	FMed	614
Economos, Katherine (NY)	GO	454
Eddleman, Keith (NY)	MF	210
Edelman, Bruce (NJ)	Oto	845
Edelman, Robert (NY)	U	589
Edelson, Charles (NY)	OrS	685
Edelson, David (NY)	IM	547
Edelson, Richard (CT)	D	1004
Edelstein, Barbara (NY)	DR	158
Edelstein, David (NY)	Oto	289
Edelstein, Gary (NY)	Ped	320
Edelstein, Martin (NY)	FMed	540
Eden, Edward (NY)	Pul	354
Edwards, Bruce (NY)	A&I	527
Edwards, Wendy (NY)	H & PM	192
Effron, Charles (NJ)	N	745
Efthimiou, Petros (NY)	Rhu	434
Eggers, Howard (NY)	Oph	257
Eglinton, Gary (NY)	MF	497
Egol, Kenneth (NY)	OrS	273
Ehrenkranz, Richard (CT)	NP	1013
Ehrlich, Amy (NY)	Ger	413
Ehrlich, Conrad (CT)	DR	949
Ehrlich, James (NY)	Ge	659
Ehrlich, Martin (NY)	IM	200
Ehrlich, Paul (NY)	PA&I	303
Eichenbaum, Joseph (NY)	Oph	257
Eichenfield, Andrew (NY)	PRhu	316
Eichler, Joel (NJ)	Oph	790
Eichman, Gerard (NJ)	Cv	724
Eilbott, David (CT)	IM	1009
Eilen, Bonnie (NY)	ObG	680
Einstein, Mark (NY)	GO	414
Eisenberg, Mark (NY)	NS	553
Eisenberg, Richard (NJ)	D	918
Eisenberg, Sheldon (NJ)	Cv	724
Eisenstat, Steven (NJ)	FMed	919
Eisenstat, Theodore (NJ)	CRS	833
Eitan, Noam (NY)	Psyc	476
El Baba, Fadi (NY)	Oph	624
El-Sadr, Wafaa (NY)	Inf	193
El-Tamer, Mahmoud (NY)	S	374
Elahi, Ebrahim (NY)	Oph	257
Elamir, Mazhar (NJ)	Pul	811

Alphabetical Listing of Doctors

Name	Specialty	Pg
Elefteriades, John (CT)	T&CS	1031
Elias, Steven (NJ)	VascS	770
Elkind, Barry (NJ)	Cv	807
Elkind, Mitchell (NY)	N	236
Elkowitz, Marc (NY)	PlS	576
Elkwood, Andrew (NJ)	PlS	866
Ellenson, Lora (NY)	Path	301
Elliott, Andrew (NY)	OrS	273
Ellis, Earl (NY)	IM	456
Ellman, Matthew (CT)	IM	1009
Ellozy, Sharif (NY)	VascS	398
Elmann, Elie (NJ)	T&CS	767
Emami, Arash (NJ)	OrS	896
Emond, Jean (NY)	S	374
Emre, Sukru (CT)	S	1030
Ende, Leigh (NJ)	HS	877
Eng, Margaret (NJ)	Inf	860
Engel, Harry (NY)	Oph	257
Engel, J. Mark (NJ)	Oph	843
Engel, Lenore (NY)	ChAP	447
Engel, Mark (NJ)	Oph	863
Engel, Murray (NY)	ChiN	143
Engelhardt, Martin (NY)	IM	667
Engler, Mitchell (NJ)	Pul	762
Englert, Christopher (NJ)	ObG	747
Ennis, David (NY)	IM	667
Ennis, Francis (CT)	OrS	976
Ennis, Ronald (NY)	RadRO	358
Epstein, Lawrence (NY)	PM	298
Epstein, Marcia (NY)	Inf	545
Epstein, Nancy (NY)	NS	554
Epstein, Robert (NJ)	DR	834
Erb, Markus (NY)	PCd	690
Erber, William (NY)	Ge	451
Erlebacher, Jay (NJ)	Cv	725
Ernberg, Lauren (CT)	DR	949
Ernst, Jerome (NY)	IM	416
Errico, Thomas (NY)	OrS	273
Errico, Vito (CT)	NRad	1015
Escalera, Sandra (CT)	PGe	1022
Escher, Jeffrey (NY)	Ger	663
Esformes, Ira (NJ)	OrS	750
Eshghi, A. Majid (NY)	U	710
Eskreis, David (NY)	Ge	541
Esposito, Donna (NY)	Oph	257
Esposito, Michael (NY)	Path	567
Esposito, Michael (NJ)	U	768
Esposito, Rick (NY)	T&CS	588
Esposito, Stephen (NY)	Ge	493
Estabrook, Alison (NY)	S	374
Esteban-Cruciani, Nora (NY)	Ped	429
Etingin, Orli (NY)	IM	200
Ettinger, Alan (NY)	N	555
Evanko, John (NY)	ObG	248
Evans, Andrew (NY)	RadRO	358
Evans, Lydia (NY)	D	652
Evans, Mark (NY)	ObG	248
Evans, Steven (NY)	CE	528
Ezratty, Ari (NY)	Cv	530

F

Name	Specialty	Pg
Faber, Mark (NJ)	Psyc	799
Fafalak, Robert (NY)	IM	200
Fagin, James (NY)	PA&I	567
Fagin, James (NY)	EDM	164
Fahey, Thomas (NY)	S	375
Fahn, Stanley (NY)	N	236
Fahoum, Bashar (NY)	S	482
Fakharzadeh, Frederick (NJ)	HS	736
Falco, Thomas (NY)	Cv	608
Falcon, Ronald (NY)	D	535
Falk, Theodore (NJ)	A&I	723
Falkoff, Alan (CT)	FMed	951
Faller, Jason (NY)	Rhu	365
Fallon, Brian (NY)	Psyc	341
Fang, Bruno (NJ)	Onc	907
Fang, Deborah (CT)	RadRO	989
Fantasia, Michele (NJ)	PMR	849
Farber, Bruce (NY)	Inf	546
Farber, Charles (NY)	Ge	541
Farber, Charles (NJ)	Onc	879
Farhath, Sabeena (NJ)	PGe	825
Faries, Peter (NY)	VascS	398
Farkas, Edward (NJ)	Psyc	761
Farkas, John (NJ)	Ge	894
Farmer, James (NY)	OrS	273
Farrell, Matthew (CT)	FMed	951
Farrell, Robert (NY)	U	505

Name	Specialty	Pg
Farrer, William (NJ)	Inf	921
Fass, Arthur (NY)	Cv	644
Fass, Daniel (NY)	RadRO	704
Fastenberg, David (NY)	Oph	559
Fateh, Majid (NY)	RE	362
Fath, Robert (NY)	Ge	659
Faust, Glenn (NY)	VascS	592
Faust, Michael (NY)	Ge	170
Faust, Michael (NJ)	ObG	747
Fazio, Nelson (NY)	IM	667
Fazio, Richard (NY)	Ge	512
Fealy, Stephen (NY)	OrS	273
Federbush, Richard (NY)	IM	547
Federico, John (CT)	T&CS	1031
Federman, Alex (NY)	IM	200
Fefferman, Nancy (NY)	DR	158
Feghali, Joseph (NY)	Oto	424
Feher, Laszlo (NY)	Ger	180
Feigenbaum, Howard (NJ)	S	899
Fein, Alan (NY)	Pul	580
Fein, Deborah (NJ)	Nep	743
Fein, Frederick (NY)	Cv	530
Feinberg, Joseph (NY)	PMR	325
Feinberg, Joseph (NY)	PlS	577
Feinberg, Todd (NY)	N	236
Feingold, Daniel (NY)	CRS	146
Feinstein, Neil (NY)	Oph	466
Feinstein, Ronald (NY)	AM	526
Feintzeig, Irwin (CT)	Nep	965
Feit, Alan (NY)	Cv	444
Feit, David (NJ)	Ge	920
Feit, Frederick (NY)	IC	208
Feld, Michael (NY)	Cv	645
Felderman, Lenora (NY)	D	150
Feldman, Darren (NY)	Onc	214
Feldman, David (NJ)	SM	888
Feldman, David (NY)	OrS	274
Feldman, Eric (NY)	Onc	214
Feldman, Jeffrey (NJ)	IM	921
Feldman, Philip (NY)	D	449
Feldman, Sheldon (NY)	S	375
Feldman, Steven (CT)	Oto	979
Feldman, Stuart (NY)	Onc	672
Feldman, Tatyana (NJ)	Hem	737
Feldstein, Neil (NY)	NS	230
Fellman, Damon (NJ)	N	745
Fellus, Jonathan (NJ)	N	880
Felsenstein, Jerome (NY)	D	652
Feltheimer, Seth (NY)	IM	200
Feng, William (CT)	T&CS	994
Fennell, Gail (CT)	IM	958
Fennelly, Bryan (NJ)	Psyc	887
Fennoy, Ilene (NY)	PEn	306
Fenster, Mitchell (NY)	IM	667
Ferges, Mitchell (NJ)	Ge	905
Ferguson, Kevin (CT)	Ped	983
Fern, Craig (NY)	Oph	682
Fernandes, David (NY)	Ped	475
Fernandes, John (NJ)	PCd	793
Fernandez, Harold (NY)	T&CS	588
Fernandez, Jacinto (NJ)	ObG	747
Fernbach, Barry (NJ)	Hem	737
Ferran, Elena (NY)	Ge	171
Ferran, Ernesto (NY)	Psyc	341
Ferrante, Maurice (NJ)	IM	906
Ferrick, Kevin (NY)	CE	404
Ferrier, Genevieve (NY)	Ped	320
Ferrone, Philip (NY)	Oph	559
Ferrucci, Leonard (CT)	ObG	970
Ferrucci, Vito (CT)	ObG	970
Festa, Robert (NY)	Ped	629
Feteiha, Muhammad (NJ)	S	931
Feuer, Martin (NY)	IM	200
Fey, Christopher (CT)	DR	949
Fialk, Mark (NY)	Onc	672
Fiedler, Robert (NY)	IM	200
Fiel, Stanley (NJ)	Pul	887
Field, Barry (NY)	Ge	659
Fields, Suzanne (NY)	Ger	616
Fields, Theodore (NY)	Rhu	366
Fiest, Thomas (NJ)	Ge	859
Figgie, Mark (NY)	OrS	274
Figlia, Paul (NJ)	PlS	898
Filiberto, Cosmo (CT)	FMed	951
Filippone, Mark (NJ)	PMR	811
Filor, Caroline (CT)	ObG	970
Filsoufi, Farzan (NY)	T&CS	383
Fine, Emily (CT)	ObG	1016
Fine, Eugene (NY)	U	389
Fine, Howard (NY)	Onc	214

Alphabetical Listing of Doctors

Name	Specialty	Pg
Fine, Jonathan (CT)	Pul	988
Fine, Paul (NJ)	Nep	880
Fine, Robert (NY)	Onc	215
Finegold, Jonathan (NY)	Ge	659
Finger, Paul (NY)	Oph	258
Fink, Candida (NY)	ChAP	648
Fink, Matthew (NY)	N	236
Finkel, Jay (NY)	Psyc	341
Finkelstein, Martin (NY)	Ger	180
Finkelstein, Warren (NJ)	Ge	781
Finlay, Alexis (CT)	Oph	972
Fiore, Amory (CT)	NS	966
Fiore, John (NY)	Onc	620
Fiorella, David (NY)	NRad	622
Fiorentino, Thomas (NY)	IM	667
First, Michael (NY)	Psyc	342
Fisch, Arthur (NJ)	Cv	874
Fisch, Harry (NY)	U	389
Fischbach, Neal (CT)	Onc	963
Fischer, Harry (NY)	Rhu	366
Fish, Bernard (NY)	PCd	690
Fishbach, Mitchell (NY)	Cv	645
Fishbane-Mayer, Jill (NY)	ObG	248
Fisher, George (NY)	FMed	493
Fisher, Laura (NY)	IM	200
Fisher, Lawrence (CT)	Cv	944
Fisher, Margaret (NJ)	PInf	865
Fisher, Martin (NY)	AM	526
Fisher, Rosemarie (CT)	Ge	1006
Fisher, Yale (NY)	Oph	258
Fishkin, Michael (NY)	FMed	614
Fishman, Allen (NY)	Oph	499
Fishman, David (NY)	GO	184
Fishman, Donald (NY)	Pul	354
Fishman, Eric (NY)	VascS	713
Fishman, Miriam (NJ)	D	729
Fishman, Robert (CT)	IC	961
Fiske, Steven (NJ)	Ge	781
Fitzgerald, Denis (NJ)	Onc	861
FitzGibbons, James (CT)	OrS	976
Flamm, Eugene (NY)	NS	419
Flanagan, Michael (CT)	U	1032
Flanagan, Steven (NY)	PMR	325
Flanzman, Susan (NJ)	IM	739
Flatow, Evan (NY)	OrS	274
Fleischer, Adiel (NY)	MF	549
Fleischer, Lee (NY)	S	603
Fleischer, Marian (NY)	CRS	448
Fleischman, Jay (NY)	Oph	682
Fleischman, Jean (NY)	Pul	502
Fleisher, Michael (NJ)	Ped Uro	848
Fleming, Gregory (NJ)	Oto	883
Fletcher, H. Stephen (NJ)	S	801
Flis, Raymond (NJ)	Nep	862
Floch, Neil (CT)	S	993
Flood, Mary (NY)	Inf	194
Florakis, George (NY)	Oph	258
Flores, Raja (NY)	T&CS	383
Florio, Philip (NY)	ObG	680
Flug, Frances (NJ)	PHO	755
Flynn, Maryirene (NY)	OrS	516
Flynn, Patrick (NY)	PCd	304
Flynn, William (CT)	OrS	1018
Fochios, Steven (NY)	Ge	171
Fogel, Joyce (NY)	Ger	181
Fogel, Mitchell (CT)	Nep	965
Fogler, Richard (NY)	S	482
Fojas, Antonio (NY)	IM	416
Foley, Carmel (NY)	ChAP	533
Folman, Robert (CT)	Onc	963
Fomberstein, Barry (NY)	Rhu	434
Fonacier, Luz (NY)	A&I	527
Fong, Raymond (NY)	Oph	258
Fong, Yuman (NY)	S	375
Fontana, Gregory (NY)	T&CS	383
Foo, Sun-Hoo (NY)	N	236
Foong, Anthony (NY)	Ge	171
Ford, Robert (NJ)	DR	834
Forlenza, Thomas (NY)	Onc	513
Forley, Bryan (NY)	PlS	331
Forman, Mark (NJ)	T&CS	802
Forman, Robert (NY)	Cv	404
Forman, Scott (NY)	Oph	682
Formenti, Silvia (NY)	RadRO	359
Formica, Richard (CT)	Nep	1014
Fornari, Victor (NY)	ChAP	491
Fornier, Monica (NY)	Onc	215
Forte, Francis (NJ)	Onc	741
Fortunato, Franklin (NJ)	IM	785
Foss, Francine (CT)	Onc	1011

Alphabetical Listing of Doctors

Name	Specialty	Pg
From, Stuart (NJ)	A&I	723
Fromer, Mark (NY)	Oph	259
Frost, James (NJ)	S	931
Fruchtman, Steven (NY)	Hem	189
Fuchs, Richard (NY)	Cv	132
Fuchs, Wayne (NY)	Oph	259
Fuhrman, Robert (NJ)	EDM	918
Fukilman, Oscar (NY)	IM	496
Fuks, Joachim (NY)	Onc	417
Fulop, Robert (NY)	IM	513
Funt, David (NY)	PlS	577
Fuqua, James (NY)	DR	159
Furie, Richard (NY)	Rhu	584
Fuster, Valentin (NY)	Cv	132
Fyer, Abby (NY)	Psyc	342
Fyer, Minna (NY)	Psyc	342

G

Name	Specialty	Pg
Gabbay, Vilma (NY)	ChAP	141
Gabel, Richard (NY)	Psyc	700
Gabelman, Gary (NY)	Cv	645
Gabrilove, Janice (NY)	Onc	215
Gaffney, Joseph (NJ)	PCd	846
Gaglio, Paul (NY)	Ge	411
Gagne, Paul (CT)	VascS	996
Gainey, Patrick (NJ)	N	862
Gajdos, Robert (NJ)	IM	895
Galanter, I Marc (NY)	AdP	123
Galetta, Steven (NY)	N	237
Galinkin, Lawrence (NY)	Ped	573
Gallagher, Mary (NY)	PEn	306
Gallagher, Pamela (NY)	PlS	577
Galland, Leo (NY)	IM	201
Galler, Marilyn (NY)	Nep	498
Gallick, Gregory (NJ)	OrS	925
Gallin, Pamela (NY)	Oph	259
Gallina, Gregory (NJ)	CRS	727
Gallousis, Francene (NY)	MF	671
Galloway, Aubrey (NY)	T&CS	383
Gallucci, John (NJ)	PS	848
Gamache, Francis (NY)	NS	230
Gambarin, Boris (NY)	IM	456
Gammon, G. Davis (CT)	ChAP	1002
Gamss, Jeffrey (NY)	Ge	451
Ganchi, Parham (NJ)	PlS	898
Gandhi, Lajpat (NY)	ChAP	609
Gandhi, Rajinder (NJ)	PS	757
Gannon, Christopher (NJ)	S	827
Gannon, Jennifer (NY)	ObG	680
Garan, Hasan (NY)	CE	128
Garay, Kenneth (NJ)	Oto	810
Garay, Stuart (NY)	Pul	354
Garcia, Mario (NY)	Cv	405
Gardenswartz, Mark (NY)	Nep	227
Gardin, Julius (NJ)	Cv	725
Gardner, James (NJ)	PlS	929
Gardner, Sharon (NY)	PHO	310
Garfein, Evan (NY)	PlS	431
Garfinkel, Matthew (NJ)	OrS	844
Garg, Madhur (NY)	RadRO	434
Gargano, Robert (NY)	Oto	626
Gargiulo, Juan (NY)	PM	626
Garner, Bruce (NY)	Rhu	480
Garner, Steven (NY)	DR	449
Garrett, Leila (CT)	ObG	970
Garrick, Renee (NY)	Nep	675
Garvey, Michael (NY)	Nep	227
Garvey, Richard (CT)	S	993
Garvey, Richard (NY)	PlS	698
Garvin, James (NY)	PHO	310
Garzon, Maria (NY)	D	150
Gass, Alan (NY)	Cv	645
Gayle, Lloyd (NY)	PlS	331
Gaynor, Mitchell (NY)	Onc	215
Gazzara, Paul (NY)	IM	513
Gecelter, Gary (NY)	S	586
Geders, Jane (NY)	Ge	659
Geer-Yan, Lisa (CT)	ObG	970
Gehrmann, Robin (NJ)	SM	801
Gejerman, Glen (NJ)	RadRO	763
Gekowski, Kathleen (NJ)	Inf	819
Gelato, Marie (NY)	EDM	613
Gelb, Bruce (NY)	PCd	304
Gelbard, Sandra (NY)	IM	201
Gelberg, Burt (NY)	IM	547
Gelbfish, Joseph (NY)	Cv	444
Gelbman, Brian (NY)	Pul	354
Gelfand, Janice (NY)	Psyc	432

Alphabetical Listing of Doctors

Name	Specialty	Pg
Glaser, Morton (NY)	Pul	632
Glashow, Jonathan (NY)	OrS	274
Glassman, Charles (NY)	U	711
Glassman, Charles (NY)	IM	597
Glassman, Lawrence (NY)	T&CS	588
Glassman, Mark (CT)	PGe	981
Glassman, Morris (NY)	Oph	682
Glatt, Herbert (NJ)	Oph	790
Glazer, Steven (CT)	IM	958
Gleckel, Louis (NY)	Cv	530
Gleicher, Norbert (NY)	RE	362
Glesby, Marshall (NY)	Inf	194
Glick, Sharon (NY)	D	449
Glickel, Steven (NY)	HS	186
Glicksman, Caroline (NJ)	PlS	866
Glickstein, Shari (NY)	IM	668
Gliedman, Paul (NY)	RadRO	479
Gliklich, Jerry (NY)	Cv	132
Glowacki, Jan (NJ)	IM	860
Gluck, Ian (NJ)	ObG	881
Gluck, Robert (NY)	HS	544
Glusac, Earl (CT)	Path	1021
Gmyrek, Robyn (NY)	D	151
Gobin, Y Pierre (NY)	NRad	244
Gochfeld, Michael (NJ)	OM	843
Godfrey, Norman (NY)	PlS	331
Godfrey, Philip (NY)	PlS	332
Godin, David (NY)	Oto	289
Goff, Donald (NY)	Psyc	342
Goland, Robin (NY)	EDM	164
Golbe, Lawrence (NJ)	N	841
Gold, Alan (NY)	PlS	577
Gold, David (NY)	PGe	627
Gold, Jeffrey (NJ)	IM	895
Gold, Joan (NY)	PMR	326
Gold, Jonathan (NJ)	D	893
Gold, Julie (NY)	Onc	673
Gold, Marji (NY)	FMed	410
Gold, Scott (NY)	Oto	289
Goldberg, Arthur (NY)	Onc	215
Goldberg, Daniel (NJ)	Oph	863
Goldberg, David (NY)	D	151
Goldberg, Gary (NY)	GO	414
Goldberg, Harvey (NY)	Cv	132
Goldberg, Jeffrey (NY)	Psyc	476
Goldberg, Jonathan (NY)	Onc	673
Goldberg, Jory (NJ)	Pul	850
Goldberg, Joseph (CT)	Psyc	986
Goldberg, Leslie (NY)	Oph	560
Goldberg, Marc (NJ)	Rhu	899
Goldberg, Michael (NJ)	GO	836
Goldberg, Myron (NY)	Ge	172
Goldberg, Neil (NY)	D	652
Goldberg, Nieca (NY)	Cv	132
Goldberg, Robert (NY)	Onc	597
Goldberg, Roy (NY)	Ger	413
Goldberg, Steven (NY)	Cv	530
Goldberg, Stuart (NJ)	Onc	741
Goldberg-Berman, Judith (CT)	EDM	950
Goldblatt, Kenneth (NJ)	Pul	850
Goldblatt, Robert (NY)	Ge	660
Goldblum, Lester (NY)	Ge	541
Golden, Flavia (NY)	IM	201
Goldenberg, Alan (NY)	EDM	614
Goldenberg, Alec (NY)	Hem	189
Goldenberg, Bruce (NJ)	T&CS	803
Goldenberg, David (NJ)	Ge	920
Goldenberg, David (CT)	PlS	985
Goldenberg, David (NY)	Psyc	342
Goldfarb, Alisan (NY)	S	375
Goldfarb, C. Richard (NY)	NuM	246
Goldfarb, Joel (NJ)	Ge	734
Goldfarb, Michael (NJ)	S	868
Goldfischer, Mindy (NJ)	DR	730
Goldin, Daniel (NY)	IM	201
Goldin, Howard (NY)	Ge	172
Goldman, Gary (NY)	ObG	249
Goldman, Jack (NY)	IM	668
Goldman, Joel (NY)	EDM	450
Goldman, Kenneth (NJ)	VascS	854
Goldman, Martin (NY)	Cv	132
Goldman, Michael (NJ)	EDM	732
Goldman, Neil (NY)	Psyc	342
Goldman, Neil (NY)	A&I	642
Goldschmidt, Howard (NJ)	Cv	725
Goldsmith, Ari (NY)	PO	473
Goldsmith, Stanley (NY)	NuM	246
Goldstein, Carl (NJ)	Nep	922
Goldstein, Daniel (NY)	T&CS	436
Goldstein, Jeffrey (NY)	OrS	274

Name	Specialty	Pg
Goldstein, Jonathan (NJ)	IC	785
Goldstein, Jonathan (NY)	N	237
Goldstein, Judith (NY)	Ped	320
Goldstein, Marc (NY)	U	389
Goldstein, Mark (NY)	Rhu	519
Goldstein, Martin (NY)	ObG	249
Goldstein, Michael (NY)	Oph	259
Goldstein, Paul (NY)	IM	201
Goldstein, Robert (NY)	PlS	431
Goldstein, Stanley (NY)	A&I	527
Goldstein, Steven (NY)	Oto	424
Goldstein, Steven (NJ)	ObG	863
Goldstein, Steven (NY)	Ped	501
Goldstein, Steven (NY)	ObG	249
Goldstein, Susanna (NY)	Psyc	343
Goldweit, Richard (NJ)	Cv	725
Golfinos, John (NY)	NS	230
Golombek, Sergio (NY)	NP	675
Goltzman, Carey (NY)	PCCM	690
Gomes, Joseph (NY)	CE	128
Gomez, Henry (NY)	Cv	530
Gomez, William (NJ)	OrS	824
Gomolin, Irving (NY)	Ger	543
Gonter, Neil (NJ)	Rhu	764
Gonzalez, David (NJ)	MF	861
Goodgold, Abraham (NJ)	IM	921
Goodman, Alan (NJ)	A&I	916
Goodman, Dennis (NY)	Cv	133
Goodman, Karyn (NY)	RadRO	359
Goodman, Kenneth (NY)	DR	537
Goodman, Mark (NY)	Cv	530
Goodman, Michael (NY)	IM	547
Goodman, Robert (NY)	NS	231
Goodman, Robert (NJ)	RadRO	812
Goodman, Susan (NY)	Rhu	366
Goodman, Wayne (NY)	Psyc	343
Goodstein, Carolyn (NJ)	A&I	723
Goodwin, Charles (NY)	OrS	275
Gordon, James (NY)	Oph	682
Gordon, Jeffrey (NY)	EDM	538
Gordon, Marc (NY)	N	555
Gordon, Mark (NY)	S	708
Gordon, Marsha (NY)	D	151
Gordon, Michael (NY)	Oto	564
Gordon, Neil (CT)	Oto	979
Gordon, Richard (NJ)	Rhu	827
Gordon, Richard (NY)	Pul	581
Gorecki, Piotr (NY)	S	482
Gorenstein, Lyall (NY)	T&CS	383
Gorevic, Peter (NY)	Rhu	366
Gorfine, Stephen (NY)	CRS	146
Gorkin, Janet (NY)	Nep	419
Gorlick, Richard (NY)	PHO	426
Gorman, Lauren (NY)	Psyc	343
Gorman, Robert (NJ)	FMed	781
Gorski, Lydia (NY)	IM	547
Gotfried, Fern (NJ)	Ped	885
Gotkin, Robert (NY)	PlS	577
Gotlin, Robert (NY)	PMR	326
Gottesfeld, Peter (NY)	FMed	657
Gottesman, Malcolm (NY)	N	555
Gottlieb, Beth (NY)	PRhu	572
Gottridge, Joanne (NY)	IM	547
Gouge, Thomas (NY)	S	375
Gould, Elaine (NY)	DR	612
Gould, Eric (NY)	Ped	574
Gould, Perry (NY)	Ge	541
Gould, Richard (NY)	Ge	660
Goy, Andre (NJ)	Onc	741
Goyal, Arun (NY)	VascS	713
Goydos, James (NJ)	S	852
Grabowski, Wayne (NJ)	Oph	844
Grace, William (NY)	Onc	215
Graff, Michael (NJ)	NP	861
Graham, Alan (NJ)	VascS	854
Grajower, Martin (NY)	EDM	409
Granatir, Charles (NJ)	OrS	810
Granet, Kenneth (NJ)	IM	860
Granick, Mark (NJ)	PlS	798
Grann, Alison (NJ)	RadRO	800
Grano, Vanessa (NY)	ObG	680
Granowetter, Linda (NY)	PHO	310
Grant, John (NY)	NS	554
Grant, Linda (CT)	PMR	984
Grant, Robert (NY)	PlS	332
Grasso, Cono (NY)	Oph	500
Grasso, Michael (NY)	U	389
Grasso, Michael (NJ)	Nep	787
Grauer, Jonathan (CT)	OrS	1018
Graver, L. Michael (NY)	T&CS	505

Alphabetical Listing of Doctors

Name	Specialty	Pg
Gray, William (NY)	IC	208
Grayson, Douglas (NY)	Oph	259
Grazi, Richard (NY)	RE	480
Greaney, Edward (NY)	IM	201
Grecco, Dominic (NY)	ObG	680
Greeley, John (CT)	FMed	951
Greeley, Norman (NY)	A&I	443
Green, Abraham (NY)	Ped	574
Green, Jeffrey (CT)	Cv	944
Green, Mark (NY)	N	237
Green, Michele (NY)	D	151
Green, Peter (NY)	Ge	172
Green, Richard (NY)	VascS	398
Green, Robert (NY)	Oto	289
Green, Stephen (NY)	Cv	530
Green, Steven (NY)	OrS	275
Green, Stuart (NY)	Rhu	480
Greenbaum, Allen (NY)	Oph	682
Greenberg, Harly (NY)	Pul	581
Greenberg, Howard (NY)	Onc	498
Greenberg, Mark (NY)	Cv	405
Greenberg, Martin (NJ)	Pul	799
Greenberg, Robert (NY)	GerPsy	454
Greenberg, Ronald (NY)	Ge	541
Greenberg, Rosalie (NJ)	ChAP	917
Greenberg, Steven (NY)	Oph	683
Greenberg, Susan (NJ)	Onc	861
Greenblatt, Louis (NY)	FMed	615
Greene, Jeffrey (NY)	Inf	194
Greene, Loren (NY)	EDM	164
Greenfield, Martin (NY)	EDM	538
Greengart, Alvin (NY)	Cv	445
Greenhill, Laurence (NY)	ChAP	648
Greenman, James (NJ)	Inf	921
Greenspan, Alan (NY)	D	151
Greenstein, Bruce (NY)	PlS	431
Greenstein, Stuart (NY)	S	435
Greenwald, Blaine (NY)	GerPsy	494
Greenwald, Brian (NJ)	PMR	849
Greenwald, Bruce (NY)	PCCM	306
Greenwald, David (NY)	Ge	411
Greenwald, Joshua (NY)	PlS	698
Greenwald, Marc (NY)	CRS	534
Greenwald, Robert (NY)	Rhu	584
Greer, David (CT)	N	1015
Greer, Jeannete (NJ)	DR	904
Greif, Richard (NY)	Cv	645
Greisberg, Justin (NY)	OrS	275
Greisman, Stewart (NY)	Rhu	366
Grelsamer, Ronald (NY)	OrS	275
Grendell, James (NY)	Ge	541
Grenell, Steven (NY)	N	420
Grenis, Michael (NJ)	OrS	824
Gress, Francis (NY)	Ge	172
Gretz, Herbert (NY)	GO	663
Gribbin, Dorota (NJ)	PMR	825
Gribbon, John (NJ)	IM	785
Gribetz, Michael (NY)	U	389
Grice, Dorothy (NY)	ChAP	141
Grieco, Michael (NY)	S	586
Grifo, James (NY)	RE	362
Grijnsztein, Jacob (NY)	Ped	574
Grimshaw, Robert (NY)	Ger	663
Grizzanti, Joseph (NJ)	Pul	898
Grodberg, Michele (NJ)	D	729
Grodman, Richard (NY)	Cv	509
Groeger, William (NY)	PlS	577
Groff, Walter (NJ)	CRS	918
Gropper, David (CT)	Ped	983
Gross, Dennis (NY)	D	151
Gross, Elliott (NY)	N	677
Gross, Gary (NJ)	A&I	857
Gross, Harvey (NJ)	FMed	733
Gross, Ian (CT)	NP	1013
Gross, Jay (NY)	CE	404
Gross, Jeffrey (CT)	N	967
Gross, Jeffrey (NY)	IM	668
Gross, Joshua (NJ)	DR	730
Grossbard, Michael (NY)	Onc	215
Grossi, Eugene (NY)	T&CS	384
Grossi, Robert (NY)	VascS	398
Grossman, Bernard (NJ)	Onc	820
Grossman, Edward (CT)	Ge	952
Grossman, Elliot (NJ)	ChiN	875
Grossman, Kenneth (NJ)	D	858
Grossman, Marc (NY)	D	652
Grossman, Melanie (NY)	D	151
Grossman, Robert (NJ)	OrS	864
Grossman, Susan (NY)	Nep	514
Grosso, John (NY)	Oto	564

H

Alphabetical Listing of Doctors

Name	Specialty	Pg
Hammer, Glenn (NY)	Inf	194
Hammer, Scott (NY)	Inf	194
Hammerman, Hillel (NY)	Ge	172
Hammers, Lynwood (CT)	DR	1004
Hammerschlag, Paul (NY)	Oto	289
Hamner, Daniel (NY)	SM	370
Hand, Ivan (NY)	NP	498
Handelsman, Dan (NY)	PEn	691
Handelsman, Richard (NY)	IM	597
Handler, Robert (NJ)	Ped	885
Hankin, Dorie (NY)	Ped	574
Hanley, Gerard (NY)	Cv	445
Hanna, Moneer (NY)	U	590
Hannafin, Jo (NY)	OrS	275
Hanon, Samuel (NY)	CE	128
Hanson, Matthew (NY)	Oto	470
Har-El, Gady (NY)	Oto	290
Haramati, Linda (NY)	DR	408
Haramati, Nogah (NY)	DR	408
Harangozo, Andrea (NJ)	Pul	851
Harary, Albert (NY)	Ge	172
Haratz-Rubinstein, Natan (NY)	ObG	465
Hardart, Anne (NY)	ObG	249
Harden, Cynthia (NY)	N	555
Harish, Ziv (NJ)	A&I	723
Harlam, Dean (NY)	Psyc	700
Harlow, Paul (NJ)	Ped	758
Harman, John (NJ)	IM	820
Harmon, Gregory (NY)	Oph	260
Harnick, David (NY)	CE	128
Harooni, Robert (NY)	Ge	493
Harpaz, Noam (NY)	Path	301
Harper, Harry (NJ)	Onc	741
Harrington, Elizabeth (NY)	VascS	398
Harrington, Martin (NY)	VascS	398
Harris, Dena (NY)	ObG	249
Harris, Leon (NY)	Pul	602
Harris, Loren (NY)	T&CS	483
Harris, Michael (NJ)	S	766
Harris, Michael (NJ)	PHO	755
Harris, Steven (NY)	U	590
Harrison, Aaron (NY)	Ge	615
Harrison, Louis (NY)	RadRO	359
Hart, Catherine (NY)	IM	201
Hart, Sidney (CT)	Psyc	986
Hartl, Roger (NY)	NS	231
Hartman, Alan (NY)	T&CS	635
Hartman, Barry (NY)	Inf	194
Hartz, Cindi (NY)	Ped	696
Hartzband, Mark (NJ)	OrS	750
Harwin, Steven (NY)	OrS	276
Hasapis, Peter (CT)	IM	958
Haselkorn, Joan (NY)	ObG	557
Hashim, Sabet (CT)	T&CS	1032
Hassoun, Hani (NY)	Onc	216
Hatcher, Virgil (NY)	D	152
Hatsis, Alexander (NY)	Oph	560
Hauptman, Allen (NY)	IM	202
Hausman, Michael (NY)	OrS	276
Havens, Jennifer (NY)	ChAP	141
Hayes, Leslie (NY)	AM	443
Hayworth, Robin (NY)	Oph	422
Hayworth, Scott (NY)	ObG	680
Healey, John (NY)	OrS	276
Heary, Robert (NJ)	NS	787
Hecht, Alan (NY)	Cv	133
Hecht, Andrew (NY)	OrS	276
Hedrick, David (CT)	Ped	983
Heerdt, Alexandra (NY)	S	375
Hefter, Harold (NY)	D	536
Heftler, Jeffrey (CT)	PMR	985
Heier, Stephen (NY)	Ge	660
Heim, John (NJ)	T&CS	853
Heiman, Mark (CT)	Cv	944
Heiman, Peter (NY)	Psyc	432
Heinemann, Murk (NY)	Oph	260
Heisman, Alexander (NY)	Psyc	477
Heitner, John (NY)	Cv	445
Helbraun, Mark (NJ)	CRS	728
Heldman, Jay (NJ)	D	729
Helfet, David (NY)	OrS	276
Helfgott, David (NY)	Inf	194
Hellenbrand, William (CT)	PCd	1022
Heller, Debra (NJ)	Path	793
Heller, Keith (NY)	S	375
Heller, Paul (NJ)	GO	877
Heller, Stanley (NY)	Psyc	343
Hellerman, James (NY)	EDM	656
Hemmers, Philip (CT)	A&I	941
Hen, Jacob (CT)	PPul	982

Name	Specialty	Pg
Henderson, Cassandra (NY)	MF	417
Henick, David (NJ)	Oto	751
Hennessy, William (CT)	U	995
Henry, Glen (CT)	IC	1010
Henschke, Claudia (NY)	DR	159
Henshaw, D. Ross (CT)	OrS	976
Hensle, Terry (NJ)	U	769
Heptulla, Rubina (NY)	PEn	426
Herbert, Joseph (NY)	N	237
Herbert, Joshua (CT)	FMed	951
Herbin, Joseph (CT)	Inf	956
Herbst, Roy (CT)	Onc	1012
Herbstein, Diego (NY)	N	237
Herbstman, Robert (NJ)	PlS	849
Herman, David (NJ)	Inf	906
Herman, Martin (NJ)	N	841
Herman, Zeva (NY)	DR	159
Hermele, Herbert (CT)	OrS	976
Herold, Betsy (NY)	PInf	427
Herr, Harry (NY)	U	390
Herron, Daniel (NY)	S	375
Hersh, Peter (NJ)	Oph	749
Hershlag, Avner (NY)	RE	583
Hershman, Dawn (NY)	Onc	216
Hershman, Elliott (NY)	SM	370
Hershman, Ronnie (NY)	Cv	531
Herskovitz, Steven (NY)	N	420
Hertan, Hilary (NY)	Ge	412
Hertz, Marc (NY)	DR	654
Hertz, Steven (NJ)	VascS	804
Herzlinger, Robert (CT)	NP	965
Herzog, David (NY)	IM	668
Herzog, Ronit (NY)	PA&I	303
Herzog, Thomas (NY)	GO	184
Hes, Dyan (NY)	Ped	320
Hetzler, Peter (NJ)	PlS	866
Heublum, Michael (NY)	N	237
Hiatt, I Mark (NJ)	NP	840
Hibbard, Claire (NY)	DR	654
Hicks, Patricia (NJ)	PA&I	753
Hidalgo, David (NY)	PlS	332
Hiesiger, Emile (NY)	N	237
Higgins, Susan (CT)	RadRO	1028
Higgins, William (NY)	IM	668
Hillman, Deborah (NY)	Ge	660
Hiltebeitel, Carolyn (NY)	Ped	320
Hindenburg, Alexander (NY)	Onc	550
Hindin, Lee (NJ)	Psyc	898
Hindman, Steven (CT)	OrS	977
Hines, Brian (CT)	ObG	970
Hines, William (CT)	Nep	966
Hiotis, Spiros (NY)	S	376
Hirmand, Haideh (NY)	PlS	332
Hirsch, Andrew (NJ)	A&I	857
Hirsch, Bruce (NY)	Inf	546
Hirsch, Glenn (NY)	ChAP	141
Hirsch, Lawrence (CT)	N	1015
Hirsch, Lissa (NY)	ObG	250
Hirschman, Alan (NY)	Ped	429
Hirschman, Richard (NY)	Onc	216
Hirshaut, Yashar (NY)	Onc	216
Hirt, Paula (NY)	ObG	623
Hisler, Barbara (NY)	D	536
Hjemdahl-Monsen, Craig (NY)	IC	671
Ho, Bryan (NJ)	Oto	752
Ho, Sammy (NY)	Ge	412
Ho, Sharon (NY)	Ped	320
Hochman, Herbert (NY)	D	152
Hochstein, Martin (NJ)	EDM	732
Hochster, Howard (CT)	Onc	1012
Hockstein, Steven (NY)	ObG	250
Hoda, Syed (NY)	Path	301
Hodes, David (NY)	Pul	602
Hodes, Steven (NJ)	Ge	836
Hodges, David (NJ)	Cv	725
Hodges, Laura (CT)	VIR	996
Hodosh, Richard (NJ)	NS	923
Hoffman, Darryl (NY)	T&CS	384
Hoffman, Eileen (NY)	IM	202
Hoffman, Janet (NY)	DR	537
Hoffman, Joel (NY)	Psyc	343
Hoffman, Lloyd (NY)	PlS	332
Hoffman, Michael (NY)	Rhu	584
Hoffman, Pamela (CT)	IM	958
Hoffman, Richard (NY)	EDM	511
Hoffman, Robert (NY)	PrM	338
Hoffman, Ronald (NY)	Oto	290
Holcomb, Kevin (NY)	GO	184
Holcombe, Randall (NY)	Onc	216
Holder, Jonathan (NY)	OrS	686

Alphabetical Listing of Doctors

Name	Specialty	Pg
Holland, Claudia (NY)	ObG	250
Holland, Elbridge (NJ)	FMed	876
Holland, James (NY)	Onc	216
Holland, Neil (NJ)	N	862
Hollander, Eric (NY)	Psyc	343
Hollander, Gerald (NY)	Cv	445
Holliday, Roy (NY)	DR	159
Hollister, Dickerman (CT)	Onc	964
Holodny, Andrei (NY)	NRad	244
Holtzman, Robert (NY)	NS	554
Holzer, Barry (NY)	ChAP	447
Holzman, Ian (NY)	NP	225
Hon, Man (NY)	VIR	592
Hong, Andrew (NY)	PS	572
Honig, Stephen (NY)	Rhu	366
Hopkins, Arthur (NY)	IM	668
Horbar, Gary (NY)	IM	202
Horn, Corinne (NY)	Oto	290
Horn, Evelyn (NY)	Cv	133
Horn, Jay (CT)	IM	959
Horner, Neil (NJ)	NRad	924
Hornyak, Stephen (NY)	S	519
Horovitz, Len (NY)	IM	202
Horowitz, Harold (NY)	Inf	195
Horowitz, Marc (NY)	Oph	683
Horowitz, Mark (NY)	Ped Uro	517
Horowitz, Mark (NY)	Rhu	366
Horowitz, Steven (CT)	Cv	944
Horvath, Susanna (NY)	N	238
Horwitz, Steven (NY)	Onc	217
Hostin, Helen (NY)	ObG	599
Hotchkiss, Edward (NY)	IM	547
Hotchkiss, Robert (NY)	HS	186
Housman, Arno (NY)	U	711
Howanitz, Nancy (NY)	D	652
Howes, Christopher (CT)	IC	961
Hricak, Hedvig (NY)	DR	159
Hsu, Daphne (NY)	PCd	425
Hsueh, John (NY)	Cv	490
Hsuih, Terence (NY)	IM	457
Hu, Kenneth (NY)	RadRO	359
Huang, Russel (NY)	OrS	276
Hubbard, Christopher (NY)	OrS	276
Hubschmann, Otakar (NJ)	NS	788
Hudis, Clifford (NY)	Onc	217
Hug, Eugen (NJ)	RadRO	910
Hughes, Peter (CT)	OrS	977
Huh, Julie (NY)	D	611
Hunt, William (CT)	Nep	966
Hunter, John (NY)	PlS	332
Huo, Jerry (NY)	Oto	500
Hupart, Kenneth (NY)	EDM	539
Huprikar, Shirish (NY)	Inf	195
Huribal, Marsel (CT)	VascS	996
Hurst, Lawrence (NY)	HS	616
Hurst, Wendy (NJ)	ObG	748
Hurwitz, Diana (NY)	D	652
Hurwitz, Joshua (CT)	RE	991
Huston, Jan (NJ)	S	802
Hutchinson, Gordon (CT)	Rhu	1029
Hutson, J. Milton (NY)	MF	211
Hwang, Cheng-hong (NJ)	Pul	930
Hyans, Peter (NJ)	PlS	929
Hyler, Irene (NY)	ChAP	649
Hyman, David (NY)	CG	610
Hyman, George (NY)	Oph	466
Hyman, Jeffrey (NY)	IM	457
Hyman, Joshua (NY)	OrS	277
Hyman, Kevin (NY)	T&CS	588
Hyman, Martin (NJ)	ObG	924
Hymes, Kenneth (NY)	Hem	189
Hyun, Grace (NY)	Ped Uro	318

I

Name	Specialty	Pg
Iammatteo, Matthew (NJ)	ObG	881
Iannuzzi, Christopher (CT)	RadRO	990
Ibelli, Vincent (NY)	FMed	596
Igel, Gerard (NY)	Ped	429
Ilan, Doron (NY)	HS	664
Ilowite, Norman (NY)	PRhu	428
Ilson, David (NY)	Onc	217
Imber, Gerald (NY)	PlS	332
Implicito, Dante (NJ)	OrS	751
Imundo, Lisa (NY)	PRhu	316
Inabnet, William (NY)	S	376
Inamdar, Sarla (NY)	Ped	320
Indio, Lillian (NY)	IM	668
Ingenito, Anthony (NJ)	RadRO	763

Name	Specialty	Pg
Inglis, Steven (NY)	MF	497
Ingrassia, Joseph (NY)	FMed	596
Innella, Robin (NJ)	OrS	926
Innerfield, Michael (NY)	IC	597
Inra, Lawrence (NY)	Cv	133
Inwald, Gary (NY)	PMR	431
Inzucchi, Silvio (CT)	EDM	1005
Iorio, Richard (NY)	OrS	277
Ipp, Lisa (NY)	AM	124
Isaacs, Ellen (NY)	IM	668
Isaacson, Steven (NY)	RadRO	359
Islam, Sohel (CT)	PlS	985
Isola, Luis (NY)	Hem	189
Isom, O. Wayne (NY)	T&CS	384
Israel, Alan (NJ)	Hem	737
Israel, Gary (CT)	DR	1005
Israel, Jessica (NJ)	Ger	859
Israel, Shara (CT)	IM	959
Israeli, Ron (NY)	PlS	577
Issenberg, Henry (NY)	PCd	690
Istrico, Richard (NY)	FMed	493
Iswara, Kadirawelpillai (NY)	Ge	452
Itzkowitz, Steven (NY)	Ge	172
Iwai, Sei (NY)	CE	643

J

Name	Specialty	Pg
Jabs, Douglas (NY)	Oph	260
Jackson, Rosemary (NY)	Ped	475
Jacob, Brian (NY)	S	376
Jacob, Jessica (NY)	ObG	558
Jacobowitz, Glenn (NY)	VascS	398
Jacobowitz, Marilyn (NY)	Pul	703
Jacobs, Elliot (NY)	PlS	333
Jacobs, Jonathan (NY)	Inf	195
Jacobs, Joseph (NY)	Oto	290
Jacobs, Laurie (NY)	Ger	413
Jacobs, Michael (NY)	D	152
Jacobs, Morton (NY)	DR	159
Jacobs, Thomas (NY)	EDM	165
Jacobson, Edward (CT)	ObG	970
Jacobson, Ira (NY)	Ge	173
Jacobson, Marc (NY)	AM	526
Jacobson, Ronald (NY)	ChiN	650
Jacoby, Jacob (NJ)	Psyc	811
Jacono, Andrew (NY)	Oto	564
Jacowitz, Joel (NJ)	Cv	725
Jadonath, Ram (NY)	CE	528
Jafar, Jafar (NY)	NS	231
Jaffe, Alan (NY)	Ge	660
Jaffe, Fredrick (NY)	OrS	277
Jaffe, Herbert (NY)	Oph	466
Jaffin, Barry (NY)	Ge	173
Jagannath, Sundar (NY)	Onc	217
John, Anthony (NY)	Oto	290
Jahre, Caren (NY)	NRad	244
Jaile-Marti, Jesus (NY)	NP	675
Jain, Dhanpat (CT)	Path	1021
Jain, Subhash (NY)	PM	298
Jakubowski, Ann (NY)	Onc	217
Jamidar, Priya (CT)	Ge	1006
Jan, Dominique (NY)	PS	428
Jarnagin, William (NY)	S	376
Jarowski, Charles (NY)	Onc	217
Jarrett, Mark (NY)	Rhu	585
Jauhar, Rajiv (NY)	Cv	531
Javit, Daniel (NY)	VIR	395
Jawetz, Harold (NJ)	IM	895
Jayaram, Nadubeethi (NY)	OrS	516
Jazrawi, Laith (NY)	OrS	277
Jelin, Abraham (NY)	PGe	471
Jelveh, Mansoor (NY)	Cv	531
Jenkins, Arthur (NY)	NS	231
Jennis, Andrew (NJ)	Onc	742
Jeremias, Allen (NY)	Cv	608
Jeshion, Wendy (NJ)	PGe	754
Jessurun, Jose (NY)	Path	301
John, Sylvia (NY)	PMR	630
Johns, William (CT)	NuM	968
Johnson, Alan (NY)	NRad	557
Johnson, Diane (NY)	Inf	546
Johnson, Michele (CT)	NRad	1016
Johnson, Robert (NJ)	AM	776
Johnson, Sabrina (NY)	FMed	615
Johnson, Valerie (NY)	PNep	313
Johnson Miller, Denise (NJ)	S	868
Jokl, Peter (CT)	OrS	1018
Jones, David (NY)	T&CS	384
Jones, Frank (NJ)	Psyc	850

Name	Specialty	Pg
Jones, Jacqueline (NY)	Oto	290
Jones, Stephen (CT)	Ger	954
Jonna, Siva (NJ)	PCCM	846
Jordan, Barry (NY)	N	678
Jordan, Lawrence (NJ)	S	852
Jorde, Ulrich (NY)	Cv	133
Joseph, John (NY)	IM	496
Joseph, Patricia (NY)	S	603
Joseph, Rosy (NJ)	Nep	744
Josephson, Jordan (NY)	Oto	290
Josephson, Lynn (NY)	S	708
Joy, Mark (NY)	IM	457
Juan, Paul (CT)	Ped	983
Judson, Benjamin (CT)	Oto	1019
Julie, Edward (NJ)	Cv	893
Jumper, Robert (CT)	IC	961
Jurcic, Joseph (NY)	Hem	190
Jutkowitz, Robert (NY)	N	514
Juvan, Luci (CT)	PMR	1026

K

Name	Specialty	Pg
Kabis, Suzanne (NJ)	Nep	907
Kabnick, Lowell (NJ)	VascS	890
Kacker, Ashutosh (NY)	Oto	290
Kadan-Lottick, Nina (CT)	PHO	1023
Kafantaris, Vivian (NY)	ChAP	491
Kagan, Peter (NJ)	VascS	771
Kahaleh, Michel (NY)	Ge	173
Kahn, David (NY)	Psyc	343
Kahn, Jeffrey (NY)	Psyc	700
Kahn, Leonard (NY)	Path	567
Kahn, Max (NY)	Ped	321
Kahn, Oren (NY)	Ge	660
Kahn, Stuart (NY)	PM	298
Kairam, Indira (NY)	Ge	173
Kairam, Ram (NY)	ChiN	143
Kaiser, Michael (NY)	NS	231
Kaiser, Paul (NJ)	N	822
Kaiser, Stephen (NY)	IM	457
Kalapatapu, Kumar (NY)	IC	671
Kalash, Glenn (NY)	Psyc	501
Kalchthaler, Thomas (NY)	Ger	663
Kaleya, Ronald (NY)	S	482
Kalikow, Kevin (NY)	ChAP	649
Kalinich, Lila (NY)	Psyc	343
Kalischer, Alan (NJ)	Cv	917
Kalish, Robin (NY)	MF	211
Kalman, Arlene (CT)	Psyc	986
Kalman, Jill (NY)	Cv	133
Kalnicki, Shalom (NY)	RadRO	434
Kamalakar, Peri (NJ)	PHO	795
Kamen, Mazen (NY)	Cv	133
Kaminer, Ruth (NY)	Ped	429
Kaminetsky, Jed (NY)	U	390
Kaminsky, Donald (NY)	IM	202
Kamler, Kenneth (NY)	HS	495
Kanengiser, Steven (NJ)	PPul	756
Kang, Harriet (NY)	ChiN	650
Kang, Pritpal (NY)	Cv	445
Kanner, Ronald (NY)	N	555
Kanter, Alan (NJ)	Ped	758
Kantor, Alan (NY)	EDM	656
Kanumury, Sunita (NJ)	A&I	873
Kapel, Robert (CT)	Ge	953
Kaplan, Barry (NY)	Cv	531
Kaplan, Gabriel (NJ)	Psyc	929
Kaplan, Jeffrey (CT)	Oph	973
Kaplan, Jonathan (NY)	EDM	539
Kaplan, Kenneth (NY)	Cv	645
Kaplan, Martin (NY)	Ped	629
Kaplan, Matthew (NY)	PNep	473
Kaplan, Rana (NY)	Pul	354
Kaplan, Ronald (NY)	PM	298
Kaplan, Sherri (NY)	D	652
Kaplan, Steven (NY)	U	390
Kaplovitz, Harry (NY)	PCd	470
Kapo, Jennifer (CT)	H & PM	1009
Kapoor, Satish (NY)	IM	668
Kaporis, Athena (NY)	D	652
Kappel, Bruce (NY)	Onc	550
Kapur, Sandip (NY)	S	376
Karamitsos, Harry (NY)	ObG	250
Karanfilian, Richard (NY)	VascS	713
Karas, David (CT)	PO	1024
Karas, Evan (NY)	OrS	686
Karasu, Sylvia (NY)	Psyc	343
Karasu, T Byram (NY)	Psyc	344
Karatoprak, Ohan (NJ)	FMed	733

Name	Specialty	Pg
Karetzky, Monroe (NY)	Pul	433
Karlsrud, Katherine (NY)	Ped	321
Karmen, Carol (NY)	IM	668
Karp, Adam (NY)	Ger	181
Karp, George (NJ)	Hem	837
Karp, Nolan (NY)	PlS	333
Karpeh, Martin (NY)	S	376
Kasabian, Armen (NY)	PlS	577
Kase, Steven (NY)	Oto	688
Kaskel, Frederick (NY)	PNep	427
Kasper, William (NY)	Oph	560
Kass, Lewis (NY)	PPul	693
Kassapidis, Sotirios (NY)	Pul	502
Kassotis, John (NY)	CE	443
Kates, Matthew (NY)	Oto	688
Kato, Tomoaki (NY)	S	376
Kattan, Meyer (NY)	PPul	315
Katus, Eli (NY)	Psyc	579
Katz, Aaron (NY)	U	590
Katz, Alan (NY)	RadRO	503
Katz, Amiram (CT)	N	1015
Katz, Andrea (NJ)	Ped	909
Katz, Bruce (NY)	D	152
Katz, Edward (NY)	Cv	134
Katz, Harry (NJ)	Oto	752
Katz, Henry (NY)	Ge	660
Katz, Herbert (NJ)	U	812
Katz, Jack (NY)	Psyc	579
Katz, Jeffrey (NJ)	U	803
Katz, Lester Brian (NY)	S	376
Katz, Martin (CT)	Hem	1008
Katz, Seymour (NY)	Ge	542
Katz, Steven (NJ)	U	769
Katz, Stuart (NY)	Cv	134
Katz, Susan (NY)	D	152
Katzenelenbogen, Moshe (NY)	IM	457
Katzenstein, Martin (NY)	Ped	601
Kaufman, Alan (NY)	A&I	403
Kaufman, Andrew (NJ)	PM	792
Kaufman, David (NY)	Cv	405
Kaufman, David (NY)	ChiN	143
Kaufman, David (NY)	N	420
Kaufman, Matthew (NJ)	PlS	850
Kaufman, Richard (CT)	A&I	1001
Kaufmann, Charles (NY)	Psyc	344

Name	Specialty	Pg
Kaul, Ashutosh (NY)	S	708
Kaushik, Raj (NJ)	T&CS	900
Kauvar, Arielle (NY)	D	152
Kavaler, Elizabeth (NY)	U	390
Kavanagh, Brian (CT)	OrS	977
Kavookjian, Haik (CT)	HS	955
Kavoussi, Louis (NY)	U	590
Kay, Arthur (NY)	N	463
Kay, Richard (NY)	Cv	646
Kay, Scott (NJ)	Oto	845
Kaynan, Ayal (NJ)	U	890
Kazam, Ezra (NJ)	Oph	882
Kazim, Michael (NY)	Oph	260
Kazlow, Philip (NY)	PGe	308
Kearney, Thomas (NJ)	S	853
Keefe, David (NY)	RE	362
Keilson, Marshall (NY)	N	463
Keiser, Harold (NY)	Rhu	434
Keith, Marie (NY)	Ped	321
Kelemen, John (NY)	N	555
Keller, Adina (NY)	ObG	680
Keller, Andrew (CT)	Cv	944
Keller, Irwin (NJ)	NRad	842
Keller, Jeffrey (NY)	PO	693
Keller, Peter (NY)	Cv	405
Keller, Steven (NY)	T&CS	436
Kellner, Charles (NY)	Psyc	344
Kelly, Anna (NY)	NRad	244
Kelly, Bryan (NY)	OrS	277
Kelly, Michael (NJ)	OrS	751
Kelly, Stephen (NY)	Oph	260
Kelsen, David (NY)	Onc	217
Keltz, Martin (NY)	RE	362
Keltz, Theodore (NY)	Cv	646
Kemeny, M Margaret (NY)	S	504
Kemeny, Nancy (NY)	Onc	217
Kempin, Sanford (NY)	Hem	190
Kenan, Samuel (NY)	OrS	562
Kenet, Barney (NY)	D	152
Kenigsberg, Daniel (NY)	RE	633
Kenler, Andrew (CT)	S	993
Kennedy, Gary (NY)	GerPsy	414
Kennedy, James (NY)	IM	202
Kennedy, Timothy (NY)	S	435
Kennish, Arthur (NY)	IM	202

Alphabetical Listing of Doctors

Name	Specialty	Pg
Kenny, Raymond (NJ)	Ge	782
Kent, Jennifer (NY)	IM	202
Kent, Joan (NY)	ObG	250
Kepecs, Gilbert (NJ)	Rhu	765
Kernan, Nancy (NY)	PHO	310
Kernan, Walter (CT)	IM	1010
Kerner, Michael (NJ)	Ge	920
Kerns, John (NJ)	U	769
Kerr, Alicia (CT)	ObG	970
Kerr, Leslie (NY)	Rhu	367
Kerstein, Joshua (NY)	Cv	445
Kesarwala, Hemant (NJ)	A&I	831
Kesh, Sandra (NY)	Inf	665
Kessler, Alan (NY)	ObG	250
Kessler, Bradley (NY)	PGe	627
Kessler, Edmund (NY)	PS	474
Kessler, Jeffrey (NY)	N	556
Kessler, Leonard (NY)	Onc	551
Kessler, Martin (NY)	PlS	578
Kessler, William (NJ)	Hem	920
Kett, Kevin (CT)	IC	1010
Khabie, Victor (NY)	OrS	686
Khaghan, Neda (CT)	Ge	953
Khakoo, Yasmin (NY)	ChiN	143
Khalife, Michael (NY)	S	587
Khan, Arfa (NY)	DR	537
Khandji, Alexander (NY)	NRad	244
Khilnani, Neil (NY)	VIR	395
Khimani, Karim (NJ)	Ger	920
Khokhar, Asim (NY)	Ge	616
Khosh, Maurice (NY)	Oto	291
Khoury, F. Frederic (NY)	PlS	698
Khoury, Paul (NY)	DR	654
Khulpateea, Neekianund (NY)	GO	454
Kier, Catherine (NY)	PPul	628
Kiernan, Howard (NY)	OrS	277
Kim, Heakyung (NY)	PMR	326
Kim, Joyce (NY)	ObG	250
Kim, Matthew (CT)	MF	962
Kim, Michelle (NY)	Ge	173
Kim, Tae Ho (NY)	PlS	699
Kim-Schluger, Hyung (NY)	Ge	173
Kimball, Annetta (NY)	Ge	173
Kimmelstiel, Fred (NY)	S	376
Kimura, Yukiko (NJ)	PRhu	756
King, Michael (CT)	DR	949
King, William (NY)	HS	186
Kini, Subhash (NY)	S	377
Kinkhabwala, Milan (NY)	S	435
Kinzler, Wendy (NY)	MF	549
Kipen, Howard (NJ)	OM	843
Kipnis, James (NY)	OrS	562
Kirchoff, Kathryn (NY)	N	420
Kirschenbaum, Alexander (NY)	U	390
Kirshblum, Steven (NJ)	PMR	798
Kirshbom, Paul (CT)	T&CS	1032
Kirshy, David (NY)	DR	613
Kirtane, Sanjay (NY)	Cv	490
Kizelshteyn, Grigory (NY)	PM	689
Klafter, Robert (NY)	Onc	218
Klagsbrun, Samuel (NY)	Psyc	701
Klapholz, Ari (NY)	Pul	354
Klapholz, Marc (NJ)	Cv	777
Klapper, Daniel (NY)	Oph	260
Klapper, Philip (NY)	Pul	433
Klar, Tobi (NY)	D	652
Klares, Scott (NY)	Pul	703
Klarsfeld, Jay (CT)	Oto	979
Klausner, Stanley (NY)	S	634
Kleber, Herbert (NY)	AdP	123
Klecz, Robert (NJ)	PMR	886
Kleeman, Harris (NY)	Cv	446
Klein, George (NY)	U	390
Klein, James (NJ)	T&CS	767
Klein, Janice (NY)	NP	225
Klein, Jeffrey (NY)	RE	705
Klein, Michael (NY)	Nep	676
Klein, Natalie (NY)	Inf	546
Klein, Neil (CT)	IM	959
Klein, Norman (NY)	A&I	443
Klein, Patricia (NJ)	N	745
Klein, Paula (NY)	Onc	218
Klein, Robert (NJ)	A&I	893
Klein, Victor (NY)	MF	549
Klein, Walter (NJ)	Ge	734
Kleinbaum, Jerry (NY)	EDM	656
Kleinberg, David (NY)	EDM	165
Kleiner, Morton (NY)	Nep	514
Kleinman, Andrew (NY)	PlS	699
Kleinman, Gary (CT)	ObG	971

Name	Specialty	Pg
Kleinman, Paul (NY)	OrS	423
Klenk, Rosemary (CT)	Ped	983
Klenoff, Bruce (CT)	Oto	979
Kliger, Alan (CT)	Nep	1014
Kligfield, Paul (NY)	Cv	134
Kligler, Benjamin (NY)	FMed	167
Klimstra, David (NY)	Path	301
Kline, Gary (NJ)	T&CS	588
Kline, Mitchell (NY)	D	152
Klos, Andrzej (NJ)	Ped	810
Kloss, Robert (CT)	Onc	964
Klyde, Barry (NY)	EDM	165
Knackmuhs, Gary (NJ)	Inf	738
Knapp, Albert (NY)	Ge	173
Knep, Stanley (NJ)	N	895
Knightly, John (NJ)	NS	880
Knisely, Jonathan (NY)	RadRO	583
Knopp, Edmond (NY)	NRad	244
Kobren, Steven (NY)	Cv	531
Kocher, Jeffrey (NJ)	Inf	738
Kocsis, James (NY)	Psyc	344
Kodali, Susheel (NY)	IC	208
Kodsi, Sylvia (NY)	Oph	560
Kofinas, George (NY)	RE	480
Kohan, Darius (NY)	Oto	291
Kohn, Brenda (NY)	PEn	306
Kohn, Gary (NJ)	PPul	927
Kolenik, Steven (CT)	D	947
Kolitz, Jonathan (NY)	Hem	545
Kolker, Adam (NY)	PlS	333
Kolker, Dov (NY)	OrS	468
Kolker, Harvey (NY)	Ped	629
Kolodny, Erwin (NY)	Pul	355
Kolsky, Neil (NJ)	Ped	758
Komarynsky, Irene (CT)	ObG	971
Komisar, Arnold (NY)	Oto	291
Kon, Shulamite (NY)	Ped	321
Kondziolka, Douglas (NY)	NS	231
Koniaris, Soula (NJ)	PGe	847
Konka, Sudarsanam (NY)	Cv	446
Koo, Harry (NJ)	Ped Uro	757
Kopec, Anna (NJ)	D	807
Kopelman, Rima (NJ)	Rhu	765
Kopf, Gary (CT)	T&CS	1032
Koplewicz, Harold (NY)	ChAP	141
Koplin, Richard (NY)	Oph	261
Koppel, Barbara (NY)	N	238
Korc-Grodzicki, Beatriz (NY)	Ger	181
Koreen, Amy (NY)	Psyc	631
Korenstein, Deborah (NY)	IM	202
Kornbluth, Arthur (NY)	Ge	174
Kornel, Ezriel (NY)	NS	676
Korovin, Gwen (NY)	Oto	291
Korsten, Mark (NY)	Ge	412
Korval, Arnold (CT)	Ped	983
Kosinski, Edward (CT)	Cv	944
Kosofsky, Barry (NY)	ChiN	144
Kososky, Charles (NJ)	N	822
Koss, Jerome (NY)	Cv	531
Kostis, John (NJ)	Cv	831
Kotin, Neal (NY)	Ped	321
Kotkes, Herschel (NY)	PM	299
Kotler, Donald (NY)	Ge	174
Kotler, Lisa (NJ)	ChAP	727
Kottler, William (NJ)	PPul	796
Kottmeier, Stephen (NY)	OrS	625
Koufman, Jamie (NY)	Oto	291
Koulos, John (NY)	GO	184
Kowallis, George (NY)	Psyc	344
Kozel, Joseph (NJ)	IM	809
Kozicky, Orest (NY)	Ge	661
Kozin, Arthur (NY)	Nep	598
Kozlowski, Jeffrey (NJ)	Nep	744
Kozuch, Peter (NY)	Onc	218
Krakovitz, Evan (NY)	CRS	651
Kramer, David (CT)	OrS	977
Kramer, Kim (NY)	PHO	310
Kramer, Mitchell (NY)	ObG	623
Kramer, Neil (NJ)	Rhu	931
Kramer, Philip (NY)	Oph	515
Kranzler, Elliot (NY)	Psyc	344
Kranzler, L Stephan (NY)	N	678
Kraus, Dennis (NY)	Oto	291
Krause, Cynthia (NY)	ObG	250
Kraushaar, Barry (NY)	SM	603
Kreitzer, Joel (NY)	PM	299
Kreitzer, Paula (NY)	PEn	569
Krellenstein, Daniel (NY)	T&CS	384
Kremberg, M Roy (NY)	Psyc	344
Krespi, Yosef (NY)	Oto	291

Name	Specialty	Pg
Kressner, Michael (NY)	Ge	661
Krevitt, Lane (NY)	Oto	291
Kriegel, David (NY)	D	152
Krieger, Ana (NY)	Pul	355
Krieger, Karl (NY)	T&CS	384
Krieger, Richard (NJ)	Inf	877
Krieger, Sharon (NY)	IM	669
Krilov, Leonard (NY)	PInf	571
Krim, Eileen (NY)	ObG	558
Krinick, Ronald (NY)	SM	371
Krinsky, Glenn (NJ)	DR	730
Krinsley, James (CT)	Pul	988
Kris, Mark (NY)	Onc	218
Krishnan, Sankaran (NY)	PPul	694
Kristal, Leonard (NY)	D	611
Kristan, Ronald (NJ)	Oph	863
Krol, Kristine (NJ)	A&I	903
Kron, Leo (NY)	ChAP	141
Kronn, David (NY)	CG	651
Kronzon, Itzhak (NY)	Cv	134
Krotowski, Mark (NY)	FMed	451
Krueger, Richard (NY)	Psyc	344
Krug, Lee (NY)	Onc	218
Kruger, Bernard (NY)	Onc	218
Krumerman, Andrew (NY)	CE	404
Krumholz, Michael (NY)	Ge	174
Krutchik, Allan (NJ)	Onc	742
Kubersky, Steven (NY)	IM	669
Kudelka, Andrzej (NY)	Onc	620
Kuflik, Paul (NY)	OrS	277
Kuhel, William (NY)	Oto	292
Kula, Roger (NY)	N	556
Kulick, Roy (NY)	HS	414
Kulkarni, Rachana (NJ)	Cv	903
Kulpa, Jolanta (NY)	PHO	472
Kulsakdinun, Chaiyaporn (NY)	OrS	423
Kumar, Mark (NJ)	VascS	933
Kummer, Bart (NY)	Ge	174
Kunkes, Steven (CT)	Cv	944
Kupersmith, Andrew (NY)	Cv	646
Kupersmith, Mark (NY)	Oph	261
Kupfer, Gary (CT)	PHO	1023
Kupfer, Yizhak (NY)	Pul	478
Kurani, Devendra (NJ)	Psyc	811
Kurer, Cheryl (NJ)	PCd	846
Kurfist, Lee (NY)	Ped	630
Kuriloff, Daniel (NY)	Oto	292
Kurlan, Roger (NJ)	N	923
Kurtz, Caroline (CT)	Pul	988
Kurtz, Lewis (NY)	S	587
Kurtz, Robert (NY)	Ge	174
Kurtzman, Scott (CT)	S	1030
Kurucz, Oliver (NY)	Rhu	602
Kushner, Brian (NY)	PHO	311
Kushner, Evan (NJ)	IM	739
Kushner, Susan (NJ)	Ped	758
Kutcher, Rosalyn (NY)	DR	654
Kutnick, Richard (NY)	Cv	134
Kutscher, Martin (NY)	ChiN	650
Kuzniecky, Ruben (NY)	N	238
Kveton, John (CT)	Oto	1019
Kwartler, Jed (NJ)	Oto	926

L

Name	Specialty	Pg
La Bagnara, James (NJ)	Oto	897
La Gamma, Edmund (NY)	NP	675
La Marca, Charles (NY)	Oto	500
La Quaglia, Michael (NY)	PS	317
Laban-Grant, Olgica (NY)	N	678
Labar, Douglas (NY)	N	238
Labow, Daniel (NY)	S	377
LaBruna, Anthony (NY)	PIS	333
Lachman, Reid (NJ)	Oto	883
Lachmann, Elisabeth (NY)	PMR	326
Lachs, Mark (NY)	Ger	181
Lacqua, Frank (NY)	CRS	510
Lacy, Jill (CT)	Onc	1012
Lafaro, Rocco (NY)	T&CS	709
Lafferty, James (NY)	Cv	509
Lagmay, Victor (NY)	Oto	470
Lahita, Robert (NJ)	Rhu	800
Laifer, Steven (CT)	MF	962
Laitman, Robert (NY)	Nep	419
LaJoie, Josiane (NY)	ChiN	534
Laks, Mitchell (NY)	DR	408
Lalli, Corradino (NY)	IM	618
Lalwani, Anil (NY)	Oto	292
Lamanna, Nicole (NY)	Onc	218

Name	Specialty	Pg
Lambroza, Arnon (NY)	Ge	174
Lamm, Carin (NY)	PPul	315
Lamm, Steven (NY)	IM	203
Lampert, Rachel (CT)	CE	1001
Lan, Vivian (NJ)	IM	739
Landau, Alan (CT)	Ge	953
Landau, Leon (NY)	Hem	415
Landau, Steven (NY)	Ge	661
Landers, David (NJ)	Cv	725
Landesman, Sheldon (NY)	Inf	455
Landis, Gregg (NY)	VascS	592
Landrigan, Philip (NY)	OM	253
Landzberg, Joel (NJ)	Cv	726
Lane, Edward (CT)	Oto	979
Lane, Joseph (NY)	OrS	278
Lane, Lewis (NY)	HS	544
Lanfranchi, Angela (NJ)	S	911
Lang, Paul (NY)	A&I	527
Lang, Samuel (NY)	T&CS	505
Lange, Dale (NY)	N	238
Lange, David (NJ)	PlS	886
Langer, David (NY)	NS	231
Langer, Paul (NJ)	Oph	790
Langsner, Alan (NY)	PCd	794
Lanman, Geraldine (NY)	Ger	543
Lannin, Donald (CT)	S	1030
Lans, David (NY)	Rhu	706
Lansing, Martha (NJ)	FMed	818
Lansman, Steven (NY)	T&CS	709
Lanteri, Vincent (NJ)	U	769
Lantis, John (NY)	VascS	399
Lara, Jonathan (NJ)	Path	793
Laraque, Danielle (NY)	Ped	475
Larsen, John (NY)	PInf	312
Larson, Signe (NY)	Ped	321
Lasala, Johanna (CT)	Onc	1012
LaSala, Patrick (NY)	NS	420
Lassman, Andrew (NY)	N	238
Latov, Norman (NY)	N	238
Lau, Har Chi (NY)	S	708
Laudone, Vincent (NY)	U	390
Lauer, Simeon (NY)	Oph	261
Lauricella, Joseph (NJ)	IM	739
Lavaia-Marzano, Maria (NJ)	Ped	885
Laver, Joseph (NY)	PHO	628
Lavine, Joel (NY)	PGe	308
Lavyne, Michael (NY)	NS	232
Lawson, William (NY)	Oto	292
Lawson, William (NY)	IC	619
Lax, James (NY)	Ge	174
Layne, Jeffrey (NY)	U	590
Lazar, Amy (NJ)	Oto	908
Lazar, Lorraine (NJ)	ChiN	875
Lazar, Mark (NJ)	N	841
Lazar, Robert (NY)	Ge	616
Lazarus, George (NY)	Ped	321
Lazarus, Herbert (NY)	PRhu	316
Lazarus, Laura (CT)	S	993
Lazzaro, Douglas (NY)	Oph	466
Lazzaro, Richard (NY)	T&CS	384
Leach, Thomas (NJ)	PlS	826
Leavens-Maurer, Jill (NY)	Ped	574
Leb, Alvin (NY)	Ge	452
LeBenger, Kerry (NJ)	A&I	916
Lebinger, Martin (NY)	Psyc	432
Lebofsky, Martin (NY)	IM	669
Lebovics, Edward (NY)	Ge	661
Lebovics, Robert (NY)	Oto	292
Lebowicz, Joseph (NY)	Onc	459
Lebowitz, Mark (NY)	Oph	467
Lebwohl, Mark (NY)	D	153
Lebwohl, Oscar (NY)	Ge	174
Lechner, Michael (NY)	IM	669
Leckman, James (CT)	ChAP	1002
Lederer, David (NY)	Pul	355
Lederman, Jeffrey (NY)	Inf	665
Lederman, Josiane (NY)	D	510
Lederman, Martin (NY)	Oph	683
Lederman, Sanford (NY)	ObG	465
Lee, Alexander (NY)	PMR	326
Lee, Alfred (CT)	Hem	1008
Lee, April (NY)	AM	509
Lee, Carol (NY)	Oph	261
Lee, Donna (NJ)	PPul	756
Lee, Douglas (NY)	ObG	623
Lee, Francis (NY)	OrS	278
Lee, Haesoon (NY)	PPul	474
Lee, Huey-Jen (NJ)	DR	780
Lee, James (NY)	S	377
Lee, Kwang (NY)	Psyc	631

Name	Specialty	Pg
Lee, Leonard (NJ)	T&CS	853
Lee, Lucille (NY)	RadRO	583
Lee, Marjorie (NY)	Pul	355
Lee, Merlin (CT)	Onc	964
Lee, Nancy (NY)	RadRO	359
Lee, Paul (NY)	T&CS	505
Lee, Richard (CT)	A&I	941
Lee, Roberta (NY)	IM	203
Lee, Ronald (CT)	DR	949
Lee, Sang (NY)	CRS	146
Lee, Sang (NY)	Ge	661
Lee, Sicy (NY)	Rhu	367
Lee, Steve (NY)	HS	187
Lee, Sun (NJ)	NS	840
Lee, Thomas (NY)	PS	628
Lee, Thomas (NY)	NS	677
Leeman, Benjamin (NY)	Pul	581
Leffell, David (CT)	D	1004
Lefkovitz, Zvi (NY)	DR	654
Lefkowitz, Mathew (NY)	PM	470
Lefton, Daniel (NY)	NRad	244
Legato, Marianne (NY)	IM	203
Lehach, Joan (NY)	A&I	403
Lehman, Thomas (NY)	PRhu	316
Lehrhoff, Bernard (NJ)	U	932
Lehrman, Gary (NY)	Pul	703
Lehrman, Stuart (NY)	Pul	703
Leib, Martin (NY)	Oph	261
Leibner, Donald (NJ)	A&I	831
Leiboff, Arnold (NY)	CRS	610
Leibowitz, Evan (NJ)	Rhu	765
Leibowitz, Jonas (NY)	EDM	656
Leichter, Donald (NJ)	PCd	927
Leifer, Bennett (NJ)	Ger	736
Leifer, Marvin (NJ)	Psyc	826
Leipsner, George (NJ)	FMed	733
Leipzig, Rosanne (NY)	Ger	181
Leipziger, Lyle (NY)	PlS	578
Leiter, Gila (NY)	ObG	250
Leitman, I Michael (NY)	S	377
Leitner, Stuart (NJ)	Onc	786
Lemercier, Maud (NY)	S	708
Lenci, Margaret (NY)	Rhu	706
Lense, Lloyd (NY)	Cv	609
Lent, David (NY)	OrS	686
Lenzo, Salvatore (NY)	HS	187
Leon, Martin (NY)	IC	208
Leon, Steven (NY)	NS	621
Leonard, Daniel (NY)	Cv	646
Leonard, John (NY)	Hem	190
Leondires, Mark (CT)	RE	991
Leong, Mary (NY)	ObG	558
Leong, Pauline (NY)	IM	547
Lepor, Herbert (NY)	U	390
Lepore, Frederick (NJ)	N	841
Lerma, Pauline (NJ)	Onc	820
Lerman, Bruce (NY)	CE	128
Lerman, Jay (NY)	D	407
Lerman, Jay (NY)	DR	449
Lerner, Chester (NY)	Inf	195
Lerner, Elliot (NJ)	NRad	746
Lerner, Seth (NY)	U	711
Lerner, William (NJ)	Hem	860
Lescale, Keith (NY)	MF	672
Leslie, Denise (NY)	DR	655
Lesorgen, Philip (NJ)	RE	764
Lesser, Robert (NY)	Rhu	480
Lesser, Robert (CT)	Oph	1017
Lessing, Jeffrey (NY)	U	520
Lester, Mitchell (CT)	A&I	941
Lester, Thomas (NY)	Hem	664
Lettera, James (CT)	T&CS	994
Levchuck, Sean (NY)	PCd	568
Leventhal, Bennett (NY)	ChAP	595
Levey, Kenneth (NY)	ObG	251
Levey, Robert (NY)	IM	457
Levin, Alexander (NJ)	PM	846
Levin, Andrew (NY)	Psyc	701
Levin, David (NJ)	Nep	744
Levin, Frances (NY)	AdP	123
Levin, Kenneth (NJ)	N	746
Levin, Richard (CT)	Oto	980
Levin, Sheryl (NY)	PMR	431
Levine, Alice (NY)	EDM	165
Levine, David (NY)	N	238
Levine, David (NY)	OrS	278
Levine, Dorothy (CT)	Ped	983
Levine, Evan (NY)	Cv	646
Levine, Jeremiah (NY)	PGe	308
Levine, Joseph (NY)	CE	528

Alphabetical Listing of Doctors

Name	Specialty	Pg
Lipton, Brian (NY)	Psyc	345
Lipton, Jeffrey (NY)	PHO	570
Lipton, Mark (NY)	IM	203
Lipton, Richard (NY)	N	420
Lis, Eric (NY)	NRad	245
Lisman, Richard (NY)	Oph	261
Liss, Donald (NJ)	PMR	759
Liss, Howard (NJ)	PMR	759
Liss, Mark (NY)	Ge	661
Lisser, Steven (NJ)	HS	860
Litchman, Charisse (CT)	N	967
Litchman, Mark (CT)	A&I	942
Liteplo, Ronald (NY)	D	407
Litman, Nathan (NY)	PInf	427
Litman, Richard (NY)	Oto	626
Litman, Steven (NY)	PM	626
Littlejohn, Charles (CT)	CRS	946
Lituchy, Andrew (NY)	Cv	531
Litvin, Y. Samuel (NJ)	U	869
Liu, David (NY)	Nep	227
Liu, DeLong (NY)	Onc	673
Liu, George (NY)	IM	204
Liva, Douglas (NJ)	Oph	749
Lizza, Eli (NY)	U	390
Lo, K.M. Steve (CT)	Onc	964
Lobritto, Steven (NY)	PGe	308
Lodge, Henry (NY)	IM	204
Lodish, Stephanie (NJ)	Ped	885
LoGalbo, Peter (NY)	A&I	595
Logan, Bruce (NY)	IM	204
Loganathan, Raghunandan (NY)	Pul	433
Lois, William (NY)	S	482
Lomasky, Steven (NY)	EDM	539
Lombardi, Joseph (NJ)	OrS	844
Lombardo, Gerard (NY)	Pul	478
Lombardo, James (NY)	Oph	467
Lombardo, Peter (NY)	D	153
Lomnitz, David (CT)	Cv	945
Lomonaco, Salvatore (NY)	ChAP	649
Lonberg, Mathew (NY)	Onc	598
London, Ronald (NY)	Ped	697
Longo, Walter (CT)	CRS	1004
Lonner, Baron (NY)	OrS	278
Loo, Marcus (NY)	U	391
Lookstein, Robert (NY)	VIR	395
Lopez, Clark (NY)	FMed	451
Lopez, Ralph (NY)	AM	124
Lorber, Daniel (NY)	EDM	492
Lorefice, Laurence (CT)	Psyc	987
Loren, Gary (NJ)	PM	824
Loria, Jeffrey (NY)	Ge	175
Lorich, Dean (NY)	OrS	278
LoRusso, Diane (NY)	DR	655
Loughlin, Gerald (NY)	PPul	315
Louie, Eddie (NY)	Inf	195
Louis, Elan (NY)	N	239
Loulmet, Didier (NY)	T&CS	384
Love, Barry (NY)	PCd	304
Lovecchio, John (NY)	GO	543
LoVerme, Paul (NJ)	PlS	798
Low, Ronald (NJ)	Oto	752
Lowe, Franklin (NY)	U	391
Lowell, Barry (NJ)	Cv	874
Lowenthal, Dennis (NJ)	Onc	922
Lowenthal, Diana (NY)	PPul	694
Lowy, Joseph (NY)	Pul	355
Lozner, Jerrold (NJ)	S	932
Lu, Bing (NY)	IM	457
Lu, Gabriel (NY)	PM	689
Lu, Stanley (NJ)	NRad	863
Lubat, Edward (NJ)	DR	731
Lubell, Harry (NY)	Ped	697
Lubitz, Arthur (NY)	A&I	127
Lublin, Fred (NY)	N	239
Lubliner, Jerry (NY)	OrS	278
Lucak, Susan (NY)	Ge	175
Lucariello, Richard (NY)	Cv	405
Luchs, Jonathan (NY)	DR	537
Luciani, Richard (NJ)	ObG	789
Luciano, Daniel (NY)	N	239
Ludwig, Shelly (NJ)	Ge	859
Lukash, Barbara (NY)	D	653
Lukash, Frederick (NY)	PlS	578
Luks, Howard (NY)	SM	707
Lundberg, Walter (CT)	Onc	1012
Lunt, John (CT)	HS	955
Lusman, Paul (NY)	A&I	607
Lustbader, Andrew (CT)	ChAP	946
Lustbader, Ian (NY)	Ge	175
Lutchman, Gordon (NY)	S	519

Name	Specialty	Pg
Lutz, Christopher (NY)	PMR	326
Lutz, Gregory (NY)	PMR	326
Lutzker, Letty (NJ)	NuM	788
Lux, Michael (NJ)	IC	922
Luxenberg, Douglas (NY)	PCd	568
Lyden, John (NY)	OrS	278
Lydic, Michael (NY)	RE	633
Lyman, Neil (NJ)	Nep	880
Lynch, Michael (CT)	OrS	977
Lynch, Thomas (CT)	Onc	1012
Lynch, Vincent (CT)	ObG	1016
Lynn, Robert (NY)	Nep	419
Lyon, Valerie (NY)	FMed	167

M

Name	Specialty	Pg
Ma, Dong (NY)	PMR	326
Macaulay, William (NY)	OrS	279
Maccabee, Paul (NY)	N	463
Maccia, Clement (NJ)	A&I	916
Macher, Mark (NJ)	RadRO	852
Machler, Brian (NJ)	D	875
Macina, Lucy (NY)	Ger	543
Mack, Laurence (NY)	ObG	558
MacKay, Cynthia (NY)	Oph	262
MacKenzie, C Ronald (NY)	Rhu	367
Mackessy, Richard (NJ)	OrS	926
Mackler, Karen (NY)	D	653
Mackool, Richard (NY)	Oph	500
Maclaren, Noel (NY)	EDM	165
MacMillan, William (NJ)	MF	839
Maddalo, Anthony (NY)	OrS	686
Madigan, Janet (CT)	ChAP	1003
Maggio, William (NJ)	NS	862
Magid, Steven (NY)	Rhu	367
Magill, Richard (NY)	HS	664
Maglaras, Nicholas (NJ)	IM	921
Magner, Joan (CT)	Ped	983
Magramm, Irene (NY)	Oph	262
Magriples, Urania (CT)	MF	1011
Magro, Cynthia (NY)	Path	301
Magun, Arthur (NY)	Ge	175
Mahal, Pradeep (NJ)	Ge	920
Mahalingam, Banu (NJ)	Cv	817
Maharam, Lewis (NY)	SM	371
Maher, Elizabeth (NY)	Oph	262
Maher, John (NY)	ObG	465
Maheshwari, Vivek (NJ)	S	802
Mahnensmith, Rex (CT)	Nep	1014
Mahoney, Maurice (CT)	CG	1003
Maier, Herbert (NJ)	D	894
Mailloux, Lionel (NY)	Nep	553
Maiman, Mitchell (NY)	GO	512
Maiocco, Kenneth (CT)	D	947
Maizel, Barry (NY)	Ge	452
Maki, Robert (NY)	Onc	218
Malach, Barbara (NY)	IM	513
Malamud, Stephen (NY)	Onc	219
Malanga, Gerard (NJ)	PMR	928
Malaspina, Dolores (NY)	Psyc	345
Maldonado, Thomas (NY)	VascS	399
Malefatto, Jerry (CT)	Onc	964
Malik, Asim (NY)	IM	457
Malik, Rubina (NY)	Ger	413
Malik, Sajid (NY)	Oph	560
Malison, Robert (CT)	AdP	1001
Malits, Bella (NY)	PM	689
Mallozzi, Angelo (CT)	FMed	951
Mally, Pradeep (NY)	NP	225
Maloney, Patrick (NY)	A&I	642
Malovany, Robert (NJ)	Pul	763
Malpeso, James (NY)	IC	513
Maman, Arie (NJ)	EDM	835
Manasseh, Donna-Marie (NY)	S	482
Mancini, Donna (NY)	Cv	134
Mandava, Suresh (CT)	Oph	973
Mandel, Eric (NY)	Oph	262
Mandel, Marc (NJ)	S	932
Mandel, Michael (NY)	Pul	703
Mandelbaum, Sidney (NY)	Oph	262
Manevitz, Alan (NY)	Psyc	345
Mangi, Abeel (CT)	T&CS	1032
Manginello, Frank (NJ)	NP	743
Mani, John (NY)	OrS	468
Mani, Susan (CT)	Cv	945
Maniatis, Theodore (NY)	Pul	518
Maniscalco, Anthony (NY)	N	463
Manjoney, Delia (CT)	Oph	973
Mankes, Seth (NY)	DR	613

Alphabetical Listing of Doctors

Name	Specialty	Pg
Mann, J. John (NY)	Psyc	345
Mann, Ronald (NY)	OrS	686
Mann, Samuel (NY)	IM	204
Manners, Richard (NY)	Ped	630
Manning, Eric (NJ)	Nep	862
Manno, Joseph (NJ)	VascS	771
Manolas, Panagiotis (NY)	S	504
Mansouri, Hormoz (NY)	S	587
Marchetta, Paula (NY)	Rhu	367
Marcus, Judith (NY)	PHO	311
Marcus, Michael (NY)	PPul	474
Marcus, Norman (NY)	PM	299
Marcus, Ralph (NJ)	Rhu	765
Marcus, Richard (NJ)	Ped	797
Marder, Karen (NY)	N	239
Marghoob, Ashfaq (NY)	D	611
Margolis, Eric (NJ)	U	769
Margulies, Paul (NY)	EDM	539
Margulis, Elynne (NJ)	ObG	925
Margulis, Stephen (NJ)	Ge	734
Margulis, Steven (NY)	IM	669
Marienberg, Evelyn (NY)	RadRO	583
Marin, Deborah (NY)	Psyc	345
Marin, Geobel (NJ)	Ge	818
Marin, Michael (NY)	VascS	399
Marino, A. Michael (CT)	Pul	988
Marino, John (NY)	Onc	551
Marino, Ronald (NY)	Ped	574
Marion, James (NY)	Ge	175
Marion, Robert (NY)	CG	406
Markell, Mariana (NY)	Nep	460
Markenson, Joseph (NY)	Rhu	367
Markovics, Sharon (NY)	A&I	527
Markowitz, Arlene (NY)	Oto	292
Markowitz, Arnold (NY)	Ge	175
Markowitz, David (NY)	Ge	176
Markowitz, James (NY)	PGe	570
Markowitz, John (NY)	Psyc	345
Markowitz, Steven (NY)	CE	129
Marks, Alan (NY)	Oph	560
Marks, Andrea (NY)	AM	125
Marks, David (NJ)	N	788
Marks, Jon (NY)	U	391
Marks, Laura (CT)	Ped	983
Marks, Stephen (NY)	N	678
Marmur, Ellen (NY)	D	153
Marmur, Jonathan (NY)	IC	458
Marmur, Ronen (NY)	Rhu	706
Marotta, James (NY)	PlS	631
Marottoli, Richard (CT)	Ger	1006
Marr, Brian (NY)	Oph	262
Marron-Corwin, Mary (NY)	NP	225
Marsan, Ben (CT)	VascS	997
Marsh, Franklin (NY)	Ge	176
Marsh, James (CT)	OrS	1018
Marshalko, Stephen (CT)	Cv	945
Marshall, Ian (NJ)	PEn	847
Marshall, Randolph (NY)	N	239
Martens, Mark (NJ)	ObG	863
Martimucci, William (NY)	Ger	663
Martin, Christopher (NY)	Ge	661
Martin, Jeffrey (NY)	Oph	624
Martins, Publius (NY)	Pul	518
Martz, Joseph (NY)	CRS	146
Marx, Robert (NY)	OrS	279
Masani, Naveed (NY)	Nep	553
Mascarenhas, Bento (NY)	Rhu	706
Masci, Joseph (NY)	Inf	495
Masciello, Michael (NY)	Cv	609
Maselli, Frank (NY)	FMed	410
Masino, Frank (CT)	RadRO	990
Maslak, Peter (NY)	Hem	190
Masri, Bassem (NY)	Cv	134
Massie, Mary Jane (NY)	Psyc	345
Masson, Lalitha (NJ)	ObG	810
Masterson, Raymond (NJ)	IM	861
Matalon, Robert (NY)	Nep	227
Matarasso, Alan (NY)	PlS	333
Matczuk, Agnieszka (CT)	A&I	942
Mateo, Romeo (NY)	VascS	713
Matera, Cristina (NY)	RE	362
Math, Kevin (NY)	DR	160
Mathias, Stephen (CT)	Oph	973
Matilsky, Michael (NY)	Cv	609
Matos, Jeffrey (NY)	CE	129
Matos, Marshall (NY)	Cv	646
Matossian, Cynthia (NJ)	Oph	823
Matta, Raymond (NY)	Cv	135
Mattana, Joseph (NY)	Nep	553
Mattel, Stephen (NJ)	Oto	897

Name	Specialty	Pg
Mattes, Leonard (NY)	Cv	135
Matthews, Gerald (NY)	U	711
Mattison, Timothy (NY)	D	653
Mattoo, Nirmal (NY)	Nep	498
Mattucci, Kenneth (NY)	Oto	565
Mauer, Kenneth (CT)	Ge	953
Mauri, Thomas (NY)	OrS	563
Mauskop, Alexander (NY)	N	239
Maxfield, Roger (NY)	Pul	355
May, Louis (NY)	Ge	597
Mayer, Daniel (NY)	A&I	607
Mayer, Deborah (CT)	IM	959
Mayer, Fern (CT)	D	947
Mayer, Ira (NY)	Ge	452
Mayer, Stephan (NY)	N	239
Mayers, Marguerite (NY)	Ped	430
Mayers, Martin (NY)	Oph	422
Mayerson, Adam (CT)	EDM	1005
Mayeux, Richard (NY)	N	240
Maytal, Joseph (NY)	ChiN	534
Mazur, Eric (CT)	Hem	956
Mazza, David (NY)	A&I	127
Mazzara, Carl (NJ)	Oto	845
Mc Inerney, Vincent (NJ)	OrS	896
McAbee, Gary (NJ)	ChiN	807
McAleer, Patricia (CT)	D	947
McAllister, Peter (CT)	N	968
McAnally, James (NJ)	Nep	923
McBride, Whitney (NY)	PS	694
McCain, Donald (NJ)	S	766
McCalley, Stuart (CT)	Pul	989
McCance, Sean (NY)	OrS	279
McCann, Peter (NY)	OrS	279
McCarthy, Paul (CT)	PRhu	1024
McCarton, Cecelia (NY)	Ped	321
McClane, James (CT)	CRS	946
McClelland, Shearwood (NY)	OrS	279
McClung, John (NY)	Cv	646
McConnell, Robert (NY)	EDM	165
McCormack, Patricia (NY)	D	510
McCormick, Beryl (NY)	RadRO	359
McCormick, Paul (NY)	NS	232
McCullough, Jock (NJ)	T&CS	767
McDermott, John (NY)	Oph	262
McFarlane-Ferreira, Yvonne (NY)	PGe	471
McGinn, Joseph (NY)	T&CS	520
McGinniss, George (CT)	OrS	977
McGinty, James (NY)	S	377
McGovern, Catherine (NY)	ObG	680
McGovern, Margaret (NY)	CG	610
McGovern, Patrick (NJ)	S	812
McGovern, Peter (NJ)	RE	764
McGovern, Thomas (NY)	U	391
McGowan, Charles (NY)	PMR	697
McGowan, Joseph (NY)	Inf	546
McGrath, Patrick (NY)	Psyc	345
McHugh, Margaret (NY)	Ped	322
McIlveen, Stephen (NJ)	OrS	751
McKee, Heather (NY)	Oph	683
McKenna, Michael (NJ)	RadRO	826
McKhann, Guy (NY)	NS	232
McKiernan, James (NY)	U	391
McKinley, Matthew (NY)	Ge	542
McKinsey, James (NY)	VascS	399
McLaughlin, Mark (NJ)	NS	822
McLeod, Gavin (CT)	Inf	957
McMahon, Donna-Marie (NY)	Ped	630
McManus, Edward (NJ)	Inf	878
McManus, Susan (NJ)	S	853
McMeeking, Alexander (NY)	Inf	195
McMenomey, Sean (NY)	Oto	293
McMullen, Robert (NY)	Psyc	346
McNamara, Joseph (CT)	PHO	1023
McPherson, Craig (CT)	CE	943
McWhorter, Philip (CT)	S	993
Meacham, Kevin (NY)	ObG	681
Mears, John Gregory (NY)	Hem	190
Mechanic, Laura (NY)	A&I	642
Mechanick, Jeffrey (NY)	EDM	165
Medici, Mark (NY)	OrS	600
Medina, Emma (NY)	Cv	647
Medow, Norman (NY)	Oph	422
Medvecky, Michael (CT)	OrS	1019
Meed, Steven (NY)	Rhu	367
Meere, Patrick (NY)	OrS	279
Megibow, Alec (NY)	DR	160
Mehran, Roxana (NY)	IC	208
Mehrara, Babak (NY)	PlS	333
Mehrotra, Bhoomi (NY)	Onc	551
Mehta, Davendra (NY)	CE	129

Alphabetical Listing of Doctors

Name	Specialty	Pg
Mehta, Rajeev (NJ)	NP	840
Mehta, Viplov (NY)	IM	457
Meighan, Dennis (CT)	Ge	953
Meirowitz, Natalie (NY)	MF	549
Meirowitz, Robert (NJ)	Ge	818
Meisenberg, Gene (NY)	U	483
Meisler, Susan (NY)	Ped	697
Meiteles, Lawrence (NY)	Oto	688
Meixler, Steven (NY)	Pul	704
Meizlish, Jay (CT)	Cv	945
Melamed, Jonathan (NY)	Path	301
Melillo, Nicholas (NJ)	Pul	851
Meller, Jose (NY)	Cv	135
Mellinger, Brett (NY)	U	590
Mellman, Lisa (NY)	Psyc	346
Melman, Martin (NY)	IM	669
Melnick, Hugh (NY)	ObG	251
Melone, Charles (NY)	HS	187
Melton, Roberta (NY)	Oph	262
Meltzer, Alan (NJ)	Ped	885
Melville, Gordon (NJ)	DR	904
Menchell, David (NY)	A&I	490
Mendelowitz, Alan (NY)	Psyc	502
Mendelowitz, Lawrence (NY)	ObG	681
Mendelsohn, Michael (NY)	PO	571
Mendelsohn, Sara (NY)	OM	559
Mendelson, Joel (NJ)	A&I	916
Mendes, Donna (NY)	VascS	399
Mendes, John (NJ)	OrS	791
Mendoza, Ernesto (NY)	S	504
Mendoza, Francis (NY)	OrS	279
Mendoza, Glenn (NY)	NP	598
Menegus, Mark (NY)	Cv	405
Menezes, Nelson (NY)	VascS	484
Menezes, Placido (NY)	OrS	468
Menitove, Stephen (NY)	Pul	602
Ment, Laura (CT)	ChiN	1003
Menza, Matthew (NJ)	Psyc	850
Menzin, Andrew (NY)	GO	544
Merav, Avraham (NY)	T&CS	709
Mercando, Anthony (NY)	Cv	647
Meredith, Gary (NY)	Rhu	585
Merer, David (NY)	PO	693
Merhige, Kenneth (NY)	Oph	262
Merker, Edward (NY)	FMed	657
Mermelstein, Erwin (NJ)	Cv	832
Mermelstein, Harold (NY)	D	653
Mermelstein, Steve (NY)	Pul	581
Merola, Andrew (NY)	OrS	468
Merriam, John (NY)	Oph	263
Meskin, Seth (CT)	Oph	1017
Messana, Ida (NY)	IM	496
Messerli, Franz (NY)	Cv	135
Messina, John (NJ)	PCd	754
Messinger, David (NY)	IC	671
Metz, John (NJ)	FMed	835
Metzger, Scott (NJ)	PM	865
Metzl, Jordan (NY)	SM	371
Meyer, David (NY)	T&CS	588
Meyer, Dodi (NY)	Ped	322
Meyer, Monica (NJ)	ObG	748
Meyer, Richard (NY)	Hem	190
Meyers, Barnett (NY)	Psyc	701
Meyers, Paul (NY)	PHO	311
Meyers, Philip (NY)	NRad	245
Meyers-Seifer, Cynthia (NJ)	PEn	865
Miarrostami, Rameen (NY)	Pul	478
Mich, Robert (NJ)	IC	922
Michaelides, Elias (CT)	Oto	1020
Michaelson, Richard (NJ)	Onc	786
Michaelson, Stephen (CT)	Cv	945
Michel, Ketly (NY)	ObG	251
Michelassi, Fabrizio (NY)	S	377
Michelis, Mary Ann (NJ)	A&I	723
Michelis, Michael (NY)	Nep	227
Michels, Robert (NY)	Psyc	346
Michler, Robert (NY)	T&CS	437
Mickley, Diane (CT)	IM	959
Mickley, Steven (CT)	IM	959
Middlesworth, William (NY)	PS	317
Middleton, John (NJ)	Inf	837
Midulla, Peter (NY)	PS	317
Mieszerski, Laura (NY)	ObG	681
Mignone, Biagio (NY)	Oph	683
Miguel, Eduardo (NJ)	IM	739
Mikkilineni, Sushmita (NJ)	PPul	796
Milanaik, Ruth (NY)	Ped	574
Milano, Andrew (NY)	Ge	176
Mildvan, Donna (NY)	Inf	195
Miles, Daniel (NY)	ChiN	144

Name	Specialty	Pg
Milgraum, Sandy (NJ)	D	833
Milgrim, Laurence (NJ)	Oto	752
Milite, James (NJ)	Oph	844
Miller, Aaron (NY)	N	240
Miller, Andrew (NJ)	Oto	845
Miller, Daniel (NY)	FMed	657
Miller, David (NY)	Cv	135
Miller, David (NJ)	Psyc	929
Miller, Dennis (NY)	Inf	195
Miller, Jane (NJ)	RE	764
Miller, Jeffrey (NJ)	HS	877
Miller, Kenneth (CT)	Rhu	992
Miller, Kenneth (NJ)	IC	785
Miller, Kevin (CT)	S	993
Miller, Leslie (CT)	FMed	951
Miller, Mark (NJ)	U	932
Miller, Philip (NY)	Oto	293
Miller, Rachel (NY)	Pul	355
Miller, Richard (NJ)	Pul	799
Miller, Scott (NY)	PHO	472
Miller, Seth (CT)	OrS	977
Miller, Seth (NY)	Ge	542
Miller, Theodore (NY)	DR	160
Miller-Breslow, Anne (NJ)	HS	736
Mills, Carl (NY)	U	636
Mills, Christopher (NY)	S	377
Mills, Nancy (NY)	Onc	673
Milman, Perry (NY)	Ge	542
Milone, Richard (NY)	Psyc	701
Milsom, Jeffrey (NY)	CRS	146
Milstein, David (NY)	NuM	421
Min, Albert (NY)	Ge	176
Mindel, Joel (NY)	Oph	263
Miner, Charles (CT)	IM	959
Mini, Katherine (CT)	Ped	984
Minikes, Neil (NJ)	A&I	723
Minkoff, Howard (NY)	ObG	465
Minkowitz, Susan (NY)	IM	204
Mintz, Abraham (CT)	NS	966
Mintz, Douglas (NY)	DR	160
Mintz, Guy (NY)	Cv	531
Mirra, Suzanne (NY)	Path	470
Miskovitz, Paul (NY)	Ge	176
Mitchell, John (NY)	Oph	263
Mitnick, Hal (NY)	Rhu	367
Mitnick, Julie (NY)	DR	160
Mitsumoto, Hiroshi (NY)	N	240
Mittal, Suneet (NJ)	CE	723
Mittler, Mark (NY)	NS	554
Moazed, Kambiz (NY)	Oph	263
Modi, Vikash (NY)	PO	314
Mogan, Glen (NJ)	Ge	782
Mogil, Laurey (NY)	Oph	467
Mohr, JP (NY)	N	240
Mohr, Robert (NJ)	ObG	881
Moisa, Idel (NY)	Oto	565
Mojtabai, Shaparak (NY)	IM	416
Moldover, Jonathan (NY)	PMR	327
Moldwin, Robert (NY)	U	591
Mollin, Joel (NY)	DR	492
Molloy, Edward (CT)	IM	959
Molmenti, Ernesto (NY)	S	587
Molnar, Thomas (NY)	FMed	493
Molofsky, Walter (NY)	ChiN	144
Monasebian, Douglas (NY)	PlS	333
Mondrow, Daniel (NJ)	Cv	832
Mongillo, Nicholas (CT)	Ped	984
Monrad, E. Scott (NY)	Cv	405
Montalvo-Stanton, Evelyn (NJ)	PPul	796
Montero, Carlos (NY)	OrS	563
Montgomery, Kenneth (NJ)	OrS	882
Montgomery, Leslie (NY)	S	436
Monti, Louis (NY)	Ped	322
Montoya-Iraheta, Carlos (NY)	PCd	568
Moore, Anne (NY)	Onc	219
Moore, Frank (NJ)	NS	745
Moore, Joanne (NY)	Psyc	346
Moorjani, Harish (NY)	Inf	665
Moorthy, Chitti (NY)	RadRO	704
Moorthy, Lakshmi (NJ)	PRhu	848
Mootabar, Hamid (NY)	MF	672
Moqtaderi, Farideh (NY)	PM	299
Moraille, Pascale (NJ)	Psyc	811
Moreau, Donna (NY)	ChAP	141
Morel, Kimberly (NY)	D	153
Morelli, Alan (CT)	Ped	984
Morello, Robert (NY)	Oph	683
Moreno, Pedro (NY)	IC	209
Moreta, Henry (NY)	N	622
Morgan, Charles (CT)	Psyc	987

Alphabetical Listing of Doctors

Name	Specialty	Pg
Morgan, Daniel (NY)	OrS	469
Morgan, James (CT)	Ped	1025
Moriarty, Daniel (NJ)	Onc	922
Moritz, Jacques (NY)	ObG	251
Morledge, Louis (NY)	IM	204
Morman, Manuel (NJ)	D	729
Morris, Carol (NY)	OrS	279
Morris, Elizabeth (NY)	DR	160
Morris, James (NY)	N	678
Morris, Michael (NY)	Onc	219
Morris, Robert (NY)	Oph	624
Morrison, R Sean (NY)	Ger	181
Morrison, Susan (NJ)	PA&I	793
Morrissey, Nicholas (NY)	VascS	399
Morrow, Jon (CT)	Path	1021
Morrow, Monica (NY)	S	378
Morrow, Robert (NY)	FMed	410
Morrow, Todd (NJ)	Oto	792
Mosca, Ralph (NY)	T&CS	385
Moses, Jeffrey (NY)	IC	209
Moses, Stuart (NJ)	DR	780
Moseson, Michael (NY)	CRS	535
Moshe, Solomon (NY)	ChiN	406
Moskovich, Ronald (NY)	OrS	280
Moskovits, Norbert (NY)	Cv	446
Moskovits, Tibor (NY)	Hem	191
Moskowitz, Bruce (NY)	Oph	263
Moskowitz, Craig (NY)	Onc	219
Moskowitz, George (NY)	FMed	451
Moskowitz, Richard (NJ)	CRS	875
Most, Richard (NY)	Oph	683
Motiwala, Rajeev (NY)	N	240
Motzer, Robert (NY)	Onc	219
Moucha, Calin (NY)	OrS	280
Moulton, Thomas (NY)	PHO	427
Moussa, Ghias (NJ)	Cv	807
Moynihan, Brian (NY)	FMed	540
Moynihan, Gavan (NY)	D	612
Muchnick, Richard (NY)	Oph	263
Mueller, F. Carl (CT)	Psyc	987
Mueller, Richard (NY)	Cv	135
Muensterer, Oliver (NY)	PS	694
Muggia, Franco (NY)	Onc	219
Mukherjee, Tanmoy (NY)	RE	363
Muldoon, Lawrence (CT)	U	995
Muldoon, Thomas (NY)	Oph	263
Mulford, Gregory (NJ)	PMR	886
Mulgaonkar, Shamkant (NJ)	Nep	787
Mulhall, John (NY)	U	391
Mullen, David (CT)	DR	949
Mullen, Edward (NY)	RadRO	583
Mullen, Michael (NY)	Inf	196
Multz, Alan (NY)	Pul	581
Mulvehill, Joseph (NY)	IM	204
Mulvey, Lauri (NJ)	Oph	823
Munver, Ravi (NJ)	U	769
Muraca, Glenn (NY)	FMed	493
Murali, Raj (NY)	NS	677
Murdock, Cynthia (CT)	RE	991
Murphy, Ramon (NY)	Ped	322
Murphy, Robert (NJ)	Ped	866
Murphy, Robyn (NJ)	DR	876
Murray, Henry (NY)	Inf	196
Murray, Simon (NJ)	IM	820
Muskin, Philip (NY)	Psyc	346
Musto, Anthony (CT)	Oph	973
Mutterperl, Mitchell (NJ)	IM	809
Myerson, Merle (NY)	Cv	135
Myskowski, Patricia (NY)	D	153
Myssiorek, David (NY)	Oto	293

N

Name	Specialty	Pg
Nachajon, Roberto (NJ)	PPul	897
Nachman, Sharon (NY)	PInf	628
Nackenson, Marcia (NY)	AM	642
Nadelman, Robert (NY)	Inf	665
Nadzam, Geoffrey (CT)	S	1031
Nagarsheth, Nimesh (NY)	GO	184
Nagler, Harris (NY)	U	391
Nagler, Jerry (NY)	Ge	176
Nahass, Ronald (NJ)	Inf	906
Nahm, Frederick (CT)	N	968
Naidich, David (NY)	DR	160
Naidich, Jason (NY)	VIR	592
Naidich, Thomas (NY)	NRad	245
Naidorf, Ellen (CT)	D	948
Najarian, James (NJ)	Nep	880
Najjar, Sessine (NJ)	Inf	894

Name	Specialty	Pg
Najjar, Souhel (NY)	N	515
Naka, Yoshifumi (NY)	T&CS	385
Nalbandian, Matthew (NY)	VascS	399
Namerow, David (NJ)	Ped	758
Nanus, David (NY)	Onc	219
Napolitano, Joseph (NJ)	Oph	844
Napolitano, Massimo (NJ)	VascS	771
Narayan, Deepak (CT)	PlS	1026
Narins, Rhoda (NY)	D	653
Narula, Amarjot (NJ)	Psyc	761
Narula, Pramod (NY)	PPul	474
Nascimento, Joao (CT)	Rhu	992
Nash, Bernard (NY)	Inf	617
Nash, Ira (NY)	Cv	135
Nash, Thomas (NY)	Pul	356
Nass, Jack (NY)	Psyc	631
Nass, Richard (NY)	Oto	293
Nass, Ruth (NY)	ChiN	144
Nassberg, Barton (NJ)	EDM	858
Natale, Benjamin (NJ)	Oph	925
Nath, Sunil (NY)	Pul	502
Nattis, Richard (NY)	Oph	624
Nauheim, Richard (NY)	Oph	560
Neal, Wendy (NJ)	AM	776
Nealon, Nancy (NY)	N	240
Nee, Paul (CT)	Inf	957
Needleman, Joshua (NY)	PPul	474
Neelakantappa, Kotresha (NY)	Nep	460
Neely, Michael (NY)	PMR	327
Neeson, Francis (CT)	Cv	945
Neibart, Eric (NY)	Inf	196
Neibart, Richard (NJ)	T&CS	868
Neiman, Deborah (NJ)	IM	906
Neistadt, L Daniel (NY)	DR	161
Nelson, Alan (CT)	Ge	953
Nelson, David (NY)	Oph	560
Nelson, Deena (NY)	IM	204
Nelson, John (NY)	Hem	665
Nelson, John (NY)	OrS	686
Nelson, Judith (NY)	Pul	356
Nelson, William (NY)	ObG	681
Neophytides, Andreas (NY)	N	240
Nepola, Neil (NY)	FMed	511
Nero, Thomas (CT)	IC	961
Nerwen, Clifford (NY)	Ped	575
Neschis, Ronald (NY)	Psyc	701
Neu, Natalie (NY)	PInf	312
Neuberg, Gerald (NY)	Cv	406
Neugarten, Joel (NY)	Nep	419
Neuwirth, Michael (NY)	OrS	280
Nevin, Marie (NJ)	EDM	876
New, Maria (NY)	PEn	307
Newburger, Amy (NY)	D	653
Newhouse, Jeffrey (NY)	DR	161
Newman, Elliot (NY)	S	378
Newman, Fredric (CT)	PlS	985
Newman, Lawrence (NY)	N	240
Newman, Scott (NY)	PlS	699
Newman, Stephen (NY)	N	556
Newman-Cedar, Meryl (NY)	Ped	322
Newmark, Ian (NY)	Pul	581
Newton, Michael (NY)	Oph	263
Ng, John (NY)	RadRO	359
Ngai, Pakkay (NJ)	PPul	756
Ngeow, Jeffrey (NY)	PM	299
Nguyen, Khanh (NY)	T&CS	385
Nicholas, Stephen (NY)	OrS	280
Nickerson, Katherine (NY)	Rhu	368
Nicosia, Thomas (NY)	Cv	532
Niederman, Michael (NY)	Pul	581
Nierman, David (NY)	CCM	491
Nightingale, Jeffrey (NY)	Oph	264
Nikias, George (NJ)	Ge	734
Nimaroff, Michael (NY)	ObG	550
Nini, Kevin (NJ)	PlS	850
Nininger, James (NY)	Psyc	346
Nisonson, Barton (NY)	SM	371
Nissenblatt, Michael (NJ)	Onc	839
Nitti, Victor (NY)	U	391
Nitzberg, Richard (NJ)	S	932
Nizin, Joel (NJ)	CRS	728
Nobert, Craig (NY)	U	391
Nocek, David (CT)	OrS	977
Nogueira, Mark (NY)	U	711
Norden, Richard (NJ)	Oph	749
Nori, Dattatreyudu (NY)	RadRO	360
Norton, Larry (NY)	Onc	219
Nosher, John (NJ)	VIR	854
Nosko, Michael (NJ)	NS	840
Notar-Francesco, Vincent (NY)	Ge	452

Alphabetical Listing of Doctors

Name	Specialty	Pg
Notaro, Antoinette (NY)	D	612
Noto, Richard (NY)	PEn	691
Nouri, Shahin (NY)	N	463
Novack, Stuart (CT)	Rhu	992
Novick, Brian (NY)	A&I	527
Novick, Mark (NY)	DR	161
Novitch, Richard (NY)	Pul	704
Novogroder, Michael (NJ)	PEn	754
Nowak, Eugene (NY)	S	378
Nowak-Wegrzyn, Anna (NY)	PA&I	303
Noy, Ron (NY)	SM	371
Noyes, Nicole (NY)	RE	363
Nucci, Annamaria (NJ)	Psyc	799
Nucci-Sack, Anne (NY)	AM	125
Nunes, Edward (NY)	Psyc	346
Nurzia, Michael (CT)	U	995
Nussbaum, Michel (NY)	Ge	494

O

Name	Specialty	Pg
O'Brien, Daryl (NJ)	Ped	759
O'Brien, Francis (NY)	Cv	136
O'Connell, Joseph (CT)	PIS	986
O'Connor, Brian (NJ)	PCd	794
O'Connor, Owen (NY)	Onc	220
O'Connor, Patrick (CT)	IM	1010
O'Dell, Michael (NY)	PMR	327
O'Donnell, Timothy (NJ)	Pul	888
O'Hea, Brian (NY)	S	635
O'Leary, Patrick (NY)	OrS	280
O'Malley, Grace (NY)	Oph	624
O'Malley, Martin (NY)	OrS	280
O'Regan, Simon (CT)	FMed	951
O'Reilly, Eileen (NY)	Onc	220
O'Reilly, Richard (NY)	PHO	311
O'Shaughnessy, Althea (NJ)	RE	826
Ober, David (NY)	N	599
Oberfield, Richard (NY)	Psyc	346
Oberfield, Sharon (NY)	PEn	307
Obstbaum, Stephen (NY)	Oph	264
Odaimi, Marcel (NY)	Onc	514
Odel, Jeffrey (NY)	Oph	264
Oeffinger, Kevin (NY)	Ped	322
Oestreicher, Mark (CT)	D	948
Offit, Kenneth (NY)	Onc	220
Oghia, Hady (NY)	Ped	475
Oh, William (NY)	Onc	220
Oh, Youn (NJ)	N	842
Oh, Young (NY)	OrS	686
Oko, Piotr (NJ)	Ped	811
Olanow, C Warren (NY)	N	241
Olarte, Marcelo (NY)	N	241
Olds, David (NY)	Psyc	347
Oleske, James (NJ)	PInf	795
Olichney, John (NY)	IM	205
Olin, Craig (CT)	IM	959
Oliver, Gregory (NJ)	CRS	833
Olsen, Drew (NJ)	Path	753
Olsewski, John (NY)	OrS	423
Olson, Robert (NJ)	PIS	909
Onesti, Stephen (NY)	NS	554
Ong, Lawrence (NY)	IC	619
Opler, Lewis (NY)	Psyc	701
Oppedisano, Carlyn (NY)	Ped	430
Oppenheim, Jeffrey (NY)	NS	599
Oppenheim, Jennifer (NY)	Ped	475
Oppenheimer, John (NY)	IM	618
Oratz, Ruth (NY)	Onc	220
Orazi, Attilio (NY)	Path	301
Orbe, Jessica (NY)	Ped	322
Orbuch, Philip (NY)	D	153
Ordorica, Steven (NY)	ObG	251
Orell, Jeffrey (CT)	Hem	1008
Orentreich, David (NY)	D	153
Oribe, Emilio (NY)	N	499
Orlow, Seth (NY)	D	154
Ornstein, Matthew (NY)	Rhu	368
Orsher, Stuart (NY)	IM	205
Orsini, William (NJ)	D	858
Ortiz, Orlando (NY)	NRad	557
Osei-Tutu, John (NY)	Psyc	432
Oshman, Robin (CT)	D	948
Osleeb, Craig (NY)	A&I	643
Osnoss, Kenneth (CT)	IM	959
Ossias, A Lawrence (NY)	Hem	191
Ostad, Ariel (NY)	D	154
Oster, Martin (NY)	Onc	220
Ostrer, Harry (NY)	CG	407
Ostriker, Glenn (CT)	Oph	973

Name	Specialty	Pg
Ostrow, Stanley (NY)	Onc	620
Otsuka, Norman (NY)	OrS	280
Ott, Allen (NY)	ObG	623
Ott, Casey (CT)	Ger	1007
Ottaviano, Lawrence (NY)	Ge	176
Owens, George (NY)	U	711
Oz, Mehmet (NY)	T&CS	385
Ozkaynak, Mehmet (NY)	PHO	692

P

Name	Specialty	Pg
Paccione, Jeffrey (NY)	Oph	264
Pace, Benjamin (NY)	S	504
Pachter, H Leon (NY)	S	378
Pacia, Steven (NY)	N	241
Packer, Samuel (NY)	Oph	560
Padela, Mohammad (NJ)	N	896
Padgett, Douglas (NY)	OrS	280
Padilla, Maria (NY)	Pul	356
Paget, Stephen (NY)	Rhu	368
Pahuja, Murlidhar (NY)	S	520
Paidas, Michael (CT)	MF	1011
Paiusco, Augusto (NY)	Cv	446
Pak, Jayoung (NJ)	ChiN	778
Palaia, David (NY)	PlS	699
Palatt, Terry (NY)	T&CS	636
Palese, Michael (NY)	U	392
Palestro, Christopher (NY)	NuM	557
Paley, Ari (NY)	Cv	647
Palma, Eugen (NY)	CE	404
Palsky, Glenn (NJ)	Ped	825
Paltzik, Robert (NY)	D	536
Palu, Richard (NY)	Oph	264
Pan, Cynthia (NY)	H & PM	495
Pandit-Taskar, Neeta (NY)	NuM	246
Panella, Vincent (NJ)	Ge	734
Panicek, David (NY)	DR	161
Pannone, John (NY)	Nep	460
Panush, David (NJ)	DR	731
Panza, Robert (NJ)	Ped	928
Panzner, Elizabeth (NJ)	Ped	928
Papadakos, Stylianos (NY)	IC	497
Papish, Steven (NJ)	Onc	879
Papp, Laszlo (NY)	Psyc	347
Pappas, John (NY)	CG	145
Pappas, Steven (NY)	IM	669
Pappas, Thomas (NY)	Cv	532
Pappert, Amy (NJ)	D	904
Parashar, Bhupesh (NY)	RadRO	360
Parekh, Aruna (NY)	NP	621
Parikh, Manish (NY)	IC	209
Paris, Barbara (NY)	Ger	453
Park, Bernard (NJ)	T&CS	767
Park, Kenneth (NJ)	PM	753
Park, Tae (NY)	RadRO	633
Parker, Andrew (CT)	Oto	980
Parker, Robert (NY)	PHO	628
Parks, Michael (NY)	OrS	281
Parles, James (NY)	Ped	630
Parnell, Vincent (NY)	PS	573
Parnes, Eliezer (NY)	Nep	461
Parness, Ira (NY)	PCd	305
Parrish, Edward (NY)	Rhu	368
Parry, Michael (CT)	Inf	957
Pascal, Mark (NJ)	Onc	742
Pasik, Deborah (NJ)	Rhu	888
Pasmantier, Mark (NY)	Onc	220
Pasquale, Jack (NY)	IM	496
Pasquariello, Palmo (NY)	Ped	322
Pass, Harvey (NY)	T&CS	385
Pass, Helen (CT)	S	993
Pass, Robert (NY)	PCd	425
Passarelli, Marianne (CT)	U	1033
Passaretti, David (CT)	PlS	986
Passeri, Daniel (CT)	S	993
Pastore, Doris (NY)	AM	125
Pastorek, Norman (NY)	Oto	293
Patchell, Roy (NJ)	N	822
Patel, Aman (NY)	NS	232
Patel, Amit (NJ)	VascS	804
Patel, Bhavesh (CT)	PMR	1026
Patel, Jitendra (NY)	Rhu	481
Pathare, Pradip (CT)	RadRO	990
Patrick, Sharon (NY)	MF	211
Patrizio, Pasquale (CT)	RE	1029
Patterson, Francis (NJ)	OrS	791
Pattner, Austin (NJ)	Nep	744
Paty, Philip (NY)	S	378
Paul, Edward (NY)	AdP	123

Alphabetical Listing of Doctors

Name	Specialty	Pg
Paul, Elliot (NY)	U	591
Paul, Matthew (CT)	Oph	973
Pavlakis, Steven (NY)	ChiN	447
Pavlick, Anna (NY)	Onc	221
Pavlov, Helene (NY)	DR	161
Pawel, Michael (NY)	Psyc	347
Pearl, Adam (CT)	Oto	980
Pearl, Michael (NY)	GO	616
Pearle, Andrew (NY)	OrS	281
Pechman, Karen (NY)	PMR	698
Peck, Valerie (NY)	EDM	166
Pecker, Mark (NY)	IM	205
Pecora, Andrew (NJ)	Onc	742
Pedinoff, Andrew (NJ)	A&I	903
Pegler, Cynthia (NY)	AM	125
Pelavin, Martin (NJ)	IM	739
Pellicci, Paul (NY)	OrS	281
Pellicone, John (NY)	Pul	602
Peng, Benjamin (NY)	U	392
Penzer, Jason (NY)	CRS	146
Pepe, John (NY)	Nep	514
Pereira, Frederick (NY)	D	492
Pereira, Stephen (NJ)	S	766
Perelstein, Eduardo (NY)	PNep	313
Perez-Soler, Roman (NY)	Onc	418
Perin, Noel (NY)	NS	232
Perin, Patrick (NJ)	A&I	723
Perl, Harold (NJ)	NP	743
Perlman, Barry (NY)	Psyc	701
Perlman, David (NY)	Inf	196
Perlman, Donald (NJ)	A&I	776
Perlman, Fern (CT)	Ped	984
Perlman, Jeffrey (NY)	NP	225
Perlman, Philip (NY)	Oto	565
Perron, Reed (NJ)	N	746
Perrotti, John (NY)	PlS	334
Perry, Arthur (NJ)	PlS	909
Perry, Bradford (NY)	Psyc	701
Perry, Henry (NY)	Oph	561
Perry, Richard (NY)	ChAP	142
Perry-Bottinger, Lynne (NY)	Cv	647
Persing, John (CT)	PlS	1026
Persky, Mark (NY)	Oto	293
Pesce, Joseph (CT)	D	948
Peschel, Richard (CT)	RadRO	1028
Peterson, Monte (NY)	Ger	181
Peterson, Stephen (NY)	IM	457
Petito, Frank (NY)	N	241
Petrone, Sylvia (NJ)	S	802
Petrossian, George (NY)	IC	549
Petrotos, Athanassios (CT)	S	994
Petrylak, Daniel (CT)	Onc	1013
Pettei, Michael (NY)	PGe	570
Peyster, Robert (NY)	NRad	622
Pfaff, H Charles (NY)	DR	161
Pfeffer, Cynthia (NY)	Psyc	347
Pfeifer, Tracy (NY)	PlS	334
Pfister, David (NY)	Onc	221
Philipp, Claire (NJ)	Hem	837
Phillips, Elizabeth (NY)	Onc	673
Phillips, Howard (NY)	Oph	684
Phillips, John (NY)	U	711
Phillips, Malcolm (NY)	Cv	406
Phillips, Robin (NY)	ObG	251
Pianka, George (NY)	HS	664
Picciano, Anne (NJ)	FMed	835
Piccione, Paul (NY)	Ge	452
Piccirilli, Dora (NY)	FMed	657
Pici, Ralph (NY)	PMR	698
Picone, Frank (NJ)	A&I	857
Pidoriano, Arthur (NY)	OrS	686
Pieczara, Beata (NJ)	Onc	742
Piepmeier, Joseph (CT)	NS	1014
Pierce, Sean (NJ)	NRad	746
Pietanza, Maria (NY)	Onc	221
Pilchik, Robert (NY)	Cv	647
Pile-Spellman, John (NY)	NRad	557
Pincus, Emile (NJ)	ChAP	727
Pincus, Robert (NY)	Oto	293
Pines, Jeffrey (NY)	Psyc	347
Pinke, James (CT)	Oph	974
Pinke, Robert (NJ)	Oph	882
Pinney, Sean (NY)	Cv	136
Pinsky, Steven (NY)	PM	566
Pinto, Marguerite (CT)	Path	981
Pipia, Paul (NY)	PMR	476
Piro, Philip (CT)	Oph	974
Pirzada, Melodi (NY)	PPul	572
Pisani, Margaret (CT)	Pul	1027
Piskun, Andrew (NJ)	OrS	844

Name	Specialty	Pg
Pitchumoni, Capecomorin (NJ)	Ge	836
Pitman, Gerald (NY)	PlS	334
Pittaro, Michael (CT)	CE	943
Piwoz, Julia (NJ)	PInf	755
Pizzarello, Louis (NY)	Oph	624
Pizzurro, Joseph (NJ)	OrS	751
Plancher, Kevin (NY)	OrS	281
Plestis, Konstadinos (NY)	T&CS	385
Plumser, Allan (NJ)	Ge	836
Pochapin, Mark (NY)	Ge	176
Podell, Richard (NJ)	FMed	919
Podwal, Mark (NY)	D	154
Pogo, Gustave (NY)	T&CS	588
Polatsch, Daniel (NY)	HS	187
Polifroni, Nicholas (CT)	OrS	977
Polin, Richard (NY)	NP	225
Polis, Laurie (NY)	D	154
Politsky, Jeffrey (NJ)	N	924
Polkow, Melvin (NJ)	Pul	763
Poll, Joan (CT)	ChAP	946
Pollack, Brian (CT)	Cv	945
Pollack, Geoffrey (NY)	Oto	293
Pollack, Jed (NY)	RadRO	633
Pollack, Shoshannah (NJ)	D	894
Pollak, Harvey (NY)	IM	547
Pollak, Jeffrey (CT)	VIR	1033
Pollina, Robert (NY)	VascS	636
Pollock, Alan (NY)	Inf	196
Pollock, Jeffrey (NJ)	N	924
Pollock, Roger (NJ)	OrS	751
Pollowitz, James (NY)	A&I	643
Polsky, Bruce (NY)	Inf	196
Pomerantz, Daniel (NY)	IM	669
Pomeroy, John (NY)	ChAP	610
Pomp, Alfons (NY)	S	378
Ponamgi, Suri (NJ)	PlS	760
Pond, William (NJ)	IM	878
Poneros, John (NY)	Ge	177
Ponterio, Jane (NY)	ObG	515
Pontoriero, Michael (NJ)	T&CS	900
Poole, John (NJ)	S	766
Poon, Eric (NY)	Ped	322
Poon, Michael (NY)	Cv	136
Poplausky, Maurice (NY)	DR	655
Popp, Beth (NY)	H & PM	455
Poppas, Dix (NY)	Ped Uro	318
Popper, Laura (NY)	Ped	323
Porder, Joseph (NY)	IM	205
Poretsky, Leonid (NY)	EDM	166
Porges, Andrew (NY)	Rhu	585
Port, Abraham (NY)	DR	537
Port, Elisa (NY)	S	378
Port, Jeffrey (NY)	T&CS	385
Portenoy, Russell (NY)	H & PM	193
Portlock, Carol (NY)	Onc	221
Portnay, Edward (CT)	IC	961
Portnoy, William (NY)	Oto	294
Porto, Anthony (CT)	PGe	1022
Porwancher, Richard (NJ)	Inf	819
Posada, Roberto (NY)	PInf	313
Posner, David (NY)	Pul	356
Posner, Jerome (NY)	N	241
Posner, Marshall (NY)	Onc	221
Possick, Paul (NJ)	D	729
Post, Kalmon (NY)	NS	232
Post, Martin (NY)	Cv	136
Postley, John (NY)	IM	205
Potenza, Marc (CT)	AdP	1001
Pothuri, Bhavana (NY)	GO	184
Potter, Hollis (NY)	DR	161
Potter, William (CT)	Oph	974
Potters, Louis (NY)	RadRO	583
Powell, Charles (NY)	Pul	356
Powell, Jeffrey (NY)	EDM	656
Poynor, Elizabeth (NY)	GO	184
Prabhu, H Sudhakar (NY)	Cv	446
Prager, Kenneth (NY)	Pul	356
Prakash, Anaka (NJ)	Ge	808
Preis, Oded (NY)	Ped	475
Preminger, Mark (NJ)	CE	724
Prenner, Jonathan (NJ)	Oph	844
Press, Robert (NY)	Inf	196
Presti, Salvatore (NY)	PCd	305
Pretto, Zorayda (NY)	EDM	656
Preven, David (NY)	Psyc	347
Prezant, David (NY)	Pul	433
Prezioso, Paula (NY)	Ped	323
Price, Andrew (NY)	OrS	281
Price, Gary (CT)	PlS	1027
Price, Thomas (NY)	Cv	647

Alphabetical Listing of Doctors

Name	Specialty	Pg
Primas, Ronald (NY)	IM	205
Prince, Alice (NY)	PInf	313
Prince, Andrew (NY)	Oph	264
Prince, Martin (NY)	DR	161
Principe, David (NJ)	MF	741
Prine, Linda (NY)	FMed	167
Prioleau, Philip (NY)	D	154
Procaccino, John (NY)	CRS	535
Proctor, Deborah (CT)	Ge	1006
Proskin, Wendy (NY)	Ped	697
Provenzano, Anthony (NY)	Onc	673
Provet, John (NY)	U	392
Pruzan-Clain, Debra (CT)	D	948
Pruzansky, Mark (NY)	HS	187
Pryor, Aurora (NY)	S	635
Prystowsky, Janet (NY)	D	154
Prywes, Arnold (NY)	Oph	561
Przybylski, Gregory (NJ)	NS	841
Puccio, Carmelo (NY)	Onc	673
Pucillo, Anthony (NY)	Cv	647
Puder, Douglas (NY)	Ped	601
Puglisi, Jeffrey (CT)	IM	960
Pujol-Morato, Fernando (NY)	Inf	455
Pumill, Rick (NJ)	Cv	726
Purtill, William (NY)	VascS	592
Pusztai, Lajos (CT)	Onc	1013
Putman, Donald (NJ)	PCd	794
Putterman, Eric (NY)	SM	634
Pyo, Daniel (NJ)	PIS	887

Q

Name	Specialty	Pg
Qadir, Shuja (NY)	Cv	446
Quaegebeur, Jan (NY)	PS	317
Quagliarello, John (NY)	RE	363
Quagliarello, Vincent (CT)	Inf	1009
Quartell, Anthony (NJ)	ObG	789
Queler, Seth (NJ)	OrS	791
Quest, Donald (NY)	NS	232
Quinn, Joseph (NY)	Ped	630
Quinn, Leslie (NY)	Ped	630
Quittell, Lynne (NY)	PPul	315
Qureshi, Sheeraz (NY)	OrS	281

R

Name	Specialty	Pg
Raab, Edward (NY)	Oph	264
Rabin, Aaron (NJ)	N	746
Rabinowicz, Morris (NY)	Ped	575
Rabinowitz, Arnold (NJ)	Ped	759
Rabinowitz, Ilene (NY)	ChAP	649
Rabinowitz, Simon (NY)	PGe	471
Rabinowitz, Stephen (CT)	Oph	974
Raboy, Adley (NY)	U	520
Rackoff, Paula (NY)	Rhu	368
Raden, Mark (NY)	NRad	515
Radhakrishnan, Jai (NY)	Nep	227
Radin, Alan (CT)	IM	960
Radwaner, Bradley (NY)	Cv	136
Raffalli, John (NY)	Inf	665
Rafizadeh, Farhad (NJ)	PIS	887
Ragnarsson, Kristjan (NY)	PMR	327
Ragno, Philip (NY)	Cv	532
Rago, Thomas (CT)	HS	955
Ragone, Philip (NY)	N	556
Ragukonis, Thomas (NJ)	PM	753
Rahaman, Jamal (NY)	GO	185
Rahmin, Michael (NJ)	Ge	735
Rai, Kanti (NY)	Hem	545
Raia, Carolyn (NY)	DR	511
Rajdeo, Heena (NY)	S	708
Rajpal, Sanjeev (NY)	S	482
Rakos, Gerald (CT)	NP	965
Rakow, Joel (NJ)	DR	731
Rakowski, Thomas (NJ)	Onc	742
Raman, Bharathi (NY)	Ger	181
Ramaswamy, Prema (NY)	PCd	471
Rambler, Louis (NJ)	DR	731
Ramgopal, Mekala (NY)	Ge	494
Ramirez, Mark (NY)	Onc	418
Ramsay, David (NY)	D	154
Ranawat, Amar (NY)	OrS	281
Rand, James (NY)	Ge	494
Randazzo, Jean (NJ)	IM	878
Randolph, Audrey (NY)	PMR	698
Randolph, Christopher (CT)	PA&I	1021
Rangraj, Madhu (NY)	S	708
Raniolo, Robert (NY)	S	709
Ransom, Mark (NJ)	RE	899

Name	Specialty	Pg
Ranta, Jeffrey (CT)	U	995
Rao, Yalamanchi (NY)	A&I	443
Rao, Yalamanchili (NY)	A&I	509
Raoof, Suhail (NY)	Pul	478
Rapaport, Jeffrey (NJ)	D	729
Rapaport, Robert (NY)	PEn	307
Raphael, Bruce (NY)	Hem	191
Rapoport, Samuel (NY)	N	241
Raptis, George (NY)	Onc	551
Rashba, Eric (NY)	CE	607
Rashbaum, Ira (NY)	PMR	327
Raska, Karel (NJ)	Cv	874
Raskin, Elsa (CT)	PlS	986
Raskin, Jonathan (NY)	Pul	356
Raskin, Keith (NY)	HS	187
Rathauser, Robert (NJ)	ObG	843
Ratner, Desiree (NY)	D	154
Ratner, Lloyd (NY)	S	378
Ratner, Lynn (NY)	Onc	221
Raucher, Harold (NY)	Ped	323
Ravitz, Alan (NY)	ChAP	142
Rawlins, Bernard (NY)	OrS	282
Ray, Audell (NY)	Oph	684
Rayfield, Elliot (NY)	EDM	166
Raymond, Gerald (NJ)	Ped	825
Raza, Azra (NY)	Onc	221
Razaboni, Rosa (NY)	PlS	334
Rebarber, Andrei (NY)	MF	211
Recht, Michael (NY)	DR	162
Rechter, Lesley (NY)	FMed	540
Reckler, Jon (NY)	U	392
Reda, Dominick (NY)	Nep	676
Reda, Edward (NY)	Ped Uro	695
Reddy, Mallikarjuna (NY)	FMed	493
Reddy, Vivek (NY)	CE	129
Reding, Michael (NY)	N	678
Redlich, Carrie (CT)	Pul	1028
Redner, Arlene (NY)	PHO	570
Rednor, Jeffrey (NJ)	FMed	818
Rees, Ellen (NY)	Psyc	347
Regard, Monique (NY)	ObG	681
Reich, Raymond (NY)	Oph	467
Reich, Steven (NJ)	OrS	845
Reicher, Oscar (NJ)	OrS	897
Reichstein, Robert (NY)	Cv	136

Name	Specialty	Pg
Reid, Malcolm (NY)	PMR	327
Reiffel, Robert (NY)	PlS	699
Reilly, James (NY)	ObG	515
Reilly, John (NY)	OrS	516
Reiner, Dan (NY)	S	587
Reiner, Mark (NY)	S	378
Reinitz, Elizabeth (NY)	Rhu	706
Reisberg, Barry (NY)	GerPsy	182
Reisner, Michelle (NJ)	Ger	808
Reison, Dennis (NJ)	Cv	726
Reizis, Igal (NY)	ObG	465
Rekate, Harold (NY)	NS	554
Relkin, Norman (NY)	N	241
Relland, Maureen (NY)	Oph	264
Remy, Prospere (NY)	Ge	412
Rennert, Nancy (CT)	EDM	950
Rentrop, K. Peter (NY)	Cv	136
Repice, Michael (NY)	Rhu	634
Reppucci, Vincent (CT)	Oph	974
Resmovits, Marvin (NY)	Ped	575
Resor, Louise (CT)	N	968
Respler, Don (NJ)	PO	756
Resta, Christine (NY)	EDM	450
Restifo, Richard (CT)	PlS	1027
Rettig, Michael (NY)	HS	187
Reuter, Victor (NY)	Path	302
Rezac, Craig (NJ)	CRS	833
Reznik, Alan (CT)	OrS	1019
Rezvani, Fred (NJ)	ObG	748
Rho, Dae (NY)	PMR	327
Ribakove, Greg (NY)	T&CS	483
Riccio, Gioia (CT)	DR	949
Rice, Stephen (NJ)	SM	868
Rich, Daniel (NY)	OrS	563
Rich, Glenn (CT)	EDM	950
Richards, Steven (NJ)	U	853
Richardson, William (NJ)	Psyc	929
Richel, Peter (NY)	Ped	697
Richheimer, Michael (NY)	A&I	607
Richlin, Spencer (CT)	RE	991
Richman, Daniel (NY)	PM	299
Richstone, Lee (NY)	U	591
Richter, Edwin (CT)	PMR	985
Ricketti, Anthony (NJ)	A&I	817
Ridge, Gerald (NY)	IM	669

Alphabetical Listing of Doctors

Name	Specialty	Pg
Rie, Jonathan (NY)	Nep	676
Rieber, Jonathan (NY)	Ge	177
Riechers, Roger (NY)	U	711
Rieder, Jessica (NY)	AM	403
Rieger, Kenneth (NJ)	OrS	882
Rieger, Mark (NJ)	OrS	883
Rifkin, Matthew (NY)	DR	537
Rigel, Darrell (NY)	D	155
Rigolosi, Robert (NJ)	Nep	744
Rigtrup, Edward (NJ)	Ped	797
Riina, Howard (NY)	NS	232
Riley, David (NJ)	Pul	851
Rimm, David (CT)	Path	1021
Ring, Kenneth (NJ)	U	932
Ritch, Robert (NY)	Oph	265
Ritterband, David (NY)	Oph	265
Rivadeneira, David (NY)	CRS	610
Rivera, Jeanette (CT)	ObG	971
Rivera, Yadyra (NJ)	Onc	742
Riviello, James (NY)	ChiN	144
Rizk, Nabil (NY)	T&CS	385
Rizk, Samieh (NY)	Oto	294
Rizvi, Hasan (NY)	Onc	620
Rizvi, Naiyer (NY)	Onc	221
Robbins, Kim (CT)	Oph	974
Robbins, Michael (NY)	Cv	490
Robbins, Michael (CT)	PM	1020
Robbins, Noah (NY)	Inf	415
Robert, Marie (CT)	Ped	1025
Roberti, M. Isabel (NJ)	PNep	795
Roberts, J Kirk (NY)	N	241
Roberts, Kenneth (CT)	RadRO	1029
Roberts, Larry (NY)	U	711
Roberts, Matthew (NY)	OrS	282
Robilotti, James (NY)	Ge	177
Robinson, Michael (NY)	PMR	601
Robinson, Newell (NY)	T&CS	589
Roboz, Gail (NY)	Onc	222
Robson, Mark (NY)	Onc	222
Roca, Dominic (CT)	Pul	989
Rochelson, Burton (NY)	MF	549
Rochester, Carolyn (CT)	Pul	1028
Rochford, Joseph (NJ)	Psyc	910
Rockman, Caron (NY)	VascS	400
Rodeo, Scott (NY)	SM	371
Rodgers, I Rand (NY)	Oph	265
Rodino, William (NY)	VascS	521
Rodke, Gae (NY)	ObG	251
Rodriguez, Jose (NY)	OrS	282
Rodriguez, Lorna (NJ)	GO	836
Rodriguez-Sains, Rene (NY)	Oph	265
Roelke, Marc (NJ)	CE	777
Rogal, Gary (NJ)	Cv	777
Rogers, David (NY)	VIR	506
Rohr, Michele (CT)	ObG	971
Rokhsar, Cameron (NY)	D	155
Rokito, Andrew (NY)	SM	371
Roland, J Thomas (NY)	Oto	294
Roland, Robert (NJ)	Inf	921
Rolandelli, Rolando (NJ)	S	889
Romagnoli, Mario (NY)	Inf	196
Roman, Ashley (NY)	MF	211
Romanelli, John (NY)	Oph	624
Romanello, Paul (NY)	Cv	136
Romano, Alicia (NY)	PEn	691
Romano, Angela (NY)	PCd	568
Romano, John (NY)	D	155
Romano, Rosario (NY)	IM	618
Romas, Nicholas (NY)	U	392
Romero, Carlos (NY)	S	587
Romeu, Jose (NY)	Ge	177
Romita, Mauro (NY)	PlS	334
Rommer, James (NJ)	IM	785
Romo, Thomas (NY)	Oto	294
Roose, Steven (NY)	Psyc	347
Root, Barry (NY)	PMR	575
Rosa, Joseph (CT)	EDM	950
Rosa, Richard (NJ)	OrS	791
Rosch, Elliott (NY)	IM	670
Rose, Donald (NY)	OrS	282
Rose, Elliott (NY)	PlS	334
Rose, Howard (NY)	OrS	282
Rose, John (NJ)	U	869
Rose, Michael (NJ)	PlS	867
Rose, Roberta (CT)	Rhu	992
Rosell, Frank (NY)	T&CS	520
Rosello, Lori (NY)	Ped	323
Roseman, Bruce (NY)	ChiN	650
Rosemarin, Jack (NY)	Ge	661
Rosen, Allen (NJ)	PlS	798

Name	Specialty	Pg
Rosen, Arie (NJ)	Oto	752
Rosen, Arnold (NY)	Psyc	348
Rosen, Bruce (NY)	Psyc	632
Rosen, Douglas (NY)	D	407
Rosen, Evelyn (NY)	GerPsy	454
Rosen, Jeffrey (NY)	SM	504
Rosen, Michael (NY)	Nep	676
Rosen, Nedra (NY)	IM	205
Rosen, Norman (NY)	Onc	674
Rosen, Robert (NY)	VIR	395
Rosen, Tove (NY)	NP	226
Rosenbaum, Alfred (NY)	RadRO	360
Rosenbaum, Daniel (NY)	N	463
Rosenbaum, Jeffrey (NJ)	Oto	845
Rosenbaum, Marlon (NY)	Cv	137
Rosenbaum, Michael (NY)	Ped	323
Rosenbaum, Pearl (NY)	Oph	422
Rosenbaum, Robert (NJ)	EDM	919
Rosenberg, Craig (NY)	PMR	630
Rosenberg, David (NY)	Oto	294
Rosenberg, Gene (NJ)	U	769
Rosenberg, Howard (NY)	Inf	197
Rosenberg, Kenneth (NY)	AdP	123
Rosenberg, Michael (NY)	PlS	699
Rosenberg, Michael (NJ)	N	842
Rosenberg, Vladimiro (NY)	S	379
Rosenberg, Zehava (NY)	DR	162
Rosenblatt, Joshua (NJ)	Ped	797
Rosenblatt, Ruth (NY)	DR	162
Rosenblatt, William (NY)	PlS	334
Rosenblum, Bruce (NJ)	NS	862
Rosenblum, David (CT)	PMR	1026
Rosenblum, Marc (NY)	Path	302
Rosenfeld, Alvin (CT)	ChAP	946
Rosenfeld, David (NJ)	Psyc	761
Rosenfeld, David (NJ)	DR	834
Rosenfeld, Richard (NY)	PO	473
Rosenfeld, Stanley (NY)	DR	162
Rosenfeld, Suzanne (NY)	Ped	323
Rosenfeld, Walter (NJ)	AM	873
Rosenkilde, Carl (NY)	N	678
Rosenn, Barak (NY)	MF	211
Rosenstein, Elliot (NJ)	Rhu	931
Rosenstein, Roger (NJ)	HS	737
Rosenstock, Arthur (CT)	PlS	986
Rosenstreich, David (NY)	A&I	403
Rosenthal, David (NY)	EDM	539
Rosenthal, Jeanne (NY)	Oph	265
Rosenthal, Jesse (NY)	Psyc	348
Rosenthal, Kenneth (NY)	Oph	561
Rosenthal, Richard (NY)	Psyc	348
Rosenthal, Sheldon (NY)	U	483
Rosenwaks, Zev (NY)	RE	363
Rosenwasser, Melvin (NY)	HS	187
Roses, Daniel (NY)	S	379
Rosewater, Karen (NY)	AM	125
Rosh, Joel (NJ)	PGe	884
Rosman, Lawrence (NY)	EDM	492
Rosner, Bruce (NJ)	Ge	819
Rosner, Louis (NY)	Oto	565
Rosner, Richard (NY)	Psyc	348
Rosner, Saran (NY)	NS	677
Ross, Douglas (CT)	Oto	980
Ross, Marc (NY)	PMR	476
Ross, Steven (NY)	Psyc	348
Rossakis, Constantine (NJ)	Cv	726
Rossi, Dennis (NY)	DR	537
Rossman, Barry (NJ)	U	827
Rossos, Apostolos (NJ)	Oto	864
Roston, Alfred (NY)	Ge	662
Roth, Alan (NY)	FMed	493
Roth, Andrew (NY)	Psyc	348
Roth, Douglas (NY)	PlS	699
Roth, Jeffrey (NY)	D	155
Roth, Joseph (NJ)	Ge	735
Roth, Neil (NY)	SM	372
Roth, Patrick (NJ)	NS	745
Roth, Philip (NY)	NP	514
Roth, Richard (NY)	Cv	595
Rothberg, Charles (NY)	Oph	624
Rothberg, Robert (NJ)	CRS	779
Rothman, Howard (NJ)	Cv	726
Rothman, Jeffrey (NY)	EDM	511
Rothschild, Michael (NY)	PO	314
Rothschild, Rachel (CT)	Ped	984
Rothstein, Stephen (NY)	Oto	294
Rotman, Marvin (NY)	RadRO	480
Rotolo, James (NJ)	U	869
Roubin, Gary (NY)	IC	209
Rowley, Scott (NJ)	Hem	737

Name	Specialty	Pg
Roychowdhury, Sudipta (NJ)	NRad	842
Roye, David (NY)	OrS	282
Rozanski, Alan (NY)	Cv	137
Rozanski, Reuben (NJ)	D	779
Rozbruch, Jacob (NY)	OrS	282
Rozbruch, S Robert (NY)	OrS	283
Rozenblit, Alla (NY)	DR	408
Rozenblit, Grigory (NY)	VIR	712
Rubenstein, Andrew (NJ)	ObG	748
Rubenstein, Jack (NY)	IM	548
Rubin, Cheryl (NY)	OrS	600
Rubin, David (NY)	CE	643
Rubin, Kenneth (NJ)	Psyc	867
Rubin, Kenneth (NJ)	Ge	735
Rubin, Laurence (NY)	Oph	561
Rubin, Lorry (NY)	PInf	571
Rubin, Marc (NJ)	Ge	819
Rubin, Moshe (NY)	Ge	177
Rubin, Steven (NY)	Oph	561
Rubinoff, Mitchell (NJ)	Ge	735
Rubinstein, Arye (NY)	A&I	404
Rubinstein, Boris (NY)	ChAP	649
Rubinstein, Morton (NY)	Psyc	348
Rucker, Steve (NY)	IM	548
Ruddy, Michael (NJ)	Nep	821
Ruderman, Marvin (NJ)	N	788
Rudick, Albert (NY)	Oph	265
Rudikoff, Donald (NY)	D	407
Rudin, Eric (NY)	EDM	657
Rudman, Michael (NJ)	PM	883
Rudolph, Daniel (CT)	Pul	989
Rudolph, Steven (NY)	N	463
Rudy, Bret (NY)	AM	125
Ruggiero, Joseph (NY)	Onc	222
Ruiz, Carlos (NY)	Cv	137
Rundback, John (NJ)	VIR	770
Ruoff, Michael (NY)	Ge	177
Rusch, Valerie (NY)	T&CS	386
Rush, Thomas (NY)	Inf	665
Rusk, Alice (CT)	N	968
Russakoff, L. Mark (NY)	Psyc	702
Russell, Linda (NY)	Rhu	368
Russell, Robin (NY)	Ger	413
Russell, Shereen (NY)	ObG	251
Russo, John (NJ)	IM	785
Russo, Paul (NY)	U	392
Rutenberg, Kathryn (NY)	ObG	251
Rutherford, Thomas (CT)	GO	1007
Rutkovsky, Edward (NY)	Cv	532
Rutkovsky, Lisa (NY)	PCd	501
Ruzal-Shapiro, Carrie (NY)	DR	162
Ryan, Sheryl (CT)	AM	1001
Ryback, Hyman (NY)	Oto	688
Rydzinski, Mayer (NY)	Cv	490

S

Name	Specialty	Pg
Saada, Simon (NY)	U	483
Saal, Stuart (NY)	Nep	228
Sabatino, Dominick (NY)	PHO	570
Sabbath, Kert (CT)	Hem	1008
Sabbatini, Paul (NY)	Onc	222
Saberski, Lloyd (CT)	PM	1020
Sabetta, James (CT)	Inf	957
Sabharwal, Sanjeev (NJ)	OrS	792
Sable, Robert (NY)	Ge	412
Sabnani, Indu (NJ)	Hem	783
Saboeiro, Gregory (NY)	VIR	395
Sabry, M. Zakir (NY)	PIS	334
Sacco, Margaret (NJ)	S	932
Sachar, David (NY)	Ge	177
Sachs, Paul (CT)	Pul	989
Sachs, R. Gregory (NJ)	Cv	917
Sachs, Ronald (NJ)	Oph	882
Sachs, Stephen (NJ)	N	924
Sacker, Ira (NY)	Ped	323
Sacks, Michael (NY)	Psyc	348
Sacks, Steven (NY)	Oto	294
Sacks-Berg, Anne (NY)	Inf	617
Sadan, Sara (NY)	Onc	674
Sadanandan, Swayam (NY)	PHO	472
Sadarangani, Balvinder (NY)	ObG	252
Sadeghi, Hooshang (NJ)	N	809
Sadeghi, Hossein (CT)	PPul	982
Sadeghi-Nejad, Hossein (NJ)	U	769
Sadiq, Saud (NY)	N	241
Sadock, Virginia (NY)	Psyc	348
Sadovsky, Richard (NY)	FMed	451
Saenger, Paul (NY)	PEn	691

Name	Specialty	Pg
Safai, Bijan (NY)	D	155
Safdieh, Joseph (NY)	N	242
Saffra, Norman (NY)	Oph	467
Safirstein, Benjamin (NJ)	Pul	799
Safran, Steven (NJ)	Oph	823
Sage, Jacob (NJ)	N	842
Sagorin, Charles (NJ)	Onc	786
Sagy, Mayer (NY)	PCCM	306
Saha, Prantik (NY)	Ped	323
Sahar, David (NY)	Cv	406
Saidi, James (NJ)	U	803
Saiman, Lisa (NY)	PInf	313
Saland, Jeffrey (NY)	PNep	313
Salas, Max (NJ)	PEn	847
Salazer, Thomas (NJ)	Nep	744
Saleh, Anthony (NY)	Pul	479
Salem, Noel (NJ)	Rhu	765
Salem, Ronald (CT)	S	1031
Salerno, William (NJ)	Cv	726
Sales, Clifford (NJ)	VascS	933
Salgado, Miran (NY)	N	464
Salifu, Moro (NY)	Nep	461
Salik, Erez (CT)	DR	949
Salik, James (NY)	Ge	177
Salimi, Mostafa (NJ)	Cv	893
Salky, Barry (NY)	S	379
Salmon, Jane (NY)	Rhu	368
Salsitz, Edwin (NY)	IM	205
Saltz, Leonard (NY)	Onc	222
Saltzman, Daniel (NY)	MF	211
Saltzman, Martin (NY)	Nep	676
Saltzman-Gabelman, Lori (NY)	IM	670
Salvati, Eduardo (NY)	OrS	283
Salwitz, James (NJ)	Onc	907
Salz, Alan (NJ)	Oph	908
Salzer, Richard (NJ)	OrS	751
Salzer, Stephen (CT)	Oto	980
Salzman, Jacqueline (NY)	Oph	684
Salzman, Ronnie (NY)	ObG	558
Sama, Andrew (NY)	OrS	283
Samach, Michael (NJ)	Ge	876
Samadi, David (NY)	U	392
Samadi, Sharyar (NJ)	PO	756
Samberg, Eslee (NY)	Psyc	349
Sami, Sherif (NY)	Psyc	580
Sampson, Hugh (NY)	PA&I	303
Sampson, Steven (NY)	OrS	626
Samra, Said (NJ)	PlS	867
Samson, C Michael (NY)	Oph	265
Samsonov, Dmitry (NY)	PNep	692
Samuels, Jonathan (NY)	Rhu	368
Samuels, Steven (NY)	Inf	617
Samuels, Steven (NJ)	Psyc	761
Samuelson, Robert (CT)	ObG	971
San Roman, Gerardo (NY)	ObG	623
Sanacora, Gerard (CT)	Psyc	1027
Sanchez, Miguel (NJ)	Path	753
Sanchez-Catanese, Betty (NJ)	IM	906
Sander, Howard (NY)	N	242
Sander, Norbert (NY)	IM	416
Sanders, Abraham (NY)	Pul	357
Sanders, Leslie (NJ)	AM	916
Sanders, Linda (NJ)	DR	780
Sanderson, Rhonda (NJ)	ObG	908
Sanderson, Scott (CT)	NS	967
Sandhaus, Jeffrey (NY)	U	505
Sandhu, Fatejeet (CT)	VIR	996
Sandhu, Harvinder (NY)	OrS	283
Sandler, Benjamin (NY)	ObG	252
Sandoval, Claudio (NY)	PHO	692
Sands, Andrew (NY)	OrS	283
Sanelli, Pina (NY)	NRad	245
Sanford, Marie (NY)	Ped	323
Sanger, Joseph (NY)	NuM	246
Sanghavi, Seema (CT)	RadRO	990
Santamaria, Jaime (NJ)	Oph	844
Santarosa, Richard (CT)	U	995
Santilli, John (CT)	A&I	942
Santin, Alessandro (CT)	GO	1007
Santos, Elmer (NY)	NuM	246
Saponara, Eduardo (NY)	Onc	674
Sara, Gabriel (NY)	Onc	222
Saraiya, Narendra (NJ)	Ped	928
Sarnelle, James (CT)	S	994
Sarnoff, Deborah (NY)	D	536
Saroff, Alan (NJ)	Cv	777
Sarokhan, Alan (NJ)	OrS	926
Sas, Norman (NY)	S	436
Sasaki, Clarence (CT)	Oto	1020
Sasso, Louis (NY)	Pul	519

Alphabetical Listing of Doctors

Name	Specialty	Pg
Schob, Clifford (NJ)	OrS	792
Schoen, Robert (CT)	Rhu	1030
Schoeneman, Morris (NY)	PNep	473
Schoenfeld, Mark (CT)	CE	1002
Schonfeld, Steven (NJ)	NRad	842
Schor, Joshua (NJ)	Ger	782
Schottenstein, Douglas (NY)	PM	299
Schrager, Alan (NY)	U	712
Schreiber, Carl (NY)	Cv	532
Schreiber, Klaus (NY)	ChAP	649
Schreiber, Michael (NY)	Pul	704
Schrier, Amilia (NY)	Oph	266
Schroeder, Karl (NY)	Psyc	601
Schubach, Scott (NY)	T&CS	589
Schubert, Hermann (NY)	Oph	266
Schubert, Romaine (NY)	ChiN	447
Schulam, Peter (CT)	U	1033
Schulder, Michael (NY)	NS	554
Schulhafer, Edwin (NJ)	A&I	903
Schulman, Ira (NY)	Cv	137
Schulman, Matthew (NY)	PlS	335
Schulman, Norman (NY)	PlS	335
Schulster, Rita (NY)	Pul	581
Schultz, Barbara (NY)	Pul	357
Schultz, Neal (NY)	D	155
Schulze, Ruth (NJ)	ObG	748
Schuss, Steven (NJ)	Ped	759
Schuster, Edward (CT)	Cv	945
Schuster, Joseph (NJ)	IM	739
Schuster, Michael (NY)	Hem	617
Schwab, Frank (NY)	OrS	283
Schwarcz, Robert (NY)	Oph	266
Schwartz, Allan (NY)	Cv	137
Schwartz, Amit (NY)	NS	462
Schwartz, Bruce (NY)	Psyc	432
Schwartz, Charles (NY)	Cv	509
Schwartz, David (NY)	RadRO	519
Schwartz, Evan (NY)	OrS	500
Schwartz, Gary (NY)	Ge	542
Schwartz, Jeffrey (NY)	OrS	284
Schwartz, Joel (NY)	NRad	599
Schwartz, Joseph (NJ)	EDM	732
Schwartz, Judith (NY)	ObG	252
Schwartz, Lawrence (NY)	DR	162
Schwartz, Louis (NJ)	RadRO	930
Schwartz, Michael (NY)	Psyc	632
Schwartz, Myron (NY)	S	379
Schwartz, Paula (NY)	Onc	551
Schwartz, Peter (CT)	GO	1007
Schwartz, Robert (NJ)	D	779
Schwartz, Theodore (NY)	NS	233
Schwartz, William (NY)	Cv	137
Schwartzberg, Mori (NJ)	Rhu	867
Schwartzfarb, Lanny (NY)	Rhu	369
Schwartzman, Alexander (NY)	S	482
Schwartzman, Sergio (NY)	Rhu	369
Schwarz, Steven (NY)	PGe	471
Schweiger, Eric (NY)	D	155
Schweitzer, Mark (NY)	DR	613
Schweitzer, Philip (NY)	Ge	412
Schweizer, William (NY)	ObG	252
Schwinn, Hans (NY)	FMed	615
Scibetta, Maria (NJ)	IM	739
Scigliano, Eileen (NY)	Hem	191
Scimeca, Michael (NY)	AdP	124
Sciortino, Patrick (NY)	Oph	467
Sclafani, Anthony (NY)	Oto	295
Sclafani, Lisa (NY)	S	635
Sclafani, Michael (NJ)	SM	868
Sclafani, Salvatore (NY)	VIR	484
Scofield, Lisa (NJ)	Ped	898
Scoppetuolo, Michael (NJ)	Onc	787
Scott, David (NY)	Nep	499
Scott, John (NY)	Oto	688
Scott, Richard (NJ)	RE	911
Scott, Susan (NY)	PlS	335
Scott, W Norman (NY)	OrS	284
Scoutt, Leslie (CT)	DR	1005
Scriven, Richard (NY)	PS	629
Scuderi, Giles (NY)	OrS	284
Sculco, Thomas (NY)	OrS	284
Scully, Brian (NY)	Inf	197
Seaman, Cheryl (NY)	Psyc	349
Seashore, Margretta (CT)	CG	1004
Seaver, Robert (NY)	ChAP	649
Seebacher, J Robert (NY)	OrS	687
Seedor, John (NY)	Oph	266
Seelagy, Marc (NJ)	Pul	826
Segal-Maurer, Sorana (NY)	Inf	496
Segarra, Pedro (NY)	ObG	623

Name	Specialty	Pg
Seideman, Bruce (NY)	OrS	563
Seidenberg, Roy (NY)	D	155
Seidenstein, Michael (NJ)	OrS	792
Seidman, Barry (NJ)	U	932
Seidman, Mitchell (NY)	Oph	467
Seifer, David (NY)	RE	480
Seigel, Mark (NJ)	ObG	863
Seinfeld, David (NY)	Cv	137
Seinfeld, Fredric (NJ)	T&CS	827
Seiter, Karen (NY)	Onc	674
Selesnick, Samuel (NY)	Oto	295
Seliger, Glenn (NY)	N	599
Selinger, Sharon (NJ)	EDM	919
Selman, Jay (NY)	N	678
Selter, Jared (CT)	IC	961
Seltzer, Terry (NY)	EDM	166
Selwyn, Peter (NY)	IM	416
Selzer, Jeffrey (NY)	Psyc	502
Seminara, Donna (NY)	Ger	512
Sen, Chandranath (NY)	NS	233
Sender, Joel (NY)	Pul	434
Seneviratne, Aruna (NY)	SM	372
Sensakovic, John (NJ)	Inf	837
Sepkowitz, Kent (NY)	Inf	197
Seplowitz, Alan (NY)	EDM	166
Serby, Michael (NY)	GerPsy	182
Sergiou, Harry (NY)	Ped	475
Serle, Janet (NY)	Oph	266
Serur, Eli (NY)	GO	454
Sethi, Paul (CT)	OrS	978
Sett, Suvro (NY)	T&CS	709
Setton, Avi (NY)	NRad	557
Setzen, Michael (NY)	Oto	565
Sgaglione, Nicholas (NY)	OrS	563
Sgouros, Anthony (NY)	Ge	662
Shaari, Christopher (NJ)	Oto	752
Shabsigh, Ridwan (NY)	U	484
Shabto, Uri (NY)	Oph	266
Shack, Robert (NJ)	S	802
Shah, Darsit (NJ)	Oto	864
Shah, Jatin (NY)	S	379
Shah, Paresh (NY)	S	379
Shah, Pritesh (NJ)	Psyc	762
Shah, Smita (NJ)	Pul	800
Shahabi, Shohreh (CT)	GO	954
Shahid, Syed (CT)	NS	967
Shahrivar, Farrokh (NY)	NP	226
Shamamian, Peter (NY)	S	436
Shamoon, Fayez (NJ)	Cv	777
Shamoon, Harry (NY)	EDM	409
Shampain, Lawrence (NJ)	ChAP	832
Shams, Joseph (NY)	VIR	396
Shanahan, Andrew (NJ)	IC	820
Shane, Elizabeth (NY)	EDM	166
Shani, Jacob (NY)	IC	458
Shapir, Yehuda (NY)	PCd	568
Shapira, Iuliana (NY)	Onc	551
Shapiro, Barry (NY)	Oto	688
Shapiro, Bruce (CT)	Psyc	987
Shapiro, Ellen (NY)	Ped Uro	318
Shapiro, Eugene (CT)	PInf	1023
Shapiro, Jeffrey (NY)	OrS	563
Shapiro, Kenneth (NY)	Nep	598
Shapiro, Lawrence (NY)	EDM	539
Shapiro, Marc (NY)	S	635
Shapiro, Mark (NJ)	DR	731
Shapiro, Martin (CT)	Oph	1017
Shapiro, Michael (NJ)	S	802
Shapiro, Michael (NY)	D	449
Shapiro, Neil (NY)	Ge	662
Shapiro, Peter (NY)	Psyc	349
Shapiro, Richard (NY)	S	379
Shapiro, Warren (NY)	Nep	461
Sharaby, Jacob (NY)	U	484
Sharan, Alok (NY)	OrS	423
Sharma, Samin (NY)	IC	209
Sharon, David (NJ)	Onc	861
Sharon, Ezra (NY)	Rhu	503
Sharpe, Arleen (NY)	FMed	658
Shatkin, Jess (NY)	ChAP	142
Shaw, Ronda (NY)	Psyc	349
Shaw-Brachfeld, Jennifer (NJ)	Ped	886
Shayani, Steven (NY)	Cv	532
Shaywitz, Bennett (CT)	ChiN	1003
Shaywitz, Sally (CT)	Ped	1026
Shear, Perry (CT)	NS	967
Shebairo, Raymond (NY)	OrS	563
Sheikh, Shahid (NY)	Cv	647
Shein, Leon (NY)	Nep	461
Sheinart, Kara (NY)	N	242

Alphabetical Listing of Doctors

Name	Specialty	Pg
Silverman, Cary (NJ)	Oph	882
Silverman, David (NY)	IM	206
Silverman, Joel (NY)	Pul	502
Silverman, Lewis (NY)	Onc	223
Silverman, Mark (NY)	D	536
Silverman, Mitchell (NJ)	EDM	919
Silverman, Robert (NJ)	PM	753
Silverman, Rubin (NY)	Cv	406
Silvermann, Ronald (NY)	N	678
Silverstone, Philip (CT)	Oph	1017
Simberkoff, Michael (NY)	Inf	197
Similon, Philippe (NY)	Ped	323
Simmons, Rache (NY)	S	379
Simon, Beth (NY)	ObG	252
Simon, Clifford (NJ)	Pul	763
Simon, Jonathan (NJ)	Rhu	800
Simon, Lloyd (NY)	IM	618
Simon, Scott (CT)	NS	967
Simon, Sheldon (NY)	OrS	284
Simon, Steven (NY)	D	449
Simon, Todd (NY)	IM	458
Simons, Grant (NJ)	CE	724
Simonson, Barry (NY)	OrS	564
Simotas, Alexander (NY)	PMR	328
Simpson, David (NY)	N	242
Simpson, Joe (NY)	ObG	681
Simpson, Lynn (NY)	MF	212
Simpson, Roger (NY)	PlS	578
Singer, Lewis (NY)	PCCM	425
Singer, Mark (NY)	IM	619
Singer, Samuel (NY)	S	380
Singh, Anup (NJ)	PNep	847
Singh, Avtar (NY)	N	679
Singh, Bhuvanesh (NY)	Oto	296
Singh, Dinesh (CT)	U	1033
Singhal, Pravin (NY)	Nep	553
Sink, Ernest (NY)	OrS	284
Sinnreich, Abraham (NY)	Oto	516
Sipzner, Robert (NJ)	Nep	787
Siris, Ethel (NY)	EDM	166
Siskind, Steven (NY)	Cv	490
Sisti, Michael (NY)	NS	233
Sivak, Mark (NY)	N	242
Sivitz, Jennifer (NJ)	PEn	794
Sklar, Charles (NY)	PEn	307
Sklar, Jeffrey (NY)	D	536
Sklarek, Howard (NY)	Pul	632
Sklarin, Nancy (NY)	Onc	223
Sklaroff, Herschel (NY)	Cv	138
Sklower, Jay (NJ)	FMed	808
Sklower Brooks, Susan (NJ)	CG	833
Skolnick, Lawrence (NJ)	NP	879
Skolnik, Richard (NY)	PlS	335
Skopicki, Hal (NY)	Cv	609
Skripkus, Aldona (NJ)	Ped	811
Skrokov, Robert (NY)	D	612
Skudlarska, Beata (CT)	Ger	954
Skupski, Daniel (NY)	MF	497
Slakter, Jason (NY)	Oph	267
Slama, Robert (NJ)	Cv	917
Slamovits, Thomas (NY)	Oph	422
Slankard, Marjorie (NY)	A&I	127
Slater, Gary (NY)	S	380
Slater, James (NY)	IC	209
Slater, Jonathan (NY)	ChAP	650
Slater, William (NY)	Cv	138
Slavin, Kevin (NJ)	PInf	755
Slavit, David (NY)	Oto	296
Slim, Jihad (NJ)	Inf	784
Sloane, Lori (NY)	Rhu	706
Slogoff, Frederick (CT)	IM	960
Slovin, Susan (NY)	Onc	223
Slupchynskyj, Oleh (NY)	Oto	296
Small, Eric (NY)	SM	707
Small, Robert (NY)	OrS	687
Small, Steven (NY)	OrS	687
Smallberg, Gerald (NY)	N	242
Smilen, Scott (NY)	ObG	252
Smiles, Stephen (NY)	Rhu	369
Smith, Brian (CT)	OrS	1019
Smith, Craig (NY)	T&CS	386
Smith, Edward (NY)	Oph	468
Smith, Harriet (NY)	GO	414
Smith, Joann (CT)	Psyc	987
Smith, Julia (NY)	Onc	223
Smith, Lee (NY)	PO	571
Smith, Leon (NJ)	MF	786
Smith, Leon (NJ)	Inf	784
Smith, Mark (NY)	PlS	335
Smith, Paul (NY)	Inf	197

Name	Specialty	Pg
Smith, Peter (NY)	Pul	479
Smith, Peter (NJ)	VIR	813
Smith, Richard (NY)	Oto	424
Smith, Robin (NY)	ChiN	534
Smith, Sharon (NY)	IM	206
Smith, Stephen (NJ)	Inf	784
Smithy, William (NY)	CRS	611
Smotkin, David (NY)	GO	414
Smotrich, Gary (NJ)	PlS	826
Snepar, Richard (NJ)	Inf	837
Snow, Robert (NY)	NS	233
Snowball, Halina (CT)	PMR	985
Snyder, Barbara (NJ)	AM	831
Snyder, David (NY)	N	243
Snyder, Gary (NY)	Oto	501
Snyder, Michael (CT)	PCd	981
Snyder, Stephen (NY)	Psyc	350
Soave, Rosemary (NY)	Inf	197
Sobel, Howard (NY)	D	156
Sobol, Norman (NY)	N	464
Sockolow, Robbyn (NY)	PGe	309
Sofair, Jane (CT)	Psyc	987
Sofer, Alfred (CT)	PlS	986
Soff, Gerald (NY)	Hem	191
Soffen, Edward (NJ)	RadRO	852
Soffer, Jeffrey (NJ)	ObG	925
Sofocleous, Constantinos (NY)	VIR	396
Softness, Barney (NY)	Ped	324
Sogani, Pramod (NY)	U	393
Sohn, Won (NY)	Ge	453
Soifer, Todd (NY)	OrS	469
Sokal, Myron (NY)	NP	460
Sokol, Sergio (NY)	Cv	532
Soletic, Raymond (NY)	Oto	565
Solitar, Bruce (NY)	Rhu	369
Sollinger, Jonathan (CT)	Ped	984
Solny, Meyer (NY)	Ge	178
Solomon, Edward (NJ)	Oph	749
Solomon, Gary (NY)	Rhu	369
Solomon, Gregory (NY)	IM	206
Solomon, Ira (NY)	Oph	684
Solomon, Jennifer (NY)	PMR	328
Solomon, Joel (NY)	Oph	267
Solomon, Michael (NJ)	U	853
Solomon, Robert (NY)	NS	233
Solomon, Robert (NJ)	Ger	920
Solomon, Sherry (NY)	Oph	684
Solomon, Stephen (NY)	VIR	396
Solomon, William (NY)	Onc	459
Soloway, Bruce (NY)	FMed	410
Soloway, Gregory (CT)	Ge	953
Solowiejczyk, David (NJ)	PCd	754
Soltren, Rafael (NY)	IM	670
Som, Peter (NY)	DR	162
Sommer, Robert (NY)	PCd	305
Somogyi, Anthony (NY)	IM	496
Sonett, Joshua (NY)	T&CS	386
Sonnenblick, Emily (NY)	DR	162
Sonoda, Toyooki (NY)	CRS	147
Sonoda, Yukio (NY)	GO	185
Sonpal, Girish (NY)	Rhu	503
Sood, Sunil (NY)	PInf	571
Sorbera, Carmine (NY)	CE	643
Soren, Karen (NY)	AM	125
Soriano, John (NJ)	Ge	876
Soroko, Theresa (NJ)	Inf	784
Sorra, Toomas (NY)	Ge	453
Soskel, Neil (NY)	FMed	540
Soslow, Robert (NY)	Path	302
Sosulski, Richard (NY)	Ped	630
Soter, Nicholas (NY)	D	156
Sotolongo, Anays (NJ)	Pul	851
Sotsky, Gerald (NJ)	Cv	727
Sousa, Rolando (NJ)	ChiN	875
Southern, Darrell (NJ)	A&I	903
Southren, David (NY)	Cv	595
Souweidane, Mark (NY)	NS	233
Spadaro, Louise (NY)	Cv	533
Spaide, Richard (NY)	Oph	267
Spak, James (CT)	OrS	978
Spandorfer, Steven (NY)	RE	364
Spanknebel, Kathryn (NY)	S	709
Spano, Frank (CT)	IM	960
Spanolios, Paris (CT)	IM	1010
Sparano, Joseph (NY)	Onc	418
Sparr, Steven (NY)	N	421
Spector, Jason (NY)	PlS	336
Speiser, Phyllis (NY)	PEn	569
Spencer, Dennis (CT)	NS	1014
Spencer, Elizabeth Kay (NY)	ChAP	142

Alphabetical Listing of Doctors

Name	Specialty	Pg
Spencer, Eric (NY)	OrS	687
Spera, John (CT)	RadRO	990
Sperber, Laurence (NY)	Oph	267
Sperber, Steven (NJ)	Inf	738
Sperling, David (NY)	VIR	396
Sperling, Neil (NY)	Oto	296
Spero, Marc (NY)	IM	206
Speyer, James (NY)	Onc	223
Spicehandler, Debra (NY)	Inf	666
Spiegel, Alan (NY)	Cv	138
Spiegel, Michael (CT)	Rhu	992
Spielberg, Alan (NY)	Ge	616
Spielman, Joel (NJ)	OrS	883
Spielvogel, David (NY)	T&CS	710
Spiera, Harry (NY)	Rhu	369
Spiera, Robert (NY)	Rhu	369
Spigland, Nitsana (NY)	PS	317
Spiler, Ira (NJ)	EDM	835
Spindola-Franco, Hugo (NY)	DR	408
Spinelli, Henry (NY)	PlS	336
Spinnell, Mitchell (NJ)	Ge	735
Spinowitz, Alan (NY)	D	536
Spinowitz, Bruce (NY)	Nep	499
Spira, Robert (NJ)	Ge	782
Spitalewitz, Samuel (NY)	Nep	461
Spitz, Henry (NY)	Psyc	350
Spitzer, Daniel (NY)	NS	599
Spivack, Julie (CT)	Ge	954
Spivak, Jeffrey (NY)	OrS	284
Spivak, William (NY)	PGe	309
Splain, Shepard (NY)	OrS	469
Spriggs, David (NY)	Onc	224
Sprotzer, Samuel (CT)	Oph	1017
Sproviero, Joseph (CT)	A&I	942
Squitieri, Rafael (CT)	T&CS	994
Staats, Peter (NJ)	PM	865
Stabile, John (NJ)	Oph	749
Staeger-Hirsch, Christine (NY)	DR	655
Staffenberg, David (NY)	PlS	336
Stafford, John (NY)	NP	675
Stafford, Perry (NJ)	PS	848
Stahl, Richard (CT)	PlS	1027
Stallone, James (NY)	IM	619
Stam, Lawrence (NY)	Nep	461
Stambuk, Hilda (NY)	NRad	245
Stanford, Paulette (NJ)	AM	776
Stangel, John (NY)	RE	705
Starc, Thomas (NY)	PCd	305
Starke, Charles (NY)	IM	670
Starker, Isaac (NJ)	PlS	887
Starker, Paul (NJ)	S	932
Starkman, Harold (NJ)	PEn	884
Starpoli, Anthony (NY)	Ge	178
Starr, Amy (NY)	PRhu	316
Starr, Christopher (NY)	Oph	267
Starr, Michael (NY)	Oph	267
Staszewski, Harry (NY)	Hem	545
Steckel, Rebecca (NJ)	FMed	905
Steele, Andrew (NY)	NP	552
Steele, Mark (NY)	Oph	267
Steer, Robert (NJ)	ObG	881
Steever, John (NY)	AM	125
Steiger, David (NY)	Pul	357
Steigman, Elliot (NJ)	U	812
Stein, Adam (NY)	PMR	575
Stein, Alan (NY)	Inf	456
Stein, Arnold (NY)	Oph	468
Stein, Barry (NY)	Ped	324
Stein, Daniel (NY)	RE	364
Stein, David (NY)	Ge	413
Stein, Jeffrey (NY)	Ge	179
Stein, Jeffrey (NY)	VascS	400
Stein, Joel (NY)	PMR	328
Stein, Lawrence (NJ)	Ge	876
Stein, Mark (NY)	U	437
Stein, Mitchell (NY)	Oph	684
Stein, Perry (NY)	PMR	476
Stein, Randy (NY)	EDM	657
Stein, Richard (NY)	Cv	138
Stein, Ruth (NY)	Ped	430
Stein, Sidney (NY)	Pul	357
Stein, Stefan (NY)	Psyc	350
Steinbaum, Suzanne (NY)	Cv	139
Steinberg, Charles (NY)	IM	206
Steinberg, Harry (NY)	Pul	582
Steinberg, L Gary (NY)	PCd	305
Steinberger, Alfred (NJ)	NS	745
Steingart, Richard (NY)	Cv	139
Steinhagen, Randolph (NY)	CRS	147
Steinherz, Laurel (NY)	PCd	305

Name	Specialty	Pg
Sweeney, Thomas (CT)	VascS	1034
Swerdlow, Michael (NY)	N	421
Swiderski, Deborah (NY)	IM	416
Swift, Richard (NY)	PlS	336
Swigart, Carrie (CT)	HS	1008
Swiller, Hillel (NY)	Psyc	350
Swistel, Alexander (NY)	S	380
Swistel, Daniel (NY)	T&CS	386
Syed, Tariqshah (NJ)	IC	740
Szabo, Albert (NY)	N	679
Sze, Gordon (CT)	NRad	1016
Szeto, Marjorie (CT)	ObG	971
Sznol, Mario (CT)	Onc	1013

T

Name	Specialty	Pg
Tabachnick, John (NJ)	FMed	919
Tabar, Viviane (NY)	NS	234
Tabbal, Nicolas (NY)	PlS	336
Tabershaw, Richard (NY)	OrS	626
Taffet, Berton (NJ)	OrS	883
Taffet, Sanford (NY)	Ge	662
Tagawa, Scott (NY)	Onc	224
Taikowski, Richard (CT)	Cv	946
Taitsman, James (NJ)	OrS	824
Takoudes, Thomas (CT)	Oto	1020
Tal, Avraham (NY)	IM	458
Talansky, Arthur (NY)	Ge	542
Talansky, Marvin (NJ)	Oph	864
Tallia, Alfred (NJ)	FMed	835
Tallman, Martin (NY)	Hem	191
Talmor, Mia (NY)	PlS	336
Tamborlane, William (CT)	PEn	1022
Tamerin, John (CT)	Psyc	987
Tan, Virak (NJ)	HS	783
Tancredi, Laurence (NY)	Psyc	350
Taneja, Samir (NY)	U	393
Tanenbaum, Diane (NY)	D	156
Tang, David (NY)	IM	670
Tank, Lisa (NJ)	Ger	736
Tanoue, Lynn (CT)	Pul	1028
Tanzer, Floyd (NJ)	D	894
Tap, William (NY)	Onc	224
Tarasuk, Albert (NY)	U	505
Tartaglia, Joseph (NY)	Cv	648
Tartell, Jay (NY)	DR	492
Tartini, Albert (NJ)	Nep	744
Tartter, Paul (NY)	S	380
Tassiopoulos, Apostolos (NY)	VascS	636
Taub, Peter (NY)	PlS	336
Taubin, Howard (CT)	Ge	954
Taubman, Lowell (NY)	IM	548
Tavassoli, Fattaneh (CT)	Path	1021
Tavill, Michael (NJ)	PO	865
Tawfik, Bernard (NY)	Oto	565
Tay, Steven (NY)	IM	206
Taylor, Howard (NJ)	Oto	883
Taylor, Hugh (CT)	RE	1029
Taylor, James (NY)	T&CS	636
Taylor, Noel (NY)	Psyc	351
Taylor, Robert (NJ)	GO	783
Te, Alexis (NY)	U	394
Tedjarati, Sean (NY)	GO	663
Teffera, Fassil (NY)	IM	416
Teichholz, Louis (NJ)	Cv	727
Tello, Celso (NY)	Oph	268
Telzak, Edward (NY)	Inf	415
Tempera, Patrick (NJ)	Ge	920
Temple, Larissa (NY)	CRS	147
Tenenbaum, Joseph (NY)	Cv	139
Tenet, William (NY)	Cv	533
Tennenbaum, Steven (NJ)	Ped Uro	757
Tenner, Michael (NY)	NRad	679
Teodorescu, Victoria (NY)	VascS	400
Teperman, Lewis (NY)	S	380
Tepler, Isidore (CT)	Onc	964
Tepler, Melvin (NY)	OrS	469
Teplitz, Glenn (NY)	HS	544
Tepper, Howard (NJ)	PlS	929
Terjanian, Terenig (NY)	Onc	514
Tessler, Sidney (NY)	Pul	479
Testa, Francine (CT)	ChiN	1003
Teusink, J. Paul (NY)	Psyc	351
Tewari, Ashutosh (NY)	U	394
Theofanidis, Stylianos (CT)	NP	965
Thomas, Byron (CT)	IM	960
Thomas, David (NY)	PMR	328
Thomas, Gary (NY)	PM	300
Thomas, Mark (NY)	PMR	431

Alphabetical Listing of Doctors

Name	Specialty	Pg
Turtel, Penny (NJ)	Ge	859
Tuttle, R Michael (NY)	EDM	167
Tyagi, Renuka (NY)	ObG	253
Tyberg, Theodore (NY)	Cv	139
Tyshkov, Michael (NJ)	PGe	927

U

Name	Specialty	Pg
Uday, Kalpana (NY)	Nep	419
Udell, Ira (NY)	Oph	562
Udelsman, Robert (CT)	S	1031
Ugol, Jay (CT)	ObG	971
Uhm, Kyudong (NJ)	Onc	895
Ullman, Joel (NY)	ObG	681
Ullman, Thomas (NY)	Ge	179
Underberg, James (NY)	IM	207
Underberg-Davis, Sharon (NJ)	DR	834
Unger, Allen (NY)	Cv	139
Unger, Walter (NY)	D	156
Unis, George (NY)	OrS	285
Unterricht, Sam (NY)	Oph	468
Urban, William (NY)	OrS	469
Urken, Mark (NY)	Oto	297
Ushay, H Michael (NY)	PCCM	425
Uy, Vena (NJ)	ObG	810

V

Name	Specialty	Pg
Vad, Vijay (NY)	PMR	328
Vahdat, Linda (NY)	Onc	224
Vaidya, Ami (NJ)	GO	736
Vaidya, Sudhir (NY)	FMed	658
Vaillancourt, Philippe (NY)	PM	626
Valda, Victor (NJ)	PS	757
Valenza, Joseph (NJ)	PMR	886
Valinoti, Anne Marie (NJ)	IM	740
Vallarino, Ramon (NY)	PMR	501
Vallone, Ambrose (NY)	PCd	568
Vambutas, Andrea (NY)	Oto	566
Van Besien, Koen (NY)	Hem	192
van Dyck, Christopher (CT)	GerPsy	1007
Van Engel, Daniel (NJ)	N	746
van Gilder, Max (NY)	Ped	324
Van Slooten, David (NJ)	N	746
Van Zee, Kimberly (NY)	S	380
Vapnek, Jonathan (NY)	U	394
Vargas-Rodriguez, Ileana (NY)	PEn	307
Varlotta, Gerard (NY)	PMR	328
Varriale, Philip (NY)	Cv	139
Varsos, George (NY)	RadRO	503
Vas, George (NY)	N	464
Vasselli, Anthony (NJ)	U	827
Vastola, A Paul (NY)	Oto	470
Vasudeva, Kusum (NY)	ObG	558
Vates, Thomas (NJ)	Ped Uro	849
Vaughan, Margaret (NY)	Ger	663
Vazquez, Marietta (CT)	PInf	1023
Vazzana, Thomas (NY)	Cv	510
Vega, Aida (NY)	IM	207
Veksler-Offengenden, Irena (CT)	A&I	942
Velcek, Francisca (NY)	PS	318
Verga, Michele (NY)	PIS	337
Verma, Rajiv (NJ)	PCd	794
Versfelt, Mary (NY)	Ped	697
Vesole, David (NJ)	Hem	737
Vester, John (NJ)	N	822
Vialotti, Charles (NJ)	RadRO	763
Vicencio, Alfin (NY)	PPul	316
Vickery, Carlin (NY)	PIS	337
Vieira, Jeffrey (NY)	IM	458
Vietorisz, Esteban (CT)	Oph	974
Vigorita, Vincent (NY)	Path	470
Villafranca, Manuel (NJ)	Psyc	930
Villamena, Patricia (NY)	Pul	358
Villongco, Raymond (NJ)	Ger	736
Vincent, Julie (NY)	PCd	305
Vincent, Miriam (NY)	FMed	451
Vinciguerra, Vincent (NY)	Onc	551
Vine, Anthony (NY)	S	380
Vine, John (NJ)	D	833
Viner, Nicholas (CT)	U	995
Vingan, Roy (NJ)	NS	745
Vining, Eugenia (CT)	Oto	1020
Vintzileos, Anthony (NY)	MF	550
Violi, Caterina (CT)	ObG	972
Visconti, Ernest (NY)	Ped	517
Viswanathan, Kusum (NY)	PHO	472
Viswanathan, Ramaswamy (NY)	Psyc	477
Vitale, Gerard (NY)	S	587

Name	Specialty	Pg
Vitale, Michael (NY)	OrS	285
Vitting, Kevin (NJ)	Nep	895
Vivek, Seeth (NY)	Psyc	502
Voellmicke, Kurt (NY)	OrS	687
Vogel, James (NY)	Hem	192
Vogel, Louis (NY)	D	156
Vogel, Mitchell (NJ)	Oph	896
Vogelman, Arthur (NY)	Ge	494
Vogiatzi, Maria (NY)	PEn	307
Vogl, Steven (NY)	Onc	418
Volcovici, Guido (NY)	Pul	704
Volm, Matthew (NY)	Onc	224
Volpe, Anthony (NJ)	IM	740
Volpi, David (NY)	Oto	297
Vukasin, Alexander (NJ)	U	828

W

Name	Specialty	Pg
Wachtel, Alan (NY)	Psyc	351
Wager, Marc (NY)	Ped	697
Wager, Steven (NY)	Psyc	351
Wagle, Sharad (NJ)	Psyc	762
Wagman, Raquel (NJ)	RadRO	800
Wagner, Ira (NY)	CCM	147
Wagner, John (NY)	Nep	553
Wagner, Rudolph (NJ)	Oph	790
Wainstein, Sasha (NY)	U	484
Waintraub, Stanley (NJ)	Onc	743
Waitze, Alan (CT)	NS	1015
Walczyk, John (NY)	D	537
Wald, Leonard (NY)	DR	655
Waldman, Seth (NY)	PM	300
Waldorf, Donald (NY)	D	596
Waldorf, Heidi (NY)	D	596
Walfish, Jacob (NY)	IM	458
Walke, Lisa (CT)	Ger	1007
Walker, Audrey (NY)	ChAP	650
Walker, Yvette (NY)	IM	417
Walkup, John (NY)	ChAP	142
Wallach, Frances (NY)	Inf	197
Wallach, Robert (NY)	GO	185
Wallack, Joel (NY)	Psyc	351
Wallack, Marc (NY)	S	380
Wallis, Joseph (NJ)	ObG	881
Walser, Lawrence (NY)	Pul	632
Walsh, B. Timothy (NY)	Psyc	351
Walsh, Christina (NJ)	Onc	861
Walsh, Christine (NY)	PCd	425
Walsh, Francis (CT)	IM	960
Walsh, Joseph (NY)	Oph	268
Walsh, Peter (NY)	ChAP	142
Walsh, Raymond (NY)	OrS	469
Walther, Robert (NY)	D	156
Waner, Milton (NY)	Oto	297
Wang, Beverly (NY)	Path	302
Wang, Edward (NY)	HS	617
Wang, Frederick (NY)	Oph	268
Wang, John (NY)	Nep	228
Wang, Julie (NY)	PA&I	303
Wang, Timothy (NY)	Ge	179
Wangenheim, Paul (NJ)	Cv	778
Wapner, Ronald (NY)	MF	212
Ward, Barbara (CT)	S	994
Ward, Robert (NY)	PO	314
Wardlaw, Sharon (NY)	EDM	167
Warman, Jacob (NY)	EDM	450
Warner, Robert (NY)	D	157
Warren, Floyd (NY)	Oph	268
Warren, Michelle (NY)	RE	364
Warren, Ronald (NJ)	IM	820
Warren, Russell (NY)	OrS	285
Warren, Wendy (NJ)	MF	786
Warshofsky, Stephen (NY)	IM	670
Warshofsky, Mark (CT)	IC	961
Wasnick, Robert (NY)	Ped Uro	629
Wasser, Kenneth (NJ)	Rhu	868
Wasserheit, Carolyn (NY)	Onc	674
Wasserman, Barry (NJ)	Oph	823
Wasserman, Eric (CT)	Oph	975
Wasserman, Gary (NJ)	U	770
Wasserman, Hal (CT)	IC	962
Wasserman, Kenneth (NJ)	IM	740
Wasserstein, Melissa (NY)	CG	145
Waters, Cheryl (NY)	N	243
Waters, Paul (CT)	T&CS	994
Waterstone, Melissa (NY)	ObG	253
Watkins, Kevin (NY)	S	635
Wattenberg, Debra (NY)	D	157
Wax, Michael (NJ)	Onc	922

Name	Specialty	Pg
Waxberg, Jonathan (CT)	U	996
Waxenbaum, Steven (NJ)	CRS	728
Waye, Jerome (NY)	Ge	179
Wayne, Peter (NY)	Ge	662
Waynik, Mark (CT)	Psyc	987
Weber, Kaare (NY)	S	709
Weber, Pamela (NY)	Oph	625
Weber, Richard (CT)	Oph	975
Wechsler, Amy (NY)	D	157
Weck, Steven (NY)	DR	538
Wedderburn, Raymond (NY)	S	381
Weg, Arnold (NY)	Ge	494
Weg, Ira (NY)	Cv	533
Wehmann, Robert (NJ)	EDM	732
Wei, Fong (NJ)	Nep	821
Weiland, Andrew (NY)	OrS	285
Weill, Terry (NY)	Psyc	351
Wein, Paul (NY)	Cv	446
Weinberg, Gerard (NY)	PS	428
Weinberg, Harlan (NY)	Pul	704
Weinberg, Harold (NY)	N	243
Weinberg, Jeffrey (NY)	PMR	517
Weinberg, Jerry (NY)	U	712
Weinberg, Marc (NY)	Cv	609
Weinberg, Martin (NJ)	Oph	749
Weinberger, George (NJ)	D	918
Weinberger, Jesse (NY)	N	243
Weinberger, Judah (NY)	IC	210
Weinberger, Michael (NY)	PM	300
Weinberger, Sylvain (NY)	Ped	324
Weinblatt, Mark (NY)	PHO	571
Weine, Gary (NJ)	IM	878
Weiner, David (NY)	U	394
Weiner, Howard (NY)	NS	234
Weiner, Kevin (NY)	PMR	518
Weiner, Lon (NY)	OrS	285
Weiner, Michael (NY)	PHO	312
Weiner, Richard (NY)	Ped	430
Weinerman, Stuart (NY)	EDM	450
Weinfeld, Steven (NY)	OrS	286
Weingarten, Phyllis (NY)	Oph	599
Weingarten-Arams, Jacqueline (NY)	PCCM	426
Weinreb, Jeffrey (CT)	DR	1005
Weinstein, David (CT)	ObG	972
Weinstein, Jay (NY)	IM	207
Weinstein, Joseph (NY)	Oph	562
Weinstein, Joshua (NY)	Rhu	435
Weinstein, Larry (NJ)	PlS	887
Weinstein, Mark (NY)	IM	548
Weinstein, Melvin (NJ)	Inf	838
Weinstein, Paul (CT)	Onc	964
Weinstein, Richard (NY)	OrS	687
Weinstein, Samuel (NY)	T&CS	437
Weinstein, Toba (NY)	PGe	570
Weinstock, Gary (NY)	A&I	528
Weintraub, Howard (NY)	Cv	139
Weintraub, Joshua (NY)	VIR	396
Weintraub, Michael (NY)	N	679
Weisbrot, Deborah (NY)	ChAP	610
Weiselberg, Lora (NY)	Onc	552
Weisenseel, Arthur (NY)	Cv	139
Weiser, Kenneth (NY)	EDM	657
Weiser, Martin (NY)	CRS	147
Weiser, Robert (NY)	VascS	485
Weiser, Todd (NY)	T&CS	710
Weisholtz, Steven (NJ)	Inf	738
Weiss, Carol (NY)	AdP	124
Weiss, Christopher (NJ)	Ped	759
Weiss, Darryl (NJ)	D	730
weiss, Deborah (NY)	IM	619
Weiss, E Michael (NJ)	Cv	893
Weiss, Gabriella (NJ)	Inf	894
Weiss, Gerson (NJ)	RE	764
Weiss, Jona (NY)	Ped	324
Weiss, Jonathan (NY)	DR	655
Weiss, Louis (NY)	Inf	416
Weiss, Lyn (NY)	PMR	575
Weiss, Lynne (NJ)	PNep	848
Weiss, Melvin (NY)	IC	671
Weiss, Michael (NY)	Oph	268
Weiss, Paul (NY)	PlS	337
Weiss, Rita (NY)	Onc	552
Weiss, Robert (NY)	Ge	179
Weiss, Robert (NJ)	U	853
Weiss, Robert (CT)	Ped Uro	1025
Weiss, Steven (NJ)	A&I	776
Weissbrot, Jay (NY)	Ped	697
Weissman, Gary (NY)	Ge	542
Weissman, Ronald (NY)	Cv	648
Weisstuch, Joseph (NY)	Nep	228

Name	Specialty	Pg
Weitzman, Steven (NY)	EDM	614
Weizman, Howard (NJ)	Nep	744
Wells, Scott (NY)	PlS	337
Welsh, Howard (NY)	Psyc	351
Welshinger, Marie (NY)	GO	495
Wenig, Bruce (NY)	Path	302
Werner, Michael (NY)	U	712
Wertheim, David (NY)	A&I	528
Wertheim, Iris (NY)	GO	664
Wertheim, William (NY)	IM	619
Wertkin, Martin (NY)	S	709
Weseley, Peter (NY)	Oph	268
Westcott, Mark (NY)	VIR	397
Westrich, Geoffrey (NY)	OrS	286
Wetmore, Robert (CT)	OrS	1019
Wetzler, Graciela (NY)	PGe	472
Wexler, Craig (NY)	EDM	614
Wexler, Leonard (NY)	PHO	312
Wexler, Patricia (NY)	D	157
Wey, Philip (NJ)	PlS	850
Whang, William (NY)	CE	129
Whelan, Richard (NY)	CRS	147
Whelan, Thomas (CT)	Ge	954
White, Ronald (NJ)	CRS	728
Whiteson, Johnathan (NY)	PMR	328
Whitley-Williams, Patricia (NJ)	PInf	847
Whitman, Eric (NJ)	S	889
Whitman, Gail (CT)	D	948
Whitman, Hendricks (NY)	Rhu	370
Whitmore, Wayne (NY)	Oph	268
Whyte, Dilys (NY)	PNep	628
Wickiewicz, Thomas (NY)	OrS	286
Wickiewicz, Thomas (NY)	SM	372
Wickremesinghe, Prasanna (NY)	Ge	512
Widmann, Mark (NJ)	T&CS	889
Widmann, Roger (NY)	OrS	286
Wiesen, Mark (NJ)	EDM	732
Wiesner, Elizabeth (CT)	Ped	1026
Wijesekera, Shirvinda (CT)	OrS	1019
Wilbur, Sabrina (NY)	CE	444
Wilchinsky, Mark (CT)	OrS	978
Wild, David (NJ)	Cv	727
Wilkenfeld, Marc (NY)	OM	559
Williams, Ann (CT)	FMed	951
Williams, Daniel (NY)	ChAP	533
Williams, Gail (NY)	Nep	228
Williams, Jill (NJ)	AdP	831
Williams, John (NY)	U	394
Williams, Marcus (NJ)	Cv	727
Williams, Mathew (NY)	T&CS	387
Williams, Riley (NY)	SM	372
Williams, Shaun (CT)	RE	991
Willner, Joseph (NJ)	N	746
Wilner, Philip (NY)	Psyc	352
Wilson, Arnold (NY)	OrS	424
Wilson, Lynn (CT)	RadRO	1029
Wilson, Thomas (NY)	PEn	627
Winant, John (NJ)	A&I	817
Winchester, James (NY)	IM	207
Windsor, Russell (NY)	OrS	286
Winfree, Christopher (NY)	NS	234
Winslow, Robert (CT)	CE	943
Winston, Jonathan (NY)	Nep	228
Winter, Robin (NJ)	FMed	836
Winter, Stephen (CT)	Pul	989
Winter, Steven (NY)	Cv	510
Winterkorn, Jacqueline (NY)	Oph	500
Winters, Richard (NY)	Psyc	352
Winters, Richard (NJ)	PlS	761
Winters, Stephen (NJ)	CE	873
Wirz, Diane (CT)	N	968
Wisch, Nathaniel (NY)	Hem	192
Wiseman, Paul (NY)	IM	207
Wishner, Jerald (NY)	CRS	651
Wisnicki, H Jay (NY)	Oph	269
Wisoff, Jeffrey (NY)	NS	234
Wisotsky, David (NJ)	Ped	759
Wistinghausen, Birte (NY)	PHO	312
Witt, Barry (CT)	RE	991
Witt, Marvin (NY)	IM	207
Witte, Arnold (NJ)	N	822
Wittig, James (NY)	OrS	286
Wiznia, Andrew (NY)	PA&I	424
Wohlberg, Gary (NY)	Pul	633
Wolchok, Jedd (NY)	Onc	224
Wolf, David (NY)	Ge	662
Wolf, David (NY)	Hem	192
Wolf, Ellen (NY)	DR	409
Wolf, Kenneth (NY)	Oph	423
Wolf, Steven (NY)	ChiN	144

Alphabetical Listing of Doctors

Name	Specialty	Pg
Wolf-Klein, Gisele (NY)	Ger	543
Wolfe, Lawrence (NY)	PHO	571
Wolfe, Mary (NY)	IM	670
Wolfe, Scott (NY)	HS	188
Wolff, Edward (NY)	IM	548
Wolff, Steven (NY)	DR	162
Wolfson, Robert (NY)	IM	670
Wolk, Michael (NY)	Cv	140
Wollack, Jan (NJ)	ChiN	832
Wolodiger, Fred (NJ)	VascS	771
Won, Christine (CT)	Pul	1028
Wong, Anthony (NY)	D	612
Wong, James (NJ)	RadRO	888
Wong, Raymond (NY)	Oph	269
Wong, Richard (NJ)	Oph	823
Wong, Richard (NY)	Oto	297
Woo, Henry (NY)	NS	621
Woo, Peak (NY)	Oto	297
Wormser, Gary (NY)	Inf	666
Worth, David (NJ)	Rhu	931
Wrone, David (NJ)	D	834
Wu, Jason (NY)	Ped	475
Wyner, Perry (NY)	Pul	582
Wysoki, Randee (NY)	ObG	681
Wysolmerski, John (CT)	EDM	1005
Wyszynski, Bernard (NY)	Psyc	432

X

Name	Specialty	Pg
Xu, Bo (CT)	Path	981

Y

Name	Specialty	Pg
Yablon, Steven (NY)	Nep	598
Yablonsky, Thaddeus (NJ)	VIR	890
Yadoo, Moshe (NY)	Ped	501
Yaffe, Bruce (NY)	IM	207
Yagoda, Arnold (NY)	Oph	269
Yahalom, Joachim (NY)	RadRO	360
Yaker, Michael (NY)	Ped	324
Yalamanchi, Krishan (NJ)	Ped	849
Yale, Suzanne (NY)	ObG	253
Yamane, Michael (NJ)	IM	820
Yancovitz, Stanley (NY)	Inf	198
Yang, Hee (NJ)	S	767
Yang, Roger (NJ)	DR	904
Yang, S Steven (NY)	HS	188
Yankelevitz, David (NY)	DR	163
Yankelowitz, Stanley (NY)	Oto	424
Yannuzzi, Lawrence (NY)	Oph	269
Yarberry-Allen, Patricia (NY)	ObG	253
Yarbrough, Wendell (CT)	Oto	1020
Yasgur, David (NY)	OrS	687
Yee, Arthur (NY)	Rhu	370
Yee, Arthur (CT)	Inf	957
Yegudin-Ash, Julia (NY)	Rhu	707
Yeh, Timothy (NJ)	PCCM	794
Yellin, Joseph (NY)	N	464
Yi, Peter (NJ)	Onc	821
Yiengpruksawan, Anusak (NJ)	S	767
Yip, Chun (NY)	Pul	358
Yoo, Jinil (NY)	Nep	419
Yoon, Sydney (NY)	DR	538
Yorke, Eric (NJ)	Ped	909
Youner, Craig (NY)	DR	492
Young, Bruce (NY)	ObG	253
Young, Constance (NY)	ObG	422
Young, George (NY)	U	394
Young, Joshua (NY)	Oph	269
Young, Nwanmegha (CT)	Oto	1020
Young, Stuart (NY)	A&I	127
Youngerman, Jay (NY)	Oto	566
Youssef-Bessler, Manal (NJ)	Inf	784
Yudin, Howard (NY)	FMed	658
Yue, James (CT)	OrS	1019
Yuh, David (CT)	T&CS	1032
Yung, Elizabeth (NY)	NuM	557
Yurt, Roger (NY)	S	381

Z

Name	Specialty	Pg
Zaccaria, Alan (NJ)	PlS	867
Zagzag, David (NY)	Path	302
Zahtz, Gerald (NY)	Oto	566
Zaidi, Syed (NJ)	Psyc	762
Zaidman, Gerald (NY)	Oph	684
Zairis, Ignatios (NJ)	T&CS	767
Zakashansky, Konstantin (NY)	GO	185

Name	Specialty	Pg
Zalkowitz, Alan (NJ)	Rhu	765
Zaloom, Robert (NY)	Cv	447
Zalvan, Craig (NY)	Oto	689
Zambetti, George (NY)	OrS	286
Zampella, Edward (NJ)	NS	880
Zapolanski, Alex (NJ)	T&CS	768
Zarbin, Marco (NJ)	Oph	790
Zaremski, Benjamin (NY)	IM	207
Zarich, Stuart (CT)	Cv	946
Zarnegar, Rasa (NY)	S	381
Zarowitz, William (NY)	IM	670
Zauber, N Peter (NJ)	Hem	783
Zbar, Lloyd (NJ)	Oto	792
Zeale, Peter (NY)	IM	207
Zeitels, Jerrold (NJ)	PlS	929
Zeitlin, Alan (NY)	S	505
Zeldis, Steven (NY)	Cv	533
Zelefsky, Michael (NY)	RadRO	360
Zelenetz, Andrew (NY)	Onc	225
Zelicof, Steven (NY)	OrS	688
Zelkowitz, Richard (CT)	Onc	965
Zellner, James (NY)	Oph	468
Zelman, Warren (NY)	Oto	566
Zelop, Carolyn (NJ)	MF	741
Zeltser, Ross (NY)	D	654
Zeltsman, Vadim (NY)	T&CS	589
Zerykier, Abraham (NY)	Oph	515
Zevon, Scott (NY)	PlS	337
Zide, Barry (NY)	PlS	337
Ziegelbaum, Michael (NY)	U	591
Ziering, Thomas (NJ)	FMed	905
Zimbalist, Eliot (NY)	Ge	453
Zimberg, Sheldon (NY)	Psyc	352
Zimbler, Marc (NY)	Oto	297
Zimmerman, Franklin (NY)	Cv	648
Zimmerman, Gary (CT)	NS	967
Zimmerman, Jerald (NJ)	PMR	760
Zimmerman, Marc (NY)	Onc	598
Zimmerman, Mark (NJ)	Pul	930
Zimmerman, Sol (NY)	Ped	324
Zingale, Robert (NY)	S	635
Zingler, Barry (NJ)	Ge	735
Zinkin, Lewis (NJ)	CRS	833
Zinkin, Noah (NY)	Ge	616
Zirvi, Monib (NJ)	D	918
Zisfein, Jerome (NY)	IC	549
Zitsman, Jeffrey (NY)	PS	694
Zlotoff, Ronald (CT)	Ge	1006
Zolkind, Neil (NY)	Psyc	702
Zolkowski-Wynne, Joanna (CT)	AM	941
Zolotnitskaya, Anna (NY)	PNep	692
Zoltan, Irving (NY)	Ped	430
Zonenshayn, Martin (NY)	NS	462
Zonszein, Joel (NY)	EDM	409
Zornitzer, Michael (NJ)	Psyc	799
Zou, Shengping (NY)	PM	300
Zubowski, Robert (NJ)	PlS	761
Zucker, Ira (NJ)	Ge	735
Zucker, Mark (NJ)	Cv	778
Zucker, Michael (CT)	IM	960
Zuckerman, Howard (CT)	U	996
Zuckerman, Joseph (NY)	OrS	287
Zuckerman, Kaye (CT)	S	1031
Zupnick, Henry (NY)	Pul	582
Zwas, Felice (CT)	Ge	954
Zweibel, Lawrence (NY)	Oph	625
Zweibel, Stuart (NY)	D	654
Zweifach, Philip (NY)	Oph	269
Zweig, Susan (NY)	EDM	167

The Best in American Medicine
www.CastleConnolly.com

Acknowledgments

The publishers would like to thank the entire staff for their many hours and days of intense and precise work on this guide in order to further its goal of assisting consumers in making the best healthcare choices.

Castle Connolly Executive Management:

Chairman	John K. Castle
President & CEO	John J. Connolly, Ed.D.
Vice President, Chief Medical & Research Officer	Jean Morgan, M.D.
Vice President, Chief Strategy & Operations Officer	William Liss-Levinson, Ph.D.

Vice President, Advertising	Mark McGinty
Senior Research & Healthcare Associate	Maryann Hynd, RN

Research Coordinators

Terysia Browne	Najette Miller
Anicia Buite	Yuliya Nagdimova
Catherine Hoffman-Freiria	Zachary Preneta
Maitry Gandhi	Maria Salvador
Samiya Ikram	Mariadiep Vu

Book Layout, Database Management	Russell Hodgson
Office Manager	Marcie Samartino
Director of Client Relations & Research Operations	Nicki Hughes
Manager, Client Relations	Adam Akmal-Gonzalez

We also would like to extend our gratitude to the American Board of Medical Specialties (ABMS) for allowing us to use excerpts, especially the descriptions of medical specialties and subspecialties, from the text of their publication "Which Medical Specialist for You?"

Other Publications from Castle Connolly Medical Ltd.:
America's Top Doctors® for Cancer*; *Top Doctors: Chicago Metro Area; Top Doctors Southern California; Top Doctors Washington-Baltimore; Cancer Made Easier: New York—Metro Area*, *Eldercare and others...
Order online at http://www.castleconnolly.com/books

Corporate Membership for Corporations & Organizations

This service enables an employer to assist employees in identifying Top Doctors to care for themselves and their families. It is a low-cost, non-intrusive service that will result in better care and, ultimately, lower healthcare costs. For as low as a few dollars per year, employees can have complete access to the Castle Connolly website and database of Top Doctors who were nominated by their peers and screened by the Castle Connolly physician-led research team.

Instead of simply choosing a doctor's name from the phone book or a plan directory, the employee can compare physician names to the Castle Connolly database of 34,000 plus Top Doctors and select from among the best doctors in the country. This will result in overall better care, lower costs and improved morale. Once an employee logs on to the Castle Connolly database, valuable background information is available on every Top Doctor such as: medical school, board certifications, fellowships, hospital affiliations, residencies and much more, to allow them to make the best informed decision they can make when selecting a doctor.

Top Doctors can have an enormous impact. For patients and their families, the value of receiving first-class medical care is great but unquantifiable – it is measured in quality and even length of life. Employers, however, can see the results in their bottom line. Faulty diagnoses and improper treatment take a toll in productivity and ripple out into higher workplace costs. No company should have to "make do" for weeks or months without a key employee or executive, when a Top Doctor may have solved the patient's problem quickly and efficiently. The effort to identify the best doctors from ordinary ones is justified by the money saved on incorrect treatments, unnecessary surgery and days lost from work.

The Corporate Membership is suited for employers of varying sizes and can also be of great value to professional, social, civic, fraternal and religious associations. Castle Connolly may also be able to adapt and tailor the presentation of the database to meet the specific corporate client's needs.

New Movers Program

The Castle Connolly New Movers Program is designed to alleviate that concern, or even fear, as well as the time-consuming struggle to identify the right – and best – doctors and hospitals in one's new community or region. The service can be provided on a family basis (those living in the household) or for a single client. The service includes identifying primary care physicians, including Pediatricians, OB/GYN's, Internists and Family Practitioners as well as other specialists that may be needed: for example, Ophthalmologists, Allergists, Endocrinologists, Surgeons or others as required.

Perhaps nothing is more challenging to a family that has relocated to a new community than finding appropriate healthcare resources, especially physicians. While they can turn to recommendations from new neighbors and friends, or select names from the phone book or a plan directory, that is hardly adequate, especially if there are special healthcare needs in the family.

A Castle Connolly Health Advisor will identify two or three recommendations for up to six different medical specialties. If, for some reason the client wishes to change doctors within two months, Castle Connolly will identify new physicians in the same specialty. After the selection process occurs, the Health Advisor will make an introductory phone call to the physician's office. This typically facilitates faster appointments.

Healthcare Solutions

Castle Connolly's Healthcare Solutions is designed to help your employees and their loved ones navigate through the healthcare system with less stress, faster service and better outcomes. It is a high touch service with a hands-on health advocate to serve as a guide and dedicated healthcare champion 24 hours a day, 7 days a week, 365 days a year. Why have your most valued employees, your most critical asset, spend their time -- and possibly company time –coping with difficult and complex medical issues they may know little about, when Castle Connolly's Healthcare Solutions professionals can resolve them quickly and expertly. With one phone call, your employees will gain priority access to a global network of best-in-class medical professionals, Castle Connolly Top Doctors™, and higher quality patient resources. Our professional staff coordinates the entire process to provide consistency and support during their time of need.

Services include, but are not limited to, the following:

» Identifying top physicians and hospitals (nationally)

» Identifying reputable non-physician providers, such as Dieticians, Physical and Occupational Therapists, etc.

» Facilitating second opinions

» Defining complex medical terminology and situations

» Providing a list of tailored questions to discuss with your medical team

» Conducting medical research on your health condition

» Navigating the healthcare system

» Assisting with medical record retrieval and/or arranging a medical record review

» Identifying and assisting with eldercare issues

» Coordinating a hospital transfer

» Arranging medical transport or evacuation for travelers

» Coordinating with the employers' other vendors for continuity of care

Healthcare Solutions can be made available to your organization as a specific number of cases during the course of the year with the option to obtain more, or as a yearly retainer. Organizations may opt to make this service available for all of their employees, or to select groups such as high level executives or partners.

For further information on Healthcare Solutions, Corporate Membership, New Movers, and Doctor-Patient Advisor Program, please contact:

Michael D. Wolf, Ph.D.
Vice President, Corporate Services Division
Castle Connolly Medical Ltd.
42 W. 24th St
New York, NY 10010
212-367-8400 Ext. 132
mwolf@castleconnolly.com

Thora Eidsdottir, Ed.D.
Account Executive
Castle Connolly Medical Ltd.
42 W. 24th St.
New York, NY 10010
teidsdottir@castleconnolly.com

Strategic Relationships

Castle Connolly Medical Ltd. has a number of strategic relationships that may be of interest to consumers and physicians.

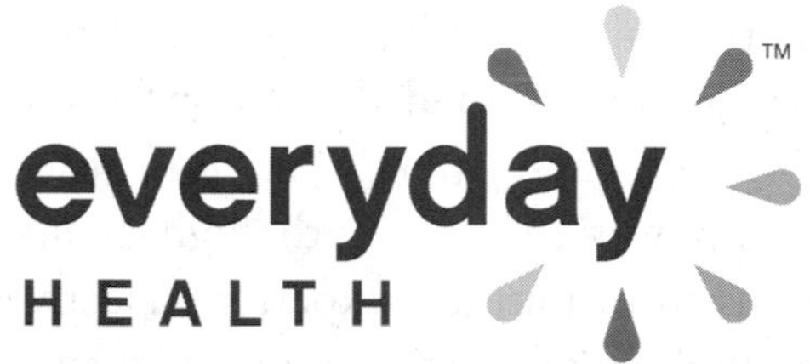

Everyday Health, Inc. comprises some of the nation's leading online health information resources. With over 25 comprehensive health websites including www.EverydayHealth.com, www.Carepages.com, PDRHealth.com and www.WhatToExpect.com, information and knowledge is accessible on a wide range of health topics such as lifestyle offerings in pregnancy, diet and fitness to in-depth medical content for condition prevention and management.

In addition to their commitment to provide consumers with health solutions that span the health spectrum, they also provide a wide range of content and advertising-based services to healthcare entities including hospitals, physicians and other healthcare professionals. Castle Connolly has formed a strategic relationship with Everyday Health to offer one of these services in particular; Reputation Management Solutions.

More than 150 million people search listings and online healthcare directories each month making it imperative for physicians and hospitals to consistently update and manage their information on local directories, reviews sites and social networks. Understandably, this is, at times, an unfeasible commitment. Everyday Health's Reputation Management Solutions provides online visibility information which shows exactly where listings appear on the web, information across hundreds of directory sites, identifying and tips on how to respond to negative reviews and much more.

For more information, please contact our Manager of Client Relations at (212) 367-8400 Ext. 123.

sharecare

Sharecare is an interactive, social Q&A platform designed to greatly simplify the search for quality healthcare information and help consumers live their healthiest life. Sharecare has enlisted the nation's leading health experts, care providers, organizations, and brands to join the health and wellness conversation and empowering users with high-quality, relevant answers to their health questions from multiple expert perspectives and with interactive health and wellness tools to take action on what they've learned.

The website was launched in 2010 by Jeff Arnold, founder of WebMD, and Emmy–award winning host, Dr. Mehmet Oz, in partnership with Harpo Studios, Sony Pictures Television and Discovery Communications.

Castle Connolly teamed up with Sharecare in 2011. Dr. John Connolly, President and CEO of CCML, is one of the featured experts on Sharecare for healthcare choice questions. Find out more at www.sharecare.com

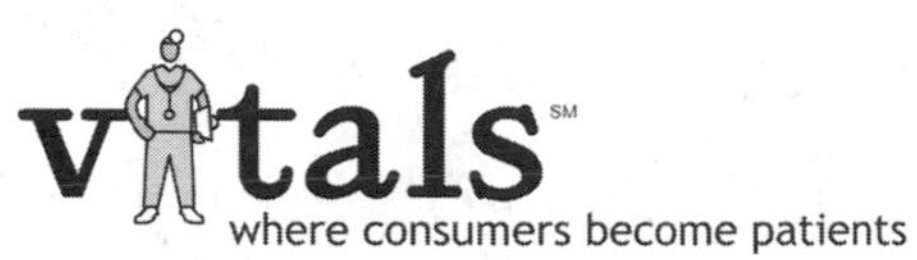

Vitals (www.vitals.com), an innovative online doctor review and comparison service from MDx Medical Inc., is the comprehensive source for vital information, peer evaluations and patient feedback on more than 700,000 doctors nationwide. Drawing upon prestigious information repositories, cutting-edge search and comparison technologies, and a robust patient feedback mechanism, Vitals has organized key information to help patients make an informed choice in their search for the right doctor. Castle Connolly and Vitals have a branding relationship in which those physicians who are Castle Connolly Top Doctors™ and appear on Vitals web sites have an icon indicating their status and recognition as a Castle Connolly Top Doctor.

In 2012, Castle Connolly will begin displaying insurance plans that are accepted by all physicians listed as Castle Connolly Top Doctors. An appointment scheduling feature will also appear on our site for those physicians who wish to participate in this feature. Additional information can be found at www.vitals.com.

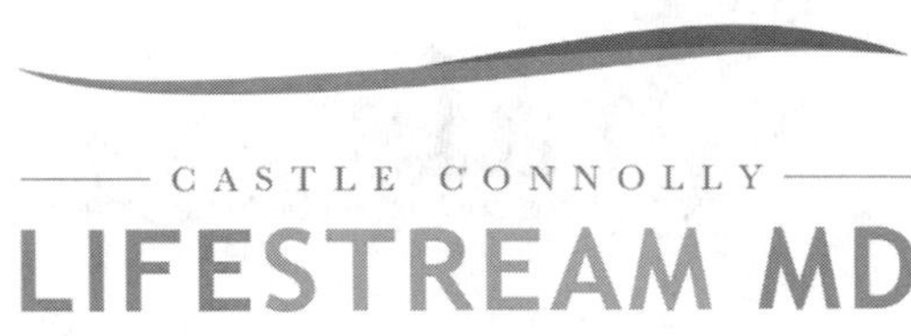

Castle Connolly Medical Ltd. has a strategic relationship with Castle Connolly LifeStream MD to provide a unique health advisory service designed for families and executives, especially those who travel regularly or may have more than one residence.

Each client is assigned a Castle Connolly LifeStream MD physician who is available to them by phone 24/7/365. A client call from anywhere in the world is answered promptly and the client is connected with their Castle Connolly LifeStream MD physician advisor.

The Castle Connolly LifeStream MD physician acts as a health manager assisting in navigation of an increasingly complex health care environment. The Castle Connolly LifeStream MD physician does not replace the member's primary physician or specialists, but provides additional independent counsel and services that provide security to our members either at home or while traveling.

In the United States, the Castle Connolly LifeStream MD physician will use the Castle Connolly database of Top Doctors to assure that the client is cared for in the best medical facilities by the top doctors. Assistance in securing timely appointments with specialists and records transfers is facilitated as needed. Outside of the United States, Castle Connolly LifeStream MD has an affiliation with International SOS, the world's largest and leading provider of travel medical assistance to assure the LifeStream MD member is cared for by the best doctors and hospitals available in that region or, if necessary, is transported to a place where that care is available.

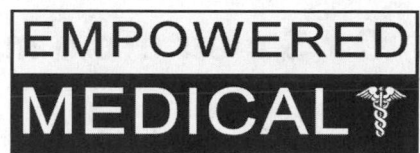

Empowered Doctor is a media, news and marketing service. Empowered Doctor produces syndicated consumer health reports. Its video and text news stories appear on major media websites, including CBS. Empowered Doctor also provides marketing services to hospitals, clinics and individual physicians by generating visibility in online search and social media. Empowered Doctor's clients benefit from the company's efficient methodologies for generating new patient referrals.

For more information call 888-333-1027 or visit www.empowereddoctor.com

DrScore.com
PATIENTS SPEAK, DOCTORS LISTEN

Founded by Steven Feldman, M.D., DrScore.com is an interactive online survey site where patients can rate their physicians, as well as find a physician based on their service level preference.

The mission of DrScore.com is to improve medical care by giving patients a forum for rating their physician and by giving doctors an affordable, objective, non-intrusive means of documenting the quality of care that they provide. Visitors on Castle Connolly's website who are searching for "top doctors" have the option to also rate these and other physicians they have been to as patients, as well as to see if these physicians have been rated previously by other consumers on DrScore.com. Visitors to DrScore.com will be able to see if their doctors and/or other doctors are Castle Connolly "top doctors."

For more information, visit www.drscore.com.

grandparents.com®
it's great to be grand.

Grandparents.com is dedicated to enhancing the lives of America's 70 million grandparents by fostering family connections, via child- and grandparent-friendly activities, travel ideas, compelling lifestyle features, expert advice, gift ideas, recipes, and more. Visitors have access to a range of tools, including groups, discussions, a homepage blog, photo sharing, and a Facebook page and Twitter feeds. Through the Grandparents.com Grand Deals page members can receive discounts and incentives they can use every day, in categories like gifts, clothes, and vitamins, plus exclusive opportunities to save on hotels, cruises, auto rentals, theme park trips, theatrical productions, and insurance. Grandparents can share their membership benefits with four extended family and household members. In 2010, Grandparents.com was ranked as the No. 3 website for seniors, boomers, and grandparents, following the U.S. Government and AARP. Castle Connolly provides access to its Top Doctors' database, its Doctor-Patient Advisor and New Movers programs for Grandparents.com members.

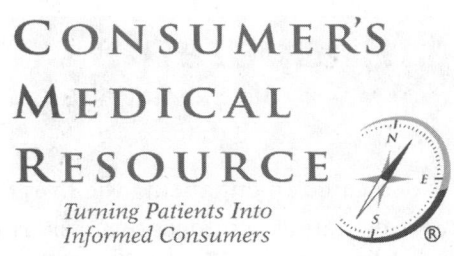

Consumer's Medical Resource was started in 1996 to offer high-quality, high-impact employee benefit programs to help employees and their dependents, and has been a pioneer in Medical Decision Support® services. CMR addresses all medical conditions at any point within the continuum of care, by providing personalized, evidence-based medical research, information, access to genuine, in-person second opinions and support services to employees who face serious, complicated, and chronic illness, or would like to become well-informed healthcare consumers.

Leveraging a state-of-the-art integrated model of web, phone, and print-based services, CMR enables employees to fully understand and evaluate their options so they can make the most informed medical decisions possible with their doctors. The company is privately held and currently provides services to more than 750,000 Americans, achieving extremely high levels of user and customer satisfaction, improved clinical quality outcomes, and generated excellent ROI.

Castle Connolly and CMR are working together to provide Castle Connolly's various corporate services to CMR client companies and their employees.

For more information, please visit: http://www.consumersmedical.com.

Gluten-Free
RESOURCE DIRECTORY

The Gluten-Free Resource Directory is a unique and easy, one-stop guide to all things Gluten-Free. Each category on this site has been carefully selected to provide you with products and services that simplify and demystify the Gluten-Free shopping experience. The Gluten-Free Resource Directory is dynamic in that it is constantly evolving, growing, changing and being updated with new products and services every day. So, be sure to check the site often to take advantage of some great promotions and new-to-market products available to you and your family.

Castle Connolly has entered into a strategic partnership with Directory Media Group, publishers of The Gluten-Free Resource Directory, to provide more than 1,900 doctors listings at www.glutenfreeresourcedirectory.com, free of charge. The listings include profiles of the nation's most distinguished gastroenterology, pediatric allergy and immunology, allergy and immunology and pediatric gastroenterology physicians.

Visitors to the Gluten-Free Resource Directory can search the more than 1,900 Castle Connolly Top Doctor profiles for each physician's contact information, specialty, training and faculty appointments, along with which medical school and residency program they attended. The profiles also include information for the insurance plans accepted by each Castle Connolly Top Doctor.

For more information, please visit: http://GlutenFreeResourceDirectory.com.

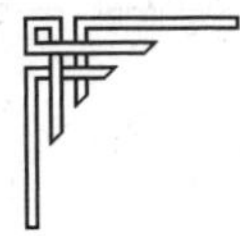

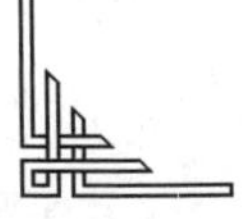

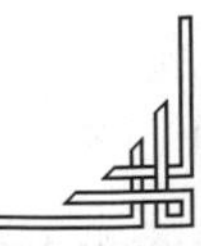

National Physician of the Year Awards

Castle Connolly Medical Ltd. proudly hosted its seventh annual ***National Physician of the Year Awards*** on March 18, 2013 at The Pierre Hotel in New York City. It was a spectacular evening which allowed us to recognize both the outstanding honorees and the excellence of the many thousands of physicians throughout the nation.

The Genesis of the National Physician of the Year Award.

Each year we receive thousands of nominations from physicians and the medical leadership of major medical centers, specialty hospitals, teaching hospitals and regional and community medical centers across the United States as an integral part of our research, screening and selection process to identify ***America's Top Doctors®***. The selected physicians, while spread across all fifty states and involved in more than 70 medical specialties and subspecialties, all share one distinguishing professional attribute: an unwavering dedication to their patients and to medicine as a whole. Each and every one of these outstanding medical professionals is a symbol of the clinical excellence that characterizes American medicine. In honor of these exemplary physicians, Castle Connolly Medical Ltd. has created the ***National Physician of the Year Awards*** to recognize the thousands of excellent, dedicated physicians across the United States. Our Medical Advisory Board selected the honorees from the hundreds nominated in a special nomination process conducted months before the event.

The honorees, Drs. Gopal Badlani, Jo A. Hannafin, and Jerry A. Shields, are superb examples of excellence in clinical medical practice. In addition to these awards for Clinical Excellence, Castle Connolly Medical Ltd. honored Drs. Michael Harrison and Sterling B. Williams for their lifetime achievement in medicine. Ms. Dawn Halfaker is a tireless fundraiser for Wounded Warrior Project and an exemplary recipient for the seventh National Health Leadership Award.

Each honoree received a beautiful and distinctive porcelain figurine created by the Boehm Porcelain Company exclusively for the National Physician of the Year Awards. The award features a golden caduceus, the symbol of the medical community, surrounded by a golden laurel wreath. Laurel wreaths were used by the ancients to crown and honor their leaders.

The caduceus and laurel rest upon a column accented by the signature Castle Connolly logo. By combining the caduceus and the laurel wreaths, the award embodies the excellence in medical achievement that the National Physician of the Year Awards celebrates each year.

2013 National Physician of the Year Awards Honorees

"Top Doctors Make a Difference™"

For Clinical Excellence

Gopal Badlani, M.D.
Professor and Vice Chair for Clinical Affairs
Department of Urology
Wake Forest Baptist Medical Center

Jo A. Hannafin, M.D., Ph.D.
Hospital for Special Surgry
Professor of Orthopaedic Surgery
Weill Cornell Medical College

Jerry A. Shields, M.D.
Professor of Ophthalmology
Thomas Jefferson University
Director, Oncology Service
Wills Eye Institute

For Lifetime Achievement

Michael R. Harrison, M.D.
Professor Emeritus of Surgery, Pediatrics,
Obstetrics, Gynecology & Reproductive Sciences
Founding Director, Fetal Treatment Center
University of California, San Francisco

Sterling Williams, M.S., M.D., Ph.D.
Clinical Professor of Obstetrics & Gynecology
George Washington University Medical School
Vice President of Education
American College of Obstetricians & Gynecologists

National Health Leadership

Dawn Halfaker
President and CEO
Halfaker and Associated, LLC
President, Board of Directors, Wounded Warrior Project

2012 National Physician of the Year Awards Honorees

"Top Doctors Make a Difference™"

For Clinical Excellence

Richard Edelson, M.D.
Aaron B. and Marguerite Lerner Professor
Chairman of the Department of Dermatology
Yale School of Medicine.

Susan Mackinnon, M.D.
Chief of Plastic and Reconstructive Surgery
Washington University School of Medicine

John M. Morton, M.D., M.P.H., F.A.C.S.
Associate Professor of Surgery
Stanford University
Chief of Minimally Invasive Surgery,
Director of Bariatric Surgery and Surgical Quality

For Lifetime Achievement

Robert L. Brent, M.D., Ph.D., D.Sc.
Distinguished Professor of Pediatrics, Radiology and Pathology
Louis and Bess Stein Professor of Pediatrics at the Jefferson Medical College
and the Nemours/Alfred I. DuPont Hospital for Children

John G. Clarkson, M.D.
Dean Emeritus and Professor of Ophthalmology
Anne Bates Leach Eye Hospital/Bascom Palmer Eye Institute
Department of Ophthalmology
Miller School of Medicine at the University of Miami

National Health Leadership

Marlo Thomas
National Outreach Director
St. Jude Children's Research Hospital

2011 National Physician of the Year Awards Honorees

"Doctors Make a Difference"

For Clinical Excellence

Armando E. Giuliano, M.D., FACS, FRCSED
Chief of Science and Medicine
John Wayne Cancer Institute at Saint John's Health Center,
Santa Monica, CA

O. Wayne Isom, M.D.
Chairman of the Dept. of Cardiothoracic Surgery
New York Presbyterian-Weill Cornell Medical College

David W. Kennedy, M.D.
Otorhinolaryngology Professor at the
University of Pennsylvania

For Lifetime Achievement

George P. Canellos, M.D.
Served as Founding Chief of Medical Oncology at
Dana-Farber Cancer Institute;

Matthew D. Davis, M.D.
University of Wisconsin Medical Center
Chair, UW Opthalmology

National Health Leadership

Evelyn H. Lauder
Chairman of The Breast Cancer Research Foundation®

2010

Clinical Excellence

John B. Buse, M.D., Ph.D.

Director of the Diabetes Care Center, Professor, Chief of the Division of Endocrinology and Executive Associate Dean for Clinical Research, University of North Carolina School of Medicine, Chapel Hill

Larry Norton, M.D.

Deputy Physician-in-Chief, Memorial Hospital, Memorial Sloan-Kettering Cancer Center, for Breast Cancer Programs
Medical Director of the MSKCC's Breast and Imaging Center, Evelyn H. Lauder Breast Center

Ching-Hon Pui, M.D.

Department Chair of Oncology, St. Jude Children's Research Hospital
Medical Director of the St. Jude International Outreach China Program, holder of the Fahad Nassar Al-Rashid Chair of Leukemia Research

Lifetime Achievement

Basil I Hirschowitz, M.D.

Director, Gastroenterology Division, The University of Alabama
Receipient of the Kettering Medal from the General Motors Cancer Foundation; Friedenwald Medal of the AGA; the Schindler Medal and the Crystal Award for lifetime contributions to Endoscopy by the ASGE; honorary doctorate of Gothenburg University; honorary fellow of the Royal Society of Medicine

Leonard Apt, M.D.

Professor of Ophthalmology Emeritus; Director Emeritus and Founder of the Division of Pediatric Opthalmology and Strabismus, and Co-Director of UCLA's Center for Child Blindness

National Health Leadership

Alexandra Reeve Givens and Matthew Reeve

Trustees, The Christopher & Dana Reeve Foundation

2009

Clinical Excellence

Carol R. Bradford, M.D.,
Professor and Chair
Department of Otolaryngology
University of Michigan Medical System

Diane E. Meier, M.D.,
Director, Center to Advance Palliative Care
Mount Sinai School of Medicine

Judd W. Moul, M.D.,
Chief of Urology
Duke University Medical Center

Lifetime Achievement

Emil J. Freireich, M.D., D. Sc. (Hon.),
Ruth Harriet Ainsworth Chair, Distinguished Teaching Professor
Director, Special Medical Education Programs
Director, Adult Leukemia Research Program
The University of Texas M.D. Anderson Cancer Center

Thomas E. Starzl, M.D., Ph.D.
Professor of Surgery, Emeritus
Distinguished Service Professor
University of Pittsburgh Medical Center

National Health Leadership

Page Morton Black
Chairman of the Board, Parkinson's Disease Foundation

****

2008

Clinical Excellence
Robert W. Carlson, M.D.
Medical Oncology
Stanford University Medical Center

Stanley Chang, M.D.
Ophthalmology
New York-Presbyterian Hospital

L. Dade Lunsford, M.D.
Neurological Surgery
University of Pittsburgh Medical Center

Lifetime Achievement
Jacqueline A. Noonan, M.D.
Pediatric Cardiology
University of Kentucky Medical Center

Robert W. Schrier, M.D.
Nephrology
University of Colorado Health Sciences Center

National Health Leadership
Suzanne and Robert Wright
Vice-Chair of the Board, General Electric Company
Co-founders of Autism Speaks™

****

2007

Clinical Excellence

Delos M. Cosgrove, M.D.
Chairman, Board of Governors
CEO and President
The Cleveland Clinic

Joseph G. McCarthy, M.D.
Lawrence D. Bell Professor of Plastic Surgery
Director, The Institute of Reconstructive Plastic Surgery
NYU Medical Center

Patrick C. Walsh, M.D.
University Distinguished Service Professor and Director of Urology
The James Buchanan Brady Urological Institute
The Johns Hopkins Hospital

Lifetime Achievement

Maria Delivoria-Papadopoulos, M.D.
Director, The Neonatal Intensive Care Unit
St. Christopher's Hospital for Children;
Professor of Pediatrics, Physiology and Obstetrics/Gynecology
Drexel University College of Medicine

National Health Leadership

The Honorable Nancy G. Brinker
Founder of Susan G. Komen for the Cure
Former U.S. Ambassador to Hungary

****

2006

Clinical Excellence

Bart Barlogie, M.D., Ph.D.
Director, Myeloma Institute for Research Therapy
University of Arkansas for Medical Services

Marilyn J. Bull, M.D.
Morris Green Professor of Pediatrics
Riley Hospital for Children

Michael J. Zinner, M.D.
Moseley Professor of Surgery
Harvard Medical School
Surgeon-in-Chief, Brigham & Women's Hospital

Lifetime Achievement

Michael E. DeBakey, M.D.
Chancellor Emeritus, Baylor College of Medicine

National Health Leadership

Princess Yasmin Aga Khan
Honorary Vice Chair
Alzheimer's Association

Castle Connolly maintains Facebook, Twitter, LinkedIn and Sharecare accounts in an effort to keep consumers informed of the latest news not only regarding Castle Connolly Medical Ltd., its Top Doctors and Top Hospitals, but also reports on various health observances and events. A live Twitter feed can also be found on the homepage of www.castleconnolly.com.

Consumers who use our print guides, online database or refer to our regional magazine features can find up-to-date information about Castle Connolly, healthcare and medical news by logging onto these social networking sites:

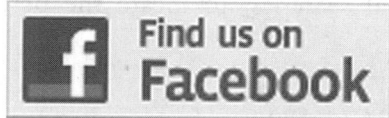

www.facebook.com/TopDoctors

Blog - Ask America's Top Doctors™
www.castleconnolly.com/blog

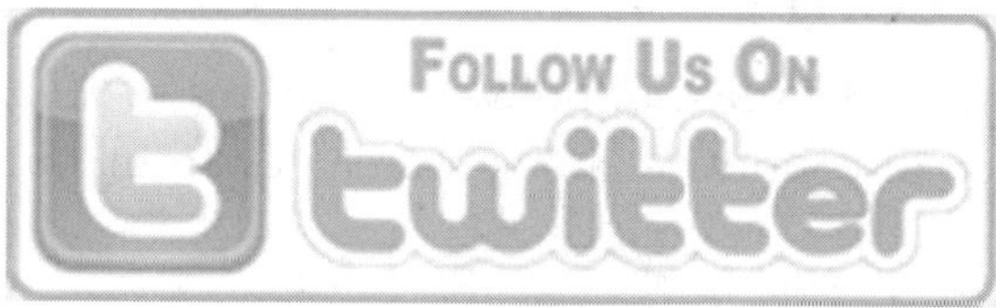

www.twitter.com/CastleConnolly

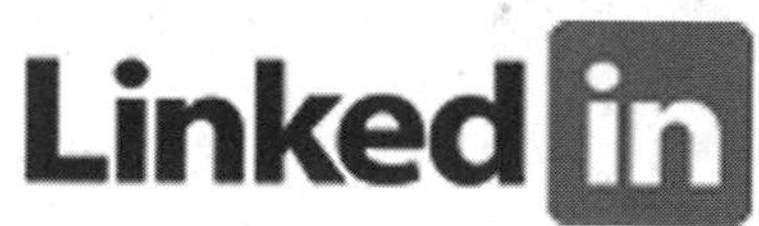

http://linkd.in/mP4Lmb (case sensitive)

Do you have a story about a Castle Connolly Top Doctor or Top Hospital that you want to share? If so, please email a link to the article to:

Nicki Hughes
Director of Client Relations & Research Operations
nhughes@castleconnolly.com

Doctor-Patient Advisor for Individual Consumers

Doctor-Patient Advisor is a Castle Connolly Medical Ltd. service providing one-on-one consultations with a physician or nurse practitioner to individuals who have serious or complex medical problems or to anyone who feels he/she needs assistance finding the right physician for any purpose. Each client will receive personalized assistance in identifying the appropriate specialists for his/her condition, utilizing the Castle Connolly Medical Ltd. database of physicians and hospitals, as well as individual searches, to locate the best resources to meet the client's needs.

Fee: $375. For further information call (212) 367-8400 x 116.

Premium Membership to www.CastleConnolly.com

Reap the benefits of membership with Castle Connolly. Gain access to ALL online top doctor listings and get discounts on book purchases from our extensive catalog.

- Search among more than 34,000 Castle Connolly Top Doctor listings
- Search among select hospitals and centers of excellence
- Receive a 30% discount on all book purchases

Membership Levels:
- One year - $24.95
- Two years - $34.95

For more information visit: www.CastleConnolly.com/membership

Other Products From Castle Connolly

Castle Connolly Guides

Titles Include:

- ***America's Top Doctors®***
- ***America's Top Doctors® for Cancer***

And Many More

To order other Castle Connolly guides at a 15% discount please visit
http://www.CastleConnolly.com/books
When ordering use discount code: **NY17DOM**

Castle Connolly's Top Doctors Available Online

- Free Access to 20 -25% of Castle Connolly's Top Doctors
- Purchase Access to the entire database of more than 34,000 doctor profiles

http://www.castleconnolly.com/membership

Customer Feedback

We appreciate your comments regarding our guides. Please email us at info@castleconnolly.com

The Best in American Medicine
www.CastleConnolly.com